OTHER PMIC TITLES OF INTEREST

CODING AND REIMBURSEMENT TITLES

Collections Made Easy!
CPT Coders Choice®, Thumb Indexed
CPT & HCPCS Coding Made Easy!
CPT Easy Links
CPT Plus!
DRG Plus!
E/M Coding Made Easy!
Getting Paid for What You Do
HCPCS Coders Choice®, Color Coded, Thumb Indexed
Health Insurance Carrier Directory
HIPAA Compliance Manual
ICD-9-CM, Coders Choice®, Thumb Indexed
ICD-9-CM Coding for Physicians' Offices
ICD-9-CM Coding Made Easy!
ICD-9-CM, Home Health Edition
Medical Fees in the United States
Medicare Compliance Manual
Medicare Rules & Regulations
Physicians Fee Guide
Reimbursement Manual for the Medical Office

PRACTICE MANAGEMENT TITLES

Accounts Receivable Management for the Medical Practice
Achieving Profitability With a Medical Office System
Encyclopedia of Practice and Financial Management
Managed Care Organizations
Managing Medical Office Personnel
Marketing Strategies for Physicians
Medical Marketing Handbook
Medical Office Policy Manual
Medical Practice Forms
Medical Practice Handbook
Medical Staff Privileges
Negotiating Managed Care Contracts
Patient Satisfaction
Performance Standards for the Laboratory
Professional and Practice Development
Promoting Your Medical Practice
Starting in Medical Practice
Working With Insurance and Managed Care Plans

**AVAILABLE FROM YOUR LOCAL MEDICAL
BOOK STORE OR CALL 1-800-MED-SHOP**

OTHER PMIC TITLES OF INTEREST

RISK MANAGEMENT TITLES
Malpractice Depositions
Medical Risk Management
Preparing for Your Deposition
Preventing Emergency Malpractice
Testifying in Court

FINANCIAL MANAGEMENT TITLES
A Physician's Guide to Financial Independence
Business Ventures for Physicians
Financial Valuation of Your Practice
Personal Money Management for Physicians
Personal Pension Plan Strategies for Physicians
Securing Your Assets

DICTIONARIES AND OTHER REFERENCE TITLES
Drugs of Abuse
Health and Medicine on the Internet
Medical Acronyms and Abbreviations
Medical Phrase Index
Medical Word Building
Medico Mnemonica
Medico-Legal Glossary
Spanish/English Handbook for Medical Professionals

MEDICAL REFERENCE AND CLINICAL TITLES
Advance Medical Directives
Clinical Research Opportunities
Gastroenterology: Problems in Primary Care
Manual of IV Therapy
Medical Care of the Adolescent Athlete
Medical Procedures for Referral
Neurology: Problems in Primary Care
Orthopaedics: Problems in Primary Care
Patient Care Emergency Handbook
Patient Care Flowchart Manual
Patient Care Procedures for Your Practice
Physician's Office Laboratory
Pulmonary Medicine: Problems in Primary Care
Questions and Answers on AIDS

**AVAILABLE FROM YOUR LOCAL MEDICAL
BOOK STORE OR CALL 1-800-MED-SHOP**

ICD·9·CM

International Classification of Diseases
9th Revision

Clinical Modification
Sixth Edition

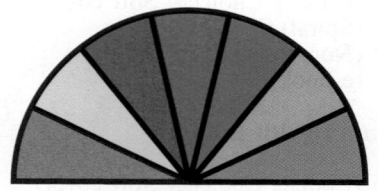

Color Coded

2010

Volumes 1 & 2 : Office Edition

ISBN 978-1-57066-609-4 (Coder's Choice® Soft cover)
ISBN 978-1-57066-610-0 (Spiral)
ISBN 978-1-57066-611-7 (Non-indexed)
ISBN 978-1-57066-602-5 (e-book)

Volumes 1, 2, & 3 : Hospital Edition

ISBN 978-1-57066-606-3 (Coder's Choice® Soft cover)
ISBN 978-1-57066-607-0 (Spiral)
ISBN 978-1-57066-608-7 (Non-indexed)
ISBN 978-1-57066-603-2 (e-book)

Volumes 1, 2, & 3 : Home Health Edition

ISBN 978-1-57066-605-6 (Coder's Choice® Soft cover)
ISBN 978-1-57066-604-9 (e-book)

Practice Management Information Corporation [PMIC]
4727 Wilshire Boulevard, Suite 300
Los Angeles, California 90010
1-800-MED-SHOP
http://www.pmiconline.com

Printed in China

Preface

Health care professionals have long used coding systems to describe procedures, services, and supplies. However, most described the reason for the procedure, service or supply with a diagnostic statement. Of those health care professionals who do code the diagnosis, either due to a requirement for a computer billing system and/or electronic claims filing, many do not code completely or accurately. With the passage of the Medicare Catastrophic Coverage Act of 1988, diagnostic coding using *ICD-9-CM* became mandatory for Medicare claims. In the area of health care reimbursement rules and regulations, the typical progression is that changes required for Medicare are followed shortly by similar changes for Medicaid and private insurance carriers.

To some professionals, the requirement to use diagnostic coding may have seemed like a burden or simply another excuse for Medicare intermediaries to delay or deny payment. However, it is important to understand that the proper use of coding systems for both procedures and diagnoses gives the professional absolute control over his or her billing and reimbursement. Accurate diagnosis coding is not easy. It requires a good working knowledge of medical terminology and a fundamental understanding of *ICD-9-CM*. In addition, the coder must know the rules and regulations required to comply with Medicare requirements for coding.

This edition of the *International Classification of Diseases, 9th Revision, Clinical Modification (ICD-9-CM)* is published by Practice Management Information Corporation in recognition of its responsibility to promulgate this classification throughout the United States for morbidity coding and billing purposes. *The International Classification of Diseases, 9th Revision*, originally published by the World Health Organization (WHO) is the foundation of the *ICD-9-CM* and continues to be the classification employed in cause-of-death coding in the United States.

The *ICD-9-CM* is recommended for use in all clinical settings, but is required for reporting diagnoses and diseases to all U.S. Public Health Service and Department of Health and Human Services programs, such as Medicare and Medicaid. This version faithfully follows and contains the same information found in the official U.S. government version of the *ICD-9-CM*.

All official authorized addenda effective October 1, 2009, have been included in this edition. A new revision will be available approximately September 15th of each year. Revised editions may be purchased from:

Practice Management Information Corporation
4727 Wilshire Boulevard, Suite 300
Los Angeles, California 90010
1-800-MED-SHOP

Or by contacting our web site at http://www.pmiconline.com.

Disclaimer

This publication includes all official ICD-9-CM codes, descriptions, annotations and guidelines as maintained by the U.S. Department of Health and Human Services with the exception that this publication includes special symbols to indicate additions and revisions from the previous edition and special symbols to facilitate identification of diagnostic codes that require 4th or 5th digit specificity, the use of color coding to alert the user to special coding considerations, and thumb indexing to make locating codes easier. This publication is revised annually so that we may present the most current information possible. Though all of the information is carefully researched and checked for accuracy and completeness, the publisher accepts no responsibility with regard to errors, omissions, misuse or misinterpretation.

Table of Contents

TABLE OF CONTENTS

[1] These listings appear only in the three volume edition

Introduction to ICD-9-CM

ICD-9-CM is an acronym for *International Classification of Diseases, 9th Revision, Clinical Modification*, published under different names since 1900. *ICD-9-CM* is a statistical classification system that arranges diseases and injuries into groups according to established criteria. Most *ICD-9-CM* codes are numeric and consist of three, four or five numbers and a description. The codes are revised approximately every 10 years by the World Health Organization and annual updates are published by Center for Medicare and Medicaid Services (CMS).

HISTORICAL PERSPECTIVE

The *International Classification of Diseases, 9th Revision, Clinical Modification (ICD-9-CM)* is based on the official version of the *World Health Organization's (WHO) 9th Revision, International Classification of Diseases (ICD-9)*. *ICD-9* is designed for the classification of morbidity and mortality information for statistical purposes, and for the indexing of medical records by disease and operations, and for data storage and retrieval. *ICD-9-CM* replaced the Eighth Revision International Classification of Diseases, Adapted for Use in the United States commonly referred to as *ICDA*.

The concept of extending the International Classification of Diseases for use in hospital indexing was originally developed in response to a need for a more efficient basis for storage and retrieval of diagnostic data. In 1950, the U.S. Public Health Service and the Veterans Administration began independent tests of the International Classification of Diseases for hospital indexing purposes. In the following year, the Columbia Presbyterian Medical Center in New York City adopted the International Classification of Diseases, 6th Revision for use in its medical record department. A few years later, the Commission on Professional and Hospital Activities adopted the International Classification of Diseases for use in hospitals participating in the Professional Activity Study (PAS).

In view of the growing interest in the use of the International Classification of Diseases for hospital indexing, a study was undertaken in 1956 by the American Medical Association and the American Medical Record Association of the relative efficiencies of coding systems for diagnostic indexing. Following this study, the major uses of the International Classification of Diseases for hospital indexing purposes consolidated their experiences and an adaptation was published in December 1959. A revision containing the first "Classification of Operations and Treatments" was published in 1962.

In 1968, following a study by the American Hospital Association, the United States Public Health Service published the Eighth Revision International Classification of Diseases, Adapted for Use in the United States. This publication became commonly known as ICDA, and served as the basis for coding diagnostic data for official morbidity and mortality statistics in the United States.

ICD-9-CM Background

In February 1977, a committee was convened by the National Center for Health Statistics to provide advice and counsel for the development of clinical modification of the ICD-9. The organizations represented on the committee included:

American Association of Health Data Systems
American Hospital Association
American Medical Record Association
Association for Health Records
Commission on Professional and Hospital Activities
Council on Clinical Classifications, sponsored by:

American Academy of Pediatrics
American College of Obstetricians and Gynecologists
American College of Physicians
American College of Surgeons
American Psychiatric Association

Health Care Financing Administration
WHO Center for Classification of Diseases

The resulting *ICD-9-CM* is a clinical modification of the *World Health Organization's International Classification of Diseases, 9th Revision (ICD-9)*. The term "clinical" is used to emphasize the modifications intent; namely, to serve as a useful tool in the area of classification of morbidity data for indexing of medical records, medical care review, ambulatory and other medical care programs, as well as for basic health statistics.

In use since January 1979, *ICD-9-CM* provides a diagnostic coding system that is more precise than those needed only for statistical groupings and trend analysis. Official addenda (updates) to *ICD-9-CM* are issued in October each year by the National Center for Health Statistics (NCHS), part of the Centers for Disease Control (CDC).

Use of ICD-9-CM Codes for Professional Billing

Until passage of the Medicare Catastrophic Coverage Act of 1988, health care professionals were not required to report *ICD-9-CM* codes when billing government or private insurance carriers for reimbursement. The exception to this requirement was for those health care professionals who filed insurance claims electronically and those who used "code driven" computer billing services or computer systems.

Most health care professionals simply included the text or description of the injury, illness, sign or symptom that was the reason for the encounter. Insurance carriers who used *ICD-9-CM* coding had to code the diagnostic statements prior to input into their computer systems for reimbursement processing.

A specific requirement of the Medicare Catastrophic Coverage Act of 1988 required health care professionals to include *ICD-9-CM* codes on their Medicare claim forms effective April 1, 1989. After a two-month grace period, the requirement was officially implemented on June 1, 1989. The Medicare Catastrophic Coverage Act was repealed in November, 1989; however the ICD-9-CM coding requirement was continued.

TERMINOLOGY

There are terms used throughout this publication that are important for a proper understanding of *ICD-9-CM*. The following terms are defined specifically as they are used for *ICD-9-CM* with the knowledge that some terms may have other definitions and meanings.

acute refers to the condition that is the primary reason for the current encounter.

addenda official updates to ICD-9-CM published continuously since 1986, that become effective on October 1st of each year.

adverse any response to a drug that is noxious and unintended and occurs with proper dosage.

aftercare an encounter for something planned in advance, for example, cast removal.

AHFS American Hospital Formulary Service.

alphabetic index the portion of ICD-9-CM that lists definitions and codes in alphabetic order. Also called Volume 2.

category refers to diagnoses codes listed within a specific three-digit category, for example category 250, Diabetes Mellitus.

cause that which brings about any condition or produces any effect.

chronic continuing over a long period of time or recurring frequently.

coding the process of transferring written or verbal descriptions of diseases, injuries and procedures into numerical designations.

combination a code that combines a diagnosis with an associated secondary process or complication.

complication the occurrence of two or more diseases in the same patient at the same time.

concurrent when a patient is being treated by more than one provider for different care conditions at the same time.

conventions refers to the use of certain abbreviations, punctuation, symbols, type faces, and other instructions that must be clearly understood in order to use ICD-9-CM.

CPT Current Procedural Terminology. Listing of codes and descriptions for procedures, services and supplies published by the American Medical Association. Used to bill insurance carriers.

diagnosis a written description of the reason(s) for the procedure, service, supply or encounter.

down coding the process where insurance carriers reduce the value of a procedure, and the resulting reimbursement, due to either 1) a mismatch of CPT code and description or 2) ICD-9-CM code does not justify the procedure or level of service.

E codes specific ICD-9-CM codes used to identify the cause of injury, poisoning and other adverse effects.

eponyms medical procedures or conditions named after a person or a place.

etiology the cause(s) or origin of a disease.

HCFA1500	Uniform health insurance claim form used for billing services to Medicare and other insurance carriers.
hierarchy	a system that ranks items one above another.
ICD-9-CM	International Classification of Diseases, 9th Revision, Clinical Modification.
ICD-10	International Classification of Diseases, 10th Revision
late effect	a residual effect (condition produced) after the acute phase of an illness or injury has ended.
main term	refers to listings in the Alphabetic Index appearing **BOLDFACE** type.
manifestation	characteristic signs or symptoms of an illness.
multiple	refers to the need to use more than one ICD-9-CM code to fully identify coding a condition.
primary code	the ICD-9-CM code that defines the main reason for the current encounter.
residual	the long-term condition(s) resulting from a previous acute illness or injury.
rule out	refers to a method used to indicate that a condition is probable, suspected, or questionable but unconfirmed. ICD-9-CM has no provisions for the use of this term.
secondary	code(s) listed after the primary code that further indicate the cause(s) code for the current encounter or define the need for higher levels of care.
sections	refers to portions of the Tabular List that are organized in groups of three-digit code numbers. For example, Malignant Neoplasm of Lip, Oral Cavity and Pharynx (140-149).
sequencing	the process of listing ICD-9-CM codes in the proper order.
specificity	refers to the requirement to code to the highest number of digits possible, 3, 4 or 5, when choosing an ICD-9-CM code.
sub term	refers to listings appearing in the Alphabetic Index under MAIN TERMS and always indented two spaces to the right.
subcategories	refers to groupings of four-digit codes listed under three-digit categories.
Tabular List	the portion of ICD-9-CM that lists codes and definitions in numeric order. Also referred to as Volume 1.
V codes	specific ICD-9-CM codes used to identify encounters for reasons other than illness or injury, for example, immunization.
Volume 1	see TABULAR LIST
Volume 2	see ALPHABETIC INDEX
Volume 3	procedure codes used only for hospital coding. Volume 3 contains both a numeric listing and an alphabetic index.

FORMAT OF ICD-9-CM

The *International Classification of Diseases, 9th Revision, Clinical Modification* was originally published as a three volume set (2nd edition). Newer versions of *ICD-9-CM* are available as two separate books containing Volume 1 and Volume 2 in one book and Volumes 1, 2 and 3 in the other. It is also now available on CD-ROM from the U.S. Government.

This edition of *ICD-9-CM* includes all official addenda from October 1986 through October 2009.

The Tabular List (Volume 1)

The Tabular List (Volume 1) is a *numeric* listing of diagnosis codes and descriptions consisting of 17 chapters that classify diseases and injuries, two sections containing supplementary codes (V codes and E codes) and four appendices.

Classification of Diseases and Injuries

The Classification of Diseases and Injuries includes the following 17 chapters:

Chapter 1   Infectious and Parasitic Diseases (001-139)

Chapter 2   Neoplasms (140-239)

Chapter 3   Endocrine, Nutritional and Metabolic Diseases, and Immunity Disorders (240-279)

Chapter 4   Diseases of the Blood and Blood-Forming Organs (280-289)

Chapter 5   Mental Disorders (290-319)

Chapter 6   Diseases of the Nervous System and Sense Organs (320-389)

Chapter 7   Diseases of the Circulatory System (390-459)

Chapter 8   Diseases of the Respiratory System (460-519)

Chapter 9   Diseases of the Digestive System (520-579)

Chapter 10   Diseases of the Genitourinary System (580-629)

Chapter 11   Complications of Pregnancy, Childbirth, and the Puerperium (630-677)

Chapter 12   Diseases of the Skin and Subcutaneous Tissue (680-709)

Chapter 13   Diseases of the Musculoskeletal System and Connective Tissue (710-739)

Chapter 14   Congenital Anomalies (740-759)

Chapter 15   Certain Conditions Originating in the Perinatal Period (760-779)

Chapter 16   Symptoms, Signs and Ill-defined Conditions (780-799)

Chapter 17   Injury and Poisoning (800-999)

Each chapter of the Tabular List (Volume 1) is structured into four components, namely:

Sections: groups of three-digit code numbers

Categories: three-digit code numbers

Subcategories: four-digit code numbers

Fifth-Digit Subclassifications: five-digit code numbers

Supplementary Classifications

There are two supplementary classifications included in the Tabular List (Volume 1). These are:

V Codes   Supplementary Classification of Factors Influencing Health Status and Contact with Health Services (V01-V89)

E Codes   Supplementary Classification of External Causes of Injury and Poisoning (E000-E999)

Appendices

The Tabular List (Volume 1) includes four appendices. These are:

Appendix A   Morphology of Neoplasms

Appendix C   Classification of Drugs by American Hospital Formulary Service List Number and Their ICD-9-CM Equivalents

Appendix D   Classification of Industrial Accidents According to Agency

Appendix E   List of Three-Digit Categories

Specifications for the Tabular List

1.   Three-digit rubrics and their contents are unchanged from *ICD-9*.

2.   The sequence of three-digit rubrics is unchanged from *ICD-9*.

3.   Three-digit rubrics are not added to the main body of the classification.

4.   Unsubdivided three-digit rubrics are subdivided where necessary to:

   a) Add clinical detail

   b) Isolate terms for clinical accuracy

5.   The modification in *ICD-9-CM* is accomplished by the addition of a fifth digit to existing *ICD-9* rubrics, except as noted under number 7 below.

6.   Four-digit rubrics are added to subdivided three-digit codes only when there is no other means of achieving desired detail. These codes, unique to *ICD-9-CM* (28 three-digit categories) are marked with the symbol in the Tabular List.

7.   The optional dual classification in *ICD-9* is modified.

   a) Duplicate rubrics are deleted:

      1) Four-digit manifestation categories duplicating etiology entries.

      2) Manifestation inclusion terms duplicating etiology entries.

   b) Manifestations of diseases are identified, to the extent possible, by creating five digit codes in the etiology rubrics.

   c) When the manifestation of a disease cannot be included in the etiology rubrics, provision for its identification is made by retaining the *ICD-9* rubrics used for classifying manifestations of disease.

8.   The format of *ICD-9-CM* is revised from that used in *ICD-9*.

   a) American spelling of medical terms is used.

   b) Inclusion terms are indented beneath the titles of codes.

   c) Codes not to be used for primary tabulation of disease are printed in italics with the notation, "code also underlying disease."

The Alphabetic Index (Volume 2)

The Alphabetic Index (Volume 2) of *ICD-9-CM* consists of an alphabetic list of terms and codes, two supplementary Sections following the alphabetic listing, plus two special tables found within the alphabetic listing. The Alphabetic Index (Volume 2) is structured as follows:

MAIN TERMS: appear in **BOLDFACE** type

SUBTERMS: are always indented two spaces to the right under main terms

CARRY-OVER   are always indented more than two spaces from the level of
LINES: the preceding line

Supplementary Sections

The supplementary sections following the Alphabetic Index are:

TABLE OF DRUGS AND CHEMICALS

This table contains a classification of drugs and other chemical substances to identify poisoning states and external causes of adverse effects.

INDEX TO EXTERNAL CAUSES OF INJURIES & POISONINGS (E-CODES)

This section contains the index to the codes that classify environmental events, circumstances, and other conditions as the cause of injury and other adverse effects.

Special Tables

The two special tables, located within the Alphabetic Index, and found under the main terms as underlined below, are:

HYPERTENSION TABLE

NEOPLASM TABLE

Specifications for the Alphabetic Index

1. Format of the Alphabetic Index follows the format of the ICD-9.

2. Main terms in the Alphabetic Index are printed in bold face type.

3. When two codes are required to indicate etiology and manifestation, the optional manifestation code appears in brackets, e.g., diabetic cataract 250.5 *[366.41]*.

Procedures: Tabular List and Alphabetic Index (Volume 3)

Volume 3 consists of two sections, a Tabular List of codes and an alphabetic index. These codes define procedures instead of diagnoses. Frequently used incorrectly by health care professionals, codes from Volume 3 are intended only for use by hospitals.

The ICD-9-CM Procedure Classification is a modification of WHO's *Fascicle V, Surgical Procedures*, and is published as Volume 3 of ICD-9-CM. It contains both a Tabular List and an Alphabetic Index. Greater detail has been added to the ICD-9-CM Procedure Classification necessitating expansion of the codes from three to four digits. Approximately 90% of the rubrics refer to surgical procedures with the remaining 10% accounting for other investigative and therapeutic procedures.

Tabular List of Procedures

The Tabular List includes 16 chapters containing codes and descriptions for surgical procedures and miscellaneous diagnostic and therapeutic procedures.

Alphabetic Index to Procedures

The Alphabetic Index provides an alphabetic index to the Tabular List of Volume 3

Specifications for the Procedure Classification

1. The ICD-9-CM Procedure Classification is published in its own volume containing both a Tabular List and an Alphabetic Index.

2. The classification is a modification of *Fascicle V Surgical Procedures* of the ICD-9 Classification of Procedures in Medicine, working from the draft dated Geneva, 30 September-6 October 1975, and labeled WHO/ICD-9/Rev. Conf. 75.4.

3. All three-digit rubrics in the range 01-86 are maintained as they appear in *Fascicle V*, whenever feasible.

4. Nonsurgical procedures are segregated from the surgical procedures and confined to the rubrics 87-99, whenever feasible.

5. Selected detail contained in the remaining fascicles of the *ICD-9 Classification of Procedures in Medicine* is accommodated where possible.

6. The structure of the classification is based on anatomy rather than surgical specialty.

7. The *ICD-9-CM* Procedure Classification is numeric only, i.e., no alphabetic characters are used.

8. The classification is based on a two-digit structure with two decimal digits where necessary.

9. Compatibility with the *ICD-9 Classification of Procedures in Medicine* was not maintained when a different axis was deemed more clinically appropriate.

CONVENTIONS USED IN THE TABULAR LIST

The *ICD-9-CM* Tabular List (Volume 1) makes use of certain abbreviations, punctuation, symbols, and other conventions that must be clearly understood. The purpose of these conventions is to first, provide special coding instructions, and second, to conserve space.

Abbreviations

NOS   Not Otherwise Specified. Equivalent to Unspecified. This abbreviation refers to a lack of sufficient detail in the statement of diagnosis to be able to assign it to a more specific sub division within the classification.

NEC   Not Elsewhere Classified. Used with ill-defined terms to alert the coder that a specified form of the condition is classified differently. The category number for the term including NEC is to be used only when the coder lacks the information necessary to code the term to a more specific category.

Punctuation

( )   PARENTHESES are used to enclose supplementary words that may be present or absent in a statement of disease without affecting the code assignment.

[ ]   SQUARE BRACKETS are used to enclose synonyms, alternate wordings or explanatory phrases.

:   COLONS are used after an incomplete phrase or term that requires one or more of the modifiers indented under it to make it assignable to a given category. EXCEPTION to this rule pertains to the abbreviation NOS.

Symbols

●   A filled BLACK CIRCLE preceding a code indicates that the code is new to this revision of ICD-9-CM. A symbol key appears on all left-hand pages of the Tabular List, Volume 1 and Volume 3.

▲   A filled BLACK TRIANGLE preceding a code indicates that there is a revision to the text of an existing code. A symbol key appears on all left-hand pages of the Tabular List, Volume 1 and Volume 3.

④ ⑤   A circle containing the number 4 or the number 5 preceding a code indicates that a fourth or fifth digit is required for coding to the highest level of specificity. Valid digits are in [brackets] under each code if the fourth- and fifth-digit codes themselves are not listed. Definitions of valid fifth digits are found under the major category.

Other conventions

Type Face:

BOLD: Bold type face is used for all codes and titles in the Tabular List.

Italics: Italicized type face is used for all exclusion notes and to identify those rubrics that are not to be used for primary tabulations of disease.

Format: ICD-9-CM uses an indented format for ease in reference.

Instructional Notations

Instructional terms define what is, or what is not, included in a given subdivision. This is accomplished by using both inclusion and exclusion terms.

INCLUDES:	Indicates separate terms, such as, modifying adjectives, sites and conditions, entered under a subdivision, such as a category, to further define or give examples of, the content of the category.
Excludes:	Exclusion terms are enclosed in a box and are printed in italics to draw attention to their presence. The importance of this instructional term is its use as a guideline to direct the coder to the proper code assignment. In other words, all terms following the word EXCLUDES: are to be coded elsewhere as indicated in each instance.
NOTES	These are used to define terms and give coding instructions. Often used to list the fifth-digit subclassifications for certain categories.
SEE	The "see" instruction following a main term in the index indicates that another term should be referenced. It is necessary to go to the main term referenced with the "see" note to locate the correct code.
SEE CATEGORY	A variation of the instructional term SEE. This refers the coder to a specific category. You must *always* follow this instructional term.
SEE ALSO	A "see also" instruction following a main term in the index instructs that there is another main term that may also be referenced that may provide additional index entries that may be useful. It is not necessary to follow the "see also" note when the original main term provides the necessary code.
CODE FIRST	This instructional note is used for those codes not intended to be used as a principal diagnosis, or not to be sequenced before the underlying disease. The note requires that the underlying disease (etiology) be coded first with the code the note is applied to being coded second. This note appears only in the Tabular List (Vol. 1).
USE ADDITIONAL CODE	This instruction is placed in the Tabular List in those categories where the coder may wish to add further information, by using an additional code, to give a more complete picture of the diagnosis or procedure.

Related terms

AND	The word "and" should be interpreted to mean either "and" or "or" when it appears in a title.
WITH	The word "with" in the alphabetic index is sequenced immediately following the main term, not in alphabetical order.

COLOR CODING

A PMIC versions of ICD-9-CM include color-coding to alert the user to special coding situations or conditions that require additional attention. The use of color-coding is found in the Tabular List of Volume 1 and the Tabular List of Volume 3. The color is applied as solid rectangular bars over the codes only so that the descriptions remain clear and legible. The color codes and definitions are printed at the bottom of all right-sided pages of Volume 1 and Volume 3.

Volume 1

Three digit codes. Coding to fourth or fifth digit specificity is required.

Unspecified code. Descriptions include the term "unspecified." Use only if a more specific diagnosis is not known or available.

Nonspecific code. Descriptions include the term "nonspecific, unspecified, other specified or other." A report *may* be required by insurance carriers.

Manifestation codes. Used only to code the manifestation of an underlying disease. Code the underlying disease first.

Medicare secondary payer (MSP) alert. Diagnoses that may trigger a post-payment review by Medicare. Medicare is usually the secondary payer for these diagnoses.

Secondary diagnosis only. V codes that may only be used as additional codes, not as first-listed codes.

Primary diagnosis only. V codes which are only acceptable as first listed codes.

Volume 3*

Noncovered operating room procedure. An operating room procedure that is not covered by Medicare.

Non-operating room procedure. A procedure that is not performed in the operating room that affects DRG assignment.

Bilateral procedure.

Valid operating room procedure. Prompts a change in DRG assignment.

Nonspecific operating room procedure. Choose a more precise code if possible.

*These colors appear only in the three-volume edition

ICD-9-CM OFFICIAL GUIDELINES FOR CODING AND REPORTING

Guidelines effective as of publication date. For updates, visit http://pmiconline.com
The guidelines include the updated V Code Table

The Centers for Medicare and Medicaid Services (CMS) and the National Center for Health Statistics (NCHS), two departments within the U.S. Federal Government's Department of Health and Human Services (DHHS) provide the following guidelines for coding and reporting using the International Classification of Diseases, 9th Revision, Clinical Modification (ICD-9-CM). These guidelines should be used as a companion document to the official version of the ICD-9CM as published on CD-ROM by the U.S. Government Printing Office (GPO).

These guidelines have been approved by the four organizations that make up the Cooperating Parties for the ICD-9-CM: the American Hospital Association (AHA), the American Health Information Management Association (AHIMA), CMS, and NCHS. These guidelines are included on the official government version of the ICD-9-CM, and also appear in "Coding Clinic for ICD-9-CM" published by the AHA.

These guidelines are a set of rules that have been developed to accompany and complement the official conventions and instructions provided within the ICD-9-CM itself. These guidelines are based on the coding and sequencing instructions in Volumes I, II and III of ICD-9-CM, but provide additional instruction. Adherence to these guidelines when assigning ICD-9-CM diagnosis and procedure codes is required under the Health Insurance Portability and Accountability Act (HIPAA). The diagnosis codes (Volumes 1-2) have been adopted under HIPAA for all healthcare settings. Volume 3 procedure codes have been adopted for inpatient procedures reported by hospitals. A joint effort between the healthcare provider and the coder is essential to achieve complete and accurate documentation, code assignment, and reporting of diagnoses and procedures. These guidelines have been developed to assist both the healthcare provider and the coder in identifying those diagnoses and procedures that are to be reported. The importance of consistent, complete documentation in the medical record cannot be overemphasized. Without such documentation accurate coding cannot be achieved. The entire record should be reviewed to determine the specific reason for the encounter and the conditions treated.

The term encounter is used for all settings, including hospital admissions. In the context of these guidelines, the term provider is used throughout the guidelines to mean physician or any qualified health care practitioner who is legally accountable for establishing the patient's diagnosis. Only this set of guidelines, approved by the Cooperating Parties, is official.

The guidelines are organized into sections. Section I includes the structure and conventions of the classification and general guidelines that apply to the entire classification, and chapter specific guidelines that correspond to the chapters as they are arranged in the classification. Section II includes guidelines for selection of principal diagnosis for non-outpatient settings. Section III includes guidelines for reporting additional diagnoses in non-outpatient settings. Section IV is for outpatient coding and reporting.

ICD-9-CM Official Guidelines for Coding and Reporting

Section I. Conventions, general coding guidelines and chapter specific guidelines.

A. Conventions for the ICD-9-CM

1. Format
2. Abbreviations
    a. Index abbreviations
    b. Tabular abbreviations
3. Punctuation
4. Includes and Excludes Notes and Inclusion terms
5. Other and Unspecified codes
    a. "Other" codes
    b   "Unspecified" codes
6. Etiology/manifestation convention ("code first", "use additional code" and "in diseases classified elsewhere" notes)
7. "And"
8. "With"
9. "See" and "See Also"

B. General Coding Guidelines

1. Use of Both Alphabetic Index and Tabular List
2. Locate each term in the Alphabetic Index
3. Level of Detail in Coding
4. Code or codes from 001.0 through V89
5. Selection of codes 001.0 through 999.9
6. Signs and symptoms
7. Conditions that are an integral part of a disease process
8. Conditions that are not an integral part of a disease process
9. Multiple coding for a single condition
10 Acute and Chronic Conditions
11 Combination Code
12 Late Effects
13 Impending or Threatened Condition
14 Reporting Same Diagnosis Code More Than Once
15 Admissions/Encounters for Rehabilitation
16 Documentation for BMI and Pressure Ulcer Stages

C. Chapter-Specific Coding Guidelines

1. Chapter 1: Infectious and Parasitic Diseases (001-139)
    a. Human Immunodeficiency Virus (HIV) Infections
    b. Septicemia, Systemic Inflammatory Response Syndrome (SIRS), Sepsis, Severe Sepsis and Septic Shock
    c. Methicillin Resistant *Staphylococcus aureus* (MRSA) Conditions
2. Chapter 2: Neoplasms (140-239)
    a. Treatment directed at the malignancy
    b. Treatment of secondary site
    c. Coding and sequencing of complications
    d. Primary malignancy previously excised
    e. Admissions/Encounters involving chemotherapy, immunotherapy and radiation therapy
    f. Admission/encounter to determine extent of malignancy

    g. Symptoms, signs, and ill-defined conditions listed in Chapter 16 associated with neoplasms.
    h. Admission/encounter for pain control/management
    i. Malignant neoplasm associated with transplanted organ

3. Chapter 3: Endocrine, Nutritional, and Metabolic Diseases and Immunity Disorders (240-279)
    a. Diabetes mellitus

4. Chapter 4: Diseases of Blood and Blood Forming Organs (280-289)
    a. Anemia of chronic disease

5. Chapter 5: Mental Disorders (290-319)
  Reserved for future guideline expansion

6. Chapter 6: Diseases of Nervous System and Sense Organs (320-389)
    a. Pain - Category 338

7. Chapter 7: Diseases of Circulatory System (390-459)
    a. Hypertension
    b. Cerebral infarction/stroke/cerebrovascular accident (CVA)
    c. Postoperative cerebrovascular accident
    d. Late Effects of Cerebrovascular Disease
    e. Acute myocardial infarction (AMI)

8. Chapter 8: Diseases of Respiratory System (460-519)
    a. Chronic Obstructive Pulmonary Disease [COPD] and Asthma
    b   Chronic Obstructive Pulmonary Disease [COPD] and Bronchitis
    c. Acute Respiratory Failure
    d. Influenza due to identified avian influenza virus (avian influenza)

9. Chapter 9: Diseases of Digestive System (520-579)
  Reserved for future guideline expansion

10. Chapter 10: Diseases of Genitourinary System (580-629)
    a. Chronic kidney disease

11. Chapter 11: Complications of Pregnancy, Childbirth, and the Puerperium (630-677)
    a. General Rules for Obstetric Cases
    b. Selection of OB Principal or First-listed Diagnosis
    c. Fetal Conditions Affecting the Management of the Mother
    d. HIV Infection in Pregnancy, Childbirth and the Puerperium
    e. Current Conditions Complicating Pregnancy
    f. Diabetes mellitus in pregnancy
    g. Gestational diabetes
    h. Normal Delivery, Code 650
    i. The Postpartum and Peripartum Periods
    j. Code 677, Late effect of complication of pregnancy
    k. Abortions

12. Chapter 12: Diseases Skin and Subcutaneous Tissue (680-709)
    a. Pressure ulcer stage codes

13. Chapter 13: Diseases of Musculoskeletal and Connective Tissue (710-739)
    a. Coding of Pathologic Fractures

14 Chapter 14: Congenital Anomalies (740-759)
    a. Codes in categories 740-759, Congenital Anomalies

15. Chapter 15: Newborn (Perinatal) Guidelines (760-779)
    a. General Perinatal Rules
    b. Use of codes V30-V39
    c. Newborn transfers
    d. Use of category V29
    e. Use of other V codes on perinatal records
    f. Maternal Causes of Perinatal Morbidity
    g. Congenital Anomalies in Newborns
    h. Coding Additional Perinatal Diagnoses
    i. Prematurity and Fetal Growth Retardation
    j. Newborn sepsis

16. Chapter 16: Signs, Symptoms and Ill-Defined Conditions (780-799)
Reserved for future guideline expansion

17. Chapter 17: Injury and Poisoning (800-999)
    a. Coding of Injuries
    b. Coding of Traumatic Fractures
    c. Coding of Burns
    d. Coding of Debridement of Wound, Infection, or Burn
    e. Adverse Effects, Poisoning and Toxic Effects
    f. Complications of care
    g. SIRS due to Non-infectious Process

18. Classification of Factors Influencing Health Status and Contact with Health Service (Supplemental V01-V89)
    a. Introduction
    b. V codes use in any healthcare setting
    c. V Codes indicate a reason for an encounter
    d. Categories of V Codes
    e. V Code Table

19. Supplemental Classification of External Causes of Injury and Poisoning (E-codes, E800-E999)
    a. General E Code Coding Guidelines
    b. Place of Occurrence Guideline
    c. Adverse Effects of Drugs, Medicinal and Biological Substances Guidelines
    d. Multiple Cause E Code Coding Guidelines
    e. Child and Adult Abuse Guideline
    f. Unknown or Suspected Intent Guideline
    g. Undetermined Cause
    h. Late Effects of External Cause Guidelines
    i. Misadventures and Complications of Care Guidelines
    j. Terrorism Guidelines

Section II. Selection of Principal Diagnosis

A. Codes for symptoms, signs, and ill-defined conditions

B. Two or more interrelated conditions, each potentially meeting the definition for principal diagnosis

C. Two or more diagnoses that equally meet the definition for principal diagnosis

D. Two or more comparative or contrasting conditions.

E. A symptom(s) followed by contrasting/comparative diagnoses

F. Original treatment plan not carried out

G. Complications of surgery and other medical care

H. Uncertain Diagnosis

I. Admission from Observation Unit
   1. Admission Following Medical Observation
   2. Admission Following Post-Operative Observation

J. Admission from Outpatient Surgery

Section III. Reporting Additional Diagnoses

A. Previous conditions .
B. Abnormal findings
C. Uncertain Diagnosis

Section IV. Diagnostic Coding and Reporting Guidelines for Outpatient Services

A. Selection of first-listed condition
   1. Outpatient Surgery
   2. Observation Stay

B. Codes from 001.0 through V89.09
C. Accurate reporting of ICD-9-CM diagnosis codes
D. Selection of codes 001.0 through 999.9
E. Codes that describe symptoms and signs
F. Encounters for circumstances other than a disease or injury

G. Level of Detail in Coding
   1. ICD-9-CM codes with 3, 4, or 5 digits
   2. Use of full number of digits required for a code

H. ICD-9-CM code for the diagnosis, condition, problem, or other reason for encounter/visit
I. Uncertain diagnosis
J. Chronic diseases
K. Code all documented conditions that coexist
L. Patients receiving diagnostic services only
M. Patients receiving therapeutic services only
N. Patients receiving preoperative evaluations only
O. Ambulatory surgery
P. Routine outpatient prenatal visits

Appendix I: Present on Admission Reporting Guidelines

SECTION I. CONVENTIONS, GENERAL CODING GUIDELINES AND CHAPTER SPECIFIC GUIDELINES

The conventions, general guidelines and chapter-specific guidelines are applicable to all health care settings unless otherwise indicated.

A. Conventions for the ICD-9-CM

The conventions for the ICD-9-CM are the general rules for use of the classification independent of the guidelines. These conventions are incorporated within the index and tabular of the ICD-9-CM as instructional notes. The conventions are as follows:

1. Format:

The ICD-9-CM uses an indented format for ease in reference

2. Abbreviations

a. Index abbreviations

NEC   "Not elsewhere classifiable"

This abbreviation in the index represents "other specified" when a specific code is not available for a condition the index directs the coder to the "other specified" code in the tabular.

b. Tabular abbreviations

NEC   "Not elsewhere classifiable"

This abbreviation in the tabular represents "other specified". When a specific code is not available for a condition the tabular includes an NEC entry under a code to identify the code as the "other specified" code.

(See Section I.A.5.a. "Other" codes").

NOS   "Not otherwise specified"

This abbreviation is the equivalent of unspecified.

(See Section I.A.5.b., "Unspecified" codes)

3. Punctuation

[ ]   Brackets are used in the tabular list to enclose synonyms, alternative wording or explanatory phrases. Brackets are used in the index to identify manifestation codes.

(See Section I.A.6. "Etiology/manifestations")

( )   Parentheses are used in both the index and tabular to enclose supplementary words that may be present or absent in the statement of a disease or procedure without affecting the code number to which it is assigned. The terms within the parentheses are referred to as nonessential modifiers.

:   Colons are used in the Tabular list after an incomplete term which needs one or more of the modifiers following the colon to make it assignable to a given category.

4. Includes and Excludes Notes and Inclusion terms

Includes: This note appears immediately under a three-digit code title to further define, or give examples of, the content of the category.

Excludes: An excludes note under a code indicates that the terms excluded from the code are to be coded elsewhere. In some cases the codes for the excluded terms should not be used in conjunction with the code from which it is excluded. An example of this is a congenital condition excluded from an acquired form of the same condition. The congenital and acquired codes should not be used together. In other cases, the excluded terms may be used together with an excluded code. An example of this is when fractures of different bones are coded to different codes. Both codes may be used together if both types of fractures are present.

Inclusion terms: List of terms is included under certain four and five digit codes. These terms are the conditions for which that code number is to be used. The terms may be synonyms of the code title, or, in the case of "other specified" codes, the terms are a list of the various conditions assigned to that code. The inclusion terms are not necessarily exhaustive. Additional terms found only in the index may also be assigned to a code.

5. Other and Unspecified codes

a. "Other" codes

Codes titled "other" or "other specified" (usually a code with a 4th digit 8 or fifth-digit 9 for diagnosis codes) are for use when the information in the medical record provides detail for which a specific code does not exist. Index entries with NEC in the line designate "other" codes in the tabular. These index entries represent specific disease entities for which no specific code exists so the term is included within an "other" code.

b. "Unspecified" codes

Codes (usually a code with a 4th digit 9 or 5th digit 0 for diagnosis codes) titled "unspecified" are for use when the information in the medical record is insufficient to assign a more specific code.

6. Etiology/manifestation convention ("code first", "use additional code" and "in diseases classified elsewhere" notes)

Certain conditions have both an underlying etiology and multiple body system manifestations due to the underlying etiology. For such conditions, the ICD-9-CM has a coding convention that requires the underlying condition be sequenced first followed by the manifestation. Wherever such a combination exists, there is a "use additional code" note at the etiology code, and a "code first" note at the manifestation code. These instructional notes indicate the proper sequencing order of the codes, etiology followed by manifestation.

In most cases the manifestation codes will have in the code title, "in diseases classified elsewhere." Codes with this title are a component of the etiology/ manifestation convention. The code title indicates that it is a manifestation code. "In diseases classified elsewhere" codes are never permitted to be used as first listed or principal diagnosis codes. They must be used in conjunction with an underlying condition code and they must be listed following the underlying condition.

There are manifestation codes that do not have "in diseases classified elsewhere" in the title. For such codes a "use additional code" note will still be present and the rules for sequencing apply.

In addition to the notes in the tabular, these conditions also have a specific index entry structure. In the index both conditions are listed together with the etiology code first followed by the manifestation codes in brackets. The code in brackets is always to be sequenced second.

The most commonly used etiology/manifestation combinations are the codes for Diabetes mellitus, category 250. For each code under category 250 there is a use additional code note for the manifestation that is specific for that particular diabetic manifestation. Should a patient have more than one manifestation of diabetes, more than one code from category 250 may be used with as many manifestation codes as are needed to fully describe the patient's complete diabetic condition. The category 250 diabetes codes should be sequenced first, followed by the manifestation codes.

"Code first" and "Use additional code" notes are also used as sequencing rules in the classification for certain codes that are not part of an etiology/ manifestation combination.

See - Section I.B.9. "Multiple coding for a single condition".

7. "And"

The word "and" should be interpreted to mean either "and" or "or" when it appears in a title.

8. "With"

The word "with" in the alphabetic index is sequenced immediately following the main term, not in alphabetical order.

9. "See" and "See Also"

The "see" instruction following a main term in the index indicates that another term should be referenced. It is necessary to go to the main term referenced with the "see" note to locate the correct code.

A "see also" instruction following a main term in the index instructs that there is another main term that may also be referenced that may provide additional index entries that may be useful. It is not necessary to follow the "see also" note when the original main term provides the necessary code.

B. General Coding Guidelines

1. Use of Both Alphabetic Index and Tabular List

Use both the Alphabetic Index and the Tabular List when locating and assigning a code. Reliance on only the Alphabetic Index or the Tabular List leads to errors in code assignments and less specificity in code selection.

2. Locate each term in the Alphabetic Index

Locate each term in the Alphabetic Index and verify the code selected in the Tabular List. Read and be guided by instructional notations that appear in both the Alphabetic Index and the Tabular List.

3. Level of Detail in Coding

Diagnosis and procedure codes are to be used at their highest number of digits available.

ICD-9-CM diagnosis codes are composed of codes with 3, 4, or 5 digits. Codes with three digits are included in ICD-9-CM as the heading of a category of codes that may be further subdivided by the use of fourth and/or fifth digits, which provide greater detail.

A three-digit code is to be used only if it is not further subdivided. Where fourth-digit subcategories and/or fifth-digit subclassifications are provided, they must be assigned. A code is invalid if it has not been coded to the full number of digits required for that code. For example, Acute myocardial infarction, code 410, has fourth digits that describe the location of the infarction (e.g., 410.2, Of inferolateral wall), and fifth digits that identify the episode of care. It would be incorrect to report a code in category 410 without a fourth and fifth digit.

ICD-9-CM Volume 3 procedure codes are composed of codes with either 3 or 4 digits. Codes with two digits are included in ICD-9-CM as the heading of a category of codes that may be further subdivided by the use of third and/or fourth digits, which provide greater detail.

4. Code or codes from 001.0 through V84.8

The appropriate code or codes from 001.0 through V84.8 must be used to identify diagnoses, symptoms, conditions, problems, complaints or other reason(s) for the encounter/visit.

5. Selection of codes 001.0 through 999.9

The selection of codes 001.0 through 999.9 will frequently be used to describe the reason for the admission/encounter. These codes are from the section of ICD-9-CM for the classification of diseases and injuries (e.g., infectious and parasitic diseases; neoplasms; symptoms, signs, and ill-defined conditions, etc.).

6. Signs and symptoms

Codes that describe symptoms and signs, as opposed to diagnoses, are acceptable for reporting purposes when a related definitive diagnosis has not been established (confirmed) by the provider. Chapter 16 of ICD-9-CM, Symptoms, Signs, and Ill-defined conditions (codes 780.0 - 799.9) contain many, but not all codes for symptoms.

7. Conditions that are an integral part of a disease process

Signs and symptoms that are associated routinely with a disease process should not be assigned as additional codes, unless otherwise instructed by the classification.

8. Conditions that are not an integral part of a disease process

Additional signs and symptoms that may not be associated routinely with a disease process should be coded when present.

9. Multiple coding for a single condition

In addition to the etiology/manifestation convention that requires two codes to fully describe a single condition that affects multiple body systems, there are other single conditions that also require more than one code. "Use additional code" notes are found in the tabular at codes that are not part of an etiology/manifestation pair where a secondary code is useful to fully describe a condition. The sequencing rule is the same as the etiology/manifestation pair - , "use additional code" indicates that a secondary code should be added.

For example, for infections that are not included in chapter 1, a secondary code from category 041, Bacterial infection in conditions classified elsewhere and of unspecified site, may be required to identify the bacterial organism causing the infection. A "use additional code" note will normally be found at the infectious disease code, indicating a need for the organism code to be added as a secondary code.

"Code first" notes are also under certain codes that are not specifically manifestation codes but may be due to an underlying cause. When a "code first" note is present and an underlying condition is present the underlying condition should be sequenced first.

"Code, if applicable, any causal condition first", notes indicate that this code may be assigned as a principal diagnosis when the causal condition is unknown or not applicable. If a causal condition is known, then the code for that condition should be sequenced as the principal or first-listed diagnosis.

Multiple codes may be needed for late effects, complication codes and obstetric codes to more fully describe a condition. See the specific guidelines for these conditions for further instruction.

10. Acute and Chronic Conditions

If the same condition is described as both acute (subacute) and chronic, and separate subentries exist in the Alphabetic Index at the same indentation level, code both and sequence the acute (subacute) code first.

11. Combination Code

A combination code is a single code used to classify: Two diagnoses, or A diagnosis with an associated secondary process (manifestation) A diagnosis with an associated complication Combination codes are identified by referring to subterm entries in the Alphabetic Index and by reading the inclusion and exclusion notes in the Tabular List.

Assign only the combination code when that code fully identifies the diagnostic conditions involved or when the Alphabetic Index so directs.

Multiple coding should not be used when the classification provides a combination code that clearly identifies all of the elements documented in the diagnosis. When the combination code lacks necessary specificity in describing the manifestation or complication, an additional code should be used as a secondary code.

12. Late Effects

A late effect is the residual effect (condition produced) after the acute phase of an illness or injury has terminated. There is no time limit on when a late effect code can be used. The residual may be apparent early, such as in cerebrovascular accident cases, or it may occur months or years later, such as that due to a previous injury. Coding of late effects generally requires two codes sequenced in the following order: The condition or nature of the late effect is sequenced first. The late effect code is sequenced second.

An exception to the above guidelines are those instances where the code for late effect is followed by a manifestation code identified in the Tabular List and title, or the late effect code has been expanded (at the fourth and fifth-digit levels) to include the manifestation(s). The code for the acute phase of an illness or injury that led to the late effect is never used with a code for the late effect.

13. Impending or Threatened Condition

Code any condition described at the time of discharge as "impending" or "threatened" as follows:

If it did occur, code as confirmed diagnosis.

If it did not occur, reference the Alphabetic Index to determine if the condition has a subentry term for "impending" or "threatened" and also reference main term entries for "Impending" and for "Threatened." If the subterms are listed, assign the given code.

If the subterms are not listed, code the existing underlying condition(s) and not the condition described as impending or threatened.

14. Reporting Same Diagnosis Code More Than Once

Each unique ICD-9-CM diagnosis code may be reported only once for an encounter. This applies to bilateral conditions or two different conditions classified to the same ICD-9-CM diagnosis code.

15. Admissions/Encounters for Rehabilitation

When the purpose for the admission/encounter is rehabilitation, sequence the appropriate V code from category V57, Care involving use of rehabilitation procedures, as the principal/first-listed diagnosis. The code for the condition for which the service is being performed should be reported as an additional diagnosis.

Only one code from category V57 is required. Code V57.89, Other specified rehabilitation procedures, should be assigned if more than one type of rehabilitation is performed during a single encounter. A procedure code should be reported to identify each type of rehabilitation therapy actually performed.

16. Documentation of BMI and Pressure Ulcer Stages

For the Body Mass Index (BMI) and pressure ulcer stage codes, code assignment may be based on medical record documentation from clinicians who are not the patient's provider (i.e., physician or otherqualified healthcare practitioner legally accountable for establishing the patient's diagnosis), since this information is typically documented by other clinicians involved in the care of the patient (e.g., a dietitian often documents the BMI and nurses often documents the pressure ulcer stages). However, the associated diagnosis (such as overweight, obesity, or pressure ulcer) must be documented by the patient's provider. If there is conflicting medical record documentation, either from the same clinician or different clinicians, the patient's attending provider should be queried for clarification.

The BMI and pressure ulcer stage codes should only be reported as secondary diagnoses. As with all other secondary diagnosis codes, the BMI and pressure ulcer stage codes should only be assigned when they meet the definition of a reportable additional diagnosis (see Section III, Reporting Additional Diagnoses).

C. Chapter-Specific Coding Guidelines

In addition to general coding guidelines, there are guidelines for specific diagnoses and/or conditions in the classification. Unless otherwise indicated, these guidelines apply to all health care settings. Please refer to Section II for guidelines on the selection of principal diagnosis.

1. Chapter 1: Infectious and Parasitic Diseases (001-139)

a. Human Immunodeficiency Virus (HIV) Infections

1) Code only confirmed cases

Code only confirmed cases of HIV infection/illness. This is an exception to the hospital inpatient guideline Section II, H. In this context, "confirmation" does not require documentation of positive serology or culture for HIV; the provider's diagnostic statement that the patient is HIV positive, or has an HIV-related illness is sufficient.

2) **Selection and sequencing of HIV codes**

(a) **Patient admitted for HIV-related condition**

If a patient is admitted for an HIV-related condition, the principal diagnosis should be 042, followed by additional diagnosis codes for all reported HIV-related conditions.

(b) **Patient with HIV disease admitted for unrelated condition**

If a patient with HIV disease is admitted for an unrelated condition (such as a traumatic injury), the code for the unrelated condition (e.g., the nature of injury code) should be the principal diagnosis. Other diagnoses would be 042 followed by additional diagnosis codes for all reported HIV-related conditions.

(c) **Whether the patient is newly diagnosed**

Whether the patient is newly diagnosed or has had previous admissions/encounters for HIV conditions is irrelevant to the sequencing decision.

(d) **Asymptomatic human immunodeficiency virus V08**

Asymptomatic human immunodeficiency virus [HIV] infection, is to be applied when the patient without any documentation of symptoms is listed as being "HIV positive," "known HIV," "HIV test positive," or similar terminology. Do not use this code if the term "AIDS" is used or if the patient is treated for any HIV-related illness or is described as having any condition(s) resulting from his/her HIV positive status; use 042 in these cases.

(e) **Patients with inconclusive HIV serology**

Patients with inconclusive HIV serology, but no definitive diagnosis or manifestations of the illness, may be assigned code 795.71, Inconclusive serologic test for Human Immunodeficiency Virus [HIV].

(f) **Previously diagnosed HIV-related illness**

Patients with any known prior diagnosis of an HIV-related illness should be coded to 042. Once a patient has developed an HIV-related illness, the patient should always be assigned code 042 on every subsequent admission/encounter. Patients previously diagnosed with any HIV illness (042) should never be assigned to 795.71 or V08.

(g) **HIV Infection in Pregnancy, Childbirth and the Puerperium**

During pregnancy, childbirth or the puerperium, a patient admitted (or presenting for a health care encounter) because of an HIV-related illness should receive a principal diagnosis code of 647.6X, Other specified infectious and parasitic diseases in the mother classifiable elsewhere, but complicating the pregnancy, childbirth or the puerperium, followed by 042 and the code(s) for the HIV-related illness(es). Codes from Chapter 15 always take sequencing priority.

Patients with asymptomatic HIV infection status admitted (or presenting for a health care encounter) during pregnancy, childbirth, or the puerperium should receive codes of 647.6X and V08.

(h) Encounters for testing for HIV

If a patient is being seen to determine his/her HIV status, use code V73.89, Screening for other specified viral disease. Use code V69.8, Other problems related to lifestyle, as a secondary code if an asymptomatic patient is in a known high risk group for HIV. Should a patient with signs or symptoms or illness, or a confirmed HIV related diagnosis be tested for HIV, code the signs and symptoms or the diagnosis. An additional counseling code V65.44 may be used if counseling is provided during the encounter for the test.

When a patient returns to be informed of his/her HIV test results use code V65.44, HIV counseling, if the results of the test are negative.

If the results are positive but the patient is asymptomatic use code V08, Asymptomatic HIV infection. If the results are positive and the patient is symptomatic use code 042, HIV infection, with codes for the HIV related symptoms or diagnosis. The HIV counseling code may also be used if counseling is provided for patients with positive test results.

b. Septicemia, Systemic Inflammatory Response Syndrome (SIRS), Sepsis, Severe Sepsis, and Septic Shock

1) SIRS, Septicemia, and Sepsis

(a) The terms septicemia and sepsis are often used interchangeably by providers, however they are not considered synonymous terms. The following descriptions are provided for reference but do not preclude querying the provider for clarification about terms used in the documentation:

   (i) Septicemia generally refers to a systemic disease associated with the presence of pathological microorganisms or toxins in the blood, which can include bacteria, viruses, fungi or other organisms.

   (ii) Systemic inflammatory response syndrome (SIRS) generally refers to the systemic response to infection, trauma/burns, or other insult (such as cancer) with symptoms including fever, tachycardia, tachypnea, and leukocytosis.

   (iii) Sepsis generally refers to SIRS due to infection.

   (iv) Severe sepsis generally refers to sepsis with associated acute organ dysfunction.

(b) The Coding of SIRS, sepsis and severe sepsis requires a minimum of 2 codes: a code for the underlying cause (such as infection or trauma) and a code from subcategory 995.9 Systemic inflammatory response syndrome (SIRS).

   (i) The code for the underlying cause (such as infection or trauma) must be sequenced before the code from subcategory 995.9 Systemic inflammatory response syndrome (SIRS).

   (ii) Sepsis and severe sepsis require a code for the systemic infection (038.xx, 112.5, etc.) and either code 995.91, Sepsis, or 995.92, Severe sepsis. If the causal organism is not documented, assign code 038.9, Unspecified septicemia.

   (iii) Severe sepsis requires additional code(s) for the associated acute organ dysfunction(s).

   (iv) If a patient has sepsis with multiple organ dysfunctions, follow the instructions for coding severe sepsis.

   (v) Either the term sepsis or SIRS must be documented to assign a code from subcategory 995.9.

   (vi) See Section I.C.17.g), Injury and poisoning, for information regarding systemic inflammatory response syndrome (SIRS) due to trauma/burns and other non-infectious processes.

(c) Due to the complex nature of sepsis and severe sepsis, some cases may require querying the provider prior to assignment of the codes.

2) Sequencing sepsis and severe sepsis

(a) Sepsis and severe sepsis as principal diagnosis

   If sepsis or severe sepsis is present on admission, and meets the definition of principal diagnosis, the systemic infection code (e.g., 038.xx, 112.5, etc) should be assigned as the principal diagnosis, followed by code 995.91, Sepsis, or 995.92, Severe sepsis, as required by the sequencing rules in the Tabular List. Codes from subcategory 995.9 can never be assigned as a principal diagnosis. A code should also be assigned for any localized infection, if present.

   If the sepsis or severe sepsis is due to a postprocedural infection, see Section I.C.10 for guidelines related to sepsis due to postprocedural infection.

(b) Sepsis and severe sepsis as secondary diagnoses

   When sepsis or severe sepsis develops during the encounter (it was not present on admission), the systemic infection code and code 995.91 or 995.92 should be assigned as secondary diagnoses.

(c) Documentation unclear as to whether sepsis or severe sepsis is present on admission

Sepsis or severe sepsis may be present on admission but the diagnosis may not be confirmed until sometime after admission. If the documentation is not clear whether the sepsis or severe sepsis was present on admission, the provider should be queried.

3) Sepsis/SIRS with Localized Infection

If the reason for admission is both sepsis, severe sepsis, or SIRS and a localized infection, such as pneumonia or cellulitis, a code for the systemic infection (038.xx, 112.5, etc) should be assigned first, then code 995.91 or 995.92, followed by the code for the localized infection. If the patient is admitted with a localized infection, such as pneumonia, and sepsis/SIRS doesn't develop until after admission, see guideline I.C.1.b.2.b).

If the localized infection is postprocedural, see Section I.C.10 for guidelines related to sepsis due to postprocedural infection.

Note: The term urosepsis is a nonspecific term. If that is the only term documented then only code 599.0 should be assigned based on the default for the term in the ICD-9-CM index, in addition to the code for the causal organism if known.

4) Bacterial Sepsis and Septicemia

In most cases, it will be a code from category 038, Septicemia, that will be used in conjunction with a code from subcategory 995.9 such as the following:

(a) Streptococcal sepsis

If the documentation in the record states streptococcal sepsis, codes 038.0, Streptococcal septicemia, and code 995.91 should be used, in that sequence.

(b) Streptococcal septicemia

If the documentation states streptococcal septicemia, only code 038.0 should be assigned, however, the provider should be queried whether the patient has sepsis, an infection with SIRS.

5) Acute organ dysfunction that is not clearly associated with the sepsis

If a patient has sepsis and an acute organ dysfunction, but the medical record documentation indicates that the acute organ dysfunction is related to a medical condition other than the sepsis, do not assign code 995.92, Severe sepsis. An acute organ dysfunction must be associated with the sepsis in order to assign the severe sepsis code. If the documentation is not clear as to whether an acute organ dysfunction is related to the sepsis or another medical condition, query the provider.

6) Septic shock

(a) Sequencing of septic shock

Septic shock generally refers to circulatory failure associated with severe sepsis, and, therefore, it represents a type of acute organ dysfunction.

For all cases of septic shock, the code for the systemic infection should be sequenced first, followed by codes 995.92 and 785.52. Any additional codes for other acute organ dysfunctions should also be assigned. As noted in the sequencing instructions in the Tabular List, the code for septic shock cannot be assigned as a principal diagnosis.

(b) Septic Shock without documentation of severe sepsis

Septic shock indicates the presence of severe sepsis.

Code 995.92, Severe sepsis, must be assigned with code 785.52, Septic shock, even if the term severe sepsis is not documented in the record. The "use additional code" note and the "code first" note in the tabular support this guideline.

7) Sepsis and septic shock complicating abortion and pregnancy

Sepsis and septic shock complicating abortion, ectopic pregnancy, and molar pregnancy are classified to category codes in Chapter 11 (630-639).

See section I.C.11.

8) Negative or inconclusive blood cultures

Negative or inconclusive blood cultures do not preclude a diagnosis of septicemia or sepsis in patients with clinical evidence of the condition, however, the provider should be queried.

9) Newborn sepsis

See Section I.C.15.j for information on the coding of newborn sepsis.

10) Sepsis due to a Postprocedural Infection

(a) Documentation of causal relationship

As with all postprocedural complications, code assign-ment is based on the provider's documentation of the relationship between the infection and the procedure.

(b) Sepsis due to postprocedural infection

In cases of postprocedural sepsis, the complication code, such as code 998.59, Other postoperative infection, or 674.3x, Other complications of obstetrical surgical wounds should be coded first followed by the appropriate sepsis codes (systemic infection code and either code 995.91or 995.92). An additional code(s) for any acute organ dysfunction should also be assigned for cases of severe sepsis.

11) External cause of injury codes with SIRS

Refer to Section I.C.19.a.7 for instruction on the use of external cause of injury codes with codes for SIRS resulting from trauma.

12) Sepsis and Severe Sepsis Associated with Noninfectious Process

In some cases, a non-infectious process, such as trauma, may lead to an infection which can result in sepsis or severe sepsis. If sepsis or severe sepsis is documented as associated with a non-infectious condition, such as a burn or serious injury, and this condition meets the definition for principal diagnosis, the code for the noninfectious condition should be sequenced first, followed by the code for the systemic infection and either code 995.91, Sepsis, or 995.92, Severe sepsis. Additional codes for any associated acute organ dysfunction(s) should also be assigned for cases of severe sepsis. If the sepsis or severe sepsis meets the definition of principal diagnosis, the systemic infection and sepsis codes should be sequenced before the non-infectious condition. When both the associated non-infectious condition and the sepsis or severe sepsis meet the definition of principal diagnosis, either may be assigned as principal diagnosis.

See Section I.C.1.b.2)(a) for guidelines pertaining to sepsis or severe sepsis as the principal diagnosis.

Only one code from subcategory 995.9 should be assigned. Therefore, when a non-infectious condition leads to an infection resulting in sepsis or severe sepsis, assign either code 995.91 or 995.92. Do not additionally assign code 995.93, Systemic inflammatory response syndrome due to non-infectious process without acute organ dysfunction, or 995.94, Systemic inflammatory response syndrome with acute organ dysfunction.

See Section I.C.17.g for information on the coding of SIRS due to trauma/burns or other non-infectious disease processes.

c. Methicillin Resistant Staphylococcus aureus (MRSA) Conditions

1) Selection and sequencing of MRSA codes

(a) Combination codes for MRSA infection

When a patient is diagnosed with an infection that is due to methicillin resistant Staphylococcus aureus (MRSA), and that infection has a combination code that includes the causal organism (e.g., septicemia, pneumonia) assign the appropriate code for the condition (e.g., code 038.12, Methicillin resistant Staphylococcus aureus septicemia or code 482.42, Methicillin resistant pneumonia due to Staphylococcus aureus). Do not assign code 041.12, Methicillin resistant Staphylococcus aureus, as an additional code because the code includes the type of infection and the MRSA organism. Do not assign a code from subcategory V09.0, Infection with microorganisms resistant to penicillins, as an additional diagnosis.

See Section C.1.b.1 for instructions on coding and sequencing of septicemia.

(b) Other codes for MRSA infection

When there is documentation of a current infection (e.g., wound infection, stitch abscess, urinary tract infection) due to MRSA, and that infection does not have a combination code that includes the causal organism, select the appropriate code to identify the condition along with code 041.12, Methicillin resistant Staphylococcus aureus, for the MRSA infection. Do not assign a code from subcategory V09.0, Infection with microorganisms resistant to penicillins.

(c) Methicillin susceptible Staphylococcus aureus (MSSA) and MRSA colonization

The condition or state of being colonized or carrying MSSA or MRSA is called colonization or carriage, while an individual person is described as being colonized or being a carrier. Colonization means that MSSA or MSRA is present on or in the body without necessarily causing illness. A positive MRSA colonization test might be documented by the provider as "MRSA screen positive" or "MRSA nasal swab positive".

Assign code V02.54, Carrier or suspected carrier, Methicillin resistant Staphylococcus aureus, for patients documented as having MRSA colonization. Assign code V02.53, Carrier or suspected carrier, Methicillin susceptible Staphylococcus aureus, for patient documented as having MSSA colonization. Colonization is not necessarily indicative of a disease process or as the cause of a specific condition the patient may have unless documented as such by the provider.

Code V02.59, Other specified bacterial diseases, should be assigned for other types of staphylococcal colonization (e.g., S. epidermidis, S. saprophyticus). Code V02.59 should not be assigned for colonization with any type of Staphylococcus aureus (MRSA, MSSA).

(d) MRSA colonization and infection

If a patient is documented as having both MRSA colonization and infection during a hospital admission, code V02.54, Carrier or suspected carrier, Methicillin resistant Staphylococcus aureus, and a code for the MRSA infection may both be assigned.

2. **Chapter 2: Neoplasms (140-239)**

General guidelines

Chapter 2 of the ICD-9-CM contains the codes for most benign and all malignant neoplasms. Certain benign neoplasms, such as prostatic adenomas, may be found in the specific body system chapters. To properly code a neoplasm it is necessary to determine from the record if the neoplasm is benign, in-situ, malignant, or of uncertain histologic behavior. If malignant, any secondary (metastatic) sites should also be determined.

The neoplasm table in the Alphabetic Index should be referenced first. However, if the histological term is documented, that term should be referenced first, rather than going immediately to the Neoplasm Table, in order to determine which column in the Neoplasm Table is appropriate. For example, if the documentation indicates "adenoma," refer to the term in the Alphabetic Index to review the entries under this term and the instructional note to "see also neoplasm, by site, benign." The table provides the proper code based on the type of neoplasm and the site. It is important to select the proper column in the table that corresponds to the type of neoplasm. The tabular should then be referenced to verify that the correct code has been selected from the table and that a more specific site code does not exist.

See Section I. C. 18.d.4. for information regarding V codes for genetic susceptibility to cancer.

a. Treatment directed at the malignancy

If the treatment is directed at the malignancy, designate the malignancy as the principal diagnosis.

The only exception to this guideline is if a patient admission/encounter is solely for the administration of chemotherapy, immunotherapy or radiation therapy, assign the appropriate V58.x code as the first-listed or principal diagnosis, and the diagnosis or problem for which the service is being performed as a secondary diagnosis.

b. Treatment of secondary site

When a patient is admitted because of a primary neoplasm with metastasis and treatment is directed toward the secondary site only, the secondary neoplasm is designated as the principal diagnosis even though the primary malignancy is still present.

c. Coding and sequencing of complications

Coding and sequencing of complications associated with the malignancies or with the therapy thereof are subject to the following guidelines:

1) Anemia associated with malignancy

When admission/encounter is for management of an anemia associated with the malignancy, and the treatment is only for anemia, the appropriate anemia code (such as code 285.22, Anemia in neoplastic disease) is designated as the principal diagnosis and is followed by the appropriate code(s) for the malignancy.

Code 285.22 may also be used as a secondary code if the patient suffers from anemia and is being treated for the malignancy.

2) **Anemia associated with chemotherapy, immunotherapy and radiation therapy**

When the admission/encounter is for management of an anemia associated with chemotherapy, immunotherapy or radiotherapy and the only treatment is for the anemia, the anemia is sequenced first followed by code E933.1. The appropriate neoplasm code should be assigned as an additional code.

3) **Management of dehydration due to the malignancy**

When the admission/encounter is for management of dehydration due to the malignancy or the therapy, or a combination of both, and only the dehydration is being treated (intravenous rehydration), the dehydration is sequenced first, followed by the code(s) for the malignancy.

4) **Treatment of a complication resulting from a surgical procedure**

When the admission/encounter is for treatment of a complication resulting from a surgical procedure, designate the complication as the principal or first-listed diagnosis if treatment is directed at resolving the complication.

d. **Primary malignancy previously excised**

When a primary malignancy has been previously excised or eradicated from its site and there is no further treatment directed to that site and there is no evidence of any existing primary malignancy, a code from category V10, Personal history of malignant neoplasm, should be used to indicate the former site of the malignancy. Any mention of extension, invasion, or metastasis to another site is coded as a secondary malignant neoplasm to that site. The secondary site may be the principal or first-listed with the V10 code used as a secondary code.

e. **Admissions/Encounters involving chemotherapy, immunotherapy and radiation therapy**

1) **Episode of care involves surgical removal of neoplasm**

When an episode of care involves the surgical removal of a neoplasm, primary or secondary site, followed by adjunct chemotherapy or radiation treatment during the same episode of care, the neoplasm code should be assigned as principal or first-listed diagnosis, using codes in the 140-198 series or where appropriate in the 200-203 series.

2) **Patient admission/encounter solely for administration of chemotherapy, immunotherapy and radiation therapy**

If a patient admission/encounter is solely for the administration of chemotherapy, immunotherapy or radiation therapy assign code V58.0, Encounter for radiation therapy, or V58.11, Encounter for antineoplastic chemotherapy, or V58.12, Encounter for antineoplastic immunotherapy as the first-listed or principal diagnosis. If a patient receives more than one of these therapies during the same admission more than one of these codes may be assigned, in any sequence.

The malignancy for which the therapy is being administered should be assigned as a secondary diagnosis.

3) Patient admitted for radiotherapy/chemotherapy and immunotherapy and develops complications

When a patient is admitted for the purpose of radiotherapy, immunotherapy or chemotherapy and develops complications such as uncontrolled nausea and vomiting or dehydration, the principal or first-listed diagnosis is V58.0, Encounter for radiotherapy, or V58.11, Encounter for antineoplastic chemotherapy, or V58.12, Encounter for antineoplastic immunotherapy followed by any codes for the complications.

f. Admission/encounter to determine extent of malignancy

When the reason for admission/encounter is to determine the extent of the malignancy, or for a procedure such as paracentesis or thoracentesis, the primary malignancy or appropriate metastatic site is designated as the principal or first-listed diagnosis, even though chemotherapy or radiotherapy is administered.

g. Symptoms, signs, and ill-defined conditions listed in Chapter 16 associated with neoplasms

Symptoms, signs, and ill-defined conditions listed in Chapter 16 characteristic of, or associated with, an existing primary or secondary site malignancy cannot be used to replace the malignancy as principal or first-listed diagnosis, regardless of the number of admissions or encounters for treatment and care of the neoplasm.

See section I.C.18.d.14, Encounter for prophylactic organ removal.

h. Admission/encounter for pain control/management

A malignant neoplasm of a transplanted organ should be coded as a transplant complication. Assign first the appropriate code from subcategory 996.8, Complications of transplanted organ, followed by code 199.2, Malignant neoplasm associated with transplanted organ. Use an additional code for the specific malignancy.

3. Chapter 3: Endocrine, Nutritional, and Metabolic Diseases and Immunity Disorders (240-279)

a. Diabetes mellitus

Codes under category 250, Diabetes mellitus, identify complications/ manifestations associated with diabetes mellitus. A fifth-digit is required for all category 250 codes to identify the type of diabetes mellitus and whether the diabetes is controlled or uncontrolled.

See I.C.3.a.7 for secondary diabetes.

1) **Fifth-digits for category 250:**
The following are the fifth-digits for the codes under category 250:

0   type II or unspecified type, not stated as uncontrolled
1   type I, [juvenile type], not stated as uncontrolled
2   type II or unspecified type, uncontrolled
3   type I, [juvenile type], uncontrolled

The age of a patient is not the sole determining factor, though most type I diabetics develop the condition before reaching puberty. For this reason type I diabetes mellitus is also referred to as juvenile diabetes.

2) **Type of diabetes mellitus not documented**

If the type of diabetes mellitus is not documented in the medical record the default is type II.

3) **Diabetes mellitus and the use of insulin**

All type I diabetics must use insulin to replace what their bodies do not produce. However, the use of insulin does not mean that a patient is a type I diabetic. Some patients with type II diabetes mellitus are unable to control their blood sugar through diet and oral medication alone and do require insulin. If the documentation in a medical record does not indicate the type of diabetes but does indicate that the patient uses insulin, the appropriate fifth-digit for type II must be used. For type II patients who routinely use insulin, code V58.67, Long-term (current) use of insulin, should also be assigned to indicate that the patient uses insulin. Code V58.67 should not be assigned if insulin is given temporarily to bring a type II patient's blood sugar under control during an encounter.

4) **Assigning and sequencing diabetes codes and associated conditions**

When assigning codes for diabetes and its associated conditions, the code(s) from category 250 must be sequenced before the codes for the associated conditions. The diabetes codes and the secondary codes that correspond to them are paired codes that follow the etiology/manifestation convention of the classification (See Section I.A.6., Etiology/manifestation convention). Assign as many codes from category 250 as needed to identify all of the associated conditions that the patient has. The corresponding secondary codes are listed under each of the diabetes codes.

(a) Diabetic retinopathy/diabetic macular edema

Diabetic macular edema, code 362.07, is only present with diabetic retinopathy. Another code from subcategory 362.0, Diabetic retinopathy, must be used with code 362.07. Codes under subcategory 362.0 are diabetes manifestation codes, so they must be used following the appropriate diabetes code.

5) Diabetes mellitus in pregnancy and gestational diabetes

(a) For diabetes mellitus complicating pregnancy, see Section I.C.11.f., Diabetes mellitus in pregnancy.

(b) For gestational diabetes, see Section I.C.11, g., Gestational diabetes.

6) Insulin pump malfunction

(a) Underdose of insulin due insulin pump failure

An underdose of insulin due to an insulin pump failure should be assigned 996.57, Mechanical complication due to insulin pump, as the principal or first listed code, followed by the appropriate diabetes mellitus code based on documentation.

(b) Overdose of insulin due to insulin pump failure

The principal or first listed code for an encounter due to an insulin pump malfunction resulting in an overdose of insulin, should also be 996.57, Mechanical complication due to insulin pump, followed by code 962.3, Poisoning by insulins and antidiabetic agents, and the appropriate diabetes mellitus code based on documentation.

7) Secondary Diabetes Mellitus

Codes under category 249, Secondary diabetes mellitus, identify complications/manifestations associated with secondary diabetes mellitus. Secondary diabetes is always caused by another condition or event (e.g., cystic fibrosis, malignant neoplasm of pancreas, pancreatectomy, adverse effect of drug, or poisoning).

(a) Fifth-digits for category 249:

A fifth-digit is required for all category 249 codes to identify whether the diabetes is controlled or uncontrolled.

(b) Secondary diabetes mellitus and the use of insulin

For patients who routinely use insulin, code V58.67, Long-term (current) use of insulin, should also be assigned. Code V58.67 should not be assigned if insulin is given temporarily to bring a patient's blood sugar under control during an encounter.

(c) Assigning and sequencing secondary diabetes codes and associated conditions

When assigning codes for secondary diabetes and its associated conditions (e.g. renal manifestations), the code(s) from category 249 must be sequenced before the codes for the associated conditions. The secondary diabetes codes and the diabetic manifestation codes that correspond to them are paired codes that follow the etiology/manifestation convention of the classification. Assign as many codes from category 249 as needed to identify all of the associated conditions that the patient has. The corresponding codes for the associated conditions are listed under each of the secondary diabetes codes. For example, secondary diabetes with diabetic nephrosis is assigned to code 249.40, followed by 581.81.

(d)   Assigning and sequencing secondary diabetes codes and its causes

The sequencing of the secondary diabetes codes in relationship to codes for the cause of the diabetes is based on the reason for the encounter, applicable ICD-9-CM sequencing conventions, and chapter-specific guidelines.

If a patient is seen for treatment of the secondary diabetes or one of its associated conditions, a code from category 249 is sequenced as the principal or first-listed diagnosis, with the cause of the secondary diabetes (e.g. cystic fibrosis) sequenced as an additional diagnosis.

If, however, the patient is seen for the treatment of the condition causing the secondary diabetes (e.g., malignant neoplasm of pancreas), the code for the cause of the secondary diabetes should be sequenced as the principal or first-listed diagnosis followed by a code from category 249.

(i)   Secondary diabetes mellitus due to pancreatectomy

For postpancreatectomy diabetes mellitus (lack of insulin due to the surgical removal of all or part of the pancreas), assign code 251.3, Postsurgical hypoinsulinemia. A code from subcategory 249 should not be assigned for secondary diabetes mellitus due to pancreatectomy. Code also any diabetic manifestations (e.g. diabetic nephrosis 581.81).

(ii)   Secondary diabetes due to drugs

Secondary diabetes may be caused by an adverse effect of correctly administered medications, poisoning or late effect of poisoning.

See section I.C.17.e for coding of adverse effects and poisoning, and section I.C.19 for E code reporting.

4.   **Chapter 4: Diseases of Blood and Blood Forming Organs (280-289)**

a. **Anemia of chronic disease**

Subcategory 285.2, Anemia in chronic illness, has codes for anemia in chronic kidney disease, code 285.21; anemia in neoplastic disease, code 285.22; and anemia in other chronic illness, code 285.29. These codes can be used as the principal/first listed code if the reason for the encounter is to treat the anemia. They may also be used as secondary codes if treatment of the anemia is a component of an encounter, but not the primary reason for the encounter. When using a code from subcategory 285 it is also necessary to use the code for the chronic condition causing the anemia.

1) Anemia in chronic kidney disease

When assigning code 285.21, Anemia in chronic kidney disease, it is also necessary to assign a code from category 585, Chronic kidney disease, to indicate the stage of chronic kidney disease.
See I.C.10.a. Chronic kidney disease (CKD).

2) Anemia in neoplastic disease

When assigning code 285.22, Anemia in neoplastic disease, it is also necessary to assign the neoplasm code that is responsible for the anemia. Code 285.22 is for use for anemia that is due to the malignancy, not for anemia due to antineoplastic chemotherapy drugs, which is an adverse effect.

See I.C.2.c.1 Anemia associated with malignancy. See I.C.2.c.2 Anemia associated with chemotherapy, immunotherapy and radiation therapy. See I.C.17.e.1. Adverse effects.

5. Chapter 5: Mental Disorders (290-319)

Reserved for future guideline expansion

6. Chapter 6: Diseases of Nervous System and Sense Organs (320-389)

a. Pain - Category 338

1) General coding information

Codes in category 338 may be used in conjunction with codes from other categories and chapters to provide more detail about acute or chronic pain and neoplasm-related pain, unless otherwise indicated below.

If the pain is not specified as acute or chronic, do not assign codes from category 338, except for post-thoracotomy pain, postoperative pain, neoplasm related pain, or central pain syndrome.

A code from subcategories 338.1 and 338.2 should not be assigned if the underlying (definitive) diagnosis is known, unless the reason for the encounter is pain control/ management and not management of the underlying condition.

(a) Category 338 Codes as Principal or First-Listed Diagnosis

Category 338 codes are acceptable as principal diagnosis or the first-listed code:

- When pain control or pain management is the reason for the admission/encounter (e.g., a patient with displaced intervertebral disc, nerve impingement and severe back pain presents for injection of steroid into the spinal canal). The underlying cause of the pain should be reported as an additional diagnosis, if known.

- When an admission or encounter is for a procedure aimed at treating the underlying condition (e.g., spinal fusion, kyphoplasty), a code for the underlying condition (e.g., vertebral fracture, spinal stenosis) should be assigned as the principal diagnosis. No code from category 338 should be assigned.

- When a patient is admitted for the insertion of a neurostimulator for pain control, assign the appropriate pain code as the principal or first listed diagnosis. When an admission or encounter is for a procedure aimed at treating the underlying condition and a neurostimulator is inserted for pain control during the same admission/encounter, a code for the underlying condition should be assigned as the principal diagnosis and the appropriate pain code should be assigned as a secondary diagnosis.

(b) Use of Category 338 Codes in Conjunction with Site-Specific Pain Codes

(i) Assigning Category 338 Codes and Site Specific Pain Codes

Codes from category 338 may be used in conjunction with codes that identify the site of pain (including codes from chapter 16) if the category 338 code provides additional information. For example, if the code describes the site of the pain, but does not fully describe whether the pain is acute or chronic, then both codes should be assigned.

(ii) Sequencing of Category 338 Codes with Site Specific Pain Codes

The sequencing of category 338 codes with site specific pain codes (including chapter 16 codes), is dependent on the circumstances of the encounter/admission as follows:

- If the encounter is for pain control or pain management, assign the code from category 338 followed by the code identifying the specific site of pain (e.g., encounter for pain management for acute neck pain from trauma is assigned code 338.11, Acute pain due to trauma, followed by code 723.1, Cervicalgia, to identify the site of pain).

- If the encounter is for any other reason except pain control or pain management, and a related definitive diagnosis has not been established (confirmed) by the provider, assign the code for the specific site of pain first, followed by the appropriate code from category 338.

2) **Pain due to devices, implants and grafts**

Pain associated with devices, implants or grafts left in a surgical site (for example painful hip prosthesis) is assigned to the appropriate code(s) found in Chapter 17, Injury and Poisoning. Use additional code(s) from category 338 to identify acute or chronic pain due to presence of the device, implant or graft (338.18-338.19 or 338.28-338.29).

3) **Postoperative Pain**

Post-thoracotomy pain and other postoperative pain are classified to subcategories 338.1 and 338.2, depending on whether the pain is acute or chronic. The default for post-thoracotomy and other postoperative pain not specified as acute or chronic is the code for the acute form.

Routine or expected postoperative pain immediately after surgery should not be coded.

(a) Postoperative pain not associated with specific postoperative complication

Postoperative pain not associated with a specific postoperative complication is assigned to the appropriate postoperative pain code in category 338.

(b) Postoperative pain associated with specific postoperative complication

Postoperative pain associated with a specific postoperative complication (such as painful wire sutures) is assigned to the appropriate code(s) found in Chapter 17, Injury and Poisoning. If appropriate, use additional code(s) from category 338 to identify acute or chronic pain (338.18 or 338.28). If pain control/management is the reason for the encounter, a code from category 338 should be assigned as the principal or first-listed diagnosis in accordance with Section I.C.6.a.1.a above.

(c) Postoperative pain as principal or first-listed diagnosis

Postoperative pain may be reported as the principal or first-listed diagnosis when the stated reason for the admission/encounter is documented as postoperative pain control/management.

(d) Postoperative pain as secondary diagnosis

Postoperative pain may be reported as a secondary diagnosis code when a patient presents for outpatient surgery and develops an unusual or inordinate amount of postoperative pain.

The provider's documentation should be used to guide the coding of postoperative pain, as well as Section III. Reporting Additional Diagnoses and Section IV. Diagnostic Coding and Reporting in the Outpatient Setting.

See Section II.I.2 for information on sequencing of diagnoses for patients admitted to hospital inpatient care following post-operative observation.

See Section II.J for information on sequencing of diagnoses for patients admitted to hospital inpatient care from outpatient surgery.

See Section IV.A.2 for information on sequencing of diagnoses for patients admitted for observation.

4) Chronic pain

Chronic pain is classified to subcategory 338.2. There is no time frame defining when pain becomes chronic pain. The provider's documentation should be used to guide use of these codes.

5) Neoplasm Related Pain

Code 338.3 is assigned to pain documented as being related, associated or due to cancer, primary or secondary malignancy, or tumor. This code is assigned regardless of whether the pain is acute or chronic.

This code may be assigned as the principal or first listed code when the stated reason for the admission/encounter is documented as pain control/pain management. The underlying neoplasm should be reported as an additional diagnosis.

When the reason for the admission/encounter is management of the neoplasm and the pain associated with the neoplasm is also documented, code 338.3 may be assigned as an additional diagnosis.

See Section I.C.2 for instructions on the sequencing of neoplasms for all other stated reasons for the admission/encounter (except for pain control/pain management).

6) Chronic pain syndrome

This condition is different than the term "chronic pain," and therefore this code should only be used when the provider has specifically documented this condition.

7. Chapter 7: Diseases of Circulatory System (390-459)

a. Hypertension

Hypertension Table

The Hypertension Table, found under the main term, "Hypertension", in the Alphabetic Index, contains a complete listing of all conditions due to or associated with hypertension and classifies them according to malignant, benign, and unspecified.

1) Hypertension, Essential, or NOS

Assign hypertension (arterial) (essential) (primary) (systemic) (NOS) to category code 401 with the appropriate fourth digit to indicate malignant (.0), benign (.1), or unspecified (.9). Do not use either .0 malignant or .1 benign unless medical record documentation supports such a designation.

2) Hypertension with Heart Disease

Heart conditions (425.8, 429.0-429.3, 429.8, 429.9) are assigned to a code from category 402 when a causal relationship is stated (due to hypertension) or implied (hypertensive). Use an additional code from category 428 to identify the type of heart failure in those patients with heart failure. More than one code from category 428 may be assigned if the patient has systolic or diastolic failure and congestive heart failure.

The same heart conditions (425.8, 429.0-429.3, 429.8, 429.9) with hypertension, but without a stated causal relationship, are coded separately. Sequence according to the circumstances of the admission/encounter.

3) Hypertensive Chronic Kidney Disease

Assign codes from category 403, Hypertensive chronic kidney disease, when conditions classified to categories 585-587 are present. Unlike hypertension with heart disease, ICD-9-CM presumes a cause-and-effect relationship and classifies chronic kidney disease (CKD) with hypertension as hypertensive chronic kidney disease.

Fifth digits for category 403 should be assigned as follows:

0 with CKD stage I through stage IV, or unspecified.

1 with CKD stage V or end stage renal disease.

The appropriate code from category 585, Chronic kidney disease, should be used as a secondary code with a code from category 403 to identify the stage of chronic kidney disease.

See Section I.C.10.a for information on the coding of chronic kidney disease.

4) Hypertensive Heart and Chronic Kidney Disease

Assign codes from combination category 404, Hypertensive heart and chronic kidney disease, when both hypertensive kidney disease and hypertensive heart disease are stated in the diagnosis. Assume a relationship between the hypertension and the chronic kidney disease, whether or not the condition is so designated. Assign an additional code from category 428, to identify the type of heart failure. More than one code from category 428 may be assigned if the patient has systolic or diastolic failure and congestive heart failure.

Fifth digits for category 404 should be assigned as follows:

0 without heart failure and with chronic kidney disease (CKD) stage I through stage IV, or unspecified

1 with heart failure and with CKD stage I through stage IV, or unspecified

2 without heart failure and with CKD stage V or end stage renal disease

3 with heart failure and with CKD stage V or end stage renal disease

The appropriate code from category 585, Chronic kidney disease, should be used as a secondary code with a code from category 404 to identify the stage of kidney disease.

See Section I.C.10.a for information on the coding of chronic kidney disease.

5) **Hypertensive Cerebrovascular Disease**

First assign codes from 430-438, Cerebrovascular disease, then the appropriate hypertension code from categories 401-405.

6) **Hypertensive Retinopathy**

Two codes are necessary to identify the condition. First assign the code from subcategory 362.11, Hypertensive retinopathy, then the appropriate code from categories 401-405 to indicate the type of hypertension.

7) **Hypertension, Secondary**

Two codes are required: one to identify the underlying etiology and one from category 405 to identify the hypertension. Sequencing of codes is determined by the reason for admission/encounter.

8) **Hypertension, Transient**

Assign code 796.2, Elevated blood pressure reading without diagnosis of hypertension, unless patient has an established diagnosis of hypertension. Assign code 642.3x for transient hypertension of pregnancy.

9) **Hypertension, Controlled**

Assign appropriate code from categories 401-405. This diagnostic statement usually refers to an existing state of hypertension under control by therapy.

10) **Hypertension, Uncontrolled**

Uncontrolled hypertension may refer to untreated hypertension or hypertension not responding to current therapeutic regimen. In either case, assign the appropriate code from categories 401-405 to designate the stage and type of hypertension. Code to the type of hypertension.

11) **Elevated Blood Pressure**

For a statement of elevated blood pressure without further specificity, assign code 796.2, Elevated blood pressure reading without diagnosis of hypertension, rather than a code from category 401.

b. Cerebral infarction/stroke/cerebrovascular accident (CVA)

The terms stroke and CVA are often used interchangeably to refer to a cerebral infarction. The terms stroke, CVA, and cerebral infarction NOS are all indexed to the default code 434.91, Cerebral artery occlusion, unspecified, with infarction. Code 436, Acute, but ill-defined, cerebrovascular disease, should not be used when the documentation states stroke or CVA.

See Section I.C.18.d.3 for information on coding status post administration of tPA in a different facility within the last 24 hours.

c. Postoperative cerebrovascular accident

A cerebrovascular hemorrhage or infarction that occurs as a result of medical intervention is coded to 997.02, Iatrogenic cerebrovascular infarction or hemorrhage. Medical record documentation should clearly specify the cause- and-effect relationship between the medical intervention and the cerebrovascular accident in order to assign this code. A secondary code from the code range 430-432 or from a code from subcategories 433 or 434 with a fifth digit of "1" should also be used to identify the type of hemorrhage or infarct.

This guideline conforms to the use additional code note instruction at category 997. Code 436, Acute, but ill-defined, cerebrovascular disease, should not be used as a secondary code with code 997.02.

d. Late Effects of Cerebrovascular Disease

1) Category 438, Late Effects of Cerebrovascular disease

Category 438 is used to indicate conditions classifiable to categories 430-437 as the causes of late effects (neurologic deficits), themselves classified elsewhere. These "late effects" include neurologic deficits that persist after initial onset of conditions classifiable to 430-437. The neurologic deficits caused by cerebrovascular disease may be present from the onset or may arise at any time after the onset of the condition classifiable to 430-437.

2) Codes from category 438 with codes from 430-437

Codes from category 438 may be assigned on a health care record with codes from 430-437, if the patient has a current cerebrovascular accident (CVA) and deficits from an old CVA.

3) Code V12.54

Assign code V12.54, Transient ischemic attack (TIA), and cerebral infarction without residual deficits (and not a code from category 438) as an additional code for history of cerebrovascular disease when no neurologic deficits are present.

e. **Acute myocardial infarction (AMI)**

1) **ST elevation myocardial infarction (STEMI) and non ST elevation myocardial infarction (NSTEMI)**

The ICD-9-CM codes for acute myocardial infarction (AMI) identify the site, such as anterolateral wall or true posterior wall. Subcategories 410.0-410.6 and 410.8 are used for ST elevation myocardial infarction (STEMI). Subcategory 410.7, Subendo-cardial infarction, is used for non ST elevation myocardial infarction (NSTEMI) and nontransmural MIs.

2) **Acute myocardial infarction, unspecified**

Subcategory 410.9 is the default for the unspecified term acute myocardial infarction. If only STEMI or transmural MI without the site is documented, query the provider as to the site, or assign a code from subcategory 410.9.

3) **AMI documented as nontransmural or subendocardial but site provided**

If an AMI is documented as nontransmural or subendocardial, but the site is provided, it is still coded as a subendocardial AMI. If NSTEMI evolves to STEMI, assign the STEMI code. If STEMI converts to NSTEMI due to thrombolytic therapy, it is still coded as STEMI.

See Section I.C.18.d.3 for information on coding status post administration of tPA in a different facility within the last 24 hours.

8. **Chapter 8: Diseases of Respiratory System (460-519)**

a. **Chronic Obstructive Pulmonary Disease [COPD] and Asthma**

1) **Conditions that comprise COPD and Asthma**

The conditions that comprise COPD are obstructive chronic bronchitis, subcategory 491.2, and emphysema, category 492. All asthma codes are under category 493, Asthma. Code 496, Chronic airway obstruction, not elsewhere classified, is a nonspecific code that should only be used when the documentation in a medical record does not specify the type of COPD being treated.

2) **Acute exacerbation of chronic obstructive bronchitis and asthma**

The codes for chronic obstructive bronchitis and asthma distinguish between uncomplicated cases and those in acute exacerbation. An acute exacerbation is a worsening or a decompensation of a chronic condition. An acute exacerbation is not equivalent to an infection superimposed on a chronic condition, though an exacerbation may be triggered by an infection.

3) Overlapping nature of the conditions that comprise COPD and asthma

Due to the overlapping nature of the conditions that make up COPD and asthma, there are many variations in the way these conditions are documented. Code selection must be based on the terms as documented. When selecting the correct code for the documented type of COPD and asthma, it is essential to first review the index, and then verify the code in the tabular list. There are many instructional notes under the different COPD subcategories and codes. It is important that all such notes be reviewed to assure correct code assignment.

4) Acute exacerbation of asthma and status asthmaticus

An acute exacerbation of asthma is an increased severity of the asthma symptoms, such as wheezing and shortness of breath. Status asthmaticus refers to a patient's failure to respond to therapy administered during an asthmatic episode and is a life threatening complication that requires emergency care. If status asthmaticus is documented by the provider with any type of COPD or with acute bronchitis, the status asthmaticus should be sequenced first. It supersedes any type of COPD including that with acute exacerbation or acute bronchitis. It is inappropriate to assign an asthma code with 5th digit 2, with acute exacerbation, together with an asthma code with 5th digit 1, with status asthmatics. Only the 5th digit 1 should be assigned.

b. Chronic Obstructive Pulmonary Disease [COPD] and Bronchitis

1) Acute bronchitis with COPD

Acute bronchitis, code 466.0, is due to an infectious organism. When acute bronchitis is documented with COPD, code 491.22, Obstructive chronic bronchitis with acute bronchitis, should be assigned. It is not necessary to also assign code 466.0. If a medical record documents acute bronchitis with COPD with acute exacerbation, only code 491.22 should be assigned. The acute bronchitis included in code 491.22 supersedes the acute exacerbation. If a medical record documents COPD with acute exacerbation without mention of acute bronchitis, only code 491.21 should be assigned.

c. Acute Respiratory Failure

1) Acute respiratory failure as principal diagnosis

Code 518.81, Acute respiratory failure, may be assigned as a principal diagnosis when it is the condition established after study to be chiefly responsible for occasioning the admission to the hospital, and the selection is supported by the Alphabetic Index and Tabular List. However, chapter-specific coding guidelines (such as obstetrics, poisoning, HIV, newborn) that provide sequencing direction take precedence.

2) Acute respiratory failure as secondary diagnosis

Respiratory failure may be listed as a secondary diagnosis if it occurs after admission, or if it is present on admission, but does not meet the definition of principal diagnosis.

3) Sequencing of acute respiratory failure and another acute condition

When a patient is admitted with respiratory failure and another acute condition, (e.g., myocardial infarction, cerebrovascular accident, aspiration pneumonia), the principal diagnosis will not be the same in every situation. This applies whether the other acute condition is a respiratory or nonrespiratory condition. Selection of the principal diagnosis will be dependent on the circumstances of admission. If both the respiratory failure and the other acute condition are equally responsible for occasioning the admission to the hospital, and there are no chapter-specific sequencing rules, the guideline regarding two or more diagnoses that equally meet the definition for principal diagnosis (Section II, C.) may be applied in these situations.

If the documentation is not clear as to whether acute respiratory failure and another condition are equally responsible for occasioning the admission, query the provider for clarification.

d. Influenza due to identified avian influenza virus (avian influenza)

Code only confirmed cases of avian influenza. This is an exception to the hospital inpatient guideline Section II, H. (Uncertain Diagnosis).

In this context, "confirmation" does not require documentation of positive laboratory testing specific for avian influenza. However, coding should be based on the provider's diagnostic statement that the patient has avian influenza.

If the provider records "suspected or possible or probable avian influenza," the appropriate influenza code from category 487 should be assigned. Code 488, Influenza due to identified avian influenza virus, should not be assigned.

9. Chapter 9: Diseases of Digestive System (520-579)

Reserved for future guideline expansion

10. Chapter 10: Diseases of Genitourinary System (580-629)

a. Chronic kidney disease

1) Stages of chronic kidney disease (CKD)

The ICD-9-CM classifies CKD based on severity. The severity of CKD is designated by stages I-V. Stage II, code 585.2, equates to mild CKD; stage III, code 585.3, equates to moderate CKD; and stage IV, code 585.4, equates to severe CKD. Code 585.6, End stage renal disease (ESRD), is assigned when the provider has documented end-stage-renal disease (ESRD).

If both a stage of CKD and ESRD are documented, assign code 585.6 only.

2) **Chronic kidney disease and kidney transplant status**

Patients who have undergone kidney transplant may still have some form of CKD, because the kidney transplant may not fully restore kidney function. Therefore, the presence of CKD alone does not constitute a transplant complication. Assign the appropriate 585 code for the patient's stage of CKD and code V42.0. If a transplant complication such as failure or rejection is documented, see section I.C.17.f.1.b for information on coding complications of a kidney transplant. If the documentation is unclear as to whether the patient has a complication of the transplant, query the provider.

3) **Chronic kidney disease with other conditions**

Patients with CKD may also suffer from other serious conditions, most commonly diabetes mellitus and hypertension. The sequencing of the CKD code in relationship to codes for other contributing conditions is based on the conventions in the tabular list.

See I.C.3.a.4 for sequencing instructions for diabetes. See I.C.4.a.1 for anemia in CKD. See I.C.7.a.3 for hypertensive chronic kidney disease. See I.C.17.f.1.b, Kidney transplant complications, for instructions on coding of documented rejection or failure.

11. **Chapter 11: Complications of Pregnancy, Childbirth, and the Puerperium (630-677)**

a. **General Rules for Obstetric Cases**

1) **Codes from chapter 11 and sequencing priority**

Obstetric cases require codes from chapter 11, codes in the range 630-677, Complications of Pregnancy, Childbirth, and the Puerperium. Chapter 11 codes have sequencing priority over codes from other chapters. Additional codes from other chapters may be used in conjunction with chapter 11 codes to further specify conditions. Should the provider document that the pregnancy is incidental to the encounter, then code V22.2 should be used in place of any chapter 11 codes. It is the provider's responsibility to state that the condition being treated is not affecting the pregnancy.

2) **Chapter 11 codes used only on the maternal record**

Chapter 11 codes are to be used only on the maternal record, never on the record of the newborn.

3) **Chapter 11 fifth-digits**

Categories 640-648, 651-676 have required fifth-digits, which indicate whether the encounter is antepartum, postpartum and whether a delivery has also occurred.

4) Fifth-digits, appropriate for each code

The fifth-digits, which are appropriate for each code number, are listed in brackets under each code. The fifth-digits on each code should all be consistent with each other. That is, should a delivery occur all of the fifth-digits should indicate the delivery.

b. Selection of OB Principal or First-listed Diagnosis

1) Routine outpatient prenatal visits

For routine outpatient prenatal visits when no complications are present codes V22.0, Supervision of normal first pregnancy, and V22.1, Supervision of other normal pregnancy, should be used as the first-listed diagnoses. These codes should not be used in conjunction with chapter 11 codes.

2) Prenatal outpatient visits for high-risk patients

For prenatal outpatient visits for patients with high-risk pregnancies, a code from category V23, Supervision of high-risk pregnancy, should be used as the first-listed diagnosis. Secondary chapter 11 codes may be used in conjunction with these codes if appropriate.

3) Episodes when no delivery occurs

In episodes when no delivery occurs, the principal diagnosis should correspond to the principal complication of the pregnancy, which necessitated the encounter. Should more than one complication exist, all of which are treated or monitored, any of the complications codes may be sequenced first.

4) When a delivery occurs

When a delivery occurs, the principal diagnosis should correspond to the main circumstances or complication of the delivery. In cases of cesarean delivery, the selection of the principal diagnosis should correspond to the reason the cesarean delivery was performed unless the reason for admission/encounter was unrelated to the condition resulting in the cesarean delivery.

5) Outcome of delivery

An outcome of delivery code, V27.0-V27.9, should be included on every maternal record when a delivery has occurred. These codes are not to be used on subsequent records or on the newborn record.

c. Fetal Conditions Affecting the Management of the Mother

1) Codes from category 655

Known or suspected fetal abnormality affecting management of the mother, and category 656, Other fetal and placental problems affecting the management of the mother, are assigned only when the fetal condition is actually responsible for modifying the management of the mother, i.e., by requiring diagnostic studies, additional observation, special care, or termination of pregnancy. The fact that the fetal condition exists does not justify assigning a code from this series to the mother's record. See I.C.18.d. for suspected maternal and fetal conditions not found.

2) **In utero surgery**

In cases when surgery is performed on the fetus, a diagnosis code from category 655, Known or suspected fetal abnormalities affecting management of the mother, should be assigned identifying the fetal condition. Procedure code 75.36, Correction of fetal defect, should be assigned on the hospital inpatient record.

No code from Chapter 15, the perinatal codes, should be used on the mother's record to identify fetal conditions. Surgery performed in utero on a fetus is still to be coded as an obstetric encounter.

d. **HIV Infection in Pregnancy, Childbirth and the Puerperium**

During pregnancy, childbirth or the puerperium, a patient admitted because of an HIV-related illness should receive a principal diagnosis of 647.6X, Other specified infectious and parasitic diseases in the mother classifiable elsewhere, but complicating the pregnancy, childbirth or the puerperium, followed by 042 and the code(s) for the HIV-related illness(es).

Patients with asymptomatic HIV infection status admitted during pregnancy, childbirth, or the puerperium should receive codes of 647.6X and V08.

e. **Current Conditions Complicating Pregnancy**

Assign a code from subcategory 648.x for patients that have current conditions when the condition affects the management of the pregnancy, childbirth, or the puerperium. Use additional secondary codes from other chapters to identify the conditions, as appropriate.

f. **Diabetes mellitus in pregnancy**

Diabetes mellitus is a significant complicating factor in pregnancy. Pregnant women who are diabetic should be assigned code 648.0x, Diabetes mellitus complicating pregnancy, and a secondary code from category 250, Diabetes mellitus, or category 249, Secondary diabetes, to identify the type of diabetes.

Code V58.67, Long-term (current) use of insulin, should also be assigned if the diabetes mellitus is being treated with insulin.

g. **Gestational diabetes**

Gestational diabetes can occur during the second and third trimester of pregnancy in women who were not diabetic prior to pregnancy. Gestational diabetes can cause complications in the pregnancy similar to those of pre-existing diabetes mellitus. It also puts the woman at greater risk of developing diabetes after the pregnancy. Gestational diabetes is coded to 648.8x, Abnormal glucose tolerance. Codes 648.0x and 648.8x should never be used together on the same record.

Code V58.67, Long-term (current) use of insulin, should also be assigned if the gestational diabetes is being treated with insulin.

h. Normal Delivery, Code 650

1) Normal delivery

Code 650 is for use in cases when a woman is admitted for a full-term normal delivery and delivers a single, healthy infant without any complications antepartum, during the delivery, or postpartum during the delivery episode. Code 650 is always a principal diagnosis. It is not to be used if any other code from chapter 11 is needed to describe a current complication of the antenatal, delivery, or perinatal period. Additional codes from other chapters may be used with code 650 if they are not related to or are in any way complicating the pregnancy.

2) Normal delivery with resolved antepartum complication

Code 650 may be used if the patient had a complication at some point during her pregnancy, but the complication is not present at the time of the admission for delivery.

3) V27.0, Single liveborn, outcome of delivery

V27.0, Single liveborn, is the only outcome of delivery code appropriate for use with 650.

i. The Postpartum and Peripartum Periods

1) Postpartum and peripartum periods

The postpartum period begins immediately after delivery and continues for six weeks following delivery. The peripartum period is defined as the last month of pregnancy to five months postpartum.

2) Postpartum complication

A postpartum complication is any complication occurring within the six-week period.

3) Pregnancy-related complications after 6 week period

Chapter 11 codes may also be used to describe pregnancy-related complications after the six-week period should the provider document that a condition is pregnancy related.

4) Postpartum complications occurring during the same admission as delivery

Postpartum complications that occur during the same admission as the delivery are identified with a fifth digit of "2." Subsequent admissions/encounters for postpartum complications should be identified with a fifth digit of "4."

5) Admission for routine postpartum care following delivery outside hospital

When the mother delivers outside the hospital prior to admission and is admitted for routine postpartum care and no complications are noted, code V24.0, Postpartum care and examination immediately after delivery, should be assigned as the principal diagnosis.

6) Admission following delivery outside hospital with postpartum conditions

A delivery diagnosis code should not be used for a woman who has delivered prior to admission to the hospital. Any postpartum conditions and/or postpartum procedures should be coded.

j. Code 677, Late effect of complication of pregnancy

1) Code 677

Code 677, Late effect of complication of pregnancy, childbirth, and the puerperium is for use in those cases when an initial complication of a pregnancy develops a sequelae requiring care or treatment at a future date.

2) After the initial postpartum period

This code may be used at any time after the initial postpartum period.

3) Sequencing of Code 677

This code, like all late effect codes, is to be sequenced following the code describing the sequelae of the complication.

k. Abortions

1) Fifth-digits required for abortion categories

Fifth-digits are required for abortion categories 634-637. Fifth-digit 1, incomplete, indicates that all of the products of conception have not been expelled from the uterus. Fifth-digit 2, complete, indicates that all products of conception have been expelled from the uterus prior to the episode of care.

2) Code from categories 640-648 and 651-659

A code from categories 640-648 and 651-659 may be used as additional codes with an abortion code to indicate the complication leading to the abortion.

Fifth digit 3 is assigned with codes from these categories when used with an abortion code because the other fifth digits will not apply. Codes from the 660-669 series are not to be used for complications of abortion.

3) Code 639 for complications

Code 639 is to be used for all complications following abortion. Code 639 cannot be assigned with codes from categories 634-638.

4) Abortion with Liveborn Fetus

When an attempted termination of pregnancy results in a liveborn fetus assign code 644.21, Early onset of delivery, with an appropriate code from category V27, Outcome of Delivery. The procedure code for the attempted termination of pregnancy should also be assigned.

5) Retained Products of Conception following an abortion

Subsequent admissions for retained products of conception following a spontaneous or legally induced abortion are assigned the appropriate code from category 634, Spontaneous abortion, or 635 Legally induced abortion, with a fifth digit of "1" (incomplete). This advice is appropriate even when the patient was discharged previously with a discharge diagnosis of complete abortion.

12. Chapter 12: Diseases Skin and Subcutaneous Tissue (680-709)

a. Pressure ulcer stage codes

1) Pressure ulcer stages

Two codes are needed to completely describe a pressure ulcer: A code from subcategory 707.0, Pressure ulcer, to identify the site of the pressure ulcer and a code from subcategory 707.2, Pressure ulcer stages.

The codes in subcategory 707.2, Pressure ulcer stages, are to be used as an additional diagnosis with a code(s) from subcategory 707.0, Pressure Ulcer. Codes from 707.2, Pressure ulcer stages, may not be assigned as a principal or first-listed diagnosis. The pressure ulcer stage codes should only be used with pressure ulcers and not with other types of ulcers (e.g., stasis ulcer).

The ICD-9-CM classifies pressure ulcer stages based on severity, which is designated by stages I-IV and unstageable.

2) Unstageable pressure ulcers

Assignment of code 707.25, Pressure ulcer, unstageable, should be based on the clinical documentation. Code 707.25 is used for pressure ulcers whose stage cannot be clinically determined (e.g., the ulcer is covered by eschar or has been treated with a skin or muscle graft) and pressure ulcers that are documented as deep tissue injury but not documented as due to trauma. This code should not be confused with code 707.20, Pressure ulcer, stage unspecified. Code 707.20 should be assigned when there is no documentation regarding the stage of the pressure ulcer.

3) Documented pressure ulcer stage

Assignment of the pressure ulcer stage code should be guided by clinical documentation of the stage or documentation of the terms found in the index. For clinical terms describing the stage that are not found in the index,and there is no documentation of the stage, the provider should be queried.

4) Bilateral pressure ulcers with same stage

When a patient has bilateral pressure ulcers (e.g., both buttocks) and both pressure ulcers are documented as being the same stage, only the code for the site and one code for the stage should be reported.

5) Bilateral pressure ulcers with different stages

When a patient has bilateral pressure ulcers at the same site (e.g., both buttocks) and each pressure ulcer is documented as being at a different stage, assign one code for the site and the appropriate codes for the pressure ulcer stage.

6) Multiple pressure ulcers of different sites and stages

When a patient has multiple pressure ulcers at different sites (e.g., buttock, heel, shoulder) and each pressure ulcer is documented as being at different stages (e.g., stage 3 and stage 4), assign the appropriate codes for each different site and a code for each different pressure ulcer stage.

7) Patients admitted with pressure ulcers documented as healed

No code is assigned if the documentation states that the pressure ulcer is completely healed.

8) Patients admitted with pressure ulcers documented as healing

Pressure ulcers described as healing should be assigned the appropriate pressure ulcer stage code based on the documentation in the medical record. If the documentation does not provide information about the stage of the healing pressure ulcer, assign code 707.20, Pressure ulcer stage, unspecified.

If the documentation is unclear as to whether the patient has a current (new) pressure ulcer or if the patient is being treated for a healing pressure ulcer, query the provider.

9) Patient admitted with pressure ulcer evolving into another stage during the admission

If a patient is admitted with a pressure ulcer at one stage and it progresses to a higher stage, assign the code for highest stage reported for that site.

13. Chapter 13: Diseases of Musculoskeletal and Connective Tissue (710-739)

a. Coding of Pathologic Fractures

1) Acute Fractures vs. Aftercare

Pathologic fractures are reported using subcategory 733.1, when the fracture is newly diagnosed. Subcategory 733.1 may be used while the patient is receiving active treatment for the fracture. Examples of active treatment are: surgical treatment, emergency department encounter, evaluation and treatment by a new physician.

Fractures are coded using the aftercare codes (subcategories V54.0, V54.2, V54.8 or V54.9) for encounters after the patient has completed active treatment of the fracture and is receiving routine care for the fracture during the healing or recovery phase. Examples of fracture aftercare are: cast change or removal, removal of external or internal fixation device, medication adjustment, and follow up visits following fracture treatment.

Care for complications of surgical treatment for fracture repairs during the healing or recovery phase should be coded with the appropriate complication codes.

Care of complications of fractures, such as malunion and nonunion, should be reported with the appropriate codes. See Section I. C. 17.b for information on the coding of traumatic fractures.

14. Chapter 14: Congenital Anomalies (740-759)

a. Codes in categories 740-759, Congenital Anomalies

Assign an appropriate code(s) from categories 740-759, Congenital Anomalies, when an anomaly is documented. A congenital anomaly may be the principal/first listed diagnosis on a record or a secondary diagnosis.

When a congenital anomaly does not have a unique code assignment, assign additional code(s) for any manifestations that may be present.

When the code assignment specifically identifies the congenital anomaly, manifestations that are an inherent component of the anomaly should not be coded separately. Additional codes should be assigned for manifestations that are not an inherent component.

Codes from Chapter 14 may be used throughout the life of the patient. If a congenital anomaly has been corrected, a personal history code should be used to identify the history of the anomaly. Although present at birth, a congenital anomaly may not be identified until later in life. Whenever the condition is diagnosed by the physician, it is appropriate to assign a code from codes 740-759.

For the birth admission, the appropriate code from category V30, Liveborn infants, according to type of birth should be sequenced as the principal diagnosis, followed by any congenital anomaly codes, 740-759.

15. Chapter 15: Newborn (Perinatal) Guidelines (760-779)

For coding and reporting purposes the perinatal period is defined as before birth through the 28th day following birth. The following guidelines are provided for reporting purposes. Hospitals may record other diagnoses as needed for internal data use.

a. General Perinatal Rules

1) Chapter 15 Codes

They are never for use on the maternal record. Codes from Chapter 11, the obstetric chapter, are never permitted on the newborn record. Chapter 15 code may be used throughout the life of the patient if the condition is still present.

2) Sequencing of perinatal codes

Generally, codes from Chapter 15 should be sequenced as the principal/first-listed diagnosis on the newborn record, with the exception of the appropriate V30 code for the birth episode, followed by codes from any other chapter that provide additional detail. The "use additional code" note at the beginning of the chapter supports this guideline. If the index does not provide a specific code for a perinatal condition, assign code 779.89, Other specified conditions originating in the perinatal period, followed by the code from another chapter that specifies the condition. Codes for signs and symptoms may be assigned when a definitive diagnosis has not been established.

3) Birth process or community acquired conditions

If a newborn has a condition that may be either due to the birth process or community acquired and the documentation does not indicate which it is, the default is due to the birth process and the code from Chapter 15 should be used. If the condition is community-acquired, a code from Chapter 15 should not be assigned.

4) Code all clinically significant conditions

All clinically significant conditions noted on routine newborn examination should be coded. A condition is clinically significant if it requires:

- clinical evaluation; or

- therapeutic treatment; or

- diagnostic procedures; or

- extended length of hospital stay; or

- increased nursing care and/or monitoring; or

- has implications for future health care needs

Note: The perinatal guidelines listed above are the same as the general coding guidelines for "additional diagnoses", except for the final point regarding implications for future health care needs. Codes should be assigned for conditions that have been specified by the provider as having implications for future health care needs. Codes from the perinatal chapter should not be assigned unless the provider has established a definitive diagnosis.

b. **Use of codes V30-V39**

When coding the birth of an infant, assign a code from categories V30-V39, according to the type of birth. A code from this series is assigned as a principal diagnosis, and assigned only once to a newborn at the time of birth.

c. **Newborn transfers**

If the newborn is transferred to another institution, the V30 series is not used at the receiving hospital.

d. **Use of category V29**

1) **Assigning a code from category V29**

    Assign a code from category V29, Observation and evaluation of newborns and infants for suspected conditions not found, to identify those instances when a healthy newborn is evaluated for a suspected condition that is determined after study not to be present. Do not use a code from category V29 when the patient has identified signs or symptoms of a suspected problem; in such cases, code the sign or symptom.

    A code from category V29 may also be assigned as a principal code for readmissions or encounters when the V30 code no longer applies. Codes from category V29 are for use only for healthy newborns and infants for which no condition after study is found to be present.

2) **V29 code on a birth record**

    A V29 code is to be used as a secondary code after the V30, Outcome of delivery, code.

e. **Use of other V codes on perinatal records**

V codes other than V30 and V29 may be assigned on a perinatal or newborn record code. The codes may be used as a principal or first listed diagnosis for specific types of encounters or for readmissions or encounters when the V30 code no longer applies.

See Section I.C.18 for information regarding the assignment of V codes.

f. **Maternal Causes of Perinatal Morbidity**

Codes from categories 760-763, Maternal causes of perinatal morbidity and mortality, are assigned only when the maternal condition has actually affected the fetus or newborn. The fact that the mother has an associated medical condition or experiences some complication of pregnancy, labor or delivery does not justify the routine assignment of codes from these categories to the newborn record.

g. **Congenital Anomalies in Newborns**

For the birth admission, the appropriate code from category V30, Liveborn infants according to type of birth, should be used, followed by any congenital anomaly codes, categories 740-759. Use additional secondary codes from other chapters to specify conditions associated with the anomaly, if applicable.

Also, see Section I.C.14 for information on the coding of congenital anomalies.

h. **Coding Additional Perinatal Diagnoses**

1) **Assigning codes for conditions that require treatment**

Assign codes for conditions that require treatment or further investigation, prolong the length of stay, or require resource utilization.

2) **Codes for conditions specified as having implications for future health care needs**

Assign codes for conditions that have been specified by the provider as having implications for future health care needs.

Note: This guideline should not be used for adult patients.

3) **Codes for newborn conditions originating in the perinatal period**

Assign a code for newborn conditions originating in the perinatal period (categories 760-779), as well as complications arising during the current episode of care classified in other chapters, only if the diagnoses have been documented by the responsible provider at the time of transfer or discharge as having affected the fetus or newborn.

i. **Prematurity and Fetal Growth Retardation**

Providers utilize different criteria in determining prematurity. A code for prematurity should not be assigned unless it is documented. The 5th digit assignment for codes from category 764 and subcategories 765.0 and 765.1 should be based on the recorded birth weight and estimated gestational age.

A code from subcategory 765.2, Weeks of gestation, should be assigned as an additional code with category 764 and codes from 765.0 and 765.1 to specify weeks of gestation as documented by the provider in the record.

j. **Newborn sepsis**

Code 771.81, Septicemia [sepsis] of newborn, should be assigned with a secondary code from category 041, Bacterial infections in conditions classified elsewhere and of unspecified site, to identify the organism.

A code from category 038, Septicemia, should not be used on a newborn record. Do not assign code 995.91, Sepsis, as code 771.81 describes the sepsis. If applicable, use additional codes to identify severe sepsis (995.92) and any associated acute organ dysfunction.

16. Chapter 16: Signs, Symptoms and Ill-Defined Conditions (780-799)

Reserved for future guideline expansion

17. Chapter 17: Injury and Poisoning (800-999)

a. Coding of Injuries

When coding injuries, assign separate codes for each injury unless a combination code is provided, in which case the combination code is assigned. Multiple injury codes are provided in ICD-9-CM, but should not be assigned unless information for a more specific code is not available. These codes are not to be used for normal, healing surgical wounds or to identify complications of surgical wounds.

The code for the most serious injury, as determined by the provider and the focus of treatment, is sequenced first.

1) Superficial injuries

Superficial injuries such as abrasions or contusions are not coded when associated with more severe injuries of the same site.

2) Primary injury with damage to nerves/blood vessels

When a primary injury results in minor damage to peripheral nerves or blood vessels, the primary injury is sequenced first with additional code(s) from categories 950-957, Injury to nerves and spinal cord, and/or 900-904, Injury to blood vessels. When the primary injury is to the blood vessels or nerves, that injury should be sequenced first.

b. Coding of Traumatic Fractures

The principles of multiple coding of injuries should be followed in coding fractures. Fractures of specified sites are coded individually by site in accordance with both the provisions within categories 800-829 and the level of detail furnished by medical record content.

Combination categories for multiple fractures are provided for use when there is insufficient detail in the medical record (such as trauma cases transferred to another hospital), when the reporting form limits the number of codes that can be used in reporting pertinent clinical data, or when there is insufficient specificity at the fourth-digit or fifth-digit level. More specific guidelines are as follows:

1) Acute Fractures vs. Aftercare

Traumatic fractures are coded using the acute fracture codes (800-829) while the patient is receiving active treatment for the fracture. Examples of active treatment are: surgical treatment, emergency department encounter, and evaluation and treatment by a new physician.

Fractures are coded using the aftercare codes (subcategories V54.0, V54.1, V54.8, or V54.9) for encounters after the patient has completed active treatment of the fracture and is receiving routine care for the fracture during the healing or recovery phase. Examples of fracture aftercare are: cast change or removal, removal of external or internal fixation device, medication adjustment, and follow up visits following fracture treatment.

Care for complications of surgical treatment for fracture repairs during the healing or recovery phase should be coded with the appropriate complication codes.

Care of complications of fractures, such as malunion and nonunion, should be reported with the appropriate codes.

Pathologic fractures are not coded in the 800-829 range, but instead are assigned to subcategory 733.1. See Section I.C.13.a for additional information.

2) **Multiple fractures of same limb**

Multiple fractures of same limb classifiable to the same three-digit or four-digit category are coded to that category.

3) **Multiple unilateral or bilateral fractures of same bone**

Multiple unilateral or bilateral fractures of same bone(s) but classified to different fourth-digit subdivisions (bone part) within the same three-digit category are coded individually by site.

4) **Multiple fracture categories 819 and 828**

Multiple fracture categories 819 and 828 classify bilateral fractures of both upper limbs (819) and both lower limbs (828), but without any detail at the fourth-digit level other than open and closed type of fractures.

5) **Multiple fractures sequencing**

Multiple fractures are sequenced in accordance with the severity of the fracture. The provider should be asked to list the fracture diagnoses in the order of severity.

c. **Coding of Burns**

Current burns (940-948) are classified by depth, extent and by agent (E code). Burns are classified by depth as first degree (erythema), second degree (blistering), and third degree (full-thickness involvement).

1) **Sequencing of burn and related condition codes**

Sequence first the code that reflects the highest degree of burn when more than one burn is present.

(a.) When the reason for the admission or encounter is for treatment of external multiple burns, sequence first the code that reflects the burn of the highest degree.

(b.) When a patient has both internal and external burns, the circumstances of admission govern the selection of the principal diagnosis or first-listed diagnosis.

(c.) When a patient is admitted for burn injuries and other related conditions such as smoke inhalation and/or respiratory failure, the circumstances of admission govern the selection of the principal or first-listed diagnosis.

2) Burns of the same local site

Classify burns of the same local site (three-digit category level, 940-947) but of different degrees to the subcategory identifying the highest degree recorded in the diagnosis.

3) Non-healing burns

Non-healing burns are coded as acute burns. Necrosis of burned skin should be coded as a non-healed burn.

4) Code 958.3, Posttraumatic wound infection

Assign code 958.3, Posttraumatic wound infection, not elsewhere classified, as an additional code for any documented infected burn site.

5) Assign separate codes for each burn site

When coding burns, assign separate codes for each burn site. Category 946 Burns of Multiple specified sites, should only be used if the location of the burns are not documented.

Category 949, Burn, unspecified, is extremely vague and should rarely be used.

6) Assign codes from category 948, Burns

Burns classified according to extent of body surface involved, when the site of the burn is not specified or when there is a need for additional data. It is advisable to use category 948 as additional coding when needed to provide data for evaluating burn mortality, such as that needed by burn units. It is also advisable to use category 948 as an additional code for reporting purposes when there is mention of a third-degree burn involving 20 percent or more of the body surface.

In assigning a code from category 948:

■ Fourth-digit codes are used to identify the percentage of total body surface involved in a burn (all degree).

■ Fifth-digits are assigned to identify the percentage of body surface involved in third-degree burn.

■ Fifth-digit zero (0) is assigned when less than 10 percent or when no body surface is involved in a third-degree burn.

Category 948 is based on the classic "rule of nines" in estimating body surface involved: head and neck are assigned nine percent, each arm nine percent, each leg 18 percent, the anterior trunk 18 percent, posterior trunk 18 percent, and genitalia one percent. Providers may change these percentage assignments where necessary to accommodate infants and children who have proportionately larger heads than adults and patients who have large buttocks, thighs, or abdomen that involve burns.

7) **Encounters for treatment of late effects of burns**

Encounters for the treatment of the late effects of burns (i.e., scars or joint contractures) should be coded to the residual condition (sequelae) followed by the appropriate late effect code (906.5-906.9). A late effect E code may also be used, if desired.

8) **Sequelae with a late effect code and current burn**

When appropriate, both a sequelae with a late effect code, and a current burn code may be assigned on the same record (when both a current burn and sequelae of an old burn exist).

d. **Coding of Debridement of Wound, Infection, or Burn**

Excisional debridement involves surgical removal or cutting away, as opposed to a mechanical (brushing, scrubbing, washing) debridement.

For coding purposes, excisional debridement is assigned to code 86.22. Nonexcisional debridement is assigned to code 86.28.

e. **Adverse Effects, Poisoning and Toxic Effects**

The properties of certain drugs, medicinal and biological substances or combinations of such substances, may cause toxic reactions. The occurrence of drug toxicity is classified in ICD-9-CM as follows:

1) **Adverse Effect**

When the drug was correctly prescribed and properly administered, code the reaction plus the appropriate code from the E930-E949 series. Codes from the E930-E949 series must be used to identify the causative substance for an adverse effect of drug, medicinal and biological substances, correctly prescribed and properly administered. The effect, such as tachycardia, delirium, gastrointestinal hemorrhaging, vomit-ing, hypokalemia, hepatitis, renal failure, or respiratory failure, is coded and followed by the appropriate code from the E930-E949 series.

Adverse effects of therapeutic substances correctly prescribed and properly administered (toxicity, synergistic reaction, side effect, and idiosyncratic reaction) may be due to (1) differences among patients, such as age, sex, disease, and genetic factors, and (2) drug-related factors, such as type of drug, route of administration, duration of therapy, dosage, and bioavailability.

2) Poisoning

(a) Error was made in drug prescription

Errors made in drug prescription or in the administration of the drug by provider, nurse, patient, or other person, use the appropriate poisoning code from the 960-979 series.

(b) Overdose of a drug intentionally taken

If an overdose of a drug was intentionally taken or administered and resulted in drug toxicity, it would be coded as a poisoning (960-979 series).

(c) Nonprescribed drug taken with correctly prescribed and properly administered drug

If a nonprescribed drug or medicinal agent was taken in combination with a correctly prescribed and properly administered drug, any drug toxicity or other reaction resulting from the interaction of the two drugs would be classified as a poisoning.

(d) Interaction of drug(s) and alcohol

When a reaction results from the interaction of a drug(s) and alcohol, this would be classified as poisoning.

(e) Sequencing of poisoning

When coding a poisoning or reaction to the improper use of a medication (e.g., wrong dose, wrong substance, wrong route of administration) the poisoning code is sequenced first, followed by a code for the manifestation. If there is also a diagnosis of drug abuse or dependence to the substance, the abuse or dependence is coded as an additional code.

See Section I.C.3.a.6.b. if poisoning is the result of insulin pump malfunctions and Section I.C.19 for general use of E-codes.

3) Toxic Effects

(a) Toxic effect codes

When a harmful substance is ingested or comes in contact with a person, this is classified as a toxic effect. The toxic effect codes are in categories 980-989.

(b) Sequencing toxic effect codes

A toxic effect code should be sequenced first, followed by the code(s) that identify the result of the toxic effect.

(c) External cause codes for toxic effects

An external cause code from categories E860-E869 for accidental exposure, codes E950.6 or E950.7 for intentional self-harm, category E962 for assault, or categories E980-E982, for undetermined, should also be assigned to indicate intent.

f. Complications of care

1) Complications of care

(a) Documentation of complications of care

As with all procedural or postprocedural complications, code assignment is based on the provider's documentation of the relationship between the condition and the procedure.

2) Transplant complications

(a) Transplant complications other than kidney

Codes under subcategory 996.8, Complications of transplanted organ, are for use for both complications and rejection of transplanted organs. A transplant complication code is only assigned if the complication affects the function of the transplanted organ. Two codes are required to fully describe a transplant complication, the appropriate code from subcategory 996.8 and a secondary code that identifies the complication.

Pre-existing conditions or conditions that develop after the transplant are not coded as complications unless they affect the function of the transplanted organs.

See I.C.18.d.3) for transplant organ removal status. See I.C.2.i for malignant neoplasm associated with transplanted organ.

(b) Chronic kidney disease and kidney transplant complications

Patients who have undergone kidney transplant may still have some form of chronic kidney disease (CKD) because the kidney transplant may not fully restore kidney function. Code 996.81 should be assigned for documented complications of a kidney transplant, such as transplant failure or rejection or other transplant complication. Code 996.81 should not be assigned for post kidney transplant patients who have chronic kidney (CKD) unless a transplant complication such as transplant failure or rejection is documented. If the documentation is unclear as to whether the patient has a complication of the transplant, query the provider.

For patients with CKD following a kidney transplant, but who do not have a complication such as failure or rejection, see section I.C.10.a.2, Chronic kidney disease and kidney transplant status.

3) **Ventilator associated pneumonia**

(a) **Documentation of Ventilator associated pneumonia**

As with all procedural or postprocedural complications, code assignment is based on the provider's documentation of the relationship between the condition and the procedure.

Code 997.31, Ventilator associated pneumonia, should be assigned only when the provider has documented ventilator associated pneumonia (VAP). An additional code to identify the organism (e.g., Pseudomonas aeruginosa, code 041.7) should also be assigned. Do not assign an additional code from categories 480-484 to identify the type of pneumonia.

Code 997.31 should not be assigned for cases where the patient has pneumonia and is on a mechanical ventilator but the provider has not specifically stated that the pneumonia is ventilator-associated pneumonia.

If the documentation is unclear as to whether the patient has a pneumonia that is a complication attributable to the mechanical ventilator, query the provider.

(b) **Patient admitted with pneumonia and develops VAP**

A patient may be admitted with one type of pneumonia (e.g., code 481, Pneumococcal pneumonia) and subsequently develop VAP. In this instance, the principal diagnosis would be the appropriate code from categories 480-484 for the pneumonia diagnosed at the time of admission. Code 997.31, Ventilator associated pneumonia, would be assigned as an additional diagnosis when the provider has also documented the presence of ventilator associated pneumonia.

g. **SIRS due to Non-infectious Process**

The systemic inflammatory response syndrome (SIRS) can develop as a result of certain non-infectious disease processes, such as trauma, malignant neoplasm, or pancreatitis. When SIRS is documented with a noninfectious condition, and no subsequent infection is documented, the code for the underlying condition, such as an injury, should be assigned, followed by code 995.93, Systemic inflammatory response syndrome due to noninfectious process without acute organ dysfunction, or 995.94, Systemic inflammatory response syndrome due to non-infectious process with acute organ dysfunction. If an acute organ dysfunction is documented, the appropriate code(s) for the associated acute organ dysfunction(s) should be assigned in addition to code 995.94. If acute organ dysfunction is documented, but it cannot be determined if the acute organ dysfunction is associated with SIRS or due to another condition (e.g., directly due to the trauma), the provider should be queried.

When the non-infectious condition has led to an infection that results in SIRS, see Section I.C.1.b.12 for the guideline for sepsis and severe sepsis associated with a non-infectious process.

18. Classification of Factors Influencing Health Status and Contact with Health Service (Supplemental V01-V89)

Note: The chapter specific guidelines provide additional information about the use of V codes for specified encounters.

a. Introduction

ICD-9-CM provides codes to deal with encounters for circumstances other than a disease or injury. The Supplementary Classification of Factors Influencing Health Status and Contact with Health Services (V01.0 - V89.09) is provided to deal with occasions when circumstances other than a disease or injury (codes 001-999) are recorded as a diagnosis or problem.

There are four primary circumstances for the use of V codes:

1) A person who is not currently sick encounters the health services for some specific reason, such as to act as an organ donor, to receive prophylactic care, such as inoculations or health screenings, or to receive counseling on health related issues.

2) A person with a resolving disease or injury, or a chronic, long term condition requiring continuous care, encounters the health care system for specific aftercare of that disease or injury (e.g., dialysis for renal disease; chemotherapy for malignancy; cast change). A diagnosis/symptom code should be used whenever a current, acute, diagnosis is being treated or a sign or symptom is being studied.

3) Circumstances or problems influence a person's health status but are not in themselves a current illness or injury.

4) Newborns, to indicate birth status

b. V codes use in any healthcare setting

V codes are for use in any healthcare setting. V codes may be used as either a first listed (principal diagnosis code in the inpatient setting) or secondary code, depending on the circumstances of the encounter. Certain V codes may only be used as first listed, others only as secondary codes.

See Section I.C.18.e, V Code Table.

c. V Codes indicate a reason for an encounter

They are not procedure codes. A corresponding procedure code must accompany a V code to describe the procedure performed.

d. Categories of V Codes

1) Contact/Exposure

Category V01 indicates contact with or exposure to communicable diseases. These codes are for patients who do not show any sign or symptom of a disease but have been exposed to it by close personal contact with an infected individual or are in an area where a disease is epidemic. These codes may be used as a first listed code to explain an encounter for testing, or, more commonly, as a secondary code to identify a potential risk.

2) Inoculations and vaccinations

Categories V03-V06 are for encounters for inoculations and vaccinations. They indicate that a patient is being seen to receive a prophylactic inoculation against a disease. The injection itself must be represented by the appropriate procedure code. A code from V03-V06 may be used as a secondary code if the inoculation is given as a routine part of preventive health care, such as a well-baby visit.

3) Status

Status codes indicate that a patient is either a carrier of a disease or has the sequelae or residual of a past disease or condition. This includes such things as the presence of prosthetic or mechanical devices resulting from past treatment. A status code is informative, because the status may affect the course of treatment and its outcome. A status code is distinct from a history code. The history code indicates that the patient no longer has the condition.

A status code should not be used with a diagnosis code from one of the body system chapters, if the diagnosis code includes the information provided by the status code. For example, code V42.1, Heart transplant status, should not be used with code 996.83, Complications of transplanted heart. The status code does not provide additional information. The complication code indicates that the patient is a heart transplant patient.

The status V codes/categories are:

V02   Carrier or suspected carrier of infectious diseases

        Carrier status indicates that a person harbors the specific organisms of a disease without manifest symptoms and is capable of transmitting the infection.

V07.5x Prophylactic use of agents affecting estrogen receptors and estrogen level

        This code indicates when a patient is receiving a drug that affects estrogen receptors adn estrogen levels for prevention of cancer.

V08   Asymptomatic HIV infection status

        This code indicates that a patient has tested positive for HIV but has manifested no signs or symptoms of the disease.

V09   Infection with drug-resistant microorganisms

        This category indicates that a patient has an infectionthat is resistant to drug treatment. Sequence the infection code first.

V21   Constitutional states in development

V22.2   Pregnant state, incidental

This code is a secondary code only for use when the pregnancy is in no way complicating the reason for visit. Otherwise, a code from the obstetric chapter is required.

V26.5x Sterilization status

V42   Organ or tissue replaced by transplant

V43   Organ or tissue replaced by other means

V44   Artificial opening status

V45   Other postsurgical states

Assign code V45.87, Transplant organ removal status, to indicate that a transplanted organ has been previously removed. This code should not be assigned for the encounter in which the transplanted organ is removed. The complication necessitating removal of the transplant organ should be assigned for that encounter. *See section I.C17.f.2. for information on the coding of organ transplant complications.*

Assign code V45.88, Status post administration of tPA (rtPA) in a different facility within the last 24 hours prior to admission to the current facility, as a secondary diagnosis when a patient is received by transfer into a facility and documentation indicates they were administered tissue plasminogen activator (tPA) within the last 24 hours prior to admission to the current facility.

This guideline applies even if the patient is still receiving the tPA at the time they are received into the current facility.

The appropriate code for the condition for which the tPA was administered (such as cerebrovascular disease or myocardial infarction) should be assigned first.

Code V45.88 is only applicable to the receiving facility record and not to the transferring facility record.

V46   Other dependence on machines

V49.6   Upper limb amputation status

V49.7   Lower limb amputation status

Note: Categories V42-V46, and subcategories V49.6, V49.7 are for use only if there are no complications or malfunctions of the organ or tissue replaced, the amputation site or the equipment on which the patient is dependent.

V49.81   Postmenopausal status

V49.82   Dental sealant status

V49.83   Awaiting organ transplant status

V58.6x   Long-term (current) drug use

> Codes from this subcategory indicate a patient's continuous use of a prescribed drug (including such things as aspirin therapy) for the long-term treatment of a condition or for prophylactic use. It is not for use for patients who have addictions to drugs. This subcategory is not for use of medications for detoxification or maintenance programs to prevent withdrawal symptoms in patients with drug dependence (e.g., methadone maintenance for opiate dependence). Assign the appropriate code for the drug dependence instead.
>
> Assign a code from subcategory V58.6, Long-term (current) drug use, if the patient is receiving a medication for an extended period as a prophylactic measure (such as for the prevention of deep vein thrombosis) or as treatment of a chronic condition (such as arthritis) or a disease requiring a lengthy course of treatment (such as cancer). Do not assign a code from subcategory V58.6 for medication being administered for a brief period of time to treat an acute illness or injury (such as a course of antibiotics to treat acute bronchitis).

V83   Genetic carrier status

> Genetic carrier status indicates that a person carries a gene, associated with a particular disease, which may be passed to offspring who may develop that disease. The person does not have the disease and is not at risk of developing the disease.

V84   Genetic susceptibility status

> Genetic susceptibility indicates that a person has a gene that increases the risk of that person developing the disease.
>
> Codes from category V84, Genetic susceptibility to disease, should not be used as principal or first listed codes. If the patient has the condition to which he/she is susceptible, and that condition is the reason for the encounter, the code for the current condition should be sequenced first. If the patient is being seen for follow-up after completed treatment for this condition, and the condition no longer exists, a follow-up code should be sequenced first, followed by the appropriate personal history and genetic susceptibility codes. If the purpose of the encounter is genetic counseling associated with procreative management, a code from subcategory V26.3, Genetic counseling and

testing, should be assigned as the first-listed code, followed by a code from category V84. Additional codes should be assigned for any applicable family or personal history.

See Section I.C. 18.d.14 for information on prophylactic organ removal due to a genetic susceptibility.

V86   Estrogen receptor status

V88   Acquired absence of other organs and tissue

4) **History (of)**

There are two types of history V codes, personal and family. Personal history codes explain a patient's past medical condition that no longer exists and is not receiving any treatment, but that has the potential for recurrence, and therefore may require continued monitoring. The exceptions to this general rule are category V14, Personal history of allergy to medicinal agents, and subcategory V15.0, Allergy, other than to medicinal agents. A person who has had an allergic episode to a substance or food in the past should always be considered allergic to the substance.

Family history codes are for use when a patient has a family member(s) who has had a particular disease that causes the patient to be at higher risk of also contracting the disease.

Personal history codes may be used in conjunction with followup codes and family history codes may be used in conjunction with screening codes to explain the need for a test or procedure. History codes are also acceptable on any medical record regardless of the reason for visit. A history of an illness, even if no longer present, is important information that may alter the type of treatment ordered.

The history V code categories are:

V10   Personal history of malignant neoplasm

V12   Personal history of certain other diseases

V13   Personal history of other diseases

Except: V13.4, Personal history of arthritis, and V13.6, Personal history of congenital malformations. These conditions are life-long so are not true history codes.

V14   Personal history of allergy to medicinal agents

V15   Other personal history presenting hazards to health
Except: V15.7, Personal history of contraception.

V16   Family history of malignant neoplasm

V17   Family history of certain chronic disabling diseases

V18   Family history of certain other specific diseases

V19   Family history of other conditions

V87   Other specified personal exposure and history presenting hazards to health

5) Screening

Screening is the testing for disease or disease precursors in seemingly well individuals so that early detection and treatment can be provided for those who test positive for the disease. Screenings that are recommended for many subgroups in a population include: routine mammograms for women over 40, a fecal occult blood test for everyone over 50, an amniocentesis to rule out a fetal anomaly for pregnant women over 35, because the incidence of breast cancer and colon cancer in these subgroups is higher than in the general population, as is the incidence of Down's syndrome in older mothers.

The testing of a person to rule out or confirm a suspected diagnosis because the patient has some sign or symptom is a diagnostic examination, not a screening. In these cases, the sign or symptom is used to explain the reason for the test. A screening code may be a first listed code if the reason for the visit is specifically the screening exam. It may also be used as an additional code if the screening is done during an office visit for other health problems. A screening code is not necessary if the screening is inherent to a routine examination, such as a pap smear done during a routine pelvic examination.

Should a condition be discovered during the screening then the code for the condition may be assigned as an additional diagnosis.

The V code indicates that a screening exam is planned. A procedure code is required to confirm that the screening was performed.

The screening V code categories:

V28   Antenatal screening

V73-V82 Special screening examinations

6) Observation

There are three observation V code categories. They are for use in very limited circumstances when a person is being observed for a suspected condition that is ruled out. The observation codes are not for use if an injury or illness or any signs or symptoms related to the suspected condition are present. In such cases the diagnosis/symptom code is used with the corresponding E code to identify any external cause.

The observation codes are to be used as principal diagnosis only. The only exception to this is when the principal diagnosis is required to be a code from the V30, Live born infant, category. Then the V29 observation code is sequenced after the V30 code. Additional codes may be used in addition to the observation code but only if they are unrelated to the suspected condition being observed.

Codes from subcategory V89.0, Suspected maternal and fetal conditions not found, may either be used as a first listed or as an additional code assignment depending on the case. They are for use in very limited circumstances on a maternal record when an encounter is for a suspected maternal or fetal condition that is ruled out during that encounter (for example, a maternal or fetal condition may be suspected due to an abnormal test result). These codes should not be used when the condition is confirmed. In those cases, the confirmed condition should be coded. In addition, these codes are not for use if an illness or any signs or symptoms related to the suspected condition or problem are present. In such cases the diagnosis/symptom code is used.

Additional codes may be used in addition to the code from subcategory V89.0, but only if they are unrelated to the suspected condition being evaluated.

Codes from subcategory V89.0 may not be used for encounters for antenatal screening of mother. See Section I.C.18.d., Screening).

For encounters for suspected fetal condition that are inconclusive following testing and evaluation, assign the appropriate code from category 655, 656, 657 or 658.

The observation V code categories:

V29   Observation and evaluation of newborns for suspected condition not found

        For the birth encounter, a code from category V30 should be sequenced before the V29 code.

V71   Observation and evaluation for suspected condition not found

V89   Suspected maternal and fetal conditions not found

7) **Aftercare**

Aftercare visit codes cover situations when the initial treatment of a disease or injury has been performed and the patient requires continued care during the healing or recovery phase, or for the long-term consequences of the disease. The aftercare V code should not be used if treatment is directed at a current, acute disease or injury. The diagnosis code is to be used in these cases. Exceptions to this rule are codes V58.0, Radiotherapy, and codes from subcategory V58.1, Encounter for chemotherapy and immunotherapy for neoplastic conditions. These codes are to be first listed, followed by the diagnosis code when a patient's encounter is solely to receive radiation therapy or chemotherapy for the treatment of a neoplasm. Should a patient receive both chemotherapy and radiation therapy during the same encounter code V58.0 and V58.1 may be used together on a record with either one being sequenced first.

The aftercare codes are generally first listed to explain the specific reason for the encounter. An aftercare code may be used as an additional code when some type of aftercare is provided in addition to the reason for admission and no diagnosis code is applicable. An example of this would be the closure of a colostomy during an encounter for treatment of another condition.

Aftercare codes should be used in conjunction with any other aftercare codes or other diagnosis codes to provide better detail on the specifics of an aftercare encounter visit, unless otherwise directed by the classification. The sequencing of multiple aftercare codes is discretionary.

Certain aftercare V code categories need a secondary diagnosis code to describe the resolving condition or sequelae, for others, the condition is inherent in the code title.

Additional V code aftercare category terms include, fitting and adjustment, and attention to artificial openings.

Status V codes may be used with aftercare V codes to indicate the nature of the aftercare. For example code V45.81, Aortocoronary bypass status, may be used with code V58.73, Aftercare following surgery of the circulatory system, NEC, to indicate the surgery for which the aftercare is being performed. Also, a transplant status code may be used following code V58.44, Aftercare following organ transplant, to identify the organ transplanted. A status code should not be used when the aftercare code indicates the type of status, such as using V55.0, Attention to tracheostomy with V44.0, Tracheostomy status.

See Section I. B.16 Admissions/Encounter for Rehabilitation

The aftercare V category/codes:

V51.0　Encounter for breast reconstruction following mastectomy

V52　Fitting and adjustment of prosthetic device and implant

V53　Fitting and adjustment of other device

V54　Other orthopedic aftercare

V55　Attention to artificial openings

V56　Encounter for dialysis and dialysis catheter care

V57　Care involving the use of rehabilitation procedures

V58.0　Radiotherapy

V58.11　Encounter for antineoplastic chemotherapy

V58.12　Encounter for antineoplastic immunotherapy

V58.3x　Attention to dressings and sutures

V58.41　Encounter for planned post-operative wound closure

V58.42　Aftercare, surgery, neoplasm

V58.43　Aftercare, surgery, trauma

V58.44　Aftercare involving organ transplant

V58.49 Other specified aftercare following surgery

V58.7x Aftercare following surgery

V58.81 Fitting and adjustment of vascular catheter

V58.82 Fitting and adjustment of non-vascular catheter

V58.83 Monitoring therapeutic drug

V58.89 Other specified aftercare

8) Follow-up

The follow-up codes are used to explain continuing surveillance following completed treatment of a disease, condition, or injury. They imply that the condition has been fully treated and no longer exists. They should not be confused with aftercare codes that explain current treatment for a healing condition or its sequelae. Follow-up codes may be used in conjunction with history codes to provide the full picture of the healed condition and its treatment. The follow-up code is sequenced first, followed by the history code.

A follow-up code may be used to explain repeated visits.

Should a condition be found to have recurred on the follow-up visit, then the diagnosis code should be used in place of the follow-up code.

The follow-up V code categories:

V24   Postpartum care and evaluation

V67   Follow-up examination

9) Donor

Category V59 is the donor codes. They are used for living individuals who are donating blood or other body tissue. These codes are only for individuals donating for others, not for self donations. They are not for use to identify cadaveric donations.

10) Counseling

Counseling V codes are used when a patient or family member receives assistance in the aftermath of an illness or injury, or when support is required in coping with family or social problems. They are not necessary for use in conjunction with a diagnosis code when the counseling component of care is considered integral to standard treatment.

The counseling V categories/codes:

V25.0   General counseling and advice for contraceptive management

V26.3   Genetic counseling

V26.4   General counseling and advice for procreative management

V61.x   Other family circumstances

V65.1   Person consulted on behalf of another person

V65.3   Dietary surveillance and counseling

V65.4   Other counseling, not elsewhere classified

11) Obstetrics and related conditions

See Section I.C.11., the Obstetrics guidelines for further instruction on the use of these codes.

V codes for pregnancy are for use in those circumstances when none of the problems or complications included in the codes from the Obstetrics chapter exist (a routine prenatal visit or postpartum care). Codes V22.0, Supervision of normal first pregnancy, and V22.1, Supervision of other normal pregnancy, are always first listed and are not to be used with any other code from the OB chapter.

The outcome of delivery, category V27, should be included on all maternal delivery records. It is always a secondary code.

V codes for family planning (contraceptive) or procreative management and counseling should be included on an obstetric record either during the pregnancy or the postpartum stage, if applicable.

Obstetrics and related conditions V code categories:

V22   Normal pregnancy

V23   Supervision of high-risk pregnancy

       Except: V23.2, Pregnancy with history of abortion. Code 646.3, Habitual aborter, from the OB chapter is required to indicate a history of abortion during a pregnancy.

V24   Postpartum care and evaluation

V25   Encounter for contraceptive management

       Except V25.0x
       (See Section I.C.18.d.11, Counseling)

V26   Procreative management

       Except V26.5x, Sterilization status, V26.3 and V26.4
       (See Section I.C.18.d.11., Counseling)

V27   Outcome of delivery

V28   Antenatal screening

       (See Section I.C.18.d.6., Screening)

12) Newborn, infant and child

See Section I.C.15, the Newborn guidelines for further instruction on the use of these codes.

Newborn V code categories:

V20   Health supervision of infant or child

V29   Observation and evaluation of newborns for suspected condition not found
(See Section I.C.18.d.7, Observation)

V30-V39 Liveborn infant according to type of birth

13) Routine and administrative examinations

The V codes allow for the description of encounters for routine examinations, such as, a general check-up, or, examinations for administrative purposes, such as, a pre-employment physical. The codes are not to be used if the examination is for diagnosis of a suspected condition or for treatment purposes. In such cases the diagnosis code is used. During a routine exam, should a diagnosis or condition be discovered, it should be coded as an additional code. Pre-existing and chronic conditions and history codes may also be included as additional codes as long as the examination is for administrative purposes and not focused on any particular condition.

Pre-operative examination V codes are for use only in those situations when a patient is being cleared for surgery and no treatment is given.

The V codes categories/code for routine and administrative examinations:

V20.2   Routine infant or child health check

           Any injections given should have a corresponding procedure code.

V70   General medical examination

V72   Special investigations and examinations

Codes V72.5 and V72.6 may be used if the reason for the patient encounter is for routine laboratory/radiology testing in the absence of any signs, symptoms, or associated diagnosis. If routine testing is performed during the same encounter as a test to evaluate a sign, symptom, or diagnosis, it is appropriate to assign both the V code and the code describing the reason for the non-routine test.

14) Miscellaneous V codes

The miscellaneous V codes capture a number of other health care encounters that do not fall into one of the other categories. Certain of these codes identify the reason for the encounter, others are for use as additional codes that provide useful information on circumstances that may affect a patient's care and treatment.

Prophylactic Organ Removal

For encounters specifically for prophylactic removal of breasts, ovaries, or another organ due to a genetic susceptibility to cancer or a family history of cancer, the principal or first listed code should be a code from subcategory V50.4, Prophylactic organ removal, followed by the appropriate genetic susceptibility code and the appropriate family history code.

If the patient has a malignancy of one site and is having prophylactic removal at another site to prevent either a new primary malignancy or metastatic disease, a code for the malignancy should also be assigned in addition to a code from subcategory V50.4. A V50.4 code should not be assigned if the patient is having organ removal for treatment of a malignancy, such as the removal of the testes for the treatment of prostate cancer.

Miscellaneous V code categories/codes:

V07   Need for isolation and other prophylactic measures

        Except V07.5, Prophylactic use of agents affecting estrogen receptors and estrogen levels.

V50   Elective surgery for purposes other than remedying health states

V58.5   Orthodontics

V60   Housing, household, and economic circumstances

V62   Other psychosocial circumstances

V63   Unavailability of other medical facilities for care

V64   Persons encountering health services for specific procedures, not carried out

V66   Convalescence and Palliative Care

V68   Encounters for administrative purposes

V69   Problems related to lifestyle

V85   Body Mass Index

15) Nonspecific V codes

Certain V codes are so non-specific, or potentially redundant with other codes in the classification, that there can be little justification for their use in the inpatient setting. Their use in the outpatient setting should be limited to those instances when there is no further documentation to permit more precise coding. Otherwise, any sign or symptom or any other reason for visit that is captured in another code should be used.

Nonspecific V code categories/codes:

V11   Personal history of mental disorder

A code from the mental disorders chapter, with an in remission fifth-digit, should be used.

V13.4   Personal history of arthritis

V13.6   Personal history of congenital malformations

V15.7   Personal history of contraception

V23.2   Pregnancy with history of abortion

V40   Mental and behavioral problems

V41   Problems with special senses and other special functions

V47   Other problems with internal organs

V48   Problems with head, neck, and trunk

V49   Problems with limbs and other problems

Exceptions:

V49.6   Upper limb amputation status

V49.7   Lower limb amputation status

V49.81   Postmenopausal status

V49.82   Dental sealant status

V49.83   Awaiting organ transplant status

V51.8   Other aftercare involving the use of plastic surgery

V58.2   Blood transfusion, without reported diagnosis

V58.9   Unspecified aftercare

See Section IV.K. and Section IV.L. of the Outpatient guidelines.

V CODE TABLE

October 1, 2008 (FY2009)

The V code table below contains columns for 1st listed, 1st or additional, additional only, and non-specific. Each code or category is listed on the left hand column and the allowable sequencing of the code or codes within the category is noted under the appropriate column.

As indicated by the footnote in the "1st Dx Only" column, the V codes designated as first-listed only are generally intended to be limited for use as a first-listed only diagnosis, but may be reported as an additional diagnosis in those situations when the patient has more than one encounter on a single day and the codes for the multiple encounters are combined, or when there is more than one V code that meets the definition of principal diagnosis (e.g., a patient is admitted to home healthcare for both aftercare and rehabilitation and they equally meet the definition of principal diagnosis). The V codes designated as first-listed only should not be reported if they do not meet the definition of principal or first-listed diagnosis.

See Section II and Section IV.A for information on selection of principal and first-listed diagnosis.

See Section II.C for information on two or more diagnoses that equally meet the definition for principal diagnosis.

Codes	Description	1st Dx Only[1]	1st or Add'l Dx[2]	Add'l Dx Only[3]	Non-specific Dx[4]
V01.X	Contact with or exposure to communicable diseases		X		
V02.X	Carrier or suspected carrier of infectious diseases		X		
V03.X	Need for prophylactic vaccination and inoculation against bacterial diseases		X		
V04.X	Need for prophylactic vaccination and inoculation against certain diseases		X		
V05.X	Need for prophylactic vaccination and inoculation against single diseases		X		
V06.X	Need for prophylactic vaccination and inoculation against combinations of diseases -		X		
V07.0	Isolation		X		
V07.1	Desensitization to allergens		X		
V07.2	Prophylactic immunotherapy		X		
V07.3X	Other prophylactic chemotherapy		X		
V07.4	Hormone replacement therapy (postmenopausal)			X	

[1] Generally for use as first listed only but may be used as additional if patient has more than one encounter on one day or there is more than one reason for the encounter.

[2] These codes may be used as first listed or additional codes

[3] These codes are only for use as additional codes

[4] These codes are primarily for use in the nonacute setting and should be limited to encounters for which no sign or symptom or reason for visit is documented in the record. Their use may be as either a first listed or additional code.

Codes	Description	1st Dx Only[1]	1st or Add'l Dx[2]	Add'l Dx Only[3]	Non-specific Dx[4]
V07.5X	Prophylactic use of agents affecting estrogen receptors and estrogen levels			X	
V07.8	Other specified prophylactic measure		X		
V07.9	Unspecified prophylactic measure				X
V08	Asymptomatic HIV infection status		X		
V09.X	Infection with drug resistant organisms			X	
V10.X	Personal history of malignant neoplasm		X		
V11.X	Personal history of mental disorder				X
V12.X	Personal history of certain other diseases		X		
V13.0X	Personal history of other disorders of urinary system		X		
V13.1	Personal history of trophoblastic disease		X		
V13.2X	Personal history of other genital system and obstetric disorders		X		
V13.3	Personal history of diseases of skin and subcutaneous tissue		X		
V13.4	Personal history of arthritis				X
V13.5X	Personal history of other musculoskeletal disorders		X		
V13.61	Personal history of hypospadias			X	
V13.69	Personal history of congenital malformations				X
V13.7	Personal history of perinatal problems		X		

[1] Generally for use as first listed only but may be used as additional if patient has more than one encounter on one day or there is more than one reason for the encounter.

[2] These codes may be used as first listed or additional codes

[3] These codes are only for use as additional codes

[4] These codes are primarily for use in the nonacute setting and should be limited to encounters for which no sign or symptom or reason for visit is documented in the record. Their use may be as either a first listed or additional code.

Codes	Description	1st Dx Only[1]	1st or Add'l Dx[2]	Add'l Dx Only[3]	Non-specific Dx[4]
V13.8	Personal history of other specified diseases		X		
V13.9	Personal history of unspecified disease				X
V14.X	Personal history of allergy to medicinal agents			X	
V15.0X	Personal history of allergy, other than to medicinal agents			X	
V15.1	Personal history of surgery to heart and great vessels			X	
V15.2X	Personal history of surgery to other organs			X	
V15.3	Personal history of irradiation			X	
V15.4X	Personal history of psychological trauma			X	
V15.5X	Personal history of injury			X	
V15.6	Personal history of poisoning			X	
V15.7	Personal history of contraception				X
V15.81	Personal history of noncompliance with medical treatment			X	
V15.82	Personal history of tobacco use			X	
V15.84	Personal history of exposure to asbestos			X	
V15.85	Personal history of exposure to potentially hazardous body fluids			X	
V15.86	Personal history of exposure to lead			X	
V15.87	Personal history of extracorporeal membrane oxygenation [ECMO]			X	
V15.88	History of fall		X		

[1] Generally for use as first listed only but may be used as additional if patient has more than one encounter on one day or there is more than one reason for the encounter.

[2] These codes may be used as first listed or additional codes

[3] These codes are only for use as additional codes

[4] These codes are primarily for use in the nonacute setting and should be limited to encounters for which no sign or symptom or reason for visit is documented in the record. Their use may be as either a first listed or additional code.

Codes	Description	1st Dx Only[1]	1st or Add'l Dx[2]	Add'l Dx Only[3]	Non-specific Dx[4]
V15.89	Other specified personal history presenting hazards to health			X	
V16.X	Family history of malignant neoplasm		X		
V17.X	Family history of certain chronic disabling diseases		X		
V18.X	Family history of certain other specific conditions		X		
V19.X	Family history of other conditions		X		
V20.X	Health supervision of infant or child	X			
V21.X	Constitutional states in development			X	
V22.0	Supervision of normal first pregnancy	X			
V22.1	Supervision of other normal pregnancy	X			
V22.2	Pregnancy state, incidental			X	
V23.X	Supervision of high-risk pregnancy		X		
V24.X	Postpartum care and examination	X			
V25.X	Encounter for contraceptive management		X		
V26.0	Tuboplasty or vasoplasty after previous sterilization		X		
V26.1	Artificial insemination		X		
V26.2X	Procreative management investigation and testing		X		
V26.3X	Procreative management, genetic counseling and testing		X		
V26.4X	Procreative management, genetic counseling and advice		X		

[1] Generally for use as first listed only but may be used as additional if patient has more than one encounter on one day or there is more than one reason for the encounter.

[2] These codes may be used as first listed or additional codes

[3] These codes are only for use as additional codes

[4] These codes are primarily for use in the nonacute setting and should be limited to encounters for which no sign or symptom or reason for visit is documented in the record. Their use may be as either a first listed or additional code.

Codes	Description	1st Dx Only[1]	1st or Add'l Dx[2]	Add'l Dx Only[3]	Non-specific Dx[4]
V26.5X	Procreative management, sterilization status			X	
V26.81	Encounter for assisted reproductive fertility procedure cycle	X			
V26.89	Other specified procreative management		X		
V26.9	Unspecified procreative management		X		
V27.X	Outcome of delivery			X	
V28.X	Encounter for antenatal screening of mother		X		
V29.X	Observation and evaluation of newborns for suspected condition not found		X		
V30.X	Single liveborn	X			
V31.X	Twin, mate liveborn	X			
V32.X	Twin, mate stillborn	X			
V33.X	Twin, unspecified	X			
V34.X	Other multiple, mates all liveborn	X			
V35.X	Other multiple, mates all stillborn	X			
V36.X	Other multiple, mates live- and stillborn	X			
V37.X	Other multiple, unspecified	X			
V39.X	Unspecified	X			
V40.X	Mental and behavioral problems				X
V41.X	Problems with special senses and other special functions				X

[1] Generally for use as first listed only but may be used as additional if patient has more than one encounter on one day or there is more than one reason for the encounter.

[2] These codes may be used as first listed or additional codes

[3] These codes are only for use as additional codes

[4] These codes are primarily for use in the nonacute setting and should be limited to encounters for which no sign or symptom or reason for visit is documented in the record. Their use may be as either a first listed or additional code.

Codes	Description	1st Dx Only[1]	1st or Add'l Dx[2]	Add'l Dx Only[3]	Non-specific Dx[4]
V42.X	Organ or tissue replaced by transplant			X	
V43.0	Organ or tissue replaced by other means, eye globe			X	
V43.1	Organ or tissue replaced by other means, lens			X	
V43.21	Organ or tissue replaced by other means, heart assist device			X	
V43.22	Fully implantable artificial heart status		X		
V43.3	Organ or tissue replaced by other means, heart valve			X	
V43.4	Organ or tissue replaced by other means, blood vessel			X	
V43.5	Organ or tissue replaced by other means, bladder			X	
V43.6X	Organ or tissue replaced by other means, joint			X	
V43.7	Organ or tissue replaced by other means, limb			X	
V43.8X	Other organ or tissue replaced by other means			X	
V44.X	Artificial opening status			X	
V45.0X	Cardiac device in situ			X	
V45.1X	Renal dialysis status			X	
V45.2	Presence of cerebrospinal fluid drainage device			X	
V45.3	Intestinal bypass or anastomosis status			X	
V45.4	Arthrodesis status			X	

[1] Generally for use as first listed only but may be used as additional if patient has more than one encounter on one day or there is more than one reason for the encounter.

[2] These codes may be used as first listed or additional codes

[3] These codes are only for use as additional codes

[4] These codes are primarily for use in the nonacute setting and should be limited to encounters for which no sign or symptom or reason for visit is documented in the record. Their use may be as either a first listed or additional code.

Codes	Description	1st Dx Only[1]	1st or Add'l Dx[2]	Add'l Dx Only[3]	Non-specific Dx[4]
V45.5X	Presence of contraceptive device			X	
V45.6X	States following surgery of eye and adnexa			X	
V45.7X	Acquired absence of organ		X		
V45.8X	Other postprocedural status			X	
V46.0	Other dependence on machines, aspirator			X	
V46.11	Dependence on respiratory, status			X	
V46.12	Encounter for respirator dependence during power failure	X			
V46.13	Encounter for weaning from respirator [ventilator]	X			
V46.14	Mechanical complication of respirator [ventilator]		X		
V46.2	Other dependence on machines, supplemental oxygen			X	
V46.3	Wheelchair dependence			X	
V46.8	Other dependence on other enabling machines			X	
V46.9	Unspecified machine dependence				X
V47.X	Other problems with internal organs				X
V48.X	Problems with head, neck and trunk				X
V49.0	Deficiencies of limbs				X
V49.1	Mechanical problems with limbs				X
V49.2	Motor problems with limbs				X
V49.3	Sensory problems with limbs				X
V49.4	Disfigurements of limbs				X

[1] Generally for use as first listed only but may be used as additional if patient has more than one encounter on one day or there is more than one reason for the encounter.

[2] These codes may be used as first listed or additional codes

[3] These codes are only for use as additional codes

[4] These codes are primarily for use in the nonacute setting and should be limited to encounters for which no sign or symptom or reason for visit is documented in the record. Their use may be as either a first listed or additional code.

Codes	Description	1st Dx Only[1]	1st or Add'l Dx[2]	Add'l Dx Only[3]	Non-specific Dx[4]
V49.5	Other problems with limbs				X
V49.6X	Upper limb amputation status		X		
V49.7X	Lower limb amputation status		X		
V49.81	Asymptomatic postmenopausal status (age-related) (natural)		X		
V49.82	Dental sealant status			X	
V49.83	Awaiting organ transplant status			X	
V49.84	Bed confinement status		X		
V49.85	Dual sensory impairment			X	
V49.89	Other specified conditions influencing health status		X		
V49.9	Unspecified condition influencing health status				X
V50.X	Elective surgery for purposes other than remedying health states		X		
V51.0	Encounter for breast reconstruction following mastectomy	X			
V51.8	Other aftercare involving the use of plastic surgery				X
V52.X	Fitting and adjustment of prosthetic device and implant		X		
V53.X	Fitting and adjustment of other device		X		
V54.X	Other orthopedic aftercare		X		
V55.X	Attention to artificial openings		X		
V56.0	Extracorporeal dialysis	X			
V56.1	Encounter for fitting and adjustment of extracorporeal dialysis catheter		X		

[1] Generally for use as first listed only but may be used as additional if patient has more than one encounter on one day or there is more than one reason for the encounter.

[2] These codes may be used as first listed or additional codes

[3] These codes are only for use as additional codes

[4] These codes are primarily for use in the nonacute setting and should be limited to encounters for which no sign or symptom or reason for visit is documented in the record. Their use may be as either a first listed or additional code.

Codes	Description	1st Dx Only[1]	1st or Add'l Dx[2]	Add'l Dx Only[3]	Non-specific Dx[4]
V56.2	Encounter for fitting and adjustment of peritoneal dialysis catheter		X		
V56.3X	Encounter for adequacy testing for dialysis		X		
V56.8	Encounter for other dialysis and dialysis catheter care		X		
V57.X	Care involving use of rehabilitation procedures	X			
V58.0	Radiotherapy	X			
V58.11	Encounter for antineoplastic chemotherapy	X			
V58.12	Encounter for antineoplastic immunotherapy	X			
V58.2	Blood transfusion without reported diagnosis				X
V58.3X	Attention to dressings and sutures		X		
V58.4X	Other aftercare following surgery		X		
V58.5	Encounter for orthodontics				X
V58.6X	Long term (current) drug use			X	
V58.7X	Aftercare following surgery to specified body systems, not elsewhere classified-		X		
V58.8X	Other specified procedures and aftercare		X		
V58.9	Unspecified aftercare				X
V59.X	Donors	X			
V60.X	Housing, household, and economic circumstances			X	
V61.X	Other family circumstances		X		

[1] Generally for use as first listed only but may be used as additional if patient has more than one encounter on one day or there is more than one reason for the encounter.

[2] These codes may be used as first listed or additional codes

[3] These codes are only for use as additional codes

[4] These codes are primarily for use in the nonacute setting and should be limited to encounters for which no sign or symptom or reason for visit is documented in the record. Their use may be as either a first listed or additional code.

Codes	Description	1st Dx Only[1]	1st or Add'l Dx[2]	Add'l Dx Only[3]	Non-specific Dx[4]
V62.X	Other psychosocial circumstances			X	
V63.X	Unavailability of other medical facilities for care		X		
V64.X	Persons encountering health services for specified procedure, not carried out			X	
V65.X	Other persons seeking consultation without complaint or sickness		X		
V66.0	Convalescence and palliative care following surgery	X			
V66.1	Convalescence and palliative care following radiotherapy	X			
V66.2	Convalescence and palliative care following chemotherapy	X			
V66.3	Convalescence and palliative care following psychotherapy and other treatment for mental disorder	X			
V66.4	Convalescence and palliative care following treatment of fracture	X			
V66.5	Convalescence and palliative care following other treatment	X			
V66.6	Convalescence and palliative care following combined treatment	X			
V66.7	Encounter for palliative care			X	
V66.9	Unspecified convalescence	X			
V67.X	Follow-up examination		X		
V68.X	Encounters for administrative purposes	X			
V69.X	Problems related to lifestyle		X		

[1] Generally for use as first listed only but may be used as additional if patient has more than one encounter on one day or there is more than one reason for the encounter.

[2] These codes may be used as first listed or additional codes

[3] These codes are only for use as additional codes

[4] These codes are primarily for use in the nonacute setting and should be limited to encounters for which no sign or symptom or reason for visit is documented in the record. Their use may be as either a first listed or additional code.

Codes	Description	1st Dx Only[1]	1st or Add'l Dx[2]	Add'l Dx Only[3]	Non-specific Dx[4]
V70.0	Routine general medical examination at a health care facility	X			
V70.1	General psychiatric examination, requested by the authority	X			
V70.2	General psychiatric examination, other and unspecified	X			
V70.3	Other medical examination for administrative purposes	X			
V70.4	Examination for medicolegal reasons	X			
V70.5	Health examination of defined subpopulations	X			
V70.6	Health examination in population surveys	X			
V70.7	Examination of participant in clinical trial		X		
V70.8	Other specified general medical examinations	X			
V70.9	Unspecified general medical examination	X			
V71.X	Observation and evaluation for suspected conditions not found	X			
V72.0	Examination of eyes and vision		X		
V72.1X	Examination of ears and hearing		X		
V72.2	Dental examination		X		
V72.3X	Gynecological examination		X		
V72.4X	Pregnancy examination or test		X		
V72.5	Radiological examination, NEC		X		
V72.6	Laboratory examination		X		

[1] Generally for use as first listed only but may be used as additional if patient has more than one encounter on one day or there is more than one reason for the encounter.

[2] These codes may be used as first listed or additional codes

[3] These codes are only for use as additional codes

[4] These codes are primarily for use in the nonacute setting and should be limited to encounters for which no sign or symptom or reason for visit is documented in the record. Their use may be as either a first listed or additional code.

Codes	Description	1st Dx Only[1]	1st or Add'l Dx[2]	Add'l Dx Only[3]	Non-specific Dx[4]
V72.7	Diagnostic skin and sensitization tests		X		
V72.81	Preoperative cardiovascular examination		X		
V72.82	Preoperative respiratory examination		X		
V72.83	Other specified preoperative examination		X		
V72.84	Preoperative examination, unspecified		X		
V72.85	Other specified examination		X		
V72.86	Encounter for blood typing		X		
V72.9	Unspecified examination				X
V73.X	Special screening examination for viral and chlamydial diseases		X		
V74.X	Special screening examination for bacterial and spirochetal diseases		X		
V75.X	Special screening examination for other infectious diseases		X		
V76.X	Special screening examination for malignant neoplasms		X		
V77.X	Special screening examination for endocrine, nutritional, metabolic and immunity disorders		X		
V78.X	Special screening examination for disorders of blood and blood-forming organs		X		
V79.X	Special screening examination for mental disorders and developmental handicaps		X		
V80.X	Special screening examination for neurological, eye, and ear diseases		X		

[1] Generally for use as first listed only but may be used as additional if patient has more than one encounter on one day or there is more than one reason for the encounter.

[2] These codes may be used as first listed or additional codes

[3] These codes are only for use as additional codes

[4] These codes are primarily for use in the nonacute setting and should be limited to encounters for which no sign or symptom or reason for visit is documented in the record. Their use may be as either a first listed or additional code.

Codes	Description	1st Dx Only[1]	1st or Add'l Dx[2]	Add'l Dx Only[3]	Non-specific Dx[4]
V81.X	Special screening examination for cardiovascular, respiratory, and genitourinary diseases		X		
V82.X	Special screening examination for other conditions		X		
V83.X	Genetic carrier status		X		
V84.X	Genetic susceptibility to disease			X	
V85	Body mass index			X	
V86	Estrogen receptor status			X	
V87.0X	Contact with and (suspected) exposure to hazardous metals		X		
V87.1X	Contact with and (suspected) exposure to hazardous aromatic compounds		X		
V87.2	Contact with and (suspected) exposure to other potentially hazardous chemicals		X		
V87.3X	Contact with and (suspected) exposure to other potentially hazardous substances		X		
V87.4X	Personal history of drug therapy			X	
V88.0X	Acquired absence of cervix and uterus			X	
V89.0X	Suspected maternal and fetal anomalies not found		X		

[1] Generally for use as first listed only but may be used as additional if patient has more than one encounter on one day or there is more than one reason for the encounter.

[2] These codes may be used as first listed or additional codes

[3] These codes are only for use as additional codes

[4] These codes are primarily for use in the nonacute setting and should be limited to encounters for which no sign or symptom or reason for visit is documented in the record. Their use may be as either a first listed or additional code.

19. Supplemental Classification of External Causes of Injury and Poisoning (E-codes, E800-E999)

Introduction: These guidelines are provided for those who are currently collecting E codes in order that there will be standardization in the process. If your institution plans to begin collecting E codes, these guidelines are to be applied. The use of E codes is supplemental to the application of ICD-9-CM diagnosis codes. E codes are never to be recorded as principal diagnoses (first-listed in non-inpatient setting) and are not required for reporting to CMS.

External causes of injury and poisoning codes (E codes) are intended to provide data for injury research and evaluation of injury prevention strategies. E codes capture how the injury or poisoning happened (cause), the intent (unintentional or accidental; or intentional, such as suicide or assault), and the place where the event occurred.

Some major categories of E codes include:

transport accidents
poisoning and adverse effects of drugs, medicinal substances and biologicals
accidental falls
accidents caused by fire and flames
accidents due to natural and environmental factors
late effects of accidents, assaults or self injury
assaults or purposely inflicted injury
suicide or self inflicted injury

These guidelines apply for the coding and collection of E codes from records in hospitals, outpatient clinics, emergency departments, other ambulatory care settings and provider offices, and nonacute care settings, except when other specific guidelines apply.

a. General E Code Coding Guidelines

1) Used with any code in the range of 001-V84.8

An E code may be used with any code in the range of 001-V84.8, which indicates an injury, poisoning, or adverse effect due to an external cause.

2) Assign the appropriate E code for all initial treatments

Assign the appropriate E code for the initial encounter of an injury, poisoning, or adverse effect of drugs, not for subsequent treatment.

External cause of injury codes (E-codes) may be assigned while the acute fracture codes are still applicable.

See Section I.C.17.b.1 for coding of acute fractures.

3) Use the full range of E codes

Use the full range of E codes to completely describe the cause, the intent and the place of occurrence, if applicable, for all injuries, poisonings, and adverse effects of drugs.

4) Assign as many E codes as necessary

Assign as many E codes as necessary to fully explain each cause. If only one E code can be recorded, assign the E code most related to the principal diagnosis.

5) The selection of the appropriate E code

The selection of the appropriate E code is guided by the Index to External Causes, which is located after the alphabetical index to diseases and by Inclusion and Exclusion notes in the Tabular List.

6) E code can never be a principal diagnosis

An E code can never be a principal (first listed) diagnosis.

7) External cause code(s) with systemic inflammatory response syndrome (SIRS)

An external cause code is not appropriate with a code from subcategory 995.9, unless the patient also has an injury, poisoning, or adverse effect of drugs.

b. Place of Occurrence Guideline

Use an additional code from category E849 to indicate the Place of Occurrence for injuries and poisonings. The Place of Occurrence describes the place where the event occurred and not the patient's activity at the time of the event.

Do not use E849.9 if the place of occurrence is not stated.

c. Adverse Effects of Drugs, Medicinal and Biological Substances Guidelines

1) Do not code directly from the Table of Drugs

Do not code directly from the Table of Drugs and Chemicals. Always refer back to the Tabular List.

2) Use as many codes as necessary to describe

Use as many codes as necessary to describe completely all drugs, medicinal or biological substances.

3) If the same E code would describe the causative agent

If the same E code would describe the causative agent for more than one adverse reaction, assign the code only once.

4) If two or more drugs, medicinal or biological substances

If two or more drugs, medicinal or biological substances are reported, code each individually unless the combination code is listed in the Table of Drugs and Chemicals. In that case, assign the E code for the combination.

5) **When a reaction results from the interaction of a drug(s)**

When a reaction results from the interaction of a drug(s) and alcohol, use poisoning codes and E codes for both.

6) **If the reporting format limits the number of E codes**

If the reporting format limits the number of E codes that can be used in reporting clinical data, code the one most related to the principal diagnosis. Include at least one from each category (cause, intent, place) if possible.

If there are different fourth digit codes in the same three digit category, use the code for "Other specified" of that category. If there is no "Other specified" code in that category, use the appropriate "Unspecified" code in that category.

If the codes are in different three digit categories, assign the appropriate E code for other multiple drugs and medicinal substances.

7) **Codes from the E930-E949 series**

Codes from the E930-E949 series must be used to identify the causative substance for an adverse effect of drug, medicinal and biological substances, correctly prescribed and properly administered. The effect, such as tachycardia, delirium, gastrointestinal hemorrhaging, vomiting, hypokalemia, hepatitis, renal failure, or respiratory failure, is coded and followed by the appropriate code from the E930-E949 series.

d. **Multiple Cause E Code Coding Guidelines**

If two or more events cause separate injuries, an E code should be assigned for each cause. The first listed E code will be selected in the following order:

E codes for child and adult abuse take priority over all other E codes. See Section I.C.19.e., Child and Adult abuse guidelines.

E codes for terrorism events take priority over all other E codes except child and adult abuse

E codes for cataclysmic events take priority over all other E codes except child and adult abuse and terrorism.

E codes for transport accidents take priority over all other E codes except cataclysmic events and child and adult abuse and terrorism.

The first-listed E code should correspond to the cause of the most serious diagnosis due to an assault, accident, or self-harm, following the order of hierarchy listed above.

e. Child and Adult Abuse Guideline

1) Intentional injury

When the cause of an injury or neglect is intentional child or adult abuse, the first listed E code should be assigned from categories E960-E968, Homicide and injury purposely inflicted by other persons, (except category E967). An E code from category E967, Child and adult battering and other maltreatment, should be added as an additional code to identify the perpetrator, if known.

2) Accidental intent

In cases of neglect when the intent is determined to be accidental E code E904.0, Abandonment or neglect of infant and helpless person, should be the first listed E code.

f. Unknown or Suspected Intent Guideline

1) If the intent (accident, self-harm, assault) of the cause of an injury or poisoning is unknown

If the intent (accident, self-harm, assault) of the cause of an injury or poisoning is unknown or unspecified, code the intent as undetermined E980-E989.

2) If the intent (accident, self-harm, assault) of the cause of an injury or poisoning is questionable

If the intent (accident, self-harm, assault) of the cause of an injury or poisoning is questionable, probable or suspected, code the intent as undetermined E980-E989.

g. Undetermined Cause

When the intent of an injury or poisoning is known, but the cause is unknown, use codes: E928.9, Unspecified accident, E958.9, Suicide and self-inflicted injury by unspecified means, and E968.9, Assault by unspecified means.

These E codes should rarely be used, as the documentation in the medical record, in both the inpatient outpatient and other settings, should normally provide sufficient detail to determine the cause of the injury.

h. Late Effects of External Cause Guidelines

1) Late effect E codes

Late effect E codes exist for injuries and poisonings but not for adverse effects of drugs, misadventures and surgical complications.

2) Late effect E codes (E929, E959, E969, E977, E989, or E999.1)

A late effect E code (E929, E959, E969, E977, E989, or E999.1) should be used with any report of a late effect or sequela resulting from a previous injury or poisoning (905-909).

3) Late effect E code with a related current injury

A late effect E code should never be used with a related current nature of injury code.

4) Use of late effect E codes for subsequent visits

Use a late effect E code for subsequent visits when a late effect of the initial injury or poisoning is being treated. There is no late effect E code for adverse effects of drugs.

Do not use a late effect E code for subsequent visits for followup care (e.g., to assess healing, to receive rehabilitative therapy) of the injury or poisoning when no late effect of the injury has been documented.

i. Misadventures and Complications of Care Guidelines

1) Code range E870-E876

Assign a code in the range of E870-E876 if misadventures are stated by the provider.

2) Code range E878-E879

Assign a code in the range of E878-E879 if the provider attributes an abnormal reaction or later complication to a surgical or medical procedure, but does not mention misadventure at the time of the procedure as the cause of the reaction.

j. Terrorism Guidelines

1) Cause of injury identified by the Federal Government (FBI) as terrorism

When the cause of an injury is identified by the Federal Government (FBI) as terrorism, the first-listed E-code should be a code from category E979, Terrorism. The definition of terrorism employed by the FBI is found at the inclusion note at E979. The terrorism E-code is the only E-code that should be assigned. Additional E codes from the assault categories should not be assigned.

2) Cause of an injury is suspected to be the result of terrorism

When the cause of an injury is suspected to be the result of terrorism a code from category E979 should not be assigned. Assign a code in the range of E codes based circumstances on the documentation of intent and mechanism.

3) Code E979.9, Terrorism, secondary effects

Assign code E979.9, Terrorism, secondary effects, for conditions occurring subsequent to the terrorist event. This code should not be assigned for conditions that are due to the initial terrorist act.

4) Statistical tabulation of terrorism codes

For statistical purposes these codes will be tabulated within the category for assault, expanding the current category from E960-E969 to include E979 and E999.1.

SECTION II. SELECTION OF PRINCIPAL DIAGNOSIS

The circumstances of inpatient admission always govern the selection of principal diagnosis. The principal diagnosis is defined in the Uniform Hospital Discharge Data Set (UHDDS) as "that condition established after study to be chiefly responsible for occasioning the admission of the patient to the hospital for care."

The UHDDS definitions are used by hospitals to report inpatient data elements in a standardized manner. These data elements and their definitions can be found in the July 31, 1985, Federal Register (Vol. 50, No, 147), pp. 31038-40. Since that time the application of the UHDDS definitions has been expanded to include all nonoutpatient settings (acute care, short term, long term care and psychiatric hospitals; home health agencies; rehab facilities; nursing homes, etc). In determining principal diagnosis the coding conventions in the ICD-9-CM, Volumes I and II take precedence over these official coding guidelines.

(See Section I.A., Conventions for the ICD-9-CM)

The importance of consistent, complete documentation in the medical record cannot be overemphasized. Without such documentation the application of all coding guidelines is a difficult, if not impossible, task.

A. Codes for symptoms, signs, and ill-defined conditions

Codes for symptoms, signs, and ill-defined conditions from Chapter 16 are not to be used as principal diagnosis when a related definitive diagnosis has been established.

B. Two or more interrelated conditions, each potentially meeting the definition for principal diagnosis.

When there are two or more interrelated conditions (such as diseases in the same ICD-9-CM chapter or manifestations characteristically associated with a certain disease) potentially meeting the definition of principal diagnosis, either condition may be sequenced first, unless the circumstances of the admission, the therapy provided, the Tabular List, or the Alphabetic Index indicate otherwise.

C. Two or more diagnoses that equally meet the definition for principal diagnosis

In the unusual instance when two or more diagnoses equally meet the criteria for principal diagnosis as determined by the circumstances of admission, diagnostic workup and/or therapy provided, and the Alphabetic Index, Tabular List, or another coding guidelines does not provide sequencing direction, any one of the diagnoses may be sequenced first.

D. Two or more comparative or contrasting conditions.

In those rare instances when two or more contrasting or comparative diagnoses are documented as "either/or" (or similar terminology), they are coded as if the diagnoses were confirmed and the diagnoses are sequenced according to the circumstances of the admission. If no further determination can be made as to which diagnosis should be principal, either diagnosis may be sequenced first.

E. A symptom(s) followed by contrasting/comparative diagnoses

When a symptom(s) is followed by contrasting/comparative diagnoses, the symptom code is sequenced first. All the contrasting/comparative diagnoses should be coded as additional diagnoses.

F. Original treatment plan not carried out

Sequence as the principal diagnosis the condition, which after study occasioned the admission to the hospital, even though treatment may not have been carried out due to unforeseen circumstances.

G. Complications of surgery and other medical care

When the admission is for treatment of a complication resulting from surgery or other medical care, the complication code is sequenced as the principal diagnosis. If the complication is classified to the 996-999 series and the code lacks the necessary specificity in describing the complication, an additional code for the specific complication should be assigned.

H. Uncertain Diagnosis

If the diagnosis documented at the time of discharge is qualified as "probable", "suspected", "likely", "questionable", "possible", or "still to be ruled out", or other similar terms indicating uncertainty, code the condition as if it existed or was established. The bases for these guidelines are the diagnostic workup, arrangements for further workup or observation, and initial therapeutic approach that correspond most closely with the established diagnosis.

Note: This guideline is applicable only to inpatient admissions to short-term, acute, long-term care and psychiatric hospitals.

I. Admission from Observation Unit

1. Admission Following Medical Observation

When a patient is admitted to an observation unit for a medical condition, which either worsens or does not improve, and is subsequently admitted as an inpatient of the same hospital for this same medical condition, the principal diagnosis would be the medical condition which led to the hospital admission.

2. Admission Following Post-Operative Observation

When a patient is admitted to an observation unit to monitor a condition (or complication) that develops following outpatient surgery, and then is subsequently admitted as an inpatient of the same hospital, hospitals should apply the Uniform Hospital Discharge Data Set (UHDDS) definition of principal diagnosis as "that condition established after study to be chiefly responsible for occasioning the admission of the patient to the hospital for care."

J. Admission from Outpatient Surgery

When a patient receives surgery in the hospital's outpatient surgery department and is subsequently admitted for continuing inpatient care at the same hospital, the following guidelines should be followed in selecting the principal diagnosis for the inpatient admission:

■ If the reason for the inpatient admission is a complication, assign the complication as the principal diagnosis.

■ If no complication, or other condition, is documented as the reason for the inpatient admission, assign the reason for the outpatient surgery as the principal diagnosis.

■ If the reason for the inpatient admission is another condition unrelated to the surgery, assign the unrelated condition as the principal diagnosis.

SECTION III. REPORTING ADDITIONAL DIAGNOSES

General Rules For Other (Additional) Diagnoses

For reporting purposes the definition for "other diagnoses" is interpreted as additional conditions that affect patient care in terms of requiring:

clinical evaluation; or
therapeutic treatment; or
diagnostic procedures; or
extended length of hospital stay; or
increased nursing care and/or monitoring.

The UHDDS item #11-b defines Other Diagnoses as "all conditions that coexist at the time of admission, that develop subsequently, or that affect the treatment received and/or the length of stay. Diagnoses that relate to an earlier episode which have no bearing on the current hospital stay are to be excluded." UHDDS definitions apply to inpatients in acute care, short-term, long term care and psychiatric hospital setting. The UHDDS definitions are used by acute care short term hospitals to report inpatient data elements in a standardized manner. These data elements and their definitions can be found in the July 31, 1985, Federal Register (Vol. 50, No, 147), pp. 31038-40.

Since that time the application of the UHDDS definitions has been expanded to include all nonoutpatient settings (acute care, short term, long term care and psychiatric hospitals; home health agencies; rehab facilities; nursing homes, etc).

The following guidelines are to be applied in designating "other diagnoses" when neither the Alphabetic Index nor the Tabular List in ICD-9-CM provide direction. The listing of the diagnoses in the patient record is the responsibility of the attending provider.

A. Previous conditions

If the provider has included a diagnosis in the final diagnostic statement, such as the discharge summary or the face sheet, it should ordinarily be coded. Some providers include in the diagnostic statement resolved conditions or diagnoses and status-post procedures from previous admission that have no bearing on the current stay. Such conditions are not to be reported and are coded only if required by hospital policy.

However, history codes (V10-V19) may be used as secondary codes if the historical condition or family history has an impact on current care or influences treatment.

B. Abnormal findings

Abnormal findings (laboratory, x-ray, pathologic, and other diagnostic results) are not coded and reported unless the provider indicates their clinical significance. If the findings are outside the normal range and the attending provider has ordered other tests to evaluate the condition or prescribed treatment, it is appropriate to ask the provider whether the abnormal finding should be added.

Please note: This differs from the coding practices in the outpatient setting for coding encounters for diagnostic tests that have been interpreted by a provider.

C. Uncertain Diagnosis

If the diagnosis documented at the time of discharge is qualified as "probable", "suspected", "likely", "questionable", "possible", or "still to be ruled out" or other similar terms indicating uncertainty, code the condition as if it existed or was established. The bases for these guidelines are the diagnostic workup, arrangements for further workup or observation, and initial therapeutic approach that correspond most closely with the established diagnosis.

Note: This guideline is applicable only to inpatient admissions to short-term, acute, long-term care and psychiatric hospitals.

SECTION IV. DIAGNOSTIC CODING AND REPORTING GUIDELINES FOR OUTPATIENT SERVICES

These coding guidelines for outpatient diagnoses have been approved for use by hospitals/providers in coding and reporting hospital-based outpatient services and provider-based office visits.

Information about the use of certain abbreviations, punctuation, symbols, and other conventions used in the ICD-9-CM Tabular List (code numbers and titles), can be found in Section IA of these guidelines, under "Conventions Used in the Tabular List." Information about the correct sequence to use in finding a code is also described in Section I.

The terms encounter and visit are often used interchangeably in describing outpatient service contacts and, therefore, appear together in these guidelines without distinguishing one from the other.

Though the conventions and general guidelines apply to all settings, coding guidelines for outpatient and provider reporting of diagnoses will vary in a number of instances from those for inpatient diagnoses, recognizing that:

The Uniform Hospital Discharge Data Set (UHDDS) definition of principal diagnosis applies only to inpatients in acute, short-term, long-term care and psychiatric hospitals.

Coding guidelines for inconclusive diagnoses (probable, suspected, rule out, etc.) were developed for inpatient reporting and do not apply to outpatients.

A. Selection of first-listed condition

In the outpatient setting, the term first-listed diagnosis is used in lieu of principal diagnosis.

In determining the first-listed diagnosis the coding conventions of ICD-9-CM, as well as the general and disease specific guidelines take precedence over the outpatient guidelines.

Diagnoses often are not established at the time of the initial encounter/visit. It may take two or more visits before the diagnosis is confirmed.

The most critical rule involves beginning the search for the correct code assignment through the Alphabetic Index. Never begin searching initially in the Tabular List as this will lead to coding errors.

1. Outpatient Surgery

When a patient presents for outpatient surgery, code the reason for the surgery as the first-listed diagnosis (reason for the encounter), even if the surgery is not performed due to a contraindication.

2. Observation Stay

When a patient is admitted for observation for a medical condition, assign a code for the medical condition as the first-listed diagnosis.

When a patient presents for outpatient surgery and develops complications requiring admission to observation, code the reason for the surgery as the first reported diagnosis (reason for the encounter), followed by codes for the complications as secondary diagnoses.

B. Codes from 001.0 through V89

The appropriate code or codes from 001.0 through V89 must be used to identify diagnoses, symptoms, conditions, problems, complaints, or other reason(s) for the encounter/visit.

C. Accurate reporting of ICD-9-CM diagnosis codes

For accurate reporting of ICD-9-CM diagnosis codes, the documentation should describe the patient's condition, using terminology which includes specific diagnoses as well as symptoms, problems, or reasons for the encounter. There are ICD-9-CM codes to describe all of these.

D. Selection of codes 001.0 through 999.9

The selection of codes 001.0 through 999.9 will frequently be used to describe the reason for the encounter. These codes are from the section of ICD-9-CM for the classification of diseases and injuries (e.g. infectious and parasitic diseases; neoplasms; symptoms, signs, and ill-defined conditions, etc.).

E. Codes that describe symptoms and signs

Codes that describe symptoms and signs, as opposed to diagnoses, are acceptable for reporting purposes when a diagnosis has not been established (confirmed) by the provider. Chapter 16 of ICD-9-CM, Symptoms, Signs, and Ill-defined conditions (codes 780.0 - 799.9) contain many, but not all codes for symptoms.

F. Encounters for circumstances other than a disease or injury

ICD-9-CM provides codes to deal with encounters for circumstances other than a disease or injury. The Supplementary Classification of factors Influencing Health Status and Contact with Health Services (V01.0- V89) is provided to deal with occasions when circumstances other than a disease or injury are recorded as diagnosis or problems. See Section I.C. 18 for information on V-codes

G. Level of Detail in Coding

1. ICD-9-CM codes with 3, 4, or 5 digits

ICD-9-CM is composed of codes with either 3, 4, or 5 digits. Codes with three digits are included in ICD-9-CM as the heading of a category of codes that may be further subdivided by the use of fourth and/or fifth digits, which provide greater specificity.

2. Use of full number of digits required for a code

A three-digit code is to be used only if it is not further subdivided. Where fourth-digit subcategories and/or fifth-digit subclassifications are provided, they must be assigned. A code is invalid if it has not been coded to the full number of digits required for that code.

See also discussion under Section I.b.3., General Coding Guidelines, Level of Detail in Coding.

H. ICD-9-CM code for the diagnosis, condition, problem, or other reason for encounter/visit

List first the ICD-9-CM code for the diagnosis, condition, problem, or other reason for encounter/visit shown in the medical record to be chiefly responsible for the services provided. List additional codes that describe any coexisting conditions. In some cases the first-listed diagnosis may be a symptom when a diagnosis has not been established (confirmed) by the physician.

I. Uncertain diagnosis

Do not code diagnoses documented as "probable", "suspected," "questionable," "rule out," or "working diagnosis" or other similar terms indicating uncertainty. Rather, code the condition(s) to the highest degree of certainty for that encounter/visit, such as symptoms, signs, abnormal test results, or other reason for the visit.

Please note: This differs from the coding practices used by short-term, acute care, long-term care and psychiatric hospitals.

J. Chronic diseases

Chronic diseases treated on an ongoing basis may be coded and reported as many times as the patient receives treatment and care for the condition(s)

K. Code all documented conditions that coexist

Code all documented conditions that coexist at the time of the encounter/visit, and require or affect patient care treatment or management. Do not code conditions that were previously treated and no longer exist. However, history codes (V10-V19) may be used as secondary codes if the historical condition or family history has an impact on current care or influences treatment.

L. Patients receiving diagnostic services only

For patients receiving diagnostic services only during an encounter/visit, sequence first the diagnosis, condition, problem, or other reason for encounter/visit shown in the medical record to be chiefly responsible for the outpatient services provided during the encounter/visit. Codes for other diagnoses (e.g., chronic conditions) may be sequenced as additional diagnoses.

For encounters for routine laboratory/radiology testing in the absence of any signs, symptoms, or associated diagnosis, assign V72.5 and V72.6. If routine testing is performed during the same encounter as a test to evaluate a sign, symptom, or diagnosis, it is appropriate to assign both the V code and the code describing the reason for the non-routine test.

For outpatient encounters for diagnostic tests that have been interpreted by a physician, and the final report is available at the time of coding, code any confirmed or definitive diagnosis(es) documented in the interpretation. Do not code related signs and symptoms as additional diagnoses.

Please note: This differs from the coding practice in the hospital inpatient setting regarding abnormal findings on test results.

M. Patients receiving therapeutic services only

For patients receiving therapeutic services only during an encounter/visit, sequence first the diagnosis, condition, problem, or other reason for encounter/visit shown in the medical record to be chiefly responsible for the outpatient services provided during the encounter/visit. Codes for other diagnoses (e.g., chronic conditions) may be sequenced as additional diagnoses.

The only exception to this rule is that when the primary reason for the admission/encounter is chemotherapy, radiation therapy, or rehabilitation, the appropriate V code for the service is listed first, and the diagnosis or problem for which the service is being performed listed second.

N. Patients receiving preoperative evaluations only

For patients receiving preoperative evaluations only, sequence first a code from category V72.8, Other specified examinations, to describe the pre-op consultations. Assign a code for the condition to describe the reason for the surgery as an additional diagnosis. Code also any findings related to the pre-op evaluation.

O. Ambulatory surgery

For ambulatory surgery, code the diagnosis for which the surgery was performed. If the postoperative diagnosis is known to be different from the preoperative diagnosis at the time the diagnosis is confirmed, select the postoperative diagnosis for coding, since it is the most definitive.

P. Routine outpatient prenatal visits

For routine outpatient prenatal visits when no complications are present, codes V22.0, Supervision of normal first pregnancy, or V22.1, Supervision of other normal pregnancy, should be used as the principal diagnosis. These codes should not be used in conjunction with chapter 11 codes.

APPENDIX I

Present On Admission (POA) Reporting Guidelines

Introduction

These guidelines are to be used as a supplement to the ICD-9-CM Official Guidelines for Coding and Reporting to facilitate the assignment of the Present on Admission (POA) indicator for each diagnosis and external cause of injury code reported on claim forms (UB-04 and 837Institutional).

These guidelines are not intended to replace any guidelines in the main body of the ICD-9-CM Official Guidelines for Coding and Reporting. The POA guidelines are not intended to provide guidance on when a condition should be coded, but rather, how to apply the POA indicator to the final set of diagnosis codes that have been assigned in accordance with Sections I, II, and III of the official coding guidelines. Subsequent to the assignment of the ICD-9-CM codes, the POA indicator should then be assigned to those conditions that have been coded.

As stated in the Introduction to the ICD-9-CM Official Guidelines for Coding and Reporting, a joint effort between the healthcare provider and the coder is essential to achieve complete and accurate documentation, code assignment, and reporting of diagnoses and procedures. The importance of consistent, complete documentation in the medical record cannot be overemphasized. Medical record documentation from any provider involved in the care and treatment of the patient may be used to support the determination of whether a condition was present on admission or not. In the context of the official coding guidelines, the term "provider" means a physician or any qualified healthcare practitioner who is legally accountable for establishing the patient's diagnosis.

These guidelines are not a substitute for the provider's clinical judgment as to the determination of whether a condition was/was not present on admission. The provider should be queried regarding issues related to the linking of signs/symptoms, timing of test results, and the timing of findings.

General Reporting Requirements

All claims involving inpatient admissions to general acute care hospitals or other facilities that are subject to a law or regulation mandating collection of present on admission information.

Present on admission is defined as present at the time the order for inpatient admission occurs -- conditions that develop during an outpatient encounter, including emergency department, observation, or outpatient surgery, are considered as present on admission.

POA indicator is assigned to principal and secondary diagnoses (as defined in Section II of the Official Guidelines for Coding and Reporting) and the external cause of injury codes.

Issues related to inconsistent, missing, conflicting or unclear documentation must still be resolved by the provider.

If a condition would not be coded and reported based on UHDDS definitions and current official coding guidelines, then the POA indicator would not be reported.

Reporting Options

Y - Yes
N - No
U - Unknown
W - Clinically undetermined
Unreported/Not used (or "1" for Medicare usage) - (Exempt from POA reporting)

For more specific instructions on Medicare POA indicator reporting options, refer to http://www.cms.hhs.gov/HospitalAcqCond/02_Statute_Regulations_Program_Instru ctions.asp#TopOfPage

Reporting Definitions

Y = present at the time of inpatient admission

N = not present at the time of inpatient admission

U = documentation is insufficient to determine if condition is present on admission

W = provider is unable to clinically determine whether condition was present on admission or not

Timeframe for POA Identification and Documentation

There is no required timeframe as to when a provider (per the definition of "provider" used in these guidelines) must identify or document a condition to be present on admission. In some clinical situations, it may not be possible for a provider to make a definitive diagnosis (or a condition may not be recognized or reported by the patient) for a period of time after admission. In some cases it may be several days before the provider arrives at a definitive diagnosis. This does not mean that the condition was not present on admission. Determination of whether the condition was present on admission or not will be based on the applicable POA guideline as identified in this document, or on the provider's best clinical judgment.

If at the time of code assignment the documentation is unclear as to whether a condition was present on admission or not, it is appropriate to query the provider for clarification.

Assigning The POA Indicator

Condition is on the "Exempt from Reporting" list

Leave the "present on admission" field blank if the condition is on the list of ICD-9-CM codes for which this field is not applicable. This is the only circumstance in which the field may be left blank.

POA Explicitly Documented

Assign Y for any condition the provider explicitly documents as being present on admission.

Assign N for any condition the provider explicitly documents as not present at the time of admission.

Conditions diagnosed prior to inpatient admission

Assign "Y" for conditions that were diagnosed prior to admission (example: hypertension, diabetes mellitus, asthma)

Conditions diagnosed during the admission but clearly present before admission

Assign "Y" for conditions diagnosed during the admission that were clearly present but not diagnosed until after admission occurred.

Diagnoses subsequently confirmed after admission are considered present on admission if at the time of admission they are documented as suspected, possible, rule out, differential diagnosis, or constitute an underlying cause of a symptom that is present at the time of admission.

Condition develops during outpatient encounter prior to inpatient admission

Assign Y for any condition that develops during an outpatient encounter prior to a written order for inpatient admission.

Documentation does not indicate whether condition was present on admission

Assign "U" when the medical record documentation is unclear as to whether the condition was present on admission. "U" should not be routinely assigned and used only in very limited circumstances. Coders are encouraged to query the providers when the documentation is unclear.

Documentation states that it cannot be determined whether the condition was or was not present on admission

Assign "W" when the medical record documentation indicates that it cannot be clinically determined whether or not the condition was present on admission.

Chronic condition with acute exacerbation during the admission

If the code is a combination code that identifies both the chronic condition and the acute exacerbation, see POA guidelines pertaining to combination codes.

If the combination code only identifies the chronic condition and not the acute exacerbation (e.g., acute exacerbation of CHF), assign "Y."

Conditions documented as possible, probable, suspected, or rule out at the time of discharge

If the final diagnosis contains a possible, probable, suspected, or rule out diagnosis, and this diagnosis was suspected at the time of inpatient admission, assign "Y."

If the final diagnosis contains a possible, probable, suspected, or rule out diagnosis, and this diagnosis was based on symptoms or clinical findings that were not present on admission, assign "N".

Conditions documented as impending or threatened at the time of discharge

If the final diagnosis contains an impending or threatened diagnosis, and this diagnosis is based on symptoms or clinical findings that were present on admission, assign "Y".

If the final diagnosis contains an impending or threatened diagnosis, and this diagnosis is based on symptoms or clinical findings that were not present on admission, assign "N".

Acute and Chronic Conditions

Assign "Y" for acute conditions that are present at time of admission and N for acute conditions that are not present at time of admission.

Assign "Y" for chronic conditions, even though the condition may not be diagnosed until after admission.

If a single code identifies both an acute and chronic condition, see the POA guidelines for combination codes.

Combination Codes

Assign "N" if any part of the combination code was not present on admission (e.g., obstructive chronic bronchitis with acute exacerbation and the exacerbation was not present on admission; gastric ulcer that does not start bleeding until after admission; asthma patient develops status asthmaticus after admission)

Assign "Y" if all parts of the combination code were present on admission (e.g., patient with diabetic nephropathy is admitted with uncontrolled diabetes)

If the final diagnosis includes comparative or contrasting diagnoses, and both were present, or suspected, at the time of admission, assign "Y".

For infection codes that include the causal organism, assign "Y" if the infection (or signs of the infection) was present on admission, even though the culture results may not be known until after admission (e.g., patient is admitted with pneumonia and the provider documents pseudomonas as the causal organism a few days later).

Same Diagnosis Code for Two or More Conditions

When the same ICD-9-CM diagnosis code applies to two or more conditions during the same encounter (e.g. bilateral condition, or two separate conditions classified to the same ICD-9-CM diagnosis code):

Assign "Y" if all conditions represented by the single ICD-9-CM code were present on admission (e.g. bilateral fracture of the same bone, same site, and both fractures were present on admission)

Assign "N" if any of the conditions represented by the single ICD-9-CM code was not present on admission (e.g. dehydration with hyponatremia is assigned to code 276.1, but only one of these conditions was present on admission).

Obstetrical conditions

Whether or not the patient delivers during the current hospitalization does not affect assignment of the POA indicator. The determining factor for POA assignment is whether the pregnancy complication or obstetrical condition described by the code was present at the time of admission or not.

If the pregnancy complication or obstetrical condition was present on admission (e.g., patient admitted in preterm labor), assign "Y".

If the pregnancy complication or obstetrical condition was not present on admission (e.g., 2nd degree laceration during delivery, postpartum hemorrhage that occurred during current hospitalization, fetal distress develops after admission), assign "N".

If the obstetrical code includes more than one diagnosis and any of the diagnoses identified by the code were not present on admission assign "N". (e.g., Code 642.7, Pre-eclampsia or eclampsia superimposed on pre- existing hypertension).

If the obstetrical code includes information that is not a diagnosis, do not consider that information in the POA determination. (e.g. Code 652.1x, Breech or other malpresentation successfully converted to cephalic presentation should be reported as present on admission if the fetus was breech on admission but was converted to cephalic presentation after admission (since the conversion to cephalic presentation does not represent a diagnosis, the fact that the conversion occurred after admission has no bearing on the POA determination).

Perinatal conditions

Newborns are not considered to be admitted until after birth. Therefore, any condition present at birth or that developed in utero is considered present at admission and should be assigned "Y". This includes conditions that occur during delivery (e.g., injury during delivery, meconium aspiration, exposure to streptococcus B in the vaginal canal).

Congenital conditions and anomalies

Assign "Y" for congenital conditions and anomalies. Congenital conditions are always considered present on admission.

External cause of injury codes

Assign "Y" for any E code representing an external cause of injury or poisoning that occurred prior to inpatient admission (e.g., patient fell out of bed at home, patient fell out of bed in emergency room prior to admission)

Assign "N" for any E code representing an external cause of injury or poisoning that occurred during inpatient hospitalization (e.g., patient fell out of hospital bed during hospital stay, patient experienced an adverse reaction to a medication administered after inpatient admission)

Categories and Codes Exempt from Diagnosis Present on Admission Requirement (Effective Oct. 1, 2008)

Note: "Diagnosis present on admission" for these code categories are exempt because they represent circumstances regarding the healthcare encounter or factors influencing health status that do not represent a current disease or injury or are always present on admission

137-139	Late effects of infectious and parasitic diseases
268.1	Rickets, late effect
326	Late effects of intracranial abscess or pyogenic infection
412	Old myocardial infarction
438	Late effects of cerebrovascular disease
650	Normal delivery
660.7	Failed forceps or vacuum extractor, unspecified
677	Late effect of complication of pregnancy, childbirth, and the puerperium
905-909	Late effects of injuries, poisonings, toxic effects, and other external causes
V02	Carrier or suspected carrier of infectious diseases
V03	Need for prophylactic vaccination and inoculation against bacterial diseases
V04	Need for prophylactic vaccination and inoculation against certain viral diseases
V05	Need for other prophylactic vaccination and inoculation against single diseases

V06	Need for prophylactic vaccination and inoculation against combinations of diseases
V07	Need for isolation and other prophylactic measures
V10	Personal history of malignant neoplasm
V11	Personal history of mental disorder
V12	Personal history of certain other diseases
V13	Personal history of other diseases
V14	Personal history of allergy to medicinal agents
V15.01-V15.09	Other personal history, Allergy, other than to medicinal agents
V15.1	Other personal history, Surgery to heart and great vessels
V15.2	Other personal history, Surgery to other major organs
V15.3	Other personal history, Irradiation
V15.4	Other personal history, Psychological trauma
V15.5	Other personal history, Injury
V15.6	Other personal history, Poisoning
V15.7	Other personal history, Contraception
V15.81	Other personal history, Noncompliance with medical treatment
V15.82	Other personal history, History of tobacco use
V15.88	Other personal history, History of fall
V15.89	Other personal history, Other
V15.9	Unspecified personal history presenting hazards to health
V16	Family history of malignant neoplasm
V17	Family history of certain chronic disabling diseases
V18	Family history of certain other specific conditions
V19	Family history of other conditions
V20	Health supervision of infant or child
V21	Constitutional states in development
V22	Normal pregnancy
V23	Supervision of high-risk pregnancy
V24	Postpartum care and examination
V25	Encounter for contraceptive management
V26	Procreative management
V27	Outcome of delivery
V28	Antenatal screening
V29	Observation and evaluation of newborns for suspected condition not found
V30-V39	Liveborn infants according to type of birth
V42	Organ or tissue replaced by transplant
V43	Organ or tissue replaced by other means
V44	Artificial opening status
V45	Other postprocedural states
V46	Other dependence on machines
V49.60-V49.77	Upper and lower limb amputation status
V49.81-V49.84	Other specified conditions influencing health status
V50	Elective surgery for purposes other than remedying health states
V51	Aftercare involving the use of plastic surgery
V52	Fitting and adjustment of prosthetic device and implant
V53	Fitting and adjustment of other device
V54	Other orthopedic aftercare
V55	Attention to artificial openings
V56	Encounter for dialysis and dialysis catheter care
V57	Care involving use of rehabilitation procedures
V58	Encounter for other and unspecified procedures and aftercare
V59	Donors
V60	Housing, household, and economic circumstances
V61	Other family circumstances
V62	Other psychosocial circumstances

V64	Persons encountering health services for specific procedures, not carried out
V65	Other persons seeking consultation
V66	Convalescence and palliative care
V67	Follow-up examination
V68	Encounters for administrative purposes
V69	Problems related to lifestyle
V70	General medical examination
V71	Observation and evaluation for suspected condition not found
V72	Special investigations and examinations
V73	Special screening examination for viral and chlamydial diseases
V74	Special screening examination for bacterial and spirochetal diseases
V75	Special screening examination for other infectious diseases
V76	Special screening for malignant neoplasms
V77	Special screening for endocrine, nutritional, metabolic, and immunity disorders
V78	Special screening for disorders of blood and blood-forming organs
V79	Special screening for mental disorders and developmental handicaps
V80	Special screening for neurological, eye, and ear diseases
V81	Special screening for cardiovascular, respiratory, and genitourinary diseases
V82	Special screening for other conditions
V83	Genetic carrier status
V84	Genetic susceptibility to disease
V85	Body Mass Index
V86	Estrogen receptor status
V87.4	Personal history of drug therapy
V88	Acquired absence of cervix and uterus
V89	Suspected maternal and fetal conditions not found
E800-E807	Railway accidents
E810-E819	Motor vehicle traffic accidents
E820-E825	Motor vehicle nontraffic accidents
E826-E829	Other road vehicle accidents
E830-E838	Water transport accidents
E840-E845	Air and space transport accidents
E846-E848	Vehicle accidents not elsewhere classifiable
E849.0-E849.6	Place of occurrence
E849.8-E849.9	Place of occurrence
E883.1	Accidental fall into well
E883.2	Accidental fall into storm drain or manhole
E884.0	Fall from playground equipment
E884.1	Fall from cliff
E885.0	Fall from (nonmotorized) scooter
E885.1	Fall from roller skates
E885.2	Fall from skateboard
E885.3	Fall from skis
E885.4	Fall from snowboard
E886.0	Fall on same level from collision, pushing, or shoving, by or with other person, In sports
E890.0-E890.9	Conflagration in private dwelling
E893.0	Accident caused by ignition of clothing, from controlled fire in private dwelling
E893.2	Accident caused by ignition of clothing, from controlled fire not in building or structure
E894	Ignition of highly inflammable material
E895	Accident caused by controlled fire in private dwelling
E897	Accident caused by controlled fire not in building or structure
E898.0-E898.1	Accident caused by other specified fire and flames

E917.0	Striking against or struck accidentally by objects or persons, in sports without subsequent fall
E917.1	Striking against or struck accidentally by objects or persons, caused by a crowd, by collective fear or panic without subsequent fall
E917.2	Striking against or struck accidentally by objects or persons, in running water without subsequent fall
E917.5	Striking against or struck accidentally by objects or persons, object in sports with subsequent fall
E917.6	Striking against or struck accidentally by objects or persons, caused by a crowd, by collective fear or panic with subsequent fall
E919.0-E919.1	Accidents caused by machinery
E919.3-E919.9	Accidents caused by machinery
E921.0-E921.9	Accident caused by explosion of pressure vessel
E922.0-E922.9	Accident caused by firearm and air gun missile
E924.1	Caustic and corrosive substances
E926.2	Visible and ultraviolet light sources
E928.0-E928.8	Other and unspecified environmental and accidental causes
E929.0-E929.9	Late effects of accidental injury
E959	Late effects of self-inflicted injury
E970-E978	Legal intervention
E979	Terrorism
E981.0-E981.8	Poisoning by gases in domestic use, undetermined whether accidentally or purposely inflicted
E982.0-E982.9	Poisoning by other gases, undetermined whether accidentally or purposely inflicted
E985.0-E985.7	Injury by firearms, air guns and explosives, undetermined whether accidentally or purposely inflicted
E987.0	Falling from high place, undetermined whether accidentally or purposely inflicted, residential premises
E987.2	Falling from high place, undetermined whether accidentally or purposely inflicted, natural sites
E989	Late effects of injury, undetermined whether accidentally or purposely inflicted
E990-E999	Injury resulting from operations of war

POA EXAMPLES

General Medical Surgical

1. Patient is admitted for diagnostic work-up for cachexia. The final diagnosis is malignant neoplasm of lung with metastasis.

    Assign "Y" on the POA field for the malignant neoplasm. The malignant neoplasm was clearly present on admission, although it was not diagnosed until after the admission occurred.

2. A patient undergoes outpatient surgery. During the recovery period, the patient develops atrial fibrillation and the patient is subsequently admitted to the hospital as an inpatient.

    Assign "Y" on the POA field for the atrial fibrillation since it developed prior to a written order for inpatient admission.

3. A patient is treated in observation and while in Observation, the patient falls out of bed and breaks a hip. The patient is subsequently admitted as an inpatient to treat the hip fracture.

Assign "Y" on the POA field for the hip fracture since it developed prior to a written order for inpatient admission.

4. A patient with known congestive heart failure is admitted to the hospital after he develops decompensated congestive heart failure.

    Assign "Y" on the POA field for the congestive heart failure. The ICD-9-CM code identifies the chronic condition and does not specify the acuteexacerbation.

5. A patient undergoes inpatient surgery. After surgery, the patient develops fever and is treated aggressively. The physician's final diagnosis documents "possible postoperative infection following surgery."

    Assign "N" on the POA field for the postoperative infection since final diagnoses that contain the terms "possible", "probable", "suspected" or "rule out" and that are based on symptoms or clinical findings that were not present on admission should be reported as "N".

6. A patient with severe cough and difficulty breathing was diagnosed during his hospitalization to have lung cancer.

    Assign "Y" on the POA field for the lung cancer. Even though the cancer was not diagnosed until after admission, it is a chronic condition that was clearly present before the patient's admission.

7. A patient is admitted to the hospital for a coronary artery bypass surgery. Postoperatively he developed a pulmonary embolism.

    Assign "N" on the POA field for the pulmonary embolism. This is an acute condition that was not present on admission.

8. A patient is admitted with a known history of coronary atherosclerosis, status post myocardial infarction five years ago is now admitted for treatment of impending myocardial infarction. The final diagnosis is documented as "impending myocardial infarction."

    Assign "Y" to the impending myocardial infarction because the condition is present on admission.

9. A patient with diabetes mellitus developed uncontrolled diabetes on day 3 of the hospitalization.

    Assign "N" to the diabetes code because the "uncontrolled" component of the code was not present on admission.

10. A patient is admitted with high fever and pneumonia. The patient rapidly deteriorates and becomes septic. The discharge diagnosis lists sepsis and pneumonia. The documentation is unclear as to whether the sepsis was present on admission or developed shortly after admission.

    Query the physician as to whether the sepsis was present on admission, developed shortly after admission, or it cannot be clinically determined as to whether it was present on admission or not.

11. A patient is admitted for repair of an abdominal aneurysm. However, the aneurysm ruptures after hospital admission.

Assign "N" for the ruptured abdominal aneurysm. Although the aneurysm was present on admission, the "ruptured" component of the code description did not occur until after admission.

12. A patient with viral hepatitis B progresses to hepatic coma after admission.

    Assign "N" for the viral hepatitis B with hepatic coma because part of the code description did not develop until after admission.

13. A patient with a history of varicose veins and ulceration of the left lower extremity strikes the area against the side of his hospital bed during an inpatient hospitalization. It bleeds profusely. The final diagnosis lists varicose veins with ulcer and hemorrhage.

    Assign "Y" for the varicose veins with ulcer. Although the hemorrhage occurred after admission, the code description for varicose veins with ulcer does not mention hemorrhage.

14. The nursing initial assessment upon admission documents the presence of a decubitus ulcer. There is no mention of the decubitus ulcer in the physician documentation until several days after admission.

    Query the physician as to whether the decubitus ulcer was present on admission, or developed after admission. Both diagnosis code assignment and determination of whether a condition was present on admission must be based on provider documentation in the medical record (per the definition of "provider" found at the beginning of these POA guidelines and in the introductory section of the ICD-9-CM Official Guidelines for Coding and Reporting). If it cannot be determined from the provider documentation whether or not a condition was present on admission, the provider should be queried.

15. A urine culture is obtained on admission. The provider documents urinary tract infection when the culture results become available a few days later.

    Assign "Y" to the urinary tract infection since the diagnosis is based on test results from a specimen obtained on admission. It may not be possible for a provider to make a definitive diagnosis for a period of time after admission. There is no required timeframe as to when a provider must identify or document a condition to be present on admission.

16. A patient tested positive for Methicillin resistant Staphylococcus (MRSA) on routine nasal culture on admission to the hospital. During the hospitalization, he underwent insertion of a central venous catheter and later developed an infection and was diagnosed with MRSA sepsis due to central venous catheter infection.

    Assign "Y" to the positive MRSA colonization. Assign "N" for the MRSA sepsis due to central venous catheter infection since the patient did not have a MRSA infection at the time of admission.

Obstetrics

1. A female patient was admitted to the hospital and underwent a normal delivery.

    Leave the "present on admission" (POA) field blank. Code 650, Normal delivery, is on the "exempt from reporting" list.

2. Patient admitted in late pregnancy due to excessive vomiting and dehydration. During admission patient goes into premature labor

    Assign "Y" for the excessive vomiting and the dehydration. Assign "N" for the premature labor

3. Patient admitted in active labor. During the stay, a breast abscess is noted when mother attempted to breast feed. Provider is unable to determine whether the abscess was present on admission

    Assign "W" for the breast abscess.

4. Patient admitted in active labor. After 12 hours of labor it is noted that the infant is in fetal distress and a Cesarean section is performed

    Assign "N" for the fetal distress.

5. Pregnant female was admitted in labor and fetal nuchal cord entanglement was diagnosed. Physician is queried, but is unable to determine whether the cord entanglement was present on admission or not.

    Assign "W" for the fetal nuchal cord entanglement.

Newborn

1. A single liveborn infant was delivered in the hospital via Cesarean section. The physician documented fetal bradycardia during labor in the final diagnosis in the newborn record.

    Assign " Y" because the bradycardia developed prior to the newborn admission (birth).

2. A newborn developed diarrhea which was believed to be due to the hospital baby formula.

    Assign " N" because the diarrhea developed after admission.

3. A newborn born in the hospital, birth complicated by nuchal cord entanglement. *Assign "Y" for the nuchal cord entanglement on the baby's record. Any condition that is present at birth or that developed in utero is considered present at admission, including conditions that occur during delivery.*

ICD-10

Since 1948, the World Health Organization has revised the *International Classification of Diseases* approximately every 10 years, with a modified version appearing in the United States about one to three years following the WHO publication. Based on the regular schedule, *ICD-10* should have been released in 1987. However, due to difficulties in coordinating the international committees, the first volume of *ICD-10*, the Tabular List, was not published until June of 1992.

Implementation of ICD-10 in the United States

Prior to being implemented in the United States, *ICD-10* must be converted to "American" English and pass through a variety of private and government committees, agencies, associations and organizations. As of this printing, the official position of the CMS is that *ICD-10* will be mandated as of October 1, 2013.

WHERE TO GET ANSWERS TO QUESTIONS ABOUT ICD-9-CM

Questions regarding the use and interpretation of the *International Classification of Diseases, 9th Revision, Clinical Modification* should be directed in writing to any of the organizations listed below.

Coding Advice/Central Office on ICD-9-CM
American Hospital Association
One North Franklin
Chicago, Illinois 60606
Vols. 1 and 2: kayala@aha.org

World Health Organization Collaborating Center
    for Classification of Diseases in North America
National Center for Health Statistics
Department of Health and Human Services
6525 Belcrest Road
Hyattsville, Maryland 20782

Morbidity Classification Branch
National Center for Health Statistics
Department of Health and Human Services
6525 Belcrest Road, Room 1100
Hyattsville, Maryland 20782

Center for Medicare and Medicaid Services (CMS)
Division of Prospective Payment
Mail Stop C5-06-27
7500 Security Blvd.
Baltimore, MD   21244-1850
Vol. 3: pbrooks@cms.hhs.gov

Comments, questions or suggestions regarding the PMIC version of ICD-9-CM should be directed in writing to:

Managing Editor
Practice Management Information Corporation
4727 Wilshire Boulevard, Suite 300
Los Angeles, California 90010
http://www.pmiconline.com

Anatomical Illustrations

A fundamental knowledge and understanding of basic human anatomy and physiology is a prerequisite for accurate diagnosis coding. While a comprehensive treatment of anatomy and physiology is beyond the scope of this text, the large scale, full color anatomical illustrations on the following pages are designed to facilitate the diagnosis coding process for both beginning and experienced coders.

The illustrations provide an anatomical perspective of diagnosis coding by providing a side-by-side view of the major systems of the human body and a corresponding list of the most common diagnoses categories used to support medical, surgical and diagnostic services performed on the illustrated system.

The diagnostic categories listed on the left facing page of each anatomical illustration are three-digit categories and may not be used for coding. These categories are provided as "pointers" to the appropriate section of the ICD-9-CM Volume 1 where the complete listings, including 4th and 5th digits if appropriate, may be found.

PLATE 1. SKIN AND SUBCUTANEOUS TISSUE — MALE

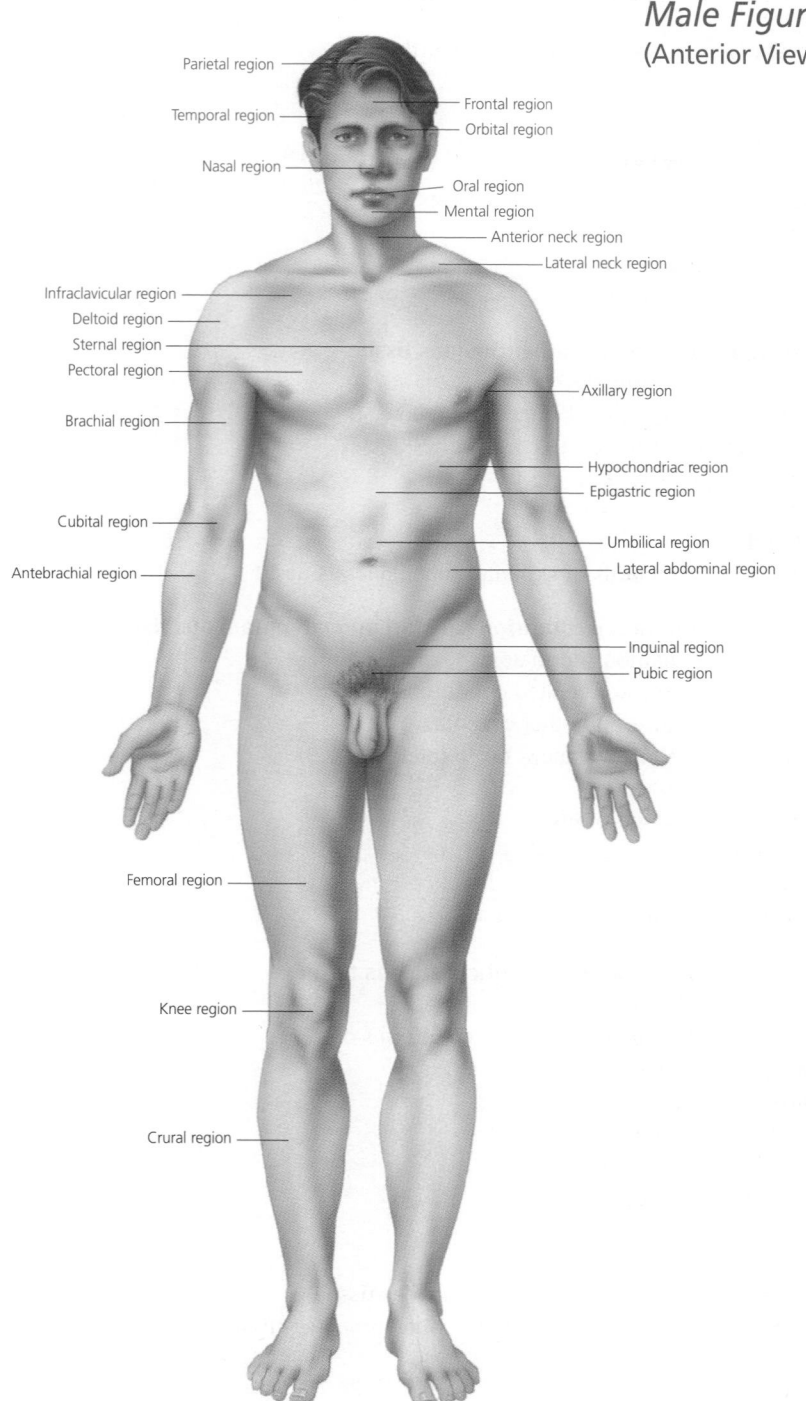

Male Figure
(Anterior View)

Parietal region

Temporal region

Nasal region

Frontal region

Orbital region

Oral region

Mental region

Anterior neck region

Lateral neck region

Infraclavicular region

Deltoid region

Sternal region

Pectoral region

Brachial region

Axillary region

Hypochondriac region

Epigastric region

Cubital region

Antebrachial region

Umbilical region

Lateral abdominal region

Inguinal region

Pubic region

Femoral region

Knee region

Crural region

PLATE 2. SKIN AND SUBCUTANEOUS TISSUE — FEMALE

Female Figure
(Anterior View)

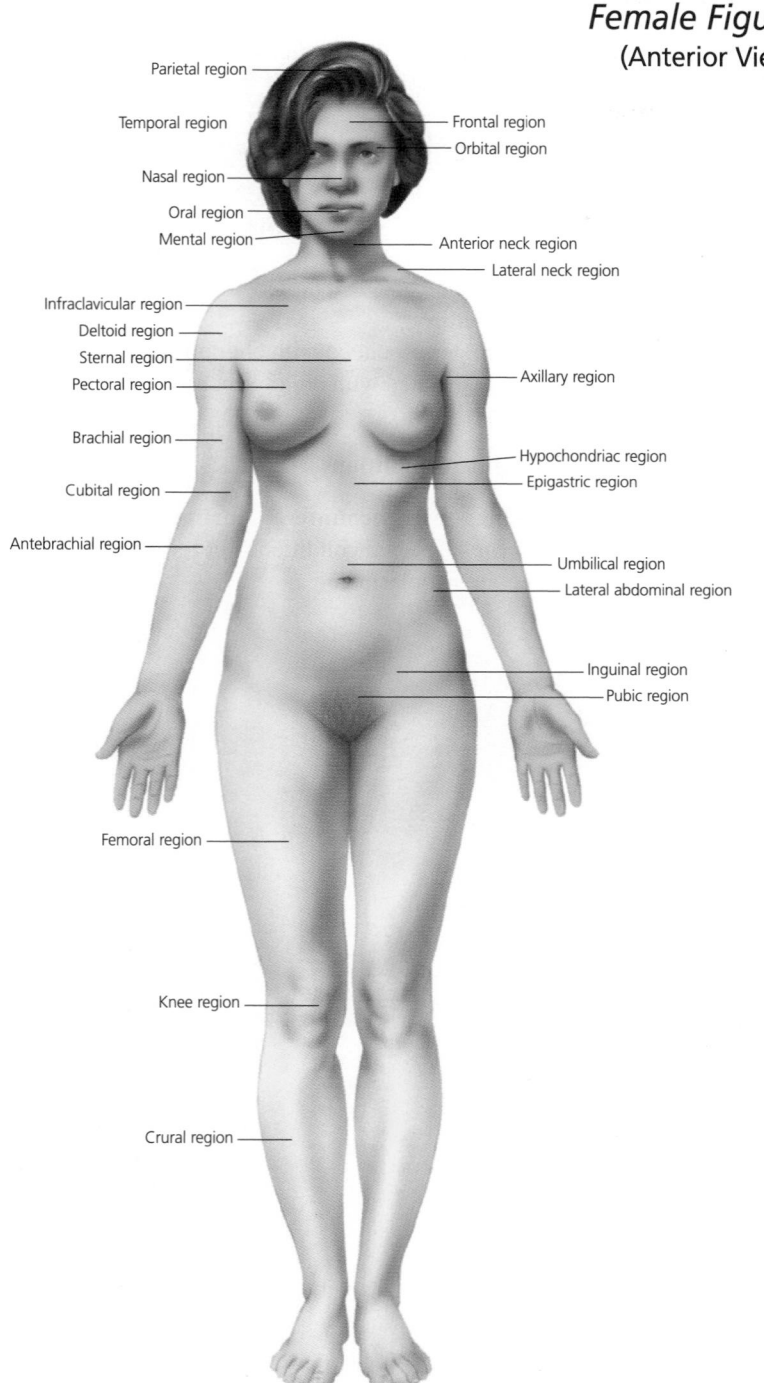

Parietal region

Temporal region

Frontal region
Orbital region

Nasal region

Oral region

Mental region

Anterior neck region

Lateral neck region

Infraclavicular region

Deltoid region

Sternal region

Pectoral region

Axillary region

Brachial region

Cubital region

Hypochondriac region

Epigastric region

Antebrachial region

Umbilical region

Lateral abdominal region

Inguinal region

Pubic region

Femoral region

Knee region

Crural region

PLATE 3. FEMALE BREAST

Female Breast

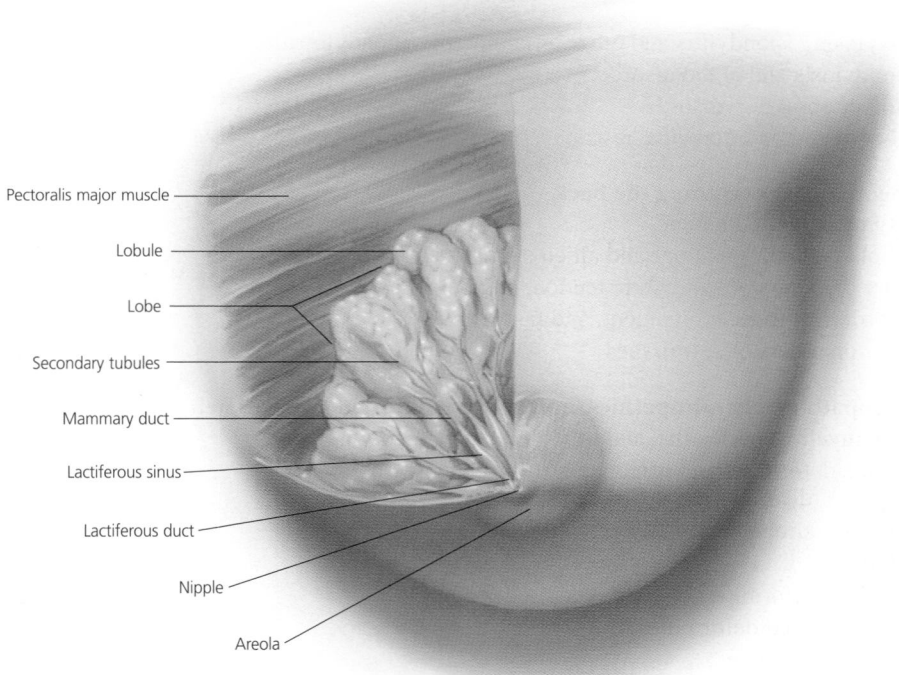

Pectoralis major muscle

Lobule

Lobe

Secondary tubules

Mammary duct

Lactiferous sinus

Lactiferous duct

Nipple

Areola

PLATE 4. MUSCULAR SYSTEM AND CONNECTIVE TISSUE — ANTERIOR VIEW

Muscular System
(Anterior View)

Temporalis m.
Orbicularis oculi m.
Masseter m.
Sternocleidomastoid m.
Trapezius m.
Levator scapulae m.

Frontalis m.
Buccinator
Orbicularis oris m.
Depressor anguli oris m.

Deltoid m.
Pectoralis major m.

Serratus anterior m.
Biceps m.
External abdominal oblique m.
Brachialis m.
Brachioradialis m.
Extensor carpi radialis longus m.
Palmaris longus m.
Flexor carpi radialis m.
Superficial inguinal ring
Tensor fasciae latae m.
Sartorius m.
Rectus femoris m.
Adductor longus m.
Vastus lateralis m.

Pectoralis minor m.
Internal intercostal m.
Coracobrachialis m.
Brachialis m.
Rectus sheath
Rectus abdominis m.
Linea alba
Internal abdominal oblique m.
Transversus abdominis m.
Flexor digitorum superficialis m.
Flexor pollicis longus m.
Abductor digiti minimi m.
Abductor pollicis brevis m.
Flexor pollicis brevis m.
Iliopsoas m.
Pectineus m.
Adductor brevis m.

Iliotibial tract
Vastus medialis m.

Gracilis m.
Adductor magnus m.
Vastus medialis m.
Vastus lateralis m.

Lateral patellar retinaculum

Sartorius m.

Patella
Patellar ligament
Medial patellar retinaculum

Tibialis anterior m.
Gastrocnemius m.
Extensor digitorum longus m.
Peroneus longus m.
Soleus m.
Peroneus brevis m.
Extensor hallucis longus m.
Extensor hallucis brevis m.
Extensor digitorum brevis m.

Gastrocnemius m.
Soleus m.
Tibia
Flexor digitorum longus m.
Extensor hallucis brevis m.
Abductor hallucis m.

PLATE 5. MUSCULAR SYSTEM AND CONNECTIVE TISSUE — POSTERIOR VIEW

Muscular System
(Posterior View)

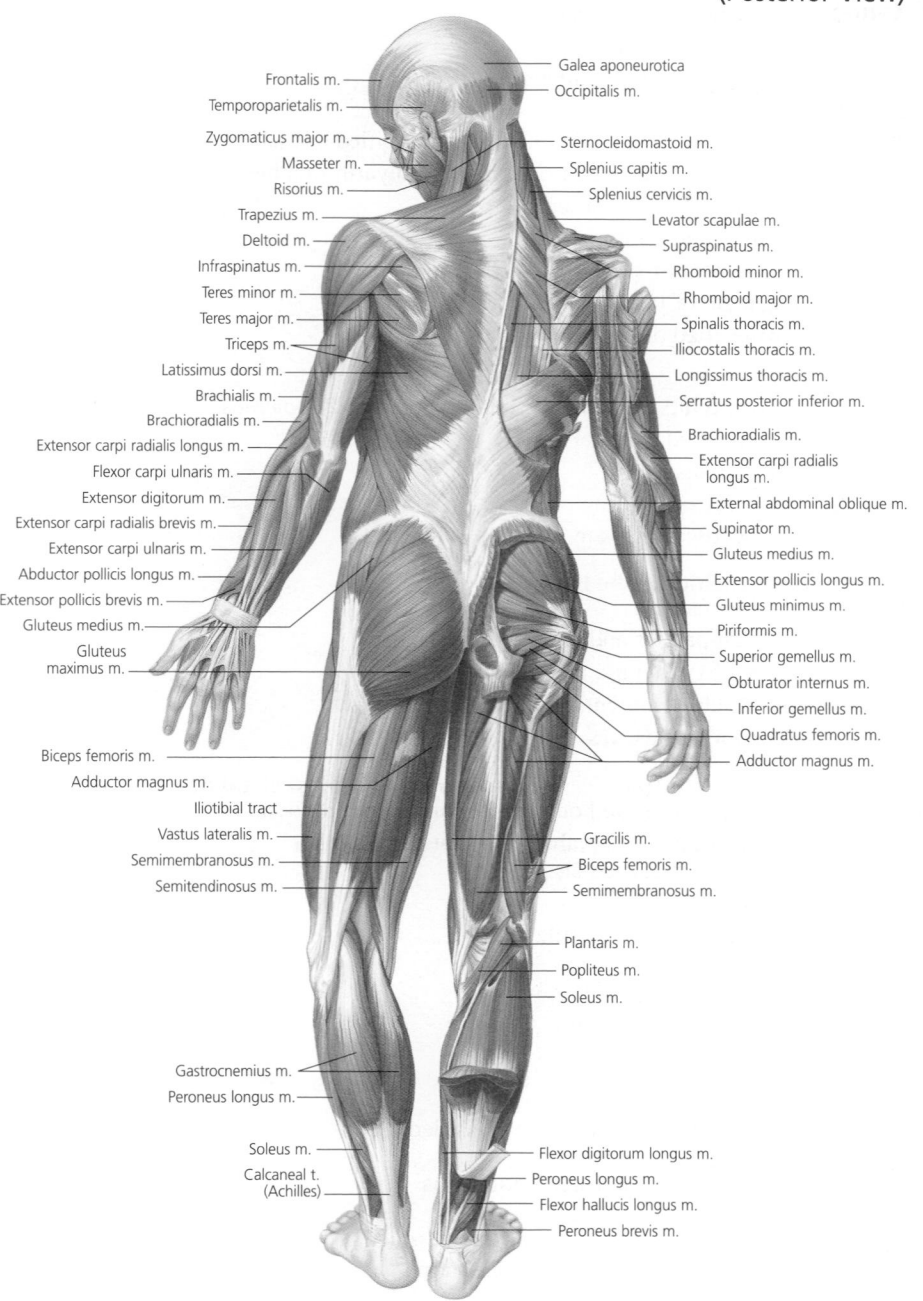

Galea aponeurotica
Occipitalis m.
Frontalis m.
Temporoparietalis m.
Zygomaticus major m.
Masseter m.
Risorius m.
Trapezius m.
Deltoid m.
Infraspinatus m.
Teres minor m.
Teres major m.
Triceps m.
Latissimus dorsi m.
Brachialis m.
Brachioradialis m.
Extensor carpi radialis longus m.
Flexor carpi ulnaris m.
Extensor digitorum m.
Extensor carpi radialis brevis m.
Extensor carpi ulnaris m.
Abductor pollicis longus m.
Extensor pollicis brevis m.
Gluteus medius m.
Gluteus maximus m.
Biceps femoris m.
Adductor magnus m.
Iliotibial tract
Vastus lateralis m.
Semimembranosus m.
Semitendinosus m.
Gastrocnemius m.
Peroneus longus m.
Soleus m.
Calcaneal t. (Achilles)

Sternocleidomastoid m.
Splenius capitis m.
Splenius cervicis m.
Levator scapulae m.
Supraspinatus m.
Rhomboid minor m.
Rhomboid major m.
Spinalis thoracis m.
Iliocostalis thoracis m.
Longissimus thoracis m.
Serratus posterior inferior m.
Brachioradialis m.
Extensor carpi radialis longus m.
External abdominal oblique m.
Supinator m.
Gluteus medius m.
Extensor pollicis longus m.
Gluteus minimus m.
Piriformis m.
Superior gemellus m.
Obturator internus m.
Inferior gemellus m.
Quadratus femoris m.
Adductor magnus m.
Gracilis m.
Biceps femoris m.
Semimembranosus m.
Plantaris m.
Popliteus m.
Soleus m.
Flexor digitorum longus m.
Peroneus longus m.
Flexor hallucis longus m.
Peroneus brevis m.

PLATE 6. MUSCULAR SYSTEM — SHOULDER AND ELBOW

Shoulder and Elbow
(Anterior View)

Coracoclavicular ligament
Acromioclavicular ligament
Coracoacromial ligament
Supraspinatus tendon
Coracohumeral ligament
Transverse humeral ligament
Tendon of long head of biceps muscle
Subscapularis tendon
Articular capsule

Acromion
Clavicle

Coracoid process
Scapular notch
Subscapular fossa
Head of humerus
Lesser tubercle
Greater tubercle
Scapula
Nutrient foramen
Humerus
Deltoid tuberosity

Articular capsule
Radial collateral ligament
Annular ligament

Ulnar collateral ligament

Interosseous membrane
Radius
Ulna

Lateral epicondyle
Capitulum
Coronoid fossa
Medial epicondyle
Trochlea
Coronoid process
Head of radius
Ulnar tuberosity
Radial tuberosity

PLATE 7. MUSCULAR SYSTEM — HAND AND WRIST

Hand and Wrist

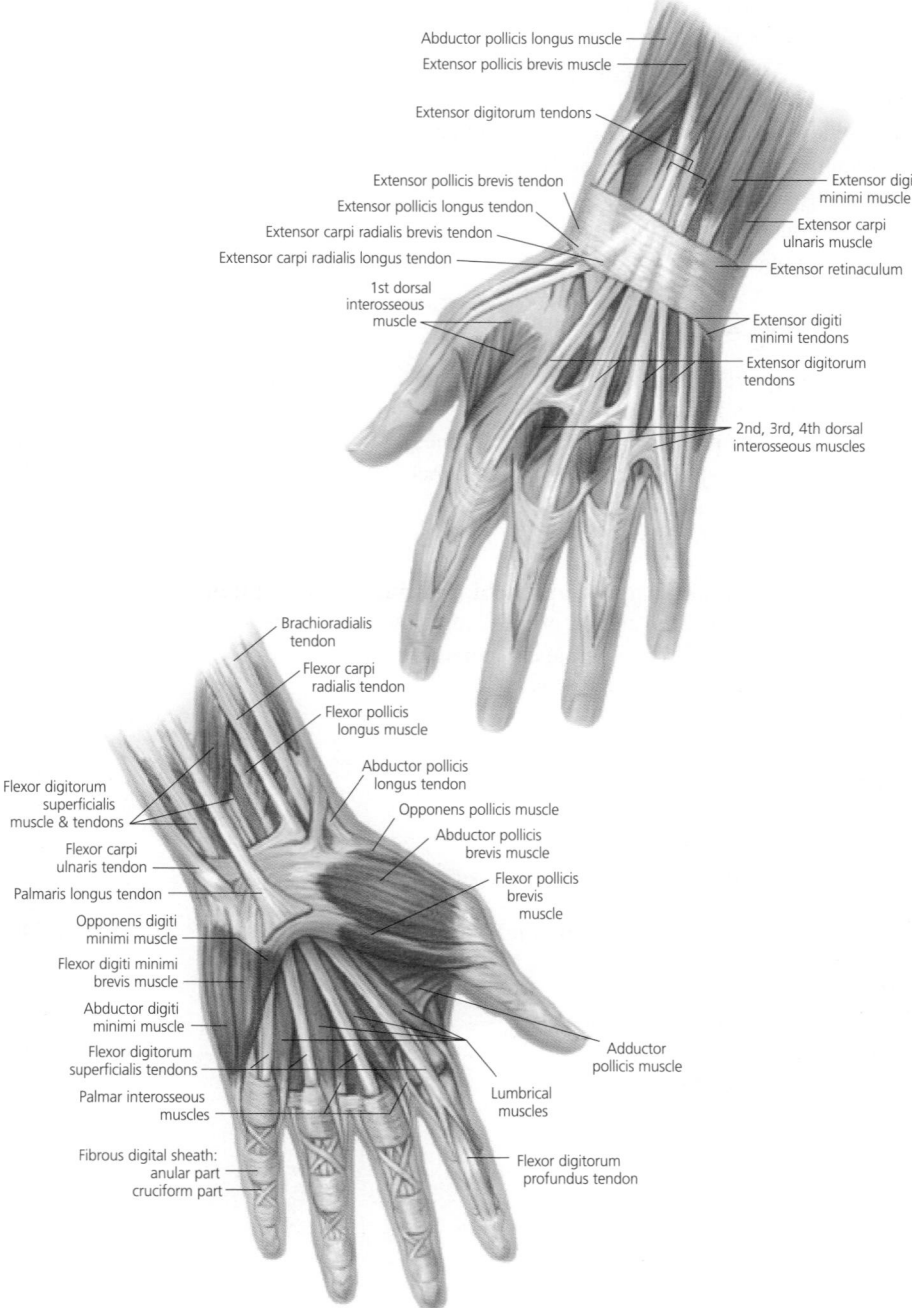

Abductor pollicis longus muscle

Extensor pollicis brevis muscle

Extensor digitorum tendons

Extensor pollicis brevis tendon

Extensor pollicis longus tendon

Extensor carpi radialis brevis tendon

Extensor carpi radialis longus tendon

1st dorsal interosseous muscle

Extensor digiti minimi muscle

Extensor carpi ulnaris muscle

Extensor retinaculum

Extensor digiti minimi tendons

Extensor digitorum tendons

2nd, 3rd, 4th dorsal interosseous muscles

Brachioradialis tendon

Flexor carpi radialis tendon

Flexor pollicis longus muscle

Abductor pollicis longus tendon

Opponens pollicis muscle

Abductor pollicis brevis muscle

Flexor pollicis brevis muscle

Flexor digitorum superficialis muscle & tendons

Flexor carpi ulnaris tendon

Palmaris longus tendon

Opponens digiti minimi muscle

Flexor digiti minimi brevis muscle

Abductor digiti minimi muscle

Flexor digitorum superficialis tendons

Palmar interosseous muscles

Fibrous digital sheath:
anular part
cruciform part

Adductor pollicis muscle

Lumbrical muscles

Flexor digitorum profundus tendon

PLATE 8. MUSCULOSKELETAL SYSTEM — HIP AND KNEE

Hip and Knee
(Anterior View)

Sacral promontory
Sacrum
Iliac crest
Ilium
Anterior superior iliac spine
Spine of ischium
Anterior inferior iliac spine
Head of femur
Greater trochanter
Obturator foramen
Pubis
Lesser trochanter

Anterior longitudinal ligament
Iliolumbar ligament
Anterior sacroiliac ligament
Coccyx
Sacrotuberous ligament
Sacrospinous ligament
Inguinal ligament
Iliofemoral ligament
Pubofemoral ligament
Obturator membrane
Pubic symphysis
Femur

Medial epicondyle
Lateral epicondyle
Patella
Lateral condyles
Head of fibula
Tibial tuberosity
Medial condyles
Tibia
Fibula

Quadriceps femoris tendon
Medial patellar retinaculum
Fibular collateral ligament
Tibial collateral ligament
Lateral patellar retinaculum
Patellar ligament
Interosseous membrane

PLATE 9. MUSCULOSKELETAL SYSTEM — FOOT AND ANKLE

Foot and Ankle

Soleus muscle

Tibia

Flexor digitorum longus muscle

Flexor hallucis tendon

Achilles tendon

Medial malleolus

Tibialis posterior tendon

Retinaculum

Tibialis anterior muscle

Peroneus brevis muscle

Peroneus longus tendon

Extensor digitorum longus muscle

Tibia

Fibula

Extensor hallucis longus muscle

Lateral malleous

Retinaculum

Peroneus longus tendon

Extensor digitorum brevis muscle

Calcaneus

Peroneus brevis tendon

Peroneus tertius tendon

Opponens digiti minimi muscle

Dorsal interosseous muscles

Extensor hallucis longus tendon

Extensor hallucis brevis muscle

Extensor digitorum longus tendons

Tibialis posterior tendon

Tibialis anterior tendon

Extensor hallucis brevis muscle

Abductor hallucis muscle

PLATE 10. SKELETAL SYSTEM — ANTERIOR VIEW

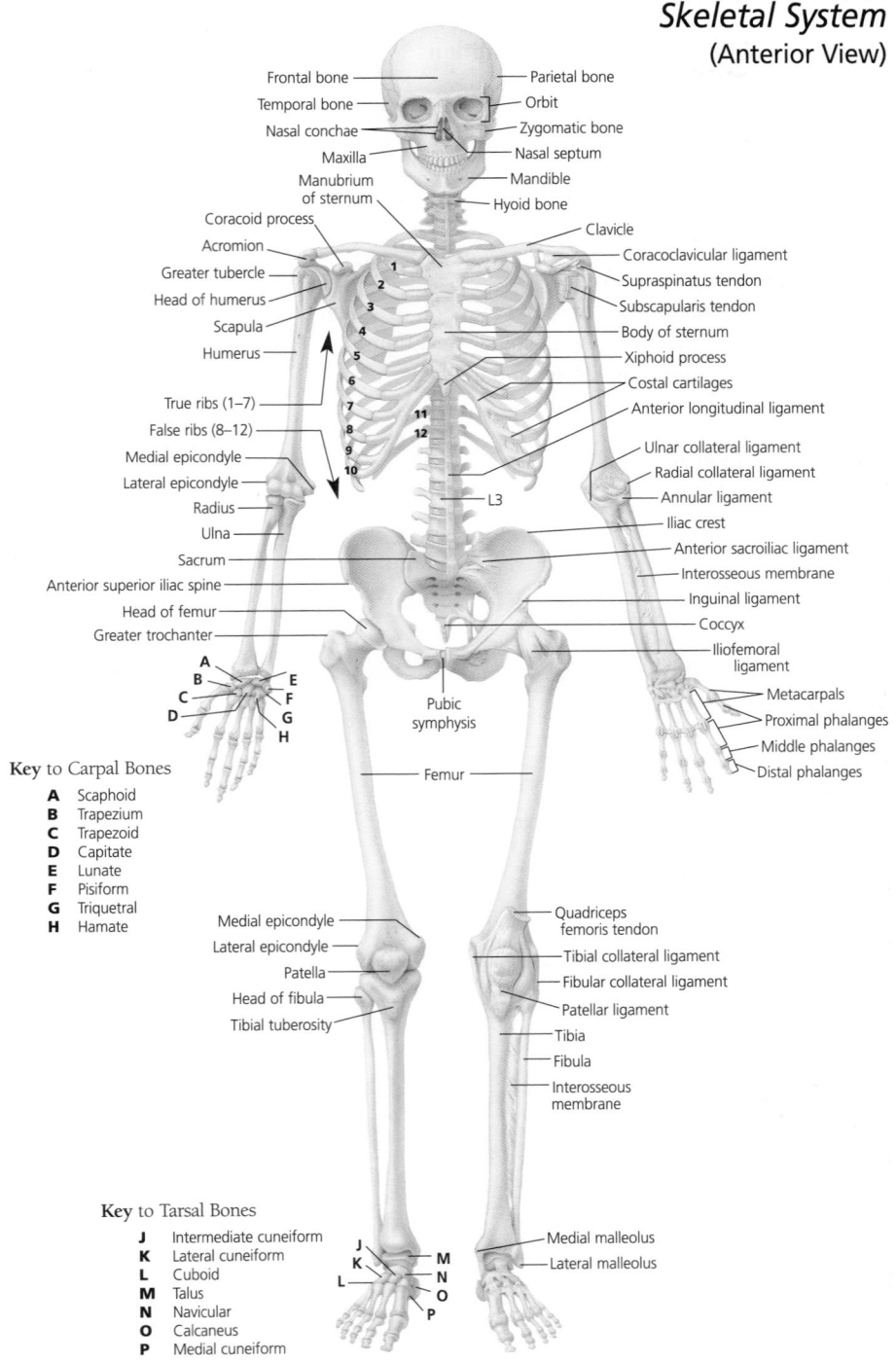

Skeletal System
(Anterior View)

Frontal bone — Parietal bone
Temporal bone — Orbit
Nasal conchae — Zygomatic bone
Maxilla — Nasal septum
Manubrium of sternum — Mandible
— Hyoid bone
Coracoid process — Clavicle
Acromion — Coracoclavicular ligament
Greater tubercle — Supraspinatus tendon
Head of humerus — Subscapularis tendon
Scapula — Body of sternum
Humerus — Xiphoid process
— Costal cartilages
True ribs (1–7) — Anterior longitudinal ligament
False ribs (8–12) —
Medial epicondyle — Ulnar collateral ligament
Lateral epicondyle — Radial collateral ligament
Radius — Annular ligament
Ulna — L3 — Iliac crest
Sacrum — Anterior sacroiliac ligament
Anterior superior iliac spine — Interosseous membrane
Head of femur — Inguinal ligament
Greater trochanter — Coccyx
— Iliofemoral ligament
A — Metacarpals
B — E — Proximal phalanges
C — F — Pubic — Middle phalanges
D — G — symphysis — Distal phalanges
— H
Femur

Key to Carpal Bones

A	Scaphoid
B	Trapezium
C	Trapezoid
D	Capitate
E	Lunate
F	Pisiform
G	Triquetral
H	Hamate

Medial epicondyle — Quadriceps femoris tendon
Lateral epicondyle — Tibial collateral ligament
Patella — Fibular collateral ligament
Head of fibula — Patellar ligament
Tibial tuberosity — Tibia
— Fibula
— Interosseous membrane

Key to Tarsal Bones

J	Intermediate cuneiform	
K	Lateral cuneiform	
L	Cuboid	Medial malleolus
M	Talus	Lateral malleolus
N	Navicular	
O	Calcaneus	
P	Medial cuneiform	

PLATE 11. SKELETAL SYSTEM — POSTERIOR VIEW

Skeletal System
(Posterior View)

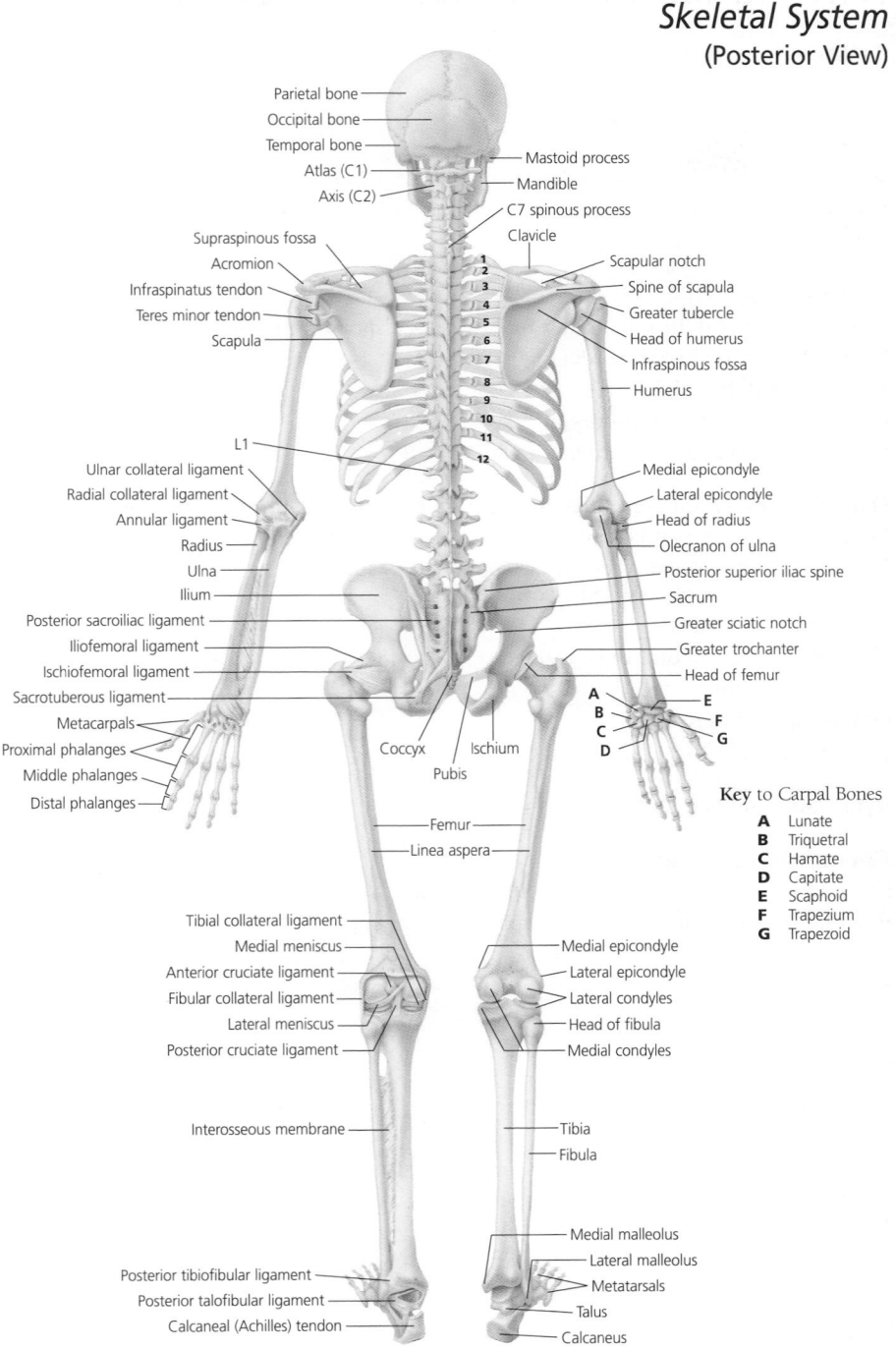

Parietal bone
Occipital bone
Temporal bone
Atlas (C1)
Axis (C2)
Mastoid process
Mandible
C7 spinous process
Supraspinous fossa
Clavicle
Acromion
Scapular notch
Infraspinatus tendon
Spine of scapula
Teres minor tendon
Greater tubercle
Scapula
Head of humerus
Infraspinous fossa
Humerus
L1
Ulnar collateral ligament
Medial epicondyle
Radial collateral ligament
Lateral epicondyle
Annular ligament
Head of radius
Radius
Olecranon of ulna
Ulna
Posterior superior iliac spine
Ilium
Sacrum
Posterior sacroiliac ligament
Greater sciatic notch
Iliofemoral ligament
Greater trochanter
Ischiofemoral ligament
Head of femur
Sacrotuberous ligament
Metacarpals
Proximal phalanges
Coccyx   Ischium
Middle phalanges
Pubis
Distal phalanges

A   E
B   F
C   G
D

Key to Carpal Bones

A	Lunate
B	Triquetral
C	Hamate
D	Capitate
E	Scaphoid
F	Trapezium
G	Trapezoid

Femur
Linea aspera
Tibial collateral ligament
Medial epicondyle
Medial meniscus
Lateral epicondyle
Anterior cruciate ligament
Lateral condyles
Fibular collateral ligament
Head of fibula
Lateral meniscus
Medial condyles
Posterior cruciate ligament

Interosseous membrane
Tibia
Fibula

Medial malleolus
Lateral malleolus
Posterior tibiofibular ligament
Metatarsals
Posterior talofibular ligament
Talus
Calcaneal (Achilles) tendon
Calcaneus

©Scientific Publishing Ltd., Rolling Meadows, IL

PLATE 12. SKELETAL SYSTEM — VERTEBRAL COLUMN

Vertebral Column
(Lateral View)

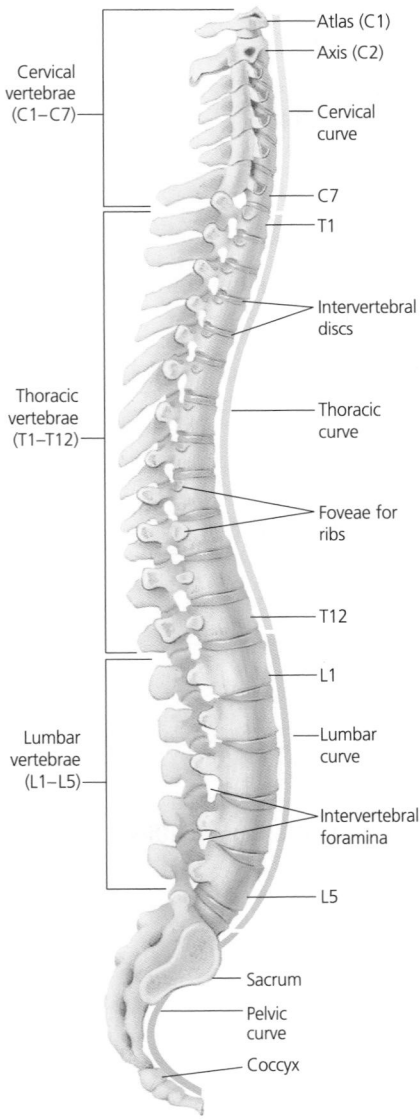

Atlas (C1)

Axis (C2)

Cervical
vertebrae
(C1–C7)

Cervical
curve

C7

T1

Intervertebral
discs

Thoracic
vertebrae
(T1–T12)

Thoracic
curve

Foveae for
ribs

T12

L1

Lumbar
vertebrae
(L1–L5)

Lumbar
curve

Intervertebral
foramina

L5

Sacrum

Pelvic
curve

Coccyx

PLATE 13. RESPIRATORY SYSTEM

Respiratory System

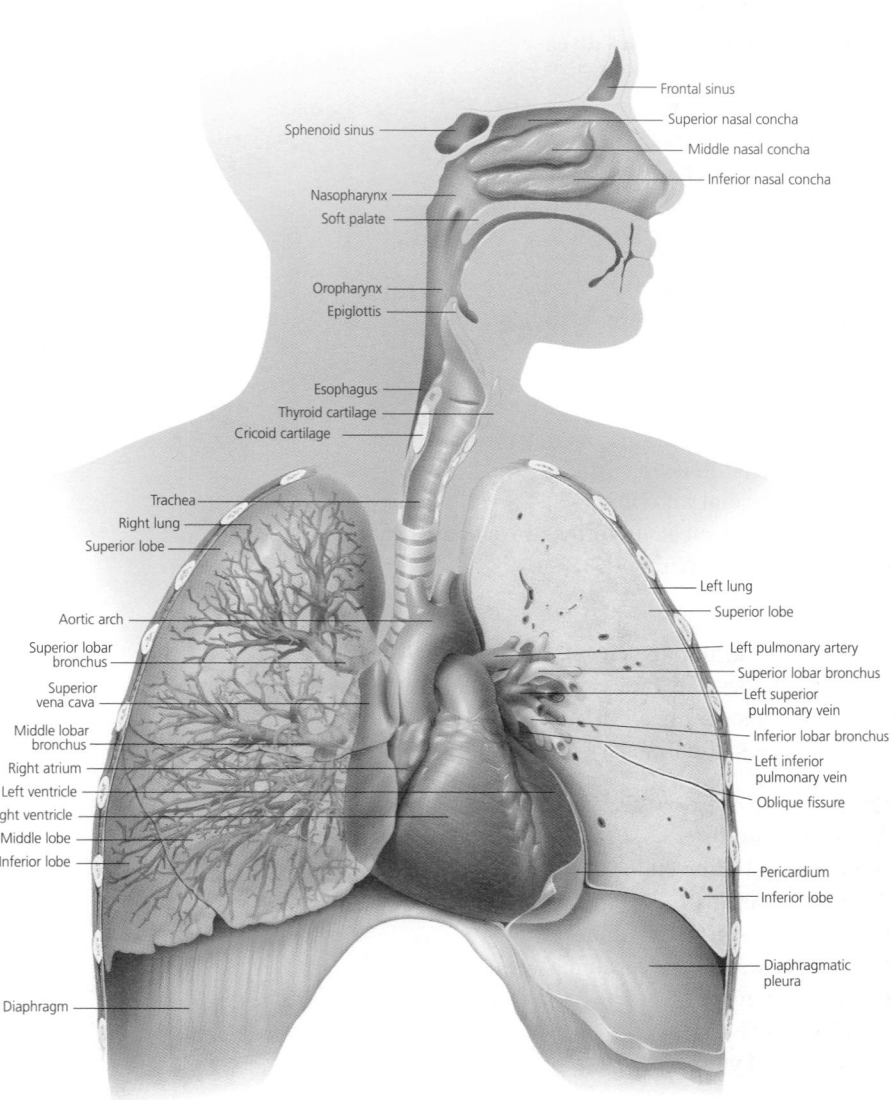

Frontal sinus

Superior nasal concha

Sphenoid sinus

Middle nasal concha

Inferior nasal concha

Nasopharynx

Soft palate

Oropharynx

Epiglottis

Esophagus

Thyroid cartilage

Cricoid cartilage

Trachea

Right lung

Superior lobe

Left lung

Superior lobe

Aortic arch

Left pulmonary artery

Superior lobar bronchus

Superior lobar bronchus

Superior vena cava

Left superior pulmonary vein

Middle lobar bronchus

Inferior lobar bronchus

Right atrium

Left inferior pulmonary vein

Left ventricle

Right ventricle

Oblique fissure

Middle lobe

Inferior lobe

Pericardium

Inferior lobe

Diaphragmatic pleura

Diaphragm

PLATE 14. HEART AND PERICARDIUM

Heart
(External View)

Left common carotid artery
Brachiocephalic artery
Left subclavian artery
Aortic arch
Ligamentum arteriosum
Superior vena cava
Left pulmonary artery
Ascending aorta
Pulmonary trunk
Left auricle
Right coronary artery
Circumflex artery
Right atrium
Great cardiac vein
Right ventricle
Anterior descending (interventricular) artery
Anterior cardiac vein
Left ventricle
Right marginal artery
Small cardiac vein
Apex

Heart
(Internal View)

Superior vena cava
Right pulmonary artery branches
Left pulmonary artery
Aorta
Pulmonary trunk
Left pulmonary veins
Right pulmonary veins
Left atrium
Pulmonary semilunar valve
Aortic semilunar valve
Right atrium
Bicuspid (left AV) valve
Tricuspid (right AV) valve
Left ventricle
Papillary muscle
Chordae tendineae
Interventricular septum
Inferior vena cava
Myocardium
Right ventricle
Trabeculae carneae

PLATE 15. CIRCULATORY SYSTEM

Vascular System

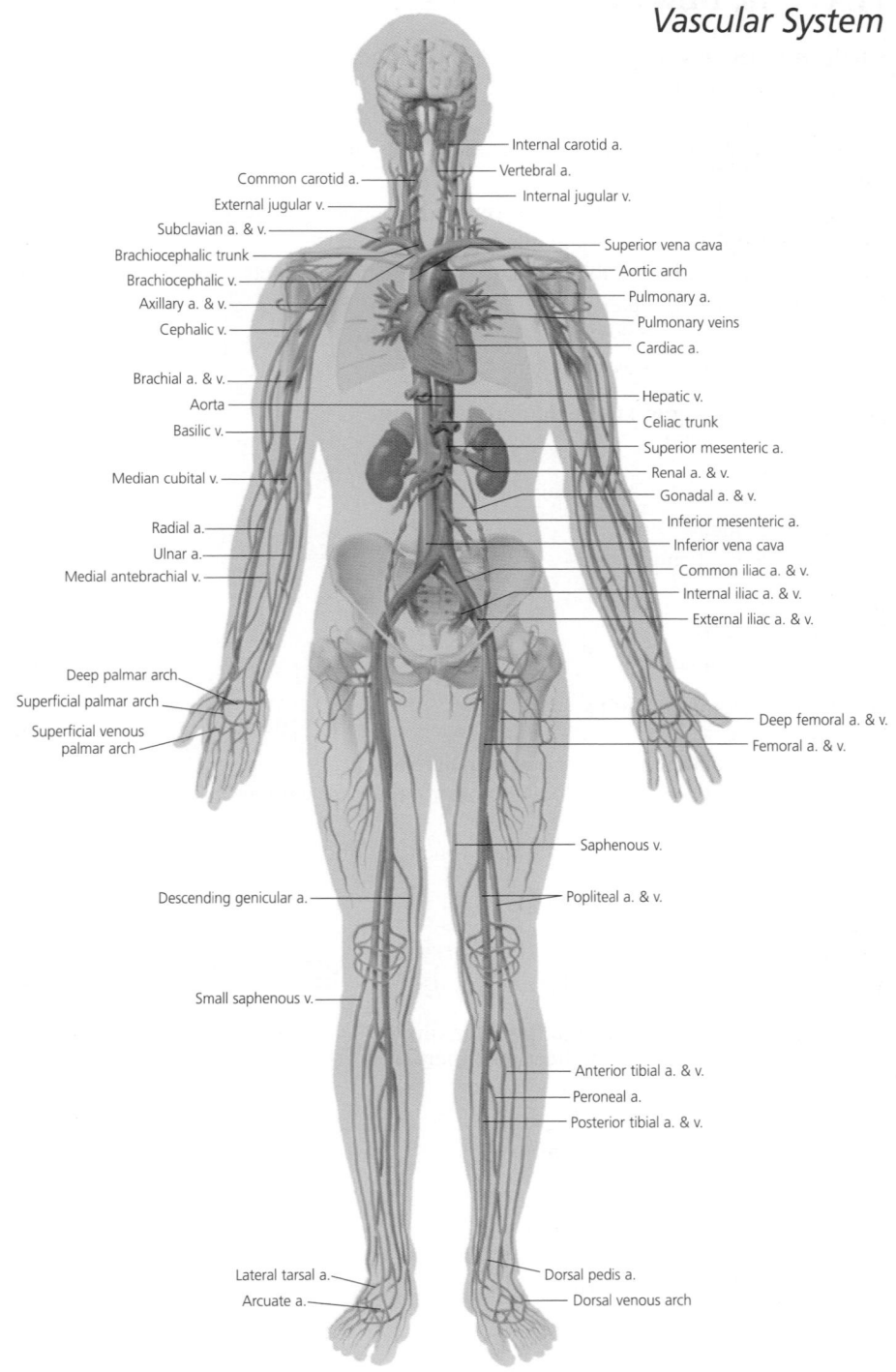

Internal carotid a.
Vertebral a.
Common carotid a.
Internal jugular v.
External jugular v.
Subclavian a. & v.
Brachiocephalic trunk
Superior vena cava
Brachiocephalic v.
Aortic arch
Axillary a. & v.
Pulmonary a.
Cephalic v.
Pulmonary veins
Cardiac a.
Brachial a. & v.
Hepatic v.
Aorta
Celiac trunk
Basilic v.
Superior mesenteric a.
Median cubital v.
Renal a. & v.
Gonadal a. & v.
Radial a.
Inferior mesenteric a.
Ulnar a.
Inferior vena cava
Medial antebrachial v.
Common iliac a. & v.
Internal iliac a. & v.
External iliac a. & v.
Deep palmar arch
Superficial palmar arch
Superficial venous palmar arch
Deep femoral a. & v.
Femoral a. & v.
Saphenous v.
Descending genicular a.
Popliteal a. & v.
Small saphenous v.
Anterior tibial a. & v.
Peroneal a.
Posterior tibial a. & v.
Lateral tarsal a.
Dorsal pedis a.
Arcuate a.
Dorsal venous arch

PLATE 16. DIGESTIVE SYSTEM

Digestive System

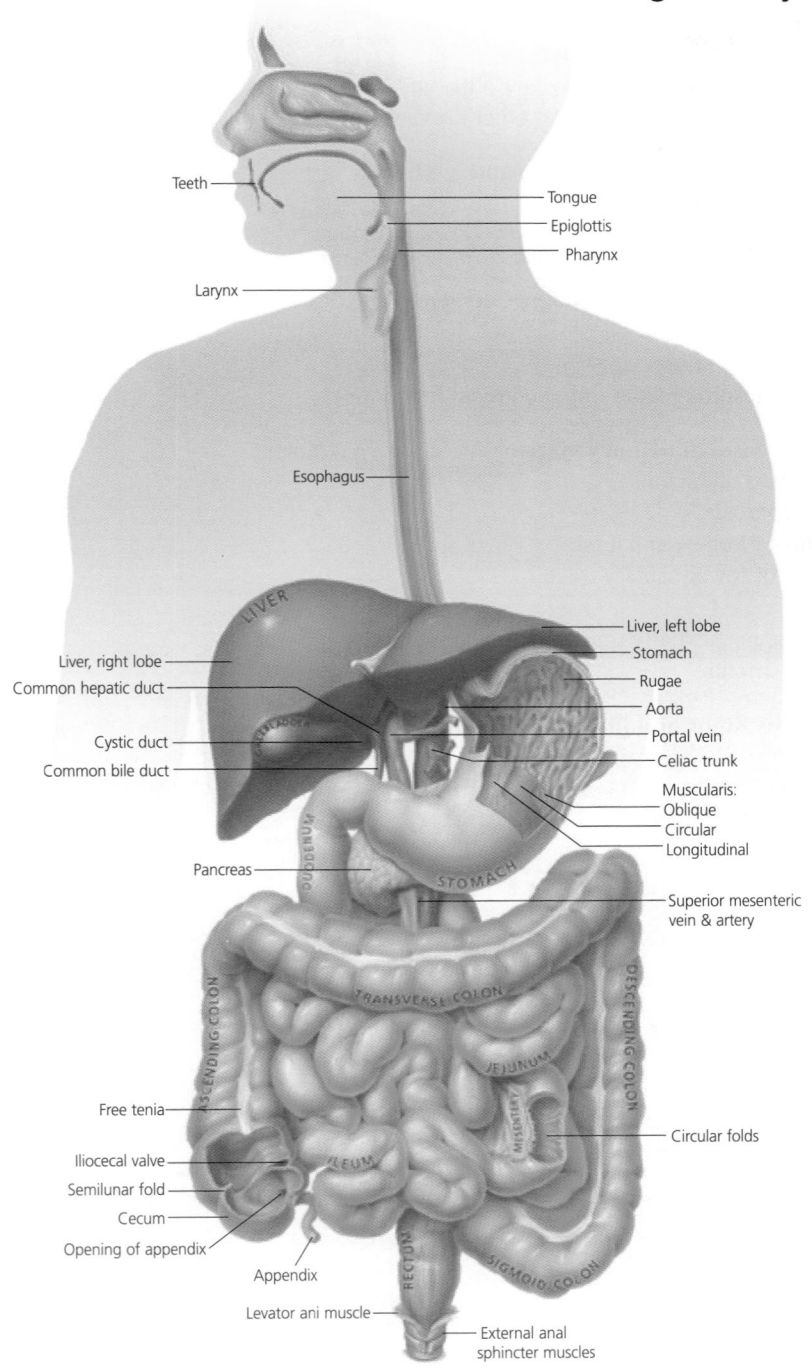

PLATE 17. GENITOURINARY SYSTEM

Urinary System

PLATE 18. MALE REPRODUCTIVE SYSTEM

Male Reproductive System

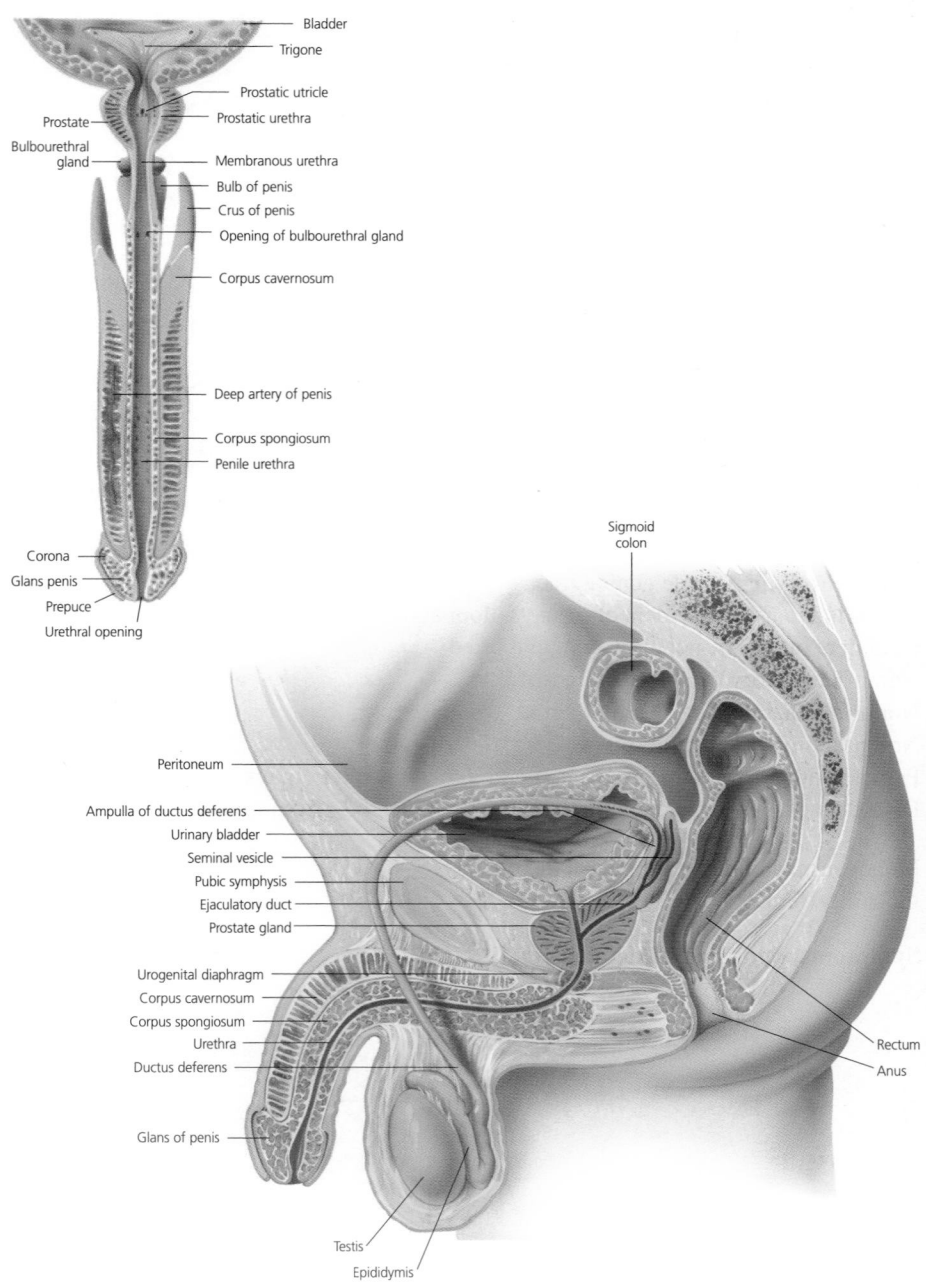

Bladder
Trigone
Prostatic utricle
Prostate
Prostatic urethra
Bulbourethral gland
Membranous urethra
Bulb of penis
Crus of penis
Opening of bulbourethral gland
Corpus cavernosum
Deep artery of penis
Corpus spongiosum
Penile urethra
Corona
Glans penis
Prepuce
Urethral opening

Sigmoid colon
Peritoneum
Ampulla of ductus deferens
Urinary bladder
Seminal vesicle
Pubic symphysis
Ejaculatory duct
Prostate gland
Urogenital diaphragm
Corpus cavernosum
Corpus spongiosum
Urethra
Ductus deferens
Glans of penis
Testis
Epididymis
Rectum
Anus

PLATE 19. FEMALE REPRODUCTIVE SYSTEM

Female Reproductive System

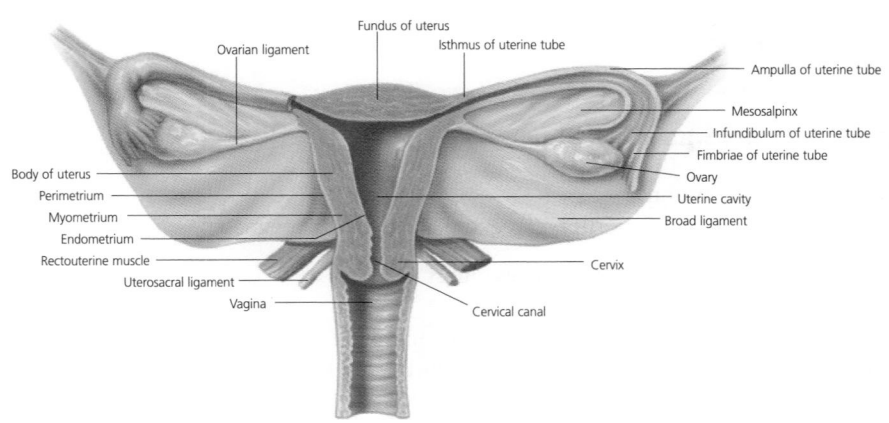

Ovarian ligament
Fundus of uterus
Isthmus of uterine tube
Ampulla of uterine tube
Mesosalpinx
Infundibulum of uterine tube
Fimbriae of uterine tube
Ovary
Body of uterus
Perimetrium
Myometrium
Endometrium
Rectouterine muscle
Uterosacral ligament
Vagina
Uterine cavity
Broad ligament
Cervix
Cervical canal

Sacrum
Suspensory ligament of ovary
Sigmoid colon
Uterine tube
Rectouterine pouch
Ovary
Round ligament of uterus
Uterus
Urinary bladder
Pubic symphysis
Cervix
Urethra
Rectum
Clitoris
Vagina
Anus
Labium minus
Labium majus
Vaginal opening

PLATE 20. PREGNANCY, CHILDBIRTH AND THE PUERPERIUM

Female Reproductive System: Pregnancy
(Lateral View)

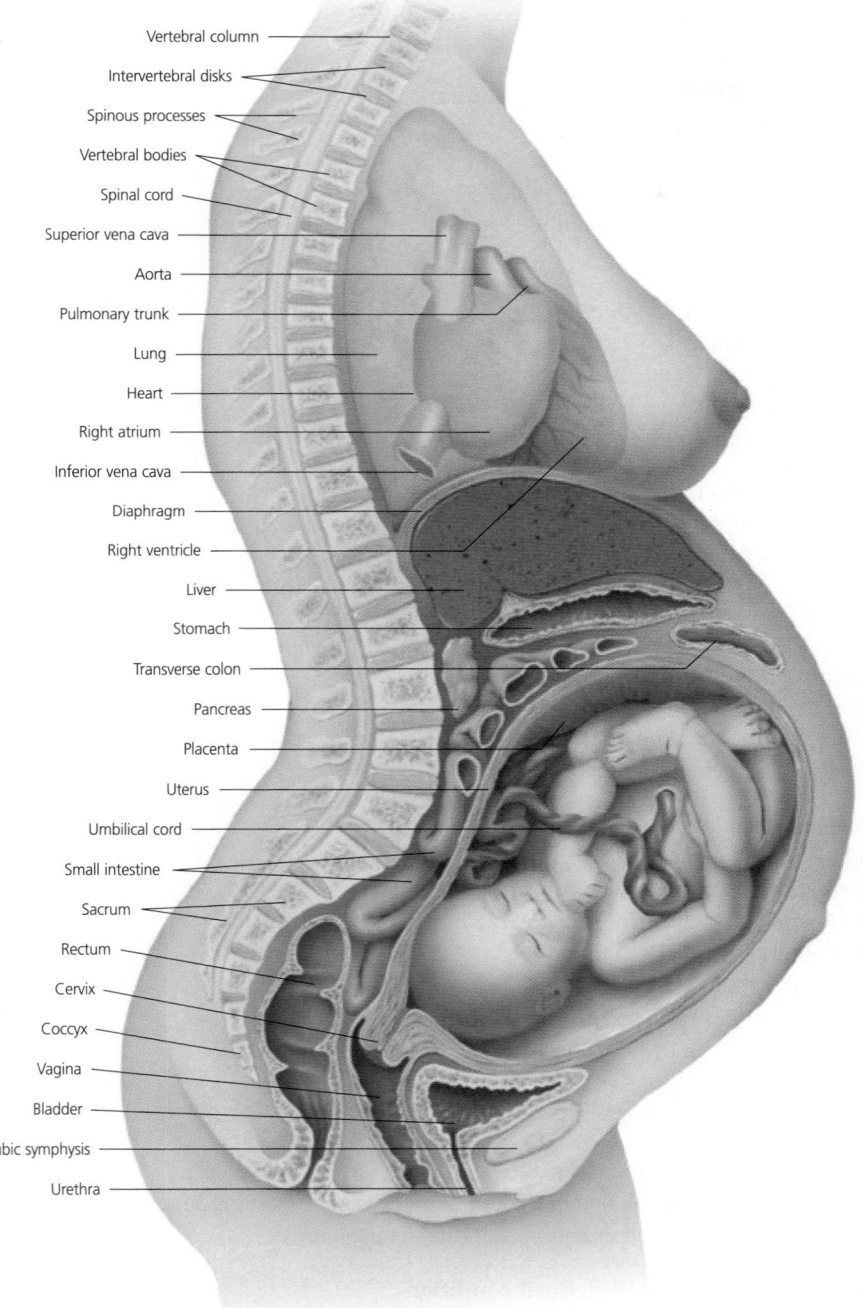

Vertebral column
Intervertebral disks
Spinous processes
Vertebral bodies
Spinal cord
Superior vena cava
Aorta
Pulmonary trunk
Lung
Heart
Right atrium
Inferior vena cava
Diaphragm
Right ventricle
Liver
Stomach
Transverse colon
Pancreas
Placenta
Uterus
Umbilical cord
Small intestine
Sacrum
Rectum
Cervix
Coccyx
Vagina
Bladder
Pubic symphysis
Urethra

PLATE 21. NERVOUS SYSTEM — BRAIN

Brain
(Base View)

Cerebrum

Anterior communicating artery

Anterior cerebral artery

Middle cerebral artery

Posterior communicating artery

Posterior cerebral artery

Superior cerebellar artery

Basilar artery

Abducens nerve

Hypoglossal nerve (XII)

Accessory nerve (XI)

Vertebral artery

Anterior spinal artery

Spinal cord

Olfactory bulb

Olfactory tract (I)

Optic nerve (II)

Optic chiasm

Internal carotid artery

Pituitary gland

Oculomotor nerve (III)

Troclear nerve (IV)

Trigeminal nerve (V)

Pons

Abducens nerve (VI)

Facial nerve (VII)

Vestibulocochlear nerve (VIII)

Glossopharyngeal nerve (IX)

Vagus nerve (X)

Anterior inferior cerebellar artery

Medulla oblongata

Cerebellum

Posterior inferior cerebellar artery

PLATE 22. NERVOUS SYSTEM

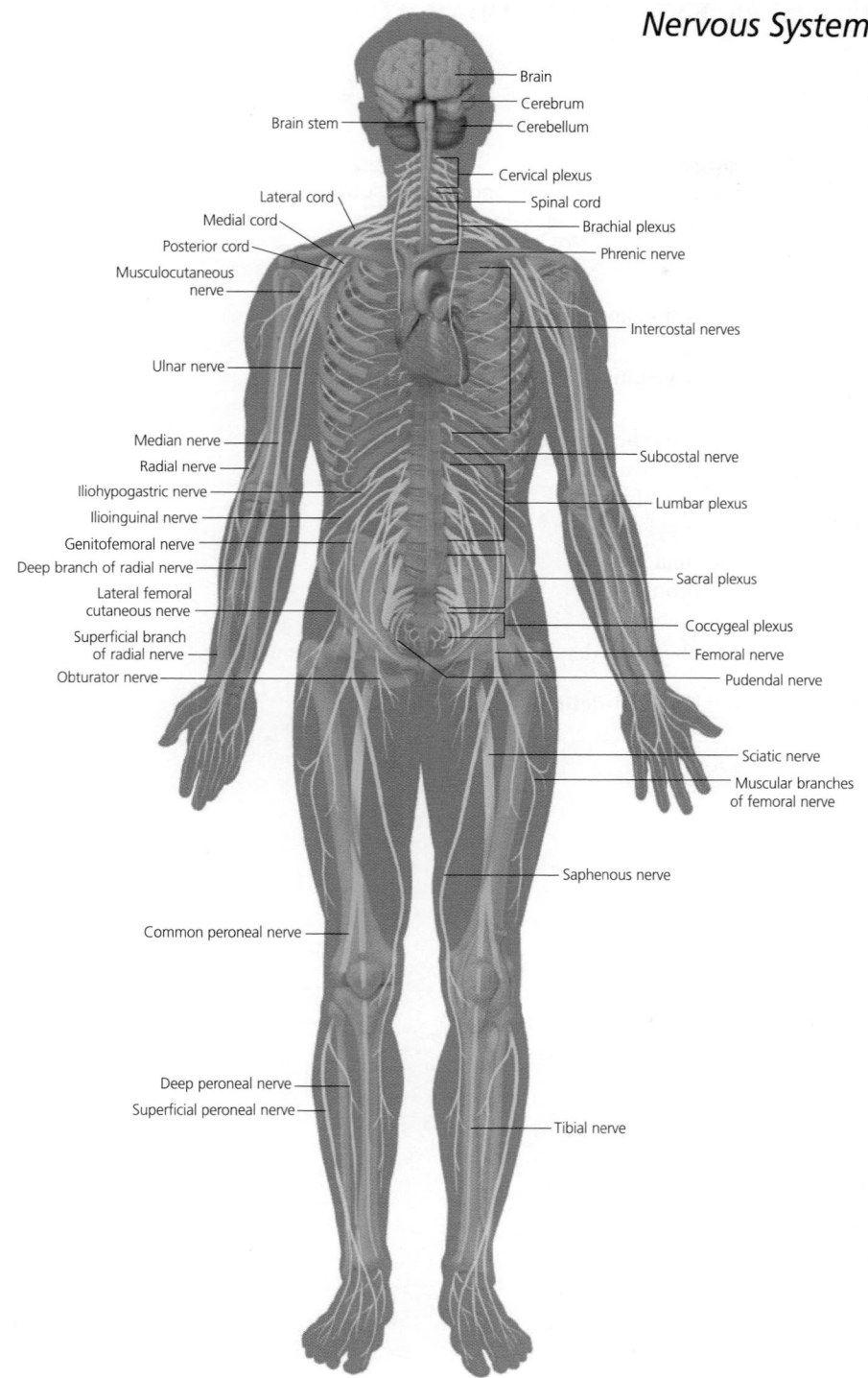

Nervous System

PLATE 23. EYE AND OCULAR ADNEXA

Right Eye
(Horizontal Section)

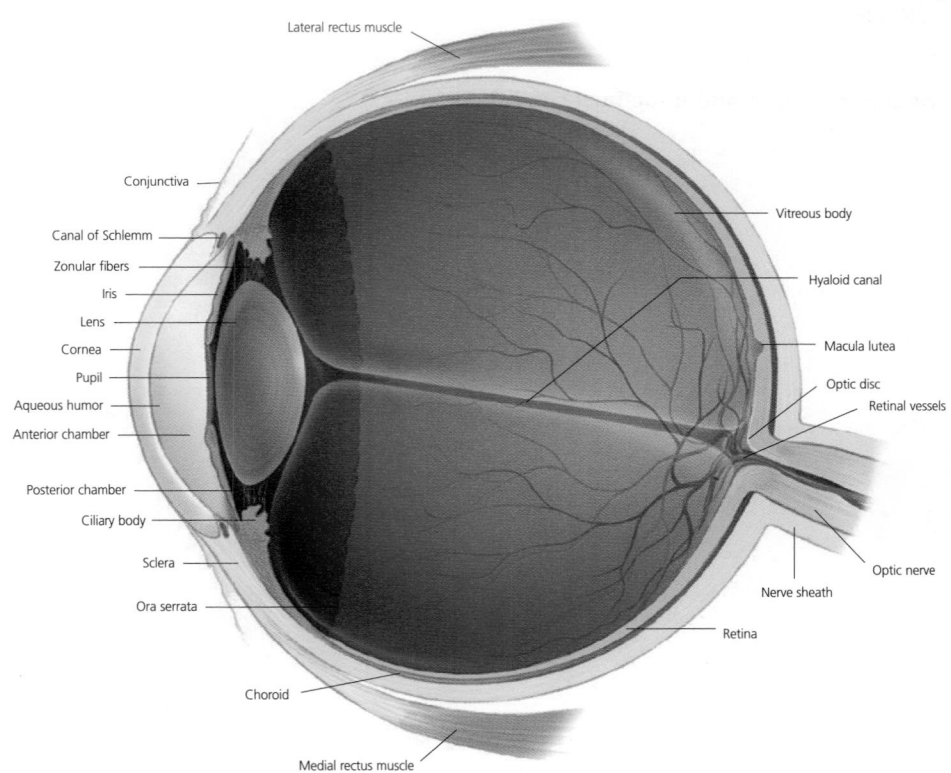

Lateral rectus muscle

Conjunctiva

Canal of Schlemm

Zonular fibers

Iris

Lens

Cornea

Pupil

Aqueous humor

Anterior chamber

Posterior chamber

Ciliary body

Sclera

Ora serrata

Choroid

Medial rectus muscle

Vitreous body

Hyaloid canal

Macula lutea

Optic disc

Retinal vessels

Optic nerve

Nerve sheath

Retina

PLATE 24. AUDITORY SYSTEM

The Ear

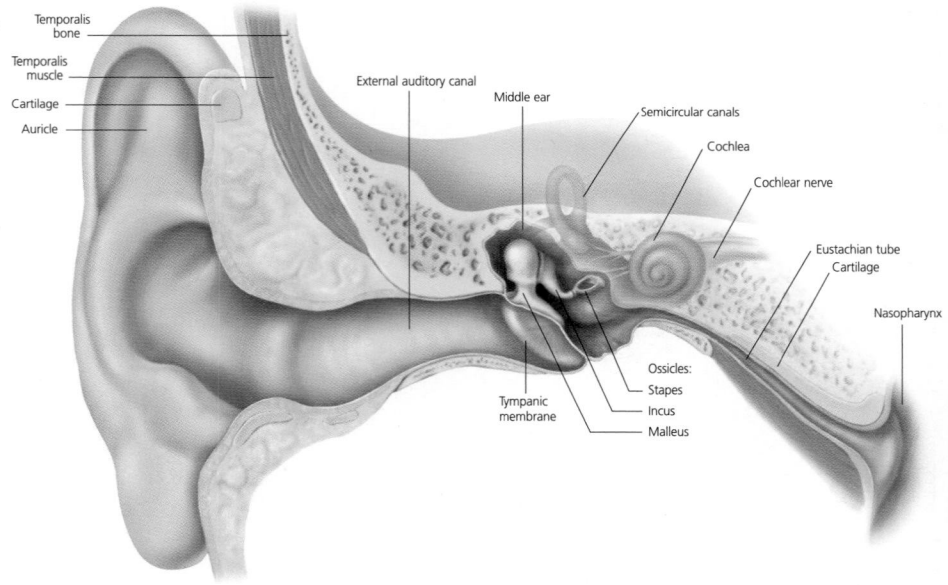

Temporalis
bone

Temporalis
muscle

Cartilage

Auricle

External auditory canal

Middle ear

Semicircular canals

Cochlea

Cochlear nerve

Eustachian tube
Cartilage

Nasopharynx

Ossicles:
Stapes
Incus
Malleus

Tympanic
membrane

DISEASES: TABULAR LIST

VOLUME 1

1. INFECTIOUS AND PARASITIC DISEASES (001-139)

Note: Categories for "late effects" of infectious and parasitic diseases are to be found at 137-139.

Includes: diseases generally recognized as communicable or transmissible as well as a few diseases of unknown but possibly infectious origin

Excludes: acute respiratory infections (460-466)
carrier or suspected carrier of infectious organism (V02.0-V02.9)
certain localized infections
influenza (487.0-487.8, 488.0-488.1)

INTESTINAL INFECTIOUS DISEASES (001-009)

Excludes: helminthiases (120.0-129)

001 Cholera

001.0 Due to Vibrio cholerae

001.1 Due to Vibrio cholerae el tor

001.9 Cholera, unspecified

002 Typhoid and paratyphoid fevers

002.0 Typhoid fever
Typhoid (fever) (infection) [any site]

002.1 Paratyphoid fever A

002.2 Paratyphoid fever B

002.3 Paratyphoid fever C

002.9 Paratyphoid fever, unspecified

003 Other salmonella infections
Includes: infection or food poisoning by Salmonella [any serotype]

003.0 Salmonella gastroenteritis
Salmonellosis

003.1 Salmonella septicemia

⑤ **003.2 Localized salmonella infections**

003.20 Localized salmonella infection, unspecified

003.21 Salmonella meningitis

003.22 Salmonella pneumonia

003.23 Salmonella arthritis

003.24 Salmonella osteomyelitis

003.29 Other

003.8 Other specified salmonella infections

003.9 Salmonella infection, unspecified

004 Shigellosis
Includes: bacillary dysentery

004.0 Shigella dysenteriae
Infection by group A Shigella (Schmitz) (Shiga)

004.1 Shigella flexneri
Infection by group B Shigella

004.2 Shigella boydii
Infection by group C Shigella

004.3 Shigella sonnei
Infection by group D Shigella

004.8 Other specified shigella infections

004.9 Shigellosis, unspecified

005 Other food poisoning (bacterial)

Excludes: salmonella infections (003.0-003.9)
toxic effect of:
food contaminants (989.7)
noxious foodstuffs (988.0-988.9)

005.0 Staphylococcal food poisoning
Staphylococcal toxemia specified as due to food

Add 4th or 5th digit | Nonspecific code | Unspecified code | Manifestation code

005.1 Botulism food poisoning
Botulism NOS
Food poisoning due to Clostridium botulinum

Excludes: *infant botulism (040.41)*
wound botulism (040.42)

005.2 Food poisoning due to Clostridium perfringens [C. welchii]
Enteritis necroticans

005.3 Food poisoning due to other Clostridia

005.4 Food poisoning due to Vibrio parahaemolyticus

⑤ **005.8 Other bacterial food poisoning**

Excludes: *salmonella food poisoning (003.0-003.9)*

　　　005.81 Food poisoning due to Vibrio vulnificus

　　　005.89 Other bacterial food poisoning
　　　Food poisoning due to Bacillus cereus

005.9 Food poisoning, unspecified

006 Amebiasis
Includes:　infection due to Entamoeba histolytica

Excludes: *amebiasis due to organisms other than Entamoeba histolytica (007.8)*

006.0 Acute amebic dysentery without mention of abscess
Acute amebiasis

006.1 Chronic intestinal amebiasis without mention of abscess
Chronic:
amebiasis
amebic dysentery

006.2 Amebic nondysenteric colitis

006.3 Amebic liver abscess
Hepatic amebiasis

006.4 Amebic lung abscess
Amebic abscess of lung (and liver)

006.5 Amebic brain abscess
Amebic abscess of brain (and liver) (and lung)

006.6 Amebic skin ulceration
Cutaneous amebiasis

006.8 Amebic infection of other sites
Amebic:　　　　　　　　　Ameboma
appendicitis
balanitis

Excludes: *specific infections by free-living amebae (136.21-136.29)*

006.9 Amebiasis, unspecified
Amebiasis NOS

007 Other protozoal intestinal diseases
Includes:　protozoal:
colitis
diarrhea
dysentery

007.0 Balantidiasis
Infection by Balantidium coli

007.1 Giardiasis
Infection by Giardia lamblia
Lambliasis

007.2 Coccidiosis
Infection by Isospora belli and Isospora hominis
Isosporiasis

007.3 Intestinal trichomoniasis

007.4 Cryptosporidiosis

007.5 Cyclosporiasis

007.8 Other specified protozoal intestinal diseases
Amebiasis due to organisms other than Entamoeba histolytica

007.9 Unspecified protozoal intestinal disease
Flagellate diarrhea　　　　　　Protozoal dysentery NOS

● Code new
　to this edition　　　　　▲ Revision of
　　　　　　　　　　　　　　existing code　　　　④ ⑤ Fourth or fifth
　　　　　　　　　　　　　　　　　　　　　　　digit required

008 **Intestinal infections due to other organisms**
Includes: any condition classifiable to 009.0-009.3 with mention of the responsible organisms

Excludes: food poisoning by these organisms (005.0-005.9)

⑤ **008.0** **Escherichia coli [E. coli]**

008.00 **E. coli, unspecified**
E. coli enteritis NOS

008.01 **Enteropathogenic E. coli**

008.02 **Enterotoxigenic E. coli**

008.03 **Enteroinvasive E. coli**

008.04 **Enterohemorrhagic E. coli**

008.09 **Other intestinal E. coli infections**

008.1 **Arizona group of paracolon bacilli**

008.2 **Aerobacter aerogenes**
Enterobacter aerogenes

008.3 **Proteus (mirabilis) (morganii)**

⑤ **008.4** **Other specified bacteria**

008.41 **Staphylococcus**
Staphylococcal enterocolitis

008.42 **Pseudomonas**

008.43 **Campylobacter**

008.44 **Yersinia enterocolitica**

008.45 **Clostridium difficile**
Pseudomembranous colitis

008.46 **Other anaerobes**
Anaerobic enteritis NOS
Bacteroides (fragilis)
Gram-negative anaerobes

008.47 **Other Gram-negative bacteria**
Gram-negative enteritis NOS

Excludes: Gram-negative anaerobes (008.46)

008.49 **Other**

008.5 **Bacterial enteritis, unspecified**

⑤ **008.6** **Enteritis due to specified virus**

008.61 **Rotavirus**

008.62 **Adenovirus**

008.63 **Norwalk virus**
Norovirus
Norwalk-like agent

008.64 **Other small round viruses [SRV's]**
Small round virus NOS

▲ **008.65** **Calicivirus**

008.66 **Astrovirus**

008.67 **Enterovirus NEC**
Coxsackie virus
Echovirus

Excludes: poliovirus (045.0-045.9)

008.69 **Other viral enteritis**
Torovirus

008.8 **Other organism, not elsewhere classified**
Viral:
enteritis NOS
gastroenteritis

Excludes: influenza with involvement of gastrointestinal tract (487.8)

| | Add 4th or 5th digit | | Nonspecific code | | Unspecified code | | Manifestation code |

009 **Ill-defined intestinal infections**

Excludes: *diarrheal disease or intestinal infection due to specified organism (001.0-008.8)*
diarrhea following gastrointestinal surgery (564.4)
intestinal malabsorption (579.0-579.9)
ischemic enteritis (557.0-557.9)
other noninfectious gastroenteritis and colitis (558.1-558.9)
regional enteritis (555.0-555.9)
ulcerative colitis (556)

009.0 **Infectious colitis, enteritis, and gastroenteritis**

Colitis, septic	Dysentery:
Enteritis, septic	NOS
Gastroenteritis, septic	catarrhal
	hemorrhagic

009.1 **Colitis, enteritis, and gastroenteritis of presumed infectious origin**

Excludes: *colitis NOS (558.9)*
enteritis NOS (558.9)
gastroenteritis NOS (558.9)

009.2 **Infectious diarrhea**

Diarrhea: Infectious diarrheal disease NOS
dysenteric
epidemic

009.3 **Diarrhea of presumed infectious origin**

Excludes: *diarrhea NOS (787.91)*

TUBERCULOSIS (010-018)

Includes: infection by Mycobacterium tuberculosis (human) (bovine)

Excludes: *congenital tuberculosis (771.2)*
late effects of tuberculosis (137.0-137.4)

The following fifth-digit subclassification is for use with categories 010-018:

0 **unspecified**
1 **bacteriological or histological examination not done**
2 **bacteriological or histological examination unknown (at present)**
3 **tubercle bacilli found (in sputum) by microscopy**
4 **tubercle bacilli not found (in sputum) by microscopy, but found by bacterial culture**
5 **tubercle bacilli not found by bacteriological examination, but tuberculosis confirmed histologically**
6 **tubercle bacilli not found by bacteriological or histological examination but tuberculosis confirmed by other methods [inoculation of animals]**

⑤ **010** **Primary tuberculous infection**

Excludes: *nonspecific reaction to tuberculin skin test without active tuberculosis (795.5)*
positive PPD (795.5)
positive tuberculin skin test without active tuberculosis (795.5)

⑤ **010.0** **Primary tuberculous complex**
[0-6]

⑤ **010.1** **Tuberculous pleurisy in primary progressive tuberculosis**
[0-6]

⑤ **010.8** **Other primary progressive tuberculosis**
[0-6]

Excludes: *tuberculous erythema nodosum (017.1)*

⑤ **010.9** **Primary tuberculous infection, unspecified**
[0-6]

⑤ **011** **Pulmonary tuberculosis**
Use additional code, if desired, to identify any associated silicosis (502)

⑤ **011.0** **Tuberculosis of lung, infiltrative**
[0-6]

⑤ **011.1** **Tuberculosis of lung, nodular**
[0-6]

⑤ **011.2** **Tuberculosis of lung with cavitation**
[0-6]

⑤ **011.3** **Tuberculosis of bronchus**
[0-6]

> Excludes: *isolated bronchial tuberculosis (012.2)*

⑤ **011.4** **Tuberculous fibrosis of lung**
[0-6]

⑤ **011.5** **Tuberculous bronchiectasis**
[0-6]

⑤ **011.6** **Tuberculous pneumonia [any form]**
[0-6]

⑤ **011.7** **Tuberculous pneumothorax**
[0-6]

⑤ **011.8** **Other specified pulmonary tuberculosis**
[0-6]

⑤ **011.9** **Pulmonary tuberculosis, unspecified**
[0-6] Respiratory tuberculosis NOS
Tuberculosis of lung NOS

⑤ **012** **Other respiratory tuberculosis**

> Excludes: *respiratory tuberculosis, unspecified (011.9)*

⑤ **012.0** **Tuberculous pleurisy**
[0-6] Tuberculosis of pleura
Tuberculous empyema
Tuberculous hydrothorax

> Excludes: *pleurisy with effusion without mention of cause (511.9)*
> *tuberculous pleurisy in primary progressive tuberculosis (010.1)*

⑤ **012.1** **Tuberculosis of intrathoracic lymph nodes**
[0-6] Tuberculosis of lymph nodes:
hilar
mediastinal
tracheobronchial
Tuberculous tracheobronchial adenopathy

> Excludes: *that specified as primary (010.0-010.9)*

⑤ **012.2** **Isolated tracheal or bronchial tuberculosis**
[0-6]

⑤ **012.3** **Tuberculous laryngitis**
[0-6] Tuberculosis of glottis

⑤ **012.8** **Other specified respiratory tuberculosis**
[0-6] Tuberculosis of: Tuberculosis of:
mediastinum   nose (septum)
nasopharynx   sinus [any nasal]

⑤ **013** **Tuberculosis of meninges and central nervous system**

⑤ **013.0** **Tuberculous meningitis**
[0-6] Tuberculosis of meninges   Tuberculous:
(cerebral) (spinal)   leptomeningitis
meningoencephalitis

> Excludes: *tuberculoma of meninges (013.1)*

⑤ **013.1** **Tuberculoma of meninges**
[0-6]

⑤ **013.2** **Tuberculoma of brain**
[0-6] Tuberculosis of brain (current disease)

⑤ **013.3** **Tuberculous abscess of brain**
[0-6]

⑤ **013.4** **Tuberculoma of spinal cord**
[0-6]

⑤ **013.5** **Tuberculous abscess of spinal cord**
[0-6]

⑤ **013.6** **Tuberculous encephalitis or myelitis**
[0-6]

⑤ **013.8** **Other specified tuberculosis of central nervous system**
[0-6]

	Add 4th or 5th digit		Nonspecific code		Unspecified code		Manifestation code

⑤ **013.9 Unspecified tuberculosis of central nervous system**
[0-6]   Tuberculosis of central nervous system NOS

⑤ **014 Tuberculosis of intestines, peritoneum, and mesenteric glands**

   ⑤ **014.0 Tuberculous peritonitis**
   [0-6]   Tuberculous ascites

   ⑤ **014.8 Other**
   [0-6]   Tuberculosis (of):   Tuberculous enteritis
                  anus
                  intestine (large) (small)
                  mesenteric glands
                  rectum
                  retroperitoneal (lymph nodes)

⑤ **015 Tuberculosis of bones and joints**
     Use additional code, if desired, to identify manifestation, as:
       tuberculous:
         arthropathy (711.4)
         necrosis of bone (730.8)
         osteitis (730.8)
         osteomyelitis (730.8)
         synovitis (727.01)
         tenosynovitis (727.01)

   ⑤ **015.0 Vertebral column**
   [0-6]   Pott's disease
     Use additional code, if desired, to identify manifestation, as:
         curvature of spine [Pott's] (737.4)
         kyphosis (737.4)
         spondylitis (720.81)

   ⑤ **015.1 Hip**
   [0-6]

   ⑤ **015.2 Knee**
   [0-6]

   ⑤ **015.5 Limb bones**
   [0-6]   Tuberculous dactylitis

   ⑤ **015.6 Mastoid**
   [0-6]   Tuberculous mastoiditis

   ⑤ **015.7 Other specified bone**
   [0-6]

   ⑤ **015.8 Other specified joint**
   [0-6]

   ⑤ **015.9 Tuberculosis of unspecified bones and joints**
   [0-6]

⑤ **016 Tuberculosis of genitourinary system**

   ⑤ **016.0 Kidney**
   [0-6]   Renal tuberculosis
     Use additional code, if desired, to identify manifestation, as:
         tuberculous:
           nephropathy (583.81)
           pyelitis (590.81)
           pyelonephritis (590.81)

   ⑤ **016.1 Bladder**
   [0-6]

   ⑤ **016.2 Ureter**
   [0-6]

   ⑤ **016.3 Other urinary organs**
   [0-6]

   ⑤ **016.4 Epididymis**
   [0-6]

   ⑤ **016.5 Other male genital organs**
   [0-6]
     Use additional code, if desired, to identify manifestation, as:
         tuberculosis of:
           prostate (601.4)
           seminal vesicle (608.81)
           testis (608.81)

● Code new   ▲ Revision of   ④ ⑤ Fourth or fifth
   to this edition   existing code   digit required

⑤ **016.6 Tuberculous oophoritis and salpingitis**
[0-6]

⑤ **016.7 Other female genital organs**
[0-6]   Tuberculous:
             cervicitis
             endometritis

⑤ **016.9 Genitourinary tuberculosis, unspecified**
[0-6]

⑤ **017 Tuberculosis of other organs**

⑤ **017.0 Skin and subcutaneous cellular tissue**
[0-6]   Lupus: Tuberculosis:
             exedens   colliquativa
             vulgaris   cutis
         Scrofuloderma   lichenoides
                                           papulonecrotica
                                           verrucosa cutis

   Excludes: lupus erythematosus (695.4)
                disseminated (710.0)
                lupus NOS (710.0)
                nonspecific reaction to tuberculin skin test without active tuberculosis (795.5)
                positive PPD (795.5)
                positive tuberculin skin test without active tuberculosis (795.5)

⑤ **017.1 Erythema nodosum with hypersensitivity reaction in tuberculosis**
[0-6]   Bazin's disease   Tuberculosis indurativa
         Erythema:
             induratum
             nodosum, tuberculous

   Excludes: erythema nodosum NOS (695.2)

⑤ **017.2 Peripheral lymph nodes**
[0-6]   Scrofula   Tuberculous adenitis
         Scrofulous abscess

   Excludes: tuberculosis of lymph nodes:
                bronchial and mediastinal (012.1)
                mesenteric and retroperitoneal (014.8)
                tuberculous tracheobronchial adenopathy (012.1)

⑤ **017.3 Eye**
[0-6]

Use additional code, if desired, to identify manifestation, as:
             tuberculous:
                 chorioretinitis, disseminated (363.13)
                 episcleritis (379.09)
                 interstitial keratitis (370.59)
                 iridocyclitis, chronic (364.11)
                 keratoconjunctivitis (phlyctenular) (370.31)

⑤ **017.4 Ear**
[0-6]   Tuberculosis of ear
         Tuberculous otitis media

   Excludes: tuberculous mastoiditis (015.6)

⑤ **017.5 Thyroid gland**
[0-6]

⑤ **017.6 Adrenal glands**
[0-6]   Addison's disease, tuberculous

⑤ **017.7 Spleen**
[0-6]

⑤ **017.8 Esophagus**
[0-6]

⑤ **017.9 Other specified organs**
[0-6]

Use additional code, if desired, to identify manifestation, as:
             tuberculosis of:
                 endocardium [any valve] (424.91)
                 myocardium (422.0)
                 pericardium (420.0)

| | Add 4th or 5th digit | | Nonspecific code | | Unspecified code | | Manifestation code |

⑤ **018** **Miliary tuberculosis**
  Includes: tuberculosis:
    disseminated
    generalized
    miliary, whether of a single specified site, multiple sites, or unspecified site
    polyserositis

⑤ **018.0** **Acute miliary tuberculosis**
  [0-6]

⑤ **018.8** **Other specified miliary tuberculosis**
  [0-6]

⑤ **018.9** **Miliary tuberculosis, unspecified**
  [0-6]

ZOONOTIC BACTERIAL DISEASES (020-027)

020 **Plague**
  Includes: infection by Yersinia [Pasteurella] pestis

  020.0 **Bubonic**

  020.1 **Cellulocutaneous**

  020.2 **Septicemic**

  020.3 **Primary pneumonic**

  020.4 **Secondary pneumonic**

  020.5 **Pneumonic, unspecified**

  020.8 **Other specified types of plague**
    Abortive plague   Pestis minor
    Ambulatory plague

  020.9 **Plague, unspecified**

021 **Tularemia**
  Includes: deerfly fever
    infection by Francisella [Pasteurella] tularensis
    rabbit fever

  021.0 **Ulceroglandular tularemia**

  021.1 **Enteric tularemia**
    Tularemia:
      cryptogenic
      intestinal
      typhoidal

  021.2 **Pulmonary tularemia**
    Bronchopneumonic tularemia

  021.3 **Oculoglandular tularemia**

  021.8 **Other specified tularemia**
    Tularemia:
      generalized or disseminated
      glandular

  021.9 **Unspecified tularemia**

022 **Anthrax**

  022.0 **Cutaneous anthrax**
    Malignant pustule

  022.1 **Pulmonary anthrax**
    Respiratory anthrax
    Wool-sorters' disease

  022.2 **Gastrointestinal anthrax**

  022.3 **Anthrax septicemia**

  022.8 **Other specified manifestations of anthrax**

  022.9 **Anthrax, unspecified**

023 **Brucellosis**
  Includes: fever:
    Malta
    Mediterranean
    undulant

  023.0 **Brucella melitensis**

  023.1 **Brucella abortus**

● Code new   ▲ Revision of   ④ ⑤ Fourth or fifth
   to this edition   existing code   digit required

023.2 Brucella suis

023.3 Brucella canis

023.8 Other brucellosis
Infection by more than one organism

023.9 Brucellosis, unspecified

024 Glanders
Infection by: Farcy
  Actinobacillus mallei   Malleus
  Malleomyces mallei
  Pseudomonas mallei

025 Melioidosis
Infection by:
  Malleomyces pseudomallei
  Pseudomonas pseudomallei
  Whitmore's bacillus
  Pseudoglanders

026 Rat-bite fever

026.0 Spirillary fever
Rat-bite fever due to Spirillum minor [S. minus]
Sodoku

026.1 Streptobacillary fever
Epidemic arthritic erythema
Haverhill fever
Rat-bite fever due to Streptobacillus moniliformis

026.9 Unspecified rat-bite fever

027 Other zoonotic bacterial diseases

027.0 Listeriosis
Infection by Listeria monocytogenes
Septicemia by Listeria monocytogenes

Use additional code to identify manifestations, as meningitis (320.7)

> *Excludes:* congenital listeriosis (771.2)

027.1 Erysipelothrix infection
Erysipeloid (of Rosenbach)
Infection by Erysipelothrix insidiosa [E. rhusiopathiae]
Septicemia by Erysipelothrix insidiosa [E. rhusiopathiae]

027.2 Pasteurellosis
Pasteurella pseudotuberculosis infection
Mesenteric adenitis by Pasteurella multocida [P. septica]
Septic infection (cat bite) (dog bite) by Pasteurella multocida [P. septica]

> *Excludes:* infection by:
>   Francisella [Pasteurella] tularensis (021.0-021.9)
>   Yersinia [Pasteurella] pestis (020.0-020.9)

027.8 Other specified zoonotic bacterial diseases

027.9 Unspecified zoonotic bacterial disease

OTHER BACTERIAL DISEASES (030-041)

> *Excludes:* bacterial venereal diseases (098.0-099.9)
>   bartonellosis (088.0)

030 Leprosy
Includes: Hansen's disease
    infection by Mycobacterium leprae

030.0 Lepromatous [type L]
Lepromatous leprosy (macular) (diffuse) (infiltrated) (nodular) (neuritic)

030.1 Tuberculoid [type T]
Tuberculoid leprosy (macular) (maculoanesthetic) (major) (minor) (neuritic)

030.2 Indeterminate [group I]
Indeterminate [uncharacteristic] leprosy (macular) (neuritic)

030.3 Borderline [group B]
Borderline or dimorphous leprosy (infiltrated) (neuritic)

030.8 Other specified leprosy

030.9 Leprosy, unspecified

	Add 4th or 5th digit		Nonspecific code		Unspecified code		Manifestation code

031 **Diseases due to other mycobacteria**

031.0 **Pulmonary**
Infection by Mycobacterium:
avium
intracellulare [Battey bacillus]
kansasii
Battey disease

031.1 **Cutaneous**
Buruli ulcer
Infection by Mycobacterium:
marinum [M. balnei]
ulcerans

031.2 **Disseminated**
Disseminated mycobacterium avium-intracellulare complex (DMAC)
Mycobacterium avium-intracellulare complex (MAC) bacteremia

031.8 **Other specified mycobacterial diseases**

031.9 **Unspecified diseases due to mycobacteria**
Atypical mycobacterium infection NOS

032 **Diphtheria**
Includes: infection by Corynebacterium diphtheriae

032.0 **Faucial diphtheria**
Membranous angina, diphtheritic

032.1 **Nasopharyngeal diphtheria**

032.2 **Anterior nasal diphtheria**

032.3 **Laryngeal diphtheria**
Laryngotracheitis, diphtheritic

⑤ **032.8** **Other specified diphtheria**

    032.81 **Conjunctival diphtheria**
        Pseudomembranous diphtheritic conjunctivitis

    032.82 **Diphtheritic myocarditis**

    032.83 **Diphtheritic peritonitis**

    032.84 **Diphtheritic cystitis**

    032.85 **Cutaneous diphtheria**

    032.89 **Other**

032.9 **Diphtheria, unspecified**

033 **Whooping cough**
Includes: pertussis

Use additional code, if desired, to identify any associated pneumonia (484.3)

033.0 **Bordetella pertussis [B. pertussis]**

033.1 **Bordetella parapertussis [B. parapertussis]**

033.8 **Whooping cough due to other specified organism**
Bordetella bronchiseptica [B. bronchiseptica]

033.9 **Whooping cough, unspecified organism**

034 **Streptococcal sore throat and scarlet fever**

034.0 **Streptococcal sore throat**
Septic: Streptococcal:
angina   angina
sore throat   laryngitis
                          pharyngitis
                          tonsillitis

034.1 **Scarlet fever**
Scarlatina

Excludes: *parascarlatina (057.8)*

035 **Erysipelas**

Excludes: *postpartum or puerperal erysipelas (670.8)*

● Code new
to this edition   ▲ Revision of
existing code   ④ ⑤ Fourth or fifth
digit required

036 **Meningococcal infection**

036.0 **Meningococcal meningitis**
Cerebrospinal fever
(meningococcal)

Meningitis:
cerebrospinal
epidemic

036.1 **Meningococcal encephalitis**

036.2 **Meningococcemia**
Meningococcal septicemia

036.3 **Waterhouse-Friderichsen syndrome, meningococcal**
Meningococcal hemorrhagic adrenalitis
Meningococcic adrenal syndrome
Waterhouse-Friderichsen syndrome NOS

⑤ **036.4** **Meningococcal carditis**

036.40 **Meningococcal carditis, unspecified**

036.41 **Meningococcal pericarditis**

036.42 **Meningococcal endocarditis**

036.43 **Meningococcal myocarditis**

⑤ **036.8** **Other specified meningococcal infections**

036.81 **Meningococcal optic neuritis**

036.82 **Meningococcal arthropathy**

036.89 **Other**

036.9 **Meningococcal infection, unspecified**
Meningococcal infection NOS

037 **Tetanus**
Excludes: *tetanus:*
complicating:
abortion (634-638 with .0, 639.0)
ectopic or molar pregnancy (639.0)
neonatorum (771.3)
puerperal (670.8)

038 **Septicemia**
Excludes: *bacteremia (790.7)*
during labor (659.3)
following ectopic or molar pregnancy (639.0)
following infusion, injection, transfusion, or vaccination (999.3)
postpartum, puerperal (670)
septicemia (sepsis) of newborn (771.81)
that complicating abortion (634-638 with .0, 639.0)

Use additional code for systemic inflammatory response syndrome (SIRS) (995.91-995.92)

038.0 **Streptococcal septicemia**

⑤ **038.1** **Staphylococcal septicemia**

038.10 **Staphylococcal septicemia, unspecified**

038.11 **Methicillin susceptible Staphylococcus aureus septicemia**
MSSA septicemia
Staphylococcus aureus septicemia NOS

038.12 **Methicillin resistant Staphylococcus aureus septicemia**

038.19 **Other staphylococcal septicemia**

038.2 **Pneumococcal septicemia**

038.3 **Septicemia due to anaerobes**
Septicemia due to bacteroides
Excludes: *gas gangrene (040.0)*
that due to anaerobic streptococci (038.0)

⑤ **038.4** **Septicemia due to other gram-negative organisms**

038.40 **Gram-negative organism, unspecified**
Gram-negative septicemia NOS

038.41 **Hemophilus influenzae [H. influenzae]**

038.42 **Escherichia coli [E. coli]**

038.43 **Pseudomonas**

038.44 **Serratia**

Add 4th or
5th digit

Nonspecific
code

Unspecified
code

Manifestation
code

038.49 Other

038.8 Other specified septicemias

> *Excludes:* septicemia (due to):
>> anthrax (022.3)
>> gonococcal (098.89)
>> herpetic (054.5)
>> meningococcal (036.2)
>> septicemic plague (020.2)

038.9 Unspecified septicemia
   Septicemia NOS

> *Excludes:* bacteremia NOS (790.7)

039 Actinomycotic infections
   Includes: actinomycotic mycetoma
      infection by Actinomycetales, such as species of Actinomyces, Actinomadura,
         Nocardia, Streptomyces
      maduromycosis (actinomycotic)
      schizomycetoma (actinomycotic)

039.0 Cutaneous
   Erythrasma   Trichomycosis axillaris

039.1 Pulmonary
   Thoracic actinomycosis

039.2 Abdominal

039.3 Cervicofacial

039.4 Madura foot

> *Excludes:* madura foot due to mycotic infection (117.4)

039.8 Of other specified sites

039.9 Of unspecified site
   Actinomycosis NOS   Nocardiosis NOS
   Maduromycosis NOS

040 Other bacterial diseases

> *Excludes:* bacteremia NOS (790.7)
> bacterial infection NOS (041.9)

040.0 Gas gangrene
   Gas bacillus infection   Malignant edema
      or gangrene   Myonecrosis, clostridial
   Infection by Clostridium: Myositis, clostridial
      histolyticum
      oedematiens
      perfringens [welchii]
      septicum
      sordellii

040.1 Rhinoscleroma

040.2 Whipple's disease
   Intestinal lipodystrophy

040.3 Necrobacillosis

⑤ **040.4** Other specified botulism
   Non-foodborne intoxication due to toxins of Clostridium botulinum [*C. botulinum*]

> *Excludes:* botulism NOS (005.1)
> food poisoning due to toxins of Clostridium botulinum (005.1)

040.41 Infant botulism

040.42 Wound botulism
   Non-foodborne botulism NOS

Use additional code to identify complicated open wound

⑤ **040.8** Other specified bacterial diseases

040.81 Tropical pyomyositis

040.82 Toxic shock syndrome
   Use additional code to identify the organism

040.89 Other

● Code new   ▲ Revision of   ④ ⑤ Fourth or fifth
   to this edition   existing code   digit required

041 **Bacterial infection in conditions classified elsewhere and of unspecified site**

Note: This category is provided to be used as an additional code where it is desired to identify the bacterial agent in diseases classified elsewhere. This category will also be used to classify bacterial infections of unspecified nature or site.

Excludes: *septicemia (038.0-038.9)*

⑤ **041.0 Streptococcus**

    041.00 **Streptococcus, unspecified**

    041.01 **Group A**

    041.02 **Group B**

    041.03 **Group C**

    041.04 **Group D [Enterococcus]**

    041.05 **Group G**

    041.09 **Other Streptococcus**

⑤ **041.1 Staphylococcus**

    041.10 **Staphylococcus, unspecified**

    041.11 **Methicillin susceptible Staphylococcus aureus**
        MSSA
        Staphylococcus aureus NOS

    041.12 **Methicillin resistant Staphylococcus aureus**
        Methicillin-resistant Staphylococcus aureus (MRSA)

    041.19 **Other Staphylococcus**

  041.2 Pneumococcus

▲ **041.3 Klebsiella pneumoniae**

  041.4 Escherichia coli [E. coli]

  041.5 Hemophilus influenzae [H. influenzae]

  041.6 Proteus (mirabilis) (morganii)

  041.7 Pseudomonas

⑤ **041.8 Other specified bacterial infections**

    041.81 **Mycoplasma**
        Eaton's agent
        Pleuropneumonia-like organisms [PPLO]

    041.82 **Bacteroides fragilis**

    041.83 **Clostridium perfringens**

    041.84 **Other anaerobes**
        Gram-negative anaerobes

    Excludes: *Helicobacter pylori (041.86)*

    041.85 **Other Gram-negative organisms**
        Aerobacter aerogenes
        Gram-negative bacteria NOS
        Mima polymorpha
        Serratia

    Excludes: *Gram-negative anaerobes (041.84)*

  ▲ 041.86 **Helicobacter pylori [H. pylori]**

    041.89 **Other specified bacteria**

  041.9 Bacterial infection, unspecified

	Add 4th or 5th digit		Nonspecific code		Unspecified code		Manifestation code

HUMAN IMMUNODEFICIENCY VIRUS (HIV) INFECTION (042)

042 Human immunodeficiency virus [HIV] disease
Acquired immune deficiency syndrome
Acquired immunodeficiency syndrome
AIDS
AIDS-like syndrome
AIDS-related complex
ARC
HIV infection, symptomatic

Use additional code(s) to identify all manifestations of HIV

Use additional code, if desired, to identify HIV-2 infection (079.53)

> Excludes: *asymptomatic HIV infection status (V08)*
> *exposure to HIV virus (V01.79)*
> *nonspecific serologic evidence of HIV (795.71)*

POLIOMYELITIS AND OTHER NON-ARTHROPOD-BORNE VIRAL DISEASES AND PRION DISEASES OF CENTRAL NERVOUS SYSTEM (045-049)

⑤ **045 Acute poliomyelitis**

> Excludes: *late effects of acute poliomyelitis (138)*

The following fifth-digit subclassification is for use with category 045:

0 poliovirus, unspecified type

1 poliovirus type I

2 poliovirus type II

3 poliovirus type III

⑤ **045.0 Acute paralytic poliomyelitis specified as bulbar**
[0-3] Infantile paralysis (acute) specified as bulbar
Poliomyelitis (acute) (anterior) specified as bulbar
Polioencephalitis (acute) (bulbar)
Polioencephalomyelitis (acute) (anterior) (bulbar)

⑤ **045.1 Acute poliomyelitis with other paralysis**
[0-3] Paralysis:
  acute atrophic, spinal
  infantile, paralytic
Poliomyelitis (acute):
  anterior, with paralysis except bulbar
  epidemic, with paralysis except bulbar

⑤ **045.2 Acute nonparalytic poliomyelitis**
[0-3] Poliomyelitis (acute):
  anterior, specified as nonparalytic
  epidemic, specified as nonparalytic

⑤ **045.9 Acute poliomyelitis, unspecified**
[0-3] Infantile paralysis, unspecified whether paralytic or nonparalytic
Poliomyelitis (acute):
  anterior, unspecified whether paralytic or nonparalytic
  epidemic, unspecified whether paralytic or nonparalytic

046 Slow virus infections and prion diseases of central nervous system

046.0 Kuru

⑤ **046.1 Jakob-Creutzfeldt disease**
Use additional code to identify dementia:
  with behavioral disturbance (294.11)
  without behavioral disturbance (294.10)

046.11 Variant Creutzfeldt-Jakob disease
vCJD

046.19 Other and unspecified Creutzfeldt-Jakob disease
CJD
Familial Creutzfeldt-Jakob disease
Iatrogenic Creutzfeldt-Jakob disease
Jakob-Creutzfeldt disease, unspecified
Sporadic Creutzfeldt-Jakob disease
Subacute spongiform encephalopathy

> Excludes: *variant Creutzfeldt-Jakob disease (vCJD) (046.11)*

046.2 Subacute sclerosing panencephalitis
Dawson's inclusion body encephalitis
Van Bogaert's sclerosing leukoencephalitis

● Code new
  to this edition
▲ Revision of
  existing code
④ ⑤ Fourth or fifth
  digit required

046.3 Progressive multifocal leukoencephalopathy
Multifocal leukoencephalopathy NOS

⑤ **046.7 Other specified prion diseases of central nervous system**

Excludes: *Creutzfeldt-Jakob disease (046.11-046.19)*
Jakob-Creutzfeldt disease (046.11-046.19)
kuru (046.0)
variant Creutzfeldt-Jakob disease (vCJD) (046.11)

046.71 Gerstmann-Straussler-Scheinker syndrome
GSS syndrome

046.72 Fatal familial insomnia
FFI

046.79 Other and unspecified prion disease of central nervous system

046.8 Other specified slow virus infection of central nervous system

046.9 Unspecified slow virus infection of central nervous system

047 Meningitis due to enterovirus
Includes: meningitis:
abacterial
aseptic
viral

Excludes: *meningitis due to:*
adenovirus (049.1)
arthropod-borne virus (060.0-066.9)
leptospira (100.81)
virus of:
herpes simplex (054.72)
herpes zoster (053.0)
lymphocytic choriomeningitis (049.0)
mumps (072.1)
poliomyelitis (045.0-045.9)
any other infection specifically classified elsewhere

047.0 Coxsackie virus

047.1 ECHO virus
Meningo-eruptive syndrome

047.8 Other specified viral meningitis

047.9 Unspecified viral meningitis
Viral meningitis NOS

048 Other enterovirus diseases of central nervous system
Boston exanthem

049 Other non-arthropod-borne viral diseases of central nervous system

Excludes: *late effects of viral encephalitis (139.0)*

049.0 Lymphocytic choriomeningitis
Lymphocytic:
meningitis (serous) (benign)
meningoencephalitis (serous) (benign)

049.1 Meningitis due to adenovirus

049.8 Other specified non-arthropod-borne viral diseases of central nervous system

Encephalitis:	Encephalitis:
acute:	lethargica
inclusion body	Rio Bravo
necrotizing	von Economo's disease
epidemic	

Excludes: *human herpesvirus 6 encephalitis (058.21)*
other human herpesvirus encephalitis (058.29)

049.9 Unspecified non-arthropod-borne viral diseases of central nervous system
Viral encephalitis NOS

VIRAL DISEASES GENERALLY ACCOMPANIED BY EXANTHEM (050-059)

Excludes: *arthropod-borne viral diseases (060.0-066.9)*
Boston exanthem (048)

050 Smallpox

183

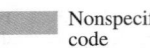 Add 4th or
5th digit

 Nonspecific
code

Unspecified
code

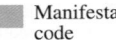 Manifestation
code

050.0 Variola major
Hemorrhagic (pustular)   Malignant smallpox
    smallpox   Purpura variolosa

050.1 Alastrim
Variola minor

050.2 Modified smallpox
Varioloid

050.9 Smallpox, unspecified

051 Cowpox and paravaccinia

⑤ **051.0 Cowpox and vaccinia not from vaccination**

    051.01 Cowpox

    051.02 Vaccinia not from vaccination

    Excludes: vaccinia *(generalized) (from vaccination) (999.0)*

051.1 Pseudocowpox
Milkers' node

051.2 Contagious pustular dermatitis
Ecthyma contagiosum   Orf

051.9 Paravaccinia, unspecified

052 Chickenpox

052.0 Postvaricella encephalitis
Postchickenpox encephalitis

052.1 Varicella (hemorrhagic) pneumonitis

052.2 Postvaricella myelitis
Postchickenpox myelitis

052.7 With other specified complications

052.8 With unspecified complication

052.9 Varicella without mention of complication
Chickenpox NOS
Varicella NOS

053 Herpes zoster
Includes: shingles
          zona

053.0 With meningitis

⑤ **053.1 With other nervous system complications**

    053.10 With unspecified nervous system complication

    053.11 Geniculate herpes zoster
        Herpetic geniculate ganglionitis

    053.12 Postherpetic trigeminal neuralgia

    053.13 Postherpetic polyneuropathy

    053.14 Herpes zoster myelitis

    053.19 Other

⑤ **053.2 With ophthalmic complications**

    053.20 Herpes zoster dermatitis of eyelid
        Herpes zoster ophthalmicus

    053.21 Herpes zoster keratoconjunctivitis

    053.22 Herpes zoster iridocyclitis

    053.29 Other

⑤ **053.7 With other specified complications**

    053.71 Otitis externa due to herpes zoster

    053.79 Other

053.8 With unspecified complication

053.9 Herpes zoster without mention of complication
Herpes zoster NOS

054 Herpes simplex

    Excludes: congenital herpes simplex *(771.2)*

● Code new
   to this edition
▲ Revision of
   existing code
④ ⑤ Fourth or fifth
      digit required

054.0 Eczema herpeticum
Kaposi's varicelliform eruption

⑤ **054.1 Genital herpes**

054.10 Genital herpes, unspecified
Herpes progenitalis

054.11 Herpetic vulvovaginitis

054.12 Herpetic ulceration of vulva

054.13 Herpetic infection of penis

054.19 Other

054.2 Herpetic gingivostomatitis

054.3 Herpetic meningoencephalitis
Herpes encephalitis
Simian B disease

Excludes: *human herpesvirus 6 encephalitis (058.21)*
other human herpesvirus encephalitis (058.29)

⑤ **054.4 With ophthalmic complications**

054.40 With unspecified ophthalmic complication

054.41 Herpes simplex dermatitis of eyelid

054.42 Dendritic keratitis

054.43 Herpes simplex disciform keratitis

054.44 Herpes simplex iridocyclitis

054.49 Other

054.5 Herpetic septicemia

054.6 Herpetic whitlow
Herpetic felon

⑤ **054.7 With other specified complications**

054.71 Visceral herpes simplex

054.72 Herpes simplex meningitis

054.73 Herpes simplex otitis externa

054.74 Herpes simplex myelitis

054.79 Other

054.8 With unspecified complication

054.9 Herpes simplex without mention of complication

055 Measles
Includes: morbilli
rubeola

055.0 Postmeasles encephalitis

055.1 Postmeasles pneumonia

055.2 Postmeasles otitis media

⑤ **055.7 With other specified complications**

055.71 Measles keratoconjunctivitis
Measles keratitis

055.79 Other

055.8 With unspecified complication

055.9 Measles without mention of complication

056 Rubella
Includes: German measles

Excludes: *congenital rubella (771.0)*

⑤ **056.0 With neurological complications**

056.00 With unspecified neurological complication

056.01 Encephalomyelitis due to rubella
Encephalitis due to rubella
Meningoencephalitis due to rubella

056.09 Other

⑤ **056.7 With other specified complications**

	Add 4th or 5th digit		Nonspecific code		Unspecified code		Manifestation code

056.71   **Arthritis due to rubella**

056.79   **Other**

056.8   **With unspecified complications**

056.9   **Rubella without mention of complication**

057   **Other viral exanthemata**

057.0   **Erythema infectiosum [fifth disease]**

057.8   **Other specified viral exanthemata**
Dukes (-Filatow) disease   Parascarlatina
Fourth disease   Pseudoscarlatina

Excludes: *exanthema subitum [sixth disease] (058.10-058.12)*
roseola infantum (058.10-058.12)

057.9   **Viral exanthem, unspecified**

⑤ **058**   **Other human herpesvirus**

Excludes: *congenital herpes (771.2)*
cytomegalovirus (078.5)
Epstein-Barr virus (075)
herpes NOS (054.0-054.9)
herpes simplex (054.0-054.9)
herpes zoster (053.0-053.9)
human herpesvirus NOS (054.0-054.9)
human herpesvirus 1 (054.0-054.9)
human herpesvirus 2 (054.0-054.9)
human herpesvirus 3 (052.0-053.9)
human herpesvirus 4 (075)
human herpesvirus 5 (078.5)
varicella (052.0-052.9)
varicella-zoster virus (052.0-053.9)

⑤ **058.1**   **Roseola infantum**
Exanthema subitum [sixth disease]

058.10   **Roseola infantum, unspecified**
Exanthema subitum [sixth disease], unspecified

058.11   **Roseola infantum due to human herpesvirus 6**
Exanthema subitum [sixth disease] due to human herpesvirus 6

058.12   **Roseola infantum due to human herpesvirus 7**
Exanthema subitum [sixth disease] due to human herpesvirus 7

⑤ **058.2**   **Other human herpesvirus encephalitis**

Excludes: *herpes encephalitis NOS (054.3)*
herpes simplex encephalitis (054.3)
human herpesvirus encephalitis NOS (054.3)
simian B herpes virus encephalitis (054.3)

058.21   **Human herpesvirus 6 encephalitis**

058.29   **Other human herpesvirus encephalitis**
Human herpesvirus 7 encephalitis

⑤ **058.8**   **Other human herpesvirus infections**

058.81   **Human herpesvirus 6 infection**

058.82   **Human herpesvirus 7 infection**

058.89   **Other human herpesvirus infection**
Human herpesvirus 8 infection
Kaposi's sarcoma-associated herpesvirus infection

059   **Other poxvirus infections**

Excludes: *contagious pustular dermatitis (051.2)*
cowpox (051.01)
ecthyma contagiosum (051.2)
milker's nodule (051.1)
orf (051.2)
paravaccinia NOS (051.9)
pseudocowpox (051.1)
smallpox (050.0-050.9)
vaccinia (generalized) (from vaccination) (999.0)
vaccinia not from vaccination (051.02)

⑤ **059.0**   **Other orthopoxvirus infections**

● Code new
to this edition

▲ Revision of
existing code

④ ⑤ Fourth or fifth
digit required

059.00 Orthopoxvirus infection, unspecified

059.01 Monkeypox

059.09 Other orthopoxvirus infection

⑤ 059.1 Other parapoxvirus infections

059.10 Parapoxvirus infection, unspecified

059.11 Bovine stomatitis

059.12 Sealpox

059.19 Other parapoxvirus infections

⑤ 059.2 Yatapoxvirus infections

059.20 Yatapoxvirus infection, unspecified

059.21 Tanapox

059.22 Yaba monkey tumor virus

059.8 Other poxvirus infections

059.9 Poxvirus infections, unspecified

ARTHROPOD-BORNE VIRAL DISEASES (060-066)

Use additional code, if desired, to identify any associated meningitis (321.2)

Excludes: late effects of viral encephalitis (139.0)

060 Yellow fever

060.0 Sylvatic
Yellow fever:
jungle
sylvan

060.1 Urban

060.9 Yellow fever, unspecified

061 Dengue
Breakbone fever

Excludes: hemorrhagic fever caused by dengue virus (065.4)

062 Mosquito-borne viral encephalitis

062.0 Japanese encephalitis
Japanese B encephalitis

062.1 Western equine encephalitis

062.2 Eastern equine encephalitis

Excludes: Venezuelan equine encephalitis (066.2)

062.3 St. Louis encephalitis

062.4 Australian encephalitis
Australian arboencephalitis
Australian X disease
Murray Valley encephalitis

062.5 California virus encephalitis
Encephalitis: Tahyna fever
California
La Crosse

062.8 Other specified mosquito-borne viral encephalitis
Encephalitis by Ilheus virus

Excludes: West Nile virus (066.40-066.49)

062.9 Mosquito-borne viral encephalitis, unspecified

063 Tick-borne viral encephalitis
Includes: diphasic meningoencephalitis

063.0 Russian spring-summer [taiga] encephalitis

063.1 Louping ill

063.2 Central European encephalitis

063.8 Other specified tick-borne viral encephalitis
Langat encephalitis
Powassan encephalitis

063.9 Tick-borne viral encephalitis, unspecified

Add 4th or   Nonspecific   Unspecified   Manifestation
5th digit   code   code   code

064 Viral encephalitis transmitted by other and unspecified arthropods
Arthropod-borne viral encephalitis, vector unknown
Negishi virus encephalitis

> *Excludes:* viral encephalitis NOS (049.9)

065 Arthropod-borne hemorrhagic fever

065.0 Crimean hemorrhagic fever [CHF Congo virus]
Central Asian hemorrhagic fever

065.1 Omsk hemorrhagic fever

065.2 Kyasanur Forest disease

065.3 Other tick-borne hemorrhagic fever

065.4 Mosquito-borne hemorrhagic fever
Chikungunya hemorrhagic fever
Dengue hemorrhagic fever

> *Excludes:* Chikungunya fever (066.3)
> dengue (061)
> yellow fever (060.0-060.9)

065.8 Other specified arthropod-borne hemorrhagic fever
Mite-borne hemorrhagic fever

065.9 Arthropod-borne hemorrhagic fever, unspecified
Arbovirus hemorrhagic fever NOS

066 Other arthropod-borne viral diseases

066.0 Phlebotomus fever
Changuinola fever
Sandfly fever

066.1 Tick-borne fever
Nairobi sheep disease
Tick fever:
  American mountain
  Colorado
Tick fever:
  Kemerovo
  Quaranfil

066.2 Venezuelan equine fever
Venezuelan equine encephalitis

066.3 Other mosquito-borne fever
Fever (viral):
  Bunyamwera
  Bwamba
  Chikungunya
  GuamaR Mayaro
  Mucambo
  O'nyong-nyong
Fever (viral):
  Oropouche
  Pixuna
  Rift valley
  Ross river
  Wesselsbron
  Zika

> *Excludes:* dengue (061)
> yellow fever (060.0-060.9)

⑤ **066.4 West Nile fever**

066.40 West Nile fever, unspecified
West Nile fever NOS
West Nile fever without complications
West Nile virus NOS

066.41 West Nile fever with encephalitis
West Nile encephalitis
West Nile encephalomyelitis

066.42 West Nile fever with other neurologic manifestation
Use additional code to specify the neurologic manifestation

066.49 West Nile fever with other complications
Use additional code to specify the other conditions

066.8 Other specified arthropod-borne viral diseases
Chandipura fever
Piry fever

066.9 Arthropod-borne viral disease, unspecified
Arbovirus infection NOS

● Code new to this edition   ▲ Revision of existing code   ④ ⑤ Fourth or fifth digit required

OTHER DISEASES DUE TO VIRUSES AND CHLAMYDIAE (070-079)

070 Viral hepatitis
Includes: viral hepatitis (acute) (chronic)

Excludes: *cytomegalic inclusion virus hepatitis (078.5)*

The following fifth-digit subclassification is for use with categories 070.2 and 070.3:

    0   **acute or unspecified, without mention of hepatitis delta**

    1   **acute or unspecified, with hepatitis delta**

    2   **chronic, without mention of hepatitis delta**

    3   **chronic, with hepatitis delta**

070.0 Viral hepatitis A with hepatic coma

070.1 Viral hepatitis A without mention of hepatic coma
Infectious hepatitis

⑤ **070.2 Viral hepatitis B with hepatic coma**
[0-3]

⑤ **070.3 Viral hepatitis B without mention of hepatic coma**
[0-3]   Serum hepatitis

⑤ **070.4 Other specified viral hepatitis with hepatic coma**

    070.41 Acute hepatitis C with hepatic coma

    070.42 Hepatitis delta without mention of active hepatitis B disease with hepatic coma
        Hepatitis delta with hepatitis B carrier state

    070.43 Hepatitis E with hepatic coma

    070.44 Chronic hepatitis C with hepatic coma

    070.49 Other specified viral hepatitis with hepatic coma

⑤ **070.5 Other specified viral hepatitis without mention of hepatic coma**

    070.51 Acute hepatitis C without mention of hepatic coma

    070.52 Hepatitis delta without mention of active hepatitis B disease or hepatic coma

    070.53 Hepatitis E without mention of hepatic coma

    070.54 Chronic hepatitis C without mention of hepatic coma

    070.59 Other specified viral hepatitis without mention of hepatic coma

070.6 Unspecified viral hepatitis with hepatic coma

Excludes: *unspecified viral hepatitis C with hepatic coma (070.71)*

⑤ **070.7 Unspecified viral hepatitis C**

    070.70 Unspecified viral hepatitis C without hepatic coma
        Unspecified viral hepatitis C NOS

    070.71 Unspecified viral hepatitis C with hepatic coma

070.9 Unspecified viral hepatitis without mention of hepatic coma
Viral hepatitis NOS

Excludes: *unspecified viral hepatitis C without hepatic coma (070.70)*

071 Rabies
Hydrophobia
Lyssa

072 Mumps

072.0 Mumps orchitis

072.1 Mumps meningitis

072.2 Mumps encephalitis
Mumps meningoencephalitis

072.3 Mumps pancreatitis

⑤ **072.7 Mumps with other specified complications**

    072.71 Mumps hepatitis

    072.72 Mumps polyneuropathy

    072.79 Other

072.8 Mumps with unspecified complication

	Add 4th or 5th digit		Nonspecific code		Unspecified code		Manifestation code

072.9 Mumps without mention of complication
Epidemic parotitis
Infectious parotitis

073 Ornithosis
Includes: parrot fever
psittacosis

073.0 With pneumonia
Lobular pneumonitis due to ornithosis

073.7 With other specified complications

073.8 With unspecified complication

073.9 Ornithosis, unspecified

074 Specific diseases due to Coxsackie virus

Excludes: *Coxsackie virus:*
infection NOS (079.2)
meningitis (047.0)

074.0 Herpangina
Vesicular pharyngitis

074.1 Epidemic pleurodynia
Bornholm disease   Epidemic:
Devil's grip   myalgia
myositis

⑤ **074.2 Coxsackie carditis**

074.20   Coxsackie carditis, unspecified

074.21   Coxsackie pericarditis

074.22   Coxsackie endocarditis

074.23   Coxsackie myocarditis
Aseptic myocarditis of newborn

074.3 Hand, foot, and mouth disease
Vesicular stomatitis and exanthem

074.8 Other specified diseases due to Coxsackie virus
Acute lymphonodular pharyngitis

075 Infectious mononucleosis
Glandular fever   Pfeiffer's disease
Monocytic angina

076 Trachoma

Excludes: *late effect of trachoma (139.1)*

076.0 Initial stage
Trachoma dubium

076.1 Active stage
Granular conjunctivitis (trachomatous)
Trachomatous:
follicular conjunctivitis
pannus

076.9 Trachoma, unspecified
Trachoma NOS

077 Other diseases of conjunctiva due to viruses and Chlamydiae

Excludes: *ophthalmic complications of viral diseases classified elsewhere*

077.0 Inclusion conjunctivitis
Paratrachoma
Swimming pool conjunctivitis

Excludes: *inclusion blennorrhea (neonatal) (771.6)*

077.1 Epidemic keratoconjunctivitis
Shipyard eye

077.2 Pharyngoconjunctival fever
Viral pharyngoconjunctivitis

077.3 Other adenoviral conjunctivitis
Acute adenoviral follicular conjunctivitis

● Code new   ▲ Revision of   ④ ⑤ Fourth or fifth
to this edition   existing code   digit required

077.4 Epidemic hemorrhagic conjunctivitis
Apollo:
  conjunctivitis
  disease
Conjunctivitis due to enterovirus type 70
Hemorrhagic conjunctivitis (acute) (epidemic)

077.8 Other viral conjunctivitis
Newcastle conjunctivitis

⑤ **077.9 Unspecified diseases of conjunctiva due to viruses and Chlamydiae**

077.98 Due to Chlamydiae

077.99 Due to viruses
Viral conjunctivitis NOS

078 Other diseases due to viruses and Chlamydiae
Excludes: viral infection NOS (079.0-079.9)
    viremia NOS (790.8)

078.0 Molluscum contagiosum

⑤ **078.1 Viral warts**
Viral warts due to Human papillomavirus

078.10 Viral warts, unspecified
Verruca vulgaris
Warts (infectious)

078.11 Condyloma acuminatum
Condyloma NOS
Genital warts NOS

078.12 Plantar wart
Verruca plantaris

078.19 Other specified viral warts
Common wart
Flat wart
Verruca plana

078.2 Sweating fever
Miliary fever
Sweating disease

078.3 Cat-scratch disease
Benign lymphoreticulosis (of inoculation)
Cat-scratch fever

078.4 Foot and mouth disease
Aphthous fever
Epizootic:
  aphthae
  stomatitis

078.5 Cytomegaloviral disease
Cytomegalic inclusion disease
Salivary gland virus disease
Use additional code, if desired, to identify manifestation, as:
  cytomegalic inclusion virus:
    hepatitis (573.1)
    pneumonia (484.1)
Excludes: congenital cytomegalovirus infection (771.1)

078.6 Hemorrhagic nephrosonephritis
Hemorrhagic fever: Hemorrhagic fever:
  epidemic   Russian
  Korean   with renal syndrome

078.7 Arenaviral hemorrhagic fever
Hemorrhagic fever: Hemorrhagic fever:
  Argentine   Junin virus
  Bolivian   Machupo virus

⑤ **078.8 Other specified diseases due to viruses and Chlamydiae**
Excludes: epidemic diarrhea (009.2)
    lymphogranuloma venereum (099.1)

078.81 Epidemic vertigo

078.82 Epidemic vomiting syndrome
Winter vomiting disease

Add 4th or 5th digit   Nonspecific code   Unspecified code   Manifestation code

`078.88` **Other specified diseases due to Chlamydiae**

`078.89` **Other specified diseases due to viruses**
Epidemic cervical myalgia
Marburg disease

`079` **Viral and Chlamydial infection in conditions classified elsewhere and of unspecified site**

Note: This category is provided to be used as an additional code where it is desired to identify the viral agent in diseases classifiable elsewhere. This category will also be used to classify virus infection of unspecified nature or site.

079.0 Adenovirus

079.1 ECHO virus

079.2 Coxsackievirus

079.3 Rhinovirus

079.4 Human papillomavirus

⑤ **079.5 Retrovirus**

Excludes: *human immunodeficiency virus, type 1 [HIV-1] (042)*
human T-cell lymphotrophic virus, type III [HTLV-III] (042)
lymphadenopathy-associated virus [LAV] (042)

079.50 Retrovirus, unspecified

079.51 Human T-cell lymphotrophic virus, type I [HTLV-I]

079.52 Human T-cell lymphotrophic virus, type II [HTLV-II]

079.53 Human immunodeficiency virus, type 2 [HIV-2]

`079.59` **Other specified retrovirus**

079.6 Respiratory syncytial virus (RSV)

⑤ **079.8 Other specified viral and chlamydial infections**

079.81 Hantavirus

079.82 SARS-associated coronavirus

079.83 Parvovirus B19
Human parvovirus
Parvovirus NOS

Excludes: *erythema infectiosum [fifth disease] (057.0)*

`079.88` **Other specified chlamydial infection**

`079.89` **Other specified viral infection**

⑤ **079.9 Unspecified viral and chlamydial infections**

Excludes: *viremia NOS (790.8)*

`079.98` **Unspecified chlamydial infection**
Chlamydial infection NOS

`079.99` **Unspecified viral infection**
Viral infection NOS

RICKETTSIOSES AND OTHER ARTHROPOD-BORNE DISEASES (080-088)

Excludes: *arthropod-borne viral diseases (060.0-066.9)*

080 Louse-borne [epidemic] typhus
Typhus (fever):   Typhus (fever):
  classical   exanthematic NOS
  epidemic   louse-borne

`081` **Other typhus**

081.0 Murine [endemic] typhus
Typhus (fever):
  endemic
  flea-borne

081.1 Brill's disease
Brill-Zinsser disease
Recrudescent typhus (fever)

081.2 Scrub typhus
Japanese river fever   Mite-borne typhus
Kedani fever   Tsutsugamushi

`081.9` **Typhus, unspecified**
Typhus (fever) NOS

  ● Code new   ▲ Revision of   ④ ⑤ Fourth or fifth
     to this edition   existing code   digit required

082 Tick-borne rickettsioses

082.0 Spotted fevers
Rocky mountain spotted fever
São Paulo fever

082.1 Boutonneuse fever
African tick typhus   Marseilles fever
India tick typhus   Mediterranean tick fever
Kenya tick typhus

082.2 North Asian tick fever
Siberian tick typhus

082.3 Queensland tick typhus

⑤ **082.4 Ehrlichiosis**

082.40 Ehrlichiosis, unspecified

082.41 Ehrlichiosis chafeensis (E. chafeensis)

082.49 Other ehrlichiosis

082.8 Other specified tick-borne rickettsioses
Lone star fever

082.9 Tick-borne rickettsiosis, unspecified
Tick-borne typhus NOS

083 Other rickettsioses

083.0 Q fever

083.1 Trench fever
Quintan fever
Wolhynian fever

083.2 Rickettsialpox
Vesicular rickettsiosis

083.8 Other specified rickettsioses

083.9 Rickettsiosis, unspecified

084 Malaria
Note: Subcategories 084.0-084.6 exclude the listed conditions with mention of pernicious
complications (084.8-084.9).

Excludes: *congenital malaria (771.2)*

084.0 Falciparum malaria [malignant tertian]
Malaria (fever):
by Plasmodium falciparum
subtertian

084.1 Vivax malaria [benign tertian]
Malaria (fever) by Plasmodium vivax

084.2 Quartan malaria
Malaria (fever) by Plasmodium malariae
Malariae malaria

084.3 Ovale malaria
Malaria (fever) by Plasmodium ovale

084.4 Other malaria
Monkey malaria

084.5 Mixed malaria
Malaria (fever) by more than one parasite

084.6 Malaria, unspecified
Malaria (fever) NOS

084.7 Induced malaria
Therapeutically induced malaria

Excludes: *accidental infection from syringe, blood transfusion, etc. (084.0-084.6, above,*
according to parasite species)
transmission from mother to child during delivery (771.2)

084.8 Blackwater fever
Hemoglobinuric: Malarial hemoglobinuria
fever (bilious)
malaria

Add 4th or 5th digit	Nonspecific code	Unspecified code	Manifestation code

084.9 Other pernicious complications of malaria
Algid malaria
Cerebral malaria
Use additional code, if desired, to identify complication, as:
malarial:
hepatitis (573.2)
nephrosis (581.81)

085 Leishmaniasis

085.0 Visceral [kala-azar]
Dumdum fever
Infection by Leishmania:
donovani
infantum
Leishmaniasis:
dermal, post-kala-azar
Mediterranean
visceral (Indian)

085.1 Cutaneous, urban
Aleppo boil
Baghdad boil
Delhi boil
Infection by Leishmania
tropica (minor)
Leishmaniasis, cutaneous:
dry form
late
recurrent
ulcerating
Oriental sore

085.2 Cutaneous, Asian desert
Infection by Leishmania tropica major
Leishmaniasis, cutaneous:
acute necrotizing
rural
wet form
zoonotic form

085.3 Cutaneous, Ethiopian
Infection by Leishmania ethiopica
Leishmaniasis, cutaneous:
diffuse
lepromatous

085.4 Cutaneous, American
Chiclero ulcer
Infection by Leishmania mexicana
Leishmaniasis tegumentaria diffusa

085.5 Mucocutaneous (American)
Espundia
Infection by Leishmania braziliensis
Uta

085.9 Leishmaniasis, unspecified

086 Trypanosomiasis
Use additional code, if desired, to identify manifestations, as:
trypanosomiasis:
encephalitis (323.2)
meningitis (321.3)

086.0 Chagas' disease with heart involvement
American trypanosomiasis with heart involvement
Infection by Trypanosoma cruzi with heart involvement
Any condition classifiable to 086.2 with heart involvement

086.1 Chagas' disease with other organ involvement
American trypanosomiasis with involvement of organ other than heart
Infection by Trypanosoma cruzi with involvement of organ other than heart
Any condition classifiable to 086.2 with involvement of organ other than heart

086.2 Chagas' disease without mention of organ involvement
American trypanosomiasis
Infection by Trypanosoma cruzi

086.3 Gambian trypanosomiasis
Gambian sleeping sickness
Infection by Trypanosoma gambiense

086.4 Rhodesian trypanosomiasis
Infection by Trypanosoma rhodesiense
Rhodesian sleeping sickness

086.5 African trypanosomiasis, unspecified
Sleeping sickness NOS

● Code new
to this edition
▲ Revision of
existing code
④ ⑤ Fourth or fifth
digit required

086.9 **Trypanosomiasis, unspecified**

087 **Relapsing fever**
Includes: recurrent fever

087.0 **Louse-borne**

087.1 **Tick-borne**

087.9 **Relapsing fever, unspecified**

088 **Other arthropod-borne diseases**

088.0 **Bartonellosis**
Carrión's disease   Verruga peruana
Oroya fever

⑤ **088.8** **Other specified arthropod-borne diseases**

    088.81 **Lyme Disease**
Erythema chronicum migrans

    088.82 **Babesiosis**
Babesiasis

    088.89 **Other**

088.9 **Arthropod-borne disease, unspecified**

SYPHILIS AND OTHER VENEREAL DISEASES (090-099)

Excludes: *nonvenereal endemic syphilis (104.0)*
urogenital trichomoniasis (131.0)

090 **Congenital syphilis**

090.0 **Early congenital syphilis, symptomatic**
Congenital syphilitic: Syphilitic (congenital):
  choroiditis   epiphysitis
  coryza (chronic)   osteochondritis
  hepatomegaly   pemphigus
  mucous patches   Any congenital syphilitic condition specified as early or
  periostitis   manifest less than two years after birth
  splenomegaly

090.1 **Early congenital syphilis, latent**
Congenital syphilis without clinical manifestations, with positive serological reaction
and negative spinal fluid test, less than two years after birth

090.2 **Early congenital syphilis, unspecified**
Congenital syphilis NOS, less than two years after birth

090.3 **Syphilitic interstitial keratitis**
Syphilitic keratitis:
  parenchymatous
  punctata profunda
Excludes: *interstitial keratitis NOS (370.50)*

⑤ **090.4** **Juvenile neurosyphilis**
Use additional code, if desired, to identify any associated mental disorder

    090.40 **Juvenile neurosyphilis, unspecified**
Congenital neurosyphilis
Dementia paralytica juvenilis
Juvenile:
  general paresis
  tabes
  taboparesis

    090.41 **Congenital syphilitic encephalitis**

    090.42 **Congenital syphilitic meningitis**

    090.49 **Other**

090.5 **Other late congenital syphilis, symptomatic**
Gumma due to congenital syphilis
Hutchinson's teeth
Syphilitic saddle nose
Any congenital syphilitic condition specified as late or manifest two years or more after
birth

090.6 **Late congenital syphilis, latent**
Congenital syphilis without clinical manifestations, with positive serological reaction
and negative spinal fluid test, two years or more after birth

---

| | Add 4th or 5th digit | | Nonspecific code | | Unspecified code | | Manifestation code |

090.7 **Late congenital syphilis, unspecified**
Congenital syphilis NOS, two years or more after birth

090.9 **Congenital syphilis, unspecified**

091 **Early syphilis, symptomatic**

> Excludes: *early cardiovascular syphilis (093.0-093.9)*
> *early neurosyphilis (094.0-094.9)*

091.0 **Genital syphilis (primary)**
Genital chancre

091.1 **Primary anal syphilis**

091.2 **Other primary syphilis**

Primary syphilis of:	Primary syphilis of:
breast	lip
fingers	tonsils

091.3 **Secondary syphilis of skin or mucous membranes**

Condyloma latum	Secondary syphilis of:
Secondary syphilis of:	skin
anus	tonsils
mouth	vulva
pharynx	

091.4 **Adenopathy due to secondary syphilis**
Syphilitic adenopathy (secondary)
Syphilitic lymphadenitis (secondary)

⑤ **091.5** **Uveitis due to secondary syphilis**

   091.50 **Syphilitic uveitis, unspecified**

   091.51 **Syphilitic chorioretinitis (secondary)**

   091.52 **Syphilitic iridocyclitis (secondary)**

⑤ **091.6** **Secondary syphilis of viscera and bone**

   091.61 **Secondary syphilitic periostitis**

   091.62 **Secondary syphilitic hepatitis**
   Secondary syphilis of liver

   091.69 **Other viscera**

091.7 **Secondary syphilis, relapse**
Secondary syphilis, relapse (treated) (untreated)

⑤ **091.8** **Other forms of secondary syphilis**

   091.81 **Acute syphilitic meningitis (secondary)**

   091.82 **Syphilitic alopecia**

   091.89 **Other**

091.9 **Unspecified secondary syphilis**

092 **Early syphilis, latent**
Includes: syphilis (acquired) without clinical manifestations, with positive serological reaction and negative spinal fluid test, less than two years after infection

092.0 **Early syphilis, latent, serological relapse after treatment**

092.9 **Early syphilis, latent, unspecified**

093 **Cardiovascular syphilis**

093.0 **Aneurysm of aorta, specified as syphilitic**
Dilatation of aorta, specified as syphilitic

093.1 **Syphilitic aortitis**

⑤ **093.2** **Syphilitic endocarditis**

   093.20 **Valve, unspecified**
   Syphilitic ostial coronary disease

   093.21 **Mitral valve**

   093.22 **Aortic valve**
   Syphilitic aortic incompetence or stenosis

   093.23 **Tricuspid valve**

   093.24 **Pulmonary valve**

⑤ **093.8** **Other specified cardiovascular syphilis**

   093.81 **Syphilitic pericarditis**

   093.82 **Syphilitic myocarditis**

● Code new
to this edition
▲ Revision of
existing code
④ ⑤ Fourth or fifth
digit required

093.89 Other

093.9 Cardiovascular syphilis, unspecified

094 Neurosyphilis

Use additional code, if desired, to identify any associated mental disorder

094.0 **Tabes dorsalis**
Locomotor ataxia (progressive)
Posterior spinal sclerosis (syphilitic)
Tabetic neurosyphilis
Use additional code, if desired, to identify manifestation, as:
neurogenic arthropathy [Charcot's joint disease] (713.5)

094.1 **General paresis**
Dementia paralytica
General paralysis (of the insane) (progressive)
Paretic neurosyphilis
Taboparesis

094.2 **Syphilitic meningitis**
Meningovascular syphilis

Excludes: *acute syphilitic meningitis (secondary) (091.81)*

094.3 **Asymptomatic neurosyphilis**

⑤ **094.8** **Other specified neurosyphilis**

094.81 Syphilitic encephalitis

094.82 Syphilitic Parkinsonism

094.83 Syphilitic disseminated retinochoroiditis

094.84 Syphilitic optic atrophy

094.85 Syphilitic retrobulbar neuritis

094.86 Syphilitic acoustic neuritis

094.87 Syphilitic ruptured cerebral aneurysm

094.89 Other

094.9 **Neurosyphilis, unspecified**
Gumma (syphilitic) of central nervous system NOS
Syphilis (early) (late) of central nervous system NOS
Syphiloma of central nervous system NOS

095 Other forms of late syphilis, with symptoms
Includes: gumma (syphilitic)
syphilis, late, tertiary, or unspecified stage

095.0 **Syphilitic episcleritis**

095.1 **Syphilis of lung**

095.2 **Syphilitic peritonitis**

095.3 **Syphilis of liver**

095.4 **Syphilis of kidney**

095.5 **Syphilis of bone**

095.6 **Syphilis of muscle**
Syphilitic myositis

095.7 **Syphilis of synovium, tendon, and bursa**
Syphilitic:
bursitis
synovitis

095.8 Other specified forms of late symptomatic syphilis

Excludes: *cardiovascular syphilis (093.0-093.9)*
neurosyphilis (094.0-094.9)

095.9 Late symptomatic syphilis, unspecified

096 Late syphilis, latent
Syphilis (acquired) without clinical manifestations, with positive serological reaction and negative spinal fluid test, two years or more after infection

097 Other and unspecified syphilis

097.0 Late syphilis, unspecified

097.1 Latent syphilis, unspecified
Positive serological reaction for syphilis

| | Add 4th or 5th digit | | Nonspecific code | | Unspecified code | | Manifestation code |

097.9 Syphilis, unspecified
Syphilis (acquired) NOS

Excludes: *syphilis NOS causing death under two years of age (090.9)*

098 Gonococcal infections

098.0 Acute, of lower genitourinary tract
Gonococcal: Gonorrhea (acute):
  Bartholinitis (acute)   NOS
  urethritis (acute)   genitourinary (tract) NOS
  vulvovaginitis (acute)

⑤ **098.1 Acute, of upper genitourinary tract**

098.10 Gonococcal infection (acute) of upper genitourinary tract, site unspecified

098.11 Gonococcal cystitis (acute)
Gonorrhea (acute) of bladder

098.12 Gonococcal prostatitis (acute)

098.13 Gonococcal epididymo-orchitis (acute)
Gonococcal orchitis (acute)

098.14 Gonococcal seminal vesiculitis (acute)
Gonorrhea (acute) of seminal vesicle

098.15 Gonococcal cervicitis (acute)
Gonorrhea (acute) of cervix

098.16 Gonococcal endometritis (acute)
Gonorrhea (acute) of uterus

098.17 Gonococcal salpingitis, specified as acute

098.19 Other

098.2 Chronic, of lower genitourinary tract
Gonococcal:
  Bartholinitis specified as chronic or with duration of two months or more
  urethritis specified as chronic or with duration of two months or more
  vulvovaginitis specified as chronic or with duration of two months or more
Gonorrhea:
  NOS specified as chronic or with duration of two months or more
  genitourinary (tract) specified as chronic or with duration of two months or more
Any condition classifiable to 098.0 specified as chronic or with duration of two months or more

⑤ **098.3 Chronic, of upper genitourinary tract**
Includes: any condition classifiable to 098.1 stated as chronic or with a duration of two months or more

098.30 Chronic gonococcal infection of upper genitourinary tract, site unspecified

098.31 Gonococcal cystitis, chronic
Any condition classifiable to 098.11, specified as chronic
Gonorrhea of bladder, chronic

098.32 Gonococcal prostatitis, chronic
Any condition classifiable to 098.12, specified as chronic

098.33 Gonococcal epididymo-orchitis, chronic
Any condition classifiable to 098.13, specified as chronic
Chronic gonococcal orchitis

098.34 Gonococcal seminal vesiculitis, chronic
Any condition classifiable to 098.14, specified as chronic
Gonorrhea of seminal vesicle, chronic

098.35 Gonococcal cervicitis, chronic
Any condition classifiable to 098.15, specified as chronic
Gonorrhea of cervix, chronic

098.36 Gonococcal endometritis, chronic
Any condition classifiable to 098.16, specified as chronic

098.37 Gonococcal salpingitis (chronic)

098.39 Other

⑤ **098.4 Gonococcal infection of eye**

098.40 Gonococcal conjunctivitis (neonatorum)
Gonococcal ophthalmia (neonatorum)

098.41 Gonococcal iridocyclitis

098.42 Gonococcal endophthalmia

● Code new to this edition   ▲ Revision of existing code   ④ ⑤ Fourth or fifth digit required

098.43 Gonococcal keratitis

098.49 Other

⑤ **098.5 Gonococcal infection of joint**

098.50 Gonococcal arthritis
Gonococcal infection of joint NOS

098.51 Gonococcal synovitis and tenosynovitis

098.52 Gonococcal bursitis

098.53 Gonococcal spondylitis

098.59 Other
Gonococcal rheumatism

098.6 Gonococcal infection of pharynx

098.7 Gonococcal infection of anus and rectum
Gonococcal proctitis

⑤ **098.8 Gonococcal infection of other specified sites**

098.81 Gonococcal keratosis (blennorrhagica)

098.82 Gonococcal meningitis

098.83 Gonococcal pericarditis

098.84 Gonococcal endocarditis

098.85 Other gonococcal heart disease

098.86 Gonococcal peritonitis

098.89 Other
Gonococcemia

099 Other venereal diseases

099.0 Chancroid

Bubo (inguinal):	Chancre:
chancroidal	Ducrey's
due to Hemophilus ducreyi	simple
	soft
	Ulcus molle (cutis) (skin)

099.1 Lymphogranuloma venereum

Climatic or tropical bubo	Esthiomene
(Durand-) Nicolas- Favre disease	Lymphogranuloma inguinale

099.2 Granuloma inguinale

Donovanosis	Granuloma venereum
Granuloma pudendi (ulcerating)	Pudendal ulcer

099.3 Reiter's disease
Reiter's syndrome
Use additional code for associated:
   arthropathy (711.1)
   conjunctivitis (372.33)

⑤ **099.4 Other nongonococcal urethritis [NGU]**

099.40 Unspecified
Nonspecific urethritis

099.41 Chlamydia trachomatis

099.49 Other specified organism

⑤ **099.5 Other venereal diseases due to Chlamydia trachomatis**

Excludes: *Chlamydia trachomatis infection of conjunctiva (076.0-076.9, 077.0, 077.9)*
Lymphogranuloma venereum (099.1)

099.50 Unspecified site

099.51 Pharynx

099.52 Anus and rectum

099.53 Lower genitourinary sites

Excludes: *urethra (099.41)*
Use additional code, if desired, to specify site of infection, such as:
   bladder (595.4)
   cervix (616.0)
   vagina and vulva (616.11)

Add 4th or 5th digit	Nonspecific code	Unspecified code	Manifestation code

099.54 Other genitourinary sites
Use additional code, if desired, to specify site of infection, such as:
pelvic inflammatory disease NOS (614.9)
testis and epididymis (604.91)

099.55 Unspecified genitourinary site

099.56 Peritoneum
Perihepatitis

099.59 Other specified site

099.8 Other specified venereal diseases

099.9 Venereal disease, unspecified

OTHER SPIROCHETAL DISEASES (100-104)

100 Leptospirosis

100.0 Leptospirosis icterohemorrhagica
Leptospiral or spirochetal jaundice (hemorrhagic)
Weil's disease

⑤ **100.8** Other specified leptospiral infections

100.81 Leptospiral meningitis (aseptic)

100.89 Other

Fever:	Infection by Leptospira:
Fort Bragg	australis
pretibial	bataviae
swamp	pyrogenes

100.9 Leptospirosis, unspecified

101 Vincent's angina

Acute necrotizing ulcerative:	Spirochetal stomatitis
gingivitis	Trench mouth
stomatitis	Vincent's:
Fusospirochetal pharyngitis	gingivitis
	infection [any site]

102 Yaws
Includes: frambesia
pian

102.0 Initial lesions

Chancre of yaws	Initial frambesial ulcer
Frambesia, initial or primary	Mother yaw

102.1 Multiple papillomata and wet crab yaws

Butter yaws	Planter or palmer papilloma of yaws
Frambesioma	
Pianoma	

102.2 Other early skin lesions
Early yaws (cutaneous) (macular) (papular) (maculopapular) (micropapular)
Frambeside of early yaws
Cutaneous yaws, less than five years after infection

102.3 Hyperkeratosis
Ghoul hand
Hyperkeratosis, palmer or plantar (early) (late) due to yaws
Worm-eaten soles

102.4 Gummata and ulcers
Nodular late yaws (ulcerated)
Gummatous frambeside

102.5 Gangosa
Rhinopharyngitis mutilans

102.6 Bone and joint lesions
Goundou, of yaws (late)
Gumma, bone, of yaws (late)
Gummatous osteitis or periostitis, of yaws (late)
Hydrarthrosis, of yaws (early) (late)
Osteitis, of yaws (early) (late)
Periostitis (hypertrophic), of yaws (early) (late)

102.7 Other manifestations
Juxta-articular nodules of yaws
Mucosal yaws

● Code new to this edition	▲ Revision of existing code	④ ⑤ Fourth or fifth digit required

102.8 Latent yaws
Yaws without clinical manifestations, with positive serology

102.9 Yaws, unspecified

103 Pinta

103.0 Primary lesions
Chancre (primary) of pinta [carate]
Papule (primary) of pinta [carate]
Pintid of pinta [carate]

103.1 Intermediate lesions
Erythematous plaques of pinta [carate]
Hyperchromic lesions of pinta [carate]
Hyperkeratosis of pinta [carate]

103.2 Late lesions
Cardiovascular lesions, of pinta [carate]
Skin lesions:
 achromic of pinta [carate]
 cicatricial of pinta [carate]
 dyschromic of pinta [carate]
Vitiligo of pinta [carate]

103.3 Mixed lesions
Achromic and hyperchromic skin lesions of pinta [carate]

103.9 Pinta, unspecified

104 Other spirochetal infection

104.0 Nonvenereal endemic syphilis
Bejel   Njovera

104.8 Other specified spirochetal infections
Excludes: *relapsing fever (087.0-087.9)*
              syphilis (090.0-097.9)

104.9 Spirochetal infection, unspecified

MYCOSES (110-118)

Use additional code, if desired, to identify manifestation, as:
 arthropathy (711.6)
 meningitis (321.0-321.1)
 otitis externa (380.15)

Excludes: *infection by Actinomycetales, such as species of Actinomyces, Actinomadura,*
              Nocardia, Streptomyces (039.0-039.9)

110 Dermatophytosis
Includes: infection by species of Epidermophyton, Microsporum, and Trichophyton
              tinea, any type except those in 111

110.0 Of scalp and beard
Kerion
Sycosis, mycotic
Trichophytic tinea [black dot tinea], scalp

110.1 Of nail
Dermatophytic onychia   Tinea unguium
Onychomycosis

110.2 Of hand
Tinea manuum

110.3 Of groin and perianal area
Dhobie itch   Tinea cruris
Eczema marginatum

110.4 Of foot
Athlete's foot   Tinea pedis

110.5 Of the body
Herpes circinatus
Tinea imbricata [Tokelau]

110.6 Deep seated dermatophytosis
Granuloma trichophyticum
Majocchi's granuloma

110.8 Of other specified sites

Add 4th or   Nonspecific   Unspecified   Manifestation
5th digit   code   code   code

110.9 Of unspecified site
Favus NOS   Ringworm NOS
Microsporic tinea NOS

111 Dermatomycosis, other and unspecified

111.0 Pityriasis versicolor
Infection by Malassezia [Pityrosporum] furfur
Tinea flava
Tinea versicolor

111.1 Tinea nigra
Infection by   Microsporosis nigra
    Cladosporium species   Pityriasis nigra
Keratomycosis nigricans   Tinea palmaris nigra

111.2 Tinea blanca
Infection by Trichosporon (beigelii) cutaneum
White piedra

111.3 Black piedra
Infection by Piedraia hortai

111.8 Other specified dermatomycoses

111.9 Dermatomycosis, unspecified

112 Candidiasis
Includes: infection by Candida species
           moniliasis

Excludes: *neonatal monilial infection (771.7)*

112.0 Of mouth
Thrush (oral)

112.1 Of vulva and vagina
Candidal vulvovaginitis   Monilial vulvovaginitis

112.2 Of other urogenital sites
Candidal balanitis

112.3 Of skin and nails
Candidal intertrigo   Candidal perionyxis [paronychia]
Candidal onychia

112.4 Of lung
Candidal pneumonia

112.5 Disseminated
Systemic candidiasis

⑤ **112.8 Of other specified sites**

    112.81 Candidal endocarditis

    112.82 Candidal otitis externa
Otomycosis in moniliasis

    112.83 Candidal meningitis

    112.84 Candidal esophagitis

    112.85 Candidal enteritis

    112.89 Other

112.9 Of unspecified site

114 Coccidioidomycosis
Includes: infection by Coccidioides (immitis)
           Posada-Wernicke disease

114.0 Primary coccidioidomycosis (pulmonary)
Acute pulmonary coccidioidomycosis
Coccidioidomycotic pneumonitis
Desert rheumatism
Pulmonary coccidioidomycosis
San Joaquin Valley fever

114.1 Primary extrapulmonary coccidioidomycosis
Chancriform syndrome
Primary cutaneous coccidioidomycosis

114.2 Coccidioidal meningitis

114.3 Other forms of progressive coccidioidomycosis
Coccidioidal granuloma
Disseminated coccidioidomycosis

● Code new   ▲ Revision of   ④ ⑤ Fourth or fifth
  to this edition   existing code   digit required

114.4 Chronic pulmonary coccidioidomycosis

114.5 Pulmonary coccidioidomycosis, unspecified

114.9 Coccidioidomycosis, unspecified

⑤ **115 Histoplasmosis**

The following fifth-digit subclassification is for use with category 115:

  0 **without mention of manifestation**

  1 **meningitis**

  2 **retinitis**

  3 **pericarditis**

  4 **endocarditis**

  5 **pneumonia**

  9 **other**

⑤ **115.0 Infection by Histoplasma capsulatum**
[0-5, 9] American histoplasmosis
Darling's disease
Reticuloendothelial cytomycosis
Small form histoplasmosis

⑤ **115.1 Infection by Histoplasma duboisii**
[0-5, 9] African histoplasmosis
Large form histoplasmosis

⑤ **115.9 Histoplasmosis, unspecified**
[0-5, 9] Histoplasmosis NOS

116 Blastomycotic infection

116.0 Blastomycosis
Blastomycotic dermatitis
Chicago disease
Cutaneous blastomycosis
Disseminated blastomycosis
Gilchrist's disease
Infection by Blastomyces [Ajellomyces] dermatitidis
North American blastomycosis
Primary pulmonary blastomycosis

116.1 Paracoccidioidomycosis
Brazilian blastomycosis
Infection by Paracoccidioides [Blastomyces] brasiliensis
Lutz-Splendore-Almeida disease
Mucocutaneous-lymphangitic paracoccidioidomycosis
Pulmonary paracoccidioidomycosis
South American blastomycosis
Visceral paracoccidioidomycosis

116.2 Lobomycosis
Infections by Loboa [Blastomyces] loboi
Keloidal blastomycosis
Lobo's disease

117 Other mycoses

117.0 Rhinosporidiosis
Infection by Rhinosporidium seeberi

117.1 Sporotrichosis
Cutaneous sporotrichosis
Disseminated sporotrichosis
Infection by Sporothrix [Sporotrichum] schenckii
Lymphocutaneous sporotrichosis
Pulmonary sporotrichosis
Sporotrichosis of the bones

117.2 Chromoblastomycosis
Chromomycosis
Infection by Cladosporidium carrionii, Fonsecaea compactum, Fonsecaea pedrosoi, Phialophora verrucosa

117.3 Aspergillosis
Infection by Aspergillus species, mainly A. fumigatus, A. flavus group, A. terreus group

| Add 4th or 5th digit | Nonspecific code | Unspecified code | Manifestation code |

117.4 Mycotic mycetomas
Infection by various genera and species of Ascomycetes and Deuteromycetes, such as Acremonium [Cephalosporium] falciforme, Neotestudina rosatii, Madurella grisea, Madurella mycetomii, Pyrenochaeta romeroi, Zopfia [Leptosphaeria] senegalensis
Madura foot, mycotic
Maduromycosis, mycotic

Excludes: *actinomycotic mycetomas (039.0-039.9)*

117.5 Cryptococcosis
Busse-Buschke's disease	Pulmonary cryptococcosis
European cryptococcosis	Systemic cryptococcosis
Infection by Cryptococcus neoformans	Torula

117.6 Allescheriosis [Petriellidosis]
Infections by Allescheria [Petriellidium] boydii [Monosporium apiospermum]

Excludes: *mycotic mycetoma (117.4)*

117.7 Zygomycosis [Phycomycosis or Mucormycosis]
Infection by species of Absidia, Basidiobolus, Conidiobolus, Cunninghamella, Entomophthora, Mucor, Rhizopus, Saksenaea

117.8 Infection by dematiacious fungi, [Phaehyphomycosis]
Infection by dematiacious fungi, such as Cladosporium trichoides [bantianum], Dreschlera hawaiiensis, Phialophora gougerotii, Phialophora jeanselmi

117.9 Other and unspecified mycoses

118 Opportunistic mycoses
Infection of skin, subcutaneous tissues, and/or organs by a wide variety of fungi generally considered to be pathogenic to compromised hosts only (e.g., infection by species of Alternaria, Dreschlera, Fusarium)

Use additional code to identify manifestation, such as:
keratitis (370.8)

HELMINTHIASES (120-129)

120 Schistosomiasis [bilharziasis]

120.0 Schistosoma haematobium
Vesical schistosomiasis NOS

120.1 Schistosoma mansoni
Intestinal schistosomiasis NOS

120.2 Schistosoma japonicum
Asiatic schistosomiasis NOS
Katayama disease or fever

120.3 Cutaneous
Cercarial dermatitis	Schistosome dermatitis
Infection by cercariae of Schistosoma	Swimmers' itch

120.8 Other specified schistosomiasis
Infection by Schistosoma:	Infection by Schistosoma spindale
bovis	Schistosomiasis chestermani
intercalatum	
mattheii	

120.9 Schistosomiasis, unspecified
Blood flukes NOS	Hemic distomiasis

121 Other trematode infections

121.0 Opisthorchiasis
Infection by:
cat liver fluke
Opisthorchis (felineus) (tenuicollis) (viverrini)

121.1 Clonorchiasis
Biliary cirrhosis due to clonorchiasis
Chinese liver fluke disease
Hepatic distomiasis due to Clonorchis sinensis
Oriental liver fluke disease

121.2 Paragonimiasis
Infection by Paragonimus	Pulmonary distomiasis
Lung fluke disease (oriental)	

● Code new to this edition ▲ Revision of existing code ④ ⑤ Fourth or fifth digit required

121.3 Fascioliasis
Infection by Fasciola: Liver flukes NOS
 gigantica   Sheep liver fluke infection
 hepatica

121.4 Fasciolopsiasis
Infection by Fasciolopsis [buski]
Intestinal distomiasis

121.5 Metagonimiasis
Infection by Metagonimus yokogawai

121.6 Heterophyiasis
Infection by:
 Heterophyes heterophyes
 Stellantchasmus falcatus

121.8 Other specified trematode infections
Infection by:
 Dicrocoelium dendriticum
 Echinostoma ilocanum
 Gastrodiscoides hominis

121.9 Trematode infection, unspecified
Distomiasis NOS   Fluke disease NOS

122 Echinococcosis
Includes: echinococciasis
 hydatid disease
 hydatidosis

122.0 Echinococcus granulosus infection of liver

122.1 Echinococcus granulosus infection of lung

122.2 Echinococcus granulosus infection of thyroid

122.3 Echinococcus granulosus infection, other

122.4 Echinococcus granulosus infection, unspecified

122.5 Echinococcus multilocularis infection of liver

122.6 Echinococcus multilocularis infection, other

122.7 Echinococcus multilocularis infection, unspecified

122.8 Echinococcosis, unspecified, of liver

122.9 Echinococcosis, other and unspecified

123 Other cestode infection

123.0 Taenia solium infection, intestinal form
Pork tapeworm (adult) (infection)

123.1 Cysticercosis
Cysticerciasis
Infection by Cysticercus cellulosae [larval form of Taenia solium]

123.2 Taenia saginata infection
Beef tapeworm (infection)
Infection by Taeniarhynchus saginatus

123.3 Taeniasis, unspecified

123.4 Diphyllobothriasis, intestinal
Diphyllobothrium (adult) (latum) (pacificum) infection
Fish tapeworm (infection)

123.5 Sparganosis [larval diphyllobothriasis]
Infection by:
 Diphyllobothrium larvae
 Sparganum (mansoni) (proliferum)
 Spirometra larvae

123.6 Hymenolepiasis
Dwarf tapeworm (infection)
Hymenolepis (diminuta) (nana) infection
Rat tapeworm (infection)

123.8 Other specified cestode infection
Diplogonoporus (grandis) infection
Dipylidium (caninum) infection
Dog tapeworm (infection) infection

205

Add 4th or   Nonspecific   Unspecified   Manifestation
5th digit   code   code   code

123.9 Cestode infection, unspecified
    Tapeworm (infection) NOS

124 Trichinosis
    Trichinella spiralis infection
    Trichinellosis
    Trichiniasis

125 Filarial infection and dracontiasis

125.0 Bancroftian filariasis
    Chyluria due to Wuchereria bancrofti
    Elephantiasis due to Wuchereria bancrofti
    Infection due to Wuchereria bancrofti
    Lymphadenitis due to Wuchereria bancrofti
    Lymphangitis due to Wuchereria bancrofti
    Wuchereriasis

125.1 Malayan filariasis
    Brugia filariasis due to Brugia [Wuchereria] malayi
    Chyluria due to Brugia [Wuchereria] malayi
    Elephantiasis due to Brugia [Wuchereria] malayi
    Infection due to Brugia [Wuchereria] malayi
    Lymphadenitis due to Brugia [Wuchereria] malayi
    Lymphangitis due to Brugia [Wuchereria] malayi

125.2 Loiasis
    Eyeworm disease of Africa
    Loa loa infection

125.3 Onchocerciasis
    Onchocerca volvulus infection
    Onchocercosis

125.4 Dipetalonemiasis
    Infection by:
        Acanthocheilonema perstans
        Dipetalonema perstans

125.5 Mansonella ozzardi infection
    Filariasis ozzardi

125.6 Other specified filariasis
    Dirofilaria infection
    Infection by:
        Acanthocheilonema streptocerca
        Dipetalonema streptocerca

125.7 Dracontiasis
    Guinea-worm infection
    Infection by Dracunculus medinensis

125.9 Unspecified filariasis

126 Ancylostomiasis and necatoriasis
    Includes: cutaneous larva migrans due to Ancylostoma
               hookworm (disease) (infection)
               uncinariasis

126.0 Ancylostoma duodenale

126.1 Necator americanus

126.2 Ancylostoma braziliense

126.3 Ancylostoma ceylanicum

126.8 Other specified Ancylostoma

126.9 Ancylostomiasis and necatoriasis, unspecified
    Creeping eruption NOS
    Cutaneous larva migrans NOS

127 Other intestinal helminthiases

127.0 Ascariasis
    Ascaridiasis
    Infection by Ascaris lumbricoides
    Roundworm infection

127.1 Anisakiasis
    Infection by Anisakis larva

● Code new   ▲ Revision of   ④ ⑤ Fourth or fifth
       to this edition   existing code   digit required

127.2 Strongyloidiasis
Infection by Strongyloides stercoralis

Excludes: *trichostrongyliasis (127.6)*

127.3 Trichuriasis
Infection by Trichuris trichiuria
Trichocephaliasis
Whipworm (disease) (infection)

127.4 Enterobiasis
Infection by Enterobius vermicularis
Oxyuriasis
Oxyuris vermicularis infection
Pinworm (disease) (infection)
Threadworm infection

127.5 Capillariasis
Infection by Capillaria philippinensis

Excludes: *infection by Capillaria hepatica (128.8)*

127.6 Trichostrongyliasis
Infection by Trichostrongylus species

127.7 Other specified intestinal helminthiasis
Infection by:
 Oesophagostomum apiostomum and related species
 Ternidens diminutus
 other specified intestinal helminth
 Physalopteriasis

127.8 Mixed intestinal helminthiasis
Infection by intestinal helminths classified to more than one of the categories
 120.0-127.7
Mixed helminthiasis NOS

127.9 Intestinal helminthiasis, unspecified

128 Other and unspecified helminthiases

128.0 Toxocariasis
Larva migrans visceralis
Toxocara (canis) (cati) infection
Visceral larva migrans syndrome

128.1 Gnathostomiasis
Infection by Gnathostoma spinigerum and related species

128.8 Other specified helminthiasis
Infection by:
 Angiostrongylus cantonensis
 Capillaria hepatica
 other specified helminth

128.9 Helminth infection, unspecified
Helminthiasis NOS
Worms NOS

129 Intestinal parasitism, unspecified

OTHER INFECTIOUS AND PARASITIC DISEASES (130-136)

130 Toxoplasmosis
Includes: infection by toxoplasma gondii
 toxoplasmosis (acquired)

Excludes: *congenital toxoplasmosis (771.2)*

130.0 Meningoencephalitis due to toxoplasmosis
Encephalitis due to acquired toxoplasmosis

130.1 Conjunctivitis due to toxoplasmosis

130.2 Chorioretinitis due to toxoplasmosis
Focal retinochoroiditis due to acquired toxoplasmosis

130.3 Myocarditis due to toxoplasmosis

130.4 Pneumonitis due to toxoplasmosis

130.5 Hepatitis due to toxoplasmosis

130.7 Toxoplasmosis of other specified sites

130.8 Multisystemic disseminated toxoplasmosis
Toxoplasmosis of multiple sites

	Add 4th or 5th digit		Nonspecific code		Unspecified code		Manifestation code

130.9 Toxoplasmosis, unspecified

131 Trichomoniasis
Includes: infection due to Trichomonas (vaginalis)

⑤ **131.0 Urogenital trichomoniasis**

    131.00 Urogenital trichomoniasis, unspecified
        Fluor (vaginalis) trichomonal or due to Trichomonas (vaginalis)
        Leukorrhea (vaginalis) trichomonal or due to Trichomonas (vaginalis)

    131.01 Trichomonal vulvovaginitis
        Vaginitis, trichomonal or due to Trichomonas (vaginalis)

    131.02 Trichomonal urethritis

    131.03 Trichomonal prostatitis

    131.09 Other

131.8 Other specified sites
Excludes: *intestinal (007.3)*

131.9 Trichomoniasis, unspecified

132 Pediculosis and phthirus infestation

132.0 Pediculus capitis [head louse]

132.1 Pediculus corporis [body louse]

132.2 Phthirus pubis [pubic louse]
Pediculus pubis

132.3 Mixed infestation
Infestation classifiable to more than one of the categories 132.0-132.2

132.9 Pediculosis, unspecified

133 Acariasis

133.0 Scabies
Infestation by Sarcoptes scabiei
Norwegian scabies
Sarcoptic itch

133.8 Other acariasis
Chiggers
Infestation by:
    Demodex folliculorum
    Trombicula

133.9 Acariasis, unspecified
Infestation by mites NOS

134 Other infestation

134.0 Myiasis
Infestation by: Infestation by:
    Dermatobia (hominis)   maggots
    fly larvae   Oestrus ovis
    Gasterophilus (intestinalis)

134.1 Other arthropod infestation
Infestation by: Jigger disease
    chigoe   Scarabiasis
    sand flea   Tungiasis
    Tunga penetrans

134.2 Hirudiniasis
Hirudiniasis (external) (internal)
Leeches (aquatic) (land)

134.8 Other specified infestations

134.9 Infestation, unspecified
Infestation (skin) NOS
Skin parasites NOS

135 Sarcoidosis
Besnier-Boeck- Schaumann disease   Sarcoid (any site):
Lupoid (miliary) of Boeck   NOS
Lupus pernio (Besnier)   Boeck
Lymphogranulomatosis, benign   Darier-Roussy
    (Schaumann's)   Uveoparotid fever

● Code new
    to this edition
▲ Revision of
    existing code
④ ⑤ Fourth or fifth
    digit required

136 **Other and unspecified infectious and parasitic diseases**

136.0 **Ainhum**
Dactylolysis spontanea

136.1 **Behçet's syndrome**

⑤ **136.2** **Specific infections by free-living amebae**

136.21 **Specific infection due to acanthamoeba**
Use additional code to identify manifestation, such as:
keratitis (370.8)

136.29 **Other specific infections by free-living amebae**
Meningoencephalitis due to Naegleria

136.3 **Pneumocystosis**
Pneumonia due to Pneumocystis carinii
Pneumonia due to Pneumocystis jiroveci

136.4 **Psorospermiasis**

136.5 **Sarcosporidiosis**
Infection by Sarcocystis lindemanni

136.8 **Other specified infectious and parasitic diseases**
Candiru infestation

136.9 **Unspecified infectious and parasitic diseases**
Infectious disease NOS
Parasitic disease NOS

LATE EFFECTS OF INFECTIOUS AND PARASITIC DISEASES (137-139)

137 **Late effects of tuberculosis**
Note: This category is to be used to indicate conditions classifiable to 010-018 as the cause of
late effects, which are themselves classified elsewhere. The "late effects" include those
specified as such, as sequelae, or as due to old or inactive tuberculosis, without evidence
of active disease.

137.0 **Late effects of respiratory or unspecified tuberculosis**

137.1 **Late effects of central nervous system tuberculosis**

137.2 **Late effects of genitourinary tuberculosis**

137.3 **Late effects of tuberculosis of bones and joints**

137.4 **Late effects of tuberculosis of other specified organs**

138 **Late effects of acute poliomyelitis**
Note: This category is to be used to indicate conditions classifiable to 045 as the cause of late
effects, which are themselves classified elsewhere. The "late effects" include conditions
specified as such, or as sequelae, or as due to old or inactive poliomyelitis, without
evidence of active disease.

139 **Late effects of other infectious and parasitic diseases**
Note: This category is to be used to indicate conditions classifiable to categories 001-009,
020-041, 046-136 as the cause of late effects, which are themselves classified elsewhere.
The "late effects" include conditions specified as such; they also include sequela of
diseases classifiable to the above categories if there is evidence that the disease itself is no
longer present.

139.0 **Late effects of viral encephalitis**
Late effects of conditions classifiable to 049.8-049.9, 062-064

139.1 **Late effects of trachoma**
Late effects of conditions classifiable to 076

139.8 **Late effects of other and unspecified infectious and parasitic diseases**

▬	Add 4th or 5th digit	▬	Nonspecific code	▬	Unspecified code	▬	Manifestation code

● Code new
to this edition

▲ Revision of
existing code

④ ⑤ Fourth or fifth
digit required

2. NEOPLASMS (140-239)

Notes:

1. Content
This chapter contains the following broad groups:

140-195 Malignant neoplasms, stated or presumed to be primary, of specified sites, except of lymphatic and hematopoietic tissue

196-198 Malignant neoplasms, stated or presumed to be secondary, of specified sites

199 Malignant neoplasms, without specification of site

200-208 Malignant neoplasms, stated or presumed to be primary, of lymphatic and hematopoietic tissue

209 Neuroendocrine tumors

210-229 Benign neoplasms

230-234 Carcinoma in situ

235-238 Neoplasms of uncertain behavior

239 Neoplasms of unspecified nature

2. Functional activity
All neoplasms are classified in this chapter, whether or not functionally active. An additional code from Chapter 3 may be used, if desired, to identify such functional activity associated with any neoplasm, e.g.:
> catecholamine-producing malignant pheochromocytoma of adrenal:
>> code 194.0, additional code 255.6
> basophil adenoma of pituitary with Cushing's syndrome:
>> code 227.3, additional code 255.0

3. Morphology [Histology]
For those wishing to identify the histological type of neoplasms, a comprehensive coded nomenclature, which comprises the morphology rubrics of the ICD-Oncology, is given in Appendix A.

4. Malignant neoplasms overlapping site boundaries
Categories 140-195 are for the classification of primary malignant neoplasms according to their point of origin. A malignant neoplasm that overlaps two or more subcategories within a three-digit rubric and whose point of origin cannot be determined should be classified to the subcategory .8 "Other." For example, "carcinoma involving tip and ventral surface of tongue" should be assigned to 141.8. On the other hand, "carcinoma of tip of tongue, extending to involve the ventral surface" should be coded to 141.2, as the point of origin, the tip, is known. Three subcategories (149.8, 159.8, 165.8) have been provided for malignant neoplasms that overlap the boundaries of three-digit rubrics within certain systems. Overlapping malignant neoplasms that cannot be classified as indicated above should be assigned to the appropriate subdivision of category 195 (Malignant neoplasm of other and ill-defined sites).

MALIGNANT NEOPLASM OF LIP, ORAL CAVITY, AND PHARYNX (140-149)

> *Excludes:* carcinoma in situ (230.0)

140 Malignant neoplasm of lip
> *Excludes:* skin of lip (173.0)

140.0 Upper lip, vermilion border
Upper lip:
   NOS
   external
   lipstick area

140.1 Lower lip, vermilion border
Lower lip:
   NOS
   external
   lipstick area

140.3 Upper lip, inner aspect
Upper lip   Upper lip:
   buccal aspect   mucosa
   frenulum   oral aspect

140.4 Lower lip, inner aspect
Lower lip: Lower lip:
   buccal aspect   mucosa
   frenulum   oral aspect

140.5 Lip, unspecified, inner aspect
Lip, not specified whether upper or lower:
   buccal aspect   frenulum
   mucosa   oral aspect

Add 4th or 5th digit | Nonspecific code | Unspecified code | Manifestation code

140.6 Commissure of lip
Labial commissure

140.8 Other sites of lip
Malignant neoplasm of contiguous or overlapping sites of lip whose point of origin cannot be determined

140.9 Lip, unspecified, vermilion border
Lip, not specified as upper or lower:
NOS
external
lipstick area

141 Malignant neoplasm of tongue

141.0 Base of tongue
Dorsal surface of base of tongue
Fixed part of tongue NOS

141.1 Dorsal surface of tongue
Anterior two-thirds of tongue, dorsal surface
Dorsal tongue NOS
Midline of tongue

Excludes: dorsal surface of base of tongue (141.0)

141.2 Tip and lateral border of tongue

141.3 Ventral surface of tongue
Anterior two-thirds of tongue, ventral surface
Frenulum linguae

141.4 Anterior two-thirds of tongue, part unspecified
Mobile part of tongue NOS

141.5 Junctional zone
Border of tongue at junction of fixed and mobile parts at insertion of anterior tonsillar pillar

141.6 Lingual tonsil

141.8 Other sites of tongue
Malignant neoplasm of contiguous or overlapping sites of tongue whose point of origin cannot be determined

141.9 Tongue, unspecified
Tongue NOS

142 Malignant neoplasm of major salivary glands
Includes: salivary ducts

Excludes: malignant neoplasm of minor salivary glands:
NOS (145.9)
buccal mucosa (145.0)
soft palate (145.3)
tongue (141.0-141.9)
tonsil, palatine (146.0)

142.0 Parotid gland

142.1 Submandibular gland
Submaxillary gland

142.2 Sublingual gland

142.8 Other major salivary glands
Malignant neoplasm of contiguous or overlapping sites of salivary glands and ducts whose point of origin cannot be determined

142.9 Salivary gland, unspecified
Salivary gland (major) NOS

143 Malignant neoplasm of gum
Includes: alveolar (ridge) mucosa
gingiva (alveolar) (marginal)
interdental papillae

Excludes: malignant odontogenic neoplasms (170.0-170.1)

143.0 Upper gum

143.1 Lower gum

143.8 Other sites of gum
Malignant neoplasm of contiguous or overlapping sites of gum whose point of origin cannot be determined

● Code new to this edition   ▲ Revision of existing code   ④ ⑤ Fourth or fifth digit required

143.9 Gum, unspecified

144 **Malignant neoplasm of floor of mouth**

144.0 Anterior portion
Anterior to the premolar-canine junction

144.1 Lateral portion

144.8 Other sites of floor of mouth
Malignant neoplasm of contiguous or overlapping sites of floor of mouth whose point of origin cannot be determined

144.9 Floor of mouth, part unspecified

145 **Malignant neoplasm of other and unspecified parts of mouth**
Excludes: mucosa of lips (140.0-140.9)

145.0 Cheek mucosa
Buccal mucosa   Cheek, inner aspect

145.1 Vestibule of mouth
Buccal sulcus (upper) (lower)
Labial sulcus (upper) (lower)

145.2 Hard palate

145.3 Soft palate
Excludes: nasopharyngeal [posterior] [superior] surface of soft palate (147.3)

145.4 Uvula

145.5 Palate, unspecified
Junction of hard and soft palate
Roof of mouth

145.6 Retromolar area

145.8 Other specified parts of mouth
Malignant neoplasm of contiguous or overlapping sites of mouth whose point of origin cannot be determined

145.9 Mouth, unspecified
Buccal cavity NOS
Minor salivary gland, unspecified site
Oral cavity NOS

146 **Malignant neoplasm of oropharynx**

146.0 Tonsil
Tonsil:
NOS
faucial
palatine
Excludes: lingual tonsil (141.6)
pharyngeal tonsil (147.1)

146.1 Tonsillar fossa

146.2 Tonsillar pillars (anterior) (posterior)
Faucial pillar   Palatoglossal arch
Glossopalatine fold   Palatopharyngeal arch

146.3 Vallecula
Anterior and medial surface of the pharyngoepiglottic fold

146.4 Anterior aspect of epiglottis
Epiglottis, free border [margin]
Glossoepiglottic fold(s)
Excludes: epiglottis:
NOS (161.1)
suprahyoid portion (161.1)

146.5 Junctional region
Junction of the free margin of the epiglottis, the aryepiglottic fold, and the pharyngoepiglottic fold

146.6 Lateral wall of oropharynx

146.7 Posterior wall of oropharynx

146.8 Other specified sites of oropharynx
Branchial cleft
Malignant neoplasm of contiguous or overlapping sites of oropharynx whose point of origin cannot be determined

Add 4th or 5th digit | Nonspecific code | Unspecified code | Manifestation code

146.9 Oropharynx, unspecified

147 Malignant neoplasm of nasopharynx

147.0 Superior wall
Roof of nasopharynx

147.1 Posterior wall
Adenoid   Pharyngeal tonsil

147.2 Lateral wall
Fossa of Rosenmüller   Pharyngeal recess
Opening of auditory tube

147.3 Anterior wall
Floor of nasopharynx
Nasopharyngeal [posterior] [superior] surface of soft palate
Posterior margin of nasal septum and choanae

147.8 Other specified sites of nasopharynx
Malignant neoplasm of contiguous or overlapping sites of nasopharynx whose point of
origin cannot be determined

147.9 Nasopharynx, unspecified
Nasopharyngeal wall NOS

148 Malignant neoplasm of hypopharynx

148.0 Postcricoid region

148.1 Pyriform sinus
Pyriform fossa

148.2 Aryepiglottic fold, hypopharyngeal aspect
Aryepiglottic fold or interarytenoid fold:
NOS
marginal zone

Excludes: *aryepiglottic fold or interarytenoid fold, laryngeal aspect (161.1)*

148.3 Posterior hypopharyngeal wall

148.8 Other specified sites of hypopharynx
Malignant neoplasm of contiguous or overlapping sites of hypopharynx whose point of
origin cannot be determined

148.9 Hypopharynx, unspecified
Hypopharyngeal wall NOS   Hypopharynx NOS

149 Malignant neoplasm of other and ill-defined sites within the lip, oral cavity, and pharynx

149.0 Pharynx, unspecified

149.1 Waldeyer's ring

149.8 Other
Malignant neoplasms of lip, oral cavity, and pharynx whose point of origin cannot be
assigned to any one of the categories 140-148

Excludes: *"book leaf" neoplasm [ventral surface of tongue and floor of mouth] (145.8)*

149.9 Ill-defined

MALIGNANT NEOPLASM OF DIGESTIVE ORGANS AND PERITONEUM (150-159)

Excludes: *carcinoma in situ (230.1-230.9)*

150 Malignant neoplasm of esophagus

150.0 Cervical esophagus

150.1 Thoracic esophagus

150.2 Abdominal esophagus

Excludes: *adenocarcinoma (151.0)*
cardio-esophageal junction (151.0)

150.3 Upper third of esophagus
Proximal third of esophagus

150.4 Middle third of esophagus

150.5 Lower third of esophagus
Distal third of esophagus

Excludes: *adenocarcinoma (151.0)*
cardio-esophageal junction (151.0)

● Code new   ▲ Revision of   ④ ⑤ Fourth or fifth
   to this edition   existing code   digit required

150.8 **Other specified part**
Malignant neoplasm of contiguous or overlapping sites of esophagus whose point of origin cannot be determined

150.9 **Esophagus, unspecified**

151 **Malignant neoplasm of stomach**

> *Excludes:* benign carcinoid tumor of stomach (209.63)
> malignant carcinoid tumor of stomach (209.23)

151.0 **Cardia**
Cardiac orifice   Cardio-esophageal junction

> *Excludes:* squamous cell carcinoma (150.2, 150.5)

151.1 **Pylorus**
Prepylorus   Pyloric canal

151.2 **Pyloric antrum**
Antrum of stomach NOS

151.3 **Fundus of stomach**

151.4 **Body of stomach**

151.5 **Lesser curvature, unspecified**
Lesser curvature, not classifiable to 151.1-151.4

151.6 **Greater curvature, unspecified**
Greater curvature, not classifiable to 151.0-151.4

151.8 **Other specified sites of stomach**
Anterior wall, not classifiable to 151.0-151.4
Posterior wall, not classifiable to 151.0-151.4
Malignant neoplasm of contiguous or overlapping sites of stomach whose point of origin cannot be determined

151.9 **Stomach, unspecified**
Carcinoma ventriculi   Gastric cancer

152 **Malignant neoplasm of small intestine, including duodenum**

> *Excludes:* benign carcinoid tumor of small intestine and duodenum (209.40-209.43)
> malignant carcinoid tumor of small intestine and duodenum (209.00-209.03)

152.0 **Duodenum**

152.1 **Jejunum**

152.2 **Ileum**

> *Excludes:* ileocecal valve (153.4)

152.3 **Meckel's diverticulum**

152.8 **Other specified sites of small intestine**
Duodenojejunal junction
Malignant neoplasm of contiguous or overlapping sites of small intestine whose point of origin cannot be determined

152.9 **Small intestine, unspecified**

153 **Malignant neoplasm of colon**

> *Excludes:* benign carcinoid tumor of colon (209.50-209.56)
> malignant carcinoid tumor of colon (209.10-209.16)

153.0 **Hepatic flexure**

153.1 **Transverse colon**

153.2 **Descending colon**
Left colon

153.3 **Sigmoid colon**
Sigmoid (flexure)

> *Excludes:* rectosigmoid junction (154.0)

153.4 **Cecum**
Ileocecal valve

153.5 **Appendix**

153.6 **Ascending colon**
Right colon

153.7 **Splenic flexure**

	Add 4th or 5th digit		Nonspecific code		Unspecified code		Manifestation code

153.8 Other specified sites of large intestine
Malignant neoplasm of contiguous or overlapping sites of colon whose point of origin cannot be determined

Excludes: *ileocecal valve (153.4)*
rectosigmoid junction (154.0)

153.9 Colon, unspecified
Large intestine NOS

154 Malignant neoplasm of rectum, rectosigmoid junction, and anus

Excludes: *benign carcinoid tumor of rectum (209.57)*
malignant carcinoid tumor of rectum (209.17)

154.0 Rectosigmoid junction
Colon with rectum   Rectosigmoid (colon)

154.1 Rectum
Rectal ampulla

154.2 Anal canal
Anal sphincter

Excludes: *skin of anus (172.5, 173.5)*

154.3 Anus, unspecified

Excludes: *anus:*
margin (172.5, 173.5)
skin (172.5, 173.5)
perianal skin (172.5, 173.5)

154.8 Other
Anorectum
Cloacogenic zone
Malignant neoplasm of contiguous or overlapping sites of rectum, rectosigmoid junction, and anus whose point of origin cannot be determined

155 Malignant neoplasm of liver and intrahepatic bile ducts

155.0 Liver, primary
Carcinoma:
liver, specified as primary
hepatocellular
liver cell
Hepatoblastoma

155.1 Intrahepatic bile ducts
Canaliculi biliferi   Intrahepatic:
Interlobular: biliary passages
bile ducts   canaliculi
biliary canals   gall duct

Excludes: *hepatic duct (156.1)*

155.2 Liver, not specified as primary or secondary

156 Malignant neoplasm of gallbladder and extrahepatic bile ducts

156.0 Gallbladder

156.1 Extrahepatic bile ducts
Biliary duct or passage NOS   Cystic duct
Common bile duct   Hepatic duct
                                     Sphincter of Oddi

156.2 Ampulla of Vater

156.8 Other specified sites of gallbladder and extrahepatic bile ducts
Malignant neoplasm of contiguous or overlapping sites of gallbladder and extrahepatic bile ducts whose point of origin cannot be determined

156.9 Biliary tract, part unspecified
Malignant neoplasm involving both intrahepatic and extrahepatic bile ducts

157 Malignant neoplasm of pancreas

157.0 Head of pancreas

157.1 Body of pancreas

157.2 Tail of pancreas

● Code new
to this edition

▲ Revision of
existing code

④ ⑤ Fourth or fifth
digit required

157.3 Pancreatic duct
Duct of:
Santorini
Wirsung

157.4 Islets of Langerhans
Islets of Langerhans, any part of pancreas

Use additional code, if desired, to identify any functional activity

157.8 Other specified sites of pancreas
Ectopic pancreatic tissue
Malignant neoplasm of contiguous or overlapping sites of pancreas whose point of origin cannot be determined

157.9 Pancreas, part unspecified

158 Malignant neoplasm of retroperitoneum and peritoneum

158.0 Retroperitoneum

Periadrenal tissue	Perirenal tissue
Perinephric tissue	Retrocecal tissue

158.8 Specified parts of peritoneum
Cul-de-sac (of Douglas)
Mesentery
Mesocolon
Omentum
Peritoneum:
parietal
pelvic
Rectouterine pouch
Malignant neoplasm of contiguous or overlapping sites of retroperitoneum and peritoneum whose point of origin cannot be determined

158.9 Peritoneum, unspecified

159 Malignant neoplasm of other and ill-defined sites within the digestive organs and peritoneum

159.0 Intestinal tract, part unspecified
Intestine NOS

159.1 Spleen, not elsewhere classified
Angiosarcoma of spleen
Fibrosarcoma of spleen

Excludes: *Hodgkin's disease (201.0-201.9)*
lymphosarcoma (200.1)
reticulosarcoma (200.0)

159.8 Other sites of digestive system and intra-abdominal organs
Malignant neoplasm of digestive organs and peritoneum whose point of origin cannot be assigned to any one of the categories 150-158

Excludes: *anus and rectum (154.8)*
cardio-esophageal junction (151.0)
colon and rectum ORANGE (154.0)

159.9 Ill-defined
Alimentary canal or tract NOS
Gastrointestinal tract NOS

Excludes: *abdominal NOS (195.2)*
intra-abdominal NOS (195.2)

MALIGNANT NEOPLASM OF RESPIRATORY AND INTRATHORACIC ORGANS (160-165)

Excludes: *carcinoma in situ (231.0-231.9)*

160 Malignant neoplasm of nasal cavities, middle ear, and accessory sinuses

160.0 Nasal cavities

Cartilage of nose	Septum of nose
Conchae, nasal	Vestibule of nose
Internal nose	

Excludes: *nasal bone (170.0)*
nose NOS (195.0)
olfactory bulb (192.0)
posterior margin of septum and choanae (147.3)
skin of nose (172.3, 173.3)
turbinates (170.0)

	Add 4th or 5th digit		Nonspecific code		Unspecified code		Manifestation code

160.1 Auditory tube, middle ear, and mastoid air cells
Antrum tympanicum   Tympanic cavity
Eustachian tube

Excludes: *auditory canal (external) (172.2, 173.2)*
bone of ear (meatus) (170.0)
cartilage of ear (171.0)
ear (external) (skin) (172.2, 173.2)

160.2 Maxillary sinus
Antrum (Highmore) (maxillary)

160.3 Ethmoidal sinus

160.4 Frontal sinus

160.5 Sphenoidal sinus

160.8 Other
Malignant neoplasm of contiguous or overlapping sites of nasal cavities, middle ear, and accessory sinuses whose point of origin cannot be determined

160.9 Accessory sinus, unspecified

161 Malignant neoplasm of larynx

161.0 Glottis
Intrinsic larynx   True vocal cord
Laryngeal commissure   Vocal cord NOS
(anterior) (posterior)

161.1 Supraglottis
Aryepiglottic fold or interarytenoid fold, laryngeal aspect
Epiglottis (suprahyoid portion) NOS
Extrinsic larynx
False vocal cords
Posterior (laryngeal) surface of epiglottis
Ventricular bands

Excludes: *anterior aspect of epiglottis (146.4)*
aryepiglottic fold or interarytenoid fold:
NOS (148.2)
hypopharyngeal aspect (148.2)
marginal zone (148.2)

161.2 Subglottis

161.3 Laryngeal cartilages
Cartilage: Cartilage:
arytenoid   cuneiform
cricoid   thyroid

161.8 Other specified sites of larynx
Malignant neoplasm of contiguous or overlapping sites of larynx whose point of origin cannot be determined

161.9 Larynx, unspecified

162 Malignant neoplasm of trachea, bronchus, and lung

Excludes: *benign carcinoid tumor of bronchus (209.61)*
malignant carcinoid tumor of bronchus (209.21)

162.0 Trachea
Cartilage of trachea
Mucosa of trachea

162.2 Main bronchus
Carina   Hilus of lung

162.3 Upper lobe, bronchus or lung

162.4 Middle lobe, bronchus or lung

162.5 Lower lobe, bronchus or lung

162.8 Other parts of bronchus or lung
Malignant neoplasm of contiguous or overlapping sites of bronchus or lung whose point of origin cannot be determined

162.9 Bronchus and lung, unspecified

163 Malignant neoplasm of pleura

163.0 Parietal pleura

163.1 Visceral pleura

● Code new to this edition   ▲ Revision of existing code   ④ ⑤ Fourth or fifth digit required

163.8 Other specified sites of pleura
Malignant neoplasm of contiguous or overlapping sites of pleura whose point of origin cannot be determined

163.9 Pleura, unspecified

164 Malignant neoplasm of thymus, heart, and mediastinum

164.0 Thymus
Excludes: benign carcinoid tumor of thymus (209.62)
malignant carcinoid tumor of thymus (209.22)

164.1 Heart
Endocardium	Myocardium
Epicardium	Pericardium

Excludes: great vessels (171.4)

164.2 Anterior mediastinum

164.3 Posterior mediastinum

164.8 Other
Malignant neoplasm of contiguous or overlapping sites of thymus, heart, and mediastinum whose point of origin cannot be determined

164.9 Mediastinum, part unspecified

165 Malignant neoplasm of other and ill-defined sites within the respiratory system and intrathoracic organs

165.0 Upper respiratory trace, part unspecified

165.8 Other
Malignant neoplasm of respiratory and intrathoracic organs whose point of origin cannot be assigned to any one of the categories 160-164

165.9 Ill-defined sites within the respiratory system
Respiratory tract NOS

Excludes: intrathoracic NOS (195.1)
thoracic NOS (195.1)

MALIGNANT NEOPLASM OF BONE, CONNECTIVE TISSUE, SKIN, AND BREAST (170-176)

Excludes: carcinoma in situ:
breast (233.0)
skin (232.0-232.9)

170 Malignant neoplasm of bone and articular cartilage
Includes: cartilage (articular) (joint)
periosteum

Excludes: bone marrow NOS (202.9)

cartilage:
ear (171.0)
eyelid (171.0)
larynx (161.3)
nose (160.0)
synovia (171.0-171.9)

170.0 Bones of skull and face, except mandible
Bone:	Bone:
ethmoid	sphenoid
frontal	temporal
malar	zygomatic
nasal	Maxilla (superior)
occipital	Turbinate
orbital	Upper jaw bone
parietal	Vomer

Excludes: carcinoma, any type except intraosseous or odontogenic:
maxilla, maxillary (sinus) (160.2)
upper jaw bone (143.0)
jaw bone (lower) (170.1)

	Add 4th or 5th digit		Nonspecific code		Unspecified code		Manifestation code

170.1 Mandible
Inferior maxilla   Lower jaw bone
Jaw bone NOS

Excludes: *carcinoma, any type except intraosseous or odontogenic:*
jaw bone NOS (143.9)
lower (143.1)
upper jaw bone (170.0)

170.2 Vertebral column, excluding sacrum and coccyx
Spinal column   Vertebra
Spine

Excludes: *sacrum and coccyx (170.6)*

170.3 Ribs, sternum, and clavicle
Costal cartilage   Xiphoid process
Costovertebral joint

170.4 Scapula and long bones of upper limb
Acromion   Radius
Bones NOS of upper limb   Ulna
Humerus

170.5 Short bones of upper limb
Carpal   Scaphoid (of hand)
Cuneiform, wrist   Semilunar or lunate
Metacarpal   Trapezium
Navicular, of hand   Trapezoid
Phalanges of hand   Unciform
Pisiform

170.6 Pelvic bones, sacrum, and coccyx
Coccygeal vertebra   Pubic bone
Ilium   Sacral vertebra
Ischium

170.7 Long bones of lower limb
Bones NOS of lower limb   Fibula
Femur   Tibia

170.8 Short bones of lower limb
Astragalus [talus]   Navicular (of ankle)
Calcaneus   Patella
Cuboid   Phalanges of foot
Cuneiform, ankle   Tarsal
Metatarsal

170.9 Bone and articular cartilage, site unspecified

171 Malignant neoplasm of connective and other soft tissue
Includes: blood vessel
bursa
fascia
fat
ligament, except uterine
muscle
peripheral, sympathetic, and parasympathetic nerves and ganglia
synovia
tendon (sheath)

Excludes: *cartilage (of):*
articular (170.0-170.9)
larynx (161.3)
nose (160.0)
connective tissue:
breast (174.0-175.9)
internal organs—code to malignant neoplasm of the site [e.g., leiomyosarcoma
of stomach, 151.9]
heart (164.1)
uterine ligament (183.4)

171.0 Head, face, and neck
Cartilage of:
ear
eyelid

171.2 Upper limb, including shoulder
Arm   Forearm
Finger   Hand

● Code new   ▲ Revision of   ④ ⑤ Fourth or fifth
to this edition   existing code   digit required

171.3 Lower limb, including hip
Foot
Leg
Popliteal space
Thigh
Toe

171.4 Thorax
Axilla
Diaphragm
Great vessels

Excludes: *heart (164.1)*
mediastinum (164.2-164.9)
thymus (164.0)

171.5 Abdomen
Abdominal wall
Hypochondrium

Excludes: *peritoneum (158.8)*
retroperitoneum (158.0)

171.6 Pelvis
Buttock
Groin
Inguinal region
Perineum

Excludes: *pelvic peritoneum (158.8)*
retroperitoneum (158.0)
uterine ligament, any (183.3-183.5)

171.7 Trunk, unspecified
Back NOS
Flank NOS

171.8 Other specified sites of connective and other soft tissue
Malignant neoplasm of contiguous or overlapping sites of connective tissue whose point of origin cannot be determined

171.9 Connective and other soft tissue, site unspecified

172 Malignant melanoma of skin
Includes: melanocarcinoma
melanoma in situ of skin
melanoma (skin) NOS

Excludes: *skin of genital organs (184.0-184.9, 187.1-187.9)*
sites other than skin—code to malignant neoplasm of the site

172.0 Lip

Excludes: *vermilion border of lip (140.0-140.1, 140.9)*

172.1 Eyelid, including canthus

172.2 Ear and external auditory canal
Auricle (ear)
Auricular canal, external
External [acoustic] meatus
Pinna

172.3 Other and unspecified parts of face
Cheek (external)
Chin
Eyebrow
Forehead
Nose, external
Temple

172.4 Scalp and neck

172.5 Trunk, except scrotum
Axilla
Breast
Buttock
Groin
Perianal skin
Perineum
Umbilicus

Excludes: *anal canal (154.2)*
anus NOS (154.3)
scrotum (187.7)

172.6 Upper limb, including shoulder
Arm
Finger
Forearm
Hand

Add 4th or 5th digit   Nonspecific code   Unspecified code   Manifestation code

172.7 Lower limb, including hip

Ankle	Leg
Foot	Popliteal area
Heel	Thigh
Knee	Toe

172.8 Other specified sites of skin
Malignant melanoma of contiguous or overlapping sites of skin whose point of origin cannot be determined

172.9 Melanoma of skin, site unspecified

173 Other malignant neoplasm of skin
Includes: malignant neoplasm of:
sebaceous glands
sudoriferous, sudoriparous glands
sweat glands

Excludes: *Kaposi's sarcoma (176.0-176.9)*
malignant melanoma of skin (172.0-172.9)
skin of genital organs (184.0-184.9, 187.1-187.9)

173.0 Skin of lip

Excludes: *vermilion border of lip (140.0-140.1, 140.9)*

173.1 Eyelid, including canthus

Excludes: *cartilage of eyelid (171.0)*

173.2 Skin of ear and external auditory canal

Auricle (ear)	External meatus
Auricular canal, external	Pinna

Excludes: *cartilage of ear (171.0)*

173.3 Skin of other and unspecified parts of face

Cheek, external	Forehead
Chin	Nose, external
Eyebrow	Temple

173.4 Scalp and skin of neck

173.5 Skin of trunk, except scrotum

Axillary fold	Skin of:
Perianal skin	buttock
Skin of:	chest wall
abdominal wall	groin
anus	perineum
back	Umbilicus
breast	

Excludes: *anal canal (154.2)*
anus NOS (154.3)
skin of scrotum (187.7)

173.6 Skin of upper limb, including shoulder

Arm	Forearm
Finger	Hand

173.7 Skin of lower limb, including hip

Ankle	Leg
Foot	Popliteal area
Heel	Thigh
Knee	Toe

173.8 Other specified sites of skin
Malignant neoplasm of contiguous or overlapping sites of skin whose point of origin cannot be determined

173.9 Skin, site unspecified

● Code new
to this edition   ▲ Revision of
existing code   ④ ⑤ Fourth or fifth
digit required

174 Malignant neoplasm of female breast
Use additional code to identify estrogen receptor status (V86.0,V86.1)
  Includes: breast (female)
        connective tissue
        soft parts
        Paget's disease of:
          breast
          nipple

Excludes: *skin of breast (172.5, 173.5)*

174.0 **Nipple and areola**

174.1 **Central portion**

174.2 **Upper-inner quadrant**

174.3 **Lower-inner quadrant**

174.4 **Upper-outer quadrant**

174.5 **Lower-outer quadrant**

174.6 **Axillary tail**

174.8 **Other specified sites of female breast**
        Ectopic sites
        Inner breast
        Lower breast
        Midline of breast
        Outer breast
        Upper breast
        Malignant neoplasm of contiguous or overlapping sites of breast whose point of origin
          cannot be determined

174.9 **Breast (female), unspecified**

175 Malignant neoplasm of male breast
Use additional code to identify estrogen receptor status (V86.0,V86.1)

Excludes: *skin of breast (172.5, 173.5)*

175.0 **Nipple and areola**

175.9 **Other and unspecified sites of male breast**
        Ectopic breast tissue, male

176 Kaposi's sarcoma

176.0 **Skin**

176.1 **Soft tissue**
        Includes: Blood vessel
              Connective tissue
              Fascia
              Ligament
              Lymphatic(s) NEC
              Muscle

Excludes: *lymph glands and nodes (176.5)*

176.2 **Palate**

176.3 **Gastrointestinal sites**

176.4 **Lung**

176.5 **Lymph nodes**

176.8 **Other specified sites**
        Includes: Oral cavity NEC

176.9 **Unspecified**
        Viscera NOS

MALIGNANT NEOPLASM OF GENITOURINARY ORGANS (179-189)

Excludes: *carcinoma in situ (233.1-233.9)*

179 Malignant neoplasm of uterus, part unspecified

180 Malignant neoplasm of cervix uteri
        Includes: invasive malignancy [carcinoma]

Excludes: *carcinoma in situ (233.1)*

| Add 4th or 5th digit | Nonspecific code | Unspecified code | Manifestation code |

180.0 Endocervix
    Cervical canal NOS   Endocervical gland
    Endocervical canal

180.1 Exocervix

180.8 Other specified sites of cervix
    Cervical stump
    Squamocolumnar junction of cervix
    Malignant neoplasm of contiguous or overlapping sites of cervix uteri whose point of
        origin cannot be determined

180.9 Cervix uteri, unspecified

181 Malignant neoplasm of placenta
    Choriocarcinoma NOS
    Chorioepithelioma NOS

    Excludes: *chorioadenoma (destruens) (236.1)*
           hydatidiform mole (630)
             malignant (236.1)
           invasive mole (236.1)
           male choriocarcinoma NOS (186.0-186.9)

182 Malignant neoplasm of body of uterus
    Excludes: *carcinoma in situ (233.2)*

182.0 Corpus uteri, except isthmus
    Cornu   Fundus
    Endometrium   Myometrium

182.1 Isthmus
    Lower uterine segment

182.8 Other specified sites of body of uterus
    Malignant neoplasm of contiguous or overlapping sites of body of uterus whose point
        of origin cannot be determined
    Excludes: *uterus NOS (179)*

183 Malignant neoplasm of ovary and other uterine adnexa
    Excludes: *Douglas' cul-de-sac (158.8)*

183.0 Ovary
Use additional code, if desired, to identify any functional activity

183.2 Fallopian tube
    Oviduct
    Uterine tube

183.3 Broad ligament
    Mesovarium
    Parovarian region

183.4 Parametrium
    Uterine ligament NOS
    Uterosacral ligament

183.5 Round ligament

183.8 Other specified sites of uterine adnexa
    Tubo-ovarian
    Utero-ovarian
    Malignant neoplasm of contiguous or overlapping sites of ovary and other uterine
        adnexa whose point of origin cannot be determined

183.9 Uterine adnexa, unspecified

184 Malignant neoplasm of other and unspecified female genital organs
    Excludes: *carcinoma in situ (233.30-233.39)*

184.0 Vagina
    Gartner's duct
    Vaginal vault

184.1 Labia majora
    Greater vestibular [Bartholin's] gland

184.2 Labia minora

184.3 Clitoris

● Code new   ▲ Revision of   ④ ⑤ Fourth or fifth
  to this edition   existing code   digit required

184.4 Vulva, unspecified
External female genitalia NOS
Pudendum

184.8 Other specified sites of female genital organs
Malignant neoplasm of contiguous or overlapping sites of female genital organs whose point of origin cannot be determined

184.9 Female genital organ, site unspecified
Female genitourinary tract NOS

185 Malignant neoplasm of prostate

Excludes: *seminal vesicles (187.8)*

186 Malignant neoplasm of testis
Use additional code, if desired, to identify any functional activity

186.0 Undescended testis
Ectopic testis
Retained testis

186.9 Other and unspecified testis
Testis:
NOS
descended
scrotal

187 Malignant neoplasm of penis and other male genital organs

187.1 Prepuce
Foreskin

187.2 Glans penis

187.3 Body of penis
Corpus cavernosum

187.4 Penis, part unspecified
Skin of penis NOS

187.5 Epididymis

187.6 Spermatic cord
Vas deferens

187.7 Scrotum
Skin of scrotum

187.8 Other specified sites of male genital organs
Seminal vesicle
Tunica vaginalis
Malignant neoplasm of contiguous or overlapping sites of penis and other male genital organs whose point of origin cannot be determined

187.9 Male genital organ, site unspecified
Male genital organ or tract NOS

188 Malignant neoplasm of bladder

Excludes: *carcinoma in situ (233.7)*

188.0 Trigone of urinary bladder

188.1 Dome of urinary bladder

188.2 Lateral wall of urinary bladder

188.3 Anterior wall of urinary bladder

188.4 Posterior wall of urinary bladder

188.5 Bladder neck
Internal urethral orifice

188.6 Ureteric orifice

188.7 Urachus

188.8 Other specified sites of bladder
Malignant neoplasm of contiguous or overlapping sites of bladder whose point of origin cannot be determined

188.9 Bladder, part unspecified
Bladder wall NOS

189 Malignant neoplasm of kidney and other and unspecified urinary organs

Excludes: *benign carcinoid tumor of kidney (209.64)*
malignant carcinoid tumor of kidney (209.24)

| ▬ | Add 4th or 5th digit | ▬ | Nonspecific code | ▬ | Unspecified code | ▬ | Manifestation code |

189.0 Kidney, except pelvis
Kidney NOS
Kidney parenchyma

189.1 Renal pelvis
Renal calyces
Ureteropelvic junction

189.2 Ureter
Excludes: ureteric orifice of bladder (188.6)

189.3 Urethra
Excludes: urethral orifice of bladder (188.5)

189.4 Paraurethral glands

189.8 Other specified sites of urinary organs
Malignant neoplasm of contiguous or overlapping sites of kidney and other urinary organs whose point of origin cannot be determined

189.9 Urinary organ, site unspecified
Urinary system NOS

MALIGNANT NEOPLASM OF OTHER AND UNSPECIFIED SITES (190-199)

Excludes: carcinoma in situ (234.0-234.9)

190 Malignant neoplasm of eye
Excludes: carcinoma in situ (234.0)
dark area on retina and choroid (239.81)
eyelid (skin) (172.1, 173.1)
    cartilage (171.0)
optic nerve (192.0)
orbital bone (170.0)
retinal freckle (239.81)

190.0 Eyeball, except conjunctiva, cornea, retina, and choroid
Ciliary body   Sclera
Crystalline lens   Uveal tract
Iris

190.1 Orbit
Connective tissue of orbit
Extraocular muscle
Retrobulbar
Excludes: bone of orbit (170.0)

190.2 Lacrimal gland

190.3 Conjunctiva

190.4 Cornea

190.5 Retina

190.6 Choroid

190.7 Lacrimal duct
Lacrimal sac
Nasolacrimal duct

190.8 Other specified sites of eye
Malignant neoplasm of contiguous or overlapping sites of eye whose point of origin cannot be determined

190.9 Eye, part unspecified

191 Malignant neoplasm of brain
Excludes: cranial nerves (192.0)
retrobulbar area (190.1)

191.0 Cerebrum, except lobes and ventricles
Basal ganglia   Globus pallidus
Cerebral cortex   Hypothalamus
Corpus striatum   Thalamus

191.1 Frontal lobe

191.2 Temporal lobe
Hippocampus
Uncus

191.3 Parietal lobe

● Code new
   to this edition   ▲ Revision of
                              existing code   ④ ⑤ Fourth or fifth
                                                          digit required

191.4 Occipital lobe

191.5 Ventricles
Choroid plexus
Floor of ventricle

191.6 Cerebellum NOS
Cerebellopontine angle

191.7 Brain stem
Cerebral peduncle   Midbrain
Medulla oblongata   Pons

191.8 Other parts of brain
Corpus callosum
Tapetum
Malignant neoplasm of contiguous or overlapping sites of brain whose point of origin
  cannot be determined

191.9 Brain, unspecified
Cranial fossa NOS

192 Malignant neoplasm of other and unspecified parts of nervous system

> *Excludes:* *peripheral, sympathetic, and parasympathetic nerves and ganglia (171.0-171.9)*

192.0 Cranial nerves
Olfactory bulb

192.1 Cerebral meninges
Dura (mater)   Meninges NOS
Falx (cerebelli) (cerebri) Tentorium

192.2 Spinal cord
Cauda equina

192.3 Spinal meninges

192.8 Other specified sites of nervous system
Malignant neoplasm of contiguous or overlapping sites of other parts of nervous system
  whose point of origin cannot be determined

192.9 Nervous system, part unspecified
Nervous system (central) NOS

> *Excludes:* *meninges NOS (192.1)*

193 Malignant neoplasm of thyroid gland
Thyroglossal duct

Use additional code, if desired, to identify any functional activity

194 Malignant neoplasm of other endocrine glands and related structures

> *Excludes:* *islets of Langerhans (157.4)*
> *neuroendocrine tumors (209.00-209.69)*
> *ovary (183.0)*
> *testis (186.0-186.9)*
> *thymus (164.0)*

194.0 Adrenal gland
Adrenal cortex   Suprarenal gland
Adrenal medulla

194.1 Parathyroid gland

194.3 Pituitary gland and craniopharyngeal duct
Craniobuccal pouch   Rathke's pouch
Hypophysis   Sella turcica

194.4 Pineal gland

194.5 Carotid body

194.6 Aortic body and other paraganglia
Coccygeal body   Para-aortic body
Glomus jugulare

194.8 Other
Pluriglandular involvement NOS

Note: If the sites of multiple involvements are known, they should be coded separately.

194.9 Endocrine gland, site unspecified

Add 4th or   Nonspecific   Unspecified   Manifestation
5th digit   code   code   code

195 **Malignant neoplasm of other and ill-defined sites**
  Includes: malignant neoplasms of contiguous sites, not elsewhere classified, whose point of
        origin cannot be determined

  Excludes: *malignant neoplasm:*
        lymphatic and hematopoietic tissue (200.0-208.9)
        secondary sites (196.0-198.8)
        unspecified site (199.0-199.1)

  195.0 **Head, face, and neck**
        Cheek NOS   Nose NOS
        Jaw NOS   Supraclavicular region NOS

  195.1 **Thorax**
        Axilla   Intrathoracic NOS
        Chest (wall) NOS

  195.2 **Abdomen**
        Intra-abdominal NOS

  195.3 **Pelvis**
        Groin
        Inguinal region NOS
        Presacral region
        Sacrococcygeal region
        Sites overlapping systems within pelvis, as:
          rectovaginal (septum)
          rectovesical (septum)

  195.4 **Upper limb**

  195.5 **Lower limb**

  195.8 **Other specified sites**
        Back NOS   Trunk NOS
        Flank NOS

196 **Secondary and unspecified malignant neoplasm of lymph nodes**

  Excludes: *any malignant neoplasm of lymph nodes, specified as primary (200.0-202.9)*
        Hodgkin's disease (201.0-201.9)
        lymphosarcoma (200.1)
        reticulosarcoma (200.0)
        other forms of lymphoma (202.0-202.9)
        secondary neuroendocrine tumor of (distant) lymph nodes (209.71)

  196.0 **Lymph nodes of head, face, and neck**
        Cervical   Scalene
        Cervicofacial   Supraclavicular

  196.1 **Intrathoracic lymph nodes**
        Bronchopulmonary   Mediastinal
        Intercostal   Tracheobronchial

  196.2 **Intra-abdominal lymph nodes**
        Intestinal   Retroperitoneal
        Mesenteric

  196.3 **Lymph nodes of axilla and upper limb**
        Brachial   Infraclavicular
        Epitrochlear   Pectoral

  196.5 **Lymph nodes of inguinal region and lower limb**
        Femoral   Popliteal
        Groin   Tibial

  196.6 **Intrapelvic lymph nodes**
        Hypogastric   Obturator
        Iliac   Parametrial

  196.8 **Lymph nodes of multiple sites**

  196.9 **Site unspecified**
        Lymph nodes NOS

197 **Secondary malignant neoplasm of respiratory and digestive systems**

  Excludes: *lymph node metastasis (196.0-196.9)*
        secondary neuroendocrine tumor of liver (209.72)
        secondary neuroendocrine tumor of respiratory organs (209.79)

  197.0 **Lung**
        Bronchus

● Code new   ▲ Revision of   ④ ⑤ Fourth or fifth
        to this edition   existing code   digit required

197.1 Mediastinum

197.2 Pleura

197.3 Other respiratory organs
Trachea

197.4 Small intestine, including duodenum

197.5 Large intestine and rectum

197.6 Retroperitoneum and peritoneum

197.7 Liver, specified as secondary

197.8 Other digestive organs and spleen

198 Secondary malignant neoplasm of other specified sites

Excludes: *lymph node metastasis (196.0-196.9)*
secondary neuroendocrine tumor of other specified sites (209.79)

198.0 Kidney

198.1 Other urinary organs

198.2 Skin
Skin of breast

198.3 Brain and spinal cord

198.4 Other parts of nervous system
Meninges (cerebral) (spinal)

198.5 Bone and bone marrow

198.6 Ovary

198.7 Adrenal gland
Suprarenal gland

⑤ **198.8 Other specified sites**

198.81 Breast

Excludes: *skin of breast (198.2)*

198.82 Genital organs

198.89 Other

Excludes: *retroperitoneal lymph nodes (196.2)*

199 Malignant neoplasm without specification of site

Excludes: *malignant carcinoid tumor of unknown primary site (209.20)*
malignant (poorly differentiated) neuroendocrine carcinoma, any site (209.30)
malignant (poorly differentiated) neuroendocrine tumor, any site (209.30)
neuroendocrine carcinoma (high grade), any site (209.30)

199.0 Disseminated
Carcinomatosis unspecified site (primary) (secondary)
Generalized:
  cancer unspecified site (primary) (secondary)
  malignancy unspecified site (primary) (secondary)
Multiple cancer unspecified site (primary) (secondary)

199.1 Other
Cancer unspecified site (primary) (secondary)
Carcinoma unspecified site (primary) (secondary)
Malignancy unspecified site (primary) (secondary)

199.2 Malignant neoplasm associated with transplanted organ
Code first complication of transplanted organ (996.80-996.89)

Use additional code for specific malignancy

MALIGNANT NEOPLASM OF LYMPHATIC AND HEMATOPOIETIC TISSUE (200-208)

Excludes: *autoimmune lymphoproliferative syndrome (279.41)*
secondary neoplasm of:
  bone marrow (198.5)
  spleen (197.8)
secondary and unspecified neoplasm of lymph nodes (196.0-196.9)

The following fifth-digit subclassification is for use with categories 200-202:

0 **unspecified site, extranodal and solid organ sites**

1 **lymph nodes of head, face, and neck**

2 **intrathoracic lymph nodes**

| | Add 4th or 5th digit | | Nonspecific code | | Unspecified code | | Manifestation code |

3 intra-abdominal lymph nodes

4 lymph nodes of axilla and upper limb

5 lymph nodes of inguinal region and lower limb

6 intrapelvic lymph nodes

7 spleen

8 lymph nodes of multiple sites

⑤ **200** Lymphosarcoma and reticulosarcoma and other specified malignant tumors of lymphatic tissue

⑤ **200.0 Reticulosarcoma**
[0-8]   Lymphoma (malignant):
          histiocytic (diffuse):
            nodular
            pleomorphic cell type
          reticulum cell type
        Reticulum cell sarcoma:
          NOS
          pleomorphic cell type

⑤ **200.1 Lymphosarcoma**
[0-8]   Lymphoblastoma (diffuse)
        Lymphoma (malignant):   Lymphosarcoma:
          lymphoblastic (diffuse)   NOS
          lymphocytic (cell type)   diffuse NOS
            (diffuse)   lymphoblastic (diffuse)
          lymphosarcoma type   lymphocytic (diffuse)
                                      prolymphocytic

        Excludes: lymphosarcoma:
                   follicular or nodular (202.0)
                   mixed cell type (200.8)
                   lymphosarcoma cell leukemia (207.8)

⑤ **200.2 Burkitt's tumor or lymphoma**
[0-8]   Malignant lymphoma, Burkitt's type

⑤ **200.3 Marginal zone lymphoma**
[0-8]   Extranodal marginal zone B-cell lymphoma
        Mucosa associated lymphoid tissue [MALT]
        Nodal marginal zone B-cell lymphoma
        Splenic marginal zone B-cell lymphoma

⑤ **200.4 Mantle cell lymphoma**
[0-8]

⑤ **200.5 Primary central nervous system lymphoma**
[0-8]

⑤ **200.6 Anaplastic large cell lymphoma**
[0-8]

⑤ **200.7 Large cell lymphoma**
[0-8]

⑤ **200.8 Other named variants**
[0-8]   Lymphoma (malignant):
          lymphoplasmacytoid type
          mixed lymphocytic-histiocytic (diffuse)
        Lymphosarcoma, mixed cell type (diffuse)
        Reticulolymphosarcoma (diffuse)

⑤ **201** Hodgkin's disease

⑤ **201.0 Hodgkin's paragranuloma**
[0-8]

⑤ **201.1 Hodgkin's granuloma**
[0-8]

⑤ **201.2 Hodgkin's sarcoma**
[0-8]

⑤ **201.4 Lymphocytic-histiocytic predominance**
[0-8]

⑤ **201.5 Nodular sclerosis**
[0-8]   Hodgkin's disease, nodular sclerosis:
          NOS
          cellular phase

● Code new
  to this edition
▲ Revision of
  existing code
④ ⑤ Fourth or fifth
  digit required

⑤ **201.6 Mixed cellularity**
[0-8]

⑤ **201.7 Lymphocytic depletion**
[0-8]   Hodgkin's disease, lymphocytic depletion:
        NOS
        diffuse fibrosis
        reticular type

⑤ **201.9 Hodgkin's disease, unspecified**
[0-8]   Hodgkin's: Malignant:
            disease NOS   lymphogranuloma
            lymphoma NOS   lymphogranulomatosis

⑤ **202**   **Other malignant neoplasms of lymphoid and histiocytic tissue**

⑤ **202.0 Nodular lymphoma**
[0-8]   Brill-Symmers disease
        Lymphoma: Lymphosarcoma:
            follicular (giant) (large cell)   follicular (giant)
            lymphocytic, nodular   nodular

⑤ **202.1 Mycosis fungoides**
[0-8]

> *Excludes:* peripheral T-cell lymphoma (202.7)

⑤ **202.2 Sézary's disease**
[0-8]

⑤ **202.3 Malignant histiocytosis**
[0-8]   Histiocytic medullary reticulosis
        Malignant:
            reticuloendotheliosis
            reticulosis

⑤ **202.4 Leukemic reticuloendotheliosis**
[0-8]   Hairy-cell leukemia

⑤ **202.5 Letterer-Siwe disease**
[0-8]   Acute:
            differentiated progressive histiocytosis
            histiocytosis X (progressive)
            infantile reticuloendotheliosis
            reticulosis of infancy

> *Excludes:* Hand-Schüller-Christian disease (277.89)
>   histiocytosis (acute) (chronic) (277.89)
>   histiocytosis X (chronic) (277.89)

⑤ **202.6 Malignant mast cell tumors**
[0-8]   Malignant: Mast cell sarcoma
            mastocytoma   Systemic tissue mast cell disease
            mastocytosis

> *Excludes:* mast cell leukemia (207.8)

⑤ **202.7 Peripheral T-cell lymphoma**
[0-8]

⑤ **202.8 Other lymphomas**
[0-8]   Lymphoma (malignant):
            NOS
            diffuse

> *Excludes:* benign lymphoma (229.0)

⑤ **202.9 Other and unspecified malignant neoplasms of lymphoid and histiocytic tissue**
[0-8]   Follicular dendritic cell sarcoma
        Interdigitating dendritic cell sarcoma
        Langerhans cell sarcoma
        Malignant neoplasm of bone marrow NOS

Add 4th or   Nonspecific   Unspecified   Manifestation
5th digit   code   code   code

⑤ **203** **Multiple myeloma and immunoproliferative neoplasms**
The following fifth-digit subclassification is for use with category 203

    0 **without mention of having achieved remission**
        failed remission

    1 **in remission**

    2 **in relapse**

⑤ **203.0** **Multiple myeloma**
[0-2]   Kahler's disease
        Myelomatosis

    Excludes: *solitary myeloma (238.6)*

⑤ **203.1** **Plasma cell leukemia**
[0-2]   Plasmacytic leukemia

⑤ **203.8** **Other immunoproliferative neoplasms**
[0-2]

⑤ **204** **Lymphoid leukemia**
    Includes: leukemia:
            lymphatic
            lymphoblastic
            lymphocytic
            lymphogenous

The following fifth-digit subclassification is for use with category 204

    0 **without mention of having achieved remission**
        failed remission

    1 **in remission**

    2 **in relapse**

⑤ **204.0** **Acute**
[0-2]

    Excludes: *acute exacerbation of chronic lymphoid leukemia (204.1)*

⑤ **204.1** **Chronic**
[0-2]

⑤ **204.2** **Subacute**
[0-2]

⑤ **204.8** **Other lymphoid leukemia**
[0-2]   Aleukemic leukemia:
      lymphatic
      lymphocytic
      lymphoid

⑤ **204.9** **Unspecified lymphoid leukemia**
[0-2]

⑤ **205** **Myeloid leukemia**
    Includes: leukemia:
            granulocytic   myelomonocytic
            myeloblastic   myelosclerotic
            myelocytic   myelosis
            myelogenous

The following fifth-digit subclassification is for use with category 205

    0 **without mention of having achieved remission**
        failed remission

    1 **in remission**

    2 **in relapse**

⑤ **205.0** **Acute**
[0-2]   Acute promyelocytic leukemia

    Excludes: *acute exacerbation of chronic myeloid leukemia (205.1)*

⑤ **205.1** **Chronic**
[0-2]   Eosinophilic leukemia   Neutrophilic leukemia

⑤ **205.2** **Subacute**
[0-2]

⑤ **205.3** **Myeloid sarcoma**
[0-2]   Chloroma
        Granulocytic sarcoma

  ● Code new   ▲ Revision of   ④ ⑤ Fourth or fifth
          to this edition   existing code   digit required

⑤ **205.8 Other myeloid leukemia**
[0-2]   Aleukemic leukemia:
          granulocytic
          myelogenous
          myeloid
        Aleukemic myelosis

⑤ **205.9 Unspecified myeloid leukemia**
[0-2]

⑤ **206 Monocytic leukemia**
        Includes: leukemia:
                   histiocytic
                   monoblastic
                   monocytoid

        The following fifth-digit subclassification is for use with category 206

        0   without mention of having achieved remission
              failed remission

        1   in remission

        2   in relapse

⑤ **206.0 Acute**
[0-2]
        | Excludes: | *acute exacerbation of chronic monocytic leukemia (206.1)* |

⑤ **206.1 Chronic**
[0-2]

⑤ **206.2 Subacute**
[0-2]

⑤ **206.8 Other monocytic leukemia**
[0-2]   Aleukemic:
          monocytic leukemia
          monocytoid leukemia

⑤ **206.9 Unspecified monocytic leukemia**
[0-2]

⑤ **207 Other specified leukemia**
        | Excludes: | *leukemic reticuloendotheliosis (202.4)* |
        | | *plasma cell leukemia (203.1)* |

        The following fifth-digit subclassification is for use with category 207

        0   without mention of having achieved remission
              failed remission

        1   in remission

        2   in relapse

⑤ **207.0 Acute erythremia and erythroleukemia**
[0-2]   Acute erythremic myelosis
          Di Guglielmo's disease
          Erythremic myelosis

⑤ **207.1 Chronic erythremia**
[0-2]   Heilmeyer-Schöner disease

⑤ **207.2 Megakaryocytic leukemia**
[0-2]   Megakaryocytic myelosis   Thrombocytic leukemia

⑤ **207.8 Other specified leukemia**
[0-2]   Lymphosarcoma cell leukemia

⑤ **208 Leukemia of unspecified cell type**
        The following fifth-digit subclassification is for use with category 208

        0   without mention of having achieved remission
              failed remission

        1   in remission

        2   in relapse

⑤ **208.0 Acute**
[0-2]   Acute leukemia NOS
          Blast cell leukemia
          Stem cell leukemia

        | Excludes: | *acute exacerbation of chronic unspecified leukemia (208.1)* |

Add 4th or   Nonspecific   Unspecified   Manifestation
5th digit   code   code   code

233

⑤ **208.1 Chronic**
[0-2]   Chronic leukemia NOS

⑤ **208.2 Subacute**
[0-2]   Subacute leukemia NOS

⑤ **208.8 Other leukemia of unspecified cell type**
[0-2]

⑤ **208.9 Unspecified leukemia**
[0-2]   Leukemia NOS

NEUROENDOCRINE TUMORS (209)

⑤ **209 Neuroendocrine tumors**
Code first any associated multiple endocrine neoplasia syndrome (258.01-258.03)
Use additional code to identify associated endocrine syndrome, such as: carcinoid syndrome (259.2)

> *Excludes:* *benign pancreatic islet cell tumors (211.7)*
> *malignant pancreatic islet cell tumors (157.4)*

⑤ **209.0 Malignant carcinoid tumors of the small intestine**

209.00 Malignant carcinoid tumor of the small intestine, unspecified portion

209.01 Malignant carcinoid tumor of the duodenum

209.02 Malignant carcinoid tumor of the jejunum

209.03 Malignant carcinoid tumor of the ileum

⑤ **209.1 Malignant carcinoid tumors of the appendix, large intestine, and rectum**

209.10 Malignant carcinoid tumor of the large intestine, unspecified portion
Malignant carcinoid tumor of the colon NOS

209.11 Malignant carcinoid tumor of the appendix

209.12 Malignant carcinoid tumor of the cecum

209.13 Malignant carcinoid tumor of the ascending colon

209.14 Malignant carcinoid tumor of the transverse colon

209.15 Malignant carcinoid tumor of the descending colon

209.16 Malignant carcinoid tumor of the sigmoid colon

209.17 Malignant carcinoid tumor of the rectum

⑤ **209.2 Malignant carcinoid tumors of other and unspecified sites**

209.20 Malignant carcinoid tumor of unknown primary site

209.21 Malignant carcinoid tumor of the bronchus and lung

209.22 Malignant carcinoid tumor of the thymus

209.23 Malignant carcinoid tumor of the stomach

209.24 Malignant carcinoid tumor of the kidney

209.25 Malignant carcinoid tumor of the foregut NOS

209.26 Malignant carcinoid tumor of the midgut NOS

209.27 Malignant carcinoid tumor of the hindgut NOS

209.29 Malignant carcinoid tumors of other sites

⑤ **209.3 Malignant poorly differentiated neuroendocrine tumors**

209.30 Malignant poorly differentiated neuroendocrine carcinoma, any site
High grade neuroendocrine carcinoma, any site
Malignant poorly differentiated neuroendocrine tumor NOS

> *Excludes:* *Merkel cell carcinoma (209.31-209.36)*

● **209.31 Merkel cell carcinoma of the face**
Merkel cell carcinoma of the ear
Merkel cell carcinoma of the eyelid, including canthus
Merkel cell carcinoma of the lip

● **209.32 Merkel cell carcinoma of the scalp and neck**

● **209.33 Merkel cell carcinoma of the upper limb**

● **209.34 Merkel cell carcinoma of the lower limb**

● **209.35 Merkel cell carcinoma of the trunk**

● Code new   ▲ Revision of   ④ ⑤ Fourth or fifth
    to this edition   existing code   digit required

● **209.36** **Merkel cell carcinoma of other sites**
Merkel cell carcinoma of the buttock
Merkel cell carcinoma of the genitals
Merkel cell carcinoma NOS

⑤ **209.4** **Benign carcinoid tumors of the small intestine**

209.40 **Benign carcinoid tumor of the small intestine, unspecified portion**

209.41 **Benign carcinoid tumor of the duodenum**

209.42 **Benign carcinoid tumor of the jejunum**

209.43 **Benign carcinoid tumor of the ileum**

⑤ **209.5** **Benign carcinoid tumors of the appendix, large intestine, and rectum**

209.50 **Benign carcinoid tumor of the large intestine, unspecified portion**
Benign carcinoid tumor of the colon NOS

209.51 **Benign carcinoid tumor of the appendix**

209.52 **Benign carcinoid tumor of the cecum**

209.53 **Benign carcinoid tumor of the ascending colon**

209.54 **Benign carcinoid tumor of the transverse colon**

209.55 **Benign carcinoid tumor of the descending colon**

209.56 **Benign carcinoid tumor of the sigmoid colon**

209.57 **Benign carcinoid tumor of the rectum**

⑤ **209.6** **Benign carcinoid tumors of other and unspecified sites**

209.60 **Benign carcinoid tumor of unknown primary site**
Carcinoid tumor NOS
Neuroendocrine tumor NOS

209.61 **Benign carcinoid tumor of the bronchus and lung**

209.62 **Benign carcinoid tumor of the thymus**

209.63 **Benign carcinoid tumor of the stomach**

209.64 **Benign carcinoid tumor of the kidney**

209.65 **Benign carcinoid tumor of the foregut NOS**

209.66 **Benign carcinoid tumor of the midgut NOS**

209.67 **Benign carcinoid tumor of the hindgut NOS**

209.69 **Benign carcinoid tumors of other sites**

● **209.7** **Secondary neuroendocrine tumors**
Secondary carcinoid tumors

● **209.70** **Secondary neuroendocrine tumor, unspecified site**

● **209.71** **Secondary neuroendocrine tumor of distant lymph nodes**
Mesentery metastasis of neuroendocrine tumor

● **209.72** **Secondary neuroendocrine tumor of liver**

● **209.73** **Secondary neuroendocrine tumor of bone**

● **209.74** **Secondary neuroendocrine tumor of peritoneum**

● **209.75** **Secondary Merkel cell carcinoma**
Merkel cell carcinoma nodal presentation
Merkel cell carcinoma visceral metastatic presentation
Secondary Merkel cell carcinoma, any site

● **209.79** **Secondary neuroendocrine tumor of other sites**

BENIGN NEOPLASMS (210-229)

210 **Benign neoplasm of lip, oral cavity, and pharynx**
Excludes: cyst (of):
jaw (526.0-526.2, 526.89)
oral soft tissue (528.4)
radicular (522.8)

210.0 **Lip**
Frenulum labii
Lip (inner aspect) (mucosa) (vermilion border)
Excludes: labial commissure (210.4)
skin of lip (216.0)

210.1 **Tongue**
Lingual tonsil

| | Add 4th or 5th digit | | Nonspecific code | | Unspecified code | | Manifestation code |

210.2 Major salivary glands
Gland:
parotid
sublingual
submandibular

Excludes: *benign neoplasms of minor salivary glands:*
NOS (210.4)
buccal mucosa (210.4)
lips (210.0)
palate (hard) (soft) (210.4)
tongue (210.1)
tonsil, palatine (210.5)

210.3 Floor of mouth

210.4 Other and unspecified parts of mouth
Gingiva   Oral mucosa
Gum (upper) (lower)   Palate (hard) (soft)
Labial commissure   Uvula
Oral cavity NOS

Excludes: *benign odontogenic neoplasms of bone (213.0-213.1)*
developmental odontogenic cysts (526.0)
mucosa of lips (210.0)
nasopharyngeal [posterior] [superior] surface of soft palate (210.7)

210.5 Tonsil
Tonsil (faucial) (palatine)

Excludes: *lingual tonsil (210.1)*
pharyngeal tonsil (210.7)
tonsillar:
fossa (210.6)
pillars (210.6)

210.6 Other parts of oropharynx
Branchial cleft or vestiges
Epiglottis, anterior aspect
Fauces NOS
Mesopharynx NOS
Tonsillar:
fossa
pillars
Vallecula

Excludes: *epiglottis:*
NOS (212.1)
suprahyoid portion (212.1)

210.7 Nasopharynx
Adenoid tissue   Pharyngeal tonsil
Lymphadenoid tissue   Posterior nasal septum

210.8 Hypopharynx
Arytenoid fold   Postcricoid region
Laryngopharynx   Pyriform fossa

210.9 Pharynx, unspecified
Throat NOS

211 Benign neoplasm of other parts of digestive system

Excludes: *benign stromal tumors of digestive system (215.5)*

211.0 Esophagus

211.1 Stomach
Body of stomach   Cardiac orifice
Cardia of stomach   Pylorus
Fundus of stomach

Excludes: *benign carcinoid tumors of the stomach (209.63)*

211.2 Duodenum, jejunum, and ileum
Small intestine NOS

Excludes: *ampulla of Vater (211.5)*
benign carcinoid tumors of the small intestine (209.40-209.43)
ileocecal valve (211.3)

● Code new
to this edition

▲ Revision of
existing code

④ ⑤ Fourth or fifth
digit required

211.3 Colon

Appendix	Ileocecal valve
Cecum	Large intestine NOS

Excludes: benign carcinoid tumors of the large intestine (209.50-209.56)
    rectosigmoid junction (211.4)

211.4 Rectum and anal canal

Anal canal or sphincter	Rectosigmoid junction
Anus NOS	

Excludes: anus:
        margin (216.5)
        skin (216.5)
    benign carcinoid tumors of the rectum (209.57)
    perianal skin (216.5)

211.5 Liver and biliary passages

Ampulla of Vater	Gallbladder
Common bile duct	Hepatic duct
Cystic duct	Sphincter of Oddi

211.6 Pancreas, except islets of Langerhans

211.7 Islets of Langerhans
    Islet cell tumor

Use additional code, if desired, to identify any functional activity

211.8 Retroperitoneum and peritoneum

Mesentery	Omentum
Mesocolon	Retroperitoneal tissue

211.9 Other and unspecified site

Alimentary tract NOS	Intestinal tract NOS
Digestive system NOS	Intestine NOS
Gastrointestinal tract NOS	Spleen, not elsewhere classified

212 Benign neoplasm of respiratory and intrathoracic organs

212.0 Nasal cavities, middle ear, and accessory sinuses

Cartilage of nose	Sinus:
Eustachian tube	ethmoidal
Nares	frontal
Septum of nose	maxillary
	sphenoidal

Excludes: auditory canal (external) (216.2)
        bone of:
          ear (213.0)
          nose [turbinates] (213.0)
        cartilage of ear (215.0)
        ear (external) (skin) (216.2)
        nose NOS (229.8)
          skin (216.3)
        olfactory bulb (225.1)
        polyp of:
          accessory sinus (471.8)
          ear (385.30-385.35)
          nasal cavity (471.0)
        posterior margin of septum and choanae (210.7)

212.1 Larynx

Cartilage:	Epiglottis (suprahyoid portion) NOS
arytenoid	Glottis
cricoid	Vocal cords (false) (true)
cuneiform	
thyroid	

Excludes: epiglottis, anterior aspect (210.6)
    polyp of vocal cord or larynx (478.4)

212.2 Trachea

212.3 Bronchus and lung
    Carina
    Hilus of lung

Excludes: benign carcinoid tumors of bronchus and lung (209.61)

Add 4th or 5th digit	Nonspecific code	Unspecified code	Manifestation code

212.4 Pleura

212.5 Mediastinum

212.6 Thymus

> *Excludes:* benign carcinoid tumors of thymus (209.62)

212.7 Heart

> *Excludes:* great vessels (215.4)

212.8 Other specified sites

212.9 Site unspecified
Respiratory organ NOS
Upper respiratory tract NOS

> *Excludes:* intrathoracic NOS (229.8)
> thoracic NOS (229.8)

213 Benign neoplasm of bone and articular cartilage
Includes: cartilage (articular) (joint)
periosteum

> *Excludes:* cartilage of:
> ear (215.0)
> eyelid (215.0)
> larynx (212.1)
> nose (212.0)
> exostosis NOS (726.91)
> synovia (215.0-215.9)

213.0 Bones of skull and face

> *Excludes:* lower jaw bone (213.1)

213.1 Lower jaw bone

213.2 Vertebral column, excluding sacrum and coccyx

213.3 Ribs, sternum, and clavicle

213.4 Scapula and long bones of upper limb

213.5 Short bones of upper limb

213.6 Pelvic bones, sacrum, and coccyx

213.7 Long bones of lower limb

213.8 Short bones of lower limb

213.9 Bone and articular cartilage, site unspecified

214 Lipoma
Includes: angiolipoma
fibrolipoma
hibernoma
lipoma (fetal) (infiltrating) (intramuscular)
myelolipoma
myxolipoma

214.0 Skin and subcutaneous tissue of face

214.1 Other skin and subcutaneous tissue

214.2 Intrathoracic organs

214.3 Intra-abdominal organs

214.4 Spermatic cord

214.8 Other specified sites

214.9 Lipoma, unspecified site

● Code new
to this edition
▲ Revision of
existing code
④ ⑤ Fourth or fifth
digit required

215 **Other benign neoplasm of connective and other soft tissue**
Includes: blood vessel
bursa
fascia
ligament
muscle
peripheral, sympathetic, and parasympathetic nerves and ganglia
synovia
tendon (sheath)

Excludes: *cartilage:*
    articular (213.0-213.9)
    larynx (212.1)
    nose (212.0)
  connective tissue of:
    breast (217)
    internal organ, except lipoma and hemangioma — code to benign neoplasm of
      the site
  lipoma (214.0-214.9)

215.0 **Head, face, and neck**

215.2 **Upper limb, including shoulder**

215.3 **Lower limb, including hip**

215.4 **Thorax**
Excludes: *heart (212.7)*
    mediastinum (212.5)
    thymus (212.6)

215.5 **Abdomen**
Abdominal wall
Benign stromal tumors of abdomen
Hypochondrium

215.6 **Pelvis**
Buttock   Inguinal region
Groin   Perineum
Excludes: *uterine:*
    leiomyoma (218.0-218.9)
    ligament, any (221.0)

215.7 **Trunk, unspecified**
Back NOS
Flank NOS

215.8 **Other specified sites**

215.9 **Site unspecified**

216 **Benign neoplasm of skin**
Includes: blue nevus
dermatofibroma
hydrocystoma
pigmented nevus
syringoadenoma
syringoma

Excludes: *skin of genital organs (221.0-222.9)*

216.0 **Skin of lip**
Excludes: *vermilion border of lip (210.0)*

216.1 **Eyelid, including canthus**
Excludes: *cartilage of eyelid (215.0)*

216.2 **Ear and external auditory canal**
Auricle (ear)   External meatus
Auricular canal, external   Pinna
Excludes: *cartilage of ear (215.0)*

216.3 **Skin of other and unspecified parts of face**
Cheek, external   Nose, external
Eyebrow   Temple

216.4 **Scalp and skin of neck**

Add 4th or
5th digit
     Nonspecific
code
     Unspecified
code
     Manifestation
code

216.5 Skin of trunk, except scrotum
Axillary fold
Perianal skin
Skin of:
  abdominal wall
  anus
  back
  breast

Skin of:
  buttock
  chest wall
  groin
  perineum
Umbilicus

> Excludes: anal canal (211.4)
> anus NOS (211.4)
> skin of scrotum (222.4)

216.6 Skin of upper limb, including shoulder

216.7 Skin of lower limb, including hip

216.8 Other specified sites of skin

216.9 Skin, site unspecified

217 Benign neoplasm of breast
Breast (male) (female)
  connective tissue
  glandular tissue
  soft parts

> Excludes: adenofibrosis (610.2)
> benign cyst of breast (610.0)
> fibrocystic disease (610.1)
> skin of breast (216.5)

218 Uterine leiomyoma
Includes: fibroid (bleeding) (uterine)
  uterine:
    fibromyoma
    myoma

218.0 Submucous leiomyoma of uterus

218.1 Intramural leiomyoma of uterus
Interstitial leiomyoma of uterus

218.2 Subserous leiomyoma of uterus
Subperitoneal leiomyoma of uterus

218.9 Leiomyoma of uterus, unspecified

219 Other benign neoplasm of uterus

219.0 Cervix uteri

219.1 Corpus uteri
Endometrium   Myometrium
Fundus

219.8 Other specified parts of uterus

219.9 Uterus, part unspecified

220 Benign neoplasm of ovary
Use additional code, if desired, to identify any functional activity (256.0-256.1)

> Excludes: cyst:
> corpus albicans (620.2)
> corpus luteum (620.1)
> endometrial (617.1)
> follicular (atretic) (620.0)
> graafian follicle (620.0)
> ovarian NOS (620.2)
> retention (620.2)

221 Benign neoplasm of other female genital organs
Includes: adenomatous polyp
  benign teratoma

> Excludes: cyst:
> epoophoron (752.11)
> fimbrial (752.11)
> Gartner's duct (752.11)
> parovarian (752.11)

● Code new
  to this edition   ▲ Revision of
       existing code   ④ ⑤ Fourth or fifth
          digit required

221.0 Fallopian tube and uterine ligaments
Oviduct   Uterine ligament (broad) (round) (uterosacral)
Parametrium   Uterine tube

221.1 Vagina

221.2 Vulva
Clitoris
External female genitalia NOS
Greater vestibular [Bartholin's] gland
Labia (majora) (minora)
Pudendum

Excludes: Bartholin's (duct) (gland) cyst (616.2)

221.8 Other specified sites of female genital organs

221.9 Female genital organ, site unspecified
Female genitourinary tract NOS

222 Benign neoplasm of male genital organs

222.0 Testis
Use additional code, if desired, to identify any functional activity

222.1 Penis
Corpus cavernosum   Prepuce
Glans penis

222.2 Prostate

Excludes: adenomatous hyperplasia of prostate (600.20-600.21)
           prostatic:
             adenoma (600.20-600.21)
             enlargement (600.00-600.01)
             hypertrophy (600.00-600.01)

222.3 Epididymis

222.4 Scrotum
Skin of scrotum

222.8 Other specified sites of male genital organs
Seminal vesicle
Spermatic cord

222.9 Male genital organ, site unspecified
Male genitourinary tract NOS

223 Benign neoplasm of kidney and other urinary organs

223.0 Kidney, except pelvis
Kidney NOS

Excludes: benign carcinoid tumors of kidney (209.64)
           renal:
             calyces (223.1)
             pelvis (223.1)

223.1 Renal pelvis

223.2 Ureter

Excludes: ureteric orifice of bladder (223.3)

223.3 Bladder

⑤ **223.8 Other specified sites of urinary organs**

   223.81 Urethra

Excludes: urethral orifice of bladder (223.3)

      223.89 Other
         Paraurethral glands

223.9 Urinary organ, site unspecified
Urinary system NOS

224 Benign neoplasm of eye

Excludes: cartilage of eyelid (215.0)
           eyelid (skin) (216.1)
           optic nerve (225.1)
           orbital bone (213.0)

241

| | Add 4th or 5th digit | | Nonspecific code | | Unspecified code | | Manifestation code |

224.0 Eyeball, except conjunctiva, cornea, retina, and choroid
Ciliary body   Sclera
Iris   Uveal tract

224.1 Orbit
Excludes: bone of orbit (213.0)

224.2 Lacrimal gland

224.3 Conjunctiva

224.4 Cornea

224.5 Retina
Excludes: hemangioma of retina (228.03)

224.6 Choroid

224.7 Lacrimal duct
Lacrimal sac
Nasolacrimal duct

224.8 Other specified parts of eye

224.9 Eye, part unspecified

225 Benign neoplasm of brain and other parts of nervous system
Excludes: hemangioma (228.02)
neurofibromatosis (237.7)
peripheral, sympathetic, and parasympathetic nerves and ganglia (215.0-215.9)
retrobulbar (224.1)

225.0 Brain

225.1 Cranial nerves

225.2 Cerebral meninges
Meninges NOS
Meningioma (cerebral)

225.3 Spinal cord
Cauda equina

225.4 Spinal meninges
Spinal meningioma

225.8 Other specified sites of nervous system

225.9 Nervous system, part unspecified
Nervous system (central) NOS
Excludes: meninges NOS (225.2)

226 Benign neoplasm of thyroid glands
Use additional code, if desired, to identify any functional activity

227 Benign neoplasm of other endocrine glands and related structures
Use additional code, if desired, to identify any functional activity
Excludes: ovary (220)
pancreas (211.6)
testis (222.0)

227.0 Adrenal gland
Suprarenal gland

227.1 Parathyroid gland

227.3 Pituitary gland and craniopharyngeal duct (pouch)
Craniobuccal pouch   Rathke's pouch
Hypophysis   Sella turcica

227.4 Pineal gland
Pineal body

227.5 Carotid body

227.6 Aortic body and other paraganglia
Coccygeal body   Para-aortic body
Glomus jugulare

227.8 Other

227.9 Endocrine gland, site unspecified

● Code new   ▲ Revision of   ④ ⑤ Fourth or fifth
to this edition   existing code   digit required

228 **Hemangioma and lymphangioma, any site**
Includes: angioma (benign) (cavernous) (congenital) NOS
cavernous nevus
glomus tumor
hemangioma (benign) (congenital)

Excludes: *benign neoplasm of spleen, except hemangioma and lymphangioma (211.9)*
glomus jugulare (227.6)
nevus:
NOS (216.0-216.9)
blue or pigmented (216.0-216.9)
vascular (757.32)

⑤ **228.0** **Hemangioma, any site**

228.00 **Of unspecified site**

228.01 **Of skin and subcutaneous tissue**

228.02 **Of intracranial structures**

228.03 **Of retina**

228.04 **Of intra-abdominal structures**
Peritoneum
Retroperitoneal tissue

228.09 **Of other sites**
Systemic angiomatosis

228.1 **Lymphangioma, any site**
Congenital lymphangioma
Lymphatic nevus

229 **Benign neoplasm of other and unspecified sites**

229.0 **Lymph nodes**
Excludes: *lymphangioma (228.1)*

229.8 **Other specified sites**
Intrathoracic NOS
Thoracic NOS

229.9 **Site unspecified**

CARCINOMA IN SITU (230-234)

Includes: Bowen's disease
erythroplasia
Queyrat's erythroplasia

Excludes: *leukoplakia—see Alphabetic Index*

230 **Carcinoma in situ of digestive organs**

230.0 **Lip, oral cavity, and pharynx**
Gingiva   Oropharynx
Hypopharynx   Salivary gland or duct
Mouth [any part]   Tongue
Nasopharynx

Excludes: *aryepiglottic fold or interarytenoid fold, laryngeal aspect (231.0)*
epiglottis:
NOS (231.0)
suprahyoid portion (231.0)
skin of lip (232.0)

230.1 **Esophagus**

230.2 **Stomach**
Body of stomach   Cardiac orifice
Cardia of stomach   Pylorus
Fundus of stomach

230.3 **Colon**
Appendix   Ileocecal valve
Cecum   Large intestine NOS

Excludes: *rectosigmoid junction (230.4)*

230.4 **Rectum**
Rectosigmoid junction

230.5 **Anal canal**
Anal sphincter

Add 4th or
5th digit   Nonspecific
code   Unspecified
code   Manifestation
code

230.6 Anus, unspecified

Excludes: anus:
  margin (232.5)
  skin (232.5)
  perianal skin (232.5)

230.7 Other and unspecified parts of intestine
Duodenum   Jejunum
Ileum   Small intestine NOS

Excludes: ampulla of Vater (230.8)

230.8 Liver and biliary system
Ampulla of Vater   Gallbladder
Common bile duct   Hepatic duct
Cystic duct   Sphincter of Oddi

230.9 Other and unspecified digestive organs
Digestive organ NOS   Pancreas
Gastrointestinal tract NOS Spleen

231 Carcinoma in situ of respiratory system

231.0 Larynx
Cartilage: Epiglottis:
  arytenoid   NOS
  cricoid   posterior surface
  cuneiform   suprahyoid portion
  thyroid   Vocal cords (false) (true)

Excludes: aryepiglottic fold or interarytenoid fold:
  NOS (230.0)
  hypopharyngeal aspect (230.0)
  marginal zone (230.0)

231.1 Trachea

231.2 Bronchus and lung
Carina
Hilus of lung

231.8 Other specified parts of respiratory system
Accessory sinuses   Nasal cavities
Middle ear   Pleura

Excludes: ear (external) (skin) (232.2)
  nose NOS (234.8)
  skin (232.3)

231.9 Respiratory system, part unspecified
Respiratory organ NOS

232 Carcinoma in situ of skin
Includes: pigment cells

Excludes: melanoma in situ of skin (172.0-172.9)

232.0 Skin of lip

Excludes: vermilion border of lip (230.0)

232.1 Eyelid, including canthus

232.2 Ear and external auditory canal

232.3 Skin of other and unspecified parts of face

232.4 Scalp and skin of neck

232.5 Skin of trunk, except scrotum
Anus, margin   Skin of:
Axillary fold   breast
Perianal skin   buttock
Skin of: chest wall
  abdominal wall   groin
  anus   perineum
  back   Umbilicus

Excludes: anal canal (230.5)
  anus NOS (230.6)
  skin of genital organs (233.30-233.39, 233.5-233.6)

● Code new to this edition   ▲ Revision of existing code   ④ ⑤ Fourth or fifth digit required

232.6 Skin of upper limb, including shoulder

232.7 Skin of lower limb, including hip

232.8 Other specified sites of skin

232.9 Skin, site unspecified

233 Carcinoma in situ of breast and genitourinary system

233.0 Breast

> *Excludes:* Paget's disease (174.0-174.9)
> skin of breast (232.5)

233.1 Cervix uteri
Adenocarcinoma in situ of cervix
Cervical intraepithelial glandular neoplasia, grade III
Cervical intraepithelial neoplasia III [CIN III]
Severe dysplasia of cervix

> *Excludes:* cervical intraepithelial neoplasia II [CIN II] (622.12)
> cytologic evidence of malignancy without histologic confirmation (795.06)
> high grade squamous intraepithelial lesion (HGSIL) (795.04)
> moderate dysplasia of cervix (622.12)

233.2 Other and unspecified parts of uterus

⑤ 233.3 Other and unspecified female genital organs

    233.30 Unspecified female genital organ

    233.31 Vagina
    Severe dysplasia of vagina
    Vaginal intraepithelial neoplasia III [VAIN III]

    233.32 Vulva
    Severe dysplasia of vulva
    Vulvar intraepithelial neoplasia III [VIN III]

    233.39 Other female genital organ

233.4 Prostate

233.5 Penis

233.6 Other and unspecified male genital organs

233.7 Bladder

233.9 Other and unspecified urinary organs

234 Carcinoma in situ of other and unspecified sites

234.0 Eye

> *Excludes:* cartilage of eyelid (234.8)
> eyelid (skin) (232.1)
> optic nerve (234.8)
> orbital bone (234.8)

234.8 Other specified sites
Endocrine gland [any]

234.9 Site unspecified
Carcinoma in situ NOS

NEOPLASMS OF UNCERTAIN BEHAVIOR (235-238)

Note: Categories 235-238 classify by site certain histo-morphologically well-defined neoplasms, the subsequent behavior of which cannot be predicted from the present appearance.

235 Neoplasm of uncertain behavior of digestive and respiratory systems

> *Excludes:* stromal tumors of uncertain behavior of digestive system (238.1)

235.0 Major salivary glands
Gland:
    parotid
    sublingual
    submandibular

> *Excludes:* minor salivary glands (235.1)

| ▓ Add 4th or 5th digit | ▒ Nonspecific code | ░ Unspecified code | ▓ Manifestation code |

235.1 Lip, oral cavity, and pharynx

Gingiva	Nasopharynx
Hypopharynx	Oropharynx
Minor salivary glands	Tongue
Mouth	

Excludes: aryepiglottic fold or interarytenoid fold, laryngeal aspect (235.6)
    epiglottis:
      NOS (235.6)
      suprahyoid portion (235.6)
    skin of lip (238.2)

235.2 Stomach, intestines, and rectum

235.3 Liver and biliary passages

Ampulla of Vater	Gallbladder
Bile ducts [any]	Liver

235.4 Retroperitoneum and peritoneum

235.5 Other and unspecified digestive organs

Anal:	Esophagus
canal	Pancreas
sphincter	Spleen
Anus NOS	

Excludes: anus:
    margin (238.2)
    skin (238.2)
    perianal skin (238.2)

235.6 Larynx

Excludes: aryepiglottic fold or interarytenoid fold:
    NOS (235.1)
    hypopharyngeal aspect (235.1)
    marginal zone (235.1)

235.7 Trachea, bronchus, and lung

235.8 Pleura, thymus, and mediastinum

235.9 Other and unspecified respiratory organs

Accessory sinuses	Nasal cavities
Middle ear	Respiratory organ NOS

Excludes: ear (external) (skin) (238.2)
    nose (238.8)
    skin (238.2)

236 Neoplasm of uncertain behavior of genitourinary organs

236.0 Uterus

236.1 Placenta
Chorioadenoma (destruens)
Invasive mole
Malignant hydatid(iform) mole

236.2 Ovary
Use additional code, if desired, to identify any functional activity

236.3 Other and unspecified female genital organs

236.4 Testis
Use additional code, if desired, to identify any functional activity

236.5 Prostate

236.6 Other and unspecified male genital organs

236.7 Bladder

⑤ **236.9 Other and unspecified urinary organs**

    236.90 Urinary organ, unspecified

    236.91 Kidney and ureter

    236.99 Other

237 Neoplasm of uncertain behavior of endocrine glands and nervous system

237.0 Pituitary gland and craniopharyngeal duct
Use additional code, if desired, to identify any functional activity

237.1 Pineal gland

● Code new to this edition   ▲ Revision of existing code   ④ ⑤ Fourth or fifth digit required

237.2 Adrenal gland
Suprarenal gland

Use additional code, if desired, to identify any functional activity

237.3 Paraganglia
Aortic body
Carotid body
Coccygeal body
Glomus jugulare

237.4 Other and unspecified endocrine glands
Parathyroid gland
Thyroid gland

237.5 Brain and spinal cord

237.6 Meninges
Meninges:
NOS
cerebral
spinal

⑤ **237.7 Neurofibromatosis**
von Recklinghausen's disease

237.70 Neurofibromatosis, unspecified

237.71 Neurofibromatosis, Type I [von Recklinghausen's disease]

237.72 Neurofibromatosis, Type II [acoustic neurofibromatosis]

237.9 Other and unspecified parts of nervous system
Cranial nerves

Excludes: *peripheral, sympathetic, and parasympathetic nerves and ganglia (238.1)*

238 Neoplasm of uncertain behavior of other and unspecified sites and tissues

238.0 Bone and articular cartilage

Excludes: *cartilage:*
ear (238.1)
eyelid (238.1)
larynx (235.6)
nose (235.9)
synovia (238.1)

238.1 Connective and other soft tissue
Peripheral, sympathetic, and parasympathetic nerves and ganglia
Stromal tumors of digestive system

Excludes: *cartilage (of):*
articular (238.0)
larynx (235.6)
nose (235.9)
connective tissue of breast (238.3)

238.2 Skin

Excludes: *anus NOS (235.5)*
skin of genital organs (236.3, 236.6)
vermilion border of lip (235.1)

238.3 Breast

Excludes: *skin of breast (238.2)*

238.4 Polycythemia vera

238.5 Histiocytic and mast cells
Mast cell tumor NOS
Mastocytoma NOS

238.6 Plasma cells
Plasmacytoma NOS
Solitary myeloma

	Add 4th or 5th digit		Nonspecific code		Unspecified code		Manifestation code

⑤ **238.7 Other lymphatic and hematopoietic tissues**

Excludes: acute myelogenous leukemia (205.0)
chronic myelomonocytic leukemia (205.1)
myelosclerosis NOS (289.89)
myelosis:
NOS (205.9)
megakaryocytic (207.2)

238.71 Essential thrombocythemia
Essential hemorrhagic thrombocythemia
Essential thrombocytosis
Idiopathic (hemorrhagic) thrombocythemia
Primary thrombocytosis

238.72 Low grade myelodysplastic syndrome lesions
Refractory anemia (RA)
Refractory anemia (RA) with excess blasts-1 (RAEB-1)
Refractory anemia with ringed sideroblasts (RARS)
Refractory cytopenia with multilineage dysplasia (RCMD)
Refractory cytopenia with multilineage dysplasia and ringed sideroblasts (RCMD-RS)

238.73 High grade myelodysplastic syndrome lesions
Refractory anemia with excess blasts-2 (RAEB-2)

238.74 Myelodysplastic syndrome with 5q deletion
5q minus syndrome NOS

Excludes: constitutional 5q deletion (758.39)
high grade myelodysplastic syndrome with 5q deletion (238.73)

238.75 Myelodysplastic syndrome, unspecified

238.76 Myelofibrosis with myeloid metaplasia
Agnogenic myeloid metaplasia
Idiopathic myelofibrosis (chronic)
Myelosclerosis with myeloid metaplasia
Primary myelofibrosis

Excludes: myelofibrosis NOS (289.83)
myelophthisic anemia (284.2)
myelophthisis (284.2)
secondary myelofibrosis (289.83)

238.77 Post-transplant lymphoproliferative disorder (PTLD)
Code first complications of transplant (996.80-996.89)

238.79 Other lymphatic and hematopoietic tissues
Lymphoproliferative disease (chronic) NOS
Megakaryocytic myelosclerosis
Myeloproliferative disease (chronic) NOS
Panmyelosis (acute)

238.8 Other specified sites
Eye
Heart

Excludes: eyelid (skin) (238.2)
cartilage (238.1)

238.9 Site unspecified

NEOPLASMS OF UNSPECIFIED NATURE (239)

239 Neoplasms of unspecified nature
Note: Category 239 classifies by site neoplasms of unspecified morphology and behavior. The term "mass," unless otherwise stated, is not to be regarded as a neoplastic growth.
Includes: "growth" NOS
neoplasm NOS
new growth NOS
tumor NOS

239.0 Digestive system

Excludes: anus:
margin (239.2)
skin (239.2)
perianal skin (239.2)

239.1 Respiratory system

● Code new
to this edition

▲ Revision of
existing code

④ ⑤ Fourth or fifth
digit required

239.2 Bone, soft tissue, and skin

Excludes: *anal canal (239.0)*
anus NOS (239.0)
bone marrow (202.9)
cartilage:
  larynx (239.1)
  nose (239.1)
connective tissue of breast (239.3)
skin of genital organs (239.5)
vermilion border of lip (239.0)

239.3 Breast

Excludes: *skin of breast (239.2)*

239.4 Bladder

239.5 Other genitourinary organs

239.6 Brain

Excludes: *cerebral meninges (239.7)*
cranial nerves (239.7)

239.7 Endocrine glands and other parts of nervous system

Excludes: *peripheral, sympathetic, and parasympathetic nerves and ganglia (239.2)*

⑤ **239.8 Other specified sites**

Excludes: *eyelids (skin) (239.2)*
cartilage (239.2)
great vessels (239.2)
optic nerve (239.7)

● **239.81 Retina and choroid**
Dark area on retina
Retinal freckle

● **239.89 Other specified sites**

239.9 Site unspecified

● Code new
to this edition

▲ Revision of
existing code

④ ⑤ Fourth or fifth
digit required

3. ENDOCRINE, NUTRITIONAL AND METABOLIC DISEASES, AND IMMUNITY DISORDERS (240-279)

> **Excludes:** *endocrine and metabolic disturbances specific to the fetus and newborn (775.0-775.9)*

Note: All neoplasms, whether functionally active or not, are classified in Chapter 2. Codes in Chapter 3 (i.e., 242.8, 246.0, 251-253, 255-259) may be used, if desired, to identify such functional activity associated with any neoplasm, or by ectopic endocrine tissue.

DISORDERS OF THYROID GLAND (240-246)

240 Simple and unspecified goiter

240.0 Goiter, specified as simple
Any condition classifiable to 240.9, specified as simple

240.9 Goiter, unspecified
Enlargement of thyroid
Goiter or struma:
  NOS
  diffuse colloid
  endemic
Goiter or struma:
  hyperplastic
  nontoxic (diffuse)
  parenchymatous
  sporadic

> **Excludes:** *congenital (dyshormonogenic) goiter (246.1)*

241 Nontoxic nodular goiter

> **Excludes:** *adenoma of thyroid (226)*
> *cystadenoma of thyroid (226)*

241.0 Nontoxic uninodular goiter
Thyroid nodule
Uninodular goiter (nontoxic)

241.1 Nontoxic multinodular goiter
Multinodular goiter (nontoxic)

241.9 Unspecified nontoxic nodular goiter
Adenomatous goiter
Nodular goiter (nontoxic) NOS
Struma nodosa (simplex)

⑤ 242 Thyrotoxicosis with or without goiter

> **Excludes:** *neonatal thyrotoxicosis (775.3)*

The following fifth-digit subclassification is for use with category 242:

0 without mention of thyrotoxic crisis or storm

1 with mention of thyrotoxic crisis or storm

⑤ 242.0 Toxic diffuse goiter
[0-1] Basedow's disease
Exophthalmic or toxic goiter NOS
Graves' disease
Primary thyroid hyperplasia

⑤ 242.1 Toxic uninodular goiter
[0-1] Thyroid nodule, toxic or with hyperthyroidism
Uninodular goiter, toxic or with hyperthyroidism

⑤ 242.2 Toxic multinodular goiter
[0-1] Secondary thyroid hyperplasia

⑤ 242.3 Toxic nodular goiter, unspecified
[0-1] Adenomatous goiter, toxic or with hyperthyroidism
Nodular goiter, toxic or with hyperthyroidism
Struma nodosa, toxic or with hyperthyroidism
Any condition classifiable to 241.9 specified as toxic or with hyperthyroidism

⑤ 242.4 Thyrotoxicosis from ectopic thyroid nodule
[0-1]

⑤ 242.8 Thyrotoxicosis of other specified origin
[0-1] Overproduction of thyroid-stimulating hormone [TSH]
Thyrotoxicosis:
  factitia
  from ingestion of excessive thyroid material
Use additional E code to identify cause, if drug-induced

⑤ 242.9 Thyrotoxicosis without mention of goiter or other cause
[0-1] Hyperthyroidism NOS
Thyrotoxicosis NOS

	Add 4th or 5th digit		Nonspecific code		Unspecified code		Manifestation code

251

243　Congenital hypothyroidism
Congenital thyroid insufficiency
Cretinism (athyrotic) (endemic)

Use additional code to identify associated mental retardation

Excludes: *congenital (dyshormonogenic) goiter (246.1)*

244　Acquired hypothyroidism
Includes:　athyroidism (acquired)
hypothyroidism (acquired)
myxedema (adult) (juvenile)
thyroid (gland) insufficiency (acquired)

244.0　Postsurgical hypothyroidism

244.1　Other postablative hypothyroidism
Hypothyroidism following therapy, such as irradiation

244.2　Iodine hypothyroidism
Hypothyroidism resulting from administration or ingestion of iodide

Use additional E code to identify drug

244.3　Other iatrogenic hypothyroidism
Hypothyroidism resulting from:
P-aminosalicylic acid [PAS]
Phenylbutazone
Resorcinol
Iatrogenic hypothyroidism NOS

Use additional E code to identify drug

244.8　Other specified acquired hypothyroidism
Secondary hypothyroidism NEC

244.9　Unspecified hypothyroidism
Hypothyroidism, primary or NOS
Myxedema, primary or NOS

245　Thyroiditis

245.0　Acute thyroiditis
Abscess of thyroid
Thyroiditis:
nonsuppurative, acute
pyogenic
suppurative

Use additional code to identify organism

245.1　Subacute thyroiditis
Thyroiditis:　　　　　　　　Thyroiditis:
de Quervain's　　　　　　　granulomatous
giant cell　　　　　　　　　viral

245.2　Chronic lymphocytic thyroiditis
Hashimoto's disease　　　　Thyroiditis:
Struma lymphomatosa　　　　autoimmune
lymphocytic (chronic)

245.3　Chronic fibrous thyroiditis
Struma fibrosa
Thyroiditis:
invasive (fibrous)
ligneous
Riedel's

245.4　Iatrogenic thyroiditis
Use additional code to identify cause

245.8　Other and unspecified chronic thyroiditis
Chronic thyroiditis:
NOS
nonspecific

245.9　Thyroiditis, unspecified
Thyroiditis NOS

246　Other disorders of thyroid

246.0　Disorders of thyrocalcitonin secretion
Hypersecretion of calcitonin or thyrocalcitonin

● Code new
to this edition
▲ Revision of
existing code
④ ⑤ Fourth or fifth
digit required

246.1 Dyshormonogenic goiter
Congenital (dyshormonogenic) goiter
Goiter due to enzyme defect in synthesis of thyroid hormone
Goitrous cretinism (sporadic)

246.2 Cyst of thyroid

Excludes: cystadenoma of thyroid (226)

246.3 Hemorrhage and infarction of thyroid

246.8 Other specified disorders of thyroid
Abnormality of	Hyper-TBG-nemia
thyroid-binding globulin	Hypo-TBG-nemia
Atrophy of thyroid	

246.9 Unspecified disorder of thyroid

DISEASES OF OTHER ENDOCRINE GLANDS (249-259)

⑤ **249 Secondary diabetes mellitus**
Includes: diabetes mellitus (due to) (in) (secondary) (with):
drug-induced or chemical induced
infection

Excludes: gestational diabetes (648.8)
hyperglycemia NOS (790.29)
neonatal diabetes mellitus (775.1)
nonclinical diabetes (790.29)
Type I diabetes - see category 250
Type II diabetes - see category 250

The following fifth-digit subclassification is for use with category 249:

0   not stated as uncontrolled, or unspecified

1   uncontrolled

Use additional code to identify any associated insulin use (V58.67)

⑤ **249.0   Secondary diabetes mellitus without mention of complication**
[0-1]   Secondary diabetes mellitus without mention of complication or manifestation
classifiable to 249.1-249.9
Secondary diabetes mellitus NOS

⑤ **249.1   Secondary diabetes mellitus with ketoacidosis**
[0-1]   Secondary diabetes mellitus with diabetic acidosis without mention of coma
Secondary diabetes mellitus with diabetic ketosis without mention of coma

⑤ **249.2   Secondary diabetes mellitus with hyperosmolarity**
[0-1]   Secondary diabetes mellitus with hyperosmolar (nonketotic) coma

⑤ **249.3   Secondary diabetes mellitus with other coma**
[0-1]   Secondary diabetes mellitus with diabetic coma (with ketoacidosis)
Secondary diabetes mellitus with diabetic hypoglycemic coma
Secondary diabetes mellitus with insulin coma NOS

Excludes: secondary diabetes mellitus with hyperosmolar coma (249.2)

⑤ **249.4   Secondary diabetes mellitus with renal manifestations**
[0-1]
Use additional code to identify manifestation, as:
chronic kidney disease (585.1-585.9)
diabetic nephropathy NOS (583.81)
diabetic nephrosis (581.81)
intercapillary glomerulosclerosis (581.81)
Kimmelstiel-Wilson syndrome (581.81)

⑤ **249.5   Secondary diabetes mellitus with ophthalmic manifestations**
[0-1]
Use additional code to identify manifestation, as:
diabetic blindness (369.00-369.9)
diabetic cataract (366.41)
diabetic glaucoma (365.44)
diabetic macular edema (362.07)
diabetic retinal edema (362.07)
diabetic retinopathy (362.01-362.07)

| Add 4th or 5th digit | Nonspecific code | Unspecified code | Manifestation code |

⑤ **249.6 Secondary diabetes mellitus with neurological manifestations**
[0-1]
Use additional code to identify manifestation, as:
diabetic amyotrophy (353.5)
diabetic gastroparalysis (536.3)
diabetic gastroparesis (536.3)
diabetic mononeuropathy (354.0-355.9)
diabetic neurogenic arthropathy (713.5)
diabetic peripheral autonomic neuropathy (337.1)
diabetic polyneuropathy (357.2)

⑤ **249.7 Secondary diabetes mellitus with peripheral circulatory disorders**
[0-1]
Use additional code to identify manifestation, as:
diabetic gangrene (785.4)
diabetic peripheral angiopathy (443.81)

⑤ **249.8 Secondary diabetes mellitus with other specified manifestations**
[0-1]   Secondary diabetic hypoglycemia in diabetes mellitus
Secondary hypoglycemic shock in diabetes mellitus
Use additional code to identify manifestation, as:
any associated ulceration (707.10-707.9)
diabetic bone changes (731.8)

⑤ **249.9 Secondary diabetes mellitus with unspecified complication**
[0-1]

⑤ **250 Diabetes mellitus**
Excludes: *gestational diabetes (648.8)*
hyperglycemia NOS (790.29)
neonatal diabetes mellitus (775.1)
nonclinical diabetes (790.29)
secondary diabetes (249.0-249.9)
The following fifth-digit subclassification is for use with category 250:
0   type II or unspecified type, not stated as uncontrolled
Fifth-digit 0 is for use with type II patients, even if the patient requires insulin
Use additional code, if applicable, for associated long-term (current) insulin use V58.67
1   type I [juvenile type], not stated as uncontrolled
2   type II or unspecified type, uncontrolled
Fifth-digit 2 is for use with type II patients, even if the patient requires insulin
Use additional code, if applicable, for associated long-term (current) insulin use V58.67
3   type I [juvenile type], uncontrolled

⑤ **250.0 Diabetes mellitus without mention of complication**
[0-3]   Diabetes mellitus without mention of complication or manifestation classifiable to
250.1-250.9
Diabetes (mellitus) NOS

⑤ **250.1 Diabetes with ketoacidosis**
[0-3]   Diabetic:
acidosis without mention of coma
ketosis without mention of coma

⑤ **250.2 Diabetes with hyperosmolarity**
[0-3]   Hyperosmolar (nonketotic) coma

⑤ **250.3 Diabetes with other coma**
[0-3]   Diabetic coma (with ketoacidosis)
Diabetic hypoglycemic coma
Insulin coma NOS

Excludes: *diabetes with hyperosmolar coma (250.2)*

⑤ **250.4 Diabetes with renal manifestations**
[0-3]
Use additional code to identify manifestation, as:
chronic kidney disease (585.1-585.9)
diabetic:
nephropathy NOS (583.81)
nephrosis (581.81)
intercapillary glomerulosclerosis (581.81)
Kimmelstiel-Wilson syndrome (581.81)

● Code new   ▲ Revision of   ④ ⑤ Fourth or fifth
to this edition   existing code   digit required

⑤ **250.5 Diabetes with ophthalmic manifestations**
[0-3]

Use additional code to identify manifestation, as:
  diabetic:
    blindness (369.00-369.9)
    cataract (366.41)
    glaucoma (365.44)
    macular edema (362.07)
    retinal edema (362.07)
    retinopathy (362.01-362.07)

⑤ **250.6 Diabetes with neurological manifestations**
[0-3]

Use additional code to identify manifestation, as:
  diabetic:
    amyotrophy (353.5)
    gastroparalysis (536.3)
    gastroparesis (536.3)
    mononeuropathy (354.0-355.9)
    neurogenic arthropathy (713.5)
    peripheral autonomic neuropathy (337.1)
    polyneuropathy (357.2)

⑤ **250.7 Diabetes with peripheral circulatory disorders**
[0-3]

Use additional code to identify manifestation, as:
  diabetic:
    gangrene (785.4)
    peripheral angiopathy (443.81)

⑤ **250.8 Diabetes with other specified manifestations**
[0-3]   Diabetic hypoglycemia NOS
         Hypoglycemic shock NOS

Use additional code to identify manifestation, as:
    any associated ulceration (707.10-707.9)
    diabetic bone changes (731.8)

⑤ **250.9 Diabetes with unspecified complication**
[0-3]

251 **Other disorders of pancreatic internal secretion**

251.0 Hypoglycemic coma
         Iatrogenic hyperinsulinism
         Non-diabetic insulin coma

Use additional E code to identify cause, if drug-induced

Excludes: *hypoglycemic coma in diabetes mellitus (249.3, 250.3)*

251.1 Other specified hypoglycemia
         Hyperinsulinism:
           NOS
           ectopic
           functional
         Hyperplasia of pancreatic islet beta cells NOS

Excludes: *hypoglycemia in diabetes mellitus (249.8, 250.8)*
           hypoglycemia in infant of diabetic mother (775.0)
           hypoglycemic coma (251.0)
           neonatal hypoglycemia (775.6)

Use additional E code to identify cause, if drug-induced

251.2 Hypoglycemia, unspecified
         Hypoglycemia:
           NOS
           reactive
           spontaneous

Excludes: *hypoglycemia:*
           with coma (251.0)
           in diabetes mellitus (249.8, 250.8)
           leucine-induced (270.3)

	Add 4th or 5th digit		Nonspecific code		Unspecified code		Manifestation code

251.3 Postsurgical hypoinsulinemia
Hypoinsulinemia following complete or partial pancreatectomy
Postpancreatectomy hyperglycemia

Use additional code to identify (any associated):
acquired absence of pancreas (V45.79)
insulin use (V58.67)
secondary diabetes mellitus (249.00-249.91)

Excludes: *transient hyperglycemia post procedure (790.29)*
transient hypoglycemia post procedure (251.2)

251.4 Abnormality of secretion of glucagon
Hyperplasia of pancreatic islet alpha cells with glucagon excess

251.5 Abnormality of secretion of gastrin
Hyperplasia of pancreatic alpha cells with gastrin excess
Zollinger-Ellison syndrome

251.8 Other specified disorders of pancreatic internal secretion

251.9 Unspecified disorder of pancreatic internal secretion
Islet cell hyperplasia NOS

252 Disorders of parathyroid gland

Excludes: *hungry bone syndrome (275.5)*

⑤ **252.0 Hyperparathyroidism**

Excludes: *ectopic hyperparathyroidism (259.3)*

252.00 Hyperparathyroidism, unspecified

252.01 Primary hyperparathyroidism
Hyperplasia of parathyroid

252.02 Secondary hyperparathyroidism, non-renal

Excludes: *secondary hyperparathyroidism (of renal origin) (588.81)*

252.08 Other hyperparathyroidism
Tertiary hyperparathyroidism

252.1 Hypoparathyroidism
Parathyroiditis (autoimmune)
Tetany:
parathyroid
parathyroprival

Excludes: *pseudohypoparathyroidism (275.4)*
pseudo-pseudohypoparathyroidism (275.4)
tetany NOS (781.7)
transitory neonatal hypoparathyroidism (775.4)

252.8 Other specified disorders of parathyroid gland
Cyst of parathyroid gland
Hemorrhage of parathyroid gland

252.9 Unspecified disorder of parathyroid gland

253 Disorders of the pituitary gland and its hypothalamic control
Includes: the listed conditions whether the disorder is in the pituitary or the hypothalamus

Excludes: *Cushing's syndrome (255.0)*

253.0 Acromegaly and gigantism
Overproduction of growth hormone

253.1 Other and unspecified anterior pituitary hyperfunction
Forbes-Albright syndrome

Excludes: *overproduction of:*
ACTH (255.3)
thyroid-stimulating hormone [TSH] (242.8)

253.2 Panhypopituitarism
Cachexia, pituitary   Sheehan's syndrome
Necrosis of pituitary   Simmonds' disease
(postpartum)
Pituitary insufficiency NOS

Excludes: *iatrogenic hypopituitarism (253.7)*

253.3 Pituitary dwarfism
Isolated deficiency of (human) growth hormone [HGH]
Lorain-Levi dwarfism

● Code new
to this edition

▲ Revision of
existing code

④ ⑤ Fourth or fifth
digit required

253.4 Other anterior pituitary disorders
Isolated or partial deficiency of an anterior pituitary hormone, other than growth hormone
Prolactin deficiency

253.5 Diabetes insipidus
Vasopressin deficiency
Excludes: nephrogenic diabetes insipidus (588.1)

253.6 Other disorders of neurohypophysis
Syndrome of inappropriate secretion of antidiuretic hormone [ADH]
Excludes: ectopic antidiuretic hormone secretion (259.3)

253.7 Iatrogenic pituitary disorders
Hypopituitarism:
hormone-induced
hypophysectomy-induced
postablative
radiotherapy-induced
Use additional E code to identify cause

253.8 Other disorders of the pituitary and other syndromes of diencephalohypophyseal origin
Abscess of pituitary
Adiposogenital dystrophy
Cyst of Rathke's pouch
Fröhlich's syndrome
Excludes: craniopharyngioma (237.0)

253.9 Unspecified
Dyspituitarism

254 Diseases of thymus gland
Excludes: aplasia or dysplasia with immunodeficiency (279.2)
hypoplasia with immunodeficiency (279.2)
myasthenia gravis (358.00-358.01)

254.0 Persistent hyperplasia of thymus
Hypertrophy of thymus

254.1 Abscess of thymus

254.8 Other specified diseases of thymus gland
Atrophy of thymus
Cyst of thymus
Excludes thymoma (212.6)

254.9 Unspecified disease of thymus gland

255 Disorders of adrenal glands
Includes: the listed conditions whether the basic disorder is in the adrenals or is pituitary-induced

255.0 Cushing's syndrome
Adrenal hyperplasia due to excess ACTH
Cushing's syndrome:
NOS
iatrogenic
idiopathic
pituitary-dependent
Ectopic ACTH syndrome
Iatrogenic syndrome of excess cortisol
Overproduction of cortisol
Excludes: congenital adrenal hyperplasia (255.2)
Use additional E code to identify cause, if drug-induced

⑤ **255.1 Hyperaldosteronism**

255.10 Hyperaldosteronism, unspecified
Aldosteronism NOS
Primary aldosteronism, unspecified
Excludes: Conn's syndrome (255.12)

255.11 Glucocorticoid-remediable aldosteronism
Familial aldosteronism type I
Excludes: Conn's syndrome (255.12)

255.12 Conn's syndrome

255.13 Bartter's syndrome

255.14 Other secondary aldosteronism

| | Add 4th or 5th digit | | Nonspecific code | | Unspecified code | | Manifestation code |

TABULAR LIST

255.2 Adrenogenital disorders
Adrenogenital syndromes, virilizing or feminizing, whether acquired or associated with congenital adrenal hyperplasia consequent on inborn enzyme defects in hormone synthesis
Achard-Thiers syndrome
Congenital adrenal hyperplasia
Female adrenal pseudohermaphroditism
Male:
    macrogenitosomia praecox
    sexual precocity with adrenal hyperplasia
Virilization (female) (suprarenal)

Excludes: *adrenal hyperplasia due to excess ACTH (255.0)*
    isosexual virilization (256.4)

255.3 Other corticoadrenal overactivity
Acquired benign adrenal androgenic overactivity
Overproduction of ACTH

⑤ 255.4 Corticoadrenal insufficiency

Excludes: *tuberculous Addison's disease (017.6)*

255.41 Glucocorticoid deficiency
Addisonian crisis
Addison's disease NOS
Adrenal atrophy (autoimmune)
Adrenal calcification
Adrenal crisis
Adrenal hemorrhage
Adrenal infarction
Adrenal insufficiency NOS
Combined glucocorticoid and mineralocorticoid deficiency
Corticoadrenal insufficiency NOS

255.42 Mineralocorticoid deficiency
Hypoaldosteronism

Excludes: *combined glucocorticoid and mineralocorticoid deficiency (255.41)*

255.5 Other adrenal hypofunction
Adrenal medullary insufficiency

Excludes: *Waterhouse-Friderichsen syndrome (meningococcal) (036.3)*

255.6 Medulloadrenal hyperfunction
Catecholamine secretion by pheochromocytoma

255.8 Other specified disorders of adrenal glands
Abnormality of cortisol-binding globulin

255.9 Unspecified disorder of adrenal glands

256 Ovarian dysfunction

256.0 Hyperestrogenism

256.1 Other ovarian hyperfunction
Hypersecretion of ovarian androgens

256.2 Postablative ovarian failure
Use additional code for states associated with artifical menopause (627.4)
Ovarian failure:
    iatrogenic
    postirradiation
    postsurgical

Excludes: *asymptomatic age-related (natural) postmenopausal status (V49.81)*
    acquired absence of ovary (V45.77)

⑤ 256.3 Other ovarian failure
Use additional code for states associated with natural menopause (627.2)

Excludes: *asymptomatic age-related (natural) postmenopausal status (V49.81)*

256.31 Premature menopause

256.39 Other ovarian failure
Delayed menarche
Ovarian hypofunction
Primary ovarian failure NOS

● Code new to this edition   ▲ Revision of existing code   ④ ⑤ Fourth or fifth digit required

256.4 Polycystic ovaries
Isosexual virilization
Stein-Leventhal syndrome

256.8 Other ovarian dysfunction

256.9 Unspecified ovarian dysfunction

257 Testicular dysfunction

257.0 Testicular hyperfunction
Hypersecretion of testicular hormones

257.1 Postablative testicular hypofunction
Testicular hypofunction:
iatrogenic
postirradiation
postsurgical

257.2 Other testicular hypofunction
Defective biosynthesis of testicular androgen
Eunuchoidism:
NOS
hypogonadotropic
Failure:
Leydig's cell, adult
seminiferous tubule, adult
Testicular hypogonadism
Excludes: azoospermia (606.0)

257.8 Other testicular dysfunction
Excludes: androgen insensitivity syndromes (259.50-259.52)

257.9 Unspecified testicular dysfunction

258 Polyglandular dysfunction and related disorders

⑤ **258.0 Polyglandular activity in multiple endocrine adenomatosis**
Multiple endocrine neoplasia [MEN] syndromes
Use additional codes to identify any malignancies and other conditions associated with the syndromes

258.01 Multiple endocrine neoplasia [MEN] type I
Wermer's syndrome

258.02 Multiple endocrine neoplasia [MEN] type IIA
Sipple's syndrome

258.03 Multiple endocrine neoplasia [MEN] type IIB

258.1 Other combinations of endocrine dysfunction
Lloyd's syndrome   Schmidt's syndrome

258.8 Other specified polyglandular dysfunction

258.9 Polyglandular dysfunction, unspecified

259 Other endocrine disorders

259.0 Delay in sexual development and puberty, not elsewhere classified
Delayed puberty

259.1 Precocious sexual development and puberty, not elsewhere classified
Sexual precocity:
NOS
constitutional
cryptogenic
idiopathic

259.2 Carcinoid syndrome
Hormone secretion by carcinoid tumors

259.3 Ectopic hormone secretion, not elsewhere classified
Ectopic:
antidiuretic hormone secretion [ADH]
hyperparathyroidism
Excludes: ectopic ACTH syndrome (255.0)

Add 4th or 5th digit | Nonspecific code | Unspecified code | Manifestation code

259.4 Dwarfism, not elsewhere classified
Dwarfism:
NOS
constitutional

Excludes: *dwarfism:*
achondroplastic (756.4)
intrauterine (759.7)
nutritional (263.2)
pituitary (253.3)
renal (588.0)
progeria (259.8)

⑤ **259.5 Androgen insensitivity syndrome**

259.50 Androgen insensitivity, unspecified

259.51 Androgen insensitivity syndrome
Complete androgen insensitivity
de Quervain's syndrome
Goldberg-Maxwell Syndrome

259.52 Partial androgen insensitivity
Partial androgen insensitivity syndrome
Reifenstein syndrome

259.8 Other specified endocrine disorders
Pineal gland dysfunction
Progeria

259.9 Unspecified endocrine disorder
Disturbance: Infantilism NOS
endocrine NOS
hormone NOS

NUTRITIONAL DEFICIENCIES (260-269)

Excludes: *deficiency anemias (280.0-281.9)*

260 Kwashiorkor
Nutritional edema with dyspigmentation of skin and hair

261 Nutritional marasmus
Nutritional atrophy   Severe malnutrition NOS
Severe calorie deficiency

262 Other severe protein-calorie malnutrition
Nutritional edema without mention of dyspigmentation of skin and hair

263 Other and unspecified protein-calorie malnutrition

263.0 Malnutrition of moderate degree

263.1 Malnutrition of mild degree

263.2 Arrested development following protein-calorie malnutrition
Nutritional dwarfism   Physical retardation due to malnutrition

263.8 Other protein-calorie malnutrition

263.9 Unspecified protein-calorie malnutrition
Dystrophy due to malnutrition
Malnutrition (calorie) NOS

Excludes: *nutritional deficiency NOS (269.9)*

264 Vitamin A deficiency

264.0 With conjunctival xerosis

264.1 With conjunctival xerosis and Bitot's spot
Bitot's spot in the young child

264.2 With corneal xerosis

264.3 With corneal ulceration and xerosis

264.4 With keratomalacia

264.5 With night blindness

264.6 With xerophthalmic scars of cornea

264.7 Other ocular manifestations of vitamin A deficiency
Xerophthalmia due to vitamin A deficiency

264.8 Other manifestations of vitamin A deficiency
Follicular keratosis due to vitamin A deficiency
Xeroderma due to vitamin A deficiency

● Code new
to this edition

▲ Revision of
existing code

④ ⑤ Fourth or fifth
digit required

264.9 Unspecified vitamin A deficiency
Hypovitaminosis A NOS

265 Thiamine and niacin deficiency states

265.0 Beriberi

265.1 Other and unspecified manifestations of thiamine deficiency
Other vitamin B_1 deficiency states

265.2 Pellagra
Deficiency:
  niacin (-tryptophan)
  nicotinamide
  nicotinic acid
  vitamin PP
Pellagra (alcoholic)

266 Deficiency of B-complex components

266.0 Ariboflavinosis
Riboflavin [vitamin B_2] deficiency

266.1 Vitamin B_6 deficiency
Deficiency: Vitamin B_6 deficiency syndrome
  pyridoxal
  pyridoxamine
  pyridoxine

Excludes: *vitamin B_6-responsive sideroblastic anemia (285.0)*

266.2 Other B-complex deficiencies
Deficiency:
  cyanocobalamin
  folic acid
  vitamin B_{12}

Excludes: *combined system disease with anemia (281.0-281.1)*
deficiency anemias (281.0-281.9)
subacute degeneration of spinal cord with anemia (281.0-281.1)

266.9 Unspecified vitamin B deficiency

267 Ascorbic acid deficiency
Deficiency of vitamin C
Scurvy

Excludes: *scorbutic anemia (281.8)*

268 Vitamin D deficiency

Excludes: *vitamin D-resistant:*
osteomalacia (275.3)
rickets (275.3)

268.0 Rickets, active

Excludes: *celiac rickets (579.0)*
renal rickets (588.0)

268.1 Rickets, late effect
Any condition specified as due to rickets and stated to be a late effect or sequela of rickets
Code first the nature of late effect

268.2 Osteomalacia, unspecified

268.9 Unspecified vitamin D deficiency
Avitaminosis D

269 Other nutritional deficiencies

269.0 Deficiency of vitamin K

Excludes: *deficiency of coagulation factor due to vitamin K deficiency (286.7)*
vitamin K deficiency of newborn (776.0)

269.1 Deficiency of other vitamins
Deficiency:
  vitamin E
  vitamin P

269.2 Unspecified vitamin deficiency
Multiple vitamin deficiency NOS

| | Add 4th or 5th digit | | Nonspecific code | | Unspecified code | | Manifestation code |

269.3 Mineral deficiency, not elsewhere classified
Deficiency:
calcium, dietary
iodine

Excludes: *deficiency:*
calcium NOS (275.4)
potassium (276.8)
sodium (276.1)

269.8 Other nutritional deficiency
Excludes: *adult failure to thrive (783.7)*
failure to thrive in childhood (783.41)
feeding problems (783.3)
newborn (779.31-779.34)

269.9 Unspecified nutritional deficiency

OTHER METABOLIC AND IMMUNITY DISORDERS (270-279)
Use additional code to identify any associated mental retardation

270 Disorders of amino-acid transport and metabolism
Excludes: *abnormal findings without manifest disease (790.0-796.9)*
disorders of purine and pyrimidine metabolism (277.1-277.2)
gout (274.00-274.9)

270.0 Disturbances of amino-acid transport
Cystinosis
Cystinuria
Fanconi (-de Toni) (-Debré) syndrome
Glycinuria (renal)
Hartnup disease

270.1 Phenylketonuria [PKU]
Hyperphenylalaninemia

270.2 Other disturbances of aromatic amino-acid metabolism
Albinism
Alkaptonuria
Alkaptonuric ochronosis
Disturbances of metabolism
of tyrosine and
tryptophan
Homogentisic acid defects
Hydroxykynureninuria
Hypertyrosinemia
Indicanuria
Kynureninase defects
Oasthouse urine disease
Ochronosis
Tyrosinosis
Tyrosinuria
Waardenburg syndrome

Excludes: *vitamin B$_6$-deficiency syndrome (266.1)*

270.3 Disturbances of branched-chain amino-acid metabolism
Disturbances of metabolism of leucine, isoleucine, and valine
Hypervalinemia
Intermittent branched-chain ketonuria
Leucine-induced hypoglycemia
Leucinosis
Maple syrup urine disease

270.4 Disturbances of sulphur-bearing amino-acid metabolism
Cystathioninemia
Cystathioninuria
Disturbances of metabolism of methionine, homocystine, and cystathionine
Homocystinuria
Hypermethioninemia
Methioninemia

270.5 Disturbances of histidine metabolism
Carnosinemia
Histidinemia
Hyperhistidinemia
Imidazole aminoaciduria

270.6 Disorders of urea cycle metabolism
Argininosuccinic aciduria
Citrullinemia
Disturbances of metabolism of ornithine, citrulline, argininosuccinic acid, arginine, and
ammonia
Hyperammonemia
Hyperornithinemia

● Code new
to this edition
▲ Revision of
existing code
④ ⑤ Fourth or fifth
digit required

270.7 Other disturbances of straight-chain amino-acid metabolism
Glucoglycinuria
Glycinemia (with methyl-
  malonic acidemia)
Hyperglycinemia
Hyperlysinemia
Pipecolic acidemia

Saccharopinuria
Other disturbances of metabolism of glycine, threonine,
  serine, glutamine, and lysine

270.8 Other specified disorders of amino-acid metabolism
Alaninemia
Ethanolaminuria
Glycoprolinuria
Hydroxyprolinemia
Hyperprolinemia

Iminoacidopathy
Prolinemia
Prolinuria
Sarcosinemia

270.9 Unspecified disorder of amino-acid metabolism

271 Disorders of carbohydrate transport and metabolism

Excludes: *abnormality of secretion of glucagon (251.4)*
          diabetes mellitus (249.0-249.9, 250.0-250.9)
          hypoglycemia NOS (251.2)
          mucopolysaccharidosis (277.5)

271.0 Glycogenosis
Amylopectinosis
Glucose-6-phosphatase
  deficiency
Glycogen storage disease

McArdle's disease
Pompe's disease
von Gierke's disease

271.1 Galactosemia
Galactose-1-phosphate uridyl transferase deficiency
Galactosuria

271.2 Hereditary fructose intolerance
Essential benign fructosuria
Fructosemia

271.3 Intestinal disaccharidase deficiencies and disaccharide malabsorption
Intolerance or malabsorption (congenital) (of):
  glucose-galactose
  lactose
  sucrose-isomaltose

271.4 Renal glycosuria
Renal diabetes

271.8 Other specified disorders of carbohydrate transport and metabolism
Essential benign pentosuria
Fucosidosis
Glycolic aciduria
Hyperoxaluria (primary)

Mannosidosis
Oxalosis
Xylosuria
Xylulosuria

271.9 Unspecified disorder of carbohydrate transport and metabolism

272 Disorders of lipoid metabolism

Excludes: *localized cerebral lipidoses (330.1)*

272.0 Pure hypercholesterolemia
Familial hypercholesterolemia
Fredrickson Type IIa hyperlipoproteinemia
Hyperbetalipoproteinemia
Hyperlipidemia, Group A
Low-density-lipoid-type [LDL] hyperlipoproteinemia

272.1 Pure hyperglyceridemia
Endogenous hyperglyceridemia
Frederickson Type IV hyperlipoproteinemia
Hyperlipidemia, Group B
Hyperprebetalipoproteinemia
Hypertriglyceridemia, essential
Very-low-density-lipoid-type [VLDL] hyperlipoproteinemia

| | Add 4th or 5th digit | | Nonspecific code | | Unspecified code | | Manifestation code |

272.2 **Mixed hyperlipidemia**
Broad- or floating-betalipoproteinemia
Combined hyperlipidemia
Elevated cholesterol with elevated triglycerides NEC
Fredrickson Type IIb or III hyperlipoproteinemia
Hypercholesterolemia with endogenous hyperglyceridemia
Hyperbetalipoproteinemia with prebetalipoproteinemia
Tubo-eruptive xanthoma
Xanthoma tuberosum

272.3 **Hyperchylomicronemia**
Bürger-Grütz syndrome
Fredrickson type I or V hyperlipoproteinemia
Hyperlipidemia, Group D
Mixed hyperglyceridemia

272.4 **Other and unspecified hyperlipidemia**
Alpha-lipoproteinemia
Hyperlipidemia NOS
Hyperlipoproteinemia NOS

272.5 **Lipoprotein deficiencies**
Abetalipoproteinemia
Bassen-Kornzweig syndrome
High-density lipoid deficiency
Hypoalphalipoproteinemia
Hypobetalipoproteinemia (familial)

272.6 **Lipodystrophy**
Barraquer-Simons disease
Progressive lipodystrophy
Use additional E code to identify cause, if iatrogenic
Excludes: intestinal lipodystrophy (040.2)

272.7 **Lipidoses**
Chemically-induced lipidosis
Disease:
  Anderson's
  Fabry's
  Gaucher's
  I cell [mucolipidosis I]
  lipoid storage NOS
  Neimann-Pick
  pseudo-Hurler's or
  mucolipidosis III
Disease:
  triglyceride storage, Type I or II
  Wolman's or triglyceride storage, Type III
Mucolipidosis II
Primary familial xanthomatosis
Excludes: cerebral lipidoses (330.1)
Tay-Sachs disease (330.1)

272.8 **Other disorders of lipoid metabolism**
Hoffa's disease or liposynovitis prepatellaris
Launois-Bensaude's lipomatosis
Lipoid dermatoarthritis

272.9 **Unspecified disorder of lipoid metabolism**

273 **Disorders of plasma protein metabolism**
Excludes: agammaglobulinemia and hypogammaglobulinemia (279.0 -279.2)
coagulation defects (286.0-286.9)
hereditary hemolytic anemias (282.0-282.9)

273.0 **Polyclonal hypergammaglobulinemia**
Hypergammaglobulinemic purpura:
  benign primary
  Waldenström's

273.1 **Monoclonal paraproteinemia**
Benign monoclonal hypergammaglobulinemia [BMH]
Monoclonal gammopathy:
  NOS
  associated with lymphoplasmacytic dyscrasias
  benign
Paraproteinemia:
  benign (familial)
  secondary to malignant or inflammatory disease

● Code new to this edition   ▲ Revision of existing code   ④ ⑤ Fourth or fifth digit required

273.2 **Other paraproteinemias**
Cryoglobulinemic: Mixed cryoglobulinemia
  purpura
  vasculitis

273.3 **Macroglobulinemia**
Macroglobulinemia (idiopathic) (primary)
Waldenström's macroglobulinemia

273.4 **Alpha-1-antitrypsin deficiency**
AAT deficiency

273.8 **Other disorders of plasma protein metabolism**
Abnormality of transport protein
Bisalbuminemia

273.9 **Unspecified disorder of plasma protein metabolism**

274 **Gout**
Excludes: lead gout (984.0-984.9)

⑤ **274.0** **Gouty arthropathy**

● **274.00** **Gout arthropathy, unspecified**

● **274.01** **Acute gouty arthropathy**
Acute gout
Gout attack
Gout flare
Podagra

● **274.02** **Chronic gouty arthropathy without mention of tophus (tophi)**
Chronic gout

● **274.03** **Chronic gouty arthropathy with tophus (tophi)**
Chronic tophaceous gout
Gout with tophi NOS

⑤ **274.1** **Gouty nephropathy**

274.10 **Gouty nephropathy, unspecified**

274.11 **Uric acid nephrolithiasis**

274.19 **Other**

⑤ **274.8** **Gout with other specified manifestations**

274.81 **Gouty tophi of ear**

274.82 **Gouty tophi of other sites**
Gouty tophi of heart

Excludes: gout with tophi NOS (274.03)
  gouty arthropathy with tophi (274.03)

274.89 **Other**
Use additional code to identify manifestations, as:
  gouty:
    iritis (364.11)
    neuritis (357.4)

274.9 **Gout, unspecified**

275 **Disorders of mineral metabolism**
Excludes: abnormal findings without manifest disease (790.0-796.9)

275.0 **Disorders of iron metabolism**
Bronzed diabetes   Pigmentary cirrhosis (of liver)
Hemochromatosis
Excludes: anemia:
    iron deficiency (280.0-280.9)
    sideroblastic (285.0)

275.1 **Disorders of copper metabolism**
Hepatolenticular degeneration
Wilson's disease

275.2 **Disorders of magnesium metabolism**
Hypermagnesemia
Hypomagnesemia

Add 4th or 5th digit   Nonspecific code   Unspecified code   Manifestation code

275.3 Disorders of phosphorus metabolism
Familial hypophosphatemia
Hypophosphatasia
Vitamin D-resistant:
  osteomalacia
  rickets

⑤ **275.4 Disorders of calcium metabolism**
Excludes: *hungry bone syndrome (275.5)*
        parathyroid disorders (252.00-252.9)
        vitamin D deficiency (268.0-268.9)

  275.40 Unspecified disorder of calcium metabolism

  275.41 Hypocalcemia

  275.42 Hypercalcemia

  275.49 Other disorders of calcium metabolism
    Nephrocalcinosis
    Pseudohypoparathyroidism
    Pseudopseudohypoparathyroidism

275.5 Hungry bone syndrome

275.8 Other specified disorders of mineral metabolism

275.9 Unspecified disorder of mineral metabolism

276 Disorders of fluid, electrolyte, and acid-base balance
Excludes: *diabetes insipidus (253.5)*
        familial periodic paralysis (359.3)

276.0 Hyperosmolality and/or hypernatremia
Sodium [Na] excess
Sodium [Na] overload

276.1 Hyposmolality and/or hyponatremia
Sodium [Na] deficiency

276.2 Acidosis
Acidosis:
  NOS
  lactic
  metabolic
  respiratory
Excludes: *diabetic acidosis (249.1, 250.1)*

276.3 Alkalosis
Alkalosis:
  NOS
  metabolic
  respiratory

276.4 Mixed acid-base balance disorder
Hypercapnia with mixed acid-base disorder

⑤ **276.5 Volume depletion**

  276.50 Volume depletion, unspecified

  276.51 Dehydration

  276.52 Hypovolemia
    Depletion of volume of plasma

276.6 Fluid overload
Fluid retention
Excludes: *ascites (789.51-789.59)*
        localized edema (782.3)

276.7 Hyperpotassemia
Hyperkalemia
Potassium [K]:
  excess
  intoxication
  overload

276.8 Hypopotassemia
Hypokalemia
Potassium [K] deficiency

● Code new
  to this edition
▲ Revision of
  existing code
④ ⑤ Fourth or fifth
    digit required

276.9 Electrolyte and fluid disorders not elsewhere classified
Electrolyte imbalance
Hyperchloremia
Hypochloremia

Excludes: *electrolyte imbalance:*
associated with hyperemesis gravidarum (643.1)
complicating labor and delivery (669.0)
following abortion and ectopic or molar pregnancy (634-638 with .4, 639.4)

277 Other and unspecified disorders of metabolism

⑤ **277.0 Cystic fibrosis**
Fibrocystic disease of the pancreas
Mucoviscidosis

277.00 Without mention of meconium ileus
Cystic fibrosis NOS

277.01 With meconium ileus
Meconium:
ileus (of newborn)
obstruction of intestine in mucoviscidosis

277.02 With pulmonary manifestations
Cystic fibrosis with pulmonary exacerbation

Use additional code to identify any infectious organism present, such as:
pseudomonas (041.7)

277.03 With gastrointestinal manifestations

Excludes: *with meconium ileus (277.01)*

277.09 With other manifestations

277.1 Disorders of porphyrin metabolism

Hematoporphyria	Porphyrinuria
Hematoporphyrinuria	Protocoproporphyria
Hereditary coproporphyria	Protoporphyria
Porphyria	Pyrroloporphyria

277.2 Other disorders of purine and pyrimidine metabolism
Hypoxanthine-guanine-phosphoribosyltransferase deficiency [HG-PRT deficiency]
Lesch-Nyhan syndrome
Xanthinuria

Excludes: *gout (274.00-274.9)*
orotic aciduric anemia (281.4)

⑤ **277.3 Amyloidosis**

277.30 Amyloidosis, unspecified
Amyloidosis NOS

277.31 Familial Mediterranean fever
Benign paroxysmal peritonitis
Hereditary amyloid nephropathy
Periodic familial polyserositis
Recurrent polyserositis

277.39 Other amyloidosis
Hereditary cardiac amyloidosis
Inherited systemic amyloidosis
Neuropathic (Portuguese) (Swiss) amyloidosis
Secondary amyloidosis

277.4 Disorders of bilirubin excretion
Hyperbilirubinemia:
congenital
constitutional
Syndrome:
Crigler-Najjar
Dubin-Johnson
Gilbert's
Rotor's

Excludes: *hyperbilirubinemias specific to the perinatal period (774.0-774.7)*

�	Add 4th or 5th digit	�	Nonspecific code	�	Unspecified code	�	Manifestation code

277.5 Mucopolysaccharidosis
Gargoylism
Hunter's syndrome
Hurler's syndrome
Lipochondrodystrophy
Maroteaux-Lamy syndrome
Morquio-Brailsford disease
Osteochondrodystrophy
Sanfilippo's syndrome
Scheie's syndrome

277.6 Other deficiencies of circulating enzymes
Hereditary angioedema

277.7 Dysmetabolic syndrome X
Use additional code for associated manifestation, such as:
cardiovascular disease (414.00-414.07)
obesity (278.00-278.01)

⑤ **277.8 Other specified disorders of metabolism**

    277.81 Primary carnitine deficiency

    277.82 Carnitine deficiency due to inborn errors of metabolism

    277.83 Iatrogenic carnitine deficiency
    Carnitine deficiency due to:
      hemodialysis
      valproic acid therapy

    277.84 Other secondary carnitine deficiency

    277.85 Disorders of fatty acid oxidation
    Carnitine palmitoyltransferase deficiencies (CPT1, CPT2)
    Glutaric aciduria type II (type IIA, IIB, IIC)
    Long chain 3-hydroxyacyl CoA dehydrogenase deficiency (LCHAD)
    Long chain/very long chain acyl CoA dehydrogenase deficiency (LCAD, VLCAD)
    Medium chain acyl CoA dehydrogenase deficiency (MCAD)
    Short chain acyl CoA dehydrogenase deficiency (SCAD)

Excludes: primary carnitine deficiency (277.81)

    277.86 Peroxisomal disorders
    Adrenomyeloneuropathy
    Neonatal adrenoleukodystrophy
    Rhizomelic chrondrodysplasia punctata
    X-linked adrenoleukodystrophy
    Zellweger syndrome

Excludes: infantile Refsum disease (356.3)

    277.87 Disorders of mitochondrial metabolism
    Kearns-Sayre syndrome
    Mitochondrial Encephalopathy, Lactic Acidosis and Stroke-like episodes (MELAS syndrome)
    Mitochondrial Neurogastrointestinal Encephalopathy syndrome (MNGIE)
    Myoclonus with Epilepsy and with Ragged Red Fibers (MERRF syndrome)
    Neuropathy, Ataxia and Retinitis Pigmentosa (NARP syndrome)
Use additional code for associated conditions

Excludes: disorders of pyruvate metabolism (271.8)
      Leber's optic atrophy (377.16)
      Leigh's subacute necrotizing encephalopathy (330.8)
      Reye's syndrome (331.81)

● **277.88 Tumor lysis syndrome**
    Spontaneous tumor lysis syndrome
    Tumor lysis syndrome following antineoplastic drug therapy
Use additional E code to identify cause, if drug-induced

    277.89 Other specified disorders of metabolism
    Hand-Schuller-Christian disease
    Histiocytosis (acute) (chronic)
    Histiocytosis X (chronic)

Excludes: histiocytosis:
      acute differentiatied progressive (202.5)
      X, acute (progressive) (202.5)

277.9 Unspecified disorder of metabolism
Enzymopathy NOS

  ● Code new
    to this edition
  ▲ Revision of
    existing code
  ④ ⑤ Fourth or fifth
    digit required

278 **Overweight, obesity and other hyperalimentation**
> Excludes: *hyperalimentation NOS (783.6)*
> *poisoning by vitamins NOS (963.5)*
> *polyphagia (783.6)*

Use additional code to identify Body Mass Index (BMI), if known (V85.21-V85.25, V85.30-V85.39, V85.4, V85.53, V85.54)

⑤ **278.0** **Overweight and obesity**
Use additional code to identify Body Mass Index (BMI), if known (V85.0-V85.54)
> Excludes: *adiposogenital dystrophy (253.8)*
> *obesity of endocrine origin NOS (259.9)*

278.00 **Obesity, unspecified**
Obesity NOS

278.01 **Morbid obesity**
Severe obesity

278.02 **Overweight**

278.1 **Localized adiposity**
Fat pad

278.2 **Hypervitaminosis A**

278.3 **Hypercarotinemia**

278.4 **Hypervitaminosis D**

278.8 **Other hyperalimentation**

279 **Disorders involving the immune mechanism**

⑤ **279.0** **Deficiency of humoral immunity**

279.00 **Hypogammaglobulinemia, unspecified**
Agammaglobulinemia NOS

279.01 **Selective IgA immunodeficiency**

279.02 **Selective IgM immunodeficiency**

279.03 **Other selective immunoglobulin deficiencies**
Selective deficiency of IgG

279.04 **Congenital hypogammaglobulinemia**
Agammaglobulinemia:
Bruton's type
X-linked

279.05 **Immunodeficiency with increased IgM**
Immunodeficiency with hyper-IgM:
autosomal recessive
X-linked

279.06 **Common variable immunodeficiency**
Dysgammaglobulinemia (acquired) (congenital) (primary)
Hypogammaglobulinemia:
acquired primary
congenital non-sex-linked
sporadic

279.09 **Other**
Transient hypogammaglobulinemia of infancy

⑤ **279.1** **Deficiency of cell-mediated immunity**

279.10 **Immunodeficiency with predominant T-cell defect, unspecified**

279.11 **DiGeorge's syndrome**
Pharyngeal pouch syndrome
Thymic hypoplasia

279.12 **Wiskott-Aldrich syndrome**

279.13 **Nezelof's syndrome**
Cellular immunodeficiency with abnormal immunoglobulin deficiency

279.19 **Other**
> Excludes: *ataxia-telangiectasia (334.8)*

Add 4th or 5th digit | Nonspecific code | Unspecified code | Manifestation code

279.2 Combined immunity deficiency
Agammaglobulinemia:
  autosomal recessive
  Swiss-type
  x-linked recessive
Severe combined immunodeficiency [SCID]
Thymic:
  alymphoplasia
  aplasia or dysplasia with immunodeficiency

Excludes: thymic hypoplasia (279.11)

279.3 Unspecified immunity deficiency

⑤ **279.4 Autoimmune disease, not elsewhere classified**

Excludes: transplant failure or rejection (996.80-996.89)

● **279.41 Autoimmune lymphoproliferative syndrome**
  ALPS

● **279.49 Autoimmune disease, not elsewhere classified**
  Autoimmune disease NOS

⑤ **279.5 Graft-versus-host disease**
Code first underlying cause, such as:
  complication of blood transfusion (999.89)
  complication of transplanted organ (996.80-996.89)
Use additional code to identify associated manifestations, such as:
  desquamative dermatitis (695.89)
  diarrhea (787.91)
  elevated bilirubin (782.4)
  hair loss (704.09)

279.50 Graft-versus-host disease, unspecified

279.51 Acute graft-versus-host disease

279.52 Chronic graft-versus-host disease

279.53 Acute on chronic graft-versus-host disease

279.8 Other specified disorders involving the immune mechanism
Single complement [C_1-C_9] deficiency or dysfunction

279.9 Unspecified disorder of immune mechanism

● Code new
  to this edition
▲ Revision of
  existing code
④ ⑤ Fourth or fifth
  digit required

4. DISEASES OF THE BLOOD AND BLOOD-FORMING ORGANS (280-289)

Excludes: anemia complicating pregnancy or the puerperium (648.2)

280 Iron deficiency anemias
Includes: anemia:
  asiderotic
  hypochromic-microcytic
  sideropenic

Excludes: familial microcytic anemia (282.49)

280.0 Secondary to blood loss (chronic)
  Normocytic anemia due to blood loss

Excludes: acute posthemorrhagic anemia (285.1)

280.1 Secondary to inadequate dietary iron intake

280.8 Other specified iron deficiency anemias
  Paterson-Kelly syndrome
  Plummer-Vinson syndrome
  Sideropenic dysphagia

280.9 Iron deficiency anemia, unspecified
  Anemia:
    achlorhydric
    chlorotic
    idiopathic hypochromic
    iron [Fe] deficiency NOS

281 Other deficiency anemias

281.0 Pernicious anemia
  Anemia: Congenital intrinsic factor [Castle's] deficiency
    Addison's
    Biermer's
    congenital pernicious

Excludes: combined system disease without mention of anemia (266.2)
  subacute degeneration of spinal cord without mention of anemia (266.2)

281.1 Other vitamin B_{12} deficiency anemia
  Anemia:
    vegan's
    vitamin B_{12} deficiency (dietary)
    due to selective vitamin B_{12} malabsorption with proteinuria
  Syndrome:
    Imerslund's
    Imerslund-Gräsbeck

Excludes: combined system disease without mention of anemia (266.2)
  subacute degeneration of spinal cord without mention of anemia (266.2)

281.2 Folate-deficiency anemia
  Congenital folate malabsorption
  Folate or folic acid deficiency anemia:
    NOS
    dietary
    drug-induced
  Goat's milk anemia
  Nutritional megaloblastic anemia (of infancy)
Use additional E code, if desired, to identify drug

281.3 Other specified megaloblastic anemias not elsewhere classified
  Combined B_{12} and folate-deficiency anemia
  Refractory megaloblastic anemia

281.4 Protein-deficiency anemia
  Amino-acid-deficiency anemia

281.8 Anemia associated with other specified nutritional deficiency
  Scorbutic anemia

281.9 Unspecified deficiency anemia
  Anemia: Anemia:
    dimorphic   nutritional NOS
    macrocytic   simple chronic
    megaloblastic NOS

TABULAR LIST

282 Hereditary hemolytic anemias

282.0 Hereditary spherocytosis
Acholuric (familial) jaundice
Congenital hemolytic anemia (spherocytic)
Congenital spherocytosis
Minkowski-Chauffard syndrome
Spherocytosis (familial)
Excludes: hemolytic anemia of newborn (773.0-773.5)

282.1 Hereditary elliptocytosis
Elliptocytosis (congenital)
Ovalocytosis (congenital) (hereditary)

282.2 Anemias due to disorders of glutathione metabolism
Anemia:
6-phosphogluconic dehydrogenase deficiency
enzyme deficiency, drug-induced
erythrocytic glutathione deficiency
glucose-6-phosphate dehydrogenase [G-6-PD] deficiency
glutathione-reductase deficiency
hemolytic nonspherocytic (hereditary), type I
Disorder of pentose phosphate pathway
Favism

282.3 Other hemolytic anemias due to enzyme deficiency
Anemia:
hemolytic nonspherocytic (hereditary), type II
hexokinase deficiency
pyruvate kinase [PK] deficiency
triosephosphate isomerase deficiency

⑤ **282.4 Thalassemias**
Excludes: sickle-cell:
disease (282.60-282.69)
trait (282.5)

282.41 Sickle-cell thalassemia without crisis
Sickle-cell thalassemia NOS
Thalassemia Hb-S disease without crisis

282.42 Sickle-cell thalassemia with crisis
Sickle-cell thalassemia with vaso-occlusive pain
Thalassemia Hb-S disease with crisis
Use additional code for types of crisis, such as:
acute chest syndrome (517.3)
splenic sequestration (289.52)

282.49 Other thalassemia
Cooley's anemia
Hb-Bart's disease
Hereditary leptocytosis
Mediterranean anemia (with other hemoglobinopathy)
Microdrepanocytosis
Thalassemia (alpha) (beta) (intermedia) (major) (minima) (minor) (mixed) (trait) (with other hemoglobinopathy)
Thalassemia NOS

282.5 Sickle-cell trait
Hb-AS genotype   Heterozygous:
Hemoglobin S [Hb-S] trait   hemoglobin S
Hb-S
Excludes: that with other hemoglobinopathy (282.60-282.69)
that with thalassemia (282.49)

⑤ **282.6 Sickle-cell disease**
Sickle-cell anemia
Excludes: sickle-cell thalassemia (282.41-282.42)
sickle-cell trait (282.5)

282.60 Sickle-cell disease, unspecified
Sickle-cell anemia NOS

282.61 Hb-SS disease without crisis

● Code new to this edition   ▲ Revision of existing code   ④ ⑤ Fourth or fifth digit required

282.62   Hb-SS disease with crisis
Hb-SS disease with vaso-occlusive pain
Sickle-cell crisis NOS

Use additional code for type of crisis, such as:
acute chest syndrome (517.3)
splenic sequestration (289.52)

282.63   Sickle-cell/Hb-C disease without crisis
Hb-S/Hb-C disease without crisis

282.64   Sickle-cell/Hb-C disease with crisis
Hb-S/Hb-C disease with crisis
Sickle-cell/Hb-C disease with vaso-occlusive pain

Use additional code for type of crisis, such as:
acute chest syndrome (517.3)
splenic sequestration (289.52)

282.68   Other sickle-cell disease without crisis
Hb-S/Hb-D disease without crisis
Hb-S/Hb-E disease without crisis
Sickle-cell/Hb-D disease without crisis
Sickle-cell/Hb-E disease without crisis

282.69   Other sickle-cell disease with crisis
Hb-S/Hb-D disease with crisis
Hb-S/Hb-E disease with crisis
Other sickle-cell disease with vaso-occlusive pain
Sickle-cell/Hb-D disease with crisis
Sickle-cell/Hb-E disease with crisis

Use additional code for type of crisis, such as:
acute chest syndrome (517.3)
splenic sequestration (289.52)

282.7   Other hemoglobinopathies
Abnormal hemoglobin NOS
Congenital Heinz-body anemia
Disease:
hemoglobin C [Hb-C]
hemoglobin D [Hb-D]
hemoglobin E [Hb-E]
hemoglobin Zurich [Hb-Zurich]
Hemoglobinopathy NOS
Hereditary persistence of fetal hemoglobin [HPFH]
Unstable hemoglobin hemolytic disease

Excludes: *familial polycythemia (289.6)*
hemoglobin M [Hb-M] disease (289.7)
high-oxygen-affinity hemoglobin (289.0)

282.8   Other specified hereditary hemolytic anemias
Stomatocytosis

282.9   Hereditary hemolytic anemia, unspecified
Hereditary hemolytic anemia NOS

283   Acquired hemolytic anemias

283.0   Autoimmune hemolytic anemias
Autoimmune hemolytic anemias (cold type) (warm type)
Chronic cold hemagglutinin disease
Cold agglutinin disease or hemoglobinuria
Hemolytic anemia:
cold type (secondary) (symptomatic)
drug-induced
warm type (secondary) (symptomatic)

Use additional E code, if desired, to identify cause, if drug-induced

Excludes: *Evans' syndrome (287.32)*
hemolytic disease of newborn (773.0-773.5)

⑤ **283.1   Non-autoimmune hemolytic anemias**

283.10   Non-autoimmune hemolytic anemia, unspecified

283.11   Hemolytic-uremic syndrome

Add 4th or   Nonspecific   Unspecified   Manifestation
5th digit   code   code   code

283.19 **Other non-autoimmune hemolytic anemias**
Hemolytic anemia:
mechanical
microangiopathic
toxic

Use additional E code, if desired, to identify cause

283.2 **Hemoglobinuria due to hemolysis from external causes**
Acute intravascular hemolysis
Hemoglobinuria:
from exertion
march
paroxysmal (cold) (nocturnal)
due to other hemolysis
Marchiafava-Micheli syndrome

Use additional E code, if desired, to identify cause

283.9 **Acquired hemolytic anemia, unspecified**
Acquired hemolytic anemia NOS
Chronic idiopathic hemolytic anemia

284 **Aplastic anemia and other bone marrow failure syndromes**

⑤ **284.0** **Constitutional aplastic anemia**

    284.01 **Constitutional red blood cell aplasia**
Aplasia, (pure) red cell:
congenital
of infants
primary
Blackfan-Diamond syndrome
Familial hypoplastic anemia

    284.09 **Other constitutional aplastic anemia**
Fanconi's anemia
Pancytopenia with malformations

284.1 **Pancytopenia**
Excludes: *pancytopenia (due to) (with):*
aplastic anemia NOS (284.9)
bone marrow infiltration (284.2)
constitutional red blood cell aplasia (284.01)
drug induced (284.89)
hairy cell leukemia (202.4)
human immunodeficiency virus disease (042)
leukoerythroblastic anemia (284.2)
malformations (284.09)
myelodysplastic syndromes (238.72-238.75)
myeloproliferative disease (238.79)
other constitutional aplastic anemia (284.09)

284.2 **Myelophthisis**
Leukoerythroblastic anemia
Myelophthisic anemia

Code first the underlying disorder, such as:
malignant neoplasm of breast (174.0-174.9, 175.0-175.9)
tuberculosis (015.0-015.9)

Excludes: *idiopathic myelofibrosis (238.76)*
myelofibrosis NOS (289.83)
myelofibrosis with myeloid metaplasia (238.76)
primary myelofibrosis (238.76)
secondary myelofibrosis (289.83)

⑤ **284.8** **Other specified aplastic anemias**

    284.81 **Red cell aplasia (acquired) (adult) (with thymoma)**
Red cell aplasia NOS

    284.89 **Other specified aplastic anemias**
Aplastic anemia (due to):
chronic systemic disease
drugs
infection
radiation
toxic (paralytic)

Use additional E code to identify cause

● Code new
to this edition

▲ Revision of
existing code

④ ⑤ Fourth or fifth
digit required

284.9 Aplastic anemia, unspecified
Anemia:
  aplastic (idiopathic) NOS
  aregenerative
  hypoplastic NOS

Anemia:
  nonregenerative
Medullary hypoplasia

Excludes: refractory anemia (238.72)

285 Other and unspecified anemias

285.0 Sideroblastic anemia
Anemia:
  hypochromic with iron loading
  sideroachrestic
  sideroblastic:
    acquired
    congenital
    hereditary
    primary
    secondary (drug-induced) (due to disease)
    sex-linked hypochromic
    vitamin B_6-responsive
Pyridoxine-responsive (hypochromic) anemia
Use additional E code, if desired, to identify cause, if drug induced

Excludes: refractory sideroblastic anemia (238.72)

285.1 Acute posthemorrhagic anemia
Anemia due to acute blood loss

Excludes: anemia due to chronic blood loss (280.0)
    blood loss anemia NOS (280.0)

⑤ 285.2 Anemia of chronic disease
Anemia in (due to) (with) chronic illness

  285.21 Anemia in chronic kidney disease
  Anemia in end stage renal disease
  Erythropoietin-resistant anemia (EPO resistant anemia)

  285.22 Anemia in neoplastic disease

Excludes: anemia due to antineoplastic chemotherapy (285.3)

  285.29 Anemia of other chronic disease
  Anemia in other chronic illness

● 285.3 Antineoplastic chemotherapy induced anemia
Anemia due to antineoplastic chemotherapy

Excludes: anemia due to drug NEC – code to type of anemia
    anemia in neoplastic disease (285.22)
    aplastic anemia due to antineoplastic chemotherapy (284.89)

285.8 Other specified anemias
Anemia:
  dyserythropoietic (congenital)
  dyshematopoietic (congenital)
  von Jaksch's
Infantile pseudoleukemia

285.9 Anemia, unspecified
Anemia:
  NOS
  essential
  normocytic, not due to blood
    loss

Anemia:
  profound
  progressive
  secondary
Oligocythemia

Excludes: anemia (due to):
  blood loss:
    acute (285.1)
    chronic or unspecified (280.0)
  iron deficiency (280.0-280.9)

Add 4th or 5th digit | Nonspecific code | Unspecified code | Manifestation code

286 Coagulation defects

286.0 Congenital factor VIII disorder
Antihemophilic globulin [AHG] deficiency
Factor VIII (functional) deficiency
Hemophilia:
NOS
A
classical
familial
hereditary
Subhemophilia

Excludes: factor VIII deficiency with vascular defect (286.4)

286.1 Congenital factor IX disorder
Christmas disease
Deficiency:
factor IX (functional)
plasma thromboplastin component [PTC]
Hemophilia B

286.2 Congenital factor XI deficiency
Hemophilia C
Plasma thromboplastin antecedent [PTA] deficiency
Rosenthal's disease

286.3 Congenital deficiency of other clotting factors
Congenital afibrinogenemia
Deficiency:
AC globulin factor:
I [fibrinogen]
II [prothrombin]
V [labile]
VII [stable]
X [Stuart-Prower]
XII [Hageman]
XIII [fibrin stabilizing]
Deficiency:
Laki-Lorand factor
proaccelerin
Disease:
Owren's
Stuart-Prower
Dysfibrinogenemia (congenital)
Dysprothrombinemia (constitutional)
Hypoproconvertinemia
Hypoprothrombinemia (hereditary)
Parahemophilia

286.4 von Willebrand's disease
Angiohemophilia (A) (B)
Constitutional thrombopathy
Factor VIII deficiency with vascular defect
Pseudohemophilia type B
Vascular hemophilia
von Willebrand's (-Jürgens') disease

Excludes: factor VIII deficiency:
NOS (286.0)
with functional defect (286.0)
hereditary capillary fragility (287.8)

286.5 Hemorrhagic disorder due to intrinsic circulating anticoagulants
Antithrombinemia
Antithromboplastinemia
Antithromboplastinogenemia
Hyperheparinemia
Increase in:
anti-VIIIa
anti-IXa
Increase in:
anti-Xa
anti-XIa
antithrombin
Secondary hemophilia
Systemic lupus erythematosus [SLE] inhibitor

286.6 Defibrination syndrome
Afibrinogenemia, acquired
Consumption coagulopathy
Diffuse or disseminated intravascular coagulation [DIC syndrome]
Fibrinolytic hemorrhage, acquired
Hemorrhagic fibrinogenolysis
Pathologic fibrinolysis
Purpura:
fibrinolytic
fulminans

Excludes: that complicating:
abortion (634-638 with .1, 639.1)
pregnancy or the puerperium (641.3, 666.3)
disseminated intravascular coagulation in newborn (776.2)

● Code new   ▲ Revision of   ④ ⑤ Fourth or fifth
to this edition   existing code   digit required

286.7 Acquired coagulation factor deficiency
Deficiency of coagulation factor due to:
liver disease
vitamin K deficiency
Hypoprothrombinemia, acquired

Excludes: vitamin K deficiency of newborn (776.0)

Use additional E-code, if desired, to identify cause, if drug induced

286.9 Other and unspecified coagulation defects
Defective coagulation NOS
Deficiency, coagulation factor NOS
Delay, coagulation
Disorder:
coagulation
hemostasis

Excludes: abnormal coagulation profile (790.92)
hemorrhagic disease of newborn (776.0)
that complicating:
abortion (634-638 with .1, 639.1)
pregnancy or the puerperium (641.3, 666.3)

287 Purpura and other hemorrhagic conditions

Excludes: hemorrhagic thrombocythemia (238.79)
purpura fulminans (286.6)

287.0 Allergic purpura
Peliosis rheumatica
Purpura:
anaphylactoid
autoimmune
Henoch's
Purpura:
nonthrombocytopenic:
hemorrhagic
idiopathic
rheumatica
Schönlein-Henoch
vascular
Vasculitis, allergic

Excludes: hemorrhagic purpura (287.39)
purpura annularis telangiectodes (709.1)

287.1 Qualitative platelet defects
Thrombasthenia (hemorrhagic) (hereditary)
Thrombocytasthenia
Thrombocytopathy (dystrophic)
Thrombopathy (Bernard-Soulier)

Excludes: von Willebrand's disease (286.4)

287.2 Other nonthrombocytopenic purpuras
Purpura:
NOS
senile
simplex

⑤ **287.3 Primary thrombocytopenia**

287.30 Primary thrombocytopenia, unspecified
Megakaryocytic hypoplasia

287.31 Immune thrombocytopenic purpura
Idiopathic thrombocytopenic purpura
Tidal platelet dysgenesis

287.32 Evans' syndrome

287.33 Congenital and hereditary thrombocytopenic purpura
Congenital and hereditary thrombocytopenia
Thrombocytopenia with absent radii (TAR) syndrome

Excludes: Wiskott-Aldrich syndrome (279.12)

287.39 Other primary thrombocytopenia

Add 4th or 5th digit   Nonspecific code   Unspecified code   Manifestation code

287.4 Secondary thrombocytopenia
Posttransfusion purpura
Thrombocytopenia (due to):
 dilutional
 drugs
 extracorporeal circulation of blood
 massive blood transfusion
 platelet alloimmunization

Use additional E code, if desired, to identify cause

Excludes: *heparin-induced thrombocytopenia (HIT) (289.84)*
 transient thrombocytopenia of newborn (776.1)

287.5 Thrombocytopenia, unspecified

287.8 Other specified hemorrhagic conditions
Capillary fragility (hereditary)
Vascular pseudohemophilia

287.9 Unspecified hemorrhagic conditions
Hemorrhagic diathesis (familial)

288 Diseases of white blood cells

Excludes: *leukemia (204.0-208.9)*

⑤ **288.0 Neutropenia**
Decreased Absolute Neutrophil Count (ANC)

Use additional code for any associated:
 fever (780.61)
 mucositis (478.11, 528.00-528.09, 538, 616.81)

Excludes: *neutropenic splenomegaly (289.53)*
 transitory neonatal neutropenia (776.7)

 288.00 Neutropenia, unspecified

 288.01 Congenital neutropenia
 Congenital agranulocytosis
 Infantile genetic agranulocytosis
 Kostmann's syndrome

 288.02 Cyclic neutropenia
 Cyclic hematopoiesis
 Periodic neutropenia

 288.03 Drug induced neutropenia
 Use additional E code to identify drug

 288.04 Neutropenia due to infection

 288.09 Other neutropenia
 Agranulocytosis
 Neutropenia:
  immune
  toxic

288.1 Functional disorders of polymorphonuclear neutrophils
Chronic (childhood) granulomatous disease
Congenital dysphagocytosis
Job's syndrome
Lipochrome histiocytosis (familial)
Progressive septic granulomatosis

288.2 Genetic anomalies of leukocytes
Anomaly (granulation) (granulocyte) or syndrome:
 Alder's (-Reilly)
 Chédiak-Steinbrinck (-Higashi)
 Jordan's
 May-Hegglin
 Pelger-Huet
Hereditary:
 hypersegmentation
 hyposegmentation
 leukomelanopathy

● Code new
  to this edition

▲ Revision of
  existing code

④ ⑤ Fourth or fifth
  digit required

288.3 Eosinophilia
Eosinophilia
   allergic
   hereditary
   idiopathic
   secondary
Eosinophilic leukocytosis

Excludes: *Löffler's syndrome (518.3)*
          pulmonary eosinophilia (518.3)

288.4 Hemophagocytic syndromes
Familial hemophagocytic lymphohistiocytosis
Familial hemophagocytic reticulosis
Hemophagocytic syndrome, infection-associated
Histiocytic syndromes
Macrophage activation syndrome

⑤ **288.5 Decreased white blood cell count**

Excludes: *neutropenia (288.01-288.09)*

   288.50   Leukocytopenia, unspecified
   Decreased leukocytes, unspecified
   Decreased white blood cell count, unspecified
   Leukopenia NOS

   288.51   Lymphocytopenia
   Decreased lymphocytes

   288.59   Other decreased white blood cell count
   Basophilic leukopenia
   Eosinophilic leukopenia
   Monocytopenia
   Plasmacytopenia

⑤ **288.6 Elevated white blood cell count**

Excludes: *eosinophilia (288.3)*

   288.60   Leukocytosis, unspecified
   Elevated leukocytes, unspecified
   Elevated white blood cell count, unspecified

   288.61   Lymphocytosis (symptomatic)
   Elevated lymphocytes

   288.62   Leukemoid reaction
   Basophilic leukemoid reaction
   Lymphocytic leukemoid reaction
   Monocytic leukemoid reaction
   Myelocytic leukemoid reaction
   Neutrophilic leukemoid reaction

   288.63   Monocytosis (symptomatic)

   Excludes: *infectious mononucleosis (075)*

   288.64   Plasmacytosis

   288.65   Basophilia

   288.66   Bandemia
   Bandemia without diagnosis of specific infection

   Excludes: *confirmed infection – code to infection leukemia (204.00-208.9)*

   288.69   Other elevated white blood cell count

288.8 Other specified disease of white blood cells

   Excludes: *decreased white blood cell counts (288.50-288.59)*
             elevated white blood cell counts (288.60-288.69)
             immunity disorders (279.0-279.9)

288.9 Unspecified disease of white blood cells

289 Other diseases of blood and blood-forming organs

■ Add 4th or   ■ Nonspecific   ■ Unspecified   ■ Manifestation
  5th digit   code   code   code

289.0 Polycythemia, secondary
High-oxygen-affinity
  hemoglobin
Polycythemia:
  acquired
  benign
  due to:
    fall in plasma volume
    high altitude

Polycythemia:
  emotional
  erythropoietin
  hypoxemic
  nephrogenous
  relative
  spurious
  stress

Excludes: polycythemia:
  neonatal (776.4)
  primary (238.4)
  vera (238.4)

289.1 Chronic lymphadenitis
Chronic:
  adenitis, any lymph node except mesenteric
  lymphadenitis, any lymph node except mesenteric

Excludes: *acute lymphadenitis (683)*
    mesenteric (289.2)
    enlarged glands NOS (785.6)

289.2 Nonspecific mesenteric lymphadenitis
Mesenteric lymphadenitis (acute) (chronic)

289.3 Lymphadenitis, unspecified, except mesenteric

289.4 Hypersplenism
"Big spleen" syndrome   Hypersplenia
Dyssplenism

Excludes: *primary splenic neutropenia (289.53)*

⑤ **289.5 Other diseases of spleen**

    289.50 Disease of spleen, unspecified

    289.51 Chronic congestive splenomegaly

    289.52 Splenic sequestration
    Code first sickle-cell disease in crisis (282.42, 282.62, 282.64, 282.69)

    289.53 Neutropenic splenomegaly

    289.59 Other
    Lien migrans
    Perisplenitis
    Splenic:
      abscess
      atrophy
      cyst

    Splenic:
      fibrosis
      infarction
      rupture, nontraumatic
    Splenitis
    Wandering spleen

    Excludes: *bilharzial splenic fibrosis (120.0-120.9)*
      hepatolienal fibrosis (571.5)
      splenomegaly NOS (789.2)

289.6 Familial polycythemia
Familial benign polycythemia
Familial erythrocytosis

289.7 Methemoglobinemia
Congenital NADH [DPNH]-methemoglobin-reductase deficiency
Hemoglobin M [Hb-M] disease
Methemoglobinemia:
  NOS
  acquired (with sulfhemoglobinemia)
  hereditary
  toxic
Stokvis' disease
Sulfhemoglobinemia
Use additional E code, if desired, to identify cause

⑤ **289.8 Other specified diseases of blood and blood-forming organs**

● Code new   ▲ Revision of   ④ ⑤ Fourth or fifth
  to this edition   existing code   digit required

289.81 Primary hypercoagulable state
Activated protein C resistance
Antithrombin III deficiency
Factor V Leiden mutation
Lupus anticoagulant
Protein C deficiency
Protein S deficiency
Prothrombin gene mutation

289.82 Secondary hypercoagulable state

Excludes: *heparin-induced thrombocytopenia (HIT) (289.84)*

289.83 Myelofibrosis
Myelofibrosis NOS
Secondary myelofibrosis

Code first the underlying disorder, such as:
malignant neoplasm of breast (174.0-174.9, 175.0-175.9)

Use additional code for associated therapy-related
myelodysplastic syndrome, if applicable (238.72, 238.73)

Use additional external cause code if due to anti-neoplastic chemotherapy (E933.1)

Excludes: *idiopathic myelofibrosis (238.76)*
leukoerythroblastic anemia (284.2)
myelofibrosis with myeloid metaplasia (238.76)
myelophthisic anemia (284.2)
myelophthisis (284.2)
primary myelofibrosis (238.76)

289.84 Heparin-induced thrombocytopenia (HIT)

289.89 Other specified diseases of blood and blood-forming organs
Hypergammaglobulinemia
Pseudocholinesterase deficiency

289.9 Unspecified diseases of blood and blood-forming organs
Blood dyscrasia NOS
Erythroid hyperplasia

Add 4th or
5th digit

Nonspecific
code

Unspecified
code

Manifestation
code

● Code new
  to this edition

▲ Revision of
  existing code

④ ⑤ Fourth or fifth
  digit required

5. MENTAL DISORDERS (290-319)

PSYCHOSES (290-299)

> *Excludes:* mental retardation (317-319)

ORGANIC PSYCHOTIC CONDITIONS (290-294)

Includes: psychotic organic brain syndrome

> *Excludes:* nonpsychotic syndromes of organic etiology (310.0-310.9)
>
> psychoses classifiable to 295-298 and without impairment of orientation, comprehension, calculation, learning capacity, and judgement, but associated with physical disease, injury, or condition affecting the brain [e.g., following childbirth] (295.0-298.8)

290 Dementias

Code first the associated neurological condition

> *Excludes:* dementia due to alcohol (291.0-291.2)
>
> dementia due to drugs (292.82)
>
> dementia not classified as senile, presenile, or arteriosclerotic (294.10-294.11)
>
> psychoses classifiable to 295-298 occurring in the senium without dementia or delirium (295.0-298.8)
>
> senility with mental changes of nonpsychotic severity (310.1)
>
> transient organic psychotic conditions (293.0-293.9)

290.0 Senile dementia, uncomplicated

Senile dementia:
NOS
simple type

> *Excludes:* mild memory disturbances, not amounting to dementia, associated with senile brain disease (310.8)
>
> senile dementia with:
> delirium or confusion (290.3)
> delusional [paranoid] features (290.20)
> depressive features (290.21)

⑤ **290.1 Presenile dementia**

Brain syndrome with presenile brain disease

> *Excludes:* arteriosclerotic dementia (290.40-290.43)
>
> dementia associated with other cerebral conditions (294.10-294.11)

290.10 Presenile dementia, uncomplicated

Presenile dementia:
NOS
simple type

290.11 Presenile dementia with delirium

Presenile dementia with acute confusional state

290.12 Presenile dementia with delusional features

Presenile dementia, paranoid type

290.13 Presenile dementia with depressive features

Presenile dementia, depressed type

⑤ **290.2 Senile dementia with delusional or depressive features**

> *Excludes:* senile dementia:
> NOS (290.0)
> with delirium and/or confusion (290.3)

290.20 Senile dementia with delusional features

Senile dementia, paranoid type
Senile psychosis NOS

290.21 Senile dementia with depressive features

290.3 Senile dementia with delirium

Senile dementia with acute confusional state

> *Excludes:* senile:
> dementia NOS (290.0)
> psychosis NOS (290.20)

⑤ **290.4 Vascular dementia**

Multi-infarct dementia or psychosis

Use additional code to identify cerebral atherosclerosis (437.0)

> *Excludes:* suspected cases with no clear evidence of arteriosclerosis (290.9)

| | Add 4th or 5th digit | | Nonspecific code | | Unspecified code | | Manifestation code |

290.40 Vascular dementia, uncomplicated
Arteriosclerotic dementia:
NOS
simple type

290.41 Vascular dementia with delirium
Arteriosclerotic dementia with acute confusional state

290.42 Vascular dementia with delusions
Arteriosclerotic dementia, paranoid type

290.43 Vascular dementia with depressed mood
Arteriosclerotic dementia, depressed type

290.8 Other specified senile psychotic conditions
Presbyophrenic psychosis

290.9 Unspecified senile psychotic condition

291 Alcohol-induced mental disorders

Excludes: alcoholism without psychosis (303.0-303.9)

291.0 Alcohol withdrawal delirium
Alcoholic delirium
Delirium tremens

Excludes: alcohol withdrawal (291.81)

291.1 Alcohol-induced persisting amnestic disorder
Alcoholic polyneuritic psychosis
Korsakoff's psychosis, alcoholic
Wernicke-Korsakoff syndrome (alcoholic)

291.2 Alcohol-induced persisting dementia
Alcoholic dementia NOS
Alcoholism associated with dementia NOS
Chronic alcoholic brain syndrome

291.3 Alcohol-induced psychotic disorder with hallucinations
Alcoholic:
hallucinosis (acute)
psychosis with hallucinosis

Excludes: alcohol withdrawal with delirium (291.0)
schizophrenia (295.0-295.9) and paranoid states (297.0-297.9) taking the form of chronic hallucinosis with clear consciousness in an alcoholic

291.4 Idiosyncratic alcohol intoxication
Pathologic:
alcohol intoxication
drunkenness

Excludes: acute alcohol intoxication (305.0)
in alcoholism (303.0)
simple drunkenness (305.0)

291.5 Alcohol-induced psychotic disorder with delusions
Alcoholic:
paranoia
psychosis, paranoid type

Excludes: nonalcoholic paranoid states (297.0-297.9)
schizophrenia, paranoid type (295.3)

⑤ **291.8 Other specified alcohol induced mental disorders**

291.81 Alcohol withdrawal
Alcohol:
withdrawal syndrome or symptoms
abstinence syndrome or symptoms

Excludes: alcohol withdrawal:
delirium (291.0)
hallucinosis (291.3)
delirium tremens (291.0)

291.82 Alcohol induced sleep disorders
Alcohol induced circadian rhythm sleep disorders
Alcohol induced hypersomnia
Alcohol induced insomnia
Alcohol induced parasomnia

● Code new
to this edition

▲ Revision of
existing code

④ ⑤ Fourth or fifth
digit required

291.89 **Other**
Alcohol induced anxiety disorder
Alcohol induced mood disorder
Alcohol induced sexual dysfunction

291.9 **Unspecified alcohol-induced mental disorders**
Alcohol-related disorder NOS
Alcoholic:
mania NOS
psychosis NOS
Alcoholism (chronic) with psychosis

292 **Drug induced mental disorders**
Includes: organic brain syndrome associated with consumption of drugs
Use additional code for any associated drug dependence (304.0-304.9)
Use additional E code, if desired, to identify drug

292.0 **Drug withdrawal**
Drug:
abstinence syndrome or symptoms
withdrawal syndrome or symptoms

⑤ **292.1** **Drug-induced psychotic disorders**

292.11 **Drug-induced psychotic disorder with delusions**
Paranoid state induced by drugs

292.12 **Drug-induced psychotic disorder with hallucinations**
Hallucinatory state induced by drugs

Excludes: *states following LSD or other hallucinogens, lasting only a few days or less ["bad trips"] (305.3)*

292.2 **Pathological drug intoxication**
Drug reaction:
NOS resulting in brief psychotic states
idiosyncratic resulting in brief psychotic states
pathologic resulting in brief psychotic states

Excludes: *expected brief psychotic reactions to hallucinogens ["bad trips"] (305.3)*
physiological side-effects of drugs (e.g., dystonias)

⑤ **292.8** **Other specified drug induced mental disorders**

292.81 **Drug induced delirium**

292.82 **Drug induced persisting dementia**

292.83 **Drug induced persisting amnestic disorder**

292.84 **Drug induced mood disorder**
Depressive state induced by drugs

292.85 **Drug induced sleep disorders**
Drug induced circadian rhythm sleep disorder
Drug induced hypersomnia
Drug induced insomnia
Drug induced parasomnia

292.89 **Other**
Drug induced anxiety disorder
Drug induced organic personality syndrome
Drug induced sexual dysfunction
Drug intoxication

292.9 **Unspecified drug-induced mental disorder**
Drug-related disorder NOS
Organic psychosis NOS due to or associated with drugs

293 **Transient mental disorders due to conditions classified elsewhere**
Includes: transient organic mental disorders not associated with alcohol or drugs
Code first the associated physical or neurological condition

Excludes: *confusional state or delirium superimposed on senile dementia (290.3)*
dementia due to:
alcohol (291.0-291.9)
arteriosclerosis (290.40-290.43)
drugs (292.82)
senility (290.0)

| | Add 4th or 5th digit | | Nonspecific code | | Unspecified code | | Manifestation code |

293.0 *Delirium due to conditions classified elsewhere*
Acute:
   confusional state
   infective psychosis
   organic reaction
   posttraumatic organic psychosis
   psycho-organic syndrome
Acute psychosis associated with endocrine, metabolic, or cerebrovascular disorder
Epileptic:
   confusional state
   twilight state

293.1 *Subacute delirium*
Subacute:
   confusional state
   infective psychosis
   organic reaction
   posttraumatic organic psychosis
   psycho-organic syndrome
   psychosis associated with endocrine or metabolic disorder

⑤ **293.8** *Other specified transient mental disorders due to conditions classified elsewhere*

  293.81 *Psychotic disorder with delusions in conditions classified elsewhere*
    Transient organic psychotic condition, paranoid type

  293.82 *Psychotic disorder with hallucinations in conditions classified elsewhere*
    Transient organic psychotic condition, hallucinatory type

  293.83 *Mood disorder in conditions classified elsewhere*
    Transient organic psychotic condition, depressive type

  293.84 *Anxiety disorder in conditions classified elsewhere*

  293.89 *Other*
    Catatonic disorder in conditions classified elsewhere

293.9 *Unspecified transient mental disorder in conditions classified elsewhere*
Organic psychosis:
   infective NOS
   posttraumatic NOS
   transient NOS
Psycho-organic syndrome

294 **Persistent mental disorders due to conditions classified elsewhere**
Includes: organic psychotic brain syndromes (chronic), not elsewhere classified

294.0 *Amnestic disorder in conditions classified elsewhere*
Code first underlying condition
Korsakoff's psychosis or syndrome (nonalcoholic)
Excludes: alcoholic:
    amnestic syndrome (291.1)
    Korsakoff's psychosis (291.1)

⑤ **294.1** *Dementia in conditions classified elsewhere*
Dementia of the Alzheimer's type
Code first any underlying physical condition, as:
dementia in:
   Alzheimer's disease (331.0)
   cerebral lipidoses (330.1)
   dementia with Lewy bodies (331.82)
   dementia with Parkinsonism (331.82)
   epilepsy (345.0-345.9)
   frontal dementia (331.19)
   frontotemporal dementia (331.19)
   general paresis [syphilis] (094.1)
   hepatolenticular degeneration (275.1)
   Huntington's chorea (333.4)
   Jakob-Creutzfeldt disease (046.11-046.19)
   multiple sclerosis (340)
   Pick's disease of the brain (331.11)
   polyarteritis nodosa (446.0)
   syphilis (094.1)
Excludes: dementia:
    arteriosclerotic (290.40-290.43)
    presenile (290.10-290.13)
    senile (290.0)
    epileptic psychosis NOS (294.8)

● Code new to this edition   ▲ Revision of existing code   ④ ⑤ Fourth or fifth digit required

294.10 *Dementia in conditions classified elsewhere without behavioral disturbance*
Dementia in conditions classified elsewhere NOS

294.11 *Dementia in conditions classified elsewhere with behavioral disturbance*
Aggressive behavior
Combative behavior
Violent behavior
Wandering off

294.8 *Other persistent mental disorders due to conditions classified elsewhere*
Amnestic disorder NOS
Dementia NOS
Epileptic psychosis NOS
Mixed paranoid and affective organic psychotic states
Use additional code for associated epilepsy (345.0-345.9)

Excludes: *mild memory disturbances, not amounting to dementia (310.8)*

294.9 *Unspecified persistent mental disorders due to conditions classified elsewhere*
Cognitive disorder NOS
Organic psychosis (chronic)

OTHER PSYCHOSES (295-299)

Use additional code to identify any associated physical disease, injury, or condition affecting the brain with psychoses classifiable to 295-298

⑤ **295** **Schizophrenic disorders**
Includes: schizophrenia of the types described in 295.0-295.9 occurring in children

Excludes: *childhood type schizophrenia (299.9)*
infantile autism (299.0)

The following fifth-digit subclassification is for use with category 295:

0 **unspecified**

1 **subchronic**

2 **chronic**

3 **subchronic with acute exacerbation**

4 **chronic with acute exacerbation**

5 **in remission**

⑤ **295.0** **Simple type**
[0-5]   Schizophrenia simplex

Excludes: *latent schizophrenia (295.5)*

⑤ **295.1** **Disorganized type**
[0-5]   Hebephrenia
Hebephrenic type schizophrenia

⑤ **295.2** **Catatonic type**
[0-5]   Catatonic (schizophrenia):   Schizophrenic:
agitation   catalepsy
excitation   catatonia
excited type   flexibilitas cerea
stupor
withdrawn type

⑤ **295.3** **Paranoid type**
[0-5]   Paraphrenic schizophrenia

Excludes: *involutional paranoid state (297.2)*
paranoia (297.1)
paraphrenia (297.2)

⑤ **295.4** **Schizophreniform disorder**
[0-5]   Oneirophrenia
Schizophreniform:
attack
psychosis, confusional type

Excludes: *acute forms of schizophrenia of:*
catatonic type (295.2)
hebephrenic type (295.1)
paranoid type (295.3)
simple type (295.0)
undifferentiated type (295.8)

| | Add 4th or 5th digit | | Nonspecific code | | Unspecified code | | Manifestation code |

⑤ **295.5 Latent schizophrenia**
[0-5]   Latent schizophrenic reaction
           Schizophrenia:
             borderline
             incipient
           Schizophrenia:
             prepsychotic
             prodromal
             pseudoneurotic
             pseudopsychopathic

           Excludes: schizoid personality (301.20-301.22)

⑤ **295.6 Residual type**
[0-5]   Chronic undifferentiated schizophrenia
           Restzustand (schizophrenic)
           Schizophrenic residual state

⑤ **295.7 Schizoaffective disorder**
[0-5]   Cyclic schizophrenia
           Mixed schizophrenic and affective psychosis
           Schizoaffective psychosis
           Schizophreniform psychosis, affective type

⑤ **295.8 Other specified types of schizophrenia**
[0-5]   Acute (undifferentiated) schizophrenia
           Atypical schizophrenia
           Cenesthopathic schizophrenia

           Excludes: infantile autism (299.0)

⑤ **295.9 Unspecified schizophrenia**
[0-5]   Schizophrenia: Schizophrenic reaction NOS
             NOS   Schizophreniform psychosis NOS
             mixed NOS
             undifferentiated NOS
             undifferentiated type

296 Episodic mood disorders
           Includes: episodic affective disorders

           Excludes: neurotic depression (300.4)
                     reactive depressive psychosis (298.0)
                     reactive excitation (298.1)

The following fifth-digit subclassification is for use with categories 296.0-296.6:

   0 unspecified

   1 mild

   2 moderate

   3 severe, without mention of psychotic behavior

   4 severe, specified as with psychotic behavior

   5 in partial or unspecified remission

   6 in full remission

⑤ **296.0 Bipolar I disorder, single manic episode**
[0-6]   Hypomania (mild) NOS, single episode or unspecified
           Hypomanic psychosis, single episode or unspecified
           Mania (monopolar) NOS, single episode or unspecified
           Manic-depressive psychosis or reaction:
             hypomanic, single episode or unspecified
             manic, single episode or unspecified

           Excludes: circular type, if there was a previous attack of depression (296.4)

⑤ **296.1 Manic disorder, recurrent episode**
[0-6]   Any condition classifiable to 296.0, stated to be recurrent

           Excludes: circular type, if there was a previous attack of depression (296.4)

● Code new   ▲ Revision of   ④ ⑤ Fourth or fifth
        to this edition   existing code   digit required

⑤ **296.2 Major depressive disorder, single episode**
[0-6]   Depressive psychosis, single episode or unspecified
Endogenous depression, single episode or unspecified
Involutional melancholia, single episode or unspecified
Manic-depressive psychosis or reaction, depressed type, single episode or unspecified
Monopolar depression, single episode or unspecified
Psychotic depression, single episode or unspecified

Excludes: *circular type, if previous attack was of manic type (296.5)*
depression NOS (311)
reactive depression (neurotic) (300.4)
psychotic (298.0)

⑤ **296.3 Major depressive disorder, recurrent episode**
[0-6]   Any condition classifiable to 296.2, stated to be recurrent

Excludes: *circular type, if previous attack was of manic type (296.5)*
depression NOS (311)
reactive depression (neurotic) (300.4)
psychotic (298.0)

⑤ **296.4 Bipolar I disorder, most recent episode (or current) manic**
[0-6]   Bipolar disorder, now manic
Manic-depressive psychosis, circular type but currently manic

Excludes: *brief compensatory or rebound mood swings (296.99)*

⑤ **296.5 Bipolar I disorder, most recent episode (or current) depressed**
[0-6]   Bipolar disorder, now depressed
Manic-depressive psychosis, circular type but currently depressed

Excludes: *brief compensatory or rebound mood swings (296.99)*

⑤ **296.6 Bipolar I disorder, most recent episode (or current) mixed**
[0-6]   Manic-depressive psychosis, circular type, mixed

296.7 Bipolar I disorder, most recent episode (or current) unspecified
Atypical bipolar affective disorder NOS
Manic-depressive psychosis, circular type, current condition not specified as either manic or depressive

⑤ **296.8 Other and unspecified bipolar disorders**

296.80 Bipolar disorder, unspecified
Bipolar disorder NOS
Manic-depressive:
reaction NOS
syndrome NOS

296.81 Atypical manic disorder

296.82 Atypical depressive disorder

296.89 Other
Bipolar II disorder
Manic-depressive psychosis, mixed type

⑤ **296.9 Other and unspecified episodic mood disorder**

Excludes: *psychogenic affective psychoses (298.0-298.8)*

296.90 Unspecified episodic mood disorder
Affective psychosis NOS
Melancholia NOS
Mood disorder NOS

296.99 Other specified episodic mood disorder
Mood swings:
brief compensatory
rebound

297 Delusional disorders
Includes: paranoid disorders

Excludes: *acute paranoid reaction (298.3)*
alcoholic jealousy or paranoid state (291.5)
paranoid schizophrenia (295.3)

297.0 Paranoid state, simple

| | Add 4th or 5th digit | | Nonspecific code | | Unspecified code | | Manifestation code |

297.1 Delusional disorder
Chronic paranoid psychosis
Sander's disease
Systematized delusions

Excludes: *paranoid personality disorder (301.0)*

297.2 Paraphrenia
Involutional paranoid state
Late paraphrenia
Paraphrenia (involutional)

297.3 Shared psychotic disorder
Folie à deux
Induced psychosis or paranoid disorder

297.8 Other specified paranoid states
Paranoia querulans
Sensitiver Beziehungswahn

Excludes: *acute paranoid reaction or state (298.3)*
senile paranoid state (290.20)

297.9 Unspecified paranoid state

Paranoid:	Paranoid:
disorder NOS	reaction NOS
psychosis	state NOS

298 Other nonorganic psychoses
Includes: psychotic conditions due to or provoked by:
emotional stress
environmental factors as major part of etiology

298.0 Depressive type psychosis
Psychogenic depressive psychosis
Psychotic reactive depression
Reactive depressive psychosis

Excludes: *manic-depressive psychosis, depressed type (296.2-296.3)*
neurotic depression (300.4)
reactive depression NOS (300.4)

298.1 Excitative type psychosis
Acute hysterical psychosis   Reactive excitation
Psychogenic excitation

Excludes: *manic-depressive psychosis, manic type (296.0-296.1)*

298.2 Reactive confusion
Psychogenic confusion
Psychogenic twilight state

Excludes: *acute confusional state (293.0)*

298.3 Acute paranoid reaction
Acute psychogenic paranoid psychosis
Bouffée délirante

Excludes: *paranoid states (297.0-297.9)*

298.4 Psychogenic paranoid psychosis
Protracted reactive paranoid psychosis

298.8 Other and unspecified reactive psychosis
Brief psychotic disorder
Brief reactive psychosis NOS
Hysterical psychosis
Psychogenic psychosis NOS
Psychogenic stupor

Excludes: *acute hysterical psychosis (298.1)*

298.9 Unspecified psychosis
Atypical psychosis
Psychosis NOS
Psychotic disorder NOS

● Code new
to this edition

▲ Revision of
existing code

④ ⑤ Fourth or fifth
digit required

⑤ **299** **Pervasive developmental disorders**

Excludes: *adult type psychoses occurring in childhood, as:*
affective disorders (296.0-296.9)
manic-depressive disorders (296.0-296.9)
schizophrenia (295.0-295.9)

The following fifth-digit subclassification is for use with category 299:

0 current or active state

1 residual state

⑤ **299.0 Autistic disorder**
[0-1] Childhood autism
Infantile psychosis
Kanner's syndrome

Excludes: *disintegrative psychosis (299.1)*
Heller's syndrome (299.1)
schizophrenic syndrome of childhood (299.9)

⑤ **299.1 Childhood disintegrative disorder**
[0-1] Heller's syndrome
Use additional code to identify any associated neurological disorder

Excludes: *infantile autism (299.0)*
schizophrenic syndrome of childhood (299.9)

⑤ **299.8** **Other specified pervasive developmental disorders**
[0-1] Asperger's disorder
Atypical childhood psychosis
Borderline psychosis of childhood

Excludes: *simple stereotypies without psychotic disturbance (307.3)*

⑤ **299.9 Unspecified pervasive developmental disorder**
[0-1] Child psychosis NOS
Pervasive developmental disorder NOS
Schizophrenia, childhood type NOS
Schizophrenic syndrome of childhood NOS

Excludes: *schizophrenia of adult type occurring in childhood (295.0-295.9)*

NEUROTIC DISORDERS, PERSONALITY DISORDERS, AND OTHER NONPSYCHOTIC MENTAL DISORDERS (300-316)

300 Anxiety, dissociative and somatoform disorders

⑤ **300.0 Anxiety states**

Excludes: *anxiety in:*
acute stress reaction (308.0)
transient adjustment reaction (309.24)
neurasthenia (300.5)
psychophysiological disorders (306.0-306.9)
separation anxiety (309.21)

300.00 **Anxiety state, unspecified**
Anxiety:
neurosis
reaction
state (neurotic)
Atypical anxiety disorder

300.01 **Panic disorder without agoraphobia**
Panic:
attack
state

Excludes: *panic disorder with agoraphobia (300.21)*

300.02 **Generalized anxiety disorder**

300.09 **Other**

⑤ **300.1 Dissociative, conversion and factitious disorders**

Excludes: *adjustment reaction (309.0-309.9)*
anorexia nervosa (307.1)
gross stress reaction (308.0-308.9)
hysterical personality (301.50-301.59)
psychophysiologic disorders (306.0-306.9)

Add 4th or 5th digit   Nonspecific code   Unspecified code   Manifestation code

300.10 Hysteria, unspecified

300.11 Conversion disorder
Astasia-abasia, hysterical
Conversion hysteria or reaction
Hysterical:
blindness
deafness
paralysis

300.12 Dissociative amnesia
Hysterical amnesia

300.13 Dissociative fugue
Hysterical fugue

300.14 Dissociative identity disorder

300.15 Dissociative disorder or reaction, unspecified

300.16 Factitious disorder with predominantly psychological signs and symptoms
Compensation neurosis
Ganser's syndrome, hysterical

300.19 Other and unspecified factitious illness
Factitious disorder (with combined psychological and physical signs and symptoms) (with predominantly physical signs and symptoms) NOS

Excludes: multiple operations or hospital addiction syndrome (301.51)

⑤ **300.2 Phobic disorders**

Excludes: anxiety state not associated with a specific situation or object (300.0-300.09)
obsessional phobias (300.3)

300.20 Phobia, unspecified
Anxiety-hysteria NOS
Phobia NOS

300.21 Agoraphobia with panic disorder
Fear of:
open spaces with panic attacks
streets with panic attacks
travel with panic attacks
Panic disorder with agoraphobia

Excludes: agoraphobia without panic disorder (300.22)
panic disorder without agoraphobia (300.01)

300.22 Agoraphobia without mention of panic attacks
Any condition classifiable to 300.21 without mention of panic attacks

300.23 Social phobia
Fear of:
eating in public
public speaking
washing in public

300.29 Other isolated or specific phobias
Acrophobia   Claustrophobia
Animal phobias   Fear of crowds

300.3 Obsessive-compulsive disorders
Anancastic neurosis   Obsessional phobia [any]
Compulsive neurosis

Excludes: obsessive-compulsive symptoms occurring in:
endogenous depression (296.2-296.3)
organic states (e.g., encephalitis)
schizophrenia (295.0-295.9)

300.4 Dysthymic disorder
Anxiety depression   Neurotic depressive state
Depression with anxiety   Reactive depression
Depressive reaction

Excludes: adjustment reaction with depressive symptoms (309.0-309.1)
depression NOS (311)
manic-depressive psychosis, depressed type (296.2-296.3)
reactive depressive psychosis (298.0)

● Code new   ▲ Revision of   ④ ⑤ Fourth or fifth
to this edition   existing code   digit required

300.5 Neurasthenia
> Fatigue neurosis
> Nervous debility
> Psychogenic:
>> asthenia
>> general fatigue

Use additional code to identify any associated physical disorder

> Excludes: *anxiety state (300.00-300.09)*
>> *neurotic depression (300.4)*
>> *psychophysiological disorders (306.0-306.9)*
>> *specific nonpsychotic mental disorders following organic brain damage (310.0-310.9)*

300.6 Depersonalization disorder
> Derealization (neurotic)
> Neurotic state with depersonalization episode

> Excludes: *depersonalization associated with:*
>> *anxiety (300.00-300.09)*
>> *depression (300.4)*
>> *manic-depressive disorder or psychosis (296.0-296.9)*
>> *schizophrenia (295.0-295.9)*

300.7 Hypochondriasis
> Body dysmorphic disorder

> Excludes: *hypochondriasis in:*
>> *hysteria (300.10-300.19)*
>> *manic-depressive psychosis, depressed type (296.2-296.3)*
>> *neurasthenia (300.5)*
>> *obsessional disorder (300.3)*
>> *schizophrenia (295.0-295.9)*

⑤ **300.8 Somatoform disorders**

> **300.81 Somatization disorder**
>> Briquet's disorder
>> Severe somatoform disorder

> **300.82 Undifferentiated somatoform disorder**
>> Atypical somatoform disorder
>> Somatoform disorder NOS

> **300.89 Other somatoform disorders**
>> Occupational neurosis, including writers' cramp
>> Psychasthenia
>> Psychasthenic neurosis

300.9 Unspecified nonpsychotic mental disorder
> Psychoneurosis NOS

301 Personality disorders
> Includes: character neurosis

Use additional code to identify any associated neurosis or psychosis, or physical condition

> Excludes: *nonpsychotic personality disorder associated with organic brain syndromes (310.0-310.9)*

301.0 Paranoid personality disorder
> Fanatic personality
> Paranoid personality (disorder)
> Paranoid traits

> Excludes: *acute paranoid reaction (298.3)*
>> *alcoholic paranoia (291.5)*
>> *paranoid schizophrenia (295.3)*
>> *paranoid states (297.0-297.9)*

⑤ **301.1 Affective personality disorder**

> Excludes: *affective psychotic disorders (296.0-296.9)*
>> *neurasthenia (300.5)*
>> *neurotic depression (300.4)*

> **301.10 Affective personality disorder, unspecified**

> **301.11 Chronic hypomanic personality disorder**
>> Chronic hypomanic disorder
>> Hypomanic personality

| | Add 4th or 5th digit | | Nonspecific code | | Unspecified code | | Manifestation code |

301.12 Chronic depressive personality disorder
Chronic depressive disorder
Depressive character or personality

301.13 Cyclothymic disorder
Cycloid personality
Cyclothymia
Cyclothymic personality

⑤ **301.2 Schizoid personality disorder**

Excludes: *schizophrenia (295.0-295.9)*

301.20 Schizoid personality disorder, unspecified

301.21 Introverted personality

301.22 Schizotypal personality disorder

301.3 Explosive personality disorder

Aggressive:	Emotional instability (excessive)
personality	Pathological emotionality
reaction	Quarrelsomeness
Aggressiveness	

Excludes: *dyssocial personality (301.7)*
hysterical neurosis (300.10-300.19)

301.4 Obsessive-compulsive personality disorder
Anancastic personality
Obsessional personality

Excludes: *obsessive-compulsive disorder (300.3)*
phobic state (300.20-300.29)

⑤ **301.5 Histrionic personality disorder**

Excludes: *hysterical neurosis (300.10-300.19)*

301.50 Histrionic personality disorder, unspecified
Hysterical personality NOS

301.51 Chronic factitious illness with physical symptoms
Hospital addiction syndrome
Multiple operations syndrome
Munchausen syndrome

301.59 Other histrionic personality disorder
Personality:
emotionally unstable
labile
psychoinfantile

301.6 Dependent personality disorder

Asthenic personality	Passive personality
Inadequate personality	

Excludes: *neurasthenia (300.5)*
passive-aggressive personality (301.84)

301.7 Antisocial personality disorder
Amoral personality
Asocial personality
Dyssocial personality
Personality disorder with predominantly sociopathic or asocial manifestation

Excludes: *disturbance of conduct without specifiable personality disorder (312.0-312.9)*
explosive personality (301.3)

⑤ **301.8 Other personality disorders**

301.81 Narcissistic personality disorder

301.82 Avoidant personality disorder

301.83 Borderline personality disorder

301.84 Passive-aggressive personality

301.89 Other

Personality:	Personality:
eccentric	masochistic
"haltlose" type	psychoneurotic
immature	

Excludes: *psychoinfantile personality (301.59)*

● Code new
to this edition

▲ Revision of
existing code

④ ⑤ Fourth or fifth
digit required

301.9 Unspecified personality disorder
Pathological personality Psychopathic:
NOS   constitutional state
Personality disorder NOS   personality (disorder)

302 Sexual and gender identity disorders

Excludes: *sexual disorder manifest in:*
  organic brain syndrome (290.0-294.9, 310.0-310.9)
  psychosis (295.0-298.9)

302.0 Ego-dystonic sexual orientation
Ego-dystonic lesbianism
Sexual orientation conflict disorder

Excludes: *homosexual pedophilia (302.2)*

302.1 Zoophilia
Bestiality

302.2 Pedophilia

302.3 Transvestic fetishism

Excludes: *trans-sexualism (302.5)*

302.4 Exhibitionism

⑤ **302.5 Trans-sexualism**
Sex reassignment surgery status

Excludes: *transvestism (302.3)*

302.50 With unspecified sexual history

302.51 With asexual history

302.52 With homosexual history

302.53 With heterosexual history

302.6 Gender identity disorder in children
Feminism in boys
Gender identity disorder NOS

Excludes: *gender identity disorder in adult (302.85)*
  trans-sexualism (302.50-302.53)
  transvestism (302.3)

⑤ **302.7 Psychosexual dysfunction**

Excludes: *impotence of organic origin (607.84)*
  normal transient symptoms from ruptured hymen
  transient or occasional failures of erection due to fatigue, anxiety, alcohol, or
  drugs

302.70 Psychosexual dysfunction, unspecified
Sexual dysfunction NOS

302.71 Hypoactive sexual desire disorder

Excludes: *decreased sexual desire NOS (799.81)*

302.72 With inhibited sexual excitement
Female sexual arousal disorder
Frigidity
Impotence
Male erectile disorder

302.73 Female orgasmic disorder

302.74 Male orgasmic disorder

302.75 Premature ejaculation

302.76 Dyspareunia, psychogenic

302.79 With other specified psychosexual dysfunctions
Sexual aversion disorder

⑤ **302.8 Other specified psychosexual disorders**

302.81 Fetishism

302.82 Voyeurism

302.83 Sexual masochism

302.84 Sexual sadism

| | Add 4th or 5th digit | | Nonspecific code | | Unspecified code | | Manifestation code |

302.85 Gender identity disorder in adolescents or adults
Use additional code to identify sex reassignment surgery status (302.5)

Excludes: *gender identity disorder NOS (302.6)*
gender identity disorder in children (302.6)

302.89 Other
Frotteurism
Nymphomania
Satyriasis

302.9 Unspecified psychosexual disorder
Paraphilia NOS
Pathologic sexuality NOS
Sexual deviation NOS
Sexual disorder NOS

5 303 Alcohol dependence syndrome
Use additional code to identify any associated condition, as:
alcoholic psychoses (291.0-291.9)
drug dependence (304.0-304.9)
physical complications of alcohol, such as:
cerebral degeneration (331.7)
cirrhosis of liver (571.2)
epilepsy (345.0-345.9)
gastritis (535.3)
hepatitis (571.1)
liver damage NOS (571.3)

Excludes: *drunkenness NOS (305.0)*

The following fifth-digit subclassification is for use with category 303:

0 unspecified

1 continuous

2 episodic

3 in remission

⑤ **303.0 Acute alcoholic intoxication**
[0-3]   Acute drunkenness in alcoholism

⑤ **303.9 Other and unspecified alcohol dependence**
[0-3]   Chronic alcoholism
Dipsomania

5 304 Drug dependence
Excludes: *nondependent abuse of drugs (305.1-305.9)*

The following fifth-digit subclassification is for use with category 304:

0 unspecified

1 continuous

2 episodic

3 in remission

⑤ **304.0 Opioid type dependence**
[0-3]   Heroin
Meperidine
Methadone
Morphine
Opium
Opium alkaloids and their derivatives
Synthetics with morphine-like effects

⑤ **304.1 Sedative, hypnotic or anxiolytic dependence**
[0-3]   Barbiturates
Nonbarbiturate sedatives and tranquilizers with a similar effect:
chlordiazepoxide
diazepam
glutethimide
meprobamate
methaqualone

● Code new   ▲ Revision of   ④ ⑤ Fourth or fifth
     to this edition   existing code   digit required

⑤ **304.2 Cocaine dependence**
[0-3]   Coca leaves and derivatives

⑤ **304.3 Cannabis dependence**
[0-3]   Hashish
          Hemp
          Marihuana

⑤ **304.4 Amphetamine and other psychostimulant dependence**
[0-3]   Methylphenidate
          Phenmetrazine

⑤ **304.5 Hallucinogen dependence**
[0-3]   Dimethyltryptamine [DMT]
          Lysergic acid diethylamide [LSD] and derivatives
          Mescaline
          Psilocybin

⑤ **304.6 Other specified drug dependence**
[0-3]   Absinthe addiction
          Glue sniffing
          Inhalant dependence
          Phencyclidine dependence

Excludes: tobacco dependence (305.1)

⑤ **304.7 Combinations of opioid type drug with any other**
[0-3]

⑤ **304.8 Combinations of drug dependence excluding opioid type drug**
[0-3]

⑤ **304.9 Unspecified drug dependence**
[0-3]   Drug addiction NOS
          Drug dependence NOS

305 Nondependent abuse of drugs
     Note: Includes cases where a person, for whom no other diagnosis is possible, has come under medical care because of the maladaptive effect of a drug on which he is not dependent and that he has taken on his own initiative to the detriment of his health or social functioning.

Excludes: alcohol dependence syndrome (303.0-303.9)
           drug dependence (304.0-304.9)
           drug withdrawal syndrome (292.0)
           poisoning by drugs or medicinal substances (960.0-979.9)

The following fifth-digit subclassification is for use with codes 305.0, 305.2-305.9:

   0 unspecified

   1 continuous

   2 episodic

   3 in remission

⑤ **305.0 Alcohol abuse**
[0-3]   Drunkenness NOS
          Excessive drinking of alcohol NOS
          "Hangover" (alcohol)
          Inebriety NOS

Excludes: acute alcohol intoxication in alcoholism (303.0)
           alcoholic psychoses (291.0-291.9)

305.1 Tobacco use disorder
          Tobacco dependence

Excludes: history of tobacco use (V15.82)
           smoking complicating pregnancy (649.0)
           tobacco use disorder complicating pregnancy (649.0)

⑤ **305.2 Cannabis abuse**
[0-3]

⑤ **305.3 Hallucinogen abuse**
[0-3]   Acute intoxication from hallucinogens ["bad trips"]
          LSD reaction

⑤ **305.4 Sedative, hypnotic or anxiolytic abuse**
[0-3]

⑤ **305.5 Opioid abuse**
[0-3]

297

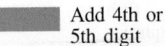 Add 4th or 5th digit   Nonspecific code   Unspecified code   Manifestation code

⑤ **305.6 Cocaine abuse**
[0-3]

⑤ **305.7 Amphetamine or related acting sympathomimetic abuse**
[0-3]

⑤ **305.8 Antidepressant type abuse**
[0-3]

⑤ **305.9 Other, mixed, or unspecified drug abuse**
[0-3] Caffeine intoxication
       Inhalant abuse
       "Laxative habit"
       Misuse of drugs NOS
       Nonprescribed use of drugs or patent medicinals
       Phencyclidine abuse

306 Physiological malfunction arising from mental factors
       Includes: psychogenic:
                  physical symptoms not involving tissue damage
                  physiological manifestation not involving tissue damage

       Excludes: *hysteria (300.11-300.19)*

                  physical symptoms secondary to a psychiatric disorder classified elsewhere
                  psychic factors associated with physical conditions involving tissue damage
                  *   classified elsewhere (316)*
                  specific nonpsychotic mental disorders following organic brain damage
                  *   (310.0-310.9)*

306.0 Musculoskeletal
       Psychogenic paralysis
       Psychogenic torticollis

       Excludes: *Gilles de la Tourette's syndrome (307.23)*

                  paralysis as hysterical or conversion reaction (300.11)
                  tics (307.20-307.22)

306.1 Respiratory
       Psychogenic: Psychogenic:
       air hunger   hyperventilation
       cough   yawning
       hiccough

       Excludes: *psychogenic asthma (316 and 493.9)*

306.2 Cardiovascular
       Cardiac neurosis
       Cardiovascular neurosis
       Neurocirculatory asthenia
       Psychogenic cardiovascular disorder

       Excludes: *psychogenic paroxysmal tachycardia (316 and 427.2)*

306.3 Skin
       Psychogenic pruritus

       Excludes: *psychogenic:*

                  alopecia (316 and 704.00)
                  dermatitis (316 and 692.9)
                  eczema (316 and 691.8 or 692.9)
                  urticaria (316 and 708.0-708.9)

306.4 Gastrointestinal
       Aerophagy   Diarrhea, psychogenic
       Cyclical vomiting,   Nervous gastritis
          psychogenic   Psychogenic dyspepsia

       Excludes: *cyclical vomiting NOS (536.2)*

                  associated with migraine (346.2)
                  globus hystericus (300.11)
                  mucous colitis (316 and 564.9)
                  psychogenic:
                  * cardiospasm (316 and 530.0)*
                  * duodenal ulcer (316 and 532.0-532.9)*
                  * gastric ulcer (316 and 531.0-531.9)*
                  * peptic ulcer NOS (316 and 533.0-533.9)*
                  * vomiting NOS (307.54)*

● Code new   ▲ Revision of   ④ ⑤ Fourth or fifth
  to this edition   existing code   digit required

⑤ **306.5 Genitourinary**

> Excludes: *enuresis, psychogenic (307.6)*
> *frigidity (302.72)*
> *impotence (302.72)*
> *psychogenic dyspareunia (302.76)*

306.50 Psychogenic genitourinary malfunction, unspecified

306.51 Psychogenic vaginismus
Functional vaginismus

306.52 Psychogenic dysmenorrhea

306.53 Psychogenic dysuria

306.59 Other

306.6 Endocrine

306.7 Organs of special sense

> Excludes: *hysterical blindness or deafness (300.11)*
> *psychophysical visual disturbances (368.16)*

306.8 Other specified psychophysiological malfunction
Bruxism
Teeth grinding

306.9 Unspecified psychophysiological malfunction
Psychophysiologic disorder NOS
Psychosomatic disorder NOS

307 Special symptoms or syndromes, not elsewhere classified
Note: This category is intended for use if the psychopathology is manifested by a single specific symptom or group of symptoms which is not part of an organic illness or other mental disorder classifiable elsewhere.

> Excludes: *those due to mental disorders classified elsewhere*
> *those of organic origin*

307.0 Stuttering

> Excludes: *dysphasia (784.59)*
> *lisping or lalling (307.9)*
> *retarded development of speech (315.31-315.39)*
> *stuttering (fluency disorder) due to late effect of cerebrovascular accident (438.14)*

307.1 Anorexia nervosa

> Excludes: *eating disturbance NOS (307.50)*
> *feeding problem (783.3)*
> *of nonorganic origin (307.59)*
> *loss of appetite (783.0)*
> *of nonorganic origin (307.59)*

⑤ **307.2 Tics**

> Excludes: *nail-biting or thumb-sucking (307.9)*
> *stereotypies occurring in isolation (307.3)*
> *tics of organic origin (333.3)*

307.20 Tic disorder, unspecified
Tic disorder NOS

307.21 Transient tic disorder

307.22 Chronic motor or vocal tic disorder

307.23 Tourette's disorder
Motor-verbal tic disorder

307.3 Stereotypic movement disorder
Body-rocking   Spasmus nutans
Head banging   Stereotypies NOS

> Excludes: *tics (307.20-307.23)*
> *of organic origin (333.3)*

⑤ **307.4 Specific disorders of sleep of nonorganic origin**

> Excludes: *narcolepsy (347.00-347.11)*
> *organic hypersomnia (327.10-327.19)*
> *organic insomnia (327.00-327.09)*
> *those of unspecified cause (780.50-780.59)*

307.40 Nonorganic sleep disorder, unspecified

| | Add 4th or 5th digit | | Nonspecific code | | Unspecified code | | Manifestation code |

307.41 Transient disorder of initiating or maintaining sleep
Adjustment insomnia
Hyposomnia associated with acute or intermittent emotional reactions or
    conflicts
Insomnia associated with acute or intermittent emotional reactions or conflicts
Sleeplessness associated with acute or intermittent emotional reactions or
    conflicts

307.42 Persistent disorder of initiating or maintaining sleep
Hyposomnia, insomnia, or sleeplessness associated with:
    anxiety
    conditioned arousal
    depression (major) (minor)
    psychosis
Idiopathic insomnia
Paradoxical insomnia
Primary insomnia
Psychophysiological insomnia

307.43 Transient disorder of initiating or maintaining wakefulness
Hypersomnia associated with acute or intermittent emotional reactions or
    conflicts

307.44 Persistent disorder of initiating or maintaining wakefulness
Hypersomnia associated with depression (major) (minor)
Insufficient sleep syndrome
Primary hypersomnia

> Excludes: *sleep deprivation (V69.4)*

307.45 Circadian rhythm sleep disorder of nonorganic origin

307.46 Sleep arousal disorder
Night terror disorder
Night terrors
Sleep terror disorder
Sleepwalking
Somnambulism

307.47 Other dysfunctions of sleep stages or arousal from sleep
Dyssomnia NOS
Nightmare disorder
Nightmares:
    NOS
    REM-sleep type
Parasomnia NOS
Sleep drunkenness

307.48 Repetitive intrusions of sleep
Repetitive intrusion of sleep with:
    atypical polysomnographic features
    environmental disturbances
    repeated REM-sleep interruptions

307.49 Other
"Short-sleeper"
Subjective insomnia complaint

⑤ **307.5 Other and unspecified disorders of eating**

> Excludes: *anorexia:*
>   *nervosa (307.1)*
>   *of unspecified cause (783.0)*
>   *overeating, of unspecified cause (783.6)*
>   *vomiting:*
>   *NOS (787.03)*
>   *cyclical (536.2)*
>   *associated with migraine (346.2)*
>   *psychogenic (306.4)*

307.50 Eating disorder, unspecified
Eating disorder NOS

307.51 Bulimia nervosa
Overeating of nonorganic origin

307.52 Pica
Perverted appetite of nonorganic origin

● ˙Code new
  to this edition
▲ Revision of
  existing code
④ ⑤ Fourth or fifth
     digit required

307.53 Rumination disorder
Regurgitation, of nonorganic origin, of food with reswallowing

Excludes: *obsessional rumination (300.3)*

307.54 Psychogenic vomiting

307.59 Other
Feeding disorder of infancy or early childhood of nonorganic origin
Infantile feeding disturbances of nonorganic origin
Loss of appetite of nonorganic origin

307.6 Enuresis
Enuresis (primary) (secondary) of nonorganic origin

Excludes: *enuresis of unspecified cause (788.3)*

307.7 Encopresis
Encopresis (continuous) (discontinuous) of nonorganic origin

Excludes: *encopresis of unspecified cause (787.6)*

⑤ **307.8 Pain disorders related to psychological factors**

307.80 Psychogenic pain, site unspecified

307.81 Tension headache

Excludes: *headache:*
NOS (784.0)
migraine (346.0-346.9)
syndromes (339.00-339.89)
tension type (339.10-339.12)

307.89 Other
Code first to type or site of pain

Excludes: *pain disorder exclusively attributed to psychological factors (307.80)*
psychogenic pain (307.80)

307.9 Other and unspecified special symptoms or syndromes, not elsewhere classified
Communication disorder NOS
Hair plucking
Lalling
Lisping
Masturbation
Nail-biting
Thumb-sucking

308 Acute reaction to stress
Includes: catastrophic stress
combat fatigue
gross stress reaction (acute)
transient disorders in response to exceptional physical or mental stress which
usually subside within hours or days

Excludes: *adjustment reaction or disorder (309.0-309.9)*
chronic stress reaction (309.1-309.9)

308.0 Predominant disturbance of emotions
Anxiety as acute reaction to exceptional [gross] stress
Emotional crisis as acute reaction to exceptional [gross] stress
Panic state as acute reaction to exceptional [gross] stress

308.1 Predominant disturbance of consciousness
Fugues as acute reaction to exceptional [gross] stress

308.2 Predominant psychomotor disturbance
Agitation states as acute reaction to exceptional [gross] stress
Stupor as acute reaction to exceptional [gross] stress

308.3 Other acute reactions to stress
Acute situational disturbance
Acute stress disorder

Excludes: *prolonged posttraumatic emotional disturbance (309.81)*

308.4 Mixed disorders as reaction to stress

308.9 Unspecified acute reaction to stress

	Add 4th or 5th digit		Nonspecific code		Unspecified code		Manifestation code

309 Adjustment reaction
Includes: adjustment disorders
reaction (adjustment) to chronic stress

Excludes: *acute reaction to major stress (308.0-308.9)*
neurotic disorders (300.0-300.9)

309.0 Adjustment disorder with depressed mood
Grief reaction

Excludes: *affective psychoses (296.0-296.9)*
neurotic depression (300.4)
prolonged depressive reaction (309.1)
psychogenic depressive psychosis (298.0)

309.1 Prolonged depressive reaction

Excludes: *affective psychoses (296.0-296.9)*
brief depressive reaction (309.0)
neurotic depression (300.4)
psychogenic depressive psychosis (298.0)

⑤ **309.2 With predominant disturbance of other emotions**

309.21 Separation anxiety disorder

309.22 Emancipation disorder of adolescence and early adult life

309.23 Specific academic or work inhibition

309.24 Adjustment disorder with anxiety

309.28 Adjustment disorder with mixed anxiety and depressed mood
Adjustment reaction with anxiety and depression

309.29 Other
Culture shock

309.3 Adjustment disorder with disturbance of conduct
Conduct disturbance as adjustment reaction
Destructiveness as adjustment reaction

Excludes: *destructiveness in child (312.9)*
disturbance of conduct NOS (312.9)
dyssocial behavior without manifest psychiatric disorder (V71.01-V71.02)
personality disorder with predominantly sociopathic or asocial manifestations (301.7)

309.4 Adjustment disorder with mixed disturbance of emotions and conduct

⑤ **309.8 Other specified adjustment reactions**

309.81 Posttraumatic stress disorder
Chronic posttraumatic stress disorder
Concentration camp syndrome
Posttraumatic stress disorder NOS
Post-Traumatic Stress Disorder (PTSD)

Excludes: *acute stress disorder (308.3)*
posttraumatic brain syndrome:
nonpsychotic (310.2)
psychotic (293.0-293.9)

309.82 Adjustment reaction with physical symptoms

309.83 Adjustment reaction with withdrawal
Elective mutism as adjustment reaction
Hospitalism (in children) NOS

309.89 Other

309.9 Unspecified adjustment reaction
Adaptation reaction NOS
Adjustment reaction NOS

310 Specific nonpsychotic mental disorders due to brain damage

Excludes: *neuroses, personality disorders, or other nonpsychotic conditions occurring in a form similar to that seen with functional disorders but in association with a physical condition (300.0-300.9, 301.0-301.9)*

310.0 Frontal lobe syndrome
Lobotomy syndrome
Postleucotomy syndrome [state]

Excludes: *postcontusion syndrome (310.2)*

● Code new to this edition   ▲ Revision of existing code   ④ ⑤ Fourth or fifth digit required

310.1 Personality change due to conditions classified elsewhere
Cognitive or personality change of other type, of nonpsychotic severity
Organic psychosyndrome of nonpsychotic severity
Presbyophrenia NOS
Senility with mental changes of nonpsychotic severity

Excludes: *mild cognitive impairment (331.83)*
postconcussion syndrome (310.2)
signs and symptoms involving emotional state (799.21-799.29)

310.2 Postconcussion syndrome
Postcontusion syndrome or encephalopathy
Posttraumatic brain syndrome, nonpsychotic
Status postcommotio cerebri

Use additional code to identify associated post-traumatic headache, if applicable (339.20-339.22)

Excludes: *frontal lobe syndrome (310.0)*
postencephalitic syndrome (310.8)
any organic psychotic conditions following head injury (293.0—294.0)

310.8 Other specified nonpsychotic mental disorders following organic brain damage
Mild memory disturbance
Postencephalitic syndrome
Other focal (partial) organic psychosyndromes

Excludes: *memory loss of unknown cause (780.93)*

310.9 Unspecified nonpsychotic mental disorder following organic brain damage

311 Depressive disorder, not elsewhere classified
Depressive disorder NOS
Depressive state NOS
Depression NOS

Excludes: *acute reaction to major stress with depressive symptoms (308.0)*
affective personality disorder (301.10-301.13)
affective psychoses (296.0-296.9)
brief depressive reaction (309.0)
depressive states associated with stressful events (309.0-309.1)
disturbance of emotions specific to childhood and adolescence, with misery and
*   unhappiness (313.1)*
mixed adjustment reaction with depressive symptoms (309.4)
neurotic depression (300.4)
prolonged depressive adjustment reaction (309.1)
psychogenic depressive psychosis (298.0)

312 Disturbance of conduct, not elsewhere classified

Excludes: *adjustment reaction with disturbance of conduct (309.3)*
drug dependence (304.0-304.9)
dyssocial behavior without manifest psychiatric disorder (V71.01-V71.02)
personality disorder with predominantly sociopathic or asocial manifestations
*   (301.7)*
sexual deviations (302.0-302.9)

The following fifth-digit subclassification is for use with categories 312.0-312.2:

0 unspecified

1 mild

2 moderate

3 severe

⑤ **312.0 Undersocialized conduct disorder, aggressive type**
[0-3] Aggressive outburst
Anger reaction
Unsocialized aggressive disorder

⑤ **312.1 Undersocialized conduct disorder, unaggressive type**
[0-3] Childhood truancy,   Solitary stealing
unsocialized   Tantrums

⑤ **312.2 Socialized conduct disorder**
[0-3] Childhood truancy, socialized
Group delinquency

Excludes: *gang activity without manifest psychiatric disorder (V71.01)*

⑤ **312.3 Disorders of impulse control, not elsewhere classified**

312.30 Impulse control disorder, unspecified

| | Add 4th or 5th digit | | Nonspecific code | | Unspecified code | | Manifestation code |

312.31 **Pathological gambling**

312.32 **Kleptomania**

312.33 **Pyromania**

312.34 **Intermittent explosive disorder**

312.35 **Isolated explosive disorder**

`312.39` **Other**
Trichotillomania

312.4 **Mixed disturbance of conduct and emotions**
Neurotic delinquency

`Excludes:` *compulsive conduct disorder (312.3)*

⑤ 312.8 **Other specified disturbances of conduct, not elsewhere classified**

312.81 **Conduct disorder, childhood onset type**

312.82 **Conduct disorder, adolescent onset type**

`312.89` **Other conduct disorder**
Conduct disorder of unspecified onset

312.9 **Unspecified disturbance of conduct**
Delinquency (juvenile)
Disruptive behavior disorder NOS

`313` **Disturbance of emotions specific to childhood and adolescence**

`Excludes:` *adjustment reaction (309.0-309.9)*
emotional disorder of neurotic type (300.0-300.9)
masturbation, nail-biting, thumb-sucking, and other isolated symptoms (307.0-307.9)

313.0 **Overanxious disorder**
Anxiety and fearfulness of childhood and adolescence
Overanxious disorder of childhood and adolescence

`Excludes:` *abnormal separation anxiety (309.21)*
anxiety states (300.00-300.09)
hospitalism in children (309.83)
phobic state (300.20-300.29)

313.1 **Misery and unhappiness disorder**

`Excludes:` *depressive neurosis (300.4)*

⑤ 313.2 **Sensitivity, shyness, and social withdrawal disorder**

`Excludes:` *infantile autism (299.0)*
schizoid personality (301.20-301.22)
schizophrenia (295.0-295.9)

313.21 **Shyness disorder of childhood**
Sensitivity reaction of childhood or adolescence

313.22 **Introverted disorder of childhood**
Social withdrawal of childhood and adolescence
Withdrawal reaction of childhood and adolescence

313.23 **Selective mutism**

`Excludes:` *elective mutism as adjustment reaction (309.83)*

313.3 **Relationship problems**
Sibling jealousy

`Excludes:` *relationship problems associated with aggression, destruction, or other forms of conduct disturbance (312.0-312.9)*

⑤ 313.8 **Other or mixed emotional disturbances of childhood or adolescence**

313.81 **Oppositional defiant disorder**

313.82 **Identity disorder**
Identity problem

313.83 **Academic underachievement disorder**

`313.89` **Other**
Reactive attachment disorder of infancy or early childhood

313.9 **Unspecified emotional disturbance of childhood or adolescence**
Mental disorder of infancy, childhood or adolescence NOS

`314` **Hyperkinetic syndrome of childhood**

`Excludes:` *hyperkinesis as symptom of underlying disorder—code the underlying disorder*

● Code new
to this edition

▲ Revision of
existing code

④ ⑤ Fourth or fifth
digit required

⑤ **314.0 Attention deficit disorder**
Adult
Child

314.00 Without mention of hyperactivity
Predominantly inattentive type

314.01 With hyperactivity
Combined type
Overactivity NOS
Predominantly hyperactive/impulsive type
Simple disturbance of attention with overactivity

314.1 Hyperkinesis with developmental delay
Developmental disorder of hyperkinesis

Use additional code to identify any associated neurological disorder

314.2 Hyperkinetic conduct disorder
Hyperkinetic conduct disorder without developmental delay

Excludes: hyperkinesis with significant delays in specific skills (314.1)

314.8 Other specified manifestations of hyperkinetic syndrome

314.9 Unspecified hyperkinetic syndrome
Hyperkinetic reaction of childhood or adolescence NOS
Hyperkinetic syndrome NOS

315 Specific delays in development

Excludes: that due to a neurological disorder (320.0-389.9)

⑤ **315.0 Specific reading disorder**

315.00 Reading disorder, unspecified

315.01 Alexia

315.02 Developmental dyslexia

315.09 Other
Specific spelling difficulty

315.1 Mathematics disorder
Dyscalculia

315.2 Other specific learning difficulties
Disorder of written expression

Excludes: specific arithmetical disorder (315.1)
specific reading disorder (315.00-315.09)

⑤ **315.3 Developmental speech or language disorder**

315.31 Expressive language disorder
Developmental aphasia
Word deafness

Excludes: acquired aphasia (784.3)
elective mutism (309.83, 313.0, 313.23)

315.32 Mixed receptive-expressive language disorder
Central auditory processing disorder

Excludes: acquired auditory processing disorder (388.45)

315.34 Speech and language developmental delay due to hearing loss

315.39 Other
Developmental articulation disorder
Dyslalia
Phonological disorder

Excludes: lisping and lalling (307.9)
stammering and stuttering (307.0)

315.4 Developmental coordination disorder
Clumsiness syndrome
Dyspraxia syndrome
Specific motor development disorder

315.5 Mixed development disorder

315.8 Other specified delays in development

315.9 Unspecified delay in development
Developmental disorder NOS
Learning disorder NOS

| | Add 4th or 5th digit | | Nonspecific code | | Unspecified code | | Manifestation code |

316 Psychic factors associated with diseases classified elsewhere
Psychologic factors in physical conditions classified elsewhere

Use additional code to identify the associated physical condition, as:
psychogenic:
asthma (493.9)
dermatitis (692.9)
duodenal ulcer (532.0-532.9)
eczema (691.8, 692.9)
gastric ulcer (531.0-531.9)
mucous colitis (564.9)
paroxysmal tachycardia (427.2)
ulcerative colitis (556)
urticaria (708.0-708.9)
psychosocial dwarfism (259.4)

> Excludes: *physical symptoms and physiological malfunctions, not involving tissue damage, of mental origin (306.0-306.9)*

MENTAL RETARDATION (317-319)

Use additional code(s) to identify any associated psychiatric or physical condition(s)

317 Mild mental retardation
High-grade defect   Mild mental subnormality
IQ 50-70

318 Other specified mental retardation

    318.0 Moderate mental retardation
IQ 35-49
Moderate mental subnormality

    318.1 Severe mental retardation
IQ 20-34
Severe mental subnormality

    318.2 Profound mental retardation
IQ under 20
Profound mental subnormality

319 Unspecified mental retardation
Mental deficiency NOS
Mental subnormality NOS

6. DISEASES OF THE NERVOUS SYSTEM AND SENSE ORGANS (320-389)

INFLAMMATORY DISEASES OF THE CENTRAL NERVOUS SYSTEM (320-326)

320 **Bacterial meningitis**
Includes: arachnoiditis, bacterial
leptomeningitis, bacterial
meningitis, bacterial
meningoencephalitis, bacterial
meningomyelitis, bacterial
pachymeningitis, bacterial

320.0 Hemophilus meningitis
Meningitis due to Hemophilus influenzae [H. influenzae]

320.1 Pneumococcal meningitis

320.2 Streptococcal meningitis

320.3 Staphylococcal meningitis

320.7 *Meningitis in other bacterial diseases classified elsewhere*
Code first underlying disease, as:
actinomycosis (039.8)
listeriosis (027.0)
typhoid fever (002.0)
whooping cough (033.0-033.9)

Excludes: *meningitis (in):*
epidemic (036.0)
gonococcal (098.82)
meningococcal (036.0)
salmonellosis (003.21)
syphilis:
NOS (094.2)
congenital (090.42)
meningovascular (094.2)
secondary (091.81)
tuberculous (013.0)

⑤ **320.8 Meningitis due to other specified bacteria**

320.81 **Anaerobic meningitis**
Bacteroides (fragilis)
Gram-negative anaerobes

320.82 **Meningitis due to Gram-negative bacteria, not elsewhere classified**
Aerobacter aerogenes
Escherichia coli [E. coli]
Friedlander bacillus
Klebsiella pneumoniae
Proteus morganii
Pseudomonas

Excludes: *Gram-negative anaerobes (320.81)*

320.89 **Meningitis due to other specified bacteria**
Bacillus pyocyaneus

320.9 Meningitis due to unspecified bacterium

Meningitis:	Meningitis:
bacterial NOS	pyogenic NOS
purulent NOS	suppurative NOS

321 **Meningitis due to other organisms**
Includes: arachnoiditis due to organisms other than bacteria
leptomeningitis due to organisms other than bacteria
meningitis due to organisms other than bacteria
pachymeningitis due to organisms other than bacteria

321.0 *Cryptococcal meningitis*
Code first underlying disease (117.5)

321.1 *Meningitis in other fungal diseases*
Code first underlying disease (110.0-118)

Excludes: *meningitis in:*
candidiasis (112.83)
coccidioidomycosis (114.2)
histoplasmosis (115.01, 115.11, 115.91)

	Add 4th or 5th digit		Nonspecific code		Unspecified code		Manifestation code

321.2 Meningitis due to viruses not elsewhere classified
 Code first underlying disease, as:
  meningitis due to arbovirus (060.0-066.9)

 Excludes: *meningitis (due to):*
   abacterial (047.0-047.9)
   adenovirus (049.1)
   aseptic NOS (047.9)
   Coxsackie (virus) (047.0)
   ECHO virus (047.1)
   enterovirus (047.0-047.9)
   herpes simplex virus (054.72)
   herpes zoster virus (053.0)
   lymphocytic choriomeningitis virus (049.0)
   mumps (072.1)
   viral NOS (047.9)
   meningo-eruptive syndrome (047.1)

321.3 Meningitis due to trypanosomiasis
 Code first underlying disease (086.0-086.9)

321.4 Meningitis in sarcoidosis
 Code first underlying disease (135)

321.8 Meningitis due to other nonbacterial organisms classified elsewhere
 Code first underlying disease

 Excludes: *leptospiral meningitis (100.81)*

322 Meningitis of unspecified cause
 Includes: arachnoiditis with no organism specified as cause
   leptomeningitis with no organism specified as cause
   meningitis with no organism specified as cause
   pachymeningitis with no organism specified as cause

322.0 Nonpyogenic meningitis
 Meningitis with clear cerebrospinal fluid

322.1 Eosinophilic meningitis

322.2 Chronic meningitis

322.9 Meningitis, unspecified

323 Encephalitis, myelitis, and encephalomyelitis
 Includes: acute disseminated encephalomyelitis
   meningoencephalitis, except bacterial
   meningomyelitis, except bacterial
   myelitis:
    ascending
    transverse

 Excludes: *acute transverse myelitis NOS (341.20)*
   acute transverse myelitis in conditions classified elsewhere (341.21)
   bacterial:
    meningoencephalitis (320.0-320.9)
    meningomyelitis (320.0-320.9)
    idiopathic transverse myelitis (341.22)
   idiopathic transverse myelitis (341.22)

⑤ **323.0 Encephalitis, myelitis, and encephalomyelitis in viral diseases classified elsewhere**
 Code first underlying disease, as:
  cat-scratch disease (078.3)
  infectious mononucleosis (075)
  ornithosis (073.7)

 323.01 Encephalitis and encephalomyelitis in viral diseases classified elsewhere
 Excludes: *encephalitis (in):*
   arthropod-borne viral (062.0-064)
   herpes simplex (054.3)
   mumps (072.2)
   other viral diseases of central nervous system (049.8-049.9)
   poliomyelitis (045.0-045.9)
   rubella (056.01)
   slow virus infections of central nervous system (046.0-046.9)
   viral NOS (049.9)
   West Nile (066.41)

● Code new
 to this edition

▲ Revision of
 existing code

④ ⑤ Fourth or fifth
 digit required

323.02 *Myelitis in viral diseases classified elsewhere*

Excludes: *myelitis (in):*
> *herpes simplex (054.74)*
> *herpes zoster (053.14)*
> *poliomyelitis (045.0-045.9)*
> *rubella (056.01)*
> *other viral diseases of central nervous system (049.8-049.9)*

323.1 *Encephalitis, myelitis, and encephalomyelitis in rickettsial diseases classified elsewhere*
> *Code first underlying disease (080-083.9)*

323.2 *Encephalitis, myelitis, and encephalomyelitis in protozoal diseases classified elsewhere*
> *Code first underlying disease, as:*
> malaria (084.0-084.9)
> trypanosomiasis (086.0-086.9)

⑤ **323.4 *Other encephalitis, myelitis, and encephalomyelitis due to infection classified elsewhere***
> *Code first underlying disease*

323.41 *Other encephalitis and encephalomyelitis due to infection classified elsewhere*

Excludes: *encephalitis (in):*
> *meningococcal (036.1)*
> *syphilis:*
> > *NOS (094.81)*
> > *congenital (090.41)*
> *toxoplasmosis (130.0)*
> *tuberculosis (013.6)*
> *meningoencephalitis due to free-living ameba [Naegleria] (136.29)*

323.42 *Other myelitis due to infection classified elsewhere*

Excludes: *myelitis (in):*
> *syphilis (094.89)*
> *tuberculosis (013.6)*

⑤ **323.5 Encephalitis, myelitis, and encephalomyelitis following immunization procedures**
Use additional E code, if desired, to identify vaccine

323.51 Encephalitis and encephalomyelitis following immunization procedures
> Encephalitis postimmunization or postvaccinal
> Encephalomyelitis postimmunization or postvaccinal

323.52 Myelitis following immunization procedures
> Myelitis postimmunization or postvaccinal

⑤ **323.6 *Postinfectious encephalitis, myelitis, and encephalomyelitis***
> *Code first underlying disease*

323.61 *Infectious acute disseminated encephalomyelitis (ADEM)*
> Acute necrotizing hemorrhagic encephalopathy

Excludes: *noninfectious acute disseminated encephalomyelitis (ADEM) (323.81)*

323.62 *Other postinfectious encephalitis and encephalomyelitis*

Excludes: *encephalitis:*
> *postchickenpox (052.0)*
> *postmeasles (055.0)*

323.63 *Postinfectious myelitis*

Excludes: *postchickenpox myelitis (052.2)*
> *herpes simplex myelitis (054.74)*
> *herpes zoster myelitis (053.14)*

⑤ **323.7 *Toxic encephalitis, myelitis, and encephalomyelitis***
> *Code first underlying cause, as:*
> carbon tetrachloride (982.1)
> hydroxyquinoline derivatives (961.3)
> lead (984.0-984.9)
> mercury (985.0)
> thallium (985.8)

323.71 *Toxic encephalitis and encephalomyelitis*

323.72 *Toxic myelitis*

⑤ **323.8 Other causes of encephalitis, myelitis, and encephalomyelitis**

323.81 Other causes of encephalitis and encephalomyelitis
> Noninfectious acute disseminated encephalomyelitis (ADEM)

	Add 4th or 5th digit		Nonspecific code		Unspecified code		Manifestation code

323.82 Other causes of myelitis
Transverse myelitis NOS

323.9 Unspecified causes of encephalitis, myelitis, and encephalomyelitis

324 Intracranial and intraspinal abscess

324.0 Intracranial abscess
Abscess (embolic):
  cerebellar
  cerebral

Abscess (embolic) of brain [any part]:
  epidural
  extradural
  otogenic
  subdural

Excludes: tuberculous (013.3)

324.1 Intraspinal abscess
Abscess (embolic) of spinal cord [any part]:
  epidural
  extradural
  subdural

Excludes: tuberculous (013.5)

324.9 Of unspecified site
Extradural or subdural abscess NOS

325 Phlebitis and thrombophlebitis of intracranial venous sinuses
Embolism, of cavernous, lateral, or other intracranial or unspecified intracranial venous sinus
Endophlebitis, of cavernous, lateral, or other intracranial or unspecified intracranial venous sinus
Phlebitis, septic or suppurative, of cavernous, lateral, or other intracranial or unspecified intracranial venous sinus
Thrombophlebitis of cavernous, lateral, or other intracranial or unspecified intracranial venous sinus
Thrombosis of cavernous, lateral, or other intracranial or unspecified intracranial venous sinus

Excludes: that specified as:
  complicating pregnancy, childbirth, or the puerperium (671.5)
  of nonpyogenic origin (437.6)

326 Late effects of intracranial abscess or pyogenic infection
Note: This category is to be used to indicate conditions whose primary classification is to 320-325 [excluding 320.7, 321.0-321.8, 323.01-323.42, 323.61-323.72] as the cause of late effects, themselves classifiable elsewhere. The "late effects" include conditions specified as such, or as sequelae, which may occur at any time after the resolution of the causal condition.

Use additional code, if desired, to identify condition, as:
hydrocephalus (331.4)
paralysis (342.0-342.9, 344.0-344.9)

ORGANIC SLEEP DISORDERS (327)

327 Organic sleep disorders

⑤ **327.0** Organic disorders of initiating and maintaining sleep [Organic insomnia]

Excludes: insomnia NOS (780.52)
  insomnia not due to a substance or known physiological condition (307.41-307.42)
  insomnia with sleep apnea NOS (780.51)

327.00 Organic insomnia, unspecified

327.01 Insomnia due to medical condition classified elsewhere
Code first underlying condition

Excludes: insomnia due to mental disorder (327.02)

327.02 Insomnia due to mental disorder
Code first mental disorder

Excludes: alcohol induced insomnia (291.82)
  drug induced insomnia (292.85)

327.09 Other organic insomnia

⑤ **327.1** Organic disorder of excessive somnolence [Organic hypersomnia]

Excludes: hypersomnia NOS (780.54)
  hypersomnia not due to a substance or known physiological condition (307.43-307.44)
  hypersomnia with sleep apnea NOS (780.53)

327.10 Organic hypersomnia, unspecified

● Code new
to this edition

▲ Revision of
existing code

④ ⑤ Fourth or fifth
digit required

327.11   **Idiopathic hypersomnia with long sleep time**

327.12   **Idiopathic hypersomnia without long sleep time**

327.13   **Recurrent hypersomnia**
Kleine-Levin syndrome
Menstrual related hypersomnia

327.14   **Hypersomnia due to medical condition classified elsewhere**
Code first underlying condition

Excludes: *hypersomnia due to mental disorder (327.15)*

327.15   **Hypersomnia due to mental disorder**
Code first mental disorder

Excludes: *alcohol induced hypersomnia (291.82)*
drug induced hypersomnia (292.85)

327.19   **Other organic hypersomnia**

⑤ **327.2   Organic sleep apnea**

Excludes: *Cheyne-Stokes breathing (786.04)*
hypersomnia with sleep apnea NOS (780.53)
insomnia with sleep apnea NOS (780.51)
sleep apnea in newborn (770.81-770.82)
sleep apnea NOS (780.57)

327.20   **Organic sleep apnea, unspecified**

327.21   **Primary central sleep apnea**

327.22   **High altitude periodic breathing**

327.23   **Obstructive sleep apnea (adult) (pediatric)**

327.24   **Idiopathic sleep related nonobstructive alveolar hypoventilation**
Sleep related hypoxia

327.25   **Congenital central alveolar hypoventilation syndrome**

327.26   **Sleep related hypoventilation/hypoxemia in conditions classifiable elsewhere**
Code first underlying condition

327.27   **Central sleep apnea in conditions classified elsewhere**
Code first underlying condition

327.29   **Other organic sleep apnea**

⑤ **327.3   Circadian rhythm sleep disorder**
Organic disorder of sleep wake cycle
Organic disorder of sleep wake schedule

Excludes: *alcohol induced circadian rhythm sleep disorder (291.82)*
circadian rhythm sleep disorder of nonorganic origin (307.45)
disruption of 24 hour sleep wake cycle NOS (780.55)
drug induced circadian rhythm sleep disorder (292.85)

327.30   **Circadian rhythm sleep disorder, unspecified**

327.31   **Circadian rhythm sleep disorder, delayed sleep phase type**

327.32   **Circadian rhythm sleep disorder, advanced sleep phase type**

327.33   **Circadian rhythm sleep disorder, irregular sleep-wake type**

327.34   **Circadian rhythm sleep disorder, free-running type**

327.35   **Circadian rhythm sleep disorder, jet lag type**

327.36   **Circadian rhythm sleep disorder, shift work type**

327.37   **Circadian rhythm sleep disorder in conditions classified elsewhere**
Code first underlying condition

327.39   **Other circadian rhythm sleep disorder**

⑤ **327.4   Organic parasomnia**

Excludes: *alcohol induced parasomnia (291.82)*
drug induced parasomnia (292.85)
parasomnia not due to a known physiological condition (307.47)

327.40   **Organic parasomnia, unspecified**

327.41   **Confusional arousals**

327.42   **REM sleep behavior disorder**

327.43   **Recurrent isolated sleep paralysis**

327.44   **Parasomnia in conditions classified elsewhere**
Code first underlying condition

Add 4th or 5th digit	Nonspecific code	Unspecified code	Manifestation code

327.49 Other organic parasomnia

⑤ **327.5** **Organic sleep related movement disorders**

Excludes: *restless legs syndrome (333.94)*
sleep related movement disorder NOS (780.58)

327.51 **Periodic limb movement disorder**
Periodic limb movement sleep disorder

327.52 **Sleep related leg cramps**

327.53 **Sleep related bruxism**

327.59 Other organic sleep related movement disorders

327.8 Other organic sleep disorders

HEREDITARY AND DEGENERATIVE DISEASES OF THE CENTRAL NERVOUS SYSTEM (330-337)

Excludes: *hepatolenticular degeneration (275.1)*
multiple sclerosis (340)
other demyelinating diseases of central nervous system (341.0-341.9)

330 **Cerebral degenerations usually manifest in childhood**
Use additional code, if desired, to identify associated mental retardation

330.0 **Leukodystrophy**
Krabbe's disease
Leukodystrophy:
NOS
globoid cell
Leukodystrophy:
metachromatic
sudanophilic
Pelizaeus-Merzbacher disease
Sulfatide lipidosis

330.1 **Cerebral lipidoses**
Amaurotic (familial) idiocy
Disease:
Batten
Jansky-Bielschowsky
Disease:
Kufs'
Spielmeyer-Vogt
Tay-Sachs
Gangliosidosis

330.2 *Cerebral degeneration in generalized lipidoses*
Code first underlying disease, as:
Fabry's disease (272.7)
Gaucher's disease (272.7)
Neimann-Pick disease (272.7)
sphingolipidosis (272.7)

330.3 *Cerebral degeneration of childhood in other diseases classified elsewhere*
Code first underlying disease, as:
Hunter's disease (277.5)
mucopolysaccharidosis (277.5)

330.8 **Other specified cerebral degenerations in childhood**
Alpers' disease or gray-matter degeneration
Infantile necrotizing encephalomyelopathy
Leigh's disease
Subacute necrotizing encephalopathy or encephalomyelopathy

330.9 **Unspecified cerebral degeneration in childhood**

331 **Other cerebral degenerations**
Use additional code, where applicable, to identify dementia:
with behavioral disturbance (294.11)
without behavioral disturbance (294.10)

331.0 **Alzheimer's disease**

⑤ **331.1** **Frontotemporal dementia**

331.11 **Pick's disease**

331.19 **Other frontotemporal dementia**
Frontal dementia

331.2 **Senile degeneration of brain**
Excludes: *senility NOS (797)*

● Code new to this edition ▲ Revision of existing code ④ ⑤ Fourth or fifth digit required

331.3 Communicating hydrocephalus
Secondary normal pressure hydrocephalus

Excludes: *congenital hydrocephalus (742.3)*
idiopathic normal pressure hydrocephalus (331.5)
normal pressure hydrocephalus (331.5)
spina bifida with hydrocephalus (741.0)

331.4 Obstructive hydrocephalus
Acquired hydrocephalus NOS

Excludes: *congenital hydrocephalus (742.3)*
idiopathic normal pressure hydrocephalus (331.5)
normal pressure hydrocephalus (331.5)
spina bifida with hydrocephalus (741.0)

331.5 Idiopathic normal pressure hydrocephalus (INPH)
Normal pressure hydrocephalus NOS

Excludes: *congenital hydrocephalus (742.3)*
secondary normal pressure hydrocephalus (331.3)
spina bifida with hydrocephalus (741.0)

331.7 *Cerebral degeneration in diseases classified elsewhere*
Code first underlying disease, as:
alcoholism (303.0-303.9)
beriberi (265.0)
cerebrovascular disease (430-438)
congenital hydrocephalus (741.0, 742.3)
neoplastic disease (140.0-239.9)
myxedema (244.0-244.9)
vitamin B_{12} deficiency (266.2)

Excludes: *cerebral degeneration in:*
Jakob-Creutzfeldt disease (046.11-046.19)
progressive multifocal leukoencephalopathy (046.3)
subacute spongiform encephalopathy (046.1)

⑤ **331.8 Other cerebral degeneration**

331.81 Reye's syndrome

331.82 Dementia with Lewy bodies
Dementia with Parkinsonism
Lewy body dementia
Lewy body disease

331.83 Mild cognitive impairment, so stated

Excludes: *altered mental status (780.97)*
cerebral degeneration (331.0-331.9)
change in mental status (780.97)
cognitive deficits following (late effects of) cerebral hemorrhage or infarction (438.0)
cognitive impairment due to intracranial or head injury (850-854, 959.01)
cognitive impairment due to late effect of intracranial injury (907.0)
cognitive impairment due to skull fracture (800-801, 803-804)
dementia (290.0-290.43, 294.8)
mild memory disturbance (310.8)
neurologic neglect syndrome (781.8)
personality change, nonpsychotic (310.1)

331.89 Other
Cerebral ataxia

331.9 Cerebral degeneration, unspecified

332 Parkinson's disease

Excludes: *dementia with Parkinsonism (331.82)*

332.0 Paralysis agitans
Parkinsonism or Parkinson's disease:
NOS
idiopathic
primary

Add 4th or 5th digit   Nonspecific code   Unspecified code   Manifestation code

332.1 Secondary Parkinsonism
   Neuroleptic-induced Parkinsonism
   Parkinsonism due to drugs
Use additional E code, if desired, to identify drug, if drug-induced

   Excludes: *Parkinsonism (in):*
      Huntington's disease (333.4)
      progressive supranuclear palsy (333.0)
      Shy-Drager syndrome (333.0)
      syphilitic (094.82)

333 Other extrapyramidal disease and abnormal movement disorders
   Includes: other forms of extrapyramidal, basal ganglia, or striatopallidal disease

   Excludes: *abnormal movements of head NOS (781.0)*
      sleep related movement disorders (327.51-327.59)

333.0 Other degenerative diseases of the basal ganglia
   Atrophy or degeneration:
      olivopontocerebellar [Déjérine-Thomas syndrome]
      pigmentary pallidal [Hallervorden-Spatz disease]
      striatonigral
   Parkinsonian syndrome associated with:
      idiopathic orthostatic hypotension
      symptomatic orthostatic hypotension
   Progressive supranuclear ophthalmoplegia
   Shy-Drager syndrome

333.1 Essential and other specified forms of tremor
   Benign essential tremor
   Familial tremor
   Medication-induced postural tremor
Use additional E code, if desired, to identify drug, if drug-induced

   Excludes: *tremor NOS (781.0)*

333.2 Myoclonus
   Familial essential myoclonus
   Palatal myoclonus

   Excludes: *progressive myoclonic epilepsy (345.1)*
      Unverricht-Lundborg disease (345.1)
Use additional E code, if desired, to identify drug, if drug-induced

333.3 Tics of organic origin

   Excludes: *Gilles de la Tourette's syndrome (307.23)*
      habit spasm (307.22)
      tic NOS (307.20)
Use additional E code, if desired, to identify drug, if drug-induced

333.4 Huntington's chorea

333.5 Other choreas
   Hemiballism(us)
   Paroxysmal choreo-athetosis

   Excludes: *Sydenham's or rheumatic chorea (392.0-392.9)*
Use additional E code, if desired, to identify drug, if drug-induced

333.6 Genetic torsion dystonia
   Dystonia:
      deformans progressiva
      musculorum deformans
   (Schwalbe-) Ziehen-Oppenheim disease

⑤ **333.7 Acquired torsion dystonia**

   333.71 Athetoid cerebral palsy
      Double athetosis (syndrome)
      Vogt's disease

   Excludes: *infantile cerebral palsy (343.0-343.9)*

● Code new to this edition	▲ Revision of existing code	④ ⑤ Fourth or fifth digit required

333.72 Acute dystonia due to drugs
Acute dystonic reaction due to drugs
Neuroleptic induced acute dystonia

Use additional E code to identify drug

Excludes: *blepharospasm due to drugs (333.85)*
orofacial dyskinesia due to drugs (333.85)
secondary Parkinsonism (332.1)
subacute dyskinesia due to drugs (333.85)
tardive dyskinesia (333.85)

333.79 Other acquired torsion dystonia

⑤ **333.8 Fragments of torsion dystonia**
Use additional E code, if desired, to identify drug, if drug-induced

333.81 Blepharospasm

Excludes: *blepharospasm due to drugs (333.85)*

333.82 Orofacial dyskinesia

Excludes: *orofacial dyskinesia due to drugs (333.85)*

333.83 Spasmodic torticollis

Excludes: *torticollis:*
NOS (723.5)
hysterical (300.11)
psychogenic (306.0)

333.84 Organic writers' cramp

Excludes: *psychogenic (300.89)*

333.85 Subacute dyskinesia due to drugs
Blepharospasm due to drugs
Orofacial dyskinesia due to drugs
Tardive dyskinesia

Use additional E code to identify drug

Excludes: *acute dystonia due to drugs (333.72)*
acute dystonic reaction due to drugs (333.72)
secondary Parkinsonism (332.1)

333.89 Other

⑤ **333.9 Other and unspecified extrapyramidal diseases and abnormal movement disorders**

333.90 Unspecified extrapyramidal disease and abnormal movement disorder
Medication-induced movement disorders NOS
Use additional E code to identify drug, if drug-induced

333.91 Stiff-man syndrome

333.92 Neuroleptic malignant syndrome
Use additional E code to identify drug

Excludes: *neuroleptic induced Parkinsonism (332.1)*

333.93 Benign shuddering attacks

333.94 Restless legs syndrome (RLS)

333.99 Other
Neuroleptic-induced acute akathisia
Use additional E code to identify drug, if drug-induced

334 Spinocerebellar disease

Excludes: *olivopontocerebellar degeneration (333.0)*
peroneal muscular atrophy (356.1)

334.0 Friedreich's ataxia

334.1 Hereditary spastic paraplegia

334.2 Primary cerebellar degeneration
Cerebellar ataxia:
Marie's
Sanger-Brown
Dyssynergia cerebellaris myoclonica
Primary cerebellar degeneration:
NOS
hereditary
sporadic

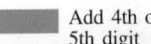

| Add 4th or 5th digit | Nonspecific code | Unspecified code | Manifestation code |

334.3 **Other cerebellar ataxia**
Cerebellar ataxia NOS

Use additional E code, if desired, to identify drug, if drug-induced

334.4 *Cerebellar ataxia in diseases classified elsewhere*
Code first underlying disease, as:
alcoholism (303.0-303.9)
myxedema (244.0-244.9)
neoplastic disease (140.0-239.9)

334.8 **Other spinocerebellar diseases**
Ataxia-telangiectasia [Louis-Bar syndrome]
Corticostriatal-spinal degeneration

334.9 **Spinocerebellar disease, unspecified**

335 **Anterior horn cell disease**

335.0 **Werdnig-Hoffmann disease**
Infantile spinal muscular atrophy
Progressive muscular atrophy of infancy

⑤ **335.1** **Spinal muscular atrophy**

335.10 **Spinal muscular atrophy, unspecified**

335.11 **Kugelberg-Welander disease**
Spinal muscular atrophy:
familial
juvenile

335.19 **Other**
Adult spinal muscular atrophy

⑤ **335.2** **Motor neuron disease**

335.20 **Amyotrophic lateral sclerosis**
Motor neuron disease (bulbar) (mixed type)

335.21 **Progressive muscular atrophy**
Duchenne-Aran muscular atrophy
Progressive muscular atrophy (pure)

335.22 **Progressive bulbar palsy**

335.23 **Pseudobulbar palsy**

335.24 **Primary lateral sclerosis**

335.29 **Other**

335.8 **Other anterior horn cell diseases**

335.9 **Anterior horn cell disease, unspecified**

336 **Other diseases of spinal cord**

336.0 **Syringomyelia and syringobulbia**

336.1 **Vascular myelopathies**
Acute infarction of spinal cord (embolic) (nonembolic)
Arterial thrombosis of spinal cord
Edema of spinal cord
Hematomyelia
Subacute necrotic myelopathy

336.2 *Subacute combined degeneration of spinal cord in diseases classified elsewhere*
Code first underlying disease, as:
pernicious anemia (281.0)
other vitamin B_{12} deficiency anemia (281.1)
vitamin B_{12} deficiency (266.2)

336.3 *Myelopathy in other diseases classified elsewhere*
Code first underlying disease, as:
myelopathy in neoplastic disease (140.0-239.9)

Excludes: *myelopathy in:*
intervertebral disc disorder (722.70-722.73)
spondylosis (721.1, 721.41-721.42, 721.91)

336.8 **Other myelopathy**
Myelopathy:
drug-induced
radiation-induced

Use additional E code, if desired, to identify cause

● Code new to this edition   ▲ Revision of existing code   ④ ⑤ Fourth or fifth digit required

336.9 Unspecified disease of spinal cord
Cord compression NOS   Myelopathy NOS
Excludes: *myelitis (323.02, 323.1, 323.2, 323.42, 323.52, 323.63, 323.72, 323.82, 323.9)*
spinal (canal) stenosis (723.0, 724.00-724.09)

337 Disorders of the autonomic nervous system
Includes: disorders of peripheral autonomic, sympathetic, parasympathetic, or vegetative
system
Excludes: *familial dysautonomia [Riley-Day syndrome] (742.8)*

⑤ **337.0 Idiopathic peripheral autonomic neuropathy**

337.00 Idiopathic peripheral autonomic neuropathy, unspecified

337.01 Carotid sinus syndrome
Carotid sinus syncope

337.09 Other idiopathic peripheral autonomic neuropathy
Cervical sympathetic dystrophy or paralysis

337.1 Peripheral autonomic neuropathy in disorders classified elsewhere
Code first underlying disease, as:
amyloidosis (277.30-277.39)
diabetes (249.6, 250.6)

⑤ **337.2 Reflex sympathetic dystrophy**

337.20 Reflex sympathetic dystrophy, unspecified
Complex regional pain syndrome type I, unspecified

337.21 Reflex sympathetic dystrophy of the upper limb
Complex regional pain syndrome type I of the upper limb

337.22 Reflex sympathetic dystrophy of the lower limb
Complex regional pain syndrome type I of the lower limb

337.29 Reflex sympathetic dystrophy of other specified site
Complex regional pain syndrome type I of other specified site

337.3 Autonomic dysreflexia
Use additional code to identify the cause, such as:
fecal impaction (560.39)
pressure ulcer (707.00-707.09)
urinary tract infection (599.0)

337.9 Unspecified disorder of autonomic nervous system

PAIN (338)

338 Pain, not elsewhere classified
Use additional code to identify:
pain associated with psychological factors (307.89)
Excludes: *generalized pain (780.96)*
headache syndromes (339.00-339.89)
localized pain, unspecified type – code to pain by site
migraines (346.0-346.9)
pain disorder exclusively attributed to psychological factors (307.80)
vulvar vestibulitis (625.71)
vulvodynia (625.70-625.79)

338.0 Central pain syndrome
Déjérine-Roussy syndrome
Myelopathic pain syndrome
Thalamic pain syndrome (hyperesthetic)

⑤ **338.1 Acute pain**

338.11 Acute pain due to trauma

338.12 Acute post-thoracotomy pain
Post-thoracotomy pain NOS

338.18 Other acute postoperative pain
Postoperative pain NOS

338.19 Other acute pain
Excludes: *neoplasm related acute pain (338.3)*

317

| | Add 4th or 5th digit | | Nonspecific code | | Unspecified code | | Manifestation code |

⑤ **338.2 Chronic pain**

> *Excludes:* *causalgia (355.9)*
>> *lower limb (355.71)*
>> *upper limb (354.4)*
>> *chronic pain syndrome (338.4)*
>> *myofascial pain syndrome (729.1)*
>> *neoplasm related chronic pain (338.3)*
>> *reflex sympathetic dystrophy (337.20-337.29)*

  338.21 Chronic pain due to trauma

  338.22 Chronic post-thoracotomy pain

  338.28 Other chronic postoperative pain

  338.29 Other chronic pain

338.3 Neoplasm related pain (acute) (chronic)
Cancer associated pain
Pain due to malignancy (primary) (secondary)
Tumor associated pain

338.4 Chronic pain syndrome
Chronic pain associated with significant psychosocial dysfunction

OTHER HEADACHE SYNDROMES (339)

339 Other headache syndromes

> *Excludes:* *headache:*
>> *NOS (784.0)*
>> *due to lumbar puncture (349.0)*
>> *migraine (346.0-346.9)*

⑤ **339.0 Cluster headaches and other trigeminal autonomic cephalgias**
TACS

  339.00 Cluster headache syndrome, unspecified
Ciliary neuralgia
Cluster headache NOS
Histamine cephalgia
Lower half migraine
Migrainous neuralgia

  339.01 Episodic cluster headache

  339.02 Chronic cluster headache

  339.03 Episodic paroxysmal hemicrania
Paroxysmal hemicrania NOS

  339.04 Chronic paroxysmal hemicrania

  339.05 Short lasting unilateral neuralgiform headache with conjunctival injection and tearing
SUNCT

  339.09 Other trigeminal autonomic cephalgias

⑤ **339.1 Tension type headache**

> *Excludes:* *tension headache NOS (307.81)*
>> *tension headache related to psychological factors (307.81)*

  339.10 Tension type headache, unspecified

  339.11 Episodic tension type headache

  339.12 Chronic tension type headache

⑤ **339.2 Post-traumatic headache**

  339.20 Post-traumatic headache, unspecified

  339.21 Acute post-traumatic headache

  339.22 Chronic post-traumatic headache

339.3 Drug induced headache not elsewhere classified
Medication overuse headache
Rebound headache

⑤ **339.4 Complicated headache syndromes**

  339.41 Hemicrania continua

  339.42 New daily persistent headache
NDPH

  339.43 Primary thunderclap headache

● Code new to this edition   ▲ Revision of existing code   ④ ⑤ Fourth or fifth digit required

339.44 Other complicated headache syndrome

⑤ **339.8** Other specified headache syndromes

339.81 Hypnic headache

339.82 Headache associated with sexual activity
Orgasmic headache
Preorgasmic headache

339.83 Primary cough headache

339.84 Primary exertional headache

339.85 Primary stabbing headache

339.89 Other specified headache syndromes

OTHER DISORDERS OF THE CENTRAL NERVOUS SYSTEM (340-349)

340 Multiple sclerosis
Disseminated or multiple sclerosis:
NOS
brain stem
cord
generalized

341 Other demyelinating diseases of central nervous system

341.0 Neuromyelitis optica

341.1 Schilder's disease
Baló's concentric sclerosis
Encephalitis periaxialis:
concentrica [Baló's]
diffusa [Schilder's]

⑤ **341.2** Acute (transverse) myelitis

Excludes: *acute (transverse)myelitis (in) (due to):*
following immunization procedures (323.52)
infection classified elsewhere (323.42)
postinfectious (323.63)
protozoal diseases classified elsewhere (323.2)
rickettsial diseases classified elsewhere (323.1)
toxic (323.72)
viral diseases classified elsewhere (323.02)
transverse myelitis NOS (323.82)

341.20 Acute (transverse) myelitis NOS

341.21 Acute (transverse) myelitis in conditions classified elsewhere
Code first underlying condition

341.22 Idiopathic transverse myelitis

341.8 Other demyelinating diseases of central nervous system
Central demyelination of corpus callosum
Central pontine myelinosis
Marchiafava (-Bignami) disease

341.9 Demyelinating disease of central nervous system, unspecified

342 Hemiplegia and hemiparesis

Excludes: *congenital (343.1)*
hemiplegia due to late effect of cerebrovascular accident (438.20-438.22)
infantile NOS (343.4)

Note: This category is to be used when hemiplegia (complete) (incomplete) is reported without further specification, or is stated to be old or long-standing but of unspecified cause. The category is also for use in multiple coding to identify these types of hemiplegia resulting from any cause.

The following fifth-digits are for use with codes 342.0-342.9

0 affecting unspecified side

1 affecting dominant side

2 affecting nondominant side

⑤ **342.0** Flaccid hemiplegia
[0-2]

⑤ **342.1** Spastic hemiplegia
[0-2]

							319
▓	Add 4th or 5th digit	▓	Nonspecific code	▓	Unspecified code	▓	Manifestation code

⑤ **342.8** **Other specified hemiplegia**
[0-2]

⑤ **342.9** **Hemiplegia, unspecified**
[0-2]

343 **Infantile cerebral palsy**
Includes: cerebral:
palsy NOS
spastic infantile paralysis
congenital spastic paralysis (cerebral)
Little's disease
paralysis (spastic) due to birth injury:
intracranial
spinal

Excludes: *athetoid cerebral palsy (333.71)*
hereditary cerebral paralysis, such as:
hereditary spastic paraplegia (334.1)
Vogt's disease (333.71)
spastic paralysis specified as noncongenital or noninfantile (344.0-344.9)

343.0 **Diplegic**
Congenital diplegia   Congenital paraplegia

343.1 **Hemiplegic**
Congenital hemiplegia

Excludes: *infantile hemiplegia NOS (343.4)*

343.2 **Quadriplegic**
Tetraplegic

343.3 **Monoplegic**

343.4 **Infantile hemiplegia**
Infantile hemiplegia (postnatal) NOS

343.8 **Other specified infantile cerebral palsy**

343.9 **Infantile cerebral palsy, unspecified**
Cerebral palsy NOS

344 **Other paralytic syndromes**
Note: This category is to be used when the listed conditions are reported without further
specification or are stated to be old or long-standing but of unspecified cause. The
category is also for use in multiple coding to identify these conditions resulting from any
cause.
Includes: paralysis (complete) (incomplete), except as classifiable to 342 and 343

Excludes: *congenital or infantile cerebral palsy (343.0-343.9)*
hemiplegia (342.0-342.9)
congenital or infantile (343.1, 343.4)

⑤ **344.0** **Quadriplegia and quadriparesis**

344.00 **Quadriplegia, unspecified**

344.01 **C1-C4, complete**

344.02 **C1-C4, incomplete**

344.03 **C5-C7, complete**

344.04 **C5-C7, incomplete**

344.09 **Other**

344.1 **Paraplegia**
Paralysis of both lower limbs
Paraplegia (lower)

344.2 **Diplegia of upper limbs**
Diplegia (upper)
Paralysis of both upper limbs

⑤ **344.3** **Monoplegia of lower limb**
Paralysis of lower limb

Excludes: *monoplegia of lower limb due to late effect of cerebrovascular accident*
(438.40-438.42)

344.30 **affecting unspecified side**

344.31 **affecting dominant side**

344.32 **affecting nondominant side**

● Code new
to this edition   ▲ Revision of
existing code   ④ ⑤ Fourth or fifth
digit required

⑤ **344.4 Monoplegia of upper limb**
Paralysis of upper limb

Excludes: *monoplegia of upper limb due to late effect of cerebrovascular accident (438.30-438.32)*

344.40 affecting unspecified side

344.41 affecting dominant side

344.42 affecting nondominant side

344.5 Unspecified monoplegia

⑤ **344.6 Cauda equina syndrome**

344.60 Without mention of neurogenic bladder

344.61 With neurogenic bladder
Acontractile bladder
Autonomic hyperreflexia of bladder
Cord bladder
Detrusor hyperreflexia

⑤ **344.8 Other specified paralytic syndromes**

344.81 Locked-in state

344.89 Other specified paralytic syndrome

344.9 Paralysis, unspecified

345 **Epilepsy and recurrent seizures**
The following fifth-digit subclassification is for use with categories 345.0, 345.1, 345.4-345.9:

0 **without mention of intractable epilepsy**

1 **with intractable epilepsy**
pharmacoresistant (pharmacologically resistant)
poorly controlled
refractory (medically)
treatment resistant

Excludes: *hippocampal sclerosis (348.81)*
mesial temporal sclerosis (348.81)
progressive myoclonic epilepsy (333.2)
temporal sclerosis (348.81)

⑤ **345.0 Generalized nonconvulsive epilepsy**
[0-1]   Absences:
atonic
typical
Minor epilepsy
Petit mal
Pykno-epilepsy
Seizures:
akinetic
atonic

⑤ **345.1 Generalized convulsive epilepsy**
[0-1]   Epileptic seizures:
clonic
myoclonic
tonic
tonic-clonic
Grand mal
Major epilepsy
Progressive myoclonic epilepsy
Unverricht-Lundborg disease

Excludes: *convulsions:*
NOS (780.39)
infantile (780.39)
newborn (779.0)
infantile spasms (345.6)

345.2 Petit mal status
Epileptic absence status

| | Add 4th or 5th digit | | Nonspecific code | | Unspecified code | | Manifestation code |

345.3 Grand mal status
Status epilepticus NOS

> Excludes: epilepsia partialis continua (345.7)
> status:
> psychomotor (345.7)
> temporal lobe (345.7)

⑤ **345.4 Localization-related (focal) (partial) epilepsy and epileptic syndromes with complex partial seizures**
[0-1] Epilepsy:
limbic system
partial:
secondarily generalized
with impairment of consciousness
with memory and ideational disturbances
psychomotor
psychosensory
temporal lobe
Epileptic automatism

⑤ **345.5 Localization-related (focal) (partial) epilepsy and epileptic syndromes with simple partial seizures**
[0-1]

Epilepsy:
Bravais-Jacksonian NOS
focal (motor) NOS
Jacksonian NOS
motor partial
partial NOS:
without impairment of consciousness

Epilepsy:
sensory-induced
somatomotor
somatosensory
visceral
visual

⑤ **345.6 Infantile spasms**
[0-1] Hypsarrhythmia
Lightning spasms
Salaam attacks

> Excludes: salaam tic (781.0)

⑤ **345.7 Epilepsia partialis continua**
[0-1] Kojevnikov's epilepsy

⑤ **345.8 Other forms of epilepsy and recurrent seizures**
[0-1] Epilepsy:
cursive [running]
gelastic

⑤ **345.9 Epilepsy, unspecified**
[0-1] Epileptic convulsions, fits, or seizures NOS
Recurrent seizures NOS
Seizure disorder NOS

> Excludes: convulsion (convulsive) disorder (780.39)
> convulsive seizure or fit NOS (780.39)
> recurrent convulsions (780.39)

⑤ **346 Migraine**

> Excludes: headache:
> NOS (784.0)
> syndromes (339.00-339.89)

The following fifth-digit subclassification is for use with category 346:

0 without mention of intractable migraine without mention of status migrainosus
1 with intractable migraine, so stated, without mention of status migrainosus
2 without mention of intractable migraine with status migrainosus
3 with intractable migraine, so stated, with status migrainosus

● Code new to this edition ▲ Revision of existing code ④ ⑤ Fourth or fifth digit required

⑤ **346.0 Migraine with aura**
[0-3]   Basilar migraine
           Classic migraine
           Migraine preceded or accompanied by transient focal neurological phenomena
           Migraine triggered seizures
           Migraine with acute-onset aura
           Migraine with aura without headache (migraine equivalents)
           Migraine with prolonged aura
           Migraine with typical aura
           Retinal migraine

Excludes: *persistent migraine aura (346.5, 346.6)*

⑤ **346.1 Migraine without aura**
[0-3]   Common migraine

⑤ **346.2 Variants of migraine, not elsewhere classified**
[0-3]   Abdominal migraine
           Cyclical vomiting associated with migraine
           Ophthalmoplegic migraine
           Periodic headache syndromes in child or adolescent

Excludes: *cyclical vomiting NOS (536.2)*
          psychogenic cyclical vomiting (306.4)

⑤ **346.3 Hemiplegic migraine**
[0-3]   Familial migraine
           Sporadic migraine

⑤ **346.4 Menstrual migraine**
[0-3]   Menstrual headache
           Menstrually related migraine
           Premenstrual headache
           Premenstrual migraine
           Pure menstrual migraine

⑤ **346.5 Persistent migraine aura without cerebral infarction**
[0-3]   Persistent migraine aura NOS

⑤ **346.6 Persistent migraine aura with cerebral infarction**
[0-3]

⑤ **346.7 Chronic migraine without aura**
[0-3]   Transformed migraine without aura

⑤ **346.8 Other forms of migraine**
[0-3]

⑤ **346.9 Migraine, unspecified**
[0-3]

347 **Cataplexy and narcolepsy**

⑤ **347.0 Narcolepsy**

   347.00   Without cataplexy
              Narcolepsy NOS

   347.01   With cataplexy

⑤ **347.1 Narcolepsy in conditions classified elsewhere**
        Code first underlying condition

   347.10 *Without cataplexy*

   347.11 *With cataplexy*

348 **Other conditions of brain**

348.0 Cerebral cysts
         Arachnoid cyst   Porencephaly, acquired
         Porencephalic cyst   Pseudoporencephaly

Excludes: *porencephaly (congenital) (742.4)*

348.1 Anoxic brain damage

Excludes: *that occurring in:*
             abortion (634-638 with .7, 639.8)
             ectopic or molar pregnancy (639.8)
             labor or delivery (668.2, 669.4)
             that of newborn (767.0, 768.0-768.9, 772.1-772.2)

Use additional E code, if desired, to identify cause

	Add 4th or 5th digit		Nonspecific code		Unspecified code		Manifestation code

348.2 Benign intracranial hypertension
Pseudotumor cerebri

Excludes: *hypertensive encephalopathy (437.2)*

⑤ **348.3 Encephalopathy, not elsewhere classified**

348.30 Encephalopathy, unspecified

348.31 Metabolic encephalopathy
Septic encephalopathy

Excludes: *toxic metabolic encephalopathy (349.82)*

348.39 Other encephalopathy

Excludes: *encephalopathy:*
alcoholic (291.2)
hepatic (572.2)
hypertensive (437.2)
toxic (349.82)

348.4 Compression of brain
Compression, brain (stem)
Herniation, brain (stem)
Posterior fossa compression syndrome

348.5 Cerebral edema

⑤ **348.8 Other conditions of brain**

● **348.81 Temporal sclerosis**
Hippocampal sclerosis
Mesial temporal sclerosis

● **348.89 Other conditions of brain**
Cerebral:
calcification
fungus

348.9 Unspecified condition of brain

349 Other and unspecified disorders of the nervous system

349.0 Reaction to spinal or lumbar puncture
Headache following lumbar puncture

349.1 Nervous system complications from surgically implanted device

349.2 Disorders of meninges, not elsewhere classified

Excludes: *immediate postoperative complications (997.00-997.09)*
mechanical complications of nervous system device (996.2)
Adhesions, meningeal (cerebral) (spinal)
Cyst, spinal meninges
Meningocele, acquired
Pseudomeningocele, acquired

⑤ **349.3 Dural tear**

349.31 Accidental puncture or laceration of dura during a procedure
Incidental (inadvertent) durotomy

349.39 Other dural tear

⑤ **349.8 Other specified disorders of nervous system**

349.81 Cerebrospinal fluid rhinorrhea

Excludes: *cerebrospinal fluid otorrhea (388.61)*

349.82 Toxic encephalopathy
Toxic metabolic encephalopathy
Use additional E code, if desired, to identify cause

349.89 Other

349.9 Unspecified disorders of nervous system
Disorder of nervous system (central) NOS

● Code new
to this edition
▲ Revision of
existing code
④ ⑤ Fourth or fifth
digit required

DISORDERS OF THE PERIPHERAL NERVOUS SYSTEM (350-359)

> Excludes: *diseases of:*
> *acoustic [8th] nerve (388.5)*
> *oculomotor [3rd, 4th, 6th] nerves (378.0-378.9)*
> *optic [2nd] nerve (377.0-377.9)*
> *peripheral autonomic nerves (337.0-337.9)*
> *neuralgia NOS or "rheumatic" (729.2)*
> *neuritis NOS or "rheumatic" (729.2)*
> *radiculitis NOS or "rheumatic" (729.2)*
> *peripheral neuritis in pregnancy (646.4)*

350 **Trigeminal nerve disorders**
Includes: disorders of 5th cranial nerve

350.1 Trigeminal neuralgia
Tic douloureux   Trigeminal neuralgia NOS
Trifacial neuralgia

> Excludes: *postherpetic (053.12)*

350.2 Atypical face pain

350.8 Other specified trigeminal nerve disorders

350.9 Trigeminal nerve disorder, unspecified

351 **Facial nerve disorders**
Includes: disorders of 7th cranial nerve

> Excludes: *that in newborn (767.5)*

351.0 Bell's palsy
Facial palsy

351.1 Geniculate ganglionitis
Geniculate ganglionitis NOS

> Excludes: *herpetic (053.11)*

351.8 Other facial nerve disorders
Facial myokymia
Melkersson's syndrome

351.9 Facial nerve disorder, unspecified

352 **Disorders of other cranial nerves**

352.0 Disorders of olfactory [1st] nerve

352.1 Glossopharyngeal neuralgia

352.2 Other disorders of glossopharyngeal [9th] nerve

352.3 Disorders of pneumogastric [10th] nerve
Disorders of vagal nerve

> Excludes: *paralysis of vocal cords or larynx (478.30-478.34)*

352.4 Disorders of accessory [11th] nerve

352.5 Disorders of hypoglossal [12th] nerve

352.6 Multiple cranial nerve palsies
Collet-Sicard syndrome
Polyneuritis cranialis

352.9 Unspecified disorder of cranial nerves

353 **Nerve root and plexus disorders**

> Excludes: *conditions due to:*
> *intervertebral disc disorders (722.0-722.9)*
> *spondylosis (720.0-721.9)*
> *vertebrogenic disorders (723.0-724.9)*

353.0 Brachial plexus lesions
Cervical rib syndrome   Scalenus anticus syndrome
Costoclavicular syndrome   Thoracic outlet syndrome

> Excludes: *brachial neuritis or radiculitis NOS (723.4)*
> *that in newborn (767.6)*

353.1 Lumbosacral plexus lesions

353.2 Cervical root lesions, not elsewhere classified

353.3 Thoracic root lesions, not elsewhere classified

353.4 Lumbosacral root lesions, not elsewhere classified

	Add 4th or 5th digit		Nonspecific code		Unspecified code		Manifestation code

353.5 Neuralgic amyotrophy
  Parsonage-Aldren-Turner syndrome
  Code first any associated underlying disease, such as:
    diabetes mellitus (249.6, 250.6)

353.6 Phantom limb (syndrome)

353.8 Other nerve root and plexus disorders

353.9 Unspecified nerve root and plexus disorder

354 Mononeuritis of upper limb and mononeuritis multiplex

354.0 Carpal tunnel syndrome
  Median nerve entrapment
  Partial thenar atrophy

354.1 Other lesion of median nerve
  Median nerve neuritis

354.2 Lesion of ulnar nerve
  Cubital tunnel syndrome
  Tardy ulnar nerve palsy

354.3 Lesion of radial nerve
  Acute radial nerve palsy

354.4 Causalgia of upper limb
  Complex regional pain syndrome type II of the upper limb

  Excludes: *causalgia:*
        NOS (355.9)
        lower limb (355.71)
        complex regional pain syndrome type II of the lower limb (355.71)

354.5 Mononeuritis multiplex
  Combinations of single conditions classifiable to 354 or 355

354.8 Other mononeuritis of upper limb

354.9 Mononeuritis of upper limb, unspecified

355 Mononeuritis of lower limb and unspecified site

355.0 Lesion of sciatic nerve
  Excludes: *sciatica NOS (724.3)*

355.1 Meralgia paresthetica
  Lateral cutaneous femoral nerve of thigh compression or syndrome

355.2 Other lesion of femoral nerve

355.3 Lesion of lateral popliteal nerve
  Lesion of common peroneal nerve

355.4 Lesion of medial popliteal nerve

355.5 Tarsal tunnel syndrome

355.6 Lesion of plantar nerve
  Morton's metatarsalgia, neuralgia, or neuroma

⑤ **355.7 Other mononeuritis of lower limb**

  355.71 Causalgia of lower limb
  Excludes: *causalgia:*
        NOS (355.9)
        upper limb (354.4)
        complex regional pain syndrome type II of upper limb (354.4)

  355.79 Other mononeuritis of lower limb

355.8 Mononeuritis of lower limb, unspecified

355.9 Mononeuritis of unspecified site
  Causalgia NOS
  Complex regional pain syndrome NOS

  Excludes: *causalgia:*
        lower limb (355.71)
        upper limb (354.4)
      complex regional pain syndrome:
        lower limb (355.71)
        upper limb (354.4)

● Code new
  to this edition
▲ Revision of
  existing code
④ ⑤ Fourth or fifth
  digit required

356 **Hereditary and idiopathic peripheral neuropathy**

356.0 **Hereditary peripheral neuropathy**
Déjérine-Sottas disease

356.1 **Peroneal muscular atrophy**
Charcot-Marie-Tooth disease
Neuropathic muscular atrophy

356.2 **Hereditary sensory neuropathy**

356.3 **Refsum's disease**
Heredopathia atactica polyneuritiformis

356.4 **Idiopathic progressive polyneuropathy**

356.8 **Other specified idiopathic peripheral neuropathy**
Supranuclear paralysis

356.9 **Unspecified**

357 **Inflammatory and toxic neuropathy**

357.0 **Acute infective polyneuritis**
Guillain-Barré syndrome
Postinfectious polyneuritis

357.1 *Polyneuropathy in collagen vascular disease*
Code first underlying disease, as:
disseminated lupus erythematosus (710.0)
polyarteritis nodosa (446.0)
rheumatoid arthritis (714.0)

357.2 *Polyneuropathy in diabetes*
Code first underlying disease (249.6, 250.6)

357.3 *Polyneuropathy in malignant disease*
Code first underlying disease (140.0-208.9)

357.4 *Polyneuropathy in other diseases classified elsewhere*
Code first underlying disease, as:
amyloidosis (277.30-277.39)
beriberi (265.0)
chronic uremia (585.9)
deficiency of B vitamins (266.0-266.9)
diphtheria (032.0-032.9)
hypoglycemia (251.2)
pellagra (265.2)
porphyria (277.1)
sarcoidosis (135)
uremia NOS (586)

Excludes: *polyneuropathy in:*
herpes zoster (053.13)
mumps (072.72)

357.5 **Alcoholic polyneuropathy**

357.6 **Polyneuropathy due to drugs**
Use additional E code, if desired, to identify drug

357.7 **Polyneuropathy due to other toxic agents**
Use additional E code, if desired, to identify toxic agent

⑤ **357.8** **Other**

357.81 **Chronic inflammatory demyelinating polyneuritis**

357.82 **Critical illness polyneuropathy**
Acute motor neuropathy

357.89 **Other inflammatory and toxic neuropathy**

357.9 **Unspecified**

358 **Myoneural disorders**

⑤ **358.0** **Myasthenia gravis**

358.00 **Myasthenia gravis without (acute) exacerbation**
Myasthenia gravis NOS

358.01 **Myasthenia gravis with (acute) exacerbation**
Myasthenia gravis in crisis

| | Add 4th or 5th digit | | Nonspecific code | | Unspecified code | | Manifestation code |

358.1 Myasthenic syndromes in diseases classified elsewhere
Eaton-Lambert syndrome from stated cause classified elsewhere
Code first underlying disease, as:
botulism (005.1, 040.41-040.42)
hypothyroidism (244.0-244.9)
malignant neoplasm (140.0-208.9)
pernicious anemia (281.0)
thyrotoxicosis (242.0-242.9)

358.2 Toxic myoneural disorders
Use additional E code, if desired, to identify toxic agent

358.8 Other specified myoneural disorders

358.9 Myoneural disorders, unspecified

359 Muscular dystrophies and other myopathies
Excludes: idiopathic polymyositis (710.4)

359.0 Congenital hereditary muscular dystrophy
Benign congenital myopathy
Central core disease
Centronuclear myopathy
Myotubular myopathy
Nemaline body disease

Excludes: arthrogryposis multiplex congenita (754.89)

359.1 Hereditary progressive muscular dystrophy
Muscular dystrophy: Muscular dystrophy:
NOS   Gower's
distal   Landouzy-Déjérine
Duchenne   limb-girdle
Erb's   ocular
fascioscapulohumeral   oculopharyngeal

⑤ **359.2 Myotonic disorders**
Excludes: periodic paralysis (359.3)

359.21 Myotonic muscular dystrophy
Dystrophia myotonica
Myotonia atrophica
Myotonic dystrophy
Proximal myotonic myopathy (PROMM)
Steinert's disease

359.22 Myotonia congenita
Acetazolamide responsive myotonia congenita
Dominant form (Thomsen's disease)
Myotonia levior
Recessive form (Becker's disease)

359.23 Myotonic chondrodystrophy
Congenital myotonic chondrodystrophy
Schwartz-Jampel disease

359.24 Drug-induced myotonia
Use additional E code to identify drug

359.29 Other specified myotonic disorder
Myotonia fluctuans
Myotonia permanens
Paramyotonia congenita (of von Eulenburg)

359.3 Periodic paralysis
Familial periodic paralysis
Hyperkalemic periodic paralysis
Hypokalemic familial periodic paralysis
Hypokalemic periodic paralysis
Potassium sensitive periodic paralysis

Excludes: paramyotonia congenita (of von Eulenburg) (359.29)

359.4 Toxic myopathy
Use additional E code, if desired, to identify toxic agent

● Code new to this edition   ▲ Revision of existing code   ④ ⑤ Fourth or fifth digit required

359.5   Myopathy in endocrine diseases classified elsewhere
Code first underlying disease, as:
Addison's disease (255.41)
Cushing's syndrome (255.0)
hypopituitarism (253.2)
myxedema (244.0-244.9)
thyrotoxicosis (242.0-242.9)

359.6   Symptomatic inflammatory myopathy in diseases classified elsewhere
Code first underlying disease, as:
amyloidosis (277.30-277.39)
disseminated lupus erythematosus (710.0)
malignant neoplasm (140.0-208.9)
polyarteritis nodosa (446.0)
rheumatoid arthritis (714.0)
sarcoidosis (135)
scleroderma (710.1)
Sjögren's disease (710.2)

● **359.7   Inflammatory and immune myopathies, NEC**

● **359.71   Inclusion body myositis**
IBM

● **359.79   Other inflammatory and immune myopathies, NEC**
Inflammatory myopathy NOS

⑤ **359.8   Other myopathies**

359.81   Critical illness myopathy
Acute necrotizing myopathy
Acute quadriplegic myopathy
Intensive care (ICU) myopathy
Myopathy of critical illness

359.89   Other myopathies

359.9   Myopathy, unspecified

DISORDERS OF THE EYE AND ADNEXA (360-379)

Use additional external cause code, if applicable, to identify the cause of the eye condition

360   Disorders of the globe
Includes: disorders affecting multiple structures of eye

⑤ **360.0   Purulent endophthalmitis**

Excludes: bleb associated endophthalmitis (379.63)

360.00   Purulent endophthalmitis, unspecified

360.01   Acute endophthalmitis

360.02   Panophthalmitis

360.03   Chronic endophthalmitis

360.04   Vitreous abscess

⑤ **360.1   Other endophthalmitis**

Excludes: bleb associated endophthalmitis (379.63)

360.11   Sympathetic uveitis

360.12   Panuveitis

360.13   Parasitic endophthalmitis NOS

360.14   Ophthalmia nodosa

360.19   Other
Phacoanaphylactic endophthalmitis

⑤ **360.2   Degenerative disorders of globe**

360.20   Degenerative disorder of globe, unspecified

360.21   Progressive high (degenerative) myopia
Malignant myopia

360.23   Siderosis

360.24   Other metallosis
Chalcosis

360.29   Other

Excludes: xerophthalmia (264.7)

| | Add 4th or 5th digit | | Nonspecific code | | Unspecified code | | Manifestation code |

⑤ **360.3 Hypotony of eye**

    360.30 Hypotony, unspecified

    360.31 Primary hypotony

    360.32 Ocular fistula causing hypotony

    360.33 Hypotony associated with other ocular disorders

    360.34 Flat anterior chamber

⑤ **360.4 Degenerated conditions of globe**

    360.40 Degenerated globe or eye, unspecified

    360.41 Blind hypotensive eye
        Atrophy of globe
        Phthisis bulbi

    360.42 Blind hypertensive eye
        Absolute glaucoma

    360.43 Hemophthalmos, except current injury

    Excludes: *traumatic (871.0-871.9, 921.0-921.9)*

    360.44 Leucocoria

⑤ **360.5 Retained (old) intraocular foreign body, magnetic**

    Excludes: *current penetrating injury with magnetic foreign body (871.5)*
              retained (old) foreign body of orbit (376.6)

    360.50 Foreign body, magnetic, intraocular, unspecified

    360.51 Foreign body, magnetic, in anterior chamber

    360.52 Foreign body, magnetic, in iris or ciliary body

    360.53 Foreign body, magnetic, in lens

    360.54 Foreign body, magnetic, in vitreous

    360.55 Foreign body, magnetic, in posterior wall

    360.59 Foreign body, magnetic, in other or multiple sites

⑤ **360.6 Retained (old) intraocular foreign body, nonmagnetic**
    Retained (old) foreign body:
        NOS
        nonmagnetic

    Excludes: *current penetrating injury with (nonmagnetic) foreign body (871.6)*
              retained (old) foreign body in orbit (376.6)

    360.60 Foreign body, intraocular, unspecified

    360.61 Foreign body in anterior chamber

    360.62 Foreign body in iris or ciliary body

    360.63 Foreign body in lens

    360.64 Foreign body in vitreous

    360.65 Foreign body in posterior wall

    360.69 Foreign body in other or multiple sites

⑤ **360.8 Other disorders of globe**

    360.81 Luxation of globe

    360.89 Other

360.9 Unspecified disorder of globe

361 Retinal detachments and defects

⑤ **361.0 Retinal detachment with retinal defect**
    Rhegmatogenous retinal detachment

    Excludes: *detachment of retinal pigment epithelium (362.42-362.43)*
              retinal detachment (serous) (without defect) (361.2)

    361.00 Retinal detachment with retinal defect, unspecified

    361.01 Recent detachment, partial, with single defect

    361.02 Recent detachment, partial, with multiple defects

    361.03 Recent detachment, partial, with giant tear

    361.04 Recent detachment, partial, with retinal dialysis
        Dialysis (juvenile) of retina (with detachment)

    361.05 Recent detachment, total or subtotal

● Code new   ▲ Revision of   ④ ⑤ Fourth or fifth
   to this edition   existing code   digit required

361.06 Old detachment, partial
Delimited old retinal detachment

361.07 Old detachment, total or subtotal

⑤ **361.1 Retinoschisis and retinal cysts**

Excludes: *juvenile retinoschisis (362.73)*
microcystoid degeneration of retina (362.62)
parasitic cyst of retina (360.13)

361.10 Retinoschisis, unspecified

361.11 Flat retinoschisis

361.12 Bullous retinoschisis

361.13 Primary retinal cysts

361.14 Secondary retinal cysts

361.19 Other
Pseudocyst of retina

361.2 Serous retinal detachment
Retinal detachment without retinal defect

Excludes: *central serous retinopathy (362.41)*
retinal pigment epithelium detachment (362.42-362.43)

⑤ **361.3 Retinal defects without detachment**

Excludes: *chorioretinal scars after surgery for detachment (363.30-363.35)*
peripheral retinal degeneration without defect (362.60-362.66)

361.30 Retinal defect, unspecified
Retinal break(s) NOS

361.31 Round hole of retina without detachment

361.32 Horseshoe tear of retina without detachment
Operculum of retina without mention of detachment

361.33 Multiple defects of retina without detachment

⑤ **361.8 Other forms of retinal detachment**

361.81 Traction detachment of retina
Traction detachment with vitreoretinal organization

361.89 Other

361.9 Unspecified retinal detachment

362 Other retinal disorders

Excludes: *chorioretinal scars (363.30-363.35)*
chorioretinitis (363.0-363.2)

⑤ *362.0 Diabetic retinopathy*
Code first diabetes (249.5, 250.5)

362.01 Background diabetic retinopathy
Diabetic retinal microaneurysms
Diabetic retinopathy NOS

362.02 Proliferative diabetic retinopathy

362.03 Nonproliferative diabetic retinopathy NOS

362.04 Mild nonproliferative diabetic retinopathy

362.05 Moderate nonproliferative diabetic retinopathy

362.06 Severe nonproliferative diabetic retinopathy

362.07 Diabetic macular edema
Diabetic retinal edema
Note: Code 362.07 must be used with a code for diabetic retinopathy (362.01-362.06)

⑤ **362.1 Other background retinopathy and retinal vascular changes**

362.10 Background retinopathy, unspecified

362.11 Hypertensive retinopathy

362.12 Exudative retinopathy
Coats' syndrome

362.13 Changes in vascular appearance
Vascular sheathing of retina

Use additional code for any associated atherosclerosis (440.8)

362.14 Retinal microaneurysms NOS

| | Add 4th or 5th digit | | Nonspecific code | | Unspecified code | | Manifestation code |

362.15 Retinal telangiectasia

362.16 Retinal neovascularization NOS
Neovascularization:
choroidal
subretinal

362.17 Other intraretinal microvascular abnormalities
Retinal varices

362.18 Retinal vasculitis

Eales' disease
Retinal:
arteritis
endarteritis

Retinal:
perivasculitis
phlebitis

⑤ **362.2 Other proliferative retinopathy**

362.20 Retinopathy of prematurity, unspecified
Retinopathy of prematurity NOS

362.21 Retrolental fibroplasia
Cicatricial retinopathy of prematurity

362.22 Retinopathy of prematurity, stage 0

362.23 Retinopathy of prematurity, stage 1

362.24 Retinopathy of prematurity, stage 2

362.25 Retinopathy of prematurity, stage 3

362.26 Retinopathy of prematurity, stage 4

362.27 Retinopathy of prematurity, stage 5

362.29 Other nondiabetic proliferative retinopathy

⑤ **362.3 Retinal vascular occlusion**

362.30 Retinal vascular occlusion, unspecified

362.31 Central retinal artery occlusion

362.32 Arterial branch occlusion

362.33 Partial arterial occlusion
Hollenhorst plaque
Retinal microembolism

362.34 Transient arterial occlusion
Amaurosis fugax

362.35 Central retinal vein occlusion

362.36 Venous tributary (branch) occlusion

362.37 Venous engorgement
Occlusion:
incipient of retinal vein
partial of retinal vein

⑤ **362.4 Separation of retinal layers**

Excludes: retinal detachment (serous) (361.2)
rhegmatogenous (361.00-361.07)

362.40 Retinal layer separation, unspecified

362.41 Central serous retinopathy

362.42 Serous detachment of retinal pigment epithelium
Exudative detachment of retinal pigment epithelium

362.43 Hemorrhagic detachment of retinal pigment epithelium

⑤ **362.5 Degeneration of macula and posterior pole**

Excludes: degeneration of optic disc (377.21-377.24)
hereditary retinal degeneration [dystrophy] (362.70-362.77)

362.50 Macular degeneration (senile), unspecified

362.51 Nonexudative senile macular degeneration
Senile macular degeneration:
atrophic
dry

362.52 Exudative senile macular degeneration
Kuhnt-Junius degeneration
Senile macular degeneration:
disciform
wet

● Code new
to this edition

▲ Revision of
existing code

④ ⑤ Fourth or fifth
digit required

362.53 Cystoid macular degeneration
Cystoid macular edema

362.54 Macular cyst, hole, or pseudohole

362.55 Toxic maculopathy
Use additional E code, if desired, to identify drug, if drug induced

362.56 Macular puckering
Preretinal fibrosis

362.57 Drusen (degenerative)

⑤ **362.6 Peripheral retinal degenerations**

Excludes: *hereditary retinal degeneration [dystrophy] (362.70-362.77)*
retinal degeneration with retinal defect (361.00-361.07)

362.60 Peripheral retinal degeneration, unspecified

362.61 Paving stone degeneration

362.62 Microcystoid degeneration
Blessig's cysts   Iwanoff's cysts

362.63 Lattice degeneration
Palisade degeneration of retina

362.64 Senile reticular degeneration

362.65 Secondary pigmentary degeneration
Pseudoretinitis pigmentosa

362.66 Secondary vitreoretinal degenerations

⑤ **362.7 Hereditary retinal dystrophies**

362.70 Hereditary retinal dystrophy, unspecified

362.71 *Retinal dystrophy in systemic or cerebroretinal lipidoses*
Code first underlying disease, as:
cerebroretinal lipidoses (330.1)
systemic lipidoses (272.7)

362.72 *Retinal dystrophy in other systemic disorders and syndromes*
Code first underlying disease, as:
Bassen-Kornzweig syndrome (272.5)
Refsum's disease (356.3)

362.73 Vitreoretinal dystrophies
Juvenile retinoschisis

362.74 Pigmentary retinal dystrophy
Retinal dystrophy, albipunctate
Retinitis pigmentosa

362.75 Other dystrophies primarily involving the sensory retina
Progressive cone (-rod) dystrophy
Stargardt's disease

362.76 Dystrophies primarily involving the retinal pigment epithelium
Fundus flavimaculatus
Vitelliform dystrophy

362.77 Dystrophies primarily involving Bruch's membrane
Dystrophy:
hyaline
pseudoinflammatory foveal
Hereditary drusen

⑤ **362.8 Other retinal disorders**

Excludes: *chorioretinal inflammations (363.0-363.2)*
chorioretinal scars (363.30-363.35)

362.81 Retinal hemorrhage
Hemorrhage:
preretinal
retinal (deep) (superficial)
subretinal

362.82 Retinal exudates and deposits

362.83 Retinal edema
Retinal:
cotton wool spots
edema (localized) (macular) (peripheral)

362.84 Retinal ischemia

| | Add 4th or 5th digit | | Nonspecific code | | Unspecified code | | Manifestation code |

362.85   **Retinal nerve fiber bundle defects**

362.89   Other retinal disorders

362.9 **Unspecified retinal disorder**

363 **Chorioretinal inflammations, scars, and other disorders of choroid**

⑤ **363.0 Focal chorioretinitis and focal retinochoroiditis**

Excludes: *focal chorioretinitis or retinochoroiditis in:*
histoplasmosis (115.02, 115.12, 115.92)
toxoplasmosis (130.2)
congenital infection (771.2)

363.00   **Focal chorioretinitis, unspecified**
Focal:
choroiditis or chorioretinitis NOS
retinitis or retinochoroiditis NOS

363.01   **Focal choroiditis and chorioretinitis, juxtapapillary**

363.03   **Focal choroiditis and chorioretinitis of other posterior pole**

363.04   **Focal choroiditis and chorioretinitis, peripheral**

363.05   **Focal retinitis and retinochoroiditis, juxtapapillary**
Neuroretinitis

363.06   **Focal retinitis and retinochoroiditis, macular or paramacular**

363.07   **Focal retinitis and retinochoroiditis of other posterior pole**

363.08   **Focal retinitis and retinochoroiditis, peripheral**

⑤ **363.1 Disseminated chorioretinitis and disseminated retinochoroiditis**

Excludes: *disseminated choroiditis or chorioretinitis in secondary syphilis (091.51)*
neurosyphilitic disseminated retinitis or retinochoroiditis (094.83)
retinal (peri)vasculitis (362.18)

363.10   **Disseminated chorioretinitis, unspecified**
Disseminated:
choroiditis or chorioretinitis NOS
retinitis or retinochoroiditis NOS

363.11   **Disseminated choroiditis and chorioretinitis, posterior pole**

363.12   **Disseminated choroiditis and chorioretinitis, peripheral**

363.13   **Disseminated choroiditis and chorioretinitis, generalized**
Code first any underlying disease, as:
tuberculosis (017.3)

363.14   **Disseminated retinitis and retinochoroiditis, metastatic**

363.15   **Disseminated retinitis and retinochoroiditis, pigment epitheliopathy**
Acute posterior multifocal placoid pigment epitheliopathy

⑤ **363.2 Other and unspecified forms of chorioretinitis and retinochoroiditis**

Excludes: *panophthalmitis (360.02)*
sympathetic uveitis (360.11)
uveitis NOS (364.3)

363.20   **Chorioretinitis, unspecified**
Choroiditis NOS
Retinitis NOS
Uveitis, posterior NOS

363.21   **Pars planitis**
Posterior cyclitis

363.22   **Harada's disease**

⑤ **363.3 Chorioretinal scars**
Scar (postinflammatory) (postsurgical) (posttraumatic):
choroid
retina

363.30   **Chorioretinal scar, unspecified**

363.31   **Solar retinopathy**

363.32   **Other macular scars**

363.33   **Other scars of posterior pole**

363.34   **Peripheral scars**

363.35   **Disseminated scars**

● Code new   ▲ Revision of   ④ ⑤ Fourth or fifth
to this edition   existing code   digit required

⑤ **363.4 Choroidal degenerations**

    363.40 Choroidal degeneration, unspecified
        Choroidal sclerosis NOS

    363.41 Senile atrophy of choroid

    363.42 Diffuse secondary atrophy of choroid

    363.43 Angioid streaks of choroid

⑤ **363.5 Hereditary choroidal dystrophies**
    Hereditary choroidal atrophy:
      partial [choriocapillaris]
      total [all vessels]

    363.50 Hereditary choroidal dystrophy or atrophy, unspecified

    363.51 Circumpapillary dystrophy of choroid, partial

    363.52 Circumpapillary dystrophy of choroid, total
        Helicoid dystrophy of choroid

    363.53 Central dystrophy of choroid, partial
        Dystrophy, choroidal:
          central areolar
          circinate

    363.54 Central choroidal atrophy, total
        Dystrophy, choroidal:
          central gyrate
          serpiginous

    363.55 Choroideremia

    363.56 Other diffuse or generalized dystrophy, partial
        Diffuse choroidal sclerosis

    363.57 Other diffuse or generalized dystrophy, total
        Generalized gyrate atrophy, choroid

⑤ **363.6 Choroidal hemorrhage and rupture**

    363.61 Choroidal hemorrhage, unspecified

    363.62 Expulsive choroidal hemorrhage

    363.63 Choroidal rupture

⑤ **363.7 Choroidal detachment**

    363.70 Choroidal detachment, unspecified

    363.71 Serous choroidal detachment

    363.72 Hemorrhagic choroidal detachment

363.8 Other disorders of choroid

363.9 Unspecified disorder of choroid

364 Disorders of iris and ciliary body

⑤ **364.0 Acute and subacute iridocyclitis**
    Anterior uveitis, acute, subacute
    Cyclitis, acute, subacute
    Iridocyclitis, acute, subacute
    Iritis, acute, subacute

    Excludes: gonococcal (098.41)
          herpes simplex (054.44)
          herpes zoster (053.22)

    364.00 Acute and subacute iridocyclitis, unspecified

    364.01 Primary iridocyclitis

    364.02 Recurrent iridocyclitis

    364.03 Secondary iridocyclitis, infectious

    364.04 Secondary iridocyclitis, noninfectious
        Aqueous:
          cells
          fibrin
          flare

    364.05 Hypopyon

⑤ **364.1 Chronic iridocyclitis**

    Excludes: posterior cyclitis (363.21)

    364.10 Chronic iridocyclitis, unspecified

	Add 4th or 5th digit		Nonspecific code		Unspecified code		Manifestation code

335

364.11 Chronic iridocyclitis in diseases classified elsewhere
Code first underlying disease, as:
sarcoidosis (135)
tuberculosis (017.3)

Excludes: syphilitic iridocyclitis (091.52)

⑤ **364.2 Certain types of iridocyclitis**

Excludes: posterior cyclitis (363.21)
sympathetic uveitis (360.11)

364.21 Fuchs' heterochromic cyclitis

364.22 Glaucomatocyclitic crises

364.23 Lens-induced iridocyclitis

364.24 Vogt-Koyanagi syndrome

364.3 Unspecified iridocyclitis
Uveitis NOS

⑤ **364.4 Vascular disorders of iris and ciliary body**

364.41 Hyphema
Hemorrhage of iris or ciliary body

364.42 Rubeosis iridis
Neovascularization of iris or ciliary body

⑤ **364.5 Degenerations of iris and ciliary body**

364.51 Essential or progressive iris atrophy

364.52 Iridoschisis

364.53 Pigmentary iris degeneration
Acquired heterochromia of iris
Pigment dispersion syndrome of iris
Translucency of iris

364.54 Degeneration of pupillary margin
Atrophy of sphincter of iris
Ectropion of pigment epithelium of iris

364.55 Miotic cysts of pupillary margin

364.56 Degenerative changes of chamber angle

364.57 Degenerative changes of ciliary body

364.59 Other iris atrophy
Iris atrophy (generalized) (sector shaped)

⑤ **364.6 Cysts of iris, ciliary body, and anterior chamber**

Excludes: miotic pupillary cyst (364.55)
parasitic cyst (360.13)

364.60 Idiopathic cysts

364.61 Implantation cysts
Epithelial down-growth, anterior chamber
Implantation cysts (surgical) (traumatic)

364.62 Exudative cysts of iris or anterior chamber

364.63 Primary cyst of pars plana

364.64 Exudative cyst of pars plana

⑤ **364.7 Adhesions and disruptions of iris and ciliary body**

Excludes: flat anterior chamber (360.34)

364.70 Adhesions of iris, unspecified
Synechiae (iris) NOS

364.71 Posterior synechiae

364.72 Anterior synechiae

364.73 Goniosynechiae
Peripheral anterior synechiae

364.74 Pupillary membranes
Iris bombé
Pupillary:
occlusion
seclusion

● Code new to this edition   ▲ Revision of existing code   ④ ⑤ Fourth or fifth digit required

364.75 Pupillary abnormalities
Deformed pupil   Rupture of sphincter, pupil
Ectopic pupil

364.76 Iridodialysis

364.77 Recession of chamber angle

⑤ **364.8 Other disorders of iris and ciliary body**

364.81 Floppy iris syndrome
Intraoperative floppy iris syndrome (IFIS)

Use additional E code to identify cause, such as:
sympatholytics [antiadrenergics] causing adverse effect in therapeutic use (E941.3)

364.82 Plateau iris syndrome

364.89 Other disorders of iris and ciliary body
Prolapse of iris NOS

Excludes: *prolapse of iris in recent wound (871.1)*

364.9 Unspecified disorder of iris and ciliary body

365 Glaucoma

Excludes: *blind hypertensive eye [absolute glaucoma] (360.42)*
congenital glaucoma (743.20-743.22)

⑤ **365.0 Borderline glaucoma [glaucoma suspect]**

365.00 Preglaucoma, unspecified

365.01 Open angle with borderline findings
Open angle with:
borderline intraocular pressure
cupping of optic discs

365.02 Anatomical narrow angle

365.03 Steroid responders

365.04 Ocular hypertension

⑤ **365.1 Open-angle glaucoma**

365.10 Open-angle glaucoma, unspecified
Wide-angle glaucoma NOS

365.11 Primary open angle glaucoma
Chronic simple glaucoma

365.12 Low tension glaucoma

365.13 Pigmentary glaucoma

365.14 Glaucoma of childhood
Infantile or juvenile glaucoma

365.15 Residual stage of open angle glaucoma

⑤ **365.2 Primary angle-closure glaucoma**

365.20 Primary angle-closure glaucoma, unspecified

365.21 Intermittent angle-closure glaucoma
Angle-closure glaucoma:
interval
subacute

365.22 Acute angle-closure glaucoma

365.23 Chronic angle-closure glaucoma

365.24 Residual stage of angle-closure glaucoma

⑤ **365.3 Corticosteroid-induced glaucoma**

365.31 Glaucomatous stage

365.32 Residual stage

⑤ **365.4 Glaucoma associated with congenital anomalies, dystrophies, and systemic syndromes**

365.41 *Glaucoma associated with chamber angle anomalies*

365.42 *Glaucoma associated with anomalies of iris*

365.43 *Glaucoma associated with other anterior segment anomalies*

365.44 *Glaucoma associated with systemic syndromes*
Code first associated disease, as:
neurofibromatosis (237.7)
Sturge-Weber (-Dimitri) syndrome (759.6)

	Add 4th or 5th digit		Nonspecific code		Unspecified code		Manifestation code

⑤ **365.5 Glaucoma associated with disorders of the lens**

    365.51 Phacolytic glaucoma

    365.52 Pseudoexfoliation glaucoma

    365.59 Glaucoma associated with other lens disorders

⑤ **365.6 Glaucoma associated with other ocular disorders**

    365.60 Glaucoma associated with unspecified ocular disorder

    365.61 Glaucoma associated with pupillary block

    365.62 Glaucoma associated with ocular inflammations

    365.63 Glaucoma associated with vascular disorders

    365.64 Glaucoma associated with tumors or cysts

    365.65 Glaucoma associated with ocular trauma

⑤ **365.8 Other specified forms of glaucoma**

    365.81 Hypersecretion glaucoma

    365.82 Glaucoma with increased episcleral venous pressure

    365.83 Aqueous misdirection
        Malignant glaucoma

    365.89 Other specified glaucoma

  365.9 Unspecified glaucoma

366 Cataract

    Excludes: *congenital cataract (743.30-743.34)*

⑤ **366.0 Infantile, juvenile, and presenile cataract**

    366.00 Nonsenile cataract, unspecified

    366.01 Anterior subcapsular polar cataract

    366.02 Posterior subcapsular polar cataract

    366.03 Cortical, lamellar, or zonular cataract

    366.04 Nuclear cataract

    366.09 Other and combined forms of nonsenile cataract

⑤ **366.1 Senile cataract**

    366.10 Senile cataract, unspecified

    366.11 Pseudoexfoliation of lens capsule

    366.12 Incipient cataract
        Cataract: Water clefts
          coronary
          immature NOS
          punctate

    366.13 Anterior subcapsular polar senile cataract

    366.14 Posterior subcapsular polar senile cataract

    366.15 Cortical senile cataract

    366.16 Nuclear sclerosis
        Cataracta brunescens
        Nuclear cataract

    366.17 Total or mature cataract

    366.18 Hypermature cataract
        Morgagni cataract

    366.19 Other and combined forms of senile cataract

⑤ **366.2 Traumatic cataract**

    366.20 Traumatic cataract, unspecified

    366.21 Localized traumatic opacities
        Vossius' ring

    366.22 Total traumatic cataract

    366.23 Partially resolved traumatic cataract

⑤ **366.3 Cataract secondary to ocular disorders**

    366.30 Cataracts complicata, unspecified

    366.31 Glaucomatous flecks (subcapsular)
        Code first underlying glaucoma (365.0-365.9)

● Code new to this edition   ▲ Revision of existing code   ④ ⑤ Fourth or fifth digit required

366.32 *Cataract in inflammatory disorders*
Code first underlying condition, as:
chronic choroiditis (363.0-363.2)

366.33 *Cataract with neovascularization*
Code first underlying condition, as:
chronic iridocyclitis (364.10)

366.34 *Cataract in degenerative disorders*
Sunflower cataract
Code first underlying condition, as:
chalcosis (360.24)
degenerative myopia (360.21)
pigmentary retinal dystrophy (362.74)

⑤ **366.4 Cataract associated with other disorders**

366.41 *Diabetic cataract*
Code first diabetes (249.5, 250.5)

366.42 *Tetanic cataract*
Code first underlying disease, as:
calcinosis (275.4)
hypoparathyroidism (252.1)

366.43 *Myotonic cataract*
Code first underlying disorder (359.21, 359.23)

366.44 *Cataract associated with other syndromes*
Code first underlying condition, as:
craniofacial dysostosis (756.0)
galactosemia (271.1)

366.45 Toxic cataract
Drug-induced cataract

Use additional E code, if desired, to identify drug or other toxic substance

366.46 Cataract associated with radiation and other physical influences
Use additional E code, if desired, to identify cause

⑤ **366.5 After-cataract**

366.50 After-cataract, unspecified
Secondary cataract NOS

366.51 Soemmering's ring

366.52 Other after-cataract, not obscuring vision

366.53 After-cataract, obscuring vision

366.8 Other cataract
Calcification of lens

366.9 Unspecified cataract

367 Disorders of refraction and accommodation

367.0 Hypermetropia
Far-sightedness
Hyperopia

367.1 Myopia
Near-sightedness

⑤ **367.2 Astigmatism**

367.20 Astigmatism, unspecified

367.21 Regular astigmatism

367.22 Irregular astigmatism

⑤ **367.3 Anisometropia and aniseikonia**

367.31 Anisometropia

367.32 Aniseikonia

367.4 Presbyopia

⑤ **367.5 Disorders of accommodation**

367.51 Paresis of accommodation
Cycloplegia

367.52 Total or complete internal ophthalmoplegia

367.53 Spasm of accommodation

⑤ **367.8 Other disorders of refraction and accommodation**

367.81 Transient refractive change

Add 4th or 5th digit	Nonspecific code	Unspecified code	Manifestation code

367.89 Other
Drug-induced disorders of refraction and accommodation
Toxic disorders of refraction and accommodation

367.9 Unspecified disorder of refraction and accommodation

368 Visual disturbances

> Excludes: *electrophysiological disturbances (794.11-794.14)*

⑤ **368.0 Amblyopia ex anopsia**

368.00 Amblyopia, unspecified

368.01 Strabismic amblyopia
Suppression amblyopia

368.02 Deprivation amblyopia

368.03 Refractive amblyopia

⑤ **368.1 Subjective visual disturbances**

368.10 Subjective visual disturbance, unspecified

368.11 Sudden visual loss

368.12 Transient visual loss
Concentric fading
Scintillating scotoma

368.13 Visual discomfort
Asthenopia   Photophobia
Eye strain

368.14 Visual distortions of shape and size
Macropsia   Micropsia
Metamorphopsia

368.15 Other visual distortions and entoptic phenomena
Photopsia   Visual halos
Refractive:
    diplopia
    polyopia

368.16 Psychophysical visual disturbances
Prosopagnosia
Visual:
    agnosia
    disorientation syndrome
    hallucinations
    object agnosia

368.2 Diplopia
Double vision

⑤ **368.3 Other disorders of binocular vision**

368.30 Binocular vision disorder, unspecified

368.31 Suppression of binocular vision

368.32 Simultaneous visual perception without fusion

368.33 Fusion with defective stereopsis

368.34 Abnormal retinal correspondence

⑤ **368.4 Visual field defects**

368.40 Visual field defect, unspecified

368.41 Scotoma involving central area
Scotoma:
    central
    centrocecal
    paracentral

368.42 Scotoma of blind spot area
Enlarged: Paracecal scotoma
    angioscotoma
    blind spot

368.43 Sector or arcuate defects
Scotoma:
    arcuate
    Bjerrum
    Seidel

● Code new   ▲ Revision of   ④ ⑤ Fourth or fifth
   to this edition   existing code   digit required

368.44 **Other localized visual field defect**
Scotoma: Visual field defect:
 NOS   nasal step
 ring   peripheral

368.45 **Generalized contraction or constriction**

368.46 **Homonymous bilateral field defects**
Hemianopsia (altitudinal) (homonymous)
Quadrant anopia

368.47 **Heteronymous bilateral field defects**
Hemianopsia:
 binasal
 bitemporal

⑤ **368.5** **Color vision deficiencies**
Color blindness

368.51 **Protan defect**
Protanomaly
Protanopia

368.52 **Deutan defect**
Deuteranomaly
Deuteranopia

368.53 **Tritan defect**
Tritanomaly
Tritanopia

368.54 **Achromatopsia**
Monochromatism (cone) (rod)

368.55 **Acquired color vision deficiencies**

368.59 **Other color vision deficiencies**

⑤ **368.6** **Night blindness**
Nyctalopia

368.60 **Night blindness, unspecified**

368.61 **Congenital night blindness**
Hereditary night blindness
Oguchi's disease

368.62 **Acquired night blindness**

Excludes: that due to vitamin A deficiency (264.5)

368.63 **Abnormal dark adaptation curve**
Abnormal threshold of cones or rods
Delayed adaptation of cones or rods

368.69 **Other night blindness**

368.8 **Other specified visual disturbances**
Blurred vision NOS

368.9 **Unspecified visual disturbance**

369 **Blindness and low vision**
Note: Visual impairment refers to a functional limitation of the eye (e.g., limited visual acuity or visual field). It should be distinguished from visual disability, indicating a limitation of the abilities of the individual (e.g., limited reading skills, vocational skills), and from visual handicap, indicating a limitation of personal and socioeconomic independence (e.g., limited mobility, limited employability.)

The levels of impairment defined in the table in this section are based on the recommendations of the WHO Study Group on Prevention of Blindness (Geneva, November 6-10, 1972; WHO Technical Report Series 518), and of the International Council of Ophthalmology (1976).
Note that definitions of blindness vary in different settings.

For international reporting WHO defines blindness as profound impairment. This definition can be applied to blindness of one eye (369.1, 369.6) and to blindness of the individual (369.0).

For determination of benefits in the U.S.A., the definition of legal blindness as severe impairment is often used. This definition applies to blindness of the individual only.

Excludes: correctable impaired vision due to refractive errors (367.0-367.9)

	Add 4th or 5th digit		Nonspecific code		Unspecified code		Manifestation code

Classification		LEVELS OF VISUAL IMPAIRMENT					Additional Descriptors
"legal"	WHO	Visual Acuity and/or Visual Field Limitation (whichever is worse)					which may be encountered
LEGAL BLINDNESS	(NEAR-) NORMAL VISION	**RANGE OF NORMAL VISION** 20/10 20/13 20/16 20/20 20/25 0.7 0.6 0.5 0.4 0.8					
		NEAR-NORMAL VISION 20/30 20/40 20/50 20/60 0.7 0.6 0.5 0.4 0.4					
	LOW VISION	**MODERATE VISUAL IMPAIRMENT** 20/70 20/80 20/100 20/125 20/160 0.25 0.20 0.16 0.12					Moderate low vision
		SEVERE VISUAL IMPAIRMENT 20/200 20/250 20/320 20/400 0.10 0.08 0.06 0.05 Visual Field: 20 degrees or less					Severe low vision, "legal blindness"
	BLINDNESS	**PROFOUND VISUAL IMPAIRMENT** 20/500 20/630 20/800 20/1000 0.04 0.03 0.025 0.02 Count Fingers at: less than 3 m (10ft) Visual Field: 10 degrees or less					Profound low vision, moderate blindness
		NEAR-TOTAL VISUAL IMPAIRMENT Visual Acuity: less than 0.02 (20/1000) Count Fingers at: 1 m (3 ft) or less Hand Movements: 5m (15ft) or less Light projection, light perception Visual Field: 5 degrees or less					Severe blindness Near-Total blindness
(USA) both eyes	(WHO) one or both eyes	**TOTAL VISUAL IMPAIRMENT** No light perception (NLP)					Total blindness

Visual acuity refers to best achievable acuity with correction
Non-listed Snellen fractions may be classified by converting to the nearest decimal equivalent, e.g., 10/200=0.05, 6/30=0.20
CF (count fingers) without designation of distance, may be classified to profound impairment
HM (hand motion) without designation of distance, may be classified to near-total impairment.
Visual field measurements refer to the largest field diameter for a 1/100 white test object.

⑤ **369.0 Profound impairment, both eyes**

     `369.00` **Impairment level not further specified**
         Blindness:
         NOS according to WHO definition
         both eyes

     369.01 **Better eye: total impairment;**
         lesser eye: total impairment

     `369.02` **Better eye: near-total impairment;**
         lesser eye: not further specified

     369.03 **Better eye: near-total impairment;**
         lesser eye: total impairment

     369.04 **Better eye: near-total impairment;**
         lesser eye: near-total impairment

     `369.05` **Better eye: profound impairment;**
         lesser eye: not further specified

     369.06 **Better eye: profound impairment;**
         lesser eye: total impairment

     369.07 **Better eye: profound impairment;**
         lesser eye: near-total impairment

     369.08 **Better eye: profound impairment;**
         lesser eye: profound impairment

● Code new   ▲ Revision of   ④ ⑤ Fourth or fifth
      to this edition   existing code   digit required

⑤ **369.1 Moderate or severe impairment, better eye, profound impairment lesser eye**

369.10 Impairment level not further specified
Blindness, one eye, low vision other eye

369.11 Better eye: severe impairment;
lesser eye: blind, not further specified

369.12 Better eye: severe impairment;
lesser eye: total impairment

369.13 Better eye: severe impairment;
lesser eye: near-total impairment

369.14 Better eye: severe impairment;
lesser eye: profound impairment

369.15 Better eye: moderate impairment;
lesser eye: blind, not further specified

369.16 Better eye: moderate impairment;
lesser eye: total impairment

369.17 Better eye: moderate impairment;
lesser eye: near-total impairment

369.18 Better eye: moderate impairment;
lesser eye: profound impairment

⑤ **369.2 Moderate or severe impairment, both eyes**

369.20 Impairment level not further specified
Low vision, both eyes NOS

369.21 Better eye: severe impairment;
lesser eye: not further specified

369.22 Better eye: severe impairment;
lesser eye: severe impairment

369.23 Better eye: moderate impairment;
lesser eye: not further specified

369.24 Better eye: moderate impairment;
lesser eye: severe impairment

369.25 Better eye: moderate impairment;
lesser eye: moderate impairment

369.3 Unqualified visual loss, both eyes

Excludes: blindness NOS:
legal [U.S.A. definition] (369.4)
WHO definition (369.00)

369.4 Legal blindness, as defined in U.S.A.
Blindness NOS according to U.S.A. definition

Excludes: legal blindness with specification of impairment level (369.01-369.08,
369.11-369.14, 369.21-369.22)

⑤ **369.6 Profound impairment, one eye**

369.60 Impairment level not further specified
Blindness, one eye

369.61 One eye: total impairment; other eye: not specified

369.62 One eye: total impairment; other eye: near-normal vision

369.63 One eye: total impairment; other eye: normal vision

369.64 One eye: near-total impairment; other eye: not specified

369.65 One eye: near-total impairment; other eye: near-normal vision

369.66 One eye: near-total impairment; other eye: normal vision

369.67 One eye: profound impairment; other eye: not specified

369.68 One eye: profound impairment; other eye: near-normal vision

369.69 One eye: profound impairment; other eye: normal vision

⑤ **369.7 Moderate or severe impairment, one eye**

369.70 Impairment level not further specified
Low vision, one eye

369.71 One eye: severe impairment; other eye: not specified

369.72 One eye: severe impairment; other eye: near-normal vision

369.73 One eye: severe impairment; other eye: normal vision

| | Add 4th or 5th digit | | Nonspecific code | | Unspecified code | | Manifestation code |

369.74	**One eye: moderate impairment; other eye: not specified**
369.75	**One eye: moderate impairment; other eye: near-normal vision**
369.76	**One eye: moderate impairment; other eye: normal vision**

369.8 **Unqualified visual loss, one eye**

369.9 **Unspecified visual loss**

370 **Keratitis**

⑤ **370.0** **Corneal ulcer**

Excludes: *that due to vitamin A deficiency (264.3)*

370.00	**Corneal ulcer, unspecified**
370.01	**Marginal corneal ulcer**
370.02	**Ring corneal ulcer**
370.03	**Central corneal ulcer**
370.04	**Hypopyon ulcer** Serpiginous ulcer
370.05	**Mycotic corneal ulcer**
370.06	**Perforated corneal ulcer**
370.07	**Mooren's ulcer**

⑤ **370.2** **Superficial keratitis without conjunctivitis**

Excludes: *dendritic [herpes simplex] keratitis (054.42)*

370.20	**Superficial keratitis, unspecified**
370.21	**Punctate keratitis** Thygeson's superficial punctate keratitis
370.22	**Macular keratitis**

Keratitis:	Keratitis:
areolar	stellate
nummular	striate

370.23	**Filamentary keratitis**
370.24	**Photokeratitis** Snow blindness Welders' keratitis

⑤ **370.3** **Certain types of keratoconjunctivitis**

370.31	**Phlyctenular keratoconjunctivitis** Phlyctenulosis

Use additional code for any associated tuberculosis (017.3)

370.32	**Limbar and corneal involvement in vernal conjunctivitis**

Use additional code for vernal conjunctivitis (372.13)

370.33	**Keratoconjunctivitis sicca, not specified as Sjögren's**

Excludes: *Sjögren's syndrome (710.2)*

370.34	**Exposure keratoconjunctivitis**
370.35	**Neurotrophic keratoconjunctivitis**

⑤ **370.4** **Other and unspecified keratoconjunctivitis**

370.40	**Keratoconjunctivitis, unspecified** Superficial keratitis with conjunctivitis NOS
370.44	***Keratitis or keratoconjunctivitis in exanthema*** *Code first underlying condition (050.0-052.9)*

Excludes: *herpes simplex (054.43)*
herpes zoster (053.21)
measles (055.71)

370.49	**Other**

Excludes: *epidemic keratoconjunctivitis (077.1)*

⑤ **370.5** **Interstitial and deep keratitis**

370.50	**Interstitial keratitis, unspecified**
370.52	**Diffuse interstitial keratitis** Cogan's syndrome
370.54	**Sclerosing keratitis**
370.55	**Corneal abscess**

● Code new to this edition	▲ Revision of existing code	④ ⑤ Fourth or fifth digit required

370.59 Other

Excludes: *disciform herpes simplex keratitis (054.43)*
syphilitic keratitis (090.3)

⑤ **370.6** **Corneal neovascularization**

370.60 Corneal neovascularization, unspecified

370.61 Localized vascularization of cornea

370.62 Pannus (corneal)

370.63 Deep vascularization of cornea

370.64 Ghost vessels (corneal)

370.8 **Other forms of keratitis**

Code first underlying condition, such as:
Acanthamoeba (136.21)
Fusarium (118)

370.9 **Unspecified keratitis**

371 **Corneal opacity and other disorders of cornea**

⑤ **371.0** **Corneal scars and opacities**

Excludes: *that due to vitamin A deficiency (264.6)*

371.00 Corneal opacity, unspecified
Corneal scar NOS

371.01 Minor opacity of cornea
Corneal nebula

371.02 Peripheral opacity of cornea
Corneal macula not interfering with central vision

371.03 Central opacity of cornea
Corneal:
leucoma interfering with central vision
macula interfering with central vision

371.04 Adherent leucoma

371.05 *Phthisical cornea*
Code first underlying tuberculosis (017.3)

⑤ **371.1** **Corneal pigmentations and deposits**

371.10 Corneal deposit, unspecified

371.11 Anterior pigmentations
Stähli's lines

371.12 Stromal pigmentations
Hematocornea

371.13 Posterior pigmentations
Krukenberg spindle

371.14 Kayser-Fleischer ring

371.15 Other deposits associated with metabolic disorders

371.16 Argentous deposits

⑤ **371.2** **Corneal edema**

371.20 Corneal edema, unspecified

371.21 Idiopathic corneal edema

371.22 Secondary corneal edema

371.23 Bullous keratopathy

371.24 Corneal edema due to wearing of contact lenses

⑤ **371.3** **Changes of corneal membranes**

371.30 Corneal membrane change, unspecified

371.31 Folds and rupture of Bowman's membrane

371.32 Folds in Descemet's membrane

371.33 Rupture in Descemet's membrane

⑤ **371.4** **Corneal degenerations**

371.40 Corneal degeneration, unspecified

	Add 4th or 5th digit		Nonspecific code		Unspecified code		Manifestation code

371.41 **Senile corneal changes**
Arcus senilis
Hassall-Henle bodies

371.42 **Recurrent erosion of cornea**

Excludes: Mooren's ulcer (370.07)

371.43 **Band-shaped keratopathy**

371.44 **Other calcerous degenerations of cornea**

371.45 **Keratomalacia NOS**

Excludes: that due to vitamin A deficiency (264.4)

371.46 **Nodular degeneration of cornea**
Salzmann's nodular dystrophy

371.48 **Peripheral degenerations of cornea**
Marginal degeneration of cornea [Terrien's]

371.49 **Other**
Discrete colliquative keratopathy

⑤ **371.5** **Hereditary corneal dystrophies**

371.50 **Corneal dystrophy, unspecified**

371.51 **Juvenile epithelial corneal dystrophy**

371.52 **Other anterior corneal dystrophies**
Corneal dystrophy:
microscopic cystic
ring-like

371.53 **Granular corneal dystrophy**

371.54 **Lattice corneal dystrophy**

371.55 **Macular corneal dystrophy**

371.56 **Other stromal corneal dystrophies**
Crystalline corneal dystrophy

371.57 **Endothelial corneal dystrophy**
Combined corneal dystrophy
Cornea guttata
Fuchs' endothelial dystrophy

371.58 **Other posterior corneal dystrophies**
Polymorphous corneal dystrophy

⑤ **371.6** **Keratoconus**

371.60 **Keratoconus, unspecified**

371.61 **Keratoconus, stable condition**

371.62 **Keratoconus, acute hydrops**

⑤ **371.7** **Other corneal deformities**

371.70 **Corneal deformity, unspecified**

371.71 **Corneal ectasia**

371.72 **Descemetocele**

371.73 **Corneal staphyloma**

⑤ **371.8** **Other corneal disorders**

371.81 **Corneal anesthesia and hypoesthesia**

371.82 **Corneal disorder due to contact lens**

Excludes: corneal edema due to contact lens (371.24)

371.89 **Other**

371.9 **Unspecified corneal disorder**

372 **Disorders of conjunctiva**

Excludes: keratoconjunctivitis (370.3-370.4)

⑤ **372.0** **Acute conjunctivitis**

372.00 **Acute conjunctivitis, unspecified**

372.01 **Serous conjunctivitis, except viral**

Excludes: viral conjunctivitis NOS (077.9)

● Code new
to this edition　　▲ Revision of
existing code　　④ ⑤ Fourth or fifth
digit required

372.02 Acute follicular conjunctivitis
Conjunctival folliculosis NOS

Excludes: *conjunctivitis:*
adenoviral (acute follicular) (077.3)
epidemic hemorrhagic (077.4)
inclusion (077.0)
Newcastle (077.8)
epidemic keratoconjunctivitis (077.1)
pharyngoconjunctival fever (077.2)

372.03 Other mucopurulent conjunctivitis
Catarrhal conjunctivitis

Excludes: *blennorrhea neonatorum (gonococcal) (098.40)*
neonatal conjunctivitis (771.6)
ophthalmia neonatorum NOS (771.6)

372.04 Pseudomembranous conjunctivitis
Membranous conjunctivitis

Excludes: *diphtheritic conjunctivitis (032.81)*

372.05 Acute atopic conjunctivitis

● **372.06 Acute chemical conjunctivitis**
Acute toxic conjunctivitis

Use addtional E code to identify the chemical or toxic agent

Excludes: *burn of eye and adnexa (940.0-940.9)*
chemical corrosion injury of eye (940.2-940.3)

⑤ **372.1 Chronic conjunctivitis**

372.10 Chronic conjunctivitis, unspecified

372.11 Simple chronic conjunctivitis

372.12 Chronic follicular conjunctivitis

372.13 Vernal conjunctivitis

372.14 Other chronic allergic conjunctivitis

372.15 *Parasitic conjunctivitis*
Code first underlying disease, as:
filariasis (125.0-125.9)
mucocutaneous leishmaniasis (085.5)

⑤ **372.2 Blepharoconjunctivitis**

372.20 Blepharoconjunctivitis, unspecified

372.21 Angular blepharoconjunctivitis

372.22 Contact blepharoconjunctivitis

⑤ **372.3 Other and unspecified conjunctivitis**

372.30 Conjunctivitis, unspecified

372.31 *Rosacea conjunctivitis*
Code first underlying rosacea dermatitis (695.3)

372.33 *Conjunctivitis in mucocutaneous disease*
Code first underlying disease, as:
erythema multiforme (695.10-695.19)
Reiter's disease (099.3)

Excludes: *ocular pemphigoid (694.61)*

372.34 Pingueculitis

Excludes: *pinguecula (372.51)*

372.39 Other

⑤ **372.4 Pterygium**

Excludes: *pseudopterygium (372.52)*

372.40 Pterygium, unspecified

372.41 Peripheral pterygium, stationary

372.42 Peripheral pterygium, progressive

372.43 Central pterygium

372.44 Double pterygium

372.45 Recurrent pterygium

| Add 4th or 5th digit | Nonspecific code | Unspecified code | Manifestation code |

⑤ **372.5 Conjunctival degenerations and deposits**

    372.50 Conjunctival degeneration, unspecified

    372.51 Pinguecula

    Excludes: *pingueculitis (372.34)*

    372.52 Pseudopterygium

    372.53 Conjunctival xerosis

    Excludes: *conjunctival xerosis due to vitamin A deficiency (264.0, 264.1, 264.7)*

    372.54 Conjunctival concretions

    372.55 Conjunctival pigmentations
        Conjunctival argyrosis

    372.56 Conjunctival deposits

⑤ **372.6 Conjunctival scars**

    372.61 Granuloma of conjunctiva

    372.62 Localized adhesions and strands of conjunctiva

    372.63 Symblepharon
        Extensive adhesions of conjunctiva

    372.64 Scarring of conjunctiva
        Contraction of eye socket (after enucleation)

⑤ **372.7 Conjunctival vascular disorders and cysts**

    372.71 Hyperemia of conjunctiva

    372.72 Conjunctival hemorrhage
        Hyposphagma
        Subconjunctival hemorrhage

    372.73 Conjunctival edema
        Chemosis of conjunctiva
        Subconjunctival edema

    372.74 Vascular abnormalities of conjunctiva
        Aneurysm(ata) of conjunctiva

    372.75 Conjunctival cysts

⑤ **372.8 Other disorders of conjunctiva**

    372.81 Conjunctivochalasis

    372.89 Other disorders of conjunctiva

  372.9 Unspecified disorder of conjunctiva

373 **Inflammation of eyelids**

⑤ **373.0 Blepharitis**

    Excludes: *blepharoconjunctivitis (372.20-372.22)*

    373.00 Blepharitis, unspecified

    373.01 Ulcerative blepharitis

    373.02 Squamous blepharitis

⑤ **373.1 Hordeolum and other deep inflammation of eyelid**

    373.11 Hordeolum externum
        Hordeolum NOS
        Stye

    373.12 Hordeolum internum
        Infection of meibomian gland

    373.13 Abscess of eyelid
        Furuncle of eyelid

  373.2 Chalazion
      Meibomian (gland) cyst

    Excludes: *infected meibomian gland (373.12)*

⑤ **373.3 Noninfectious dermatoses of eyelid**

    373.31 Eczematous dermatitis of eyelid

    373.32 Contact and allergic dermatitis of eyelid

    373.33 Xeroderma of eyelid

    373.34 Discoid lupus erythematosus of eyelid

● Code new
to this edition

▲ Revision of
existing code

④ ⑤ Fourth or fifth
digit required

373.4 *Infective dermatitis of eyelid of types resulting in deformity*
Code first underlying disease, as:
 leprosy (030.0-030.9)
 lupus vulgaris (tuberculous) (017.0)
 yaws (102.0-102.9)

373.5 *Other infective dermatitis of eyelid*
Code first underlying disease, as:
 actinomycosis (039.3)
 impetigo (684)
 mycotic dermatitis (110.0-111.9)
 vaccinia (051.0)
 postvaccination (999.0)

Excludes: *herpes:*
 simplex (054.41)
 zoster (053.20)

373.6 *Parasitic infestation of eyelid*
Code first underlying disease, as:
 leishmaniasis (085.0-085.9)
 loiasis (125.2)
 onchocerciasis (125.3)
 pediculosis (132.0)

373.8 **Other inflammations of eyelids**

373.9 **Unspecified inflammation of eyelid**

374 **Other disorders of eyelids**

⑤ **374.0** **Entropion and trichiasis of eyelid**

 374.00 **Entropion, unspecified**

 374.01 **Senile entropion**

 374.02 **Mechanical entropion**

 374.03 **Spastic entropion**

 374.04 **Cicatricial entropion**

 374.05 **Trichiasis without entropion**

⑤ **374.1** **Ectropion**

 374.10 **Ectropion, unspecified**

 374.11 **Senile ectropion**

 374.12 **Mechanical ectropion**

 374.13 **Spastic ectropion**

 374.14 **Cicatricial ectropion**

⑤ **374.2** **Lagophthalmos**

 374.20 **Lagophthalmos, unspecified**

 374.21 **Paralytic lagophthalmos**

 374.22 **Mechanical lagophthalmos**

 374.23 **Cicatricial lagophthalmos**

⑤ **374.3** **Ptosis of eyelid**

 374.30 **Ptosis of eyelid, unspecified**

 374.31 **Paralytic ptosis**

 374.32 **Myogenic ptosis**

 374.33 **Mechanical ptosis**

 374.34 **Blepharochalasis**
 Pseudoptosis

⑤ **374.4** **Other disorders affecting eyelid function**

Excludes: *blepharoclonus (333.81)*
 blepharospasm (333.81)
 facial nerve palsy (351.0)
 third nerve palsy or paralysis (378.51-378.52)
 tic (psychogenic) (307.20-307.23)
 organic (333.3)

 374.41 **Lid retraction or lag**

	Add 4th or 5th digit		Nonspecific code		Unspecified code		Manifestation code

374.43 Abnormal innervation syndrome
Jaw-blinking
Paradoxical facial movements

374.44 Sensory disorders

374.45 Other sensorimotor disorders
Deficient blink reflex

374.46 Blepharophimosis
Ankyloblepharon

⑤ **374.5 Degenerative disorders of eyelid and periocular area**

374.50 Degenerative disorder of eyelid, unspecified

374.51 *Xanthelasma*
Xanthoma (planum) (tuberosum) of eyelid
Code first underlying condition (272.0-272.9)

374.52 Hyperpigmentation of eyelid
Chloasma
Dyspigmentation

374.53 Hypopigmentation of eyelid
Vitiligo of eyelid

374.54 Hypertrichosis of eyelid

374.55 Hypotrichosis of eyelid
Madarosis of eyelid

374.56 Other degenerative disorders of skin affecting eyelid

⑤ **374.8 Other disorders of eyelid**

374.81 Hemorrhage of eyelid
Excludes: *black eye (921.0)*

374.82 Edema of eyelid
Hyperemia of eyelid

374.83 Elephantiasis of eyelid

374.84 Cysts of eyelids
Sebaceous cyst of eyelid

374.85 Vascular anomalies of eyelid

374.86 Retained foreign body of eyelid

374.87 Dermatochalasis

374.89 Other disorders of eyelid

374.9 Unspecified disorder of eyelid

375 Disorders of lacrimal system

⑤ **375.0 Dacryoadenitis**

375.00 Dacryoadenitis, unspecified

375.01 Acute dacryoadenitis

375.02 Chronic dacryoadenitis

375.03 Chronic enlargement of lacrimal gland

⑤ **375.1 Other disorders of lacrimal gland**

375.11 Dacryops

375.12 Other lacrimal cysts and cystic degeneration

375.13 Primary lacrimal atrophy

375.14 Secondary lacrimal atrophy

375.15 Tear film insufficiency, unspecified
Dry eye syndrome

375.16 Dislocation of lacrimal gland

⑤ **375.2 Epiphora**

375.20 Epiphora, unspecified as to cause

375.21 Epiphora due to excess lacrimation

375.22 Epiphora due to insufficient drainage

⑤ **375.3 Acute and unspecified inflammation of lacrimal passages**
Excludes: *neonatal dacryocystitis (771.6)*

375.30 Dacryocystitis, unspecified

● Code new
to this edition

▲ Revision of
existing code

④ ⑤ Fourth or fifth
digit required

375.31   **Acute canaliculitis, lacrimal**

375.32   **Acute dacryocystitis**
       Acute peridacryocystitis

375.33   **Phlegmonous dacryocystitis**

⑤ **375.4 Chronic inflammation of lacrimal passages**

375.41   **Chronic canaliculitis**

375.42   **Chronic dacryocystitis**

375.43   **Lacrimal mucocele**

⑤ **375.5 Stenosis and insufficiency of lacrimal passages**

375.51   **Eversion of lacrimal punctum**

375.52   **Stenosis of lacrimal punctum**

375.53   **Stenosis of lacrimal canaliculi**

375.54   **Stenosis of lacrimal sac**

375.55   **Obstruction of nasolacrimal duct, neonatal**

Excludes:	congenital anomaly of nasolacrimal duct (743.65)

375.56   **Stenosis of nasolacrimal duct, acquired**

375.57   **Dacryolith**

⑤ **375.6 Other changes of lacrimal passages**

375.61   **Lacrimal fistula**

`375.69`   **Other**

⑤ **375.8 Other disorders of lacrimal system**

375.81   **Granuloma of lacrimal passages**

`375.89`   **Other**

375.9 Unspecified disorder of lacrimal system

`376` **Disorders of the orbit**

⑤ **376.0 Acute inflammation of orbit**

`376.00`   **Acute inflammation of orbit, unspecified**

376.01   **Orbital cellulitis**
       Abscess of orbit

376.02   **Orbital periostitis**

376.03   **Orbital osteomyelitis**

376.04   **Tenonitis**

⑤ **376.1 Chronic inflammatory disorders of orbit**

`376.10`   **Chronic inflammation of orbit, unspecified**

376.11   **Orbital granuloma**
       Pseudotumor (inflammatory) of orbit

376.12   **Orbital myositis**

`376.13`   *Parasitic infestation of orbit*
       Code first underlying disease, as:
       hydatid infestation of orbit (122.3, 122.6, 122.9)
       myiasis of orbit (134.0)

⑤ **376.2 *Endocrine exophthalmos***
     Code first underlying thyroid disorder (242.0-242.9)

`376.21`   *Thyrotoxic exophthalmos*

`376.22`   *Exophthalmic ophthalmoplegia*

⑤ **376.3 Other exophthalmic conditions**

`376.30`   **Exophthalmos, unspecified**

376.31   **Constant exophthalmos**

376.32   **Orbital hemorrhage**

376.33   **Orbital edema or congestion**

376.34   **Intermittent exophthalmos**

376.35   **Pulsating exophthalmos**

376.36   **Lateral displacement of globe**

⑤ **376.4 Deformity of orbit**

	Add 4th or 5th digit		Nonspecific code		Unspecified code		Manifestation code

376.40 Deformity of orbit, unspecified

376.41 Hypertelorism of orbit

376.42 Exostosis of orbit

376.43 Local deformities due to bone disease

376.44 Orbital deformities associated with craniofacial deformities

376.45 Atrophy of orbit

376.46 Enlargement of orbit

376.47 Deformity due to trauma or surgery

⑤ 376.5 Enophthalmos

376.50 Enophthalmos, unspecified as to cause

376.51 Enophthalmos due to atrophy of orbital tissue

376.52 Enophthalmos due to trauma or surgery

376.6 Retained (old) foreign body following penetrating wound of orbit
Retrobulbar foreign body

⑤ 376.8 Other orbital disorders

376.81 Orbital cysts
Encephalocele of orbit

376.82 Myopathy of extraocular muscles

376.89 Other

376.9 Unspecified disorder of orbit

377 Disorders of optic nerve and visual pathways

⑤ 377.0 Papilledema

377.00 Papilledema, unspecified

377.01 Papilledema associated with increased intracranial pressure

377.02 Papilledema associated with decreased ocular pressure

377.03 Papilledema associated with retinal disorder

377.04 Foster-Kennedy syndrome

⑤ 377.1 Optic atrophy

377.10 Optic atrophy, unspecified

377.11 Primary optic atrophy

Excludes: neurosyphilitic optic atrophy (094.84)

377.12 Postinflammatory optic atrophy

377.13 Optic atrophy associated with retinal dystrophies

377.14 Glaucomatous atrophy [cupping] of optic disc

377.15 Partial optic atrophy
Temporal pallor of optic disc

377.16 Hereditary optic atrophy
Optic atrophy:
dominant hereditary
Leber's

⑤ 377.2 Other disorders of optic disc

377.21 Drusen of optic disc

377.22 Crater-like holes of optic disc

377.23 Coloboma of optic disc

377.24 Pseudopapilledema

⑤ 377.3 Optic neuritis

Excludes: meningococcal optic neuritis (036.81)

377.30 Optic neuritis, unspecified

377.31 Optic papillitis

377.32 Retrobulbar neuritis (acute)

Excludes: syphilitic retrobulbar neuritis (094.85)

377.33 Nutritional optic neuropathy

377.34 Toxic optic neuropathy
Toxic amblyopia

● Code new
to this edition   ▲ Revision of
existing code   ④ ⑤ Fourth or fifth
digit required

377.39 Other

Excludes: *ischemic optic neuropathy (377.41)*

⑤ **377.4** Other disorders of optic nerve

377.41 Ischemic optic neuropathy

377.42 Hemorrhage in optic nerve sheaths

377.43 Optic nerve hypoplasia

377.49 Other
Compression of optic nerve

⑤ **377.5** Disorders of optic chiasm

377.51 Associated with pituitary neoplasms and disorders

377.52 Associated with other neoplasms

377.53 Associated with vascular disorders

377.54 Associated with inflammatory disorders

⑤ **377.6** Disorders of other visual pathways

377.61 Associated with neoplasms

377.62 Associated with vascular disorders

377.63 Associated with inflammatory disorders

⑤ **377.7** Disorders of visual cortex

Excludes: *visual:*
agnosia (368.16)
hallucinations (368.16)
halos (368.15)

377.71 Associated with neoplasms

377.72 Associated with vascular disorders

377.73 Associated with inflammatory disorders

377.75 Cortical blindness

377.9 Unspecified disorder of optic nerve and visual pathways

378 Strabismus and other disorders of binocular eye movements

Excludes: *nystagmus and other irregular eye movements (379.50-379.59)*

⑤ **378.0** Esotropia
Convergent concomitant strabismus

Excludes: *intermittent esotropia (378.20-378.22)*

378.00 Esotropia, unspecified

378.01 Monocular esotropia

378.02 Monocular esotropia with A pattern

378.03 Monocular esotropia with V pattern

378.04 Monocular esotropia with other noncomitancies
Monocular esotropia with X or Y pattern

378.05 Alternating esotropia

378.06 Alternating esotropia with A pattern

378.07 Alternating esotropia with V pattern

378.08 Alternating esotropia with other noncomitancies
Alternating esotropia with X or Y pattern

⑤ **378.1** Exotropia
Divergent concomitant strabismus

Excludes: *intermittent exotropia (378.20, 378.23-378.24)*

378.10 Exotropia, unspecified

378.11 Monocular exotropia

378.12 Monocular exotropia with A pattern

378.13 Monocular exotropia with V pattern

378.14 Monocular exotropia with other noncomitancies
Monocular exotropia with X or Y pattern

378.15 Alternating exotropia

378.16 Alternating exotropia with A pattern

Add 4th or 5th digit	Nonspecific code	Unspecified code	Manifestation code

378.17   Alternating exotropia with V pattern

378.18   Alternating exotropia with other noncomitancies
Alternating exotropia with X or Y pattern

⑤ **378.2   Intermittent heterotropia**

Excludes: *vertical heterotropia (intermittent) (378.31)*

378.20   Intermittent heterotropia, unspecified
Intermittent:
     esotropia NOS
     exotropia NOS

378.21   Intermittent esotropia, monocular

378.22   Intermittent esotropia, alternating

378.23   Intermittent exotropia, monocular

378.24   Intermittent exotropia, alternating

⑤ **378.3   Other and unspecified heterotropia**

378.30   Heterotropia, unspecified

378.31   Hypertropia
Vertical heterotropia (constant) (intermittent)

378.32   Hypotropia

378.33   Cyclotropia

378.34   Monofixation syndrome
Microtropia

378.35   Accommodative component in esotropia

⑤ **378.4   Heterophoria**

378.40   Heterophoria, unspecified

378.41   Esophoria

378.42   Exophoria

378.43   Vertical heterophoria

378.44   Cyclophoria

378.45   Alternating hyperphoria

⑤ **378.5   Paralytic strabismus**

378.50   Paralytic strabismus, unspecified

378.51   Third or oculomotor nerve palsy, partial

378.52   Third or oculomotor nerve palsy, total

378.53   Fourth or trochlear nerve palsy

378.54   Sixth or abducens nerve palsy

378.55   External ophthalmoplegia

378.56   Total ophthalmoplegia

⑤ **378.6   Mechanical strabismus**

378.60   Mechanical strabismus, unspecified

378.61   Brown's (tendon) sheath syndrome

378.62   Mechanical strabismus from other musculofascial disorders

378.63   Limited duction associated with other conditions

⑤ **378.7   Other specified strabismus**

378.71   Duane's syndrome

378.72   Progressive external ophthalmoplegia

378.73   Strabismus in other neuromuscular disorders

⑤ **378.8   Other disorders of binocular eye movements**

Excludes: *nystagmus (379.50-379.56)*

378.81   Palsy of conjugate gaze

378.82   Spasm of conjugate gaze

378.83   Convergence insufficiency or palsy

378.84   Convergence excess or spasm

378.85   Anomalies of divergence

378.86   Internuclear ophthalmoplegia

● Code new
to this edition   ▲ Revision of
existing code   ④ ⑤ Fourth or fifth
digit required

`378.87` **Other dissociated deviation of eye movements**
Skew deviation

`378.9` **Unspecified disorder of eye movements**
Ophthalmoplegia NOS
Strabismus NOS

`379` **Other disorders of eye**

⑤ **379.0 Scleritis and episcleritis**

Excludes: *syphilitic episcleritis (095.0)*

`379.00` **Scleritis, unspecified**
Episcleritis NOS

`379.01` **Episcleritis periodica fugax**

`379.02` **Nodular episcleritis**

`379.03` **Anterior scleritis**

`379.04` **Scleromalacia perforans**

`379.05` **Scleritis with corneal involvement**
Scleroperikeratitis

`379.06` **Brawny scleritis**

`379.07` **Posterior scleritis**
Sclerotenonitis

`379.09` **Other**
Scleral abscess

⑤ **379.1 Other disorders of sclera**

Excludes: *blue sclera (743.47)*

`379.11` **Scleral ectasia**
Scleral staphyloma NOS

`379.12` **Staphyloma posticum**

`379.13` **Equatorial staphyloma**

`379.14` **Anterior staphyloma, localized**

`379.15` **Ring staphyloma**

`379.16` **Other degenerative disorders of sclera**

`379.19` **Other**

⑤ **379.2 Disorders of vitreous body**

`379.21` **Vitreous degeneration**
Vitreous:
cavitation
detachment
liquefaction

`379.22` **Crystalline deposits in vitreous**
Asteroid hyalitis
Synchysis scintillans

`379.23` **Vitreous hemorrhage**

`379.24` **Other vitreous opacities**
Vitreous floaters

`379.25` **Vitreous membranes and strands**

`379.26` **Vitreous prolapse**

`379.29` **Other disorders of vitreous**

Excludes: *vitreous abscess (360.04)*

⑤ **379.3 Aphakia and other disorders of lens**

Excludes: *after-cataract (366.50-366.53)*

`379.31` **Aphakia**

Excludes: *cataract extraction status (V45.61)*

`379.32` **Subluxation of lens**

`379.33` **Anterior dislocation of lens**

`379.34` **Posterior dislocation of lens**

`379.39` **Other disorders of lens**

⑤ **379.4 Anomalies of pupillary function**

	Add 4th or 5th digit		Nonspecific code		Unspecified code		Manifestation code

379.40 **Abnormal pupillary function, unspecified**

379.41 **Anisocoria**

379.42 **Miosis (persistent), not due to miotics**

379.43 **Mydriasis (persistent) not due to mydriatics**

379.45 **Argyll Robertson pupil, atypical**
Argyll Robertson phenomenon or pupil, nonsyphilitic

Excludes: *Argyll Robertson pupil (syphilitic) (094.89)*

379.46 **Tonic pupillary reaction**
Adie's pupil or syndrome

379.49 **Other**
Hippus
Pupillary paralysis

⑤ 379.5 **Nystagmus and other irregular eye movements**

379.50 **Nystagmus, unspecified**

379.51 **Congenital nystagmus**

379.52 **Latent nystagmus**

379.53 **Visual deprivation nystagmus**

379.54 **Nystagmus associated with disorders of the vestibular system**

379.55 **Dissociated nystagmus**

379.56 **Other forms of nystagmus**

379.57 **Deficiencies of saccadic eye movements**
Abnormal optokinetic response

379.58 **Deficiencies of smooth pursuit movements**

379.59 **Other irregularities of eye movements**
Opsoclonus

⑤ 379.6 **Inflammation (infection) of postprocedural bleb**
Postprocedural blebitis

379.60 **Inflammation (infection) of postprocedural bleb, unspecified**

379.61 **Inflammation (infection) of postprocedural bleb, stage 1**

379.62 **Inflammation (infection) of postprocedural bleb, stage 2**

379.63 **Inflammation (infection) of postprocedural bleb, stage 3**
Bleb associated endophthalmitis

379.8 **Other specified disorders of eye and adnexa**

⑤ 379.9 **Unspecified disorder of eye and adnexa**

379.90 **Disorder of eye, unspecified**

379.91 **Pain in or around eye**

379.92 **Swelling or mass of eye**

379.93 **Redness or discharge of eye**

379.99 **Other ill-defined disorders of eye**

Excludes: *blurred vision NOS (368.8)*

DISEASES OF THE EAR AND MASTOID PROCESS (380-389)

Use additional external cause code, if applicable, to identify the cause of the ear condition

380 **Disorders of external ear**

⑤ 380.0 **Perichondritis and chondritis of pinna**
Chondritis of auricle
Perichondritis of auricle

380.00 **Perichondritis of pinna, unspecified**

380.01 **Acute perichondritis of pinna**

380.02 **Chronic perichondritis of pinna**

380.03 **Chondritis of pinna**

⑤ 380.1 **Infective otitis externa**

● Code new
to this edition

▲ Revision of
existing code

④ ⑤ Fourth or fifth
digit required

380.10 **Infective otitis externa, unspecified**
Otitis externa (acute):
NOS
circumscribed
diffuse
hemorrhagica
infective NOS

380.11 **Acute infection of pinna**

Excludes: *furuncular otitis externa (680.0)*

380.12 **Acute swimmers' ear**
Beach ear
Tank ear

380.13 *Other acute infections of external ear*
Code first underlying disease, as:
erysipelas (035)
impetigo (684)
seborrheic dermatitis (690.10-690.18)

Excludes: *herpes simplex (054.73)*
herpes zoster (053.71)

380.14 **Malignant otitis externa**

380.15 *Chronic mycotic otitis externa*
Code first underlying disease, as:
aspergillosis (117.3)
otomycosis NOS (111.9)

Excludes: *candidal otitis externa (112.82)*

380.16 **Other chronic infective otitis externa**
Chronic infective otitis externa NOS

⑤ **380.2** **Other otitis externa**

380.21 **Cholesteatoma of external ear**
Keratosis obturans of external ear (canal)

Excludes: *cholesteatoma NOS (385.30-385.35)*
postmastoidectomy (383.32)

380.22 **Other acute otitis externa**
Acute otitis externa:
actinic
chemical
contact
eczematoid
reactive

380.23 **Other chronic otitis externa**
Chronic otitis externa NOS

⑤ **380.3** **Noninfectious disorders of pinna**

380.30 **Disorder of pinna, unspecified**

380.31 **Hematoma of auricle or pinna**

380.32 **Acquired deformities of auricle or pinna**

Excludes: *cauliflower ear (738.7)*

380.39 **Other**

Excludes: *gouty tophi of ear (274.81)*

380.4 **Impacted cerumen**
Wax in ear

⑤ **380.5** **Acquired stenosis of external ear canal**
Collapse of external ear canal

380.50 **Acquired stenosis of external ear canal, unspecified as to cause**

380.51 **Secondary to trauma**

380.52 **Secondary to surgery**

380.53 **Secondary to inflammation**

⑤ **380.8** **Other disorders of external ear**

380.81 **Exostosis of external ear canal**

380.89 **Other**

| | Add 4th or 5th digit | | Nonspecific code | | Unspecified code | | Manifestation code |

380.9 Unspecified disorder of external ear

381 Nonsuppurative otitis media and Eustachian tube disorders

⑤ **381.0 Acute nonsuppurative otitis media**
Acute tubotympanic catarrh
Otitis media, acute or subacute:
  catarrhal
  exudative
  transudative
  with effusion

Excludes: *otitic barotrauma (993.0)*

381.00 Acute nonsuppurative otitis media, unspecified

381.01 Acute serous otitis media
Acute or subacute secretory otitis media

381.02 Acute mucoid otitis media
Acute or subacute seromucinous otitis media
Blue drum syndrome

381.03 Acute sanguinous otitis media

381.04 Acute allergic serous otitis media

381.05 Acute allergic mucoid otitis media

381.06 Acute allergic sanguinous otitis media

⑤ **381.1 Chronic serous otitis media**
Chronic tubotympanic catarrh

381.10 Chronic serous otitis media, simple or unspecified

381.19 Other
Serosanguinous chronic otitis media

⑤ **381.2 Chronic mucoid otitis media**
Glue ear

Excludes: *adhesive middle ear disease (385.10-385.19)*

381.20 Chronic mucoid otitis media, simple or unspecified

381.29 Other
Mucosanguinous chronic otitis media

381.3 Other and unspecified chronic nonsuppurative otitis media
Otitis media, chronic: Otitis media, chronic:
  allergic   seromucinous
  exudative   transudative
  secretory   with effusion

381.4 Nonsuppurative otitis media, not specified as acute or chronic
Otitis media: Otitis media:
  allergic   secretory
  catarrhal   seromucinous
  exudative   serous
  mucoid   transudative
                          with effusion

⑤ **381.5 Eustachian salpingitis**

381.50 Eustachian salpingitis, unspecified

381.51 Acute Eustachian salpingitis

381.52 Chronic Eustachian salpingitis

⑤ **381.6 Obstruction of Eustachian tube**
Stenosis of Eustachian tube
Stricture of Eustachian tube

381.60 Obstruction of Eustachian tube, unspecified

381.61 Osseous obstruction of Eustachian tube
Obstruction of Eustachian tube from cholesteatoma, polyp, or other osseous lesion

381.62 Intrinsic cartilagenous obstruction of Eustachian tube

381.63 Extrinsic cartilagenous obstruction of Eustachian tube
Compression of Eustachian tube

381.7 Patulous Eustachian tube

⑤ **381.8 Other disorders of Eustachian tube**

381.81 Dysfunction of Eustachian tube

● Code new to this edition   ▲ Revision of existing code   ④ ⑤ Fourth or fifth digit required

381.89 Other

381.9 Unspecified Eustachian tube disorder

382 Suppurative and unspecified otitis media

⑤ **382.0** Acute suppurative otitis media
Otitis media, acute:
   necrotizing NOS
   purulent

382.00 Acute suppurative otitis media without spontaneous rupture of ear drum

382.01 Acute suppurative otitis media with spontaneous rupture of ear drum

382.02 *Acute suppurative otitis media in diseases classified elsewhere*
Code first underlying disease, as:
   influenza (487.8)
   scarlet fever (034.1)

Excludes: *postmeasles otitis (055.2)*

382.1 Chronic tubotympanic suppurative otitis media
Benign chronic suppurative otitis media (with anterior perforation of ear drum)
Chronic tubotympanic disease (with anterior perforation of ear drum)

382.2 Chronic atticoantral suppurative otitis media
Chronic atticoantral disease (with posterior or superior marginal perforation of ear drum)
Persistent mucosal disease (with posterior or superior marginal perforation of ear drum)

382.3 Unspecified chronic suppurative otitis media
Chronic purulent otitis media

Excludes: *tuberculous otitis media (017.4)*

382.4 Unspecified suppurative otitis media
Purulent otitis media NOS

382.9 Unspecified otitis media
Otitis media:
   NOS
   acute NOS
   chronic NOS

383 Mastoiditis and related conditions

⑤ **383.0** Acute mastoiditis
Abscess of mastoid
Empyema of mastoid

383.00 Acute mastoiditis without complications

383.01 Subperiosteal abscess of mastoid

383.02 Acute mastoiditis with other complications
Gradenigo's syndrome

383.1 Chronic mastoiditis
Caries of mastoid
Fistula of mastoid

Excludes: *tuberculous mastoiditis (015.6)*

⑤ **383.2** Petrositis
Coalescing osteitis of petrous bone
Inflammation of petrous bone
Osteomyelitis of petrous bone

383.20 Petrositis, unspecified

383.21 Acute petrositis

383.22 Chronic petrositis

⑤ **383.3** Complications following mastoidectomy

383.30 Postmastoidectomy complication, unspecified

383.31 Mucosal cyst of postmastoidectomy cavity

383.32 Recurrent cholesteatoma of postmastoidectomy cavity

383.33 Granulations of postmastoidectomy cavity
Chronic inflammation of postmastoidectomy cavity

⑤ **383.8** Other disorders of mastoid

383.81 Postauricular fistula

383.89 Other

	Add 4th or 5th digit		Nonspecific code		Unspecified code		Manifestation code

383.9 Unspecified mastoiditis

384 Other disorders of tympanic membrane

⑤ **384.0 Acute myringitis without mention of otitis media**

  384.00 Acute myringitis, unspecified
  Acute tympanitis NOS

  384.01 Bullous myringitis
  Myringitis bullosa hemorrhagica

  384.09 Other

384.1 Chronic myringitis without mention of otitis media
  Chronic tympanitis

⑤ **384.2 Perforation of tympanic membrane**
  Perforation of ear drum:
  NOS
  persistent posttraumatic
  postinflammatory

  Excludes: *otitis media with perforation of tympanic membrane (382.00-382.9)*
  traumatic perforation [current injury] (872.61)

  384.20 Perforation of tympanic membrane, unspecified

  384.21 Central perforation of tympanic membrane

  384.22 Attic perforation of tympanic membrane
  Pars flaccida

  384.23 Other marginal perforation of tympanic membrane

  384.24 Multiple perforations of tympanic membrane

  384.25 Total perforation of tympanic membrane

⑤ **384.8 Other specified disorders of tympanic membrane**

  384.81 Atrophic flaccid tympanic membrane
  Healed perforation of ear drum

  384.82 Atrophic nonflaccid tympanic membrane

384.9 Unspecified disorder of tympanic membrane

385 Other disorders of middle ear and mastoid

  Excludes: *mastoiditis (383.0-383.9)*

⑤ **385.0 Tympanosclerosis**

  385.00 Tympanosclerosis, unspecified as to involvement

  385.01 Tympanosclerosis involving tympanic membrane only

  385.02 Tympanosclerosis involving tympanic membrane and ear ossicles

  385.03 Tympanosclerosis involving tympanic membrane, ear ossicles, and middle ear

  385.09 Tympanosclerosis involving other combination of structures

⑤ **385.1 Adhesive middle ear disease**
  Adhesive otitis
  Otitis media:
  chronic adhesive
  fibrotic

  Excludes: *glue ear (381.20-381.29)*

  385.10 Adhesive middle ear disease, unspecified as to involvement

  385.11 Adhesions of drum head to incus

  385.12 Adhesions of drum head to stapes

  385.13 Adhesions of drum head to promontorium

  385.19 Other adhesions and combinations

⑤ **385.2 Other acquired abnormality of ear ossicles**

  385.21 Impaired mobility of malleus
  Ankylosis of malleus

  385.22 Impaired mobility of other ear ossicles
  Ankylosis of ear ossicles, except malleus

  385.23 Discontinuity or dislocation of ear ossicles

  385.24 Partial loss or necrosis of ear ossicles

● Code new
to this edition

▲ Revision of
existing code

④ ⑤ Fourth or fifth
digit required

⑤ **385.3 Cholesteatoma of middle ear and mastoid**
Cholesterosis of (middle) ear
Epidermosis of (middle) ear
Keratosis of (middle) ear
Polyp of (middle) ear

Excludes: cholesteatoma:
    external ear canal (380.21)
    recurrent of postmastoidectomy cavity (383.32)

    385.30 Cholesteatoma, unspecified

    385.31 Cholesteatoma of attic

    385.32 Cholesteatoma of middle ear

    385.33 Cholesteatoma of middle ear and mastoid

    385.35 Diffuse cholesteatosis

⑤ **385.8 Other disorders of middle ear and mastoid**

    385.82 Cholesterin granuloma

    385.83 Retained foreign body of middle ear

    385.89 Other

385.9 Unspecified disorder of middle ear and mastoid

386 Vertiginous syndromes and other disorders of vestibular system

    Excludes: *vertigo NOS (780.4)*

⑤ **386.0 Ménière's disease**
Endolymphatic hydrops   Ménière's syndrome or vertigo
Lermoyez's syndrome

    386.00 Ménière's disease, unspecified
        Ménière's disease (active)

    386.01 Active Ménière's disease, cochleovestibular

    386.02 Active Ménière's disease, cochlear

    386.03 Active Ménière's disease, vestibular

    386.04 Inactive Ménière's disease
        Ménière's disease in remission

⑤ **386.1 Other and unspecified peripheral vertigo**

    Excludes: *epidemic vertigo (078.81)*

    386.10 Peripheral vertigo, unspecified

    386.11 Benign paroxysmal positional vertigo
        Benign paroxysmal positional nystagmus

    386.12 Vestibular neuronitis
        Acute (and recurrent) peripheral vestibulopathy

    386.19 Other
        Aural vertigo
        Otogenic vertigo

386.2 Vertigo of central origin
Central positional nystagmus
Malignant positional vertigo

⑤ **386.3 Labyrinthitis**

    386.30 Labyrinthitis, unspecified

    386.31 Serous labyrinthitis
        Diffuse labyrinthitis

    386.32 Circumscribed labyrinthitis
        Focal labyrinthitis

    386.33 Suppurative labyrinthitis
        Purulent labyrinthitis

    386.34 Toxic labyrinthitis

    386.35 Viral labyrinthitis

⑤ **386.4 Labyrinthine fistula**

    386.40 Labyrinthine fistula, unspecified

    386.41 Round window fistula

    386.42 Oval window fistula

	Add 4th or 5th digit		Nonspecific code		Unspecified code		Manifestation code

386.43   Semicircular canal fistula

386.48   Labyrinthine fistula of combined sites

⑤ 386.5 Labyrinthine dysfunction

    386.50   Labyrinthine dysfunction, unspecified

    386.51   Hyperactive labyrinth, unilateral

    386.52   Hyperactive labyrinth, bilateral

    386.53   Hypoactive labyrinth, unilateral

    386.54   Hypoactive labyrinth, bilateral

    386.55   Loss of labyrinthine reactivity, unilateral

    386.56   Loss of labyrinthine reactivity, bilateral

    386.58   Other forms and combinations

386.8 Other disorders of labyrinth

386.9 Unspecified vertiginous syndromes and labyrinthine disorders

387 Otosclerosis
    Includes: otospongiosis

387.0 Otosclerosis involving oval window, nonobliterative

387.1 Otosclerosis involving oval window, obliterative

387.2 Cochlear otosclerosis
    Otosclerosis involving:
      otic capsule
      round window

387.8 Other otosclerosis

387.9 Otosclerosis, unspecified

388 Other disorders of ear

⑤ 388.0 Degenerative and vascular disorders of ear

    388.00   Degenerative and vascular disorders, unspecified

    388.01   Presbyacusis

    388.02   Transient ischemic deafness

⑤ 388.1 Noise effects on inner ear

    388.10   Noise effects on inner ear, unspecified

    388.11   Acoustic trauma (explosive) to ear
        Otitic blast injury

    388.12   Noise-induced hearing loss

388.2 Sudden hearing loss, unspecified

⑤ 388.3 Tinnitus

    388.30   Tinnitus, unspecified

    388.31   Subjective tinnitus

    388.32   Objective tinnitus

⑤ 388.4 Other abnormal auditory perception

    388.40   Abnormal auditory perception, unspecified

    388.41   Diplacusis

    388.42   Hyperacusis

    388.43   Impairment of auditory discrimination

    388.44   Recruitment

    388.45   Acquired auditory processing disorder
        Auditory processing disorder NOS

   Excludes: *central auditory processing disorder (315.32)*

388.5 Disorders of acoustic nerve
    Acoustic neuritis
    Degeneration of acoustic or eighth nerve
    Disorder of acoustic or eighth nerve

   Excludes: *acoustic neuroma (225.1)*
          syphilitic acoustic neuritis (094.86)

⑤ **388.6 Otorrhea**

    388.60 Otorrhea, unspecified
        Discharging ear NOS

    388.61 Cerebrospinal fluid otorrhea

    Excludes: *cerebrospinal fluid rhinorrhea (349.81)*

    388.69 Other
        Otorrhagia

⑤ **388.7 Otalgia**

    388.70 Otalgia, unspecified
        Earache NOS

    388.71 Otogenic pain

    388.72 Referred pain

  388.8 Other disorders of ear

  388.9 Unspecified disorder of ear

389 Hearing loss

⑤ **389.0 Conductive hearing loss**
    Conductive deafness

    Excludes: *mixed conductive and sensorineural hearing loss (389.20-389.22)*

    389.00 Conductive hearing loss, unspecified

    389.01 Conductive hearing loss, external ear

    389.02 Conductive hearing loss, tympanic membrane

    389.03 Conductive hearing loss, middle ear

    389.04 Conductive hearing loss, inner ear

    389.05 Conductive hearing loss, unilateral

    389.06 Conductive hearing loss, bilateral

    389.08 Conductive hearing loss of combined types

⑤ **389.1 Sensorineural hearing loss**
    Perceptive hearing loss or deafness

    Excludes: *abnormal auditory perception (388.40-388.44)*
              mixed conductive and sensorineural hearing loss (389.20-389.22)
              psychogenic deafness (306.7)

    389.10 Sensorineural hearing loss, unspecified

    389.11 Sensory hearing loss, bilateral

    389.12 Neural hearing loss, bilateral

    389.13 Neural hearing loss, unilateral

    389.14 Central hearing loss

    389.15 Sensorineural hearing loss, unilateral

    389.16 Sensorineural hearing loss, asymmetrical

    389.17 Sensory hearing loss, unilateral

    389.18 Sensorineural hearing loss, bilateral

⑤ **389.2 Mixed conductive and sensorineural hearing loss**
    Deafness or hearing loss of type classifiable to 389.00-389.08 with type classifiable to
    389.10-389.18

    389.20 Mixed hearing loss, unspecified

    389.21 Mixed hearing loss, unilateral

    389.22 Mixed hearing loss, bilateral

  389.7 Deaf nonspeaking, not elsewhere classifiable

  389.8 Other specified forms of hearing loss

  389.9 Unspecified hearing loss
    Deafness NOS

	Add 4th or 5th digit		Nonspecific code		Unspecified code		Manifestation code

7. DISEASES OF THE CIRCULATORY SYSTEM (390-459)

ACUTE RHEUMATIC FEVER (390-392)

390 Rheumatic fever without mention of heart involvement
Arthritis, rheumatic, acute or subacute
Rheumatic fever (active) (acute)
Rheumatism, articular, acute or subacute

> *Excludes:* *that with heart involvement (391.0-391.9)*

391 Rheumatic fever with heart involvement

> *Excludes:* *chronic heart diseases of rheumatic origin (393-398.99) unless rheumatic fever is also present or there is evidence of recrudescence or activity of the rheumatic process*

391.0 Acute rheumatic pericarditis
Rheumatic:
fever (active) (acute) with pericarditis
pericarditis (acute)
Any condition classifiable to 390 with pericarditis

> *Excludes:* *that not specified as rheumatic (420.0-420.9)*

391.1 Acute rheumatic endocarditis
Rheumatic:
endocarditis, acute
fever (active) (acute) with endocarditis or valvulitis
valvulitis acute
Any condition classifiable to 390 with endocarditis or valvulitis

391.2 Acute rheumatic myocarditis
Rheumatic fever (active) (acute) with myocarditis
Any condition classifiable to 390 with myocarditis

391.8 Other acute rheumatic heart disease
Rheumatic:
fever (active) (acute) with other or multiple types of heart involvement
pancarditis, acute
Any condition classifiable to 390 with other or multiple types of heart involvement

391.9 Acute rheumatic heart disease, unspecified
Rheumatic:
carditis, acute
fever (active) (acute) with unspecified type of heart involvement
heart disease, active or acute
Any condition classifiable to 390 with unspecified type of heart involvement

392 Rheumatic chorea
Includes: Sydenham's chorea

> *Excludes:* *chorea:*
> *NOS (333.5)*
> *Huntington's (333.4)*

392.0 With heart involvement
Rheumatic chorea with heart involvement of any type classifiable to 391

392.9 Without mention of heart involvement

CHRONIC RHEUMATIC HEART DISEASE (393-398)

393 Chronic rheumatic pericarditis
Adherent pericardium, rheumatic
Chronic rheumatic:
mediastinopericarditis
myopericarditis

> *Excludes:* *pericarditis NOS or not specified as rheumatic (423.0-423.9)*

394 Diseases of mitral valve

> *Excludes:* *that with aortic valve involvement (396.0-396.9)*

394.0 Mitral stenosis
Mitral (valve):
obstruction (rheumatic)
stenosis NOS

| | Add 4th or 5th digit | | Nonspecific code | | Unspecified code | | Manifestation code |

394.1 Rheumatic mitral insufficiency
Rheumatic mitral:
 incompetence
 regurgitation

Excludes: *that not specified as rheumatic (424.0)*

394.2 Mitral stenosis with insufficiency
Mitral stenosis with incompetence or regurgitation

394.9 Other and unspecified mitral valve diseases
Mitral (valve):
 disease (chronic)
 failure

395 Diseases of aortic valve

Excludes: *that not specified as rheumatic (424.1)*
  that with mitral valve involvement (396.0-396.9)

395.0 Rheumatic aortic stenosis
Rheumatic aortic (valve) obstruction

395.1 Rheumatic aortic insufficiency
Rheumatic aortic:
 incompetence
 regurgitation

395.2 Rheumatic aortic stenosis with insufficiency
Rheumatic aortic stenosis with incompetence or regurgitation

395.9 Other and unspecified rheumatic aortic diseases
Rheumatic aortic (valve) disease

396 Diseases of mitral and aortic valves
Includes: involvement of both mitral and aortic valves, whether specified as rheumatic or
not

396.0 Mitral valve stenosis and aortic valve stenosis
Atypical aortic (valve) stenosis
Mitral and aortic (valve) obstruction (rheumatic)

396.1 Mitral valve stenosis and aortic valve insufficiency

396.2 Mitral valve insufficiency and aortic valve stenosis

396.3 Mitral valve insufficiency and aortic valve insufficiency
Mitral and aortic (valve):
 incompetence
 regurgitation

396.8 Multiple involvement of mitral and aortic valves
Stenosis and insufficiency of mitral or aortic valve with stenosis or insufficiency, or
both, of the other valve

396.9 Mitral and aortic valve diseases, unspecified

397 Diseases of other endocardial structures

397.0 Diseases of tricuspid valve
Tricuspid (valve) (rheumatic):
 disease
 insufficiency
 obstruction
 regurgitation
 stenosis

397.1 Rheumatic diseases of pulmonary valve

Excludes: *that not specified as rheumatic (424.3)*

397.9 Rheumatic diseases of endocardium, valve unspecified
Rheumatic:
 endocarditis (chronic)
 valvulitis (chronic)

Excludes: *that not specified as rheumatic (424.90-424.99)*

398 Other rheumatic heart disease

398.0 Rheumatic myocarditis
Rheumatic degeneration of myocardium

Excludes: *myocarditis not specified as rheumatic (429.0)*

⑤ **398.9 Other and unspecified rheumatic heart diseases**

● Code new
 to this edition

▲ Revision of
 existing code

④ ⑤ Fourth or fifth
 digit required

398.90 Rheumatic heart disease, unspecified
Rheumatic:
   carditis
   heart disease NOS

Excludes: *carditis not specified as rheumatic (429.89)*
heart disease NOS not specified as rheumatic (429.9)

398.91 Rheumatic heart failure (congestive)
Rheumatic left ventricular failure

398.99 Other

HYPERTENSIVE DISEASE (401-405)

Excludes: *that complicating pregnancy, childbirth, or the puerperium (642.0-642.9)*
that involving coronary vessels (410.00-414.9)

401 Essential hypertension
Includes: high blood pressure
   hyperpiesia
   hyperpiesis
   hypertension (arterial) (essential) (primary) (systemic)
   hypertensive vascular:
     degeneration
     disease

Excludes: *elevated blood pressure without diagnosis of hypertension (796.2)*
pulmonary hypertension (416.0-416.9)
that involving vessels of:
   brain (430-438)
   eye (362.11)

401.0 Malignant

401.1 Benign

401.9 Unspecified

402 Hypertensive heart disease
Use additional code to specify type of heart failure (428.0-428.43), if known
Includes: hypertensive:
   cardiomegaly
   cardiopathy
   cardiovascular disease
   heart (disease) (failure)
   any condition classifiable to 429.0-429.3, 429.8, 429.9 due to hypertension

⑤ **402.0 Malignant**
   402.00 Without heart failure
   402.01 With heart failure

⑤ **402.1 Benign**
   402.10 Without heart failure
   402.11 With heart failure

⑤ **402.9 Unspecified**
   402.90 Without heart failure
   402.91 With heart failure

| | Add 4th or 5th digit | | Nonspecific code | | Unspecified code | | Manifestation code |

⑤ **403** **Hypertensive chronic kidney disease**
The following fifth-digit subclassification is for use with category 403:

    0 **with chronic kidney disease stage I through stage IV, or unspecified**

        Use additional code to identify the stage of chronic kidney disease (585.1-585.4, 585.9)

    1 **with chronic kidney disease stage V or end stage renal disease**

        Use additional code to identify the stage of chronic kidney disease (585.5, 585.6)

Includes: arteriolar nephritis
          arteriosclerosis of:
            kidney
            renal arterioles
          arteriosclerotic nephritis (chronic) (interstitial)
          hypertensive:
            nephropathy
            renal failure
            uremia (chronic)
          nephrosclerosis
          renal sclerosis with hypertension
          any condition classifiable to 585 with any condition classifiable to 401

Excludes: *acute kidney failure (584.5-584.9)*
         renal disease stated as not due to hypertension
         renovascular hypertension (405.0-405.9 with fifth-digit 1)

⑤ **403.0** **Malignant**
[0-1]

⑤ **403.1** **Benign**
[0-1]

⑤ **403.9** **Unspecified**
[0-1]

⑤ **404** **Hypertensive heart and chronic kidney disease**
Use additional code to specify type of heart failure (428.0-428.43), if known
The following fifth-digit subclassification is for use with category 404:

    0 **without heart failure and with chronic kidney disease stage I through stage IV, or unspecified**

        Use additional code to identify the stage of chronic kidney disease (585.1-585.4, 585.9)

    1 **with heart failure and with chronic kidney disease stage I through stage IV, or unspecified**

        Use additional code to identify the stage of chronic kidney disease (585.1-585.4, 585.9)

    2 **without heart failure and with chronic kidney disease stage V or end stage renal disease**

        Use additional code to identify the stage of chronic kidney disease (585.5, 585.6)

    3 **with heart failure and chronic kidney disease stage V or end stage renal disease**

        Use additional code to identify the stage of chronic kidney disease (585.5-585.6)

Includes: disease:
          cardiornal
          cardiovascular renal
          any condition classifiable to 402 with any condition classifiable to 403

⑤ **404.0** **Malignant**
[0-3]

⑤ **404.1** **Benign**
[0-3]

⑤ **404.9** **Unspecified**
[0-3]

405 **Secondary hypertension**

⑤ **405.0** **Malignant**

      405.01 **Renovascular**

      405.09 **Other**

⑤ **405.1** **Benign**

      405.11 **Renovascular**

      405.19 **Other**

● Code new to this edition   ▲ Revision of existing code   ④ ⑤ Fourth or fifth digit required

⑤ **405.9 Unspecified**

　　　　405.91　Renovascular

　　　　405.99　Other

ISCHEMIC HEART DISEASE (410-414)

　　　　Includes: that with mention of hypertension

　　　　Use additional code, if desired, to identify presence of hypertension (401.0-405.9)

⑤ **410 Acute myocardial infarction**

　　　　ST elevation (STEMI) and non-ST elevation (NSTEMI) myocardial infarction
　　　　Includes: cardiac infarction
　　　　　　　　　coronary (artery):
　　　　　　　　　　embolism
　　　　　　　　　　occlusion
　　　　　　　　　　rupture
　　　　　　　　　　thrombosis
　　　　　　　　　infarction of heart, myocardium, or ventricle
　　　　　　　　　rupture of heart, myocardium, or ventricle
　　　　　　　　　any condition classifiable to 414.1-414.9 specified as acute or with a stated
　　　　　　　　　　duration of 8 weeks or less

The following fifth-digit subclassification is for use with category 410:

　　0　episode of care unspecified
　　　　　Use when the source document does not contain sufficient information for the
　　　　　assignment of fifth digit 1 or 2.

　　1　initial episode of care
　　　　　Use fifth digit 1 to designate the first episode of care (regardless of facility site) for a
　　　　　newly diagnosed myocardial infarction. The fifth digit 1 is assigned regardless of
　　　　　the number of times a patient may be transferred during the initial episode of care

　　2　subsequent episode of care
　　　　　Use fifth digit 2 to designate an episode of care following the initial episode when the
　　　　　patient is admitted for further observation, evaluation, or treatment for a
　　　　　myocardial infarction that has received initial treatment, but is still less than 8
　　　　　weeks old.

⑤ **410.0 Of anterolateral wall**
　[0-2]　　ST elevation myocardial infarction (STEMI) of anterolateral wall

⑤ **410.1 Of other anterior wall**
　[0-2]　　ST elevation myocardial infarction (STEMI) of other anterior wall
　　　　　Infarction:
　　　　　　anterior (wall) NOS (with contiguous portion of intraventricular septum)
　　　　　　anteroapical (with contiguous portion of intraventricular septum)
　　　　　　anteroseptal (with contiguous portion of intraventricular septum)

⑤ **410.2 Of inferolateral wall**
　[0-2]　　ST elevation myocardial infarction (STEMI) of inferolateral wall

⑤ **410.3 Of inferoposterior wall**
　[0-2]　　ST elevation myocardial infarction (STEMI) of inferoposterior wall

⑤ **410.4 Of other inferior wall**
　[0-2]　　ST elevation myocardial infarction (STEMI) of other inferior wall
　　　　　Infarction:
　　　　　　diaphragmatic wall NOS (with contiguous portion of intraventricular septum)
　　　　　　inferior (wall) NOS (with contiguous portion of intraventricular septum)

⑤ **410.5 Of other lateral wall**
　[0-2]　　ST elevation myocardial infarction (STEMI) of other lateral wall
　　　　　Infarction:　　　　　　　　Infarction:
　　　　　　apical-lateral　　　　　　high lateral
　　　　　　basal-lateral　　　　　　posterolateral

⑤ **410.6 True posterior wall infarction**
　[0-2]　　ST elevation myocardial infarction (STEMI) of true posterior wall
　　　　　Infarction:
　　　　　　posterobasal
　　　　　　strictly posterior

⑤ **410.7 Subendocardial infarction**
　[0-2]　　Non-ST elevation myocardial infarction (NSTEMI)
　　　　　Nontransmural infarction

	Add 4th or 5th digit		Nonspecific code		Unspecified code		Manifestation code

⑤ **410.8** **Other specified sites**
[0-2] ST elevation myocardial infarction (STEMI) of other specified sites
Infarction of:
  atrium
  papillary muscle
  septum alone

⑤ **410.9** **Unspecified site**
[0-2] Acute myocardial infarction NOS
Coronary occlusion NOS
Myocardial infarction NOS

411 **Other acute and subacute forms of ischemic heart disease**

411.0 **Postmyocardial infarction syndrome**
Dressler's syndrome

411.1 **Intermediate coronary syndrome**
Impending infarction   Preinfarction syndrome
Preinfarction angina   Unstable angina

Excludes: angina (pectoris) (413.9)
         decubitus (413.0)

⑤ **411.8** **Other**

411.81 **Acute coronary occlusion without myocardial infarction**
Acute coronary (artery):
  embolism without or not resulting in myocardial infarction
  obstruction without or not resulting in myocardial infarction
  occlusion without or not resulting in myocardial infarction
  thrombosis without or not resulting in myocardial infarction

Excludes: obstruction without infarction due to atherosclerosis (414.00-414.07)
         occlusion without infarction due to atherosclerosis (414.00-414.07)

411.89 **Other**
Coronary insufficiency (acute)
Subendocardial ischemia

412 **Old myocardial infarction**
Healed myocardial infarction
Past myocardial infarction diagnosed on ECG [EKG] or other special investigation, but
currently presenting no symptoms

413 **Angina pectoris**

413.0 **Angina decubitus**
Nocturnal angina

413.1 **Prinzmetal angina**
Variant angina pectoris

413.9 **Other and unspecified angina pectoris**
Angina: Anginal syndrome
  equivalent   Status anginosus
  NOS   Stenocardia
  cardiac   Syncope anginosa
  of effort
Use additional code(s) for symptoms associated with angina equivalent

Excludes: preinfarction angina (411.1)

414 **Other forms of chronic ischemic heart disease**

Excludes: arteriosclerotic cardiovascular disease [ASCVD] (429.2)
         cardiovascular:
           arteriosclerosis or sclerosis (429.2)
           degeneration or disease (429.2)

● Code new   ▲ Revision of   ④ ⑤ Fourth or fifth
   to this edition   existing code   digit required

⑤ **414.0 Coronary atherosclerosis**
    Arteriosclerotic heart disease [ASHD]
    Atherosclerotic heart disease
    Coronary (artery):
        arteriosclerosis
        arteritis or endarteritis
        atheroma
        sclerosis
        stricture

Use additional code, if applicable, to identify chronic total occlusion of coronary artery (414.2)

   Excludes: *embolism of graft (996.72)*
             occlusion NOS of graft (996.72)
             thrombus of graft (996.72)

   414.00 Of unspecified type of vessel, native or graft

   414.01 Of native coronary artery

   414.02 Of autologous vein bypass graft

   414.03 Of nonautologous biological bypass graft

   414.04 Of artery bypass graft
            Internal mammary artery

   414.05 Of unspecified type of bypass graft
            Bypass graft NOS

   414.06 Of native coronary artery of transplanted heart

   414.07 Of bypass graft (artery) (vein) of transplanted heart

⑤ **414.1 Aneurysm and dissection of heart**

   414.10 Aneurysm of heart (wall)
            Aneurysm (arteriovenous):
                mural
                ventricular

   414.11 Aneurysm of coronary vessels
            Aneurysm (arteriovenous) of coronary vessels

   414.12 Dissection of coronary artery

   414.19 Other aneurysm of heart
            Arteriovenous fistula, acquired, of heart

414.2 Chronic total occlusion of coronary artery
    Complete occlusion of coronary artery
    Total occlusion of coronary artery

Code first coronary atherosclerosis (414.00-414.07)

   Excludes: *acute coronary occlusion with myocardial infarction (410.00-410.92)*
             acute coronary occlusion without myocardial infarction (411.81)

414.3 Coronary atherosclerosis due to lipid rich plaque
Code first coronary atherosclerosis (414.00-414.07)

414.8 Other specified forms of chronic ischemic heart disease
    Chronic coronary insufficiency
    Ischemia, myocardial (chronic)
    Any condition classifiable to 410 specified as chronic, or presenting with symptoms
        after 8 weeks from date of infarction

   Excludes: *coronary insufficiency (acute) (411.89)*

414.9 Chronic ischemic heart disease, unspecified
    Ischemic heart disease NOS

DISEASES OF PULMONARY CIRCULATION (415-417)

415 Acute pulmonary heart disease

   415.0 Acute cor pulmonale

      Excludes: *cor pulmonale NOS (416.9)*

| | Add 4th or 5th digit | | Nonspecific code | | Unspecified code | | Manifestation code |

⑤ **415.1 Pulmonary embolism and infarction**
　　Pulmonary (artery) (vein):
　　　apoplexy
　　　embolism
　　　infarction (hemorrhagic)
　　　thrombosis

> Excludes: *chronic pulmonary embolism (416.2)*
> 　　*personal history of pulmonary embolism (V12.51)*
> 　　*that complicating:*
> 　　　*abortion (634-638 with .6, 639.6)*
> 　　　*ectopic or molar pregnancy (639.6)*
> 　　　*pregnancy, childbirth, or the puerperium (673.0-673.8)*

　　415.11　Iatrogenic pulmonary embolism and infarction
　　Use additional code for associated septic pulmonary embolism, if applicable, 415.12

　　415.12　Septic pulmonary embolism
　　　　Septic embolism NOS

　　Code first underlying infection, such as:
　　　　septicemia (038.0-038.9)

> Excludes: *septic arterial embolism (449)*

　　415.19　Other

416　Chronic pulmonary heart disease

　416.0　Primary pulmonary hypertension
　　　Idiopathic pulmonary arteriosclerosis
　　　Pulmonary hypertension (essential) (idiopathic) (primary)

　416.1　Kyphoscoliotic heart disease

● **416.2　Chronic pulmonary embolism**
　Use additional code, if applicable, for associated long-term (current) use of anticoagulants
　　(V58.61)

> Excludes: *personal history of pulmonary embolism (V12.51)*

　416.8　Other chronic pulmonary heart diseases
　　　Pulmonary hypertension, secondary

　416.9　Chronic pulmonary heart disease, unspecified
　　　Chronic cardiopulmonary disease
　　　Cor pulmonale (chronic) NOS

417　Other diseases of pulmonary circulation

　417.0　Arteriovenous fistula of pulmonary vessels

> Excludes: *congenital arteriovenous fistula (747.3)*

　417.1　Aneurysm of pulmonary artery

> Excludes: *congenital aneurysm (747.3)*

　417.8　Other specified diseases of pulmonary circulation
　　　Pulmonary:
　　　　arteritis
　　　　endarteritis
　　　Rupture of pulmonary vessel
　　　Stricture of pulmonary vessel

　417.9　Unspecified disease of pulmonary circulation

OTHER FORMS OF HEART DISEASE (420-429)

420　Acute pericarditis
　　Includes:　acute:
　　　　　mediastinopericarditis
　　　　　myopericarditis
　　　　　pericardial effusion
　　　　　pleuropericarditis
　　　　　pneumopericarditis

> Excludes: *acute rheumatic pericarditis (391.0)*
> 　　*postmyocardial infarction syndrome [Dressler's] (411.0)*

● Code new
　to this edition

▲ Revision of
　existing code

④ ⑤ Fourth or fifth
　　digit required

420.0 *Acute pericarditis in diseases classified elsewhere*
Code first underlying disease, as:
actinomycosis (039.8)
amebiasis (006.8)
chronic uremia (585.9)
nocardiosis (039.8)
tuberculosis (017.9)
uremia NOS (586)

Excludes: *pericarditis (acute) (in):*
Coxsackie (virus) (074.21)
gonococcal (098.83)
histoplasmosis (115.0-115.9 with fifth-digit 3)
meningococcal infection (036.41)
syphilitic (093.81)

⑤ **420.9 Other and unspecified acute pericarditis**

420.90 Acute pericarditis, unspecified
Pericarditis (acute):
NOS
infective NOS
sicca

420.91 Acute idiopathic pericarditis
Pericarditis, acute:
benign
nonspecific
viral

420.99 Other

Pericarditis (acute):	Pericarditis (acute):
pneumococcal	streptococcal
purulent	suppurative
staphylococcal	Pneumopyopericardium
	Pyopericardium

Excludes: *pericarditis in diseases classified elsewhere (420.0)*

421 Acute and subacute endocarditis

421.0 Acute and subacute bacterial endocarditis

Endocarditis (acute) (chronic) (subacute):	Endocarditis (acute) (chronic) (subacute):
bacterial	septic
infective NOS	ulcerative
lenta	vegetative
malignant	Infective aneurysm
purulent	Subacute bacterial endocarditis [SBE]

Use additional code, if desired, to identify infectious organism [e.g., Streptococcus 041.0, Staphylococcus 041.1]

421.1 *Acute and subacute infective endocarditis in diseases classified elsewhere*
Code first underlying disease, as:
blastomycosis (116.0)
Q fever (083.0)
typhoid (fever) (002.0)

Excludes: *endocarditis (in):*
Coxsackie (virus) (074.22)
gonococcal (098.84)
histoplasmosis (115.0-115.9 with fifth-digit 4)
meningococcal infection (036.42)
monilial (112.81)

421.9 Acute endocarditis, unspecified
Endocarditis, acute or subacute
Myoendocarditis, acute or subacute
Periendocarditis, acute or subacute

Excludes: *acute rheumatic endocarditis (391.1)*

422 Acute myocarditis

Excludes: *acute rheumatic myocarditis (391.2)*

	Add 4th or 5th digit		Nonspecific code		Unspecified code		Manifestation code

422.0 *Acute myocarditis in diseases classified elsewhere*
　　Code first underlying disease, as:
　　　myocarditis (acute):
　　　　influenzal (487.8)
　　　　tuberculous (017.9)

　　Excludes: *myocarditis (acute) (due to):*
　　　　　aseptic, of newborn (074.23)
　　　　　Coxsackie (virus) (074.23)
　　　　　diphtheritic (032.82)
　　　　　meningococcal infection (036.43)
　　　　　syphilitic (093.82)
　　　　　toxoplasmosis (130.3)

⑤ **422.9** **Other and unspecified acute myocarditis**

　　422.90 **Acute myocarditis, unspecified**
　　　　　Acute or subacute (interstitial) myocarditis

　　422.91 **Idiopathic myocarditis**
　　　　　Myocarditis (acute or subacute):
　　　　　　Fiedler's
　　　　　　giant cell
　　　　　　isolated (diffuse) (granulomatous)
　　　　　　nonspecific granulomatous

　　422.92 **Septic myocarditis**
　　　　　Myocarditis, acute or subacute:
　　　　　　pneumococcal
　　　　　　staphylococcal

　　Use additional code, if desired, to identify infectious organism [e.g., Staphylococcus 041.1]

　　Excludes: *myocarditis, acute or subacute:*
　　　　　in bacterial diseases classified elsewhere (422.0)
　　　　　streptococcal (391.2)

　　422.93 **Toxic myocarditis**

　　422.99 **Other**

423 **Other diseases of pericardium**

　　Excludes: *that specified as rheumatic (393)*

　　423.0 **Hemopericardium**

　　423.1 **Adhesive pericarditis**
　　　　Adherent pericardium　　　　Pericarditis:
　　　　Fibrosis of pericardium　　　　　adhesive
　　　　Milk spots　　　　　　　　　　　obliterative
　　　　　　　　　　　　　　　　　　　Soldiers' patches

　　423.2 **Constrictive pericarditis**
　　　　Concato's disease
　　　　Pick's disease of heart (and liver)

　　423.3 **Cardiac tamponade**
　　Code first the underlying cause

　　423.8 **Other specified diseases of pericardium**
　　　　Calcification of pericardium
　　　　Fistula of pericardium

　　423.9 **Unspecified disease of pericardium**

424 **Other diseases of endocardium**

　　Excludes: *bacterial endocarditis (421.0-421.9)*
　　　　　rheumatic endocarditis (391.1, 394.0-397.9)
　　　　　syphilitic endocarditis (093.20-093.24)

　● Code new　　　　▲ Revision of　　④ ⑤ Fourth or fifth
　　　to this edition　　　existing code　　　digit required

424.0 Mitral valve disorders
Mitral (valve):
    incompetence NOS of specified cause, except rheumatic
    insufficiency NOS of specified cause, except rheumatic
    regurgitation NOS of specified cause, except rheumatic

Excludes: *mitral (valve):*
    disease (394.9)
    failure (394.9)
    stenosis (394.0)
    the listed conditions:
      specified as rheumatic (394.1)
      unspecified as to cause but with mention of:
        diseases of aortic valve (396.0-396.9)
        mitral stenosis or obstruction (394.2)

424.1 Aortic valve disorders
Aortic (valve):
    incompetence NOS of specified cause, except rheumatic
    insufficiency NOS of specified cause, except rheumatic
    regurgitation NOS of specified cause, except rheumatic
    stenosis NOS of specified cause, except rheumatic

Excludes: *hypertrophic subaortic stenosis (425.1)*
    that specified as rheumatic (395.0-395.9)
    that of unspecified cause but with mention of diseases of mitral valve
      (396.0-396.9)

424.2 Tricuspid valve disorders, specified as nonrheumatic
Tricuspid valve:
    incompetence of specified cause, except rheumatic
    insufficiency of specified cause, except rheumatic
    regurgitation of specified cause, except rheumatic
    stenosis of specified cause, except rheumatic

Excludes: *rheumatic or of unspecified cause (397.0)*

424.3 Pulmonary valve disorders
Pulmonic: Pulmonic:
  incompetence NOS   regurgitation NOS
  insufficiency NOS   stenosis NOS

Excludes: *that specified as rheumatic (397.1)*

⑤ 424.9 Endocarditis, valve unspecified

424.90 Endocarditis, valve unspecified, unspecified cause
Endocarditis (chronic):
  NOS
  nonbacterial thrombotic
Valvular:
  incompetence of unspecified valve, unspecified cause
  insufficiency of unspecified valve, unspecified cause
  regurgitation of unspecified valve, unspecified cause
  stenosis of unspecified valve, unspecified cause
Valvulitis (chronic)

424.91 *Endocarditis in diseases classified elsewhere*
Code first underlying disease, as:
  atypical verrucous endocarditis [Libman-Sacks] (710.0)
  disseminated lupus erythematosus (710.0)
  tuberculosis (017.9)

Excludes: *syphilitic (093.20-093.24)*

424.99 Other
Any condition classifiable to 424.90 with specified cause, except rheumatic

Excludes: *endocardial fibroelastosis (425.3)*
    that specified as rheumatic (397.9)

425 Cardiomyopathy
Includes: myocardiopathy

425.0 Endomyocardial fibrosis

425.1 Hypertrophic obstructive cardiomyopathy
Hypertrophic subaortic stenosis (idiopathic)

| | Add 4th or 5th digit | | Nonspecific code | | Unspecified code | | Manifestation code |

425.2 Obscure cardiomyopathy of Africa
Becker's disease
Idiopathic mural endomyocardial disease

425.3 Endocardial fibroelastosis
Elastomyofibrosis

425.4 Other primary cardiomyopathies

Cardiomyopathy:	Cardiomyopathy:
NOS	idiopathic
congestive	nonobstructive
constrictive	obstructive
familial	restrictive
hypertrophic	Cardiovascular collagenosis

425.5 Alcoholic cardiomyopathy

425.7 *Nutritional and metabolic cardiomyopathy*
Code first underlying disease, as:
amyloidosis (277.30-277.39)
beriberi (265.0)
cardiac glycogenosis (271.0)
mucopolysaccharidosis (277.5)
thyrotoxicosis (242.0-242.9)

Excludes: *gouty tophi of heart (274.82)*

425.8 *Cardiomyopathy in other diseases classified elsewhere*
Code first underlying disease, as:
Friedreich's ataxia (334.0)
myotonia atrophica (359.21)
progressive muscular dystrophy (359.1)
sarcoidosis (135)

Excludes: *cardiomyopathy in Chagas' disease (086.0)*

425.9 Secondary cardiomyopathy, unspecified

426 Conduction disorders

426.0 Atrioventricular block, complete
Third degree atrioventricular block

⑤ **426.1 Atrioventricular block, other and unspecified**

426.10 Atrioventricular block, unspecified
Atrioventricular [AV] block (incomplete) (partial)

426.11 First degree atrioventricular block
Incomplete atrioventricular block, first degree
Prolonged P-R interval NOS

426.12 Mobitz (type) II atrioventricular block
Incomplete atrioventricular block:
Mobitz (type) II
second degree, Mobitz (type) II

426.13 Other second degree atrioventricular block
Incomplete atrioventricular block:
Mobitz (type) I [Wenckebach's]
second degree:
NOS
Mobitz (type) I
with 2:1 atrioventricular response [block]
Wenckebach's phenomenon

426.2 Left bundle branch hemiblock
Block:
left anterior fascicular
left posterior fascicular

426.3 Other left bundle branch block
Left bundle branch block:
NOS
anterior fascicular with posterior fascicular
complete
main stem

426.4 Right bundle branch block

⑤ **426.5 Bundle branch block, other and unspecified**

426.50 Bundle branch block, unspecified

426.51 Right bundle branch block and left posterior fascicular block

● Code new to this edition   ▲ Revision of existing code   ④ ⑤ Fourth or fifth digit required

426.52 Right bundle branch block and left anterior fascicular block

426.53 Other bilateral bundle branch block
Bifascicular block NOS
Bilateral bundle branch block NOS
Right bundle branch with left bundle branch block (incomplete) (main stem)

426.54 Trifascicular block

426.6 Other heart block

Intraventricular block: Sinoatrial block
NOS   Sinoauricular block
diffuse
myofibrillar

426.7 Anomalous atrioventricular excitation
Atrioventricular conduction:
accelerated
accessory
pre-excitation
Ventricular pre-excitation
Wolff-Parkinson-White syndrome

⑤ **426.8 Other specified conduction disorders**

426.81 Lown-Ganong-Levine syndrome
Syndrome of short P-R interval, normal QRS complexes, and supraventricular tachycardias

426.82 Long QT syndrome

426.89 Other
Dissociation:
atrioventricular [AV]
interference
isorhythmic
Nonparoxysmal AV nodal tachycardia

426.9 Conduction disorder, unspecified
Heart block NOS
Stokes-Adams syndrome

427 Cardiac dysrhythmias

Excludes: that complicating:
abortion (634-638 with .7, 639.8)
ectopic or molar pregnancy (639.8)
labor or delivery (668.1, 669.4)

427.0 Paroxysmal supraventricular tachycardia
Paroxysmal tachycardia:
atrial [PAT]
atrioventricular [AV]
junctional
nodal

427.1 Paroxysmal ventricular tachycardia
Ventricular tachycardia (paroxysmal)

427.2 Paroxysmal tachycardia, unspecified
Bouveret-Hoffmann syndrome
Paroxysmal tachycardia:
NOS
essential

⑤ **427.3 Atrial fibrillation and flutter**

427.31 Atrial fibrillation

427.32 Atrial flutter

⑤ **427.4 Ventricular fibrillation and flutter**

427.41 Ventricular fibrillation

427.42 Ventricular flutter

427.5 Cardiac arrest
Cardiorespiratory arrest

| | Add 4th or 5th digit | | Nonspecific code | | Unspecified code | | Manifestation code |

⑤ **427.6 Premature beats**

427.60 Premature beats, unspecified
Ectopic beats
Extrasystoles
Extrasystolic arrhythmia
Premature contractions or systoles NOS

427.61 Supraventricular premature beats
Atrial premature beats, contractions, or systoles

427.69 Other
Ventricular premature beats, contractions, or systoles

⑤ **427.8 Other specified cardiac dysrhythmias**

427.81 Sinoatrial node dysfunction

Sinus bradycardia:	Syndrome:
persistent	sick sinus
severe	tachycardia-bradycardia

Excludes: sinus bradycardia NOS (427.89)

427.89 Other

Rhythm disorder:	Rhythm disorder:
coronary sinus	nodal
ectopic	Wandering (atrial) pacemaker

Excludes: carotid sinus syncope (337.0)
neonatal bradycardia (779.81)
neonatal tachycardia (779.82)
reflex bradycardia (337.0)
tachycardia (785.0)

427.9 Cardiac dysrhythmia, unspecified
Arrhythmia (cardiac) NOS

428 Heart failure
Code, if applicable, heart failure due to hypertension first (402.0-402.9, with fifth-digit 1 or 404.0-404.9 with fifth digit 1 or 3)

Excludes: following cardiac surgery (429.4)
rheumatic (398.91)
that complicating:
abortion (634-638 with .7, 639.8)
ectopic or molar pregnancy (639.8)
labor or delivery (668.1, 669.4)

428.0 Congestive heart failure, unspecified
Congestive heart disease
Right heart failure (secondary to left heart failure)

Excludes: fluid overload NOS (276.6)

428.1 Left heart failure
Acute edema of lung with heart disease NOS or heart failure
Acute pulmonary edema with heart disease NOS or heart failure
Cardiac asthma
Left ventricular failure

⑤ **428.2 Systolic heart failure**

Excludes: combined systolic and diastolic heart failure (428.40-428.43)

428.20 Unspecified

428.21 Acute

428.22 Chronic

428.23 Acute on chronic

⑤ **428.3 Diastolic heart failure**

Excludes: combined systolic and diastolic heart failure (428.40-428.43)

428.30 Unspecified

428.31 Acute

428.32 Chronic

428.33 Acute on chronic

⑤ **428.4 Combined systolic and diastolic heart failure**

428.40 Unspecified

428.41 Acute

● Code new
to this edition

▲ Revision of
existing code

④ ⑤ Fourth or fifth
digit required

428.42 Chronic

428.43 Acute on chronic

428.9 Heart failure, unspecified
Cardiac failure NOS   Myocardial failure NOS
Heart failure NOS   Weak heart

429 Ill-defined descriptions and complications of heart disease

429.0 Myocarditis, unspecified
Myocarditis:
NOS (with mention of arteriosclerosis)
chronic (interstitial) (with mention of arteriosclerosis)
fibroid (with mention of arteriosclerosis)
senile (with mention of arteriosclerosis)
Use additional code, if desired, to identify presence of arteriosclerosis

Excludes: *acute or subacute (422.0-422.9)*
rheumatic (398.0)
acute (391.2)
that due to hypertension (402.0-402.9)

429.1 Myocardial degeneration
Degeneration of heart or myocardium:
fatty (with mention of arteriosclerosis)
mural (with mention of arteriosclerosis)
muscular (with mention of arteriosclerosis)
Myocardial:
degeneration (with mention of arteriosclerosis)
disease (with mention of arteriosclerosis)
Use additional code, if desired, to identify presence of arteriosclerosis

Excludes: *that due to hypertension (402.0-402.9)*

429.2 Cardiovascular disease, unspecified
Arteriosclerotic cardiovascular disease [ASCVD]
Cardiovascular arteriosclerosis
Cardiovascular:
degeneration (with mention of arteriosclerosis)
disease (with mention of arteriosclerosis)
sclerosis (with mention of arteriosclerosis)
Use additional code, if desired, to identify presence of arteriosclerosis

Excludes: *that due to hypertension (402.0-402.9)*

429.3 Cardiomegaly
Cardiac: Ventricular dilatation
dilatation
hypertrophy

Excludes: *that due to hypertension (402.0-402.9)*

429.4 Functional disturbances following cardiac surgery
Cardiac insufficiency following cardiac surgery or due to prosthesis
Heart failure following cardiac surgery or due to prosthesis
Postcardiotomy syndrome
Postvalvulotomy syndrome

Excludes: *cardiac failure in the immediate postoperative period (997.1)*

429.5 Rupture of chordae tendineae

429.6 Rupture of papillary muscle

⑤ **429.7 Certain sequelae of myocardial infarction, not elsewhere classified**
Use additional code to identify the associated myocardial infarction:
with onset of 8 weeks or less (410.00-410.92)
with onset of more than 8 weeks (414.8)

Excludes: *congenital defects of heart (745, 746)*
coronary aneurysm (414.11)
disorders of papillary muscle (429.6, 429.81)
postmyocardial infarction syndrome (411.0)
rupture of chordae tendineae (429.5)

429.71 Acquired cardiac septal defect

Excludes: *acute septal infarction (410.00-410.92)*

| | Add 4th or 5th digit | | Nonspecific code | | Unspecified code | | Manifestation code |

429.79 **Other**
Mural thrombus (atrial) (ventricular), acquired, following myocardial infarction

⑤ **429.8** **Other ill-defined heart diseases**

429.81 **Other disorders of papillary muscle**

Papillary muscle:
atrophy
degeneration
dysfunction

Papillary muscle:
incompetence
incoordination
scarring

429.82 **Hyperkinetic heart disease**

429.83 **Takotsubo syndrome**
Broken heart syndrome
Reversible left ventricular dysfunction following sudden emotional stress
Stress induced cardiomyopathy
Transient left ventricular apical ballooning syndrome

429.89 **Other**
Carditis

Excludes: that due to hypertension (402.0-402.9)

429.9 **Heart disease, unspecified**
Heart disease (organic) NOS
Morbus cordis NOS

Excludes: that due to hypertension (402.0-402.9)

CEREBROVASCULAR DISEASE (430-438)

Includes: with mention of hypertension (conditions classifiable to 401-405)
Use additional code, if desired, to identify presence of hypertension

Excludes: any condition classifiable to 430-434, 436, 437 occurring during pregnancy,
childbirth, or the puerperium, or specified as puerperal (674.0)
iatrogenic cerebrovascular infarction or hemorrhage (997.02)

430 **Subarachnoid hemorrhage**
Meningeal hemorrhage
Ruptured:
berry aneurysm
(congenital) cerebral aneurysm NOS

Excludes: syphilitic ruptured cerebral aneurysm (094.87)

431 **Intracerebral hemorrhage**

Hemorrhage (of):
basilar
bulbar
cerebellar
cerebral
cerebromeningeal
cortical
internal capsule

Hemorrhage (of):
intrapontine
pontine
subcortical
ventricular
Rupture of blood vessel in brain

432 **Other and unspecified intracranial hemorrhage**

432.0 **Nontraumatic extradural hemorrhage**
Nontraumatic epidural hemorrhage

432.1 **Subdural hemorrhage**
Subdural hematoma, nontraumatic

432.9 **Unspecified intracranial hemorrhage**
Intracranial hemorrhage NOS

⑤ **433** **Occlusion and stenosis of precerebral arteries**
Use additional code, if applicable, to identify status post administration of tPA (rtPA) in a
different facility within the last 24 hours prior to admission to current facility (V45.88)

The following fifth-digit subclassification is for use with category 433:

0 **without mention of cerebral infarction**

1 **with cerebral infarction**

Includes: embolism of basilar, carotid, and vertebral arteries
narrowing of basilar, carotid, and vertebral arteries
obstruction of basilar, carotid, and vertebral arteries
thrombosis of basilar, carotid, and vertebral arteries

Excludes: insufficiency NOS of precerebral arteries (435.0-435.9)

● Code new
to this edition

▲ Revision of
existing code

④ ⑤ Fourth or fifth
digit required

⑤ **433.0** **Basilar artery**
[0-1]

⑤ **433.1** **Carotid artery**
[0-1]

⑤ **433.2** **Vertebral artery**
[0-1]

⑤ **433.3** **Multiple and bilateral**
[0-1]

⑤ **433.8** **Other specified precerebral artery**
[0-1]

⑤ **433.9** **Unspecified precerebral artery**
[0-1]   Precerebral artery NOS

⑤ **434** **Occlusion of cerebral arteries**
Use additional code, if applicable, to identify status post administration of tPA (rtPA) in a
different facility within the last 24 hours prior to admission to current facility (V45.88)

The following fifth-digit subclassification is for use with category 434:

    0 **without mention of cerebral infarction**

    1 **with cerebral infarction**

⑤ **434.0** **Cerebral thrombosis**
[0-1]   Thrombosis of cerebral arteries

⑤ **434.1** **Cerebral embolism**
[0-1]

⑤ **434.9** **Cerebral artery occlusion, unspecified**
[0-1]

435 **Transient cerebral ischemia**
    Includes: cerebrovascular insufficiency (acute) with transient focal neurological signs and
symptoms
insufficiency of basilar, carotid, and vertebral arteries
spasm of cerebral arteries

    Excludes: *acute cerebrovascular insufficiency NOS (437.1)*
        that due to any condition classifiable to 433 (433.0-433.9)

435.0 **Basilar artery syndrome**

435.1 **Vertebral artery syndrome**

435.2 **Subclavian steal syndrome**

435.3 **Vertebrobasilar artery syndrome**

435.8 **Other specified transient cerebral ischemias**

435.9 **Unspecified transient cerebral ischemia**
    Impending cerebrovascular accident
    Intermittent cerebral ischemia
    Transient ischemic attack [TIA]

436 **Acute, but ill-defined, cerebrovascular disease**
    Apoplexy, apoplectic:
      NOS
      attack
      cerebral
      seizure
    Cerebral seizure

    Excludes: *any condition classifiable to categories 430-435*
        cerebrovascular accident (434.91)
        CVA (ischemic) (434.91)
         embolic (434.11)
         hemorrhagic (430, 431, 432.0-432.9)
         thrombotic (434.01)
        postoperative cerebrovascular accident (997.02)
        stroke (ischemic) (434.91)
         embolic (434.11)
         hemorrhagic (430, 431, 432.0-432.9)
         thrombotic (434.01)

437 **Other and ill-defined cerebrovascular disease**

437.0 **Cerebral atherosclerosis**
    Atheroma of cerebral arteries
    Cerebral arteriosclerosis

| | Add 4th or 5th digit | | Nonspecific code | | Unspecified code | | Manifestation code |

TABULAR LIST

437.1 **Other generalized ischemic cerebrovascular disease**
Acute cerebrovascular insufficiency NOS
Cerebral ischemia (chronic)

437.2 **Hypertensive encephalopathy**

437.3 **Cerebral aneurysm, nonruptured**
Internal carotid artery, intracranial portion
Internal carotid artery NOS

Excludes: congenital cerebral aneurysm, nonruptured (747.81)
internal carotid artery, extracranial portion (442.81)

437.4 **Cerebral arteritis**

437.5 **Moyamoya disease**

437.6 **Nonpyogenic thrombosis of intracranial venous sinus**

Excludes: pyogenic (325)

437.7 **Transient global amnesia**

437.8 **Other**

437.9 **Unspecified**
Cerebrovascular disease or lesion NOS

438 **Late effects of cerebrovascular disease**
Note: This category is to be used to indicate conditions in 430-437 as the cause of late effects. The "late effects" include conditions specified as such, as sequelae, which may occur at any time after the onset of the causal condition.

Excludes: personal history of:
cerebral infarction without residual deficits (V12.54)
PRIND (Prolonged reversible ischemic neurologic deficit) (V12.54)
RIND (Reversible ischemic neurological deficit) (V12.54)
transient ischemic attack (TIA) (V12.54)

438.0 **Cognitive deficits**

⑤ **438.1** **Speech and language deficits**

438.10 **Speech and language deficit, unspecified**

438.11 **Aphasia**

438.12 **Dysphasia**

● **438.13** **Dysarthria**

● **438.14** **Fluency disorder**
Stuttering

438.19 **Other speech and language deficits**

⑤ **438.2** **Hemiplegia/hemiparesis**

438.20 **Hemiplegia affecting unspecified side**

438.21 **Hemiplegia affecting dominant side**

438.22 **Hemiplegia affecting nondominant side**

⑤ **438.3** **Monoplegia of upper limb**

438.30 **Monoplegia of upper limb affecting unspecified side**

438.31 **Monoplegia of upper limb affecting dominant side**

438.32 **Monoplegia of upper limb affecting nondominant side**

⑤ **438.4** **Monoplegia of lower limb**

438.40 **Monoplegia of lower limb affecting unspecified side**

438.41 **Monoplegia of lower limb affecting dominant side**

438.42 **Monoplegia of lower limb affecting nondominant side**

⑤ **438.5** **Other paralytic syndrome**
Use additional code to identify type of paralytic syndrome, such as:
locked-in state (344.81)
quadriplegia (344.00-344.09)

Excludes: late effects of cerebrovascular accident with:
hemiplegia/hemiparesis (438.20-438.22)
monoplegia of lower limb (438.40-438.42)
monoplegia of upper limb (438.30-438.32)

438.50 **Other paralytic syndrome affecting unspecified side**

438.51 **Other paralytic syndrome affecting dominant side**

● Code new
to this edition
▲ Revision of
existing code
④ ⑤ Fourth or fifth
digit required

438.52　Other paralytic syndrome affecting nondominant side

438.53　Other paralytic syndrome, bilateral

438.6　Alterations of sensations
Use additional code to identify the altered sensation

438.7　Disturbances of vision
Use additional code to identify the visual disturbance

⑤ **438.8　Other late effects of cerebrovascular disease**

438.81　Apraxia

438.82　Dysphagia
Use additional code to identify the type of dysphagia, if known (787.20-787.29)

438.83　Facial weakness
Facial droop

438.84　Ataxia

438.85　Vertigo

438.89　Other late effects of cerebrovascular disease
Use additional code to identify the late effect

438.9　Unspecified late effects of cerebrovascular disease

DISEASES OF ARTERIES, ARTERIOLES, AND CAPILLARIES (440-449)

440　Atherosclerosis
Includes:　arteriolosclerosis
arteriosclerosis (obliterans) (senile)
arteriosclerotic vascular disease
atheroma
degeneration:
　arterial
　arteriovascular
　vascular
endarteritis deformans or obliterans
senile arteritis
senile endarteritis

Excludes:　atheroembolism (445.01-445.89)
atherosclerosis of bypass graft of the extremities (440.30-440.32)

440.0　Of aorta

440.1　Of renal artery

Excludes:　atherosclerosis of renal arterioles (403.00-403.91)

⑤ **440.2　Of native arteries of the extremities**
Use additional code, if applicable, to identify chronic total occlusion of artery of the extremities (440.4)

Excludes:　atherosclerosis of bypass graft of the extremities (440.30-440.32)

440.20　Atherosclerosis of the extremities, unspecified

440.21　Atherosclerosis of the extremities with intermittent claudication

440.22　Atherosclerosis of the extremities with rest pain
Any condition classifiable to 440.21

440.23　Atherosclerosis of the extremities with ulceration
Any condition classifiable to 440.21 and 440.22
Use additional code for any associated ulceration (707.10-707.9)

440.24　Atherosclerosis of the extremities with gangrene
Any condition classifiable to 440.21, 440.22, and 440.23 with ischemic
gangrene 785.4
Use additional code for any associated ulceration (707.10-707.9)

Excludes:　gas gangrene 040.0

440.29　Other

⑤ **440.3　Of bypass graft of the extremities**

Excludes:　atherosclerosis of native artery of the extremity (440.21-440.24)
embolism [occlusion NOS] [thrombus]
of graft (996.74)

440.30　Of unspecified graft

440.31　Of autologous vein bypass graft

440.32 Of nonautologous biological bypass graft

440.4 Chronic total occlusion of artery of the extremities
Complete occlusion of artery of the extremities
Total occlusion of artery of the extremities

Code first atherosclerosis of arteries of the extremities (440.20-440.29, 440.30-440.32)

> *Excludes:* acute occlusion of artery of extremity (444.21- 444.22)

440.8 Of other specified arteries

> *Excludes:* basilar (433.0)
> carotid (433.1)
> cerebral (437.0)
> coronary (414.00-414.07)
> mesenteric (557.1)
> precerebral (433.0-433.9)
> pulmonary (416.0)
> vertebral (433.2)

440.9 Generalized and unspecified atherosclerosis
Arteriosclerotic vascular disease NOS

> *Excludes:* arteriosclerotic cardiovascular disease [ASCVD] (429.2)

441 Aortic aneurysm and dissection

> *Excludes:* syphilitic aortic aneurysm (093.0)
> traumatic aortic aneurysm (901.0, 902.0)

⑤ **441.0 Dissection of aorta**

441.00 Unspecified site

441.01 Thoracic

441.02 Abdominal

441.03 Thoracoabdominal

441.1 Thoracic aneurysm, ruptured

441.2 Thoracic aneurysm without mention of rupture

441.3 Abdominal aneurysm, ruptured

441.4 Abdominal aneurysm without mention of rupture

441.5 Aortic aneurysm of unspecified site, ruptured
Rupture of aorta NOS

441.6 Thoracoabdominal aneurysm, ruptured

441.7 Thoracoabdominal aneurysm, without mention of rupture

441.9 Aortic aneurysm of unspecified site without mention of rupture
Aneurysm
Dilatation of aorta
Hyaline necrosis of aorta

442 Other aneurysm
Includes: aneurysm (ruptured) (cirsoid) (false) (varicose)
aneurysmal varix

> *Excludes:* arteriovenous aneurysm or fistula:
> acquired (447.0)
> congenital (747.60-747.69)
> traumatic (900.0-904.9)

442.0 Of artery of upper extremity

442.1 Of renal artery

442.2 Of iliac artery

442.3 Of artery of lower extremity
Aneurysm:
femoral artery
popliteal artery

⑤ **442.8 Of other specified artery**

442.81 Artery of neck
Aneurysm of carotid artery (common) (external) (internal, extracranial portion)

> *Excludes:* internal carotid artery, intracranial portion (437.3)

442.82 Subclavian artery

442.83 Splenic artery

● Code new
to this edition
▲ Revision of
existing code
④ ⑤ Fourth or fifth
digit required

442.84 Other visceral artery
Aneurysm:
celiac artery
gastroduodenal artery
gastroepiploic artery
hepatic artery
pancreaticoduodenal artery
superior mesenteric artery

442.89 Other
Aneurysm:
mediastinal artery
spinal artery

Excludes: *cerebral (nonruptured) (437.3)*
congenital (747.81)
ruptured (430)
coronary (414.11)
heart (414.10)
pulmonary (417.1)

442.9 Of unspecified site

443 Other peripheral vascular disease

443.0 Raynaud's syndrome
Raynaud's:
disease
phenomenon (secondary)
Use additional code, if desired, to identify gangrene (785.4)

443.1 Thromboangiitis obliterans [Buerger's disease]
Presenile gangrene

⑤ **443.2 Other arterial dissection**
Excludes: *dissection of aorta (441.00-441.03)*
dissection of coronary arteries (414.12)

443.21 Dissection of carotid artery

443.22 Dissection of iliac artery

443.23 Dissection of renal artery

443.24 Dissection of vertebral artery

443.29 Dissection of other artery

⑤ **443.8 Other specified peripheral vascular diseases**

443.81 Peripheral angiopathy in diseases classified elsewhere
Code first underlying disease, as:
diabetes mellitus (249.7, 250.7)

443.82 Erythromelalgia

443.89 Other
Acrocyanosis
Acroparesthesia:
simple [Schultze's type]
vasomotor [Nothnagel's type]
Erythrocyanosis

Excludes: *chilblains (991.5)*
frostbite (991.0-991.3)
immersion foot (991.4)

443.9 Peripheral vascular disease, unspecified
Intermittent claudication NOS
Peripheral:
angiopathy NOS
vascular disease NOS
Spasm of artery

Excludes: *atherosclerosis of the arteries of the extremities (440.20-440.22)*
spasm of cerebral artery (435.0-435.9)

	Add 4th or 5th digit		Nonspecific code		Unspecified code		Manifestation code

TABULAR LIST

444 **Arterial embolism and thrombosis**
Includes: infarction:
embolic
thrombotic
occlusion

Excludes: *atheroembolism (445.01-445.89)*
septic arterial embolism (449)
that complicating:
abortion (634-638 with .6, 639.6)
ectopic or molar pregnancy (639.6)
pregnancy, childbirth, or the puerperium (673.0-673.8)

444.0 **Of abdominal aorta**
Aortic bifurcation syndrome   Leriche's syndrome
Aortoiliac obstruction   Saddle embolus

444.1 **Of thoracic aorta**
Embolism or thrombosis of aorta (thoracic)

⑤ **444.2** **Of arteries of the extremities**

444.21 **Upper extremity**

444.22 **Lower extremity**
Arterial embolism or thrombosis:
femoral
peripheral NOS
popliteal

Excludes: *iliofemoral (444.81)*

⑤ **444.8** **Of other specified artery**

444.81 **Iliac artery**

444.89 **Other**

Excludes: *basilar (433.0)*
carotid (433.1)
cerebral (434.0-434.9)
coronary (410.00-410.92)
mesenteric (557.0)
ophthalmic (362.30-362.34)
precerebral (433.0-433.9)
pulmonary (415.19)
renal (593.81)
retinal (362.30-362.34)
vertebral (433.2)

444.9 **Of unspecified artery**

445 **Atheroembolism**
Includes: Atherothrombotic microembolism
Cholesterol embolism

⑤ **445.0** **Of extremities**

445.01 **Upper extremity**

445.02 **Lower extremity**

⑤ **445.8** **Of other sites**

445.81 **Kidney**
Use additional code for any associated acute kidney failure or chronic kidney disease (584, 585)

445.89 **Other site**

446 **Polyarteritis nodosa and allied conditions**

446.0 **Polyarteritis nodosa**
Disseminated necrotizing periarteritis
Necrotizing angiitis
Panarteritis (nodosa)
Periarteritis (nodosa)

446.1 **Acute febrile mucocutaneous lymph node syndrome [MLNS]**
Kawasaki disease

⑤ **446.2** **Hypersensitivity angiitis**

Excludes: *antiglomerular basement membrane disease without pulmonary hemorrhage (583.89)*

● Code new to this edition   ▲ Revision of existing code   ④ ⑤ Fourth or fifth digit required

446.20 Hypersensitivity angiitis, unspecified

446.21 Goodpasture's syndrome
Antiglomerular basement membrane antibody-mediated nephritis with
pulmonary hemorrhage

Use additional code, if desired, to identify renal disease (583.81)

446.29 Other specified hypersensitivity angiitis

446.3 Lethal midline granuloma
Malignant granuloma of face

446.4 Wegener's granulomatosis
Necrotizing respiratory granulomatosis
Wegener's syndrome

446.5 Giant cell arteritis
Cranial arteritis   Temporal arteritis
Horton's disease

446.6 Thrombotic microangiopathy
Moschcowitz's syndrome
Thrombotic thrombocytopenic purpura

446.7 Takayasu's disease
Aortic arch arteritis
Pulseless disease

447 Other disorders of arteries and arterioles

447.0 Arteriovenous fistula, acquired
Arteriovenous aneurysm, acquired

Excludes: *cerebrovascular (437.3)*
coronary (414.19)
pulmonary (417.0)
surgically created arteriovenous shunt or fistula:
complication (996.1, 996.61-996.62)
status or presence (V45.11)
traumatic (900.0-904.9)

447.1 Stricture of artery

447.2 Rupture of artery
Erosion of artery
Fistula, except arteriovenous of artery
Ulcer of artery

Excludes: *traumatic rupture of artery (900.0-904.9)*

447.3 Hyperplasia of renal artery
Fibromuscular hyperplasia of renal artery

447.4 Celiac artery compression syndrome
Celiac axis syndrome
Marable's syndrome

447.5 Necrosis of artery

447.6 Arteritis, unspecified
Aortitis NOS
Endarteritis NOS

Excludes: *arteritis, endarteritis:*
aortic arch (446.7)
cerebral (437.4)
coronary (414.00-414.07)
deformans (440.0-440.9)
obliterans (440.0-440.9)
pulmonary (417.8)
senile (440.0-440.9)
polyarteritis NOS (446.0)
syphilitic aortitis (093.1)

447.8 Other specified disorders of arteries and arterioles
Fibromuscular hyperplasia of arteries, except renal

447.9 Unspecified disorders of arteries and arterioles

448 Disease of capillaries

448.0 Hereditary hemorrhagic telangiectasia
Rendu-Osler-Weber disease

	Add 4th or 5th digit		Nonspecific code		Unspecified code		Manifestation code

448.1 Nevus, non-neoplastic
> Nevus: Nevus:
>   araneus   spider
>   senile   stellar

> Excludes: *neoplastic (216.0-216.9)*
>   *port wine (757.32)*
>   *strawberry (757.32)*

448.9 Other and unspecified capillary diseases
> Capillary:
>   hemorrhage
>   hyperpermeability
>   thrombosis

> Excludes: *capillary fragility (hereditary) (287.8)*

449 Septic arterial embolism
Code first underlying infection, such as:
   infective endocarditis (421.0)
   lung abscess (513.0)
Use additional code to identify the site of the embolism (433.0-433.9, 444.0-444.9)

> Excludes: *septic pulmonary embolism (415.12)*

DISEASES OF VEINS AND LYMPHATICS, AND OTHER DISEASES OF CIRCULATORY SYSTEM (451-459)

451 Phlebitis and thrombophlebitis
> Includes: endophlebitis
>   inflammation, vein
>   periphlebitis
>   suppurative phlebitis

Use additional E Code, if desired, to identify drug, if drug-induced

> Excludes: *that complicating:*
>   *abortion (634-638 with .7, 639.8)*
>   *ectopic or molar pregnancy (639.8)*
>   *pregnancy, childbirth, or the puerperium (671.0-671.9)*
>   *that due to or following:*
>   *implant or catheter device (996.61-996.62)*
>   *infusion, perfusion, or transfusion (999.2)*

451.0 Of superficial vessels of lower extremities
> Saphenous vein (greater) (lesser)

⑤ **451.1 Of deep vessels of lower extremities**

      451.11 Femoral vein (deep) (superficial)

      451.19 Other
>   Femoropopliteal vein
>   Popliteal vein
>   Tibial vein

451.2 Of lower extremities, unspecified

⑤ **451.8 Of other sites**

> Excludes: *intracranial venous sinus (325)*
>   *nonpyogenic (437.6)*
>   *portal (vein) (572.1)*

      451.81 Iliac vein

      451.82 Of superficial veins of upper extremities
>   Antecubital vein
>   Basilic vein
>   Cephalic vein

      451.83 Of deep veins of upper extremities
>   Brachial vein
>   Radial vein
>   Ulnar vein

      451.84 Of upper extremities, unspecified

      451.89 Other
>   Axillary vein
>   Jugular vein
>   Subclavian vein
>   Thrombophlebitis of breast (Mondor's disease)

● Code new   ▲ Revision of   ④ ⑤ Fourth or fifth
   to this edition   existing code   digit required

451.9 Of unspecified site

452 Portal vein thrombosis
Portal (vein) obstruction

Excludes: hepatic vein thrombosis (453.0)
phlebitis of portal vein (572.1)

453 Other venous embolism and thrombosis

Excludes: that complicating:
abortion (634-638 with .7, 639.8)
ectopic or molar pregnancy (639.8)
pregnancy, childbirth, or the puerperium (671.0-671.9)

453.0 Budd-Chiari syndrome
Hepatic vein thrombosis

453.1 Thrombophlebitis migrans

▲ **453.2 Of inferior vena cava**

453.3 Of renal vein

▲ **453.4 Acute venous embolism and thrombosis of deep vessels of lower extremity**

▲ **453.40** Acute venous embolism and thrombosis of unspecified deep vessels of lower extremity
Deep vein thrombosis NOS
DVT NOS

▲ **453.41** Acute venous embolism and thrombosis of deep vessels of proximal lower extremity
Femoral
Iliac
Popliteal
Thigh
Upper leg NOS

▲ **453.42** Acute venous embolism and thrombosis of deep vessels of distal lower extremity
Calf
Lower leg NOS
Peroneal
Tibial

● **453.5 Chronic venous embolism and thrombosis of deep vessels of lower extremity**
Use additional code, if applicable, for associated long-term (current) use of anticoagulants (V58.61)

Excludes: personal history of venous thrombosis and embolism (V12.51)

● **453.50** Chronic venous embolism and thrombosis of unspecified deep vessels of lower extremity

● **453.51** Chronic venous embolism and thrombosis of deep vessels of proximal lower extremity

● **453.52** Chronic venous embolism and thrombosis of deep vessels of distal lower extremity

● **453.6 Venous embolism and thrombosis of superficial vessels of lower extremity**
Saphenous vein (greater) (lesser)

● **453.7 Chronic venous embolism and thrombosis of other specified vessels**
Use additional code, if applicable, for associated long-term (current) use of anticoagulants (V58.61)

Excludes: personal history of venous thrombosis and embolism (V12.51)

● **453.71** Chronic venous embolism and thrombosis of superficial veins of upper extremity
Antecubital vein
Basilic vein
Cephalic vein

● **453.72** Chronic venous embolism and thrombosis of deep veins of upper extremity
Brachial vein
Radial vein
Ulnar vein

● **453.73** Chronic venous embolism and thrombosis of upper extremity, unspecified

● **453.74** Chronic venous embolism and thrombosis of axillary veins

● **453.75** Chronic venous embolism and thrombosis of subclavian veins

	Add 4th or 5th digit		Nonspecific code		Unspecified code		Manifestation code

● **453.76** **Chronic venous embolism and thrombosis of internal jugular veins**

● 453.77 **Chronic venous embolism and thrombosis of other thoracic veins**
　　　Brachiocephalic (innominate)
　　　Superior vena cava

● 453.79 **Chronic venous embolism and thrombosis of other specified veins**

▲ 453.8 **Acute venous embolism and thrombosis of other specified veins**

　Excludes: *cerebral (434.0-434.9)*
　　　　coronary (410.00-410.92)
　　　　intracranial venous sinus (325)
　　　　　nonpyogenic (437.6)
　　　　mesenteric (557.0)
　　　　portal (452)
　　　　precerebral (433.0-433.9)
　　　　pulmonary (415.19)

● **453.81** **Acute venous embolism and thrombosis of superficial veins of upper extremity**
　　　Antecubital vein
　　　Basilic vein
　　　Cephalic vein

● **453.82** **Acute venous embolism and thrombosis of deep veins of upper extremity**
　　　Brachial vein
　　　Radial vein
　　　Ulnar vein

● 453.83 **Acute venous embolism and thrombosis of upper extremity, unspecified**

● **453.84** **Acute venous embolism and thrombosis of axillary veins**

● **453.85** **Acute venous embolism and thrombosis of subclavian veins**

● **453.86** **Acute venous embolism and thrombosis of internal jugular veins**

● 453.87 **Acute venous embolism and thrombosis of other thoracic veins**
　　　Brachiocephalic (innominate)
　　　Superior vena cava

● 453.89 **Acute venous embolism and thrombosis of other specified veins**

　453.9 **Of unspecified site**
　　　Embolism of vein
　　　Thrombosis (vein)

454 **Varicose veins of lower extremities**

　Excludes: *that complicating pregnancy, childbirth, or the puerperium (671.0)*

　454.0 **With ulcer**
　　　Varicose ulcer (lower extremity, any part)
　　　Varicose veins with ulcer of lower extremity [any part] or of unspecified site
　　　Any condition classifiable to 454.9 with ulcer or specified as ulcerated

　454.1 **With inflammation**
　　　Stasis dermatitis
　　　Varicose veins with inflammation of lower extremity [any part] or of unspecified site
　　　Any condition classifiable to 454.9 with inflammation or specified as inflamed

　454.2 **With ulcer and inflammation**
　　　Varicose veins with ulcer and inflammation of lower extremity [any part] or of
　　　　unspecified site
　　　Any condition classifiable to 454.9 with ulcer and inflammation

　454.8 **With other complications**
　　　Edema
　　　Pain
　　　Swelling

　454.9 **Asymptomatic varicose veins**
　　　Phlebectasia of lower extremity [any part] or of unspecified site
　　　Varicose veins NOS
　　　Varicose veins of lower extremity [any part] or of unspecified site
　　　Varix of lower extremity [any part] or of unspecified site

455 **Hemorrhoids**
　　　Includes: hemorrhoids (anus) (rectum)
　　　　　piles
　　　　　varicose veins, anus or rectum

　Excludes: *that complicating pregnancy, childbirth or the puerperium (671.8)*

● Code new
　to this edition
　　　　▲ Revision of
　　　　　existing code
　　　　　　　④ ⑤ Fourth or fifth
　　　　　　　　digit required

455.0 Internal hemorrhoids without mention of complication

455.1 Internal thrombosed hemorrhoids

455.2 Internal hemorrhoids with other complication
Internal hemorrhoids: Internal hemorrhoids:
  bleeding   strangulated
  prolapsed   ulcerated

455.3 External hemorrhoids without mention of complication

455.4 External thrombosed hemorrhoids

455.5 External hemorrhoids with other complication
External hemorrhoids: External hemorrhoids:
  bleeding   strangulated
  prolapsed   ulcerated

455.6 Unspecified hemorrhoids without mention of complication
Hemorrhoids NOS

455.7 Unspecified thrombosed hemorrhoids
Thrombosed hemorrhoids, unspecified whether internal or external

455.8 Unspecified hemorrhoids with other complication
Hemorrhoids, unspecified whether internal or external:
  bleeding
  prolapsed
  strangulated
  ulcerated

455.9 Residual hemorrhoidal skin tags
Skin tags, anus or rectum

456 Varicose veins of other sites

456.0 Esophageal varices with bleeding

456.1 Esophageal varices without mention of bleeding

⑤ *456.2 Esophageal varices in diseases classified elsewhere*
Code first underlying cause, as:
  cirrhosis of liver (571.0-571.9)
  portal hypertension (572.3)

    456.20 With bleeding

    456.21 Without mention of bleeding

456.3 Sublingual varices

456.4 Scrotal varices
Varicocele

456.5 Pelvic varices
Varices of broad ligament

456.6 Vulval varices
Varices of perineum

  Excludes: *that complicating pregnancy, childbirth, or the puerperium (671.1)*

456.8 Varices of other sites
Varicose veins of nasal septum (with ulcer)

  Excludes: *placental varices (656.7)*
     retinal varices (362.17)
     varicose ulcer of unspecified site (454.0)
     varicose veins of unspecified site (454.9)

457 Noninfectious disorders of lymphatic channels

457.0 Postmastectomy lymphedema syndrome
Elephantiasis due to mastectomy
Obliteration of lymphatic vessel due to mastectomy

| ▨ | Add 4th or 5th digit | ▨ | Nonspecific code | ▨ | Unspecified code | ▨ | Manifestation code |

457.1 **Other lymphedema**
Elephantiasis (nonfilarial) NOS
Lymphangiectasis
Lymphedema:
  acquired (chronic)
  praecox
  secondary
Obliteration, lymphatic vessel

Excludes: *elephantiasis (nonfilarial):*
    congenital (757.0)
    eyelid (374.83)
    vulva (624.8)

457.2 **Lymphangitis**
Lymphangitis:
  NOS
  chronic
  subacute

Excludes: *acute lymphangitis (682.0-682.9)*

457.8 **Other noninfectious disorders of lymphatic channels**
Chylocele (nonfilarial)   Lymph node or vessel:
Chylous: fistula
  ascites   infarction
  cyst   rupture

Excludes: *chylocele:*
    filarial (125.0-125.9)
    tunica vaginalis (nonfilarial) (608.84)

457.9 **Unspecified noninfectious disorder of lymphatic channels**

458 **Hypotension**
Includes: hypopiesis

Excludes: *cardiovascular collapse (785.50)*
    maternal hypotension syndrome (669.2)
    shock (785.50-785.59)
    Shy-Drager syndrome (333.0)

458.0 **Orthostatic hypotension**
Hypotension:
  orthostatic (chronic)
  postural

458.1 **Chronic hypotension**
Permanent idiopathic hypotension

⑤ **458.2** **Iatrogenic hypotension**

    458.21 **Hypotension of hemodialysis**
        Intra-dialytic hypotension

    458.29 **Other iatrogenic hypotension**
        Postoperative hypotension

458.8 **Other specified hypotension**

458.9 **Hypotension, unspecified**
Hypotension (arterial) NOS

459 **Other disorders of circulatory system**

459.0 **Hemorrhage, unspecified**
Rupture of blood vessel NOS
Spontaneous hemorrhage NEC

Excludes: *hemorrhage:*
    gastrointestinal NOS (578.9)
    in newborn NOS (772.9)
    secondary or recurrent following trauma (958.2)
    nontraumatic hematoma of soft tissue (729.92)
    traumatic rupture of blood vessel (900.0-904.9)

⑤ **459.1** **Postphlebitic syndrome**
Chronic venous hypertension due to deep vein thrombosis

Excludes: *chronic venous hypertertension without deep vein thrombosis (459.30-459.39)*

    459.10 **Postphlebetic syndrome without complications**
        Asymptomatic postphlebetic syndrome
        Postphlebetic syndrome NOS

  ● Code new   ▲ Revision of   ④ ⑤ Fourth or fifth
     to this edition   existing code   digit required

459.11 Postphlebetic syndrome with ulcer

459.12 Postphlebetic syndrome with inflammation

459.13 Postphlebetic syndrome with ulcer and inflammation

459.19 Postphlebetic syndrome with other complication

459.2 Compression of vein
Stricture of vein
Vena cava syndrome (inferior) (superior)

⑤ **459.3 Chronic venous hypertension (idiopathic)**
Statis edema

Excludes: *chronic venous hypertension due to deep vein thrombosis (459.10-459.19)*
varicose veins (454.0-454.9)

459.30 Chronic venous hypertension without complications
Asymptomatic chronic venous hypertension
Chronic venous hypertension NOS

459.31 Chronic venous hypertension with ulcer

459.32 Chronic venous hypertension with inflammation

459.33 Chronic venous hypertension with ulcer and inflammation

459.39 Chronic venous hypertension with other complication

⑤ **459.8 Other specified disorders of circulatory system**

459.81 Venous (peripheral) insufficiency, unspecified
Chronic venous insufficiency NOS

Use additional code for any associated ulceration (707.10-707.9)

459.89 Other
Collateral circulation (venous), any site
Phlebosclerosis
Venofibrosis

459.9 Unspecified circulatory system disorder

	Add 4th or 5th digit		Nonspecific code		Unspecified code		Manifestation code

● Code new
to this edition

▲ Revision of
existing code

④ ⑤ Fourth or fifth
digit required

8. DISEASES OF THE RESPIRATORY SYSTEM (460-519)

Use additional code, if desired, to identify infectious organism

ACUTE RESPIRATORY INFECTIONS (460-466)

Excludes: pneumonia and influenza (480.0-488)

460 Acute nasopharyngitis [common cold]
Coryza (acute)   Rhinitis:
Nasal catarrh, acute   acute
Nasopharyngitis: infective
  NOS
  acute
  infective NOS

Excludes: nasopharyngitis, chronic (472.2)
   pharyngitis:
     acute or unspecified (462)
     chronic (472.1)
   rhinitis:
     allergic (477.0-477.9)
     chronic or unspecified (472.0)
   sore throat:
     acute or unspecified (462)
     chronic (472.1)

461 Acute sinusitis
Includes: abscess acute, of sinus (accessory) (nasal)
     empyema acute, of sinus (accessory) (nasal)
     infection acute, of sinus (accessory) (nasal)
     inflammation acute, of sinus (accessory) (nasal)
     suppuration acute, of sinus (accessory) (nasal)

Excludes: chronic or unspecified sinusitis (473.0-473.9)

461.0 Maxillary
Acute antritis

461.1 Frontal

461.2 Ethmoidal

461.3 Sphenoidal

461.8 Other acute sinusitis
Acute pansinusitis

461.9 Acute sinusitis, unspecified
Acute sinusitis NOS

462 Acute pharyngitis
Acute sore throat NOS   Pharyngitis (acute):
Pharyngitis (acute):   staphylococcal
  NOS   suppurative
  gangrenous   ulcerative
  infective   Sore throat (viral) NOS
  phlegmonous   Viral pharyngitis
  pneumococcal

Excludes: abscess:
     peritonsillar [quinsy] (475)
     pharyngeal NOS (478.29)
     retropharyngeal (478.24)
   chronic pharyngitis (472.1)
   infectious mononucleosis (075)
   that specified as (due to):
     Coxsackie (virus) (074.0)
     gonococcus (098.6)
     herpes simplex (054.79)
     influenza (487.1)
     septic (034.0)
     streptococcal (034.0)

Add 4th or 5th digit   Nonspecific code   Unspecified code   Manifestation code

463 Acute tonsillitis

Tonsillitis (acute):
  NOS
  follicular
  gangrenous
  infective
  pneumococcal

Tonsillitis (acute):
  septic
  staphylococcal
  suppurative
  ulcerative
  viral

Excludes: *chronic tonsillitis (474.0)*
  hypertrophy of tonsils (474.1)
  peritonsillar abscess [quinsy] (475)
  sore throat:
    acute or NOS (462)
    septic (034.0)
  streptococcal tonsillitis (034.0)

464 Acute laryngitis and tracheitis

Excludes: *that associated with influenza (487.1)*
  that due to Streptococcus (034.0)

⑤ **464.0 Acute laryngitis**

Laryngitis (acute):
  NOS
  edematous
  Hemophilus influenza
  [H. influenzae]

Laryngitis (acute):
  pneumococcal
  septic
  suppurative
  ulcerative

Excludes: *chronic laryngitis (476.0-476.1)*
  influenzal laryngitis (487.1)

464.00   Without mention of obstruction

464.01   With obstruction

⑤ **464.1 Acute tracheitis**

Tracheitis (acute):
  NOS
  catarrhal
  viral

Excludes: *chronic tracheitis (491.8)*

464.10   Without mention of obstruction

464.11   With obstruction

⑤ **464.2 Acute laryngotracheitis**

Laryngotracheitis (acute)
Tracheitis (acute) with laryngitis (acute)

Excludes: *chronic laryngotracheitis (476.1)*

464.20   Without mention of obstruction

464.21   With obstruction

⑤ **464.3 Acute epiglottitis**

Viral epiglottitis

Excludes: *epiglottitis, chronic (476.1)*

464.30   Without mention of obstruction

464.31   With obstruction

464.4 Croup

Croup syndrome

⑤ **464.5 Supraglottitis, unspecified**

464.50   Without mention of obstruction

464.51   With obstruction

465 Acute upper respiratory infections of multiple or unspecified sites

Excludes: *upper respiratory infection due to:*
  influenza (487.1)
  Streptococcus (034.0)

465.0 Acute laryngopharyngitis

465.8 Other multiple sites

Multiple URI

● Code new   ▲ Revision of   ④ ⑤ Fourth or fifth
  to this edition   existing code   digit required

465.9 Unspecified site
Acute URI NOS
Upper respiratory infection (acute)

466 Acute bronchitis and bronchiolitis
Includes: that with:
bronchospasm
obstruction

466.0 Acute bronchitis
Bronchitis, acute or subacute:
fibrinous
membranous
pneumococcal
purulent
septic
viral
with tracheitis
Croupous bronchitis
Tracheobronchitis, acute

Excludes: acute bronchitis with chronic obstructive pulmonary disease (491.22)

⑤ **466.1 Acute bronchiolitis**
Bronchiolitis (acute)
Capillary pneumonia

> **466.11 Acute bronchiolitis due to respiratory syncytial virus (RSV)**

> **466.19 Acute bronchiolitis due to other infectious organisms**
> Use additional code to identify organism

OTHER DISEASES OF THE UPPER RESPIRATORY TRACT (470-478)

470 Deviated nasal septum
Deflected septum (nasal) (acquired)

Excludes: congenital (754.0)

471 Nasal polyps

Excludes: adenomatous polyps (212.0)

471.0 Polyp of nasal cavity
Polyp:
choanal
nasopharyngeal

471.1 Polypoid sinus degeneration
Woakes' syndrome or ethmoiditis

471.8 Other polyp of sinus
Polyp of sinus: Polyp of sinus:
accessory   maxillary
ethmoidal   sphenoidal

471.9 Unspecified nasal polyp
Nasal polyp NOS

472 Chronic pharyngitis and nasopharyngitis

472.0 Chronic rhinitis
Ozena   Rhinitis:
Rhinitis: hypertrophic
NOS   obstructive
atrophic   purulent
granulomatous   ulcerative

Excludes: allergic rhinitis (477.0-477.9)

472.1 Chronic pharyngitis
Chronic sore throat
Pharyngitis:
atrophic
granular (chronic)
hypertrophic

472.2 Chronic nasopharyngitis

Excludes: acute or unspecified nasopharyngitis (460)

Add 4th or 5th digit	Nonspecific code	Unspecified code	Manifestation code

473 **Chronic sinusitis**
    Includes: abscess (chronic) of sinus (accessory) (nasal)
                 empyema (chronic) of sinus (accessory) (nasal)
                 infection (chronic) of sinus (accessory) (nasal)
                 suppuration (chronic) of sinus (accessory) (nasal)
    Excludes: *acute sinusitis (461.0-461.9)*

   473.0 **Maxillary**
       Antritis (chronic)

   473.1 **Frontal**

   473.2 **Ethmoidal**
       Excludes: *Woakes' ethmoiditis (471.1)*

   473.3 **Sphenoidal**

   473.8 **Other chronic sinusitis**
       Pansinusitis (chronic)

   473.9 **Unspecified sinusitis (chronic)**
       Sinusitis (chronic) NOS

474 **Chronic disease of tonsils and adenoids**
  ⑤ **474.0** **Chronic tonsillitis and adenoiditis**
      Excludes: *acute or unspecified tonsillitis (463)*

       474.00 **Chronic tonsillitis**

       474.01 **Chronic adenoiditis**

       474.02 **Chronic tonsillitis and adenoiditis**

  ⑤ **474.1** **Hypertrophy of tonsils and adenoids**
       Enlargement of tonsils or adenoids
       Hyperplasia of tonsils or adenoids
       Hypertrophy of tonsils or adenoids
      Excludes: *that with adenoiditis (474.01)*
              that with adenoiditis and tonsillitis (474.02)
              that with tonsillitis (474.00)

       474.10 **Tonsils with adenoids**

       474.11 **Tonsils alone**

       474.12 **Adenoids alone**

   474.2 **Adenoid vegetations**

   474.8 **Other chronic disease of tonsils and adenoids**
       Amygdalolith
       Calculus, tonsil
       Cicatrix of tonsil (and adenoid)
       Tonsillar tag
       Ulcer, tonsil

   474.9 **Unspecified chronic disease of tonsils and adenoids**
       Disease (chronic) of tonsils (and adenoids)

475 **Peritonsillar abscess**
       Abscess of tonsil
       Peritonsillar cellulitis
       Quinsy
    Excludes: *tonsillitis:*
          acute or NOS (463)
          chronic (474.0)

476 **Chronic laryngitis and laryngotracheitis**
   476.0 **Chronic laryngitis**
       Laryngitis:
        catarrhal
        hypertrophic
        Sicca

   476.1 **Chronic laryngotracheitis**
       Laryngitis, chronic, with tracheitis (chronic)
       Tracheitis, chronic, with laryngitis
      Excludes: *chronic tracheitis (491.8)*
          laryngitis and tracheitis, acute or unspecified (464.00-464.51)

● Code new   ▲ Revision of   ④ ⑤ Fourth or fifth
   to this edition   existing code   digit required

477 **Allergic rhinitis**
Includes: allergic rhinitis (nonseasonal) (seasonal)
hay fever
spasmodic rhinorrhea

Excludes: *allergic rhinitis with asthma (bronchial) (493.0)*

477.0 **Due to pollen**
Pollinosis

477.1 **Due to food**

477.2 **Due to animal (cat) (dog) hair and dander**

477.8 **Due to other allergen**

477.9 **Cause unspecified**

478 **Other diseases of upper respiratory tract**

478.0 **Hypertrophy of nasal turbinates**

⑤ **478.1** **Other diseases of nasal cavity and sinuses**

Excludes: *varicose ulcer of nasal septum (456.8)*

478.11 **Nasal mucositis (ulcerative)**
Use additional E code to identify adverse effects of therapy, such as:
antineoplastic and immunosuppressive drugs (E930.7, E933.1)
radiation therapy (E879.2)

478.19 **Other disease of nasal cavity and sinuses**
Abscess of nose (septum)
Necrosis of nose (septum)
Ulcer of nose (septum)
Cyst or mucocele of sinus (nasal)
Rhinolith

⑤ **478.2** **Other diseases of pharynx, not elsewhere classified**

478.20 **Unspecified disease of pharynx**

478.21 **Cellulitis of pharynx or nasopharynx**

478.22 **Parapharyngeal abscess**

478.24 **Retropharyngeal abscess**

478.25 **Edema of pharynx or nasopharynx**

478.26 **Cyst of pharynx or nasopharynx**

478.29 **Other**
Abscess of pharynx or nasopharynx

Excludes: *ulcerative pharyngitis (462)*

⑤ **478.3** **Paralysis of vocal cords or larynx**

478.30 **Paralysis, unspecified**
Laryngoplegia
Paralysis of glottis

478.31 **Unilateral, partial**

478.32 **Unilateral, complete**

478.33 **Bilateral, partial**

478.34 **Bilateral, complete**

478.4 **Polyp of vocal cord or larynx**

Excludes: *adenomatous polyps (212.1)*

478.5 **Other diseases of vocal cords**
Abscess of vocal cords
Cellulitis of vocal cords
Granuloma of vocal cords
Leukoplakia of vocal cords
Chorditis (fibrinous) (nodosa) (tuberosa)
Singers' nodes

478.6 **Edema of larynx**
Edema (of):
glottis
subglottic
supraglottic

⑤ **478.7** **Other diseases of larynx, not elsewhere classified**

478.70 **Unspecified disease of larynx**

	Add 4th or 5th digit		Nonspecific code		Unspecified code		Manifestation code

478.71 **Cellulitis and perichondritis of larynx**

478.74 **Stenosis of larynx**

478.75 **Laryngeal spasm**
Laryngismus (stridulus)

478.79 **Other**
Abscess of larynx
Necrosis of larynx
Obstruction of larynx
Pachyderma of larynx
Ulcer of larynx

Excludes: *ulcerative laryngitis (464.00-464.01)*

478.8 **Upper respiratory tract hypersensitivity reaction, site unspecified**

Excludes: *hypersensitivity reaction of lower respiratory tract, as:*
extrinsic allergic alveolitis (495.0-495.9)
pneumoconiosis (500-505)

478.9 **Other and unspecified diseases of upper respiratory tract**
Abscess of trachea
Cicatrix of trachea

PNEUMONIA AND INFLUENZA (480-488)

Excludes: *pneumonia:*
allergic or eosinophilic (518.3)
aspiration:
NOS (507.0)
newborn (770.18)
solids and liquids (507.0-507.8)
congenital (770.0)
lipoid (507.1)
passive (514)
rheumatic (390)
ventilator-associated (997.31)

480 **Viral pneumonia**

480.0 **Pneumonia due to adenovirus**

480.1 **Pneumonia due to respiratory syncytial virus**

480.2 **Pneumonia due to parainfluenza virus**

480.3 **Pneumonia due to SARS-associated coronavirus**

480.8 **Pneumonia due to other virus not elsewhere classified**

Excludes: *congenital rubella pneumonitis (771.0)*
influenza with pneumonia, any form (487.0)
pneumonia complicating viral diseases classified elsewhere (484.1-484.8)

480.9 **Viral pneumonia, unspecified**

481 **Pneumococcal pneumonia [*Streptococcus pneumoniae* pneumonia]**
Lobar pneumonia, organism unspecified

482 **Other bacterial pneumonia**

482.0 **Pneumonia due to Klebsiella pneumoniae**

482.1 **Pneumonia due to Pseudomonas**

482.2 **Pneumonia due to Hemophilus influenzae [H. influenzae]**

⑤ 482.3 **Pneumonia due to Streptococcus**

Excludes: *Streptococcus pneumoniae pneumonia (481)*

482.30 **Streptococcus, unspecified**

482.31 **Group A**

482.32 **Group B**

482.39 **Other Streptococcus**

⑤ 482.4 **Pneumonia due to Staphylococcus**

482.40 **Pneumonia due to Staphylococcus, unspecified**

482.41 **Methicillin susceptible pneumonia due to Staphylococcus aureus**
MSSA pneumonia
Pneumonia due to Staphylococcus aureus NOS

482.42 **Methicillin resistant pneumonia due to Staphylococcus aureus**

● Code new
to this edition
▲ Revision of
existing code
④ ⑤ Fourth or fifth
digit required

482.49   Other Staphylococcus pneumonia

⑤ **482.8**   **Pneumonia due to other specified bacteria**

> *Excludes:*   *pneumonia complicating infectious disease classified elsewhere (484.1-484.8)*

482.81   **Anaerobes**
Bacteroides (melaninogenicus)
Gram-negative anaerobes

482.82   **Escherichia coli [E. coli]**

482.83   **Other gram-negative bacteria**
Gram-negative pneumonia NOS
Proteus
Serratia marcescens

> *Excludes:*   *Gram-negative anaerobes (482.81)*
> *Legionnaires' disease (482.84)*

482.84   **Legionnaires' disease**

482.89   **Other specified bacteria**

482.9   **Bacterial pneumonia unspecified**

483   **Pneumonia due to other specified organism**

483.0   **Mycoplasma pneumoniae**
Eaton's agent
Pleuropneumonia-like organism [PPLO]

483.1   **Chlamydia**

483.8   **Other specified organism**

484   **Pneumonia in infectious diseases classified elsewhere**

> *Excludes:*   *influenza with pneumonia, any form (487.0)*

484.1   *Pneumonia in cytomegalic inclusion disease*
Code first underlying disease (078.5)

484.3   *Pneumonia in whooping cough*
Code first underlying disease (033.0-033.9)

484.5   *Pneumonia in anthrax*
Code first underlying disease (022.1)

484.6   *Pneumonia in aspergillosis*
Code first underlying disease (117.3)

484.7   *Pneumonia in other systemic mycoses*
Code first underlying disease

> *Excludes:*   *pneumonia in:*
> *candidiasis (112.4)*
> *coccidioidomycosis (114.0)*
> *histoplasmosis (115.0-115.9 with fifth-digit 5)*

484.8   *Pneumonia in other infectious diseases classified elsewhere*
Code first underlying disease, as:
Q fever (083.0)
typhoid fever (002.0)

> *Excludes:*   *pneumonia in:*
> *actinomycosis (039.1)*
> *measles (055.1)*
> *nocardiosis (039.1)*
> *ornithosis (073.0)*
> *Pneumocystis carinii (136.3)*
> *salmonellosis (003.22)*
> *toxoplasmosis (130.4)*
> *tuberculosis (011.6)*
> *tularemia (021.2)*
> *varicella (052.1)*

485   **Bronchopneumonia, organism unspecified**

Bronchopneumonia:	Pneumonia:
hemorrhagic	lobular
terminal	segmental

Pleurobronchopneumonia

> *Excludes:*   *bronchiolitis (acute) (466.11-466.19)*
> *chronic (491.8)*
> *lipoid pneumonia (507.1)*

Add 4th or 5th digit	Nonspecific code	Unspecified code	Manifestation code

486 Pneumonia, organism unspecified

> | Excludes: | *hypostatic or passive pneumonia (514)*
> | | *influenza with pneumonia, any form (487.0)*
> | | *inhalation or aspiration pneumonia due to foreign materials (507.0-507.8)*
> | | *pneumonitis due to fumes and vapors (506.0)*

487 Influenza

Influenza caused by unspecified influenza virus

> | Excludes: | *Hemophilus influenzae [H. influenzae]:*
> | | *infection NOS (041.5)*
> | | *laryngitis (464.00-464.01)*
> | | *meningitis (320.0)*
> | | *influenza due to 2009 H1N1 [swine] influenza virus (488.1)*
> | | *influenza due to identified avian influenza virus (488.0)*
> | | *influenza due to identified novel H1N1 influenza virus (488.1)*

487.0 With pneumonia

Influenza with pneumonia, any form
Influenzal:
  bronchopneumonia
  pneumonia
Use additional code to identify the type of pneumonia (480.0-480.9, 481, 482.0-482.9, 483.0-483.8, 485)

487.1 With other respiratory manifestations

Influenza NOS
Influenzal:
  laryngitis
  pharyngitis
  respiratory infection (upper) (acute)

487.8 With other manifestations

Encephalopathy due to influenza
Influenza with involvement of gastrointestinal tract

> | Excludes: | *"intestinal flu" [viral gastroenteritis] (008.8)*

▲ **488 Influenza due to certain identified influenza viruses**

> | Excludes: | *influenza caused by unspecified influenza viruses (487.0-487.8)*

● **488.0 Influenza due to identified avian influenza virus**

Avian influenza
Bird flu
Influenza A/H5N1

● **488.1 Influenza due to identified novel H1N1 influenza virus**

2009 H1N1 [swine] influenza virus
Novel 2009 influenza H1N1
Novel H1N1 influenza
Novel influenza A/H1N1
Swine flu

CHRONIC OBSTRUCTIVE PULMONARY DISEASE AND ALLIED CONDITIONS (490-496)

490 Bronchitis, not specified as acute or chronic

Bronchitis NOS: Tracheobronchitis NOS
  catarrhal
  with tracheitis NOS

> | Excludes: | *bronchitis:*
> | | *allergic NOS (493.9)*
> | | *asthmatic NOS (493.9)*
> | | *due to fumes and vapors (506.0)*

491 Chronic bronchitis

> | Excludes: | *chronic obstructive asthma (493.2)*

491.0 Simple chronic bronchitis

Catarrhal bronchitis, chronic
Smokers' cough

491.1 Mucopurulent chronic bronchitis

Bronchitis (chronic) (recurrent):
  fetid
  mucopurulent
  purulent

● Code new
  to this edition   ▲ Revision of
                           existing code   ④ ⑤ Fourth or fifth
                                                  digit required

⑤ **491.2 Obstructive chronic bronchitis**
Bronchitis:
  emphysematous
  obstructive (chronic) (diffuse)
Bronchitis with:
  chronic airway obstruction
  emphysema

Excludes: *asthmatic bronchitis (acute) NOS (493.9)*
     chronic obstructive asthma (493.2)

  491.20 Without exacerbation
    Emphysema with chronic bronchitis

  491.21 With (acute) exacerbation
    Acute exacerbation of chronic obstructive pulmonary disease [COPD]
    Decompensated chronic obstructive pulmonary disease [COPD]
    Decompensated chronic obstructive pulmonary disease [COPD] with
      exacerbation

Excludes: *chronic obstructive asthma with acute exacerbation (493.22)*

  491.22 With acute bronchitis

491.8 Other chronic bronchitis
Chronic:
  tracheitis
  tracheobronchitis

491.9 Unspecified chronic bronchitis

492 Emphysema

492.0 Emphysematous bleb
Giant bullous emphysema
Ruptured emphysematous bleb
Tension pneumatocele
Vanishing lung

492.8 Other emphysema
Emphysema (lung or
  pulmonary):
  NOS
  centriacinar
  centrilobular
  obstructive
  panacinar
Emphysema (lung or pulmonary):
  panlobular
  unilateral
  vesicular
MacLeod's syndrome
Swyer-James syndrome
Unilateral hyperlucent lung

Excludes: *emphysema:*
    compensatory (518.2)
    due to fumes and vapors (506.4)
    interstitial (518.1)
      newborn (770.2)
    mediastinal (518.1)
    surgical (subcutaneous) (998.81)
    traumatic (958.7)
    with chronic bronchitis (491.20-491.22)

493 Asthma
Excludes: *wheezing NOS (786.07)*

The following fifth-digit subclassification is for use with codes 493.0-493.2, 493.9:

  0 unspecified

  1 with status asthmaticus

  2 with (acute) exacerbation

⑤ **493.0 extrinsic asthma**
[0-2] Asthma:
    allergic with stated cause
    atopic
    childhood
    hay
    platinum
  Hay fever with asthma

Excludes: *asthma:*
    allergic NOS (493.9)
    detergent (507.8)
    miners' (500)
    wood (495.8)

⑤ **493.1 Intrinsic asthma**
[0-2]   Late-onset asthma

⑤ **493.2 Chronic obstructive asthma**
[0-2]   Asthma with chronic obstructive pulmonary disease [COPD]
          Chronic asthmatic bronchitis

> Excludes: *chronic obstructive bronchitis (491.20-491.22)*
>   *acute bronchitis (466.0)*

⑤ **493.8 Other forms of asthma**

　　　493.81 Exercise induced bronchospasm

　　　493.82 Cough variant asthma

⑤ **493.9 Asthma, unspecified**
[0-2]   Asthma (bronchial) (allergic NOS)
          Bronchitis:
            allergic
            asthmatic

494 Bronchiectasis
     Bronchiectasis (fusiform) (postinfectious) (recurrent)
     Bronchiolectasis

> Excludes: *congenital (748.61)*
>   *tuberculous bronchiectasis (current disease) (011.5)*

494.0 Bronchiectasis without acute exacerbation

494.1 Bronchiectasis with acute exacerbation

495 Extrinsic allergic alveolitis
     Includes: allergic alveolitis and pneumonitis due to inhaled organic dust particles of fungal,
                thermophilic actinomycete, or other origin

495.0 Farmers' lung

495.1 Bagassosis

495.2 Bird-fanciers' lung
     Budgerigar-fanciers' disease or lung
     Pigeon-fanciers' disease or lung

495.3 Suberosis
     Cork-handlers' disease or lung

495.4 Malt workers' lung
     Alveolitis due to Aspergillus clavatus

495.5 Mushroom workers' lung

495.6 Maple bark-strippers' lung
     Alveolitis due to Cryptostroma corticale

495.7 "Ventilation" pneumonitis
     Allergic alveolitis due to fungal, thermophilic actinomycete, and other organisms
     growing in ventilation [air conditioning] systems

495.8 Other specified allergic alveolitis and pneumonitis

Cheese-washers' lung	Pituitary snuff-takers' disease
Coffee workers' lung	Sequoiosis or red-cedar asthma
Fish-meal workers' lung	Wood asthma
Furriers' lung	
Grain-handlers' disease or lung	

495.9 Unspecified allergic alveolitis and pneumonitis
     Alveolitis, allergic (extrinsic)
     Hypersensitivity pneumonitis

● Code new   ▲ Revision of   ④ ⑤ Fourth or fifth
  to this edition   existing code   digit required

496 Chronic airway obstruction, not elsewhere classified

Note: This code is not to be used with any code from categories 491-493

Chronic:
nonspecific lung disease
obstructive lung disease
obstructive pulmonary disease [COPD] NOS

Excludes: *chronic obstructive lung disease [COPD] specified (as) (with):*
allergic alveolitis (495.0-495.9)
asthma (493.2)
bronchiectasis (494.0-494.1)
bronchitis (491.20-491.22)
with emphysema (491.20-491.22)
decompensated (491.21)
emphysema (492.0-492.8)

PNEUMOCONIOSES AND OTHER LUNG DISEASES DUE TO EXTERNAL AGENTS (500-508)

500 Coal workers' pneumoconiosis

Anthracosilicosis	Coal workers' lung
Anthracosis	Miner's asthma
Black lung disease	

501 Asbestosis

502 Pneumoconiosis due to other silica or silicates
Pneumoconiosis due to talc
Silicotic fibrosis (massive) of lung
Silicosis (simple) (complicated)

503 Pneumoconiosis due to other inorganic dust

Aluminosis (of lung)	Graphite fibrosis (of lung)
Bauxite fibrosis (of lung)	Siderosis
Berylliosis	Stannosis

504 Pneumonopathy due to inhalation of other dust

Byssinosis	Flax-dressers' disease
Cannabinosis	

Excludes: *allergic alveolitis (495.0-495.9)*
asbestosis (501)
bagassosis (495.1)
farmers' lung (495.0)

505 Pneumoconiosis, unspecified

506 Respiratory conditions due to chemical fumes and vapors
Use additional E code, if desired, to identify cause

506.0 Bronchitis and pneumonitis due to fumes and vapors
Chemical bronchitis (acute)

506.1 Acute pulmonary edema due to fumes and vapors
Chemical pulmonary edema (acute)

Excludes: *acute pulmonary edema NOS (518.4)*
chronic or unspecified pulmonary edema (514)

506.2 Upper respiratory inflammation due to fumes and vapors

506.3 Other acute and subacute respiratory conditions due to fumes and vapors

506.4 Chronic respiratory conditions due to fumes and vapors
Emphysema (diffuse) (chronic) due to inhalation of chemical fumes and vapors
Obliterative bronchiolitis (chronic) (subacute) due to inhalation of chemical fumes and vapors
Pulmonary fibrosis (chronic) due to inhalation of chemical fumes and vapors

506.9 Unspecified respiratory conditions due to fumes and vapors
Silo-fillers' disease

507 Pneumonitis due to solids and liquids

Excludes: *fetal aspiration pneumonitis (770.18)*

Add 4th or 5th digit	Nonspecific code	Unspecified code	Manifestation code

507.0 Due to inhalation of food or vomitus
Aspiration pneumonia (due to):
NOS
food (regurgitated)
gastric secretions
milk
saliva
vomitus

507.1 Due to inhalation of oils and essences
Lipoid pneumonia (exogenous)

Excludes: *endogenous lipoid pneumonia (516.8)*

507.8 Due to other solids and liquids
Detergent asthma

508 Respiratory conditions due to other and unspecified external agents
Use additional E code, if desired, to identify cause

508.0 Acute pulmonary manifestations due to radiation
Radiation pneumonitis

508.1 Chronic and other pulmonary manifestations due to radiation
Fibrosis of lung following radiation

508.8 Respiratory conditions due to other specified external agents

508.9 Respiratory conditions due to unspecified external agent

OTHER DISEASES OF RESPIRATORY SYSTEM (510-519)

510 Empyema
Use additional code, if desired, to identify infectious organism (041.0-041.9)

Excludes: *abscess of lung (513.0)*

510.0 With fistula

Fistula:	Fistula:
bronchocutaneous	mediastinal
bronchopleural	pleural
hepatopleural	thoracic

Any condition classifiable to 510.9 with fistula

510.9 Without mention of fistula

Abscess:	Pleurisy:
pleura	purulent
thorax	septic
Empyema (chest) (lung)	seropurulent
(pleura)	suppurative
Fibrinopurulent pleurisy	Pyopneumothorax
	Pyothorax

511 Pleurisy

Excludes: *pleurisy with mention of tuberculosis, current disease (012.0)*

511.0 Without mention of effusion or current tuberculosis

Adhesion, lung or pleura	Pleurisy:
Calcification of pleura	NOS
Pleurisy (acute) (sterile):	pneumococcal
diaphragmatic	staphylococcal
fibrinous	streptococcal
interlobar	Thickening of pleura

511.1 With effusion, with mention of a bacterial cause other than tuberculosis
Pleurisy with effusion (exudative) (serous):
pneumococcal
staphylococcal
streptococcal
other specified nontuberculous bacterial cause

⑤ **511.8 Other specified forms of effusion, except tuberculous**

Excludes: *traumatic (860.2-860.5, 862.29, 862.39)*

511.81 Malignant pleural effusion
Code first malignant neoplasm, if known

● Code new
to this edition

▲ Revision of
existing code

④ ⑤ Fourth or fifth
digit required

511.89 **Other specified forms of effusion, except tuberculous**
Encysted pleurisy
Hemopneumothorax
Hemothorax
Hydropneumothorax
Hydrothorax

511.9 **Unspecified pleural effusion**
Pleural effusion NOS   Pleurisy:
Pleurisy: serous
  exudative   with effusion NOS
  serofibrinous

512 Pneumothorax

512.0 **Spontaneous tension pneumothorax**

512.1 **Iatrogenic pneumothorax**
Postoperative pneumothorax

512.8 **Other spontaneous pneumothorax**
Pneumothorax:
  NOS
  acute
  chronic

Excludes: *pneumothorax:*
  congenital (770.2)
  traumatic (860.0-860.1, 860.4-860.5)
  tuberculous, current disease (011.7)

513 Abscess of lung and mediastinum

513.0 **Abscess of lung**
Abscess (multiple) of lung
Gangrenous or necrotic pneumonia
Pulmonary gangrene or necrosis

513.1 **Abscess of mediastinum**

514 Pulmonary congestion and hypostasis
Hypostatic:
  bronchopneumonia
  pneumonia
Passive pneumonia
Pulmonary congestion (chronic) (passive)
Pulmonary edema:
  NOS
  chronic

Excludes: *acute pulmonary edema:*
  NOS (518.4)
  with mention of heart disease or failure (428.1)
  hypostatic pneumonia due to or specified as a specific type of pneumonia – code
    to the type of pneumonia (480.0-480.9, 481, 482.0-482.49, 483.0-483.8, 485,
    486, 487.0)

515 Postinflammatory pulmonary fibrosis
Cirrhosis of lung, chronic or unspecified
Fibrosis of lung (atrophic) (confluent) (massive) (perialveolar) (peribronchial), chronic or
  unspecified
Induration of lung, chronic or unspecified

516 Other alveolar and parietoalveolar pneumonopathy

516.0 **Pulmonary alveolar proteinosis**

516.1 *Idiopathic pulmonary hemosiderosis*
Essential brown induration of lung
Code first underlying disease (275.0)

516.2 **Pulmonary alveolar microlithiasis**

516.3 **Idiopathic fibrosing alveolitis**
Alveolar capillary block
Diffuse (idiopathic) (interstitial) pulmonary fibrosis
Hamman-Rich syndrome

516.8 **Other specified alveolar and parietoalveolar pneumonopathies**
Endogenous lipoid pneumonia
Interstitial pneumonia (desquamative) (lymphoid)

Excludes: *lipoid pneumonia, exogenous or unspecified (507.1)*

	Add 4th or 5th digit		Nonspecific code		Unspecified code		Manifestation code

516.9 Unspecified alveolar and parietoalveolar pneumonopathy

517 Lung involvement in conditions classified elsewhere

Excludes: rheumatoid lung (714.81)

517.1 *Rheumatic pneumonia*
Code first underlying disease (390)

517.2 *Lung involvement in systemic sclerosis*
Code first underlying disease (710.1)

517.3 *Acute chest syndrome*
Code first sickle-cell disease in crisis (282.42, 282.62, 282.64, 282.69)

517.8 *Lung involvement in other diseases classified elsewhere*
Code first underlying disease, as:
amyloidosis (277.30-277.39)
polymyositis (710.4)
sarcoidosis (135)
Sjögren's disease (710.2)
systemic lupus erythematosus (710.0)

Excludes: syphilis (095.1)

518 Other diseases of lung

518.0 Pulmonary collapse
Atelectasis
Collapse of lung
Middle lobe syndrome

Excludes: atelectasis:
congenital (partial) (770.5)
primary (770.4)
tuberculous, current disease (011.8)

518.1 Interstitial emphysema
Mediastinal emphysema

Excludes: surgical (subcutaneous) emphysema (998.81)
that in fetus or newborn (770.2)
traumatic emphysema (958.7)

518.2 Compensatory emphysema

518.3 Pulmonary eosinophilia
Eosinophilic asthma   Tropical eosinophilia
Löffler's syndrome
Pneumonia:
allergic
eosinophilic

518.4 Acute edema of lung, unspecified
Acute pulmonary edema NOS
Pulmonary edema, postoperative

Excludes: pulmonary edema:
acute, with mention of heart disease or failure (428.1)
chronic or unspecified (514)
due to external agents (506.0-508.9)

518.5 Pulmonary insufficiency following trauma and surgery
Adult respiratory distress syndrome
Pulmonary insufficiency following:
shock
surgery
trauma
Shock lung

Excludes: adult respiratory distress syndrome associated with other conditions (518.82)
pneumonia:
aspiration (507.0)
hypostatic (514)
respiratory failure in other conditions (518.81, 518.83-518.84)

518.6 Allergic bronchopulmonary aspergillosis

518.7 Transfusion related acute lung injury (TRALI)

⑤ **518.8** Other diseases of lung

● Code new to this edition   ▲ Revision of existing code   ④ ⑤ Fourth or fifth digit required

518.81 Acute respiratory failure
Respiratory failure NOS

Excludes: *acute and chronic respiratory failure (518.84)*
acute respiratory distress (518.82)
chronic respiratory failure (518.83)
respiratory arrest (799.1)
respiratory failure, newborn (770.84)

518.82 Other pulmonary insufficiency, not elsewhere classified
Acute respiratory distress
Acute respiratory insufficiency
Adult respiratory distress syndrome NEC

Excludes: *adult respiratory distress syndrome associated with trauma and surgery (518.5)*
pulmonary insufficiency following trauma and surgery (518.5)
respiratory distress:
NOS (786.09)
newborn (770.89)
syndrome, newborn (769)
shock lung (518.5)

518.83 Chronic respiratory failure

518.84 Acute and chronic respiratory failure
Acute or chronic respiratory failure

518.89 Other diseases of lung, not elsewhere classified
Broncholithiasis   Lung disease NOS
Calcification of lung   Pulmolithiasis

519 Other diseases of respiratory system

⑤ **519.0 Tracheostomy complications**

519.00 Tracheostomy complication, unspecified

519.01 Infection of tracheostomy
Use additional code to identify type of infection, such as:
abscess or cellulitis of neck (682.1)
septicemia (038.0-038.9)
Use additional code to identify organism (041.00-041.9)

519.02 Mechanical complication of tracheostomy
Tracheal stenosis due to tracheostomy

519.09 Other tracheostomy complications
Hemorrhage due to tracheostomy
Tracheoesophageal fistula due to tracheostomy

⑤ **519.1 Other diseases of trachea and bronchus, not elsewhere classified**

519.11 Acute bronchospasm
Bronchospasm NOS

Excludes: *acute bronchitis with bronchospasm (466.0)*
asthma (493.00-493.92)
exercise induced bronchospasm (493.81)

519.19 Other diseases of trachea and bronchus
Calcification of bronchus or trachea
Stenosis of bronchus or trachea
Ulcer of bronchus or trachea

519.2 Mediastinitis

519.3 Other diseases of mediastinum, not elsewhere classified
Fibrosis of mediastinum
Hernia of mediastinum
Retraction of mediastinum

519.4 Disorders of diaphragm
Diaphragmitis
Paralysis of diaphragm
Relaxation of diaphragm

Excludes: *congenital defect of diaphragm (756.6)*
diaphragmatic hernia (551-553 with .3)
congenital (756.6)

519.8 Other diseases of respiratory system, not elsewhere classified

519.9 Unspecified disease of respiratory system
Respiratory disease (chronic) NOS

Add 4th or 5th digit	Nonspecific code	Unspecified code	Manifestation code

● Code new
to this edition

▲ Revision of
existing code

④ ⑤ Fourth or fifth
digit required

9. **DISEASES OF THE DIGESTIVE SYSTEM (520-579)**

DISEASES OF ORAL CAVITY, SALIVARY GLANDS, AND JAWS (520-529)

520 Disorders of tooth development and eruption

520.0 Anodontia
Absence of teeth (complete) (congenital) (partial)
Hypodontia
Oligodontia
Excludes: acquired absence of teeth (525.10-525.19)

520.1 Supernumerary teeth
Distomolar   Paramolar
Fourth molar   Supplemental teeth
Mesiodens
Excludes: supernumerary roots (520.2)

520.2 Abnormalities of size and form
Concrescence of teeth   Macrodontia
Fusion of teeth   Microdontia
Gemination of teeth   Peg-shaped [conical] teeth
Dens evaginatus   Supernumerary roots
Dens in dente   Taurodontism
Dens invaginatus   Tuberculum paramolare
Enamel pearls
Excludes: that due to congenital syphilis (090.5)
  tuberculum Carabelli, which is regarded as a normal variation

520.3 Mottled teeth
Dental fluorosis
Mottling of enamel
Nonfluoride enamel opacities

520.4 Disturbances of tooth formation
Aplasia and hypoplasia of cementum   Horner's teeth
Dilaceration of tooth   Hypocalcification of teeth
Enamel hypoplasia (neonatal) (postnatal)   Regional odontodysplasia
  (prenatal)   Turner's tooth
Excludes: Hutchinson's teeth and mulberry molars in congenital syphilis (090.5)
  mottled teeth (520.3)

520.5 Hereditary disturbances in tooth structure, not elsewhere classified
Amelogenesis imperfecta
Dentinogenesis imperfecta
Odontogenesis imperfecta
Dentinal dysplasia
Shell teeth

520.6 Disturbances of tooth eruption
Teeth: Tooth eruption:
  embedded   late
  impacted   obstructed
  natal   premature
  neonatal
  prenatal
  primary [deciduous]:
    persistent
    shedding, premature
Excludes: exfoliation of teeth (attributable to disease of surrounding tissues) (525.0-525.19)

520.7 Teething syndrome

520.8 Other specified disorders of tooth development and eruption
Color changes during tooth formation
Pre-eruptive color changes
Excludes: posteruptive color changes (521.7)

520.9 Unspecified disorder of tooth development and eruption

521 Diseases of hard tissue of teeth

⑤ **521.0 Dental caries**

521.00 Dental caries, unspecified

Add 4th or 5th digit   Nonspecific code   Unspecified code   Manifestation code

521.01 Dental caries limited to enamel
Initial caries
White spot lesion

521.02 Dental caries extending into dentine

521.03 Dental caries extending into pulp

521.04 Arrested dental caries

521.05 Odontoclasia
Infantile melanodontia
Melanodontoclasia

Excludes: *internal and external resorption of teeth (521.40-521.49)*

521.06 Dental caries pit and fissure
Primary dental caries, pit and fissure origin

521.07 Dental caries of smooth surface
Primary dental caries, smooth surface origin

521.08 Dental caries of root surface
Primary dental caries, root surface

521.09 Other dental caries

⑤ **521.1 Excessive attrition (approximal wear) (occlusal wear)**

521.10 Excessive attrition, unspecified

521.11 Excessive attrition, limited to enamel

521.12 Excessive attrition, extending into dentine

521.13 Excessive attrition, extending into pulp

521.14 Excessive attrition, localized

521.15 Excessive attrition, generalized

⑤ **521.2 Abrasion**
Abrasion of teeth:
  dentifrice
  habitual
  occupational
  ritual
  traditional
Wedge defect NOS of teeth

521.20 Abrasion, unspecified

521.21 Abrasion, limited to enamel

521.22 Abrasion, extending into dentine

521.23 Abrasion, extending into pulp

521.24 Abrasion, localized

521.25 Abrasion, generalized

⑤ **521.3 Erosion**
Erosion of teeth: Erosion of teeth:
  NOS   idiopathic
  due to: occupational
    medicine
    persistent vomiting

521.30 Erosion, unspecified

521.31 Erosion, limited to enamel

521.32 Erosion, extending into dentine

521.33 Erosion, extending into pulp

521.34 Erosion, localized

521.35 Erosion, generalized

⑤ **521.4 Pathological resorption**

521.40 Pathological resorption, unspecified

521.41 Pathological resorption, internal

521.42 Pathological resorption, external

521.49 Other pathological resorption
Internal granuloma of pulp

521.5 Hypercementosis
Cementation hyperplasia

● Code new   ▲ Revision of   ④ ⑤ Fourth or fifth
  to this edition   existing code   digit required

521.6 Ankylosis of teeth

521.7 Intrinsic posteruptive color changes
  Staining [discoloration] of teeth:
    NOS
    due to:
      drugs
      metals
      pulpal bleeding

  Excludes: *accretions [deposits] on teeth (523.6)*
    extrinsic color changes (523.6)
    pre-eruptive color changes (520.8)

⑤ **521.8 Other specific diseases of hard tissues of teeth**

  521.81 Cracked tooth

  Excludes: *asymptomatic craze lines in enamel – omit code*
    broken tooth due to trauma (873.63, 873.73)
    fractured tooth due to trauma (873.63, 873.73)

  521.89 Other specific diseases of hard tissues of teeth
      Irradiated enamel
      Sensitive dentin

521.9 Unspecified disease of hard tissues of teeth

522 Diseases of pulp and periapical tissues

  522.0 Pulpitis
    Pulpal: Pulpitis:
      abscess   acute
      polyp   chronic (hyperplastic) (ulcerative)
                                 suppurative

  522.1 Necrosis of the pulp
    Pulp gangrene

  522.2 Pulp degeneration
    Denticles
    Pulp calcifications
    Pulp stones

  522.3 Abnormal hard tissue formation in pulp
    Secondary or irregular dentin

  522.4 Acute apical periodontitis of pulpal origin

  522.5 Periapical abscess without sinus
    Abscess:
      dental
      dentoalveolar

  Excludes: *periapical abscess with sinus (522.7)*

  522.6 Chronic apical periodontitis
    Apical or periapical granuloma
    Apical periodontitis NOS

  522.7 Periapical abscess with sinus
    Fistula:
      alveolar process
      dental

  522.8 Radicular cyst
    Cyst:
      apical (periodontal)
      periapical
      radiculodental
      residual radicular

  Excludes: *lateral developmental or lateral periodontal cyst (526.0)*

  522.9 Other and unspecified diseases of pulp and periapical tissues

523 Gingival and periodontal diseases

⑤ **523.0 Acute gingivitis**

  Excludes: *acute necrotizing ulcerative gingivitis (101)*
    herpetic gingivostomatitis (054.2)

  523.00 Acute gingivitis, plaque induced
      Acute gingivitis NOS

  523.01 Acute gingivitis, non-plaque induced

413

| Add 4th or 5th digit | Nonspecific code | Unspecified code | Manifestation code |

⑤ **523.1 Chronic gingivitis**
Gingivitis (chronic):   Gingivitis (chronic):
  desquamative   simple marginal
  hyperplastic   ulcerative

Excludes: herpetic gingivostomatitis (054.2)

    523.10 Chronic gingivitis, plaque induced
        Chronic gingivitis NOS
        Gingivitis NOS

    523.11 Chronic gingivitis, non-plaque induced

⑤ **523.2 Gingival recession**
Gingival recession (postinfective) (postoperative)

    523.20 Gingival recession, unspecified
    523.21 Gingival recession, minimal
    523.22 Gingival recession, moderate
    523.23 Gingival recession, severe
    523.24 Gingival recession, localized
    523.25 Gingival recession, generalized

⑤ **523.3 Aggressive and acute periodontitis**
Acute:
  pericementitis
  pericoronitis

Excludes: acute apical periodontitis (522.4)
        periapical abscess (522.5, 522.7)

    523.30 Aggressive periodontitis, unspecified
    523.31 Aggressive periodontitis, localized
        Periodontal abscess
    523.32 Aggressive periodontitis, generalized
    523.33 Aggressive periodontitis

⑤ **523.4 Chronic periodontitis**
Chronic pericoronitis
Pericementitis (chronic)
Periodontitis:
  NOS
  complex
  simplex

Excludes: chronic apical periodontitis (522.6)

    523.40 Chronic periodontitis, unspecified
    523.41 Chronic periodontitis, localized
    523.42 Chronic periodontitis, generalized

523.5 Periodontosis

523.6 Accretions on teeth
Dental calculus:
  subgingival
  supragingival
Deposits on teeth:
  betel
  materia alba
  soft
  tartar
  tobacco
Extrinsic discoloration of teeth

Excludes: intrinsic discoloration of teeth (521.7)

● Code new to this edition   ▲ Revision of existing code   ④ ⑤ Fourth or fifth digit required

523.8 Other specified periodontal diseases
Giant cell: Gingival polyp
    epulis   Periodontal lesions due to traumatic occlusion
    peripheral granuloma   Peripheral giant cell granuloma
Gingival:
    cysts
    enlargement NOS
    fibromatosis

Excludes: leukoplakia of gingiva (528.6)

523.9 Unspecified gingival and periodontal disease

524 Dentofacial anomalies, including malocclusion

⑤ **524.0 Major anomalies of jaw size**

Excludes: hemifacial atrophy or hypertrophy (754.0)
    unilateral condylar hyperplasia or hypoplasia of mandible (526.89)

524.00 Unspecified anomaly

524.01 Maxillary hyperplasia

524.02 Mandibular hyperplasia

524.03 Maxillary hypoplasia

524.04 Mandibular hypoplasia

524.05 Macrogenia

524.06 Microgenia

524.07 Excessive tuberosity of jaw
Entire maxillary tuberosity

524.09 Other specified anomaly

⑤ **524.1 Anomalies of relationship of jaw to cranial base**

524.10 Unspecified anomaly
prognathism
retrognathism

524.11 Maxillary asymmetry

524.12 Other jaw asymmetry

524.19 Other specified anomaly

⑤ **524.2 Anomalies of dental arch relationship**
Anomaly of dental arch

Excludes: hemifacial atrophy or hypertrophy (754.0)
    soft tissue impingement (524.81-524.82)
    unilateral condylar hyperplasia or hypoplasia of mandible (526.89)

524.20 Unspecified anomaly of dental arch relationship

524.21 Malocclusion, Angle's class I
Neutro-occlusion

524.22 Malocclusion, Angle's class II
Disto-occlusion Division I
Disto-occlusion Division II

524.23 Malocclusion, Angle's class III
Mesio-occlusion

524.24 Open anterior occlusal relationship
Anterior open bite

524.25 Open posterior occlusal relationship
Posterior open bite

524.26 Excessive horizontal overlap
Excessive horizontal overjet

524.27 Reverse articulation
Anterior articulation
Crossbite
Posterior articulation

524.28 Anomalies of interarch distance
Excessive interarch distance
Inadequate interarch distance

524.29 Other anomalies of dental arch relationship
Other anomalies of dental arch

Add 4th or 5th digit   Nonspecific code   Unspecified code   Manifestation code

⑤ **524.3 Anomalies of tooth position of fully erupted teeth**

 Excludes: *impacted or embedded teeth with abnormal position of such teeth or adjacent teeth (520.6)*

524.30 Unspecified anomaly of tooth position
Diastema of teeth NOS
Displacement of teeth NOS
Transposition of teeth NOS

524.31 Crowding of teeth

524.32 Excessive spacing of teeth

524.33 Horizontal displacement of teeth
Tipped teeth
Tipping of teeth

524.34 Vertical displacement of teeth
Extruded tooth
Infraeruption of teeth
Intruded tooth
Supraeruption of teeth

524.35 Rotation of tooth/teeth

524.36 Insufficient interocclusal distance of teeth (ridge)
Lack of adequate intermaxillary vertical dimension

524.37 Excessive interocclusal distance of teeth
Excessive intermaxillary vertical dimension
Loss of occlusal vertical dimension

524.39 Other anomalies of tooth position

524.4 Malocclusion, unspecified

⑤ **524.5 Dentofacial functional abnormalities**

524.50 Dentofacial functional abnormality, unspecified

524.51 Abnormal jaw closure

524.52 Limited mandibular range of motion

524.53 Deviation in opening and closing of the mandible

524.54 Insufficient anterior guidance
Insufficient anterior occlusal guidance

524.55 Centric occlusion maximum intercuspation discrepancy
Centric occlusion of teeth discrepancy

524.56 Non-working side interference
Balancing side interference

524.57 Lack of posterior occlusal support

524.59 Other dentofacial functional abnormalities
Abnormal swallowing
Mouth breathing
Sleep postures
Tongue, lip, or finger habits

⑤ **524.6 Temporomandibular joint disorders**

 Excludes: *current temporomandibular joint:*
dislocation (830.0-830.1)
strain (848.1)

524.60 Temporomandibular joint disorders, unspecified
Temporomandibular joint-pain-dysfunction syndrome [TMJ]

524.61 Adhesions and ankylosis (bony or fibrous)

524.62 Arthralgia of temporomandibular joint

524.63 Articular disc disorder (reducing or non-reducing)

524.64 Temporomandibular joint sounds on opening and/or closing the jaw

524.69 Other specified temporomandibular joint disorders

⑤ **524.7 Dental alveolar anomalies**

524.70 Unspecified alveolar anomaly

524.71 Alveolar maxillary hyperplasia

524.72 Alveolar mandibular hyperplasia

524.73 Alveolar maxillary hypoplasia

524.74 Alveolar mandibular hypoplasia

● Code new
to this edition

▲ Revision of
existing code

④ ⑤ Fourth or fifth
digit required

524.75 **Vertical displacement of alveolus and teeth**
Extrusion of alveolus and teeth

524.76 **Occlusal plane deviation**

524.79 **Other specified alveolar anomaly**

⑤ 524.8 **Other specified dentofacial anomalies**

524.81 **Anterior soft tissue impingement**

524.82 **Posterior soft tissue impingement**

524.89 **Other specified dentofacial anomalies**

524.9 **Unspecified dentofacial anomalies**

525 **Other diseases and conditions of the teeth and supporting structures**

525.0 **Exfoliation of teeth due to systemic causes**

⑤ 525.1 **Loss of teeth due to trauma, extraction, or periodontal disease**
Code first class of edentulism (525.40-525.44, 525.50-525.54)

525.10 **Acquired absence of teeth, unspecified**
Tooth extraction status, NOS

525.11 **Loss of teeth due to trauma**

525.12 **Loss of teeth due to periodontal disease**

525.13 **Loss of teeth due to caries**

525.19 **Other loss of teeth**

⑤ 525.2 **Atrophy of edentulous alveolar ridge**

525.20 **Unspecified atrophy of edentulous alveolar ridge**
Atrophy of the mandible NOS
Atrophy of the maxilla NOS

525.21 **Minimal atrophy of the mandible**

525.22 **Moderate atrophy of the mandible**

525.23 **Severe atrophy of the mandible**

525.24 **Minimal atrophy of the maxilla**

525.25 **Moderate atrophy of the maxilla**

525.26 **Severe atrophy of the maxilla**

525.3 **Retained dental root**

⑤ 525.4 **Complete edentulism**
Use additional code to identify cause of edentulism (525.10-525.19)

525.40 **Complete edentulism, unspecified**
Edentulism NOS

525.41 **Complete edentulism, class I**

525.42 **Complete edentulism, class II**

525.43 **Complete edentulism, class III**

525.44 **Complete edentulism, class IV**

⑤ 525.5 **Partial edentulism**
Use additional code to identify cause of edentulism (525.10-525.19)

525.50 **Partial edentulism, unspecified**

525.51 **Partial edentulism, class I**

525.52 **Partial edentulism, class II**

525.53 **Partial edentulism, class III**

525.54 **Partial edentulism, class IV**

⑤ 525.6 **Unsatisfactory restoration of tooth**
Defective bridge, crown, fillings
Defective dental restoration

Excludes: *dental restoration status (V45.84)*
unsatisfactory endodontic treatment (526.61-526.69)

525.60 **Unspecified unsatisfactory restoration of tooth**
Unspecified defective dental restoration

525.61 **Open restoration margins**
Dental restoration failure of marginal integrity
Open margin on tooth restoration

| | Add 4th or 5th digit | | Nonspecific code | | Unspecified code | | Manifestation code |

525.62 Unrepairable overhanging of dental restorative materials
Overhanging of tooth restoration

525.63 Fractured dental restorative material without loss of material
Excludes: *cracked tooth (521.81)*
fractured tooth (873.63, 873.73)

525.64 Fractured dental restorative material with loss of material
Excludes: *cracked tooth (521.81)*
fractured tooth (873.63, 873.73)

525.65 Contour of existing restoration of tooth biologically incompatible with oral health
Dental restoration failure of periodontal anatomical integrity
Unacceptable contours of existing restoration
Unacceptable morphology of existing restoration

525.66 Allergy to existing dental restorative material
Use additional code to identify the specific type of allergy

525.67 Poor aesthetics of existing restoration
Dental restoration aesthetically inadequate or displeasing

525.69 Other unsatisfactory restoration of existing tooth

⑤ **525.7 Endosseous dental implant failure**

525.71 Osseointegration failure of dental implant
Failure of dental implant due to infection
Failure of dental implant due to unintentional loading
Failure of dental implant osseointegration due to premature loading
Failure of dental implant to osseointegrate prior to intentional prosthetic loading
Hemorrhagic complications of dental implant placement
Iatrogenic osseointegration failure of dental implant
Osseointegration failure of dental implant due to complications of systemic disease
Osseointegration failure of dental implant due to poor bone quality
Pre-integration failure of dental implant NOS
Pre-osseointegration failure of dental implant

525.72 Post-osseointegration biological failure of dental implant
Failure of dental implant due to lack of attached gingiva
Failure of dental implant due to occlusal trauma (caused by poor prosthetic design)
Failure of dental implant to osseointegrate following intentional prosthetic loading
Failure of dental implant due to parafunctional habits
Failure of dental implant due to periodontal infection (peri-implantitis)
Failure of dental implant due to poor oral hygiene
Iatrogenic post-osseointegration failure of dental implant
Post-osseointegration failure of dental implant due to complications of systemic disease

525.73 Post-osseointegration mechanical failure of dental implant
Failure of dental prosthesis causing loss of dental implant
Fracture of dental implant
Mechanical failure of dental implant NOS
Excludes: *cracked tooth (521.81)*
fractured dental restorative material with loss of material (525.64)
fractured dental restorative material without loss of material (525.63)
fractured tooth (873.63, 873.73)

525.79 Other endosseous dental implant failure
Dental implant failure NOS

525.8 Other specified disorders of the teeth and supporting structures
Enlargement of alveolar ridge NOS
Irregular alveolar process

525.9 Unspecified disorder of the teeth and supporting structures

● Code new to this edition   ▲ Revision of existing code   ④ ⑤ Fourth or fifth digit required

526 Diseases of the jaws

526.0 Developmental odontogenic cysts

Cyst:
  dentigerous
  eruption
  follicular
  lateral developmental

Cyst:
  lateral periodontal
  primordial
  Keratocyst

Excludes: radicular cyst (522.8)

526.1 Fissural cysts of jaw

Cyst:
  globulomaxillary
  incisor canal
  median anterior maxillary
  median palatal
  nasopalatine
  palatine of papilla

Excludes: cysts of oral soft tissues (528.4)

526.2 Other cysts of jaws

Cyst of jaw:
  NOS
  aneurysmal

Cyst of jaw:
  hemorrhagic
  traumatic

526.3 Central giant cell (reparative) granuloma

Excludes: peripheral giant cell granuloma (523.8)

526.4 Inflammatory conditions

Abscess of jaw (acute) (chronic) (suppurative)
Osteitis of jaw (acute) (chronic) (suppurative)
Osteomyelitis (neonatal) of jaw (acute) (chronic) (suppurative)
Periostitis of jaw (acute) (chronic) (suppurative)
Sequestrum of jaw bone

Excludes: alveolar osteitis (526.5)
          osteonecrosis of jaw (733.45)

526.5 Alveolitis of jaw

Alveolar osteitis
Dry socket

⑤ **526.6 Periradicular pathology associated with previous endodontic treatment**

526.61 Perforation of root canal space

526.62 Endodontic overfill

526.63 Endodontic underfill

526.69 Other periradicular pathology associated with previous endodontic treatment

⑤ **526.8 Other specified diseases of the jaws**

526.81 Exostosis of jaw
  Torus mandibularis
  Torus palatinus

526.89 Other
  Cherubism of jaw(s)
  Fibrous dysplasia of jaw(s)
  Latent bone cyst of jaw(s)
  Osteoradionecrosis of jaw(s)
  Unilateral condylar hyperplasia or hypoplasia of mandible

526.9 Unspecified disease of the jaws

527 Diseases of the salivary glands

527.0 Atrophy

527.1 Hypertrophy

527.2 Sialoadenitis

Parotitis:
  NOS
  allergic
  toxic

Sialoangitis
Sialodochitis

Excludes: epidemic or infectious parotitis (072.0-072.9)
          uveoparotid fever (135)

| | Add 4th or 5th digit | | Nonspecific code | | Unspecified code | | Manifestation code |

527.3 Abscess

527.4 Fistula
Excludes: *congenital fistula of salivary glands (750.24)*

527.5 Sialolithiasis
Calculus of salivary gland or duct
Stone of salivary gland or duct
Sialodocholithiasis

527.6 Mucocele
Mucous:
 extravasation cyst of salivary gland
 retention cyst of salivary gland
Ranula

527.7 Disturbance of salivary secretion
Hyposecretion   Sialorrhea
Ptyalism   Xerostomia

527.8 Other specified diseases of the salivary glands
Benign lymphoepithelial lesion of salivary gland
Sialectasia
Sialosis
Stenosis of salivary duct
Stricture of salivary duct

527.9 Unspecified disease of the salivary glands

528 Diseases of the oral soft tissues, excluding lesions specific for gingiva and tongue

⑤ **528.0 Stomatitis and mucositis (ulcerative)**
Excludes: *cellulitis and abscess of mouth (528.3)*
 diphtheritic stomatitis (032.0)
 epizootic stomatitis (078.4)
 gingivitis (523.0-523.1)
 oral thrush (112.0)
 Stevens-Johnson syndrome (695.13)
 stomatitis:
  acute necrotizing ulcerative (101)
  aphthous (528.2)
  gangrenous (528.1)
  herpetic (054.2)
  Vincent's (101)

 528.00 Stomatitis and mucositis, unspecified
 Mucositis NOS
 Ulcerative mucositis NOS
 Ulcerative stomatitis NOS
 Vesicular stomatitis NOS

 528.01 Mucositis (ulcerative) due to antineoplastic therapy
Use additional E code to identify adverse effects of therapy, such as:
 antineoplastic and immunosuppressive drugs (E930.7, E933.1)
 radiation therapy (E879.2)

 528.02 Mucositis (ulcerative) due to other drugs
Use additional E code to identify drug

 528.09 Other stomatitis and mucositis (ulcerative)

528.1 Cancrum oris
Gangrenous stomatitis
Noma

528.2 Oral aphthae
Aphthous stomatitis   Recurrent aphthous ulcer
Canker sore   Stomatitis herpetiformis
Periadenitis mucosa necrotica recurrens
Excludes: *herpetic stomatitis (054.2)*

● Code new to this edition   ▲ Revision of existing code   ④ ⑤ Fourth or fifth digit required

528.3 Cellulitis and abscess
Cellulitis of mouth (floor)
Ludwig's angina
Oral fistula

Excludes: abscess of tongue (529.0)
  cellulitis or abscess of lip (528.5)
  fistula (of):
    dental (522.7)
    lip (528.5)
  gingivitis (523.00-523.11)

528.4 Cysts
Dermoid cyst of mouth
Epidermoid cyst of mouth
Epstein's pearl of mouth
Lymphoepithelial cyst of mouth
Nasoalveolar cyst of mouth
Nasolabial cyst of mouth

Excludes: cyst:
  gingiva (523.8)
  tongue (529.8)

528.5 Diseases of lips
Abscess of lip(s)   Cheilitis:
Cellulitis of lip(s)   NOS
Fistula of lip(s)   angular
Hypertrophy of lip(s)   Cheilodynia
                                    Cheilosis

Excludes: actinic cheilitis (692.79)
  congenital fistula of lip (750.25)
  leukoplakia of lips (528.6)

528.6 Leukoplakia of oral mucosa, including tongue
Leukokeratosis of oral mucosa
Leukoplakia of:
  gingiva
  lips
  tongue

Excludes: carcinoma in situ (230.0, 232.0)
  leukokeratosis nicotina palati (528.79)

⑤ **528.7 Other disturbances of oral epithelium, including tongue**
Excludes: carcinoma in situ (230.0, 232.0)
  leukokeratosis NOS (702.8)

528.71 Minimal keratinized residual ridge mucosa
Minimal keratinization of alveolar ridge mucosa

528.72 Excessive keratinized residual ridge mucosa
Excessive keratinization of alveolar ridge mucosa

528.79 Other disturbances of oral epithelium, including tongue
Erythroplakia of mouth or tongue
Focal epithelial hyperplasia of mouth or tongue
Leukoedema of mouth or tongue
Leukokeratosis nicotina palate
Other oral epithelium disturbances

528.8 Oral submucosal fibrosis, including of tongue

528.9 Other and unspecified diseases of the oral soft tissues
Cheek and lip biting
Denture sore mouth
Denture stomatitis
Melanoplakia
Papillary hyperplasia of palate
Eosinophilic granuloma of oral mucosa
Irritative hyperplasia of oral mucosa
Pyogenic granuloma of oral mucosa
Ulcer (traumatic) of oral mucosa

529 Diseases and other conditions of the tongue

Add 4th or 5th digit | Nonspecific code | Unspecified code | Manifestation code

529.0 Glossitis
Abscess of tongue
Ulceration (traumatic) of tongue

Excludes: glossitis:
benign migratory (529.1)
Hunter's (529.4)
median rhomboid (529.2)
Moeller's (529.4)

529.1 Geographic tongue
Benign migratory glossitis
Glossitis areata exfoliativa

529.2 Median rhomboid glossitis

529.3 Hypertrophy of tongue papillae
Black hairy tongue
Coated tongue
Hypertrophy of foliate papillae
Lingua villosa nigra

529.4 Atrophy of tongue papillae
Bald tongue   Glossodynia exfoliativa
Glazed tongue   Smooth atrophic tongue
Glossitis:
Hunter's
Moeller's

529.5 Plicated tongue
Fissured tongue
Furrowed tongue
Scrotal tongue

Excludes: fissure of tongue, congenital (750.13)

529.6 Glossodynia
Glossopyrosis
Painful tongue

Excludes: glossodynia exfoliativa (529.4)

529.8 Other specified conditions of the tongue
Atrophy (of) tongue
Crenated (of) tongue
Enlargement (of) tongue
Hypertrophy (of) tongue
Glossocele
Glossoptosis

Excludes: erythroplasia of tongue (528.79)
leukoplakia of tongue (528.6)
macroglossia (congenital) (750.15)
microglossia (congenital) (750.16)
oral submucosal fibrosis (528.8)

529.9 Unspecified condition of the tongue

DISEASES OF ESOPHAGUS, STOMACH, AND DUODENUM (530-538)

530 Diseases of esophagus

Excludes: esophageal varices (456.0-456.2)

530.0 Achalasia and cardiospasm
Achalasia (of cardia)
Aperistalsis of esophagus
Megaesophagus

Excludes: congenital cardiospasm (750.7)

⑤ **530.1 Esophagitis**
Esophagitis:
chemical
peptic
postoperative
regurgitant

Use additional E code, if desired, to identify cause, if induced by chemical

Excludes: tuberculous esophagitis (017.8)

● Code new   ▲ Revision of   ④ ⑤ Fourth or fifth
  to this edition   existing code   digit required

530.10 Esophagitis, unspecified
Esophagitis NOS

530.11 Reflux esophagitis

530.12 Acute esophagitis

530.13 Eosinophilic esophagitis

530.19 Other esophagitis
Abscess of esophagus

⑤ **530.2 Ulcer of esophagus**
Ulcer of esophagus
fungal
peptic
Ulcer of esophagus due to ingestion of:
aspirin
chemicals
medicines

Use additional E code, if desired, to identify cause, if induced by chemical or drug

530.20 Ulcer of esophagus without bleeding
Ulcer of esophagus NOS

530.21 Ulcer of esophagus with bleeding

Excludes: *bleeding esophageal varices (456.0, 456.20)*

530.3 Stricture and stenosis of esophagus
Compression of esophagus
Obstruction of esophagus

Excludes: *congenital stricture of esophagus (750.3)*

530.4 Perforation of esophagus
Rupture of esophagus

Excludes: *traumatic perforation of esophagus (862.22, 862.32, 874.4-874.5)*

530.5 Dyskinesia of esophagus
Corkscrew esophagus   Esophagospasm
Curling esophagus   Spasm of esophagus

Excludes: *cardiospasm (530.0)*

530.6 Diverticulum of esophagus, acquired
Diverticulum, acquired:
epiphrenic
pharyngoesophageal
pulsion
subdiaphragmatic
traction
Zenker's (hypopharyngeal)
Esophageal pouch, acquired
Esophagocele, acquired

Excludes: *congenital diverticulum of esophagus (750.4)*

530.7 Gastroesophageal laceration-hemorrhage syndrome
Mallory-Weiss syndrome

⑤ **530.8 Other specified disorders of esophagus**

530.81 Esophageal reflux
Gastroesophageal reflux

Excludes: *reflux esophagitis (530.11)*

530.82 Esophageal hemorrhage

Excludes: *hemorrhage due to esophageal varices (456.0-456.2)*

530.83 Esophageal leukoplakia

530.84 Tracheoesophageal fistula

Excludes: *congenital tracheoesophageal fistula (750.3)*

530.85 Barrett's esophagus

530.86 Infection of esophagostomy
Use additional code to specify infection

530.87 Mechanical complication of esophagostomy
Malfunction of esophagostomy

	Add 4th or 5th digit		Nonspecific code		Unspecified code		Manifestation code

530.89   Other
[Excludes:] *Paterson-Kelly syndrome (280.8)*

530.9   **Unspecified disorder of esophagus**

⑤ **531**   **Gastric ulcer**
　　Includes: ulcer (peptic):
　　　　　　　　prepyloric
　　　　　　　　pylorus
　　　　　　　　stomach

Use additional E code, if desired, to identify drug, if drug-induced
　　[Excludes:] *peptic ulcer NOS (533.0-533.9)*
The following fifth-digit subclassification is for use with category 531:

　　0   **without mention of obstruction**
　　1   **with obstruction**

⑤ **531.0**   **Acute with hemorrhage**
　　[0-1]

⑤ **531.1**   **Acute with perforation**
　　[0-1]

⑤ **531.2**   **Acute with hemorrhage and perforation**
　　[0-1]

⑤ **531.3**   **Acute without mention of hemorrhage or perforation**
　　[0-1]

⑤ **531.4**   **Chronic or unspecified with hemorrhage**
　　[0-1]

⑤ **531.5**   **Chronic or unspecified with perforation**
　　[0-1]

⑤ **531.6**   **Chronic or unspecified with hemorrhage and perforation**
　　[0-1]

⑤ **531.7**   **Chronic without mention of hemorrhage or perforation**
　　[0-1]

⑤ **531.9**   **Unspecified as acute or chronic, without mention of hemorrhage or perforation**
　　[0-1]

⑤ **532**   **Duodenal ulcer**
　　Includes: erosion (acute) of duodenum
　　　　　　　　ulcer (peptic):
　　　　　　　　duodenum
　　　　　　　　postpyloric

Use additional E code, if desired, to identify drug, if drug-induced
　　[Excludes:] *peptic ulcer NOS (533.0-533.9)*
The following fifth-digit subclassification is for use with category 532:

　　0   **without mention of obstruction**
　　1   **with obstruction**

⑤ **532.0**   **Acute with hemorrhage**
　　[0-1]

⑤ **532.1**   **Acute with perforation**
　　[0-1]

⑤ **532.2**   **Acute with hemorrhage and perforation**
　　[0-1]

⑤ **532.3**   **Acute without mention of hemorrhage or perforation**
　　[0-1]

⑤ **532.4**   **Chronic or unspecified with hemorrhage**
　　[0-1]

⑤ **532.5**   **Chronic or unspecified with perforation**
　　[0-1]

⑤ **532.6**   **Chronic or unspecified with hemorrhage and perforation**
　　[0-1]

⑤ **532.7**   **Chronic without mention of hemorrhage or perforation**
　　[0-1]

⑤ **532.9**   **Unspecified as acute or chronic, without mention of hemorrhage or perforation**
　　[0-1]

　　● Code new　　　　▲ Revision of　　　　④ ⑤ Fourth or fifth
　　　　to this edition　　　　existing code　　　　digit required

⑤ **533 Peptic ulcer, site unspecified**
Includes: gastroduodenal ulcer NOS
peptic ulcer NOS
stress ulcer NOS

Use additional E code, if desired, to identify drug, if drug-induced

Excludes: *peptic ulcer:*
duodenal (532.0-532.9)
gastric (531.0-531.9)

The following fifth-digit subclassification is for use with category 533:

0 without mention of obstruction

1 with obstruction

⑤ **533.0 Acute with hemorrhage**
[0-1]

⑤ **533.1 Acute with perforation**
[0-1]

⑤ **533.2 Acute with hemorrhage and perforation**
[0-1]

⑤ **533.3 Acute without mention of hemorrhage and perforation**
[0-1]

⑤ **533.4 Chronic or unspecified with hemorrhage**
[0-1]

⑤ **533.5 Chronic or unspecified with perforation**
[0-1]

⑤ **533.6 Chronic or unspecified with hemorrhage and perforation**
[0-1]

⑤ **533.7 Chronic without mention of hemorrhage or perforation**
[0-1]

⑤ **533.9 Unspecified as acute or chronic, without mention of hemorrhage or perforation**
[0-1]

⑤ **534 Gastrojejunal ulcer**
Includes: ulcer (peptic) or erosion:
anastomotic
gastrocolic
gastrointestinal
gastrojejunal
jejunal
marginal
stomal

Excludes: *primary ulcer of small intestine (569.82)*
The following fifth-digit subclassification is for use with category 534:

0 without mention of obstruction

1 with obstruction

⑤ **534.0 Acute with hemorrhage**
[0-1]

⑤ **534.1 Acute with perforation**
[0-1]

⑤ **534.2 Acute with hemorrhage and perforation**
[0-1]

⑤ **534.3 Acute without mention of hemorrhage or perforation**
[0-1]

⑤ **534.4 Chronic or unspecified with hemorrhage**
[0-1]

⑤ **534.5 Chronic or unspecified with perforation**
[0-1]

⑤ **534.6 Chronic or unspecified with hemorrhage and perforation**
[0-1]

⑤ **534.7 Chronic without mention of hemorrhage or perforation**
[0-1]

⑤ **534.9 Unspecified as acute or chronic, without mention of hemorrhage or perforation**
[0-1]

Add 4th or 5th digit | Nonspecific code | Unspecified code | Manifestation code

⑤ 535 **Gastritis and duodenitis**
The following fifth-digit subclassification is for use with category 535

       0 without mention of hemorrhage

       1 with hemorrhage

⑤ **535.0 Acute gastritis**
[0-1]

⑤ **535.1 Atrophic gastritis**
[0-1]   Gastritis:
       atrophic-hyperplastic
       chronic (atrophic)

⑤ **535.2 Gastric mucosal hypertrophy**
[0-1]   Hypertrophic gastritis

⑤ **535.3 Alcoholic gastritis**
[0-1]

⑤ **535.4 Other specified gastritis**
[0-1]   Gastritis:
       allergic
       bile induced
       irritant
       superficial
       toxic

    Excludes: eosinophilic gastritis (535.7)

⑤ **535.5 Unspecified gastritis and gastroduodenitis**
[0-1]

⑤ **535.6 Duodenitis**
[0-1]

⑤ **535.7 Eosinophilic gastritis**
[0-1]

536 **Disorders of function of stomach**

    Excludes: functional disorders of stomach specified as psychogenic (306.4)

536.0 Achlorhydria

536.1 Acute dilatation of stomach
    Acute distention of stomach

536.2 Persistent vomiting
    Cyclical vominting
    Habit vomiting
    Persistent vomiting [not of pregnancy]
    Uncontrollable vomiting

    Excludes: bilious emesis (vomiting) (787.04)
       excessive vomiting in pregnancy (643.0-643.9)
       vomiting NOS (787.03)
        cyclical, associated with migraine (346.2)
       vomiting of fecal matter (569.87)

536.3 Gastroparesis
    Gastroparalysis
Code first underlying disease, such as:
    diabetes mellitus (249.6, 250.6)

⑤ **536.4 Gastrostomy complications**

    536.40 Gastrostomy complications, unspecified

    536.41 Infection of gastrostomy
    Use additional code to specify type of infection, such as:
       abscess or cellulitis of abdomen (682.2)
       septicemia (038.0-038.9)
    Use additional code to identify organism (041.00-041.9)

    536.42 Mechanical complication of gastrostomy

    536.49 Other gastrostomy complications

● Code new to this edition   ▲ Revision of existing code   ④ ⑤ Fourth or fifth digit required

536.8 Dyspepsia and other specified disorders of function of stomach
Achylia gastrica
Hourglass contraction of
stomach
Hyperacidity
Hyperchlorhydria
Hypochlorhydria
Indigestion
Tachygastria

Excludes: achlorhydria (536.0)
heartburn (787.1)

536.9 Unspecified functional disorder of stomach
Functional gastrointestinal:
disorder
disturbance
irritation

537 Other disorders of stomach and duodenum

537.0 Acquired hypertrophic pyloric stenosis
Constriction of pylorus, acquired or adult
Obstruction of pylorus, acquired or adult
Stricture of pylorus, acquired or adult

Excludes: congenital or infantile pyloric stenosis (750.5)

537.1 Gastric diverticulum

Excludes: congenital diverticulum of stomach (750.7)

537.2 Chronic duodenal ileus

537.3 Other obstruction of duodenum
Cicatrix of duodenum
Stenosis of duodenum
Stricture of duodenum
Volvulus of duodenum

Excludes: congenital obstruction of duodenum (751.1)

537.4 Fistula of stomach or duodenum
Gastrocolic fistula
Gastrojejunocolic fistula

537.5 Gastroptosis

537.6 Hourglass stricture or stenosis of stomach
Cascade stomach

Excludes: congenital hourglass stomach (750.7)
hourglass contraction of stomach (536.8)

⑤ **537.8 Other specified disorders of stomach and duodenum**

537.81 Pylorospasm

Excludes: congenital pylorospasm (750.5)

537.82 Angiodysplasia of stomach and duodenum without mention of hemorrhage

537.83 Angiodysplasia of stomach and duodenum with hemorrhage

537.84 Dieulafoy lesion (hemorrhagic) of stomach and duodenum

537.89 Other
Gastric or duodenal:
prolapse
rupture
Intestinal metaplasia of gastric mucosa
Passive congestion of stomach

Excludes: diverticula of duodenum (562.00-562.01)
gastrointestinal hemorrhage (578.0-578.9)

537.9 Unspecified disorder of stomach and duodenum

538 Gastrointestinal mucositis (ulcerative)
Use additional E code to identify adverse effects of therapy, such as:
antineoplastic and immunosuppressive drugs (E930.7, E933.1)
radiation therapy (E879.2)

Excludes: mucositis (ulcerative) of mouth and oral soft tissue (528.00-528.09)

Add 4th or 5th digit   Nonspecific code   Unspecified code   Manifestation code

APPENDICITIS (540-543)

540 Acute appendicitis

540.0 With generalized peritonitis
Appendicitis (acute):
fulminating with: perforation, peritonitis (generalized), rupture
gangrenous with: perforation, peritonitis (generalized), rupture
obstructive with: perforation, peritonitis (generalized), rupture
Cecitis (acute) with: perforation peritonitis (generalized) rupture
Rupture of appendix

Excludes: acute appendicitis with peritoneal abscess (540.1)

540.1 With peritoneal abscess
Abscess of appendix
With generalized peritonitis

540.9 Without mention of peritonitis
Acute:
appendicitis:
fulminating without mention of perforation, peritonitis, or rupture
gangrenous without mention of perforation, peritonitis, or rupture
inflamed without mention of perforation, peritonitis, or rupture
obstructive without mention of perforation, peritonitis, or rupture
cecitis without mention of perforation, peritonitis, or rupture

541 Appendicitis, unqualified

542 Other appendicitis
Appendicitis: Appendicitis:
chronic   relapsing
recurrent   subacute

Excludes: hyperplasia (lymphoid) of appendix (543.0)

543 Other diseases of appendix

543.0 Hyperplasia of appendix (lymphoid)

543.9 Other and unspecified diseases of appendix
Appendicular or appendiceal:
colic
concretion
fistula
Diverticulum of appendix
Fecalith of appendix
Intussusception of appendix
Mucocele of appendix
Stercolith of appendix

HERNIA OF ABDOMINAL CAVITY (550-553)

Includes: hernia:
acquired
congenital, except diaphragmatic or hiatal

⑤ **550** Inguinal hernia
Includes: bubonocele
inguinal hernia (direct) (double) (indirect) (oblique) (sliding)
scrotal hernia

The following fifth-digit subclassification is for use with category 550:

0 unilateral or unspecified (not specified as recurrent)
Unilateral NOS

1 unilateral or unspecified, recurrent

2 bilateral (not specified as recurrent)
Bilateral NOS

3 bilateral, recurrent

⑤ **550.0 Inguinal hernia, with gangrene**
[0-3]   Inguinal hernia with gangrene (and obstruction)

⑤ **550.1 Inguinal hernia, with obstruction, without mention of gangrene**
[0-3]   Inguinal hernia with mention of incarceration, irreducibility, or strangulation

⑤ **550.9 Inguinal hernia, without mention of obstruction or gangrene**
[0-3]   Inguinal hernia NOS

● Code new   ▲ Revision of   ④ ⑤ Fourth or fifth
to this edition   existing code   digit required

551 **Other hernia of abdominal cavity, with gangrene**
   Includes: that with gangrene (and obstruction)

⑤ **551.0** **Femoral hernia with gangrene**

   551.00 **Unilateral or unspecified (not specified as recurrent)**
      Femoral hernia NOS with gangrene

   551.01 **Unilateral or unspecified, recurrent**

   551.02 **Bilateral (not specified as recurrent)**

   551.03 **Bilateral, recurrent**

551.1 **Umbilical hernia with gangrene**
   Parumbilical hernia specified as gangrenous

⑤ **551.2** **Ventral hernia with gangrene**

   551.20 **Ventral, unspecified, with gangrene**

   551.21 **Incisional, with gangrene**
      Hernia:
         postoperative specified as gangrenous
         recurrent, ventral specified as gangrenous

   551.29 **Other**
      Epigastric hernia specified as gangrenous

551.3 **Diaphragmatic hernia with gangrene**
   Hernia:
      hiatal (esophageal) (sliding) specified as gangrenous
      paraesophageal specified as gangrenous
   Thoracic stomach specified as gangrenous

   Excludes: congenital diaphragmatic hernia (756.6)

551.8 **Hernia of other specified sites, with gangrene**
   Any condition classifiable to 553.8 if specified as gangrenous

551.9 **Hernia of unspecified site, with gangrene**
   Any condition classifiable to 553.9 if specified as gangrenous

552 **Other hernia of abdominal cavity, with obstruction, but without mention of gangrene**

   Excludes: that with mention of gangrene (551.0-551.9)

⑤ **552.0** **Femoral hernia with obstruction**
   Femoral hernia specified as incarcerated, irreducible, strangulated, or causing obstruction

   552.00 **Unilateral or unspecified (not specified as recurrent)**

   552.01 **Unilateral or unspecified, recurrent**

   552.02 **Bilateral (not specified as recurrent)**

   552.03 **Bilateral, recurrent**

552.1 **Umbilical hernia with obstruction**
   Parumbilical hernia specified as incarcerated, irreducible, strangulated, or causing obstruction

⑤ **552.2** **Ventral hernia with obstruction**
   Ventral hernia specified as incarcerated, irreducible, strangulated, or causing obstruction

   552.20 **Ventral, unspecified, with obstruction**

   552.21 **Incisional, with obstruction**
      Hernia:
         postoperative specified as incarcerated, irreducible, strangulated, or causing
            obstruction
         recurrent, ventral specified as incarcerated, irreducible, strangulated, or
            causing obstruction

   552.29 **Other**
      Epigastric hernia specified as incarcerated, irreducible, strangulated, or causing
         obstruction

552.3 **Diaphragmatic hernia with obstruction**
   Hernia:
      hiatal (esophageal) (sliding), specified as incarcerated, irreducible, strangulated, or
         causing obstruction
      paraesophageal, specified as incarcerated, irreducible, strangulated, or causing
         obstruction
   Thoracic stomach, specified as incarcerated, irreducible, strangulated, or causing
      obstruction

   Excludes: congenital diaphragmatic hernia (756.6)

| | Add 4th or 5th digit | | Nonspecific code | | Unspecified code | | Manifestation code |

552.8 Hernia of other specified sites, with obstruction
Any condition classifiable to 553.8 if specified as incarcerated, irreducible, strangulated, or causing obstruction

Excludes: *hernia due to adhesion with obstruction (560.81)*

552.9 Hernia of unspecified site, with obstruction
Any condition classifiable to 553.9 if specified as incarcerated, irreducible, strangulated, or causing obstruction

553 Other hernia of abdominal cavity without mention of obstruction or gangrene

Excludes: *the listed conditions with mention of:*
gangrene (and obstruction) (551.0-551.9)
obstruction (552.0-552.9)

⑤ **553.0 Femoral hernia**

553.00 Unilateral or unspecified (not specified as recurrent)
Femoral hernia NOS

553.01 Unilateral or unspecified, recurrent

553.02 Bilateral (not specified as recurrent)

553.03 Bilateral, recurrent

553.1 Umbilical hernia
Parumbilical hernia

⑤ **553.2 Ventral hernia**

553.20 Ventral, unspecified

553.21 Incisional
Hernia:
postoperative
recurrent, ventral

553.29 Other
Hernia:
epigastric
spigelian

553.3 Diaphragmatic hernia
Hernia:
hiatal (esophageal) (sliding)
paraesophageal
Thoracic stomach

Excludes: *congenital:*
diaphragmatic hernia (756.6)
hiatal hernia (750.6)
esophagocele (530.6)

553.8 Hernia of other specified sites
Hernia:
ischiatic
ischiorectal
lumbar
obturator
pudendal

Hernia:
retroperitoneal
sciatic
Other abdominal hernia of specified site

Excludes: *vaginal enterocele (618.6)*

553.9 Hernia of unspecified site
Enterocele
Epiplocele
Hernia:
NOS
interstitial

Hernia:
intestinal
intra-abdominal
Rupture (nontraumatic)
Sarcoepiplocele

NONINFECTIOUS ENTERITIS AND COLITIS (555-558)

555 Regional enteritis
Includes: Crohn's disease
Granulomatous enteritis

Excludes: *ulcerative colitis (556)*

555.0 Small intestine
Ileitis:
regional
segmental
terminal

Regional enteritis or Crohn's disease of:
duodenum
ileum
jejunum

● Code new
to this edition

▲ Revision of
existing code

④ ⑤ Fourth or fifth
digit required

555.1 Large intestine
Colitis:
  granulomatous
  regional
  transmural

Regional enteritis or Crohn's disease of:
  colon
  large bowel
  rectum

555.2 Small intestine with large intestine
Regional ileocolitis

555.9 Unspecified site
Crohn's disease NOS
Regional enteritis NOS

556 Ulcerative colitis

556.0 Ulcerative (chronic) enterocolitis

556.1 Ulcerative (chronic) ileocolitis

556.2 Ulcerative (chronic) proctitis

556.3 Ulcerative (chronic) proctosigmoiditis

556.4 Pseudopolyposis of colon

556.5 Left-sided ulcerative (chronic) colitis

556.6 Universal ulcerative (chronic) colitis
Pancolitis

556.8 Other ulcerative colitis

556.9 Ulcerative colitis, unspecified
Ulcerative enteritis NOS

557 Vascular insufficiency of intestine

> *Excludes:* necrotizing enterocolitis of the newborn (777.50-777.53)

557.0 Acute vascular insufficiency of intestine
Acute:
  hemorrhagic enterocolitis
  ischemic colitis, enteritis, or enterocolitis
  massive necrosis of intestine
Bowel infarction
Embolism of mesenteric artery
Fulminant enterocolitis
Hemorrhagic necrosis of intestine
Infarction of appendices epiploicae
Intestinal gangrene
Intestinal infarction (acute) (agnogenic) (hemorrhagic) (nonocclusive)
Mesenteric infarction (embolic) (thrombotic)
Necrosis of intestine
Terminal hemorrhagic enteropathy
Thrombosis of mesenteric artery

557.1 Chronic vascular insufficiency of intestine
Angina, abdominal
Chronic ischemic colitis, enteritis, or enterocolitis
Ischemic stricture of intestine
Mesenteric:
  angina
  artery syndrome (superior)
  vascular insufficiency

557.9 Unspecified vascular insufficiency of intestine
Alimentary pain due to vascular insufficiency
Ischemic colitis, enteritis, or enterocolitis NOS

558 Other and unspecified noninfectious gastroenteritis and colitis

> *Excludes:* infectious:
>   colitis, enteritis, or gastroenteritis (009.0-009.1)
>   diarrhea (009.2-009.3)

558.1 Gastroenteritis and colitis due to radiation
Radiation enterocolitis

558.2 Toxic gastroenteritis and colitis
Use additional E code, if desired, to identify cause

558.3 Allergic gastroenteritis and colitis
Use additional code to identify type of food allergy (V15.01-V15.05)

⑤ **558.4 Eosinophilic gastroenteritis and colitis**

       558.41 Eosinophilic gastroenteritis
           Eosinophilic enteritis

       558.42 Eosinophilic colitis

558.9 Other and unspecified noninfectious gastroenteritis and colitis
       Colitis NOS, dietetic, or noninfectious
       Enteritis NOS, dietetic, or noninfectious
       Gastroenteritis NOS, dietetic, or noninfectious
       Ileitis NOS, dietetic, or noninfectious
       Jejunitis NOS, dietetic, or noninfectious
       Sigmoiditis NOS, dietetic, or noninfectious

OTHER DISEASES OF INTESTINES AND PERITONEUM (560-569)

560 Intestinal obstruction without mention of hernia

    Excludes: *duodenum (537.2-537.3)*
             inguinal hernia with obstruction (550.1)
             intestinal obstruction complicating hernia (552.0-552.9)
             mesenteric:
                 embolism (557.0)
                 infarction (557.0)
                 thrombosis (557.0)
             neonatal intestinal obstruction (277.01, 777.1-777.2, 777.4)

    560.0 Intussusception
       Intussusception (colon) (intestine) (rectum)
       Invagination of intestine or colon

       Excludes: *intussusception of appendix (543.9)*

    560.1 Paralytic ileus
       Adynamic ileus
       Ileus (of intestine) (of bowel) (of colon)
       Paralysis of intestine or colon

       Excludes: *gallstone ileus (560.31)*

    560.2 Volvulus
       Knotting of intestine, bowel, or colon
       Strangulation of intestine, bowel, or colon
       Torsion of intestine, bowel, or colon
       Twist of intestine, bowel, or colon

⑤ **560.3 Impaction of intestine**

       560.30 Impaction of intestine, unspecified
           Impaction of colon

       560.31 Gallstone ileus
           Obstruction of intestine by gallstone

       560.39 Other
           Concretion of intestine
           Enterolith
           Fecal impaction

⑤ **560.8 Other specified intestinal obstruction**

       560.81 Intestinal or peritoneal adhesions with obstruction (postoperative)
           (postinfection)

       Excludes: *adhesions without obstruction (568.0)*

       560.89 Other
           Acute pseudo-obstruction of intestine
           Mural thickening causing obstruction

       Excludes: *ischemic stricture of intestine (557.1)*

    560.9 Unspecified intestinal obstruction
       Enterostenosis
       Obstruction of intestine or colon
       Occlusion of intestine or colon
       Stenosis of intestine or colon
       Stricture of intestine or colon

       Excludes: *congenital stricture or stenosis of intestine (751.1-751.2)*

   ● Code new   ▲ Revision of   ④ ⑤ Fourth or fifth
      to this edition   existing code   digit required

562 **Diverticula of intestine**
Use additional code, if desired, to identify any associated:
peritonitis (567.0-567.9)

Excludes: *congenital diverticulum of colon (751.5)*
diverticulum of appendix (543.9)
Meckel's diverticulum (751.0)

⑤ **562.0 Small intestine**

562.00 Diverticulosis of small intestine (without mention of hemorrhage)
Diverticulosis:
duodenum without mention of diverticulitis
ileum without mention of diverticulitis
jejunum without mention of diverticulitis

562.01 Diverticulitis of small intestine (without mention of hemorrhage)
Diverticulitis (with diverticulosis):
duodenum
ileum
jejunum
small intestine

562.02 Diverticulosis of small intestine with hemorrhage

562.03 Diverticulitis of small intestine with hemorrhage

⑤ **562.1 Colon**

562.10 Diverticulosis of colon (without mention of hemorrhage)
Diverticulosis:
NOS without mention of diverticulitis
intestine (large) without mention of diverticulitis
Diverticular disease (colon) without mention of diverticulitis

562.11 Diverticulitis of colon (without mention of hemorrhage)
Diverticulitis (with diverticulosis):
NOS
colon
intestine (large)

562.12 Diverticulosis of colon with hemorrhage

562.13 Diverticulitis of colon with hemorrhage

564 **Functional digestive disorders, not elsewhere classified**

Excludes: *functional disorders of stomach (536.0-536.9)*
those specified as psychogenic (306.4)

⑤ **564.0 Constipation**

564.00 Constipation, unspecified

564.01 Slow transit constipation

564.02 Outlet dysfunction constipation

564.09 Other constipation

564.1 Irritable bowel syndrome
Irritable colon   Spastic colon

564.2 Postgastric surgery syndromes
Dumping syndrome   Postgastrectomy syndrome
Jejunal syndrome   Postvagotomy syndrome

Excludes: *malnutrition following gastrointestinal surgery (579.3)*
postgastrojejunostomy ulcer (534.0-534.9)

564.3 Vomiting following gastrointestinal surgery
Vomiting (bilious) following gastrointestinal surgery

564.4 Other postoperative functional disorders
Diarrhea following gastrointestinal surgery

Excludes: *colostomy and enterostomy complications (569.60-569.69)*

564.5 Functional diarrhea

Excludes: *diarrhea:*
NOS (787.91)
psychogenic (306.4)

564.6 Anal spasm
Proctalgia fugax

| Add 4th or 5th digit | Nonspecific code | Unspecified code | Manifestation code |

564.7 Megacolon, other than Hirschsprung's
Dilatation of colon

Excludes: *megacolon:*
congenital [Hirschsprung's] (751.3)
toxic (556)

⑤ **564.8 Other specified functional disorders of intestine**

Excludes: *malabsorption (579.0-579.9)*

564.81 Neurogenic bowel

564.89 Other functional disorders of intestine
Atony of colon

564.9 Unspecified functional disorder of intestine

565 Anal fissure and fistula

565.0 Anal fissure

Excludes: *anal sphincter tear (healed) (non-traumatic) (old) (569.43)*
traumatic (863.89, 863.99)

565.1 Anal fistula
Fistula:
anorectal
rectal
rectum to skin

Excludes: *fistula of rectum to internal organs—see Alphabetic Index*
ischiorectal fistula (566)
rectovaginal fistula (619.1)

566 Abscess of anal and rectal regions
Abscess: Cellulitis:
ischiorectal   anal
perianal   perirectal
perirectal   rectal
                                   Ischiorectal fistula

567 Peritonitis and retroperitoneal infections

Excludes: *peritonitis:*
benign paroxysmal (277.31)
pelvic, female (614.5, 614.7)
periodic familial (277.31)
puerperal (670.8)
with or following:
abortion (634-638 with .0, 639.0)
appendicitis (540.0-540.1)
ectopic or molar pregnancy (639.0)

567.0 Peritonitis in infectious diseases classified elsewhere
Code first underlying disease

Excludes: *peritonitis:*
gonococcal (098.86)
syphilitic (095.2)
tuberculous (014.0)

567.1 Pneumococcal peritonitis

⑤ **567.2 Other suppurative peritonitis**

567.21 Peritonitis (acute) generalized
Pelvic peritonitis, male

567.22 Peritoneal abscess
Abscess (of):   Abscess (of):
abdominopelvic   retrocecal
mesenteric   subdiaphragmatic
omentum   subhepatic
peritoneum   subphrenic

567.23 Spontaneous bacterial peritonitis

Excludes: *bacterial peritonitis NOS (567.29)*

567.29 Other suppurative peritonitis
Subphrenic peritonitis

⑤ **567.3 Retroperitoneal infections**

567.31 Psoas muscle abscess

● Code new to this edition   ▲ Revision of existing code   ④ ⑤ Fourth or fifth digit required

567.38 Other retroperitoneal abscess

567.39 Other retroperitoneal infections

⑤ **567.8** Other specified peritonitis

567.81 Choleperitonitis
Peritonitis due to bile

567.82 Sclerosing mesenteritis
Fat necrosis of peritoneum
(Idiopathic) sclerosing mesenteric fibrosis
Mesenteric lipodystrophy
Mesenteric panniculitis
Retractile mesenteritis

567.89 Other specified peritonitis
Chronic proliferative peritonitis
Mesenteric saponification
Peritonitis due to urine

567.9 Unspecified peritonitis
Peritonitis:
NOS
of unspecified cause

568 Other disorders of peritoneum

568.0 Peritoneal adhesions (postoperative) (postinfection)

Adhesions (of):	Adhesions (of):
abdominal (wall)	mesenteric
diaphragm	omentum
intestine	stomach
male pelvis	Adhesive bands

Excludes: *adhesions:*

pelvic, female (614.6)
with obstruction:
duodenum (537.3)
intestine (560.81)

⑤ **568.8** Other specified disorders of peritoneum

568.81 Hemoperitoneum (nontraumatic)

568.82 Peritoneal effusion (chronic)

Excludes: *ascites NOS (789.51-789.59)*

568.89 Other
Peritoneal:
cyst
granuloma

568.9 Unspecified disorder of peritoneum

569 Other disorders of intestines

569.0 Anal and rectal polyp
Anal and rectal polyp NOS

Excludes: *adenomatous anal and rectal polyp (211.4)*

569.1 Rectal prolapse

Procidentia:	Prolapse:
anus (sphincter)	anal canal
rectum (sphincter)	rectal mucosa
Proctoptosis	

Excludes: *prolapsed hemorrhoids (455.2, 455.5)*

569.2 Stenosis of rectum and anus
Stricture of anus (sphincter)

569.3 Hemorrhage of rectum and anus

Excludes: *gastrointestinal bleeding NOS (578.9)*
melena (578.1)

⑤ **569.4** Other specified disorders of rectum and anus

569.41 Ulcer of anus and rectum
Solitary ulcer of anus (sphincter) or rectum (sphincter)
Stercoral ulcer of anus (sphincter) or rectum (sphincter)

569.42 Anal or rectal pain

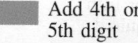

569.43 Anal sphincter tear (healed) (old)
Tear of anus, nontraumatic

Use additional code for any associated fecal incontinence (787.6)

Excludes: *anal fissure (565.0)*
anal sphincter tear (healed) (old) complicating delivery (654.8)

569.44 Dysplasia of anus
Anal intraepithelial neoplasia I and II (AIN I and II) (histologically confirmed)
Dysplasia of anus NOS
Mild and moderate dysplasia of anus (histologically confirmed)

Excludes: *abnormal results from anal cytologic examination without histologic confirmation*
(796.70-796.79)
anal intraepithelial neoplasia III (230.5, 230.6)
carcinoma in situ of anus (230.5, 230.6)
HGSIL of anus (796.74)
severe dysplasia of anus (230.5, 230.6)

569.49 Other
Granuloma of rectum (sphincter)
Rupture of rectum (sphincter)
Hypertrophy of anal papillae
Proctitis NOS

Excludes: *fistula of rectum to:*
internal organs—see Alphabetic Index
skin (565.1)
hemorrhoids (455.0-455.9)
incontinence of sphincter ani (787.6)

569.5 Abscess of intestine

Excludes: *appendiceal abscess (540.1)*

⑤ **569.6 Colostomy and enterostomy complications**

569.60 Colostomy and enterostomy complication, unspecified

569.61 Infection of colostomy or enterostomy
Use additional code to specify type of infection, such as:
abscess or cellulitis of abdomen (682.2)
septicemia (038.0-038.9)

Use additional code to identify organism (041.00-041.9)

569.62 Mechanical complication of colostomy and enterostomy
Malfunction of colostomy and enterostomy

569.69 Other complication
Fistula
Hernia
Prolapse

● **569.7 Complications of intestinal pouch**

● **569.71 Pouchitis**
Inflammation of internal ileoanal pouch

● **569.79 Other complications of intestinal pouch**

⑤ **569.8 Other specified disorders of intestine**

569.81 Fistula of intestine, excluding rectum and anus
Fistula: Fistula:
abdominal wall   enteroenteric
enterocolic   ileorectal

Excludes: *fistula of intestine to internal organs —see Alphabetic Index*
persistent postoperative fistula (998.6)

569.82 Ulceration of intestine
Primary ulcer of intestine
Ulceration of colon

Excludes: *that with perforation (569.83)*

569.83 Perforation of intestine

569.84 Angiodysplasia of intestine (without mention of hemorrhage)

569.85 Angiodysplasia of intestine with hemorrhage

569.86 Dieulafoy lesion (hemorrhagic) of intestine

● **569.87 Vomiting of fecal matter**

● Code new   ▲ Revision of   ④ ⑤ Fourth or fifth
   to this edition   existing code   digit required

569.89 Other
Enteroptosis
Granuloma of intestine
Prolapse of intestine
Pericolitis
Perisigmoiditis
Visceroptosis

Excludes: gangrene of intestine, mesentery, or omentum (557.0)
hemorrhage of intestine NOS (578.9)
obstruction of intestine (560.0-560.9)

569.9 Unspecified disorder of intestine

OTHER DISEASES OF DIGESTIVE SYSTEM (570-579)

570 Acute and subacute necrosis of liver
Acute hepatic failure
Acute or subacute hepatitis, not specified as infective
Necrosis of liver (acute) (diffuse) (massive) (subacute)
Parenchymatous degeneration of liver
Yellow atrophy (liver) (acute) (subacute)

Excludes: icterus gravis of newborn (773.0-773.2)
serum hepatitis (070.2-070.3)
that with:
  abortion (634-638 with .7, 639.8)
  ectopic or molar pregnancy (639.8)
  pregnancy, childbirth, or the puerperium (646.7)
viral hepatitis (070.0-070.9)

571 Chronic liver disease and cirrhosis

571.0 Alcoholic fatty liver

571.1 Acute alcoholic hepatitis
Acute alcoholic liver disease

571.2 Alcoholic cirrhosis of liver
Florid cirrhosis
Laennec's cirrhosis (alcoholic)

571.3 Alcoholic liver damage, unspecified

⑤ **571.4 Chronic hepatitis**

Excludes: viral hepatitis (acute) (chronic) (070.0-070.9)

571.40 Chronic hepatitis, unspecified

571.41 Chronic persistent hepatitis

571.42 Autoimmune hepatitis

571.49 Other
Chronic hepatitis:
  active
  aggressive
Recurrent hepatitis

571.5 Cirrhosis of liver without mention of alcohol
Cirrhosis of liver:
  NOS
  cryptogenic
  macronodular
  micronodular
Cirrhosis of liver:
  posthepatitic
  postnecrotic
  Healed yellow atrophy (liver)
  Portal cirrhosis
Code first, if applicable, viral hepatitis (acute) (chronic) (070.0-070.9)

571.6 Biliary cirrhosis
Chronic nonsuppurative destructive cholangitis
Cirrhosis:
  cholangitic
  cholestatic

571.8 Other chronic nonalcoholic liver disease
Chronic yellow atrophy (liver)
Fatty liver, without mention of alcohol

571.9 Unspecified chronic liver disease without mention of alcohol

572 Liver abscess and sequelae of chronic liver disease

572.0 Abscess of liver

Excludes: amebic liver abscess (006.3)

| | Add 4th or 5th digit | | Nonspecific code | | Unspecified code | | Manifestation code |

572.1 Portal pyemia
Phlebitis of portal vein   Pylephlebitis
Portal thrombophlebitis   Pylethrombophlebitis

▲ **572.2 Hepatic encephalopathy**
Hepatic coma
Hepatocerebral intoxication
Portal-systemic encephalopathy

Excludes: *hepatic coma associated with viral hepatitis – see category 070*

572.3 Portal hypertension

572.4 Hepatorenal syndrome

Excludes: *that following delivery (674.8)*

572.8 Other sequelae of chronic liver disease

573 Other disorders of liver

Excludes: *amyloid or lardaceous degeneration of liver (277.39)*
congenital cystic disease of liver (751.62)
glycogen infiltration of liver (271.0)
hepatomegaly NOS (789.1)
portal vein obstruction (452)

573.0 Chronic passive congestion of liver

573.1 Hepatitis in viral diseases classified elsewhere
Code first underlying disease as:
Coxsackie virus disease (074.8)
cytomegalic inclusion virus disease (078.5)
infectious mononucleosis (075)

Excludes: *hepatitis (in):*
mumps (072.71)
viral (070.0-070.9)
yellow fever (060.0-060.9)

573.2 Hepatitis in other infectious diseases classified elsewhere
Code first underlying disease, as:
malaria (084.9)

Excludes: *hepatitis in:*
late syphilis (095.3)
secondary syphilis (091.62)
toxoplasmosis (130.5)

573.3 Hepatitis, unspecified
Toxic (noninfectious) hepatitis
Use additional E code, if desired, to identify cause

573.4 Hepatic infarction

573.8 Other specified disorders of liver
Hepatoptosis

573.9 Unspecified disorder of liver

⑤ **574 Cholelithiasis**
The following fifth-digit subclassification is for use with category 574:

  0 without mention of obstruction

  1 with obstruction

⑤ **574.0 Calculus of gallbladder with acute cholecystitis**
[0-1] Biliary calculus with acute cholecystitis
Calculus of cystic duct with acute cholecystitis
Cholelithiasis with acute cholecystitis
Any condition classifiable to 574.2 with acute cholecystitis

⑤ **574.1 Calculus of gallbladder with other cholecystitis**
[0-1] Biliary calculus with cholecystitis
Calculus of cystic duct with cholecystitis
Cholelithiasis with cholecystitis
Cholecystitis with cholelithiasis NOS
Any condition classifiable to 574.2 with cholecystitis (chronic)

● Code new to this edition   ▲ Revision of existing code   ④ ⑤ Fourth or fifth digit required

⑤ **574.2 Calculus of gallbladder without mention of cholecystitis**
[0-1]   Biliary:
            calculus NOS
            colic NOS
          Calculus of cystic duct
          Cholelithiasis NOS
          Colic (recurrent) of
          gallbladder
          Gallstone (impacted)

⑤ **574.3 Calculus of bile duct with acute cholecystitis**
[0-1]   Calculus of bile duct [any] with acute cholecystitis
          Choledocholithiasis with acute cholecystitis
          Any condition classifiable to 574.5 with acute cholecystitis

⑤ **574.4 Calculus of bile duct with other cholecystitis**
[0-1]   Calculus of bile duct [any] with cholecystitis (chronic)
          Choledocholithiasis with cholecystitis (chronic)
          Any condition classifiable to 574.5 with cholecystitis (chronic)

⑤ **574.5 Calculus of bile duct without mention of cholecystitis**
[0-1]   Calculus of:
            bile duct [any]
            common duct
            hepatic duct
          Choledocholithiasis
          Hepatic:
            colic (recurrent)
            lithiasis

⑤ **574.6 Calculus of gallbladder and bile duct with acute cholecystitis**
[0-1]   Any condition classifiable to 574.0 and 574.3

⑤ **574.7 Calculus of gallbladder and bile duct with other cholecystitis**
[0-1]   Any condition classifiable to 574.1 and 574.4

⑤ **574.8 Calculus of gallbladder and bile duct with acute and chronic cholecystitis**
[0-1]   Any condition classifiable to 574.6 and 574.7

⑤ **574.9 Calculus of gallbladder and bile duct without cholecystitis**
[0-1]   Any condition classifiable to 574.2 and 574.5

575 **Other disorders of gallbladder**

  575.0 Acute cholecystitis
          Abscess of gallbladder without mention of calculus
          Angiocholecystitis without mention of calculus
          Cholecystitis without mention of calculus:
            emphysematous (acute)
            gangrenous
            suppurative
          Empyema of gallbladder without mention of calculus
          Gangrene of gallbladder without mention of calculus

          Excludes: *that with:*
                    acute and chronic cholecystitis (575.12)
                    choledocholithiasis (574.3)
                    choledocholithiasis and cholelithiasis (574.6)
                    cholelithiasis (574.0)

⑤ **575.1 Other cholecystitis**
          Cholecystitis:
            NOS without mention of calculus
            chronic without mention of calculus

          Excludes: *that with:*
                    choledocholithiasis (574.4)
                    choledocholithiasis and cholelithiasis (574.8)
                    cholelithiasis (574.1)

    575.10 Cholecystitis, unspecified
              Cholecystitis NOS

    575.11 Chronic cholecystitis

    575.12 Acute and chronic cholecystits

Add 4th or   Nonspecific   Unspecified   Manifestation
5th digit   code   code   code

575.2 Obstruction of gallbladder
Occlusion of cystic duct or gallbladder without mention of calculus
Stenosis of cystic duct or gallbladder without mention of calculus
Stricture of cystic duct or gallbladder without mention of calculus

Excludes: *that with calculus (574.0-574.2 with fifth-digit 1)*

575.3 Hydrops of gallbladder
Mucocele of gallbladder

575.4 Perforation of gallbladder
Rupture of cystic duct or gallbladder

575.5 Fistula of gallbladder
Fistula:
cholecystoduodenal
cholecystoenteric

575.6 Cholesterolosis of gallbladder
Strawberry gallbladder

575.8 Other specified disorders of gallbladder
Adhesions (of) cystic duct or gallbladder
Atrophy (of) cystic duct or gallbladder
Cyst (of) cystic duct or gallbladder
Hypertrophy (of) cystic duct or gallbladder
Nonfunctioning (of) cystic duct or gallbladder
Ulcer (of) cystic duct or gallbladder
Biliary dyskinesia

Excludes: *nonvisualization of gallbladder (793.3)*
Hartmann's pouch of intestine (V44.3)

575.9 Unspecified disorder of gallbladder

576 Other disorders of biliary tract

Excludes: *that involving the:*
cystic duct (575.0-575.9)
gallbladder (575.0-575.9)

576.0 Postcholecystectomy syndrome

576.1 Cholangitis

Cholangitis:
NOS
acute
ascending
chronic
primary

Cholangitis:
recurrent
sclerosing
secondary
stenosing
suppurative

576.2 Obstruction of bile duct
Occlusion of bile duct, except cystic duct, without mention of calculus
Stenosis of bile duct, except cystic duct, without mention of calculus
Stricture of bile duct, except cystic duct, without mention of calculus

Excludes: *congenital (751.61)*
that with calculus (574.3-574.5 with fifth-digit 1)

576.3 Perforation of bile duct
Rupture of bile duct, except cystic duct

576.4 Fistula of bile duct
Choledochoduodenal fistula

576.5 Spasm of sphincter of Oddi

576.8 Other specified disorders of biliary tract
Adhesions of bile duct [any]
Atrophy of bile duct [any]
Cyst of bile duct [any]
Hypertrophy of bile duct [any]
Stasis of bile duct [any]
Ulcer of bile duct [any]

Excludes: *congenital choledochal cyst (751.69)*

576.9 Unspecified disorder of biliary tract

● Code new
to this edition

▲ Revision of
existing code

④ ⑤ Fourth or fifth
digit required

577 **Diseases of pancreas**

577.0 Acute pancreatitis

Abscess of pancreas
Necrosis of pancreas:
  acute
  infective

Pancreatitis:
  NOS
  acute (recurrent)
  apoplectic
  hemorrhagic
  subacute
  suppurative

Excludes: mumps pancreatitis (072.3)

577.1 Chronic pancreatitis

Chronic pancreatitis:
  NOS
  infectious
  interstitial

Pancreatitis:
  painless
  recurrent
  relapsing

577.2 Cyst and pseudocyst of pancreas

577.8 Other specified diseases of pancreas

Atrophy of pancreas
Calculus of pancreas
Cirrhosis of pancreas
Fibrosis of pancreas

Pancreatic:
  infantilism
  necrosis:
    NOS
    aseptic
    fat
Pancreatolithiasis

Excludes: fibrocystic disease of pancreas (277.00-277.09)
islet cell tumor of pancreas (211.7)
pancreatic steatorrhea (579.4)

577.9 Unspecified disease of pancreas

578 **Gastrointestinal hemorrhage**

Excludes: that with mention of:
angiodysplasia of stomach and duodenum (537.83)
angiodysplasia of intestine (569.85)
diverticulitis, intestine:
  large (562.13)
  small (562.03)
diverticulosis, intestine:
  large (562.12)
  small (562.02)
gastritis and duodenitis (535.0-535.6)
ulcer:
  duodenal (532.0-532.9)
  gastric (531.0-531.9)
  gastrojejunal (534.0-534.9)
  peptic (533.0-533.9)

578.0 Hematemesis

Vomiting of blood

578.1 Blood in stool

Melena

Excludes: occult blood (792.1)

578.9 Hemorrhage of gastrointestinal tract, unspecified

Gastric hemorrhage
Intestinal hemorrhage

579 **Intestinal malabsorption**

579.0 Celiac disease

Celiac:
  crisis
  infantilism
  rickets

Gee (-Herter) disease
Gluten enteropathy
Idiopathic steatorrhea
Nontropical sprue

579.1 Tropical sprue

Sprue:
  NOS
  tropical

Tropical steatorrhea

441

 Add 4th or
5th digit

 Nonspecific
code

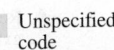 Unspecified
code

Manifestation
code

579.2 Blind loop syndrome
Postoperative blind loop syndrome

579.3 Other and unspecified postsurgical nonabsorption
Hypoglycemia following gastrointestinal surgery
Malnutrition following gastrointestinal surgery

579.4 Pancreatic steatorrhea

579.8 Other specified intestinal malabsorption
Enteropathy: Steatorrhea (chronic)
exudative
protein-losing

579.9 Unspecified intestinal malabsorption
Malabsorption syndrome NOS

● Code new to this edition   ▲ Revision of existing code   ④ ⑤ Fourth or fifth digit required

10. DISEASES OF THE GENITOURINARY SYSTEM (580-629)

NEPHRITIS, NEPHROTIC SYNDROME, AND NEPHROSIS (580-589)

Excludes: *hypertensive chronic kidney disease (403.00-403.91, 404.00-404.93)*

580 Acute glomerulonephritis
Includes: acute nephritis

580.0 With lesion of proliferative glomerulonephritis
Acute (diffuse) proliferative glomerulonephritis
Acute poststreptococcal glomerulonephritis

580.4 With lesion of rapidly progressive glomerulonephritis
Acute nephritis with lesion of necrotizing glomerulitis

⑤ **580.8 With other specified pathological lesion in kidney**

580.81 *Acute glomerulonephritis in diseases classified elsewhere*
Code first underlying disease, as:
infectious hepatitis (070.0-070.9)
mumps (072.79)
subacute bacterial endocarditis (421.0)
typhoid fever (002.0)

580.89 Other
Glomerulonephritis, acute, with lesion of:
exudative nephritis
interstitial (diffuse) (focal) nephritis

580.9 Acute glomerulonephritis with unspecified pathological lesion in kidney
Glomerulonephritis:
NOS specified as acute
hemorrhagic specified as acute
Nephritis specified as acute
Nephropathy specified as acute

581 Nephrotic syndrome

581.0 With lesion of proliferative glomerulonephritis

581.1 With lesion of membranous glomerulonephritis
Epimembranous nephritis
Idiopathic membranous glomerular disease
Nephrotic syndrome with lesion of:
focal glomerulosclerosis
sclerosing membranous glomerulonephritis
segmental hyalinosis

581.2 With lesion of membranoproliferative glomerulonephritis
Nephrotic syndrome with lesion (of):
endothelial glomerulonephritis
hypocomplementemic persistent glomerulonephritis
lobular glomerulonephritis
mesangiocapillary glomerulonephritis
mixed membranous and proliferative glomerulonephritis

581.3 With lesion of minimal change glomerulonephritis
Foot process disease
Lipoid nephrosis
Minimal change:
glomerular disease
glomerulitis
nephrotic syndrome

⑤ **581.8 With other specified pathological lesion in kidney**

581.81 *Nephrotic syndrome in diseases classified elsewhere*
Code first underlying disease, as:
amyloidosis (277.30-277.39)
diabetes mellitus (249.4, 250.4)
malaria (084.9)
polyarteritis (446.0)
systemic lupus erythematosus (710.0)

Excludes: *nephrosis in epidemic hemorrhagic fever (078.6)*

581.89 Other
Glomerulonephritis with edema and lesion of:
exudative nephritis
interstitial (diffuse) (focal) nephritis

▮ Add 4th or 5th digit	▮ Nonspecific code	▮ Unspecified code	▮ Manifestation code	

581.9 Nephrotic syndrome with unspecified pathological lesion in kidney
Glomerulonephritis with edema NOS
Nephritis:
   nephrotic NOS
   with edema NOS
Nephrosis NOS
Renal disease with edema NOS

582 Chronic glomerulonephritis
Includes: chronic nephritis

582.0 With lesion of proliferative glomerulonephritis
Chronic (diffuse) proliferative glomerulonephritis

582.1 With lesion of membranous glomerulonephritis
Chronic glomerulonephritis:
   membranous
   sclerosing
Focal glomerulosclerosis
Segmental hyalinosis

582.2 With lesion of membranoproliferative glomerulonephritis
Chronic glomerulonephritis:
   endothelial
   hypocomplementemic persistent
   lobular
   membranoproliferative
   mesangiocapillary
   mixed membranous and proliferative

582.4 With lesion of rapidly progressive glomerulonephritis
Chronic nephritis with lesion of necrotizing glomerulitis

⑤ **582.8 With other specified pathological lesion in kidney**

  582.81 *Chronic glomerulonephritis in diseases classified elsewhere*
    Code first underlying disease, as:
    amyloidosis (277.30-277.39)
    systemic lupus erythematosus (710.0)

  582.89 **Other**
    Chronic glomerulonephritis with lesion of:
     exudative nephritis
     interstitial (diffuse) (focal) nephritis

582.9 Chronic glomerulonephritis with unspecified pathological lesion in kidney
Glomerulonephritis:
   NOS specified as chronic
   hemorrhagic specified as chronic
Nephritis specified as chronic
Nephropathy specified as chronic

583 Nephritis and nephropathy, not specified as acute or chronic
Includes: "renal disease" so stated, not specified as acute or chronic but with stated
         pathology or cause

583.0 With lesion of proliferative glomerulonephritis
Proliferative:
   glomerulonephritis (diffuse) NOS
   nephritis NOS
   nephropathy NOS

583.1 With lesion of membranous glomerulonephritis
Membranous: Membranous nephropathy NOS
   glomerulonephritis NOS
   nephritis NOS

583.2 With lesion of membranoproliferative glomerulonephritis
Membranoproliferative:
   glomerulonephritis NOS
   nephritis NOS
   nephropathy NOS
Nephritis NOS, with lesion of:
   hypocomplementemic persistent glomerulonephritis
   lobular glomerulonephritis
   mesangiocapillary glomerulonephritis
   mixed membranous and proliferative glomerulonephritis

● Code new
  to this edition
▲ Revision of
  existing code
④ ⑤ Fourth or fifth
     digit required

583.4 With lesion of rapidly progressive glomerulonephritis
Necrotizing or rapidly progressive:
glomerulitis NOS
glomerulonephritis NOS
nephritis NOS
nephropathy NOS
Nephritis, unspecified, with lesion of necrotizing glomerulitis

583.6 With lesion of renal cortical necrosis
Nephritis NOS with (renal) cortical necrosis
Nephropathy NOS with (renal) cortical necrosis
Renal cortical necrosis NOS

583.7 With lesion of renal medullary necrosis
Nephritis NOS with (renal) medullary [papillary] necrosis
Nephropathy NOS with (renal) medullary [papillary] necrosis

⑤ **583.8 With other specified pathological lesion in kidney**

583.81 *Nephritis and nephropathy, not specified as acute or chronic, in diseases classified elsewhere*
Code first underlying disease, as:
amyloidosis (277.30-277.39)
diabetes mellitus (249.4, 250.4)
gonococcal infection (098.19)
Goodpasture's syndrome (446.21)
systemic lupus erythematosus (710.0)
tuberculosis (016.0)

Excludes: *gouty nephropathy (274.10)*
syphilitic nephritis (095.4)

583.89 **Other**
Glomerulitis with lesion of:
exudative nephritis
interstitial nephritis
Glomerulonephritis with lesion of:
exudative nephritis
interstitial nephritis
Nephritis with lesion of:
exudative nephritis
interstitial nephritis
Nephropathy with lesion of:
exudative nephritis
interstitial nephritis
Renal disease with lesion of:
exudative nephritis
interstitial nephritis

583.9 With unspecified pathological lesion in kidney
Glomerulitis NOS
Glomerulonephritis NOS
Nephritis NOS
Nephropathy NOS

Excludes: *nephropathy complicating pregnancy, labor, or the puerperium (642.0-642.9, 646.2)*
renal disease NOS with no stated cause (593.9)

▲ **584 Acute kidney failure**
Includes: Acute renal failure

Excludes: *following labor and delivery (669.3)*
posttraumatic (958.5)
that complicating:
abortion (634-638 with .3, 639.3)
ectopic or molar pregnancy (639.3)

▲ **584.5 Acute kidney failure with lesion of tubular necrosis**
Lower nephron nephrosis
Renal failure with (acute) tubular necrosis
Tubular necrosis:
NOS
acute

▲ **584.6 Acute kidney failure with lesion of renal cortical necrosis**

▲ **584.7 Acute kidney failure with lesion of renal medullary [papillary] necrosis**
Necrotizing renal papillitis

▲ **584.8 Acute kidney failure with other specified pathological lesion in kidney**

| | Add 4th or 5th digit | | Nonspecific code | | Unspecified code | | Manifestation code |

▲ **584.9 Acute kidney failure, unspecified**
Acute kidney injury (nontraumatic)

Excludes: *traumatic kidney injury (866.00-866.13)*

585 Chronic kidney disease (CKD)
Code first hypertensive chronic kidney disease, if applicable, (403.00-403.91, 404.00-404.93)
Use additional code to identify kidney transplant status, if applicable (V42.0)

585.1 Chronic kidney disease, Stage I

585.2 Chronic kidney disease, Stage II (mild)

585.3 Chronic kidney disease, Stage III (moderate)

585.4 Chronic kidney disease, Stage IV (severe)

585.5 Chronic kidney disease, Stage V

Excludes: *chronic kidney disease, stage V requiring chronic dialysis (585.6)*

585.6 End stage renal disease
Chronic kidney disease requiring chronic dialysis

585.9 Chronic kidney disease, unspecified
Chronic renal disease
Chronic renal failure NOS
Chronic renal insufficiency

586 Renal failure, unspecified
Uremia NOS

Excludes: *following labor and delivery (669.3)*
posttraumatic renal failure (958.5)
that complicating:
abortion (634-638 with .3, 639.3)
ectopic or molar pregnancy (639.3)
uremia:
extrarenal (788.9)
prerenal (788.9)

587 Renal sclerosis, unspecified
Includes: Atrophy of kidney
Contracted kidney
Renal:
cirrhosis
fibrosis

588 Disorders resulting from impaired renal function

588.0 Renal osteodystrophy

Azotemic osteodystrophy	Renal:
Phosphate-losing tubular	dwarfism
disorders	infantilism
	rickets

588.1 Nephrogenic diabetes insipidus

Excludes: *diabetes insipidus NOS (253.5)*

⑤ **588.8 Other specified disorders resulting from impaired renal function**

Excludes: *secondary hypertension (405.0-405.9)*

588.81 Secondary hyperparathyroidism (of renal origin)
Secondary hyperparathyroidism NOS

588.89 Other specified disorders resulting from impaired renal function
Hypokalemic nephropathy

588.9 Unspecified disorder resulting from impaired renal function

589 Small kidney of unknown cause

589.0 Unilateral small kidney

589.1 Bilateral small kidneys

589.9 Small kidney, unspecified

● Code new
to this edition

▲ Revision of
existing code

④ ⑤ Fourth or fifth
digit required

OTHER DISEASES OF URINARY SYSTEM (590-599)

590 **Infections of kidney**

Use additional code, if desired, to identify organism, such as Escherichia coli [E. coli] (041.4)

⑤ **590.0** **Chronic pyelonephritis**
Chronic pyelitis
Chronic pyonephrosis

Code, if applicable, any causal condition first

590.00 **Without lesion of renal medullary necrosis**

590.01 **With lesion of renal medullary necrosis**

⑤ **590.1** **Acute pyelonephritis**
Acute pyelitis
Acute pyonephrosis

590.10 **Without lesion of renal medullary necrosis**

590.11 **With lesion of renal medullary necrosis**

590.2 **Renal and perinephric abscess**
Abscess: Carbuncle of kidney
kidney
nephritic
perirenal

590.3 **Pyeloureteritis cystica**
Infection of renal pelvis and ureter
Ureteritis cystica

⑤ **590.8** **Other pyelonephritis or pyonephrosis, not specified as acute or chronic**

590.80 **Pyelonephritis, unspecified**
Pyelitis NOS
Pyelonephritis NOS

590.81 *Pyelitis or pyelonephritis in diseases classified elsewhere*
Code first underlying disease, as:
tuberculosis (016.0)

590.9 **Infection of kidney, unspecified**
Excludes: *urinary tract infection NOS (599.0)*

591 **Hydronephrosis**
Hydrocalycosis   Hydroureteronephrosis
Hydronephrosis
Excludes: *congenital hydronephrosis (753.29)*
hydroureter (593.5)

592 **Calculus of kidney and ureter**
Excludes: *nephrocalcinosis (275.4)*

592.0 **Calculus of kidney**
Nephrolithiasis NOS   Staghorn calculus
Renal calculus or stone   Stone in kidney
Excludes: *uric acid nephrolithiasis (274.11)*

592.1 **Calculus of ureter**
Ureteric stone
Ureterolithiasis

592.9 **Urinary calculus, unspecified**

593 **Other disorders of kidney and ureter**

593.0 **Nephroptosis**
Floating kidney
Mobile kidney

593.1 **Hypertrophy of kidney**

593.2 **Cyst of kidney, acquired**
Cyst (multiple) (solitary) of kidney, not congenital
Peripelvic (lymphatic) cyst
Excludes: *calyceal or pyelogenic cyst of kidney (591)*
congenital cyst of kidney (753.1)
polycystic (disease of) kidney (753.1)

Add 4th or 5th digit   Nonspecific code   Unspecified code   Manifestation code

593.3 Stricture or kinking of ureter
Angulation of ureter (postoperative)
Constriction of ureter (postoperative)
Stricture of pelviureteric junction

593.4 Other ureteric obstruction
Idiopathic retroperitoneal fibrosis
Occlusion NOS of ureter

Excludes: *that due to calculus (592.1)*

593.5 Hydroureter
Excludes: *congenital hydroureter (753.22)*
hydroureteronephrosis (591)

593.6 Postural proteinuria
Benign postural proteinuria
Orthostatic proteinuria

Excludes: *proteinuria NOS (791.0)*

⑤ 593.7 Vesicoureteral reflux

593.70 Unspecified or without reflux nephropathy

593.71 With reflux nephropathy, unilateral

593.72 With reflux nephropathy, bilateral

593.73 With reflux nephropathy NOS

⑤ 593.8 Other specified disorders of kidney and ureter

593.81 Vascular disorders of kidney
Renal (artery):   Renal infarction
  embolism
  hemorrhage
  thrombosis

593.82 Ureteral fistula
Intestinoureteral fistula

Excludes: *fistula between ureter and female genital tract (619.0)*

593.89 Other
Adhesions, kidney or ureter
Periureteritis
Polyp of ureter
Pyelectasia
Ureterocele

Excludes: *tuberculosis of ureter (016.2)*
ureteritis cystica (590.3)

593.9 Unspecified disorder of kidney and ureter
Acute renal disease
Acute renal insufficiency
Renal disease NOS
Salt-losing nephritis or syndrome

Excludes: *chronic renal insufficiency (585.9)*
cystic kidney disease (753.1)
nephropathy, so stated (583.0-583.9)
renal disease:
  arising in pregnancy or the puerperium (642.1-642.2, 642.4-642.7, 646.2)
  not specified as acute or chronic, but with stated pathology or cause (583.0-583.9)

594 Calculus of lower urinary tract

594.0 Calculus in diverticulum of bladder

594.1 Other calculus in bladder
Urinary bladder stone

Excludes: *staghorn calculus (592.0)*

594.2 Calculus in urethra

594.8 Other lower urinary tract calculus

594.9 Calculus of lower urinary tract, unspecified

Excludes: *calculus of urinary tract NOS (592.9)*

● Code new to this edition   ▲ Revision of existing code   ④ ⑤ Fourth or fifth digit required

595 **Cystitis**

> *Excludes:* prostatocystitis (601.3)

Use additional code, if desired, to identify organism, such as Escherichia coli [E. coli] (041.4)

595.0 Acute cystitis

> *Excludes:* trigonitis (595.3)

595.1 Chronic interstitial cystitis

Hunner's ulcer   Submucous cystitis
Panmural fibrosis of bladder

595.2 Other chronic cystitis

Chronic cystitis NOS
Subacute cystitis

> *Excludes:* trigonitis (595.3)

595.3 Trigonitis

Follicular cystitis
Trigonitis (acute) (chronic)
Urethrotrigonitis

595.4 Cystitis in diseases classified elsewhere

Code first underlying disease, as:
actinomycosis (039.8)
amebiasis (006.8)
bilharziasis (120.0-120.9)
Echinococcus infestation (122.3, 122.6)

> *Excludes:* cystitis:
> diphtheritic (032.84)
> gonococcal (098.11, 098.31)
> monilial (112.2)
> trichomonal (131.09)
> tuberculous (016.1)

⑤ **595.8 Other specified types of cystitis**

595.81 Cystitis cystica

595.82 Irradiation cystitis

Use additional E code, if desired, to identify cause

595.89 Other

Abscess of bladder
Cystitis:
bullous
emphysematous
glandularis

595.9 Cystitis, unspecified

596 **Other disorders of bladder**

Use additional code, if desired, to identify urinary incontinence (625.6, 788.30-788.39)

596.0 Bladder neck obstruction

Contracture (acquired) of bladder neck or vesicourethral orifice
Obstruction (acquired) of bladder neck or vesicourethral orifice
Stenosis (acquired) of bladder neck or vesicourethral orifice

> *Excludes:* congenital (753.6)

596.1 Intestinovesical fistula

Fistula: Fistula:
enterovesical   vesicoenteric
vesicocolic   vesicorectal

596.2 Vesical fistula, not elsewhere classified

Fistula: Fistula:
bladder NOS   vesicocutaneous
urethrovesical   vesicoperineal

> *Excludes:* fistula between bladder and female genital tract (619.0)

596.3 Diverticulum of bladder

Diverticulitis of bladder
Diverticulum (acquired) (false) of bladder

> *Excludes:* that with calculus in diverticulum of bladder (594.0)

| | Add 4th or 5th digit | | Nonspecific code | | Unspecified code | | Manifestation code |

596.4 Atony of bladder
High compliance bladder, of bladder
Hypotonicity of bladder
Inertia of bladder

Excludes: neurogenic bladder (596.54)

⑤ **596.5 Other functional disorders of bladder**

Excludes: cauda equina syndrome
with neurogenic bladder (344.61)

596.51 Hypertonicity of bladder
Hyperactivity
Overactive bladder

596.52 Low bladder compliance

596.53 Paralysis of bladder

596.54 Neurogenic bladder NOS

596.55 Detrusor sphincter dyssynergia

596.59 Other functional disorder of bladder
Detrusor instability

596.6 Rupture of bladder, nontraumatic

596.7 Hemorrhage into bladder wall
Hyperemia of bladder

Excludes: acute hemorrhagic cystitis (595.0)

596.8 Other specified disorders of bladder

Bladder:	Bladder:
calcified	hemorrhage
contracted	hypertrophy

Excludes: cystocele, female (618.01-618.02, 618.09, 618.2-618.4)
hernia or prolapse of bladder, female (618.01-618.02, 618.09, 618.2-618.4)

596.9 Unspecified disorder of bladder

597 Urethritis, not sexually transmitted, and urethral syndrome

Excludes: nonspecific urethritis, so stated (099.4)

597.0 Urethral abscess

Abscess of:	Abscess:
bulbourethral gland	periurethral
Cowper's gland	urethral (gland)
Littré's gland	Periurethral cellulitis

Excludes: urethral caruncle (599.3)

⑤ **597.8 Other urethritis**

597.80 Urethritis, unspecified

597.81 Urethral syndrome NOS

597.89 Other

Adenitis, Skene's	Meatitis, urethral
glands	Ulcer, urethra (meatus)
Cowperitis	Verumontanitis

Excludes: trichomonal (131.02)

598 Urethral stricture
Includes: pinhole meatus
stricture of urinary meatus

Excludes: congenital stricture of urethra and urinary meatus (753.6)
Use additional code to identify urinary incontinence (625.6, 788.30-788.39)

⑤ **598.0 Urethral stricture due to infection**

598.00 Due to unspecified infection

598.01 Due to infective diseases classified elsewhere
Code first underlying disease, as:
gonococcal infection (098.2)
schistosomiasis (120.0-120.9)
syphilis (095.8)

● Code new
to this edition

▲ Revision of
existing code

④ ⑤ Fourth or fifth
digit required

598.1 Traumatic urethral stricture
Stricture of urethra:
late effect of injury
postobstetric

Excludes: *postoperative following surgery on genitourinary tract (598.2)*

598.2 Postoperative urethral stricture
Postcatheterization stricture of urethra

598.8 Other specified causes of urethral stricture

598.9 Urethral stricture, unspecified

599 Other disorders of urethra and urinary tract

599.0 Urinary tract infection, site not specified
Pyuria

Excludes: *candidiasis of urinary tract (112.2)*
urinary tract infection of newborn (771.82)

Use additional code to identify organism, such as Escherichia coli [E. coli] (041.4)

599.1 Urethral fistula
Fistula: Urinary fistula NOS
urethroperineal
urethrorectal

Excludes: *fistula:*
urethroscrotal (608.89)
urethrovaginal (619.0)
urethrovesicovaginal (619.0)

599.2 Urethral diverticulum

599.3 Urethral caruncle
Polyp of urethra

599.4 Urethral false passage

599.5 Prolapsed urethral mucosa
Prolapse of urethra
Urethrocele

Excludes: *urethrocele, female (618.03, 618.09, 618.2-618.4)*

⑤ **599.6 Urinary obstruction**

599.60 Urinary obstruction, unspecified
Obstructive uropathy NOS
Urinary (tract) obstruction NOS

599.69 Urinary obstruction, not elsewhere classified
Code, if applicable, any causal condition first, such as:
hyperplasia of prostate (600.0-600.9 with fifth-digit 1)

⑤ **599.7 Hematuria**
Hematuria (benign) (essential)

Excludes: *hemoglobinuria (791.2)*

599.70 Hematuria, unspecified

599.71 Gross hematuria

599.72 Microscopic hematuria

⑤ **599.8 Other specified disorders of urethra and urinary tract**

Excludes: *symptoms and other conditions classifiable to 788.0-788.9, 791.0-791.9*
Use additional code, if desired, to identify urinary incontinence (625.6, 788.30-788.39)

599.81 Urethral hypermobility

599.82 Intrinsic (urethral) sphincter deficiency [ISD]

599.83 Urethral instability

599.84 Other specified disorders of urethra
Rupture of urethra (nontraumatic)
Urethral:
cyst
granuloma

599.89 Other specified disorders of urinary tract

599.9 Unspecified disorder of urethra and urinary tract

▮ Add 4th or 5th digit	▮ Nonspecific code	▮ Unspecified code	▮ Manifestation code

DISEASES OF MALE GENITAL ORGANS (600-608)

600 **Hyperplasia of prostate**
Includes: enlarged prostate

⑤ **600.0** **Hypertrophy (benign) of prostate**
Benign prostatic hypertrophy
Enlargement of prostate
Smooth enlarged prostate
Soft enlarged prostate

600.00 **Hypertrophy (benign) of prostate without urinary obstruction and other lower urinary tract symptoms (LUTS)**
Hypertrophy (benign) of prostate NOS

600.01 **Hypertrophy (benign) of prostate with urinary obstruction and other lower urinary tract symptoms (LUTS)**
Hypertrophy (benign) of prostate with urinary retention

Use additional code to identify symptoms:
incomplete bladder emptying (788.21)
nocturia (788.43)
straining on urination (788.65)
urinary frequency (788.41)
urinary hesitancy (788.64)
urinary incontinence (788.30-788.39)
urinary obstruction (599.69)
urinary retention (788.20)
urinary urgency (788.63)
weak urinary stream (788.62)

⑤ **600.1** **Nodular prostate**
Hard, firm prostate
Multinodular prostate

Excludes: *malignant neoplasm of prostate (185)*

600.10 **Nodular prostate without urinary obstruction**
Nodular prostate NOS

600.11 **Nodular prostate with urinary obstruction**
Nodular prostate with urinary retention

⑤ **600.2** **Benign localized hyperplasia of prostate**
Adenofibromatous hypertrophy of prostate
Adenoma of prostate
Fibroadenoma of prostate
Fibroma of prostate
Myoma of prostate
Polyp of prostate

Excludes: *benign neoplasms of prostate (222.2)*
hypertrophy of prostate (600.00-600.01)
malignant neoplasm of prostate (185)

600.20 **Benign localized hyperplasia of prostate without urinary obstruction and other lower urinary tract symptoms (LUTS)**
Benign localized hyperplasia of prostate NOS

600.21 **Benign localized hyperplasia of prostate with urinary obstruction and other lower urinary tract symptoms (LUTS)**
Benign localized hyperplasia of prostate with urinary retention

Use additional code to identify symptoms:
incomplete bladder emptying (788.21)
nocturia (788.43)
straining on urination (788.65)
urinary frequency (788.41)
urinary hesitancy (788.64)
urinary incontinence (788.30-788.39)
urinary obstruction (599.69)
urinary retention (788.20)
urinary urgency (788.63)
weak urinary stream (788.62)

600.3 **Cyst of prostate**

⑤ **600.9** **Hyperplasia of prostate, unspecified**
Median bar
Prostatic obstruction NOS

● Code new
to this edition
▲ Revision of
existing code
④ ⑤ Fourth or fifth
digit required

600.90 Hyperplasia of prostate, unspecified, without urinary obstruction and other lower urinary symptoms (LUTS)
Hyperplasia of prostate NOS

600.91 Hyperplasia of prostate, unspecified, with urinary obstruction and other lower urinary symptoms (LUTS)
Hyperplasia of prostate, unspecified, with urinary retention

Use additional code to identify symptoms:
incomplete bladder emptying (788.21)
nocturia (788.43)
straining on urination (788.65)
urinary frequency (788.41)
urinary hesitancy (788.64)
urinary incontinence (788.30-788.39)
urinary obstruction (599.69)
urinary retention (788.20)
urinary urgency (788.63)
weak urinary stream (788.62)

601 Inflammatory diseases of prostate
Use additional code, if desired, to identify organism, such as Staphylococcus (041.1), or Streptococcus (041.0)

601.0 Acute prostatitis

601.1 Chronic prostatitis

601.2 Abscess of prostate

601.3 Prostatocystitis

601.4 *Prostatitis in diseases classified elsewhere*
Code first underlying disease, as:
actinomycosis (039.8)
blastomycosis (116.0)
syphilis (095.8)
tuberculosis (016.5)

Excludes: *prostatitis:*
gonococcal (098.12, 098.32)
monilial (112.2)
trichomonal (131.03)

601.8 Other specified inflammatory diseases of prostate
Prostatitis:
cavitary
diverticular
granulomatous

601.9 Prostatitis, unspecified
Prostatitis NOS

602 Other disorders of prostate

602.0 Calculus of prostate
Prostatic stone

602.1 Congestion or hemorrhage of prostate

602.2 Atrophy of prostate

602.3 Dysplasia of prostate
Prostatic intraepithelial neoplasia I (PIN I)
Prostatic intraepithelial neoplasia II (PIN II)
Excludes: *Prostatic intraepithelial neoplasia III (PIN III) (233.4)*

602.8 Other specified disorders of prostate
Fistula of prostate
Infarction of prostate
Stricture of prostate
Periprostatic adhesions

602.9 Unspecified disorder of prostate

603 Hydrocele
Includes: hydrocele of spermatic cord, testis, or tunica vaginalis
Excludes: *congenital (778.6)*

603.0 Encysted hydrocele

603.1 Infected hydrocele
Use additional code, if desired, to identify organism

Add 4th or 5th digit | Nonspecific code | Unspecified code | Manifestation code

603.8 Other specified types of hydrocele

603.9 Hydrocele, unspecified

604 Orchitis and epididymitis

Use additional code, if desired, to identify organism, such as Escherichia coli [E. coli] (041.4), Staphylococcus (041.1), or Streptococcus (041.0)

604.0 Orchitis, epididymitis, and epididymo-orchitis, with abscess
Abscess of epididymis or testis

⑤ **604.9** Other orchitis, epididymitis, and epididymo-orchitis, without mention of abscess

604.90 Orchitis and epididymitis, unspecified

604.91 *Orchitis and epididymitis in diseases classified elsewhere*
Code first underlying disease, as:
diphtheria (032.89)
filariasis (125.0-125.9)
syphilis (095.8)

Excludes: *orchitis:*
gonococcal (098.13, 098.33)
mumps (072.0)
tuberculous (016.5)
tuberculous epididymitis (016.4)

604.99 Other

605 Redundant prepuce and phimosis
Adherent prepuce   Phimosis (congenital)
Paraphimosis   Tight foreskin

606 Infertility, male

606.0 Azoospermia
Absolute infertility
Infertility due to:
germinal (cell) aplasia
spermatogenic arrest (complete)

606.1 Oligospermia
Infertility due to:
germinal cell desquamation
hypospermatogenesis
incomplete spermatogenic arrest

606.8 Infertility due to extratesticular causes
Infertility due to:
drug therapy
infection
obstruction of efferent ducts
radiation
systemic disease

606.9 Male infertility, unspecified

607 Disorders of penis

Excludes: *phimosis (605)*

607.0 Leukoplakia of penis
Kraurosis of penis

Excludes: *carcinoma in situ of penis (233.5)*
erythroplasia of Queyrat (233.5)

607.1 Balanoposthitis
Balanitis

Use additional code, if desired, to identify organism

607.2 Other inflammatory disorders of penis
Abscess of corpus cavernosum or penis
Boil of corpus cavernosum or penis
Carbuncle of corpus cavernosum or penis
Cellulitis of corpus cavernosum or penis
Cavernitis (penis)

Use additional code, if desired, to identify organism

Excludes: *herpetic infection (054.13)*

607.3 Priapism
Painful erection

⑤ **607.8** Other specified disorders of penis

● Code new
to this edition
▲ Revision of
existing code
④ ⑤ Fourth or fifth
digit required

607.81   Balanitis xerotica obliterans
Induratio penis plastica

607.82   Vascular disorders of penis
Embolism of corpus cavernosum or penis
Hematoma (nontraumatic) of corpus cavernosum or penis
Hemorrhage of corpus cavernosum or penis
Thrombosis of corpus cavernosum or penis

607.83   Edema of penis

607.84   Impotence of organic origin

Excludes: nonorganic (302.72)

607.85   Peyronie's disease

607.89   Other
Atrophy of corpus cavernosum or penis
Fibrosis of corpus cavernosum or penis
Hypertrophy of corpus cavernosum or penis
Ulcer (chronic) of corpus cavernosum or penis

607.9   Unspecified disorder of penis

608   Other disorders of male genital organs

608.0   Seminal vesiculitis
Abscess of seminal vesicle
Cellulitis of seminal vesicle
Vesiculitis (seminal)

Use additional code, if desired, to identify organism

Excludes: gonococcal infection (098.14, 098.34)

608.1   Spermatocele

⑤ **608.2   Torsion of testis**

608.20   Torsion of testis, unspecified

608.21   Extravaginal torsion of spermatic cord

608.22   Intravaginal torsion of spermatic cord
Torsion of spermatic cord NOS

608.23   Torsion of appendix testis

608.24   Torsion of appendix epididymis

608.3   Atrophy of testis

608.4   Other inflammatory disorders of male genital organs
Abscess of scrotum, spermatic cord, testis [except abscess], tunica vaginalis, or vas deferens
Boil of scrotum, spermatic cord, testis [except abscess], tunica vaginalis, or vas deferens
Carbuncle of scrotum, spermatic cord, testis [except abscess], tunica vaginalis, or vas deferens
Cellulitis of scrotum, spermatic cord, testis [except abscess], tunica vaginalis, or vas deferens
Vasitis

Use additional code, if desired, to identify organism

Excludes: abscess of testis (604.0)

⑤ **608.8   Other specified disorders of male genital organs**

608.81   Disorders of male genital organs in diseases classified elsewhere
Code first underlying disease, as:
filariasis (125.0-125.9)
tuberculosis (016.5)

608.82   Hematospermia

608.83   Vascular disorders
Hematoma (nontraumatic) of seminal vesicle, spermatic cord, testis, scrotum, tunica vaginalis, or vas deferens
Hemorrhage of seminal vesicle, spermatic cord, testis, scrotum, tunica vaginalis, or vas deferens
Thrombosis of seminal vesicle, spermatic cord, testis, scrotum, tunica vaginalis, or vas deferens
Hematocele NOS, male

608.84   Chylocele of tunica vaginalis

608.85   Stricture
Stricture of:
spermatic cord
tunica vaginalis
vas deferens

608.86   Edema

| | Add 4th or 5th digit | | Nonspecific code | | Unspecified code | | Manifestation code |

608.87 **Retrograde ejaculation**

608.89 **Other**
Atrophy of seminal vesicle, spermatic cord, testis, scrotum, tunica vaginalis, or vas deferens
Fibrosis of seminal vesicle, spermatic cord, testis, scrotum, tunica vaginalis, or vas deferens
Hypertrophy of seminal vesicle, spermatic cord, testis, scrotum, tunica vaginalis, or vas deferens
Ulcer of seminal vesicle, spermatic cord, testis, scrotum, tunica vaginalis, or vas deferens

Excludes: atrophy of testis (608.3)

608.9 **Unspecified disorder of male genital organs**

DISORDERS OF BREAST (610-612)

610 **Benign mammary dysplasias**

610.0 **Solitary cyst of breast**
Cyst (solitary) of breast

610.1 **Diffuse cystic mastopathy**
Chronic cystic mastitis   Fibrocystic disease of breast
Cystic breast

610.2 **Fibroadenosis of breast**
Fibroadenosis of breast: Fibroadenosis of breast:
 NOS   diffuse
 chronic   periodic
 cystic   segmental

610.3 **Fibrosclerosis of breast**

610.4 **Mammary duct ectasia**
Comedomastitis   Mastitis:
Dust ectasia   periductal
                          plasma cell

610.8 **Other specified benign mammary dysplasias**
Mazoplasia
Sebaceous cyst of breast

610.9 **Benign mammary dysplasia, unspecified**

611 **Other disorders of breast**

Excludes: that associated with lactation or the puerperium (675.0-676.9)

611.0 **Inflammatory disease of breast**
Abscess (acute) (chronic) (nonpuerperal) of:
 areola
 breast
Mammillary fistula
Mastitis (acute) (subacute) (nonpuerperal):
 NOS
 infective
 retromammary
 submammary

Excludes: carbuncle of breast (680.2)
          chronic cystic mastitis (610.1)
          neonatal infective mastitis (771.5)
          thrombophlebitis of breast [Mondor's disease] (451.89)

611.1 **Hypertrophy of breast**
Gynecomastia
Hypertrophy of breast:
 NOS
 massive pubertal

Excludes: breast engorgement in newborn (778.7)
          disproportion of reconstructed breast (612.1)

611.2 **Fissure of nipple**

611.3 **Fat necrosis of breast**
Fat necrosis (segmental) of breast
Code first breast necrosis due to breast graft (996.79)

611.4 **Atrophy of breast**

611.5 **Galactocele**

● Code new   ▲ Revision of   ④ ⑤ Fourth or fifth
  to this edition   existing code   digit required

611.6 Galactorrhea not associated with childbirth

⑤ **611.7 Signs and symptoms in breast**

611.71 Mastodynia
Pain in breast

611.72 Lump or mass in breast

611.79 Other
Induration of breast   Nipple discharge
Inversion of nipple   Retraction of nipple

⑤ **611.8 Other specified disorders of breast**

611.81 Ptosis of breast

Excludes: *ptosis of native breast in relation to reconstructed breast (612.1)*

611.82 Hypoplasia of breast
Micromastia

Excludes: *congenital absence of breast (757.6)*
hypoplasia of native breast in relation to reconstructed breast (612.1)

611.83 Capsular contracture of breast implant

611.89 Other specified disorders of breast
Hematoma (nontraumatic) of breast
Infarction of breast
Occlusion of breast duct
Subinvolution of breast (postlactational) (postpartum)

611.9 Unspecified breast disorder

612 Deformity and disproportion of reconstructed breast

612.0 Deformity of reconstructed breast
Contour irregularity in reconstructed breast
Excess tissue in reconstructed breast
Misshapen reconstructed breast

612.1 Disproportion of reconstructed breast
Breast asymmetry between native breast and reconstructed breast
Disproportion between native breast and reconstructed breast

INFLAMMATORY DISEASE OF FEMALE PELVIC ORGANS (614-616)

Use additional code, if desired, to identify organism, such as Staphylococcus (041.1), or Streptococcus (041.0)

Excludes: *that associated with pregnancy, abortion, childbirth, or the puerperium (630-676.9)*

614 Inflammatory disease of ovary, fallopian tube, pelvic cellular tissue, and peritoneum

Excludes: *endometritis (615.0-615.9)*
major infection following delivery (670.0-670.8)
that complicating:
abortion (634-638 with .0, 639.0)
ectopic or molar pregnancy (639.0)
pregnancy or labor (646.6)

614.0 Acute salpingitis and oophoritis
Any condition classifiable to 614.2, specified as acute or subacute

614.1 Chronic salpingitis and oophoritis
Hydrosalpinx
Salpingitis:
follicularis
isthmica nodosa
Any condition classifiable to 614.2, specified as chronic

614.2 Salpingitis and oophoritis not specified as acute, subacute, or chronic
Abscess (of):   Perisalpingitis
fallopian tube   Pyosalpinx
ovary   Salpingitis
tubo-ovarian   Salpingo-oophoritisRTubo-ovarian inflammatory disease
Oophoritis
Perioophoritis

Excludes: *gonococcal infection (chronic) (098.37)*
acute (098.17)
tuberculous (016.6)

	Add 4th or 5th digit		Nonspecific code		Unspecified code		Manifestation code

614.3 Acute parametritis and pelvic cellulitis
Acute inflammatory pelvic disease
Any condition classifiable to 614.4, specified as acute

614.4 Chronic or unspecified parametritis and pelvic cellulitis
Abscess (of):
broad ligament, chronic or NOS
parametrium, chronic or NOS
pelvis, female, chronic or NOS
pouch of Douglas, chronic or NOS
Chronic inflammatory pelvic disease
Pelvic cellulitis, female
Excludes: tuberculous (016.7)

614.5 Acute or unspecified pelvic peritonitis, female

614.6 Pelvic peritoneal adhesions, female (postoperative) (postinfection)
Adhesions:
peritubal
tubo-ovarian
Use additional code, if desired, to identify any associated infertility (628.2)

614.7 Other chronic pelvic peritonitis, female
Excludes: tuberculous (016.7)

614.8 Other specified inflammatory disease of female pelvic organs and tissues

614.9 Unspecified inflammatory disease of female pelvic organs and tissues
Pelvic infection or inflammation, female NOS
Pelvic inflammatory disease [PID]

615 Inflammatory diseases of uterus, except cervix
Excludes: following delivery (670.0-670.8)
hyperplastic endometritis (621.30-621.35)
that complicating:
abortion (634-638 with .0, 639.0)
ectopic or molar pregnancy (639.0)
pregnancy or labor (646.6)

615.0 Acute
Any condition classifiable to 615.9, specified as acute or subacute

615.1 Chronic
Any condition classifiable to 615.9, specified as chronic

615.9 Unspecified inflammatory disease of uterus
Endometritis   Perimetritis
Endomyometritis   Pyometra
Metritis   Uterine abscess
Myometritis

616 Inflammatory disease of cervix, vagina, and vulva
Excludes: that complicating:
abortion (634-638 with .0, 639.0)
ectopic or molar pregnancy (639.0)
pregnancy, childbirth, or the puerperium (646.6)

616.0 Cervicitis and endocervicitis
Cervicitis with or without mention of erosion or ectropion
Endocervicitis with or without mention of erosion or ectropion
Nabothian (gland) cyst or follicle
Excludes: erosion or ectropion without mention of cervicitis (622.0)

⑤ **616.1 Vaginitis and vulvovaginitis**
Excludes: vulvar vestibulitis (625.71)

616.10 Vaginitis and vulvovaginitis, unspecified
Vaginitis:
NOS
postirradiation
Vulvitis NOS
Vulvovaginitis NOS
Use additional code, if desired, to identify organism, such as Escherichia coli [E. coli] (041.4), Staphylococcus (041.1), or Streptococcus (041.0)
Excludes: noninfective leukorrhea (623.5)
postmenopausal or senile vaginitis (627.3)

● Code new to this edition   ▲ Revision of existing code   ④ ⑤ Fourth or fifth digit required

616.11 *Vaginitis and vulvovaginitis in diseases classified elsewhere*
Code first underlying disease, as:
pinworm vaginitis (127.4)

Excludes:	*herpetic vulvovaginitis (054.11)*
	monilial vulvovaginitis (112.1)
	trichomonal vaginitis or vulvovaginitis (131.01)

616.2 Cyst of Bartholin's gland
Bartholin's duct cyst

616.3 Abscess of Bartholin's gland
Vulvovaginal gland abscess

616.4 Other abscess of vulva
Abscess of vulva
Carbuncle of vulva
Furuncle of vulva

⑤ **616.5 Ulceration of vulva**

616.50 Ulceration of vulva, unspecified
Ulcer NOS of vulva

616.51 *Ulceration of vulva in diseases classified elsewhere*
Code first underlying disease, as:
Behçet's syndrome (136.1)
tuberculosis (016.7)

Excludes:	*vulvar ulcer (in):*
	gonococcal (098.0)
	herpes simplex (054.12)
	syphilitic (091.0)

⑤ **616.8 Other specified inflammatory diseases of cervix, vagina, and vulva**

Excludes:	*noninflammatory disorders of:*
	cervix (622.0-622.9)
	vagina (623.0-623.9)
	vulva (624.0-624.9)

616.81 Mucositis (ulcerative) of cervix, vagina, and vulva
Use additional E code to identify adverse effects of therapy, such as:
antineoplastic and immunosuppressive drugs (E930.7, E933.1)
radiation therapy (E879.2)

616.89 Other inflammatory disease of cervix, vagina and vulva
Caruncle, vagina or labium
Ulcer, vagina

616.9 Unspecified inflammatory disease of cervix, vagina, and vulva

OTHER DISORDERS OF FEMALE GENITAL TRACT (617-629)

617 Endometriosis

617.0 Endometriosis of uterus
Adenomyosis
Endometriosis:
cervix
internal
myometrium

Excludes:	*stromal endometriosis (236.0)*

617.1 Endometriosis of ovary
Chocolate cyst of ovary
Endometrial cystoma of ovary

617.2 Endometriosis of fallopian tube

617.3 Endometriosis of pelvic peritoneum
Endometriosis: Endometriosis:
broad ligament   parametrium
cul-de-sac (Douglas')   round ligament

617.4 Endometriosis of rectovaginal septum and vagina

617.5 Endometriosis of intestine
Endometriosis:
appendix
colon
rectum

Add 4th or 5th digit	Nonspecific code	Unspecified code	Manifestation code

617.6 Endometriosis in scar of skin

617.8 Endometriosis of other specified sites
Endometriosis: Endometriosis:
   bladder   umbilicus
   lung   vulva

617.9 Endometriosis, site unspecified

618 Genital prolapse
Use additional code, if desired, to identify urinary incontinence (625.6, 788.31, 788.33-788.39)

    Excludes: that complicating pregnancy, labor, or delivery (654.4)

⑤ **618.0 Prolapse of vaginal walls without mention of uterine prolapse**

    Excludes: that with uterine prolapse (618.2-618.4)
            enterocele (618.6)
            vaginal vault prolapse following hysterectomy (618.5)

    618.00 Unspecified prolapse of vaginal walls
        Vaginal prolapse NOS

    618.01 Cystocele, midline
        Cystocele NOS

    618.02 Cystocele, lateral
        Paravaginal

    618.03 Urethrocele

    618.04 Rectocele
        Proctocele

    618.05 Perineocele

    618.09 Other prolapse of vaginal walls without mention of uterine prolapse
        Cystourethrocele

618.1 Uterine prolapse without mention of vaginal wall prolapse
Descensus uteri   Uterine prolapse:
Uterine prolapse: first degree
   NOS   second degree
   complete   third degree

    Excludes: that with mention of cystocele, urethrocele, or rectocele (618.2-618.4)

618.2 Uterovaginal prolapse, incomplete

618.3 Uterovaginal prolapse, complete

618.4 Uterovaginal prolapse, unspecified

618.5 Prolapse of vaginal vault after hysterectomy

618.6 Vaginal enterocele, congenital or acquired
    Pelvic enterocele, congenital or acquired

618.7 Old laceration of muscles of pelvic floor

⑤ **618.8 Other specified genital prolapse**

    618.81 Incompetence or weakening of pubocervical tissue

    618.82 Incompetence or weakening of rectovaginal tissue

    618.83 Pelvic muscle wasting
        Disuse atrophy of pelvic muscles and anal sphincter

    618.84 Cervical stump prolapse

    618.89 Other specified genital prolapse

618.9 Unspecified genital prolapse

619 Fistula involving female genital tract

    Excludes: vesicorectal and intestinovesical fistula (596.1)

619.0 Urinary-genital tract fistula, female
Fistula: Fistula:
   cervicovesical   uteroureteric
   ureterovaginal   uterovesical
   urethrovaginal   vesicocervicovaginal
   urethrovesicovaginal   vesicovaginal

619.1 Digestive-genital tract fistula, female
Fistula: Fistula:
   intestinouterine   rectovulval
   intestinovaginal   sigmoidovaginal
   rectovaginal   uterorectal

● Code new   ▲ Revision of   ④ ⑤ Fourth or fifth
  to this edition   existing code   digit required

619.2 Genital tract-skin fistula, female
Fistula:
uterus to abdominal wall
vaginoperinea

619.8 Other specified fistulas involving female genital tract
Fistula: Fistula:
cervix   uterus
cul-de-sac (Douglas')   vagina

619.9 Unspecified fistula involving female genital tract

620 Noninflammatory disorders of ovary, fallopian tube, and broad ligament
Excludes: hydrosalpinx (614.1)

620.0 Follicular cyst of ovary
Cyst of graafian follicle

620.1 Corpus luteum cyst or hematoma
Corpus luteum hemorrhage or rupture
Lutein cyst

620.2 Other and unspecified ovarian cyst
Cyst of ovary:
NOS
corpus albicans
retention NOS
serous
theca-lutein
Simple cystoma of ovary

Excludes: cystadenoma (benign) (serous) (220)
developmental cysts (752.0)
neoplastic cysts (220)
polycystic ovaries (256.4)
Stein-Leventhal syndrome (256.4)

620.3 Acquired atrophy of ovary and fallopian tube
Senile involution of ovary

620.4 Prolapse or hernia of ovary and fallopian tube
Displacement of ovary and fallopian tube
Salpingocele

620.5 Torsion of ovary, ovarian pedicle, or fallopian tube
Torsion:
accessory tube
hydatid of Morgagni

620.6 Broad ligament laceration syndrome
Masters-Allen syndrome

620.7 Hematoma of broad ligament
Hematocele, broad ligament

620.8 Other noninflammatory disorders of ovary, fallopian tube, and broad ligament
Cyst of broad ligament or fallopian tube
Polyp of broad ligament or fallopian tube
Infarction of ovary or fallopian tube
Rupture of ovary or fallopian tube
Hematosalpinx of ovary or fallopian tube

Excludes: hematosalpinx in ectopic pregnancy (639.2)
peritubal adhesions (614.6)
torsion of ovary, ovarian pedicle, or fallopian tube (620.5)

620.9 Unspecified noninflammatory disorder of ovary, fallopian tube, and broad ligament

621 Disorders of uterus, not elsewhere classified

621.0 Polyp of corpus uteri
Polyp:
endometrium
uterus NOS

Excludes: cervical polyp NOS (622.7)

621.1 Chronic subinvolution of uterus

Excludes: puerperal (674.8)

461

| | Add 4th or 5th digit | | Nonspecific code | | Unspecified code | | Manifestation code |

621.2 Hypertrophy of uterus
Bulky or enlarged uterus

Excludes: puerperal (674.8)

⑤ **621.3 Endometrial hyperplasia**

621.30 Endometrial hyperplasia, unspecified
Endometrial hyperplasia NOS
Hyperplasia (adenomatous) (cystic) (glandular) of endometrium
Hyperplastic endometritis

621.31 Simple endometrial hyperplasia without atypia

Excludes: benign endometrial hyperplasia (621.34)

621.32 Complex endometrial hyperplasia without atypia

Excludes: benign endometrial hyperplasia (621.34)

621.33 Endometrial hyperplasia with atypia

Excludes: endometrial intraepithelial neoplasia [EIN] (621.35)

● **621.34 Benign endometrial hyperplasia**

● **621.35 Endometrial intraepithelial neoplasia [EIN]**

Excludes: malignant neoplasm of endometrium with endometrial intraepithelial neoplasia [EIN] (182.0)

621.4 Hematometra
Hemometra

Excludes: that in congenital anomaly (752.2-752.3)

621.5 Intrauterine synechiae
Adhesions of uterus
Band(s) of uterus

621.6 Malposition of uterus
Anteversion of uterus
Retroflexion of uterus
Retroversion of uterus

Excludes: malposition complicating pregnancy, labor, or delivery (654.3-654.4)
prolapse of uterus (618.1-618.4)

621.7 Chronic inversion of uterus

Excludes: current obstetrical trauma (665.2)
prolapse of uterus (618.1-618.4)

621.8 Other specified disorders of uterus, not elsewhere classified
Atrophy, acquired of uterus
Cyst of uterus
Fibrosis NOS of uterus
Old laceration (postpartum) of uterus
Ulcer of uterus

Excludes: bilharzial fibrosis (120.0-120.9)
endometriosis (617.0)
fistulas (619.0-619.8)
inflammatory diseases (615.0-615.9)

621.9 Unspecified disorder of uterus

622 Noninflammatory disorders of cervix

Excludes: abnormality of cervix complicating pregnancy, labor, or delivery (654.5-654.6)
fistula (619.0-619.8)

622.0 Erosion and ectropion of cervix
Eversion of cervix
Ulcer of cervix

Excludes: that in chronic cervicitis (616.0)

⑤ **622.1 Dysplasia of cervix (uteri)**

Excludes: abnormal results from cervical cytologic examination without histologic confirmation (795.00-795.09)
carcinoma in situ of cervix (233.1)
cervical intraepithelial neoplasia III [CIN III] (233.1)
HGSIL of cervix (795.04)

● Code new
to this edition

▲ Revision of
existing code

④ ⑤ Fourth or fifth
digit required

622.10 Dysplasia of cervix, unspecified
    Anaplasia of cervix
    Cervical atypism
    Cervical dysplasia NOS

622.11 Mild dysplasia of cervix
    Cervical intraepithelial neoplasia I [CIN I]

622.12 Moderate dysplasia of cervix
    Cervical intraepithelial neoplasia II [CIN II]

Excludes: *carcinoma in situ of cervix (233.1)*
    cervical intraepithelial neoplasia III [CIN III] (233.1)
    severe dysplasia (233.1)

622.2 Leukoplakia of cervix (uteri)

Excludes: *carcinoma in situ of cervix (233.1)*

622.3 Old laceration of cervix
    Adhesions of cervix
    Band(s) of cervix
    Cicatrix (postpartum) of cervix

Excludes: *current obstetrical trauma (665.3)*

622.4 Stricture and stenosis of cervix
    Atresia (acquired) of cervix
    Contracture of cervix
    Occlusion of cervix
    Pinpoint os uteri

Excludes: *congenital (752.49)*
    that complicating labor (654.6)

622.5 Incompetence of cervix

Excludes: *complicating pregnancy (654.5)*
    that affecting fetus or newborn (761.0)

622.6 Hypertrophic elongation of cervix

622.7 Mucous polyp of cervix
    Polyp NOS of cervix

Excludes: *adenomatous polyp of cervix (219.0)*

622.8 Other specified noninflammatory disorders of cervix
    Atrophy (senile) of cervix
    Cyst of cervix
    Fibrosis of cervix
    Hemorrhage of cervix

Excludes: *endometriosis (617.0)*
    fistula (619.0-619.8)
    inflammatory diseases (616.0)

622.9 Unspecified noninflammatory disorder of cervix

623 Noninflammatory disorders of vagina

Excludes: *abnormality of vagina complicating pregnancy, labor, or delivery (654.7)*
    congenital absence of vagina (752.49)
    congenital diaphragm or bands (752.49)
    fistulas involving vagina (619.0-619.8)

623.0 Dysplasia of vagina
    Mild and moderate dysplasia of vagina
    Vaginal intraepithelial neoplasia I and II [VAIN I and II]

Excludes: *abnormal results from vaginal cytological examination without histologic*
    confirmation (795.10-795.19)
    carcinoma in situ of vagina (233.31)
    HGSIL of vagina (795.14)
    severe dysplasia of vagina (233.31)
    vaginal intraepithelial neoplasia III [VAIN III] (233.31)

623.1 Leukoplakia of vagina

| Add 4th or 5th digit | Nonspecific code | Unspecified code | 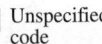 Manifestation code |

623.2 Stricture or atresia of vagina
Adhesions (postoperative) (postradiation) of vagina
Occlusion of vagina
Stenosis, vagina

Use additional E code, if desired, to identify any external cause

Excludes: *congenital atresia or stricture (752.49)*

623.3 Tight hymenal ring
Rigid hymen acquired or congenital
Tight hymenal ring acquired or congenital
Tight introitus acquired or congenital

Excludes: *imperforate hymen (752.42)*

623.4 Old vaginal laceration

Excludes: *old laceration involving muscles of pelvic floor (618.7)*

623.5 Leukorrhea, not specified as infective
Leukorrhea NOS of vagina
Vaginal discharge NOS

Excludes: *trichomonal (131.00)*

623.6 Vaginal hematoma

Excludes: *current obstetrical trauma (665.7)*

623.7 Polyp of vagina

623.8 Other specified noninflammatory disorders of vagina
Cyst of vagina
Hemorrhage of vagina

623.9 Unspecified noninflammatory disorder of vagina

624 Noninflammatory disorders of vulva and perineum

Excludes: *abnormality of vulva and perineum complicating pregnancy, labor, or delivery*
(654.8)
condyloma acuminatum (078.11)
fistulas involving:
perineum—see Alphabetic Index
vulva (619.0-619.8)
vulval varices (456.6)
vulvar involvement in skin conditions (690-709.9)

⑤ **624.0 Dystrophy of vulva**

Excludes: *carcinoma in situ of vulva (233.32)*
severe dysplasia of vulva (233.32)
vulvar intraepithelial neoplasia III [VIN III] (233.32)

624.01 Vulvar intraepithelial neoplasia I [VIN I]
Mild dysplasia of vulva

624.02 Vulvar intraepithelial neoplasia II [VIN II]
Moderate dysplasia of vulva

624.09 Other dystrophy of vulva
Kraurosis of vulva
Leukoplakia of vulva

624.1 Atrophy of vulva

624.2 Hypertrophy of clitoris

Excludes: *that in endocrine disorders (255.2, 256.1)*

624.3 Hypertrophy of labia
Hypertrophy of vulva NOS

624.4 Old laceration or scarring of vulva

624.5 Hematoma of vulva

Excludes: *that complicating delivery (664.5)*

624.6 Polyp of labia and vulva

624.8 Other specified noninflammatory disorders of vulva and perineum
Cyst of vulva
Edema of vulva
Stricture of vulva

624.9 Unspecified noninflammatory disorder of vulva and perineum

● Code new
to this edition

▲ Revision of
existing code

④ ⑤ Fourth or fifth
digit required

625 **Pain and other symptoms associated with female genital organs**

625.0 Dyspareunia
> *Excludes:* psychogenic dyspareunia (302.76)

625.1 Vaginismus
Colpospasm
Vulvismus
> *Excludes:* psychogenic vaginismus (306.51)

625.2 Mittelschmerz
Intermenstrual pain
Ovulation pain

625.3 Dysmenorrhea
Painful menstruation
> *Excludes:* psychogenic dysmenorrhea (306.52)

625.4 Premenstrual tension syndromes
Menstrual molimen
Premenstrual dysphoric disorder
Premenstrual syndrome
Premenstrual tension NOS
> *Excludes:* menstrual migraine (346.4)

625.5 Pelvic congestion syndrome
Congestion-fibrosis syndrome
Taylor's syndrome

625.6 Stress incontinence, female
> *Excludes:* mixed incontinence (788.33)
> stress incontinence, male (788.32)

⑤ **625.7 Vulvodynia**

625.70 Vulvodynia, unspecified
Vulvodynia NOS

625.71 Vulvar vestibulitis

625.79 Other vulvodynia

625.8 Other specified symptoms associated with female genital organs

625.9 Unspecified symptom associated with female genital organs

626 **Disorders of menstruation and other abnormal bleeding from female genital tract**
> *Excludes:* menopausal and premenopausal bleeding (627.0)
> pain and other symptoms associated with menstrual cycle (625.2-625.4)
> postmenopausal bleeding (627.1)

626.0 Absence of menstruation
Amenorrhea (primary) (secondary)

626.1 Scanty or infrequent menstruation
Hypomenorrhea
Oligomenorrhea

626.2 Excessive or frequent menstruation
Heavy periods   Menorrhagia
Menometrorrhagia   Polymenorrhea
> *Excludes:* premenopausal (627.0)
> that in puberty (626.3)

626.3 Puberty bleeding
Excessive bleeding associated with onset of menstrual periods
Pubertal menorrhagia

626.4 Irregular menstrual cycle
Irregular:
   bleeding NOS
   menstruation
   periods

626.5 Ovulation bleeding
Regular intermenstrual bleeding

626.6 Metrorrhagia
Bleeding unrelated to menstrual cycle
Irregular intermenstrual bleeding

| | Add 4th or 5th digit | | Nonspecific code | | Unspecified code | | Manifestation code |

626.7 Postcoital bleeding

626.8 Other
Dysfunctional or functional uterine hemorrhage NOS
Menstruation:
retained
suppression of

626.9 Unspecified

627 Menopausal and postmenopausal disorders
Excludes: *asymptomatic age-related (natural) postmenopausal status (V49.81)*

627.0 Premenopausal menorrhagia
Excessive bleeding associated with onset of menopause
Menorrhagia:
climacteric
menopausal
preclimacteric

627.1 Postmenopausal bleeding

627.2 Symptomatic menopausal or female climacteric states
Symptoms, such as flushing, sleeplessness, headache, lack of concentration, associated
with the menopause

627.3 Postmenopausal atrophic vaginitis
Senile (atrophic) vaginitis

627.4 Symptomatic states associated with artificial menopause
Postartificial menopause syndromes
Any condition classifiable to 627.1, 627.2, or 627.3 which follows induced menopause

627.8 Other specified menopausal and postmenopausal disorders
Excludes: *premature menopause NOS (256.31)*

627.9 Unspecified menopausal and postmenopausal disorder

628 Infertility, female
Includes: primary and secondary sterility

628.0 Associated with anovulation
Anovulatory cycle
Use additional code for any associated Stein-Leventhal syndrome (256.4)

628.1 *Of pituitary-hypothalamic origin*
Code first underlying cause, as:
adiposogenital dystrophy (253.8)
anterior pituitary disorder (253.0-253.4)

628.2 Of tubal origin
Infertility associated with congenital anomaly of tube
Tubal:
block
occlusion
stenosis
Use additional code for any associated peritubal adhesions (614.6)

628.3 Of uterine origin
Infertility associated with congenital anomaly of uterus
Nonimplantation
Use additional code for any associated tuberculous endometritis (016.7)

628.4 Of cervical or vaginal origin
Infertility associated with:
anomaly of cervical mucus
congenital structural anomaly
dysmucorrhea

628.8 Of other specified origin

628.9 Of unspecified origin

629 Other disorders of female genital organs

● Code new
to this edition
▲ Revision of
existing code
④ ⑤ Fourth or fifth
digit required

629.0 Hematocele, female, not elsewhere classified

Excludes: hematocele or hematoma:
>   broad ligament (620.7)
>   fallopian tube (620.8)
>   that associated with ectopic pregnancy (633.00-633.91)
>   uterus (621.4)
>   vagina (623.6)
>   vulva (624.5)

629.1 Hydrocele, canal of Nuck
Cyst of canal of Nuck (acquired)

Excludes: congenital (752.41)

⑤ **629.2 Female genital mutilation status**
Female circumcision status
Female genital cutting

> **629.20 Female genital mutilation status, unspecified**
> Female genital cutting status, unspecified
> Female genital mutilation status NOS
> Female genital mutilation status, type 4

> **629.21 Female genital mutilation Type I status**
> Clitorectomy status
> Female genital cutting Type I status

> **629.22 Female genital mutilation Type II status**
> Clitorectomy with excision of labia minor status
> Female genital cutting Type II status

> **629.23 Female genital mutilation Type III status**
> Female genital cutting Type III status
> Infibulation status

> **629.29 Other female genital mutilation status**
> Female genital cutting Type IV status
> Female genital mutilation Type IV status
> Other female genital cutting status

⑤ **629.8 Other specified disorders of female genital organs**

> **629.81 Habitual aborter without current pregnancy**

Excludes: habitual aborter with current pregnancy (646.3)

> **629.89 Other specified disorders of female genital organs**

629.9 Unspecified disorder of female genital organs

Add 4th or
5th digit

Nonspecific
code

Unspecified
code

Manifestation
code

11. COMPLICATIONS OF PREGNANCY, CHILDBIRTH, AND THE PUERPERIUM (630-679)

ECTOPIC AND MOLAR PREGNANCY (630-633)

Use additional code from category 639 to identify any complications

630 Hydatidiform mole
Trophoblastic disease NOS
Vesicular mole

> Excludes: *chorioadenoma (destruens) (236.1)*
> *chorionepithelioma (181)*
> *malignant hydatidiform mole (236.1)*

631 Other abnormal product of conception

Blighted ovum
Mole:
  NOS
  carneous

Mole:
  fleshy
  stone

632 Missed abortion
Early fetal death before completion of 22 weeks' gestation with retention of dead fetus
Retained products of conception, not following spontaneous or induced abortion or delivery

> Excludes: *failed induced abortion (638.0-638.9)*
> *fetal death (intrauterine) (late) (656.4)*
> *missed delivery (656.4)*
> *that with abnormal product of conception (630, 631)*

633 Ectopic pregnancy
Includes: ruptured ectopic pregnancy

⑤ **633.0 Abdominal pregnancy**
Intraperitoneal pregnancy

    633.00 Abdominal pregnancy without intrauterine pregnancy

    633.01 Abdominal pregnancy with intrauterine pregnancy

⑤ **633.1 Tubal pregnancy**
Fallopian pregnancy
Rupture of (fallopian) tube due to pregnancy
Tubal abortion

    633.10 Tubal pregnancy without intrauterine pregnancy

    633.11 Tubal pregnancy with intrauterine pregnancy

⑤ **633.2 Ovarian pregnancy**

    633.20 Ovarian pregnancy without intrauterine pregnancy

    633.21 Ovarian pregnancy with intrauterine pregnancy

⑤ **633.8 Other ectopic pregnancy**

Pregnancy:
  cervical
  combined
  cornual

Pregnancy:
  intraligamentous
  mesometric
  mural

    633.80 Other ectopic pregnancy without intrauterine pregnancy

    633.81 Other ectopic pregnancy with intrauterine pregnancy

⑤ **633.9 Unspecified ectopic pregnancy**

    633.90 Unspecified ectopic pregnancy without intrauterine pregnancy

    633.91 Unspecified ectopic pregnancy with intrauterine pregnancy

| | Add 4th or 5th digit | | Nonspecific code | | Unspecified code | | Manifestation code |

OTHER PREGNANCY WITH ABORTIVE OUTCOME (634-639)

Note: Use the following fifth-digit subclassification with categories 634-637:

0 Unspecified

1 Incomplete

2 Complete

The following fourth-digit subdivisions are for use with categories 634-638:

.0 Complicated by genital tract and pelvic infection
  Endometritis
  Salpingo-oophoritis
  Sepsis NOS
  Septicemia NOS
  Any condition classifiable to 639.0, with condition classifiable to 634-638

Excludes: urinary tract infection (634-638 with .7)

.1 Complicated by delayed or excessive hemorrhage
  Afibrinogenemia
  Defibrination syndrome
  Intravascular hemolysis
  Any condition classifiable to 639.1, with condition classifiable to 634-638

.2 Complicated by damage to pelvic organs and tissues
  Laceration, perforation, or tear of:
    bladder
    uterus
  Any condition classifiable to 639.2, with condition classifiable to 634-638

.3 Complicated by renal failure
  Oliguria
  Uremia
  Any condition classifiable to 639.3, with condition classifiable to 634-638

.4 Complicated by metabolic disorder
  Electrolyte imbalance with conditions classifiable to 634-638

.5 Complicated by shock
  Circulatory collapse
  Shock (postoperative) (septic)
  Any condition classifiable to 639.5, with condition classifiable to 634-638

.6 Complicated by embolism
  Embolism:
    NOS
    amniotic fluid
    pulmonary
  Any condition classifiable to 639.6, with condition classifiable to 634-638

.7 With other specified complications
  Cardiac arrest or failure
  Urinary tract infection
  Any condition classifiable to 639.8, with condition classifiable to 634-638

.8 With unspecified complication

.9 Without mention of complication

⑤ **634 Spontaneous abortion**
  Includes: miscarriage
      spontaneous abortion

⑤ **634.0 Complicated by genital tract and pelvic infection**
  [0-2]

⑤ **634.1 Complicated by delayed or excessive hemorrhage**
  [0-2]

⑤ **634.2 Complicated by damage to pelvic organs or tissues**
  [0-2]

⑤ **634.3 Complicated by renal failure**
  [0-2]

⑤ **634.4 Complicated by metabolic disorder**
  [0-2]

⑤ **634.5 Complicated by shock**
  [0-2]

⑤ **634.6 Complicated by embolism**
  [0-2]

● Code new
  to this edition

▲ Revision of
  existing code

④ ⑤ Fourth or fifth
  digit required

⑤ **634.7** With other specified complications
[0-2]

⑤ **634.8** With unspecified complication
[0-2]

⑤ 634.9 Without mention of complication
[0-2]

⑤ **635** Legally induced abortion
Includes: abortion or termination of pregnancy:
elective
legal
therapeutic

Excludes: *menstrual extraction or regulation (V25.3)*

⑤ 635.0 Complicated by genital tract and pelvic infection
[0-2]

⑤ 635.1 Complicated by delayed or excessive hemorrhage
[0-2]

⑤ 635.2 Complicated by damage to pelvic organs or tissues
[0-2]

⑤ 635.3 Complicated by renal failure
[0-2]

⑤ 635.4 Complicated by metabolic disorder
[0-2]

⑤ 635.5 Complicated by shock
[0-2]

⑤ 635.6 Complicated by embolism
[0-2]

⑤ **635.7** With other specified complications
[0-2]

⑤ **635.8** With unspecified complication
[0-2]

⑤ 635.9 Without mention of complication
[0-2]

⑤ **636** Illegally induced abortion
Includes: abortion:
criminal
illegal
self-induced

⑤ 636.0 Complicated by genital tract and pelvic infection
[0-2]

⑤ 636.1 Complicated by delayed or excessive hemorrhage
[0-2]

⑤ 636.2 Complicated by damage to pelvic organs or tissues
[0-2]

⑤ 636.3 Complicated by renal failure
[0-2]

⑤ 636.4 Complicated by metabolic disorder
[0-2]

⑤ 636.5 Complicated by shock
[0-2]

⑤ 636.6 Complicated by embolism
[0-2]

⑤ **636.7** With other specified complications
[0-2]

⑤ **636.8** With unspecified complication
[0-2]

⑤ 636.9 Without mention of complication
[0-2]

⑤ **637** Unspecified abortion
Includes: abortion NOS
retained products of conception following abortion, not classifiable elsewhere

⑤ 637.0 Complicated by genital tract and pelvic infection
[0-2]

	Add 4th or 5th digit		Nonspecific code		Unspecified code		Manifestation code

⑤ **637.1 Complicated by delayed or excessive hemorrhage**
[0-2]

⑤ **637.2 Complicated by damage to pelvic organs or tissues**
[0-2]

⑤ **637.3 Complicated by renal failure**
[0-2]

⑤ **637.4 Complicated by metabolic disorder**
[0-2]

⑤ **637.5 Complicated by shock**
[0-2]

⑤ **637.6 Complicated by embolism**
[0-2]

⑤ **637.7 With other specified complications**
[0-2]

⑤ **637.8 With unspecified complication**
[0-2]

⑤ **637.9 Without mention of complication**
[0-2]

638 Failed attempted abortion
    Includes: failure of attempted induction of (legal) abortion

    Excludes: incomplete abortion (634.0-637.9)

638.0 Complicated by genital tract and pelvic infection

638.1 Complicated by delayed or excessive hemorrhage

638.2 Complicated by damage to pelvic organs or tissues

638.3 Complicated by renal failure

638.4 Complicated by metabolic disorder

638.5 Complicated by shock

638.6 Complicated by embolism

638.7 With other specified complications

638.8 With unspecified complication

638.9 Without mention of complication

639 Complications following abortion and ectopic and molar pregnancies
    Note: This category is provided for use when it is required to classify separately the
        complications classifiable to the fourth-digit level in categories 634-638; for example:
        a) when the complication itself was responsible for an episode of medical care, the
            abortion, ectopic or molar pregnancy itself having been dealt with at a previous
            episode
        b) when these conditions are immediate complications of ectopic or molar pregnancies
            classifiable to 630-633 where they cannot be identified at fourth-digit level.

639.0 Genital tract and pelvic infection
    Endometritis following conditions classifiable to 630-638
    Parametritis following conditions classifiable to 630-638
    Pelvic peritonitis following conditions classifiable to 630-638
    Salpingitis following conditions classifiable to 630-638
    Salpingo-oophoritis following conditions classifiable to 630-638
    Sepsis NOS following conditions classifiable to 630-638
    Septicemia NOS following conditions classifiable to 630-638

    Excludes: urinary tract infection (639.8)

639.1 Delayed or excessive hemorrhage
    Afibrinogenemia following conditions classifiable to 630-638
    Defibrination syndrome following conditions classifiable to 630-638
    Intravascular hemolysis following conditions classifiable to 630-638

639.2 Damage to pelvic organs and tissues
    Laceration, perforation, or tear of:
        bladder following conditions classifiable to 630-638
        bowel following conditions classifiable to 630-638
        broad ligament following conditions classifiable to 630-638
        cervix following conditions classifiable to 630-638
        periurethral tissue following conditions classifiable to 630-638
        uterus following conditions classifiable to 630-638
        vagina following conditions classifiable to 630-638

● Code new   ▲ Revision of   ④ ⑤ Fourth or fifth
          to this edition   existing code   digit required

▲ 639.3 Kidney failure
Oliguria following conditions classifiable to 630-638
Renal (kidney):
    failure (acute) following conditions classifiable to 630-638
    shutdown following conditions classifiable to 630-638
    tubular necrosis following conditions classifiable to 630-638
Uremia following conditions classifiable to 630-638

639.4 Metabolic disorders
Electrolyte imbalance following conditions classifiable to 630-638

639.5 Shock
Circulatory collapse following conditions classifiable to 630-638
Shock (postoperative) (septic) following conditions classifiable to 630-638

639.6 Embolism
Embolism:
    NOS following conditions classifiable to 630-638
    air following conditions classifiable to 630-638
    amniotic fluid following conditions classifiable to 630-638
    blood-clot following conditions classifiable to 630-638
    fat following conditions classifiable to 630-638
    pulmonary following conditions classifiable to 630-638
    pyemic following conditions classifiable to 630-638
    septic following conditions classifiable to 630-638
    soap following conditions classifiable to 630-638

639.8 Other specified complications following abortion or ectopic and molar pregnancy
Acute yellow atrophy or necrosis of liver following conditions classifiable to 630-638
Cardiac arrest or failure following conditions classifiable to 630-638
Cerebral anoxia following conditions classifiable to 630-638
Urinary tract infection following conditions classifiable to 630-638

639.9 Unspecified complication following abortion or ectopic and molar pregnancy
Complication(s) not further specified following conditions classifiable to 630-638

COMPLICATIONS MAINLY RELATED TO PREGNANCY (640-649)

Includes: the listed conditions even if they arose or were present during labor, delivery, or the puerperium

The following fifth-digit subclassification is for use with categories 640-649 to denote the current episode of care:

0   **unspecified as to episode of care or not applicable**

1   **delivered, with or without mention of antepartum condition**
Antepartum condition with delivery
Delivery NOS (with mention of antepartum complication during current episode of care)
Intrapartum obstetric condition (with mention of antepartum complication during current episode of care)
Pregnancy, delivered (with mention of antepartum complication during current episode of care)

2   **delivered, with mention of postpartum complication**
Delivery with mention of puerperal complication during current episode of care

3   **antepartum condition or complication**
Antepartum obstetric condition, not delivered during the current episode of care

4   **postpartum condition or complication**
Postpartum or puerperal obstetric condition or complication following delivery that occurred:
    during previous episode of care
    outside hospital, with subsequent admission for observation or care

⑤ **640 Hemorrhage in early pregnancy**
Includes: hemorrhage before completion of 22 weeks' gestation

Requires fifth digit; valid digits are in [brackets] under each code. See beginning of section 640-649 for definitions.

⑤ **640.0 Threatened abortion**
[0,1,3]

⑤ **640.8 Other specified hemorrhage in early pregnancy**
[0,1,3]

⑤ **640.9 Unspecified hemorrhage in early pregnancy**
[0,1,3]

	Add 4th or 5th digit		Nonspecific code		Unspecified code		Manifestation code

⑤ **641** **Antepartum hemorrhage, abruptio placentae, and placenta previa**
Requires fifth digit; valid digits are in [brackets] under each code. See beginning of section 640-649 for definitions.

⑤ **641.0** **Placenta previa without hemorrhage**
[0,1,3] Low implantation of placenta without hemorrhage
Placenta previa noted:
during pregnancy without hemorrhage
before labor (and delivered by cesarean delivery) without hemorrhage

⑤ **641.1** **Hemorrhage from placenta previa**
[0,1,3] Low-lying placenta NOS or with hemorrhage (intrapartum)
Placenta previa:
incomplete NOS or with hemorrhage (intrapartum)
marginal NOS or with hemorrhage (intrapartum)
partial NOS or with hemorrhage (intrapartum)
total NOS or with hemorrhage (intrapartum)

Excludes: hemorrhage from vasa previa (663.5)

⑤ **641.2** **Premature separation of placenta**
[0,1,3] Ablatio placentae
Abruptio placentae
Accidental antepartum hemorrhage
Couvelaire uterus
Detachment of placenta (premature)
Premature separation of normally implanted placenta

⑤ **641.3** **Antepartum hemorrhage associated with coagulation defects**
[0,1,3] Antepartum or intrapartum hemorrhage associated with:
afibrinogenemia
hyperfibrinolysis
hypofibrinogenemia

Excludes: coagulation defects not associated with antepartum hemorrhage (649.3)

⑤ **641.8** **Other antepartum hemorrhage**
[0,1,3] Antepartum or intrapartum hemorrhage associated with:
trauma
uterine leiomyoma

⑤ **641.9** **Unspecified antepartum hemorrhage**
[0,1,3] Hemorrhage:
antepartum NOS
intrapartum NOS
of pregnancy NOS

⑤ **642** **Hypertension complicating pregnancy, childbirth, and the puerperium**
Requires fifth digit; valid digits are in [brackets] under each code. See beginning of section 640-649 for definitions.

⑤ **642.0** **Benign essential hypertension complicating pregnancy, childbirth, and the puerperium**
[0-4] Hypertension:
benign essential specified as complicating, or as a reason for obstetric care during pregnancy, childbirth, or the puerperium
chronic NOS specified as complicating, or as a reason for obstetric care during pregnancy, childbirth, or the puerperium
essential specified as complicating, or as a reason for obstetric care during pregnancy, childbirth, or the puerperium
pre-existing NOS specified as complicating, or as a reason for obstetric care during pregnancy, childbirth, or the puerperium

⑤ **642.1** **Hypertension secondary to renal disease, complicating pregnancy, childbirth, and the puerperium**
[0-4] Hypertension secondary to renal disease, specified as complicating, or as a reason for obstetric care during pregnancy, childbirth, or the puerperium

⑤ **642.2** **Other pre-existing hypertension complicating pregnancy, childbirth, and the puerperium**
[0-4] Hypertensive:
chronic kidney disease specified as complicating, or as a reason for obstetric care during pregnancy, childbirth, or the puerperium
heart and chronic kidney disease specified as complicating, or as a reason for obstetric care during pregnancy, childbirth, or the puerperium
heart disease specified as complicating, or as a reason for obstetric care during pregnancy, childbirth, or the puerperium
Malignant hypertension specified as complicating, or as a reason for obstetric care during pregnancy, childbirth, or the puerperium

● Code new
to this edition
▲ Revision of
existing code
④ ⑤ Fourth or fifth
digit required

⑤ **642.3　Transient hypertension of pregnancy**
[0-4]　　Gestational hypertension
　　　　Transient hypertension, so described, in pregnancy, childbirth, or the puerperium

⑤ **642.4　Mild or unspecified pre-eclampsia**
[0-4]　　Hypertension in pregnancy, childbirth, or the puerperium, not specified as pre-existing,
　　　　　with either albuminuria or edema, or both; mild or unspecified
　　　　Pre-eclampsia:　　　　　　　　Toxemia (pre-eclamptic):
　　　　　NOS　　　　　　　　　　　　NOS
　　　　　mild　　　　　　　　　　　　mild

　　　　Excludes: albuminuria in pregnancy, without mention of hypertension (646.2)
　　　　　　　　　　edema in pregnancy, without mention of hypertension (646.1)

⑤ **642.5　Severe pre-eclampsia**
[0-4]　　Hypertension in pregnancy, childbirth, or the puerperium, not specified as pre-existing,
　　　　　with either albuminuria or edema, or both; specified as severe
　　　　Pre-eclampsia, severe
　　　　Toxemia (pre-eclamptic), severe

⑤ **642.6　Eclampsia**
[0-4]　　Toxemia:
　　　　　eclamptic
　　　　　with convulsions

⑤ **642.7　Pre-eclampsia or eclampsia superimposed on pre-existing hypertension**
[0-4]　　Conditions classifiable to 642.4-642.6, with conditions classifiable to 642.0-642.2

⑤ **642.9　Unspecified hypertension complicating pregnancy, childbirth, or the puerperium**
[0-4]　　Hypertension NOS, without mention of albuminuria or edema, complicating pregnancy,
　　　　　childbirth, or the puerperium

⑤ **643　Excessive vomiting in pregnancy**
　　　　Includes:　hyperemesis arising during pregnancy
　　　　　　　　　vomiting:
　　　　　　　　　　persistent arising during pregnancy
　　　　　　　　　　vicious arising during pregnancy
　　　　　　　　　hyperemesis gravidarum

　　　　Requires fifth digit; valid digits are in [brackets] under each code. See beginning of section
　　　　　640-649 for definitions.

⑤ **643.0　Mild hyperemesis gravidarum**
[0,1,3]　　Hyperemesis gravidarum, mild or unspecified, starting before the end of the 22nd week
　　　　　of gestation

⑤ **643.1　Hyperemesis gravidarum with metabolic disturbance**
[0,1,3]　　Hyperemesis gravidarum, starting before the end of the 22nd week of gestation, with
　　　　　metabolic disturbance, such as:
　　　　　carbohydrate depletion
　　　　　dehydration
　　　　　electrolyte imbalance

⑤ **643.2　Late vomiting of pregnancy**
[0,1,3]　　Excessive vomiting starting after 22 completed weeks of gestation

⑤ **643.8　Other vomiting complicating pregnancy**
[0,1,3]　　Vomiting due to organic disease or other cause, specified as complicating pregnancy, or
　　　　　as a reason for obstetric care during pregnancy
　　　　Use additional code, if desired, to specify cause

⑤ **643.9　Unspecified vomiting of pregnancy**
[0,1,3]　　Vomiting as a reason for care during pregnancy, length of gestation unspecified

⑤ **644　Early or threatened labor**
　　　　Requires fifth digit; valid digits are in [brackets] under each code. See beginning of section
　　　　　640-649 for definitions.

⑤ **644.0　Threatened premature labor**
[0,3]　　Premature labor after 22 weeks, but before 37 completed weeks of gestation without
　　　　　delivery

　　　　Excludes: that occurring before 22 completed weeks of gestation (640.0)

⑤ **644.1　Other threatened labor**
[0,3]　　False labor:
　　　　　NOS without delivery
　　　　　after 37 completed weeks of gestation without delivery
　　　　Threatened labor NOS without delivery

| ▮ Add 4th or 5th digit | ▮ Nonspecific code | ▮ Unspecified code | ▮ Manifestation code |

⑤ **644.2 Early onset of delivery**
[0,1]   Onset (spontaneous) of delivery before 37 completed weeks of gestation
          Premature labor with onset of delivery before 37 completed weeks of gestation

⑤ **645 Late pregnancy**
          Requires fifth digit; valid digits are in [brackets] under each code. See beginning of section
          640-649 for definitions.

⑤ **645.1 Post term pregnancy**
[0,1,3]   Pregnancy over 40 completed weeks to 42 completed weeks gestation

⑤ **645.2 Prolonged pregnancy**
[0,1,3]   Pregnancy which has advanced beyond 42 completed weeks gestation

⑤ **646 Other complications of pregnancy, not elsewhere classified**
          Requires fifth digit; valid digits are in [brackets] under each code. See beginning of section
          640-649 for definitions.

          Use additional code(s) to further specify complication

⑤ **646.0 Papyraceous fetus**
[0,1,3]

⑤ **646.1 Edema or excessive weight gain in pregnancy, without mention of hypertension**
[0-4]   Gestational edema
          Maternal obesity syndrome

          | Excludes: | that with mention of hypertension (642.0-642.9) |

⑤ **646.2 Unspecified renal disease in pregnancy, without mention of hypertension**
[0-4]   Albuminuria in pregnancy or the puerperium, without mention of hypertension
          Nephropathy NOS in pregnancy or the puerperium, without mention of hypertension
          Renal disease NOS in pregnancy or the puerperium, without mention of hypertension
          Uremia in pregnancy or the puerperium, without mention of hypertension
          Gestational proteinuria in pregnancy or the puerperium, without mention of hypertension

          | Excludes: | that with mention of hypertension (642.0-642.9) |

⑤ **646.3 Habitual aborter**
[0,1,3]

          | Excludes: | with current abortion (634.0-634.9) |
          | | without current pregnancy (629.81) |

⑤ **646.4 Peripheral neuritis in pregnancy**
[0-4]

⑤ **646.5 Asymptomatic bacteriuria in pregnancy**
[0-4]

⑤ **646.6 Infections of genitourinary tract in pregnancy**
[0-4]   Conditions classifiable to 590, 595, 597, 599.0, 616 complicating pregnancy, childbirth,
          or the puerperium
          Conditions classifiable to (614.0-614.5, 617.7-614.9, 615) complicating pregnancy or
          labor

          | Excludes: | major puerperal infection (670.0-670.8) |

⑤ **646.7 Liver disorders in pregnancy**
[0,1,3]   Acute yellow atrophy of liver (obstetric) (true) of pregnancy
          Icterus gravis of pregnancy
          Necrosis of liver of pregnancy

          | Excludes: | hepatorenal syndrome following delivery (674.8) |
          | | viral hepatitis (647.6) |

⑤ **646.8 Other specified complications of pregnancy**
[0-4]   Fatigue during pregnancy
          Herpes gestationis
          Insufficient weight gain of pregnancy

⑤ **646.9 Unspecified complication of pregnancy**
[0,1,3]

⑤ **647 Infectious and parasitic conditions in the mother classifiable elsewhere, but complicating
          pregnancy, childbirth, or the puerperium**
          Includes: the listed conditions when complicating the pregnant state, aggravated by the
          pregnancy, or when a main reason for obstetric care

          | Excludes: | those conditions in the mother known or suspected to have affected the fetus |
          | | (655.0-655.9) |

          Requires fifth digit; valid digits are in [brackets] under each code. See beginning of section
          640-649 for definitions.

          Use additional code(s) to further specify complication

● Code new   ▲ Revision of   ④ ⑤ Fourth or fifth
       to this edition   existing code   digit required

⑤ **647.0 Syphilis**
[0-4]   Conditions classifiable to 090-097

⑤ **647.1 Gonorrhea**
[0-4]   Conditions classifiable to 098

⑤ **647.2 Other venereal diseases**
[0-4]   Conditions classifiable to 099

⑤ **647.3 Tuberculosis**
[0-4]   Conditions classifiable to 010-018

⑤ **647.4 Malaria**
[0-4]   Conditions classifiable to 084

⑤ **647.5 Rubella**
[0-4]   Conditions classifiable to 056

⑤ **647.6 Other viral diseases**
[0-4]   Conditions classifiable to 042, 050-055, 057-079, 795.05, 795.15, 795.75

⑤ **647.8 Other specified infectious and parasitic diseases**
[0-4]

⑤ **647.9 Unspecified infection or infestation**
[0-4]

⑤ **648 Other current conditions in the mother classifiable elsewhere, but complicating pregnancy, childbirth, or the puerperium**
Includes: the listed conditions when complicating the pregnant state, aggravated by the pregnancy, or when a main reason for obstetric care

Excludes: *those conditions in the mother known or suspected to have affected the fetus (655.0-655.9)*

Requires fifth digit; valid digits are in [brackets] under each code. See beginning of section 640-649 for definitions.

Use additional code(s) to identify the condition

⑤ **648.0 Diabetes mellitus**
[0-4]   Conditions classifiable to 249, 250

Excludes: *gestational diabetes (648.8)*

⑤ **648.1 Thyroid dysfunction**
[0-4]   Conditions classifiable to 240-246

⑤ **648.2 Anemia**
[0-4]   Conditions classifiable to 280-285

⑤ **648.3 Drug dependence**
[0-4]   Conditions classifiable to 304

⑤ **648.4 Mental disorders**
[0-4]   Conditions classifiable to 290-303, 305.0, 305.2-305.9, 306-316, 317-319

⑤ **648.5 Congenital cardiovascular disorders**
[0-4]   Conditions classifiable to 745-747

⑤ **648.6 Other cardiovascular diseases**
[0-4]   Conditions classifiable to 390-398, 410-429

Excludes: *cerebrovascular disorders in the puerperium (674.0)*
peripartum cardiomyopathy (674.5)
venous complications (671.0-671.9)

⑤ **648.7 Bone and joint disorders of back, pelvis, and lower limbs**
[0-4]   Conditions classifiable to 720-724, and those classifiable to 711-719 or 725-738, specified as affecting the lower limbs

⑤ **648.8 Abnormal glucose tolerance**
[0-4]   Conditions classifiable to 790.21-790.29
Gestational diabetes
Use additional code, if applicable, for associated long-term (current) insulin use (V58.67)

⑤ **648.9 Other current conditions classifiable elsewhere**
[0-4]   Conditions classifiable to 440-459, 795.01-795.04, 795.06, 795.10-795.14, 795.16, 796.70-796.74, 796.76
Nutritional deficiencies [conditions classifiable to 260-269]

	Add 4th or 5th digit		Nonspecific code		Unspecified code		Manifestation code

649 Other conditions or status of the mother complicating pregnancy, childbirth, or the puerperium

The following fifth-digit subclassification is for use with categories 640-649 to denote the current episode of care:

0 unspecified as to episode of care or not applicable

1 delivered, with or without mention of antepartum condition
Antepartum condition with delivery
Delivery NOS (with mention of antepartum complication during current episode of care)
Intrapartum obstetric condition (with mention of antepartum complication during current episode of care)
Pregnancy, delivered (with mention of antepartum complication during current episode of care)

2 delivered, with mention of postpartum complication
Delivery with mention of puerperal complication during current episode of care

3 antepartum condition or complication
Antepartum obstetric condition, not delivered during the current episode of care

4 postpartum condition or complication
Postpartum or puerperal obstetric condition or complication following delivery that occurred:
during previous episode of care
outside hospital, with subsequent admission for observation or care

⑤ **649.0** Tobacco use disorder complicating pregnancy, childbirth, or the puerperium
[0-4] Smoking complicating pregnancy, childbirth, or the puerperium

⑤ **649.1** Obesity complicating pregnancy, childbirth, or the puerperium
[0-4]
Use additional code to identify the obesity (278.00, 278.01)

⑤ **649.2** Bariatric surgery status complicating pregnancy, childbirth, or the puerperium
[0-4] Gastric banding status complicating pregnancy, childbirth, or the puerperium
Gastric bypass status for obesity complicating pregnancy, childbirth, or the puerperium
Obesity surgery status complicating pregnancy, childbirth, or the puerperium

⑤ **649.3** Coagulation defects complicating pregnancy, childbirth, or the puerperium
[0-4] Conditions classifiable to 286, 287, 289
Use additional code to identify the specific coagulation defect (286.0-286.9, 287.0-287.9, 289.0-289.9)
Excludes: coagulation defects causing antepartum hemorrhage (641.3)
postpartum coagulation defects (666.3)

⑤ **649.4** Epilepsy complicating pregnancy, childbirth, or the puerperium
[0-4] Conditions classifiable to 345
Use additional code to identify the specific type of epilepsy (345.00-345.91)
Excludes: eclampsia (642.6)

⑤ **649.5** Spotting complicating pregnancy
[0,1,3]
Excludes: antepartum hemorrhage (641.0-641.9)
hemorrhage in early pregnancy (640.0-640.9)

⑤ **649.6** Uterine size date discrepancy
[0-4]
Excludes: suspected problem with fetal growth not found (V89.04)

⑤ **649.7** Cervical shortening
[0,1,3]
Excludes: suspected cervical shortening not found (V89.05)

● Code new to this edition ▲ Revision of existing code ④ ⑤ Fourth or fifth digit required

NORMAL DELIVERY, AND OTHER INDICATIONS FOR CARE IN PREGNANCY, LABOR, AND DELIVERY (650-659)

650 Normal delivery

Delivery requiring minimal or no assistance, with or without episiotomy, without fetal manipulation [e.g., rotation version] or instrumentation [forceps] of spontaneous, cephalic, vaginal, full-term, single, live born infant. This code is for use as a single diagnosis code and is not to be used with any other code in the range 630-676.

> Excludes: *breech delivery (assisted) (spontaneous) NOS (652.2)*
>
> *delivery by vacuum extractor, forceps, cesarean section, or breech extraction, without specified complication (669.5-669.7)*

Use additional code to indicate outcome of delivery (V27.0)

The following fifth-digit subclassification is for use with categories 651-659 to denote the current episode of care:

0 unspecified as to episode of care or not applicable

1 delivered, with or without mention of antepartum condition

2 delivered, with mention of postpartum complication

3 antepartum condition or complication

4 postpartum condition or complication

⑤ **651 Multiple gestation**

  ⑤ **651.0 Twin pregnancy**
[0,1,3]
> Excludes: *fetal conjoined twins (678.1)*

  ⑤ **651.1 Triplet pregnancy**
[0,1,3]

  ⑤ **651.2 Quadruplet pregnancy**
[0,1,3]

  ⑤ **651.3 Twin pregnancy with fetal loss and retention of one fetus**
[0,1,3]

  ⑤ **651.4 Triplet pregnancy with fetal loss and retention of one or more fetus(es)**
[0,1,3]

  ⑤ **651.5 Quadruplet pregnancy with fetal loss and retention of one or more fetus(es)**
[0,1,3]

  ⑤ **651.6 Other multiple pregnancy with fetal loss and retention of one or more fetus(es)**
[0,1,3]

  ⑤ **651.7 Multiple gestation following (elective) fetal reduction**
Fetal reduction of multiple fetuses reduced to single fetus

    651.70 Multiple gestation following (elective) fetal reduction, unspecified as to episode of care or not applicable

    651.71 Multiple gestation following (elective) fetal reduction, delivered, with or without mention of antepartum condition

    651.73 Multiple gestation following (elective) fetal reduction, antepartum condition or complication

  ⑤ **651.8 Other specified multiple gestation**
[0,1,3]

  ⑤ **651.9 Unspecified multiple gestation**
[0,1,3]

⑤ **652 Malposition and malpresentation of fetus**
Code first any associated obstructed labor (660.0)

  ⑤ **652.0 Unstable lie**
[0,1,3]

  ⑤ **652.1 Breech or other malpresentation successfully converted to cephalic presentation**
[0,1,3] Cephalic version NOS

| ▬ Add 4th or 5th digit | ▬ Nonspecific code | ▬ Unspecified code | ▬ Manifestation code |

⑤ **652.2 Breech presentation without mention of version**
[0,1,3] Breech delivery (assisted) (spontaneous) NOS
Buttocks presentation
Complete breech
Frank breech

> Excludes: *footling presentation (652.8)*
> *incomplete breech (652.8)*

⑤ **652.3 Transverse or oblique presentation**
[0,1,3] Oblique lie   Transverse lie

> Excludes: *transverse arrest of fetal head (660.3)*

⑤ **652.4 Face or brow presentation**
[0,1,3] Mentum presentation

⑤ **652.5 High head at term**
[0,1,3] Failure of head to enter pelvic brim

⑤ **652.6 Multiple gestation with malpresentation of one fetus or more**
[0,1,3]

⑤ **652.7 Prolapsed arm**
[0,1,3]

⑤ **652.8 Other specified malposition or malpresentation**
[0,1,3] Compound presentation

⑤ **652.9 Unspecified malposition or malpresentation**
[0,1,3]

⑤ **653 Disproportion**
Code first any associated obstructed labor (660.1)

⑤ **653.0 Major abnormality of bony pelvis, not further specified**
[0,1,3] Pelvic deformity NOS

⑤ **653.1 Generally contracted pelvis**
[0,1,3] Contracted pelvis NOS

⑤ **653.2 Inlet contraction of pelvis**
[0,1,3] Inlet contraction (pelvis)

⑤ **653.3 Outlet contraction of pelvis**
[0,1,3] Outlet contraction (pelvis)

⑤ **653.4 Fetopelvic disproportion**
[0,1,3] Cephalopelvic disproportion NOS
Disproportion of mixed maternal and fetal origin, with normally formed fetus

⑤ **653.5 Unusually large fetus causing disproportion**
[0,1,3] Disproportion of fetal origin with normally formed fetus
Fetal disproportion NOS

> Excludes: *that when the reason for medical care was concern for the fetus (656.6)*

⑤ **653.6 Hydrocephalic fetus causing disproportion**
[0,1,3]

> Excludes: *that when the reason for medical care was concern for the fetus (655.0)*

⑤ **653.7 Other fetal abnormality causing disproportion**
[0,1,3]   Fetal:
ascites
hydrops
myelomeningocele
sacral teratoma
tumor

> Excludes: *conjoined twins causing disproportion (678.1)*

⑤ **653.8 Disproportion of other origin**
[0,1,3]

> Excludes: *shoulder (girdle) dystocia (660.4)*

⑤ **653.9 Unspecified disproportion**
[0,1,3]

● Code new
to this edition

▲ Revision of
existing code

④ ⑤ Fourth or fifth
digit required

⑤ **654** **Abnormality of organs and soft tissues of pelvis**
    Includes: the listed conditions during pregnancy, childbirth, or the puerperium
    Code first any associated obstructed labor (660.2)

    Excludes: trauma to perineum and vulva complicating current delivery (664.0-664.9)

⑤ **654.0** **Congenital abnormalities of uterus**
[0-4]   Double uterus   Uterus bicornis

⑤ **654.1** **Tumors of body of uterus**
[0-4]   Uterine fibroids

⑤ **654.2** **Previous cesarean delivery NOS**
[0,1,3]   Uterine scar from previous cesarean delivery

⑤ **654.3** **Retroverted and incarcerated gravid uterus**
[0-4]

⑤ **654.4** **Other abnormalities in shape or position of gravid uterus and of neighboring structures**
[0-4]   Cystocele
         Pelvic floor repair
         Pendulous abdomen
         Prolapse of gravid uterus
         Rectocele
         Rigid pelvic floor

⑤ **654.5** **Cervical incompetence**
[0-4]   Presence of Shirodkar suture with or without mention of cervical incompetence

⑤ **654.6** **Other congenital or acquired abnormality of cervix**
[0-4]   Cicatricial cervix
         Polyp of cervix
         Previous surgery to cervix
         Rigid cervix (uteri)
         Stenosis or stricture of cervix
         Tumor of cervix

⑤ **654.7** **Congenital or acquired abnormality of vagina**
[0-4]   Previous surgery to vagina
         Septate vagina
         Stenosis of vagina (acquired) (congenital)
         Stricture of vagina
         Tumor of vagina

⑤ **654.8** **Congenital or acquired abnormality of vulva**
[0-4]   Anal sphincter tear (healed) (old) complicating delivery
         Fibrosis of perineum
         Persistent hymen
         Previous surgery to perineum or vulva
         Rigid perineum
         Tumor of vulva

    Excludes: anal sphincter tear (healed) (old) not associated with delivery (569.43)
            varicose veins of vulva (671.1)

⑤ **654.9** **Other and unspecified**
[0-4]   Uterine scar NEC

⑤ **655** **Known or suspected fetal abnormality affecting management of mother**
    Includes: the listed conditions in the fetus as a reason for observation or obstetrical care of the mother, or for termination of pregnancy

⑤ **655.0** **Central nervous system malformation in fetus**
[0,1,3]   Fetal or suspected fetal:
         anencephaly
         hydrocephalus
         spina bifida (with myelomeningocele)

⑤ **655.1** **Chromosomal abnormality in fetus**
[0,1,3]

⑤ **655.2** **Hereditary disease in family possibly affecting fetus**
[0,1,3]

⑤ **655.3** **Suspected damage to fetus from viral disease in the mother**
[0,1,3]   Suspected damage to fetus from maternal rubella

⑤ **655.4** **Suspected damage to fetus from other disease in the mother**
[0,1,3]   Suspected damage to fetus from maternal:
         alcohol addiction
         listeriosis
         toxoplasmosis

	Add 4th or 5th digit		Nonspecific code		Unspecified code		Manifestation code

481

⑤ **655.5 Suspected damage to fetus from drugs**
[0,1,3]

⑤ **655.6 Suspected damage to fetus from radiation**
[0,1,3]

⑤ **655.7 Decreased fetal movements**
[0,1,3]

⑤ **655.8 Other known or suspected fetal abnormality, not elsewhere classified**
[0,1,3] Suspected damage to fetus from:
environmental toxins
intrauterine contraceptive device

⑤ **655.9 Unspecified**
[0,1,3]

⑤ **656 Other known or suspected fetal and placental problems affecting management of mother**
Excludes: *fetal hematologic conditions (678.0)*
suspected placental problems not found (V89.02)

⑤ **656.0 Fetal-maternal hemorrhage**
[0,1,3] Leakage (microscopic) of fetal blood into maternal circulation

⑤ **656.1 Rhesus isoimmunization**
[0,1,3] Anti-D [Rh] antibodies
Rh incompatibility

⑤ **656.2 Isoimmunization from other and unspecified blood-group incompatibility**
[0,1,3] ABO isoimmunization

⑤ **656.3 Fetal distress**
[0,1,3] Fetal metabolic acidemia

Excludes: *abnormal fetal acid-base balance (656.8)*
abnormality in fetal heart rate or rhythm (659.7)
fetal bradycardia (659.7)
fetal tachycardia (659.7)
meconium in liquor (656.8)

⑤ **656.4 Intrauterine death**
[0,1,3] Fetal death:
NOS
after completion of 22 weeks' gestation
late
Missed delivery
Excludes: *missed abortion (632)*

⑤ **656.5 Poor fetal growth**
[0,1,3] "Light-for-dates"   "Small-for-dates"
"Placental insufficiency"

⑤ **656.6 Excessive fetal growth**
[0,1,3] "Large-for-dates"

⑤ **656.7 Other placental conditions**
[0,1,3] Abnormal placenta   Placental infarct
Excludes: *placental polyp (674.4)*
placentitis (658.4)

⑤ **656.8 Other specified fetal and placental problems**
[0,1,3] Abnormal acid-base balance
Intrauterine acidosis
Lithopedian
Meconium in liquor
Subchorionic hematoma

⑤ **656.9 Unspecified fetal and placental problem**
[0,1,3]

⑤ **657 Polyhydramnios**
[0,1,3] Hydramnios
Excludes: *suspected polyhydramnios not found (V89.01)*

Use 0 as fourth-digit for this category

● Code new to this edition   ▲ Revision of existing code   ④ ⑤ Fourth or fifth digit required

⑤ **658** **Other problems associated with amniotic cavity and membranes**

> *Excludes:* amniotic fluid embolism (673.1)
>
> suspected problems with amniotic cavity and membranes not found (V89.01)

⑤ **658.0** **Oligohydramnios**
[0,1,3]   Oligohydramnios without mention of rupture of membranes

⑤ **658.1** **Premature rupture of membranes**
[0,1,3]   Rupture of amniotic sac less than 24 hours prior to the onset of labor

⑤ **658.2** **Delayed delivery after spontaneous or unspecified rupture of membranes**
[0,1,3]   Prolonged rupture of membranes NOS
        Rupture of amniotic sac 24 hours or more prior to the onset of labor

⑤ **658.3** **Delayed delivery after artificial rupture of membranes**
[0,1,3]

⑤ **658.4** **Infection of amniotic cavity**
[0,1,3]   Amnionitis
        Chorioamnionitis
        Membranitis
        Placentitis

⑤ **658.8** **Other**
[0,1,3]   Amnion nodosum
        Amniotic cyst

⑤ **658.9** **Unspecified**
[0,1,3]

⑤ **659** **Other indications for care or intervention related to labor and delivery, not elsewhere classified**

⑤ **659.0** **Failed mechanical induction**
[0,1,3]   Failure of induction of labor by surgical or other instrumental methods

⑤ **659.1** **Failed medical or unspecified induction**
[0,1,3]   Failed induction NOS
        Failure of induction of labor by medical methods, such as oxytocic drugs

⑤ **659.2** **Maternal pyrexia during labor, unspecified**
[0,1,3]

⑤ **659.3** **Generalized infection during labor**
[0,1,3]   Septicemia during labor

⑤ **659.4** **Grand multiparity**
[0,1,3]

> *Excludes:* supervision only, in pregnancy (V23.3)
>
> without current pregnancy (V61.5)

⑤ **659.5** **Elderly primigravida**
[0,1,3]   First pregnancy in a woman who will be 35 years of age or older at expected date of delivery

> *Excludes:* supervision only, in pregnancy (V23.81)

⑤ **659.6** **Elderly multigravida**
[0,1,3]   Second or more pregnancy in a woman who will be 35 years of age or older at expected date of delivery

> *Excludes:* elderly primigravida 659.5
>
> supervision only, in pregnancy (V23.82)

⑤ **659.7** **Abnormality in fetal heart rate or rhythm**
[0,1,3]   Depressed fetal heart tones
        Fetal:
          bradycardia
          tachycardia
        Fetal heart rate decelerations
        Non-reassuring fetal heart rate or rhythm

⑤ **659.8** **Other specified indications for care or intervention related to labor and delivery**
[0,1,3]   Pregnancy in female less than 16 years old at expected date of delivery
        Very young maternal age

⑤ **659.9** **Unspecified indication for care or intervention related to labor and delivery**
[0,1,3]

| | Add 4th or 5th digit | | Nonspecific code | | Unspecified code | | Manifestation code |

COMPLICATIONS OCCURRING MAINLY IN THE COURSE OF LABOR AND DELIVERY (660-669)

The following fifth-digit subclassification is for use with categories 660-669 to denote the current episode of care:

0 unspecified as to episode of care or not applicable

1 delivered, with or without mention of antepartum condition

2 delivered, with mention of postpartum complication

3 antepartum condition or complication

4 postpartum condition or complication

⑤ **660 Obstructed labor**

  ⑤ **660.0 Obstruction caused by malposition of fetus at onset of labor**
    [0,1,3]   Any condition classifiable to 652, causing obstruction during labor
    Use additional code from 652.0-652.9, if desired, to identify condition

  ⑤ **660.1 Obstruction by bony pelvis**
    [0,1,3]   Any condition classifiable to 653, causing obstruction during labor
    Use additional code from 653.0-653.9, if desired, to identify condition

  ⑤ **660.2 Obstruction by abnormal pelvic soft tissues**
    [0,1,3]   Prolapse of anterior lip of cervix
            Any condition classifiable to 654, causing obstruction during labor
    Use additional code from 654.0-654.9, if desired, to identify condition

  ⑤ **660.3 Deep transverse arrest and persistent occipitoposterior position**
    [0,1,3]

  ⑤ **660.4 Shoulder (girdle) dystocia**
    [0,1,3]   Impacted shoulders

  ⑤ **660.5 Locked twins**
    [0,1,3]

  ⑤ **660.6 Failed trial of labor, unspecified**
    [0,1,3]   Failed trial of labor, without mention of condition or suspected condition

  ⑤ **660.7 Failed forceps or vacuum extractor, unspecified**
    [0,1,3]   Application of ventouse or forceps, without mention of condition

  ⑤ **660.8 Other causes of obstructed labor**
    [0,1,3]   Use additional code to identify condition

  ⑤ **660.9 Unspecified obstructed labor**
    [0,1,3]   Dystocia:
            NOS
            fetal NOS
            maternal NOS

⑤ **661 Abnormality of forces of labor**

  ⑤ **661.0 Primary uterine inertia**
    [0,1,3]   Failure of cervical dilation
            Hypotonic uterine dysfunction, primary
            Prolonged latent phase of labor

  ⑤ **661.1 Secondary uterine inertia**
    [0,1,3]   Arrested active phase of labor
            Hypotonic uterine dysfunction, secondary

  ⑤ **661.2 Other and unspecified uterine inertia**
    [0,1,3]   Atony of uterus without hemorrhage
            Desultory labor   Poor contractions
            Irregular labor   Slow slope active phase of labor

    Excludes: *atony of uterus with hemorrhage (666.1)*
               postpartum atony of uterus without hemorrhage (669.8)

  ⑤ **661.3 Precipitate labor**
    [0,1,3]

● Code new
   to this edition

▲ Revision of
   existing code

④ ⑤ Fourth or fifth
   digit required

⑤ **661.4 Hypertonic, incoordinate, or prolonged uterine contractions**
[0,1,3] Cervical spasm
Contraction ring (dystocia)
Dyscoordinate labor
Hourglass contraction of uterus
Hypertonic uterine dysfunction
Incoordinate uterine action
Retraction ring (Bandl's) (pathological)
Tetanic contractions
Uterine dystocia NOS
Uterine spasm

⑤ **661.9 Unspecified abnormality of labor**
[0,1,3]

⑤ **662 Long labor**

⑤ **662.0 Prolonged first stage**
[0,1,3]

⑤ **662.1 Prolonged labor, unspecified**
[0,1,3]

⑤ **662.2 Prolonged second stage**
[0,1,3]

⑤ **662.3 Delayed delivery of second twin, triplet, etc.**
[0,1,3]

⑤ **663 Umbilical cord complications**

⑤ **663.0 Prolapse of cord**
[0,1,3] Presentation of cord

⑤ **663.1 Cord around neck, with compression**
[0,1,3] Cord tightly around neck

⑤ **663.2 Other and unspecified cord entanglement, with compression**
[0,1,3] Entanglement of cords of twins in mono-amniotic sac
Knot in cord (with compression)

⑤ **663.3 Other and unspecified cord entanglement, without mention of compression**
[0,1,3]

⑤ **663.4 Short cord**
[0,1,3]

⑤ **663.5 Vasa previa**
[0,1,3]

⑤ **663.6 Vascular lesions of cord**
[0,1,3] Bruising of cord
Hematoma of cord
Thrombosis of vessels of cord

⑤ **663.8 Other umbilical cord complications**
[0,1,3] Velamentous insertion of umbilical cord

⑤ **663.9 Unspecified umbilical cord complication**
[0,1,3]

⑤ **664 Trauma to perineum and vulva during delivery**
Includes: damage from instruments
that from extension of episiotomy

⑤ **664.0 First-degree perineal laceration**
[0,1,4] Perineal laceration, rupture, or tear involving:
fourchette
hymen
labia
skin
vagina
vulva

⑤ **664.1 Second-degree perineal laceration**
[0,1,4] Perineal laceration, rupture, or tear (following episiotomy) involving:
pelvic floor
perineal muscles
vaginal muscles

Excludes: *that involving anal sphincter (664.2)*

Add 4th or 5th digit   Nonspecific code   Unspecified code   Manifestation code

⑤ **664.2 Third-degree perineal laceration**
[0,1,4]   Perineal laceration, rupture, or tear (following episiotomy) involving:
      anal sphincter
      rectovaginal septum
      sphincter NOS

      Excludes: *anal sphincter tear during delivery not associated with third-degree perineal*
         laceration (664.6)
         that with anal or rectal mucosal laceration (664.3)

⑤ **664.3 Fourth-degree perineal laceration**
[0,1,4]   Perineal laceration, rupture, or tear as classifiable to 664.2 and involving also:
      anal mucosa
      rectal mucosa

⑤ **664.4 Unspecified perineal laceration**
[0,1,4]   Central laceration

⑤ **664.6 Anal sphincter tear complicating delivery, not associated with third-degree perineal laceration**
[0,1,4]

      Excludes: *third-degree perineal laceration (664.2)*

⑤ **664.5 Vulval and perineal hematoma**
[0,1,4]

⑤ **664.8 Other specified trauma to perineum and vulva**
[0,1,4]

⑤ **664.9 Unspecified trauma to perineum and vulva**
[0,1,4]

⑤ **665 Other obstetrical trauma**
    Includes: damage from instruments

⑤ **665.0 Rupture of uterus before onset of labor**
[0,1,3]

⑤ **665.1 Rupture of uterus during labor**
[0,1]   Rupture of uterus NOS

⑤ **665.2 Inversion of uterus**
[0,2,4]

⑤ **665.3 Laceration of cervix**
[0,1,4]

⑤ **665.4 High vaginal laceration**
[0,1,4]   Laceration of vaginal wall or sulcus without mention of perineal laceration

⑤ **665.5 Other injury to pelvic organs**
[0,1,4]   Injury to:
      bladder
      urethra

⑤ **665.6 Damage to pelvic joints and ligaments**
[0,1,4]   Avulsion of inner symphyseal cartilage
      Damage to coccyx
      Separation of symphysis (pubis)

⑤ **665.7 Pelvic hematoma**
[0,1,2,4]   Hematoma of vagina

⑤ **665.8 Other specified obstetrical trauma**
[0-4]

⑤ **665.9 Unspecified obstetrical trauma**
[0-4]

⑤ **666 Postpartum hemorrhage**

⑤ **666.0 Third-stage hemorrhage**
[0,2,4]   Hemorrhage associated with retained, trapped, or adherent placenta
      Retained placenta NOS

⑤ **666.1 Other immediate postpartum hemorrhage**
[0,2,4]   Atony of uterus with hemorrhage
      Hemorrhage within the first 24 hours following delivery of placenta
      Postpartum atony of uterus with hemorrhage
      Postpartum hemorrhage (atonic) NOS

      Excludes: *atony of uterus without hemorrhage (661.2)*
         postpartum atony of uterus without hemorrhage (669.8)

● Code new to this edition   ▲ Revision of existing code   ④ ⑤ Fourth or fifth digit required

⑤ **666.2 Delayed and secondary postpartum hemorrhage**
[0,2,4]   Hemorrhage:
        after the first 24 hours following delivery
        associated with retained portions of placenta or membranes
    Postpartum hemorrhage specified as delayed or secondary
    Retained products of conception NOS, following delivery

⑤ **666.3 Postpartum coagulation defects**
[0,2,4]   Postpartum afibrinogenemia
    Postpartum fibrinolysis

⑤ **667 Retained placenta or membranes, without hemorrhage**

⑤ **667.0 Retained placenta without hemorrhage**
[0,2,4]   Placenta accreta without hemorrhage
    Retained placenta: without hemorrhage
      NOS without hemorrhage
      total without hemorrhage

⑤ **667.1 Retained portions of placenta or membranes, without hemorrhage**
[0,2,4]   Retained products of conception following delivery, without hemorrhage

⑤ **668 Complications of the administration of anesthetic or other sedation in labor and delivery**
    Includes: complications arising from the administration of a general or local anesthetic,
          analgesic, or other sedation in labor and delivery

    Excludes: *reaction to spinal or lumbar puncture (349.0)*
               spinal headache (349.0)

    Use additional code(s) to further specify complication

⑤ **668.0 Pulmonary complications**
[0-4]   Inhalation [aspiration] of stomach contents or secretions following anesthesia or other
        sedation in labor or delivery
    Mendelson's syndrome following anesthesia or other sedation in labor or delivery
    Pressure collapse of lung following anesthesia or other sedation in labor or delivery

⑤ **668.1 Cardiac complications**
[0-4]   Cardiac arrest or failure following anesthesia or other sedation in labor and delivery

⑤ **668.2 Central nervous system complications**
[0-4]   Cerebral anoxia following anesthesia or other sedation in labor and delivery

⑤ **668.8 Other complications of anesthesia or other sedation in labor and delivery**
[0-4]

⑤ **668.9 Unspecified complication of anesthesia and other sedation**
[0-4]

⑤ **669 Other complications of labor and delivery, not elsewhere classified**

⑤ **669.0 Maternal distress**
[0-4]   Metabolic disturbance in labor and delivery

⑤ **669.1 Shock during or following labor and delivery**
[0-4]   Obstetric shock

⑤ **669.2 Maternal hypotension syndrome**
[0-4]

▲ **669.3 Acute kidney failure following labor and delivery**
[0,2,4]

⑤ **669.4 Other complications of obstetrical surgery and procedures**
[0-4]   Cardiac:
        arrest following cesarean or other obstetrical surgery or procedure, including delivery NOS
        failure following cesarean or other obstetrical surgery or procedure, including delivery NOS
    Cerebral anoxia following cesarean or other obstetrical surgery or procedure, including
        delivery NOS

    Excludes: *complications of obstetrical surgical wounds (674.1-674.3)*

⑤ **669.5 Forceps or vacuum extractor delivery without mention of indication**
[0,1]   Delivery by ventouse, without mention of indication

⑤ **669.6 Breech extraction, without mention of indication**
[0,1]

    Excludes: *breech delivery NOS (652.2)*

⑤ **669.7 Cesarean delivery, without mention of indication**
[0,1]

⑤ **669.8 Other complications of labor and delivery**
[0-4]

	Add 4th or 5th digit		Nonspecific code		Unspecified code		Manifestation code

⑤ **669.9** **Unspecified complication of labor and delivery**
[0-4]

COMPLICATIONS OF THE PUERPERIUM (670-677)

Note: Categories 671 and 673-676 include the listed conditions even if they occur during pregnancy or childbirth.

The following fifth-digit subclassification is for use with categories 670-676 to denote the current episode of care:

0 **unspecified as to episode of care or not applicable**

1 **delivered, with or without mention of antepartum condition**

2 **delivered, with mention of postpartum complication**

3 **antepartum condition or complication**

4 **postpartum condition or complication**

⑤ **670** **Major puerperal infection**

Excludes: infection following abortion (639.0)
minor genital tract infection following delivery (646.6)
puerperal pyrexia NOS (672)
puerperal fever NOS (672)
puerperal pyrexia of unknown origin (672)
urinary tract infection following delivery (646.6)

▲ **670.0** **Major puerperal infection, unspecified**
[0,2,4]

● **670.1** **Puerperal endometritis**
[0,2,4]

● **670.2** **Puerperal sepsis**
[0,2,4] Puerperal pyemia

● **670.3** **Puerperal septic thrombophlebitis**
[0,2,4]

● **670.8** **Other major puerperal infection**
[0,2,4] Puerperal:
pelvic cellulitis
peritonitis
salpingitis

⑤ **671** **Venous complications in pregnancy and the puerperium**

Excludes: personal history of venous complications prior to pregnancy, such as:
thrombophlebitis (V12.52)
thrombosis and embolism (V12.51)

⑤ **671.0** **Varicose veins of legs**
[0-4] Varicose veins NOS

⑤ **671.1** **Varicose veins of vulva and perineum**
[0-4]

⑤ **671.2** **Superficial thrombophlebitis**
[0-4] Phlebitis NOS
Thrombophlebitis (superficial)
Thrombosis NOS

⑤ **671.3** **Deep phlebothrombosis, antepartum**
[0,1,3] Deep-vein thrombosis, antepartum

Use additional code to identify the deep vein thrombosis (453.40-453.42, 453.50-453.52, 453.72-453.79, 453.82-453.89)

Use additional code for long term (current) use of anticoagulants, if applicable (V58.61)

⑤ **671.4** **Deep phlebothrombosis, postpartum**
[0,2,4] Deep-vein thrombosis, postpartum
Pelvic thrombophlebitis, postpartum
Phlegmasia alba dolens (puerperal)

Use additional code to identify the deep vein thrombosis (453.40-453.42, 453.50-453.52, 453.72-453.79, 453.82-453.89)

Use additional code for long term (current) use of anticoagulants, if applicable (V58.61)

⑤ **671.5** **Other phlebitis and thrombosis**
[0-4] Cerebral venous thrombosis
Thrombosis of intracranial venous sinus

● Code new to this edition   ▲ Revision of existing code   ④ ⑤ Fourth or fifth digit required

⑤ **671.8** **Other venous complications**
[0-4]   Hemorrhoids

⑤ **671.9** **Unspecified venous complication**
[0-4]

⑤ **672** **Pyrexia of unknown origin during the puerperium**
[0,2,4]   Puerperal fever NOS
          Postpartum fever NOS

Use 0 as fourth-digit for this category

⑤ **673** **Obstetrical pulmonary embolism**
        Includes: pulmonary emboli in pregnancy, childbirth, or the puerperium, or specified as
                  puerperal

        Excludes: *embolism following abortion (639.6)*

⑤ **673.0** **Obstetrical air embolism**
[0-4]

⑤ **673.1** **Amniotic fluid embolism**
[0-4]

⑤ **673.2** **Obstetrical blood-clot embolism**
[0-4]   Puerperal pulmonary embolism NOS

⑤ **673.3** **Obstetrical pyemic and septic embolism**
[0-4]

⑤ **673.8** **Other pulmonary embolism**
[0-4]   Fat embolism

⑤ **674** **Other and unspecified complications of the puerperium, not elsewhere classified**

⑤ **674.0** **Cerebrovascular disorders in the puerperium**
[0-4]   Any condition classifiable to 430-434, 436-437 occurring during pregnancy, childbirth,
         or the puerperium, or specified as puerperal

        Excludes: *intracranial venous sinus thrombosis (671.5)*

⑤ **674.1** **Disruption of cesarean wound**
[0,2,4]   Dehiscence or disruption of uterine wound

        Excludes: *uterine rupture before onset of labor (665.0)*
                 uterine rupture during labor (665.1)

⑤ **674.2** **Disruption of perineal wound**
[0,2,4]   Breakdown of perineum
          Disruption of wound of:
             episiotomy
             perineal laceration
          Secondary perineal tear

⑤ **674.3** **Other complications of obstetrical surgical wounds**
[0,2,4]   Hematoma of cesarean section or perineal wound
          Hemorrhage of cesarean section or perineal wound
          Infection of cesarean section or perineal wound

        Excludes: *damage from instruments in delivery (664.0-665.9)*

⑤ **674.4** **Placental polyp**
[0,2,4]

⑤ **674.5** **Peripartum cardiomyopathy**
[0-4]   Postpartum cardiomyopathy

⑤ **674.8** **Other**
[0,2,4]   Hepatorenal syndrome, following delivery
          Postpartum:
             subinvolution of uterus
             uterine hypertrophy

⑤ **674.9** **Unspecified**
[0,2,4]   Sudden death of unknown cause during the puerperium

⑤ **675** **Infections of the breast and nipple associated with childbirth**
        Includes: the listed conditions during pregnancy, childbirth, or the puerperium

⑤ **675.0** **Infections of nipple**
[0-4]   Abscess of nipple

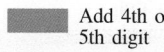 Add 4th or
5th digit

 Nonspecific
code

 Unspecified
code

 Manifestation
code

⑤ **675.1 Abscess of breast**
[0-4]   Abscess:
             mammary
             subareolar
             submammary
           Mastitis:
             purulent
             retromammary
             submammary

⑤ **675.2 Nonpurulent mastitis**
[0-4]   Lymphangitis of breast
           Mastitis:
             NOS
             interstitial
             parenchymatous

⑤ **675.8 Other specified infections of the breast and nipple**
[0-4]

⑤ **675.9 Unspecified infection of the breast and nipple**
[0-4]

⑤ **676 Other disorders of the breast associated with childbirth and disorders of lactation**
       Includes: the listed conditions during pregnancy, the puerperium, or lactation

⑤ **676.0 Retracted nipple**
[0-4]

⑤ **676.1 Cracked nipple**
[0-4]   Fissure of nipple

⑤ **676.2 Engorgement of breasts**
[0-4]

⑤ **676.3 Other and unspecified disorder of breast**
[0-4]

⑤ **676.4 Failure of lactation**
[0-4]   Agalactia

⑤ **676.5 Suppressed lactation**
[0-4]

⑤ **676.6 Galactorrhea**
[0-4]

       Excludes: galactorrhea not associated with childbirth (611.6)

⑤ **676.8 Other disorders of lactation**
[0-4]   Galactocele

⑤ **676.9 Unspecified disorder of lactation**
[0-4]

677 Late effect of complication of pregnancy, childbirth, and the puerperium
       Note: This category is to be used to indicate conditions in 632-648.9 and 651-676.9 as the cause
           of the late effect, themselves classifiable elsewhere. The "late effects" include conditions
           specified as such, or as sequelae, which may occur at any time after the puerperium.
           Code first any sequelae

OTHER MATERNAL AND FETAL COMPLICATIONS (678-679)

       The following fifth-digit subclassification is for use with categories 678-679 to denote the
           current episode of care:

       0   unspecified as to episode of care or not applicable

       1   delivered, with or without mention of antepartum condition

       2   delivered, with mention of postpartum complication

       3   antepartum condition or complication

       4   postpartum condition or complication

⑤ **678 Other fetal conditions**
       Requires fifth digit; valid digits are in [brackets] under each code. See beginning of section
           678-679 for definitions.

● Code new   ▲ Revision of   ④ ⑤ Fourth or fifth
  to this edition   existing code   digit required

⑤ **678.0 Fetal hematologic conditions**
[0,1,3]   Fetal anemia
            Fetal thrombocytopenia
            Fetal twin to twin transfusion

>   Excludes: *fetal and neonatal hemorrhage (772.0-772.9)*
>   *fetal hematologic disorders affecting newborn (776.0-776.9)*
>   *fetal-maternal hemorrhage (656.00-656.03)*
>   *isoimmunization incompatibility (656.10-656.13, 656.20-656.23)*

⑤ **678.1 Fetal conjoined twins**
[0,1,3]

⑤ **679 Complications of in utero procedures**
    Requires fifth digit; valid digits are in [brackets] under each code. See beginning of section
        678-679 for definitions.

⑤ **679.0 Maternal complications from in utero procedure**
[0-4]

>   Excludes: *maternal history of in utero procedure during previous pregnancy (V23.86)*

⑤ **679.1 Fetal complications from in utero procedure**
[0-4]   Fetal complications from amniocentesis

>   Excludes: *newborn affected by in utero procedure (760.61-760.64)*

	Add 4th or 5th digit		Nonspecific code		Unspecified code		Manifestation code

● Code new
to this edition

▲ Revision of
existing code

④ ⑤ Fourth or fifth
digit required

12. DISEASES OF THE SKIN AND SUBCUTANEOUS TISSUE (680-709)

INFECTIONS OF SKIN AND SUBCUTANEOUS TISSUE (680-686)

> Excludes: *certain infections of skin classified under "Infectious and Parasitic Diseases," such as:*
> *erysipelas (035)*
> *erysipeloid of Rosenbach (027.1)*
> *herpes:*
> *simplex (054.0-054.9)*
> *zoster (053.0-053.9)*
> *molluscum contagiosum (078.0)*
> *viral warts (078.10-078.19)*

680 Carbuncle and furuncle
Includes: boil
furunculosis

680.0 Face
Ear [any part]
Face [any part, except eye]
Nose (septum)
Temple (region)

> Excludes: *eyelid (373.13)*
> *lacrimal apparatus (375.31)*
> *orbit (376.01)*

680.1 Neck

680.2 Trunk

Abdominal wall	Flank
Back [any part, except	Groin
buttocks]	Pectoral region
Breast	Perineum
Chest wall	Umbilicus

> Excludes: *buttocks (680.5)*
> *external genital organs:*
> *female (616.4)*
> *male (607.2, 608.4)*

680.3 Upper arm and forearm
Arm [any part, except hand]
Axilla
Shoulder

680.4 Hand

Finger [any]	Wrist
Thumb	

680.5 Buttock
Anus
Gluteal region

680.6 Leg, except foot

Ankle	Knee
Hip	Thigh

680.7 Foot
Heel
Toe

680.8 Other specified sites
Head [any part, except face]
Scalp

> Excludes: *external genital organs:*
> *female (616.4)*
> *male (607.2, 608.4)*

680.9 Unspecified site

Boil NOS	Furuncle NOS
Carbuncle NOS	

681 Cellulitis and abscess of finger and toe
Includes: that with lymphangitis

Use additional code, if desired, to identify organism, such as Staphylococcus (041.1)

⑤ **681.0 Finger**

681.00 Cellulitis and abscess, unspecified

Add 4th or 5th digit	Nonspecific code	Unspecified code	Manifestation code

681.01 Felon
Pulp abscess
Whitlow

Excludes: herpetic whitlow (054.6)

681.02 Onychia and paronychia of finger
Panaritium of finger
Perionychia of finger

⑤ **681.1 Toe**

681.10 Cellulitis and abscess, unspecified

681.11 Onychia and paronychia of toe
Panaritium of toe
Perionychia of toe

681.9 Cellulitis and abscess of unspecified digit
Infection of nail NOS

682 Other cellulitis and abscess
Includes: abscess (acute) (with lymphangitis) except of finger or toe
cellulitis (diffuse) (with lymphangitis) except of finger or toe
lymphangitis, acute (with lymphangitis) except of finger or toe

Use additional code, if desired, to identify organism, such as Staphylococcus (041.1)

Excludes: lymphangitis (chronic) (subacute) (457.2)

682.0 Face
Cheek, external   Nose, external
Chin   Submandibular
Forehead   Temple (region)

Excludes: ear [any part] (380.10-380.16)
eyelid (373.13)
lacrimal apparatus (375.31)
lip (528.5)
mouth (528.3)
nose (internal) (478.1)
orbit (376.01)

682.1 Neck

682.2 Trunk
Abdominal wall   Groin
Back [any part, except   Pectoral region
  buttock]   Perineum
Chest wall   Umbilicus, except newborn
Flank

Excludes: anal and rectal regions (566)
breast:
NOS (611.0)
puerperal (675.1)
external genital organs:
female (616.3-616.4)
male (604.0, 607.2, 608.4)
umbilicus, newborn (771.4)

682.3 Upper arm and forearm
Arm [any part, except hand]
Axilla
Shoulder

Excludes: hand (682.4)

682.4 Hand, except fingers and thumb
Wrist

Excludes: finger and thumb (681.00-681.02)

682.5 Buttock
Gluteal region

Excludes: anal and rectal regions (566)

682.6 Leg, except foot
Ankle   Knee
Hip   Thigh

● Code new to this edition   ▲ Revision of existing code   ④ ⑤ Fourth or fifth digit required

682.7 Foot, except toes
Heel

Excludes: toe (681.10-681.11)

682.8 Other specified sites
Head [except face]
Scalp

Excludes: face (682.0)

682.9 Unspecified site
Abscess NOS
Cellulitis NOS
Lymphangitis, acute NOS

Excludes: lymphangitis NOS (457.2)

683 Acute lymphadenitis
Abscess (acute), lymph gland or node, except mesenteric
Adenitis, acute, lymph gland or node, except mesenteric
Lymphadenitis, acute, lymph gland or node, except mesenteric
Use additional code, if desired, to identify organism, such as Staphylococcus (041.1)

Excludes: enlarged glands NOS (785.6)
lymphadenitis:
chronic or subacute, except mesenteric (289.1)
mesenteric (acute) (chronic) (subacute) (289.2)
unspecified (289.3)

684 Impetigo
Impetiginization of other dermatoses
Impetigo (contagiosa) [any site] [any organism]:
bullous
circinate
neonatorum
simplex
Pemphigus neonatorum

Excludes: impetigo herpetiformis (694.3)

685 Pilonidal cyst
Includes:
fistula, coccygeal or pilonidal
sinus, coccygeal or pilonidal

685.0 With abscess

685.1 Without mention of abscess

686 Other local infections of skin and subcutaneous tissue
Use additional code, if desired, to identify any infectious organism (041.0-041.8)

⑤ **686.0 Pyoderma**
Dermatitis:
purulent
septic
suppurative

686.00 Pyoderma, unspecified

686.01 Pyoderma gangrenosum

686.09 Other pyoderma

686.1 Pyogenic granuloma
Granuloma:
septic
suppurative
telangiecticum

Excludes: pyogenic granuloma of oral mucosa (528.9)

686.8 Other specified local infections of skin and subcutaneous tissue
Bacterid (pustular)
Dermatitis vegetans
Ecthyma
Perlèche

Excludes: dermatitis infectiosa eczematoides (690.8)
panniculitis (729.30-729.39)

686.9 Unspecified local infection of skin and subcutaneous tissue
Fistula of skin NOS
Skin infection NOS

Excludes: fistula to skin from internal organs—see Alphabetic Index

Add 4th or
5th digit

Nonspecific
code

Unspecified
code

Manifestation
code

OTHER INFLAMMATORY CONDITIONS OF SKIN AND SUBCUTANEOUS TISSUE (690-698)

Excludes: *panniculitis (729.30-729.39)*

690 **Erythematosquamous dermatosis**

Excludes: *eczematous dermatitis of eyelid (373.31)*
parakeratosis variegata (696.2)
psoriasis (696.0-696.1)
seborrheic keratosis (702.11-702.19)

⑤ **690.1** **Seborrheic dermatitis**

690.10 **Seborrheic dermatitis, unspecified**
Seborrheic dermatitis NOS

690.11 **Seborrhea capitis**
Cradle cap

690.12 **Seborrheic infantile dermatitis**

690.18 **Other seborrheic dermatitis**

690.8 **Other erythematosquamous dermatosis**

691 **Atopic dermatitis and related conditions**

691.0 **Diaper or napkin rash**
Ammonia dermatitis
Diaper or napkin:
dermatitis
erythema
rash
Psoriasiform napkin eruption

691.8 **Other atopic dermatitis and related conditions**
Atopic dermatitis
Besnier's prurigo
Eczema:
atopic
flexural
intrinsic (allergic)

Neurodermatitis:
atopic
diffuse (of Brocq)

692 **Contact dermatitis and other eczema**
Includes:

dermatitis:
NOS
contact
occupational
venenata

eczema (acute) (chronic):
NOS
allergic
erythematous
occupational

Excludes: *allergy NOS (995.3)*
contact dermatitis of eyelids (373.32)
dermatitis due to substances taken internally (693.0-693.9)
eczema of external ear (380.22)
perioral dermatitis (695.3)
urticarial reactions (708.0-708.9, 995.1)

692.0 **Due to detergents**

692.1 **Due to oils and greases**

692.2 **Due to solvents**
Dermatitis due to solvents of:
chlorocompound group
cyclohexane group
ester group
glycol group
hydrocarbon group
ketone group

● Code new
  to this edition

▲ Revision of
  existing code

④ ⑤ Fourth or fifth
  digit required

692.3 Due to drugs and medicines in contact with skin
Dermatitis (allergic) (contact) due to:
  arnica
  fungicides
  iodine
  keratolytics
  mercurials
  neomycin
  pediculocides
  phenols
  scabicides
  any drug applied to skin
Dermatitis medicamentosa due to drug applied to skin

Use additional E code, if desired, to identify drug

Excludes: *allergy NOS due to drugs (995.27)*
         dermatitis due to ingested drugs (693.0)
         dermatitis medicamentosa NOS (693.0)

692.4 Due to other chemical products

Dermatitis due to:	Dermatitis due to:
acids	insecticide
adhesive plaster	nylon
alkalis	plastic
caustics	rubber
dichromate	

692.5 Due to food in contact with skin

Dermatitis, contact, due to:	Dermatitis, contact, due to:
cereals	fruit
fish	meat
flour	milk

Excludes: *dermatitis due to:*
         dyes (692.89)
         ingested foods (693.1)
         preservatives (692.89)

692.6 Due to plants [except food]
Dermatitis due to:
  lacquer tree [Rhus verniciflua]
  poison ivy [Rhus toxicodendron]
  poison oak [Rhus diversiloba]
  poison sumac [Rhus venenata]
  poison vine [Rhus radicans]
  primrose [Primula]
  ragweed [Senecio jacobae]
  other plants in contact with the skin

Excludes: *allergy NOS due to pollen (477.0)*
         nettle rash (708.8)

⑤ **692.7 Due to solar radiation**

Excludes: *sunburn due to other ultraviolet radiation exposure (692.82)*

692.70 Unspecified dermatitis due to sun

692.71 Sunburn
First degree sunburn
Sunburn NOS

692.72 Acute dermatitis due to solar radiation
Berloque dermatitis
Photoallergic response
Phototoxic response
Polymorphus light eruption
Acute solar skin damage NOS

Excludes: *sunburn (692.71, 692.76-692.77)*
Use additional E code, if desired, to identify drug, if drug induced

692.73 Actinic reticuloid and actinic granuloma

692.74 Other chronic dermatitis due to solar radiation
Solar elastosis
Chronic solar skin damage NOS

Excludes: *actinic [solar] keratosis (702.0)*

	Add 4th or 5th digit		Nonspecific code		Unspecified code		Manifestation code

692.75 **Disseminated superficial actinic porokeratosis (DSAP)**

692.76 **Sunburn of second degree**

692.77 **Sunburn of third degree**

692.79 **Other dermatitis due to solar radiation**
Hydroa aestivale
Photodermatitis due to sun
Photosensitiveness due to sun
Solar skin damage NOS

⑤ **692.8 Due to other specified agents**

692.81 **Dermatitis due to cosmetics**

692.82 **Dermatitis due to other radiation**
Infrared rays
Light, except from sun
Radiation NOS
Ultraviolet rays, except from sun
X-rays
Tanning bed

Excludes: *that due to solar radiation (692.70-692.79)*

692.83 **Dermatitis due to metals**
Jewelry

692.84 **Due to animal (cat) (dog) dander**
Due to animal (cat) (dog) hair

692.89 **Other**
Dermatitis due to:
cold weather
dyes
hot weather
preservatives

Excludes: *allergy (NOS) (rhinitis) due to animal hair or dander (477.2)*
allergy to dust (477.8)
sunburn (692.71, 692.76-692.77)

692.9 Unspecified cause
Dermatitis: Eczema NOS
NOS
contact NOS
venenata NOS

693 Dermatitis due to substances taken internally

Excludes: *adverse effect NOS of drugs and medicines (995.20)*
allergy NOS (995.3)
contact dermatitis (692.0-692.9)
urticarial reactions (708.0-708.9, 995.1)

693.0 Due to drugs and medicines
Dermatitis medicamentosa NOS
Use additional E code, if desired, to identify drug
Excludes: *that due to drugs in contact with skin (692.3)*

693.1 Due to food

693.8 Due to other specified substances taken internally

693.9 Due to unspecified substance taken internally
Excludes: *dermatitis NOS (692.9)*

694 Bullous dermatoses

694.0 Dermatitis herpetiformis
Dermatosis herpetiformis
Duhring's disease
Hydroa herpetiformis

Excludes: *herpes gestationis (646.8)*
dermatitis herpetiformis:
juvenile (694.2)
senile (694.5)

694.1 Subcorneal pustular dermatosis
Sneddon-Wilkinson disease or syndrome

● Code new
to this edition
▲ Revision of
existing code
④ ⑤ Fourth or fifth
digit required

694.2 Juvenile dermatitis herpetiformis
Juvenile pemphigoid

694.3 Impetigo herpetiformis

694.4 Pemphigus

Pemphigus:
  NOS
  erythematosus
  foliaceus

Pemphigus:
  malignant
  vegetans
  vulgaris

Excludes: *pemphigus neonatorum (684)*

694.5 Pemphigoid
Benign pemphigus NOS
Bullous pemphigoid
Herpes circinatus bullosus
Senile dermatitis herpetiformis

⑤ **694.6 Benign mucous membrane pemphigoid**
Cicatricial pemphigoid
Mucosynechial atrophic bullous dermatitis

694.60 Without mention of ocular involvement

694.61 With ocular involvement
Ocular pemphigus

694.8 Other specified bullous dermatoses

Excludes: *herpes gestationis (646.8)*

694.9 Unspecified bullous dermatoses

695 Erythematous conditions

695.0 Toxic erythema
Erythema venenatum

⑤ **695.1 Erythema multiforme**
Use additional code to identify associated manifestations, such as:
  arthropathy associated with dermatological disorders (713.3)
  conjunctival edema (372.73)
  conjunctivitis (372.04, 372.33)
  corneal scars and opacities (371.00-371.05)
  corneal ulcer (370.00-370.07)
  edema of eyelid (374.82)
  inflammation of eyelid (373.8)
  keratoconjunctivitis sicca (370.33)
  mechanical lagophthalmos (374.22)
  mucositis (478.11, 528.00, 538, 616.81)
  stomatitis (528.00)
  symblepharon (372.63)
Use additional E-code to identify drug, if drug-induced
Use additional code to identify percentage of skin exfoliation (695.50-695.59)

Excludes: *(staphylococcal) scalded skin syndrome (695.81)*

695.10 Erythema multiforme, unspecified
Erythema iris
Herpes iris

695.11 Erythema multiforme minor

695.12 Erythema multiforme major

695.13 Stevens-Johnson syndrome

695.14 Stevens-Johnson syndrome-toxic epidermal
necrolysis overlap syndrome
SJS-TEN overlap syndrome

695.15 Toxic epidermal necrolysis
Lyell's syndrome

695.19 Other erythema multiforme

695.2 Erythema nodosum

Excludes: *tuberculous erythema nodosum (017.1)*

695.3 Rosacea

Acne:
  erythematosa
  rosacea

Perioral dermatitis
Rhinophyma

	Add 4th or 5th digit		Nonspecific code		Unspecified code		Manifestation code

695.4 Lupus erythematosus
Lupus:
erythematodes (discoid)
erythematosus (discoid), not disseminated

Excludes: lupus (vulgaris) NOS (017.0)
systemic [disseminated] lupus erythematosus (710.0)

⑤ **695.5 Exfoliation due to erythematous conditions according to extent of body surface involved**
Code first erythematous condition causing exfoliation, such as:
Ritter's disease (695.81)
(Staphylococcal) scalded skin syndrome (695.81)
Stevens-Johnson syndrome (695.13)
Stevens-Johnson syndrome-toxic epidermal necrolysis overlap syndrome (695.14)
Toxic epidermal necrolysis (695.15)

695.50 Exfoliation due to erythematous condition involving less than 10 percent of body surface
Exfoliation due to erythematous condition NOS

695.51 Exfoliation due to erythematous condition involving 10-19 percent of body surface

695.52 Exfoliation due to erythematous condition involving 20-29 percent of body surface

695.53 Exfoliation due to erythematous condition involving 30-39 percent of body surface

695.54 Exfoliation due to erythematous condition involving 40-49 percent of body surface

695.55 Exfoliation due to erythematous condition involving 50-59 percent of body surface

695.56 Exfoliation due to erythematous condition involving 60-69 percent of body surface

695.57 Exfoliation due to erythematous condition involving 70-79 percent of body surface

695.58 Exfoliation due to erythematous condition involving 80-89 percent of body surface

695.59 Exfoliation due to erythematous condition involving 90 percent or more of body surface

⑤ **695.8 Other specified erythematous conditions**

695.81 Ritter's disease
Dermatitis exfoliativa neonatorum
(Staphylococcal) Scalded skin syndrome
Use additional code to identify percentage of skin exfoliation (695.50-695.59)

695.89 Other
Erythema intertrigo
Intertrigo
Pityriasis rubra (Hebra)

Excludes: mycotic intertrigo (111.0-111.9)

695.9 Unspecified erythematous condition
Erythema NOS
Erythroderma (secondary)

696 Psoriasis and similar disorders

696.0 Psoriatic arthropathy

696.1 Other psoriasis
Acrodermatitis continua
Dermatitis repens
Psoriasis:
NOS
any type, except arthropathic

Excludes: psoriatic arthropathy (696.0)

696.2 Parapsoriasis
Parakeratosis variegata
Parapsoriasis lichenoides chronica
Pityriasis lichenoides et varioliformis

696.3 Pityriasis rosea
Pityriasis circinata (et maculata)

● Code new to this edition   ▲ Revision of existing code   ④ ⑤ Fourth or fifth digit required

696.4 Pityriasis rubra pilaris
Devergie's disease
Lichen ruber acuminatus

Excludes: *pityriasis rubra (Hebra) (695.89)*

696.5 Other and unspecified pityriasis
Pityriasis:
NOS
alba
streptogenes

Excludes: *pityriasis simplex (690.18)*
pityriasis versicolor (111.0)

696.8 Other

697 Lichen

Excludes: *lichen:*
obtusus corneus (698.3)
pilaris (congenital) (757.39)
ruber acuminatus (696.4)
sclerosus et atrophicus (701.0)
scrofulosus (017.0)
simplex chronicus (698.3)
spinulosus (congenital) (757.39)
urticatus (698.2)

697.0 Lichen planus
Lichen:
planopilaris
ruber planus

697.1 Lichen nitidus
Pinkus' disease

697.8 Other lichen, not elsewhere classified
Lichen:
ruber moniliforme
striata

697.9 Lichen, unspecified

698 Pruritus and related conditions

Excludes: *pruritus specified as psychogenic (306.3)*

698.0 Pruritus ani
Perianal itch

698.1 Pruritus of genital organs

698.2 Prurigo
Lichen urticatus
Prurigo:
NOS
Hebra's
mitis
simplex
Urticaria papulosa (Hebra)

Excludes: *prurigo nodularis (698.3)*

698.3 Lichenification and lichen simplex chronicus
Hyde's disease
Neurodermatitis (circumscripta) (local)
Prurigo nodularis

Excludes: *neurodermatitis, diffuse (of Brocq) (691.8)*

698.4 Dermatitis factitia [artefacta]
Dermatitis ficta
Neurotic excoriation

Use additional code, if desired, to identify any associated mental disorder

698.8 Other specified pruritic conditions
Pruritus:
hiemalis
senilis
Winter itch

| | Add 4th or 5th digit | | Nonspecific code | | Unspecified code | | Manifestation code |

698.9 Unspecified pruritic disorder
Itch NOS
Pruritus NOS

OTHER DISEASES OF SKIN AND SUBCUTANEOUS TISSUE (700-709)

Excludes: *conditions confined to eyelids (373.0-374.9)*
congenital conditions of skin, hair, and nails (757.0-757.9)

700 Corns and callosities
Callus
Clavus

701 Other hypertrophic and atrophic conditions of skin

Excludes: *dermatomyositis (710.3)*
hereditary edema of legs (757.0)
scleroderma (generalized) (710.1)

701.0 Circumscribed scleroderma
Addison's keloid
Dermatosclerosis, localized
Lichen sclerosus et atrophicus
Morphea
Scleroderma, circumscribed or localized

701.1 Keratoderma, acquired
Acquired:
ichthyosis
keratoderma palmaris et plantaris
Elastosis perforans serpiginosa
Hyperkeratosis:
NOS
follicularis in cutem penetrans
palmoplantaris climacterica
Keratoderma:
climactericum
tylodes, progressive
Keratosis (blennorrhagica)

Excludes: *Darier's disease [keratosis follicularis] (congenital) (757.39)*
keratosis:
arsenical (692.4)
gonococcal (098.81)

701.2 Acquired acanthosis nigricans
Keratosis nigricans

701.3 Striae atrophicae
Atrophic spots of skin
Atrophoderma maculatum
Atrophy blanche (of Milian)
Degenerative colloid atrophy
Senile degenerative atrophy
Striae distensae

701.4 Keloid scar
Cheloid
Hypertrophic scar
Keloid

701.5 Other abnormal granulation tissue
Excessive granulation

701.8 Other specified hypertrophic and atrophic conditions of skin
Acrodermatitis atrophicans chronica
Atrophia cutis senilis
Atrophoderma neuriticum
Confluent and reticulate papillomatosis
Cutis laxa senilis
Elastosis senilis
Folliculitis ulerythematosa reticulata
Gougerot-Carteaud syndrome or disease

701.9 Unspecified hypertrophic and atrophic conditions of skin
Atrophoderma

● Code new
to this edition

▲ Revision of
existing code

④ ⑤ Fourth or fifth
digit required

702 **Other dermatoses**

Excludes: *carcinoma in situ (232.0-232.9)*

702.0 **Actinic keratosis**

⑤ **702.1** **Seborrheic keratosis**

> **702.11** **Inflamed seborrheic keratosis**
>
> **702.19** **Other seborrheic keratosis**
> Seborrheic keratosis NOS

702.8 **Other specified dermatoses**

703 **Diseases of nail**

Excludes: *congenital anomalies (757.5)*
onychia and paronychia (681.02, 681.11)

703.0 **Ingrowing nail**
Ingrowing nail with infection
Unguis incarnatus

Excludes: *infection, nail NOS (681.9)*

703.8 **Other specified diseases of nail**
Dystrophia unguium   Onychauxis
Hypertrophy of nail   Onychogryposis
Koilonychia   Onycholysis
Leukonychia (punctata) (striata)

703.9 **Unspecified disease of nail**

704 **Diseases of hair and hair follicles**

Excludes: *congenital anomalies (757.4)*

⑤ **704.0** **Alopecia**

Excludes: *madarosis (374.55)*
syphilitic alopecia (091.82)

> **704.00** **Alopecia, unspecified**
> Baldness
> Loss of hair
>
> **704.01** **Alopecia areata**
> Ophiasis
>
> **704.02** **Telogen effluvim**
>
> **704.09** **Other**
> Folliculitis decalvans
> Hypotrichosis:
>   NOS
>   postinfectional NOS
> Pseudopelade

704.1 **Hirsutism**
Hypertrichosis:
  NOS
  lanuginosa, acquired
Polytrichia

Excludes: *hypertrichosis of eyelid (374.54)*

704.2 **Abnormalities of the hair**
Atrophic hair   Trichiasis:
Clastothrix   NOS
Fragilitas crinium   cicatrical
                              Trichorrhexis (nodosa)

Excludes: *trichiasis of eyelid (374.05)*

704.3 **Variations in hair color**
Canities (premature)   Poliosis:
Grayness, hair (premature)   NOS
Heterochromia of hair   circumscripta, acquired

	Add 4th or 5th digit		Nonspecific code		Unspecified code		Manifestation code

704.8 **Other specified diseases of hair and hair follicles**

Folliculitis:
NOS
abscedens et suffodiens
pustular
Perifolliculitis:
NOS
capitis abscedens et suffodiens
scalp

Sycosis:
NOS
barbae [not parasitic]
lupoid
vulgaris

704.9 **Unspecified disease of hair and hair follicles**

705 **Disorders of sweat glands**

705.0 **Anhidrosis**
Hypohidrosis
Oligohidrosis

705.1 **Prickly heat**
Heat rash
Miliaria rubra (tropicalis)
Sudamina

⑤ **705.2** **Focal hyperhidrosis**

Excludes: generalized (secondary) hyperhidrosis (780.8)

    705.21 **Primary focal hyperhidrosis**
Focal hyperhidrosis NOS
Hyperhidrosis NOS
Hyperhidrosis of:
axilla
face
palms
soles

    705.22 **Secondary focal hyperhidrosis**
Frey's syndrome

⑤ **705.8** **Other specified disorders of sweat glands**

    705.81 **Dyshidrosis**
Cheiropompholyx
Pompholyx

    705.82 **Fox-Fordyce disease**

    705.83 **Hidradenitis**
Hidradenitis suppurativa

    705.89 **Other**
Bromhidrosis
Chromhidrosis

Granulosis rubra nasi
Urhidrosis

Excludes: generalized hyperhidrosis (780.8)
hidrocystoma (216.0-216.9)

705.9 **Unspecified disorder of sweat glands**
Disorder of sweat glands NOS

706 **Diseases of sebaceous glands**

706.0 **Acne varioliformis**
Acne:
frontalis
necrotica

706.1 **Other acne**
Acne:
NOS
conglobata
cystic
pustular
vulgaris

Blackhead
Comedo

Excludes: acne rosacea (695.3)

706.2 **Sebaceous cyst**
Atheroma, skin
Keratin cyst
Wen

● Code new
to this edition

▲ Revision of
existing code

④ ⑤ Fourth or fifth
digit required

706.3 Seborrhea

Excludes: *seborrhea:*
> *capitis (690.11)*
> *sicca (690.18)*
> *seborrheic dermatitis (690.11)*
> *seborrheic keratosis (702.11-702.19)*

706.8 Other specified diseases of sebaceous glands
Asteatosis (cutis)
Xerosis cutis

706.9 Unspecified disease of sebaceous glands

707 Chronic ulcer of skin
Includes: non-infected sinus of skin
non-healing ulcer

Excludes: *varicose ulcer (454.0, 454.2)*

⑤ **707.0 Pressure ulcer**
Bed sore
Decubitus ulcer
Plaster ulcer

Use additional code to identify pressure ulcer stage (707.20 -707.25)

707.00 Unspecified site

707.01 Elbow

707.02 Upper back
Shoulder blades

707.03 Lower back
Coccyx
Sacrum

707.04 Hip

707.05 Buttock

707.06 Ankle

707.07 Heel

707.09 Other site
Head

⑤ **707.1 Ulcer of lower limbs, except pressure ulcer**
Ulcer, chronic, of lower limb:
neurogenic of lower limb
trophic of lower limb

Code, if applicable, any causal condition first:
atherosclerosis of the extremities with ulceration (440.23)
chronic venous hypertension with ulcer (459.31)
chronic venous hypertension with ulcer and inflammation (459.33)
diabetes mellitus (249.80-249.81, 250.80-250.83)
postphlebetic syndrome with ulcer (459.11)
postphlebetic syndrome with ulcer and inflammation (459.13)

707.10 Ulcer of lower limb, unspecified

707.11 Ulcer of thigh

707.12 Ulcer of calf

707.13 Ulcer of ankle

707.14 Ulcer of heel and midfoot
Plantar surface of midfoot

707.15 Ulcer of other part of foot
Toes

707.19 Ulcer of other part of lower limb

⑤ **707.2 Pressure ulcer stages**
Code first site of pressure ulcer (707.00-707.09)

707.20 Pressure ulcer, unspecified stage
Healing pressure ulcer NOS
Healing pressure ulcer, unspecified stage

707.21 Pressure ulcer stage I
Healing pressure ulcer, stage I
Pressure pre-ulcer skin changes limited to persistent focal erythema

| | Add 4th or 5th digit | | Nonspecific code | | Unspecified code | | Manifestation code |

707.22 Pressure ulcer stage II
Healing pressure ulcer, stage II
Pressure ulcer with abrasion, blister, partial thickness skin loss involving epidermis and/or dermis

707.23 Pressure ulcer stage III
Healing pressure ulcer, stage III
Pressure ulcer with full thickness skin loss involving damage or necrosis of subcutaneous tissue

707.24 Pressure ulcer stage IV
Healing pressure ulcer, stage IV
Pressure ulcer with necrosis of soft tissues through to underlying muscle, tendon, or bone

707.25 Pressure ulcer, unstageable

707.8 Chronic ulcer of other specified sites
Ulcer, chronic, of other specified sites:
neurogenic of other specified sites
trophic of other specified sites

707.9 Chronic ulcer of unspecified site
Chronic ulcer NOS   Tropical ulcer NOS
Trophic ulcer NOS   Ulcer of skin NOS

708 Urticaria
Excludes: edema:
angioneurotic (995.1)
Quincke's (995.1)
hereditary angioedema (277.6)
urticaria:
giant (995.1)
papulosa (Hebra) (698.2)
pigmentosa (juvenile) (congenital) (757.33)

708.0 Allergic urticaria

708.1 Idiopathic urticaria

708.2 Urticaria due to cold and heat
Thermal urticaria

708.3 Dermatographic urticaria
Dermatographia
Factitial urticaria

708.4 Vibratory urticaria

708.5 Cholinergic urticaria

708.8 Other specified urticaria
Nettle rash
Urticaria:
chronic
recurrent periodic

708.9 Urticaria, unspecified
Hives NOS

709 Other disorders of skin and subcutaneous tissue

⑤ **709.0 Dyschromia**
Excludes: albinism (270.2)
pigmented nevus (216.0-216.9)
that of eyelid (374.52-374.53)

709.00 Dyschromia, unspecified

709.01 Vitiligo

709.09 Other

709.1 Vascular disorders of skin
Angioma serpiginosum
Purpura (primary) annularis telangiectodes

● Code new to this edition   ▲ Revision of existing code   ④ ⑤ Fourth or fifth digit required

709.2 **Scar conditions and fibrosis of skin**
Adherent scar (skin)
Cicatrix
Disfigurement (due to scar)
Fibrosis, skin NOS
Scar NOS

Excludes: keloid scar (701.4)

709.3 **Degenerative skin disorders**

Calcinosis: Degeneration, skin
  circumscripta   Deposits, skin
  cutis   Senile dermatosis NOS
Colloid milium   Subcutaneous calcification

709.4 **Foreign body granuloma of skin and subcutaneous tissue**

Excludes: residual foreign body without granuloma of skin and subcutaneous tissue (729.6)
        that of muscle (728.82)

709.8 **Other specified disorders of skin**
Epithelial hyperplasia
Menstrual dermatosis
Vesicular eruption

709.9 **Unspecified disorder of skin and subcutaneous tissue**
Dermatosis NOS

Add 4th or   Nonspecific   Unspecified   Manifestation
5th digit   code   code   code

● Code new
to this edition

▲ Revision of
existing code

④ ⑤ Fourth or fifth
digit required

13. DISEASES OF THE MUSCULOSKELETAL SYSTEM AND CONNECTIVE TISSUE (710-739)

Use additional external cause code, if applicable, to identify the cause of the musculoskeletal condition

The following fifth-digit subclassification is for use with categories 711-712, 715-716, 718-719, and 730:

0 site unspecified

1 shoulder region
   Acromioclavicular joint(s)
   Glenohumeral joint(s)
   Sternoclavicular joint(s)
   Clavicle
   Scapula

2 upper arm
   Elbow joint   Humerus

3 forearm
   Radius   Wrist joint
   Ulna

4 hand
   Carpus   Phalanges [fingers]
   Metacarpus

5 pelvic region and thigh
   Buttock   Hip (joint)
   Femur

6 lower leg
   Fibula   Patella
   Knee joint   Tibia

7 ankle and foot
   Ankle joint   Phalanges, foot
   Digits [toes]   Tarsus
   Metatarsus   Other joints in foot

8 other specified sites
   Head   Skull
   Neck   Trunk
   Ribs   Vertebral column

9 multiple sites

ARTHROPATHIES AND RELATED DISORDERS (710-719)

   Excludes: disorders of spine (720.0-724.9)

710 Diffuse diseases of connective tissue
   Includes: all collagen diseases whose effects are not mainly confined to a single system

   Excludes: those affecting mainly the cardiovascular system, i.e., polyarteritis nodosa and allied conditions (446.0-446.7)

710.0 Systemic lupus erythematosus
   Disseminated lupus erythematosus
   Libman-Sacks disease

Use additional code, if desired, to identify manifestation, as:
   endocarditis (424.91)
   nephritis (583.81)
      chronic (582.81)
      nephrotic syndrome (581.81)

   Excludes: lupus erythematosus (discoid) NOS (695.4)

710.1 Systemic sclerosis
   Acrosclerosis
   CRST syndrome
   Progressive systemic sclerosis
   Scleroderma

Use additional code, if desired, to identify manifestation, as:
   lung involvement (517.2)
   myopathy (359.6)

   Excludes: circumscribed scleroderma (701.0)

710.2 Sicca syndrome
   Keratoconjunctivitis sicca
   Sjögren's disease

710.3 Dermatomyositis
Poikilodermatomyositis
Polymyositis with skin involvement

710.4 Polymyositis

710.5 Eosinophilia myalgia syndrome
Toxic oil syndrome

Use additional E code, if desired, to identify drug, if drug induced

710.8 Other specified diffuse diseases of connective tissue
Multifocal fibrosclerosis (idiopathic) NEC
Systemic fibrosclerosing syndrome

710.9 Unspecified diffuse connective tissue disease
Collagen disease NOS

⑤ **711 Arthropathy associated with infections**
Includes: arthritis associated with conditions classifiable below
arthropathy associated with conditions classifiable below
polyarthritis associated with conditions classifiable below
polyarthropathy associated with conditions classifiable below

Excludes: rheumatic fever (390)

The following fifth-digit subclassification is for use with category 711; valid digits are in [brackets] under each code. For definitions, see the beginning of this chapter:

  0 site unspecified
  1 shoulder region
  2 upper arm
  3 forearm
  4 hand
  5 pelvic region and thigh
  6 lower leg
  7 ankle and foot
  8 other specified sites
  9 multiple sites

⑤ **711.0 Pyogenic arthritis**
[0-9] Arthritis or polyarthritis (due to):
coliform [Escherichia coli]
Hemophilus influenzae [H. influenzae]
pneumococcal
Pseudomonas
staphylococcal
streptococcal
Pyarthrosis

Use additional code, if desired, to identify infectious organism (041.0-041.8)

⑤ **711.1 Arthropathy associated with Reiter's disease and nonspecific urethritis**
[0-9] Code first underlying disease, as:
nonspecific urethritis (099.4)
Reiter's disease (099.3)

⑤ **711.2 Arthropathy in Behçet's syndrome**
[0-9] Code first underlying disease (136.1)

⑤ **711.3 Postdysenteric arthropathy**
[0-9] Code first underlying disease, as:
dysentery (009.0)
enteritis, infectious (008.0-009.3)
paratyphoid fever (002.1-002.9)
typhoid fever (002.0)

Excludes: salmonella arthritis (003.23)

⑤ **711.4 Arthropathy associated with other bacterial diseases**
[0-9] Code first underlying disease, as:
diseases classifiable to 010-040, 090-099, except as in 711.1, 711.3, and 713.5
leprosy (030.0-030.9)
tuberculosis (015.0-015.9)

Excludes: gonococcal arthritis (098.50)
meningococcal arthritis (036.82)

● Code new to this edition   ▲ Revision of existing code   ④ ⑤ Fourth or fifth digit required

⑤ **711.5** *Arthropathy associated with other viral diseases*
[0-9]   *Code first underlying disease, as:*
          diseases classifiable to 045-049, 050-079, 480, 487
          O'nyong nyong (066.3)

   Excludes: *that due to rubella (056.71)*

⑤ **711.6** *Arthropathy associated with mycoses*
[0-9]   *Code first underlying disease (110.0-118)*

⑤ **711.7** *Arthropathy associated with helminthiasis*
[0-9]   *Code first underlying disease, as:*
          filariasis (125.0-125.9)

⑤ **711.8** *Arthropathy associated with other infectious and parasitic diseases*
[0-9]   *Code first underlying disease, as:*
          diseases classifiable to 080-088, 100-104, 130-136

   Excludes: *arthropathy associated with sarcoidosis (713.7)*

⑤ **711.9** **Unspecified infective arthritis**
[0-9]   Infective arthritis or polyarthritis (acute) (chronic) (subacute) NOS

⑤ **712** **Crystal arthropathies**
          Includes: crystal-induced arthritis and synovitis

   Excludes: *gouty arthropathy (274.00-274.03)*

The following fifth-digit subclassification is for use with category 712; valid digits are in
   [brackets] under each code. See beginning of this chapter for definitions:

   0 **site unspecified**

   1 **shoulder region**

   2 **upper arm**

   3 **forearm**

   4 **hand**

   5 **pelvic region and thigh**

   6 **lower leg**

   7 **ankle and foot**

   8 **other specified sites**

   9 **multiple sites**

⑤ **712.1** *Chondrocalcinosis due to dicalcium phosphate crystals*
[0-9]   Chondrocalcinosis due to dicalcium phosphate crystals (with other crystals)
          Code first underlying disease (275.4)

⑤ **712.2** *Chondrocalcinosis due to pyrophosphate crystals*
[0-9]   *Code first underlying disease (275.4)*

⑤ **712.3** *Chondrocalcinosis, unspecified*
[0-9]   *Code first underlying disease (275.4)*

⑤ **712.8** **Other specified crystal arthropathies**
[0-9]

⑤ **712.9** **Unspecified crystal arthropathy**
[0-9]

713 **Arthropathy associated with other disorders classified elsewhere**
          Includes: arthritis associated with conditions classifiable below
                     arthropathy associated with conditions classifiable below
                     polyarthritis associated with conditions classifiable below
                     polyarthropathy associated with conditions classifiable below

| | Add 4th or 5th digit | | Nonspecific code | | Unspecified code | | Manifestation code |

713.0 *Arthropathy associated with other endocrine and metabolic disorders*
   Code first underlying disease, as:
   acromegaly (253.0)
   hemochromatosis (275.0)
   hyperparathyroidism (252.00-252.08)
   hypogammaglobulinemia (279.00-279.09)
   hypothyroidism (243-244.9)
   lipoid metabolism disorder (272.0-272.9)
   ochronosis (270.2)

   | Excludes: | *arthropathy associated with:*

   amyloidosis (713.7)
   crystal deposition disorders, except gout (712.1-712.9)
   diabetic neuropathy (713.5)
   gout (274.00-274.03)

713.1 *Arthropathy associated with gastrointestinal conditions other than infections*
   Code first underlying disease, as:
   regional enteritis (555.0-555.9)
   ulcerative colitis (556)

713.2 *Arthropathy associated with hematological disorders*
   Code first underlying disease, as:
   hemoglobinopathy (282.4-282.7)
   hemophilia (286.0-286.2)
   leukemia (204.0-208.9)
   malignant reticulosis (202.3)
   multiple myelomatosis (203.0)

   | Excludes: | *arthropathy associated with Henoch-Schönlein purpura (713.6)*

713.3 *Arthropathy associated with dermatological disorders*
   Code first underlying disease, as:
   erythema multiforme (695.10-695.19)
   erythema nodosum (695.2)

   | Excludes: | *psoriatic arthropathy (696.0)*

713.4 *Arthropathy associated with respiratory disorders*
   Code first underlying disease, as:
   diseases classifiable to 490-519

   | Excludes: | *arthropathy associated with respiratory infections (711.0, 711.4-711.8)*

713.5 *Arthropathy associated with neurological disorders*
   Charcot's arthropathy associated with diseases classifiable elsewhere
   Neuropathic arthritis associated with diseases classifiable elsewhere
   Code first underlying disease, as:
   neuropathic joint disease [Charcot's joints]:
     NOS (094.0)
     diabetic (249.6, 250.6)
     syringomyelic (336.0)
     tabetic [syphilitic] (094.0)

713.6 *Arthropathy associated with hypersensitivity reaction*
   Code first underlying disease, as:
   Henoch (-Schönlein) purpura (287.0)
   serum sickness (999.5)

   | Excludes: | *allergic arthritis NOS (716.2)*

713.7 *Other general diseases with articular involvement*
   Code first underlying disease, as:
   amyloidosis (277.30-277.39)
   familial Mediterranean fever (277.31)
   sarcoidosis (135)

713.8 *Arthropathy associated with other conditions classifiable elsewhere*
   Code first underlying disease, as:
   conditions classifiable elsewhere except as in 711.1-711.8, 712, and 713.0-713.7

714 **Rheumatoid arthritis and other inflammatory polyarthropathies**
   | Excludes: | *rheumatic fever (390)*
   rheumatoid arthritis of spine NOS (720.0)

● Code new   ▲ Revision of   ④ ⑤ Fourth or fifth
  to this edition   existing code   digit required

714.0 Rheumatoid arthritis
Arthritis or polyarthritis:
atrophic
rheumatic (chronic)
Use additional code, if desired, to identify manifestation, as:
myopathy (359.6)
polyneuropathy (357.1)

> Excludes: *juvenile rheumatoid arthritis NOS (714.30)*

714.1 Felty's syndrome
Rheumatoid arthritis with splenoadenomegaly and leukopenia

714.2 Other rheumatoid arthritis with visceral or systemic involvement
Rheumatoid carditis

⑤ **714.3 Juvenile chronic polyarthritis**

> **714.30 Polyarticular juvenile rheumatoid arthritis, chronic or unspecified**
> Juvenile rheumatoid arthritis NOS
> Still's disease

> **714.31 Polyarticular juvenile rheumatoid arthritis, acute**

> **714.32 Pauciarticular juvenile rheumatoid arthritis**

> **714.33 Monoarticular juvenile rheumatoid arthritis**

714.4 Chronic postrheumatic arthropathy
Chronic rheumatoid nodular fibrositis
Jaccoud's syndrome

⑤ **714.8 Other specified inflammatory polyarthropathies**

> **714.81 Rheumatoid lung**
> Caplan's syndrome
> Diffuse interstitial rheumatoid disease of lung
> Fibrosing alveolitis, rheumatoid

> **714.89 Other**

714.9 Unspecified inflammatory polyarthropathy
Inflammatory polyarthropathy or polyarthritis NOS

> Excludes: *polyarthropathy NOS (716.5)*

⑤ **715 Osteoarthrosis and allied disorders**
Note: Localized, in the subcategories below, includes bilateral involvement of the same site.
Includes: arthritis or polyarthritis:
degenerative
hypertrophic
degenerative joint disease
osteoarthritis

> Excludes: *Marie-Strümpell spondylitis (720.0)*
> *osteoarthrosis [osteoarthritis] of spine (721.0-721.9)*

The following fifth-digit subclassification is for use with category 715; valid digits are in [brackets] under each code. See beginning of this chapter for definitions:

0 site unspecified
1 shoulder region
2 upper arm
3 forearm
4 hand
5 pelvic region and thigh
6 lower leg
7 ankle and foot
8 other specified sites
9 multiple sites

⑤ **715.0 Osteoarthrosis, generalized**
[0,4,9]   Degenerative joint disease, involving multiple joints
Primary generalized hypertrophic osteoarthrosis

⑤ **715.1 Osteoarthrosis, localized, primary**
[0-8]   Localized osteoarthropathy, idiopathic

⑤ **715.2 Osteoarthrosis, localized, secondary**
[0-8]   Coxae malum senilis

▰ Add 4th or 5th digit	▰ Nonspecific code	▰ Unspecified code	▰ Manifestation code

⑤ **715.3 Osteoarthrosis, localized, not specified whether primary or secondary**
[0-8]   Otto's pelvis

⑤ **715.8 Osteoarthrosis involving, or with mention of more than one site, but not specified as**
[0,9]   **generalized**

⑤ **715.9 Osteoarthrosis, unspecified whether generalized or localized**
[0-8]

⑤ **716** **Other and unspecified arthropathies**

> Excludes: *cricoarytenoid arthropathy (478.79)*

The following fifth-digit subclassification is for use with category 716; valid digits are in [brackets] under each code. See beginning of this chapter for definitions:

  0 site unspecified

  1 shoulder region

  2 upper arm

  3 forearm

  4 hand

  5 pelvic region and thigh

  6 lower leg

  7 ankle and foot

  8 other specified sites

  9 multiple sites

⑤ **716.0 Kaschin-Beck disease**
[0-9]   Endemic polyarthritis

⑤ **716.1 Traumatic arthropathy**
[0-9]

⑤ **716.2 Allergic arthritis**
[0-9]

> Excludes: *arthritis associated with Henoch-Schönlein purpura or serum sickness (713.6)*

⑤ **716.3 Climacteric arthritis**
[0-9]   Menopausal arthritis

⑤ **716.4 Transient arthropathy**
[0-9]

> Excludes: *palindromic rheumatism (719.3)*

⑤ **716.5 Unspecified polyarthropathy or polyarthritis**
[0-9]

⑤ **716.6 Unspecified monoarthritis**
[0-8]   Coxitis

⑤ **716.8 Other specified arthropathy**
[0-9]

⑤ **716.9 Arthropathy, unspecified**
[0-9]   Arthritis (acute) (chronic) (subacute)
          Arthropathy (acute) (chronic) (subacute)
          Articular rheumatism (chronic)
          Inflammation of joint NOS

717 **Internal derangement of knee**
     Includes: degeneration of articular cartilage or meniscus of knee
               rupture, old, of articular cartilage or meniscus of knee
               tear, old, of articular cartilage or meniscus of knee

> Excludes: *acute derangement of knee (836.0-836.6)*
>   *ankylosis (718.5)*
>   *contracture (718.4)*
>   *current injury (836.0-836.6)*
>   *deformity (736.4-736.6)*
>   *recurrent dislocation (718.3)*

717.0 Old bucket handle tear of medial meniscus
     Old bucket handle tear of unspecified cartilage

717.1 Derangement of anterior horn of medial meniscus

717.2 Derangement of posterior horn of medial meniscus

717.3 Other and unspecified derangement of medial meniscus
     Degeneration of internal semilunar cartilage

● Code new   ▲ Revision of   ④ ⑤ Fourth or fifth
       to this edition   existing code   digit required

⑤ **717.4 Derangement of lateral meniscus**

    717.40 Derangement of lateral meniscus, unspecified

    717.41 Bucket handle tear of lateral meniscus

    717.42 Derangement of anterior horn of lateral meniscus

    717.43 Derangement of posterior horn of lateral meniscus

    717.49 Other

717.5 Derangement of meniscus, not elsewhere classified
    Congenital discoid meniscus
    Cyst of semilunar cartilage
    Derangement of semilunar cartilage NOS

717.6 Loose body in knee
    Joint mice, knee
    Rice bodies, knee (joint)

717.7 Chondromalacia of patella
    Chondromalacia patellae
    Degeneration [softening] of articular cartilage of patella

⑤ **717.8 Other internal derangement of knee**

    717.81 Old disruption of lateral collateral ligament

    717.82 Old disruption of medial collateral ligament

    717.83 Old disruption of anterior cruciate ligament

    717.84 Old disruption of posterior cruciate ligament

    717.85 Old disruption of other ligaments of knee
        Capsular ligament of knee

    717.89 Other
        Old disruption of ligaments of knee NOS

717.9 Unspecified internal derangement of knee
    Derangement NOS of knee

⑤ **718 Other derangement of joint**

    Excludes: *current injury (830.0-848.9)*
              jaw (524.60-524.69)

The following fifth-digit subclassification is for use with category 718; valid digits are in [brackets] under each code. See beginning of this chapter for definitions:

    0 site unspecified

    1 shoulder region

    2 upper arm

    3 forearm

    4 hand

    5 pelvic region and thigh

    6 lower leg

    7 ankle and foot

    8 other specified sites

    9 multiple sites

⑤ **718.0 Articular cartilage disorder**
    [0-5, 7-9] Meniscus:
        disorder
        rupture, old
        tear, old
    Old rupture of ligament(s) of joint NOS

    Excludes: *articular cartilage disorder:*
        in ochronosis (270.2)
        knee (717.0-717.9)
        chondrocalcinosis (275.4)
        metastatic calcification (275.4)

⑤ **718.1 Loose body in joint**
    [0-5, 7-9] Joint mice

    Excludes: *knee (717.6)*

⑤ **718.2 Pathological dislocation**
    [0-9] Dislocation or displacement of joint, not recurrent and not current injury
        Spontaneous dislocation (joint)

	Add 4th or 5th digit		Nonspecific code		Unspecified code		Manifestation code

⑤ **718.3 Recurrent dislocation of joint**
[0-9]

⑤ **718.4 Contracture of joint**
[0-9]

⑤ **718.5 Ankylosis of joint**
[0-9]   Ankylosis of joint (fibrous) (osseous)

   Excludes: spine (724.9)
            stiffness of joint without mention of ankylosis (719.5)

⑤ **718.6 Unspecified intrapelvic protrusion of acetabulum**
[0, 5]   Protrusio acetabuli, unspecified

⑤ **718.7 Developmental dislocation of joint**
[0-9]

   Excludes: congenital dislocation of joint (754.0-755.8)
            traumatic dislocation of joint (830-839)

⑤ **718.8 Other joint derangement, not elsewhere classified**
[0-9]   Flail joint (paralytic)   Instability of joint

   Excludes: deformities classifiable to 736 (736.0-736.9)

⑤ **718.9 Unspecified derangement of joint**
[0-5, 7-9]

   Excludes: knee (717.9)

719 Other and unspecified disorders of joint

   Excludes: jaw (524.60-524.69)

   The following fifth-digit subclassification is for use with codes 719.0-719.6, 719.8-719.9; valid
      digits are in [brackets] under each code. See list at beginning of chapter for definitions:

   0 site unspecified

   1 shoulder region

   2 upper arm

   3 forearm

   4 hand

   5 pelvic region and thigh

   6 lower leg

   7 ankle and foot

   8 other specified sites

   9 multiple sites

⑤ **719.0 Effusion of joint**
[0-9]   Hydrarthrosis
         Swelling of joint, with or without pain

   Excludes: intermittent hydrarthrosis (719.3)

⑤ **719.1 Hemarthrosis**
[0-9]

   Excludes: current injury (840.0-848.9)

⑤ **719.2 Villonodular synovitis**
[0-9]

⑤ **719.3 Palindromic rheumatism**
[0-9]   Hench-Rosenberg syndrome
         Intermittent hydrarthrosis

⑤ **719.4 Pain in joint**
[0-9]   Arthralgia

⑤ **719.5 Stiffness of joint, not elsewhere classified**
[0-9]

⑤ **719.6 Other symptoms referable to joint**
[0-9]   Joint crepitus   Snapping hip

   719.7 Difficulty in walking

   Excludes: abnormality of gait (781.2)

● Code new   ▲ Revision of   ④ ⑤ Fourth or fifth
   to this edition   existing code   digit required

⑤ **719.8** **Other specified disorders of joint**
[0-9]   Calcification of joint   Fistula of joint

Excludes: *temporomandibular joint-pain-dysfunction syndrome [Costen's syndrome] (524.60)*

⑤ **719.9** **Unspecified disorder of joint**
[0-9]

DORSOPATHIES (720-724)

Excludes: *curvature of spine (737.0-737.9)*
osteochondrosis of spine (juvenile) (732.0)
adult (732.8)

720 **Ankylosing spondylitis and other inflammatory spondylopathies**

720.0 **Ankylosing spondylitis**
Rheumatoid arthritis of spine NOS
Spondylitis:
Marie-Strümpell
rheumatoid

720.1 **Spinal enthesopathy**
Disorder of peripheral ligamentous or muscular attachments of spine
Romanus lesion

720.2 **Sacroiliitis, not elsewhere classified**
Inflammation of sacroiliac joint NOS

⑤ **720.8** **Other inflammatory spondylopathies**

720.81 *Inflammatory spondylopathies in diseases classified elsewhere*
Code first underlying disease, as:
tuberculosis (015.0)

720.89 **Other**

720.9 **Unspecified inflammatory spondylopathy**
Spondylitis NOS

721 **Spondylosis and allied disorders**

721.0 **Cervical spondylosis without myelopathy**
Cervical or cervicodorsal:
arthritis
osteoarthritis
spondylarthritis

721.1 **Cervical spondylosis with myelopathy**
Anterior spinal artery compression syndrome
Spondylogenic compression of cervical spinal cord
Vertebral artery compression syndrome

721.2 **Thoracic spondylosis without myelopathy**
Thoracic:
arthritis
osteoarthritis
spondylarthritis

721.3 **Lumbosacral spondylosis without myelopathy**
Lumbar or lumbosacral:
arthritis
osteoarthritis
spondylarthritis

⑤ **721.4** **Thoracic or lumbar spondylosis with myelopathy**

721.41 **Thoracic region**
Spondylogenic compression of thoracic spinal cord

721.42 **Lumbar region**
Spondylogenic compression of lumbar spinal cord

721.5 **Kissing spine**
Baastrup's syndrome

721.6 **Ankylosing vertebral hyperostosis**

721.7 **Traumatic spondylopathy**
Kümmell's disease or spondylitis

721.8 **Other allied disorders of spine**

⑤ **721.9** **Spondylosis of unspecified site**

517

▮ Add 4th or 5th digit	▮ Nonspecific code	▮ Unspecified code	▮ Manifestation code

721.90 Without mention of myelopathy
Spinal:
   arthritis (deformans) (degenerative) (hypertrophic)
   osteoarthritis NOS
Spondylarthrosis NOS

721.91 With myelopathy
Spondylogenic compression of spinal cord NOS

722 Intervertebral disc disorders

722.0 Displacement of cervical intervertebral disc without myelopathy
Neuritis (brachial) or radiculitis due to displacement or rupture of cervical intervertebral disc
Any condition classifiable to 722.2 of the cervical or cervicothoracic intervertebral disc

⑤ **722.1 Displacement of thoracic or lumbar intervertebral disc without myelopathy**

722.10 Lumbar intervertebral disc without myelopathy
Lumbago or sciatica due to displacement of intervertebral disc
Neuritis or radiculitis due to displacement or rupture of lumbar intervertebral disc
Any condition classifiable to 722.2 of the lumbar or lumbosacral intervertebral disc

722.11 Thoracic intervertebral disc without myelopathy
Any condition classifiable to 722.2 of thoracic intervertebral disc

722.2 Displacement of intervertebral disc, site unspecified, without myelopathy
Discogenic syndrome NOS
Herniation of nucleus pulposus NOS
Intervertebral disc NOS:
   extrusion
   prolapse
   protrusion
   rupture
Neuritis or radiculitis due to displacement or rupture of intervertebral disc

⑤ **722.3 Schmorl's nodes**

722.30 Unspecified region

722.31 Thoracic region

722.32 Lumbar region

722.39 Other

722.4 Degeneration of cervical intervertebral disc
Degeneration of cervicothoracic intervertebral disc

⑤ **722.5 Degeneration of thoracic or lumbar intervertebral disc**

722.51 Thoracic or thoracolumbar intervertebral disc

722.52 Lumbar or lumbosacral intervertebral disc

722.6 Degeneration of intervertebral disc, site unspecified
Degenerative disc disease NOS
Narrowing of intervertebral disc or space NOS

⑤ **722.7 Intervertebral disc disorder with myelopathy**

722.70 Unspecified region

722.71 Cervical region

722.72 Thoracic region

722.73 Lumbar region

⑤ **722.8 Postlaminectomy syndrome**

722.80 Unspecified region

722.81 Cervical region

722.82 Thoracic region

722.83 Lumbar region

⑤ **722.9 Other and unspecified disc disorder**
Calcification of intervertebral cartilage or disc
Discitis

722.90 Unspecified region

722.91 Cervical region

722.92 Thoracic region

722.93 Lumbar region

● Code new to this edition   ▲ Revision of existing code   ④ ⑤ Fourth or fifth digit required

723 Other disorders of cervical region

> *Excludes:* conditions due to:
> > intervertebral disc disorders (722.0-722.9)
> > spondylosis (721.0-721.9)

723.0 Spinal stenosis in cervical region

723.1 Cervicalgia
Pain in neck

723.2 Cervicocranial syndrome
Barré-Liéou syndrome
Posterior cervical sympathetic syndrome

723.3 Cervicobrachial syndrome (diffuse)

723.4 Brachial neuritis or radiculitis NOS
Cervical radiculitis
Radicular syndrome of upper limbs

723.5 Torticollis, unspecified
Contracture of neck

> *Excludes:* congenital (754.1)
> > due to birth injury (767.8)
> > hysterical (300.11)
> > ocular torticollis (781.93)
> > psychogenic (306.0)
> > spasmodic (333.83)
> > traumatic, current (847.0)

723.6 Panniculitis specified as affecting neck

723.7 Ossification of posterior longitudinal ligament in cervical region

723.8 Other syndromes affecting cervical region
Cervical syndrome NEC
Klippel's disease
Occipital neuralgia

723.9 Unspecified musculoskeletal disorders and symptoms referable to neck
Cervical (region) disorder NOS

724 Other and unspecified disorders of back

> *Excludes:* collapsed vertebra (code to cause, e.g., osteoporosis, 733.00-733.09)
> > conditions due to:
> > > intervertebral disc disorders (722.0-722.9)
> > > spondylosis (721.0-721.9)

⑤ **724.0** Spinal stenosis, other than cervical

> **724.00** Spinal stenosis, unspecified region
>
> **724.01** Thoracic region
>
> **724.02** Lumbar region
>
> **724.09** Other

724.1 Pain in thoracic spine

724.2 Lumbago
Low back pain
Low back syndrome
Lumbalgia

724.3 Sciatica
Neuralgia or neuritis of sciatic nerve

> *Excludes:* specified lesion of sciatic nerve (355.0)

724.4 Thoracic or lumbosacral neuritis or radiculitis, unspecified
Radicular syndrome of lower limbs

724.5 Backache, unspecified
Vertebrogenic (pain) syndrome NOS

724.6 Disorders of sacrum
Ankylosis, lumbosacral or sacroiliac (joint)
Instability, lumbosacral or sacroiliac (joint)

⑤ **724.7** Disorders of coccyx

> **724.70** Unspecified disorder of coccyx
>
> **724.71** Hypermobility of coccyx

	Add 4th or 5th digit		Nonspecific code		Unspecified code		Manifestation code

724.79 Other
Coccygodynia

724.8 **Other symptoms referable to back**
Ossification of posterior longitudinal ligament NOS
Panniculitis specified as sacral or affecting back

724.9 **Other unspecified back disorders**
Ankylosis of spine NOS
Compression of spinal nerve root NEC
Spinal disorder NOS

Excludes: *sacroiliitis (720.2)*

RHEUMATISM, EXCLUDING THE BACK (725-729)

Includes: disorders of muscles and tendons and their attachments, and of other soft tissues

725 **Polymyalgia rheumatica**

726 **Peripheral enthesopathies and allied syndromes**
Note: Enthesopathies are disorders of peripheral ligamentous or muscular attachments.

Excludes: *spinal enthesopathy (720.1)*

726.0 **Adhesive capsulitis of shoulder**

⑤ **726.1** **Rotator cuff syndrome of shoulder and allied disorders**

   726.10 **Disorders of bursae and tendons in shoulder region, unspecified**
   Rotator cuff syndrome NOS
   Supraspinatus syndrome NOS

   726.11 **Calcifying tendinitis of shoulder**

   726.12 **Bicipital tenosynovitis**

   726.19 **Other specified disorders**

Excludes: *complete rupture of rotator cuff, nontraumatic (727.61)*

726.2 **Other affections of shoulder region, not elsewhere classified**
Periarthritis of shoulder
Scapulohumeral fibrositis

⑤ **726.3** **Enthesopathy of elbow region**

   726.30 **Enthesopathy of elbow, unspecified**

   726.31 **Medial epicondylitis**

   726.32 **Lateral epicondylitis**
   Epicondylitis NOS
   Golfers' elbow
   Tennis elbow

   726.33 **Olecranon bursitis**
   Bursitis of elbow

   726.39 **Other**

726.4 **Enthesopathy of wrist and carpus**
Bursitis of hand or wrist
Periarthritis of wrist

726.5 **Enthesopathy of hip region**
Bursitis of hip   Psoas tendinitis
Gluteal tendinitis   Trochanteric tendinitis
Iliac crest spur

⑤ **726.6** **Enthesopathy of knee**

   726.60 **Enthesopathy of knee, unspecified**
   Bursitis of knee NOS

   726.61 **Pes anserinus tendinitis or bursitis**

   726.62 **Tibial collateral ligament bursitis**
   Pellegrini-Stieda syndrome

   726.63 **Fibular collateral ligament bursitis**

   726.64 **Patellar tendinitis**

   726.65 **Prepatellar bursitis**

   726.69 **Other**
   Bursitis:
      infrapatellar
      subpatellar

● Code new   ▲ Revision of   ④ ⑤ Fourth or fifth
      to this edition   existing code   digit required

⑤ **726.7 Enthesopathy of ankle and tarsus**

726.70 Enthesopathy of ankle and tarsus, unspecified
Metatarsalgia NOS

| Excludes: | Morton's metatarsalgia (355.6) |

726.71 Achilles bursitis or tendinitis

726.72 Tibialis tendinitis
Tibialis (anterior) (posterior) tendinitis

726.73 Calcaneal spur

726.79 Other
Peroneal tendinitis

726.8 Other peripheral enthesopathies

⑤ **726.9 Unspecified enthesopathy**

726.90 Enthesopathy of unspecified site
Capsulitis NOS
Periarthritis NOS
Tendinitis NOS

726.91 Exostosis of unspecified site
Bone spur NOS

727 Other disorders of synovium, tendon, and bursa

⑤ **727.0 Synovitis and tenosynovitis**

727.00 Synovitis and tenosynovitis, unspecified
Synovitis NOS
Tenosynovitis NOS

727.01 Synovitis and tenosynovitis in diseases classified elsewhere
Code first underlying disease, as:
tuberculosis (015.0-015.9)

Excludes:	crystal-induced (275.4)
	gonococcal (098.51)
	gout (274.00-274.03)
	syphilitic (095.7)

727.02 Giant cell tumor of tendon sheath

727.03 Trigger finger (acquired)

727.04 Radial styloid tenosynovitis
de Quervain's disease

727.05 Other tenosynovitis of hand and wrist

727.06 Tenosynovitis of foot and ankle

727.09 Other

727.1 Bunion

727.2 Specific bursitides often of occupational origin
Beat:
elbow
hand
knee
Chronic crepitant synovitis of wrist
Miners':
elbow
knee

727.3 Other bursitis
Bursitis NOS

Excludes:	bursitis:
	gonococcal (098.52)
	subacromial (726.19)
	subcoracoid (726.19)
	subdeltoid (726.19)
	syphilitic (095.7)
	"frozen shoulder" (726.0)

⑤ **727.4 Ganglion and cyst of synovium, tendon, and bursa**

727.40 Synovial cyst, unspecified

| Excludes: | that of popliteal space (727.51) |

727.41 Ganglion of joint

| | Add 4th or 5th digit | | Nonspecific code | | Unspecified code | | Manifestation code |

727.42 **Ganglion of tendon sheath**

727.43 **Ganglion, unspecified**

727.49 **Other**
Cyst of bursa

⑤ 727.5 **Rupture of synovium**

727.50 **Rupture of synovium, unspecified**

727.51 **Synovial cyst of popliteal space**
Baker's cyst (knee)

727.59 **Other**

⑤ 727.6 **Rupture of tendon, nontraumatic**

727.60 **Nontraumatic rupture of unspecified tendon**

727.61 **Complete rupture of rotator cuff**

727.62 **Tendons of biceps (long head)**

727.63 **Extensor tendons of hand and wrist**

727.64 **Flexor tendons of hand and wrist**

727.65 **Quadriceps tendon**

727.66 **Patellar tendon**

727.67 **Achilles tendon**

727.68 **Other tendons of foot and ankle**

727.69 **Other**

⑤ 727.8 **Other disorders of synovium, tendon, and bursa**

727.81 **Contracture of tendon (sheath)**
Short Achilles tendon (acquired)

727.82 **Calcium deposits in tendon and bursa**
Calcification of tendon NOS
Calcific tendinitis NOS

Excludes: *peripheral ligamentous or muscular attachments (726.0-726.9)*

727.83 **Plica syndrome**
Plica knee

727.89 **Other**
Abscess of bursa or tendon

Excludes: *xanthomatosis localized to tendons (272.7)*

727.9 **Unspecified disorder of synovium, tendon, and bursa**

728 **Disorders of muscle, ligament, and fascia**

Excludes: *enthesopathies (726.0-726.9)*
muscular dystrophies (359.0-359.1)
myoneural disorders (358.00-358.9)
myopathies (359.2-359.9)
nontraumatic hematoma of muscle (729.92)
old disruption of ligaments of knee (717.81-717.89)

728.0 **Infective myositis**
Myositis:
purulent
suppurative

Excludes: *myositis:*
epidemic (074.1)
interstitial (728.81)
syphilitic (095.6)
tropical (040.81)

⑤ 728.1 **Muscular calcification and ossification**

728.10 **Calcification and ossification, unspecified**
Massive calcification (paraplegic)

728.11 **Progressive myositis ossificans**

728.12 **Traumatic myositis ossificans**
Myositis ossificans (circumscripta)

728.13 **Postoperative heterotopic calcification**

728.19 **Other**
Polymyositis ossificans

● Code new
to this edition

▲ Revision of
existing code

④ ⑤ Fourth or fifth
digit required

728.2 Muscular wasting and disuse atrophy, not elsewhere classified
Amyotrophia NOS
Myofibrosis

Excludes:	*neuralgic amyotrophy (353.5)*
	pelvic muscle wasting and disuse atrophy (618.83)
	progressive muscular atrophy (335.0-335.9)

728.3 Other specific muscle disorders
Arthrogryposis
Immobility syndrome (paraplegic)

Excludes:	*arthrogryposis multiplex congenita (754.89)*
	stiff-man syndrome (333.91)

728.4 Laxity of ligament

728.5 Hypermobility syndrome

728.6 Contracture of palmar fascia
Dupuytren's contracture

⑤ **728.7 Other fibromatoses**

    728.71 Plantar fascial fibromatosis
    Contracture of plantar fascia
    Plantar fasciitis (traumatic)

    728.79 Other
    Garrod's or knuckle pads
    Nodular fasciitis
    Pseudosarcomatous fibromatosis (proliferative) (subcutaneous)

⑤ **728.8 Other disorders of muscle, ligament, and fascia**

    728.81 Interstitial myositis

    728.82 Foreign body granuloma of muscle
    Talc granuloma of muscle

    728.83 Rupture of muscle, nontraumatic

    728.84 Diastasis of muscle
    Diastasis recti (abdomen)

Excludes:	*diastasis recti complicating pregnancy, labor, and delivery (665.8)*

    728.85 Spasm of muscle

    728.86 Necrotizing fasciitis
    Use additional code to identify:
    infectious organism (041.00 - 041.89)
    gangrene (785.4), if applicable

    728.87 Muscle weakness (generalized)

Excludes:	*generalized weakness (780.79)*

    728.88 Rhabdomyolysis

    728.89 Other
    Eosinophilic fasciitis
    Use additional E code, if desired, to identify drug, if drug induced

728.9 Unspecified disorder of muscle, ligament, and fascia

729 Other disorders of soft tissues

Excludes:	*acroparesthesia (443.89)*
	carpal tunnel syndrome (354.0)
	disorders of the back (720.0-724.9)
	entrapment syndromes (354.0-355.9)
	palindromic rheumatism (719.3)
	periarthritis (726.0-726.9)
	psychogenic rheumatism (306.0)

729.0 Rheumatism, unspecified and fibrositis

729.1 Myalgia and myositis, unspecified
Fibromyositis NOS

Add 4th or 5th digit	Nonspecific code	Unspecified code	Manifestation code

729.2 Neuralgia, neuritis, and radiculitis, unspecified

Excludes: *brachial radiculitis (723.4)*
cervical radiculitis (723.4)
lumbosacral radiculitis (724.4)
mononeuritis (354.0-355.9)
radiculitis due to intervertebral disc involvement (722.0-722.2, 722.7)
sciatica (724.3)

⑤ **729.3 Panniculitis, unspecified**

729.30 Panniculitis, unspecified site
Weber-Christian disease

729.31 Hypertrophy of fat pad, knee
Hypertrophy of infrapatellar fat pad

729.39 Other site

Excludes: *panniculitis specified as (affecting):*
back (724.8)
neck (723.6)
sacral (724.8)

729.4 Fasciitis, unspecified

Excludes: *necrotizing fasciitis (728.86)*
nodular fasciitis (728.79)

729.5 Pain in limb

729.6 Residual foreign body in soft tissue

Excludes: *foreign body granuloma:*
muscle (728.82)
skin and subcutaneous tissue (709.4)

⑤ **729.7 Nontraumatic compartment syndrome**
Code first, if applicable, postprocedural complication (998.89)

Excludes: *compartment syndrome NOS (958.90)*
traumatic compartment syndrome (958.90-958.99)

729.71 Nontraumatic compartment syndrome of upper extremity
Nontraumatic compartment syndrome of shoulder, arm, forearm, wrist, hand and fingers

729.72 Nontraumatic compartment syndrome of lower extremity
Nontraumatic compartment syndrome of hip, buttock, thigh, leg, foot and toes

729.73 Nontraumatic compartment syndrome of abdomen

729.79 Nontraumatic compartment syndrome of other sites

⑤ **729.8 Other musculoskeletal symptoms referable to limbs**

729.81 Swelling of limb

729.82 Cramp

729.89 Other

Excludes: *abnormality of gait (781.2)*
tetany (781.7)
transient paralysis of limb (781.4)

⑤ **729.9 Other and unspecified disorders of soft tissue**

729.90 Disorders of soft tissue, unspecified

729.91 Post-traumatic seroma

Excludes: *seroma complicating a procedure (998.13)*

729.92 Nontraumatic hematoma of soft tissue
Nontraumatic hematoma of muscle

729.99 Other disorders of soft tissue
Polyalgia

OSTEOPATHIES, CHONDROPATHIES, AND ACQUIRED MUSCULOSKELETAL DEFORMITIES (730-739)

⑤ **730 Osteomyelitis, periostitis, and other infections involving bone**

Excludes: *jaw (526.4-526.5)*
petrous bone (383.2)

Use additional code, if desired, to identify organism, such as Staphylococcus (041.1)

● Code new
to this edition

▲ Revision of
existing code

④ ⑤ Fourth or fifth
digit required

The following fifth-digit subclassification is for use with category 730; valid digits are in [brackets] under each code. See beginning of this chapter for definitions:

0 site unspecified

1 shoulder region

2 upper arm

3 forearm

4 hand

5 pelvic region and thigh

6 lower leg

7 ankle and foot

8 other specified sites

9 multiple sites

⑤ **730.0 Acute osteomyelitis**
[0-9] Abscess of any bone except accessory sinus, jaw, or mastoid
Acute or subacute osteomyelitis, with or without mention of periostitis
Use additional code to identify major osseous defect, if applicable (731.3)

⑤ **730.1 Chronic osteomyelitis**
[0-9] Brodie's abscess
Chronic or old osteomyelitis, with or without mention of periostitis
Sequestrum of bone
Sclerosing osteomyelitis of Garré
Use additional code to identify major osseous defect, if applicable (731.3)
Excludes: *aseptic necrosis of bone (733.40-733.49)*

⑤ **730.2 Unspecified osteomyelitis**
[0-9] Osteitis or osteomyelitis NOS, with or without mention of periostitis
Use additional code to identify major osseous defect, if applicable (731.3)

⑤ **730.3 Periostitis without mention of osteomyelitis**
[0-9] Abscess of periosteum without mention of osteomyelitis
Periostosis without mention of osteomyelitis
Excludes: *that in secondary syphilis (091.61)*

⑤ **730.7 *Osteopathy resulting from poliomyelitis***
[0-9] *Code first underlying disease (045.0-045.9)*

⑤ **730.8 *Other infections involving bone in diseases classified elsewhere***
[0-9] *Code first underlying disease, as:*
tuberculosis (015.0-015.9)
typhoid fever (002.0)
Excludes: *syphilis of bone NOS (095.5)*

⑤ **730.9 Unspecified infection of bone**
[0-9]

731 Osteitis deformans and osteopathies associated with other disorders classified elsewhere

731.0 Osteitis deformans without mention of bone tumor
Paget's disease of bone

731.1 *Osteitis deformans in diseases classified elsewhere*
Code first underlying disease, as:
malignant neoplasm of bone (170.0-170.9)

731.2 Hypertrophic pulmonary osteoarthropathy
Bamberger-Marie disease

731.3 Major osseous defects
Code first underlying disease, if known, such as:
aseptic necrosis (733.40-733.49)
malignant neoplasm of bone (170.0-170.9)
osteomyelitis (730.00-730.29)
osteoporosis (733.00-733.09)
peri-prosthetic osteolysis (996.45)

731.8 *Other bone involvement in diseases classified elsewhere*
Code first underlying disease, as:
diabetes mellitus (249.8, 250.8)
Use additional code to specify bone condition, such as:
acute osteomyelitis (730.00-730.09)

| Add 4th or 5th digit | Nonspecific code | Unspecified code | Manifestation code |

`732` Osteochondropathies

732.0 Juvenile osteochondrosis of spine
Juvenile osteochondrosis (of):
    marginal or vertebral epiphysis (of Scheuermann)
    spine NOS
Vertebral epiphysitis

> Excludes: *adolescent postural kyphosis (737.0)*

732.1 Juvenile osteochondrosis of hip and pelvis
Coxa plana
Ischiopubic synchondrosis (of van Neck)
Osteochondrosis (juvenile) of:
    acetabulum
    head of femur (of Legg-Calvé-Perthes)
    iliac crest (of Buchanan)
    symphysis pubis (of Pierson)
Pseudocoxalgia

732.2 Nontraumatic slipped upper femoral epiphysis
Slipped upper femoral epiphysis NOS

732.3 Juvenile osteochondrosis of upper extremity
Osteochondrosis (juvenile) of:
    capitulum of humerus (of Panner)
    carpal lunate (of Kienbock)
    hand NOS
    head of humerus (of Haas)
    heads of metacarpals (of Mauclaire)
    lower ulna (of Burns)
    radial head (of Brailsford)
    upper extremity NOS

732.4 Juvenile osteochondrosis of lower extremity, excluding foot
Osteochondrosis (juvenile) of:
    lower extremity NOS
    primary patellar center (of Köhler)
    proximal tibia (of Blount)
    secondary patellar center (of Sinding-Larsen)
    tibial tubercle (of Osgood-Schlatter)
Tibia vara

732.5 Juvenile osteochondrosis of foot
Calcaneal apophysitis
Epiphysitis, os calcis
Osteochondrosis (juvenile) of:
    astragalus (of Diaz)
    calcaneum (of Sever)
    foot NOS
    metatarsal
        second (of Freiberg)
        fifth (of Iselin)
    os tibiale externum (Haglund)
    tarsal navicular (of Köhler)

732.6 Other juvenile osteochondrosis
Apophysitis specified as juvenile, of other site, or site NOS
Epiphysitis specified as juvenile, of other site, or site NOS
Osteochondritis specified as juvenile, of other site, or site NOS
Osteochondrosis specified as juvenile, of other site, or site NOS

732.7 Osteochondritis dissecans

732.8 Other specified forms of osteochondropathy
Adult osteochondrosis of spine

● Code new   ▲ Revision of   ④ ⑤ Fourth or fifth
       to this edition   existing code   digit required

732.9 Unspecified osteochondropathy
  Apophysitis
  NOS
  not specified as adult or juvenile, of unspecified site
  Epiphysitis
  NOS
  not specified as adult or juvenile, of unspecified site
  Osteochondritis
  NOS
  not specified as adult or juvenile, of unspecified site
  Osteochondrosis
  NOS
  not specified as adult or juvenile, of unspecified site

733 Other disorders of bone and cartilage

  Excludes: *bone spur (726.91)*
       cartilage of, or loose body in, joint (717.0-717.9, 718.0-718.9)
       giant cell granuloma of jaw (526.3)
       osteitis fibrosa cystica generalisata (252.01)
       osteomalacia (268.2)
       polyostotic fibrous dysplasia of bone (756.54)
       prognathism, retrognathism (524.1)
       xanthomatosis localized to bone (272.7)

⑤ **733.0 Osteoporosis**
  Use additional code to identify major osseous defect, if applicable (731.3)
  Use additional code to identify personal history of pathologic (healed) fracture (V13.51)

  733.00 Osteoporosis, unspecified
      Wedging of vertebra NOS

  733.01 Senile osteoporosis
      Postmenopausal osteoporosis

  733.02 Idiopathic osteoporosis

  733.03 Disuse osteoporosis

  733.09 Other
      Drug-induced osteoporosis
  Use additional E code, if desired, to identify drug

⑤ **733.1 Pathologic fracture**
  Chronic fracture
  Spontaneous fracture

  Excludes: *traumatic fracture (800-829)*
       stress fracture (733.93-733.95)

  733.10 Pathologic fracture, unspecified site

  733.11 Pathologic fracture of humerus

  733.12 Pathologic fracture of distal radius and ulna
      Wrist NOS

  733.13 Pathologic fracture of vertebrae
      Collapse of vertebra NOS

  733.14 Pathologic fracture of neck of femur
      Femur NOS
      Hip NOS

  733.15 Pathologic fracture of other specified part of femur

  733.16 Pathologic fracture of tibia or fibula
      Ankle NOS

  733.19 Pathologic fracture of other specified site

⑤ **733.2 Cyst of bone**

  733.20 Cyst of bone (localized), unspecified

  733.21 Solitary bone cyst
      Unicameral bone cyst

  733.22 Aneurysmal bone cyst

  733.29 Other
      Fibrous dysplasia (monostotic)

  Excludes: *cyst of jaw (526.0-526.2, 526.89)*
       osteitis fibrosa cystica (252.01)
       polyostotic fibrous dysplasia of bone (756.54)

| | Add 4th or 5th digit | | Nonspecific code | | Unspecified code | | Manifestation code |

733.3 Hyperostosis of skull
Hyperostosis interna frontalis
Leontiasis ossium

⑤ **733.4 Aseptic necrosis of bone**
Use additional code to identify major osseous defect, if applicable (731.3)
Excludes: *osteochondropathies (732.0-732.9)*

733.40 Aseptic necrosis of bone, site unspecified

733.41 Head of humerus

733.42 Head and neck of femur
Femur NOS
Excludes: *Legg-Calvé-Perthes disease (732.1)*

733.43 Medial femoral condyle

733.44 Talus

733.45 Jaw
Use additional E code to identify drug, if drug-induced
Excludes: *osteoradionecrosis of jaw (526.89)*

733.49 Other

733.5 Osteitis condensans
Piriform sclerosis of ilium

733.6 Tietze's disease
Costochondral junction syndrome
Costochondritis

733.7 Algoneurodystrophy
Disuse atrophy of bone
Sudeck's atrophy

⑤ **733.8 Malunion and nonunion of fracture**

733.81 Malunion of fracture

733.82 Nonunion of fracture
Pseudoarthrosis (bone)

⑤ **733.9 Other and unspecified disorders of bone and cartilage**

733.90 Disorder of bone and cartilage, unspecified

733.91 Arrest of bone development or growth
Epiphyseal arrest

733.92 Chondromalacia
Chondromalacia:
  NOS
  localized, except patella
  systemic
  tibial plateau
Excludes: *chondromalacia of patella (717.7)*

733.93 Stress fracture of tibia or fibula
Stress reaction of tibia or fibula
Use additional external cause code(s) to identify the cause of the stress fracture

733.94 Stress fracture of the metatarsals
Stress reaction of metatarsals
Use additional external cause code(s) to identify the cause of the stress fracture

733.95 Stress fracture of other bone
Stress reaction of other bone
Use additional external cause code(s) to identify the cause of the stress fracture
Excludes: *stress fracture of:*
  femoral neck (733.96)
  fibula (733.93)
  metatarsals (733.94)
  pelvis (733.98)
  shaft of femur (733.97)
  tibia (733.93)

733.96 Stress fracture of femoral neck
Stress reaction of femoral neck
Use additional external cause code(s) to identify the cause of the stress fracture

● Code new to this edition   ▲ Revision of existing code   ④ ⑤ Fourth or fifth digit required

733.97 Stress fracture of shaft of femur
Stress reaction of shaft of femur

Use additional external cause code(s) to identify the cause of the stress fracture

733.98 Stress fracture of pelvis
Stress reaction of pelvis

Use additional external cause code(s) to identify the cause of the stress fracture

733.99 Other
Diaphysitis
Hypertrophy of bone
Relapsing polychondritis

734 Flat foot
Pes planus (acquired)
Talipes planus (acquired)

Excludes: congenital (754.61)
rigid flat foot (754.61)
spastic (everted) flat foot (754.61)

735 Acquired deformities of toe

Excludes: congenital (754.60-754.69, 755.65-755.66)

735.0 Hallux valgus (acquired)

735.1 Hallux varus (acquired)

735.2 Hallux rigidus

735.3 Hallux malleus

735.4 Other hammer toe (acquired)

735.5 Claw toe (acquired)

735.8 Other acquired deformities of toe

735.9 Unspecified acquired deformity of toe

736 Other acquired deformities of limbs

Excludes: congenital (754.3-755.9)

⑤ **736.0 Acquired deformities of forearm, excluding fingers**

736.00 Unspecified deformity
Deformity of elbow, forearm, hand, or wrist (acquired) NOS

736.01 Cubitus valgus (acquired)

736.02 Cubitus varus (acquired)

736.03 Valgus deformity of wrist (acquired)

736.04 Varus deformity of wrist (acquired)

736.05 Wrist drop (acquired)

736.06 Claw hand (acquired)

736.07 Club hand, acquired

736.09 Other

736.1 Mallet finger

⑤ **736.2 Other acquired deformities of finger**

736.20 Unspecified deformity
Deformity of finger (acquired) NOS

736.21 Boutonniere deformity

736.22 Swan-neck deformity

736.29 Other

Excludes: trigger finger (727.03)

⑤ **736.3 Acquired deformities of hip**

736.30 Unspecified deformity
Deformity of hip (acquired) NOS

736.31 Coxa valga (acquired)

736.32 Coxa vara (acquired)

736.39 Other

⑤ **736.4 Genu valgum or varum (acquired)**

736.41 Genu valgum (acquired)

	Add 4th or 5th digit		Nonspecific code		Unspecified code		Manifestation code

736.42 Genu varum (acquired)

736.5 Genu recurvatum (acquired)

736.6 Other acquired deformities of knee
Deformity of knee (acquired) NOS

⑤ **736.7 Other acquired deformities of ankle and foot**
Excludes: deformities of toe (acquired) (735.0-735.9)
pes planus (acquired) (734)

736.70 Unspecified deformity of ankle and foot, acquired

736.71 Acquired equinovarus deformity
Clubfoot, acquired
Excludes: clubfoot not specified as acquired (754.5-754.7)

736.72 Equinus deformity of foot, acquired

736.73 Cavus deformity of foot
Excludes: that with claw foot (736.74)

736.74 Claw foot, acquired

736.75 Cavovarus deformity of foot, acquired

736.76 Other calcaneus deformity

736.79 Other
Acquired:
pes not elsewhere classified
talipes not elsewhere classified

⑤ **736.8 Acquired deformities of other parts of limbs**

736.81 Unequal leg length (acquired)

736.89 Other
Deformity (acquired):
arm or leg, not elsewhere classified
shoulder

736.9 Acquired deformity of limb, site unspecified

737 Curvature of spine
Excludes: congenital (754.2)

737.0 Adolescent postural kyphosis
Excludes: osteochondrosis of spine (juvenile) (732.0)
adult (732.8)

⑤ **737.1 Kyphosis (acquired)**

737.10 Kyphosis (acquired) (postural)

737.11 Kyphosis due to radiation

737.12 Kyphosis, postlaminectomy

737.19 Other
Excludes: that associated with conditions classifiable elsewhere (737.41)

⑤ **737.2 Lordosis (acquired)**

737.20 Lordosis (acquired) (postural)

737.21 Lordosis, postlaminectomy

737.22 Other postsurgical lordosis

737.29 Other
Excludes: that associated with conditions classifiable elsewhere (737.42)

⑤ **737.3 Kyphoscoliosis and scoliosis**

737.30 Scoliosis [and kyphoscoliosis], idiopathic

737.31 Resolving infantile idiopathic scoliosis

737.32 Progressive infantile idiopathic scoliosis

737.33 Scoliosis due to radiation

737.34 Thoracogenic scoliosis

737.39 Other
Excludes: that associated with conditions classifiable elsewhere (737.43)
that in kyphoscoliotic heart disease (416.1)

● Code new to this edition   ▲ Revision of existing code   ④ ⑤ Fourth or fifth digit required

⑤ **737.4** *Curvature of spine associated with other conditions*
Code first associated condition, as:
Charcot-Marie-Tooth disease (356.1)
mucopolysaccharidosis (277.5)
neurofibromatosis (237.7)
osteitis deformans (731.0)
osteitis fibrosa cystica (252.01)
osteoporosis (733.00-733.09)
poliomyelitis (138)
tuberculosis [Pott's curvature] (015.0)

737.40 *Curvature of spine, unspecified*

737.41 *Kyphosis*

737.42 *Lordosis*

737.43 *Scoliosis*

737.8 **Other curvatures of spine**

737.9 **Unspecified curvature of spine**
Curvature of spine (acquired) (idiopathic) NOS
Hunchback, acquired

Excludes: *deformity of spine NOS (738.5)*

738 **Other acquired deformity**

Excludes: *congenital (754.0-756.9, 758.0-759.9)*
dentofacial anomalies (524.0-524.9)

738.0 **Acquired deformity of nose**
Deformity of nose (acquired)
Overdevelopment of nasal bones

Excludes: *deflected or deviated nasal septum (470)*

⑤ **738.1** **Other acquired deformity of head**

738.10 **Unspecified deformity**

738.11 **Zygomatic hyperplasia**

738.12 **Zygomatic hypoplasia**

738.19 **Other specified deformity**

738.2 **Acquired deformity of neck**

738.3 **Acquired deformity of chest and rib**
Deformity: Pectus:
  chest (acquired)   carinatum, acquired
  rib (acquired)   excavatum, acquired

738.4 **Acquired spondylolisthesis**
Degenerative spondylolisthesis
Spondylolysis, acquired

Excludes: *congenital (756.12)*

738.5 **Other acquired deformity of back or spine**
Deformity of spine NOS

Excludes: *curvature of spine (737.0-737.9)*

738.6 **Acquired deformity of pelvis**
Pelvic obliquity

Excludes: *intrapelvic protrusion of acetabulum (718.6)*
that in relation to labor and delivery (653.0-653.4, 653.8-653.9)

738.7 **Cauliflower ear**

738.8 **Acquired deformity of other specified site**
Deformity of clavicle

738.9 **Acquired deformity of unspecified site**

739 **Nonallopathic lesions, not elsewhere classified**
Includes: segmental dysfunction
           somatic dysfunction

739.0 **Head region**
Occipitocervical region

739.1 **Cervical region**
Cervicothoracic region

	Add 4th or 5th digit		Nonspecific code		Unspecified code		Manifestation code

739.2 Thoracic region
Thoracolumbar region

739.3 Lumbar region
Lumbosacral region

739.4 Sacral region
Sacrococcygeal region
Sacroiliac region

739.5 Pelvic region
Hip region
Pubic region

739.6 Lower extremities

739.7 Upper extremities
Acromioclavicular region
Sternoclavicular region

739.8 Rib cage
Costochondral region   Sternochondral region
Costovertebral region

739.9 Abdomen and other

● Code new to this edition   ▲ Revision of existing code   ④ ⑤ Fourth or fifth digit required

14. CONGENITAL ANOMALIES (740-759)

740 Anencephalus and similar anomalies

740.0 Anencephalus

Acrania	Hemianencephaly
Amyelencephalus	Hemicephaly

740.1 Craniorachischisis

740.2 Iniencephaly

⑤ **741 Spina bifida**

Excludes: *spina bifida occulta (756.17)*

The following fifth-digit subclassification is for use with category 741:

0 unspecified region

1 cervical region

2 dorsal [thoracic] region

3 lumbar region

⑤ **741.0 With hydrocephalus**
[0-3]   Arnold-Chiari syndrome, type II
Any condition classifiable to 741.9 with any condition classifiable to 742.3
Chiari malformation, type II

⑤ **741.9 Without mention of hydrocephalus**
[0-3]   Hydromeningocele (spinal)

Hydromyelocele	Myelocystocele
Meningocele (spinal)	Rachischisis
Meningomyelocele	Spina bifida (aperta)
Myelocele	Syringomyelocele

742 Other congenital anomalies of nervous system

Excludes: *congenital central alveolar hypoventilation syndrome (327.25)*

742.0 Encephalocele

Encephalocystocele	Meningocele, cerebral
Encephalomyelocele	Meningoencephalocele
Hydroencephalocele	
Hydromeningocele, cranial	

742.1 Microcephalus
Hydromicrocephaly
Micrencephaly

742.2 Reduction deformities of brain
Absence of part of brain
Agenesis of part of brain
Agyria
Aplasia of part of brain
Arhinencephaly
Hypoplasia of part of brain
Holoprosencephaly
Microgyria

742.3 Congenital hydrocephalus
Aqueduct of Sylvius:
   anomaly
   obstruction, congenital
   stenosis
Atresia of foramina of Magendie and Luschka
Hydrocephalus in newborn

Excludes: *hydrocephalus:*
   acquired (331.3-331.4)
   due to congenital toxoplasmosis (771.2)
   with any condition classifiable to 741.9 (741.0)

742.4 Other specified anomalies of brain

Congenital cerebral cyst	Multiple anomalies of brain NOS
Macroencephaly	Porencephaly
Macrogyria	Ulegyria
Megalencephaly	

⑤ **742.5 Other specified anomalies of spinal cord**

742.51 Diastematomyelia

				533
Add 4th or 5th digit	Nonspecific code	Unspecified code	Manifestation code	

742.53 Hydromyelia
Hydrorhachis

742.59 Other
Amyelia
Atelomyelia
Congenital anomaly of spinal meninges
Defective development of cauda equina
Hypoplasia of spinal cord
Myelatelia
Myelodysplasia

742.8 Other specified anomalies of nervous system

Agenesis of nerve
Displacement of brachial
  plexus
Familial dysautonomia

Jaw-winking syndrome
Marcus-Gunn syndrome
Riley-Day syndrome

Excludes: *neurofibromatosis (237.7)*

742.9 Unspecified anomaly of brain, spinal cord, and nervous system
Anomaly of brain, nervous system, and spinal cord
Congenital:
  disease of brain, nervous system, and spinal cord
  lesion of brain, nervous system, and spinal cord
Deformity of brain, nervous system, and spinal cord

743 Congenital anomalies of eye

⑤ **743.0 Anophthalmos**

743.00 Clinical anophthalmos, unspecified
Agenesis of eye
Congenital absence of eye
Anophthalmos NOS

743.03 Cystic eyeball, congenital

743.06 Cryptophthalmos

⑤ **743.1 Microphthalmos**
Dysplasia of eye
Hypoplasia of eye
Rudimentary eye

743.10 Microphthalmos, unspecified

743.11 Simple microphthalmos

743.12 Microphthalmos associated with other anomalies of eye and adnexa

⑤ **743.2 Buphthalmos**
Glaucoma: Hydrophthalmos
  congenital
  newborn

Excludes: *glaucoma of childhood (365.14)*
         traumatic glaucoma due to birth injury (767.8)

743.20 Buphthalmos, unspecified

743.21 Simple buphthalmos

743.22 Buphthalmos associated with other ocular anomalies
Keratoglobus, congenital associated with buphthalmos
Megalocornea associated with buphthalmos

⑤ **743.3 Congenital cataract and lens anomalies**

Excludes: *infantile cataract (366.00-366.09)*

743.30 Congenital cataract, unspecified

743.31 Capsular and subcapsular cataract

743.32 Cortical and zonular cataract

743.33 Nuclear cataract

743.34 Total and subtotal cataract, congenital

743.35 Congenital aphakia
Congenital absence of lens

743.36 Anomalies of lens shape
Microphakia
Spherophakia

743.37 Congenital ectopic lens

● Code new
  to this edition
▲ Revision of
  existing code
④ ⑤ Fourth or fifth
     digit required

743.39 Other

⑤ **743.4** Coloboma and other anomalies of anterior segment

    743.41 Anomalies of corneal size and shape
        Microcornea

    Excludes: *that associated with buphthalmos (743.22)*

    743.42 Corneal opacities, interfering with vision, congenital

    743.43 Other corneal opacities, congenital

    743.44 Specified anomalies of anterior chamber, chamber angle, and related structures
        Anomaly:
          Axenfeld's
          Peters'
          Rieger's

    743.45 Aniridia

    743.46 Other specified anomalies of iris and ciliary body
        Anisocoria, congenital
        Atresia of pupil
        Coloboma of iris
        Corectopia

    743.47 Specified anomalies of sclera

    743.48 Multiple and combined anomalies of anterior segment

    743.49 Other

⑤ **743.5** Congenital anomalies of posterior segment

    743.51 Vitreous anomalies
        Congenital vitreous opacity

    743.52 Fundus coloboma

    743.53 Chorioretinal degeneration, congenital

    743.54 Congenital folds and cysts of posterior segment

    743.55 Congenital macular changes

    743.56 Other retinal changes, congenital

    743.57 Specified anomalies of optic disc
        Coloboma of optic disc (congenital)

    743.58 Vascular anomalies
        Congenital retinal aneurysm

    743.59 Other

⑤ **743.6** Congenital anomalies of eyelids, lacrimal system, and orbit

    743.61 Congenital ptosis

    743.62 Congenital deformities of eyelids
        Ablepharon   Congenital:
        Absence of eyelid   ectropion
        Accessory eyelid   entropion

    743.63 Other specified congenital anomalies of eyelid
        Absence, agenesis, of cilia

    743.64 Specified congenital anomalies of lacrimal gland

    743.65 Specified congenital anomalies of lacrimal passages
        Absence, agenesis of:
          lacrimal apparatus
          punctum lacrimale
        Accessory lacrimal canal

    743.66 Specified congenital anomalies of orbit

    743.69 Other
        Accessory eye muscles

743.8 Other specified anomalies of eye

    Excludes: *congenital nystagmus (379.51)*
          ocular albinism (270.2)
          optic nerve hypoplasia (377.43)
          retinitis pigmentosa (362.74)

| ▓ Add 4th or 5th digit | ▓ Nonspecific code | ▓ Unspecified code | ▓ Manifestation code |

743.9 Unspecified anomaly of eye
Congenital:
  anomaly NOS of eye [any part]
  deformity NOS of eye [any part]

744 Congenital anomalies of ear, face, and neck
Excludes: anomaly of:
    cervical spine (754.2, 756.10-756.19)
    larynx (748.2-748.3)
    nose (748.0-748.1)
    parathyroid gland (759.2)
    thyroid gland (759.2)
  cleft lip (749.10-749.25)

⑤ **744.0 Anomalies of ear causing impairment of hearing**
Excludes: congenital deafness without mention of cause (389.0-389.9)

744.00 Unspecified anomaly of ear with impairment of hearing

744.01 Absence of external ear
Absence of:
  auditory canal (external)
  auricle (ear) (with stenosis or atresia of auditory canal)

744.02 Other anomalies of external ear with impairment of hearing
Atresia or stricture of auditory canal (external)

744.03 Anomaly of middle ear, except ossicles
Atresia or stricture of osseous meatus (ear)

744.04 Anomalies of ear ossicles
Fusion of ear ossicles

744.05 Anomalies of inner ear
Congenital anomaly of:
  membranous labyrinth
  organ of Corti

744.09 Other
Absence of ear, congenital

744.1 Accessory auricle
Accessory tragus   Supernumerary:
Polyotia   ear
Preauricular appendage lobule

⑤ **744.2 Other specified anomalies of ear**
Excludes: that with impairment of hearing (744.00-744.09)

744.21 Absence of ear lobe, congenital

744.22 Macrotia

744.23 Microtia

744.24 Specified anomalies of Eustachian tube
Absence of Eustachian tube

744.29 Other
Bat ear   Prominence of auricle
Darwin's tubercle   Ridge ear
Pointed ear

Excludes: preauricular sinus (744.46)

744.3 Unspecified anomaly of ear
Congenital:
  anomaly NOS of ear, not elsewhere classified
  deformity NOS of ear, not elsewhere classified

⑤ **744.4 Branchial cleft cyst or fistula; preauricular sinus**

744.41 Branchial cleft sinus or fistula
Branchial:
  sinus (external) (internal)
  vestige

744.42 Branchial cleft cyst

744.43 Cervical auricle

744.46 Preauricular sinus or fistula

744.47 Preauricular cyst

● Code new to this edition   ▲ Revision of existing code   ④ ⑤ Fourth or fifth digit required

744.49 **Other**
Fistula (of):
  auricle, congenital
  cervicoaural

744.5 **Webbing of neck**
Pterygium colli

⑤ **744.8** **Other specified anomalies of face and neck**

744.81 **Macrocheilia**
Hypertrophy of lip, congenital

744.82 **Microcheilia**

744.83 **Macrostomia**

744.84 **Microstomia**

744.89 **Other**

Excludes: *congenital fistula of lip (750.25)*
    musculoskeletal anomalies (754.0-754.1, 756.0)

744.9 **Unspecified anomalies of face and neck**
Congenital:
  anomaly NOS of face [any part] or neck [any part]
  deformity NOS of face [any part] or neck [any part]

745 **Bulbus cordis anomalies and anomalies of cardiac septal closure**

745.0 **Common truncus**
Absent septum between aorta and pulmonary artery
Communication (abnormal) between aorta and pulmonary artery
Aortic septal defect
Common aortopulmonary trunk
Persistent truncus arteriosus

⑤ **745.1** **Transposition of great vessels**

745.10 **Complete transposition of great vessels**
Transposition of great vessels:
  NOS
  classical

745.11 **Double outlet right ventricle**
Dextratransposition of aorta
Incomplete transposition of great vessels
Origin of both great vessels from right ventricle
Taussig-Bing syndrome or defect

745.12 **Corrected transposition of great vessels**

745.19 **Other**

745.2 **Tetralogy of Fallot**
Fallot's pentalogy
Ventricular septal defect with pulmonary stenosis or atresia, dextraposition of aorta, and
  hypertrophy of right ventricle

Excludes: *Fallot's triad (746.09)*

745.3 **Common ventricle**
Cor triloculare biatriatum
Single ventricle

745.4 **Ventricular septal defect**
Eisenmenger's defect or complex
Gerbode defect
Interventricular septal defect
Left ventricular-right atrial communication
Roger's disease

Excludes: *common atrioventricular canal type (745.69)*
    single ventricle (745.3)

745.5 **Ostium secundum type atrial septal defect**
Defect: Patent or persistent:
  atrium secundum   foramen ovale
  fossa ovalis   ostium secundum
  Lutembacher's syndrome

⑤ **745.6** **Endocardial cushion defects**

745.60 **Endocardial cushion defect, unspecified type**

| | Add 4th or 5th digit | | Nonspecific code | | Unspecified code | | Manifestation code |

745.61 Ostium primum defect
Persistent ostium primum

745.69 Other
Absence of atrial septum
Atrioventricular canal type ventricular septal defect
Common atrioventricular canal
Common atrium

745.7 Cor biloculare
Absence of atrial and ventricular septa

745.8 Other

745.9 Unspecified defect of septal closure
Septal defect NOS

746 Other congenital anomalies of heart

Excludes: *endocardial fibroelastosis (425.3)*

⑤ **746.0 Anomalies of pulmonary valve**

Excludes: *infundibular or subvalvular pulmonic stenosis (746.83)*
tetralogy of Fallot (745.2)

746.00 Pulmonary valve anomaly, unspecified

746.01 Atresia, congenital
Congenital absence of pulmonary valve

746.02 Stenosis, congenital

746.09 Other
Congenital insufficiency of pulmonary valve
Fallot's triad or trilogy

746.1 Tricuspid atresia and stenosis, congenital
Absence of tricuspid valve

746.2 Ebstein's anomaly

746.3 Congenital stenosis of aortic valve
Congenital aortic stenosis

Excludes: *congenital:*
subaortic stenosis (746.81)
supravalvular aortic stenosis (747.22)

746.4 Congenital insufficiency of aortic valve
Bicuspid aortic valve
Congenital aortic insufficiency

746.5 Congenital mitral stenosis
Fused commissure of mitral valve
Parachute deformity of mitral valve
Supernumerary cusps of mitral valve

746.6 Congenital mitral insufficiency

746.7 Hypoplastic left heart syndrome
Atresia, or marked hypoplasia, of aortic orifice or valve, with hypoplasia of ascending aorta and defective development of left ventricle (with mitral valve atresia)

⑤ **746.8 Other specified anomalies of heart**

746.81 Subaortic stenosis

746.82 Cor triatriatum

746.83 Infundibular pulmonic stenosis
Subvalvular pulmonic stenosis

746.84 Obstructive anomalies of heart, not elsewhere classified
Shone's syndrome
Uhl's disease

Use additional code for associated anomalies, such as:
coarctation of aorta (747.10)
congenital mitral stenosis (746.5)
subaortic stenosis (746.81)

746.85 Coronary artery anomaly
Anomalous origin or communication of coronary artery
Arteriovenous malformation of coronary artery
Coronary artery:
absence
arising from aorta or pulmonary trunk
single

● Code new
to this edition

▲ Revision of
existing code

④ ⑤ Fourth or fifth
digit required

746.86 Congenital heart block
Complete or incomplete atrioventricular [AV] block

746.87 Malposition of heart and cardiac apex
Abdominal heart   Levocardia (isolated)
Dextrocardia   Mesocardia
Ectopia cordis

Excludes: *dextrocardia with complete transposition of viscera (759.3)*

746.89 Other
Atresia of cardiac vein
Hypoplasia of cardiac vein
Congenital:
  cardiomegaly
  diverticulum, left ventricle
  pericardial defect

746.9 Unspecified anomaly of heart
Congenital:
  anomaly of heart NOS
  heart disease NOS

747 Other congenital anomalies of circulatory system

747.0 Patent ductus arteriosus
Patent ductus Botalli
Persistent ductus arteriosus

⑤ **747.1 Coarctation of aorta**

747.10 Coarctation of aorta (preductal) (postductal)
Hypoplasia of aortic arch

747.11 Interruption of aortic arch

⑤ **747.2 Other anomalies of aorta**

747.20 Anomaly of aorta, unspecified

747.21 Anomalies of aortic arch
Anomalous origin, right subclavian artery
Dextraposition of aorta
Double aortic arch
Kommerell's diverticulum
Overriding aorta
Persistent:
  convolutions, aortic arch
  right aortic arch
Vascular ring

Excludes: *hypoplasia of aortic arch (747.10)*

747.22 Atresia and stenosis of aorta
Absence of aorta
Aplasia of aorta
Hypoplasia of aorta
Stricture of aorta
Supra (valvular)-aortic stenosis

Excludes: *congenital aortic (valvular) stenosis or stricture, so stated (746.3)*
hypoplasia of aorta in hypoplastic left heart syndrome (746.7)

747.29 Other
Aneurysm of sinus of Valsalva
Congenital:
  aneurysm of aorta
  dilation of aorta

747.3 Anomalies of pulmonary artery
Agenesis of pulmonary artery
Anomaly of pulmonary artery
Atresia of pulmonary artery
Coarctation of pulmonary artery
Hypoplasia of pulmonary artery
Stenosis of pulmonary artery
Pulmonary arteriovenous aneurysm

⑤ **747.4 Anomalies of great veins**

747.40 Anomaly of great veins, unspecified
Anomaly NOS of:
  pulmonary veins
  vena cava

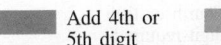 Add 4th or 5th digit

 Nonspecific code

 Unspecified code

Manifestation code

539

747.41 Total anomalous pulmonary venous connection
Total anomalous pulmonary venous return [TAPVR]:
subdiaphragmatic
supradiaphragmatic

747.42 Partial anomalous pulmonary venous connection
Partial anomalous pulmonary venous return

747.49 Other anomalies of great veins
Absence of vena cava (inferior) (superior)
Congenital stenosis of vena cava (inferior) (superior)
Persistent:
left posterior cardinal vein
left superior vena cava
Scimitar syndrome
Transposition of pulmonary veins NOS

747.5 Absence or hypoplasia of umbilical artery
Single umbilical artery

⑤ **747.6 Other anomalies of peripheral vascular system**
Absence of artery or vein, not elsewhere classified
Anomaly of artery or vein, not elsewhere classified
Atresia of artery or vein, not elsewhere classified
Arteriovenous aneurysm (peripheral)
Arteriovenous malformation of the peripheral vascular system
Congenital:
aneurysm (peripheral)
phlebectasia
stricture, artery
varix
Multiple renal arteries

Excludes: anomalies of:
cerebral vessels (747.81)
pulmonary artery (747.3)
congenital retinal aneurysm (743.58)
hemangioma (228.00-228.09)
lymphangioma (228.1)

747.60 Anomaly of the peripheral vascular system, unspecified site
747.61 Gastrointestinal vessel anomaly
747.62 Renal vessel anomaly
747.63 Upper limb vessel anomaly
747.64 Lower limb vessel anomaly
747.69 Anomalies of other specified sites of peripheral vascular system

⑤ **747.8 Other specified anomalies of circulatory system**

747.81 Anomalies of cerebrovascular system
Arteriovenous malformation of brain
Cerebral arteriovenous aneurysm, congenital
Congenital anomalies of cerebral vessels

Excludes: ruptured cerebral (arteriovenous) aneurysm (430)

747.82 Spinal vessel anomaly
Arteriovenous malformation of spinal vessel

747.83 Persistent fetal circulation
Persistent pulmonary hypertension
Primary pulmonary hypertension of newborn

747.89 Other
Aneurysm, congenital, specified site not elsewhere classified

Excludes: congenital aneurysm:
coronary (746.85)
peripheral (747.6)
pulmonary (747.3)
retinal (743.58)

747.9 Unspecified anomaly of circulatory system
748 Congenital anomalies of respiratory system

Excludes: congenital central alveolar hypoventilation syndrome (327.25)
congenital defect of diaphragm (756.6)

● Code new to this edition   ▲ Revision of existing code   ④ ⑤ Fourth or fifth digit required

748.0 Choanal atresia
Atresia of nares (anterior) (posterior)
Congenital stenosis of nares (anterior) (posterior)

748.1 Other anomalies of nose
Absent nose
Accessory nose
Cleft nose
Deformity of wall of nasal
sinus

Congenital:
deformity of nose
notching of tip of nose
perforation of wall of nasal sinus

Excludes: congenital deviation of nasal septum (754.0)

748.2 Web of larynx
Web of larynx:
NOS
glottic
subglottic

748.3 Other anomalies of larynx, trachea, and bronchus
Absence or agenesis of:
bronchus
larynx
trachea
Anomaly (of):
cricoid cartilage
epiglottis
thyroid cartilage
tracheal cartilage
Atresia (of):
epiglottis
glottis
larynx
trachea
Cleft thyroid, cartilage,
congenital

Congenital:
dilation, trachea
stenosis:
larynx
trachea
tracheocele
Diverticulum:
bronchus
trachea
Fissure of epiglottis
Laryngocele
Posterior cleft of cricoid cartilage (congenital)
Rudimentary tracheal bronchus
Stridor, laryngeal, congenital

748.4 Congenital cystic lung
Disease, lung:
cystic, congenital
polycystic, congenital

Honeycomb lung, congenital

Excludes: acquired or unspecified cystic lung (518.89)

748.5 Agenesis, hypoplasia, and dysplasia of lung
Absence of lung (fissures) (lobe)
Aplasia of lung
Hypoplasia of lung (lobe)
Sequestration of lung

⑤ **748.6 Other anomalies of lung**

748.60 Anomaly of lung, unspecified

748.61 Congenital bronchiectasis

748.69 Other
Accessory lung (lobe)
Azygos lobe (fissure), lung

748.8 Other specified anomalies of respiratory system
Abnormal communication between pericardial and pleural sacs
Anomaly, pleural folds
Atresia of nasopharynx
Congenital cyst of mediastinum

748.9 Unspecified anomaly of respiratory system
Anomaly of respiratory system NOS

749 Cleft palate and cleft lip
⑤ **749.0 Cleft palate**

749.00 Cleft palate, unspecified

749.01 Unilateral, complete

749.02 Unilateral, incomplete
Cleft uvula

749.03 Bilateral, complete

749.04 Bilateral, incomplete

Add 4th or 5th digit | Nonspecific code | Unspecified code | Manifestation code

⑤ **749.1 Cleft lip**
    Cheiloschisis   Harelip
    Congenital fissure of lip   Labium leporinum

    749.10   **Cleft lip, unspecified**

    749.11   **Unilateral, complete**

    749.12   **Unilateral, incomplete**

    749.13   **Bilateral, complete**

    749.14   **Bilateral, incomplete**

⑤ **749.2 Cleft palate with cleft lip**
    Cheilopalatoschisis

    749.20   **Cleft palate with cleft lip, unspecified**

    749.21   **Unilateral, complete**

    749.22   **Unilateral, incomplete**

    749.23   **Bilateral, complete**

    749.24   **Bilateral, incomplete**

    749.25   **Other combinations**

750 **Other congenital anomalies of upper alimentary tract**

    Excludes: dentofacial anomalies (524.0-524.9)

  750.0 Tongue tie
    Ankyloglossia

⑤ **750.1 Other anomalies of tongue**

    750.10   **Anomaly of tongue, unspecified**

    750.11   **Aglossia**

    750.12   **Congenital adhesions of tongue**

    750.13   **Fissure of tongue**
          Bifid tongue
          Double tongue

    750.15   **Macroglossia**
          Congenital hypertrophy of tongue

    750.16   **Microglossia**
          Hypoplasia of tongue

    750.19   **Other**

⑤ **750.2 Other specified anomalies of mouth and pharynx**

    750.21   **Absence of salivary gland**

    750.22   **Accessory salivary gland**

    750.23   **Atresia, salivary duct**
          Imperforate salivary duct

    750.24   **Congenital fistula of salivary gland**

    750.25   **Congenital fistula of lip**
          Congenital (mucus) lip pits

    750.26   **Other specified anomalies of mouth**
          Absence of uvula

    750.27   **Diverticulum of pharynx**
          Pharyngeal pouch

    750.29   **Other specified anomalies of pharynx**
          Imperforate pharynx

  750.3 Tracheoesophageal fistula, esophageal atresia and stenosis
    Absent esophagus   Congenital fistula:
    Atresia of esophagus   esophagobronchial
    Congenital: esophagotracheal
      esophageal ring   Imperforate esophagus
      stenosis of esophagus   Webbed esophagus
      stricture of esophagus

● Code new   ▲ Revision of   ④ ⑤ Fourth or fifth
  to this edition   existing code   digit required

750.4 Other specified anomalies of esophagus
Dilatation, congenital (of) esophagus
Displacement, congenital (of) esophagus
Diverticulum (of) esophagus
Duplication (of) esophagus
Giant esophagus
Esophageal pouch

Excludes: *congenital hiatus hernia (750.6)*

750.5 Congenital hypertrophic pyloric stenosis
Congenital or infantile:
constriction of pylorus
hypertrophy of pylorus
spasm of pylorus
stenosis of pylorus
stricture of pylorus

750.6 Congenital hiatus hernia
Displacement of cardia through esophageal hiatus

Excludes: *congenital diaphragmatic hernia (756.6)*

750.7 Other specified anomalies of stomach

Congenital:	Duplication of stomach
cardiospasm	Megalogastria
hourglass stomach	Microgastria
Displacement of stomach	Transposition of stomach
Diverticulum of stomach, congenital	

750.8 Other specified anomalies of upper alimentary tract

750.9 Unspecified anomaly of upper alimentary tract
Congenital:
anomaly NOS of upper alimentary tract [any part, except tongue]
deformity NOS of upper alimentary tract [any part, except tongue]

751 Other congenital anomalies of digestive system

751.0 Meckel's diverticulum
Meckel's diverticulum (displaced) (hypertrophic)
Persistent:
omphalomesenteric duct
vitelline duct

751.1 Atresia and stenosis of small intestine
Atresia of:
duodenum
ileum
intestine NOS
Congenital:
absence of small intestine or intestine NOS
obstruction of small intestine or intestine NOS
stenosis of small intestine or intestine NOS
stricture of small intestine or intestine NOS
Imperforate jejunum

751.2 Atresia and stenosis of large intestine, rectum, and anal canal

Absence:	Congenital or infantile:
anus (congenital)	obstruction of large intestine
appendix, congenital	occlusion of anus
large intestine, congenital	stricture of anus
rectum	Imperforate:
Atresia of:	anus
anus	rectum
colon	Stricture of rectum, congenital
rectum	

751.3 Hirschsprung's disease and other congenital functional disorders of colon

Aganglionosis	Congenital megacolon
Congenital dilation of colon	Macrocolon

751.4 Anomalies of intestinal fixation

Congenital adhesions:	Rotation of cecum or colon:
omental, anomalous	failure of
peritoneal	incomplete
Jackson's membrane	insufficient
Malrotation of colon	Universal mesentery

Add 4th or 5th digit	Nonspecific code	Unspecified code	Manifestation code

751.5 Other anomalies of intestine
Congenital diverticulum,   Megaloappendix
  colon   Megaloduodenum
Dolichocolon   Microcolon
Duplication of: Persistent cloaca
  anus   Transposition of:
  appendix   appendix
  cecum   colon
  intestine   intestine
Ectopic anus

⑤ **751.6 Anomalies of gallbladder, bile ducts, and liver**

751.60 Unspecified anomaly of gallbladder, bile ducts, and liver

751.61 Biliary atresia
Congenital:
  absence of bile duct (common) or passage
  hypoplasia of bile duct (common) or passage
  obstruction of bile duct (common) or passage
  stricture of bile duct (common) or passage

751.62 Congenital cystic disease of liver
Congenital polycystic disease of liver
Fibrocystic disease of liver

751.69 Other anomalies of gallbladder, bile ducts, and liver
Absence of: Duplication of:
  gallbladder, congenital   biliary duct
  liver (lobe)   cystic duct
Accessory: gallbladder
  hepatic ducts   liver
  liver   Floating:
Congenital: gallbladder
  choledochal cyst   liver
  hepatomegaly   Intrahepatic gallbladder

751.7 Anomalies of pancreas
Absence of pancreas
Accessory pancreas
Agenesis of pancreas
Annular pancreas
Ectopic pancreatic tissue
Hypoplasia of pancreas
Pancreatic heterotopia

Excludes: *diabetes mellitus (249.0-249.9, 250.0-250.9)*
fibrocystic disease of pancreas (277.00-277.09)
neonatal diabetes mellitus (775.1)

751.8 Other specified anomalies of digestive system
Absence (complete) (partial) of alimentary tract NOS
Duplication of digestive organs NOS
Malposition, congenital of digestive organs NOS

Excludes: *congenital diaphragmatic hernia (756.6)*
congenital hiatus hernia (750.6)

751.9 Unspecified anomaly of digestive system
Congenital:
  anomaly NOS of digestive system NOS
  deformity NOS of digestive system NOS

752 Congenital anomalies of genital organs

Excludes: *syndromes associated with anomalies in the number and form of chromosomes (758.0-758.9)*

752.0 Anomalies of ovaries
Absence, congenital (of) ovary
Accessory ovary
Ectopic ovary
Streak of ovary

⑤ **752.1 Anomalies of fallopian tubes and broad ligaments**

752.10 Unspecified anomaly of fallopian tubes and broad ligaments

● Code new to this edition   ▲ Revision of existing code   ④ ⑤ Fourth or fifth digit required

752.11 Embryonic cyst of fallopian tubes and broad ligaments
Cyst:
epoophoron
fimbrial
parovarian

752.19 Other
Absence of fallopian tube or broad ligament
Accessory fallopian tube or broad ligament
Atresia of fallopian tube or broad ligament

752.2 Doubling of uterus
Didelphic uterus
Doubling of uterus [any degree] (associated with doubling of cervix and vagina)

752.3 Other anomalies of uterus
Absence, congenital, of uterus
Agenesis of uterus
Aplasia of uterus
Bicornuate uterus
Uterus unicornis
Uterus with only one functioning horn

⑤ **752.4 Anomalies of cervix, vagina, and external female genitalia**

752.40 Unspecified anomaly of cervix, vagina, and external female genitalia

752.41 Embryonic cyst of cervix, vagina, and external female genitalia
Cyst of: Cyst of:
canal of Nuck, congenital   vagina, embryonal
Gartner's duct   vulva, congenital

752.42 Imperforate hymen

752.49 Other anomalies of cervix, vagina, and external female genitalia
Absence of cervix, clitoris, vagina, or vulva
Agenesis of cervix, clitoris, vagina, or vulva
Congenital stenosis or stricture of:
cervical canal
vagina

Excludes: double vagina associated with total duplication (752.2)

⑤ **752.5 Undescended and retractile testicle**

752.51 Undescended testis
Cryptorchism
Ectopic testis

752.52 Retractile testis

⑤ **752.6 Hypospadias and epispadias and other penile anomalies**

752.61 Hypospadias

752.62 Epispadias
Anaspadias

752.63 Congenital chordee

752.64 Micropenis

752.65 Hidden penis

752.69 Other penile anomalies

752.7 Indeterminate sex and pseudohermaphroditism
Gynandrism   Pseudohermaphroditism (male) (female)
Hermaphroditism   Pure gonadal dysgenesis
Ovotestis

Excludes: androgen insensitivity (259.50-259.52)
pseudohermaphroditism:
female, with adrenocortical disorder (255.2)
male, with gonadal disorder (257.8)
with specified chromosomal anomaly (758.0-758.9)
testicular feminization syndrome (259.50-259.72)

⑤ **752.8 Other specified anomalies of genital organs**
Excludes: congenital hydrocele (778.6)
penile anomalies (752.61-752.69)
phimosis or paraphimosis (605)

752.81 Scrotal transposition

Add 4th or 5th digit | Nonspecific code | Unspecified code | Manifestation code

752.89 **Other specified anomalies of genital organs**
Absence of:
  prostate
  spermatic cord
  vas deferens
Anorchism
Aplasia (congenital) of:
  prostate
  round ligament
  testicle
Atresia of:
  ejaculatory duct
  vas deferens
Fusion of testes
Hypoplasia of testes
Monorchism
Polyorchism

752.9 **Unspecified anomaly of genital organs**
Congenital:
  anomaly NOS of genital organ, NEC
  deformity NOS of genital organ, NEC

753 **Congenital anomalies of urinary system**

753.0 **Renal agenesis and dysgenesis**

Atrophy of kidney:	Congenital absence of kidney(s)
congenital	Hypoplasia of kidney(s)
infantile	

⑤ **753.1** **Cystic kidney disease**

Excludes: *acquired cyst of kidney (593.2)*

753.10 **Cystic kidney disease, unspecified**

753.11 **Congenital single renal cyst**

753.12 **Polycystic kidney, unspecified type**

753.13 **Polycystic kidney, autosomal dominant**

753.14 **Polycystic kidney, autosomal recessive**

753.15 **Renal dysplasia**

753.16 **Medullary cystic kidney**
Nephronopthisis

753.17 **Medullary sponge kidney**

753.19 **Other specified cystic kidney disease**
Multicystic kidney

⑤ **753.2** **Obstructive defects of renal pelvis and ureter**

753.20 **Unspecified obstructive defect of renal pelvis and ureter**

753.21 **Congenital obstruction of ureteropelvic junction**

753.22 **Congenital obstruction of ureterovesical junction**
Adynamic ureter
Congenital hydroureter

753.23 **Congenital ureterocele**

753.29 **Other**

753.3 **Other specified anomalies of kidney**

Accessory kidney	Fusion of kidneys
Congenital:	Giant kidney
calculus of kidney	Horseshoe kidney
displaced kidney	Hyperplasia of kidney
Discoid kidney	Lobulation of kidney
Double kidney with double	Malrotation of kidney
pelvis	Trifid kidney (pelvis)
Ectopic kidney	

753.4 **Other specified anomalies of ureter**

Absent ureter	Double ureter
Accessory ureter	Ectopic ureter
Deviation of ureter	Implantation, anomalous of ureter
Displaced ureteric orifice	

753.5 **Exstrophy of urinary bladder**

Ectopia vesicae	Extroversion of bladder

● Code new
to this edition

▲ Revision of
existing code

④ ⑤ Fourth or fifth
digit required

753.6 Atresia and stenosis of urethra and bladder neck
    Congenital obstruction: Imperforate urinary meatus
      bladder neck   Impervious urethra
      urethra   Urethral valve formation
    Congenital stricture of:
    urethra (valvular)
    urinary meatus
    vesicourethral orifice

753.7 Anomalies of urachus
    Cyst (of) urachus   Persistent umbilical sinus
    Fistula (of) urachus
    Patent (of) urachus

753.8 Other specified anomalies of bladder and urethra
    Absence, congenital of: Congenital urethrorectal fistula
      bladder   Congenital prolapse of:
      urethra   bladder (mucosa)
    Accessory: urethra
      bladder   Double:
      urethra   urethra
    Congenital: urinary meatus
      diverticulum of bladder
      hernia of bladder

753.9 Unspecified anomaly of urinary system
    Congenital:
    anomaly NOS of urinary system [any part, except urachus]
    deformity NOS of urinary system [any part, except urachus]

754 Certain congenital musculoskeletal deformities
    Includes: nonteratogenic deformities which are considered to be due to intrauterine malposition and pressure

754.0 Of skull, face, and jaw
    Asymmetry of face   Dolichocephaly
    Compression facies   Plagiocephaly
    Depressions in skull   Potter's facies
    Deviation of nasal   Squashed or bent nose, congenital
      septum, congenital

    Excludes: dentofacial anomalies (524.0-524.9)
              syphilitic saddle nose (090.5)

754.1 Of sternocleidomastoid muscle
    Congenital sternomastoid torticollis
    Congenital wryneck
    Contracture of sternocleidomastoid (muscle)
    Sternomastoid tumor

754.2 Of spine
    Congenital postural:
    lordosis
    scoliosis

⑤ **754.3 Congenital dislocation of hip**

    754.30 Congenital dislocation of hip, unilateral
      Congenital dislocation of hip NOS

    754.31 Congenital dislocation of hip, bilateral

    754.32 Congenital subluxation of hip, unilateral
      Congenital flexion deformity, hip or thigh
      Predislocation status of hip at birth
      Preluxation of hip, congenital

    754.33 Congenital subluxation of hip, bilateral

    754.35 Congenital dislocation of one hip with subluxation of other hip

⑤ **754.4 Congenital genu recurvatum and bowing of long bones of leg**

    754.40 Genu recurvatum

    754.41 Congenital dislocation of knee (with genu recurvatum)

    754.42 Congenital bowing of femur

    754.43 Congenital bowing of tibia and fibula

    754.44 Congenital bowing of unspecified long bones of leg

Add 4th or 5th digit   Nonspecific code   Unspecified code   Manifestation code

⑤ **754.5 Varus deformities of feet**

Excludes: *acquired (736.71, 736.75, 736.79)*

754.50 Talipes varus
Congenital varus deformity of foot, unspecified
Pes varus

754.51 Talipes equinovarus
Equinovarus (congenital)

754.52 Metatarsus primus varus

754.53 Metatarsus varus

754.59 Other
Talipes calcaneovarus

⑤ **754.6 Valgus deformities of feet**

Excludes: *valgus deformity of foot (acquired) (736.79)*

754.60 Talipes valgus
Congenital valgus deformity of foot, unspecified

754.61 Congenital pes planus
Congenital rocker bottom flat foot
Flat foot, congenital

Excludes: *pes planus (acquired) (734)*

754.62 Talipes calcaneovalgus

754.69 Other
Talipes:
  equinovalgus
  planovalgus

⑤ **754.7 Other deformities of feet**

Excludes: *acquired (736.70-736.79)*

754.70 Talipes, unspecified
Congenital deformity of foot NOS

754.71 Talipes cavus
Cavus foot (congenital)

754.79 Other
Asymmetric talipes
Talipes:
  calcaneus
  equinus

⑤ **754.8 Other specified nonteratogenic anomalies**

754.81 Pectus excavatum
Congenital funnel chest

754.82 Pectus carinatum
Congenital pigeon chest [breast]

754.89 Other
Club hand (congenital)
Congenital:
  deformity of chest wall
  dislocation of elbow
Generalized flexion contractures of lower limb joints, congenital
Spade-like hand (congenital)

755 Other congenital anomalies of limbs

Excludes: *those deformities classifiable to 754.0-754.8*

⑤ **755.0 Polydactyly**

755.00 Polydactyly, unspecified digits
Supernumerary digits

755.01 Of fingers
Accessory fingers

755.02 Of toes
Accessory toes

⑤ **755.1 Syndactyly**
Symphalangy
Webbing of digits

755.10 Of multiple and unspecified sites

● Code new
to this edition

▲ Revision of
existing code

④ ⑤ Fourth or fifth
digit required

755.11 Of fingers without fusion of bone

755.12 Of fingers with fusion of bone

755.13 Of toes without fusion of bone

755.14 Of toes with fusion of bone

⑤ **755.2 Reduction deformities of upper limb**

755.20 Unspecified reduction deformity of upper limb
Ectromelia NOS of upper limb
Hemimelia NOS of upper limb
Shortening of arm, congenital

755.21 Transverse deficiency of upper limb
Amelia of upper limb
Congenital absence of:
 fingers, all (complete or partial)
 forearm, including hand and fingers
 upper limb, complete
Congenital amputation of upper limb
Transverse hemimelia of upper limb

755.22 Longitudinal deficiency of upper limb, not elsewhere classified
Phocomelia NOS of upper limb
Rudimentary arm

755.23 Longitudinal deficiency, combined, involving humerus, radius, and ulna (complete or incomplete)
Congenital absence of arm and forearm (complete or incomplete) with or
 without metacarpal deficiency and/or phalangeal deficiency, incomplete
Phocomelia, complete, of upper limb

755.24 Longitudinal deficiency, humeral, complete or partial (with or without distal deficiencies, incomplete)
Congenital absence of humerus (with or without absence of some [but not all]
 distal elements)
Proximal phocomelia of upper limb

755.25 Longitudinal deficiency, radioulnar, complete or partial (with or without distal deficiencies, incomplete)
Congenital absence of radius and ulna (with or without absence of some [but
 not all] distal elements)
Distal phocomelia of upper limb

755.26 Longitudinal deficiency, radial, complete or partial (with or without distal deficiencies, incomplete)
Agenesis of radius
Congenital absence of radius (with or without absence of some [but not all]
 distal elements)

755.27 Longitudinal deficiency, ulnar, complete or partial (with or without distal deficiencies, incomplete)
Agenesis of ulna
Congenital absence of ulna (with or without absence of some [but not all]
 distal elements)

755.28 Longitudinal deficiency, carpals or metacarpals, complete or partial (with or without incomplete phalangeal deficiency)

755.29 Longitudinal deficiency, phalanges, complete or partial
Absence of finger, congenital
Aphalangia of upper limb, terminal, complete or partial

Excludes: *terminal deficiency of all five digits (755.21)*
 transverse deficiency of phalanges (755.21)

⑤ **755.3 Reduction deformities of lower limb**

755.30 Unspecified reduction deformity of lower limb
Ectromelia NOS of lower limb
Hemimelia NOS of lower limb
Shortening of leg, congenital

755.31 Transverse deficiency of lower limb
Amelia of lower limb
Congenital absence of:
 foot
 leg, including foot and toes
 lower limb, complete
 toes, all, complete
Transverse hemimelia of lower limb

	Add 4th or 5th digit		Nonspecific code		Unspecified code		Manifestation code

755.32 Longitudinal deficiency of lower limb, not elsewhere classified
Phocomelia NOS of lower limb

755.33 Longitudinal deficiency, combined, involving femur, tibia, and fibula (complete or incomplete)
Congenital absence of thigh and (lower) leg (complete or incomplete) with or without metacarpal deficiency and/or phalangeal deficiency, incomplete
Phocomelia, complete, of lower limb

755.34 Longitudinal deficiency, femoral, complete or partial (with or without distal deficiencies, incomplete)
Congenital absence of femur (with or without absence of some [but not all] distal elements)
Proximal phocomelia of lower limb

755.35 Longitudinal deficiency, tibiofibular, complete or partial (with or without distal deficiencies, incomplete)
Congenital absence of tibia and fibula (with or without absence of some [but not all] distal elements)
Distal phocomelia of lower limb

755.36 Longitudinal deficiency, tibia, complete or partial (with or without distal deficiencies, incomplete)
Agenesis of tibia
Congenital absence of tibia (with or without absence of some [but not all] distal elements)

755.37 Longitudinal deficiency, fibular, complete or partial (with or without distal deficiencies, incomplete)
Agenesis of fibula
Congenital absence of fibula (with or without absence of some [but not all] distal elements)

755.38 Longitudinal deficiency, tarsals or metatarsals, complete or partial (with or without incomplete phalangeal deficiency)

755.39 Longitudinal deficiency, phalanges, complete or partial
Absence of toe, congenital
Aphalangia of lower limb, terminal, complete or partial

Excludes: *terminal deficiency of all five digits (755.31)*
transverse deficiency of phalanges (755.31)

755.4 Reduction deformities, unspecified limb
Absence, congenital (complete or partial) of limb NOS
Amelia of unspecified limb
Ectromelia of unspecified limb
Hemimelia of unspecified limb
Phocomelia of unspecified limb

⑤ **755.5 Other anomalies of upper limb, including shoulder girdle**

755.50 Unspecified anomaly of upper limb

755.51 Congenital deformity of clavicle

755.52 Congenital elevation of scapula
Sprengel's deformity

755.53 Radioulnar synostosis

755.54 Madelung's deformity

755.55 Acrocephalosyndactyly
Apert's syndrome

755.56 Accessory carpal bones

755.57 Macrodactylia (fingers)

755.58 Cleft hand, congenital
Lobster-claw hand

755.59 Other
Cleidocranial dysostosis
Cubitus:
valgus, congenital
varus, congenital

Excludes: *club hand (congenital) (754.89)*
congenital dislocation of elbow (754.89)

⑤ **755.6 Other anomalies of lower limb, including pelvic girdle**

755.60 Unspecified anomaly of lower limb

755.61 Coxa valga, congenital

● Code new
to this edition

▲ Revision of
existing code

④ ⑤ Fourth or fifth
digit required

755.62   **Coxa vara, congenital**

755.63   **Other congenital deformity of hip (joint)**
Congenital anteversion of femur (neck)

Excludes: congenital dislocation of hip (754.30-754.35)

755.64   **Congenital deformity of knee (joint)**
Congenital:
absence of patella
genu valgum [knock-knee]
genu varum [bowleg]
Rudimentary patella

755.65   **Macrodactylia of toes**

755.66   **Other anomalies of toes**
Congenital:
hallux valgus
hallux varus
hammer toe

755.67   **Anomalies of foot, not elsewhere classified**
Astragaloscaphoid synostosis
Calcaneonavicular bar
Coalition of calcaneus
Talonavicular synostosis
Tarsal coalitions

755.69   **Other**
Congenital:
angulation of tibia
deformity (of):
ankle (joint)
sacroiliac (joint)
fusion of sacroiliac joint

755.8   **Other specified anomalies of unspecified limb**

755.9   **Unspecified anomaly of unspecified limb**
Congenital:
anomaly NOS of unspecified limb
deformity NOS of unspecified limb

Excludes: reduction deformity of unspecified limb (755.4)

756   **Other congenital musculoskeletal anomalies**

Excludes: congenital myotonic chondrodystrophy (359.23)
those deformities classifiable to 754.0-754.8

756.0   **Anomalies of skull and face bones**

Absence of skull bones	Imperfect fusion of skull
Acrocephaly	Oxycephaly
Congenital deformity of	Platybasia
forehead	Premature closure of cranial sutures
Craniosynostosis	Tower skull
Crouzon's disease	Trigonocephaly
Hypertelorism	

Excludes: acrocephalosyndactyly [Apert's syndrome] (755.55)
dentofacial anomalies (524.0-524.9)
skull defects associated with brain anomalies, such as:
anencephalus (740.0)
encephalocele (742.0)
hydrocephalus (742.3)
microcephalus (742.1)

⑤ 756.1   **Anomalies of spine**

756.10   **Anomaly of spine, unspecified**

756.11   **Spondylolysis, lumbosacral region**
Prespondylolisthesis (lumbosacral)

756.12   **Spondylolisthesis**

756.13   **Absence of vertebra, congenital**

756.14   **Hemivertebra**

756.15   **Fusion of spine [vertebra], congenital**

756.16   **Klippel-Feil syndrome**

756.17   Spina bifida occulta

Excludes: *spina bifida (aperta) (741.0-741.9)*

756.19   Other
  Platyspondylia
  Supernumerary vertebra

756.2   Cervical rib
  Supernumerary rib in the cervical region

756.3   Other anomalies of ribs and sternum
  Congenital absence of:
   rib
   sternum
  Congenital:
   fissure of sternum
   fusion of ribs
  Sternum bifidum

Excludes: *nonteratogenic deformity of chest wall (754.81-754.89)*

756.4   Chondrodystrophy
  Achondroplasia
  Chondrodystrophia (fetalis)
  Dyschondroplasia
  Enchondromatosis
  Ollier's disease

Excludes: *congenital myotonic chondrodystrophy (359.23)*
    lipochondrodystrophy [Hurler's syndrome] (277.5)
    Morquio's disease (277.5)

⑤ **756.5   Osteodystrophies**

756.50   Osteodystrophy, unspecified

756.51   Osteogenesis imperfecta
   Fragilitas ossium
   Osteopsathyrosis

756.52   Osteopetrosis

756.53   Osteopoikilosis

756.54   Polyostotic fibrous dysplasia of bone

756.55   Chondroectodermal dysplasia
   Ellis-van Creveld syndrome

756.56   Multiple epiphyseal dysplasia

756.59   Other
   Albright (-McCune)-Sternberg syndrome

756.6   Anomalies of diaphragm
  Absence of diaphragm
  Congenital hernia:
   diaphragmatic
   foramen of Morgagni
  Eventration of diaphragm

Excludes: *congenital hiatus hernia (750.6)*

⑤ **756.7   Anomalies of abdominal wall**

756.70   Anomaly of abdominal wall, unspecified

756.71   Prune belly syndrome
   Eagle-Barrett syndrome
   Prolapse of bladder mucosa

● **756.72   Omphalocele**
   Exomphalos

● **756.73   Gastroschisis**

756.79   Other congenital anomalies of abdominal wall

Excludes: *umbilical hernia (551-553 with .1)*

⑤ **756.8   Other specified anomalies of muscle, tendon, fascia, and connective tissue**

756.81   Absence of muscle and tendon
   Absence of muscle (pectoral)

756.82   Accessory muscle

756.83   Ehlers-Danlos syndrome

● Code new
  to this edition
▲ Revision of
  existing code
④ ⑤ Fourth or fifth
    digit required

756.89 **Other**
Amyotrophia congenita
Congenital shortening of tendon

756.9 **Other and unspecified anomalies of musculoskeletal system**
Congenital:
anomaly NOS of musculoskeletal system, not elsewhere classified
deformity NOS of musculoskeletal system, not elsewhere classified

757 **Congenital anomalies of the integument**
Includes: anomalies of skin, subcutaneous tissue, hair, nails, and breast

Excludes: *hemangioma (228.00-228.09)*
pigmented nevus (216.0-216.9)

757.0 **Hereditary edema of legs**
Congenital lymphedema   Milroy's disease
Hereditary trophedema

757.1 **Ichthyosis congenita**
Congenital ichthyosis
Harlequin fetus
Ichthyosiform erythroderma

757.2 **Dermatoglyphic anomalies**
Abnormal palmar creases

⑤ **757.3** **Other specified anomalies of skin**

757.31 **Congenital ectodermal dysplasia**

757.32 **Vascular hamartomas**
Birthmarks
Port-wine stain
Strawberry nevus

757.33 **Congenital pigmentary anomalies of skin**
Congenital poikiloderma
Urticaria pigmentosa
Xeroderma pigmentosum

Excludes: *albinism (270.2)*

757.39 **Other**
Accessory skin tags, congenital
Congenital scar
Epidermolysis bullosa
Keratoderma (congenital)

Excludes: *pilonidal cyst (685.0-685.1)*

757.4 **Specified anomalies of hair**
Congenital: Congenital:
alopecia   hypertrichosis
atrichosis   monilethrix
beaded hair   Persistent lanugo

757.5 **Specified anomalies of nails**
Anonychia   Congenital:
Congenital: leukonychia
clubnail   onychauxis
koilonychia   pachyonychia

▲ **757.6** **Specified congenital anomalies of breast**
Congenital absent breast or nipple
Accessory breast or nipple
Supernumerary breast or nipple

Excludes: *absence of pectoral muscle (756.81)*
hypoplasia of breast (611.82)
micromastia (611.82)

757.8 **Other specified anomalies of the integument**

757.9 **Unspecified anomaly of the integument**
Congenital:
anomaly NOS of integument
deformity NOS of integument

758 **Chromosomal anomalies**
Includes: syndromes associated with anomalies in the number and form of chromosomes
Use additional codes for conditions associated with the chromosomal anomalies

---

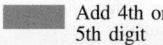 Add 4th or
5th digit

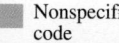 Nonspecific
code

Unspecified
code

Manifestation
code

758.0 Down's syndrome
Mongolism
Translocation Down's
  syndrome
Trisomy:
  21 or 22
  G

758.1 Patau's syndrome
Trisomy:
  13
  D_1

758.2 Edwards' syndrome
Trisomy:
  18
  E_3

⑤ **758.3 Autosomal deletion syndromes**

   758.31 Cri-du-chat syndrome
     Deletion 5p

   758.32 Velo-cardio-facial syndrome
     Deletion 22q11.2

   758.33 Other microdeletions
     Miller-Dieker syndrome
     Smith-Magenis syndrome

   758.39 Other autosomal deletions

758.4 Balanced autosomal translocation in normal individual

758.5 Other conditions due to autosomal anomalies
Accessory autosomes NEC

758.6 Gonadal dysgenesis
Ovarian dysgenesis
Turner's syndrome
XO syndrome

  Excludes: pure gonadal dysgenesis (752.7)

758.7 Klinefelter's syndrome
XXY syndrome

⑤ **758.8 Other conditions due to chromosome anomalies**

   758.81 Other conditions due to sex chromosome anomalies

   758.89 Other

758.9 Conditions due to anomaly of unspecified chromosome

759 Other and unspecified congenital anomalies

759.0 Anomalies of spleen
Aberrant spleen
Absent spleen
Accessory spleen
Congenital splenomegaly
Ectopic spleen
Lobulation of spleen

759.1 Anomalies of adrenal gland
Aberrant adrenal gland
Absent adrenal gland
Accessory adrenal gland

  Excludes: adrenogenital disorders (255.2)
     congenital disorders of steroid metabolism (255.2)

759.2 Anomalies of other endocrine glands
Absent parathyroid gland
Accessory thyroid gland
Persistent thyroglossal or thyrolingual duct
Thyroglossal (duct) cyst

  Excludes: congenital:
     goiter (246.1)
     hypothyroidism (243)

759.3 Situs inversus
Situs inversus or transversus:
  abdominalis
  thoracis
Transposition of viscera:
  abdominal
  thoracic

  Excludes: dextrocardia without mention of complete transposition (746.87)

● Code new
  to this edition

▲ Revision of
  existing code

④ ⑤ Fourth or fifth
  digit required

759.4 Conjoined twins
Craniopagus
Dicephalus
Pygopagus
Thoracopagus
Xiphopagus

759.5 Tuberous sclerosis
Bourneville's disease
Epiloia

759.6 Other hamartoses, not elsewhere classified
Syndrome:
Peutz-Jeghers
Sturge-Weber (-Dimitri)
von Hippel-Lindau

Excludes: *neurofibromatosis (237.7)*

759.7 Multiple congenital anomalies, so described
Congenital:
anomaly, multiple NOS
deformity, multiple NOS

⑤ **759.8 Other specified anomalies**

759.81 Prader-Willi syndrome

759.82 Marfan syndrome

759.83 Fragile X syndrome

759.89 Other
Congenital malformation syndromes affecting multiple systems, not elsewhere classified
Laurence-Moon-Biedl syndrome

759.9 Congenital anomaly, unspecified

| | Add 4th or 5th digit | | Nonspecific code | | Unspecified code | | Manifestation code |

● Code new
to this edition   ▲ Revision of
existing code   ④ ⑤ Fourth or fifth
digit required

15. CERTAIN CONDITIONS ORIGINATING IN THE PERINATAL PERIOD (760-779)

Includes: conditions which have their origin in the perinatal period, before birth through the first 28 days after birth, even though death or morbidity occurs later

Use additional code(s) to further specify condition

MATERNAL CAUSES OF PERINATAL MORBIDITY AND MORTALITY (760-763)

760 **Fetus or newborn affected by maternal conditions which may be unrelated to present pregnancy**
Includes: the listed maternal conditions only when specified as a cause of mortality or morbidity of the fetus or newborn

Excludes: *maternal endocrine and metabolic disorders affecting fetus or newborn (775.0-775.9)*

760.0 Maternal hypertensive disorders
Fetus or newborn affected by maternal conditions classifiable to 642

760.1 Maternal renal and urinary tract diseases
Fetus or newborn affected by maternal conditions classifiable to 580-599

760.2 Maternal infections
Fetus or newborn affected by maternal infectious disease classifiable to 001-136 and 487, but fetus or newborn not manifesting that disease

Excludes: *congenital infectious diseases (771.0-771.8)*
maternal genital tract and other localized infections (760.8)

760.3 Other chronic maternal circulatory and respiratory diseases
Fetus or newborn affected by chronic maternal conditions classifiable to 390-459, 490-519, 745-748

760.4 Maternal nutritional disorders
Fetus or newborn affected by:
maternal disorders classifiable to 260-269
maternal malnutrition NOS

Excludes: *fetal malnutrition (764.10-764.29)*

760.5 Maternal injury
Fetus or newborn affected by maternal conditions classifiable to 800-995

⑤ **760.6 Surgical operation on mother and fetus**

Excludes: *cesarean section for present delivery (763.4)*
damage to placenta from amniocentesis, cesarean section, or surgical induction (762.1)

760.61 Newborn affected by amniocentesis

Excludes: *fetal complications from amniocentesis (679.1)*

760.62 Newborn affected by other in utero procedure

Excludes: *fetal complications of in utero procedure (679.1)*

760.63 Newborn affected by other surgical operations on mother during pregnancy

Excludes: *newborn affected by previous surgical procedure on mother not associated with pregnancy (760.64)*

760.64 Newborn affected by previous surgical procedure on mother not associated with pregnancy

⑤ **760.7 Noxious influences affecting fetus or newborn via placenta or breast milk**
Fetus or newborn affected by noxious substance transmitted via placenta or breast milk

Excludes: *anesthetic and analgesic drugs administered during labor and delivery (763.5)*
drug withdrawal syndrome in newborn (779.5)

760.70 Unspecified noxious substance
Fetus or newborn affected by:
Drug NEC

760.71 Alcohol
Fetal alcohol syndrome

760.72 Narcotics

760.73 Hallucinogenic agents

760.74 Anti-infectives
Antibiotics
Antifungals

760.75 Cocaine

| Add 4th or 5th digit | Nonspecific code | Unspecified code | Manifestation code |

760.76 Diethylstilbestrol (DES)

760.77 Anticonvulsants
Carbamazepine
Phenobarbital
Phenytoin
Valproic acid

760.78 Antimetabolic agents
Methotrexate
Retinoic acid
Statins

760.79 Other
Fetus or newborn affected by:
immune sera transmitted via placenta or breast milk
medicinal agents NEC transmitted via placenta or breast milk
toxic substance NEC transmitted via placenta or breast milk

760.8 Other specified maternal conditions affecting fetus or newborn
Maternal genital tract and other localized infection affecting fetus or newborn, but fetus or newborn not manifesting that disease

Excludes: maternal urinary tract infection affecting fetus or newborn (760.1)

760.9 Unspecified maternal condition affecting fetus or newborn

761 Fetus or newborn affected by maternal complications of pregnancy
Includes: the listed maternal conditions only when specified as a cause of mortality or morbidity of the fetus or newborn

761.0 Incompetent cervix

761.1 Premature rupture of membranes

761.2 Oligohydramnios

Excludes: that due to premature rupture of membranes (761.1)

761.3 Polyhydramnios
Hydramnios (acute) (chronic)

761.4 Ectopic pregnancy
Pregnancy:
abdominal
intraperitoneal
tubal

761.5 Multiple pregnancy
Triplet (pregnancy)
Twin (pregnancy)

761.6 Maternal death

761.7 Malpresentation before labor
Breech presentation before labor
External version before labor
Oblique lie before labor
Transverse lie before labor
Unstable lie before labor

761.8 Other specified maternal complications of pregnancy affecting fetus or newborn
Spontaneous abortion, fetus

761.9 Unspecified maternal complication of pregnancy affecting fetus or newborn

762 Fetus or newborn affected by complications of placenta, cord, and membranes
Includes: the listed maternal conditions only when specified as a cause of mortality or morbidity in the fetus or newborn

762.0 Placenta previa

762.1 Other forms of placental separation and hemorrhage
Abruptio placentae
Antepartum hemorrhage
Damage to placenta from amniocentesis, cesarean section, or surgical induction
Maternal blood loss
Premature separation of placenta
Rupture of marginal sinus

762.2 Other and unspecified morphological and functional abnormalities of placenta
Placental:
dysfunction
infarction
insufficiency

● Code new
to this edition

▲ Revision of
existing code

④ ⑤ Fourth or fifth
digit required

762.3 Placental transfusion syndromes
Placental and cord abnormality resulting in twin-to-twin or other transplacental transfusion

Use additional code to indicate resultant condition in newborn:
fetal blood loss (772.0)
polycythemia neonatorum (776.4)

762.4 Prolapsed cord
Cord presentation

762.5 Other compression of umbilical cord
Cord around neck   Knot in cord
Entanglement of cord   Torsion of cord

762.6 Other and unspecified conditions of umbilical cord
Short umbilical cord
Thrombosis of umbilical cord
Varices of umbilical cord
Velamentous insertion of umbilical cord
Vasa previa

Excludes: *infection of umbilical cord (771.4)*
single umbilical artery (747.5)

762.7 Chorioamnionitis
Amnionitis
Membranitis
Placentitis

762.8 Other specified abnormalities of chorion and amnion

762.9 Unspecified abnormality of chorion and amnion

763 Fetus or newborn affected by other complications of labor and delivery
Includes: the listed conditions only when specified as a cause of mortality or morbidity in the fetus or newborn

Excludes: *newborn affected by surgical procedures on mother (760.61-760.64)*

763.0 Breech delivery and extraction

763.1 Other malpresentation, malposition, and disproportion during labor and delivery
Fetus or newborn affected by:
abnormality of bony pelvis
contracted pelvis
persistent occipitoposterior position
shoulder presentation
transverse lie
conditions classifiable to 652, 653, and 660

763.2 Forceps delivery
Fetus or newborn affected by forceps extraction

763.3 Delivery by vacuum extractor

763.4 Cesarean delivery

Excludes: *placental separation or hemorrhage from cesarean section (762.1)*

763.5 Maternal anesthesia and analgesia
Reactions and intoxications from maternal opiates and tranquilizers during labor and delivery

Excludes: *drug withdrawal syndrome in newborn (779.5)*

763.6 Precipitate delivery
Rapid second stage

763.7 Abnormal uterine contractions
Fetus or newborn affected by:
contraction ring
hypertonic labor
hypotonic uterine dysfunction
uterine inertia or dysfunction
conditions classifiable to 661, except 661.3

⑤ **763.8 Other specified complications of labor and delivery affecting fetus or newborn**

     763.81 Abnormality in fetal heart rate or rhythm before the onset of labor

     763.82 Abnormality in fetal heart rate or rhythm during labor

     763.83 Abnormality in fetal heart rate or rhythm, unspecified as to time of onset

	Add 4th or 5th digit		Nonspecific code		Unspecified code		Manifestation code

763.84 Meconium passage during delivery

Excludes: *meconium aspiration (770.11, 770.12)*
meconium staining (779.84)

763.89 Other specified complications of labor and delivery affecting fetus or newborn
Fetus or newborn affected by:
abnormality of maternal soft tissues
destructive operation on live fetus to facilitate delivery
induction of labor (medical)
other conditions classifiable to 650-669
other procedures used in labor and delivery

763.9 Unspecified complication of labor and delivery affecting fetus or newborn

OTHER CONDITIONS ORIGINATING IN THE PERINATAL PERIOD (764-779)

The following fifth-digit subclassification is for use with categories 764 and codes 765.0 and 765.1 to denote birthweight:

0 unspecified [weight]

1 less than 500 grams

2 500-749 grams

3 750-999 grams

4 1,000- 1,249 grams

5 1,250-1,499 grams

6 1,500-1,749 grams

7 1,750-1,999 grams

8 2,000-2,499 grams

9 2,500 grams and over

⑤ **764 Slow fetal growth and fetal malnutrition**

⑤ **764.0 "Light-for-dates" without mention of fetal malnutrition**
[0-9]   Infants underweight for gestational age
"Small-for-dates"

⑤ **764.1 "Light-for-dates" with signs of fetal malnutrition**
[0-9]   Infants "light-for-dates" classifiable to 764.0, who in addition show signs of fetal malnutrition, such as dry peeling skin and loss of subcutaneous tissue

⑤ **764.2 Fetal malnutrition without mention of "light-for-dates"**
[0-9]   Infants, not underweight for gestational age, showing signs of fetal malnutrition, such as dry peeling skin and loss of subcutaneous tissue
Intrauterine malnutrition

⑤ **764.9 Fetal growth retardation, unspecified**
[0-9]   Intrauterine growth retardation

765 Disorders relating to short gestation and low birthweight
Includes: the listed conditions, without further specification, as causes of mortality, morbidity, or additional care, in fetus or newborn

⑤ **765.0 Extreme immaturity**
[0-9]
Note: Usually implies a birthweight of less than 1000 grams
Use additional code for weeks of gestation (765.20-765.29)

⑤ **765.1 Other preterm infants**
[0-9]   Prematurity NOS
Prematurity or small size, not classifiable to 765.0 or as "light-for-dates" in 764
Note: Usually implies a birthweight of 1000-2499 grams
Use additional code for weeks of gestation (765.20-765.29)

⑤ **765.2 Weeks of gestation**

765.20 Unspecified weeks of gestation

765.21 Less than 24 completed weeks of gestation

765.22 24 completed weeks of gestation

765.23 25-26 completed weeks of gestation

765.24 27-28 completed weeks of gestation

765.25 29-30 completed weeks of gestation

765.26 31-32 completed weeks of gestation

● Code new to this edition   ▲ Revision of existing code   ④ ⑤ Fourth or fifth digit required

765.27 **33-34 completed weeks of gestation**

765.28 **35-36 completed weeks of gestation**

765.29 **37 or more completed weeks of gestation**

766 **Disorders relating to long gestation and high birthweight**
Includes: the listed conditions, without further specification, as causes of mortality, morbidity, or additional care, in fetus or newborn

766.0 Exceptionally large baby
Note: Usually implies a birthweight of 4500 grams or more.

766.1 Other "heavy-for-dates" infants
Other fetus or infant "heavy-" or "large-for-dates" regardless of period of gestation

⑤ **766.2 Late infant, not "heavy-for-dates"**

766.21 Post-term infant
Infant with gestation period over 40 completed weeks to 42 completed weeks

766.22 Prolonged gestation of infant
Infant with gestation period over 42 completed weeks
Postmaturity NOS

767 **Birth trauma**

767.0 Subdural and cerebral hemorrhage
Subdural and cerebral hemorrhage, whether described as due to birth trauma or to intrapartum anoxia or hypoxia
Subdural hematoma (localized)
Tentorial tear

Use additional code, if desired, to identify cause

Excludes: *intraventricular hemorrhage (772.10-772.14)*
subarachnoid hemorrhage (772.2)

⑤ **767.1 Injuries to scalp**

767.11 Epicranial subaponeurotic hemorrhage (massive)
Subgaleal hemorrhage

767.19 Other injuries to scalp
Caput succedaneum
Cephalhematoma
Chignon (from vacuum extraction)

767.2 Fracture of clavicle

767.3 Other injuries to skeleton
Fracture of:
long bones
skull

Excludes: *congenital dislocation of hip (754.30-754.35)*
fracture of spine, congenital (767.4)

767.4 Injury to spine and spinal cord
Dislocation of spine or spinal cord due to birth trauma
Fracture of spine or spinal cord due to birth trauma
Laceration of spine or spinal cord due to birth trauma
Rupture of spine or spinal cord due to birth trauma

767.5 Facial nerve injury
Facial palsy

767.6 Injury to brachial plexus
Palsy or paralysis:
brachial
Erb (-Duchenne)
Klumpke (-Déjérine)

767.7 Other cranial and peripheral nerve injuries
Phrenic nerve paralysis

767.8 Other specified birth trauma

Eye damage	Rupture of:
Hematoma of:	liver
liver (subcapsular)	spleen
testes	Scalpel wound
vulva	Traumatic glaucoma

Excludes: *hemorrhage classifiable to 772.0-772.9*

767.9 Birth trauma, unspecified
Birth injury NOS

Add 4th or 5th digit	Nonspecific code	Unspecified code	Manifestation code

768 **Intrauterine hypoxia and birth asphyxia**
Use only when associated with newborn morbidity classifiable elsewhere

> Excludes: *acidemia NOS of newborn (775.81)*
> *acidosis NOS of newborn (775.81)*
> *cerebral ischemia NOS (779.2)*
> *hypoxia NOS of newborn (770.88)*
> *mixed metabolic and respiratory acidosis of newborn (775.81)*
> *respiratory arrest of newborn (770.87)*

768.0 **Fetal death from asphyxia or anoxia before onset of labor or at unspecified time**

768.1 **Fetal death from asphyxia or anoxia during labor**

768.2 **Fetal distress before onset of labor, in liveborn infant**
Fetal metabolic acidemia before onset of labor, in liveborn infant

768.3 **Fetal distress first noted during labor and delivery, in liveborn infant**
Fetal metabolic acidemia first noted during labor and delivery, in liveborn infant

768.4 **Fetal distress, unspecified as to time of onset, in liveborn infant**
Fetal metabolic acidemia unspecified as to time of onset, in liveborn infant

768.5 **Severe birth asphyxia**
Birth asphyxia with neurologic involvement

> Excludes: *hypoxic-ischemic encephalopathy (HIE) (768.70-768.73)*

768.6 **Mild or moderate birth asphyxia**
Other specified birth asphyxia (without mention of neurologic involvement)

> Excludes: *hypoxic-ischemic encephalopathy (HIE) (768.70-768.73)*

⑤ 768.7 **Hypoxic-ischemic encephalopathy (HIE)**

● **768.70** **Hypoxic-ischemic encephalopathy, unspecified**

● **768.71** **Mild hypoxic-ischemic encephalopathy**

● **768.72** **Moderate hypoxic-ischemic encephalopathy**

● **768.73** **Severe hypoxic-ischemic encephalopathy**

768.9 **Unspecified birth asphyxia in liveborn infant**
Anoxia NOS, in liveborn infant
Asphyxia NOS, in liveborn infant

769 **Respiratory distress syndrome**
Cardiorespiratory distress syndrome of newborn
Hyaline membrane disease (pulmonary)
Idiopathic respiratory distress syndrome [IRDS or RDS] of newborn
Pulmonary hypoperfusion syndrome

> Excludes: *transient tachypnea of newborn (770.6)*

770 **Other respiratory conditions of fetus and newborn**

770.0 **Congenital pneumonia**
Infective pneumonia acquired prenatally

> Excludes: *pneumonia from infection acquired after birth (480.0-486)*

⑤ 770.1 **Fetal and newborn aspiration**

> Excludes: *aspiration of postnatal stomach contents (770.85, 770.86)*
> *meconium passage during delivery (763.84)*
> *meconium staining (779.84)*

770.10 **Fetal and newborn aspiration, unspecified**

770.11 **Meconium aspiration without respiratory symptoms**
Meconium aspiration NOS

770.12 **Meconium aspiration with respiratory symptoms**
Meconium aspiration pneumonia
Meconium aspiration pneumonitis
Meconium aspiration syndrome NOS
Use additional code to identify any secondary pulmonary hypertension (416.8), if applicable

770.13 **Aspiration of clear amniotic fluid without respiratory symptoms**
Aspiration of clear amniotic fluid NOS

770.14 **Aspiration of clear amniotic fluid with respiratory symptoms**
Aspiration of clear amniotic fluid with pneumonia
Aspiration of clear amniotic fluid with pneumonitis
Use additional code to identify any secondary pulmonary hypertension (416.8), if applicable

---

● Code new to this edition   ▲ Revision of existing code   ④ ⑤ Fourth or fifth digit required

770.15 Aspiration of blood without respiratory symptoms
Aspiration of blood NOS

770.16 Aspiration of blood with respiratory symptoms
Aspiration of blood with pneumonia
Aspiration of blood with pneumonitis
Use additional code to identify any secondary pulmonary hypertension (416.8), if applicable

770.17 Other fetal and newborn aspiration without respiratory symptoms

770.18 Other fetal and newborn aspiration with respiratory symptoms
Other aspiration pneumonia
Other aspiration pneumonitis
Use additional code to identify any secondary pulmonary hypertension (416.8), if applicable

770.2 Interstitial emphysema and related conditions
Pneumomediastinum originating in the perinatal period
Pneumopericardium originating in the perinatal period
Pneumothorax originating in the perinatal period

770.3 Pulmonary hemorrhage
Hemorrhage:
   alveolar (lung) originating in the perinatal period
   intra-alveolar (lung) originating in the perinatal period
   massive pulmonary originating in the perinatal period

770.4 Primary atelectasis
Pulmonary immaturity NOS

770.5 Other and unspecified atelectasis
Atelectasis:
   NOS, originating in the perinatal period
   partial, originating in the perinatal period
   secondary, originating in the perinatal period
Pulmonary collapse, originating in the perinatal period

770.6 Transitory tachypnea of newborn
Idiopathic tachypnea of newborn
Wet lung syndrome

Excludes: respiratory distress syndrome (769)

770.7 Chronic respiratory disease arising in the perinatal period
Bronchopulmonary dysplasia
Interstitial pulmonary fibrosis of prematurity
Wilson-Mikity syndrome

⑤ **770.8 Other respiratory problems after birth**

Excludes: mixed metabolic and respiratory acidosis of newborn (775.81)

770.81 Primary apnea of newborn
Apneic spells of newborn NOS
Essential apnea of newborn
Sleep apnea of newborn

770.82 Other apnea of newborn
Obstructure apnea of newborn

770.83 Cyanotic attacks of newborn

770.84 Respiratory failure of newborn

Excludes: respiratory distress syndrome (769)

770.85 Aspiration of postnatal stomach contents without respiratory symptoms
Aspiration of postnatal stomach contents NOS

770.86 Aspiration of postnatal stomach contents with respiratory symptoms
Aspiration of postnatal stomach contents with pneumonia
Aspiration of postnatal stomach contents with pneumonitis
Use additional code to identify any secondary pulmonary hypertension (416.8), if applicable

770.87 Respiratory arrest of newborn

770.88 Hypoxemia of newborn
Hypoxia NOS of newborn

770.89 Other respiratory problems after birth

770.9 Unspecified respiratory condition of fetus and newborn

	Add 4th or 5th digit		Nonspecific code		Unspecified code		Manifestation code

771 Infections specific to the perinatal period
Includes: infections acquired before or during birth via the umbilicus or during the first 28 days after birth

Excludes: *congenital pneumonia (770.0)*
congenital syphilis (090.0-090.9)
infant botulism (040.41)
maternal infectious disease as a cause of mortality or morbidity in fetus or newborn, but fetus or newborn not manifesting the disease (760.2)
ophthalmia neonatorum due to gonococcus (098.40)
other infections not specifically classified to this category

771.0 Congenital rubella
Congenital rubella pneumonitis

771.1 Congenital cytomegalovirus infection
Congenital cytomegalic inclusion disease

771.2 Other congenital infections
Congenital:
  herpes simplex
  listeriosis
  malaria
Congenital:
  toxoplasmosis
  tuberculosis

771.3 Tetanus neonatorum
Tetanus omphalitis

Excludes: *hypocalcemic tetany (775.4)*

771.4 Omphalitis of the newborn
Infection:
  navel cord
  umbilical stump

Excludes: *tetanus omphalitis (771.3)*

771.5 Neonatal infective mastitis

Excludes: *noninfective neonatal mastitis (778.7)*

771.6 Neonatal conjunctivitis and dacryocystitis
Ophthalmia neonatorum NOS

Excludes: *ophthalmia neonatorum due to gonococcus (098.40)*

771.7 Neonatal Candida infection
Neonatal moniliasis
Thrush in newborn

⑤ **771.8 Other infections specific to the perinatal period**
Use additional code to identify organism (041.00-041.9)

771.81 Septicemia [sepsis] of newborn
Use additional code(s) to identify severe sepsis (995.92) and any associated acute organ dysfunction, if applicable

771.82 Urinary tract infection of newborn

771.83 Bacteremia of newborn

771.89 Other infections specific to the perinatal period
Intra-amniotic infection of fetus NOS
Infection of newborn NOS

772 Fetal and neonatal hemorrhage

Excludes: *fetal hematologic conditions complicating pregnancy (678.0)*
hematological disorders of fetus and newborn (776.0-776.9)

▲ **772.0 Fetal blood loss affecting newborn**
Fetal blood loss from:
  cut end of co-twin's cord
  placenta
  ruptured cord
  vasa previa
Fetal exsanguination
Fetal hemorrhage into:
  co-twin
  mother's circulation

⑤ **772.1 Intraventricular hemorrhage**
Intraventricular hemorrhage from any perinatal cause

772.10 Unspecified grade

772.11 Grade I
Bleeding into germinal matrix

772.12 Grade II
Bleeding into ventricle

● Code new to this edition   ▲ Revision of existing code   ④ ⑤ Fourth or fifth digit required

772.13 Grade III
Bleeding with enlargement of ventricle

772.14 Grade IV
Bleeding into cerebral cortex

772.2 Subarachnoid hemorrhage
Subarachnoid hemorrhage from any perinatal cause

Excludes: subdural and cerebral hemorrhage (767.0)

772.3 Umbilical hemorrhage after birth
Slipped umbilical ligature

772.4 Gastrointestinal hemorrhage
Excludes: swallowed maternal blood (777.3)

772.5 Adrenal hemorrhage

772.6 Cutaneous hemorrhage
Bruising in fetus or newborn
Ecchymoses in fetus or newborn
Petechiae in fetus or newborn
Superficial hematoma in fetus or newborn

772.8 Other specified hemorrhage of fetus or newborn
Excludes: hemorrhagic disease of newborn (776.0)
pulmonary hemorrhage (770.3)

772.9 Unspecified hemorrhage of newborn

773 Hemolytic disease of fetus or newborn, due to isoimmunization

773.0 Hemolytic disease due to Rh isoimmunization
Anemia due to RH:
antibodies
isoimmunization
maternal/fetal incompatibility
Erythroblastosis (fetalis) due to RH:
antibodies
isoimmunization
maternal/fetal incompatibility
Hemolytic disease (fetus) (newborn) due to RH:
antibodies
isoimmunization
maternal/fetal incompatibility
Jaundice due to RH:
antibodies
isoimmunization
maternal/fetal incompatibility
Rh hemolytic disease
Rh isoimmunization

773.1 Hemolytic disease due to ABO isoimmunization
ABO hemolytic disease
ABO isoimmunization
Anemia due to ABO: antibodies, isoimmunization, or maternal/fetal incompatibility
Erythroblastosis (fetalis) due to ABO:
antibodies
isoimmunization
maternal/fetal incompatibility
Hemolytic disease (fetus) (newborn) due to ABO:
antibodies
isoimmunization
maternal/fetal incompatibility
Jaundice due to ABO:
antibodies
isoimmunization
maternal/fetal incompatibility

773.2 Hemolytic disease due to other and unspecified isoimmunization
Erythroblastosis (fetalis) (neonatorum) NOS
Hemolytic disease (fetus) (newborn) NOS
Jaundice or anemia due to other and unspecified blood-group incompatibility

773.3 Hydrops fetalis due to isoimmunization
Use additional code, if desired, to identify type of isoimmunization (773.0-773.2)

773.4 Kernicterus due to isoimmunization
Use additional code, if desired, to identify type of isoimmunization (773.0-773.2)

Add 4th or
5th digit

Nonspecific
code

Unspecified
code

Manifestation
code

TABULAR LIST

773.5 Late anemia due to isoimmunization

774 Other perinatal jaundice

774.0 *Perinatal jaundice from hereditary hemolytic anemias*
Code first underlying disease (282.0-282.9)

774.1 Perinatal jaundice from other excessive hemolysis
Fetal or neonatal jaundice from:
bruising
drugs or toxins transmitted from mother
infection
polycythemia
swallowed maternal blood
Use additional code, if desired, to identify cause

Excludes: jaundice due to isoimmunization (773.0-773.2)

774.2 Neonatal jaundice associated with preterm delivery
Hyperbilirubinemia of prematurity
Jaundice due to delayed conjugation associated with preterm delivery

⑤ **774.3 Neonatal jaundice due to delayed conjugation from other causes**

774.30 Neonatal jaundice due to delayed conjugation, cause unspecified

774.31 *Neonatal jaundice due to delayed conjugation in diseases classified elsewhere*
Code first underlying diseases, as:
congenital hypothyroidism (243)
Crigler-Najjar syndrome (277.4)
Gilbert's syndrome (277.4)

774.39 Other
Jaundice due to delayed conjugation from causes, such as:
breast milk inhibitors
delayed development of conjugating system

774.4 Perinatal jaundice due to hepatocellular damage
Fetal or neonatal hepatitis
Giant cell hepatitis
Inspissated bile syndrome

774.5 *Perinatal jaundice from other causes*
Code first underlying cause, as:
congenital obstruction of bile duct (751.61)
galactosemia (271.1)
mucoviscidosis (277.00-277.09)

774.6 Unspecified fetal and neonatal jaundice
Icterus neonatorum
Neonatal hyperbilirubinemia (transient)
Physiologic jaundice NOS in newborn

Excludes: that in preterm infants (774.2)

774.7 Kernicterus not due to isoimmunization
Bilirubin encephalopathy
Kernicterus of newborn NOS

Excludes: kernicterus due to isoimmunization (773.4)

775 Endocrine and metabolic disturbances specific to the fetus and newborn
Includes: transitory endocrine and metabolic disturbances caused by the infant's response to maternal endocrine and metabolic factors, its removal from them, or its adjustment to extrauterine existence

775.0 Syndrome of "infant of a diabetic mother"
Maternal diabetes mellitus affecting fetus or newborn (with hypoglycemia)

775.1 Neonatal diabetes mellitus
Diabetes mellitus syndrome in newborn infant

775.2 Neonatal myasthenia gravis

775.3 Neonatal thyrotoxicosis
Neonatal hyperthyroidism (transient)

775.4 Hypocalcemia and hypomagnesemia of newborn
Cow's milk hypocalcemia
Hypocalcemic tetany, neonatal
Neonatal hypoparathyroidism
Phosphate-loading hypocalcemia

775.5 Other transitory neonatal electrolyte disturbances
Dehydration, neonatal

● Code new to this edition   ▲ Revision of existing code   ④ ⑤ Fourth or fifth digit required

775.6 Neonatal hypoglycemia
Excludes: *infant of mother with diabetes mellitus (775.0)*

775.7 Late metabolic acidosis of newborn

⑤ **775.8 Other neonatal endocrine and metabolic disturbances**

775.81 Other acidosis of newborn
Acidemia NOS of newborn
Acidosis of newborn NOS
Mixed metabolic and respiratory acidosis of newborn

775.89 Other neonatal endocrine and metabolic disturbances
Amino-acid metabolic disorders described as transitory

775.9 Unspecified endocrine and metabolic disturbances specific to the fetus and newborn

776 Hematological disorders of newborn
Includes: disorders specific to the newborn though possibly originating in utero
Excludes: *fetal hematologic conditions (678.0)*

776.0 Hemorrhagic disease of newborn
Hemorrhagic diathesis of newborn
Vitamin K deficiency of newborn
Excludes: *fetal or neonatal hemorrhage (772.0-772.9)*

776.1 Transient neonatal thrombocytopenia
Neonatal thrombocytopenia due to:
exchange transfusion
idiopathic maternal thrombocytopenia
isoimmunization

776.2 Disseminated intravascular coagulation in newborn

776.3 Other transient neonatal disorders of coagulation
Transient coagulation defect, newborn

776.4 Polycythemia neonatorum
Plethora of newborn
Polycythemia due to:
donor twin transfusion
maternal-fetal transfusion

776.5 Congenital anemia
Anemia following fetal blood loss
Excludes: *anemia due to isoimmunization (773.0-773.2, 773.5)*
hereditary hemolytic anemias (282.0-282.9)

776.6 Anemia of prematurity

776.7 Transient neonatal neutropenia
Isoimmune neutropenia
Maternal transfer neutropenia
Excludes: *congenital neutropenia (nontransient) (288.01)*

776.8 Other specified transient hematological disorders

▲ **776.9 Unspecified hematological disorder specific to newborn**

777 Perinatal disorders of digestive system
Includes: disorders specific to the fetus and newborn
Excludes: *intestinal obstruction classifiable to 560.0-560.9*

777.1 Meconium obstruction
Congenital fecaliths
Delayed passage of meconium
Meconium ileus NOS
Meconium plug syndrome
Excludes: *meconium ileus in cystic fibrosis (277.01)*

777.2 Intestinal obstruction due to inspissated milk

777.3 Hematemesis and melena due to swallowed maternal blood
Swallowed blood syndrome in newborn
Excludes: *that not due to swallowed maternal blood (772.4)*

777.4 Transitory ileus of newborn
Excludes: *Hirschsprung's disease (751.3)*

	Add 4th or 5th digit		Nonspecific code		Unspecified code		Manifestation code

⑤ **777.5　Necrotizing enterocolitis in newborn**

    777.50　Necrotizing enterocolitis in newborn, unspecified
        Necrotizing enterocolitis in newborn, NOS

    777.51　Stage I necrotizing enterocolitis in newborn
        Necrotizing enterocolitis without pneumatosis, without perforation

    777.52　Stage II necrotizing enterocolitis in newborn
        Necrotizing enterocolitis with pneumatosis, without perforation

    777.53　Stage III necrotizing enterocolitis in newborn
        Necrotizing enterocolitis with perforation
        Necrotizing enterocolitis with pneumatosis and perforation

777.6　Perinatal intestinal perforation
    Meconium peritonitis

777.8　Other specified perinatal disorders of digestive system

777.9　Unspecified perinatal disorder of digestive system

778　Conditions involving the integument and temperature regulation of fetus and newborn

778.0　Hydrops fetalis not due to isoimmunization
    Idiopathic hydrops

    Excludes: *hydrops fetalis due to isoimmunization (773.3)*

778.1　Sclerema neonatorum
    Subcutaneous fat necrosis

778.2　Cold injury syndrome of newborn

778.3　Other hypothermia of newborn

778.4　Other disturbances of temperature regulation of newborn
    Dehydration fever in newborn
    Environmentally-induced pyrexia
    Hyperthermia in newborn
    Transitory fever of newborn

778.5　Other and unspecified edema of newborn
    Edema neonatorum

778.6　Congenital hydrocele
    Congenital hydrocele of tunica vaginalis

778.7　Breast engorgement in newborn
    Noninfective mastitis of newborn

    Excludes: *infective mastitis of newborn (771.5)*

778.8　Other specified conditions involving the integument of fetus and newborn
    Urticaria neonatorum

    Excludes: *impetigo neonatorum (684)*
        pemphigus neonatorum (684)

778.9　Unspecified condition involving the integument and temperature regulation of fetus and newborn

779　Other and ill-defined conditions originating in the perinatal period

779.0　Convulsions in newborn
    Fits in newborn
    Seizures in newborn

779.1　Other and unspecified cerebral irritability in newborn

779.2　Cerebral depression, coma, and other abnormal cerebral signs
    Cerebral ischemia NOS of newborn
    CNS dysfunction in newborn NOS

    Excludes: *cerebral ischemia due to birth trauma (767.0)*
        intrauterine cerebral ischemia (768.2-768.9)
        intraventricular hemorrhage (772.10-772.14)

▲ **779.3　Disorder of stomach function and feeding problems in newborn**

    ● **779.31　Feeding problems in newborn**
        Slow feeding in newborn

    Excludes: *feeding problem in child over 28 days old　(783.3)*

    ● **779.32　Bilious vomiting in newborn**

    Excludes: *bilious vomiting in child over 28 days old (787.04)*

● Code new
  to this edition
▲ Revision of
  existing code
④ ⑤ Fourth or fifth
    digit required

● **779.33** **Other vomiting in newborn**
Regurgitation of food in newborn

Excludes: *vomiting in child over 28 days old (536.2,787.01-787.03, 787.04)*

● **779.34** **Failure to thrive in newborn**

Excludes: *failure to thrive in child over 28 days old (783.41)*

779.4 **Drug reactions and intoxications specific to newborn**
Gray syndrome from chloramphenicol administration in newborn

Excludes: *fetal alcohol syndrome (760.71)*
reactions and intoxications from maternal opiates and tranquilizers (763.5)

779.5 **Drug withdrawal syndrome in newborn**
Drug withdrawal syndrome in infant of dependent mother

Excludes: *fetal alcohol syndrome (760.71)*

779.6 **Termination of pregnancy (fetus)**
Fetus death due to:
induced abortion
termination of pregnancy

Excludes: *spontaneous abortion (fetus) (761.8)*

779.7 **Periventricular leukomalacia**

⑤ **779.8** **Other specified conditions originating in the perinatal period**

779.81 **Neonatal bradycardia**

Excludes: *abnormality in fetal heart rate or rhythm complicating labor and delivery*
(763.81-763.83)
bradycardia due to birth asphyxia (768.5-768.9)

779.82 **Neonatal tachycardia**

Excludes: *abnormality in fetal heart rate or rhythm complicating labor and delivery*
(763.81-763.83)

779.83 **Delayed separation of umbilical cord**

779.84 **Meconium staining**

Excludes: *meconium aspiration (770.11, 770.12)*
meconium passage during delivery (763.84)

779.85 **Cardiac arrest of newborn**

779.89 **Other specified conditions originating in the perinatal period**
Use additional code to specify condition

779.9 **Unspecified condition originating in the perinatal period**
Congenital debility NOS
Stillbirth NEC

● Code new
to this edition

▲ Revision of
existing code

④ ⑤ Fourth or fifth
digit required

16.   SYMPTOMS, SIGNS, AND ILL-DEFINED CONDITIONS (780-799)

This section includes symptoms, signs, abnormal results of laboratory or other investigative procedures, and ill-defined conditions regarding which no diagnosis classifiable elsewhere is recorded.

Signs and symptoms that point rather definitely to a given diagnosis are assigned to some category in the preceding part of the classification. In general, categories 780-796 include the more ill-defined conditions and symptoms that point with perhaps equal suspicion to two or more diseases or to two or more systems of the body, and without the necessary study of the case to make a final diagnosis. Practically all categories in this group could be designated as "not otherwise specified," or as "unknown etiology," or as "transient." The Alphabetic Index should be consulted to determine which symptoms and signs are to be allocated here and which to more specific sections of the classification; the residual subcategories numbered .9 are provided for other relevant symptoms which cannot be allocated elsewhere in the classification.

The conditions and signs or symptoms included in categories 780-796 consist of: (a) cases for which no more specific diagnosis can be made even after all facts bearing on the case have been investigated; (b) signs or symptoms existing at the time of initial encounter that proved to be transient and whose causes could not be determined; (c) provisional diagnoses in a patient who failed to return for further investigation or care; (d) cases referred elsewhere for investigation or treatment before the diagnosis was made; (e) cases in which a more precise diagnosis was not available for any other reason; (f) certain symptoms which represent important problems in medical care and which it might be desired to classify in addition to a known cause.

SYMPTOMS (780-789)

780   **General symptoms**

⑤   **780.0   Alteration of consciousness**

Excludes: *alteration of consciousness due to:*
> *intracranial injuries (850.0-854.19)*
> *skull fractures (800.00-801.99, 803.00-804.99)*
> *coma:*
> > *diabetic (249.2-249.3, 250.2-250.3)*
> > *hepatic (572.2)*
> > *originating in the perinatal period (779.2)*

  780.01   Coma

  780.02   Transient alteration of awareness

  780.03   Persistent vegetative state

  780.09   Other
Drowsiness	Somnolence
Semicoma	Stupor
Unconsciousness	

780.1   Hallucinations

Hallucinations:	Hallucinations:
NOS	olfactory
auditory	tactile
gustatory	

Excludes: *those associated with mental disorders, as functional psychoses (295.0-298.9)*
> *organic brain syndromes (290.0-294.9, 310.0-310.9)*
> *visual hallucinations (368.16)*

780.2   Syncope and collapse

Blackout	(Near) (Pre) syncope
Fainting	Vasovagal attack

Excludes: *carotid sinus syncope (337.0)*
> *heat syncope (992.1)*
> *neurocirculatory asthenia (306.2)*
> *orthostatic hypotension (458.0)*
> *shock NOS (785.50)*

⑤   **780.3   Convulsions**

Excludes: *convulsions:*
> *epileptic (345.10-345.91)*
> *in newborn (779.0)*

  780.31   Febrile convulsions (simple), unspecified
  Febrile seizure NOS

▣ Add 4th or 5th digit	▣ Nonspecific code	▣ Unspecified code	▣ Manifestation code

780.32 Complex febrile convulsions
Febrile seizure:
   atypical
   complex
   complicated

Excludes: *status epilepticus (345.3)*

780.39 Other convulsions
Convulsive disorder NOS
Fit NOS
Recurrent convulsions NOS
Seizure NOS

780.4 Dizziness and giddiness
Light-headedness
Vertigo NOS

Excludes: *Ménière's disease and other specified vertiginous syndromes (386.0-386.9)*

⑤ **780.5 Sleep disturbances**

Excludes: *circadian rhythm sleep disorders (327.30-327.39)*
organic hypersomnia (327.10-327.19)
organic insomnia (327.00-327.09)
organic sleep apnea (327.20-327.29)
organic sleep related movement disorders (327.51-327.59)
parasomnias (327.40-327.49)
that of nonorganic origin (307.40-307.49)

780.50 Sleep disturbance, unspecified

780.51 Insomnia with sleep apnea, unspecified

780.52 Insomnia, unspecified

780.53 Hypersomnia with sleep apnea, unspecified

780.54 Hypersomnia, unspecified

780.55 Disruption of 24 hour sleep wake cycle, unspecified

780.56 Dysfunctions associated with sleep stages or arousal from sleep

780.57 Unspecified sleep apnea

780.58 Sleep related movement disorder, unspecified

Excludes: *restless legs syndrome (333.94)*

780.59 Other

⑤ **780.6 Fever and other physiologic disturbances of temperature regulation**

Excludes: *effects of reduced environmental temperature (991.0-991.9)*
effects of heat and light (992.0-992.9)
fever, chills or hypothermia associated with confirmed infection - code to infection

780.60 Fever, unspecified
Chills with fever
Fever NOS
Fever of unknown origin (FUO)
Hyperpyrexia NOS
Pyrexia NOS
Pyrexia of unknown origin

Excludes: *chills without fever (780.64)*
neonatal fever (778.4)
pyrexia of unknown origin (during):
in newborn (778.4)
labor (659.2)
the puerperium (672)

780.61 Fever presenting with conditions classified elsewhere
Code first underlying condition when associated fever is present, such as with:
   leukemia (conditions classifiable to 204-208)
   neutropenia (288.00-288.09)
   sickle-cell disease (282.60-282.69)

780.62 Postprocedural fever

Excludes: *postvaccination fever (780.63)*

780.63 Postvaccination fever
Postimmunization fever

● Code new
to this edition
▲ Revision of
existing code
④ ⑤ Fourth or fifth
digit required

780.64 Chills (without fever)
Chills NOS

Excludes: chills with fever (780.60)

780.65 Hypothermia not associated with low environmental temperature

Excludes: hypothermia:
associated with low environmental temperature (991.6)
due to anesthesia (995.89)
of newborn (778.2, 778.3)

⑤ **780.7 Malaise and fatigue**

Excludes: debility, unspecified (799.3)
fatigue (during):
combat (308.0-308.9)
heat (992.6)
pregnancy (646.8)
neurasthenia (300.5)
senile asthenia (797.5)

780.71 Chronic fatigue syndrome

780.72 Functional quadriplegia
Complete immobility due to severe physical disability or frailty

Excludes: hysterical paralysis (300.11)
immobility syndrome (728.3)
neurologic quadriplegia (344.00-344.09)
quadriplegia NOS (344.00)

780.79 Other malaise and fatigue
Asthenia NOS
Lethargy
Postviral (asthenic) syndrome
Tiredness

780.8 Generalized hyperhidrosis
Diaphoresis
Excessive sweating
Secondary hyperhidrosis

Excludes: focal (localized) (primary) (secondary) hyperhidrosis (705.21-705.22)
Frey's syndrome (705.22)

⑤ **780.9 Other general symptoms**

Excludes: hypothermia:
NOS (accidental) (991.6)
due to anesthesia (995.89)
of newborn (778.2-778.3)
memory disturbance as part of a pattern of mental disorder

780.91 Fussy infant (baby)

780.92 Excessive crying of infant (baby)

Excludes: excessive crying of child, adolescent or adult (780.95)

780.93 Memory loss
Amnesia (retrograde)
Memory loss NOS

Excludes: memory loss due to:
intracranial injuries (850.0-854.19)
skull fractures (800.00-801.99, 803.00-804.99)
mild memory disturbance due to organic brain damage (310.8)
transient global amnesia (437.7)

780.94 Early satiety

780.95 Excessive crying of child, adolescent, or adult

Excludes: excessive crying of infant (baby) (780.92)

780.96 Generalized pain
Pain NOS

780.97 Altered mental status
Change in mental status

Excludes: altered level of consciousness (780.01-780.09)
altered mental status due to known condition — code to condition
delirium NOS (780.09)

	Add 4th or 5th digit		Nonspecific code		Unspecified code		Manifestation code

780.99 **Other general symptoms**

781 **Symptoms involving nervous and musculoskeletal systems**

Excludes: *depression NOS (311)*

disorders specifically relating to:
back (724.0-724.9)
hearing (388.0-389.9)
joint (718.0-719.9)
limb (729.0-729.9)
neck (723.0-723.9)
vision (368.0-369.9)
pain in limb (729.5)

781.0 **Abnormal involuntary movements**
Abnormal head movements
Fasciculation
Spasms NOS
Tremor NOS

Excludes: *abnormal reflex (796.1)*
chorea NOS (333.5)
infantile spasms (345.60-345.61)
spastic paralysis (342.1, 343.0-344.9)
specified movement disorders classifiable to 333 (333.0-333.9)
that of nonorganic origin (307.2-307.3)

781.1 **Disturbances of sensation of smell and taste**
Anosmia   Parosmia
Parageusia

781.2 **Abnormality of gait**
Gait: Gait:
  ataxic   spastic
  paralytic   staggering

Excludes: *ataxia:*
NOS (781.3)
locomotor (progressive) (094.0)
difficulty in walking (719.7)

781.3 **Lack of coordination**
Ataxia NOS
Muscular incoordination

Excludes: *ataxic gait (781.2)*
cerebellar ataxia (334.0-334.9)
difficulty in walking (719.7)
vertigo NOS (780.4)

781.4 **Transient paralysis of limb**
Monoplegia, transient NOS

Excludes: *paralysis (342.0-344.9)*

781.5 **Clubbing of fingers**

781.6 **Meningismus**
Dupré's syndrome
Meningism

781.7 **Tetany**
Carpopedal spasm

Excludes: *tetanus neonatorum (771.3)*
tetany:
hysterical (300.11)
newborn (hypocalcemic) (775.4)
parathyroid (252.1)
psychogenic (306.0)

781.8 **Neurologic neglect syndrome**
Asomatognosia   Left-sided neglect
Hemi-akinesia   Sensory extinction
Hemi-inattention   Sensory neglect
Hemispatial neglect   Visuospatial neglect

⑤ **781.9** **Other symptoms involving nervous and musculoskeletal systems**

781.91 **Loss of height**

Excludes: *osteoporosis (733.00-733.09)*

● Code new   ▲ Revision of   ④ ⑤ Fourth or fifth
             to this edition   existing code   digit required

781.92 Abnormal posture

781.93 Ocular torticollis

781.94 Facial weakness
Facial droop

Excludes: facial weakness due to late effect of cerebrovascular accident (438.83)

781.99 Other symptoms involving nervous and musculoskeletal systems

782 Symptoms involving skin and other integumentary tissue

Excludes: symptoms relating to breast (611.71-611.79)

782.0 Disturbance of skin sensation

Anesthesia of skin	Hypoesthesia
Burning or prickling	Numbness
sensation	Paresthesia
Hyperesthesia	Tingling

782.1 Rash and other nonspecific skin eruption
Exanthem

Excludes: vesicular eruption (709.8)

782.2 Localized superficial swelling, mass, or lump
Subcutaneous nodules

Excludes: localized adiposity (278.1)

782.3 Edema

Anasarca	Localized edema NOS
Dropsy	

Excludes: ascites (789.51-789.59)
edema of:
newborn NOS (778.5)
pregnancy (642.0-642.9, 646.1)
fluid retention (276.6)
hydrops fetalis (773.3, 778.0)
hydrothorax (511.81-511.89)
nutritional edema (260, 262)

782.4 Jaundice, unspecified, not of newborn
Cholemia NOS
Icterus NOS

Excludes: jaundice in newborn (774.0-774.7)
due to isoimmunization (773.0-773.2, 773.4)

782.5 Cyanosis

Excludes: newborn (770.83)

⑤ **782.6 Pallor and flushing**

782.61 Pallor

782.62 Flushing
Excessive blushing

782.7 Spontaneous ecchymoses
Petechiae

Excludes: ecchymosis in fetus or newborn (772.6)
purpura (287.0-287.9)

782.8 Changes in skin texture
Induration of skin
Thickening of skin

782.9 Other symptoms involving skin and integumentary tissues

783 Symptoms concerning nutrition, metabolism, and development

783.0 Anorexia
Loss of appetite

Excludes: anorexia nervosa (307.1)
loss of appetite of nonorganic origin (307.59)

Add 4th or 5th digit	Nonspecific code	Unspecified code	Manifestation code

783.1 Abnormal weight gain

Excludes: *excessive weight gain in pregnancy (646.1)*
obesity (278.00)
morbid (278.01)

⑤ **783.2 Abnormal loss of weight and underweight**
Use additional code to identify Body Mass Index (BMI), if known (V85.0-V85.54)

783.21 Loss of weight

783.22 Underweight

783.3 Feeding difficulties and mismanagement
Feeding problem (elderly) (infant)

Excludes: *feeding disturbance or problems:*
in newborn (779.31-779.34)
of nonorganic origin (307.50-307.59)

⑤ **783.4 Lack of expected normal physiological development in childhood**

Excludes: *delay in sexual development and puberty (259.0)*
gonadal dysgenesis (758.6)
pituitary dwarfism (253.3)
slow fetal growth and fetal malnutrition (764.00-764.99)
specific delays in mental development (315.0-315.9)

783.40 Lack of normal physiological development, unspecified
Inadequate development
Lack of development

783.41 Failure to thrive
Failure to gain weight

Excludes: *failure to thrive in newborn (779.34)*

783.42 Delayed milestones
Late talker
Late walker

783.43 Short stature
Growth failure
Growth retardation
Lack of growth
Physical retardation

783.5 Polydipsia
Excessive thirst

783.6 Polyphagia
Excessive eating
Hyperalimentation NOS

Excludes: *disorders of eating of nonorganic origin (307.50-307.59)*

783.7 Adult failure to thrive

783.9 Other symptoms concerning nutrition, metabolism, and development
Hypometabolism

Excludes: *abnormal basal metabolic rate (794.7)*
dehydration (276.51)
other disorders of fluid, electrolyte, and acid-base balance (276.0-276.9)

784 Symptoms involving head and neck

Excludes: *encephalopathy NOS (348.30)*
specific symptoms involving neck classifiable to 723 (723.0-723.9)

784.0 Headache
Facial pain
Pain in head NOS

Excludes: *atypical face pain (350.2)*
migraine (346.0-346.9)
tension headache (307.81)

784.1 Throat pain

Excludes: *dysphagia (787.20-787.29)*
neck pain (723.1)
sore throat (462)
chronic (472.1)

● Code new   ▲ Revision of   ④ ⑤ Fourth or fifth
to this edition   existing code   digit required

784.2 Swelling, mass, or lump in head and neck
Space-occupying lesion, intracranial NOS

784.3 Aphasia
Excludes: *aphasia due to late effects of cerebrovascular disease (438.11)*
developmental aphasia (315.31)

▲ **784.4 Voice and resonance disorders**

▲ **784.40 Voice and resonance disorder, unspecified**

784.41 Aphonia
Loss of voice

● **784.42 Dysphonia**
Hoarseness

● **784.43 Hypernasality**

● **784.44 Hyponasality**

▲ **784.49 Other voice and resonance disorders**
Change in voice

⑤ **784.5 Other speech disturbance**
Excludes: *speech disorder due to late effect of cerebrovascular accident (438.10 - 438.19)*
stammering and stuttering (307.0)
that of nonorganic origin (307.0, 307.9)

● **784.51 Dysarthria**
Excludes: *dysarthria due to late effect of cerebrovascular accident (438.13)*

● **784.59 Other speech disturbance**
Dysphasia
Slurred speech
Speech disturbance NOS

⑤ **784.6 Other symbolic dysfunction**
Excludes: *developmental learning delays (315.0-315.9)*

784.60 Symbolic dysfunction, unspecified

784.61 Alexia and dyslexia
Alexia (with agraphia)

784.69 Other
Acalculia   Agraphia NOS
Agnosia   Apraxia

784.7 Epistaxis
Hemorrhage from nose
Nosebleed

784.8 Hemorrhage from throat
Excludes: *hemoptysis (786.3)*

⑤ **784.9 Other symptoms involving head and neck**

784.91 Postnasal drip

784.99 Other symptoms involving head and neck
Choking sensation
Feeling of foreign body in throat
Halitosis
Mouth breathing
Sneezing

Excludes: *foreign body in throat (933.0)*

785 Symptoms involving cardiovascular system
Excludes: *heart failure NOS (428.9)*

785.0 Tachycardia, unspecified
Rapid heart beat
Excludes: *neonatal tachycardia (779.82)*
paroxysmal tachycardia (427.0-427.2)

785.1 Palpitations
Awareness of heart beat
Excludes: *specified dysrhythmias (427.0-427.9)*

785.2 Undiagnosed cardiac murmurs
Heart murmur NOS

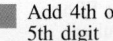

| Add 4th or 5th digit | Nonspecific code | Unspecified code | Manifestation code |

785.3 Other abnormal heart sounds
  Cardiac dullness, increased or decreased
  Friction fremitus, cardiac
  Precordial friction

785.4 Gangrene
  Gangrene NOS
  Gangrene spreading cutaneous
  Gangrenous cellulitis
  Phagedena
Code first any associated underlying condition, as:
  diabetes (250.7)
  Raynaud's syndrome (443.0)

  |Excludes:| *gangrene of certain sites—see Alphabetic Index*
           gangrene with atherosclerosis of the extremities (440.24)
           gas gangrene (040.0)

⑤ **785.5 Shock without mention of trauma**

  785.50 Shock, unspecified
      Failure of peripheral circulation

  785.51 Cardiogenic shock

  785.52 Septic shock
      endotoxic
      gram-negative
Code first systemic inflammatory response syndrome due to infectious process with organ dysfunction (995.92)

  785.59 Other
      Shock:
          hypovolemic

  |Excludes:| *shock (due to):*
           anesthetic (995.4)
           anaphylactic (995.0)
           due to serum (999.4)
           electric (994.8)
           following abortion (639.5)
           lightning (994.0)
           obstetrical (669.1)
           postoperative (998.0)
           traumatic (958.4)

785.6 Enlargement of lymph nodes
  Lymphadenopathy
  "Swollen glands"

  |Excludes:| *lymphadenitis (chronic) (289.1-289.3)*
           acute (683)

785.9 Other symptoms involving cardiovascular system
  Bruit (arterial)
  Weak pulse

786 Symptoms involving respiratory system and other chest symptoms

⑤ **786.0 Dyspnea and respiratory abnormalities**

  786.00 Respiratory abnormality, unspecified

  786.01 Hyperventilation

  |Excludes:| *hyperventilation, psychogenic (306.1)*

  786.02 Orthopnea

  786.03 Apnea

  |Excludes:| *apnea of newborn (770.81, 770.82)*
           sleep apnea (780.51, 780.53, 780.57)

  786.04 Cheyne-Stokes respiration

  786.05 Shortness of breath

  786.06 Tachypnea

  |Excludes:| *transitory tachypnea of newborn (770.6)*

  786.07 Wheezing

  |Excludes:| *asthma (493.00-493.92)*

● Code new   ▲ Revision of   ④ ⑤ Fourth or fifth
       to this edition   existing code   digit required

786.09 Other
Respiratory:
distress
insufficiency

Excludes: *respiratory distress:*
following trauma and surgery (518.5)
newborn (770.89)
syndrome (newborn) (769)
adult (518.5)
respiratory failure (518.81, 518.83-518.84)
newborn (770.84)

786.1 Stridor

Excludes: *congenital laryngeal stridor (748.3)*

786.2 Cough

Excludes: *cough:*
psychogenic (306.1)
smokers' (491.0)
with hemorrhage (786.3)

786.3 Hemoptysis
Cough with hemorrhage
Pulmonary hemorrhage NOS

Excludes: *pulmonary hemorrhage of newborn (770.3)*

786.4 Abnormal sputum
Abnormal:
amount (of) sputum
color (of) sputum
odor (of) sputum
Excessive sputum

⑤ **786.5 Chest pain**

786.50 Chest pain, unspecified

786.51 Precordial pain

786.52 Painful respiration
Pain:
anterior chest wall
pleuritic
Pleurodynia

Excludes: *epidemic pleurodynia (074.1)*

786.59 Other
Discomfort in chest
Pressure in chest
Tightness in chest

Excludes: *pain in breast (611.71)*

786.6 Swelling, mass, or lump in chest

Excludes: *lump in breast (611.72)*

786.7 Abnormal chest sounds
Abnormal percussion, chest   Rales
Friction sounds, chest   Tympany, chest

Excludes: *wheezing (786.07)*

786.8 Hiccough

Excludes: *psychogenic hiccough (306.1)*

786.9 Other symptoms involving respiratory system and chest
Breath-holding spell

787 Symptoms involving digestive system

Excludes: *constipation (564.00-564.09)*
pylorospasm (537.81)
congenital (750.5)

	Add 4th or 5th digit		Nonspecific code		Unspecified code		Manifestation code

⑤ **787.0 Nausea and vomiting**
Emesis

Excludes: *hematemesis NOS (578.0)*
vomiting:
bilious, following gastrointestinal surgery (564.3)
cyclical (536.2)
associated with migraine (346.2)
psychogenic (306.4)
excessive, in pregnancy (643.0-643.9)
fecal matter (569.87)
habit (536.2)
of newborn (779.32, 779.33)
persistent (536.2)
psychogenic NOS (307.54)

787.01 **Nausea with vomiting**

787.02 **Nausea alone**

787.03 **Vomiting alone**

● 787.04 **Bilious emesis**
Bilious vomiting

Excludes: *bilious emesis (vomiting) in newborn (779.32)*

787.1 Heartburn
Pyrosis
Waterbrash

Excludes: *dyspepsia or indigestion (536.8)*

⑤ **787.2 Dysphagia**
Code first, if applicable, dysphagia due to late effect of cerebrovascular accident (438.82)

787.20 **Dysphagia, unspecified**
Difficulty in swallowing NOS

787.21 **Dysphagia, oral phase**

787.22 **Dysphagia, oropharyngeal phase**

787.23 **Dysphagia, pharyngeal phase**

787.24 **Dysphagia, pharyngoesophageal phase**

787.29 **Other dysphagia**
Cervical dysphagia
Neurogenic dysphagia

787.3 Flatulence, eructation, and gas pain
Abdominal distention (gaseous)
Bloating
Tympanites (abdominal) (intestinal)

Excludes: *aerophagy (306.4)*

787.4 Visible peristalsis
Hyperperistalsis

787.5 Abnormal bowel sounds
Absent bowel sounds
Hyperactive bowel sounds

787.6 Incontinence of feces
Encopresis NOS
Incontinence of sphincter ani

Excludes: *that of nonorganic origin (307.7)*

787.7 Abnormal feces
Bulky stools

Excludes: *abnormal stool content (792.1)*
melena:
NOS (578.1)
newborn (772.4, 777.3)

● Code new
to this edition   ▲ Revision of
existing code   ④ ⑤ Fourth or fifth
digit required

⑤ **787.9 Other symptoms involving digestive system**

Excludes: *gastrointestinal hemorrhage (578.0-578.9)*
intestinal obstruction (560.0-560.9)
specific functional digestive disorders:
  esophagus (530.0-530.9)
  stomach and duodenum (536.0-536.9)
  those not elsewhere classified (564.00-564.9)

787.91 Diarrhea
Diarrhea NOS

787.99 Other
Change in bowel habitsTenesmus (rectal)

788 Symptoms involving urinary system

Excludes: *hematuria (599.70-599.72)*
nonspecific findings on examination of the urine (791.0-791.9)
small kidney of unknown cause (589.0-589.9)
uremia NOS (586)
urinary obstruction (599.60, 599.69)

788.0 Renal colic
Colic (recurrent) of:
  kidney
  ureter

788.1 Dysuria
Painful urination
Strangury

⑤ **788.2 Retention of urine**
Code, if applicable, any causal condition first, such as:
  hyperplasia of prostate (600.0-600.9 with fifth-digit 1)

788.20 Retention of urine, unspecified

788.21 Incomplete bladder emptying

788.29 Other specified retention of urine

⑤ **788.3 Urinary incontinence**

Excludes: *functional urinary incontinence (788.91)*
that of nonorganic origin (307.6)
urinary incontinence associated with cognitive impairment (788.91)

Code, if applicable, any causal condition first, such as:
  congenital ureterocele (753.23)
  genital prolapse (618.00-618.9)
  hyperplasia of prostate (600.0-600.9 with fifth-digit 1)

788.30 Urinary incontinence, unspecified
Enuresis NOS

788.31 Urge incontinence

788.32 Stress incontinence, male

Excludes: *stress incontinence (female) (625.6)*

788.33 Mixed incontinence (male) (female)
Urge and stress

788.34 Incontinence without sensory awareness

788.35 Post-void dribbling

788.36 Nocturnal enuresis

788.37 Continuous leakage

788.38 Overflow incontinence

788.39 Other urinary incontinence

⑤ **788.4 Frequency of urination and polyuria**
Code, if applicable, any causal condition first, such as:
  hyperplasia of prostate (600.0-600.9 with fifth-digit 1)

788.41 Urinary frequency
Frequency of micturition

788.42 Polyuria

788.43 Nocturia

	Add 4th or 5th digit		Nonspecific code		Unspecified code		Manifestation code

788.5 Oliguria and anuria
Deficient secretion of urine
Suppression of urinary secretion

Excludes: *that complicating:*
abortion (634-638 with .3, 639.3)
ectopic or molar pregnancy (639.3)
pregnancy, childbirth, or the puerperium (642.0-642.9, 646.2)

⑤ **788.6 Other abnormality of urination**
Code, if applicable, any causal condition first, such as:
hyperplasia of prostate (600.0-600.9 with fifth-digit 1)

788.61 Splitting of urinary stream
Intermittent urinary stream

788.62 Slowing of urinary stream
Weak stream

788.63 Urgency of urination

Excludes: *urge incontinence (788.31, 788.33)*

788.64 Urinary hesitancy

788.65 Straining on urination

788.69 Other

788.7 Urethral discharge
Penile discharge
Urethrorrhea

788.8 Extravasation of urine

⑤ **788.9 Other symptoms involving urinary system**

788.91 Functional urinary incontinence
Urinary incontinence due to cognitive impairment, or severe physical disability or immobility

Excludes: *urinary incontinence due to physiologic condition (788.30-788.39)*

788.99 Other symptoms involving urinary system
Extrarenal uremia
Vesical:
pain
tenesmus

789 Other symptoms involving abdomen and pelvis
The following fifth-digit subclassification is to be used for codes 789.0, 789.3, 789.4, 789.6

0 unspecified site
1 right upper quadrant
2 left upper quadrant
3 right lower quadrant
4 left lower quadrant
5 periumbilic
6 epigastric
7 generalized
9 other specified site
multiple sites

Excludes: *symptoms referable to genital organs:*
female (625.0-625.9)
male (607.0-608.9)
psychogenic (302.70-302.79)

⑤ **789.0 Abdominal pain**
[0-7,9] Cramps, abdominal

789.1 Hepatomegaly
Enlargement of liver

789.2 Splenomegaly
Enlargement of spleen

● Code new
to this edition
▲ Revision of
existing code
④ ⑤ Fourth or fifth
digit required

⑤ **789.3 Abdominal or pelvic swelling, mass, or lump**
[0-7,9]   Diffuse or generalized swelling or mass:
abdominal NOS
umbilical

Excludes: *abdominal distention (gaseous) (787.3)*
ascites (789.51-789.59)

⑤ **789.4 Abdominal rigidity**
[0-7,9]

⑤ **789.5 Ascites**
Fluid in peritoneal cavity

789.51 Malignant ascites
Code first malignancy, such as:
malignant neoplasm of ovary (183.0)
secondary malignant neoplasm of retroperitoneum and peritoneum (197.6)

789.59 Other ascites

⑤ **789.6 Abdominal tenderness**
[0-7,9]   Rebound tenderness

● **789.7 Colic**
Colic NOS
Infantile colic

Excludes: *colic in adult and child over 12 months old (789.0)*
renal colic (788.0)

789.9 Other symptoms involving abdomen and pelvis
Umbilical:
bleeding
discharge

NONSPECIFIC ABNORMAL FINDINGS (790-796)

790 Nonspecific findings on examination of blood

Excludes: *abnormalities of:*
platelets (287.0-287.9)
thrombocytes (287.0-287.9)
white blood cells (288.00-288.9)

⑤ **790.0 Abnormality of red blood cells**

Excludes: *anemia:*
congenital (776.5)
newborn, due to isoimmunization (773.0-773.2, 773.5)
of premature infant (776.6)
other specified types (280.0-285.9)
hemoglobin disorders (282.5-282.7)
polycythemia:
familial (289.6)
neonatorum (776.4)
secondary (289.0)
vera (238.4)

790.01 Precipitous drop in hematocrit
Drop in hematocrit
Drop in hemoglobin

790.09 Other abnormality of red blood cells
Abnormal red cell morphology NOS
Abnormal red cell volume NOS
Anisocytosis
Poikilocytosis

790.1 Elevated sedimentation rate

⑤ **790.2 Abnormal glucose**

Excludes: *diabetes mellitus (249.00-249.91, 250.00-250.93)*
dysmetabolic syndrome X (277.7)
gestational diabetes (648.8)
glycosuria (791.5)
hypoglycemia (251.2)
that complicating pregnancy, childbirth, or the puerperium (648.8)

790.21 Impaired fasting glucose
Elevated fasting glucose

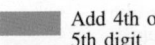

| | Add 4th or 5th digit | | Nonspecific code | | Unspecified code | | Manifestation code |

790.22 Impaired glucose tolerance test (oral)
Elevated glucose tolerance test

790.29 Other abnormal glucose
Abnormal glucose NOS
Abnormal non-fasting glucose
Hyperglycemia NOS
Pre-diabetes NOS

790.3 Excessive blood level of alcohol
Elevated blood-alcohol

790.4 Nonspecific elevation of levels of transaminase or lactic acid dehydrogenase [LDH]

790.5 Other nonspecific abnormal serum enzyme levels
Abnormal serum level of: Abnormal serum level of:
  acid phosphatase   amylase
  alkaline phosphatase   lipase

Excludes: deficiency of circulating enzymes (277.6)

790.6 Other abnormal blood chemistry
Abnormal blood level of: Abnormal blood level of:
  cobalt   lithium
  copper   magnesium
  iron   mineral
  lead   zinc

Excludes: abnormality of electrolyte or acid-base balance (276.0-276.9)
        hypoglycemia NOS (251.2)
        lead poisoning (984.0-984.9)
        specific finding indicating abnormality of:
          amino-acid transport and metabolism (270.0-270.9)
          carbohydrate transport and metabolism (271.0-271.9)
          lipid metabolism (272.0-272.9)
        uremia NOS (586)

790.7 Bacteremia

Excludes: bacteremia of newborn (771.83)
        septicemia (038)

Use additional code, if desired, to identify organism (041)

790.8 Viremia, unspecified

⑤ **790.9 Other nonspecific findings on examination of blood**

    790.91 Abnormal arterial blood gases

    790.92 Abnormal coagulation profile
      Abnormal or prolonged:
        bleeding time
        coagulation time
        partial thromboplastin time [PTT]
        prothrombin time [PT]

Excludes: coagulation (hemorrhagic) disorders (286.0-286.9)

    790.93 Elevated prostate specific antigen (PSA)

    790.94 Euthyroid sick syndrome

    790.95 Elevated C-reactive protein (CRP)

    790.99 Other

791 Nonspecific findings on examination of urine

Excludes: hematuria NOS (599.70-599.72)
        specific findings indicating abnormality of:
          amino-acid transport and metabolism (270.0-270.9)
          carbohydrate transport and metabolism (271.0-271.9)

791.0 Proteinuria
Albuminuria
Bence-Jones proteinuria

Excludes: postural proteinuria (593.6)
        that arising during pregnancy or the puerperium (642.0-642.9, 646.2)

791.1 Chyluria

Excludes: filarial (125.0-125.9)

791.2 Hemoglobinuria

● Code new   ▲ Revision of   ④ ⑤ Fourth or fifth
  to this edition   existing code   digit required

791.3 Myoglobinuria

791.4 Biliuria

791.5 Glycosuria

Excludes: *renal glycosuria (271.4)*

791.6 Acetonuria
Ketonuria

791.7 Other cells and casts in urine

791.9 Other nonspecific findings on examination of urine
Crystalluria
Elevated urine levels of:
  17-ketosteroids
  catecholamines
  indolacetic acid
  vanillylmandelic acid [VMA]
Melanuria

792 Nonspecific abnormal findings in other body substances

Excludes: *that in chromosomal analysis (795.2)*

792.0 Cerebrospinal fluid

792.1 Stool contents
Abnormal stool color
Fat in stool   Occult blood
Mucus in stool   Pus in stool

Excludes: *blood in stool [melena] (578.1)*
          newborn (772.4, 777.3)

792.2 Semen
Abnormal spermatozoa

Excludes: *azoospermia (606.0)*
          oligospermia (606.1)

792.3 Amniotic fluid

792.4 Saliva

Excludes: *that in chromosomal analysis (795.2)*

792.5 Cloudy (hemodialysis) (peritoneal) dialysis effluent

792.9 Other nonspecific abnormal findings in body substances
Peritoneal fluid   Synovial fluid
Pleural fluid   Vaginal fluids

▲ **793 Nonspecific (abnormal) findings on radiological and other examinations of body structure**
Includes: nonspecific abnormal findings of:
              thermography
              ultrasound examination [echogram]
              x-ray examination

Excludes: *abnormal results of function studies and radioisotope scans (794.0-794.9)*

793.0 Skull and head

Excludes: *nonspecific abnormal echoencephalogram (794.01)*

793.1 Lung field
Coin lesion of lung
Shadow, lung

793.2 Other intrathoracic organ
Abnormal: Mediastinal shift
  echocardiogram
  heart shadow
  ultrasound cardiogram

793.3 Biliary tract
Nonvisualization of gallbladder

793.4 Gastrointestinal tract

793.5 Genitourinary organs
Filling defect:
  bladder
  kidney
  ureter

Add 4th or 5th digit   Nonspecific code   Unspecified code   Manifestation code

793.6 **Abdominal area, including retroperitoneum**

793.7 **Musculoskeletal system**

⑤ 793.8 **Breast**

   793.80 **Abnormal mammogram, unspecified**

   793.81 **Mammographic microcalcification**

Excludes: *mammographic calcification (793.89)*
mammographic calculus (793.89)

   ● 793.82 **Inconclusive mammogram**
   Dense breasts NOS
   Inconclusive mammogram NEC
   Inconclusive mammography due to dense breasts
   Inconclusive mammography NEC

   ▲ **793.89** **Other (abnormal) findings on radiological examination of breast**
   Mammographic calcification
   Mammographic calculus

⑤ 793.9 **Other**

Excludes: *abnormal finding by radioisotope localization of placenta (794.9)*

   793.91 **Image test inconclusive due to excess body fat**
   Use additional code to identify Body Mass Index (BMI), if known
   (V85.0-V85.54)

   793.99 **Other nonspecific abnormal findings on radiological and other examinations of body structure**
   Abnormal:
       placental finding by x-ray or ultrasound method
       radiological findings in skin and subcutaneous tissue

794 **Nonspecific abnormal results of function studies**
   Includes: radioisotope:
               scans
               uptake studies
           scintiphotography

⑤ 794.0 **Brain and central nervous system**

   794.00 **Abnormal function study, unspecified**

   794.01 **Abnormal echoencephalogram**

   794.02 **Abnormal electroencephalogram [EEG]**

   794.09 **Other**
   Abnormal brain scan

⑤ 794.1 **Peripheral nervous system and special senses**

   794.10 **Abnormal response to nerve stimulation, unspecified**

   794.11 **Abnormal retinal function studies**
   Abnormal electroretinogram [ERG]

   794.12 **Abnormal electro-oculogram [EOG]**

   794.13 **Abnormal visually evoked potential**

   794.14 **Abnormal oculomotor studies**

   794.15 **Abnormal auditory function studies**

   794.16 **Abnormal vestibular function studies**

   794.17 **Abnormal electromyogram [EMG]**

Excludes: *that of eye (794.14)*

   794.19 **Other**

794.2 **Pulmonary**
   Abnormal lung scan
   Reduced:
       ventilatory capacity
       vital capacity

⑤ 794.3 **Cardiovascular**

   794.30 **Abnormal function study, unspecified**

   794.31 **Abnormal electrocardiogram [ECG] [EKG]**

Excludes: *long QT syndrome (426.82)*

● Code new   ▲ Revision of   ④ ⑤ Fourth or fifth
        to this edition   existing code   digit required

794.39 Other
Abnormal:
  ballistocardiogram
  phonocardiogram
  vectorcardiogram

794.4 Kidney
Abnormal renal function test

794.5 Thyroid
Abnormal thyroid:
  scan
  uptake

794.6 Other endocrine function study

794.7 Basal metabolism
Abnormal basal metabolic rate [BMR]

794.8 Liver
Abnormal liver scan

794.9 Other
Bladder
Pancreas
Placenta
Spleen

795 Other and nonspecific abnormal cytological, histological, immunological and DNA test findings

> Excludes: *abnormal cytologic smear of anus and anal HPV (796.70-796.79)*
> *nonspecific abnormalities of red blood cells (790.01-790.09)*

⑤ **795.0 Abnormal Papanicolaou smear of cervix and cervical HPV**
Abnormal thin preparation smear of cervix
Abnormal cervical cytology

> Excludes: *abnormal cytologic smear of vagina and vaginal HPV (795.10-795.19)*
> *carcinoma in situ of cervix (233.1)*
> *cervical intraepithelial neoplasia I [CIN I] (622.11)*
> *cervical intraepithelial neoplasia II [CIN II] (622.12)*
> *cervical intraepithelial neoplasia III [CIN III] (233.1)*
> *dysplasia (histologically confirmed) of cervix (uteri) NOS (622.10)*
> *mild cervical dysplasia (histologically confirmed) (622.11)*
> *moderate cervical dysplasia (histologically confirmed) (622.12)*
> *severe cervical dysplasia (histologically confirmed) (233.1)*

795.00 Abnormal glandular Papanicolaou smear of cervix
Atypical cervical glandular cells NOS
Atypical endocervical cells NOS
Atypical endometrial cells NOS

795.01 Papanicolaou smear of cervix with atypical squamous cells of undetermined significance (ASC-US)

795.02 Papanicolaou smear of cervix with atypical squamous cells cannot exclude high grade squamous intraepithelial lesion (ASC-H)

795.03 Papanicolaou smear of cervix with low grade squamous intraepithelial lesion (LGSIL)

795.04 Papanicolaou smear of cervix with high grade squamous intraepithelial lesion (HGSIL)

795.05 Cervical high risk human papillomavirus (HPV) DNA test positive

795.06 Papanicolaou smear of cervix with cytologic evidence of malignancy

795.07 Satisfactory cervical smear but lacking transformation zone

795.08 Unsatisfactory cervical cytology smear
Inadequate cervical cytology sample

795.09 Other abnormal Papanicolaou smear of cervix and cervical HPV
Cervical low risk human papillomavirus (HPV) DNA test positive
Papanicolaou smear of cervix with low risk human papillomavirus (HPV) DNA test positive
Use additional code for associated human papillomavirus (HPV) (079.4)

> Excludes: *encounter for Papanicolaou cervical smear to confirm findings of recent normal smear following initial abnormal smear (V72.32)*

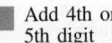

| | Add 4th or 5th digit | | Nonspecific code | | Unspecified code | | Manifestation code |

⑤ **795.1   Abnormal Papanicolaou smear of vagina and vaginal HPV**
Abnormal thin preparation smear of vagina NOS
Abnormal vaginal cytology NOS

Use additional code to identify acquired absence of uterus and cervix, if applicable
(V88.01-V88.03)

Excludes: *abnormal cytologic smear of cervix and cervical HPV (795.00-795.09)*
carcinoma in situ of vagina (233.31)
carcinoma in situ of vulva (233.32)
dysplasia (histologically confirmed) of vagina NOS (623.0, 233.31)
dysplasia (histologically confirmed) of vulva NOS (624.01, 624.02, 233.32)
mild vaginal dysplasia (histologically confirmed) (623.0)
mild vulvar dysplasia (histologically confirmed) (624.01)
moderate vaginal dysplasia (histologically confirmed) (623.0)
moderate vulvar dysplasia (histologically confirmed) (624.02)
severe vaginal dysplasia (histologically confirmed) (233.31)
severe vulvar dysplasia (histologically confirmed) (233.32)
vaginal intraepithelial neoplasia I (VAIN I) (623.0)
vaginal intraepithelial neoplasia II (VAIN II) (623.0)
vaginal intraepithelial neoplasia III (VAIN III) (233.31)
vulvar intraepithelial neoplasia I (VIN I) (624.01)
vulvar intraepithelial neoplasia II (VIN II) (624.02)
vulvar intraepithelial neoplasia III (VIN III) (233.32)

795.10   Abnormal glandular Papanicolaou smear of vagina
Atypical vaginal glandular cells NOS

795.11   Papanicolaou smear of vagina with atypical squamous cells of undetermined significance (ASC-US)

795.12   Papanicolaou smear of vagina with atypical squamous cells cannot exclude high grade squamous intraepithelial lesion (ASC-H)

795.13   Papanicolaou smear of vagina with low grade squamous intraepithelial lesion (LGSIL)

795.14   Papanicolaou smear of vagina with high grade squamous intraepithelial lesion (HGSIL)

795.15   Vaginal high risk human papillomavirus (HPV) DNA test positive

Excludes: *condyloma acuminatum (078.11)*
genital warts (078.11)

795.16   Papanicolaou smear of vagina with cytologic evidence of malignancy

795.18   Unsatisfactory vaginal cytology smear
Inadequate vaginal cytology sample

795.19   Other abnormal Papanicolaou smear of vagina and vaginal HPV
Vaginal low risk human papillomavirus (HPV) DNA test positive

Use additional code for associated human papillomavirus (079.4)

795.2   Nonspecific abnormal findings on chromosomal analysis
Abnormal karyotype

⑤ **795.3   Nonspecific positive culture findings**
Positive culture findings in:
nose
sputum
throat
wound

Excludes: *that of:*
blood (790.7-790.8)
urine (791.9)

795.31   Nonspecific positive findings for anthrax
Positive findings by nasal swab

795.39   Other nonspecific positive culture findings

Excludes: *colonization status (V02.0-V02.9)*

795.4   Other nonspecific abnormal histological findings

795.5   Nonspecific reaction to tuberculin skin test without active tuberculosis
Abnormal result of Mantoux test
PPD positive
Tuberculin (skin test):
positive
reactor

● Code new to this edition   ▲ Revision of existing code   ④ ⑤ Fourth or fifth digit required

795.6 False positive serological test for syphilis
False positive Wassermann reaction

⑤ **795.7 Other nonspecific immunological findings**

Excludes: *abnormal tumor markers (795.81-795.89)*
elevated prostate specific antigen [PSA] (790.93)
elevated tumor associated antigens (795.81-795.89)
isoimmunization, in pregnancy (656.1-656.2)
affecting fetus or newborn (773.0-773.2)

795.71 Nonspecific serologic evidence of human immunodeficiency virus [HIV]
Inconclusive human immunodeficiency virus [HIV] test (adult) (infant)

Note: This code is ONLY to be used when a test finding is reported as nonspecific.
Asymptomatic positive findings are coded to V08. If any HIV infection symptom or
condition is present, see code 042. Negative findings are not coded.

Excludes: *acquired immunodeficiency syndrome [AIDS] (042)*
asymptomatic human immunodeficiency virus, [HIV] infection status (V08)
HIV infection, symptomatic (042)
human immunodeficiency virus [HIV] disease (042)
positive (status) NOS (V08)

795.79 Other and unspecified nonspecific immunological findings
Raised antibody titer
Raised level of immunoglobulins

⑤ **795.8 Abnormal tumor markers**
Elevated tumor associated antigens [TAA]
Elevated tumor specific antigens [TSA]

Excludes: *elevated prostate specific antigen [PSA] (790.93)*

795.81 Elevated carcinoembryonic antigen (CEA)

795.82 Elevated cancer antigen 125 (CA 125)

795.89 Other abnormal tumor markers

796 Other nonspecific abnormal findings

796.0 Nonspecific abnormal toxicological findings
Abnormal levels of heavy metals or drugs in blood, urine, or other tissue

Excludes: *excessive blood level of alcohol (790.3)*

796.1 Abnormal reflex

796.2 Elevated blood pressure reading without diagnosis of hypertension
Note: This category is to be used to record an episode of elevated blood pressure in a patient in
whom no formal diagnosis of hypertension has been made, or as an incidental finding.

796.3 Nonspecific low blood pressure reading

796.4 Other abnormal clinical findings

796.5 Abnormal finding on antenatal screening

796.6 Abnormal findings on neonatal screening

Excludes: *nonspecific serologic evidence of human immunodeficiency virus [HIV] (795.71)*

⑤ **796.7 Abnormal cytologic smear of anus and anal HPV**

Excludes: *abnormal cytologic smear of cervix and cervical HPV (795.00-795.09)*
abnormal cytologic smear of vagina and vaginal HPV (795.10-795.19)
anal intraepithelial neoplasia I (AIN I) (569.44)
anal intraepithelial neoplasia II (AIN II) (569.44)
anal intraepithelial neoplasia III (AIN III) (230.5, 230.6)
carcinoma in situ of anus (230.5, 230.6)
dysplasia (histologically confirmed) of anus NOS (569.44)
mild anal dysplasia (histologically confirmed) (569.44)
moderate anal dysplasia (histologically confirmed) (569.44)
severe anal dysplasia (histologically confirmed) (230.5, 230.6)

796.70 Abnormal glandular Papanicolaou smear of anus
Atypical anal glandular cells NOS

**796.71 Papanicolaou smear of anus with atypical squamous cells of undetermined
significance (ASC-US)**

**796.72 Papanicolaou smear of anus with atypical squamous cells cannot exclude
high grade squamous intraepithelial lesion (ASC-H)**

**796.73 Papanicolaou smear of anus with low grade squamous intraepithelial lesion
(LGSIL)**

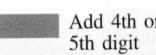

| | Add 4th or 5th digit | | Nonspecific code | | Unspecified code | | Manifestation code |

796.74 **Papanicolaou smear of anus with high grade squamous intraepithelial lesion (HGSIL)**

796.75 **Anal high risk human papillomavirus (HPV) DNA test positive**

796.76 **Papanicolaou smear of anus with cytologic evidence of malignancy**

796.77 **Satisfactory anal smear but lacking transformation zone**

796.78 **Unsatisfactory anal cytology smear**
Inadequate anal cytology sample

796.79 **Other abnormal Papanicolaou smear of anus and anal HPV**
Anal low risk human papillomavirus (HPV)
DNA test positive

Use additional code for associated human papillomavirus (079.4)

796.9 **Other**

ILL-DEFINED AND UNKNOWN CAUSES OF MORBIDITY AND MORTALITY (797-799)

797 **Senility without mention of psychosis**
Frailty
Old age
Senescence
Senile asthenia
Senile debility
Senile exhaustion

Excludes: *senile psychoses (290.0-290.9)*

798 **Sudden death, cause unknown**

798.0 **Sudden infant death syndrome**
Cot death
Crib death
Sudden death of nonspecific cause in infancy

798.1 **Instantaneous death**

798.2 **Death occurring in less than 24 hours from onset of symptoms, not otherwise explained**
Death known not to be violent or instantaneous, for which no cause could be discovered
Died without sign of disease

798.9 **Unattended death**
Death in circumstances where the body of the deceased was found and no cause could be discovered
Found dead

799 **Other ill-defined and unknown causes of morbidity and mortality**

⑤ 799.0 **Asphyxia and hypoxemia**

Excludes: *asphyxia and hypoxemia (due to)*
hypercapnia (786.09)

799.01 **Asphyxia**

799.02 **Hypoxemia**

799.1 **Respiratory arrest**
Cardiorespiratory failure

Excludes: *cardiac arrest (427.5)*
failure of peripheral circulation (785.50)
respiratory distress:
NOS (786.09)
acute (518.82)
following trauma and surgery (518.5)
newborn (770.89)
syndrome (newborn) (769)
adult (following trauma and surgery) (518.5)
other (518.82)
respiratory failure (518.81, 518.83-518.84)
newborn (770.84)
respiratory insufficiency (786.09)
acute (518.82)

▲ 799.2 **Signs and symptoms involving emotional state**

Excludes: *anxiety (293.84, 300.00-300.09)*
depression (311)

● Code new
to this edition

▲ Revision of
existing code

④ ⑤ Fourth or fifth
digit required

● **799.21 Nervousness**
Nervous

● **799.22 Irritability**
Irritable

● **799.23 Impulsiveness**
Impulsive

Excludes: *impulsive neurosis (300.3)*

● **799.24 Emotional lability**

● **799.25 Demoralization and apathy**
Apathetic

● **799.29 Other signs and symptoms involving emotional state**

799.3 Debility, unspecified

Excludes: *asthenia (780.79)*
nervous debility (300.5)
neurasthenia (300.5)
senile asthenia (797)

799.4 Cachexia
Wasting disease

Code first underlying condition, if known

⑤ **799.8 Other ill-defined conditions**

799.81 Decreased libido
Decreased sexual desire

Excludes: *psychosexual dysfunction with inhibited sexual desire (302.71)*

● **799.82 Apparent life threatening event in infant**
ALTE
Apparent life threatening event in newborn and infant

Use additional code(s) for associated signs and symptoms

Excludes: *signs and symptoms associated with a confirmed diagnosis- code to confirmed diagnosis*

799.89 Other ill-defined conditions

799.9 Other unknown and unspecified cause
Undiagnosed disease, not specified as to site or system involved
Unknown cause of morbidity or mortality

| | Add 4th or 5th digit | | Nonspecific code | | Unspecified code | | Manifestation code |

● Code new
 to this edition

▲ Revision of
 existing code

④ ⑤ Fourth or fifth
 digit required

17. INJURY AND POISONING (800-999)

Use E code(s) to identify the cause and intent of the injury or poisoning (E800-E999)

Note:

1. The principle of multiple coding of injuries should be followed wherever possible. Combination categories for multiple injuries are provided for use when there is insufficient detail as to the nature of the individual conditions, or for primary tabulation purposes when it is more convenient to record a single code; otherwise, the component injuries should be coded separately.

   Where multiple sites of injury are specified in the titles, the word "with" indicates involvement of both sites, and the word "and" indicates involvement of either or both sites. The word "finger" includes thumb.

2. Categories for "late effect" of injuries are to be found at 905-909.

FRACTURES (800-829)

> Excludes: malunion (733.81)
> nonunion (733.82)
> pathologic or spontaneous fracture (733.10-733.19)
> stress fractures (733.93-733.95)

The terms "condyle," "coronoid process," "ramus," and "symphysis" indicate the portion of the bone fractured, not the name of the bone involved.

The descriptions "closed" and "open" used in the fourth-digit subdivisions include the following terms:

closed (with or without delayed healing):

comminuted	impacted
depressed	linear
elevated	simple
fissured	slipped epiphysis
fracture NOS	spiral
greenstick	

open (with or without delayed healing):

compound	puncture
infected	with foreign body
missile	

A fracture not indicated as closed or open should be classified as closed.

FRACTURE OF SKULL (800-804)

Includes: traumatic brain injury due to fracture of skull

The following fifth-digit subclassification is for use with the appropriate codes in categories 800, 801, 803, and 804:

0 unspecified state of consciousness

1 with no loss of consciousness

2 with brief [less than one hour] loss of consciousness

3 with moderate [1-24 hours] loss of consciousness and return to pre-existing conscious level

4 with prolonged [more than 24 hours] loss of consciousness and return to pre-existing conscious level

5 with prolonged [more than 24 hours] loss of consciousness, without return to pre-existing conscious level
    Use fifth-digit 5 to designate when a patient is unconscious and dies before regaining consciousness, regardless of the duration of the loss of consciousness

6 with loss of consciousness of unspecified duration

9 with concussion, unspecified

⑤ **800** **Fracture of vault of skull**
    Includes: frontal bone
              parietal bone

⑤ **800.0** **Closed without mention of intracranial injury**
    [0-6,9]

⑤ **800.1** **Closed with cerebral laceration and contusion**
    [0-6,9]

⑤ **800.2** **Closed with subarachnoid, subdural, and extradural hemorrhage**
    [0-6,9]

⑤ **800.3** **Closed with other and unspecified intracranial hemorrhage**
    [0-6,9]

Add 4th or 5th digit	Nonspecific code	Unspecified code	Medicare secondary payer (MSP) alert

⑤ **800.4** Closed with intracranial injury of other and unspecified nature
[0-6,9]

⑤ **800.5** Open without mention of intracranial injury
[0-6,9]

⑤ **800.6** Open with cerebral laceration and contusion
[0-6,9]

⑤ **800.7** Open with subarachnoid, subdural, and extradural hemorrhage
[0-6,9]

⑤ **800.8** Open with other and unspecified intracranial hemorrhage
[0-6,9]

⑤ **800.9** Open with intracranial injury of other and unspecified nature
[0-6,9]

⑤ **801** Fracture of base of skull
Includes:

fossa:	sinus:
anterior	ethmoid
middle	frontal
posterior	sphenoid bone
occiput bone	temporal bone
orbital roof	

⑤ **801.0** Closed without mention of intracranial injury
[0-6,9]

⑤ **801.1** Closed with cerebral laceration and contusion
[0-6,9]

⑤ **801.2** Closed with subarachnoid, subdural, and extradural hemorrhage
[0-6,9]

⑤ **801.3** Closed with other and unspecified intracranial hemorrhage
[0-6,9]

⑤ **801.4** Closed with intracranial injury of other and unspecified nature
[0-6,9]

⑤ **801.5** Open without mention of intracranial injury
[0-6,9]

⑤ **801.6** Open with cerebral laceration and contusion
[0-6,9]

⑤ **801.7** Open with subarachnoid, subdural, and extradural hemorrhage
[0-6,9]

⑤ **801.8** Open with other and unspecified intracranial hemorrhage
[0-6,9]

⑤ **801.9** Open with intracranial injury of other and unspecified nature
[0-6,9]

802 Fracture of face bones

802.0 Nasal bones, closed

802.1 Nasal bones, open

⑤ **802.2** Mandible, closed
Inferior maxilla
Lower jaw (bone)

802.20 Unspecified site

802.21 Condylar process

802.22 Subcondylar

802.23 Coronoid process

802.24 Ramus, unspecified

802.25 Angle of jaw

802.26 Symphysis of body

802.27 Alveolar border of body

802.28 Body, other and unspecified

802.29 Multiple sites

⑤ **802.3** Mandible, open

802.30 Unspecified site

802.31 Condylar process

● Code new
to this edition

▲ Revision of
existing code

④ ⑤ Fourth or fifth
digit required

802.32 **Subcondylar**

802.33 **Coronoid process**

802.34 **Ramus, unspecified**

802.35 **Angle of jaw**

802.36 **Symphysis of body**

802.37 **Alveolar border of body**

802.38 **Body, other and unspecified**

802.39 **Multiple sites**

802.4 **Malar and maxillary bones, closed**
    Superior maxilla   Zygoma
    Upper jaw (bone)   Zygomatic arch

802.5 **Malar and maxillary bones, open**

802.6 **Orbital floor (blow-out), closed**

802.7 **Orbital floor (blow-out), open**

802.8 **Other facial bones, closed**
    Alveolus
    Orbit:
      NOS
      part other than roof or floor
    Palate

    Excludes: *orbital:*
        floor (802.6)
        roof (801.0-801.9)

802.9 **Other facial bones, open**

⑤ **803 Other and unqualified skull fractures**
    Includes: skull NOS
               skull multiple NOS

⑤ 803.0 **Closed without mention of intracranial injury**
    [0-6,9]

⑤ 803.1 **Closed with cerebral laceration and contusion**
    [0-6,9]

⑤ 803.2 **Closed with subarachnoid, subdural, and extradural hemorrhage**
    [0-6,9]

⑤ 803.3 **Closed with other and unspecified intracranial hemorrhage**
    [0-6,9]

⑤ 803.4 **Closed with intracranial injury of other and unspecified nature**
    [0-6,9]

⑤ 803.5 **Open without mention of intracranial injury**
    [0-6,9]

⑤ 803.6 **Open with cerebral laceration and contusion**
    [0-6,9]

⑤ 803.7 **Open with subarachnoid, subdural, and extradural hemorrhage**
    [0-6,9]

⑤ 803.8 **Open with other and unspecified intracranial hemorrhage**
    [0-6,9]

⑤ 803.9 **Open with intracranial injury of other and unspecified nature**
    [0-6,9]

⑤ **804 Multiple fractures involving skull or face with other bones**

⑤ 804.0 **Closed without mention of intracranial injury**
    [0-6,9]

⑤ 804.1 **Closed with cerebral laceration and contusion**
    [0-6,9]

⑤ 804.2 **Closed with subarachnoid, subdural, and extradural hemorrhage**
    [0-6,9]

⑤ 804.3 **Closed with other and unspecified intracranial hemorrhage**
    [0-6,9]

⑤ 804.4 **Closed with intracranial injury of other and unspecified nature**
    [0-6,9]

| | Add 4th or 5th digit | | Nonspecific code | | Unspecified code | | Medicare secondary payer (MSP) alert |

⑤ **804.5** **Open without mention of intracranial injury**
[0-6,9]

⑤ **804.6** **Open with cerebral laceration and contusion**
[0-6,9]

⑤ **804.7** **Open with subarachnoid, subdural, and extradural hemorrhage**
[0-6,9]

⑤ **804.8** **Open with other and unspecified intracranial hemorrhage**
[0-6,9]

⑤ **804.9** **Open with intracranial injury of other and unspecified nature**
[0-6,9]

FRACTURE OF NECK AND TRUNK (805-809)

805 **Fracture of vertebral column without mention of spinal cord injury**
      Includes: neural arch
                 spine
                 spinous process
                 transverse process
                 vertebra

The following fifth-digit subclassification is for use with codes 805.0-805.1:

  0 **cervical vertebra, unspecified level**

  1 **first cervical vertebra**

  2 **second cervical vertebra**

  3 **third cervical vertebra**

  4 **fourth cervical vertebra**

  5 **fifth cervical vertebra**

  6 **sixth cervical vertebra**

  7 **seventh cervical vertebra**

  8 **multiple cervical vertebrae**

⑤ **805.0** **Cervical, closed**
[0-8]   Atlas
          Axis

⑤ **805.1** **Cervical, open**
[0-8]

  805.2 **Dorsal [thoracic], closed**

  805.3 **Dorsal [thoracic], open**

  805.4 **Lumbar, closed**

  805.5 **Lumbar, open**

  805.6 **Sacrum and coccyx, closed**

  805.7 **Sacrum and coccyx, open**

  805.8 **Unspecified, closed**

  805.9 **Unspecified, open**

806 **Fracture of vertebral column with spinal cord injury**
      Includes: any condition classifiable to 805 with:
                 complete or incomplete transverse lesion (of cord)
                 hematomyelia
                 injury to:
                    cauda equina
                    nerve
                 paralysis
                 paraplegia
                 quadriplegia
                 spinal concussion

⑤ **806.0** **Cervical, closed**

    806.00 **C_1-C_4 level with unspecified spinal cord injury**
          Cervical region NOS with spinal cord injury NOS

    806.01 **C_1-C_4 level with complete lesion of cord**

    806.02 **C_1-C_4 level with anterior cord syndrome**

    806.03 **C_1-C_4 level with central cord syndrome**

    ● Code new   ▲ Revision of   ④ ⑤ Fourth or fifth
       to this edition   existing code   digit required

806.04 C_1-C_4 level with other specified spinal cord injury
C_1-C_4 level with:
  incomplete spinal cord lesion NOS
  posterior cord syndrome

806.05 C_5-C_7 level with unspecified spinal cord injury

806.06 C_5-C_7 level with complete lesion of cord

806.07 C_5-C_7 level with anterior cord syndrome

806.08 C_5-C_7 level with central cord syndrome

806.09 C_5-C_7 level with other specified spinal cord injury
C_5-C_7 level with:
  incomplete spinal cord lesion NOS
  posterior cord syndrome

⑤ **806.1 Cervical, open**

806.10 C_1-C_4 level with unspecified spinal cord injury

806.11 C_1-C_4 level with complete lesion of cord

806.12 C_1-C_4 level with anterior cord syndrome

806.13 C_1-C_4 level with central cord syndrome

806.14 C_1-C_4 level with other specified spinal cord injury
C_1-C_4 level with:
  incomplete spinal cord lesion NOS
  posterior cord syndrome

806.15 C_5-C_7 level with unspecified spinal cord injury

806.16 C_5-C_7 level with complete lesion of cord

806.17 C_5-C_7 level with anterior cord syndrome

806.18 C_5-C_7 level with central cord syndrome

806.19 C_5-C_7 level with other specified spinal cord injury
C_5-C_7 level with:
  incomplete spinal cord lesion NOS
  posterior cord syndrome

⑤ **806.2 Dorsal [thoracic], closed**

806.20 T_1-T_6 level with unspecified spinal cord injury
Thoracic region NOS with spinal cord injury NOS

806.21 T_1-T_6 level with complete lesion of cord

806.22 T_1-T_6 level with anterior cord syndrome

806.23 T_1-T_6 level with central cord syndrome

806.24 T_1-T_6 level with other specified spinal cord injury
T_1-T_6 level with:
  incomplete spinal cord lesion NOS
  posterior cord syndrome

806.25 T_7-T_{12} level with unspecified spinal cord injury

806.26 T_7-T_{12} level with complete lesion of cord

806.27 T_7-T_{12} level with anterior cord syndrome

806.28 T_7-T_{12} level with central cord syndrome

806.29 T_7-T_{12} level with other specified spinal cord injury
T_7-T_{12} level with:
  incomplete spinal cord lesion NOS
  posterior cord syndrome

⑤ **806.3 Dorsal [thoracic], open**

806.30 T_1-T_6 level with unspecified spinal cord injury

806.31 T_1-T_6 level with complete lesion of cord

806.32 T_1-T_6 level with anterior cord syndrome

806.33 T_1-T_6 level with central cord syndrome

806.34 T_1-T_6 level with other specified spinal cord injury
T_1-T_6 level with:
  incomplete spinal cord lesion NOS
  posterior cord syndrome

806.35 T_7-T_{12} level with unspecified spinal cord injury

806.36 T_7-T_{12} level with complete lesion of cord

Add 4th or 5th digit	Nonspecific code	Unspecified code	Medicare secondary payer (MSP) alert

806.37 T$_7$-T$_{12}$ level with anterior cord syndrome

806.38 T$_7$-T$_{12}$ level with central cord syndrome

806.39 T$_7$-T$_{12}$ level with other specified spinal cord injury
T$_7$-T$_{12}$ level with:
    incomplete spinal cord lesion NOS
    posterior cord syndrome

806.4 Lumbar, closed

806.5 Lumbar, open

⑤ **806.6** Sacrum and coccyx, closed

   806.60 With unspecified spinal cord injury

   806.61 With complete cauda equina lesion

   806.62 With other cauda equina injury

   806.69 With other spinal cord injury

⑤ **806.7** Sacrum and coccyx, open

   806.70 With unspecified spinal cord injury

   806.71 With complete cauda equina lesion

   806.72 With other cauda equina injury

   806.79 With other spinal cord injury

806.8 Unspecified, closed

806.9 Unspecified, open

807 Fracture of rib(s), sternum, larynx, and trachea
The following fifth-digit subclassification is for use with codes 807.0-807.1:

   0 rib(s), unspecified

   1 one rib

   2 two ribs

   3 three ribs

   4 four ribs

   5 five ribs

   6 six ribs

   7 seven ribs

   8 eight or more ribs

   9 multiple ribs, unspecified

⑤ **807.0** Rib(s), closed
[0-9]

⑤ **807.1** Rib(s), open
[0-9]

807.2 Sternum, closed

807.3 Sternum, open

807.4 Flail chest

807.5 Larynx and trachea, closed
Hyoid bone   Trachea
Thyroid cartilage

807.6 Larynx and trachea, open

808 Fracture of pelvis

808.0 Acetabulum, closed

808.1 Acetabulum, open

808.2 Pubis, closed

808.3 Pubis, open

⑤ **808.4** Other specified part, closed

   808.41 Ilium

   808.42 Ischium

   808.43 Multiple pelvic fractures with disruption of pelvic circle

   808.49 Other
Innominate bone
Pelvic rim

● Code new   ▲ Revision of   ④ ⑤ Fourth or fifth
to this edition   existing code   digit required

⑤ **808.5 Other specified part, open**

      808.51 Ilium

      808.52 Ischium

      808.53 Multiple pelvic fractures with disruption of pelvic circle

      808.59 Other

  808.8 Unspecified, closed

  808.9 Unspecified, open

809 Ill-defined fractures of bones of trunk
    Includes: bones of trunk with other bones except those of skull and face
                  multiple bones of trunk

    Excludes: *multiple fractures of:*
              pelvic bones alone (808.0-808.9)
              ribs alone (807.0-807.1, 807.4)
              ribs or sternum with limb bones (819.0-819.1, 828.0-828.1)
              skull or face with other bones (804.0-804.9)

  809.0 Fracture of bones of trunk, closed

  809.1 Fracture of bones of trunk, open

FRACTURE OF UPPER LIMB (810-819)

⑤ **810 Fracture of clavicle**
    Includes: collar bone
                  interligamentous part of clavicle

  The following fifth-digit subclassification is for use with category 810:

      0 unspecified part
            Clavicle NOS

      1 sternal end of clavicle

      2 shaft of clavicle

      3 acromial end of clavicle

  ⑤ **810.0 Closed**
    [0-3]

  ⑤ **810.1 Open**
    [0-3]

⑤ **811 Fracture of scapula**
    Includes: shoulder blade

  The following fifth-digit subclassification is for use with category 811:

      0 unspecified part

      1 acromial process
            Acromion (process)

      2 coracoid process

      3 glenoid cavity and neck of scapula

      9 other
            Scapula body

  ⑤ **811.0 Closed**
    [0-3,9]

  ⑤ **811.1 Open**
    [0-3,9]

812 Fracture of humerus

  ⑤ **812.0 Upper end, closed**

      812.00 Upper end, unspecified part
               Proximal end
               Shoulder

      812.01 Surgical neck
               Neck of humerus NOS

      812.02 Anatomical neck

      812.03 Greater tuberosity

      812.09 Other
               Head
               Upper epiphysis

  ⑤ **812.1 Upper end, open**

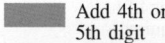

	Add 4th or 5th digit		Nonspecific code		Unspecified code		Medicare secondary payer (MSP) alert

812.10 **Upper end, unspecified part**

812.11 **Surgical neck**

812.12 **Anatomical neck**

812.13 **Greater tuberosity**

812.19 **Other**

⑤ 812.2 **Shaft or unspecified part, closed**

812.20 **Unspecified part of humerus**
Humerus NOS
Upper arm NOS

812.21 **Shaft of humerus**

⑤ 812.3 **Shaft or unspecified part, open**

812.30 **Unspecified part of humerus**

812.31 **Shaft of humerus**

⑤ 812.4 **Lower end, closed**
Distal end of humerus
Elbow

812.40 **Lower end, unspecified part**

812.41 **Supracondylar fracture of humerus**

812.42 **Lateral condyle**
External condyle

812.43 **Medial condyle**
Internal epicondyle

812.44 **Condyle(s), unspecified**
Articular process NOS
Lower epiphysis NOS

812.49 **Other**
Multiple fractures of lower end
Trochlea

⑤ 812.5 **Lower end, open**

812.50 **Lower end, unspecified part**

812.51 **Supracondylar fracture of humerus**

812.52 **Lateral condyle**

812.53 **Medial condyle**

812.54 **Condyle(s), unspecified**

812.59 **Other**

813 **Fracture of radius and ulna**

⑤ 813.0 **Upper end, closed**
Proximal end

813.00 **Upper end of forearm, unspecified**

813.01 **Olecranon process of ulna**

813.02 **Coronoid process of ulna**

813.03 **Monteggia's fracture**

813.04 **Other and unspecified fractures of proximal end of ulna (alone)**
Multiple fractures of ulna, upper end

813.05 **Head of radius**

813.06 **Neck of radius**

813.07 **Other and unspecified fractures of proximal end of radius (alone)**
Multiple fractures of radius, upper end

813.08 **Radius with ulna, upper end [any part]**

⑤ 813.1 **Upper end, open**

813.10 **Upper end of forearm, unspecified**

813.11 **Olecranon process of ulna**

813.12 **Coronoid process of ulna**

813.13 **Monteggia's fracture**

813.14 **Other and unspecified fractures of proximal end of ulna (alone)**

813.15 **Head of radius**

● Code new
to this edition

▲ Revision of
existing code

④ ⑤ Fourth or fifth
digit required

813.16　Neck of radius

813.17　Other and unspecified fractures of proximal end of radius (alone)

813.18　Radius with ulna, upper end [any part]

⑤ 813.2　Shaft, closed

813.20　Shaft, unspecified

813.21　Radius (alone)

813.22　Ulna (alone)

813.23　Radius with ulna

⑤ 813.3　Shaft, open

813.30　Shaft, unspecified

813.31　Radius (alone)

813.32　Ulna (alone)

813.33　Radius with ulna

⑤ 813.4　Lower end, closed
　　　Distal end

813.40　Lower end of forearm, unspecified

813.41　Colles' fracture
　　　Smith's fracture

813.42　Other fractures of distal end of radius (alone)
　　　Dupuytren's fracture, radius
　　　Radius, lower end

813.43　Distal end of ulna (alone)
　　　Ulna:　　　　　　　Ulna:
　　　　head　　　　　　　lower epiphysis
　　　　lower end　　　　　styloid process

813.44　Radius with ulna, lower end

▲ 813.45　Torus fracture of radius (alone)

Excludes: *Torus fracture of radius and ulna (813.47)*

● 813.46　Torus fracture of ulna (alone)

Excludes: *Torus fracture of radius and ulna (813.47)*

● 813.47　Torus fracture of radius and ulna

⑤ 813.5　Lower end, open

813.50　Lower end of forearm, unspecified

813.51　Colles' fracture

813.52　Other fractures of distal end of radius (alone)

813.53　Distal end of ulna (alone)

813.54　Radius with ulna, lower end

⑤ 813.8　Unspecified part, closed

813.80　Forearm, unspecified

813.81　Radius (alone)

813.82　Ulna (alone)

813.83　Radius with ulna

⑤ 813.9　Unspecified part, open

813.90　Forearm, unspecified

813.91　Radius (alone)

813.92　Ulna (alone)

813.93　Radius with ulna

⑤ **814**　Fracture of carpal bone(s)
　　The following fifth-digit subclassification is for use with category 814:

0　carpal bone, unspecified
　　Wrist NOS

1　navicular [scaphoid] of wrist

2　lunate [semilunar] bone of wrist

3　triquetral [cuneiform] bone of wrist

| ▨ Add 4th or 5th digit | ▨ Nonspecific code | ▨ Unspecified code | ▨ Medicare secondary payer (MSP) alert |

    4   **pisiform**

    5   **trapezium bone [larger multangular]**

    6   **trapezoid bone [smaller multangular]**

    7   **capitate bone [os magnum]**

    8   **hamate [unciform] bone**

    9   **other**

⑤ **814.0** **Closed**
[0-9]

⑤ **814.1** **Open**
[0-9]

⑤ **815** **Fracture of metacarpal bone(s)**
      Includes: hand [except finger]
                metacarpus

    The following fifth-digit subclassification is for use with category 815:

    0   **metacarpal bone(s), site unspecified**

    1   **base of thumb [first] metacarpal**
         Bennett's fracture

    2   **base of other metacarpal bone(s)**

    3   **shaft of metacarpal bone(s)**

    4   **neck of metacarpal bone(s)**

    9   **multiple sites of metacarpus**

⑤ **815.0** **Closed**
[0-4,9]

⑤ **815.1** **Open**
[0-4,9]

⑤ **816** **Fracture of one or more phalanges of hand**
      Includes: finger(s)
                thumb

    The following fifth-digit subclassification is for use with category 816:

    0   **phalanx or phalanges, unspecified**

    1   **middle or proximal phalanx or phalanges**

    2   **distal phalanx or phalanges**

    3   **multiple sites**

⑤ **816.0** **Closed**
[0-3]

⑤ **816.1** **Open**
[0-3]

817 **Multiple fractures of hand bones**
      Includes: metacarpal bone(s) with phalanx or phalanges of same hand

    817.0 **Closed**

    817.1 **Open**

818 **Ill-defined fractures of upper limb**
      Includes: arm NOS
                multiple bones of same upper limb

    Excludes: *multiple fractures of:*
            metacarpal bone(s) with phalanx or phalanges (817.0-817.1)
            phalanges of hand alone (816.0-816.1)
            radius with ulna (813.0-813.9)

    818.0 **Closed**

    818.1 **Open**

819 **Multiple fractures involving both upper limbs, and upper limb with rib(s) and sternum**
      Includes: arm(s) with rib(s) or sternum
                both arms [any bones]

    819.0 **Closed**

    819.1 **Open**

FRACTURE OF LOWER LIMB (820-829)

820 **Fracture of neck of femur**

    ● Code new   ▲ Revision of   ④ ⑤ Fourth or fifth
        to this edition   existing code   digit required

⑤ **820.0** **Transcervical fracture, closed**

    820.00 **Intracapsular section, unspecified**

    820.01 **Epiphysis (separation) (upper)**
        Transepiphyseal

    820.02 **Midcervical section**
        Transcervical NOS

    820.03 **Base of neck**
        Cervicotrochanteric section

    820.09 **Other**
        Head of femur
        Subcapital

⑤ **820.1** **Transcervical fracture, open**

    820.10 **Intracapsular section, unspecified**

    820.11 **Epiphysis (separation) (upper)**

    820.12 **Midcervical section**

    820.13 **Base of neck**

    820.19 **Other**

⑤ **820.2** **Pertrochanteric fracture, closed**

    820.20 **Trochanteric section, unspecified**
        Trochanter:
          NOS
          greater
          lesser

    820.21 **Intertrochanteric section**

    820.22 **Subtrochanteric section**

⑤ **820.3** **Pertrochanteric fracture, open**

    820.30 **Trochanteric section, unspecified**

    820.31 **Intertrochanteric section**

    820.32 **Subtrochanteric section**

    820.8 **Unspecified part of neck of femur, closed**
        Hip NOS
        Neck of femur NOS

    820.9 **Unspecified part of neck of femur, open**

821 **Fracture of other and unspecified parts of femur**

⑤ **821.0** **Shaft or unspecified part, closed**

    821.00 **Unspecified part of femur**
        Thigh
        Upper leg

    Excludes: hip NOS (820.8)

    821.01 **Shaft**

⑤ **821.1** **Shaft or unspecified part, open**

    821.10 **Unspecified part of femur**

    821.11 **Shaft**

⑤ **821.2** **Lower end, closed**
    Distal end

    821.20 **Lower end, unspecified part**

    821.21 **Condyle, femoral**

    821.22 **Epiphysis, lower (separation)**

    821.23 **Supracondylar fracture of femur**

    821.29 **Other**
        Multiple fractures of lower end

⑤ **821.3** **Lower end, open**

    821.30 **Lower end, unspecified part**

    821.31 **Condyle, femoral**

    821.32 **Epiphysis, lower (separation)**

    821.33 **Supracondylar fracture of femur**

| | Add 4th or 5th digit | | Nonspecific code | | Unspecified code | | Medicare secondary payer (MSP) alert |

821.39 Other

822 **Fracture of patella**

   822.0 **Closed**

   822.1 **Open**

823 **Fracture of tibia and fibula**

> Excludes: *Dupuytren's fracture (824.4-824.5)*
> *ankle (824.4-824.5)*
> *radius (813.42, 813.52)*
> *Pott's fracture (824.4-824.5)*
> *that involving ankle (824.0-824.9)*

The following fifth-digit subclassification is for use with category 823:

   0 **tibia alone**

   1 **fibula alone**

   2 **fibula with tibia**

⑤ **823.0** **Upper end, closed**
[0-2]   Head
        Proximal end
        Tibia:
          condyles
          tuberosity

⑤ **823.1** **Upper end, open**
[0-2]

⑤ **823.2** **Shaft, closed**
[0-2]

⑤ **823.3** **Shaft, open**
[0-2]

⑤ **823.4** **Torus fracture**
[0-2]

⑤ **823.8** **Unspecified part, closed**
[0-2]   Lower leg NOS

⑤ **823.9** **Unspecified part, open**
[0-2]

824 **Fracture of ankle**

   824.0 **Medial malleolus, closed**
        Tibia involving:
          ankle
          malleolus

   824.1 **Medial malleolus, open**

   824.2 **Lateral malleolus, closed**
        Fibula involving:
          ankle
          malleolus

   824.3 **Lateral malleolus, open**

   824.4 **Bimalleolar, closed**
        Dupuytren's fracture, fibula
        Pott's fracture

   824.5 **Bimalleolar, open**

   824.6 **Trimalleolar, closed**
        Lateral and medial malleolus with anterior or posterior lip of tibia

   824.7 **Trimalleolar, open**

   824.8 **Unspecified, closed**
        Ankle NOS

   824.9 **Unspecified, open**

825 **Fracture of one or more tarsal and metatarsal bones**

   825.0 **Fracture of calcaneus, closed**
        Heel bone
        Os calcis

   825.1 **Fracture of calcaneus, open**

⑤ **825.2** **Fracture of other tarsal and metatarsal bones, closed**

● Code new
   to this edition
	▲ Revision of
	   existing code
		④ ⑤ Fourth or fifth
		   digit required

825.20 **Unspecified bone(s) of foot [except toes]**
Instep

825.21 **Astragalus**
Talus

825.22 **Navicular [scaphoid], foot**

825.23 **Cuboid**

825.24 **Cuneiform, foot**

825.25 **Metatarsal bone(s)**

825.29 **Other**
Tarsal with metatarsal bone(s) only

Excludes: calcaneus (825.0)

⑤ 825.3 **Fracture of other tarsal and metatarsal bones, open**

825.30 **Unspecified bone(s) of foot [except toes]**

825.31 **Astragalus**

825.32 **Navicular [scaphoid], foot**

825.33 **Cuboid**

825.34 **Cuneiform, foot**

825.35 **Metatarsal bone(s)**

825.39 **Other**

826 **Fracture of one or more phalanges of foot**
Includes: toe(s)

826.0 **Closed**

826.1 **Open**

827 **Other, multiple, and ill-defined fractures of lower limb**
Includes: leg NOS
multiple bones of same lower limb

Excludes: multiple fractures of:
ankle bones alone (824.4-824.9)
phalanges of foot alone (826.0-826.1)
tarsal with metatarsal bones (825.29, 825.39)
tibia with fibula (823.0-823.9 with fifth-digit 2)

827.0 **Closed**

827.1 **Open**

828 **Multiple fractures involving both lower limbs, lower with upper limb, and lower limb(s) with rib(s) and sternum**
Includes: arm(s) with leg(s) [any bones]
both legs [any bones]
leg(s) with rib(s) or sternum

828.0 **Closed**

828.1 **Open**

829 **Fracture of unspecified bones**

829.0 **Unspecified bone, closed**

829.1 **Unspecified bone, open**

DISLOCATION (830-839)

Includes: displacement
subluxation

Excludes: congenital dislocation (754.0-755.8)
pathological dislocation (718.2)
recurrent dislocation (718.3)

The descriptions "closed" and "open", used in the fourth-digit subdivisions, include the following terms:

closed:	open:
complete	compound
dislocation NOS	infected
partial	with foreign body
simple	
uncomplicated	

A dislocation not indicated as closed or open should be classified as closed.

Add 4th or 5th digit | Nonspecific code | Unspecified code | Medicare secondary payer (MSP) alert

830 Dislocation of jaw
    Includes: jaw (cartilage) (meniscus)
                mandible
                maxilla (inferior)
                temporomandibular (joint)

  830.0 Closed dislocation

  830.1 Open dislocation

⑤ **831 Dislocation of shoulder**

    Excludes: *sternoclavicular joint (839.61, 839.71)*
                     sternum (839.61, 839.71)

  The following fifth-digit subclassification is for use with category 831:

    0 shoulder, unspecified
       Humerus NOS

    1 anterior dislocation of humerus

    2 posterior dislocation of humerus

    3 inferior dislocation of humerus

    4 acromioclavicular (joint)
       Clavicle

    9 other
       Scapula

  ⑤ **831.0 Closed dislocation**
    [0-4,9]

  ⑤ **831.1 Open dislocation**
    [0-4,9]

832 Dislocation of elbow
  The following fifth-digit subclassification is for use with subcategories 832.0 and 832.1:

    0 elbow unspecified

    1 anterior dislocation of elbow

    2 posterior dislocation of elbow

    3 medial dislocation of elbow

    4 lateral dislocation of elbow

    9 other

  ⑤ **832.0 Closed dislocation**
    [0-4,9]

  ⑤ **832.1 Open dislocation**
    [0-4,9]

  ● **832.2 Nursemaid's elbow**
    Subluxation of radial head

⑤ **833 Dislocation of wrist**
  The following fifth-digit subclassification is for use with category 833:

    0 wrist, unspecified part
       Carpal (bone)   Radius, distal end

    1 radioulnar (joint), distal

    2 radiocarpal (joint)

    3 midcarpal (joint)

    4 carpometacarpal (joint)

    5 metacarpal (bone), proximal end

    9 other
       Ulna, distal end

  ⑤ **833.0 Closed dislocation**
    [0-5,9]

  ⑤ **833.1 Open dislocation**
    [0-5,9]

● Code new to this edition   ▲ Revision of existing code   ④ ⑤ Fourth or fifth digit required

⑤ **834** **Dislocation of finger**
        Includes: finger(s)
                 phalanx of hand
                 thumb

      The following fifth-digit subclassification is for use with category 834:

          0 **finger, unspecified part**

          1 **metacarpophalangeal (joint)**
              Metacarpal (bone), distal end

          2 **interphalangeal (joint), hand**

⑤   **834.0** **Closed dislocation**
      [0-2]

⑤   **834.1** **Open dislocation**
      [0-2]

⑤ **835** **Dislocation of hip**
      The following fifth-digit subclassification is for use with category 835:

          0 **dislocation of hip, unspecified**

          1 **posterior dislocation**

          2 **obturator dislocation**

          3 **other anterior dislocation**

⑤   **835.0** **Closed dislocation**
      [0-3]

⑤   **835.1** **Open dislocation**
      [0-3]

836 **Dislocation of knee**

         | Excludes: | *dislocation of knee:*
                       old or pathological (718.2)
                       recurrent (718.3)
                 internal derangement of knee joint (717.0-717.5, 717.8-717.9)
                 old tear of cartilage or meniscus of knee (717.0-717.5, 717.8-717.9)

    836.0 **Tear of medial cartilage or meniscus of knee, current**
         Bucket handle tear:
           NOS current injury
         medial meniscus current injury

    836.1 **Tear of lateral cartilage or meniscus of knee, current**

    836.2 **Other tear of cartilage or meniscus of knee, current**
         Tear of:
           cartilage (semilunar) current injury, not specified as medial or lateral
           meniscus current injury, not specified as medial or lateral

    836.3 **Dislocation of patella, closed**

    836.4 **Dislocation of patella, open**

⑤   **836.5** **Other dislocation of knee, closed**

         836.50 **Dislocation of knee, unspecified**

         836.51 **Anterior dislocation of tibia, proximal end**
             Posterior dislocation of femur, distal end

         836.52 **Posterior dislocation of tibia, proximal end**
             Anterior dislocation of femur, distal end

         836.53 **Medial dislocation of tibia, proximal end**

         836.54 **Lateral dislocation of tibia, proximal end**

         836.59 **Other**

⑤   **836.6** **Other dislocation of knee, open**

         836.60 **Dislocation of knee, unspecified**

         836.61 **Anterior dislocation of tibia, proximal end**

         836.62 **Posterior dislocation of tibia, proximal end**

         836.63 **Medial dislocation of tibia, proximal end**

         836.64 **Lateral dislocation of tibia, proximal end**

         836.69 **Other**

| Add 4th or 5th digit | Nonspecific code | Unspecified code | Medicare secondary payer (MSP) alert |

837 Dislocation of ankle
Includes: astragalus
fibula, distal end
navicular, foot
scaphoid, foot
tibia, distal end

837.0 Closed dislocation

837.1 Open dislocation

⑤ **838 Dislocation of foot**
The following fifth-digit subclassification is for use with category 838:

0 foot, unspecified

1 tarsal (bone), joint unspecified

2 midtarsal (joint)

3 tarsometatarsal (joint)

4 metatarsal (bone), joint unspecified

5 metatarsophalangeal (joint)

6 interphalangeal (joint), foot

9 other
Phalanx of foot
Toe(s)

⑤ **838.0 Closed dislocation**
[0-6,9]

⑤ **838.1 Open dislocation**
[0-6,9]

839 Other, multiple, and ill-defined dislocations

⑤ **839.0 Cervical vertebra, closed**
Cervical spine
Neck

    839.00 Cervical vertebra, unspecified

    839.01 First cervical vertebra

    839.02 Second cervical vertebra

    839.03 Third cervical vertebra

    839.04 Fourth cervical vertebra

    839.05 Fifth cervical vertebra

    839.06 Sixth cervical vertebra

    839.07 Seventh cervical vertebra

    839.08 Multiple cervical vertebrae

⑤ **839.1 Cervical vertebra, open**

    839.10 Cervical vertebra, unspecified

    839.11 First cervical vertebra

    839.12 Second cervical vertebra

    839.13 Third cervical vertebra

    839.14 Fourth cervical vertebra

    839.15 Fifth cervical vertebra

    839.16 Sixth cervical vertebra

    839.17 Seventh cervical vertebra

    839.18 Multiple cervical vertebrae

⑤ **839.2 Thoracic and lumbar vertebra, closed**

    839.20 Lumbar vertebra

    839.21 Thoracic vertebra
Dorsal [thoracic] vertebra

⑤ **839.3 Thoracic and lumbar vertebra, open**

    839.30 Lumbar vertebra

    839.31 Thoracic vertebra

⑤ **839.4 Other vertebra, closed**

● Code new
to this edition

▲ Revision of
existing code

④ ⑤ Fourth or fifth
digit required

839.40 **Vertebra, unspecified site**
Spine NOS

839.41 **Coccyx**

839.42 **Sacrum**
Sacroiliac (joint)

839.49 **Other**

⑤ 839.5 **Other vertebra, open**

839.50 **Vertebra, unspecified site**

839.51 **Coccyx**

839.52 **Sacrum**

839.59 **Other**

⑤ 839.6 **Other location, closed**

839.61 **Sternum**
Sternoclavicular joint

839.69 **Other**
Pelvis

⑤ 839.7 **Other location, open**

839.71 **Sternum**

839.79 **Other**

839.8 **Multiple and ill-defined, closed**
Arm
Back
Hand
Multiple locations, except fingers or toes alone
Other ill-defined locations
Unspecified location

839.9 **Multiple and ill-defined, open**

SPRAINS AND STRAINS OF JOINTS AND ADJACENT MUSCLES (840-848)

Includes: avulsion of: joint capsule, ligament, muscle, tendon
hemarthrosis of: joint capsule, ligament, muscle, tendon
laceration of: joint capsule, ligament, muscle, tendon
rupture of: joint capsule, ligament, muscle, tendon
sprain of: joint capsule, ligament, muscle, tendon
strain of: joint capsule, ligament, muscle, tendon
tear of: joint capsule, ligament, muscle, tendon

Excludes: *laceration of tendon in open wounds (880-884 and 890-894 with .2)*

840 **Sprains and strains of shoulder and upper arm**

840.0 **Acromioclavicular (joint) (ligament)**

840.1 **Coracoclavicular (ligament)**

840.2 **Coracohumeral (ligament)**

840.3 **Infraspinatus (muscle) (tendon)**

840.4 **Rotator cuff (capsule)**

Excludes: *complete rupture of rotator cuff, nontraumatic (727.61)*

840.5 **Subscapularis (muscle)**

840.6 **Supraspinatus (muscle) (tendon)**

840.7 **Superior glenoid labrum lesion**
SLAP lesion

840.8 **Other specified sites of shoulder and upper arm**

840.9 **Unspecified site of shoulder and upper arm**
Arm NOS
Shoulder NOS

841 **Sprains and strains of elbow and forearm**

841.0 **Radial collateral ligament**

841.1 **Ulnar collateral ligament**

841.2 **Radiohumeral (joint)**

841.3 **Ulnohumeral (joint)**

841.8 **Other specified sites of elbow and forearm**

| | Add 4th or 5th digit | | Nonspecific code | | Unspecified code | | Medicare secondary payer (MSP) alert |

841.9 Unspecified site of elbow and forearm
Elbow NOS

842 Sprains and strains of wrist and hand

⑤ **842.0 Wrist**

842.00 Unspecified site

842.01 Carpal (joint)

842.02 Radiocarpal (joint) (ligament)

842.09 Other
Radioulnar joint, distal

⑤ **842.1 Hand**

842.10 Unspecified site

842.11 Carpometacarpal (joint)

842.12 Metacarpophalangeal (joint)

842.13 Interphalangeal (joint)

842.19 Other
Midcarpal (joint)

843 Sprains and strains of hip and thigh

843.0 Iliofemoral (ligament)

843.1 Ischiocapsular (ligament)

843.8 Other specified sites of hip and thigh

843.9 Unspecified site of hip and thigh
Hip NOS
Thigh NOS

844 Sprains and strains of knee and leg

844.0 Lateral collateral ligament of knee

844.1 Medial collateral ligament of knee

844.2 Cruciate ligament of knee

844.3 Tibiofibular (joint) (ligament), superior

844.8 Other specified sites of knee and leg

844.9 Unspecified site of knee and leg
Knee NOS
Leg NOS

845 Sprains and strains of ankle and foot

⑤ **845.0 Ankle**

845.00 Unspecified site

845.01 Deltoid (ligament), ankle
Internal collateral (ligament), ankle

845.02 Calcaneofibular (ligament)

845.03 Tibiofibular (ligament), distal

845.09 Other
Achilles tendon

⑤ **845.1 Foot**

845.10 Unspecified site

845.11 Tarsometatarsal (joint) (ligament)

845.12 Metatarsophalangeal (joint)

845.13 Interphalangeal (joint), toe

845.19 Other

846 Sprains and strains of sacroiliac region

846.0 Lumbosacral (joint) (ligament)

846.1 Sacroiliac ligament

846.2 Sacrospinatus (ligament)

846.3 Sacrotuberous (ligament)

846.8 Other specified sites of sacroiliac region

846.9 Unspecified site of sacroiliac region

847 Sprains and strains of other and unspecified parts of back

● Code new
to this edition

▲ Revision of
existing code

④ ⑤ Fourth or fifth
digit required

Excludes: *lumbosacral (846.0)*

847.0 Neck
Anterior longitudinal (ligament), cervical
Atlanto-axial (joints)
Atlanto-occipital (joints)
Whiplash injury

Excludes: *neck injury NOS (959.0)*
thyroid region (848.2)

847.1 Thoracic

847.2 Lumbar

847.3 Sacrum
Sacrococcygeal (ligament)

847.4 Coccyx

847.9 Unspecified site of back
Back NOS

848 Other and ill-defined sprains and strains

848.0 Septal cartilage of nose

848.1 Jaw
Temporomandibular (joint) (ligament)

848.2 Thyroid region
Cricoarytenoid (joint) (ligament)
Cricothyroid (joint) (ligament)
Thyroid cartilage

848.3 Ribs
Chondrocostal (joint) without mention of injury to sternum
Costal cartilage without mention of injury to sternum

⑤ **848.4 Sternum**

848.40 Unspecified site

848.41 Sternoclavicular (joint) (ligament)

848.42 Chondrosternal (joint)

848.49 Other
Xiphoid cartilage

848.5 Pelvis
Symphysis pubis

Excludes: *that in childbirth (665.6)*

848.8 Other specified sites of sprains and strains

848.9 Unspecified site of sprain and strain

INTRACRANIAL INJURY, EXCLUDING THOSE WITH SKULL FRACTURE (850-854)

Excludes: *intracranial injury with skull fracture (800-801 and 803-804, except .0 and .5)*
open wound of head without intracranial injury (870.0-873.9)
skull fracture alone (800-801 and 803-804 with .0, .5)

Includes: traumatic brain injury without skull fracture

The description "with open intracranial wound," used in the fourth-digit subdivisions, includes those specified as open or with mention of infection or foreign body.

The following fifth-digit subclassification is for use with categories 851-854:

0 **unspecified state of consciousness**

1 **with no loss of consciousness**

2 **with brief [less than one hour] loss of consciousness**

3 **with moderate [1-24 hours] loss of consciousness**

4 **with prolonged [more than 24 hours] loss of consciousness and return to pre-existing conscious level**

5 **with prolonged [more than 24 hours] loss of consciousness, without return to pre-existing conscious level**

Use fifth-digit 5 to designate when a patient is unconscious and dies before regaining consciousness, regardless of the duration of the loss of consciousness

6 **with loss of consciousness of unspecified duration**

9 **with concussion, unspecified**

	Add 4th or 5th digit		Nonspecific code		Unspecified code		Medicare secondary payer (MSP) alert

850 Concussion
Includes: commotio cerebri
Excludes: *concussion with:*
cerebral laceration or contusion (851.0-851.9)
cerebral hemorrhage (852-853)
head injury NOS (959.01)

850.0 With no loss of consciousness
Concussion with mental confusion or disorientation, without loss of consciousness

⑤ **850.1 With brief loss of consciousness**
Loss of consciousness for less than one hour

850.11 With loss of consciousness of 30 minutes or less

850.12 With loss of consciousness from 31 to 59 minutes

850.2 With moderate loss of consciousness
Loss of consciousness for 1-24 hours

850.3 With prolonged loss of consciousness and return to pre-existing conscious level
Loss of consciousness for more than 24 hours with complete recovery

850.4 With prolonged loss of consciousness, without return to pre-existing conscious level

850.5 With loss of consciousness of unspecified duration

850.9 Concussion, unspecified

⑤ **851 Cerebral laceration and contusion**

⑤ **851.0 Cortex (cerebral) contusion without mention of open intracranial wound**
[0-6,9]

⑤ **851.1 Cortex (cerebral) contusion with open intracranial wound**
[0-6,9]

⑤ **851.2 Cortex (cerebral) laceration without mention of open intracranial wound**
[0-6,9]

⑤ **851.3 Cortex (cerebral) laceration with open intracranial wound**
[0-6,9]

⑤ **851.4 Cerebellar or brain stem contusion without mention of open intracranial wound**
[0-6,9]

⑤ **851.5 Cerebellar or brain stem contusion with open intracranial wound**
[0-6,9]

⑤ **851.6 Cerebellar or brain stem laceration without mention of open intracranial wound**
[0-6,9]

⑤ **851.7 Cerebellar or brain stem laceration with open intracranial wound**
[0-6,9]

⑤ **851.8 Other and unspecified cerebral laceration and contusion, without mention of open intracranial wound**
[0-6,9] Brain (membrane) NOS

⑤ **851.9 Other and unspecified cerebral laceration and contusion, with open intracranial wound**
[0-6,9]

⑤ **852 Subarachnoid, subdural, and extradural hemorrhage, following injury**
Excludes: *Cerebral contusion or laceration (with hemorrhage) (851.0-851.9)*

⑤ **852.0 Subarachnoid hemorrhage following injury without mention of open intracranial wound**
[0-6,9] Middle meningeal hemorrhage following injury

⑤ **852.1 Subarachnoid hemorrhage following injury with open intracranial wound**
[0-6,9]

⑤ **852.2 Subdural hemorrhage following injury without mention of open intracranial wound**
[0-6,9]

⑤ **852.3 Subdural hemorrhage following injury with open intracranial wound**
[0-6,9]

⑤ **852.4 Extradural hemorrhage following injury without mention of open intracranial wound**
[0-6,9] Epidural hematoma following injury

⑤ **852.5 Extradural hemorrhage following injury with open intracranial wound**
[0-6,9]

● Code new to this edition   ▲ Revision of existing code   ④ ⑤ Fourth or fifth digit required

⑤ **853** Other and unspecified intracranial hemorrhage following injury

  ⑤ **853.0** Without mention of open intracranial wound
    [0-6,9]   Cerebral compression due to injury
           Intracranial hematoma following injury
           Traumatic cerebral hemorrhage

  ⑤ **853.1** With open intracranial wound
    [0-6,9]

⑤ **854** Intracranial injury of other and unspecified nature
    Includes: injury
               brain NOS
               intracranial
               traumatic brain NOS
               cavernous sinus

    Excludes: *any condition classifiable to 850-853*
               head injury NOS (959.01)

  ⑤ **854.0** Without mention of open intracranial wound
    [0-6,9]

  ⑤ **854.1** With open intracranial wound
    [0-6,9]

INTERNAL INJURY OF THORAX, ABDOMEN, AND PELVIS (860-869)

    Includes:
           blast injuries of internal organs
           blunt trauma of internal organs
           bruise of internal organs
           concussion injuries (except cerebral) of internal organs
           crushing of internal organs
           hematoma of internal organs
           laceration of internal organs
           puncture of internal organs
           tear of internal organs
           traumatic rupture of internal organs

    Excludes: *concussion NOS (850.0-850.9)*
               flail chest (807.4)
               foreign body entering through orifice (930.0-939.9)
               injury to blood vessels (901.0-902.9)

The description "with open wound," used in the fourth-digit subdivisions, includes those with mention of infection or foreign body.

860 Traumatic pneumothorax and hemothorax

  860.0 Pneumothorax without mention of open wound into thorax

  860.1 Pneumothorax with open wound into thorax

  860.2 Hemothorax without mention of open wound into thorax

  860.3 Hemothorax with open wound into thorax

  860.4 Pneumohemothorax without mention of open wound into thorax

  860.5 Pneumohemothorax with open wound into thorax

861 Injury to heart and lung

    Excludes: *injury to blood vessels of thorax (901.0-901.9)*

  ⑤ **861.0** Heart, without mention of open wound into thorax

    861.00 Unspecified injury

    861.01 Contusion
          Cardiac contusion
          Myocardial contusion

    861.02 Laceration without penetration of heart chambers

    861.03 Laceration with penetration of heart chambers

  ⑤ **861.1** Heart, with open wound into thorax

    861.10 Unspecified injury

    861.11 Contusion

    861.12 Laceration without penetration of heart chambers

    861.13 Laceration with penetration of heart chambers

  ⑤ **861.2** Lung, without mention of open wound into thorax

613

■ Add 4th or 5th digit	■ Nonspecific code	■ Unspecified code	■ Medicare secondary payer (MSP) alert

861.20 Unspecified injury

861.21 Contusion

861.22 Laceration

⑤ 861.3 Lung, with open wound into thorax

861.30 Unspecified injury

861.31 Contusion

861.32 Laceration

862 Injury to other and unspecified intrathoracic organs

[Excludes:] *injury to blood vessels of thorax (901.0-901.9)*

862.0 Diaphragm, without mention of open wound into cavity

862.1 Diaphragm, with open wound into cavity

⑤ 862.2 Other specified intrathoracic organs, without mention of open wound into cavity

862.21 Bronchus

862.22 Esophagus

862.29 Other
Pleura
Thymus gland

⑤ 862.3 Other specified intrathoracic organs, with open wound into cavity

862.31 Bronchus

862.32 Esophagus

862.39 Other

862.8 Multiple and unspecified intrathoracic organs, without mention of open wound into cavity
Crushed chest
Multiple intrathoracic organs

862.9 Multiple and unspecified intrathoracic organs, with open wound into cavity

863 Injury to gastrointestinal tract

[Excludes:] *anal sphincter laceration during delivery (664.2)*
bile duct (868.0-868.1 with fifth-digit 2)
gallbladder (868.0-868.1 with fifth-digit 2)

863.0 Stomach, without mention of open wound into cavity

863.1 Stomach, with open wound into cavity

⑤ 863.2 Small intestine, without mention of open wound into cavity

863.20 Small intestine, unspecified site

863.21 Duodenum

863.29 Other

⑤ 863.3 Small intestine, with open wound into cavity

863.30 Small intestine, unspecified site

863.31 Duodenum

863.39 Other

⑤ 863.4 Colon or rectum, without mention of open wound into cavity

863.40 Colon, unspecified site

863.41 Ascending [right] colon

863.42 Transverse colon

863.43 Descending [left] colon

863.44 Sigmoid colon

863.45 Rectum

863.46 Multiple sites in colon and rectum

863.49 Other

⑤ 863.5 Colon or rectum, with open wound into cavity

863.50 Colon, unspecified site

863.51 Ascending [right] colon

863.52 Transverse colon

● Code new
to this edition

▲ Revision of
existing code

④ ⑤ Fourth or fifth
digit required

863.53	Descending [left] colon
863.54	Sigmoid colon
863.55	Rectum
863.56	Multiple sites in colon and rectum
863.59	Other

⑤ **863.8 Other and unspecified gastrointestinal sites, without mention of open wound into cavity**

863.80	Gastrointestinal tract, unspecified site
863.81	Pancreas, head
863.82	Pancreas, body
863.83	Pancreas, tail
863.84	Pancreas, multiple and unspecified sites
863.85	Appendix
863.89	Other
	Intestine NOS

⑤ **863.9 Other and unspecified gastrointestinal sites, with open wound into cavity**

863.90	Gastrointestinal tract, unspecified site
863.91	Pancreas, head
863.92	Pancreas, body
863.93	Pancreas, tail
863.94	Pancreas, multiple and unspecified sites
863.95	Appendix
863.99	Other

⑤ **864 Injury to liver**

The following fifth-digit subclassification is for use with category 864:

0 unspecified injury

1 hematoma and contusion

2 laceration, minor
Laceration involving capsule only, or without significant involvement of hepatic parenchyma [i.e., less than 1 cm deep]

3 laceration, moderate
Laceration involving parenchyma but without major disruption of parenchyma [i.e., less than 10 cm long and less than 3 cm deep]

4 laceration, major
Laceration with significant disruption of hepatic parenchyma [i.e., 10 cm long and 3 cm deep]
Multiple moderate lacerations, with or without hematoma
Stellate lacerations of liver

5 laceration, unspecified

9 other

⑤ **864.0 Without mention of open wound into cavity**
[0-5,9]

⑤ **864.1 With open wound into cavity**
[0-5,9]

⑤ **865 Injury to spleen**

The following fifth-digit subclassification is for use with category 865:

0 unspecified injury

1 hematoma without rupture of capsule

2 capsular tears, without major disruption of parenchyma

3 laceration extending into parenchyma

4 massive parenchymal disruption

9 other

⑤ **865.0 Without mention of open wound into cavity**
[0-4,9]

⑤ **865.1 With open wound into cavity**
[0-4,9]

| | Add 4th or 5th digit | | Nonspecific code | | Unspecified code | | Medicare secondary payer (MSP) alert |

⑤ **866** **Injury to kidney**

> *Excludes:* *acute kidney injury (nontraumatic) (584.9)*

The following fifth-digit subclassification is for use with category 866:

    0 **unspecified injury**

    1 **hematoma without rupture of capsule**

    2 **laceration**

    3 **complete disruption of kidney parenchyma**

⑤ **866.0** **Without mention of open wound into cavity**
    [0-3]

⑤ **866.1** **With open wound into cavity**
    [0-3]

867 **Injury to pelvic organs**

> *Excludes:* *injury during delivery (664.0-665.9)*

    867.0 **Bladder and urethra, without mention of open wound into cavity**

    867.1 **Bladder and urethra, with open wound into cavity**

    867.2 **Ureter, without mention of open wound into cavity**

    867.3 **Ureter, with open wound into cavity**

    867.4 **Uterus, without mention of open wound into cavity**

    867.5 **Uterus, with open wound into cavity**

    867.6 **Other specified pelvic organs, without mention of open wound into cavity**

        Fallopian tube   Seminal vesicle
        Ovary   Vas deferens
        Prostate

    867.7 **Other specified pelvic organs, with open wound into cavity**

    867.8 **Unspecified pelvic organs, without mention of open wound into cavity**

    867.9 **Unspecified pelvic organ, with open wound into cavity**

⑤ **868** **Injury to other intra-abdominal organs**

The following fifth-digit subclassification is for use with category 868:

    0 **unspecified intra-abdominal organ**

    1 **adrenal gland**

    2 **bile duct and gallbladder**

    3 **peritoneum**

    4 **retroperitoneum**

    9 **other and multiple intra-abdominal organs**

⑤ **868.0** **Without mention of open wound into cavity**
    [0-4,9]

⑤ **868.1** **With open wound into cavity**
    [0-4,9]

869 **Internal injury to unspecified or ill-defined organs**

    Includes: internal injury NOS
                  multiple internal injury NOS

    869.0 **Without mention of open wound into cavity**

    869.1 **With open wound into cavity**

OPEN WOUNDS (870-897)

    Includes: animal bite
                  avulsion
                  cut
                  laceration
                  puncture wound
                  traumatic amputation

● Code new
  to this edition   ▲ Revision of
                existing code   ④ ⑤ Fourth or fifth
                                              digit required

> *Excludes:* *burn (940.0-949.5)*
> *crushing (925-929.9)*
> *puncture of internal organs (860.0-869.1)*
> *superficial injury (910.0-919.9)*
> *that incidental to:*
> *dislocation (830.0-839.9)*
> *fracture (800.0-829.1)*
> *internal injury (860.0-869.1)*
> *intracranial injury (851.0-854.1)*

Note: The description "complicated" used in the fourth-digit subdivisions includes those with mention of delayed healing, delayed treatment, foreign body, or infection.

OPEN WOUND OF HEAD, NECK, AND TRUNK (870-879)

870 Open wound of ocular adnexa

870.0 Laceration of skin of eyelid and periocular area

870.1 Laceration of eyelid, full-thickness, not involving lacrimal passages

870.2 Laceration of eyelid involving lacrimal passages

870.3 Penetrating wound of orbit, without mention of foreign body

870.4 Penetrating wound of orbit with foreign body

> *Excludes:* *retained (old) foreign body in orbit (376.6)*

870.8 Other specified open wounds of ocular adnexa

870.9 Unspecified open wound of ocular adnexa

871 Open wound of eyeball

> *Excludes:* *2nd cranial nerve [optic] injury (950.0-950.9)*
> *3rd cranial nerve [oculomotor] injury (951.0)*

871.0 Ocular laceration without prolapse of intraocular tissue

871.1 Ocular laceration with prolapse or exposure of intraocular tissue

871.2 Rupture of eye with partial loss of intraocular tissue

871.3 Avulsion of eye
Traumatic enucleation

871.4 Unspecified laceration of eye

871.5 Penetration of eyeball with magnetic foreign body

> *Excludes:* *retained (old) magnetic foreign body in globe (360.50-360.59)*

871.6 Penetration of eyeball with (nonmagnetic) foreign body

> *Excludes:* *retained (old) (nonmagnetic) foreign body in globe (360.60-360.69)*

871.7 Unspecified ocular penetration

871.9 Unspecified open wound of eyeball

872 Open wound of ear

⑤ **872.0** External ear, without mention of complication

872.00 External ear, unspecified site

872.01 Auricle, ear
Pinna

872.02 Auditory canal

⑤ **872.1** External ear, complicated

872.10 External ear, unspecified site

872.11 Auricle, ear

872.12 Auditory canal

⑤ **872.6** Other specified parts of ear, without mention of complication

872.61 Ear drum
Drumhead
Tympanic membrane

872.62 Ossicles

872.63 Eustachian tube

872.64 Cochlea

872.69 Other and multiple sites

| | Add 4th or 5th digit | | Nonspecific code | | Unspecified code | | Medicare secondary payer (MSP) alert |

⑤ 872.7   **Other specified parts of ear, complicated**

     872.71   **Ear drum**

     872.72   **Ossicles**

     872.73   **Eustachian tube**

     872.74   **Cochlea**

     `872.79`   **Other and multiple sites**

  `872.8`   **Ear, part unspecified, without mention of complication**
       Ear NOS

  `872.9`   **Ear, part unspecified, complicated**

`873`   **Other open wound of head**

  873.0   **Scalp, without mention of complication**

  873.1   **Scalp, complicated**

⑤ 873.2   **Nose, without mention of complication**

     `873.20`   **Nose, unspecified site**

     873.21   **Nasal septum**

     873.22   **Nasal cavity**

     873.23   **Nasal sinus**

     `873.29`   **Multiple sites**

⑤ 873.3   **Nose, complicated**

     `873.30`   **Nose, unspecified site**

     873.31   **Nasal septum**

     873.32   **Nasal cavity**

     873.33   **Nasal sinus**

     `873.39`   **Multiple sites**

⑤ 873.4   **Face, without mention of complication**

     `873.40`   **Face, unspecified site**

     873.41   **Cheek**

     873.42   **Forehead**
          Eyebrow

     873.43   **Lip**

     873.44   **Jaw**

     `873.49`   **Other and multiple sites**

⑤ 873.5   **Face, complicated**

     `873.50`   **Face, unspecified site**

     873.51   **Cheek**

     873.52   **Forehead**

     873.53   **Lip**

     873.54   **Jaw**

     `873.59`   **Other and multiple sites**

⑤ 873.6   **Internal structures of mouth, without mention of complication**

     `873.60`   **Mouth, unspecified site**

     873.61   **Buccal mucosa**

     873.62   **Gum (alveolar process)**

     873.63   **Tooth (broken) (fractured) (due to trauma)**

    | Excludes: | *cracked tooth (521.81)* |

     873.64   **Tongue and floor of mouth**

     873.65   **Palate**

     `873.69`   **Other and multiple sites**

⑤ 873.7   **Internal structures of mouth, complicated**

     `873.70`   **Mouth, unspecified site**

     873.71   **Buccal mucosa**

     873.72   **Gum (alveolar process)**

● Code new to this edition   ▲ Revision of existing code   ④ ⑤ Fourth or fifth digit required

873.73 Tooth (broken) (fractured) (due to trauma)

Excludes: cracked tooth (521.81)

873.74 Tongue and floor of mouth

873.75 Palate

873.79 Other and multiple sites

873.8 Other and unspecified open wound of head without mention of complication
Head NOS

873.9 Other and unspecified open wound of head, complicated

874 Open wound of neck

⑤ **874.0** Larynx and trachea, without mention of complication

874.00 Larynx with trachea

874.01 Larynx

874.02 Trachea

⑤ **874.1** Larynx and trachea, complicated

874.10 Larynx with trachea

874.11 Larynx

874.12 Trachea

874.2 Thyroid gland, without mention of complication

874.3 Thyroid gland, complicated

874.4 Pharynx, without mention of complication
Cervical esophagus

874.5 Pharynx, complicated

874.8 Other and unspecified parts, without mention of complication
Nape of neck　　　　　　Throat NOS
Supraclavicular region

874.9 Other and unspecified parts, complicated

875 Open wound of chest (wall)

Excludes: open wound into thoracic cavity (860.0-862.9)
traumatic pneumothorax and hemothorax (860.1, 860.3, 860.5)

875.0 Without mention of complication

875.1 Complicated

876 Open wound of back
Includes: loin
lumbar region

Excludes: open wound into thoracic cavity (860.0-862.9)
traumatic pneumothorax and hemothorax (860.1, 860.3, 860.5)

876.0 Without mention of complication

876.1 Complicated

877 Open wound of buttock
Includes: sacroiliac region

877.0 Without mention of complication

877.1 Complicated

878 Open wound of genital organs (external), including traumatic amputation

Excludes: injury during delivery (664.0-665.9)
internal genital organs (867.0-867.9)

878.0 Penis, without mention of complication

878.1 Penis, complicated

878.2 Scrotum and testes, without mention of complication

878.3 Scrotum and testes, complicated

878.4 Vulva, without mention of complication
Labium (majus) (minus)

878.5 Vulva, complicated

878.6 Vagina, without mention of complication

878.7 Vagina, complicated

878.8 Other and unspecified parts, without mention of complication

| | Add 4th or 5th digit | | Nonspecific code | | Unspecified code | | Medicare secondary payer (MSP) alert |

878.9 Other and unspecified parts, complicated

879 Open wound of other and unspecified sites, except limbs

879.0 Breast, without mention of complication

879.1 Breast, complicated

879.2 Abdominal wall, anterior, without mention of complication
Abdominal wall NOS   Pubic region
Epigastric region   Umbilical region
Hypogastric region

879.3 Abdominal wall, anterior, complicated

879.4 Abdominal wall, lateral, without mention of complication
Flank   Iliac (region)
Groin   Inguinal region
Hypochondrium

879.5 Abdominal wall, lateral, complicated

879.6 Other and unspecified parts of trunk, without mention of complication
Pelvic region   Trunk NOS
Perineum

879.7 Other and unspecified parts of trunk, complicated

879.8 Open wound(s) (multiple) of unspecified site(s) without mention of complication
Multiple open wounds NOS
Open wound NOS

879.9 Open wound(s) (multiple) of unspecified site(s), complicated

OPEN WOUND OF UPPER LIMB (880-887)

⑤ **880** Open wound of shoulder and upper arm
The following fifth-digit subclassification is for use with category 880:

    0 shoulder region

    1 scapular region

    2 axillary region

    3 upper arm

    9 multiple sites

⑤ 880.0 Without mention of complication

⑤ 880.1 Complicated

⑤ 880.2 With tendon involvement

⑤ **881** Open wound of elbow, forearm, and wrist
The following fifth-digit subclassification is for use with category 881:

    0 forearm

    1 elbow

    2 wrist

⑤ 881.0 Without mention of complication

⑤ 881.1 Complicated

⑤ 881.2 With tendon involvement

882 Open wound of hand except finger(s) alone

882.0 Without mention of complication

882.1 Complicated

882.2 With tendon involvement

883 Open wound of finger(s)
Includes: fingernail
            thumb (nail)

883.0 Without mention of complication

883.1 Complicated

883.2 With tendon involvement

884 Multiple and unspecified open wound of upper limb
Includes: arm NOS
            multiple sites of one upper limb
            upper limb NOS

  ● Code new   ▲ Revision of   ④ ⑤ Fourth or fifth
     to this edition   existing code   digit required

884.0 Without mention of complication

884.1 Complicated

884.2 With tendon involvement

885 Traumatic amputation of thumb (complete) (partial)
Includes: thumb(s) (with finger(s) of either hand)

885.0 Without mention of complication

885.1 Complicated

886 Traumatic amputation of other finger(s) (complete) (partial)
Includes: finger(s) of one or both hands, without mention of thumb(s)

886.0 Without mention of complication

886.1 Complicated

887 Traumatic amputation of arm and hand (complete) (partial)

887.0 Unilateral, below elbow, without mention of complication

887.1 Unilateral, below elbow, complicated

887.2 Unilateral, at or above elbow, without mention of complication

887.3 Unilateral, at or above elbow, complicated

887.4 Unilateral, level not specified, without mention of complication

887.5 Unilateral, level not specified, complicated

887.6 Bilateral [any level], without mention of complication
One hand and other arm

887.7 Bilateral [any level], complicated

OPEN WOUND OF LOWER LIMB (890-897)

890 Open wound of hip and thigh

890.0 Without mention of complication

890.1 Complicated

890.2 With tendon involvement

891 Open wound of knee, leg [except thigh], and ankle
Includes: leg NOS
multiple sites of leg, except thigh

Excludes: *that of thigh (890.0-890.2)*
with multiple sites of lower limb (894.0-894.2)

891.0 Without mention of complication

891.1 Complicated

891.2 With tendon involvement

892 Open wound of foot except toe(s) alone
Includes: heel

892.0 Without mention of complication

892.1 Complicated

892.2 With tendon involvement

893 Open wound of toe(s)
Includes: toenail

893.0 Without mention of complication

893.1 Complicated

893.2 With tendon involvement

894 Multiple and unspecified open wound of lower limb
Includes: lower limb NOS
multiple sites of one lower limb, with thigh

894.0 Without mention of complication

894.1 Complicated

894.2 With tendon involvement

895 Traumatic amputation of toe(s) (complete) (partial)
Includes: toe(s) of one or both feet

895.0 Without mention of complication

895.1 Complicated

	Add 4th or 5th digit		Nonspecific code		Unspecified code		Medicare secondary payer (MSP) alert

896 Traumatic amputation of foot (complete) (partial)

    896.0 Unilateral, without mention of complication

    896.1 Unilateral, complicated

    896.2 Bilateral, without mention of complication

       Excludes: one foot and other leg (897.6-897.7)

    896.3 Bilateral, complicated

897 Traumatic amputation of leg(s) (complete) (partial)

    897.0 Unilateral, below knee, without mention of complication

    897.1 Unilateral, below knee, complicated

    897.2 Unilateral, at or above knee, without mention of complication

    897.3 Unilateral, at or above knee, complicated

    897.4 Unilateral, level not specified, without mention of complication

    897.5 Unilateral, level not specified, complicated

    897.6 Bilateral [any level], without mention of complication
        One foot and other leg

    897.7 Bilateral [any level], complicated

INJURY TO BLOOD VESSELS (900-904)

    Includes: arterial hematoma of blood vessel, secondary to other injuries e.g., fracture or
            open wound
           avulsion of blood vessel, secondary to other injuries e.g., fracture or open wound
           cut of blood vessel, secondary to other injuries e.g., fracture or open wound
           laceration of blood vessel, secondary to other injuries e.g., fracture or open wound
           rupture of blood vessel, secondary to other injuries e.g., fracture or open wound
           traumatic aneurysm or fistula (arteriovenous) of blood vessel, secondary to other
            injuries e.g., fracture or open wound

       Excludes: accidental puncture or laceration during medical procedure (998.2)
                intracranial hemorrhage following injury (851.0-854.1)

900 Injury to blood vessels of head and neck

⑤ **900.0** Carotid artery

        900.00 Carotid artery, unspecified

        900.01 Common carotid artery

        900.02 External carotid artery

        900.03 Internal carotid artery

    900.1 Internal jugular vein

⑤ **900.8** Other specified blood vessels of head and neck

        900.81 External jugular vein
            Jugular vein NOS

        900.82 Multiple blood vessels of head and neck

        900.89 Other

    900.9 Unspecified blood vessel of head and neck

901 Injury to blood vessels of thorax

       Excludes: traumatic hemothorax (860.2-860.5)

    901.0 Thoracic aorta

    901.1 Innominate and subclavian arteries

    901.2 Superior vena cava

    901.3 Innominate and subclavian veins

⑤ **901.4** Pulmonary blood vessels

        901.40 Pulmonary vessel(s), unspecified

        901.41 Pulmonary artery

        901.42 Pulmonary vein

⑤ **901.8** Other specified blood vessels of thorax

        901.81 Intercostal artery or vein

        901.82 Internal mammary artery or vein

        901.83 Multiple blood vessels of thorax

    ● Code new   ▲ Revision of   ④ ⑤ Fourth or fifth
       to this edition   existing code   digit required

901.89 Other
   Azygos vein
   Hemiazygos vein

901.9 Unspecified blood vessel of thorax

902 Injury to blood vessels of abdomen and pelvis

902.0 Abdominal aorta

⑤ **902.1** Inferior vena cava

   902.10 Inferior vena cava, unspecified

   902.11 Hepatic veins

   902.19 Other

⑤ **902.2** Celiac and mesenteric arteries

   902.20 Celiac and mesenteric arteries, unspecified

   902.21 Gastric artery

   902.22 Hepatic artery

   902.23 Splenic artery

   902.24 Other specified branches of celiac axis

   902.25 Superior mesenteric artery (trunk)

   902.26 Primary branches of superior mesenteric artery
      Ileo-colic artery

   902.27 Inferior mesenteric artery

   902.29 Other

⑤ **902.3** Portal and splenic veins

   902.31 Superior mesenteric vein and primary subdivisions
      Ileo-colic vein

   902.32 Inferior mesenteric vein

   902.33 Portal vein

   902.34 Splenic vein

   902.39 Other
      Cystic vein
      Gastric vein

⑤ **902.4** Renal blood vessels

   902.40 Renal vessel(s), unspecified

   902.41 Renal artery

   902.42 Renal vein

   902.49 Other
      Suprarenal arteries

⑤ **902.5** Iliac blood vessels

   902.50 Iliac vessel(s), unspecified

   902.51 Hypogastric artery

   902.52 Hypogastric vein

   902.53 Iliac artery

   902.54 Iliac vein

   902.55 Uterine artery

   902.56 Uterine vein

   902.59 Other

⑤ **902.8** Other specified blood vessels of abdomen and pelvis

   902.81 Ovarian artery

   902.82 Ovarian vein

   902.87 Multiple blood vessels of abdomen and pelvis

   902.89 Other

902.9 Unspecified blood vessel of abdomen and pelvis

903 Injury to blood vessels of upper extremity

⑤ **903.0** Axillary blood vessels

   903.00 Axillary vessel(s), unspecified

| | Add 4th or 5th digit | | Nonspecific code | | Unspecified code | | Medicare secondary payer (MSP) alert |

903.01   Axillary artery

903.02   Axillary vein

903.1   **Brachial blood vessels**

903.2   **Radial blood vessels**

903.3   **Ulnar blood vessels**

903.4   **Palmar artery**

903.5   **Digital blood vessels**

903.8   **Other specified blood vessels of upper extremity**
Multiple blood vessels of upper extremity

903.9   **Unspecified blood vessel of upper extremity**

904   **Injury to blood vessels of lower extremity and unspecified sites**

904.0   **Common femoral artery**
Femoral artery above profunda origin

904.1   **Superficial femoral artery**

904.2   **Femoral veins**

904.3   **Saphenous veins**
Saphenous vein (greater) (lesser)

⑤ 904.4   **Popliteal blood vessels**

904.40   **Popliteal vessel(s), unspecified**

904.41   **Popliteal artery**

904.42   **Popliteal vein**

⑤ 904.5   **Tibial blood vessels**

904.50   **Tibial vessel(s), unspecified**

904.51   **Anterior tibial artery**

904.52   **Anterior tibial vein**

904.53   **Posterior tibial artery**

904.54   **Posterior tibial vein**

904.6   **Deep plantar blood vessels**

904.7   **Other specified blood vessels of lower extremity**
Multiple blood vessels of lower extremity

904.8   **Unspecified blood vessel of lower extremity**

904.9   **Unspecified site**
Injury to blood vessel NOS

LATE EFFECTS OF INJURIES, POISONINGS, TOXIC EFFECTS, AND OTHER EXTERNAL CAUSES (905-909)

Note: These categories are to be used to indicate conditions classifiable to 800-999 as the cause of late effects, which are themselves classified elsewhere. The "late effects" include those specified as such, or as sequelae, which may occur at any time after the acute injury.

905   **Late effects of musculoskeletal and connective tissue injuries**

905.0   **Late effect of fracture of skull and face bones**
Late effect of injury classifiable to 800-804

905.1   **Late effect of fracture of spine and trunk without mention of spinal cord lesion**
Late effect of injury classifiable to 805, 807-809

905.2   **Late effect of fracture of upper extremities**
Late effect of injury classifiable to 810-819

905.3   **Late effect of fracture of neck of femur**
Late effect of injury classifiable to 820

905.4   **Late effect of fracture of lower extremities**
Late effect of injury classifiable to 821-827

905.5   **Late effect of fracture of multiple and unspecified bones**
Late effect of injury classifiable to 828-829

905.6   **Late effect of dislocation**
Late effect of injury classifiable to 830-839

905.7   **Late effect of sprain and strain without mention of tendon injury**
Late effect of injury classifiable to 840-848, except tendon injury

● Code new
to this edition

▲ Revision of
existing code

④ ⑤ Fourth or fifth
digit required

905.8 Late effect of tendon injury
Late effect of tendon injury due to:
open wound [injury classifiable to 880-884 with .2, 890-894 with .2]
sprain and strain [injury classifiable to 840-848]

905.9 Late effect of traumatic amputation
Late effect of injury classifiable to 885-887, 895-897

Excludes: *late amputation stump complication (997.60-997.69)*

906 Late effects of injuries to skin and subcutaneous tissues

906.0 Late effect of open wound of head, neck, and trunk
Late effect of injury classifiable to 870-879

906.1 Late effect of open wound of extremities without mention of tendon injury
Late effect of injury classifiable to 880-884, 890-894 except .2

906.2 Late effect of superficial injury
Late effect of injury classifiable to 910-919

906.3 Late effect of contusion
Late effect of injury classifiable to 920-924

906.4 Late effect of crushing
Late effect of injury classifiable to 925-929

906.5 Late effect of burn of eye, face, head, and neck
Late effect of injury classifiable to 940-941

906.6 Late effect of burn of wrist and hand
Late effect of injury classifiable to 944

906.7 Late effect of burn of other extremities
Late effect of injury classifiable to 943 or 945

906.8 Late effect of burns of other specified sites
Late effect of injury classifiable to 942, 946-947

906.9 Late effect of burn of unspecified site
Late effect of injury classifiable to 948-949

907 Late effects of injuries to the nervous system

907.0 Late effect of intracranial injury without mention of skull fracture
Late effect of injury classifiable to 850-854

907.1 Late effect of injury to cranial nerve
Late effect of injury classifiable to 950-951

907.2 Late effect of spinal cord injury
Late effect of injury classifiable to 806, 952

907.3 Late effect of injury to nerve root(s), spinal plexus(es), and other nerves of trunk
Late effect of injury classifiable to 953-954

907.4 Late effect of injury to peripheral nerve of shoulder girdle and upper limb
Late effect of injury classifiable to 955

907.5 Late effect of injury to peripheral nerve of pelvic girdle and lower limb
Late effect of injury classifiable to 956

907.9 Late effect of injury to other and unspecified nerve
Late effect of injury classifiable to 957

908 Late effects of other and unspecified injuries

908.0 Late effect of internal injury to chest
Late effect of injury classifiable to 860-862

908.1 Late effect of internal injury to intra-abdominal organs
Late effect of injury classifiable to 863-866, 868

908.2 Late effect of internal injury to other internal organs
Late effect of injury classifiable to 867 or 869

908.3 Late effect of injury to blood vessel of head, neck, and extremities
Late effect of injury classifiable to 900, 903-904

908.4 Late effect of injury to blood vessel of thorax, abdomen, and pelvis
Late effect of injury classifiable to 901-902

908.5 Late effect of foreign body in orifice
Late effect of injury classifiable to 930-939

908.6 Late effect of certain complications of trauma
Late effect of complications classifiable to 958

908.9 Late effect of unspecified injury
Late effect of injury classifiable to 959

| | Add 4th or 5th digit | | Nonspecific code | | Unspecified code | | Medicare secondary payer (MSP) alert |

909 Late effects of other and unspecified external causes

909.0 **Late effect of poisoning due to drug, medicinal or biological substance**
Late effect of conditions classifiable to 960-979

Excludes: *late effect of adverse effect of drug, medicinal or biological substance (909.5)*

909.1 **Late effect of toxic effects of nonmedical substances**
Late effect of conditions classifiable to 980-989

909.2 **Late effect of radiation**
Late effect of conditions classifiable to 990

909.3 **Late effect of complications of surgical and medical care**
Late effect of conditions classifiable to 996-999

909.4 **Late effect of certain other external causes**
Late effect of conditions classifiable to 991-994

909.5 **Late effect of adverse effect of drug, medicinal or biological substance**

Excludes: *late effect of poisoning due to drug, medicinal or biological substance (909.0)*

909.9 **Late effect of other and unspecified external causes**

SUPERFICIAL INJURY (910-919)

Excludes: *burn (blisters) (940.0-949.5)*
contusion (920-924.9)
foreign body:
granuloma (728.82)
inadvertently left in operative wound (998.4)
residual, in soft tissue (729.6)
insect bite, venomous (989.5)
open wound with incidental foreign body (870.0-897.7)

910 Superficial injury of face, neck, and scalp except eye
Includes: cheek
ear
gum
lip
nose
throat

Excludes: *eye and adnexa (918.0-918.9)*

910.0 **Abrasion or friction burn without mention of infection**

910.1 **Abrasion or friction burn, infected**

910.2 **Blister without mention of infection**

910.3 **Blister, infected**

910.4 **Insect bite, nonvenomous, without mention of infection**

910.5 **Insect bite, nonvenomous, infected**

910.6 **Superficial foreign body (splinter) without major open wound and without mention of infection**

910.7 **Superficial foreign body (splinter) without major open wound, infected**

910.8 **Other and unspecified superficial injury of face, neck, and scalp without mention of infection**

910.9 **Other and unspecified superficial injury of face, neck, and scalp, infected**

911 Superficial injury of trunk
Includes:

abdominal wall	interscapular region
anus	labium (majus) (minus)
back	penis
breast	perineum
buttock	scrotum
chest wall	testis
flank	vagina
groin	vulva

Excludes: *hip (916.0-916.9)*
scapular region (912.0-912.9)

911.0 **Abrasion or friction burn without mention of infection**

911.1 **Abrasion or friction burn, infected**

911.2 **Blister without mention of infection**

● Code new
to this edition

▲ Revision of
existing code

④ ⑤ Fourth or fifth
digit required

911.3 Blister, infected

911.4 Insect bite, nonvenomous, without mention of infection

911.5 Insect bite, nonvenomous, infected

911.6 Superficial foreign body (splinter) without major open wound and without mention of infection

911.7 Superficial foreign body (splinter) without major open wound, infected

911.8 Other and unspecified superficial injury of trunk without mention of infection

911.9 Other and unspecified superficial injury of trunk, infected

912 Superficial injury of shoulder and upper arm
Includes: axilla   scapular region

912.0 Abrasion or friction burn without mention of infection

912.1 Abrasion or friction burn, infected

912.2 Blister without mention of infection

912.3 Blister, infected

912.4 Insect bite, nonvenomous, without mention of infection

912.5 Insect bite, nonvenomous, infected

912.6 Superficial foreign body (splinter) without major open wound and without mention of infection

912.7 Superficial foreign body (splinter) without major open wound, infected

912.8 Other and unspecified superficial injury of shoulder and upper arm without mention of infection

912.9 Other and unspecified superficial injury of shoulder and upper arm, infected

913 Superficial injury of elbow, forearm, and wrist

913.0 Abrasion or friction burn without mention of infection

913.1 Abrasion or friction burn, infected

913.2 Blister without mention of infection

913.3 Blister, infected

913.4 Insect bite, nonvenomous, without mention of infection

913.5 Insect bite, nonvenomous, infected

913.6 Superficial foreign body (splinter) without major open wound and without mention of infection

913.7 Superficial foreign body (splinter) without major open wound, infected

913.8 Other and unspecified superficial injury of elbow, forearm, and wrist without mention of infection

913.9 Other and unspecified superficial injury of elbow, forearm, and wrist, infected

914 Superficial injury of hand(s) except finger(s) alone

914.0 Abrasion or friction burn without mention of infection

914.1 Abrasion or friction burn, infected

914.2 Blister without mention of infection

914.3 Blister, infected

914.4 Insect bite, nonvenomous, without mention of infection

914.5 Insect bite, nonvenomous, infected

914.6 Superficial foreign body (splinter) without major open wound and without mention of infection

914.7 Superficial foreign body (splinter) without major open wound, infected

914.8 Other and unspecified superficial injury of hand without mention of infection

914.9 Other and unspecified superficial injury of hand, infected

915 Superficial injury of finger(s)
Includes: fingernail   thumb (nail)

915.0 Abrasion or friction burn without mention of infection

915.1 Abrasion or friction burn, infected

915.2 Blister without mention of infection

915.3 Blister, infected

915.4 Insect bite, nonvenomous, without mention of infection

	Add 4th or 5th digit		Nonspecific code		Unspecified code		Medicare secondary payer (MSP) alert

915.5 Insect bite, nonvenomous, infected

915.6 Superficial foreign body (splinter) without major open wound and without mention of infection

915.7 Superficial foreign body (splinter) without major open wound, infected

915.8 Other and unspecified superficial injury of fingers without mention of infection

915.9 Other and unspecified superficial injury of fingers, infected

916 Superficial injury of hip, thigh, leg, and ankle

916.0 Abrasion or friction burn without mention of infection

916.1 Abrasion or friction burn, infected

916.2 Blister without mention of infection

916.3 Blister, infected

916.4 Insect bite, nonvenomous, without mention of infection

916.5 Insect bite, nonvenomous, infected

916.6 Superficial foreign body (splinter) without major open wound and without mention of infection

916.7 Superficial foreign body (splinter) without major open wound, infected

916.8 Other and unspecified superficial injury of hip, thigh, leg, and ankle without mention of infection

916.9 Other and unspecified superficial injury of hip, thigh, leg, and ankle, infected

917 Superficial injury of foot and toe(s)
Includes: heel   toenail

917.0 Abrasion or friction burn without mention of infection

917.1 Abrasion or friction burn, infected

917.2 Blister without mention of infection

917.3 Blister, infected

917.4 Insect bite, nonvenomous, without mention of infection

917.5 Insect bite, nonvenomous, infected

917.6 Superficial foreign body (splinter) without major open wound and without mention of infection

917.7 Superficial foreign body (splinter) without major open wound, infected

917.8 Other and unspecified superficial injury of foot and toes without mention of infection

917.9 Other and unspecified superficial injury of foot and toes, infected

918 Superficial injury of eye and adnexa
Excludes: burn (940.0-940.9)
              foreign body on external eye (930.0-930.9)

918.0 Eyelids and periocular area
Abrasion   Superficial foreign body (splinter)
Insect bite

918.1 Cornea
Corneal abrasion
Superficial laceration
Excludes: corneal injury due to contact lens (371.82)

918.2 Conjunctiva

918.9 Other and unspecified superficial injuries of eye
Eye (ball) NOS

919 Superficial injury of other, multiple, and unspecified sites
Excludes: multiple sites classifiable to the same three-digit category (910.0-918.9)

919.0 Abrasion or friction burn without mention of infection

919.1 Abrasion or friction burn, infected

919.2 Blister without mention of infection

919.3 Blister, infected

919.4 Insect bite, nonvenomous, without mention of infection

919.5 Insect bite, nonvenomous, infected

919.6 Superficial foreign body (splinter) without major open wound and without mention of infection

● Code new
   to this edition   ▲ Revision of
                 existing code   ④ ⑤ Fourth or fifth
                                          digit required

919.7 Superficial foreign body (splinter) without major open wound, infected

919.8 Other and unspecified superficial injury without mention of infection

919.9 Other and unspecified superficial injury, infected

CONTUSION WITH INTACT SKIN SURFACE (920-924)

Includes: bruise without fracture or open wound
hematoma without fracture or open wound

Excludes: *concussion (850.0-850.9)*
hemarthrosis (840.0-848.9)
internal organs (860.0-869.1)
that incidental to:
crushing injury (925-929.9)
dislocation (830.0-839.9)
fracture (800.0-829.1)
internal injury (860.0-869.1)
intracranial injury (850.0-854.1)
nerve injury (950.0-957.9)
open wound (870.0-897.7)

920   Contusion of face, scalp, and neck except eye(s)

Cheek	Mandibular joint area
Ear (auricle)	Nose
Gum	Throat
Lip	

921 Contusion of eye and adnexa

921.0 Black eye, not otherwise specified

921.1 Contusion of eyelids and periocular area

921.2 Contusion of orbital tissues

921.3 Contusion of eyeball

921.9 Unspecified contusion of eye
Injury of eye NOS

922 Contusion of trunk

922.0 Breast

922.1 Chest wall

922.2 Abdominal wall
Flank
Groin

⑤ **922.3 Back**

Excludes: *scapular region (923.01)*

922.31   Back

Excludes: *interscapular region (922.33)*

922.32   Buttock

922.33   Interscapular region

922.4 Genital organs

Labium (majus) (minus)	Testis
Penis	Vagina
Perineum	Vulva
Scrotum	

922.8 Multiple sites of trunk

922.9 Unspecified part
Trunk NOS

923 Contusion of upper limb

⑤ **923.0 Shoulder and upper arm**

923.00   Shoulder region

923.01   Scapular region

923.02   Axillary region

923.03   Upper arm

923.09   Multiple sites

⑤ **923.1 Elbow and forearm**

923.10   Forearm

Add 4th or 5th digit	Nonspecific code	Unspecified code	Medicare secondary payer (MSP) alert

923.11   **Elbow**

⑤ **923.2   Wrist and hand(s), except finger(s) alone**

923.20   **Hand(s)**

923.21   **Wrist**

923.3   **Finger**
Fingernail
Thumb (nail)

923.8 **Multiple sites of upper limb**

923.9 **Unspecified part of upper limb**
Arm NOS

924 **Contusion of lower limb and of other and unspecified sites**

⑤ **924.0   Hip and thigh**

924.00   **Thigh**

924.01   **Hip**

⑤ **924.1   Knee and lower leg**

924.10   **Lower leg**

924.11   **Knee**

⑤ **924.2   Ankle and foot, excluding toe(s)**

924.20   **Foot**
Heel

924.21   **Ankle**

924.3   **Toe**
Toenail

924.4 **Multiple sites of lower limb**

924.5 **Unspecified part of lower limb**
Leg NOS

924.8 **Multiple sites, not elsewhere classified**

924.9 **Unspecified site**

CRUSHING INJURY (925-929)

Use additional code to identify any associated injuries, such as:
fractures (800-829)
internal injuries (860.0-869.1)
intracranial injury (850.0-854.1)

925 **Crushing injury of face, scalp, and neck**
Cheek   Pharynx
Ear   Throat
Larynx

925.1   **Crushing injury of face and scalp**
Cheek   Ear

925.2   **Crushing injury of neck**
Larynx   Throat
Pharynx

926 **Crushing injury of trunk**

926.0   **External genitalia**
Labium (majus) (minus)   Testis
Penis   Vulva
Scrotum

⑤ **926.1   Other specified sites**

926.11   **Back**

926.12   **Buttock**

926.19 **Other**
Breast

926.8 **Multiple sites of trunk**

926.9 **Unspecified site**
Trunk NOS

927 **Crushing injury of upper limb**

⑤ **927.0   Shoulder and upper arm**

● Code new
to this edition

▲ Revision of
existing code

④ ⑤ Fourth or fifth
digit required

927.00   Shoulder region

927.01   Scapular region

927.02   Axillary region

927.03   Upper arm

927.09   Multiple sites

⑤ 927.1   Elbow and forearm

927.10   Forearm

927.11   Elbow

⑤ 927.2   Wrist and hand(s), except finger(s) alone

927.20   Hand(s)

927.21   Wrist

927.3   Finger(s)

927.8   Multiple sites of upper limb

927.9   Unspecified site
    Arm NOS

928   Crushing injury of lower limb

⑤ 928.0   Hip and thigh

928.00   Thigh

928.01   Hip

⑤ 928.1   Knee and lower leg

928.10   Lower leg

928.11   Knee

⑤ 928.2   Ankle and foot, excluding toe(s) alone

928.20   Foot
    Heel

928.21   Ankle

928.3   Toe(s)

928.8   Multiple sites of lower limb

928.9   Unspecified site
    Leg NOS

929   Crushing injury of multiple and unspecified sites

929.0   Multiple sites, not elsewhere classified

929.9   Unspecified site

EFFECTS OF FOREIGN BODY ENTERING THROUGH ORIFICE (930-939)

Excludes: foreign body:
    granuloma (728.82)
    inadvertently left in operative wound (998.4, 998.7)
    in open wound (800-839, 851-897)
    residual, in soft tissues (729.6)
    superficial without major open wound (910-919 with .6 or .7)

930   Foreign body on external eye

Excludes: foreign body in penetrating wound of:
    eyeball (871.5-871.6)
    retained (old) (360.5-360.6)
    ocular adnexa (870.4)
    retained (old) (376.6)

930.0   Corneal foreign body

930.1   Foreign body in conjunctival sac

930.2   Foreign body in lacrimal punctum

930.8   Other and combined sites

930.9   Unspecified site
    External eye NOS

931   Foreign body in ear
    Auditory canal
    Auricle

| | Add 4th or 5th digit | | Nonspecific code | | Unspecified code | | Medicare secondary payer (MSP) alert |

932 Foreign body in nose
Nasal sinus
Nostril

933 Foreign body in pharynx and larynx

933.0 Pharynx
Nasopharynx
Throat NOS

933.1 Larynx
Asphyxia due to foreign body
Choking due to:
food (regurgitated)
phlegm

934 Foreign body in trachea, bronchus, and lung

934.0 Trachea

934.1 Main bronchus

934.8 Other specified parts
Bronchioles
Lung

934.9 Respiratory tree, unspecified
Inhalation of liquid or vomitus, lower respiratory tract NOS

935 Foreign body in mouth, esophagus, and stomach

935.0 Mouth

935.1 Esophagus

935.2 Stomach

936 Foreign body in intestine and colon

937 Foreign body in anus and rectum
Rectosigmoid (junction)

938 Foreign body in digestive system, unspecified
Alimentary tract NOS
Swallowed foreign body

939 Foreign body in genitourinary tract

939.0 Bladder and urethra

939.1 Uterus, any part

Excludes: intrauterine contraceptive device:
complications from (996.32, 996.65)
presence of (V45.51)

939.2 Vulva and vagina

939.3 Penis

939.9 Unspecified site

BURNS (940-949)

Includes: burns from:
electrical heating appliance
electricity
flame
hot object
lightning
radiation
chemical burns (external) (internal)
scalds

Excludes: friction burns (910-919 with .0, .1)
sunburn (692.71, 692.76-692.77)

940 Burn confined to eye and adnexa

940.0 Chemical burn of eyelids and periocular area

940.1 Other burns of eyelids and periocular area

940.2 Alkaline chemical burn of cornea and conjunctival sac

940.3 Acid chemical burn of cornea and conjunctival sac

940.4 Other burn of cornea and conjunctival sac

940.5 Burn with resulting rupture and destruction of eyeball

● Code new
to this edition
▲ Revision of
existing code
④ ⑤ Fourth or fifth
digit required

940.9 Unspecified burn of eye and adnexa

⑤ **941** **Burn of face, head, and neck**

> Excludes: mouth (947.0)

The following fifth-digit subclassification is for use with category 941:

0 face and head, unspecified site

1 ear [any part]

2 eye (with other parts of face, head, and neck)

3 lip(s)

4 chin

5 nose (septum)

6 scalp [any part]
Temple (region)

7 forehead and cheek

8 neck

9 multiple sites [except with eye] of face, head, and neck

⑤ **941.0** **Unspecified degree**
[0-9]

⑤ **941.1** **Erythema [first degree]**
[0-9]

⑤ **941.2** **Blisters, epidermal loss [second degree]**
[0-9]

⑤ **941.3** **Full-thickness skin loss [third degree NOS]**
[0-9]

⑤ **941.4** **Deep necrosis of underlying tissues [deep third degree] without mention of loss of a body part**
[0-9]

⑤ **941.5** **Deep necrosis of underlying tissues [deep third degree] with loss of a body part**
[0-9]

⑤ **942** **Burn of trunk**

> Excludes: scapular region (943.0-943.5 with fifth-digit 6)

The following fifth-digit subclassification is for use with category 942:

0 trunk, unspecified site

1 breast

2 chest wall, excluding breast and nipple

3 abdominal wall
　Flank　　　　　　　　　　　　Groin

4 back [any part]
　Buttock　　　　　　　　　　Interscapular region

5 genitalia
　Labium (majus) (minus)　　Scrotum
　Penis　　　　　　　　　　　Testis
　Perineum　　　　　　　　　Vulva

9 other and multiple sites of trunk

⑤ **942.0** **Unspecified degree**
[0-5,9]

⑤ **942.1** **Erythema [first degree]**
[0-5,9]

⑤ **942.2** **Blisters, epidermal loss [second degree]**
[0-5,9]

⑤ **942.3** **Full-thickness skin loss [third degree NOS]**
[0-5,9]

⑤ **942.4** **Deep necrosis of underlying tissues [deep third degree] without mention of loss of a body part**
[0-5,9]

⑤ **942.5** **Deep necrosis of underlying tissues [deep third degree] with loss of a body part**
[0-5,9]

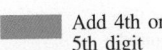

| | Add 4th or 5th digit | | Nonspecific code | | Unspecified code | | Medicare secondary payer (MSP) alert |

⑤ **943** **Burn of upper limb, except wrist and hand**

The following fifth-digit subclassification is for use with category 943:

    0   **upper limb, unspecified site**

    1   forearm

    2   elbow

    3   upper arm

    4   axilla

    5   shoulder

    6   scapular region

    9   **multiple sites of upper limb, except wrist and hand**

⑤ **943.0** **Unspecified degree**
[0-6,9]

⑤ **943.1** **Erythema [first degree]**
[0-6,9]

⑤ **943.2** **Blisters, epidermal loss [second degree]**
[0-6,9]

⑤ **943.3** **Full-thickness skin loss [third degree NOS]**
[0-6,9]

⑤ **943.4** **Deep necrosis of underlying tissues [deep third degree] without mention of loss of a body part**
[0-6,9]

⑤ **943.5** **Deep necrosis of underlying tissues [deep third degree] with loss of a body part**
[0-6,9]

⑤ **944** **Burn of wrist(s) and hand(s)**

The following fifth-digit subclassification is for use with category 944:

    0   **hand, unspecified site**

    1   single digit [finger (nail)] other than thumb

    2   thumb (nail)

    3   two or more digits, not including thumb

    4   two or more digits including thumb

    5   palm

    6   back of hand

    7   wrist

    8   **multiple sites of wrist(s) and hand(s)**

⑤ **944.0** **Unspecified degree**
[0-8]

⑤ **944.1** **Erythema [first degree]**
[0-8]

⑤ **944.2** **Blisters, epidermal loss [second degree]**
[0-8]

⑤ **944.3** **Full-thickness skin loss [third degree NOS]**
[0-8]

⑤ **944.4** **Deep necrosis of underlying tissues [deep third degree] without mention of loss of a body part**
[0-8]

⑤ **944.5** **Deep necrosis of underlying tissues [deep third degree] with loss of a body part**
[0-8]

⑤ **945** **Burn of lower limb(s)**

The following fifth-digit subclassification is for use with category 945:

    0   **lower limb [leg], unspecified site**

    1   toe(s) (nail)

    2   foot

    3   ankle

    4   lower leg

    5   knee

    6   thigh [any part]

    9   **multiple sites of lower limb(s)**

● Code new to this edition   ▲ Revision of existing code   ④ ⑤ Fourth or fifth digit required

⑤ **945.0** **Unspecified degree**
[0-6,9]

⑤ **945.1** **Erythema [first degree]**
[0-6,9]

⑤ **945.2** **Blisters, epidermal loss [second degree]**
[0-6,9]

⑤ **945.3** **Full-thickness skin loss [third degree NOS]**
[0-6,9]

⑤ **945.4** **Deep necrosis of underlying tissues [deep third degree] without mention of loss of a body part**
[0-6,9]

⑤ **945.5** **Deep necrosis of underlying tissues [deep third degree] with loss of a body part**
[0-6,9]

946 **Burns of multiple specified sites**
Includes: burns of sites classifiable to more than one three-digit category in 940-945

Excludes: *multiple burns NOS (949.0-949.5)*

946.0 **Unspecified degree**

946.1 **Erythema [first degree]**

946.2 **Blisters, epidermal loss [second degree]**

946.3 **Full-thickness skin loss [third degree NOS]**

946.4 **Deep necrosis of underlying tissues [deep third degree] without mention of loss of a body part**

946.5 **Deep necrosis of underlying tissues [deep third degree] with loss of a body part**

947 **Burn of internal organs**
Includes: burns from chemical agents (ingested)

947.0 **Mouth and pharynx**
Gum
Tongue

947.1 **Larynx, trachea, and lung**

947.2 **Esophagus**

947.3 **Gastrointestinal tract**
Colon   Small intestine
Rectum   Stomach

947.4 **Vagina and uterus**

947.8 **Other specified sites**

947.9 **Unspecified site**

⑤ **948** **Burns classified according to extent of body surface involved**

Excludes: *sunburn (692.71, 692.76-692.77)*

Note: This category is to be used when the site of the burn is unspecified, or with categories 940-947 when the site is specified.

The following fifth-digit subclassification is for use with category 948 to indicate the percent of *body surface* with *third degree burn*; valid digits are in [brackets] under each code:

0 **less than 10 percent or unspecified**

1 **10-19%**

2 **20-29%**

3 **30-39%**

4 **40-49%**

5 **50-59%**

6 **60-69%**

7 **70-79%**

8 **80-89%**

9 **90% or more of body surface**

⑤ **948.0** **Burn [any degree] involving less than 10 percent of body surface**
[0]

⑤ **948.1** **10-19 percent of body surface**
[0-1]

⑤ **948.2** **20-29 percent of body surface**
[0-2]

| | Add 4th or 5th digit | | Nonspecific code | | Unspecified code | | Medicare secondary payer (MSP) alert |

⑤ **948.3 30-39 percent of body surface**
[0-3]

⑤ **948.4 40-49 percent of body surface**
[0-4]

⑤ **948.5 50-59 percent of body surface**
[0-5]

⑤ **948.6 60-69 percent of body surface**
[0-6]

⑤ **948.7 70-79 percent of body surface**
[0-7]

⑤ **948.8 80-89 percent of body surface**
[0-8]

⑤ **948.9 90 percent or more of body surface**
[0-9]

949 Burn, unspecified
Includes: burn NOS
multiple burns NOS

Excludes: *burn of unspecified site but with statement of the extent of body surface involved (948.0-948.9)*

949.0 Unspecified degree

949.1 Erythema [first degree]

949.2 Blisters, epidermal loss [second degree]

949.3 Full-thickness skin loss [third degree NOS]

949.4 Deep necrosis of underlying tissues [deep third degree] without mention of loss of a body part

949.5 Deep necrosis of underlying tissues [deep third degree] with loss of a body part

INJURY TO NERVES AND SPINAL CORD (950-957)

Includes:

division of nerve (with open wound)
lesion in continuity (with open wound)
traumatic neuroma (with open wound)
traumatic transient paralysis (with open wound)

Excludes: *accidental puncture or laceration during medical procedure (998.2)*

950 Injury to optic nerve and pathways

950.0 Optic nerve injury
Second cranial nerve

950.1 Injury to optic chiasm

950.2 Injury to optic pathways

950.3 Injury to visual cortex

950.9 Unspecified
Traumatic blindness NOS

951 Injury to other cranial nerve(s)

951.0 Injury to oculomotor nerve
Third cranial nerve

951.1 Injury to trochlear nerve
Fourth cranial nerve

951.2 Injury to trigeminal nerve
Fifth cranial nerve

951.3 Injury to abducens nerve
Sixth cranial nerve

951.4 Injury to facial nerve
Seventh cranial nerve

951.5 Injury to acoustic nerve
Auditory nerve   Traumatic deafness NOS
Eighth cranial nerve

951.6 Injury to accessory nerve
Eleventh cranial nerve

951.7 Injury to hypoglossal nerve
Twelfth cranial nerve

● Code new
to this edition

▲ Revision of
existing code

④ ⑤ Fourth or fifth
digit required

951.8 **Injury to other specified cranial nerves**
 Glossopharyngeal [9th cranial] nerve
 Olfactory [1st cranial] nerve
 Pneumogastric [10th cranial] nerve
 Traumatic anosmia NOS
 Vagus [10th cranial] nerve

951.9 **Injury to unspecified cranial nerve**

952 **Spinal cord injury without evidence of spinal bone injury**

⑤ **952.0** **Cervical**

952.00 **C_1-C_4 level with unspecified spinal cord injury**
 Spinal cord injury, cervical region NOS

952.01 **C_1-C_4 level with complete lesion of spinal cord**

952.02 **C_1-C_4 level with anterior cord syndrome**

952.03 **C_1-C_4 level with central cord syndrome**

952.04 **C_1-C_4 level with other specified spinal cord injury**
 Incomplete spinal cord lesion at C_1-C_4 level:
  NOS
  with posterior cord syndrome

952.05 **C_5-C_7 level with unspecified spinal cord injury**

952.06 **C_5-C_7 level with complete lesion of spinal cord**

952.07 **C_5-C_7 level with anterior cord syndrome**

952.08 **C_5-C_7 level with central cord syndrome**

952.09 **C_5-C_7 level with other specified spinal cord injury**
 Incomplete spinal cord lesion at C_5-C_7 level:
  NOS
  with posterior cord syndrome

⑤ **952.1** **Dorsal [thoracic]**

952.10 **T_1-T_6 level with unspecified spinal cord injury**
 Spinal cord injury, thoracic region NOS

952.11 **T_1-T_6 level with complete lesion of spinal cord**

952.12 **T_1-T_6 level with anterior cord syndrome**

952.13 **T_1-T_6 level with central cord syndrome**

952.14 **T_1-T_6 level with other specified spinal cord injury**
 Incomplete spinal cord lesion at T_1-T_6 level:
  NOS
  with posterior cord syndrome

952.15 **T_7-T_{12} level with unspecified spinal cord injury**

952.16 **T_7-T_{12} level with complete lesion of spinal cord**

952.17 **T_7-T_{12} level with anterior cord syndrome**

952.18 **T_7-T_{12} level with central cord syndrome**

952.19 **T_7-T_{12} level with other specified spinal cord injury**
 Incomplete spinal cord lesion at T_7-T_{12} level:
  NOS
  with posterior cord syndrome

952.2 **Lumbar**

952.3 **Sacral**

952.4 **Cauda equina**

952.8 **Multiple sites of spinal cord**

952.9 **Unspecified site of spinal cord**

953 **Injury to nerve roots and spinal plexus**

953.0 **Cervical root**

953.1 **Dorsal root**

953.2 **Lumbar root**

953.3 **Sacral root**

953.4 **Brachial plexus**

953.5 **Lumbosacral plexus**

953.8 **Multiple sites**

953.9 **Unspecified site**

| | Add 4th or 5th digit | | Nonspecific code | | Unspecified code | | Medicare secondary payer (MSP) alert |

954 Injury to other nerve(s) of trunk, excluding shoulder and pelvic girdles

    954.0 Cervical sympathetic

    954.1 Other sympathetic
        Celiac ganglion or plexus   Splanchnic nerve(s)
        Inferior mesenteric plexus   Stellate ganglion

    954.8 Other specified nerve(s) of trunk

    954.9 Unspecified nerve of trunk

955 Injury to peripheral nerve(s) of shoulder girdle and upper limb

    955.0 Axillary nerve

    955.1 Median nerve

    955.2 Ulnar nerve

    955.3 Radial nerve

    955.4 Musculocutaneous nerve

    955.5 Cutaneous sensory nerve, upper limb

    955.6 Digital nerve

    955.7 Other specified nerve(s) of shoulder girdle and upper limb

    955.8 Multiple nerves of shoulder girdle and upper limb

    955.9 Unspecified nerve of shoulder girdle and upper limb

956 Injury to peripheral nerve(s) of pelvic girdle and lower limb

    956.0 Sciatic nerve

    956.1 Femoral nerve

    956.2 Posterior tibial nerve

    956.3 Peroneal nerve

    956.4 Cutaneous sensory nerve, lower limb

    956.5 Other specified nerve(s) of pelvic girdle and lower limb

    956.8 Multiple nerves of pelvic girdle and lower limb

    956.9 Unspecified nerve of pelvic girdle and lower limb

957 Injury to other and unspecified nerves

    957.0 Superficial nerves of head and neck

    957.1 Other specified nerve(s)

    957.8 Multiple nerves in several parts
        Multiple nerve injury NOS

    957.9 Unspecified site
        Nerve injury NOS

CERTAIN TRAUMATIC COMPLICATIONS AND UNSPECIFIED INJURIES (958-959)

958 Certain early complications of trauma

    Excludes: *adult respiratory distress syndrome (518.5)*
        flail chest (807.4)
        post-traumatic seroma (729.91)
        shock lung (518.5)
        that occurring during or following medical procedures (996.0-999.9)

    958.0 Air embolism
        Pneumathemia
        Excludes: *that complicating:*
           abortion (634-638 with .6, 639.6)
           ectopic or molar pregnancy (639.6)
           pregnancy, childbirth, or the puerperium (673.0)

    958.1 Fat embolism
        Excludes: *that complicating:*
           abortion (634-638 with .6, 639.6)
           pregnancy, childbirth, or the puerperium (673.8)

    958.2 Secondary and recurrent hemorrhage

    958.3 Posttraumatic wound infection, not elsewhere classified
        Excludes: *infected open wounds—code to complicated open wound of site*

● Code new to this edition   ▲ Revision of existing code   ④ ⑤ Fourth or fifth digit required

958.4 Traumatic shock
  Shock (immediate) (delayed) following injury

  Excludes: *shock:*
    anaphylactic (995.0)
      due to serum (999.4)
    anesthetic (995.4)
    electric (994.8)
    following abortion (639.5)
    lightning (994.0)
    nontraumatic NOS (785.50)
    obstetric (669.1)
    postoperative (998.0)

958.5 Traumatic anuria
  Crush syndrome
  Renal failure following crushing

  Excludes: *that due to a medical procedure (997.5)*

958.6 Volkmann's ischemic contracture
  Posttraumatic muscle contracture

958.7 Traumatic subcutaneous emphysema

  Excludes: *subcutaneous emphysema resulting from a procedure (998.81)*

958.8 Other early complications of trauma

⑤ **958.9 Traumatic compartment syndrome**

  Excludes: *nontraumatic compartment syndrome (729.71-729.79)*

  958.90 Compartment syndrome, unspecified

  958.91 Traumatic compartment syndrome of upper extremity
    Traumatic compartment syndrome of shoulder, arm, forearm, wrist, hand, and fingers

  958.92 Traumatic compartment syndrome of lower extremity
    Traumatic compartment syndrome of hip, buttock, thigh, leg, foot, and toes

  958.93 Traumatic compartment syndrome of abdomen

  958.99 Traumatic compartment syndrome of other sites

959 Injury, other and unspecified
  Includes: injury NOS

  Excludes: *injury NOS of:*
    blood vessels (900.0-904.9)
    eye (921.0-921.9)
    internal organs (860.0-869.1)
    intracranial sites (854.0-854.1)
    nerves (950.0-951.9, 953.0-957.9)
    spinal cord (952.0-952.9)

⑤ **959.0 Head, face and neck**

Cheek	Mouth
Ear	Nose
Eyebrow	Throat
Lip	

  959.01 Head injury, unspecified

  Excludes: *concussion (850.1-850.9)*
    with head injury NOS (850.1-850.9)
    head injury NOS with loss of consciousness (850.1-850.5)
    specified intracranial injuries (850.0-854.1)

  959.09 Injury of face and neck

⑤ **959.1 Trunk**

  Excludes: *scapular region (959.2)*

  959.11 Other injury of chest wall

  959.12 Other injury of abdomen

  959.13 Fracture of corpus cavernosum penis

  959.14 Other injury of external genitals

  959.19 Other injury of other sites of trunk
    Injury of trunk NOS

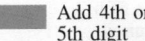

959.2 Shoulder and upper arm
Axilla
Scapular region

959.3 Elbow, forearm, and wrist

959.4 Hand, except finger

959.5 Finger
Fingernail
Thumb (nail)

959.6 Hip and thigh
Upper leg

959.7 Knee, leg, ankle, and foot

959.8 Other specified sites, including multiple
Excludes: multiple sites classifiable to the same four-digit category (959.0-959.7)

959.9 Unspecified site

POISONING BY DRUGS, MEDICINAL AND BIOLOGICAL SUBSTANCES (960-979)

Includes: overdose of these substances
wrong substances given or taken in error

Excludes: adverse effects ["hypersensitivity," "reaction," etc.] of correct substance properly
administered. Such cases are to be classified according to the nature of the
adverse effect, such as:
adverse effect NOS (995.20)
allergic lymphadenitis (289.3)
aspirin gastritis (535.4)
blood disorders (280.0-289.9)
dermatitis:
contact (692.0-692.9)
due to ingestion (693.0-693.9)
nephropathy (583.9)
[The drug giving rise to the adverse effect may be identified by use of categories
E930-E949]
drug dependence (304.0-304.9)
drug reaction and poisoning affecting the newborn (760.0-779.9)
nondependent abuse of drugs (305.0-305.9)
pathological drug intoxication (292.2)

Use additional code to specify the effects of the poisoning

960 Poisoning by antibiotics
Excludes: antibiotics:
ear, nose, and throat (976.6)
eye (976.5)
local (976.0)

960.0 Penicillins
Ampicillin   Cloxacillin
Carbenicillin   Penicillin G

960.1 Antifungal antibiotics
Amphotericin B   Nystatin
Griseofulvin   Trichomycin

Excludes: preparations intended for topical use (976.0-976.9)

960.2 Chloramphenicol group
Chloramphenicol
Thiamphenicol

960.3 Erythromycin and other macrolides
Oleandomycin
Spiramycin

960.4 Tetracycline group
Doxycycline   Oxytetracycline
Minocycline

960.5 Cephalosporin group
Cephalexin   Cephaloridine
Cephaloglycin   Cephalothin

960.6 Antimycobacterial antibiotics
Cycloserine   Rifampin
Kanamycin   Streptomycin

● Code new   ▲ Revision of   ④ ⑤ Fourth or fifth
to this edition   existing code   digit required

960.7 Antineoplastic antibiotics
Actinomycin such as:
    Cactinomycin
    Dactinomycin
Bleomycin
Daunorubicin
Mitomycin

960.8 Other specified antibiotics

960.9 Unspecified antibiotic

961 Poisoning by other anti-infectives
Excludes: anti-infectives:
    ear, nose, and throat (976.6)
    eye (976.5)
    local (976.0)

961.0 Sulfonamides
Sulfadiazine
Sulfafurazole
Sulfamethoxazole

961.1 Arsenical anti-infectives

961.2 Heavy metal anti-infectives
Compounds of:
    antimony
    bismuth
Compounds of:
    lead
    mercury

Excludes: mercurial diuretics (974.0)

961.3 Quinoline and hydroxyquinoline derivatives
Chiniofon
Diiodohydroxyquin

Excludes: antimalarial drugs (961.4)

961.4 Antimalarials and drugs acting on other blood protozoa
Chloroquine
Cycloguanil
Primaquine
Proguanil [chloroguanide]
Pyrimethamine
Quinine

961.5 Other antiprotozoal drugs
Emetine

961.6 Anthelmintics
Hexylresorcinol
Piperazine
Thiabendazole

961.7 Antiviral drugs
Methisazone

Excludes: amantadine (966.4)
    cytarabine (963.1)
    idoxuridine (976.5)

961.8 Other antimycobacterial drugs
Ethambutol
Ethionamide
Isoniazid
Para-aminosalicylic acid derivatives
Sulfones

961.9 Other and unspecified anti-infectives
Flucytosine
Nitrofuran derivatives

962 Poisoning by hormones and synthetic substitutes
Excludes: oxytocic hormones (975.0)

962.0 Adrenal cortical steroids
Cortisone derivatives
Desoxycorticosterone derivatives
Fluorinated corticosteroids

962.1 Androgens and anabolic congeners
Methandriol
Nandrolone
Oxymetholone
Testosterone

962.2 Ovarian hormones and synthetic substitutes
Contraceptives, oral
Estrogens
Estrogens and progestogens, combined
Progestogens

Add 4th or 5th digit	Nonspecific code	Unspecified code	Medicare secondary payer (MSP) alert

962.3 Insulins and antidiabetic agents
Acetohexamide Insulin
Biguanide derivatives, oral Phenformin
Chlorpropamide Sulfonylurea derivatives, oral
Glucagon Tolbutamide

962.4 Anterior pituitary hormones
Corticotropin
Gonadotropin
Somatotropin [growth hormone]

962.5 Posterior pituitary hormones
Vasopressin

Excludes: oxytocic hormones (975.0)

962.6 Parathyroid and parathyroid derivatives

962.7 Thyroid and thyroid derivatives
Dextrothyroxin Liothyronine
Levothyroxine sodium Thyroglobulin

962.8 Antithyroid agents
Iodides Thiourea
Thiouracil

962.9 Other and unspecified hormones and synthetic substitutes

963 Poisoning by primarily systemic agents

963.0 Antiallergic and antiemetic drugs
Antihistamines Diphenylpyraline
Chlorpheniramine Thonzylamine
Diphenhydramine Tripelennamine

Excludes: phenothiazine-based tranquilizers (969.1)

963.1 Antineoplastic and immunosuppressive drugs
Azathioprine Cytarabine
Busulfan Fluorouracil
Chlorambucil Mercaptopurine
Cyclophosphamide thio-TEPA

Excludes: antineoplastic antibiotics (960.7)

963.2 Acidifying agents

963.3 Alkalizing agents

963.4 Enzymes, not elsewhere classified
Penicillinase

963.5 Vitamins, not elsewhere classified
Vitamin A
Vitamin D

Excludes: nicotinic acid (972.2)
vitamin K (964.3)

963.8 Other specified systemic agents
Heavy metal antagonists

963.9 Unspecified systemic agent

964 Poisoning by agents primarily affecting blood constituents

964.0 Iron and its compounds
Ferric salts
Ferrous sulfate and other ferrous salts

964.1 Liver preparations and other antianemic agents
Folic acid

964.2 Anticoagulants
Coumarin Phenindione
Heparin Warfarin sodium

964.3 Vitamin K [phytonadione]

964.4 Fibrinolysis-affecting drugs
Aminocaproic acid Streptokinase
Streptodornase Urokinase

964.5 Anticoagulant antagonists and other coagulants
Hexadimethrine
Protamine sulfate

● Code new to this edition   ▲ Revision of existing code   ④ ⑤ Fourth or fifth digit required

964.6 Gamma globulin

964.7 Natural blood and blood products
Blood plasma   Packed red cells
Human fibrinogen   Whole blood

Excludes: transfusion reactions (999.4-999.8)

964.8 Other specified agents affecting blood constituents
Macromolecular blood substitutes
Plasma expanders

964.9 Unspecified agent affecting blood constituents

965 Poisoning by analgesics, antipyretics, and antirheumatics

Excludes: drug dependence (304.0-304.9)
nondependent abuse (305.0-305.9)

⑤ **965.0 Opiates and related narcotics**

965.00 Opium (alkaloids), unspecified

965.01 Heroin
Diacetylmorphine

965.02 Methadone

965.09 Other
Codeine [methylmorphine]
Meperidine [pethidine]
Morphine

965.1 Salicylates
Acetylsalicylic acid [aspirin]
Salicylic acid salts

965.4 Aromatic analgesics, not elsewhere classified
Acetanilid
Paracetamol [acetaminophen]
Phenacetin [acetophenetidin]

965.5 Pyrazole derivatives
Aminophenazone [aminopyrine]
Phenylbutazone

⑤ **965.6 Antirheumatics [antiphlogistics]**

Excludes: salicylates (965.1)
steroids (962.0-962.9)

965.61 Propionic acid derivatives
Fenoprofen   Ketoprofen
Flurbiprofen   Naproxen
Ibuprofen   Oxaprozin

965.69 Other antirheumatics
Gold salts
Indomethacin

965.7 Other non-narcotic analgesics
Pyrabital

965.8 Other specified analgesics and antipyretics
Pentazocine

965.9 Unspecified analgesic and antipyretic

966 Poisoning by anticonvulsants and anti-Parkinsonism drugs

966.0 Oxazolidine derivatives
Paramethadione
Trimethadione

966.1 Hydantoin derivatives
Phenytoin

966.2 Succinimides
Ethosuximide
Phensuximide

966.3 Other and unspecified anticonvulsants
Primidone

Excludes: barbiturates (967.0)
sulfonamides (961.0)

	Add 4th or 5th digit		Nonspecific code		Unspecified code		Medicare secondary payer (MSP) alert

966.4 Anti-Parkinsonism drugs
Amantadine
Ethopropazine [profenamine]
Levodopa [L-dopa]

967 Poisoning by sedatives and hypnotics

Excludes: *drug dependence (304.0-304.9)*
nondependent abuse (305.0-305.9)

967.0 Barbiturates
Amobarbital [amylobarbitone]
Barbital [barbitone]
Butabarbital [butabarbitone]
Pentobarbital [pentobarbitone]
Phenobarbital [phenobarbitone]
Secobarbital [quinalbarbitone]

Excludes: *thiobarbiturate anesthetics (968.3)*

967.1 Chloral hydrate group

967.2 Paraldehyde

967.3 Bromine compounds
Bromide
Carbromal (derivatives)

967.4 Methaqualone compounds

967.5 Glutethimide group

967.6 Mixed sedatives, not elsewhere classified

967.8 Other sedatives and hypnotics

967.9 Unspecified sedative or hypnotic
Sleeping:
drug NOS
pill NOS
tablet NOS

968 Poisoning by other central nervous system depressants and anesthetics

Excludes: *drug dependence (304.0-304.9)*
nondependent abuse (305.0-305.9)

968.0 Central nervous system muscle-tone depressants
Chlorphenesin (carbamate)   Methocarbamol
Mephenesin

968.1 Halothane

968.2 Other gaseous anesthetics
Ether
Halogenated hydrocarbon derivatives, except halothane
Nitrous oxide

968.3 Intravenous anesthetics

Excludes: *Methohexital [methohexitone]*
Thiobarbiturates, such as thiopental sodium

968.4 Other and unspecified general anesthetics

968.5 Surface [topical] and infiltration anesthetics
Cocaine   Procaine
Lidocaine [lignocaine]   Tetracaine

968.6 Peripheral nerve and plexus-blocking anesthetics

968.7 Spinal anesthetics

968.9 Other and unspecified local anesthetics

969 Poisoning by psychotropic agents

Excludes: *drug dependence (304.0-304.9)*
nondependent abuse (305.0-305.9)

⑤ **969.0 Antidepressants**

● **969.00 Antidepressant, unspecified**

● **969.01 Monoamine oxidase inhibitors**
MAOI

● **969.02 Selective serotonin and norepinephrine reuptake inhibitors**
SSNRI antidepressants

● Code new
to this edition

▲ Revision of
existing code

④ ⑤ Fourth or fifth
digit required

- ● **969.03** **Selective serotonin reuptake inhibitors**
  SSRI antidepressants

- ● **969.04** **Tetracyclic antidepressants**

- ● **969.05** **Tricyclic antidepressants**

- ● **969.09** **Other antidepressants**

969.1 Phenothiazine-based tranquilizers
Chlorpromazine   Prochlorperazine
Fluphenazine   Promazine

969.2 Butyrophenone-based tranquilizers
Haloperidol   Trifluperidol
Spiperone

969.3 Other antipsychotics, neuroleptics, and major tranquilizers

969.4 Benzodiazepine-based tranquilizers
Chlordiazepoxide   Lorazepam
Diazepam   Medazepam
Flurazepam   Nitrazepam

969.5 Other tranquilizers
Hydroxyzine
Meprobamate

969.6 Psychodysleptics [hallucinogens]
Cannabis (derivatives)   Mescaline
Lysergide [LSD]   Psilocin
Marihuana (derivatives)   Psilocybin

⑤ **969.7 Psychostimulants**

> Excludes: *central appetite depressants (977.0)*

- ● **969.70** **Psychostimulant, unspecified**

- ● **969.71** **Caffeine**

- ● **969.72** **Amphetamines**
  Methamphetamines

- ● **969.73** **Methylphenidate**

- ● **969.79** **Other psychostimulants**

969.8 Other specified psychotropic agents

969.9 Unspecified psychotropic agent

970 Poisoning by central nervous system stimulants

970.0 Analeptics
Lobeline
Nikethamide

970.1 Opiate antagonists
Levallorphan   Naloxone
Nalorphine

970.8 Other specified central nervous system stimulants

970.9 Unspecified central nervous system stimulant

971 Poisoning by drugs primarily affecting the autonomic nervous system

971.0 Parasympathomimetics [cholinergics]
Acetylcholine   Pilocarpine
Anticholinesterase:
  organophosphorus
  reversible

971.1 Parasympatholytics [anticholinergics and antimuscarinics] and spasmolytics
Atropine   Hyoscine [scopolamine]
Homatropine   Quaternary ammonium derivatives

> Excludes: *papaverine (972.5)*

971.2 Sympathomimetics [adrenergics]
Epinephrine [adrenalin]
Levarterenol [noradrenalin]

971.3 Sympatholytics [antiadrenergics]
Phenoxybenzamine
Tolazoline hydrochloride

971.9 Unspecified drug primarily affecting autonomic nervous system

---

Add 4th or   Nonspecific   Unspecified   Medicare secondary
5th digit   code   code   payer (MSP) alert

972 **Poisoning by agents primarily affecting the cardiovascular system**

972.0 Cardiac rhythm regulators
Practolol   Propranolol
Procainamide   Quinidine
Excludes: lidocaine (968.5)

972.1 Cardiotonic glycosides and drugs of similar action
Digitalis glycosides   Strophanthins
Digoxin

972.2 Antilipemic and antiarteriosclerotic drugs
Clofibrate
Nicotinic acid derivatives

972.3 Ganglion-blocking agents
Pentamethonium bromide

972.4 Coronary vasodilators
Dipyridamole   Nitrites
Nitrates [nitroglycerin]

972.5 Other vasodilators
Cyclandelate   Papaverine
Diazoxide
Excludes: nicotinic acid (972.2)

972.6 Other antihypertensive agents
Clonidine   Rauwolfia alkaloids
Guanethidine   Reserpine

972.7 Antivaricose drugs, including sclerosing agents
Sodium morrhuate
Zinc salts

972.8 Capillary-active drugs
Adrenochrome derivatives
Metaraminol

972.9 Other and unspecified agents primarily affecting the cardiovascular system

973 **Poisoning by agents primarily affecting the gastrointestinal system**

973.0 Antacids and antigastric secretion drugs
Aluminum hydroxide
Magnesium trisilicate

973.1 Irritant cathartics
Bisacodyl   Phenolphthalein
Castor oil

973.2 Emollient cathartics
Dioctyl sulfosuccinates

973.3 Other cathartics, including intestinal atonia drugs
Magnesium sulfate

973.4 Digestants
Pancreatin   Pepsin
Papain

973.5 Antidiarrheal drugs
Kaolin
Pectin
Excludes: anti-infectives (960.0-961.9)

973.6 Emetics

973.8 Other specified agents primarily affecting the gastrointestinal system

973.9 Unspecified agent primarily affecting the gastrointestinal system

974 **Poisoning by water, mineral, and uric acid metabolism drugs**

974.0 Mercurial diuretics
Chlormerodrin   Mersalyl
Mercaptomerin

974.1 Purine derivative diuretics
Theobromine
Theophylline
Excludes: aminophylline [theophylline ethylenediamine] (975.7)
caffeine (969.71)

● Code new to this edition   ▲ Revision of existing code   ④ ⑤ Fourth or fifth digit required

974.2 Carbonic acid anhydrase inhibitors
Acetazolamide

974.3 Saluretics
Benzothiadiazides
Chlorothiazide group

974.4 Other diuretics
Ethacrynic acid
Furosemide

974.5 Electrolytic, caloric, and water-balance agents

974.6 Other mineral salts, not elsewhere classified

974.7 Uric acid metabolism drugs
Allopurinol   Probenecid
Colchicine

975 Poisoning by agents primarily acting on the smooth and skeletal muscles and respiratory system

975.0 Oxytocic agents
Ergot alkaloids   Prostaglandins
Oxytocin

975.1 Smooth muscle relaxants
Adiphenine
Metaproterenol [orciprenaline]
Excludes: papaverine (972.5)

975.2 Skeletal muscle relaxants

975.3 Other and unspecified drugs acting on muscles

975.4 Antitussives
Dextromethorphan
Pipazethate

975.5 Expectorants
Acetylcysteine   Terpin hydrate
Guaifenesin

975.6 Anti-common cold drugs

975.7 Antiasthmatics
Aminophylline [theophylline ethylenediamine]

975.8 Other and unspecified respiratory drugs

976 Poisoning by agents primarily affecting skin and mucous membrane, ophthalmological, otorhinolaryngological, and dental drugs

976.0 Local anti-infectives and anti-inflammatory drugs

976.1 Antipruritics

976.2 Local astringents and local detergents

976.3 Emollients, demulcents, and protectants

976.4 Keratolytics, keratoplastics, other hair treatment drugs and preparations

976.5 Eye anti-infectives and other eye drugs
Idoxuridine

976.6 Anti-infectives and other drugs and preparations for ear, nose, and throat

976.7 Dental drugs topically applied
Excludes: anti-infectives (976.0)
          local anesthetics (968.5)

976.8 Other agents primarily affecting skin and mucous membrane
Spermicides [vaginal contraceptives]

976.9 Unspecified agent primarily affecting skin and mucous membrane

977 Poisoning by other and unspecified drugs and medicinal substances

977.0 Dietetics
Central appetite depressants

977.1 Lipotropic drugs

977.2 Antidotes and chelating agents, not elsewhere classified

977.3 Alcohol deterrents

977.4 Pharmaceutical excipients
Pharmaceutical adjuncts

| | Add 4th or 5th digit | | Nonspecific code | | Unspecified code | | Medicare secondary payer (MSP) alert |

977.8 **Other specified drugs and medicinal substances**
Contrast media used for diagnostic x-ray procedures
Diagnostic agents and kits

977.9 **Unspecified drug or medicinal substance**

978 **Poisoning by bacterial vaccines**

978.0 **BCG**

978.1 **Typhoid and paratyphoid**

978.2 **Cholera**

978.3 **Plague**

978.4 **Tetanus**

978.5 **Diphtheria**

978.6 **Pertussis vaccine, including combinations with a pertussis component**

978.8 **Other and unspecified bacterial vaccines**

978.9 **Mixed bacterial vaccines, except combinations with a pertussis component**

979 **Poisoning by other vaccines and biological substances**
Excludes: gamma globulin (964.6)

979.0 **Smallpox vaccine**

979.1 **Rabies vaccine**

979.2 **Typhus vaccine**

979.3 **Yellow fever vaccine**

979.4 **Measles vaccine**

979.5 **Poliomyelitis vaccine**

979.6 **Other and unspecified viral and rickettsial vaccines**
Mumps vaccine

979.7 **Mixed viral-rickettsial and bacterial vaccines, except combinations with a pertussis component**
Excludes: combinations with a pertussis component (978.6)

979.9 **Other and unspecified vaccines and biological substances**

TOXIC EFFECTS OF SUBSTANCES CHIEFLY NONMEDICINAL AS TO SOURCE (980-989)

Excludes: burns from chemical agents (ingested) (947.0-947.9)
localized toxic effects indexed elsewhere (001.0-799.9)
respiratory conditions due to external agents (506.0-508.9)

Use additional code to specify the nature of the toxic effect

980 **Toxic effect of alcohol**

980.0 **Ethyl alcohol**
Denatured alcohol
Ethanol
Grain alcohol
Use additional code to identify any associated:
acute alcohol intoxication (305.0)
in alcoholism (303.0)
drunkenness (simple) (305.0)
pathological (291.4)

980.1 **Methyl alcohol**
Methanol   Wood alcohol

980.2 **Isopropyl alcohol**
Dimethyl carbinol   Rubbing alcohol
Isopropanol

980.3 **Fusel oil**
Alcohol:
amyl
butyl
propyl

980.8 **Other specified alcohols**

980.9 **Unspecified alcohol**

● Code new
to this edition
▲ Revision of
existing code
④ ⑤ Fourth or fifth
digit required

981 Toxic effect of petroleum products

      Benzine   Petroleum:
      Gasoline   ether
      Kerosene   naphtha
      Paraffin wax   spirit

982 Toxic effect of solvents other than petroleum-based

982.0 Benzene and homologues

982.1 Carbon tetrachloride

982.2 Carbon disulfide
      Carbon bisulfide

982.3 Other chlorinated hydrocarbon solvents
      Tetrachloroethylene
      Trichloroethylene

      Excludes: *chlorinated hydrocarbon preparations other than solvents (989.2)*

982.4 Nitroglycol

982.8 Other nonpetroleum-based solvents
      Acetone

983 Toxic effect of corrosive aromatics, acids, and caustic alkalis

983.0 Corrosive aromatics
      Carbolic acid or phenol
      Cresol

983.1 Acids
      Acid:
        hydrochloric
        nitric
        sulfuric

983.2 Caustic alkalis
      Lye   Sodium hydroxide
      Potassium hydroxide

983.9 Caustic, unspecified

984 Toxic effect of lead and its compounds (including fumes)
      Includes: that from all sources except medicinal substances

984.0 Inorganic lead compounds
      Lead dioxide
      Lead salts

984.1 Organic lead compounds
      Lead acetate
      Tetraethyl lead

984.8 Other lead compounds

984.9 Unspecified lead compound

985 Toxic effect of other metals
      Includes: that from all sources except medicinal substances

985.0 Mercury and its compounds
      Minamata disease

985.1 Arsenic and its compounds

985.2 Manganese and its compounds

985.3 Beryllium and its compounds

985.4 Antimony and its compounds

985.5 Cadmium and its compounds

985.6 Chromium

985.8 Other specified metals
      Brass fumes   Iron compounds
      Copper salts   Nickel compounds

985.9 Unspecified metal

986 Toxic effect of carbon monoxide
      Carbon monoxide from any source

987 Toxic effect of other gases, fumes, or vapors

987.0 Liquefied petroleum gases
      Butane
      Propane

| | Add 4th or 5th digit | | Nonspecific code | | Unspecified code | | Medicare secondary payer (MSP) alert |

987.1 Other hydrocarbon gas

987.2 Nitrogen oxides
Nitrogen dioxide
Nitrous fumes

987.3 Sulfur dioxide

987.4 Freon
Dichloromonofluoromethane

987.5 Lacrimogenic gas
Bromobenzyl cyanide   Ethyliodoacetate
Chloroacetophenone

987.6 Chlorine gas

987.7 Hydrocyanic acid gas

987.8 Other specified gases, fumes, or vapors
Phosgene
Polyester fumes

987.9 Unspecified gas, fume, or vapor

988 Toxic effect of noxious substances eaten as food

> *Excludes:* *allergic reaction to food, such as:*
> *gastroenteritis (558.3)*
> *rash (692.5, 693.1)*
> *food poisoning (bacterial) (005.0-005.9)*
> *toxic effects of food contaminants, such as:*
> *aflatoxin and other mycotoxin (989.7)*
> *mercury (985.0)*

988.0 Fish and shellfish

988.1 Mushrooms

988.2 Berries and other plants

988.8 Other specified noxious substances eaten as food

988.9 Unspecified noxious substance eaten as food

989 Toxic effect of other substances, chiefly nonmedicinal as to source

989.0 Hydrocyanic acid and cyanides
Potassium cyanide
Sodium cyanide

> *Excludes:* *gas and fumes (987.7)*

989.1 Strychnine and salts

989.2 Chlorinated hydrocarbons
Aldrin   DDT
Chlordane   Dieldrin

> *Excludes:* *chlorinated hydrocarbon solvents (982.0-982.3)*

989.3 Organophosphate and carbamate
Carbaryl   Parathion
Dichlorvos   Phorate
Malathion   Phosdrin

989.4 Other pesticides, not elsewhere classified
Mixtures of insecticides

989.5 Venom
Bites of venomous snakes, lizards, and spiders
Tick paralysis

989.6 Soaps and detergents

989.7 Aflatoxin and other mycotoxin [food contaminants]

⑤ **989.8** Other substances, chiefly nonmedicinal as to source

    989.81 Asbestos

> *Excludes:* *asbestosis (501)*
> *exposure to asbestos (V15.84)*

    989.82 Latex

    989.83 Silicone

> *Excludes:* *silicone used in medical devices, implants and grafts (996.00-996.79)*

    989.84 Tobacco

● Code new to this edition   ▲ Revision of existing code   ④ ⑤ Fourth or fifth digit required

989.89   Other

989.9   Unspecified substance, chiefly nonmedicinal as to source

OTHER AND UNSPECIFIED EFFECTS OF EXTERNAL CAUSES (990-995)

990   **Effects of radiation, unspecified**
Complication of phototherapy   Radiation sickness
Complication of radiation therapy

> Excludes: specified adverse effects of radiation
> Such conditions are to be classified according to the nature of the adverse effect,
> as:
> burns (940.0-949.5)
> dermatitis (692.7-692.8)
> leukemia (204.0-208.9)
> pneumonia (508.0)
> sunburn (692.71, 692.76-692.77)
> [The type of radiation giving rise to the adverse effect may be identified by use
> of the E codes.]

991   **Effects of reduced temperature**

991.0   **Frostbite of face**

991.1   **Frostbite of hand**

991.2   **Frostbite of foot**

991.3   **Frostbite of other and unspecified sites**

991.4   **Immersion foot**
Trench foot

991.5   **Chilblains**
Erythema pernio
Perniosis

991.6   **Hypothermia**
Hypothermia (accidental)

> Excludes: hypothermia following anesthesia (995.89)
> hypothermia not associated with low environmental temperature (780.65)

991.8   **Other specified effects of reduced temperature**

991.9   **Unspecified effect of reduced temperature**
Effects of freezing or excessive cold NOS

992   **Effects of heat and light**

> Excludes: burns (940.0-949.5)
> diseases of sweat glands due to heat (705.0-705.9)
> malignant hyperpyrexia following anesthesia (995.86)
> sunburn (692.71, 692.76-692.77)

992.0   **Heat stroke and sunstroke**
Heat apoplexy   Siriasis
Heat pyrexia   Thermoplegia
Ictus solaris

992.1   **Heat syncope**
Heat collapse

992.2   **Heat cramps**

992.3   **Heat exhaustion, anhydrotic**
Heat prostration due to water depletion

> Excludes: that associated with salt depletion (992.4)

992.4   **Heat exhaustion due to salt depletion**
Heat prostration due to salt (and water) depletion

992.5   **Heat exhaustion, unspecified**
Heat prostration NOS

992.6   **Heat fatigue, transient**

992.7   **Heat edema**

992.8   **Other specified heat effects**

992.9   **Unspecified**

| | Add 4th or 5th digit | | Nonspecific code | | Unspecified code | | Medicare secondary payer (MSP) alert |

993 Effects of air pressure

993.0 **Barotrauma, otitic**
Aero-otitis media
Effects of high altitude on ears

993.1 **Barotrauma, sinus**
Aerosinusitis
Effects of high altitude on sinuses

993.2 **Other and unspecified effects of high altitude**
Alpine sickness
Andes disease
Anoxia due to high altitude
Hypobaropathy
Mountain sickness

993.3 **Caisson disease**
Bends
Compressed-air disease
Decompression sickness
Divers' palsy or paralysis

993.4 **Effects of air pressure caused by explosion**

993.8 **Other specified effects of air pressure**

993.9 **Unspecified effect of air pressure**

994 Effects of other external causes

Excludes: certain adverse effects not elsewhere classified (995.0-995.8)

994.0 **Effects of lightning**
Shock from lightning
Struck by lightning NOS

Excludes: burns (940.0-949.5)

994.1 **Drowning and nonfatal submersion**
Bathing cramp
Immersion

994.2 **Effects of hunger**
Deprivation of food
Starvation

994.3 **Effects of thirst**
Deprivation of water

994.4 **Exhaustion due to exposure**

994.5 **Exhaustion due to excessive exertion**
Exhaustion due to overexertion

994.6 **Motion sickness**
Air sickness
Seasickness
Travel sickness

994.7 **Asphyxiation and strangulation**
Suffocation (by):
bedclothes
cave-in
constriction
mechanical
Suffocation (by):
plastic bag
pressure
strangulation

Excludes: asphyxia from:
carbon monoxide (986)
inhalation of food or foreign body (932-934.9)
other gases, fumes, and vapors (987.0-987.9)

994.8 **Electrocution and nonfatal effects of electric current**
Shock from electric current
Shock from electroshock gun (taser)

Excludes: electric burns (940.0-949.5)

994.9 **Other effects of external causes**
Effects of:
abnormal gravitational [G] forces or states
weightlessness

995 Certain adverse effects not elsewhere classified

Excludes: complications of surgical and medical care (996.0-999.9)

● Code new to this edition   ▲ Revision of existing code   ④ ⑤ Fourth or fifth digit required

995.0 Other anaphylactic shock
Allergic shock NOS or due to adverse effect of correct medicinal substance properly administered
Anaphylactic reaction NOS or due to adverse effect of correct medicinal substance properly administered
Anaphylaxis NOS or due to adverse effect of correct medicinal substance properly administered

Excludes: *anaphylactic reaction to serum (999.4)*
anaphylactic shock due to adverse food reaction (995.60-995.69)

Use additional E code, if desired, to identify external cause, such as:
adverse effects of correct medicinal substance properly administered (E930-E949)

995.1 Angioneurotic edema
Giant urticaria

Excludes: *Urticaria:*
due to serum (999.5)
other specified (698.2, 708.0-708.9, 757.33)

⑤ **995.2 Other and unspecified adverse effect of drug, medicinal and biological substance**
Adverse effect to correct medicinal substance properly administered
Allergic reaction to correct medicinal substance properly administered
Hypersensitivity to correct medicinal substance properly administered
Idiosyncrasy due to correct medicinal substance properly administered
Drug:
hypersensitivity NOS
reaction NOS

Excludes: *pathological drug intoxication (292.2)*

995.20 Unspecified adverse effect of unspecified drug, medicinal and biological substance

995.21 Arthus phenomenon
Arthus reaction

995.22 Unspecified adverse effect of anesthesia

995.23 Unspecified adverse effect of insulin

● **995.24 Failed moderate sedation during procedure**
Failed conscious sedation during procedure

995.27 Other drug allergy
Drug allergy NOS
Drug hypersensitivity NOS

995.29 Unspecified adverse effect of other drug, medicinal and biological substance

995.3 Allergy, unspecified
Allergic reaction NOS   Idiosyncrasy NOS
Hypersensitivity NOS

Excludes: *allergic reaction NOS to correct medicinal substance properly administered (995.27)*
allergy to existing dental restorative materials (525.66)
specific types of allergic reaction, such as:
allergic diarrhea (558.3)
dermatitis (691.0-693.9)
hay fever (477.0-477.9)

995.4 Shock due to anesthesia
Shock due to anesthesia in which the correct substance was properly administered

Excludes: *complications of anesthesia in labor or delivery (668.0-668.9)*
overdose or wrong substance given (968.0-969.9)
postoperative shock NOS (998.0)
specified adverse effects of anesthesia classified elsewhere, such as:
anoxic brain damage (348.1)
hepatitis (070.0-070.9), etc.
unspecified adverse effect of anesthesia (995.22)

⑤ **995.5 Child maltreatment syndrome**
Use additional code(s), if applicable, to identify any associated injuries
Use additional E code to identify:
nature of abuse (E960-E968)
perpetrator (E967.0-E967.9)

995.50 Child abuse, unspecified

995.51 Child emotional/psychological abuse

Add 4th or 5th digit   Nonspecific code   Unspecified code   Medicare secondary payer (MSP) alert

995.52 **Child neglect (nutritional)**

995.53 **Child sexual abuse**

995.54 **Child physical abuse**
Battered baby or child syndrome

Excludes: *Shaken infant syndrome (995.55)*

995.55 **Shaken infant syndrome**
Use additional code(s) to identify any associated injuries

995.59 **Other child abuse and neglect**
Multiple forms of abuse

⑤ **995.6 Anaphylactic shock due to adverse food reaction**
Anaphylactic reaction due to food
Anaphylactic shock due to nonpoisonous foods

995.60 **Due to unspecified food**

995.61 **Due to peanuts**

995.62 **Due to crustaceans**

995.63 **Due to fruits and vegetables**

995.64 **Due to tree nuts and seeds**

995.65 **Due to fish**

995.66 **Due to food additives**

995.67 **Due to milk products**

995.68 **Due to eggs**

995.69 **Due to other specified food**

995.7 **Other adverse food reactions, not elsewhere classified**
Use additional code to identify the type of reaction, such as:
hives (708.0)
wheezing (786.07)

Excludes: *anaphylactic shock due to adverse food reaction (995.60-995.69)*
asthma (493.0, 493.9)
dermatitis due to food (693.1)
in contact with the skin (692.5)
gastroenteritis and colitis due to food (558.3)
rhinitis due to food (477.1)

⑤ **995.8 Other specified adverse effects, not elsewhere classified**

995.80 **Adult maltreatment, unspecified**
Abused person NOS
Use additional code to identify:
any associated injury
perpetrator (E967.0-E967.9)

995.81 **Adult physical abuse**
Battered:
person syndrome NEC
man
spouse
woman
Use additional code to identify:
any associated injury
nature of abuse (E960-E968)
perpetrator (E967.0-E967.9)

995.82 **Adult emotional/psychological abuse**
Use additional E code to identify perpetrator (E967.0-E967.9)

995.83 **Adult sexual abuse**
Use additional code to identify:
any associated injury
perpetrator (E967.0-E967.9)

995.84 **Adult neglect (nutritional)**
Use additional code to identify:
intent of neglect (E904.0, E968.4)
perpetrator (E967.0-967.9)

● Code new
to this edition

▲ Revision of
existing code

④ ⑤ Fourth or fifth
digit required

995.85 **Other adult abuse and neglect**
Multiple forms of abuse and neglect

Use additional code to identify:
any associated injury
intent of neglect (E904.0, E968.4)
nature of abuse (E960-E968)
perpetrator (E967.0-E967.9)

995.86 **Malignant hyperthermia**
Malignant hyperpyrexia due to anesthesia

995.89 **Other**
Hypothermia due to anesthesia

⑤ **995.9** **Systemic inflammatory response syndrome (SIRS)**

995.90 **Systemic inflammatory response syndrome, unspecified**
SIRS NOS

995.91 **Sepsis**
Systemic inflammatory response syndrome due to infectious process without
acute organ dysfunction

Code first underlying infection

Excludes: *sepsis with acute organ dysfunction (995.92)*
sepsis with multiple organ dysfunction (995.92)
severe sepsis (995.92)

995.92 **Severe sepsis**
Sepsis with acute organ dysfunction
Sepsis with multiple organ dysfunction (MOD)
Systemic inflammatory response syndrome due to infectious process with acute
organ dysfunction

Code first underlying infection

Use additional code to specify acute organ dysfunction, such as:
acute kidney failure (584.5-584.9)
acute respiratory failure (518.81)
critical illness myopathy (359.81)
critical illness polyneuropathy (357.82)
disseminated intravascular coagulopathy (DIC) syndrome (286.6)
encephalopathy (348.31)
hepatic failure (570)
septic shock (785.52)

995.93 **Systemic inflammatory response syndrome due to noninfectious process
without acute organ dysfunction**
Code first underlying conditions, such as:
acute pancreatitis (577.0)
trauma

Excludes: *systemic inflammatory response syndrome due to noninfectious process with acute
organ dysfunction (995.94)*

995.94 **Systemic inflammatory response syndrome due to noninfectious process with
acute organ dysfunction**
Code first underlying condition, such as:
acute pancreatitis (577.0)
trauma

Use additional code to specify acute organ dysfunction, such as:
acute kidney failure (584.5-584.9)
acute respiratory failure (518.81)
critical illness myopathy (359.81)
critical illness polyneuropathy (357.82)
disseminated intravascular coagulopathy (DIC) syndrome (286.6)
encephalopathy (348.31)
hepatic failure (570)

Excludes: *severe sepsis (995.92)*

▓	Add 4th or 5th digit	▓	Nonspecific code	▓	Unspecified code	Medicare secondary payer (MSP) alert

COMPLICATIONS OF SURGICAL AND MEDICAL CARE, NOT ELSEWHERE CLASSIFIED (996-999)

> Excludes: *adverse effects of medicinal agents (001.0-799.9, 995.0-995.8)*
> *burns from local applications and irradiation (940.0-949.5)*
> *complications of:*
> *conditions for which the procedure was performed*
> *surgical procedures during abortion, labor, and delivery (630-676.9)*
> *poisoning and toxic effects of drugs and chemicals (960.0-989.9)*
> *postoperative conditions in which no complications are present, such as:*
> *artificial opening status (V44.0-V44.9)*
> *closure of external stoma (V55.0-V55.9)*
> *fitting of prosthetic device (V52.0-V52.9)*
> *specified complications classified elsewhere*
> *anesthetic shock (995.4)*
> *electrolyte imbalance (276.0-276.9)*
> *postlaminectomy syndrome (772.80-722.83)*
> *postmastectomy lymphedema syndrome (457.0)*
> *postoperative psychosis (293.0-293.9)*
> *any other condition classified elsewhere in the Alphabetic Index when described as due to a procedure*

996 Complications peculiar to certain specified procedures

Includes: complications, not elsewhere classified, in the use of artificial substitutes [e.g., Dacron, metal, Silastic, Teflon] or natural sources [e.g., bone] involving:
anastomosis (internal)
graft (bypass) (patch)
implant
internal device:
catheter
electronic
fixation
prosthetic
reimplant
transplant

> Excludes: *accidental puncture or laceration during procedure (998.2)*
> *capsular contracture of breast implant (611.83)*
> *complications of internal anastomosis of:*
> *gastrointestinal tract (997.4)*
> *urinary tract (997.5)*
> *endosseous dental implant failures (525.71-525.79)*
> *intraoperative floppy iris syndrome (IFIS) (364.81)*
> *mechanical complication of respirator (V46.14)*
> *other specified complications classified elsewhere, such as:*
> *hemolytic anemia (283.1)*
> *functional cardiac disturbances (429.4)*
> *serum hepatitis (070.2-070.3)*

⑤ **996.0 Mechanical complication of cardiac device, implant, and graft**

Breakdown (mechanical)	Obstruction, mechanical
Displacement	Perforation
Leakage	Protrusion

996.00 Unspecified device, implant, and graft

996.01 Due to cardiac pacemaker (electrode)

996.02 Due to heart valve prosthesis

996.03 Due to coronary bypass graft

> Excludes: *atherosclerosis of graft (414.02, 414.03)*
> *embolism [occlusion NOS] [thrombus] of graft (996.72)*

996.04 Due to automatic implantable cardiac defibrillator

996.09 Other

● Code new to this edition ▲ Revision of existing code ④ ⑤ Fourth or fifth digit required

996.1 **Mechanical complication of other vascular device, implant, and graft**
Mechanical complications involving:
aortic (bifurcation) graft (replacement)
arteriovenous:
dialysis catheter
fistula surgically created
shunt surgicall created
balloon (counterpulsation) device, intra-aortic
carotid artery bypass graft
femoral-popliteal bypass graft
umbrella device, vena cava

Excludes: *atherosclerosis of biological graft (440.30-440.32)*
embolism [occlusion NOS] [thrombus] of (biological) (synthetic) graft (996.74)
peritoneal dialysis catheter (996.56)

996.2 **Mechanical complication of nervous system device, implant, and graft**
Mechanical complications involving:
dorsal column stimulator
electrodes implanted in brain [brain "pacemaker"]
peripheral nerve graft
ventricular (communicating) shunt

⑤ **996.3** **Mechanical complication of genitourinary device, implant, and graft**

996.30 **Unspecified device, implant, and graft**

996.31 **Due to urethral [indwelling] catheter**

996.32 **Due to intrauterine contraceptive device**

996.39 **Other**
Cystostomy catheter
Prosthetic reconstruction of vas deferens
Repair (graft) of ureter without mention of resection

Excludes: *complications due to:*
external stoma of urinary tract (997.5)
internal anastomosis of urinary tract (997.5)

⑤ **996.4** **Mechanical complication of internal orthopedic device, implant, and graft**
Use additional code to identify prosthetic joint with mechanical complication (V43.60-V43.69)

996.40 **Unspecified mechanical complication of internal orthopedic device, implant, and graft**

996.41 **Mechanical loosening of prosthetic joint**
Aseptic loosening

996.42 **Dislocation of prosthetic joint**
Instability of prosthetic joint
Subluxation of prosthetic joint

▲ **996.43** **Broken prosthetic joint implant**
Breakage (fracture) of prosthetic joint

996.44 **Peri-prosthetic fracture around prosthetic joint**

996.45 **Peri-prosthetic osteolysis**
Use additional code to identify major osseous defect, if applicable (731.3)

996.46 **Articular bearing surface wear of prosthetic joint**

996.47 **Other mechanical complication of prosthetic joint implant**
Mechanical complication of prosthetic joint NOS
Prosthetic joint implant failure NOS

996.49 **Other mechanical complication of other internal orthopedic device, implant, and graft**
Breakage of internal fixation device in bone
Dislocation of internal fixation device in bone

Excludes: *mechanical complication of prosthetic joint implant (996.41-996.47)*

⑤ **996.5** **Mechanical complication of other specified prosthetic device, implant, and graft**
Mechanical complications involving:
prosthetic implant in:
bile duct
breast
chin
orbit of eye
nonabsorbable surgical material NOS
other graft, implant, and internal device, not elsewhere classified

---

| | Add 4th or 5th digit | | Nonspecific code | | Unspecified code | | Medicare secondary payer (MSP) alert |

996.51 **Due to corneal graft**

996.52 **Due to graft of other tissue, not elsewhere classified**
Skin graft failure or rejection

Excludes: *failure of artificial skin graft (996.55)*
failure of decellularized allodermis (996.55)
sloughing of temporary skin allografts or xenografts (pigskin)—omit code

996.53 **Due to ocular lens prosthesis**

Excludes: *contact lenses—code to condition*

996.54 **Due to breast prosthesis**
Breast capsule (prosthesis)
Mammary implant

996.55 **Due to artificial skin graft and decellularized allodermis**
Dislodgement   Displacement
Failure   Non-adherence
Poor incorporation   Shearing

996.56 **Due to peritoneal dialysis catheter**

Excludes: *mechanical complication of arteriovenous dialysis catheter (996.1)*

996.57 **Due to insulin pump**

996.59 **Due to other implant and internal device, not elsewhere classified**
Nonabsorbable surgical material NOS
Prosthetic implant in:
  bile duct
  chin
  orbit of eye

⑤ **996.6 Infection and inflammatory reaction due to internal prosthetic device, implant, and graft**
Infection (causing obstruction) due to (presence of) any device, implant and graft classifiable to 996.0-996.5
Inflammation due to (presence of) any device, implant and graft classifiable to 996.0-996.5
Use additional code to identify specified infections

996.60 **Due to unspecified device, implant, and graft**

996.61 **Due to cardiac device, implant, and graft**
Cardiac pacemaker or defibrillator:
  electrode(s), lead(s)
  pulse generator
  subcutaneous pocket
Coronary artery bypass graft
Heart valve prosthesis

996.62 **Due to other vascular device, implant, and graft**
Arterial graft
Arteriovenous fistula or shunt
Infusion pump
Vascular catheter (arterial) (dialysis) (peripheral venous)

Excludes: *infection due to:*
central venous catheter (999.31)
Hickman catheter (999.31)
peripherally inserted central catheter (PICC) (999.31)
portacath (port-a-cath) (999.31)
triple lumen catheter (999.31)
umbilical venous catheter (999.31)

996.63 **Due to nervous system device, implant, and graft**
Electrodes implanted in brain
Peripheral nerve graft
Spinal canal catheter
Ventricular (communicating) shunt (catheter)

996.64 **Due to indwelling urinary catheter**
Use additional code to identify specified infections, such as:
  Cystitis (595.0-595.9)
  Sepsis (038.0-038.9)

996.65 **Due to other genitourinary device, implant, and graft**
Intrauterine contraceptive device

● Code new
   to this edition
▲ Revision of
   existing code
④ ⑤ Fourth or fifth
   digit required

996.66 Due to internal joint prosthesis
Use additional code to identify infected prosthetic joint (V43.60-V43.69)

996.67 Due to other internal orthopedic device, implant, and graft
Bone growth stimulator (electrode)
Internal fixation device (pin) (rod) (screw)

996.68 Due to peritoneal dialysis catheter
Exit-site infection or inflammation

996.69 Due to other internal prosthetic device, implant, and graft
Breast prosthesis
Ocular lens prosthesis
Prosthetic orbital implant

⑤ **996.7 Other complications of internal (biological) (synthetic) prosthetic device, implant, and graft**
Complication NOS due to (presence of) any device, implant, and graft classifiable to 996.0-996.5
occlusion NOS
Embolism due to (presence of) any device, implant, and graft classifiable to 996.0-996.5
Fibrosis due to (presence of) any device, implant, and graft classifiable to 996.0-996.5
Hemorrhage due to (presence of) any device, implant, and graft classifiable to 996.0-996.5
Pain due to (presence of) any device, implant, and graft classifiable to 996.0-996.5
Stenosis due to (presence of) any device, implant, and graft classifiable to 996.0-996.5
Thrombus due to (presence of) any device, implant, and graft classifiable to 996.0-996.5
Use additional code to identify complication, such as:
pain due to presence of device, implant or graft (338.18-338.19,338.28-338.29)
venous embolism and thrombosis (453.2-453.9)

Excludes: *disruption (dehiscence) of internal suture material (998.31)*
transplant rejection (996.8)

996.70 Due to unspecified device, implant, and graft

996.71 Due to heart valve prosthesis

996.72 Due to other cardiac device, implant, and graft
Cardiac pacemaker or defibrillator:
electrode(s), lead(s)
subcutaneous pocket
Coronary artery bypass (graft)

Excludes: *occlusion due to atherosclerosis (414.02-414.06)*

996.73 Due to renal dialysis device, implant, and graft

996.74 Due to other vascular device, implant, and graft

Excludes: *occlusion of biological graft due to atherosclerosis (440.30-440.32)*

996.75 Due to nervous system device, implant, and graft

996.76 Due to genitourinary device, implant, and graft

996.77 Due to internal joint prosthesis
Use additional code to identify prosthetic joint (V43.60 - V43.69)

996.78 Due to other internal orthopedic device, implant, and graft

996.79 Due to other internal prosthetic device, implant, and graft

⑤ **996.8 Complications of transplanted organ**
Use additional code, if desired, to identify nature of complication, such as:
cytomegalovirus (CMV) infection (078.5)
graft-versus-host disease (279.50-279.53)
malignancy associated with organ transplant (199.2)
post-transplant lymphoproliferative disorder (PTLD) (238.77)
transplant failure or rejection

996.80 Transplanted organ, unspecified

996.81 Kidney

996.82 Liver

996.83 Heart

996.84 Lung

996.85 Bone Marrow

996.86 Pancreas

996.87 Intestine

| | Add 4th or 5th digit | | Nonspecific code | | Unspecified code | | Medicare secondary payer (MSP) alert |

996.89 Other specified transplanted organ

⑤ **996.9** Complications of reattached extremity or body part

996.90 Unspecified extremity

996.91 Forearm

996.92 Hand

996.93 Finger(s)

996.94 Upper extremity, other and unspecified

996.95 Foot and toe(s)

996.96 Lower extremity, other and unspecified

996.99 Other specified body part

997 Complications affecting specified body systems, not elsewhere classified
Use additional code to identify complication

Excludes: *the listed conditions when specified as:*
    causing shock (998.0)
    complications of:
      anesthesia:
        adverse effect (001.0-799.9, 995.0-995.8)
        in labor or delivery (668.0-668.9)
        poisoning (968.0-969.9)
      implanted device or graft (996.0-996.9)
      obstetrical procedures (669.0-669.4)
      reattached extremity (996.90-996.96)
      transplanted organ (996.80-996.89)

⑤ **997.0** Nervous system complications

997.00 Nervous system complication, unspecified

997.01 Central nervous system complication
Anoxic brain damage
Cerebral hypoxia

Excludes: *cerebrovascular hemorrhage or infarction (997.02)*

997.02 Iatrogenic cerebrovascular infarction or hemorrhage
Postoperative stroke

997.09 Other nervous system complications

997.1 Cardiac complications
Cardiac arrest during or resulting from a procedure
Cardiac insufficiency during or resulting from a procedure
Cardiorespiratory failure during or resulting from a procedure
Heart failure during or resulting from a procedure

Excludes: *the listed conditions as long-term effects of cardiac surgery or due to the presence*
    of cardiac prosthetic device (429.4)

997.2 Peripheral vascular complications
Phlebitis or thrombophlebitis during or resulting from a procedure

Excludes: *the listed conditions due to:*
    implant or catheter device (996.62)
    infusion, perfusion, or transfusion (999.2)
    complications affecting blood vessels (997.71-997.79)

⑤ **997.3** Respiratory complications

Excludes: *iatrogenic [postoperative] pneumothorax (512.1)*
    iatrogenic pulmonary embolism (415.11)
    Mendelson's syndrome in labor and delivery (668.0)
    specified complications classified elsewhere, such as:
      adult respiratory distress syndrome (518.5)
      pulmonary edema, postoperative (518.4)
      respiratory insufficiency, acute, postoperative (518.5)
      shock lung (518.5)
      tracheostomy complications (519.00-519.09)
      transfusion related acute lung injury (TRALI) (518.7)

997.31 Ventilator associated pneumonia
Ventilator associated pneumonitis

Use additional code to identify organism

● Code new
  to this edition
▲ Revision of
  existing code
④ ⑤ Fourth or fifth
    digit required

997.39   **Other respiratory complications**
       Mendelson's syndrome resulting from a procedure
       Pneumonia (aspiration) resulting from a procedure

997.4   **Digestive system complications**
       Complications of intestinal (internal) anastomosis and bypass, not elsewhere classified,
          except that involving urinary tract
       Hepatic failure specified as due to a procedure
       Hepatorenal syndrome specified as due to a procedure
       Intestinal obstruction NOS specified as due to a procedure

    | Excludes: | specified gastrointestinal complications classified elsewhere, such as:
              blind loop syndrome (579.2)
              colostomy or enterostomy complications (569.60-569.69)
              complications of intestinal pouch (569.71-569.79)
              gastrostomy complications (536.40-536.49)
              gastrojejunal ulcer (534.0-534.9)
              infection of esophagostomy (530.86)
              infection of external stoma (569.61)
              mechanical complication of esophagostomy (530.87)
              pelvic peritoneal adhesions, female (614.6)
              peritoneal adhesions (568.0)
              peritoneal adhesions with obstruction (560.81)
              postcholecystectomy syndrome (576.0)
              postgastric surgery syndromes (564.2)
              pouchitis (569.71)
              vomiting following gastrointestinal surgery (564.3)

997.5   **Urinary complications**
       Complications of:
         external stoma of urinary tract
         internal anastomosis and bypass of urinary tract, including that involving intestinal
           tract
       Oliguria or anuria specified as due to procedure
       Renal (kidney):
         failure (acute) specified as due to procedure
         insufficiency (acute) specified as due to procedure
       Tubular necrosis (acute) specified as due to procedure

    | Excludes: | specified complications classified elsewhere, such as:
              postoperative stricture of:
                ureter (593.3)
                urethra (598.2)

⑤ **997.6**   **Amputation stump complication**

    | Excludes: | admission for treatment for a current traumatic amputation; code to complicated
              traumatic amputation
              phantom limb (syndrome) (353.6)

    997.60   **Unspecified complication**

    997.61   **Neuroma of amputation stump**

    997.62   **Infection (chronic)**
    Use additional code to identify the organism

    997.69   **Other**

⑤ **997.7**   **Vascular complications of other vessels**

    | Excludes: | peripheral vascular complications (997.2)

    997.71   **Vascular complications of mesenteric artery**

    997.72   **Vascular complications of renal artery**

    997.79   **Vascular complications of other vessels**

⑤ **997.9**   **Complications affecting other specified body systems, not elsewhere classified**

    | Excludes: | specified complications classified elsewhere, such as:
              broad ligament laceration syndrome (620.6)
              postartificial menopause syndrome (627.4)
              postoperative stricture of vagina (623.2)

    997.91   **Hypertension**
    | Excludes: | essential hypertension (401.0-401.9)

    997.99   **Other**
        Vitreous touch syndrome

| ▮ Add 4th or | ▮ Nonspecific | ▮ Unspecified | ▮ Medicare secondary |
| 5th digit | code | code | payer (MSP) alert |

998 Other complications of procedures, not elsewhere classified

998.0 Postoperative shock
Collapse NOS during or resulting from a surgical procedure
Shock (endotoxic) (hypovolemic) (septic) during or resulting from a surgical procedure

Excludes: *shock:*
anaphylactic due to serum (999.4)
anesthetic (995.4)
electric (994.8)
following abortion (639.5)
obstetric (669.1)
traumatic (958.4)

⑤ **998.1 Hemorrhage or hematoma or seroma complicating a procedure**

Excludes: *hemorrhage due to implanted device or graft (996.70-996.79)*
hemorrhage, hematoma or seroma complicating cesarean section or puerperal perineal wound (674.3)

998.11 Hemorrhage complicating a procedure

998.12 Hematoma complicating a procedure

998.13 Seroma complicating a procedure

998.2 Accidental puncture or laceration during a procedure
Accidental perforation by catheter or other instrument during a procedure on:
blood vessel
nerve
organ

Excludes: *iatrogenic [postoperative] pneumothorax (512.1)*
puncture or laceration caused by implanted device intentionally left in operation wound (996.0-996.5)
specified complications classified elsewhere, such as:
broad ligament laceration syndrome (620.6)
dural tear (349.31)
incidental durotomy (349.31)
trauma from instruments during delivery (664.0-665.9)

⑤ **998.3 Disruption of wound**
Dehiscence of operation wound
Disruption of any suture materials or other closure method
Rupture of operation wound

Excludes: *disruption of:*
cesarean wound (674.1)
perineal wound, puerperal (674.2)

998.30 Disruption of wound, unspecified
Disruption of wound NOS

998.31 Disruption of internal operation (surgical) wound
Disruption or dehiscence of closure of:
fascia, superficial or muscular
internal organ
muscle or muscle flap
ribs or rib cage
skull or craniotomy
sternum or sternotomy
tendon or ligament
Deep disruption or dehiscence of operation wound NOS

Excludes: *complications of internal anastomosis of:*
gastrointestinal tract (997.4)
urinary tract (997.5)

998.32 Disruption of external operation (surgical) wound
Disruption or dehiscence of closure of:
cornea
mucosa
skin
subcutaneous tissue
Disruption of operation wound NOS
Full-thickness skin disruption or dehiscence
Superficial disruption or dehiscence of operation wound

998.33 Disruption of traumatic injury wound repair
Disruption or dehiscence of closure of traumatic laceration (external) (internal)

● Code new
to this edition
▲ Revision of
existing code
④ ⑤ Fourth or fifth
digit required

998.4 Foreign body accidentally left during a procedure
Adhesions due to foreign body accidentally left in operative wound or body cavity during a procedure
Obstruction due to foreign body accidentally left in operative wound or body cavity during a procedure
Perforation due to foreign body accidentally left in operative wound or body cavity during a procedure

Excludes: *obstruction or perforation caused by implanted device intentionally left in body (996.0-996.5)*

⑤ **998.5 Postoperative infection**

Excludes: *bleb associated endophthalmitis (379.63)*
infection due to:
implanted device (996.60-996.69)
infusion, perfusion, or transfusion (999.31-999.39)
postoperative obstetrical wound infection (674.3)

998.51 Infected postoperative seroma
Use additional code to identify organism

998.59 Other postoperative infection
Abscess: postoperative
intra-abdominal postoperative
stitch postoperative
subphrenic postoperative
wound postoperative
Septicemia postoperative
Use additional code to identify infection

998.6 Persistent postoperative fistula

998.7 Acute reaction to foreign substance accidentally left during a procedure
Peritonitis:
aseptic
chemical

⑤ **998.8 Other specified complications of procedures, not elsewhere classified**

998.81 Emphysema (subcutaneous) (surgical) resulting from a procedure

998.82 Cataract fragments in eye following cataract surgery

998.83 Non-healing surgical wound

998.89 Other specified complications

998.9 Unspecified complication of procedure, not elsewhere classified
Postoperative complication NOS

Excludes: *complication NOS of obstetrical surgery or procedure (669.4)*

999 Complications of medical care, not elsewhere classified
Use additional code, where applicable, to identify specific complication
Includes: complications, not elsewhere classified, of:
dialysis (hemodialysis) (peritoneal) (renal)
extracorporeal circulation
hyperalimentation therapy
immunization
infusion
inhalation therapy
injection
inoculation
perfusion
transfusion
vaccination
ventilation therapy

Excludes: *specified complications classified elsewhere such as:*
complications of implanted device (996.0-996.9)
contact dermatitis due to drugs (692.3)
dementia dialysis (294.8)
transient (293.9)
dialysis disequilibrium syndrome (276.0-276.9)
poisoning and toxic effects of drugs and chemicals (960.0-989.9)
postvaccinal encephalitis (323.51)
water and electrolyte imbalance (276.0-276.9)

| | Add 4th or 5th digit | | Nonspecific code | | Unspecified code | | Medicare secondary payer (MSP) alert |

999.0 Generalized vaccinia

Excludes: *vaccinia not from vaccine (051.02)*

999.1 Air embolism
Air embolism to any site following infusion, perfusion, or transfusion

Excludes: *embolism specified as:*
  complicating:
    abortion (634-638 with .6, 639.6)
    ectopic or molar pregnancy (639.6)
    pregnancy, childbirth, or the puerperium (673.0)
  due to implanted device (996.7)
  traumatic (958.0)

999.2 Other vascular complications
Phlebitis following infusion, perfusion, or transfusion
Thromboembolism following infusion, perfusion, or transfusion
Thrombophlebitis following infusion, perfusion, or transfusion

Excludes: *extravasation of vesicant drugs (999.81, 999.82)*
  the listed conditions when specified as:
  due to implanted device (996.61-996.62, 996.72-996.74)
  postoperative NOS (997.2, 997.71-997.79)

⑤ **999.3 Other infection**
Infection following infusion, injection, transfusion, or vaccination
Sepsis following infusion, injection, transfusion, or vaccination
Septicemia following infusion, injection, transfusion, or vaccination
Use additional code to identify the specified infection, such as:
  septicemia (038.0-038.9)

Excludes: *the listed conditions when specified as:*
  due to implanted device (996.60-996.69)
  postoperative NOS (998.51-998.59)

  999.31 Infection due to central venous catheter
  Catheter-related bloodstream infection (CRBSI) NOS
  Infection due to:
    Hickman catheter
    portacath (port-a-cath)
    peripherally inserted central catheter (PICC)
    triple lumen catheter
    umbilical venous catheter

Excludes: *infection due to:*
  arterial catheter (996.62)
  catheter NOS (996.69)
  peripheral venous catheter (996.62)
  urinary catheter (996.64)

  999.39 Infection following other infusion, injection, transfusion, or vaccination

999.4 Anaphylactic shock due to serum
Anaphylactic reaction due to serum

Excludes: *shock:*
  allergic NOS (995.0)
  anaphylactic:
  NOS (995.0)
  due to drugs and chemicals (995.0)

999.5 Other serum reaction
Intoxication by serum	Serum sickness
Protein sickness	Urticaria due to serum
Serum rash	

Excludes: *serum hepatitis (070.2-070.3)*

999.6 ABO incompatibility reaction
Incompatible blood transfusion
Reaction to blood group incompatibility in infusion or transfusion

Excludes: *minor blood group antigens reactions (Duffy) (E) (K(ell)) (Kidd) (Lewis) (M) (N)*
  (P) (S) (999.89)

999.7 Rh incompatibility reaction
Reactions due to Rh factor in infusion or transfusion

⑤ **999.8 Other infusion and transfusion reaction**

> Excludes: *postoperative shock (998.0)*
> *transfusion related acute lung injury (TRALI) (518.7)*

999.81 Extravasation of vesicant chemotherapy
Infiltration of vesicant chemotherapy

999.82 Extravasation of other vesicant agent
Infiltration of other vesicant agent

999.88 Other infusion reaction

999.89 Other transfusion reaction
Transfusion reaction NOS

Use additional code to identify graft-versus-host reaction (279.5)

999.9 Other and unspecified complications of medical care, not elsewhere classified
Complications, not elsewhere classified, of:
electroshock therapy
inhalation therapy
ultrasound therapy
ventilation therapy
Unspecified misadventure of medical care

> Excludes: *unspecified complication of:*
> *phototherapy (990)*
> *radiation therapy (990)*
> *ventilator associated pneumonia (997.31)*

Add 4th or 5th digit	Nonspecific code	Unspecified code	Medicare secondary payer (MSP) alert

● Code new
to this edition

▲ Revision of
existing code

④ ⑤ Fourth or fifth
digit required

SUPPLEMENTARY CLASSIFICATION OF FACTORS INFLUENCING HEALTH STATUS AND CONTACT WITH HEALTH SERVICES (V01-V89)

This classification is provided to deal with occasions when circumstances other than a disease or injury classifiable to categories 001-999 (the main part of ICD) are recorded as "diagnoses" or "problems." This can arise mainly in three ways:

a) When a person who is not currently sick encounters the health services for some specific purpose, such as to act as a donor of an organ or tissue, to receive prophylactic vaccination, or to discuss a problem which is in itself not a disease or injury. This will be a fairly rare occurrence among hospital inpatients, but will be relatively more common among hospital outpatients and patients of family practitioners, health clinics, etc.

b) When a person with a known disease or injury, whether it is current or resolving, encounters the health care system for a specific treatment of that disease or injury (e.g., dialysis for renal disease; chemotherapy for malignancy; cast change).

c) When some circumstance or problem is present which influences the person's health status but is not in itself a current illness or injury. Such factors may be elicited during population surveys, when the person may or may not be currently sick, or be recorded as an additional factor to be borne in mind when the person is receiving care for some current illness or injury classifiable to categories 001-999.

In the latter circumstances the V code should be used only as a supplementary code and should not be the one selected for use in primary, single cause tabulations. Examples of these circumstances are a personal history of certain diseases, or a person with an artificial heart valve in situ.

PERSONS WITH POTENTIAL HEALTH HAZARDS RELATED TO COMMUNICABLE DISEASES (V01-V06)

> Excludes: family history of infectious and parasitic diseases (V18.8)
> personal history of infectious and parasitic diseases (V12.0)

V01 Contact with or exposure to communicable diseases

V01.0 Cholera
Conditions classifiable to 001

V01.1 Tuberculosis
Conditions classifiable to 010-018

V01.2 Poliomyelitis
Conditions classifiable to 045

V01.3 Smallpox
Conditions classifiable to 050

V01.4 Rubella
Conditions classifiable to 056

V01.5 Rabies
Conditions classifiable to 071

V01.6 Venereal diseases
Conditions classifiable to 090-099

⑤ V01.7 Other viral diseases
Conditions classifiable to 042-078 and V08, except as above

V01.71 Varicella
V01.79 Other viral diseases

⑤ V01.8 Other communicable diseases
Conditions classifiable to 001-136, except as above

V01.81 Anthrax
V01.82 Exposure to SARS-associated coronavirus
V01.83 Escherichia coli (E. coli)
V01.84 Meningococcus
V01.89 Other communicable diseases

V01.9 Unspecified communicable disease

V02 Carrier or suspected carrier of infectious diseases
Includes: Colonization status

V02.0 Cholera
V02.1 Typhoid
V02.2 Amebiasis
V02.3 Other gastrointestinal pathogens
V02.4 Diphtheria

Add 4th or 5th digit	Nonspecific code	Unspecific code	Secondary Dx Only	Primary Dx Only

⑤ **V02.5** Other specified bacterial diseases

    V02.51 Group B streptococcus

    V02.52 Other streptococcus

    V02.53 Methicillin susceptible Staphylococcus aureus
        MSSA colonization

    V02.54 Methicillin resistant Staphylococcus aureus
        MRSA colonization

    V02.59 Other specified bacterial diseases
        Meningococcal
        Staphylococcal

⑤ **V02.6** Viral hepatitis
    Hepatitis Australian-antigen [HAA] [SH] carrier
    Serum hepatitis carrier

    V02.60 Viral hepatitis carrier, unspecified

    V02.61 Hepatitis B carrier

    V02.62 Hepatitis C carrier

    V02.69 Other viral hepatitis carrier

V02.7 Gonorrhea

V02.8 Other venereal diseases

V02.9 Other specified infectious organism

V03 Need for prophylactic vaccination and inoculation against bacterial diseases

    Excludes: vaccination not carried out (V64.00-V64.09)
        vaccines against combinations of diseases (V06.0-V06.9)

V03.0 Cholera alone

V03.1 Typhoid-paratyphoid alone [TAB]

V03.2 Tuberculosis [BCG]

V03.3 Plague

V03.4 Tularemia

V03.5 Diphtheria alone

V03.6 Pertussis alone

V03.7 Tetanus toxoid alone

⑤ **V03.8** Other specified vaccinations against single bacterial diseases

    V03.81 Hemophilus influenza, type B [Hib]

    V03.82 Streptococcus pneumoniae [pneumococcus]

    V03.89 Other specified vaccination

V03.9 Unspecified single bacterial disease

V04 Need for prophylactic vaccination and inoculation against certain viral diseases

    Excludes: vaccines against combinations of diseases (V06.0-V06.9)

V04.0 Poliomyelitis

V04.1 Smallpox

V04.2 Measles alone

V04.3 Rubella alone

V04.4 Yellow fever

V04.5 Rabies

V04.6 Mumps alone

V04.7 Common cold

⑤ **V04.8** Other viral diseases

    V04.81 Influenza

    V04.82 Respiratory syncytial virus (RSV)

    V04.89 Other viral diseases

V05 Need for other prophylactic vaccination and inoculation against single diseases

    Excludes: vaccines against combinations of diseases (V06.0-V06.9)

V05.0 Arthropod-borne viral encephalitis

V05.1 Other arthropod-borne viral diseases

● Code new to this edition   ▲ Revision of existing code   ④ ⑤ Fourth or fifth digit required

V05.2 Leishmaniasis

V05.3 Viral hepatitis

V05.4 Varicella
Chickenpox

V05.8 Other specified disease

V05.9 Unspecified single disease

V06 Need for prophylactic vaccination and inoculation against combinations of diseases
Note: Use additional single vaccination codes from categories V03-V05 to identify any vaccinations not included in a combination code.

V06.0 Cholera with typhoid-paratyphoid [cholera + TAB]

V06.1 Diphtheria-tetanus-pertussis, combined [DTP] [DTaP]

V06.2 Diphtheria-tetanus-pertussis with typhoid-paratyphoid [DTP + TAB]

V06.3 Diphtheria-tetanus-pertussis with poliomyelitis [DTP + polio]

V06.4 Measles-mumps-rubella [MMR]

V06.5 Tetanus-diphtheria [Td] [DT]

V06.6 Streptococcus pneumoniae [pneumococcus] and influenza

V06.8 Other combinations
Excludes: multiple single vaccination codes (V03.0-V05.9)

V06.9 Unspecified combined vaccine

PERSONS WITH NEED FOR ISOLATION, OTHER POTENTIAL HEALTH HAZARDS AND PROPHYLACTIC MEASURES (V07-V09)

V07 Need for isolation and other prophylactic measures
Excludes: prophylactic organ removal (V50.41-V50.49)

V07.0 Isolation
Admission to protect the individual from his surroundings or for isolation of individual after contact with infectious diseases

V07.1 Desensitization to allergens

V07.2 Prophylactic immunotherapy
Administration of:
antivenin
immune sera [gamma globulin]
RhoGAM
tetanus antitoxin

⑤ V07.3 Other prophylactic chemotherapy

V07.31 Prophylactic fluoride administration

V07.39 Other prophylactic chemotherapy
Excludes: maintenance chemotherapy following disease (V58.11)

V07.4 Hormone replacement therapy (postmenopausal)

⑤ V07.5 Prophylactic use of agents affecting estrogen receptors and estrogen levels
Code first, if applicable:
malignant neoplasm of breast (174.0-174.9, 175.0-175.9)
malignant neoplasm of prostate (185)

Use additional code, if applicable, to identify:
estrogen receptor positive status (V86.0)
family history of breast cancer (V16.3)
genetic susceptibility to cancer (V84.01-V84.09)
personal history of breast cancer (V10.3)
personal history of prostate cancer (V10.46)
postmenopausal status (V49.81)

Excludes: hormone replacement therapy (postmenopausal) (V07.4)

V07.51 Prophylactic use of selective estrogen receptor modulators (SERMs)
Prophylactic use of:
raloxifene (Evista)
tamoxifen (Nolvadex)
toremifene (Fareston)

■ Add 4th or 5th digit	■ Nonspecific code	■ Unspecific code	■ Secondary Dx Only	■ Primary Dx Only

V07.52 **Prophylactic use of aromatase inhibitors**
Prophylactic use of:
anastrozole (Arimidex)
exemestane (Aromasin)
letrozole (Femara)

V07.59 **Prophylactic use of other agents affecting estrogen receptors and estrogen levels**
Prophylactic use of:
estrogen receptor downregulators
fulvestrant (Faslodex)
gonadotropin-releasing hormone (GnRH) agonist
goserelin acetate (Zoladex)
leuprolide acetate (leuprorelin) (Lupron)
megestrol acetate (Megace)

V07.8 **Other specified prophylactic measure**

V07.9 **Unspecified prophylactic measure**

V08 Asymptomatic human immunodeficiency virus [HIV] infection status
HIV positive NOS

Note: This code is ONLY to be used when NO HIV infection symptoms or conditions are present. If any HIV infection symptoms or conditions are present, see code 042.

Excludes: *AIDS (042)*
human immunodeficiency virus [HIV] disease (042)
exposure to HIV (V01.79)
nonspecific serologic evidence of HIV (795.71)
symptomatic human immunodeficiency virus [HIV] infection (042)

V09 Infection with drug-resistant microorganisms

Note: This category is intended for use as an additional code for infectious conditions classified elsewhere to indicate the presence of drug-resistance of the infectious organism.

V09.0 **Infection with microorganisms resistant to penicillins**

V09.1 **Infection with microorganisms resistant to cephalosporins and other B-lactam antibiotics**

V09.2 **Infection with microorganisms resistant to macrolides**

V09.3 **Infection with microorganisms resistant to tetracyclines**

V09.4 **Infection with microorganisms resistant to aminoglycosides**

⑤ **V09.5 Infection with microorganisms resistant to quinolones and fluoroquinolones**

V09.50 **Without mention of resistance to multiple quinolones and fluoroquinolones**

V09.51 **With resistance to multiple quinolones and fluoroquinolones**

V09.6 **Infection with microorganisms resistant to sulfonamides**

⑤ **V09.7 Infection with microorganisms resistant to other specified antimycobacterial agents**

Excludes: *Amikacin (V09.4)*
Kanamycin (V09.4)
Streptomycin [SM] (V09.4)

V09.70 **Without mention of resistance to multiple antimycobacterial agents**

V09.71 **With resistance to multiple antimycobacterial agents**

⑤ **V09.8 Infection with microorganisms resistant to other specified drugs**
Vancomycin (glycopeptide) intermediate staphylococcus aureus (VISA/GISA)
Vancomycin (glycopeptide) resistant enterococcus (VRE)
Vancomycin (glycopeptide) resistant staphylococcus aureus (VRSA/GRSA)

V09.80 **Without mention of resistance to multiple drugs**

V09.81 **With resistance to multiple drugs**

⑤ **V09.9 Infection with drug-resistant microorganisms, unspecified**
Drug resistance NOS

V09.90 **Without mention of multiple drug resistance**

V09.91 **With multiple drug resistance**
Multiple drug resistance NOS

● Code new to this edition   ▲ Revision of existing code   ④ ⑤ Fourth or fifth digit required

PERSONS WITH POTENTIAL HEALTH HAZARDS RELATED TO PERSONAL AND FAMILY HISTORY (V10-V19)

> *Excludes:* *obstetric patients where the possibility that the fetus might be affected is the reason for observation or management during pregnancy (655.0-655.9)*

V10 **Personal history of malignant neoplasm**

⑤ **V10.0 Gastrointestinal tract**
History of conditions classifiable to 140-159

> *Excludes:* *personal history of malignant carcinoid tumor (V10.91)*
> *personal history of malignant neuroendocrine tumor (V10.91)*

   V10.00 Gastrointestinal tract, unspecified

   V10.01 Tongue

   V10.02 Other and unspecified oral cavity and pharynx

   V10.03 Esophagus

   V10.04 Stomach

   V10.05 Large intestine

   V10.06 Rectum, rectosigmoid junction, and anus

   V10.07 Liver

   V10.09 Other

⑤ **V10.1 Trachea, bronchus, and lung**
History of conditions classifiable to 162

> *Excludes:* *personal history of malignant carcinoid tumor (V10.91)*
> *personal history of malignant neuroendocrine tumor (V10.91)*

   V10.11 Bronchus and lung

   V10.12 Trachea

⑤ **V10.2 Other respiratory and intrathoracic organs**
History of conditions classifiable to 160, 161, 163-165

   V10.20 Respiratory organ, unspecified

   V10.21 Larynx

   V10.22 Nasal cavities, middle ear, and accessory sinuses

   V10.29 Other

V10.3 Breast
History of conditions classifiable to 174 and 175

⑤ **V10.4 Genital organs**
History of conditions classifiable to 179-187

   V10.40 Female genital organ, unspecified

   V10.41 Cervix uteri

   V10.42 Other parts of uterus

   V10.43 Ovary

   V10.44 Other female genital organs

   V10.45 Male genital organ, unspecified

   V10.46 Prostate

   V10.47 Testis

   V10.48 Epididymis

   V10.49 Other male genital organs

⑤ **V10.5 Urinary organs**
History of conditions classifiable to 188 and 189

   V10.50 Urinary organ, unspecified

   V10.51 Bladder

   V10.52 Kidney

> *Excludes:* *renal pelvis (V10.53)*

   V10.53 Renal pelvis

   V10.59 Other

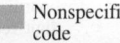

| | Add 4th or 5th digit | | Nonspecific code | | Unspecific code | | Secondary Dx Only | | Primary Dx Only |

⑤ **V10.6 Leukemia**
Conditions classifiable to 204-208

Excludes: *leukemia in remission (204-208)*

V10.60 Leukemia, unspecified

V10.61 **Lymphoid leukemia**

V10.62 **Myeloid leukemia**

V10.63 **Monocytic leukemia**

V10.69 Other

⑤ **V10.7 Other lymphatic and hematopoietic neoplasms**
Conditions classifiable to 200-203

Excludes: *listed conditions in 200-203 in remission*

V10.71 **Lymphosarcoma and reticulosarcoma**

V10.72 **Hodgkin's disease**

V10.79 Other

⑤ **V10.8 Personal history of malignant neoplasm of other sites**
History of conditions classifiable to 170-173, 190-195

Excludes: *personal history of malignant carcinoid tumor (V10.91)*
personal history of malignant neuroendocrine tumor (V10.91)

V10.81 **Bone**

V10.82 **Malignant melanoma of skin**

V10.83 Other malignant neoplasm of skin

V10.84 **Eye**

V10.85 **Brain**

V10.86 Other parts of nervous system

Excludes: *peripheral, sympathetic, and parasympathetic nerves (V10.89)*

V10.87 **Thyroid**

V10.88 Other endocrine glands and related structures

V10.89 Other

▲ **V10.9 Other and unspecified personal history of malignant neoplasm**

● **V10.90 Personal history of unspecified malignant neoplasm**
Personal history of malignant neoplasm NOS

Excludes: *personal history of malignant carcinoid tumor (V10.91)*
personal history of malignant neuroendocrine tumor (V10.91)
personal history of Merkel cell carcinoma (V10.91)

● **V10.91 Personal history of malignant neuroendocrine tumor**
Personal history of malignant carcinoid tumor NOS
Personal history of malignant neuroendocrine tumor NOS
Personal history of Merkel cell carcinoma NOS

Code first any continuing functional activity, such as: carcinoid syndrome (259.2)

V11 Personal history of mental disorder

V11.0 Schizophrenia

Excludes: *that in remission (295.0-295.9 with fifth-digit 5)*

V11.1 Affective disorders
Personal history of manic-depressive psychosis

Excludes: *that in remission (296.0-296.6 with fifth-digit 5, 6)*

V11.2 Neurosis

V11.3 Alcoholism

V11.8 Other mental disorders

V11.9 Unspecified mental disorder

V12 Personal history of certain other diseases

⑤ **V12.0 Infectious and parasitic diseases**

Excludes: *personal history of infectious diseases specific to a body system*

V12.00 Unspecified infectious and parasitic disease

V12.01 **Tuberculosis**

● Code new
to this edition

▲ Revision of
existing code

④ ⑤ Fourth or fifth
digit required

V12.02 **Poliomyelitis**

V12.03 **Malaria**

V12.04 **Methicillin resistant Staphylococcus aureus**
MRSA

V12.09 **Other**

V12.1 **Nutritional deficiency**

V12.2 **Endocrine, metabolic, and immunity disorders**
Excludes: *history of allergy (V14.0-V14.9, V15.01-V15.09)*

V12.3 **Diseases of blood and blood-forming organs**

⑤ V12.4 **Disorders of nervous system and sense organs**

V12.40 **Unspecified disorder of nervous system and sense organs**

V12.41 **Benign neoplasm of the brain**

V12.42 **Infections of the central nervous system**
Encephalitis
Meningitis

V12.49 **Other disorders of nervous system and sense organs**

⑤ V12.5 **Diseases of circulatory system**
Excludes: *old myocardial infarction (412)*
postmyocardial infarction syndrome (411.0)

V12.50 **Unspecified circulatory disease**

V12.51 **Venous thrombosis and embolism**
Pulmonary embolism

V12.52 **Thrombophlebitis**

V12.53 **Sudden cardiac arrest**
Sudden cardiac death successfully resuscitated

V12.54 **Transient ischemic attack (TIA), and cerebral infarction without residual deficits**
Prolonged reversible ischemic neurological deficit (PRIND)
Reversible ischemic neurologic deficit (RIND)
Stroke NOS without residual deficits

Excludes: *history of traumatic brain injury (V15.52)*
late effects of cerebrovascular disease (438.0-438.9)

V12.59 **Other**
Note: Assign code V12.59 (and not a code from category 438) as an additional code for history of cerebrovascular disease when no neurologic deficits are present.

⑤ V12.6 **Diseases of respiratory system**
Excludes: *tuberculosis (V12.01)*

V12.60 **Unspecified disease of respiratory system**

V12.61 **Pneumonia (recurrent)**

V12.69 **Other diseases of respiratory system**

⑤ V12.7 **Diseases of digestive system**

V12.70 **Unspecified digestive disease**

V12.71 **Peptic ulcer disease**

V12.72 **Colonic polyps**

V12.79 **Other**

V13 **Personal history of other diseases**

⑤ V13.0 **Disorders of urinary system**

V13.00 **Unspecified urinary disorder**

V13.01 **Urinary calculi**

V13.02 **Urinary (tract) infection**

V13.03 **Nephrotic syndrome**

V13.09 **Other**

V13.1 **Trophoblastic disease**
Excludes: *supervision during a current pregnancy (V23.1)*

| | Add 4th or 5th digit | | Nonspecific code | | Unspecific code | | Secondary Dx Only | | Primary Dx Only |

⑤ **V13.2 Other genital system and obstetric disorders**

> *Excludes:* *supervision during a current pregnancy of a woman with poor obstetric history*
> *(V23.0-V23.9)*
> *habitual aborter (646.3)*
> *without current pregnancy (629.81)*

V13.21 Personal history of pre-term labor

> *Excludes:* *current pregnancy with history of pre-term labor (V23.41)*

V13.22 Personal history of cervical dysplasia
  Personal history of conditions classifiable to 622.10-622.12

> *Excludes:* *personal history of malignant neoplasm of cervix uteri (V10.41)*

V13.29 Other genital system and obstetric disorders

V13.3 Diseases of skin and subcutaneous tissue

V13.4 Arthritis

⑤ **V13.5 Other musculoskeletal disorders**

V13.51 Pathologic fracture
  Healed pathologic fracture

> *Excludes:* *personal history of traumatic fracture (V15.51)*

V13.52 Stress fracture
  Healed stress fracture

> *Excludes:* *personal history of traumatic fracture (V15.51)*

V13.59 Other musculoskeletal disorders

⑤ **V13.6 Congenital malformations**

V13.61 Hypospadias

V13.69 Other congenital malformations

V13.7 Perinatal problems

> *Excludes:* *low birth weight status (V21.30-V21.35)*

V13.8 Other specified diseases

V13.9 Unspecified disease

V14 Personal history of allergy to medicinal agents

V14.0 Penicillin

V14.1 Other antibiotic agent

V14.2 Sulfonamides

V14.3 Other anti-infective agent

V14.4 Anesthetic agent

V14.5 Narcotic agent

V14.6 Analgesic agent

V14.7 Serum or vaccine

V14.8 Other specified medicinal agents

V14.9 Unspecified medicinal agent

V15 Other personal history presenting hazards to health

> *Excludes:* *personal history of drug therapy (V87.41-V87.49)*

⑤ **V15.0 Allergy, other than to medicinal agents**

> *Excludes:* *allergy to food substance used as base for medicinal agent (V14.0-V14.9)*

V15.01 Allergy to peanuts

V15.02 Allergy to milk products

> *Excludes:* *lactose intolerance (271.3)*

V15.03 Allergy to eggs

V15.04 Allergy to seafood
  Seafood (octopus) (squid) ink
  Shellfish

V15.05 Allergy to other foods
  Food additives
  Nuts other than peanuts

● Code new to this edition   ▲ Revision of existing code   ④ ⑤ Fourth or fifth digit required

▲ **V15.06** **Allergy to insects and arachnids**
Bugs
Insect bites and stings
Spiders

V15.07 **Allergy to latex**
Latex sensitivity

V15.08 **Allergy to radiographic dye**
Contrast media used for diagnostic x-ray procedures

V15.09 **Other allergy, other than to medicinal agents**

V15.1 **Surgery to heart and great vessels**

Excludes: *replacement by transplant or other means (V42.1-V42.2, V43.2-V43.4)*

⑤ **V15.2** **Surgery to other organs**

Excludes: *replacement by transplant or other means (V42.0-V43.8)*

V15.21 **Personal history of undergoing in utero procedure during pregnancy**

V15.22 **Personal history of undergoing in utero procedure while a fetus**

V15.29 **Surgery to other organs**

V15.3 **Irradiation**
Previous exposure to therapeutic or other ionizing radiation

⑤ **V15.4** **Psychological trauma**

Excludes: *history of condition classifiable to 290-316 (V11.0-V11.9)*

V15.41 **History of physical abuse**
Rape

V15.42 **History of emotional abuse**
Neglect

V15.49 **Other**

⑤ **V15.5** **Injury**

V15.51 **Traumatic fracture**
Healed traumatic fracture

Excludes: *personal history of pathologic and stress fracture (V13.51, V13.52)*

● **V15.52** **History of traumatic brain injury**

Excludes: *personal history of cerebrovascular accident (cerebral infarction) without residual deficits (V12.54)*

V15.59 **Other injury**

V15.6 **Poisoning**

V15.7 **Contraception**

Excludes: *current contraceptive management (V25.0-V25.4)*
presence of intrauterine contraceptive device as incidental finding (V45.5)

⑤ **V15.8** **Other specified personal history presenting hazards to health**

Excludes: *contact with and (suspected) exposure to:*
aromatic compounds and dyes (V87.11-V87.19)
arsenic and other metals (V87.01-V87.09)
molds (V87.31)

● **V15.80** **History of failed moderate sedation**
History of failed conscious sedation

V15.81 **Noncompliance with medical treatment**

Excludes: *noncompliance with renal dialysis (V45.12)*

V15.82 **History of tobacco use**

Excludes: *tobacco dependence (305.1)*

● **V15.83** **Underimmunization status**
Delinquent immunization status
Lapsed immunization schedule status

▲ **V15.84** **Contact with and (suspected) exposure to asbestos**

▲ **V15.85** **Contact with and (suspected) exposure to potentially hazardous body fluids**

▲ **V15.86** **Contact with and (suspected) exposure to lead**

V15.87 **History of extracorporeal membrane oxygenation [ECMO]**

| | Add 4th or 5th digit | | Nonspecific code | | Unspecific code | | Secondary Dx Only | | Primary Dx Only |

V15.88 History of fall
At risk for falling

V15.89 Other

Excludes: contact with and (suspected) exposure to other potentially hazardous chemicals
(V87.2)
contact with and (suspected) exposure to other potentially hazardous substances
(V87.39)

V15.9 Unspecified personal history presenting hazards to health

V16 Family history of malignant neoplasm

V16.0 Gastrointestinal tract
Family history of condition classifiable to 140-159

V16.1 Trachea, bronchus, and lung
Family history of condition classifiable to 162

V16.2 Other respiratory and intrathoracic organs
Family history of condition classifiable to 160-161, 163-165

V16.3 Breast
Family history of condition classifiable to 174

⑤ **V16.4 Genital organs**
Family history of condition classifiable to 179-187

V16.40 Genital organ, unspecified

V16.41 Ovary

V16.42 Prostate

V16.43 Testis

V16.49 Other

⑤ **V16.5 Urinary organs**
Family history of condition classifiable to 188-189

V16.51 Kidney

V16.52 Bladder

V16.59 Other

V16.6 Leukemia
Family history of condition classifiable to 204-208

V16.7 Other lymphatic and hematopoietic neoplasms
Family history of condition classifiable to 200-203

V16.8 Other specified malignant neoplasm
Family history of other condition classifiable to 140-199

V16.9 Unspecified malignant neoplasm

V17 Family history of certain chronic disabling diseases

V17.0 Psychiatric condition

Excludes: family history of mental retardation (V18.4)

V17.1 Stroke (cerebrovascular)

V17.2 Other neurological diseases
Epilepsy
Huntington's chorea

V17.3 Ischemic heart disease

⑤ **V17.4 Other cardiovascular diseases**

V17.41 Family history of sudden cardiac death (SCD)

Excludes: family history of ischemic heart disease (V17.3)
family history of myocardial infarction (V17.3)

V17.49 Family history of other cardiovascular diseases
Family history of cardiovascular disease NOS

V17.5 Asthma

V17.6 Other chronic respiratory conditions

V17.7 Arthritis

⑤ **V17.8 Other musculoskeletal diseases**

V17.81 Osteoporosis

V17.89 Other musculoskeletal diseases

● Code new
  to this edition

▲ Revision of
  existing code

④ ⑤ Fourth or fifth
  digit required

V18 Family history of certain other specific conditions

    V18.0 Diabetes mellitus

⑤ V18.1 Other endocrine and metabolic diseases

        V18.11 Multiple endocrine neoplasia [MEN] syndrome

        V18.19 Other endocrine and metabolic diseases

    V18.2 Anemia

    V18.3 Other blood disorders

    V18.4 Mental retardation

⑤ V18.5 Digestive disorders

        V18.51 Colonic polyps

        Excludes: *family history of malignant neoplasm of gastrointestinal tract (V16.0)*

        V18.59 Other digestive disorders

⑤ V18.6 Kidney diseases

        V18.61 Polycystic kidney

        V18.69 Other kidney diseases

    V18.7 Other genitourinary diseases

    V18.8 Infectious and parasitic diseases

    V18.9 Genetic disease carrier

V19 Family history of other conditions

    V19.0 Blindness or visual loss

    V19.1 Other eye disorders

    V19.2 Deafness or hearing loss

    V19.3 Other ear disorders

    V19.4 Skin conditions

    V19.5 Congenital anomalies

    V19.6 Allergic disorders

    V19.7 Consanguinity

    V19.8 Other condition

PERSONS ENCOUNTERING HEALTH SERVICES IN CIRCUMSTANCES RELATED TO REPRODUCTION AND DEVELOPMENT (V20-V29)

V20 Health supervision of infant or child

    V20.0 Foundling

    V20.1 Other healthy infant or child receiving care
        Medical or nursing care supervision of healthy infant in cases of:
            maternal illness, physical or psychiatric
            socioeconomic adverse condition at home
            too many children at home preventing or interfering with normal care

    V20.2 Routine infant or child health check
        Developmental testing of infant or child
        Health check for child over 28 days old
        Immunizations appropriate for age
        Routine vision and hearing testing

        Excludes: *health check for child under 29 days old (V20.31-V20.32)*
            newborn health supervision (V20.31-V20.32)
            special screening for developmental handicaps (V79.3)

    Use additional code(s) to identify:
        Special screening examination(s) performed (V73.0-V82.9)

● **V20.3** Newborn health supervision
        Health check for child under 29 days old

        Excludes: *health check for child over 28 days old (V20.2)*

    ● **V20.31** Health supervision for newborn under 8 days old
        Health check for newborn under 8 days old

    ● **V20.32** Health supervision for newborn 8 to 28 days old
        Health check for newborn 8 to 28 days old
        Newborn weight check

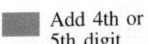 Add 4th or 5th digit
 Nonspecific code
 Unspecific code
 Secondary Dx Only
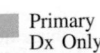 Primary Dx Only

V21 Constitutional states in development

 V21.0 Period of rapid growth in childhood

 V21.1 Puberty

 V21.2 Other adolescence

⑤ **V21.3** Low birth weight status

 Excludes: *history of perinatal problems (V13.7)*

 V21.30 Low birth weight status, unspecified

 V21.31 Low birth weight status, less than 500 grams

 V21.32 Low birth weight status, 500-999 grams

 V21.33 Low birth weight status, 1000-1499 grams

 V21.34 Low birth weight status, 1500-1999 grams

 V21.35 Low birth weight status, 2000-2500 grams

 V21.8 Other specified constitutional states in development

 V21.9 Unspecified constitutional state in development

V22 Normal pregnancy

 Excludes: *pregnancy examination or test, pregnancy unconfirmed (V72.40)*

 V22.0 Supervision of normal first pregnancy

 V22.1 Supervision of other normal pregnancy

 V22.2 Pregnant state, incidental
  Pregnant state NOS

V23 Supervision of high-risk pregnancy

 V23.0 Pregnancy with history of infertility

 V23.1 Pregnancy with history of trophoblastic disease
  Pregnancy with history of:
   hydatidiform mole
   vesicular mole

 Excludes: *that without current pregnancy (V13.1)*

 V23.2 Pregnancy with history of abortion
  Pregnancy with history of conditions classifiable to 634-638

 Excludes: *habitual aborter:*
   care during pregnancy (646.3)
   that without current pregnancy (629.81)

 V23.3 Grand multiparity

 Excludes: *care in relation to labor and delivery (659.4)*
   that without current pregnancy (V61.5)

⑤ **V23.4** Pregnancy with other poor obstetric history
  Pregnancy with history of other conditions classifiable to 630-676

 V23.41 Pregnancy with history of pre-term labor

 V23.49 Pregnancy with other poor obstetric history

 V23.5 Pregnancy with other poor reproductive history
  Pregnancy with history of stillbirth or neonatal death

 V23.7 Insufficient prenatal care
  History of little or no prenatal care

⑤ **V23.8** Other high-risk pregnancy

 V23.81 Elderly primigravida
   First pregnancy in a woman who will be 35 years of age or older at expected date of delivery

 Excludes: *elderly primigravida complicating pregnancy (659.5)*

 V23.82 Elderly multigravida
   Second or more pregnancy in a woman who will be 35 years of age or older at expected date of delivery

 Excludes: *elderly multigravida complicating pregnancy (659.6)*

 V23.83 Young primigravida
   First pregnancy in a female less than 16 years old at expected date of delivery

 Excludes: *young primigravida complicating pregnancy (659.8)*

● Code new to this edition ▲ Revision of existing code ④ ⑤ Fourth or fifth digit required

V23.84 Young multigravida
Second or more pregnancy in a female less than 16 years old at expected date of delivery

Excludes: *young multigravida complicating pregnancy (659.8)*

V23.85 Pregnancy resulting from assisted reproductive technology
Pregnancy resulting from in vitro fertilization

V23.86 Pregnancy with history of in utero procedure during previous pregnancy

Excludes: *management of pregnancy affected by in utero procedure during current pregnancy (679.0-679.1)*

V23.89 Other high-risk pregnancy

V23.9 Unspecified high-risk pregnancy

V24 Postpartum care and examination

V24.0 Immediately after delivery
Care and observation in uncomplicated cases

V24.1 Lactating mother
Supervision of lactation

V24.2 Routine postpartum follow-up

V25 Encounter for contraceptive management

⑤ **V25.0 General counseling and advice**

V25.01 Prescription of oral contraceptives

V25.02 Initiation of other contraceptive measures
Fitting of diaphragm
Prescription of foams, creams, or other agents

V25.03 Encounter for emergency contraceptive counseling and prescription
Encounter for postcoital contraceptive counseling and prescription

V25.04 Counseling and instruction in natural family planning to avoid pregnancy

V25.09 Other
Family planning advice

V25.1 Insertion of intrauterine contraceptive device

V25.2 Sterilization
Admission for interruption of fallopian tubes or vas deferens

V25.3 Menstrual extraction
Menstrual regulation

⑤ **V25.4 Surveillance of previously prescribed contraceptive methods**
Checking, reinsertion, or removal of contraceptive device
Repeat prescription for contraceptive method
Routine examination in connection with contraceptive maintenance

Excludes: *presence of intrauterine contraceptive device as incidental finding (V45.5)*

V25.40 Contraceptive surveillance, unspecified

V25.41 Contraceptive pill

V25.42 Intrauterine contraceptive device
Checking, reinsertion, or removal of intrauterine device

V25.43 Implantable subdermal contraceptive

V25.49 Other contraceptive method

V25.5 Insertion of implantable subdermal contraceptive

V25.8 Other specified contraceptive management
Postvasectomy sperm count

Excludes: *sperm count following sterilization reversal (V26.22)*
sperm count for fertility testing (V26.21)

V25.9 Unspecified contraceptive management

V26 Procreative management

V26.0 Tuboplasty or vasoplasty after previous sterilization

V26.1 Artificial insemination

⑤ **V26.2 Investigation and testing**

Excludes: *postvasectomy sperm count (V25.8)*

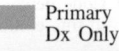

■ Add 4th or   ■ Nonspecific   □ Unspecific   ■ Secondary   ■ Primary
5th digit   code   code   Dx Only   Dx Only

V26.21 Fertility testing
　　Fallopian insufflation
　　Sperm count for fertility testing

Excludes: genetic counseling and testing (V26.31-V26.39)

V26.22 Aftercare following sterilization reversal
　　Fallopian insufflation following sterilization reversal
　　Sperm count following sterilization reversal

V26.29 Other investigation and testing

⑤ **V26.3 Genetic counseling and testing**

Excludes: fertility testing (V26.21)
　　　　nonprocreative genetic screening (V82.71, V82.79)

V26.31 Testing of female for genetic disease carrier status

V26.32 Other genetic testing of female
Use additional code to identify habitual aborter (629.81, 646.3)

V26.33 Genetic counseling

V26.34 Testing of male for genetic disease carrier status

V26.35 Encounter for testing of male partner of habitual aborter

V26.39 Other genetic testing of male

⑤ **V26.4 General counseling and advice**

V26.41 Procreative counseling and advice using natural family planning

● **V26.42 Encounter for fertility preservation counseling**
　　Encounter for fertility preservation counseling prior to cancer therapy
　　Encounter for fertility preservation counseling prior to surgical removal of gonads

V26.49 Other procreative management counseling and advice

⑤ **V26.5 Sterilization status**

V26.51 Tubal ligation status

Excludes: infertility not due to previous tubal ligation (628.0-628.9)

V26.52 Vasectomy status

⑤ **V26.8 Other specified procreative management**

V26.81 Encounter for assisted reproductive fertility procedure cycle
　　Patient undergoing in vitro fertilization cycle
Use additional code to identify the type of infertility

Excludes: pre-cycle diagnosis and testing – code to reason for encounter

● **V26.82 Encounter for fertility preservation procedure**
　　Encounter for fertility preservation procedure prior to cancer therapy
　　Encounter for fertility preservation procedure prior to surgical removal of gonads

V26.89 Other specified procreative management

V26.9 Unspecified procreative management

V27 Outcome of delivery
Note: This category is intended for the coding of the outcome of delivery on the mother's record.

V27.0 Single liveborn

V27.1 Single stillborn

V27.2 Twins, both liveborn

V27.3 Twins, one liveborn and one stillborn

V27.4 Twins, both stillborn

V27.5 Other multiple birth, all liveborn

V27.6 Other multiple birth, some liveborn

V27.7 Other multiple birth, all stillborn

V27.9 Unspecified outcome of delivery
　　Single birth, outcome to infant unspecified
　　Multiple birth, outcome to infant unspecified

V28 Encounter for antenatal screening of mother

> Excludes: *abnormal findings on screening—code to findings*
> *routine prenatal care (V22.0-V23.9)*
> *suspected fetal conditions affecting management of pregnancy (655.00-655.93, 656.00-656.93, 657.00-657.03, 658.00 -658.93)*
> *suspected fetal conditions not found (V89.01-V89.09)*

V28.0 Screening for chromosomal anomalies by amniocentesis

V28.1 Screening for raised alpha-fetoprotein levels in amniotic fluid

V28.2 Other screening based on amniocentesis

V28.3 Encounter for routine screening for malformation using ultrasonics
Encounter for routine fetal ultrasound NOS

> Excludes: *encounter for feal anatomic survey (V28.81)*
> *genetic counseling and testing (V26.31-V26.39)*

V28.4 Screening for fetal growth retardation using ultrasonics

V28.5 Screening for isoimmunization

V28.6 Screening for Streptococcus B

⑤ V28.8 Other specified antenatal screening

    V28.81 Encounter for fetal anatomic survey

    V28.82 Encounter for screening for risk of pre-term labor

    V28.89 Other specified antenatal screening
        Chorionic villus sampling
        Genomic screening
        Nuchal translucency testing
        Proteomic screening

V28.9 Unspecified antenatal screening

V29 Observation and evaluation of newborns for suspected condition not found

Note: This category is to be used for newborns, within the neonatal period, (the first 28 days of life) who are suspected of having an abnormal condition resulting from exposure from the mother or the birth process, but without signs or symptoms, and, which after examination and observation, is found not to exist.

> Excludes: *suspected fetal conditions not found (V89.01-V89.09)*

V29.0 Observation for suspected infectious condition

V29.1 Observation for suspected neurological condition

V29.2 Observation for suspected respiratory condition

V29.3 Observation for suspected genetic or metabolic condition

V29.8 Observation for other specified suspected condition

V29.9 Observation for unspecified suspected condition

LIVEBORN INFANTS ACCORDING TO TYPE OF BIRTH (V30-V39)

Note: These categories are intended for the coding of liveborn infants who are consuming health care [e.g., crib or bassinet occupancy].

The following fourth-digit subdivisions are for use with categories V30-V39:

⑤ .0 Born in hospital

.1 Born before admission to hospital

.2 Born outside hospital and not hospitalized

The following two fifth-digits are for use with the fourth-digit .0, Born in hospital:

0 delivered without mention of cesarean delivery

1 delivered by cesarean delivery

④ **V30** Single liveborn

④ **V31** Twin, mate liveborn

④ **V32** Twin, mate stillborn

④ **V33** Twin, unspecified

④ **V34** Other multiple, mates all liveborn

④ **V35** Other multiple, mates all stillborn

④ **V36** Other multiple, mates live- and stillborn

④ **V37** Other multiple, unspecified

④ **V39** Unspecified

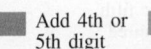

| | Add 4th or 5th digit | | Nonspecific code | | Unspecific code | | Secondary Dx Only | | Primary Dx Only |

PERSONS WITH A CONDITION INFLUENCING THEIR HEALTH STATUS (V40-V49)

Note: These categories are intended for use when these conditions are recorded as "diagnoses" or "problems."

V40 Mental and behavioral problems

V40.0 Problems with learning

V40.1 Problems with communication [including speech]

V40.2 Other mental problems

V40.3 Other behavioral problems

V40.9 Unspecified mental or behavioral problem

V41 Problems with special senses and other special functions

V41.0 Problems with sight

V41.1 Other eye problems

V41.2 Problems with hearing

V41.3 Other ear problems

V41.4 Problems with voice production

V41.5 Problems with smell and taste

V41.6 Problems with swallowing and mastication

V41.7 Problems with sexual function

Excludes: marital problems (V61.10)
psychosexual disorders (302.0-302.9)

V41.8 Other problems with special functions

V41.9 Unspecified problem with special function

V42 Organ or tissue replaced by transplant
Includes: homologous or heterologous (animal) (human) transplant organ status

V42.0 Kidney

V42.1 Heart

V42.2 Heart valve

V42.3 Skin

V42.4 Bone

V42.5 Cornea

V42.6 Lung

V42.7 Liver

⑤ **V42.8 Other specified organ or tissue**

V42.81 Bone marrow

V42.82 Peripheral stem cells

V42.83 Pancreas

V42.84 Intestines

V42.89 Other

V42.9 Unspecified organ or tissue

V43 Organ or tissue replaced by other means
Includes: organ or tissue assisted by other means
replacement of organ by:
artificial device
mechanical device
prosthesis

Excludes: cardiac pacemaker in situ (V45.01)
fitting and adjustment of prosthetic device (V52.0-V52.9)
renal dialysis status (V45.11)

V43.0 Eye globe

V43.1 Lens
Pseudophakos

⑤ **V43.2 Heart**

V43.21 Heart assist device

V43.22 Fully implantable artificial heart

V43.3 Heart valve

● Code new
to this edition

▲ Revision of
existing code

④ ⑤ Fourth or fifth
digit required

V43.4 Blood vessel

V43.5 Bladder

⑤ **V43.6** Joint

    V43.60 Unspecified joint

    V43.61 Shoulder

    V43.62 Elbow

    V43.63 Wrist

    V43.64 Hip

    V43.65 Knee

    V43.66 Ankle

    V43.69 Other

V43.7 Limb

⑤ **V43.8** Other organ or tissue

    V43.81 Larynx

    V43.82 Breast

    V43.83 Artificial skin

    V43.89 Other

V44 Artificial opening status

    Excludes: *artificial openings requiring attention or management (V55.0-V55.9)*

V44.0 Tracheostomy

V44.1 Gastrostomy

V44.2 Ileostomy

V44.3 Colostomy

V44.4 Other artificial opening of gastrointestinal tract

⑤ **V44.5** Cystostomy

    V44.50 Cystostomy, unspecified

    V44.51 Cutaneous-vesicostomy

    V44.52 Appendico-vesicostomy

    V44.59 Other cystostomy

V44.6 Other artificial opening of urinary tract
    Nephrostomy
    Ureterostomy
    Urethrostomy

V44.7 Artificial vagina

V44.8 Other artificial opening status

V44.9 Unspecified artificial opening status

V45 Other postprocedural states

    Excludes: *aftercare management (V51-V58.9)*
        malfunction or other complication—code to condition

⑤ **V45.0** Cardiac device in situ

    Excludes: *artificial heart (V43.22)*
        heart assist device (V43.21)

    V45.00 Unspecified cardiac device

    V45.01 Cardiac pacemaker

    V45.02 Automatic implantable cardiac defibrillator

    V45.09 Other specified cardiac device
        Carotid sinus pacemaker in situ

⑤ **V45.1** Renal dialysis status

    Excludes: *admission for dialysis treatment, or session (V56.0)*

    V45.11 Renal dialysis status
        Hemodialysis status
        Patient requiring intermittent renal dialysis
        Peritoneal dialysis status
        Presence of arterial-venous shunt (for dialysis)

	Add 4th or 5th digit		Nonspecific code		Unspecific code		Secondary Dx Only		Primary Dx Only

V45.12 Noncompliance with renal dialysis

V45.2 Presence of cerebrospinal fluid drainage device
Cerebral ventricle (communicating) shunt, valve, or device in situ

Excludes: malfunction (996.2)

V45.3 Intestinal bypass or anastomosis status

Excludes: bariatric surgery status (V45.86)
gastric bypass status (V45.86)
obesity surgery status (V45.86)

V45.4 Arthrodesis status

⑤ **V45.5** Presence of contraceptive device

Excludes: checking, reinsertion, or removal of device (V25.42)
complication from device (996.32)
insertion of device (V25.1)

V45.51 Intrauterine contraceptive device

V45.52 Subdermal contraceptive implant

V45.59 Other

⑤ **V45.6** States following surgery of eye and adnexa
Cataract extraction state following eye surgery
Filtering bleb state following eye surgery
Surgical eyelid adhesion state following eye surgery

Excludes: aphakia (379.31)
artificial eye globe (V43.0)

V45.61 Cataract extraction status
Use additional code for associated artificial lens status (V43.1)

V45.69 Other states following surgery of eye and adnexa

⑤ **V45.7** Acquired absence of organ

V45.71 Acquired absence of breast and nipple

Excludes: congenital absence of breast and nipple (757.6)

V45.72 Acquired absence of intestine (large) (small)

V45.73 Acquired absence of kidney

V45.74 Other parts of urinary tract
Bladder

V45.75 Stomach

V45.76 Lung

V45.77 Genital organs

Excludes: acquired absence of cervix and uterus (V88.01-V88.03)
female genital mutilation status (629.20-629.29)

V45.78 Eye

V45.79 Other acquired absence of organ

⑤ **V45.8** Other postprocedural status

V45.81 Aortocoronary bypass status

V45.82 Percutaneous transluminal coronary angioplasty status

V45.83 Breast implant removal status

V45.84 Dental restoration status
Dental crowns status
Dental fillings status

V45.85 Insulin pump status

V45.86 Bariatric surgery status
Gastric banding status
Gastric bypass status for obesity
Obesity surgery status

Excludes: bariatric surgery status complicating pregnancy, childbirth or the puerperium (649.2)
intestinal bypass or anastomosis status (V45.3)

● Code new
to this edition   ▲ Revision of
existing code   ④ ⑤ Fourth or fifth
digit required

V45.87 Transplanted organ removal status
Transplanted organ previously removed due to complication, failure, rejection or infection

Excludes: *encounter for removal of transplanted organ - code to complication of transplanted organ (996.80-996.89)*

V45.88 Status post administration of tPA (rtPA) in a different facility within the last 24 hours prior to admission to current facility
Code first condition requiring tPA administration, such as:
acute cerebral infarction (433.0-433.9 with fifth-digit 1, 434.0-434.9 with fifth digit 1)
acute myocardial infarction (410.00-410.92)

V45.89 Other
Presence of neuropacemaker or other electronic device

Excludes: *artificial heart valve in situ (V43.3)*
vascular prosthesis in situ (V43.4)

V46 Other dependence on machines and devices

V46.0 Aspirator

⑤ **V46.1 Respirator [Ventilator]**
Iron lung

V46.11 Dependence on respirator, status

V46.12 Encounter for respirator dependence during power failure

V46.13 Encounter for weaning from respirator [ventilator]

V46.14 Mechanical complication of respirator [ventilator]
Mechanical failure of respirator [ventilator]

V46.2 Supplemental oxygen
Long-term oxygen therapy

V46.3 Wheelchair dependence
Wheelchair confinement status

Code first cause of dependence, such as:
muscular dystrophy (359.1)
obesity (278.00, 278.01)

V46.8 Other enabling machines
Hyperbaric chamber
Possum [Patient-Operated-Selector-Mechanism]

Excludes: *cardiac pacemaker (V45.0)*
kidney dialysis machine (V45.11)

V46.9 Unspecified machine dependence

V47 Other problems with internal organs

V47.0 Deficiencies of internal organs

V47.1 Mechanical and motor problems with internal organs

V47.2 Other cardiorespiratory problems
Cardiovascular exercise intolerance with pain (with):
at rest
less than ordinary activity
ordinary activity

V47.3 Other digestive problems

V47.4 Other urinary problems

V47.5 Other genital problems

V47.9 Unspecified

V48 Problems with head, neck, and trunk

V48.0 Deficiencies of head

Excludes: *deficiencies of ears, eyelids, and nose (V48.8)*

V48.1 Deficiencies of neck and trunk

V48.2 Mechanical and motor problems with head

V48.3 Mechanical and motor problems with neck and trunk

V48.4 Sensory problem with head

V48.5 Sensory problem with neck and trunk

V48.6 Disfigurements of head

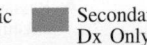

| | Add 4th or 5th digit | | Nonspecific code | | Unspecific code | | Secondary Dx Only | | Primary Dx Only |

V48.7 Disfigurements of neck and trunk

V48.8 Other problems with head, neck, and trunk

V48.9 Unspecified problem with head, neck, or trunk

V49 Other conditions influencing health status

V49.0 Deficiencies of limbs

V49.1 Mechanical problems with limbs

V49.2 Motor problems with limbs

V49.3 Sensory problems with limbs

V49.4 Disfigurements of limbs

V49.5 Other problems of limbs

⑤ V49.6 Upper limb amputation status

    V49.60 Unspecified level

    V49.61 Thumb

    V49.62 Other finger(s)

    V49.63 Hand

    V49.64 Wrist
        Disarticulation of wrist

    V49.65 Below elbow

    V49.66 Above elbow
        Disarticulation of elbow

    V49.67 Shoulder
        Disarticulation of shoulder

⑤ V49.7 Lower limb amputation status

    V49.70 Unspecified level

    V49.71 Great toe

    V49.72 Other toe(s)

    V49.73 Foot

    V49.74 Ankle
        Disarticulation of ankle

    V49.75 Below knee

    V49.76 Above knee
        Disarticulation of knee

    V49.77 Hip
        Disarticulation of hip

⑤ V49.8 Other specified conditions influencing health status

    V49.81 Asymptomatic postmenopausal status (age-related) (natural)

    Excludes: *menopausal and premenopausal disorders (627.0-627.9)*
        postsurgical menopause (256.2)
        premature menopause (256.31)
        symptomatic menopause (627.0-627.9)

    V49.82 Dental sealant status

    V49.83 Awaiting organ transplant status

    V49.84 Bed confinement status

    V49.85 Dual sensory impairment
        Blindness with deafness
        Combined visual hearing impairment

    Code first:
      hearing impairment (389.00-389.9)
      visual impairment (369.00-369.9)

    V49.89 Other specified conditions influencing health status

V49.9 Unspecified

● Code new
  to this edition

▲ Revision of
  existing code

④ ⑤ Fourth or fifth
    digit required

PERSONS ENCOUNTERING HEALTH SERVICES FOR SPECIFIC PROCEDURES AND AFTERCARE (V50-V59)

Note: Categories V51-V58 are intended for use to indicate a reason for care in patients who may have already been treated for some disease or injury not now present, but who are receiving care to consolidate the treatment, to deal with residual states, or to prevent recurrence.

Excludes: follow-up examination for medical surveillance following treatment (V67.0-V67.9)

V50 Elective surgery for purposes other than remedying health states

V50.0 Hair transplant

V50.1 Other plastic surgery for unacceptable cosmetic appearance
Breast augmentation or reduction
Face-lift

Excludes: encounter for breast reduction (611.1)
plastic surgery following healed injury or operation (V51.0-V51.8)

V50.2 Routine or ritual circumcision
Circumcision in the absence of significant medical indication

V50.3 Ear piercing

⑤ V50.4 Prophylactic organ removal

Excludes: organ donations (V59.0-V59.9)
therapeutic organ removal—code to condition

V50.41 Breast

V50.42 Ovary

V50.49 Other

V50.8 Other

V50.9 Unspecified

V51 Aftercare involving the use of plastic surgery
Plastic surgery following healed injury or operation

Excludes: cosmetic plastic surgery (V50.1)
plastic surgery as treatment for current condition or injury—code to condition or injury
repair of scarred tissue—code to scar

V51.0 Encounter for breast reconstruction following mastectomy

Excludes: deformity and disproportion of reconstructed breast (612.0-612.1)

V51.8 Other aftercare involving the use of plastic surgery

V52 Fitting and adjustment of prosthetic device and implant
Includes: removal of device

Excludes: malfunction or complication of prosthetic device (996.0-996.7)
status only, without need for care (V43.0-V43.8)

V52.0 Artificial arm (complete) (partial)

V52.1 Artificial leg (complete) (partial)

V52.2 Artificial eye

V52.3 Dental prosthetic device

V52.4 Breast prosthesis and implant
Elective implant exchange (different material) (different size)
Removal of tissue expander without synchronous insertion of permanent implant

Excludes: admission for initial breast implant insertion for breast augmentation (V50.1)
complications of breast implant (996.54, 996.69, 996.79)
encounter for breast reconstruction following mastectomy (V51.0)

V52.8 Other specified prosthetic device

V52.9 Unspecified prosthetic device

V53 **Fitting and adjustment of other device**
    Includes: removal of device
                replacement of device

    Excludes: *status only, without need for care (V45.0-V45.8)*

⑤ **V53.0** **Devices related to nervous system and special senses**
      V53.01 **Fitting and adjustment of cerebral ventricular (communicating) shunt**
      V53.02 **Neuropacemaker (brain) (peripheral nerve) (spinal cord)**
      V53.09 **Fitting and adjustment of other devices related to nervous system and special senses**
          Auditory substitution device
          Visual substitution device

    V53.1 **Spectacles and contact lenses**
    V53.2 **Hearing aid**
⑤ **V53.3** **Cardiac device**
      Reprogramming
      V53.31 **Cardiac pacemaker**

    Excludes: *mechanical complication of cardiac pacemaker (996.01)*

      V53.32 **Automatic implantable cardiac defibrillator**
      V53.39 **Other cardiac device**
    V53.4 **Orthodontic devices**
▲ **V53.5** **Other gastrointestinal appliance and device**

    Excludes: *colostomy (V55.3)*
          ileostomy (V55.2)
          other artificial opening of digestive tract (V55.4)

    ● **V53.50** **Fitting and adjustment of intestinal appliance and device**
    ● **V53.51** **Fitting and adjustment of gastric lap band**
    ● **V53.59** **Fitting and adjustment of other gastrointestinal appliance and device**
    V53.6 **Urinary devices**
      Urinary catheter

    Excludes: *cystostomy (V55.5)*
          nephrostomy (V55.6)
          ureterostomy (V55.6)
          urethrostomy (V55.6)

    V53.7 **Orthopedic devices**
      Orthopedic: Orthopedic:
        brace   corset
        cast   shoes

    Excludes: *other orthopedic aftercare (V54)*

    V53.8 **Wheelchair**
⑤ **V53.9** **Other and unspecified device**
      V53.90 **Unspecified device**
      V53.91 **Fitting and adjustment of insulin pump**
          Insulin pump titration
      V53.99 **Other device**

V54 **Other orthopedic aftercare**

    Excludes: *fitting and adjustment of orthopedic devices (V53.7)*
          malfunction of internal orthopedic device (996.40-996.49)
          other complication of nonmechanical nature (996.60-996.79)

⑤ **V54.0** **Aftercare involving internal fixation device**

    Excludes: *malfunction of internal orthopedic device (996.40-996.49)*
          removal of external fixation device (V54.89)

      V54.01 **Encounter for removal of internal fixation device**
      V54.02 **Encounter for lengthening/adjustment of growth rod**
      V54.09 **Other aftercare involving internal fixation device**

● Code new to this edition   ▲ Revision of existing code   ④ ⑤ Fourth or fifth digit required

⑤ **V54.1 Aftercare for healing traumatic fracture**

> *Excludes:* *aftercare following joint replacement (V54.81)*
> *aftercare for amputation stump (V54.89)*

    V54.10 Aftercare for healing traumatic fracture of arm, unspecified

    V54.11 Aftercare for healing traumatic fracture of upper arm

    V54.12 Aftercare for healing traumatic fracture of lower arm

    V54.13 Aftercare for healing traumatic fracture of hip

    V54.14 Aftercare for healing traumatic fracture of leg, unspecified

    V54.15 Aftercare for healing traumatic fracture of upper leg

> *Excludes:* *aftercare for healing traumatic fracture of hip (V54.13)*

    V54.16 Aftercare for healing traumatic fracture of lower leg

    V54.17 Aftercare for healing traumatic fracture of vertebrae

    V54.19 Aftercare for healing traumatic fracture of other bone

⑤ **V54.2 Aftercare for healing pathologic fracture**

> *Excludes:* *aftercare following joint replacement (V54.81)*

    V54.20 Aftercare for healing pathologic fracture of arm, unspecified

    V54.21 Aftercare for healing pathologic fracture of upper arm

    V54.22 Aftercare for healing pathologic fracture of lower arm

    V54.23 Aftercare for healing pathologic fracture of hip

    V54.24 Aftercare for healing pathologic fracture of leg, unspecified

    V54.25 Aftercare for healing pathologic fracture of upper leg

> *Excludes:* *aftercare for healing pathologic fracture of hip (V54.23)*

    V54.26 Aftercare for healing pathologic fracture of lower leg

    V54.27 Aftercare for healing pathologic fracture of vertebrae

    V54.29 Aftercare for healing pathologic fracture of other bone

⑤ **V54.8 Other orthopedic aftercare**

    V54.81 Aftercare following joint replacement
    Use additional code to identify joint replacement site (V43.60-V43.69)

    V54.89 Other orthopedic aftercare
    Aftercare for healing fracture NOS

V54.9 Unspecified orthopedic aftercare

V55 Attention to artificial openings
    Includes: adjustment or repositioning of catheter
            closure
            passage of sounds or bougies
            reforming
            removal or replacement of catheter
            toilet or cleansing

> *Excludes:* *complications of external stoma (519.00-519.09, 569.60-569.69, 997.4, 997.5)*
> *status only, without need for care (V44.0-V44.9)*

V55.0 Tracheostomy

V55.1 Gastrostomy

V55.2 Ileostomy

V55.3 Colostomy

V55.4 Other artificial opening of digestive tract

V55.5 Cystostomy

V55.6 Other artificial opening of urinary tract
    Nephrostomy   Urethrostomy
    Ureterostomy

V55.7 Artificial vagina

V55.8 Other specified artificial opening

V55.9 Unspecified artificial opening

V56 Encounter for dialysis and dialysis catheter care
    Use additional code to identify the associated condition

> *Excludes:* *dialysis preparation—code to condition*

■ Add 4th or 5th digit	■ Nonspecific code	□ Unspecific code	■ Secondary Dx Only	■ Primary Dx Only

V56.0 Extracorporeal dialysis
Dialysis (renal) NOS

Excludes: dialysis status (V45.11)

V56.1 Fitting and adjustment of extracorporeal dialysis catheter
Removal or replacement of catheter
Toilet or cleansing
Use additional code for any concurrent extracorporeal dialysis (V56.0)

V56.2 Fitting and adjustment of peritoneal dialysis catheter
Use additional code for any concurrent peritoneal dialysis (V56.8)

⑤ **V56.3 Encounter for adequacy testing for dialysis**

V56.31 Encounter for adequacy testing for hemodialysis

V56.32 Encounter for adequacy testing for peritoneal dialysis
Peritoneal equilibration test

V56.8 Other dialysis
Peritoneal dialysis

V57 Care involving use of rehabilitation procedures
Use additional code to identify underlying condition

V57.0 Breathing exercises

V57.1 Other physical therapy
Therapeutic and remedial exercises, except breathing

⑤ **V57.2 Occupational therapy and vocational rehabilitation**

V57.21 Encounter for occupational therapy

V57.22 Encounter for vocational therapy

▲ **V57.3 Speech-language therapy**

V57.4 Orthoptic training

⑤ **V57.8 Other specified rehabilitation procedure**

V57.81 Orthotic training
Gait training in the use of artificial limbs

V57.89 Other
Multiple training or therapy

V57.9 Unspecified rehabilitation procedure

V58 Encounter for other and unspecified procedures and aftercare

Excludes: convalescence and palliative care (V66)

V58.0 Radiotherapy
Encounter or admission for radiotherapy

Excludes: encounter for radioactive implant—code to condition
radioactive iodine therapy—code to condition

⑤ **V58.1 Encounter for chemotherapy and immunotherapy for neoplastic conditions**
Encounter or admission for chemotherapy

Excludes: chemotherapy and immunotherapy for nonneoplastic conditions—code to condition

V58.11 Encounter for antineoplastic chemotherapy

V58.12 Encounter for antineoplastic immunotherapy

V58.2 Blood transfusion, without reported diagnosis

⑤ **V58.3 Attention to dressings and sutures**
Change or removal of wound packing

Excludes: attention to drains (V58.49)
planned postoperative wound closure (V58.41)

V58.30 Encounter for change or removal of nonsurgical wound dressing
Encounter for change or removal of wound dressing NOS

V58.31 Encounter for change or removal of surgical wound dressing

V58.32 Encounter for removal of sutures
Encounter for removal of staples

● Code new
to this edition
▲ Revision of
existing code
④ ⑤ Fourth or fifth
digit required

⑤ **V58.4 Other aftercare following surgery**

Note: Codes from this subcategory should be used in conjunction with other aftercare codes to fully identify the reason for the aftercare encounter

Excludes: *aftercare following sterilization reversal surgery (V26.22)*
   attention to artificial openings (V55.0-V55.9)
   orthopedic aftercare (V54.0-V54.9)

V58.41 Encounter for planned postoperative wound closure

Excludes: *disruption of operative wound (998.31-998.32)*
   encounter for dressings and suture aftercare (V58.30-V58.32)

V58.42 Aftercare following surgery for neoplasm
   Conditions classifiable to 140-239

V58.43 Aftercare following surgery for injury and trauma
   Conditions classifiable to 800-999

Excludes: *aftercare for healing traumatic fracture (V54.10-V54.19)*

V58.44 Aftercare following organ transplant
Use additional code to identify the organ transplanted (V42.0-V42.9)

V58.49 Other specified aftercare following surgery
   Change or removal of drains

V58.5 Orthodontics

Excludes: *fitting and adjustment of orthodontic device (V53.4)*

⑤ **V58.6 Long-term (current) drug use**

Excludes: *drug abuse (305.00-305.93)*
   drug abuse and dependence complicating pregnancy (648.3-648.4)
   drug dependence (304.00-304.93)
   hormone replacement therapy (postmenopausal) (V07.4)
   prophylactic use of agents affecting estrogen receptors and estrogen levels (V07.51-V07.59)

V58.61 Long-term (current) use of anticoagulants
Excludes: *long-term (current) use of aspirin (V58.66)*

V58.62 Long-term (current) use of antibiotics

V58.63 Long-term (current) use of antiplatelets/antithrombotics
Excludes: *long-term (current) use of aspirin (V58.66)*

V58.64 Long-term (current) use of non-steroidal anti-inflammatories (NSAID)
Excludes: *long-term (current) use of aspirin (V58.66)*

V58.65 Long-term (current) use of steroids

V58.66 Long-term (current) use of aspirin

V58.67 Long-term (current) use of insulin

V58.69 Long-term (current) use of other medications
   Long term current use of methadone
   Long term current use of opiate analgesic
   Other high-risk medications

⑤ **V58.7 Aftercare following surgery to specified body systems, not elsewhere classified**

Note: Codes from this subcategory should be used in conjunction with other aftercare codes to fully identify the reason for the aftercare encounter

Excludes: *aftercare following organ transplant (V58.44)*
   aftercare following surgery for neoplasm (V58.42)

V58.71 Aftercare following surgery of the sense organs, NEC
   Conditions classifiable to 360-379, 380-389

V58.72 Aftercare following surgery of the nervous system, NEC
   Conditions classifiable to 320-359

Excludes: *aftercare following surgery of the sense organs, NEC (V58.71)*

V58.73 Aftercare following surgery of the circulatory system, NEC
   Conditions classifiable to 390-459

V58.74 Aftercare following surgery of the respiratory system, NEC
   Conditions classifiable to 460-519

V58.75 Aftercare following surgery of the teeth, oral cavity and digestive system, NEC
   Conditions classifiable to 520-579

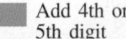 Add 4th or 5th digit   Nonspecific code   Unspecific code   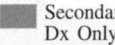 Secondary Dx Only   Primary Dx Only

V58.76 Aftercare following surgery of the genitourinary system, NEC
Conditions classifiable to 580-629

Excludes: *aftercare following sterilization reversal (V26.22)*

V58.77 Aftercare following surgery of the skin and subcutaneous tissue, NEC
Conditions classifiable to 680-709

V58.78 Aftercare following surgery of the musculoskeletal system, NEC
Conditions classifiable to 710-739

Excludes: *orthopedic aftercare (V54.01-V54.9)*

⑤ **V58.8 Other specified procedures and aftercare**

V58.81 Fitting and adjustment of vascular catheter
Removal or replacement of catheter
Toilet or cleansing

Excludes: *complication of renal dialysis catheter (996.73)*
complication of vascular catheter (996.74)
dialysis preparation — code to condition
encounter for dialysis (V56.0-V56.8)
fitting and adjustment of dialysis catheter (V56.1)

V58.82 Fitting and adjustment of non-vascular catheter NEC
Removal or replacement of catheter
Toilet or cleansing

Excludes: *fitting and adjustment of peritoneal dialysis catheter (V56.2)*
fitting and adjustment of urinary catheter (V53.6)

V58.83 Encounter for therapeutic drug monitoring
Use additional code for any associated long-term (current) drug use (V58.61-V58.69)

Excludes: *blood-drug testing for medicolegal reasons (V70.4)*

V58.89 Other specified aftercare

V58.9 Unspecified aftercare

V59 Donors

Excludes: *examination of potential donor (V70.8)*
self-donation of organ or tissue—code to condition

⑤ **V59.0 Blood**

V59.01 Whole blood

V59.02 Stem cells

V59.09 Other

V59.1 Skin

V59.2 Bone

V59.3 Bone marrow

V59.4 Kidney

V59.5 Cornea

V59.6 Liver

⑤ **V59.7 Egg (oocyte) (ovum)**

V59.70 Egg (oocyte) (ovum) donor, unspecified

V59.71 Egg (oocyte) (ovum) donor, under age 35, anonymous recipient
Egg donor, under age 35 NOS

V59.72 Egg (oocyte) (ovum) donor, under age 35, designated recipient

V59.73 Egg (oocyte) (ovum) donor, age 35 and over, anonymous recipient
Egg donor, age 35 and over NOS

V59.74 Egg (oocyte) (ovum) donor, age 35 and over, designated recipient

V59.8 Other specified organ or tissue

V59.9 Unspecified organ or tissue

● Code new
to this edition
▲ Revision of
existing code
④ ⑤ Fourth or fifth
digit required

PERSONS ENCOUNTERING HEALTH SERVICES IN OTHER CIRCUMSTANCES (V60-V69)

V60 Housing, household, and economic circumstances

V60.0 Lack of housing

Hobos	Transients
Social migrants	Vagabonds
Tramps	

V60.1 Inadequate housing
Lack of heating
Restriction of space
Technical defects in home preventing adequate care

V60.2 Inadequate material resources
Economic problem
Poverty NOS

V60.3 Person living alone

V60.4 No other household member able to render care
Person requiring care (has) (is):
family member too handicapped, ill, or otherwise unsuited to render care
partner temporarily away from home
temporarily away from usual place of abode

Excludes: *holiday relief care (V60.5)*

V60.5 Holiday relief care
Provision of health care facilities to a person normally cared for at home, to enable relatives to take a vacation

V60.6 Person living in residential institution
Boarding school resident

⑤ V60.8 Other specified housing or economic circumstances

● **V60.81** Foster care (status)

● **V60.89** Other specified housing or economic circumstances

V60.9 Unspecified housing or economic circumstance

V61 Other family circumstances
Includes: when these circumstances or fear of them, affecting the person directly involved or others, are mentioned as the reason, justified or not, for seeking or receiving medical advice or care

⑤ V61.0 Family disruption

V61.01 Family disruption due to family member on military deployment
Individual or family affected by other family member being on deployment

Excludes: *family disruption due to family member on non-military extended absence from home (V61.08)*

V61.02 Family disruption due to return of family member from military deployment
Individual or family affected by other family member having returned from deployment (current or past conflict)

V61.03 Family disruption due to divorce or legal separation

V61.04 Family disruption due to parent-child estrangement

Excludes: *other family estrangement (V61.09)*

V61.05 Family disruption due to child in welfare custody

V61.06 Family disruption due to child in foster care or in care of non-parental family member

● **V61.07** Family disruption due to death of family member

Excludes: *bereavement (V62.82)*

● **V61.08** Family disruption due to other extended absence of family member

Excludes: *family disruption due to family member on military deployment (V61.01)*

V61.09 Other family disruption
Family estrangement NOS

⑤ V61.1 Counseling for marital and partner problems

Excludes: *problems related to:*
psychosexual disorders (302.0-302.9)
sexual function (V41.7)

■	Add 4th or 5th digit	■	Nonspecific code		Unspecific code	■	Secondary Dx Only	■	Primary Dx Only

V61.10 Counseling for marital and partner problems, unspecified
Marital conflict
Marital relationship problem
Partner conflict
Partner relationship problem

V61.11 Counseling for victim of spousal and partner abuse

Excludes: encounter for treatment of current injuries due to abuse (995.80-995.85)

V61.12 Counseling for perpetrator of spousal and partner abuse

⑤ **V61.2 Parent-child problems**

V61.20 Counseling for parent-child problem, unspecified
Concern about behavior of child
Parent-child conflict
Parent-child relationship problem

V61.21 Counseling for victim of child abuse
Child battering
Child neglect

Excludes: current injuries due to abuse (995.50-995.59)

V61.22 Counseling for perpetrator of parental child abuse

Excludes: counseling for non-parental abuser (V62.83)

● **V61.23 Counseling for parent-biological child problem**
Concern about behavior of biological child
Parent-biological child conflict
Parent-biological child relationship problem

● **V61.24 Counseling for parent-adopted child problem**
Concern about behavior of adopted child
Parent-adopted child conflict
Parent-adopted child relationship problem

● **V61.25 Counseling for parent (guardian)-foster child problem**
Concern about behavior of foster child
Parent (guardian)-foster child conflict
Parent (guardian)-foster child relationship problem

▲ **V61.29 Other parent-child problems**

V61.3 Problems with aged parents or in-laws

⑤ **V61.4 Health problems within family**

V61.41 Alcoholism in family

● **V61.42 Substance abuse in family**

V61.49 Other
Care of sick or handicapped person in family or household
Presence of sick or handicapped person in family or household

V61.5 Multiparity

V61.6 Illegitimacy or illegitimate pregnancy

V61.7 Other unwanted pregnancy

V61.8 Other specified family circumstances
Problems with family members NEC
Sibling relationship problem

V61.9 Unspecified family circumstance

V62 Other psychosocial circumstances
Includes: those circumstances or fear of them, affecting the person directly involved or others, mentioned as the reason, justified or not, for seeking or receiving medical advice or care

Excludes: previous psychological trauma (V15.41-V15.49)

V62.0 Unemployment

Excludes: circumstances when main problem is economic inadequacy or poverty (V60.2)

V62.1 Adverse effects of work environment

⑤ **V62.2 Other occupational circumstances or maladjustment**

V62.21 Personal current military deployment status
Individual (civilian or military) currently deployed in theater or in support of military war, peacekeeping and humanitarian operations

● Code new
   to this edition
▲ Revision of
   existing code
④ ⑤ Fourth or fifth
       digit required

V62.22 **Personal history of return from military deployment**
Individual (civilian or military) with past history of military war, peacekeeping and humanitarian deployment (current or past conflict)

V62.29 **Other occupational circumstances or maladjustment**
Career choice problem
Dissatisfaction with employment
Occupational problem

V62.3 **Educational circumstances**
Academic problem
Dissatisfaction with school environment
Educational handicap

V62.4 **Social maladjustment**
Acculturation problem
Cultural deprivation
Political, religious, or sex
discrimination
Social:
isolation
persecution

V62.5 **Legal circumstances**
Imprisonment
Legal investigation
Litigation
Prosecution

V62.6 **Refusal of treatment for reasons of religion or conscience**

⑤ **V62.8** **Other psychological or physical stress, not elsewhere classified**

V62.81 **Interpersonal problems, not elsewhere classified**
Relational problem NOS

V62.82 **Bereavement, uncomplicated**

Excludes: *bereavement as adjustment reaction (309.0)*
family disruption due to death of family member (V61.07)

V62.83 **Counseling for perpetrator of physical/sexual abuse**

Excludes: *counseling for perpetrator of parental child abuse (V61.22)*
counseling for perpetrator of spousal and partner abuse (V61.12)

V62.84 **Suicidal ideation**

Excludes: *suicidal tendencies (300.9)*

V62.89 **Other**
Borderline intellectual functioning
Life circumstance problems
Phase of life problems
Religious or spiritual problem

V62.9 **Unspecified psychosocial circumstance**

V63 **Unavailability of other medical facilities for care**

V63.0 **Residence remote from hospital or other health care facility**

V63.1 **Medical services in home not available**

Excludes: *no other household member able to render care (V60.4)*

V63.2 **Person awaiting admission to adequate facility elsewhere**

V63.8 **Other specified reasons for unavailability of medical facilities**
Person on waiting list undergoing social agency investigation

V63.9 **Unspecified reason for unavailability of medical facilities**

V64 **Persons encountering health services for specific procedures, not carried out**

⑤ **V64.0** **Vaccination not carried out**

V64.00 **Vaccination not carried out, unspecified reason**

V64.01 **Vaccination not carried out because of acute illness**

V64.02 **Vaccination not carried out because of chronic illness or condition**

V64.03 **Vaccination not carried out because of immune compromised state**

V64.04 **Vaccination not carried out because of allergy to vaccine or component**

V64.05 **Vaccination not carried out because of caregiver refusal**
Guardian refusal
Parent refusal

Excludes: *vaccination not carried out because of caregiver refusal for religious reasons (V64.07)*

V64.06 **Vaccination not carried out because of patient refusal**

V64.07 **Vaccination not carried out for religious reasons**

Add 4th or 5th digit   Nonspecific code   Unspecific code   Secondary Dx Only   Primary Dx Only

V64.08 Vaccination not carried out because patient had disease being vaccinated against

V64.09 Vaccination not carried out for other reason

V64.1 Surgical or other procedure not carried out because of contraindication

V64.2 Surgical or other procedure not carried out because of patient's decision

V64.3 Procedure not carried out for other reasons

⑤ **V64.4** Closed surgical procedure converted to open procedure

   V64.41 Laparoscopic surgical procedure converted to open procedure

   V64.42 Thoracoscopic surgical procedure converted to open procedure

   V64.43 Arthroscopic surgical procedure converted to open procedure

V65 Other persons seeking consultation

V65.0 Healthy person accompanying sick person
   Boarder

⑤ **V65.1** Person consulting on behalf of another person
   Advice or treatment for nonattending third party

   Excludes: concern (normal) about sick person in family (V61.41-V61.49)

   ▲ **V65.11** Pediatric pre-birth visit for expectant parent(s)
      Pre-adoption visit for adoptive parent(s)

   V65.19 Other person consulting on behalf of another person

V65.2 Person feigning illness
   Malingerer
   Peregrinating patient

V65.3 Dietary surveillance and counseling
   Dietary surveillance and counseling (in):
     NOS
     colitis
     diabetes mellitus
     food allergies or intolerance
     gastritis
     hypercholesterolemia
     hypoglycemia
     obesity
   Use additional code to identify Body Mass Index (BMI), if known (V85.0-V85.54)

⑤ **V65.4** Other counseling, not elsewhere classified
   Health:
     advice
     education
     instruction

   Excludes: counseling (for):
     contraception (V25.40-V25.49)
     genetic (V26.31-V26.39)
     on behalf of third party (V65.11, V65.19)
     procreative management (V26.41-V26.49)

   V65.40 Counseling NOS

   V65.41 Exercise counseling

   V65.42 Counseling on substance use and abuse

   V65.43 Counseling on injury prevention

   V65.44 Human immunodeficiency virus [HIV] counseling

   V65.45 Counseling on other sexually transmitted diseases

   V65.46 Encounter for insulin pump training

   V65.49 Other specified counseling

V65.5 Person with feared complaint in whom no diagnosis was made
   Feared condition not demonstrated
   Problem was normal state
   "Worried well"

V65.8 Other reasons for seeking consultation

   Excludes: specified symptoms

V65.9 Unspecified reason for consultation

● Code new to this edition   ▲ Revision of existing code   ④ ⑤ Fourth or fifth digit required

V66 Convalescence and palliative care

    V66.0 Following surgery

    V66.1 Following radiotherapy

    V66.2 Following chemotherapy

    V66.3 Following psychotherapy and other treatment for mental disorder

    V66.4 Following treatment of fracture

    V66.5 Following other treatment

    V66.6 Following combined treatment

    V66.7 Encounter for palliative care
        End-of-life care
        Hospice care
        Terminal care

    Code first underlying disease

    V66.9 Unspecified convalescence

V67 Follow-up examination
    Includes: surveillance only following completed treatment
    Excludes: *surveillance of contraception (V25.40-V25.49)*

  ⑤ **V67.0 Following surgery**

      V67.00 Following surgery, unspecified

      V67.01 Follow-up vaginal pap smear
          Vaginal pap smear, status-post hysterectomy for malignant condition

    Use additional code to identify:
        acquired absence of uterus (V88.01-88.03)
        personal history of malignant neoplasm (V10.40-V10.44)

    Excludes: *vaginal pap smear status-post hysterectomy for non-malignant condition (V76.47)*

      V67.09 Following other surgery

    Excludes: *sperm count following sterilization reversal (V26.22)*
         sperm count for fertility testing (V26.21)

    V67.1 Following radiotherapy

    V67.2 Following chemotherapy
      Cancer chemotherapy follow-up

    V67.3 Following psychotherapy and other treatment for mental disorder

    V67.4 Following treatment of healed fracture

    Excludes: *current (healing) fracture aftercare (V54.0-V54.9)*

  ⑤ **V67.5 Following other treatment**

      V67.51 Following completed treatment with high-risk medication, NEC

    Excludes: *long-term (current) drug use (V58.61-V58.69)*

      V67.59 Other

    V67.6 Following combined treatment

    V67.9 Unspecified follow-up examination

V68 Encounters for administrative purposes

  ⑤ **V68.0 Issue of medical certificates**

    Excludes: *encounter for general medical examination (V70.0-V70.9)*

      V68.01 Disability examination

    Use additional code(s) to identify:
        specific examination(s), screening and testing performed (V72.0-V82.9)

      V68.09 Other issue of medical certificates

    V68.1 Issue of repeat prescriptions
      Issue of repeat prescription for:
        appliance
        glasses
        medications

    Excludes: *repeat prescription for contraceptives (V25.41-V25.49)*

    V68.2 Request for expert evidence

  ⑤ **V68.8 Other specified administrative purpose**

      V68.81 Referral of patient without examination or treatment

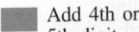

Add 4th or 5th digit	Nonspecific code	Unspecific code	Secondary Dx Only	Primary Dx Only

V68.89 Other

V68.9 Unspecified administrative purpose

V69 Problems related to lifestyle

V69.0 Lack of physical exercise

V69.1 Inappropriate diet and eating habits

Excludes: anorexia nervosa (307.1)
bulimia (783.6)
malnutrition and other nutritional deficiencies (260-269.9)
other and unspecified eating disorders (307.50-307.59)

V69.2 High-risk sexual behavior

V69.3 Gambling and betting

Excludes: pathological gambling (312.31)

V69.4 Lack of adequate sleep
Sleep deprivation

Excludes: insomnia (780.52)

V69.5 Behavioral insomnia of childhood

V69.8 Other problems related to lifestyle
Self-damaging behavior

V69.9 Problem related to lifestyle, unspecified

PERSONS WITHOUT REPORTED DIAGNOSIS ENCOUNTERED DURING EXAMINATION AND INVESTIGATION OF INDIVIDUALS AND POPULATIONS (V70-V82)

Note: Nonspecific abnormal findings disclosed at the time of these examinations are classifiable to categories 790-796.

V70 General medical examination

Use additional code(s) to identify any special screening examination(s) performed (V73.0-V82.9)

V70.0 Routine general medical examination at a health care facility
Health checkup

Excludes: health checkup of infant or child over 28 days old (V20.2)
health supervision of newborn 8 to 28 days old (V20.32)
health supervision of newborn under 8 days old (V20.31)
pre-procedural general physical examination (V72.83)

V70.1 General psychiatric examination, requested by the authority

V70.2 General psychiatric examination, other and unspecified

V70.3 Other medical examination for administrative purposes
General medical examination for:

admission to old age home	marriage
adoption	prison
camp	school admission
driving license	sports competition
immigration and naturalization	
insurance certification	

Excludes: attendance for issue of medical certificates (V68.0)
pre-employment screening (V70.5)

V70.4 Examination for medicolegal reasons
Blood-alcohol tests
Blood-drug tests
Paternity testing

Excludes: examination and observation following:
accidents (V71.3, V71.4)
assault (V71.6)
rape (V71.5)

V70.5 Health examination of defined subpopulations

Armed forces personnel	Preschool children
Inhabitants of institutions	Prisoners
Occupational health	Prostitutes
examinations	Refugees
Pre-employment screening	School children
	Students

● Code new
to this edition

▲ Revision of
existing code

④ ⑤ Fourth or fifth
digit required

V70.6 Health examination in population surveys

Excludes: special screening (V73.0-V82.9)

V70.7 Examination of participant in clinical trial
Examination of participant or control in clinical research

V70.8 Other specified general medical examinations
Examination of potential donor of organ or tissue

V70.9 Unspecified general medical examination

V71 Observation and evaluation for suspected conditions not found
Note: This category is to be used when persons without a diagnosis are suspected of having an abnormal condition, without signs or symptoms, which requires study, but after examination and observation, is found not to exist. This category is also for use for administrative and legal observation status.

Excludes: suspected maternal and fetal conditions not found (V89.01-V89.09)

⑤ **V71.0 Observation for suspected mental condition**

    V71.01 Adult antisocial behavior
    Dyssocial behavior or gang activity in adult without manifest psychiatric disorder

    V71.02 Childhood or adolescent antisocial behavior
    Dyssocial behavior or gang activity in child or adolescent without manifest psychiatric disorder

    V71.09 Other suspected mental condition

V71.1 Observation for suspected malignant neoplasm

V71.2 Observation for suspected tuberculosis

V71.3 Observation following accident at work

V71.4 Observation following other accident
Examination of individual involved in motor vehicle traffic accident

V71.5 Observation following alleged rape or seduction
Examination of victim or culprit

V71.6 Observation following other inflicted injury
Examination of victim or culprit

V71.7 Observation for suspected cardiovascular disease

⑤ **V71.8 Observation and evaluation for other specified suspected conditions**

Excludes: contact with and (suspected) exposure to (potentially) hazardous substances (V15.84-V15.86, V87.0- V87.31)

    V71.81 Abuse and neglect
Excludes: adult abuse and neglect (995.80-995.85)
child abuse and neglect (995.50-995.59)

    V71.82 Observation and evaluation for suspected exposure to anthrax

    V71.83 Observation and evaluation for suspected exposure to other biological agent

    V71.89 Other specified suspected conditions

V71.9 Observation for unspecified suspected condition

V72 Special investigations and examinations
Includes: routine examination of specific system

Excludes: general medical examination (V70.0-V70.4)
general screening examination of defined population groups (V70.5, V70.6, V70.7)
health supervision of newborn 8 to 28 days old (V20.32)
health supervision of newborn under 8 days old (V20.31)
routine examination of infant or child over 28 days old (V20.2)

Use additional code(s) to identify any special screening examination(s) performed (V73.0-V82.9)

V72.0 Examination of eyes and vision

⑤ **V72.1 Examination of ears and hearing**

    V72.11 Encounter for hearing examination following failed hearing screening

    V72.12 Encounter for hearing conservation and treatment

    V72.19 Other examination of ears and hearing

V72.2 Dental examination

| ■ Add 4th or 5th digit | ■ Nonspecific code | ■ Unspecific code | Secondary Dx Only | 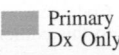 Primary Dx Only |

⑤ **V72.3 Gynecological examination**

> *Excludes:* *cervical Papanicolaou smear without general gynecological examination (V76.2)*
> *routine examination in contraceptive management (V25.40-V25.49)*

V72.31 Routine gynecological examination
General gynecological examination with or without Papanicolaou cervical smear
Pelvic examination (annual) (periodic)
Use additional code to identify routine:
human papillomavirus (HPV) screening (V73.81)
routine vaginal Papanicolaou smear (V76.47)

V72.32 Encounter for Papanicolaou cervical smear to confirm findings of recent normal smear following initial abnormal smear

⑤ **V72.4 Pregnancy examination or test**

V72.40 Pregnancy examination or test, pregnancy unconfirmed
Possible pregnancy, not (yet) confirmed

V72.41 Pregnancy examination or test, negative result

V72.42 Pregnancy examination or test, positive result

V72.5 Radiological examination, not elsewhere classified
Routine chest x-ray

> *Excludes:* *radiologic examinations as part of pre-procedural testing (V72.81-V72.84)*

⑤ **V72.6 Laboratory examination**
Encounters for blood and urine testing

● **V72.60 Laboratory examination, unspecified**

● **V72.61 Antibody response examination**
Immunity status testing

> *Excludes:* *encounter for allergy testing (V72.7)*

● **V72.62 Laboratory examination ordered as part of a routine general medical examination**
Blood tests for routine general physical examination

● **V72.63 Pre-procedural laboratory examination**
Blood tests prior to treatment or procedure
Pre-operative laboratory examination

● **V72.69 Other laboratory examination**

V72.7 Diagnostic skin and sensitization tests
Allergy tests
Skin tests for hypersensitivity

> *Excludes:* *diagnostic skin tests for bacterial diseases (V74.0-V74.9)*

⑤ **V72.8 Other specified examinations**

> *Excludes:* *pre-procedural laboratory examinations (V72.63)*

V72.81 Pre-operative cardiovascular examination
Pre-procedural cardiovascular examination

V72.82 Pre-operative respiratory examination
Pre-procedural respiratory examination

V72.83 Other specified pre-operative examination
Examination prior to chemotherapy
Other pre-procedural examination
Pre-procedural general physical examination

> *Excludes:* *routine general medical examination (V70.0)*

V72.84 Pre-operative examination, unspecified
Pre-procedural examination, unspecified

V72.85 Other specified examination

V72.86 Encounter for blood typing

V72.9 Unspecified examination

V73 **Special screening examination for viral and chlamydial diseases**
V73.0 Poliomyelitis
V73.1 Smallpox
V73.2 Measles
V73.3 Rubella

● Code new to this edition	▲ Revision of existing code	④ ⑤ Fourth or fifth digit required

V73.4 Yellow fever

V73.5 Other arthropod-borne viral diseases
  Dengue fever
  Hemorrhagic fever

  Viral encephalitis:
    mosquito-borne
    tick-borne

V73.6 Trachoma

⑤ **V73.8 Other specified viral and chlamydial diseases**

  V73.81 Human papillomavirus (HPV)

  V73.88 Other specified chlamydial diseases

  V73.89 Other specified viral diseases

⑤ **V73.9 Unspecified viral and chlamydial disease**

  V73.98 Unspecified chlamydial disease

  V73.99 Unspecified viral disease

V74 Special screening examination for bacterial and spirochetal diseases
  Includes: diagnostic skin tests for these diseases

V74.0 Cholera

V74.1 Pulmonary tuberculosis

V74.2 Leprosy [Hansen's disease]

V74.3 Diphtheria

V74.4 Bacterial conjunctivitis

V74.5 Venereal disease
  Screening for bacterial and spirochetal sexually transmitted diseases
  Screening for sexually transmitted diseases NOS

  Excludes: *special screening for nonbacterial sexually transmitted diseases (V73.81-V73.89,*
    V75.4, V75.8)

V74.6 Yaws

V74.8 Other specified bacterial and spirochetal diseases
  Brucellosis
  Leptospirosis
  Plague

  Tetanus
  Whooping cough

V74.9 Unspecified bacterial and spirochetal disease

V75 Special screening examination for other infectious diseases

V75.0 Rickettsial diseases

V75.1 Malaria

V75.2 Leishmaniasis

V75.3 Trypanosomiasis
  Chagas' disease
  Sleeping sickness

V75.4 Mycotic infections

V75.5 Schistosomiasis

V75.6 Filariasis

V75.7 Intestinal helminthiasis

V75.8 Other specified parasitic infections

V75.9 Unspecified infectious disease

V76 Special screening for malignant neoplasms

V76.0 Respiratory organs

⑤ **V76.1 Breast**

  V76.10 Breast screening, unspecified

  V76.11 Screening mammogram for high-risk patient

  V76.12 Other screening mammogram

  V76.19 Other screening breast examination

V76.2 Cervix
  Routine cervical Papanicolaou smear

  Excludes: *special screening for human papillomavirus (V73.81)*
    that as part of a general gynecological examination (V72.31)

V76.3 Bladder

701

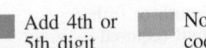 Add 4th or
5th digit

Nonspecific
code

Unspecific
code

 Secondary
Dx Only

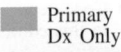 Primary
Dx Only

⑤ **V76.4 Other sites**

        V76.41 Rectum

        V76.42 Oral cavity

        V76.43 Skin

        V76.44 Prostate

        V76.45 Testis

        V76.46 Ovary

        V76.47 Vagina
          Vaginal pap smear status-post hysterectomy for non-malignant condition

     Use additional code to identify acquired absence of uterus (V88.01-V88.03)

     | Excludes: | *vaginal pap smear status-post hysterectomy for malignant condition (V67.01)*

        V76.49 Other sites

⑤ **V76.5 Intestine**

        V76.50 Intestine, unspecified

        V76.51 Colon

  | Excludes: | *rectum (V76.41)*

        V76.52 Small intestine

⑤ **V76.8 Other neoplasm**

        V76.81 Nervous system

        V76.89 Other neoplasm

   V76.9 Unspecified

V77 Special screening for endocrine, nutritional, metabolic, and immunity disorders

   V77.0 Thyroid disorders

   V77.1 Diabetes mellitus

   V77.2 Malnutrition

   V77.3 Phenylketonuria [PKU]

   V77.4 Galactosemia

   V77.5 Gout

   V77.6 Cystic fibrosis
      Screening for mucoviscidosis

   V77.7 Other inborn errors of metabolism

   V77.8 Obesity

⑤ **V77.9 Other and unspecified endocrine, nutritional, metabolic, and immunity disorders**

        V77.91 Screening for lipoid disorders
          Screening cholesterol level
          Screening for hypercholesterolemia
          Screening for hyperlipidemia

        V77.99 Other and unspecified endocrine, nutritional, metabolic, and immunity disorders

V78 Special screening for disorders of blood and blood-forming organs

   V78.0 Iron deficiency anemia

   V78.1 Other and unspecified deficiency anemia

   V78.2 Sickle-cell disease or trait

   V78.3 Other hemoglobinopathies

   V78.8 Other disorders of blood and blood-forming organs

   V78.9 Unspecified disorder of blood and blood-forming organs

V79 Special screening for mental disorders and developmental handicaps

   V79.0 Depression

   V79.1 Alcoholism

   V79.2 Mental retardation

   V79.3 Developmental handicaps in early childhood

   V79.8 Other specified mental disorders and developmental handicaps

   V79.9 Unspecified mental disorder and developmental handicap

V80 Special screening for neurological, eye, and ear diseases

| ● Code new to this edition | ▲ Revision of existing code | ④ ⑤ Fourth or fifth digit required |

⑤ **V80.0 Neurological conditions**

   ● **V80.01 Traumatic brain injury**

   ● **V80.09 Other neurological conditions**

V80.1 Glaucoma

V80.2 Other eye conditions
> Screening for:
>> cataract
>> congenital anomaly of eye
>> senile macular lesions

> [Excludes:] *general vision examination (V72.0)*

V80.3 Ear diseases
> [Excludes:] *general hearing examination (V72.11-V72.19)*

V81 Special screening for cardiovascular, respiratory, and genitourinary diseases

V81.0 Ischemic heart disease

V81.1 Hypertension

V81.2 Other and unspecified cardiovascular conditions

V81.3 Chronic bronchitis and emphysema

V81.4 Other and unspecified respiratory conditions
> [Excludes:] *screening for:*
>> *lung neoplasm (V76.0)*
>> *pulmonary tuberculosis (V74.1)*

V81.5 Nephropathy
> Screening for asymptomatic bacteriuria

V81.6 Other and unspecified genitourinary conditions

V82 Special screening for other conditions

V82.0 Skin conditions

V82.1 Rheumatoid arthritis

V82.2 Other rheumatic disorders

V82.3 Congenital dislocation of hip

V82.4 Maternal postnatal screening for chromosomal anomalies
> [Excludes:] *antenatal screening by amniocentesis (V28.0)*

V82.5 Chemical poisoning and other contamination
> Screening for:
>> heavy metal poisoning
>> ingestion of radioactive substance
>> poisoning from contaminated water supply
>> radiation exposure

V82.6 Multiphasic screening

⑤ **V82.7 Genetic screening**
> [Excludes:] *genetic testing for procreative management (V26.31-V26.39)*

   V82.71 Screening for genetic disease carrier status

   V82.79 Other genetic screening

⑤ **V82.8 Other specified conditions**

   V82.81 Osteoporosis
> Use additional code to identify:
>> hormone replacement therapy (postmenopausal) status (V07.4)
>> postmenopausal (natural) status (V49.81)

   V82.89 Other specified conditions

V82.9 Unspecified condition

GENETICS (V83-V84)

V83 Genetic carrier status

⑤ **V83.0 Hemophilia A carrier**

   V83.01 Asymptomatic hemophilia A carrier

   V83.02 Symptomatic hemophilia A carrier

⑤ **V83.8 Other genetic carrier status**

	Add 4th or 5th digit		Nonspecific code		Unspecific code		Secondary Dx Only		Primary Dx Only

V83.81 Cystic fibrosis gene carrier

V83.89 Other genetic carrier status

V84 Genetic susceptibility to disease
Includes: Confirmed abnormal gene

Use additional code, if applicable, for any associated family history of the disease (V16-V19)

⑤ **V84.0** Genetic susceptibility to malignant neoplasm
Code first, if applicable, any current malignant neoplasms (140.0-195.8, 200.0-208.9, 230.0-234.9)

Use additional code, if applicable, for any personal history of malignant neoplasm (V10.0-V10.9)

V84.01 Genetic susceptibility to malignant neoplasm of breast

V84.02 Genetic susceptibility to malignant neoplasm of ovary

V84.03 Genetic susceptibility to malignant neoplasm of prostate

V84.04 Genetic susceptibility to malignant neoplasm of endometrium

V84.09 Genetic susceptibility to other malignant neoplasm

⑤ **V84.8** Genetic susceptibility to other disease

V84.81 Genetic susceptibility to multiple endocrine neoplasia [MEN]

V84.89 Genetic susceptibility to other disease

BODY MASS INDEX (V85)

V85 Body Mass Index [BMI]
Kilograms per meters squared
Note: BMI adult codes are for use for persons over 20 years old

V85.0 Body Mass Index less than 19, adult

V85.1 Body Mass Index between 19-24, adult

⑤ **V85.2** Body Mass Index between 25-29, adult

V85.21 Body Mass Index 25.0-25.9, adult

V85.22 Body Mass Index 26.0-26.9, adult

V85.23 Body Mass Index 27.0-27.9, adult

V85.24 Body Mass Index 28.0-28.9, adult

V85.25 Body Mass Index 29.0-29.9, adult

⑤ **V85.3** Body Mass Index between 30-39, adult

V85.30 Body Mass Index 30.0-30.9, adult

V85.31 Body Mass Index 31.0-31.9, adult

V85.32 Body Mass Index 32.0-32.9, adult

V85.33 Body Mass Index 33.0-33.9, adult

V85.34 Body Mass Index 34.0-34.9, adult

V85.35 Body Mass Index 35.0-35.9, adult

V85.36 Body Mass Index 36.0-36.9, adult

V85.37 Body Mass Index 37.0-37.9, adult

V85.38 Body Mass Index 38.0-38.9, adult

V85.39 Body Mass Index 39.0-39.9, adult

V85.4 Body Mass Index 40 and over, adult

⑤ **85.5** Body Mass Index, pediatric
Note:BMI pediatric codes are for use for persons age 2-20 years old. These percentiles are based on the growth charts published by the Centers for Disease Control and Prevention (CDC)

V85.51 Body Mass Index, pediatric, less than 5th percentile for age

V85.52 Body Mass Index, pediatric, 5th percentile to less than 85th percentile for age

V85.53 Body Mass Index, pediatric, 85th percentile to less than 95th percentile for age

V85.54 Body Mass Index, pediatric, greater than or equal to 95th percentile for age

● Code new to this edition   ▲ Revision of existing code   ④ ⑤ Fourth or fifth digit required

ESTROGEN RECEPTOR STATUS (V86)

V86 Estrogen receptor status
Code first malignant neoplasm of breast (174.0-174.9, 175.0-175.9)

V86.0 Estrogen receptor positive status (ER+)

V86.1 Estrogen receptor negative status (ER−)

OTHER SPECIFIED PERSONAL EXPOSURES AND HISTORY PRESENTING HAZARDS TO HEALTH (V87)

V87 Other specified personal exposures and history presenting hazards to health

⑤ **V87.0** Contact with and (suspected) exposure to hazardous metals

Excludes: exposure to lead (V15.86)
toxic effect of metals (984.0-985.9)

V87.01 Arsenic

V87.09 Other hazardous metals
Chromium compounds
Nickel dust

⑤ **V87.1** Contact with and (suspected) exposure to hazardous aromatic compounds

Excludes: toxic effects of aromatic compounds (982.0, 983.0)

V87.11 Aromatic amines

V87.12 Benzene

V87.19 Other hazardous aromatic compounds
Aromatic dyes NOS
Polycyclic aromatic hydrocarbons

V87.2 Contact with and (suspected) exposure to other potentially hazardous chemicals
Dyes NOS

Excludes: exposure to asbestos (V15.84)
toxic effect of chemicals (980-989)

⑤ **V87.3** Contact with and (suspected) exposure to other potentially hazardous substances

Excludes: contact with and (suspected) exposure to potentially hazardous body fluids
(V15.85)
toxic effect of substances (980-989)

V87.31 Exposure to mold

● **V87.32** Contact with and (suspected) exposure to algae bloom

V87.39 Contact with and (suspected) exposure to other potentially hazardous
substances

⑤ **V87.4** Personal history of drug therapy

Excludes: long-term (current) drug use (V58.61-V58.69)

V87.41 Personal history of antineoplastic chemotherapy

V87.42 Personal history of monoclonal drug therapy

● **V87.43** Personal history of estrogen therapy

● **V87.44** Personal history of inhaled steroid therapy

● **V87.45** Personal history of systemic steroid therapy
Personal history of steroid therapy NOS

● **V87.46** Personal history of immunosuppression therapy

Excludes: personal history of steroid therapy (V87.44, V87.45)

V87.49 Personal history of other drug therapy

ACQUIRED ABSENCE OF OTHER ORGANS AND TISSUE (V88)

⑤ **V88** Acquired absence of other organs and tissue

⑤ **V88.0** Acquired absence of cervix and uterus

V88.01 Acquired absence of both cervix and uterus
Acquired absence of uterus NOS
Status post total hysterectomy

V88.02 Acquired absence of uterus with remaining cervical stump
Status post partial hysterectomy with remaining cervical stump

V88.03 Acquired absence of cervix with remaining uterus

	Add 4th or 5th digit		Nonspecific code		Unspecific code		Secondary Dx Only		Primary Dx Only

OTHER SUSPECTED CONDITIONS NOT FOUND (V89)

⑤ **V89** Other suspected conditions not found

  ⑤ **V89.0 Suspected maternal and fetal conditions not found**

> Excludes: *known or suspected fetal anomalies affecting management of mother, not ruled out (655.00, 655.93, 656.00-656.93, 657.00-657.03, 658.00-658.93)*
> *newborn and perinatal conditions - code to condition*

    V89.01 Suspected problem with amniotic cavity and membrane not found
      Suspected oligohydramnios not found
      Suspected polyhydramnios not found

    V89.02 Suspected placental problem not found

    V89.03 Suspected fetal anomaly not found

    V89.04 Suspected problem with fetal growth not found

    V89.05 Suspected cervical shortening not found

    V89.09 Other suspected maternal and fetal condition not found

● Code new to this edition ▲ Revision of existing code ④ ⑤ Fourth or fifth digit required

SUPPLEMENTARY CLASSIFICATION OF EXTERNAL CAUSES OF INJURY AND POISONING (E000-E999)

This section is provided to permit the classification of environmental events, circumstances, and conditions as the cause of injury, poisoning, and other adverse effects. Where a code from this section is applicable, it is intended that it shall be used in addition to a code from one of the main chapters of *ICD-9-CM*, indicating the nature of the condition. Certain other conditions which may be stated to be due to external causes are classified in Chapters 1 to 16 of *ICD-9-CM*. For these, the "E" code classification should be used for more detailed analysis.

Machinery accidents [other than those connected with transport] are classifiable to category E919, in which the fourth-digit allows a broad classification of the type of machinery involved.

Categories for "late effects" of accidents and other external causes are to be found at E929, E959, E969, E977, E989, and E999.

EXTERNAL CAUSE STATUS (E000)

Note: A code from category E000 should be used in conjunction with the external cause code(s) assigned to a record to indicate the status of the person at the time the event occurred. A single code from category E000 should be assigned for an encounter.

● **E000** **External cause status**

● **E000.0** **Civilian activity done for income or pay**
   Civilian activity done for financial or other compensation

   Excludes: *military activity (E000.1)*

● **E000.1** **Military activity**

   Excludes: *activity of off duty military personnel (E000.8)*

● **E000.8** **Other external cause status**
   Activity NEC
   Hobby not done for income
   Leisure activity
   Off-duty activity of military personnel
   Recreation or sport not for income or while a student
   Student activity
   Volunteer activity

   Excludes: *civilian activity done for income or compensation (E000.0)*
             military activity (E000.1)

● **E000.9** **Unspecified external cause status**

ACTIVITY (E001-E030)

Note: Categories E001 to E030 are provided for use to indicate the activity of the person seeking healthcare for an injury or health condition, such as a heart attack while shoveling snow, which resulted from, or was contributed to, by the activity. These codes are appropriate for use for both acute injuries, such as those from chapter 17, and conditions that are due to the long-term, cumulative effects of an activity, such as those from chapter 13. They are also appropriate for use with external cause codes for cause and intent if identifying the activity provides additional information on the event.

These codes should be used in conjunction with other external cause codes for external cause status (E000) and place of occurrence (E849).

This section contains the following broad activity categories:
   E001 Activities involving walking and running
   E002 Activities involving water and water craft
   E003 Activities involving ice and snow
   E004 Activities involving climbing, rappelling, and jumping off
   E005 Activities involving dancing and other rhythmic movement
   E006 Activities involving other sports and athletics played individually
   E007 Activities involving other sports and athletics played as a team or group
   E008 Activities involving other specified sports and athletics
   E009 Activity involving other cardiorespiratory exercise
   E010 Activity involving other muscle strengthening exercises
   E011 Activities involving computer technology and electronic devices
   E012 Activities involving arts and handcrafts
   E013 Activities involving personal hygiene and household maintenance
   E014 Activities involving person providing caregiving
   E015 Activities involving food preparation, cooking and grilling

	Add 4th or 5th digit		Nonspecific code		Unspecified code		Manifestation code

E016 Activities involving property and land maintenance, building and construction
E017 Activities involving roller coasters and other types of external motion
E018 Activities involving playing musical instrument
E019 Activities involving animal care
E029 Other activity
E030 Unspecified activity

● **E001** **Activities involving walking and running**

Excludes: *walking an animal (E019.0)*
walking or running on a treadmill (E009.0)

● **E001.0** **Walking, marching and hiking**
Walking, marching and hiking on level or elevated terrain

Excludes: *mountain climbing (E004.0)*

● **E001.1** **Running**

● **E002** **Activities involving water and water craft**

Excludes: *activities involving ice (E003.0-E003.9)*
boating and other watercraft transport accidents (E830-E838)

● **E002.0** **Swimming**

● **E002.1** **Springboard and platform diving**

● **E002.2** **Water polo**

● **E002.3** **Water aerobics and water exercise**

● **E002.4** **Underwater diving and snorkeling**
SCUBA diving

● **E002.5** **Rowing, canoeing, kayaking, rafting and tubing**
Canoeing, kayaking, rafting and tubing in calm and turbulent water

● **E002.6** **Water skiing and wake boarding**

● **E002.7** **Surfing, windsurfing and boogie boarding**

● **E002.8** **Water sliding**

● **E002.9** **Other activity involving water and watercraft**
Activity involving water NOS
Parasailing
Water survival training and testing

● **E003** **Activities involving ice and snow**

Excludes: *shoveling ice and snow (E016.0)*

● **E003.0** **Ice skating**
Figure skating (singles) (pairs)
Ice dancing

Excludes: *ice hockey (E003.1)*

● **E003.1** **Ice hockey**

● **E003.2** **Snow (alpine) (downhill) skiing, snow boarding, sledding, tobogganing and snow
tubing**

Excludes: *cross country skiing (E003.3)*

● **E003.3** **Cross country skiing**
Nordic skiing

● **E003.9** **Other activity involving ice and snow**
Activity involving ice and snow NOS

● **E004** **Activities involving climbing, rappelling and jumping off**

Excludes: *hiking on level or elevated terrain (E001.0)*
jumping rope (E006.5)
sky diving (E840-E844)
trampoline jumping (E005.3)

● **E004.0** **Mountain climbing, rock climbing and wall climbing**

● **E004.1** **Rappelling**

● **E004.2** **BASE jumping**
Building, Antenna, Span, Earth jumping

● **E004.3** **Bungee jumping**

● **E004.4** **Hang gliding**

● Code new
to this edition

▲ Revision of
existing code

④ ⑤ Fourth or fifth
digit required

- **E004.9** Other activity involving climbing, rappelling and jumping off
- **E005** Activities involving dancing and other rhythmic movement

  Excludes: martial arts (E008.4)

- **E005.0** Dancing
- **E005.1** Yoga
- **E005.2** Gymnastics
  Rhythmic gymnastics

  Excludes: trampoline (E005.3)

- **E005.3** Trampoline
- **E005.4** Cheerleading
- **E005.9** Other activity involving dancing and other rhythmic movements
- **E006** Activities involving other sports and athletics played individually

  Excludes: dancing (E005.0)
  gymnastic (E005.2)
  trampoline (E005.3)
  yoga (E005.1)

- **E006.0** Roller skating (inline) and skateboarding
- **E006.1** Horseback riding
- **E006.2** Golf
- **E006.3** Bowling
- **E006.4** Bike riding

  Excludes: transport accident involving bike riding (E800-E829)

- **E006.5** Jumping rope
- **E006.6** Non-running track and field events

  Excludes: running (any form) (E001.1)

- **E006.9** Other activity involving other sports and athletics played individually

  Excludes: activities involving climbing, rappelling, and jumping (E004.0-E004.9)
  activities involving ice and snow (E003.0-E003.9)
  activities involving walking and running (E001.0-E001.9)
  activities involving water and watercraft (E002.0-E002.9)

- **E007** Activities involving other sports and athletics played as a team or group

  Excludes: ice hockey (E003.1)
  water polo (E002.2)

- **E007.0** American tackle football
  Football NOS
- **E007.1** American flag or touch football
- **E007.2** Rugby
- **E007.3** Baseball
  Softball
- **E007.4** Lacrosse and field hockey
- **E007.5** Soccer
- **E007.6** Basketball
- **E007.7** Volleyball (beach) (court)
- **E007.8** Physical games generally associated with school recess, summer camp and children
  Capture the flag
  Dodge ball
  Four square
  Kickball
- **E007.9** Other activity involving other sports and athletics played as a team or group
  Cricket
- **E008** Activities involving other specified sports and athletics
- **E008.0** Boxing
- **E008.1** Wrestling

Add 4th or 5th digit   Nonspecific code   Unspecified code   Manifestation code

● **E008.2** **Racquet and hand sports**
Handball
Racquetball
Squash
Tennis

● **E008.3** **Frisbee**
Ultimate frisbee

● **E008.4** **Martial arts**
Combatives

● **E008.9** **Other specified sports and athletics activity**

Excludes: sports and athletics activities specified in categories E001-E007

●● **E009** **Activity involving other cardiorespiratory exercise**
Activity involving physical training

● **E009.0** **Exercise machines primarily for cardiorespiratory conditioning**
Elliptical and stepper machines
Stationary bike
Treadmill

● **E009.1** **Calisthenics**
Jumping jacks
Warm up and cool down

● **E009.2** **Aerobic and step exercise**

● **E009.3** **Circuit training**

● **E009.4** **Obstacle course**
Challenge course
Confidence course

● **E009.5** **Grass drills**
Guerilla drills

● **E009.9** **Other activity involving other cardiorespiratory exercise**

Excludes: activities involving cardiorespiratory exercise specified in categories E001-E008

●● **E010** **Activity involving other muscle strengthening exercises**

● **E010.0** **Exercise machines primarily for muscle strengthening**

● **E010.1** **Push-ups, pull-ups, sit-ups**

● **E010.2** **Free weights**
Barbells
Dumbbells

● **E010.3** **Pilates**

● **E010.9** **Other activity involving other muscle strengthening exercises**

Excludes: activities involving muscle strengthening specified in categories E001-E009

●● **E011** **Activities involving computer technology and electronic devices**

Excludes: electronic musical keyboard or instruments (E018.0)

● **E011.0** **Computer keyboarding**
Electronic game playing using keyboard or other stationary device

● **E011.1** **Hand held interactive electronic device**
Cellular telephone and communication device
Electronic game playing using interactive device

Excludes: electronic game playing using keyboard or other stationary device (E011.0)

● **E011.9** **Other activity involving computer technology and electronic devices**

●● **E012** **Activities involving arts and handcrafts**

Excludes: activities involving playing musical instrument (E018.0-E018.3)

● **E012.0** **Knitting and crocheting**

● **E012.1** **Sewing**

● **E012.2** **Furniture building and finishing**
Furniture repair

● **E012.9** **Activity involving other arts and handcrafts**

● Code new
to this edition   ▲ Revision of
existing code   ④ ⑤ Fourth or fifth
digit required

● **E013** **Activities involving personal hygiene and household maintenance**

> *Excludes:* activities involving cooking and grilling (E015.0-E015.9)
> activities involving property and land maintenance, building and construction (E016.0-E016.9)
> activity involving persons providing caregiving (E014.0-E014.9)
> dishwashing (E015.0)
> food preparation (E015.0)
> gardening (E016.1)

- ● E013.0 **Personal bathing and showering**
- ● E013.1 **Laundry**
- ● E013.2 **Vacuuming**
- ● E013.3 **Ironing**
- ● E013.4 **Floor mopping and cleaning**
- ● E013.5 **Residential relocation**
  Packing up and unpacking involved in moving to a new residence
- ● **E013.8** **Other personal hygiene activity**
- ● **E013.9** **Other household maintenance**

● **E014** **Activities involving person providing caregiving**

- ● E014.0 **Caregiving involving bathing**
- ● E014.1 **Caregiving involving lifting**
- ● **E014.9** **Other activity involving person providing caregiving**

● **E015** **Activities involving food preparation, cooking and grilling**

- ● E015.0 **Food preparation and clean up**
  Dishwashing
- ● E015.1 **Grilling and smoking food**
- ● E015.2 **Cooking and baking**
  Use of stove, oven and microwave oven
- ● **E015.9** **Other activity involving cooking and grilling**

● **E016** **Activities involving property and land maintenance, building and construction**

- ● E016.0 **Digging, shoveling and raking**
  Dirt digging
  Raking leaves
  Snow shoveling
- ● E016.1 **Gardening and landscaping**
  Pruning, trimming shrubs, weeding
- ● E016.2 **Building and construction**
- ● **E016.9** **Other activity involving property and land maintenance, building and construction**

● **E017** **Activities involving roller coasters and other types of external motion**

- ● E017.0 **Rollercoaster riding**
- ● **E017.9** **Other activity involving external motion**

● **E018** **Activities involving playing musical instrument**
  Activity involving playing electric musical instrument

- ● E018.0 **Piano playing**
  Musical keyboard (electronic) playing
- ● **E018.1** **Drum and other percussion instrument playing**
- ● E018.2 **String instrument playing**
- ● E018.3 **Wind and brass instrument playing**

● **E019** **Activities involving animal care**

> *Excludes:* horseback riding (E006.1)

- ● E019.0 **Walking an animal**
- ● E019.1 **Milking an animal**
- ● E019.2 **Grooming and shearing an animal**
- ● **E019.9** **Other activity involving animal care**

● **E029** **Other activity**

- ● E029.0 **Refereeing a sports activity**
- ● E029.1 **Spectator at an event**

| | Add 4th or 5th digit | | Nonspecific code | | Unspecified code | | Manifestation code |

- ● **E029.2**   **Rough housing and horseplay**
- ● **E029.9**   **Other activity**
- ● **E030** **Unspecified activity**

TRANSPORT ACCIDENTS (E800-E848)

Definitions and examples related to transport accidents

(a) A **transport accident** (E800-E848) is any accident involving a device designed primarily for, or being used at the time primarily for, conveying persons or goods from one place to another.

    Includes: accidents involving:
- aircraft and spacecraft (E840-E845)
- watercraft (E830-E838)
- motor vehicle (E810-E825)
- railway (E800-E807)
- other road vehicles (E826-E829)

In classifying accidents which involve more than one kind of transport, the above order of precedence of transport accidents should be used.

Accidents involving agriculture and construction machines, such as tractors, cranes, and bulldozers, are regarded as transport accidents only when these vehicles are under their own power on a highway [otherwise the vehicles are regarded as machinery]. Vehicles which can travel on land or water, such as hovercraft and other amphibious vehicles, are regarded as watercraft when on the water, as motor vehicles when on the highway, and as off-road motor vehicles when on land, but off the highway.

| Excludes: | *accidents:*
in sports which involve the use of transport but where the transport vehicle itself was not involved in the accident
involving vehicles which are part of industrial equipment used entirely on industrial premises
occurring during transportation but unrelated to the hazards associated with the means of transportation [e.g., injuries received in a fight on board ship; transport vehicle involved in a cataclysm such as an earthquake]
to persons engaged in the maintenance or repair of transport equipment or vehicle not in motion, unless injured by another vehicle in motion

(b) A **railway accident** is a transport accident involving a railway train or other railway vehicle operated on rails, whether in motion or not.

| Excludes: | *accidents:*
in repair shops
in roundhouse or on turntable
on railway premises but not involving a train or other railway vehicle

(c) A **railway train** or **railway vehicle** is any device with or without cars coupled to it, designed for traffic on a railway.

    Includes: interurban:
- electric car (operated chiefly on its own right-of-way, not open to other traffic)
- streetcar (operated chiefly on its own right-of-way, not open to other traffic)
- railway train, any power [diesel] [electric] [steam]
- funicular
- monorail or two-rail
- subterranean or elevated
- other vehicle designed to run on a railway track

| Excludes: | *interurban electric cars [streetcars] specified to be operating on a right-of-way that forms part of the public street or highway [definition (n)]*

(d) A **railway** or **railroad** is a right-of-way designed for traffic on rails, which is used by carriages or wagons transporting passengers or freight, and by other rolling stock, and which is not open to other public vehicular traffic.

(e) A **motor vehicle accident** is a transport accident involving a motor vehicle. It is defined as a motor vehicle traffic accident or as a motor vehicle nontraffic accident according to whether the accident occurs on a public highway or elsewhere.

| Excludes: | *injury or damage due to cataclysm*
injury or damage while a motor vehicle, not under its own power, is being loaded on, or unloaded from, another conveyance

(f) A **motor vehicle traffic accident** is any motor vehicle accident occurring on a public highway [i.e., originating, terminating, or involving a vehicle partially on the highway]. A motor vehicle accident is assumed to have occurred on the highway unless another place is specified, except in the case of accidents involving only off-road motor vehicles which are classified as nontraffic accidents unless the contrary is stated.

(g) A **motor vehicle nontraffic accident** is any motor vehicle accident which occurs entirely in any place other than a public highway.

● Code new to this edition   ▲ Revision of existing code   ④ ⑤ Fourth or fifth digit required

E CODES

(h) A **public highway [trafficway]** or **street** is the entire width between property lines [or other boundary lines] of every way or place, of which any part is open to the use of the public for purposes of vehicular traffic as a matter of right or custom. A roadway is that part of the public highway designed, improved, and ordinarily used, for vehicular travel.

Includes: approaches (public) to:
docks
public building
station

Excludes: *driveway (private)*
parking lot
ramp
roads in:
airfield
farm
industrial premises
mine
private grounds
quarry

(i) A **motor vehicle** is any mechanically or electrically powered device, not operated on rails, upon which any person or property may be transported or drawn upon a highway. Any object such as a trailer, coaster, sled, or wagon being towed by a motor vehicle is considered a part of the motor vehicle.

Includes: automobile [any type]
bus
construction machinery, farm and industrial machinery, steam roller, tractor, army tank, highway grader, or similar vehicle on wheels or treads, while in transport under own power
fire engine (motorized)
motorcycle
motorized bicycle [moped] or scooter
trolley bus not operating on rails
truck
van

Excludes: *devices used solely to move persons or materials within the confines of a building and its premises, such as:*
building elevator
coal car in mine
electric baggage or mail truck used solely within a railroad station
electric truck used solely within an industrial plant
moving overhead crane

(j) A **motorcycle** is a two-wheeled motor vehicle having one or two riding saddles and sometimes having a third wheel for the support of a sidecar. The sidecar is considered part of the motorcycle.

Includes: motorized:
bicycle [moped]
scooter
tricycle

(k) An **off-road motor vehicle** is a motor vehicle of special design, to enable it to negotiate rough or soft terrain or snow. Examples of special design are high construction, special wheels and tires, driven by treads, or support on a cushion of air.

Includes: all terrain vehicle [ATV]
army tank
hovercraft, on land or swamp
snowmobile

(l) A **driver** of a motor vehicle is the occupant of the motor vehicle operating it or intending to operate it. A **motorcyclist** is the driver of a motorcycle. Other authorized occupants of a motor vehicle are **passengers.**

(m) An **other road vehicle** is any device, except a motor vehicle, in, on, or by which any person or property may be transported on a highway.

Includes: animal carrying a person or goods
animal-drawn vehicle
animal harnessed to conveyance
bicycle [pedal cycle]
streetcar
tricycle (pedal)

Excludes: *pedestrian conveyance [definition (q)]*

| Add 4th or 5th digit | Nonspecific code | Unspecified code | Manifestation code |

(n) A **streetcar** is a device designed and used primarily for transporting persons within a municipality, running on rails, usually subject to normal traffic control signals, and operated principally on a right-of-way that forms part of the traffic way. A trailer being towed by a streetcar is considered a part of the streetcar.

    Includes: interurban or intraurban electric or streetcar, when specified to be operating on a street or public highway
           tram (car)
           trolley (car)

(o) A **pedal cycle** is any road transport vehicle operated solely by pedals.

    Includes: bicycle
           pedal cycle
           tricycle

    Excludes: *motorized bicycle [definition (i)]*

(p) A **pedal cyclist** is any person riding on a pedal cycle or in a sidecar attached to such a vehicle.

(q) A **pedestrian conveyance** is any human powered device by which a pedestrian may move other than by walking or by which a walking person may move another pedestrian.

    Includes:

baby carriage	roller skates
coaster wagon	scooter
heelies	skateboard
ice skates	skis
perambulator	sled
pushcart	wheelchair
pushchair	wheelies

(r) A **pedestrian** is any person involved in an accident who was not at the time of the accident riding in or on a motor vehicle, railroad train, streetcar, animal-drawn or other vehicle, or on a bicycle or animal.

    Includes: person:
           changing tire of vehicle
           in or operating a pedestrian conveyance
           making adjustment to motor of vehicle
           on foot

(s) A **watercraft** is any device for transporting passengers or goods on the water.

(t) A **small boat** is any watercraft propelled by paddle, oars, or small motor, with a passenger capacity of less than ten.

    Includes:

boat NOS	rowboat
canoe	rowing shell
coble	scull
dinghy	skiff
punt	small motorboat
raft	

    Excludes: *barge*
           lifeboat (used after abandoning ship)
           raft (anchored) being used as diving platform
           yacht

(u) An **aircraft** is any device for transporting passengers or goods in the air.

    Includes: airplane [any type]
           balloon
           bomber
           dirigible
           glider (hang)
           military aircraft
           parachute

(v) A **commercial transport aircraft** is any device for collective passenger or freight transportation by air, whether run on commercial lines for profit or by government authorities, with the exception of military craft.

   ● Code new
      to this edition
      ▲ Revision of
        existing code
      ④ ⑤ Fourth or fifth
        digit required

RAILWAY ACCIDENTS (E800-E807)

Note: For definitions of railway accident and related terms see definitions (a) to (d).

> Excludes: *accidents involving railway train and:*
> *aircraft (E840.0-E845.9)*
> *motor vehicle (E810.0-E825.9)*
> *watercraft (E830.0-E838.9)*

The following fourth-digit subdivisions are for use with categories E800-E807 to identify the injured person:

.0 Railway employee
Any person who by virtue of his employment in connection with a railway, whether by the railway company or not, is at increased risk of involvement in a railway accident, such as:
catering staff of train
driver
guard
porter
postal staff on train
railway fireman
shunter
sleeping car attendant

.1 Passenger on railway
Any authorized person traveling on a train, except a railway employee.

> Excludes: *intending passenger waiting at station (.8)*
> *unauthorized rider on railway vehicle (.8)*

.2 Pedestrian
See definition (r)

.3 Pedal cyclist
See definition (p)

.8 Other specified person
Intending passenger or bystander waiting at station
Unauthorized rider on railway vehicle

.9 Unspecified person

④ **E800** **Railway accident involving collision with rolling stock**
Includes: collision between railway trains or railway vehicles, any kind
collision NOS on railway
derailment with antecedent collision with rolling stock or NOS

④ **E801** **Railway accident involving collision with other object**
Includes: collision of railway train with:
buffers
fallen tree on railway
gates
platform
rock on railway
streetcar
other nonmotor vehicle
other object

> Excludes: *collision with:*
> *aircraft (E840.0-E842.9)*
> *motor vehicle (E810.0-E810.9, E820.0-E822.9)*

④ **E802** **Railway accident involving derailment without antecedent collision**

④ **E803** **Railway accident involving explosion, fire, or burning**

> Excludes: *explosion or fire, with antecedent derailment (E802.0-E802.9)*
> *explosion or fire, with mention of antecedent collision (E800.0-E801.9)*

④ **E804** **Fall in, on, or from railway train**
Includes: fall while alighting from or boarding railway train

> Excludes: *fall related to collision, derailment, or explosion of railway train (E800.0-E803.9)*

	Add 4th or 5th digit		Nonspecific code		Unspecified code		Manifestation code

TABULAR LIST

④ **E805 Hit by rolling stock**
　Includes:　crushed by railway train or part
　　　　　　injured by railway train or part
　　　　　　killed by railway train or part
　　　　　　knocked down by railway train or part
　　　　　　run over by railway train or part

　Excludes: pedestrian hit by object set in motion by railway train (E806.0-E806.9)

④ **E806 Other specified railway accident**
　Includes:　hit by object falling in railway train
　　　　　　injured by door or window on railway train
　　　　　　nonmotor road vehicle or pedestrian hit by object set in motion by railway train
　　　　　　railway train hit by falling:
　　　　　　earth NOS
　　　　　　rock
　　　　　　tree
　　　　　　other object

　Excludes: railway accident due to cataclysm (E908-E909)

④ **E807 Railway accident of unspecified nature**
　Includes:
　　　　　　found dead on railway right-of-way NOS
　　　　　　injured on railway right-of-way NOS
　　　　　　railway accident NOS

MOTOR VEHICLE TRAFFIC ACCIDENTS (E810-E819)

　Note: For definitions of motor vehicle traffic accident, and related terms, see definitions (e) to (k).

　Excludes: accidents involving motor vehicle and aircraft (E840.0-E845.9)

　The following fourth-digit subdivisions are for use with categories E810-E819 to identify the injured person:

.0 Driver of motor vehicle other than motorcycle
　See definition (l)

.1 Passenger in motor vehicle other than motorcycle
　See definition (l)

.2 Motorcyclist
　See definition (l)

.3 Passenger on motorcycle
　See definition (l)

.4 Occupant of streetcar

.5 Rider of animal; occupant of animal-drawn vehicle

.6 Pedal cyclist
　See definition (p)

.7 Pedestrian
　See definition (r)

.8 Other specified person
　Occupant of vehicle other than above
　Person in railway train involved in accident
　Unauthorized rider of motor vehicle

.9 Unspecified person

④ **E810 Motor vehicle traffic accident involving collision with train**

　Excludes: motor vehicle collision with object set in motion by railway train (E815.0-E815.9)
　　　　　　railway train hit by object set in motion by motor vehicle (E818.0-E818.9)

④ **E811 Motor vehicle traffic accident involving re-entrant collision with another motor vehicle**
　Includes:　collision between motor vehicle which accidentally leaves the roadway then re-enters the same roadway, or the opposite roadway on a divided highway, and another motor vehicle

　Excludes: collision on the same roadway when none of the motor vehicles involved have left and re-entered the roadway (E812.0-E812.9)

④ **E812 Other motor vehicle traffic accident involving collision with motor vehicle**
　Includes:　collision with another motor vehicle parked, stopped, stalled, disabled, or abandoned on the highway
　　　　　　motor vehicle collision NOS

　Excludes: collision with object set in motion by another motor vehicle (E815.0-E815.9)
　　　　　　re-entrant collision with another motor vehicle (E811.0-E811.9)

　● Code new to this edition　　▲ Revision of existing code　　④ ⑤ Fourth or fifth digit required

④ **E813** **Motor vehicle traffic accident involving collision with other vehicle**
      Includes: collision between motor vehicle, any kind, and:
               other road (nonmotor transport) vehicle, such as:
                   animal carrying a person
                   animal-drawn vehicle
                   pedal cycle
                   streetcar

    |Excludes:| *collision with:*
        object set in motion by nonmotor road vehicle (E815.0-E815.9)
        pedestrian (E814.0-E814.9)
        nonmotor road vehicle hit by object set in motion by motor vehicle (E818.0-E818.9)

④ **E814** **Motor vehicle traffic accident involving collision with pedestrian**
      Includes: collision between motor vehicle, any kind, and pedestrian
              pedestrian dragged, hit, or run over by motor vehicle, any kind

    |Excludes:| *pedestrian hit by object set in motion by motor vehicle (E818.0-E818.9)*

④ **E815** **Other motor vehicle traffic accident involving collision on the highway**
      Includes: collision (due to loss of control) (on highway) between motor vehicle, any kind, and:
              abutment (bridge) (overpass)
              animal (herded) (unattended)
              fallen stone, traffic sign, tree, utility pole
              guard rail or boundary fence
              interhighway divider
              landslide (not moving)
              object set in motion by railway train or road vehicle (motor) (nonmotor)
              object thrown in front of motor vehicle
              safety island
              temporary traffic sign or marker
              wall of cut made for road
              other object, fixed, movable, or moving

    |Excludes:| *collision with:*
        any object off the highway (resulting from loss of control) (E816.0-E816.9)
        any object which normally would have been off the highway and is not stated to have been on it (E816.0-E816.9)
        motor vehicle parked, stopped, stalled, disabled, or abandoned on highway (E812.0-E812.9)
        moving landslide (E909)
      motor vehicle hit by object:
        set in motion by railway train or road vehicle (motor) (nonmotor) (E818.0-E818.9)
        thrown into or on vehicle (E818.0-E818.9)

④ **E816** **Motor vehicle traffic accident due to loss of control, without collision on the highway**
    Includes: motor vehicle:
          failing to make curve and:
            colliding with object off the highway
            overturning
            stopping abruptly off the highway
          going out of control (due to):
            blowout and:
              colliding with object off the highway
              overturning
              stopping abruptly off the highway
            burst tire and:
              colliding with object off the highway
              overturning
              stopping abruptly off the highway
            driver falling asleep and:
              colliding with object off the highway
              overturning
              stopping abruptly off the highway
            driver inattention and:
              colliding with object off the highway
              overturning
              stopping abruptly off the highway
            excessive speed and:
              colliding with object off the highway
              overturning
              stopping abruptly off the highway
            failure of mechanical part and:
              colliding with object off the highway
              overturning
              stopping abruptly off the highway

    Excludes: *collision on highway following loss of control (E810.0-E815.9)*
          loss of control of motor vehicle following collision on the highway
           (E810.0-E815.9)

④ **E817** **Noncollision motor vehicle traffic accident while boarding or alighting**
    Includes: fall down stairs of motor bus while boarding or alighting
             fall from car in street while boarding or alighting
             injured by moving part of the vehicle while boarding or alighting
             trapped by door of motor bus while boarding or alighting

④ **E818** **Other noncollision motor vehicle traffic accident**
    Includes: accidental poisoning from exhaust gas generated by motor vehicle while in motion
             breakage of any part of motor vehicle while in motion
             explosion of any part of motor vehicle while in motion
             fall, jump, or being accidentally pushed from motor vehicle while in motion
             fire starting in motor vehicle while in motion
             hit by object thrown into or on motor vehicle while in motion
             injured by being thrown against some part of, or object in motor vehicle while in
               motion
             injury from moving part of motor vehicle while in motion
             object falling in or on motor vehicle while in motion
             object thrown on motor vehicle while in motion
             collision of railway train or road vehicle except motor vehicle, with object set in
               motion by motor vehicle
             motor vehicle hit by object set in motion by railway train or road vehicle (motor)
               (nonmotor)
             pedestrian, railway train, or road vehicle (motor) (nonmotor) hit by object set in
               motion by motor vehicle

    Excludes: *collision between motor vehicle and:*
          object set in motion by railway train or road vehicle (motor) (nonmotor)
            (E815.0-E815.9)
          object thrown towards the motor vehicle (E815.0-E815.9)
          person overcome by carbon monoxide generated by stationary motor vehicle off
           the roadway with motor running (E868.2)

④ **E819** **Motor vehicle traffic accident of unspecified nature**
    Includes: motor vehicle traffic accident NOS
             traffic accident NOS

  ● Code new   ▲ Revision of   ④ ⑤ Fourth or fifth
      to this edition   existing code   digit required

MOTOR VEHICLE NONTRAFFIC ACCIDENTS (E820-E825)

Note: For definitions of motor vehicle nontraffic accident and related terms see definitions (a) to (k).

Includes: accidents involving motor vehicles being used in recreational or sporting activities off the highway
collision and noncollision motor vehicle accidents occurring entirely off the highway

Excludes: *accidents involving motor vehicle and:*
aircraft (E840.0-E845.9)
watercraft (E830.0-E838.9)
accidents, not on the public highway, involving agricultural and construction machinery but not involving another motor vehicle (E919.0, E919.2, E919.7)

The following fourth-digit subdivisions are for use with categories E820-E825 to identify the injured person:

.0 Driver of motor vehicle other than motorcycle
See definition (l)

.1 Passenger in motor vehicle other than motorcycle
See definition (l)

.2 Motorcyclist
See definition (l)

.3 Passenger on motorcycle
See definition (l)

.4 Occupant of streetcar

.5 Rider of animal; occupant of animal-drawn vehicle

.6 Pedal cyclist
See definition (p)

.7 Pedestrian
See definition (r)

.8 Other specified person
Occupant of vehicle other than above
Person on railway train involved in accident
Unauthorized rider of motor vehicle

.9 Unspecified person

④ **E820 Nontraffic accident involving motor-driven snow vehicle**
Includes: breakage of part of motor-driven snow vehicle (not on public highway)
fall from motor-driven snow vehicle (not on public highway)
hit by motor-driven snow vehicle (not on public highway)
overturning of motor-driven snow vehicle (not on public highway)
run over or dragged by motor-driven snow vehicle (not on public highway)
collision of motor-driven snow vehicle with:
animal (being ridden) (-drawn vehicle)
another off-road motor vehicle
other motor vehicle, not on public highway
railway train
other object, fixed or movable
injury caused by rough landing of motor-driven snow vehicle (after leaving ground on rough terrain)

Excludes: *accident on the public highway involving motor driven snow vehicle (E810.0-E819.9)*

| | Add 4th or 5th digit | | Nonspecific code | | Unspecified code | | Manifestation code |

④ **E821** **Nontraffic accident involving other off-road motor vehicle**

Includes: breakage of part of off-road motor vehicle, except snow vehicle (not on public highway)

fall from off-road motor vehicle, except snow vehicle (not on public highway)

hit by off-road motor vehicle, except snow vehicle (not on public highway)

overturning of off-road motor vehicle, except snow vehicle (not on public highway)

run over or dragged by off-road motor vehicle, except snow vehicle (not on public highway)

thrown against some part of or object in off-road motor vehicle, except snow vehicle (not on public highway)

collision with:

animal (being ridden) (-drawn vehicle)

another off-road motor vehicle, except snow vehicle

other motor vehicle, not on public highway

other object, fixed or movable

Excludes: *accident on public highway involving off-road motor vehicle (E810.0-E819.9)*

collision between motor driven snow vehicle and other off-road motor vehicle (E820.0-E820.9)

hovercraft accident on water (E830.0-E838.9)

④ **E822** **Other motor vehicle nontraffic accident involving collision with moving object**

Includes: collision, not on public highway, between motor vehicle, except off-road motor vehicle and:

animal

nonmotor vehicle

other motor vehicle, except off-road motor vehicle

pedestrian

railway train

other moving object

Excludes: *collision with:*

motor-driven snow vehicle (E820.0-E820.9)

other off-road motor vehicle (E821.0-E821.9)

④ **E823** **Other motor vehicle nontraffic accident involving collision with stationary object**

Includes: collision, not on public highway, between motor vehicle, except off-road motor vehicle, and any object, fixed or movable, but not in motion

④ **E824** **Other motor vehicle nontraffic accident while boarding and alighting**

Includes: fall while boarding or alighting from motor vehicle, except off-road motor vehicle, not on public highway

injury from moving part of motor vehicle while boarding or alighting from motor vehicle, except off-road motor vehicle, not on public highway

trapped by door of motor vehicle while boarding or alighting from motor vehicle, except off-road motor vehicle, not on public highway

④ **E825** **Other motor vehicle nontraffic accident of other and unspecified nature**

Includes: accidental poisoning from carbon monoxide generated by motor vehicle while in motion, not on public highway

breakage of any part of motor vehicle while in motion, not on public highway

explosion of any part of motor vehicle while in motion, not on public highway

fall, jump, or being accidentally pushed from motor vehicle while in motion, not on public highway

fire starting in motor vehicle while in motion, not on public highway

hit by object thrown into, towards, or on motor vehicle while in motion, not on public highway

injured by being thrown against some part of, or object in motor vehicle while in motion, not on public highway

injury from moving part of motor vehicle while in motion, not on public highway

object falling in or on motor vehicle while in motion, not on public highway

motor vehicle nontraffic accident NOS

Excludes: *fall from or in stationary motor vehicle (E884.9, E885.9)*

overcome by carbon monoxide or exhaust gas generated by stationary motor vehicle off the roadway with motor running (E868.2)

struck by falling object from or in stationary motor vehicle (E916)

● Code new to this edition   ▲ Revision of existing code   ④ ⑤ Fourth or fifth digit required

OTHER ROAD VEHICLE ACCIDENTS (E826-E829)

Note: Other road vehicle accidents are transport accidents involving road vehicles other than motor vehicles. For definitions of other road vehicle and related terms see definitions (m) to (o).

Includes: accidents involving other road vehicles being used in recreational or sporting activities

Excludes: *collision of other road vehicle [any] with:*
   aircraft (E840.0-E845.9)
   motor vehicle (E813.0-E813.9, E820.0-E822.9)
   railway train (E801.0-E801.9)

The following fourth-digit subdivisions are for use with categories E826-E829 to identify the injured person:

.0 Pedestrian
   See definition (r)

.1 Pedal cyclist
   See definition (p)

.2 Rider of animal

.3 Occupant of animal-drawn vehicle

.4 Occupant of streetcar

.8 Other specified person

.9 Unspecified person

④ **E826 Pedal cycle accident**
[0-9]

Includes: breakage of any part of pedal cycle
   collision between pedal cycle and:
     animal (being ridden) (herded) (unattended)
     another pedal cycle
     nonmotor road vehicle, any
     pedestrian
     other object, fixed, movable, or moving, not set in motion by motor vehicle, railway train, or aircraft
   entanglement in wheel of pedal cycle
   fall from pedal cycle
   hit by object falling or thrown on the pedal cycle
   pedal cycle accident NOS
   pedal cycle overturned

④ **E827 Animal-drawn vehicle accident**
[0,2-4,8,9]

Includes: breakage of any part of vehicle
   collision between animal-drawn vehicle and:
     animal (being ridden) (herded) (unattended)
     nonmotor road vehicle, except pedal cycle
     pedestrian, pedestrian conveyance, or pedestrian vehicle
     other object, fixed, movable, or moving, not set in motion by motor vehicle, railway train, or aircraft
   fall from animal-drawn vehicle
   knocked down by animal-drawn vehicle
   overturning of animal-drawn vehicle
   run over by animal-drawn vehicle
   thrown from animal-drawn vehicle

Excludes: *collision of animal-drawn vehicle with pedal cycle (E826.0-E826.9)*

	Add 4th or 5th digit		Nonspecific code		Unspecified code		Manifestation code

④ **E828** **Accident involving animal being ridden**
[0,2,4,8,9]

Includes: collision between animal being ridden and:
    another animal
    nonmotor road vehicle, except pedal cycle, and animal-drawn vehicle
    pedestrian, pedestrian conveyance, or pedestrian vehicle
    other object, fixed, movable, or moving, not set in motion by motor vehicle,
        railway train, or aircraft
fall from animal being ridden
knocked down by animal being ridden
thrown from animal being ridden
trampled by animal being ridden
ridden animal stumbled and fell

Excludes: *collision of animal being ridden with:*
    animal-drawn vehicle (E827.0-E827.9)
    pedal cycle (E826.0-E826.9)

④ **E829** **Other road vehicle accidents**
[0,4,8,9]

Includes: accident while boarding or alighting from:
    streetcar
    nonmotor road vehicle not classifiable to E826-E828
blow from object in:
    streetcar
    nonmotor road vehicle not classifiable to E826-E828
breakage of any part of:
    streetcar
    nonmotor road vehicle not classifiable to E826-E828
caught in door of:
    streetcar
    nonmotor road vehicle not classifiable to E826-E828
derailment of:
    streetcar
    nonmotor road vehicle not classifiable to E826-E828
fall in, on, or from:
    streetcar
    nonmotor road vehicle not classifiable to E826-E828
fire in:
    streetcar
    nonmotor road vehicle not classifiable to E826-E828
collision between streetcar or nonmotor road vehicle, except as in E826-E828, and:
    animal (not being ridden)
    another nonmotor road vehicle not classifiable to E826-E828
    pedestrian
    other object, fixed, movable, or moving, not set in motion by motor vehicle,
        railway train, or aircraft
nonmotor road vehicle accident NOS
streetcar accident NOS

Excludes: *collision with:*
    animal being ridden (E828.0-E828.9)
    animal-drawn vehicle (E827.0-E827.9)
    pedal cycle (E826.0-E826.9)

● Code new   ▲ Revision of   ④ ⑤ Fourth or fifth
    to this edition   existing code   digit required

E CODES

WATER TRANSPORT ACCIDENTS (E830-E838)

Note: For definitions of water transport accident and related terms see definitions (a), (s), and (t).

Includes: watercraft accidents in the course of recreational activities

Excludes: *accidents involving both aircraft, including objects set in motion by aircraft, and watercraft (E840.0-E845.9)*

The following fourth-digit subdivisions are for use with categories E830-E838 to identify the injured person:

.0 Occupant of small boat, unpowered

.1 Occupant of small boat, powered
   See definition (t)

Excludes: *water skier (.4)*

.2 Occupant of other watercraft—crew
   Persons:
   engaged in operation of watercraft
   providing passenger services [cabin attendants, ship's physician, catering personnel]
   working on ship during voyage in other capacity [musician in band, operators of shops and beauty parlors]

.3 Occupant of other watercraft—other than crew
   Passenger
   Occupant of lifeboat, other than crew, after abandoning ship

.4 Water skier

.5 Swimmer

.6 Dockers, stevedores
   Longshoreman employed on the dock in loading and unloading ships

.7 Occupant of military watercraft, any type

.8 Other specified person
   Immigration and custom officials on board ship
   Person:
   accompanying passenger or member of crew
   visiting boat
   Pilot (guiding ship into port)

.9 Unspecified person

④ **E830 Accident to watercraft causing submersion**
   Includes: submersion and drowning due to:
   boat overturning
   boat submerging
   falling or jumping from burning ship
   falling or jumping from crushed watercraft
   ship sinking
   other accident to watercraft

④ **E831 Accident to watercraft causing other injury**
   Includes: any injury, except submersion and drowning, as a result of an accident to watercraft
   burned while ship on fire
   crushed between ships in collision
   crushed by lifeboat after abandoning ship
   fall due to collision or other accident to watercraft
   hit by falling object due to accident to watercraft
   injured in watercraft accident involving collision
   struck by boat or part thereof after fall or jump from damaged boat

   Excludes: *burns from localized fire or explosion on board ship (E837.0-E837.9)*

④ **E832 Other accidental submersion or drowning in water transport accident**
   Includes: submersion or drowning as a result of an accident other than accident to the watercraft, such as:
   fall:
   from gangplank
   from ship
   overboard
   thrown overboard by motion of ship
   washed overboard

   Excludes: *submersion or drowning of swimmer or diver who voluntarily jumps from boat not involved in an accident (E910.0-E910.9)*

723

	Add 4th or 5th digit		Nonspecific code		Unspecified code		Manifestation code

E833 **Fall on stairs or ladders in water transport**
    Excludes: *fall due to accident to watercraft (E831.0-E831.9)*

E834 **Other fall from one level to another in water transport**
    Excludes: *fall due to accident to watercraft (E831.0-E831.9)*

E835 **Other and unspecified fall in water transport**
    Excludes: *fall due to accident to watercraft (E831.0-E831.9)*

E836 **Machinery accident in water transport**
  Includes: injuries in water transport caused by:
      deck machinery
      engine room machinery
      galley machinery
      laundry machinery
      loading machinery

E837 **Explosion, fire, or burning in watercraft**
  Includes: explosion of boiler on steamship
      localized fire on ship
    Excludes: *burning ship (due to collision or explosion) resulting in:*
      submersion or drowning (E830.0-E830.9)
      other injury (E831.0-E831.9)

E838 **Other and unspecified water transport accident**
  Includes: accidental poisoning by gases or fumes on ship
      atomic power plant malfunction in watercraft
      crushed between ship and stationary object [wharf]
      crushed between ships without accident to watercraft
      crushed by falling object on ship or while loading or unloading
      hit by boat while water skiing
      struck by boat or part thereof (after fall from boat)
      watercraft accident NOS

AIR AND SPACE TRANSPORT ACCIDENTS (E840-E845)

Note: For definition of aircraft and related terms see definitions (u) and (v).

The following fourth-digit subdivisions are for use with categories E840-E845 to identify the injured person:

.0 **Occupant of spacecraft**

.1 **Occupant of military aircraft, any**
  Crew in military aircraft [air force] [army] [national guard] [navy]
  Passenger (civilian) (military) in military aircraft [air force] [army] [national guard] [navy]
  Troops in military aircraft [air force] [army] [national guard] [navy]
    Excludes: *occupants of aircraft operated under jurisdiction of police departments (.5)*
      parachutist (.7)

.2 **Crew of commercial aircraft (powered) in surface to surface transport**

.3 **Other occupant of commercial aircraft (powered) in surface to surface transport**
  Flight personnel:
    not part of crew
    on familiarization flight
  Passenger on aircraft (powered) NOS

.4 **Occupant of commercial aircraft (powered) in surface to air transport**
  Occupant [crew] [passenger] of aircraft (powered) engaged in activities, such as:
    aerial spraying (crops) (fire retardants)
    air drops of emergency supplies
    air drops of parachutists, except from military craft
    crop dusting
    lowering of construction material [bridge or telephone pole]
    sky writing

.5 **Occupant of other powered aircraft**
  Occupant [crew] [passenger] of aircraft [powered] engaged in activities, such as:
    aerobatic flying
    aircraft racing
    rescue operation
    storm surveillance
    traffic surveillance
  Occupant of private plane NOS

● Code new to this edition   ▲ Revision of existing code   ④ ⑤ Fourth or fifth digit required

.6 Occupant of unpowered aircraft, except parachutist
Occupant of aircraft classifiable to E842

.7 Parachutist (military) (other)
Person making voluntary descent

Excludes: *person making descent after accident to aircraft (.1-.6)*

.8 Ground crew, airline employee
Persons employed at airfields (civil) (military) or launching pads, not occupants of aircraft

.9 Other person

④ **E840 Accident to powered aircraft at takeoff or landing**
Includes: collision of aircraft with any object, fixed, movable, or moving while taking off or landing
crash while taking off or landing
explosion on aircraft while taking off or landing
fire on aircraft while taking off or landing
forced landing

④ **E841 Accident to powered aircraft, other and unspecified**
Includes: aircraft accident NOS
aircraft crash or wreck NOS
any accident to powered aircraft while in transit or when not specified whether in transit, taking off, or landing
collision of aircraft with another aircraft, bird, or any object, while in transit
explosion on aircraft while in transit
fire on aircraft while in transit

④ **E842 Accident to unpowered aircraft**
[6-9]
Includes: any accident, except collision with powered aircraft, to:
balloon
glider
hang glider
kite carrying a person
hit by object falling from unpowered aircraft

④ **E843 Fall in, on, or from aircraft**
[0-9]
Includes: accident in boarding or alighting from aircraft, any kind
fall in, on, or from aircraft [any kind], while in transit, taking off, or landing, except when as a result of an accident to aircraft

④ **E844 Other specified air transport accidents**
[0-9]
Includes: hit by:
aircraft without accident to aircraft
object falling from aircraft without accident to aircraft
injury by or from:
machinery on aircraft without accident to aircraft
rotating propeller without accident to aircraft
voluntary parachute descent without accident to aircraft
poisoning by carbon monoxide from aircraft while in transit without accident to aircraft
sucked into jet without accident to aircraft
any accident involving other transport vehicle (motor) (nonmotor) due to being hit by object set in motion by aircraft (powered)

Excludes: *air sickness (E903)*
effects of:
high altitude (E902.0-E902.1)
pressure change (E902.0-E902.1)
injury in parachute descent due to accident to aircraft (840.0-E842.9)

④ **E845 Accident involving spacecraft**
[0,8,9]
Includes: launching pad accident
Excludes: *effects of weightlessness in spacecraft (E928.0)*

	Add 4th or 5th digit		Nonspecific code		Unspecified code		Manifestation code

VEHICLE ACCIDENTS NOT ELSEWHERE CLASSIFIABLE (E846-E848)

E846 **Accidents involving powered vehicles used solely within the buildings and premises of industrial or commercial establishment**

Accident to, on, or involving:
    battery powered airport passenger vehicle
    battery powered trucks (baggage) (mail)
    coal car in mine
    logging car
    self propelled truck, industrial
    station baggage truck (powered)
    tram, truck, or tub (powered) in mine or quarry
Breakage of any part of vehicle
Collision with:
    pedestrian
    other vehicle or object within premises
Explosion of powered vehicle, industrial or commercial
Fall from powered vehicle, industrial or commercial
Overturning of powered vehicle, industrial or commercial
Struck by powered vehicle, industrial or commercial

> *Excludes:* *accidental poisoning by exhaust gas from vehicle not elsewhere classifiable*
>   *(E868.2)*
>   *injury by crane, lift (fork), or elevator (E919.2)*

E847 **Accidents involving cable cars not running on rails**

Accident to, on, or involving:
    cable car, not on rails
    ski chair-lift
    ski-lift with gondola
    téléférique
Breakage of cable
Caught or dragged by cable car, not on rails
Fall or jump from cable car, not on rails
Object thrown from or in cable car, not on rails

E848 **Accidents involving other vehicles, not elsewhere classifiable**

Accident to, on, or involving:
    ice yacht
    land yacht
    nonmotor, nonroad vehicle NOS

E849 **Place of occurrence**

The following category is for use to denote the place where the injury or poisoning occurred.

    E849.0 **Home**

Apartment	Private:
Boarding house	driveway
Farm house	garage
Home premises	garden
House (residential)	home
Noninstitutional place	walk
of residence	Swimming pool in private house or garden
	Yard of home

> *Excludes:* *home under construction but not yet occupied (E849.3)*
>   *institutional place of residence (E849.7)*

    E849.1 **Farm**

Farm:
    buildings
    land under cultivation

> *Excludes:* *farm house and home premises of farm (E849.0)*

    E849.2 **Mine and quarry**

Gravel pit	Tunnel under construction
Sand pit	

    E849.3 **Industrial place and premises**

Building under	Industrial yard
construction	Loading platform (factory) (store)
Dockyard	Plant, industrial
Dry dock	Railway yard
Factory	Shop (place of work)
building	Warehouse
premises	Workhouse
Garage (place of work)	

● Code new   ▲ Revision of   ④ ⑤ Fourth or fifth
  to this edition   existing code   digit required

E849.4 Place for recreation and sport

Amusement park
Baseball field
Basketball court
Beach resort
Cricket ground
Fives court
Football field
Golf course
Gymnasium
Hockey field
Holiday camp
Ice palace
Lake resort
Mountain resort
Playground, including
  school playground

Public park
Racecourse
Resort NOS
Riding school
Rifle range
Seashore resort
Skating rink
Sports ground
Sports palace
Stadium
Swimming pool, public
Tennis court
Vacation resort

Excludes: *that in private house or garden (E849.0)*

E849.5 Street and highway

E849.6 Public building

Building (including adjacent grounds) used by the general public or by a particular
  group of the public, such as:

airport
bank
café
casino
church
cinema
clubhouse
courthouse
dance hall
garage building (for car
  storage)
hotel
market (grocery or other
  commodity)
movie house
music hall

nightclub
office
office building
opera house
post office
public hall
radio broadcasting station
restaurant
school (state) (public) (private)
shop, commercial
station (bus) (railway)
store
theater

Excludes: *home garage (E849.0)*
  industrial building or workplace (E849.3)

E849.7 Residential institution

Children's home
Dormitory
Hospital
Jail

Old people's home
Orphanage
Prison
Reform school

E849.8 Other specified places

Beach NOS
Canal
Caravan site NOS
Derelict house
Desert
Dock
Forest
Harbor
Hill
Lake NOS
Mountain
Parking lot
Parking place

Pond or pool (natural)
Prairie
Public place NOS
Railway line
Reservoir
River
Sea
Seashore NOS
Stream
Swamp
Trailer court
Woods

E849.9 Unspecified place

ACCIDENTAL POISONING BY DRUGS, MEDICINAL SUBSTANCES, AND BIOLOGICALS (E850-E858)

Includes: accidental overdose of drug, wrong drug given or taken in error, and drug taken inadvertently

accidents in the use of drugs and biologicals in medical and surgical procedures

Excludes: *administration with suicidal or homicidal intent or intent to harm, or in circumstances classifiable to E980-E989 (E950.0-E950.5, E962.0, E980.0-E980.5)*

correct drug properly administered in therapeutic or prophylactic dosage, as the cause of adverse effect (E930.0-E949.9)

See Alphabetic Index for more complete list of specific drugs to be classified under the fourth-digit subdivisions. The American Hospital Formulary numbers can be used to classify new drugs listed by the American Hospital Formulary Service (AHFS). See appendix C.

E850   **Accidental poisoning by analgesics, antipyretics, and antirheumatics**

E850.0   **Heroin**
Diacetylmorphine

E850.1   **Methadone**

E850.2   **Other opiates and related narcotics**
Codeine [methylmorphine]   Morphine
Meperidine [pethidine]   Opium (alkaloids)

E850.3   **Salicylates**
Acetylsalicylic acid [aspirin]
Amino derivatives of salicylic acid
Salicylic acid salts

E850.4   **Aromatic analgesics, not elsewhere classified**
Acetanilid
Paracetamol [acetaminophen]
Phenacetin [acetophenetidin]

E850.5   **Pyrazole derivatives**
Aminophenazone [amidopyrine]
Phenylbutazone

E850.6   **Antirheumatics [antiphlogistics]**
Gold salts   Indomethacin

Excludes: *salicylates (E850.3)*
steroids (E858.0)

E850.7   **Other non-narcotic analgesics**
Pyrabital

E850.8   **Other specified analgesics and antipyretics**
Pentazocine

E850.9   **Unspecified analgesic or antipyretic**

E851   **Accidental poisoning by barbiturates**
Amobarbital [amylobarbitone]
Barbital [barbitone]
Butabarbital [butabarbitone]
Pentobarbital [pentobarbitone]
Phenobarbital [phenobarbitone]
Secobarbital [quinalbarbitone]

Excludes: *thiobarbiturates (E855.1)*

E852   **Accidental poisoning by other sedatives and hypnotics**

E852.0   **Chloral hydrate group**

E852.1   **Paraldehyde**

E852.2   **Bromine compounds**
Bromides   Carbromal (derivatives)

E852.3   **Methaqualone compounds**

E852.4   **Glutethimide group**

E852.5   **Mixed sedatives, not elsewhere classified**

E852.8   **Other specified sedatives and hypnotics**

● Code new to this edition   ▲ Revision of existing code   ④ ⑤ Fourth or fifth digit required

E852.9 Unspecified sedative or hypnotic
Sleeping:
   drug NOS
   pill NOS
   tablet NOS

E853 Accidental poisoning by tranquilizers

E853.0 Phenothiazine-based tranquilizers

Chlorpromazine	Prochlorperazine
Fluphenazine	Promazine

E853.1 Butyrophenone-based tranquilizers

Haloperidol	Trifluperidol
Spiperone	

E853.2 Benzodiazepine-based tranquilizers

Chlordiazepoxide	Lorazepam
Diazepam	Medazepam
Flurazepam	Nitrazepam

E853.8 Other specified tranquilizers

Hydroxyzine	Meprobamate

E853.9 Unspecified tranquilizer

E854 Accidental poisoning by other psychotropic agents

E854.0 Antidepressants

Amitriptyline	Monoamine oxidase [MAO] inhibitors
Imipramine	

E854.1 Psychodysleptics [hallucinogens]

Cannabis derivatives	Mescaline
Lysergide [LSD]	Psilocin
Marihuana (derivatives)	Psilocybin

E854.2 Psychostimulants

Amphetamine	Caffeine

Excludes: central appetite depressants (E858.8)

E854.3 Central nervous system stimulants

Analeptics	Opiate antagonists

E854.8 Other psychotropic agents

E855 Accidental poisoning by other drugs acting on central and autonomic nervous system

E855.0 Anticonvulsant and anti-Parkinsonism drugs
Amantadine
Hydantoin derivatives
Levodopa [L-dopa]
Oxazolidine derivatives [paramethadione] [trimethadione]
Succinimides

E855.1 Other central nervous system depressants

Ether	Intravenous anesthetics
Gaseous anesthetics	Thiobarbiturates, such as thiopental sodium
Halogenated hydrocarbon derivatives	

E855.2 Local anesthetics

Cocaine	Procaine
Lidocaine [lignocaine]	Tetracaine

E855.3 Parasympathomimetics [cholinergics]

Acetylcholine	Pilocarpine
Anticholinesterase:	
organophosphorus	
reversible	

E855.4 Parasympatholytics [anticholinergics and antimuscarinics] and spasmolytics

Atropine	Hyoscine [scopolamine]
Homatropine	Quaternary ammonium derivatives

E855.5 Sympathomimetics [adrenergics]
Epinephrine [adrenalin]
Levarterenol [noradrenalin]

E855.6 Sympatholytics [antiadrenergics]

Phenoxybenzamine	Tolazoline hydrochloride

Add 4th or 5th digit	Nonspecific code
Unspecified code	Manifestation code

E855.8   Other specified drugs acting on central and autonomic nervous systems

E855.9   Unspecified drug acting on central and autonomic nervous systems

E856   Accidental poisoning by antibiotics

E857   Accidental poisoning by other anti-infectives

E858   Accidental poisoning by other drugs

    E858.0   Hormones and synthetic substitutes

    E858.1   Primarily systemic agents

    E858.2   Agents primarily affecting blood constituents

    E858.3   Agents primarily affecting cardiovascular system

    E858.4   Agents primarily affecting gastrointestinal system

    E858.5   Water, mineral, and uric acid metabolism drugs

    E858.6   Agents primarily acting on the smooth and skeletal muscles and respiratory system

    E858.7   Agents primarily affecting skin and mucous membrane, ophthalmological, otorhinolaryngological, and dental drugs

    E858.8   Other specified drugs
        Central appetite depressants

    E858.9   Unspecified drug

ACCIDENTAL POISONING BY OTHER SOLID AND LIQUID SUBSTANCES, GASES, AND VAPORS (E860-E869)

> Note: Categories in this section are intended primarily to indicate the external cause of poisoning states classifiable to 980-989. They may also be used to indicate external causes of localized effects classifiable to 001-799.

E860   Accidental poisoning by alcohol, not elsewhere classified

    E860.0   Alcoholic beverages
        Alcohol in preparations intended for consumption

    E860.1   Other and unspecified ethyl alcohol and its products
        Denatured alcohol   Grain alcohol NOS
        Ethanol NOS   Methylated spirit

    E860.2   Methyl alcohol
        Methanol   Wood alcohol

    E860.3   Isopropyl alcohol
        Dimethyl carbinol   Secondary propyl alcohol
        Isopropanol
        Rubbing alcohol substitute

    E860.4   Fusel oil
        Alcohol:
          amyl
          butyl
          propyl

    E860.8   Other specified alcohols

    E860.9   Unspecified alcohol

E861   Accidental poisoning by cleansing and polishing agents, disinfectants, paints, and varnishes

    E861.0   Synthetic detergents and shampoos

    E861.1   Soap products

    E861.2   Polishes

    E861.3   Other cleansing and polishing agents
        Scouring powders

    E861.4   Disinfectants
        Household and other disinfectants not ordinarily used on the person

        Excludes: *carbolic acid or phenol (E864.0)*

    E861.5   Lead paints

    E861.6   Other paints and varnishes
        Lacquers   Paints, other than lead
        Oil colors   White washes

    E861.9   Unspecified

● Code new to this edition   ▲ Revision of existing code   ④ ⑤ Fourth or fifth digit required

E862 **Accidental poisoning by petroleum products, other solvents and their vapors, not elsewhere classified**

E862.0 **Petroleum solvents**
Petroleum:
ether
benzine
naphtha

E862.1 **Petroleum fuels and cleaners**
Antiknock additives to petroleum fuels
Gas oils
Gasoline or petrol
Kerosene

Excludes: kerosene insecticides (E863.4)

E862.2 **Lubricating oils**

E862.3 **Petroleum solids**
Paraffin wax

E862.4 **Other specified solvents**
Benzene

E862.9 **Unspecified solvent**

E863 **Accidental poisoning by agricultural and horticultural chemical and pharmaceutical preparations other than plant foods and fertilizers**

Excludes: plant foods and fertilizers (E866.5)

E863.0 **Insecticides of organochlorine compounds**
Benzene hexachloride   Dieldrin
Chlordane   Endrine
DDT   Toxaphene

E863.1 **Insecticides of organophosphorus compounds**
Demeton   Parathion
Diazinon   Phenylsulphthion
Dichlorvos   Phorate
Malathion   Phosdrin
Methyl parathion

E863.2 **Carbamates**
Aldicarb   Propoxur
Carbaryl

E863.3 **Mixtures of insecticides**

E863.4 **Other and unspecified insecticides**
Kerosene insecticides

E863.5 **Herbicides**
2, 4-Dichlorophenoxyacetic acid [2, 4-D]
2, 4, 5-Trichlorophenoxyacetic acid [2, 4, 5-T]
Chlorates
Diquat
Mixtures of plant food and fertilizers with herbicides
Paraquat

E863.6 **Fungicides**
Organic mercurials (used in seed dressing)
Pentachlorophenols

E863.7 **Rodenticides**
Fluoroacetates   Warfarin
Squill and derivatives   Zinc phosphide
Thallium

E863.8 **Fumigants**
Cyanides   Phosphine
Methyl bromide

E863.9 **Other and unspecified**

E864 **Accidental poisoning by corrosives and caustics, not elsewhere classified**

Excludes: those as components of disinfectants (E861.4)

E864.0 **Corrosive aromatics**
Carbolic acid or phenol

| | Add 4th or 5th digit | | Nonspecific code | | Unspecified code | | Manifestation code |

E864.1 Acids
Acid:
    hydrochloric
    nitric
    sulfuric

E864.2 Caustic alkalis
Lye

E864.3 Other specified corrosives and caustics

E864.4 Unspecified corrosives and caustics

E865 Accidental poisoning from poisonous foodstuffs and poisonous plants
Includes: any meat, fish, or shellfish
        plants, berries, and fungi eaten as, or in mistake for, food, or by a child

Excludes: *anaphylactic shock due to adverse food reaction (995.6)*
        food poisoning (bacterial) (005.0-005.9)
        poisoning and toxic reactions to venomous plants (E905.6-E905.7)

E865.0 Meat

E865.1 Shellfish

E865.2 Other fish

E865.3 Berries and seeds

E865.4 Other specified plants

E865.5 Mushrooms and other fungi

E865.8 Other specified foods

E865.9 Unspecified foodstuff or poisonous plant

E866 Accidental poisoning by other and unspecified solid and liquid substances

Excludes: *these substances as a component of:*
        medicines (E850.0-E858.9)
        paints (E861.5-E861.6)
        pesticides (E863.0-E863.9)
        petroleum fuels (E862.1)

E866.0 Lead and its compounds and fumes

E866.1 Mercury and its compounds and fumes

E866.2 Antimony and its compounds and fumes

E866.3 Arsenic and its compounds and fumes

E866.4 Other metals and their compounds and fumes
Beryllium (compounds)   Iron (compounds)
Brass fumes   Manganese (compounds)
Cadmium (compounds)   Nickel (compounds)
Copper salts   Thallium (compounds)

E866.5 Plant foods and fertilizers

Excludes: *mixtures with herbicides (E863.5)*

E866.6 Glues and adhesives

E866.7 Cosmetics

E866.8 Other specified solid or liquid substances

E866.9 Unspecified solid or liquid substance

E867 Accidental poisoning by gas distributed by pipeline
Carbon monoxide from incomplete combustion of piped gas
Coal gas NOS
Liquefied petroleum gas distributed through pipes (pure or mixed with air)
Piped gas (natural) (manufactured)

E868 Accidental poisoning by other utility gas and other carbon monoxide

E868.0 Liquefied petroleum gas distributed in mobile containers
Butane or carbon monoxide from incomplete combustion of this gas
Liquefied hydrocarbon gas NOS or carbon monoxide from incomplete combustion of
    this gas
Propane or carbon monoxide from incomplete combustion of this gas

● Code new   ▲ Revision of   ④ ⑤ Fourth or fifth
        to this edition   existing code   digit required

E868.1 Other and unspecified utility gas
Acetylene or or carbon monoxide from incomplete combustion of these gases
Gas NOS used for lighting, heating, cooking, or carbon monoxide from incomplete
combustion of these gases
Water gas or carbon monoxide from incomplete combustion of these gases

E868.2 Motor vehicle exhaust gas
Exhaust gas from:
farm tractor, not in transit
gas engine
motor pump
motor vehicle, not in transit
any type of combustion engine not in watercraft

Excludes: *poisoning by carbon monoxide from:*
aircraft while in transit (E844.0-E844.9)
motor vehicle while in transit (E818.0-E818.9)
watercraft whether or not in transit (E838.0-E838.9)

E868.3 Carbon monoxide from incomplete combustion of other domestic fuels
Carbon monoxide from incomplete combustion of:
coal in domestic stove or fireplace
coke in domestic stove or fireplace
kerosene in domestic stove or fireplace
wood in domestic stove or fireplace

Excludes: *carbon monoxide from smoke and fumes due to conflagration (E890.0-E893.9)*

E868.8 Carbon monoxide from other sources
Carbon monoxide from:
blast furnace gas
incomplete combustion of fuels in industrial use
kiln vapor

E868.9 Unspecified carbon monoxide

E869 Accidental poisoning by other gases and vapors

Excludes: *effects of gases used as anesthetics (E855.1, E938.2)*
fumes from heavy metals (E866.0-E866.4)
smoke and fumes due to conflagration or explosion (E890.0-E899)

E869.0 Nitrogen oxides

E869.1 Sulfur dioxide

E869.2 Freon

E869.3 Lacrimogenic gas [tear gas]
Bromobenzyl cyanide   Ethyliodoacetate
Chloroacetophenone

E869.4 Second-hand tobacco smoke

E869.8 Other specified gases and vapors
Chlorine   Hydrocyanic acid gas

E869.9 Unspecified gases and vapors

MISADVENTURES TO PATIENTS DURING SURGICAL AND MEDICAL CARE (E870-E876)

Excludes: *accidental overdose of drug and wrong drug given in error (E850.0-E858.9)*
surgical and medical procedures as the cause of abnormal reaction by the patient,
without mention of misadventure at the time of procedure (E878.0-E879.9)

E870 Accidental cut, puncture, perforation, or hemorrhage during medical care

E870.0 Surgical operation

E870.1 Infusion or transfusion

E870.2 Kidney dialysis or other perfusion

E870.3 Injection or vaccination

E870.4 Endoscopic examination

E870.5 Aspiration of fluid or tissue, puncture, and catheterization
Abdominal paracentesis   Lumbar puncture
Aspirating needle biopsy   Thoracentesis
Blood sampling

Excludes: *heart catheterization (E870.6)*

E870.6 Heart catheterization

E870.7 Administration of enema

Add 4th or   Nonspecific   Unspecified   Manifestation
5th digit   code   code   code

E870.8 Other specified medical care

E870.9 Unspecified medical care

E871 Foreign object left in body during procedure

E871.0 Surgical operation

E871.1 Infusion or transfusion

E871.2 Kidney dialysis or other perfusion

E871.3 Injection or vaccination

E871.4 Endoscopic examination

E871.5 Aspiration of fluid or tissue, puncture, and catheterization
    Abdominal paracentesis   Lumbar puncture
    Aspiration needle biopsy   Thoracentesis
    Blood sampling

    Excludes: *heart catheterization (E871.6)*

E871.6 Heart catheterization

E871.7 Removal of catheter or packing

E871.8 Other specified procedures

E871.9 Unspecified procedure

E872 Failure of sterile precautions during procedure

E872.0 Surgical operation

E872.1 Infusion or transfusion

E872.2 Kidney dialysis and other perfusion

E872.3 Injection or vaccination

E872.4 Endoscopic examination

E872.5 Aspiration of fluid or tissue, puncture, and catheterization
    Abdominal paracentesis   Lumbar puncture
    Aspirating needle biopsy   Thoracentesis
    Blood sampling

    Excludes: *heart catheterization (E872.6)*

E872.6 Heart catheterization

E872.8 Other specified procedures

E872.9 Unspecified procedure

E873 Failure in dosage

    Excludes: *accidental overdose of drug, medicinal or biological substance (E850.0-E858.9)*

E873.0 Excessive amount of blood or other fluid during transfusion or infusion

E873.1 Incorrect dilution of fluid during infusion

E873.2 Overdose of radiation in therapy

E873.3 Inadvertent exposure of patient to radiation during medical care

E873.4 Failure in dosage in electroshock or insulin-shock therapy

E873.5 Inappropriate [too hot or too cold] temperature in local application and packing

E873.6 Nonadministration of necessary drug or medicinal substance

E873.8 Other specified failure in dosage

E873.9 Unspecified failure in dosage

E874 Mechanical failure of instrument or apparatus during procedure

E874.0 Surgical operation

E874.1 Infusion and transfusion
    Air in system

E874.2 Kidney dialysis and other perfusion

E874.3 Endoscopic examination

E874.4 Aspiration of fluid or tissue, puncture, and catheterization
    Abdominal paracentesis   Lumbar puncture
    Aspirating needle biopsy   Thoracentesis
    Blood sampling

    Excludes: *heart catheterization (E874.5)*

E874.5 Heart catheterization

● Code new
to this edition
    ▲ Revision of
existing code
    ④ ⑤ Fourth or fifth
digit required

E874.8 Other specified procedures

E874.9 Unspecified procedure

E875 Contaminated or infected blood, other fluid, drug, or biological substance
Includes: presence of:
bacterial pyrogens
endotoxin-producing bacteria
serum hepatitis-producing agent

E875.0 Contaminated substance transfused or infused

E875.1 Contaminated substance injected or used for vaccination

E875.2 Contaminated drug or biological substance administered by other means

E875.8 Other

E875.9 Unspecified

E876 Other and unspecified misadventures during medical care

E876.0 Mismatched blood in transfusion

E876.1 Wrong fluid in infusion

E876.2 Failure in suture and ligature during surgical operation

E876.3 Endotracheal tube wrongly placed during anesthetic procedure

E876.4 Failure to introduce or to remove other tube or instrument
Excludes: foreign object left in body during procedure (E871.0-E871.9)

▲ **E876.5** Performance of wrong operation (procedure) on correct patient
Wrong device implanted into correct surgical site
Excludes: correct operation (procedure) performed on wrong body part (E876.7)

● **E876.6** Performance of operation (procedure) on patient not scheduled for surgery
Performance of operation (procedure) intended for another patient
Performance of operation (procedure) on wrong patient

● **E876.7** Performance of correct operation (procedure) on wrong side/body part
Performance of correct operation (procedure) on wrong side
Performance of correct operation (procedure) on wrong site

E876.8 Other specified misadventures during medical care
Performance of inappropriate treatment NEC

E876.9 Unspecified misadventure during medical care

SURGICAL AND MEDICAL PROCEDURES AS THE CAUSE OF ABNORMAL REACTION OF PATIENT OR LATER COMPLICATION, WITHOUT MENTION OF MISADVENTURE AT THE TIME OF PROCEDURE (E878-E879)

Includes: procedures as the cause of abnormal reaction, such as:
displacement or malfunction of prosthetic device
hepatorenal failure, postoperative
malfunction of external stoma
postoperative intestinal obstruction
rejection of transplanted organ

Excludes: anesthetic management properly carried out as the cause of adverse effect
(E937.0-E938.9)
infusion and transfusion, without mention of misadventure in the technique of
procedure (E930.0-E949.9)

E878 Surgical operation and other surgical procedures as the cause of abnormal reaction of
patient, or of later complication, without mention of misadventure at the time of
operation

E878.0 Surgical operation with transplant of whole organ
Transplantation of:
heart
kidney
liver

E878.1 Surgical operation with implant of artificial internal device
Cardiac pacemaker   Heart valve prosthesis
Electrodes implanted in brain   Internal orthopedic device

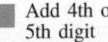 Add 4th or
5th digit

Nonspecific
code

Unspecified
code

Manifestation
code

E878.2 Surgical operation with anastomosis, bypass, or graft, with natural or artificial tissues used as implant
Anastomosis: Graft of blood vessel, tendon, or skin
  arteriovenous
  gastrojejunal

Excludes: external stoma (E878.3)

E878.3 Surgical operation with formation of external stoma
Colostomy   Gastrostomy
Cystostomy   Ureterostomy
Duodenostomy

E878.4 Other restorative surgery

E878.5 Amputation of limb(s)

E878.6 Removal of other organ (partial) (total)

E878.8 Other specified surgical operations and procedures

E878.9 Unspecified surgical operations and procedures

E879 Other procedures, without mention of misadventure at the time of procedure, as the cause of abnormal reaction of patient, or of later complication

E879.0 Cardiac catheterization

E879.1 Kidney dialysis

E879.2 Radiological procedure and radiotherapy

Excludes: radio-opaque dyes for diagnostic x-ray procedures (E947.8)

E879.3 Shock therapy
Electroshock therapy   Insulin-shock therapy

E879.4 Aspiration of fluid
Lumbar puncture   Thoracentesis

E879.5 Insertion of gastric or duodenal sound

E879.6 Urinary catheterization

E879.7 Blood sampling

E879.8 Other specified procedures
Blood transfusion

E879.9 Unspecified procedure

ACCIDENTAL FALLS (E880-E888)

Excludes: falls (in or from):
  burning building (E890.8, E891.8)
  into fire (E890.0-E899)
  into water (with submersion or drowning) (E910.0-E910.9)
  machinery (in operation) (E919.0-E919.9)
  on edged, pointed, or sharp object (E920.0-E920.9)
  transport vehicle (E800.0-E845.9)
  vehicle not elsewhere classifiable (E846-E848)

E880 Fall on or from stairs or steps

E880.0 Escalator

E880.1 Fall on or from sidewalk curb

Excludes: fall from moving sidewalk (E885.9)

E880.9 Other stairs or steps

E881 Fall on or from ladders or scaffolding

E881.0 Fall from ladder

E881.1 Fall from scaffolding

E882 Fall from or out of building or other structure
Fall from: Fall from:
  balcony   turret
  bridge   viaduct
  building   wall
  flagpole   window
  tower   Fall through roof

Excludes: collapse of a building or structure (E916)
  fall or jump from burning building (E890.8, E891.8)

● Code new to this edition   ▲ Revision of existing code   ④ ⑤ Fourth or fifth digit required

E883 **Fall into hole or other opening in surface**
Includes:

fall into:	fall into:
cavity	shaft
dock	swimming pool
hole	tank
pit	well
quarry	

Excludes: *fall into water NOS (E910.9)*
that resulting in drowning or submersion without mention of injury (E910.0-E910.9)

E883.0 **Accident from diving or jumping into water [swimming pool]**
Strike or hit:
against bottom when jumping or diving into water
wall or board of swimming pool
water surface

Excludes: *diving with insufficient air supply (E913.2)*
effects of air pressure from diving (E902.2)

E883.1 **Accidental fall into well**

E883.2 **Accidental fall into storm drain or manhole**

E883.9 **Fall into other hole or other opening in surface**

E884 **Other fall from one level to another**

E884.0 **Fall from playground equipment**

Excludes: *recreational machinery (E919.8)*

E884.1 **Fall from cliff**

E884.2 **Fall from chair**

E884.3 **Fall from wheelchair**

E884.4 **Fall from bed**

E884.5 **Fall from other furniture**

E884.6 **Fall from commode**
Toilet

E884.9 **Other fall from one level to another**

Fall from:	Fall from:
embankment	stationary vehicle
haystack	tree

E885 **Fall on same level from slipping, tripping, or stumbling**

E885.0 **Fall from (nonmotorized) scooter**

E885.1 **Fall from roller skates**
Heelies
In-line skates
Wheelies

E885.2 **Fall from skateboard**

E885.3 **Fall from skis**

E885.4 **Fall from snowboard**

E885.9 **Fall from other slipping, tripping or stumbling**
Fall on moving sidewalk

E886 **Fall on same level from collision, pushing, or shoving, by or with other person**

Excludes: *crushed or pushed by a crowd or human stampede (E917.1, E917.6)*

E886.0 **In sports**
Tackles in sports

Excludes: *kicked, stepped on, struck by object, in sports (E917.0, E917.5)*

E886.9 **Other and unspecified**
Fall from collision of pedestrian (conveyance) with another pedestrian (conveyance)

E887 **Fracture, cause unspecified**

E888 **Other and unspecified fall**
Accidental fall NOS
Fall on same level NOS

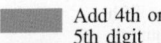 Add 4th or 5th digit   Nonspecific code   Unspecified code   Manifestation code

E888.0   **Fall resulting in striking against sharp object**
Use additional external cause code to identify object (E920)

E888.1   **Fall resulting in striking against other object**

E888.8   **Other fall**

E888.9   **Unspecified fall**
Fall NOS

ACCIDENTS CAUSED BY FIRE AND FLAMES (E890-E899)

Includes: asphyxia or poisoning due to conflagration or ignition
burning by fire
secondary fires resulting from explosion

Excludes: *arson (E968.0)*
fire in or on:
machinery (in operation) (E919.0-E919.9)
transport vehicle other than stationary vehicle (E800.0-E845.9)
vehicle not elsewhere classifiable (E846-E848)

E890   **Conflagration in private dwelling**
Includes: conflagration in:
apartment
boarding house
camping place
caravan
farmhouse
house
lodging house
mobile home
private garage
rooming house
tenement
conflagration originating from sources classifiable to E893-E898 in the above
buildings

E890.0   **Explosion caused by conflagration**

E890.1   **Fumes from combustion of polyvinylchloride [PVC] and similar material in conflagration**

E890.2   **Other smoke and fumes from conflagration**
Carbon monoxide from conflagration in private building
Fumes NOS from conflagration in private building
Smoke NOS from conflagration in private building

E890.3   **Burning caused by conflagration**

E890.8   **Other accident resulting from conflagration**
Collapse of burning private building
Fall from burning private building
Hit by object falling from burning private building
Jump from burning private building

E890.9   **Unspecified accident resulting from conflagration in private dwelling**

E891   **Conflagration in other and unspecified building or structure**

Conflagration in:	Conflagration in:
barn	farm outbuildings
church	hospital
convalescent and other	hotel
residential home	school
dormitory of educational	store
institution	theater
factory	

Conflagration originating from sources classifiable to E893-E898, in the above buildings

E891.0   **Explosion caused by conflagration**

E891.1   **Fumes from combustion of polyvinylchloride [PVC] and similar material in conflagration**

E891.2   **Other smoke and fumes from conflagration**
Carbon monoxide from conflagration in building or structure
Fumes NOS from conflagration in building or structure
Smoke NOS from conflagration in building or structure

E891.3   **Burning caused by conflagration**

● Code new to this edition   ▲ Revision of existing code   ④ ⑤ Fourth or fifth digit required

E891.8 Other accident resulting from conflagration
Collapse of burning building or structure
Fall from burning building or structure
Hit by object falling from burning building or structure
Jump from burning building or structure

E891.9 Unspecified accident resulting from conflagration of other and unspecified building or structure

E892 Conflagration not in building or structure
Fire (uncontrolled) (in) (of):
forest
grass
hay
lumber
mine
prairie
transport vehicle [any], except while in transit
tunnel

E893 Accident caused by ignition of clothing

Excludes: ignition of clothing:
from highly inflammable material (E894)
with conflagration (E890.0-E892)

E893.0 From controlled fire in private dwelling
Ignition of clothing from:
normal fire (charcoal) (coal) (electric) (gas) (wood) in:
brazier in private dwelling (as listed in E890)
fireplace in private dwelling (as listed in E890)
furnace in private dwelling (as listed in E890)
stove in private dwelling (as listed in E890)

E893.1 From controlled fire in other building or structure
Ignition of clothing from:
normal fire (charcoal) (coal) (electric) (gas) (wood) in:
brazier in other building or structure (as listed in E891)
fireplace in other building or structure (as listed in E891)
furnace in other building or structure (as listed in E891)
stove in other building or structure (as listed in E891)

E893.2 From controlled fire not in building or structure
Ignition of clothing from:
bonfire (controlled)
brazier fire (controlled), not in building or structure
trash fire (controlled)

Excludes: conflagration not in building (E892)
trash fire out of control (E892)

E893.8 From other specified sources

Ignition of clothing from:	Ignition of clothing from:
blowlamp	cigarette
blowtorch	lighter
burning bedspread	matches
candle	pipe
cigar	welding torch

E893.9 Unspecified source
Ignition of clothing (from controlled fire NOS) (in building NOS) NOS

E894 Ignition of highly inflammable material
Ignition of:
benzine (with ignition of clothing)
gasoline (with ignition of clothing)
fat (with ignition of clothing)
kerosene (with ignition of clothing)
paraffin (with ignition of clothing)
petrol (with ignition of clothing)

Excludes: ignition of highly inflammable material with:
conflagration (E890.0-E892)
explosion (E923.0-E923.9)

	Add 4th or 5th digit		Nonspecific code		Unspecified code		Manifestation code

E895 **Accident caused by controlled fire in private dwelling**
Burning by (flame of) normal fire (charcoal) (coal) (electric) (gas) (wood) in:
    brazier in private dwelling (as listed in E890)
    fireplace in private dwelling (as listed in E890)
    furnace in private dwelling (as listed in E890)
    stove in private dwelling (as listed in E890)

    Excludes: *burning by hot objects not producing fire or flames (E924.0-E924.9)*
        ignition of clothing from these sources (E893.0)
        poisoning by carbon monoxide from incomplete combustion of fuel (E867-E868.9)
        that with conflagration (E890.0-E890.9)

E896 **Accident caused by controlled fire in other and unspecified building or structure**
Burning by (flame of) normal fire (charcoal) (coal) (electric) (gas) (wood) in:
    brazier in other building or structure (as listed in E891)
    fireplace in other building or structure (as listed in E891)
    furnace in other building or structure (as listed in E891)
    stove in other building or structure (as listed in E891)

    Excludes: *burning by hot objects not producing fire or flames (E924.0-E924.9)*
        ignition of clothing from these sources (E893.1)
        poisoning by carbon monoxide from incomplete combustion of fuel (E867-E868.9)
        that with conflagration (E891.0-E891.9)

E897 **Accident caused by controlled fire not in building or structure**
Burns from flame of:
    bonfire (controlled)
    brazier fire (controlled), not in building or structure
    trash fire (controlled)

    Excludes: *ignition of clothing from these sources (E893.2)*
        trash fire out of control (E892)
        that with conflagration (E892)

E898 **Accident caused by other specified fire and flames**

    Excludes: *conflagration (E890.0-E892)*
        that with ignition of:
          clothing (E893.0-E893.9)
          highly inflammable material (E894)

E898.0 **Burning bedclothes**
    Bed set on fire NOS

E898.1 **Other**

Burning by:	Burning by:
blowlamp	lamp
blowtorch	lighter
candle	matches
cigar	pipe
cigarette	welding torch
fire in room NOS	

E899 **Accident caused by unspecified fire**
    Burning NOS

ACCIDENTS DUE TO NATURAL AND ENVIRONMENTAL FACTORS (E900-E909)

E900 **Excessive heat**

E900.0 **Due to weather conditions**
    Excessive heat as the external cause of:
        ictus solaris
        siriasis
        sunstroke

E900.1 **Of man-made origin**

Heat (in):	Heat (in):
boiler room	generated in transport vehicle
drying room	kitchen
factory	
furnace room	

E900.9 **Of unspecified origin**

● Code new to this edition   ▲ Revision of existing code   ④ ⑤ Fourth or fifth digit required

E901 **Excessive cold**

E901.0 **Due to weather conditions**
Excessive cold as the cause of:
chilblains NOS
immersion foot

E901.1 **Of man-made origin**
Contact with or inhalation of:
dry ice
liquid air
liquid hydrogen
liquid nitrogen
Prolonged exposure in:
deep freeze unit
refrigerator

E901.8 **Other specified origin**

E901.9 **Of unspecified origin**

E902 **High and low air pressure and changes in air pressure**

E902.0 **Residence or prolonged visit at high altitude**
Residence or prolonged visit at high altitude as the cause of:
Acosta syndrome
Alpine sickness
altitude sickness
Andes disease
anoxia, hypoxia
barotitis, barodontalgia, barosinusitis, otitic barotrauma
hypobarism, hypobaropathy
mountain sickness
range disease

E902.1 **In aircraft**
Sudden change in air pressure in aircraft during ascent or descent as the cause of:
aeroneurosis
aviators' disease

E902.2 **Due to diving**
High air pressure from rapid descent in water as the cause of:
caisson disease
divers' disease
divers' palsy or paralysis
Reduction in atmospheric pressure while surfacing from deep water diving as the
cause of:
caisson disease
divers' disease
divers' palsy or paralysis

E902.8 **Due to other specified causes**
Reduction in atmospheric pressure while surfacing from underground

E902.9 **Unspecified cause**

E903 **Travel and motion**

E904 **Hunger, thirst, exposure, and neglect**

Excludes: *any condition resulting from homicidal intent (E968.0-E968.9)*
*hunger, thirst, and exposure resulting from accidents connected with transport
(E800.0-E848)*

E904.0 **Abandonment or neglect of infants and helpless persons**
Exposure to weather conditions resulting from abandonment or neglect
Hunger or thirst resulting from abandonment or neglect
Desertion of newborn
Inattention at or after birth
Lack of care (helpless person) (infant)

Excludes: *criminal [purposeful] neglect (E968.4)*

E904.1 **Lack of food**
Lack of food as the cause of:
inanition
insufficient nourishment
starvation

Excludes: *hunger resulting from abandonment or neglect (E904.0)*

	Add 4th or 5th digit		Nonspecific code		Unspecified code		Manifestation code

E904.2   Lack of water
Lack of water as the cause of:
dehydration
inanition

Excludes: dehydration due to acute fluid loss (276.51)

E904.3   Exposure (to weather conditions), not elsewhere classifiable
Exposure NOS   Struck by hailstones
Humidity

Excludes: struck by lightning (E907)

E904.9   Privation, unqualified
Destitution

E905   Venomous animals and plants as the cause of poisoning and toxic reactions
Includes: chemical released by animal
insects
release of venom through fangs, hairs, spines, tentacles, and other venom
apparatus

Excludes: eating of poisonous animals or plants (E865.0-E865.9)

E905.0   Venomous snakes and lizards
Cobra   Mamba
Copperhead snake   Rattlesnake
Coral snake   Sea snake
Fer de lance   Snake (venomous)
Gila monster   Viper
Krait   Water moccasin

Excludes: bites of snakes and lizards known to be nonvenomous (E906.2)

E905.1   Venomous spiders
Black widow spider   Tarantula (venomous)
Brown spider

E905.2   Scorpion

E905.3   Hornets, wasps, and bees
Yellow jacket

E905.4   Centipede and venomous millipede (tropical)

E905.5   Other venomous arthropods
Sting of:
ant
caterpillar

E905.6   Venomous marine animals and plants
Puncture by sea urchin spine   Sting of:
Sting of: nematocysts
coral   sea anemone
jelly fish   sea cucumber
other marine animal or plant

Excludes: bites and other injuries caused by nonvenomous marine animal (E906.2-E906.8)
bite of sea snake (venomous) (E905.0)

E905.7   Poisoning and toxic reactions caused by other plants
Injection of poisons or toxins into or through skin by plant thorns, spines, or other
mechanisms

Excludes: puncture wound NOS by plant thorns or spines (E920.8)

E905.8   Other specified

E905.9   Unspecified
Sting NOS   Venomous bite NOS

E906   Other injury caused by animals

Excludes: poisoning and toxic reactions caused by venomous animals and insects
(E905.0-E905.9)
road vehicle accident involving animals (E827.0-E828.9)
tripping or falling over an animal (E885.9)

E906.0   Dog bite

E906.1   Rat bite

E906.2   Bite of nonvenomous snakes and lizards

● Code new   ▲ Revision of   ④ ⑤ Fourth or fifth
to this edition   existing code   digit required

E906.3 **Bite of other animal except arthropod**
    Cats   Rodents, except rats
    Moray eel   Shark

E906.4 **Bite of nonvenomous arthropod**
    Insect bite NOS

E906.5 **Bite by unspecified animal**
    Animal bite NOS

E906.8 **Other specified injury caused by animal**
    Butted by animal
    Fallen on by horse or other animal, not being ridden
    Gored by animal
    Implantation of quills of porcupine
    Pecked by bird
    Run over by animal, not being ridden
    Stepped on by animal, not being ridden

Excludes: *injury by animal being ridden (E828.0-E828.9)*

E906.9 **Unspecified injury caused by animal**

E907 Lightning

Excludes: *injury from:*
    fall of tree or other object caused by lightning (E916)
    fire caused by lightning (E890.0-E892)

E908 Cataclysmic storms, and floods resulting from storms

Excludes: *collapse of dam or man-made structure causing flood (E909.3)*

E908.0 **Hurricane**
    Storm surge
    "Tidal wave" caused by storm action
    Typhoon

E908.1 **Tornado**
    Cyclone
    Twisters

E908.2 **Floods**
    Torrential rainfall
    Flash flood

Excludes: *collapse of dam or man-made structure causing flood (909.3)*

E908.3 **Blizzard (snow) (ice)**

E908.4 **Dust storm**

E908.8 **Other cataclysmic storms**

E908.9 **Unspecified cataclysmic storms, and floods resulting from storms**
    Storm NOS

E909 Cataclysmic earth surface movements and eruptions

Excludes: *"tidal wave" caused by storm action (E908.0)*
    transport accident involving collision with avalanche or landslide not in motion (E800.0-E848)

E909.0 **Earthquakes**

E909.1 **Volcanic eruptions**
    Burns from lava
    Ash inhalation

E909.2 **Avalanche, landslide, or mudslide**

E909.3 **Collapse of dam or man-made structure**

E909.4 **Tidal wave caused by earthquake**
    Tidal wave NOS
    Tsunami

Excludes: *tidal wave caused by tropical storm (E908.0)*

E909.8 **Other cataclysmic earth surface movements and eruptions**

E909.9 **Unspecified cataclysmic earth surface movements and eruptions**

Add 4th or 5th digit | Nonspecific code | Unspecified code | Manifestation code

ACCIDENTS CAUSED BY SUBMERSION, SUFFOCATION, AND FOREIGN BODIES (E910-E915)

E910 Accidental drowning and submersion

Includes: immersion
swimmers' cramp

Excludes: *diving accident (NOS) (resulting in injury except drowning) (E883.0)*
diving with insufficient air supply (E913.2)
drowning and submersion due to:
cataclysm (E908-E909)
machinery accident (E919.0-E919.9)
transport accident (E800.0-E845.9)
effect of high and low air pressure (E902.2)
injury from striking against objects while in running water (E917.2)

E910.0 While water-skiing
Fall from water skis with submersion or drowning

Excludes: *accident to water-skier involving a watercraft and resulting in submersion or other*
injury (E830.4, E831.4)

E910.1 While engaged in other sport or recreational activity with diving equipment
Scuba diving NOS
Skin diving NOS
Underwater spear fishing NOS

E910.2 While engaged in other sport or recreational activity without diving equipment
Fishing or hunting, except from boat or with diving equipment
Ice skating
Playing in water
Surfboarding
Swimming NOS
Voluntarily jumping from boat, not involved in accident, for swim NOS
Wading in water

Excludes: *jumping into water to rescue another person (E910.3)*

E910.3 While swimming or diving for purposes other than recreation or sport
Marine salvage (with diving equipment)
Pearl diving (with diving equipment)
Placement of fishing nets (with diving equipment)
Rescue (attempt) of another person (with diving equipment)
Underwater construction or repairs (with diving equipment)

E910.4 In bathtub

E910.8 Other accidental drowning or submersion
Drowning in:
quenching tank
swimming pool

E910.9 Unspecified accidental drowning or submersion
Accidental fall into water NOS
Drowning NOS

E911 Inhalation and ingestion of food causing obstruction of respiratory tract or suffocation
Aspiration and inhalation of food [any] (into respiratory tract) NOS
Asphyxia by food [including bone, seed in food, regurgitated food]
Choked on food [including bone, seed in food, regurgitated food]
Suffocation by food [including bone, seed in food, regurgitated food]
Compression of trachea by food lodged in esophagus
Interruption of respiration by food lodged in esophagus
Obstruction of respiration by food lodged in esophagus
Obstruction of pharynx by food (bolus)

Excludes: *injury, except asphyxia and obstruction of respiratory passage, caused by food*
(E915)
obstruction of esophagus by food without mention of asphyxia or obstruction of
respiratory passage (E915)

● Code new
to this edition

▲ Revision of
existing code

④ ⑤ Fourth or fifth
digit required

E912 Inhalation and ingestion of other object causing obstruction of respiratory tract or suffocation

Aspiration and inhalation of foreign body except food (into respiratory tract) NOS
Foreign object [bean] [marble] in nose
Obstruction of pharynx by foreign body
Compression by foreign body in esophagus
Interruption of respiration by foreign body in esophagus
Obstruction of respiration by foreign body in esophagus

Excludes: *injury, except asphyxia and obstruction of respiratory passage, caused by foreign body (E915)*
obstruction of esophagus by foreign body without mention of asphyxia or obstruction in respiratory passage (E915)

E913 Accidental mechanical suffocation

Excludes: *mechanical suffocation from or by:*
accidental inhalation or ingestion of:
food (E911)
foreign object (E912)
cataclysm (E908-E909)
explosion (E921.0-E921.9, E923.0-E923.9)
machinery accident (E919.0-E919.9)

E913.0 In bed or cradle

Excludes: *suffocation by plastic bag (E913.1)*

E913.1 By plastic bag

E913.2 Due to lack of air (in closed place)
Accidentally closed up in refrigerator or other airtight enclosed space
Diving with insufficient air supply

Excludes: *suffocation by plastic bag (E913.1)*

E913.3 By falling earth or other substance
Cave-in NOS

Excludes: *cave-in caused by cataclysmic earth surface movements and eruptions (E909)*
struck by cave-in without asphyxiation or suffocation (E916)

E913.8 Other specified means
Accidental hanging, except in bed or cradle

E913.9 Unspecified means
Asphyxia, mechanical NOS
Strangulation NOS
Suffocation NOS

E914 Foreign body accidentally entering eye and adnexa

Excludes: *corrosive liquid (E924.1)*

E915 Foreign body accidentally entering other orifice

Excludes: *aspiration and inhalation of foreign body, any, (into respiratory tract) NOS (E911-E912)*

OTHER ACCIDENTS (E916-E928)

E916 Struck accidentally by falling object

Collapse of building, except on fire
Falling:
rock
snowslide NOS
stone
tree

Object falling from:
machine, not in operation
stationary vehicle

Code first: collapse of building on fire (E890.0-E891.9)
falling object in:
cataclysm (E908-E909)
machinery accidents (E919.0-E919.9)
transport accidents (E800.0-E845.9)
vehicle accidents not elsewhere classifiable (E846-E848)
object set in motion by:
explosion (E921.0-E921.9, E923.0-E923.9)
firearm (E922.0-E922.9)
projected object (E917.0-E917.9)

	Add 4th or 5th digit		Nonspecific code		Unspecified code		Manifestation code

E917   Striking against or struck accidentally by objects or persons
Includes: bumping into or against:
object (moving) (projected) (stationary)
pedestrian conveyance
person
colliding with:
object (moving) (projected) (stationary)
pedestrian conveyance
person
kicking against:
object (moving) (projected) (stationary)
pedestrian conveyance
person
stepping on:
object (moving) (projected) (stationary)
pedestrian conveyance
person
struck by:
object (moving) (projected) (stationary)
pedestrian conveyance
person

Excludes: *fall from collision with another person, except when caused by a crowd*
(E886.0-E886.9)
fall from stumbling over object (E885.9)
fall resulting in striking against object (E888.0, E888.1)
injury caused by:
assault (E960.0-E960.1, E967.0-E967.9)
cutting or piercing instrument (E920.0-E920.9)
explosion (E921.0-E921.9, E923.0-E923.9)
firearm (E922.0-E922.9)
machinery (E919.0-E919.9)
transport vehicle (E800.0-E845.9)
vehicle not elsewhere classifiable (E846-E848)

E917.0   In sports without subsequent fall
Kicked or stepped on during game (football) (rugby)
Struck by hit or thrown ball
Struck by hockey stick or puck

E917.1   Caused by a crowd, by collective fear or panic without subsequent fall
Crushed by crown or human stampede
Pushed by crown or human stampede
Stepped on by crown or human stampede

E917.2   In running water without subsequent fall
Excludes: *drowning or submersion (E910.0-E910.9)*
that in sports (E917.0, E917.5)

E917.3   Furniture without subsequent fall
Excludes: *fall from furniture (E884.2, E884.4-E884.5)*

E917.4   Other stationary object without subsequent fall
Bath tub
Fence
Lamp-post

E917.5   Object in sports with subsequent fall
Knocked down while boxing

E917.6   Caused by a crowd, by collective fear or panic with subsequent fall

E917.7   Furniture with subsequent fall
Excludes: *fall from furniture (E884.2, E884.4-E884.5)*

E917.8   Other stationary object with subsequent fall
Bath tub
Fence
Lamp-post

E917.9   Other striking against with or without subsequent fall

● Code new   ▲ Revision of   ④ ⑤ Fourth or fifth
   to this edition   existing code   digit required

E CODES

E918 Caught accidentally in or between objects

> Caught, crushed, jammed, or pinched in or between moving or stationary objects, such as:
> escalator
> folding object
> hand tools, appliances, or implements
> sliding door and door frame
> under packing crate
> washing machine wringer

> Excludes: injury caused by:
>> cutting or piercing instrument (E920.0-E920.9)
>> machinery (E919.0-E919.9)
>> mechanism or component of firearm and air gun (E928.7)
>> transport vehicle (E800.0-E845.9)
>> vehicle not elsewhere classifiable (E846-E848)
>> struck accidentally by:
>>> falling object (E916)
>>> object (moving) (projected) (E917.0-E917.9)

E919 Accidents caused by machinery

> Includes:
>> burned by machinery (accident)
>> caught in (moving parts of) machinery (accident)
>> collapse of machinery (accident)
>> crushed by machinery (accident)
>> cut or pierced by machinery (accident)
>> drowning or submersion caused by machinery (accident)
>> explosion of, on, in machinery (accident)
>> fall from or into moving part of machinery (accident)
>> fire starting in or on machinery (accident)
>> mechanical suffocation caused by machinery (accident)
>> object falling from, on, in motion by machinery (accident)
>> overturning of machinery (accident)
>> pinned under machinery (accident)
>> run over by machinery (accident)
>> struck by machinery (accident)
>> thrown from machinery (accident)
>> caught between machinery and other object
>> machinery accident NOS

> Excludes: accidents involving machinery, not in operation (E884.9, E916-E918)
>> injury caused by:
>>> electric current in connection with machinery (E925.0-E925.9)
>>> escalator (E880.0, E918)
>>> explosion of pressure vessel in connection with machinery (E921.0-E921.9)
>>> mechanism or component of firearm and air gun (E928.7)
>>> moving sidewalk (E885.9)
>>> powered hand tools, appliances, and implements (E916-E918, E920.0-E921.9, E923.0-E926.9)
>>> transport vehicle accidents involving machinery (E800.0-E848.9)
>> poisoning by carbon monoxide generated by machine (E868.8)

E919.0 Agriculture machines

> Animal-powered agricultural machine
> Combine
> Derrick, hay
> Farm machinery NOS
> Farm tractor
> Harvester
> Hay mower or rake
> Reaper
> Thresher

> Excludes: that in transport under own power on the highway (E810.0-E819.9)
>> that being towed by another vehicle on the highway (E810.0-E819.9, E827.0-E827.9, E829.0-E829.9)
>> that involved in accident classifiable to E820-E829 (E820.0-E829.9)

E919.1 Mining and earth-drilling machinery

> Bore or drill (land) (seabed)
> Shaft hoist
> Shaft lift
> Under-cutter

> Excludes: coal car, tram, truck, and tub in mine (E846)

Add 4th or 5th digit | Nonspecific code | Unspecified code | Manifestation code

E919.2 **Lifting machines and appliances**
Chain hoist except in agricultural or mining operations
Crane except in agricultural or mining operations
Derrick except in agricultural or mining operations
Elevator (building) (grain) except in agricultural or mining operations
Forklift truck except in agricultural or mining operations
Lift except in agricultural or mining operations
Pulley block except in agricultural or mining operations
Winch except in agricultural or mining operations

Excludes: *that being towed by another vehicle on the highway (E810.0-E819.9,*
E827.0-E827.9, E829.0-E829.9)
that in transport under own power on the highway (E810.0-E819.9)
that involved in accident classifiable to E820-E829 (E820.0-E829.9)

E919.3 **Metalworking machines**
Abrasive wheel   Metal:
Forging machine   drilling machine
Lathe   milling machine
Mechanical shears   power press
rolling-mill
sawing machine

E919.4 **Woodworking and forming machines**
Band saw   Powered saw
Bench saw   Radial saw
Circular saw   Sander
Molding machine
Overhead plane

Excludes: *hand saw (E920.1)*

E919.5 **Prime movers, except electrical motors**
Gas turbine   Steam engine
Internal combustion engine   Water driven turbine

Excludes: *that being towed by other vehicle on the highway (E810.0-E819.9, E827.0-E827.9,*
E829.0-E829.9)
that in transport under own power on the highway (E810.0-E819.9)

E919.6 **Transmission machinery**
Transmission: Transmission:
belt   pinion
cable   pulley
chain   shaft
gear

E919.7 **Earth moving, scraping, and other excavating machines**
Bulldozer   Steam shovel
Road scraper

Excludes: *that being towed by other vehicle on the highway (E810.0-E819.9, E827.0-E827.9,*
E829.0-E829.9)
that in transport under own power on the highway (E810.0-E819.9)

E919.8 **Other specified machinery**
Machines for manufacture of: Printing machine
clothing   Recreational machinery
foodstuffs and beverages   Spinning, weaving, and textile machines
paper

E919.9 **Unspecified machinery**

E920 **Accidents caused by cutting and piercing instruments or objects**
Includes: accidental injury (by) object:
edged
pointed
sharp

Excludes: *injury caused by mechanism or component of firearm and air gun (E928.7)*

E920.0 **Powered lawn mower**

● `Code new
to this edition   ▲ Revision of
existing code   ④ ⑤ Fourth or fifth
digit required

E920.1 **Other powered hand tools**
Any powered hand tool [compressed air] [electric] [explosive cartridge] [hydraulic power], such as:

drill	rivet gun
hand saw	snow blower
hedge clipper	staple gun

Excludes: *band saw (E919.4)*
bench saw (E919.4)

E920.2 **Powered household appliances and implements**

Blender	Electric:
Electric:	knife
beater or mixer	sewing machine
can opener	Garbage disposal appliance
fan	

E920.3 **Knives, swords, and daggers**

E920.4 **Other hand tools and implements**

Axe	Paper cutter
Can opener NOS	Pitchfork
Chisel	Rake
Fork	Scissors
Hand saw	Screwdriver
Hoe	Sewing machine, not powered
Ice pick	Shovel
Needle (sewing)	

E920.5 **Hypodermic needle**
Contaminated needle
Needle stick

E920.8 **Other specified cutting and piercing instruments or objects**

Arrow	Nail
Broken glass	Plant thorn
Dart	Splinter
Edge of stiff paper	Tin can lid
Lathe turnings	

Excludes: *animal spines or quills (E906.8)*
flying glass due to explosion (E921.0-E923.9)

E920.9 **Unspecified cutting and piercing instrument or object**

E921 **Accident caused by explosion of pressure vessel**
Includes: accidental explosion of pressure vessels, whether or not part of machinery

Excludes: *explosion of pressure vessel on transport vehicle (E800.0-E845.9)*

E921.0 **Boilers**

E921.1 **Gas cylinders**
Air tank   Pressure gas tank

E921.8 **Other specified pressure vessels**
Aerosol can   Pressure cooker
Automobile tire

E921.9 **Unspecified pressure vessel**

E922 **Accident caused by firearm and air gun missile**

Excludes: *injury caused by mechanism or component of firearm and air gun (E928.7)*

E922.0 **Handgun**
Pistol   Revolver

Excludes: *Verey pistol (E922.8)*

E922.1 **Shotgun (automatic)**

E922.2 **Hunting rifle**

E922.3 **Military firearms**
Army rifle   Machine gun

E922.4 **Air gun**
BB gun   Pellet gun

E922.5 **Paintball gun**

E922.8 **Other specified firearm missile**
Verey pistol [flare]

▉ Add 4th or 5th digit	▉ Nonspecific code	▉ Unspecified code	▉ Manifestation code

E922.9 Unspecified firearm missile
    Gunshot wound NOS   Shot NOS

E923 Accident caused by explosive material
    Includes: flash burns and other injuries resulting from explosion of explosive material
                ignition of highly explosive material with explosion

    Excludes: explosion:
                in or on machinery (E919.0-E919.9)
                on any transport vehicle, except stationary motor vehicle (E800.0-E848)
                with conflagration (E890.0, E891.0, E892)
                injury caused by mechanism or component of firearm and air gun (E928.7)
                secondary fires resulting from explosion (E890.0-E899)

E923.0 Fireworks

E923.1 Blasting materials
    Blasting cap   Explosive [any] used in blasting operations
    Detonator
    Dynamite

E923.2 Explosive gases
    Acetylene   Fire damp
    Butane   Gasoline fumes
    Coal gas   Methane
    Explosion in mine NOS   Propane

E923.8 Other explosive materials
    Bomb   Torpedo
    Explosive missile   Explosion in munitions:
    Grenade   dump
    Mine   factory
    Shell

E923.9 Unspecified explosive material
    Explosion NOS

E924 Accident caused by hot substance or object, caustic or corrosive material, and steam
    Excludes: *burning NOS (E899)*
                chemical burn resulting from swallowing a corrosive substance (E860.0-E864.4)
                fire caused by these substances and objects (E890.0-E894)
                radiation burns (E926.0-E926.9)
                therapeutic misadventures (E870.0-E876.9)

E924.0 Hot liquids and vapors, including steam
    Burning or scalding by:
      boiling water
      hot or boiling liquids not primarily caustic or corrosive
      liquid metal
      steam
      other hot vapor

    Excludes: *hot (boiling) tap water (E924.2)*

E924.1 Caustic and corrosive substances
    Burning by:
      acid [any kind]
      ammonia
      caustic oven cleaner or other substance
      corrosive substance
      lye
      vitriol

E924.2 Hot (boiling) tap water

E924.8 Other
    Burning by:
      heat from electric heating appliance
      hot object NOS
      light bulb
      steam pipe

E924.9 Unspecified

  ● Code new   ▲ Revision of   ④ ⑤ Fourth or fifth
        to this edition   existing code   digit required

E925 **Accident caused by electric current**
  Includes: electric current from exposed wire, faulty appliance, high voltage cable, live rail, or open electric socket as the cause of:
      burn
      cardiac fibrillation
      convulsion
      electric shock
      electrocution
      puncture wound
      respiratory paralysis

  Excludes: *burn by heat from electrical appliance (E924.8)*
        lightning (E907)

E925.0 **Domestic wiring and appliances**

E925.1 **Electric power generating plants, distribution stations, transmission lines**
  Broken power line

E925.2 **Industrial wiring, appliances, and electrical machinery**
  Conductors
  Control apparatus
  Electrical equipment and machinery
  Transformers

E925.8 **Other electric current**
  Wiring and appliances in or on:
    farm [not farmhouse]
    outdoors
    public building
    residential institutions
    schools

E925.9 **Unspecified electric current**
  Burns or other injury from electric current NOS
  Electric shock NOS
  Electrocution NOS

E926 **Exposure to radiation**

  Excludes: *abnormal reaction to or complication of treatment without mention of misadventure (E879.2)*
        atomic power plant malfunction in water transport (E838.0-E838.9)
        misadventure to patient in surgical and medical procedures (E873.2-E873.3)
        use of radiation in war operations (E996-E997.9)

E926.0 **Radiofrequency radiation**
  Overexposure to:
    microwave radiation from:
      high-powered radio and television transmitters
      industrial radiofrequency induction heaters
      radar installations
    radar radiation from:
      high-powered radio and television transmitters
      industrial radiofrequency induction heaters
      radar installations
    radiofrequency from:
      high-powered radio and television transmitters
      industrial radiofrequency induction heaters
      radar installations
    radiofrequency radiation [any] from:
      high-powered radio and television transmitters
      industrial radiofrequency induction heaters
      radar installations

E926.1 **Infra-red heaters and lamps**
  Exposure to infra-red radiation from heaters and lamps as the cause of:
    blistering
    burning
    charring
    inflammatory change

  Excludes: *physical contact with heater or lamp (E924.8)*

| | Add 4th or 5th digit | | Nonspecific code | | Unspecified code | | Manifestation code |

E926.2 **Visible and ultraviolet light sources**
Arc lamps
Black light sources
Electrical welding arc
Oxygas welding torch
Sun rays
Tanning bed

Excludes: excessive heat from these sources (E900.1-E900.9)

E926.3 **X-rays and other electromagnetic ionizing radiation**
Gamma rays   X-rays (hard) (soft)

E926.4 **Lasers**

E926.5 **Radioactive isotopes**
Radiobiologicals   Radiopharmaceuticals

E926.8 **Other specified radiation**
Artificially accelerated beams of ionized particles generated by:
betatrons
synchrotrons

E926.9 **Unspecified radiation**
Radiation NOS

E927 **Overexertion and strenuous and repetitive movements or loads**
Use additional code to identify activity (E001-E030)

E927.0 **Overexertion from sudden strenuous movement**
Sudden trauma from strenuous movement

E927.1 **Overexertion from prolonged static position**
Overexertion from maintaining prolonged positions, such as:
holding
sitting
standing

E927.2 **Excessive physical exertion from prolonged activity**

E927.3 **Cumulative trauma from repetitive motion**
Cumulative trauma from repetitive movements

E927.4 **Cumulative trauma from repetitive impact**

E927.8 **Other overexertion and strenuous and repetitive movements or loads**

E927.9 **Unspecified overexertion and strenuous and repetitive movements or loads**

E928 **Other and unspecified environmental and accidental causes**

E928.0 **Prolonged stay in weightless environment**
Weightlessness in spacecraft (simulator)

E928.1 **Exposure to noise**
Noise (pollution)
Sound waves
Supersonic waves

E928.2 **Vibration**

E928.3 **Human bite**

E928.4 **External constriction caused by hair**

E928.5 **External constriction caused by other object**

E928.6 **Environmental exposure to harmful algae and toxins**
Algae bloom NOS
Blue-green algae bloom
Brown tide
Cyanobacteria bloom
Florida red tide
Harmful algae bloom
Pfiesteria piscicida
Red tide

● **E928.7** **Mechanism or component of firearm and air gun**
Injury due to:
explosion of gun parts
recoil
Pierced, cut, crushed, or pinched by slide trigger mechanism, scope or other gun part
Powder burn from firearm or air gun

Excludes: accident caused by firearm and air gun missile (E922.0-E922.9)

E928.8 **Other**

● Code new
to this edition
▲ Revision of
existing code
④ ⑤ Fourth or fifth
digit required

E928.9 **Unspecified accident**
Accident NOS stated as accidentally inflicted
Blow NOS stated as accidentally inflicted
Casualty (not due to war), stated as accidentally inflicted, but not otherwise specified
Decapitation, stated as accidentally inflicted, but not otherwise specified
Injury [any part of body, or unspecified], stated as accidentally inflicted, but not
otherwise specified
Killed, stated as accidentally inflicted, but not otherwise specified
Knocked down, stated as accidentally inflicted, but not otherwise specified
Mangled, stated as accidentally inflicted, but not otherwise specified
Wound, stated as accidentally inflicted, but not otherwise specified

Excludes: *fracture, cause unspecified (E887)*
injuries undetermined whether accidentally or purposely inflicted (E980.0-E989)

LATE EFFECTS OF ACCIDENTAL INJURY (E929)

Note: This category is to be used to indicate accidental injury as the cause of death or disability
from late effects, which are themselves classifiable elsewhere. The "late effects" include
conditions reported as such or as sequelae which may occur at any time after the acute
injury.

E929 **Late effects of accidental injury**

Excludes: *late effects of:*
surgical and medical procedures (E870.0-E879.9)
therapeutic use of drugs and medicines (E930.0-E949.9)

E929.0 **Late effects of motor vehicle accident**
Late effects of accidents classifiable to E810-E825

E929.1 **Late effects of other transport accident**
Late effects of accidents classifiable to E800-E807, E826-E838, E840-E848

E929.2 **Late effects of accidental poisoning**
Late effects of accidents classifiable to E850-E858, E860-E869

E929.3 **Late effects of accidental fall**
Late effects of accidents classifiable to E880-E888

E929.4 **Late effects of accident caused by fire**
Late effects of accidents classifiable to E890-E899

E929.5 **Late effects of accident due to natural and environmental factors**
Late effects of accidents classifiable to E900-E909

E929.8 **Late effects of other accidents**
Late effects of accidents classifiable to E910-E928.8

E929.9 **Late effects of unspecified accident**
Late effects of accidents classifiable to E928.9

DRUGS, MEDICINAL AND BIOLOGICAL SUBSTANCES CAUSING ADVERSE EFFECTS IN THERAPEUTIC USE (E930-E949)

Includes: correct drug properly administered in therapeutic or prophylactic dosage, as the
cause of any adverse effect including allergic or hypersensitivity reactions

Excludes: *accidental overdose of drug and wrong drug given or taken in error*
(E850.0-E858.9)
accidents in the technique of administration of drug or biological substance, such
as accidental puncture during injection, or contamination of drug
(E870.0-E876.9)
administration with suicidal or homicidal intent or intent to harm, or in
circumstances classifiable to E950.0-E950.5, E962.0, E980.0-E980.5

See Alphabetic Index for more complete list of specific drugs to be classified under the
fourth-digit subdivisions. The American Hospital Formulary numbers can be used to
classify new drugs listed by the American Hospital Formulary Service (AHFS). See
appendix C.

E930 **Antibiotics**

Excludes: *that used as eye, ear, nose, and throat [ENT], and local anti-infectives*
(E946.0-E946.9)

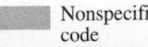 Add 4th or
5th digit   Nonspecific
code   Unspecified
code   Manifestation
code

E930.0 Penicillins
Natural
Synthetic
Semisynthetic, such as:
  ampicillin
  cloxacillin
  nafcillin
  oxacillin

E930.1 Antifungal antibiotics
Amphotericin B
Griseofulvin
Hachimycin [trichomycin]
Nystatin

E930.2 Chloramphenicol group
Chloramphenicol
Thiamphenicol

E930.3 Erythromycin and other macrolides
Oleandomycin
Spiramycin

E930.4 Tetracycline group
Doxycycline
Minocycline
Oxytetracycline

E930.5 Cephalosporin group
Cephalexin
Cephaloglycin
Cephaloridine
Cephalothin

E930.6 Antimycobacterial antibiotics
Cycloserine
Kanamycin
Rifampin
Streptomycin

E930.7 Antineoplastic antibiotics
Actinomycins, such as:
  Cactinomycin
  Dactinomycin
  Bleomycin
  Daunorubicin
  Mitomycin

Excludes: *other antineoplastic drugs (E933.1)*

E930.8 Other specified antibiotics

E930.9 Unspecified antibiotic

E931 Other anti-infectives

Excludes: *ENT, and local anti-infectives (E946.0-E946.9)*

E931.0 Sulfonamides
Sulfadiazine
Sulfafurazole
Sulfamethoxazole

E931.1 Arsenical anti-infectives

E931.2 Heavy metal anti-infectives
Compounds of:
  antimony
  bismuth
  lead
  mercury

Excludes: *mercurial diuretics (E944.0)*

E931.3 Quinoline and hydroxyquinoline derivatives
Chiniofon
Diiodohydroxyquin

Excludes: *antimalarial drugs (E931.4)*

● Code new
  to this edition

▲ Revision of
  existing code

④ ⑤ Fourth or fifth
    digit required

E931.4 Antimalarials and drugs acting on other blood protozoa
Chloroquine phosphate   Proguanil [chloroguanide]
Cycloguanil   Pyrimethamine
Primaquine   Quinine (sulphate)

E931.5 Other antiprotozoal drugs
Emetine

E931.6 Anthelmintics
Hexylresorcinol   Piperazine
Male fern oleoresin   Thiabendazole

E931.7 Antiviral drugs
Methisazone

Excludes: *amantadine (E936.4)*
cytarabine (E933.1)
idoxuridine (E946.5)

E931.8 Other antimycobacterial drugs
Ethambutol   Para-aminosalicylic acid derivatives
Ethionamide   Sulfones
Isoniazid

E931.9 Other and unspecified anti-infectives
Flucytosine   Nitrofuran derivatives

E932 Hormones and synthetic substitutes

E932.0 Adrenal cortical steroids
Cortisone derivatives
Desoxycorticosterone derivatives
Fluorinated corticosteroids

E932.1 Androgens and anabolic congeners
Nandrolone phenpropionate
Oxymetholone
Testosterone and preparations

E932.2 Ovarian hormones and synthetic substitutes
Contraceptives, oral
Estrogens
Estrogens and progestogens combined
Progestogens

E932.3 Insulins and antidiabetic agents
Acetohexamide   Insulin
Biguanide derivatives, oral   Phenformin
Chlorpropamide   Sulfonylurea derivatives, oral
Glucagon   Tolbutamide

Excludes: *adverse effect of insulin administered for shock therapy (E879.3)*

E932.4 Anterior pituitary hormones
Corticotropin   Somatotropin [growth hormone]
Gonadotropin

E932.5 Posterior pituitary hormones
Vasopressin

Excludes: *oxytocic agents (E945.0)*

E932.6 Parathyroid and parathyroid derivatives

E932.7 Thyroid and thyroid derivatives
Dextrothyroxine   Liothyronine
Levothyroxine sodium   Thyroglobulin

E932.8 Antithyroid agents
Iodides   Thiourea
Thiouracil

E932.9 Other and unspecified hormones and synthetic substitutes

E933 Primarily systemic agents

E933.0 Antiallergic and antiemetic drugs
Antihistamines   Diphenylpyraline
Chlorpheniramine   Thonzylamine
Diphenhydramine   Tripelennamine

Excludes: *phenothiazine-based tranquilizers (E939.1)*

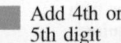 Add 4th or 5th digit   Nonspecific code   Unspecified code   Manifestation code

E933.1 **Antineoplastic and immunosuppressive drugs**
    Azathioprine   Mechlorethamine hydrochloride
    Busulfan   Mercaptopurine
    Chlorambucil   Triethylenethiophosphoramide [thio-TEPA]
    Cyclophosphamide
    Cytarabine
    Fluorouracil

    Excludes: *antineoplastic antibiotics (E930.7)*

E933.2 **Acidifying agents**

E933.3 **Alkalizing agents**

E933.4 **Enzymes, not elsewhere classified**
    Penicillinase

E933.5 **Vitamins, not elsewhere classified**
    Vitamin A
    Vitamin D

    Excludes: *nicotinic acid (E942.2)*
              vitamin K (E934.3)

E933.6 **Oral bisphosphonates**

E933.7 **Intravenous bisphosphonates**

E933.8 **Other systemic agents, not elsewhere classified**
    Heavy metal antagonists

E933.9 **Unspecified systemic agent**

E934 **Agents primarily affecting blood constituents**

E934.0 **Iron and its compounds**
    Ferric salts
    Ferrous sulphate and other ferrous salts

E934.1 **Liver preparations and other antianemic agents**
    Folic acid

E934.2 **Anticoagulants**
    Coumarin   Prothrombin synthesis inhibitor
    Heparin   Warfarin sodium
    Phenindione

E934.3 **Vitamin K [phytonadione]**

E934.4 **Fibrinolysis-affecting drugs**
    Aminocaproic acid   Streptokinase
    Streptodornase   Urokinase

E934.5 **Anticoagulant antagonists and other coagulants**
    Hexadimethrine bromide   Protamine sulfate

E934.6 **Gamma globulin**

E934.7 **Natural blood and blood products**
    Blood plasma   Packed red cells
    Human fibrinogen   Whole blood

E934.8 **Other agents affecting blood constituents**
    Macromolecular blood substitutes

E934.9 **Unspecified agent affecting blood constituents**

E935 **Analgesics, antipyretics, and antirheumatics**

E935.0 **Heroin**
    Diacetylmorphine

E935.1 **Methadone**

E935.2 **Other opiates and related narcotics**
    Codeine [methylmorphine]   Opium (alkaloids)
    Morphine   Meperidine [pethidine]

E935.3 **Salicylates**
    Acetylsalicylic acid [aspirin]
    Amino derivatives of salicylic acid
    Salicylic acid salts

E935.4 **Aromatic analgesics, not elsewhere classified**
    Acetanilid
    Paracetamol [acetaminophen]
    Phenacetin [acetophenetidin]

  ● Code new   ▲ Revision of   ④ ⑤ Fourth or fifth
        to this edition   existing code   digit required

E935.5 **Pyrazole derivatives**
Aminophenazone [aminopyrine]
Phenylbutazone

E935.6 **Antirheumatics [antiphlogistics]**
Gold salts   Indomethacin

Excludes: salicylates (E935.3)
steroids (E932.0)

E935.7 **Other non-narcotic analgesics**
Pyrabital

E935.8 **Other specified analgesics and antipyretics**
Pentazocine

E935.9 **Unspecified analgesic and antipyretic**

E936 **Anticonvulsants and anti-Parkinsonism drugs**

E936.0 **Oxazolidine derivatives**
Paramethadione
Trimethadione

E936.1 **Hydantoin derivatives**
Phenytoin

E936.2 **Succinimides**
Ethosuximide
Phensuximide

E936.3 **Other and unspecified anticonvulsants**
Beclamide
Primidone

E936.4 **Anti-Parkinsonism drugs**
Amantadine
Ethopropazine [profenamine]
Levodopa [L-dopa]

E937 **Sedatives and hypnotics**

E937.0 **Barbiturates**
Amobarbital [amylobarbitone]
Barbital [barbitone]
Butabarbital [butabarbitone]
Pentobarbital [pentobarbitone]
Phenobarbital [phenobarbitone]
Secobarbital [quinalbarbitone]

Excludes: thiobarbiturates (E938.3)

E937.1 **Chloral hydrate group**

E937.2 **Paraldehyde**

E937.3 **Bromine compounds**
Bromide
Carbromal (derivatives)

E937.4 **Methaqualone compounds**

E937.5 **Glutethimide group**

E937.6 **Mixed sedatives, not elsewhere classified**

E937.8 **Other sedatives and hypnotics**

E937.9 **Unspecified**
Sleeping:
drug NOS
pill NOS
tablet NOS

E938 **Other central nervous system depressants and anesthetics**

E938.0 **Central nervous system muscle-tone depressants**
Chlorphenesin (carbamate)   Methocarbamol
Mephenesin

E938.1 **Halothane**

E938.2 **Other gaseous anesthetics**
Ether
Halogenated hydrocarbon derivatives, except halothane
Nitrous oxide

Add 4th or
5th digit

Nonspecific
code

Unspecified
code

Manifestation
code

E938.3 Intravenous anesthetics
Ketamine
Methohexital
[methohexitone]
Thiobarbiturates, such as thiopental sodium

E938.4 Other and unspecified general anesthetics

E938.5 Surface and infiltration anesthetics
Cocaine
Lidocaine [lignocaine]
Procaine
Tetracaine

E938.6 Peripheral nerve- and plexus-blocking anesthetics

E938.7 Spinal anesthetics

E938.9 Other and unspecified local anesthetics

E939 Psychotropic agents

E939.0 Antidepressants
Amitriptyline
Imipramine
Monoamine oxidase [MAO] inhibitors

E939.1 Phenothiazine-based tranquilizers
Chlorpromazine
Fluphenazine
Phenothiazine
Prochlorperazine
Promazine

E939.2 Butyrophenone-based tranquilizers
Haloperidol
Spiperone
Trifluperidol

E939.3 Other antipsychotics, neuroleptics, and major tranquilizers

E939.4 Benzodiazepine-based tranquilizers
Chlordiazepoxide
Diazepam
Flurazepam
Lorazepam
Medazepam
Nitrazepam

E939.5 Other tranquilizers
Hydroxyzine
Meprobamate

E939.6 Psychodysleptics [hallucinogens]
Cannabis (derivatives)
Lysergide [LSD]
Marihuana (derivatives)
Mescaline
Psilocin
Psilocybin

E939.7 Psychostimulants
Amphetamine
Caffeine

Excludes: central appetite depressants (E947.0)

E939.8 Other psychotropic agents

E939.9 Unspecified psychotropic agent

E940 Central nervous system stimulants

E940.0 Analeptics
Lobeline
Nikethamide

E940.1 Opiate antagonists
Levallorphan
Nalorphine
Naloxone

E940.8 Other specified central nervous system stimulants

E940.9 Unspecified central nervous system stimulant

E941 Drugs primarily affecting the autonomic nervous system

E941.0 Parasympathomimetics [cholinergics]
Acetylcholine
Anticholinesterase:
  organophosphorus
  reversible
Pilocarpine

E941.1 Parasympatholytics [anticholinergics and antimuscarinics] and spasmolytics
Atropine
Homatropine
Hyoscine [scopolamine]
Quaternary ammonium derivatives

Excludes: papaverine (E942.5)

E941.2 Sympathomimetics [adrenergics]
Epinephrine [adrenalin]
Levarterenol [noradrenalin]

● Code new to this edition   ▲ Revision of existing code   ④ ⑤ Fourth or fifth digit required

E941.3 **Sympatholytics [antiadrenergics]**
    Phenoxybenzamine
    Tolazoline hydrochloride

E941.9 **Unspecified drug primarily affecting the autonomic nervous system**

E942 **Agents primarily affecting the cardiovascular system**

E942.0 **Cardiac rhythm regulators**
    Practolol   Propranolol
    Procainamide   Quinidine

E942.1 **Cardiotonic glycosides and drugs of similar action**
    Digitalis glycosides   Strophanthins
    Digoxin

E942.2 **Antilipemic and antiarteriosclerotic drugs**
    Cholestyramine   Nicotinic acid derivatives
    Clofibrate   Sitosterols

    Excludes: *dextrothyroxine (E932.7)*

E942.3 **Ganglion-blocking agents**
    Pentamethonium bromide

E942.4 **Coronary vasodilators**
    Dipyridamole   Nitrites
    Nitrates [nitroglycerin]   Prenylamine

E942.5 **Other vasodilators**
    Cyclandelate   Hydralazine
    Diazoxide   Papaverine

E942.6 **Other antihypertensive agents**
    Clonidine   Rauwolfia alkaloids
    Guanethidine   Reserpine

E942.7 **Antivaricose drugs, including sclerosing agents**
    Monoethanolamine   Zinc salts

E942.8 **Capillary-active drugs**
    Adrenochrome derivatives   Metaraminol
    Bioflavonoids

E942.9 **Other and unspecified agents primarily affecting the cardiovascular system**

E943 **Agents primarily affecting gastrointestinal system**

E943.0 **Antacids and antigastric secretion drugs**
    Aluminum hydroxide   Magnesium trisilicate

E943.1 **Irritant cathartics**
    Bisacodyl   Phenolphthalein
    Castor oil

E943.2 **Emollient cathartics**
    Sodium dioctyl sulfosuccinate

E943.3 **Other cathartics, including intestinal atonia drugs**
    Magnesium sulfate

E943.4 **Digestants**
    Pancreatin   Pepsin
    Papain

E943.5 **Antidiarrheal drugs**
    Bismuth subcarbonate   Pectin
    Kaolin

    Excludes: *anti-infectives (E930.0-E931.9)*

E943.6 **Emetics**

E943.8 **Other specified agents primarily affecting the gastrointestinal system**

E943.9 **Unspecified agent primarily affecting the gastrointestinal system**

E944 **Water, mineral, and uric acid metabolism drugs**

E944.0 **Mercurial diuretics**
    Chlormerodrin   Mercurophylline
    Mercaptomerin   Mersalyl

E944.1 **Purine derivative diuretics**
    Theobromine   Theophylline

    Excludes: *aminophylline [theophylline ethylenediamine] (E945.7)*

Add 4th or 5th digit	Nonspecific code	Unspecified code	Manifestation code

E944.2 Carbonic acid anhydrase inhibitors
Acetazolamide

E944.3 Saluretics
Benzothiadiazides
Chlorothiazide group

E944.4 Other diuretics
Ethacrynic acid
Furosemide

E944.5 Electrolytic, caloric, and water-balance agents

E944.6 Other mineral salts, not elsewhere classified

E944.7 Uric acid metabolism drugs
Cinchophen and congeners   Phenoquin
Colchicine   Probenecid

E945 Agents primarily acting on the smooth and skeletal muscles and respiratory system

E945.0 Oxytocic agents
Ergot alkaloids
Prostaglandins

E945.1 Smooth muscle relaxants
Adiphenine
Metaproterenol [orciprenaline]
Excludes: papaverine (E942.5)

E945.2 Skeletal muscle relaxants
Alcuronium chloride
Suxamethonium chloride

E945.3 Other and unspecified drugs acting on muscles

E945.4 Antitussives
Dextromethorphan
Pipazethate hydrochloride

E945.5 Expectorants
Acetylcysteine   Ipecacuanha
Cocillana   Terpin hydrate
Guaifenesin [glyceryl guaiacolate]

E945.6 Anti-common cold drugs

E945.7 Antiasthmatics
Aminophylline [theophylline ethylenediamine]

E945.8 Other and unspecified respiratory drugs

E946 Agents primarily affecting skin and mucous membrane, ophthalmological, otorhinolaryngological, and dental drugs

E946.0 Local anti-infectives and anti-inflammatory drugs

E946.1 Antipruritics

E946.2 Local astringents and local detergents

E946.3 Emollients, demulcents, and protectants

E946.4 Keratolytics, keratoplastics, other hair treatment drugs and preparations

E946.5 Eye anti-infectives and other eye drugs
Idoxuridine

E946.6 Anti-infectives and other drugs and preparations for ear, nose, and throat

E946.7 Dental drugs topically applied

E946.8 Other agents primarily affecting skin and mucous membrane
Spermicides

E946.9 Unspecified agent primarily affecting skin and mucous membrane

E947 Other and unspecified drugs and medicinal substances

E947.0 Dietetics

E947.1 Lipotropic drugs

E947.2 Antidotes and chelating agents, not elsewhere classified

E947.3 Alcohol deterrents

E947.4 Pharmaceutical excipients

E947.8 Other drugs and medicinal substances
Contrast media used for diagnostic x-ray procedures
Diagnostic agents and kits

● Code new to this edition   ▲ Revision of existing code   ④ ⑤ Fourth or fifth digit required

E947.9   Unspecified drug or medicinal substance

E948   Bacterial vaccines

E948.0   BCG vaccine

E948.1   Typhoid and paratyphoid

E948.2   Cholera

E948.3   Plague

E948.4   Tetanus

E948.5   Diphtheria

E948.6   Pertussis vaccine, including combinations with a pertussis component

E948.8   Other and unspecified bacterial vaccines

E948.9   Mixed bacterial vaccines, except combinations with a pertussis component

E949   Other vaccines and biological substances

> Excludes: *gamma globulin (E934.6)*

E949.0   Smallpox vaccine

E949.1   Rabies vaccine

E949.2   Typhus vaccine

E949.3   Yellow fever vaccine

E949.4   Measles vaccine

E949.5   Poliomyelitis vaccine

E949.6   Other and unspecified viral and rickettsial vaccines
Mumps vaccine

E949.7   Mixed viral-rickettsial and bacterial vaccines, except combinations with a pertussis component

> Excludes: *combinations with a pertussis component (E948.6)*

E949.9   Other and unspecified vaccines and biological substances

SUICIDE AND SELF-INFLICTED INJURY (E950-E959)

> Includes: injuries in suicide and attempted suicide
> self-inflicted injuries specified as intentional

E950   Suicide and self-inflicted poisoning by solid or liquid substances

E950.0   Analgesics, antipyretics, and antirheumatics

E950.1   Barbiturates

E950.2   Other sedatives and hypnotics

E950.3   Tranquilizers and other psychotropic agents

E950.4   Other specified drugs and medicinal substances

E950.5   Unspecified drug or medicinal substances

E950.6   Agricultural and horticultural chemical and pharmaceutical preparations other than plant foods and fertilizers

E950.7   Corrosive and caustic substances
Suicide and self-inflicted poisoning by substances classifiable to E864

E950.8   Arsenic and its compounds

E950.9   Other and unspecified solid and liquid substances

E951   Suicide and self-inflicted poisoning by gases in domestic use

E951.0   Gas distributed by pipeline

E951.1   Liquefied petroleum gas distributed in mobile containers

E951.8   Other utility gas

E952   Suicide and self-inflicted poisoning by other gases and vapors

E952.0   Motor vehicle exhaust gas

E952.1   Other carbon monoxide

E952.8   Other specified gases and vapors

E952.9   Unspecified gases and vapors

E953   Suicide and self-inflicted injury by hanging, strangulation, and suffocation

E953.0   Hanging

E953.1   Suffocation by plastic bag

	Add 4th or 5th digit		Nonspecific code		Unspecified code		Manifestation code

E953.8 Other specified means

E953.9 Unspecified means

E954 Suicide and self-inflicted injury by submersion [drowning]

E955 Suicide and self-inflicted injury by firearms, air guns and explosives

E955.0 Handgun

E955.1 Shotgun

E955.2 Hunting rifle

E955.3 Military firearms

E955.4 Other and unspecified firearm
Gunshot NOS
Shot NOS

E955.5 Explosives

E955.6 Air gun
BB gun
Pellet gun

E955.7 Paintball gun

E955.9 Unspecified

E956 Suicide and self-inflicted injury by cutting and piercing instrument

E957 Suicide and self-inflicted injuries by jumping from high place

E957.0 Residential premises

E957.1 Other man-made structures

E957.2 Natural sites

E957.9 Unspecified

E958 Suicide and self-inflicted injury by other and unspecified means

E958.0 Jumping or lying before moving object

E958.1 Burns, fire

E958.2 Scald

E958.3 Extremes of cold

E958.4 Electrocution

E958.5 Crashing of motor vehicle

E958.6 Crashing of aircraft

E958.7 Caustic substances, except poisoning
Excludes: *poisoning by caustic substance (E950.7)*

E958.8 Other specified means

E958.9 Unspecified means

E959 Late effects of self-inflicted injury
Note: This category is to be used to indicate circumstances classifiable to E950-E958 as the cause of death or disability from late effects, which are themselves classifiable elsewhere. The "late effects" include conditions reported as such or as sequelae which may occur at any time after the attempted suicide or self-inflicted injury.

HOMICIDE AND INJURY PURPOSELY INFLICTED BY OTHER PERSONS (E960-E969)

Includes: injuries inflicted by another person with intent to injure or kill, by any means
Excludes: *injuries due to:*
legal intervention (E970-E978)
operations of war (E990-E999)
terrorism (E979)

E960 Fight, brawl, rape

E960.0 Unarmed fight or brawl
Beatings NOS
Brawl or fight with hands, fists, feet
Injured or killed in fight NOS
Excludes: *homicidal:*
injury by weapons (E965.0-E966, E969)
strangulation (E963)
submersion (E964)

E960.1 Rape

● Code new to this edition ▲ Revision of existing code ④ ⑤ Fourth or fifth digit required

E961 Assault by corrosive or caustic substance, except poisoning
Injury or death purposely caused by corrosive or caustic substance, such as:
acid [any]
corrosive substance
vitriol

Excludes: burns from hot liquid (E968.3)
chemical burns from swallowing a corrosive substance (E962.0-E962.9)

E962 Assault by poisoning

E962.0 Drugs and medicinal substances
Homicidal poisoning by any drug or medicinal substance

E962.1 Other solid and liquid substances

E962.2 Other gases and vapors

E962.9 Unspecified poisoning

E963 Assault by hanging and strangulation
Homicidal (attempt):
garrotting or ligature
hanging
strangulation
suffocation

E964 Assault by submersion [drowning]

E965 Assault by firearms and explosives

E965.0 Handgun
Pistol
Revolver

E965.1 Shotgun

E965.2 Hunting rifle

E965.3 Military firearms

E965.4 Other and unspecified firearm

E965.5 Antipersonnel bomb

E965.6 Gasoline bomb

E965.7 Letter bomb

E965.8 Other specified explosive
Bomb NOS (placed in) car
Bomb NOS (placed in) house
Dynamite

E965.9 Unspecified explosive

E966 Assault by cutting and piercing instrument
Assassination (attempt), homicide (attempt) by any instrument classifiable under E920
Homicidal cut, any part of the body
Homicidal puncture, any part of the body
Homicidal stab, any part of the body
Stabbed, any part of the body

E967 Perpetrator of child and adult abuse
Note: selection of the correct perpetrator code is based on the relationship between the perpetrator and the victim

E967.0 By father, stepfather or boyfriend
Male partner of child's parent or guardian

E967.1 By other specified person

E967.2 By mother, stepmother or girlfriend
Female partner of child's parent or guardian

E967.3 By spouse or partner
Abuse of spouse or partner by ex-spouse or ex-partner

E967.4 By child

E967.5 By sibling

E967.6 By grandparent

E967.7 By other relative

E967.8 By non-related caregiver

E967.9 By unspecified person

E968 Assault by other and unspecified means

Add 4th or 5th digit   Nonspecific code   Unspecified code   Manifestation code

E968.0   Fire
Arson
Homicidal burns NOS

Excludes: *burns from hot liquid (E968.3)*

E968.1   Pushing from a high place

E968.2   Striking by blunt or thrown object

E968.3   Hot liquid
Homicidal burns by scalding

E968.4   Criminal neglect
Abandonment of child, infant, or other helpless person with intent to injure or kill

E968.5   Transport vehicle
Being struck by other vehicle or run down with intent to injure
Pushed in front of, thrown from, or dragged by moving vehicle with intent to injure

E968.6   Air gun
BB gun
Pellet gun

E968.7   Human bite

E968.8   Other specified means

E968.9   Unspecified means
Assassination (attempt) NOS   Manslaughter (nonaccidental)
Homicidal (attempt):   Murder (attempt) NOS
  injury NOS   Violence, non-accidental
  wound NOS

E969   Late effects of injury purposely inflicted by other person
Note: This category is to be used to indicate circumstances classifiable to E960-E968 as the
cause of death or disability from late effects, which are themselves classifiable elsewhere.
The "late effects" include conditions reported as such, or as sequelae which may occur at
any time after the acute injury.

LEGAL INTERVENTION (E970-E978)

Includes: injuries inflicted by the police or other law-enforcing agents, including military on
duty, in the course of arresting or attempting to arrest lawbreakers, suppressing
disturbances, maintaining order, and other legal action
legal execution

Excludes: *injuries caused by civil insurrections (E990.0-E999)*

E970   Injury due to legal intervention by firearms
Gunshot wound
Injury by:
  machine gun
  revolver
  rifle pellet or rubber bullet
  shot NOS

E971   Injury due to legal intervention by explosives
Injury by:
  dynamite
  explosive shell
  grenade
  mortar bomb

E972   Injury due to legal intervention by gas
Asphyxiation by gas
Injury by tear gas
Poisoning by gas

E973   Injury due to legal intervention by blunt object
Hit, struck by:
  baton (nightstick)
  blunt object
  stave

E974   Injury due to legal intervention by cutting and piercing instrument
Cut
Incised wound
Injured by bayonet
Stab wound

● Code new   ▲ Revision of   ④ ⑤ Fourth or fifth
  to this edition   existing code   digit required

E975 Injury due to legal intervention by other specified means
Blow
Manhandling

E976 Injury due to legal intervention by unspecified means

E977 Late effects of injuries due to legal intervention
Note: This category is to be used to indicate circumstances classifiable to E970-E976 as the cause of death or disability from late effects, which are themselves classifiable elsewhere. The "late effects" include conditions reported as such, or as sequelae which may occur at any time after the acute injury due to legal intervention.

E978 Legal execution
All executions performed at the behest of the judiciary or ruling authority [whether permanent or temporary] as:

asphyxiation by gas
beheading, decapitation
  (by guillotine)
capital punishment
electrocution

hanging
poisoning
shooting
other specified means

TERRORISM (E979)

E979 Terrorism
Injuries resulting from the unlawful use of force or violence against persons or property to intimidate or coerce a Government, the civilian population, or any segment thereof, in furtherance of political or social objective

E979.0　Terrorism involving explosion of marine weapons
Depth-charge
Marine mine
Mine NOS, at sea or in harbor
Sea-based artillery shell
Torpedo
Underwater blast

E979.1　Terrorism involving destruction of aircraft
Aircraft used as a weapon
Aircraft:
  burned
  exploded
  shot down
Crushed by falling aircraft

E979.2　Terrorism involving other explosions and fragments
Antipersonnel bomb (fragments)
Blast NOS
Explosion (of):
  artillery shell
  breech-block
  cannon block
  mortar bomb
  munitions being used in terrorism
  NOS
Fragments from:
  artillery shell
  bomb
  grenade
  guided missile
  land-mine
  rocket
  shell
  shrapnel
Mine NOS

Add 4th or
5th digit

Nonspecific
code

Unspecified
code

Manifestation
code

E979.3 **Terrorism involving fires, conflagration and hot substances**
    Burning building or structure:
      collapse of
      fall from
      hit by falling object in
      jump from
    Conflagration NOS
    Fire (causing):
      asphyxia
      burns
      NOS
      other injury
    Melting of fittings and furniture in burning
    Petrol bomb
    Smouldering building or structure

E979.4 **Terrorism involving firearms**
    Bullet:
      carbine
      machine gun
      pistol
      rifle
      rubber (rifle)
    Pellets (shotgun)

E979.5 **Terrorism involving nuclear weapons**
    Blast effects
    Exposure to ionizing radiation from nuclear weapon
    Fireball effects
    Heat from nuclear weapon
    Other direct and secondary effects of nuclear weapons

E979.6 **Terrorism involving biological weapons**
    Anthrax
    Cholera
    Smallpox

E979.7 **Terrorism involving chemical weapons**
    Gases, fumes, chemicals
    Hydrogen cyanide
    Phosgene
    Sarin

E979.8 **Terrorism involving other means**
    Drowning and submersion
    Lasers
    Piercing or stabbing instruments
    Terrorism NOS

E979.9 **Terrorism, secondary effects**
Note: This code is for use to identify conditions occuring subsequent to a terrorist attack not
    those that are due to the intial terrorist act

    Excludes: *late effect of terroist attack (E999.1)*

INJURY UNDETERMINED WHETHER ACCIDENTALLY OR PURPOSELY INFLICTED (E980-E989)

    Note: Categories E980-E989 are for use when it is unspecified or it cannot be determined
    whether the injuries are accidental (unintentional), suicide (attempted), or assault.

E980 **Poisoning by solid or liquid substances, undetermined whether accidentally or purposely inflicted**

E980.0 **Analgesics, antipyretics, and antirheumatics**

E980.1 **Barbiturates**

E980.2 **Other sedatives and hypnotics**

E980.3 **Tranquilizers and other psychotropic agents**

E980.4 **Other specified drugs and medicinal substances**

E980.5 **Unspecified drug or medicinal substance**

E980.6 **Corrosive and caustic substances**
    Poisoning, undetermined whether accidental or purposeful, by substances classifiable
      to E864

E980.7 **Agricultural and horticultural chemical and pharmaceutical preparations other than plant foods and fertilizers**

● Code new   ▲ Revision of   ④ ⑤ Fourth or fifth
    to this edition   existing code   digit required

E980.8   Arsenic and its compounds

E980.9   Other and unspecified solid and liquid substances

E981   Poisoning by gases in domestic use, undetermined whether accidentally or purposely inflicted

E981.0   Gas distributed by pipeline

E981.1   Liquefied petroleum gas distributed in mobile containers

E981.8   Other utility gas

E982   Poisoning by other gases, undetermined whether accidentally or purposely inflicted

E982.0   Motor vehicle exhaust gas

E982.1   Other carbon monoxide

E982.8   Other specified gases and vapors

E982.9   Unspecified gases and vapors

E983   Hanging, strangulation, or suffocation, undetermined whether accidentally or purposely inflicted

E983.0   Hanging

E983.1   Suffocation by plastic bag

E983.8   Other specified means

E983.9   Unspecified means

E984   Submersion [drowning], undetermined whether accidentally or purposely inflicted

E985   Injury by firearms, air guns and explosives, undetermined whether accidentally or purposely inflicted

E985.0   Handgun

E985.1   Shotgun

E985.2   Hunting rifle

E985.3   Military firearms

E985.4   Other and unspecified firearm

E985.5   Explosives

E985.6   Air gun
  BB gun
  Pellet gun

E985.7   Paintball gun

E986   Injury by cutting and piercing instruments, undetermined whether accidentally or purposely inflicted

E987   Falling from high place, undetermined whether accidentally or purposely inflicted

E987.0   Residential premises

E987.1   Other man-made structures

E987.2   Natural sites

E987.9   Unspecified site

E988   Injury by other and unspecified means, undetermined whether accidentally or purposely inflicted

E988.0   Jumping or lying before moving object

E988.1   Burns, fire

E988.2   Scald

E988.3   Extremes of cold

E988.4   Electrocution

E988.5   Crashing of motor vehicle

E988.6   Crashing of aircraft

E988.7   Caustic substances, except poisoning

E988.8   Other specified means

E988.9   Unspecified means

E989   Late effects of injury, undetermined whether accidentally or purposely inflicted

Note: This category is to be used to indicate circumstances classifiable to E980-E988 as the cause of death or disability from late effects, which are themselves classifiable elsewhere. The "late effects" include conditions reported as such or as sequelae which may occur at any time after the acute injury, undetermined whether accidentally or purposely inflicted.

	Add 4th or 5th digit		Nonspecific code		Unspecified code		Manifestation code

INJURY RESULTING FROM OPERATIONS OF WAR (E990-E999)

Includes: injuries to military personnel and civilians caused by war and civil insurrections and occurring during the time of war and insurrection, and peacekeeping missions.

Excludes: accidents during training of military personnel, manufacture of war material and transport, unless attributable to enemy action

E990 Injury due to war operations by fires and conflagrations
Includes: asphyxia, burns, or other injury originating from fire caused by a fire-producing device or indirectly by any conventional weapon

E990.0 From gasoline bomb
Incendiary bomb

● **E990.1 From flamethrower**

● **E990.2 From incendiary bullet**

● **E990.3 From fire caused indirectly from conventional weapon**
Excludes: fire aboard military aircraft (E994.3)

E990.9 From other and unspecified source

E991 Injury due to war operations by bullets and fragments
Excludes: injury due to bullets and fragments due to war operations, but occurring after cessation of hostilities (E998.0)
injury due to explosion of artillery shells and mortars (E993.2)
injury due to explosion of improvised explosive device [IED] (E993.3-E993.5)
injury due to sea-based artillery shell (E992.3)

E991.0 Rubber bullets (rifle)

E991.1 Pellets (rifle)

E991.2 Other bullets
Bullet [any, except rubber bullets and pellets]
carbine
machine gun
pistol
rifle
shotgun

E991.3 Antipersonnel bomb (fragments)

● **E991.4 Fragments from munitions**
Fragments from:
artillery shell
bombs, except antipersonnel
detonation of unexploded ordnance [UXO]
grenade
guided missile
land mine
rockets
shell

● **E991.5 Fragments from person-borne improvised explosive device [IED]**

● **E991.6 Fragments from vehicle-borne improvised explosive device [IED]**
IED borne by land, air, or water transport vehicle

● **E991.7 Fragments from other improvised explosive device [IED]**
Roadside IED

● **E991.8 Fragments from weapons**
Fragments from:
artillery
autocannons
automatic grenade launchers
missile launchers
mortars
small arms

E991.9 Other and unspecified fragments
Shrapnel NOS

E992 Injury due to war operations by explosion of marine weapons

● **E992.0 Torpedo**

● **E992.1 Depth charge**

● **E992.2 Marine mines**
Marine mines at sea or in harbor

● **E992.3 Sea-based artillery shell**

● Code new
to this edition
▲ Revision of
existing code
④ ⑤ Fourth or fifth
digit required

- **E992.8** Other by other marine weapons
- **E992.9** Unspecified marine weapon
  Underwater blast NOS

E993 Injury due to war operations by other explosion
  Injuries due to direct or indirect pressure or air blast of an explosion occurring during war operations

  > Excludes: *injury due to fragments resulting from an explosion (E991.0-E991.9)*
  > *injury due to detonation of unexploded ordnance but occurring after cessation of hostilities (E998.0-E998.9)*
  > *injury due to nuclear weapons (E996.0-E996.9)*

- **E993.0** Aerial bomb
- **E993.1** Guided missile
- **E993.2** Mortar
  Artillery shell
- **E993.3** Person-borne improvised explosive device [IED]
- **E993.4** Vehicle-borne improvised explosive device [IED]
  IED borne by land, air, or water transport vehicle
- **E993.5** Other improvised explosive device [IED]
  Roadside IED
- **E993.6** Unintentional detonation of own munitions
  Unintentional detonation of own ammunition (artillery) (mortars)
- **E993.7** Unintentional discharge of own munitions launch device
  Unintentional explosion of own:
  Autocannons
  Automatic grenade launchers
  Missile launchers
  Small arms
- **E993.8** Other specified explosion
  Bomb
  Grenade
  Land mine
- **E993.9** Unspecified explosion
  Air blast NOS
  Blast NOS
  Blast wave NOS
  Blast wind NOS
  Explosion NOS

E994 Injury due to war operations by destruction of aircraft

- **E994.0** Destruction of aircraft due to enemy fire or explosives
  Air to air missile
  Explosive device placed on aircraft
  Rocket propelled grenade [RPG]
  Small arms fire
  Surface to air missile
- **E994.1** Unintentional destruction of aircraft due to own onboard explosives
- **E994.2** Destruction of aircraft due to collision with other aircraft
- **E994.3** Destruction of aircraft due to onboard fire
- **E994.8** Other destruction of aircraft
- **E994.9** Unspecified destruction of aircraft

E995 Injury due to war operations by other and unspecified forms of conventional warfare

- **E995.0** Unarmed hand-to-hand combat

  > Excludes: *intentional restriction of airway (E995.3)*

- **E995.1** Struck by blunt object
  Baton (nightstick)
  Stave
- **E995.2** Piercing object
  Bayonet
  Knife
  Sword

	Add 4th or 5th digit		Nonspecific code		Unspecified code	Manifestation code

● **E995.3 Intentional restriction of air and airway**
Intentional submersion
Strangulation
Suffocation

● **E995.4 Unintentional drowning due to inability to surface or obtain air**
Submersion

● **E995.8 Other forms of conventional warfare**

● **E995.9 Unspecified form of conventional warfare**

E996 Injury due to war operations by nuclear weapons
Dirty bomb NOS

> Excludes: *late effects of injury due to nuclear weapons (E999.1, E999.0)*

● **E996.0 Direct blast effect of nuclear weapon**
Injury to bodily organs due to blast pressure

● **E996.1 Indirect blast effect of nuclear weapon**
Injury due to being thrown by blast
Injury due to being struck or crushed by blast debris

● **E996.2 Thermal radiation effect of nuclear weapon**
Burns due to thermal radiation
Fireball effects
Flash burns
Heat effects

● **E996.3 Nuclear radiation effects**
Acute radiation exposure
Beta burns
Fallout exposure
Radiation sickness
Secondary effects of nuclear weapons

● **E996.8 Other effects of nuclear weapons**

● **E996.9 Unspecified effect of nuclear weapon**

E997 Injury due to war operations by other forms of unconventional warfare

E997.0 Lasers

E997.1 Biological warfare

E997.2 Gases, fumes, and chemicals

● **E997.3 Weapon of mass destruction [WMD], unspecified**

E997.8 Other specified forms of unconventional warfare

E997.9 Unspecified form of unconventional warfare

E998 Injury due to war operations but occurring after cessation of hostilities
Injuries due to operations of war but occurring after cessation of hostilities by any means
classifiable under E990-E997
Injuries by explosion of bombs or mines placed in the course of operations of war, if the
explosion occurred after cessation of hostilities

● **E998.0 Explosion of mines**

● **E998.1 Explosion of bombs**

● **E998.8 Injury due to other war operations but occurring after cessation of hostilities**

● **E998.9 Injury due to unspecified war operations but occurring after cessation of hostilities**

E999 Late effect of injury due to war operations and terrorism
Note: This category is to be used to indicate circumstances classifiable to E979, E990-E998 as
the cause of death or disability from late effects, which are themselves classifiable
elsewhere. The "late effects" include conditions reported as such or as sequelae which
may occur at any time after the acute injury, resulting from operations of war or terrorism.

E999.0 Late effect of injury due to war operations

E999.1 Late effect of injury due to terrorism

● Code new
to this edition

▲ Revision of
existing code

④ ⑤ Fourth or fifth
digit required

APPENDIX A:
MORPHOLOGY OF NEOPLASMS

The World Health Organization has published an adaptation of the International Classification of Diseases for oncology (ICD-O). It contains a coded nomenclature for the morphology of neoplasms, which is reproduced here for those who wish to use it in conjunction with Chapter 2 of the *International Classification of Diseases, 9th Revision, Clinical Modification.*

The morphology code numbers consist of five digits; the first four identify the histological type of the neoplasm and the fifth indicates its behavior. The one-digit behavior code is as follows:

/0 Benign

/1 Uncertain whether benign or malignant
    Borderline malignancy

/2 Carcinoma in situ
    Intraepithelial
    Noninfiltrating
    Noninvasive

/3 Malignant, primary site

/6 Malignant, metastatic site
    Secondary site

/9 Malignant, uncertain whether primary or metastatic site

In the nomenclature below, the morphology code numbers include the behavior code appropriate to the histological type of neoplasm, but this behavior code should be changed if other reported information makes this necessary. For example, "chordoma (M9370/3)" is assumed to be malignant; the term "benign chordoma" should be coded M9370/0. Similarly, "superficial spreading adenocarcinoma (M8143/3)" described as "noninvasive" should be coded M8143/2 and "melanoma (M8720/3)" described as "secondary" should be coded M8720/6.

The following table shows the correspondence between the morphology code and the different sections of Chapter 2:

Morphology code Histology/Behavior			ICD-9-CM Chapter 2
Any	0	210-229	Benign neoplasms
M8000-M8004	1	239	Neoplasms of unspecified nature
M8010+	1	235-238	Neoplasms of uncertain behavior
Any	2	230-234	Carcinoma in situ
Any	3	140-195	Malignant neoplasms, stated or presumed to be primary
		200-208	
Any	6	196-198	Malignant neoplasms, stated or presumed to be secondary

The ICD-O behavior digit /9 is inapplicable in an ICD context, since all malignant neoplasms are presumed to be primary (/3) or secondary (/6) according to other information on the medical record.

Only the first-listed term of the full ICD-O morphology nomenclature appears against each code number in the list below. The ICD-9-CM Alphabetical Index (Volume 2), however, includes all the ICD-O synonyms as well as a number of other morphological names still likely to be encountered on medical records but omitted from ICD-O as outdated or otherwise undesirable.

A coding difficulty sometimes arises where a morphological diagnosis contains two qualifying adjectives that have different code numbers. An example is "transitional cell epidermoid carcinoma." "Transitional cell carcinoma NOS" is M8120/3 and "epidermoid carcinoma NOS" is M8070/3. In such circumstances, the higher number (M8120/3 in this example) should be used, as it is usually more specific.

CODED NOMENCLATURE FOR MORPHOLOGY OF NEOPLASMS

M800   **Neoplasms NOS**
M8000/0   *Neoplasm, benign*
M8000/1   *Neoplasm, uncertain whether benign or malignant*
M8000/3   *Neoplasm, malignant*
M8000/6   *Neoplasm, metastatic*
M8000/9   *Neoplasm, malignant, uncertain whether primary or metastatic*
M8001/0   *Tumor cells, benign*
M8001/1   *Tumor cells, uncertain whether benign or malignant*
M8001/3   *Tumor cells, malignant*
M8002/3   *Malignant tumor, small cell type*
M8003/3   *Malignant tumor, giant cell type*
M8004/3   *Malignant tumor, fusiform cell type*

M801-M804   **Epithelial neoplasms NOS**
M8010/0   *Epithelial tumor, benign*
M8010/2   *Carcinoma in situ NOS*
M8010/3   *Carcinoma NOS*
M8010/6   *Carcinoma, metastatic NOS*
M8010/9   *Carcinomatosis*
M8011/0   *Epithelioma, benign*
M8011/3   *Epithelioma, malignant*
M8012/3   *Large cell carcinoma NOS*
M8020/3   *Carcinoma, undifferentiated type NOS*
M8021/3   *Carcinoma, anaplastic type NOS*
M8022/3   *Pleomorphic carcinoma*
M8030/3   *Giant cell and spindle cell carcinoma*
M8031/3   *Giant cell carcinoma*
M8032/3   *Spindle cell carcinoma*
M8033/3   *Pseudosarcomatous carcinoma*
M8034/3   *Polygonal cell carcinoma*
M8035/3   *Spheroidal cell carcinoma*
M8040/1   *Tumorlet*
M8041/3   *Small cell carcinoma NOS*
M8042/3   *Oat cell carcinoma*
M8043/3   *Small cell carcinoma, fusiform cell type*

M805-M808   **Papillary and squamous cell neoplasms**
M8050/0   *Papilloma NOS (except Papilloma of urinary bladder M8120/1)*
M8050/2   *Papillary carcinoma in situ*
M8050/3   *Papillary carcinoma NOS*
M8051/0   *Verrucous papilloma*
M8051/3   *Verrucous carcinoma NOS*
M8052/0   *Squamous cell papilloma*
M8052/3   *Papillary squamous cell carcinoma*
M8053/0   *Inverted papilloma*
M8060/0   *Papillomatosis NOS*
M8070/2   *Squamous cell carcinoma in situ NOS*
M8070/3   *Squamous cell carcinoma NOS*
M8070/6   *Squamous cell carcinoma, metastatic NOS*
M8071/3   *Squamous cell carcinoma, keratinizing type NOS*
M8072/3   *Squamous cell carcinoma, large cell, nonkeratinizing type*
M8073/3   *Squamous cell carcinoma, small cell, nonkeratinizing type*
M8074/3   *Squamous cell carcinoma, spindle cell type*
M8075/3   *Adenoid squamous cell carcinoma*
M8076/2   *Squamous cell carcinoma in situ with questionable stromal invasion*
M8076/3   *Squamous cell carcinoma, microinvasive*
M8080/2   *Queyrat's erythroplasia*
M8081/2   *Bowen's disease*
M8082/3   *Lymphoepithelial carcinoma*

M809-M811   **Basal cell neoplasms**
M8090/1   *Basal cell tumor*
M8090/3   *Basal cell carcinoma NOS*
M8091/3   *Multicentric basal cell carcinoma*
M8092/3   *Basal cell carcinoma, morphea type*
M8093/3   *Basal cell carcinoma, fibroepithelial type*
M8094/3   *Basosquamous carcinoma*
M8095/3   *Metatypical carcinoma*
M8096/0   *Intraepidermal epithelioma of Jadassohn*
M8100/0   *Trichoepithelioma*
M8101/0   *Trichofolliculoma*

M8102/0	*Tricholemmoma*
M8110/0	*Pilomatrixoma*

M812-M813 Transitional cell papillomas and carcinomas

M8120/0	*Transitional cell papilloma NOS*
M8120/1	*Urothelial papilloma*
M8120/2	*Transitional cell carcinoma in situ*
M8120/3	*Transitional cell carcinoma NOS*
M8121/0	*Schneiderian papilloma*
M8121/1	*Transitional cell papilloma, inverted type*
M8121/3	*Schneiderian carcinoma*
M8122/3	*Transitional cell carcinoma, spindle cell type*
M8123/3	*Basaloid carcinoma*
M8124/3	*Cloacogenic carcinoma*
M8130/3	*Papillary transitional cell carcinoma*

M814-M838 Adenomas and adenocarcinomas

M8140/0	*Adenoma NOS*
M8140/1	*Bronchial adenoma NOS*
M8140/2	*Adenocarcinoma in situ*
M8140/3	*Adenocarcinoma NOS*
M8140/6	*Adenocarcinoma, metastatic NOS*
M8141/3	*Scirrhous adenocarcinoma*
M8142/3	*Linitis plastica*
M8143/3	*Superficial spreading adenocarcinoma*
M8144/3	*Adenocarcinoma, intestinal type*
M8145/3	*Carcinoma, diffuse type*
M8146/0	*Monomorphic adenoma*
M8147/0	*Basal cell adenoma*
M8150/0	*Islet cell adenoma*
M8150/3	*Islet cell carcinoma*
M8151/0	*Insulinoma NOS*
M8151/3	*Insulinoma, malignant*
M8152/0	*Glucagonoma NOS*
M8152/3	*Glucagonoma, malignant*
M8153/1	*Gastrinoma NOS*
M8153/3	*Gastrinoma, malignant*
M8154/3	*Mixed islet cell and exocrine adenocarcinoma*
M8160/0	*Bile duct adenoma*
M8160/3	*Cholangiocarcinoma*
M8161/0	*Bile duct cystadenoma*
M8161/3	*Bile duct cystadenocarcinoma*
M8170/0	*Liver cell adenoma*
M8170/3	*Hepatocellular carcinoma NOS*
M8180/0	*Hepatocholangioma, benign*
M8180/3	*Combined hepatocellular carcinoma and cholangiocarcinoma*
M8190/0	*Trabecular adenoma*
M8190/3	*Trabecular adenocarcinoma*
M8191/0	*Embryonal adenoma*
M8200/0	*Eccrine dermal cylindroma*
M8200/3	*Adenoid cystic carcinoma*
M8201/3	*Cribriform carcinoma*
M8210/0	*Adenomatous polyp NOS*
M8210/3	*Adenocarcinoma in adenomatous polyp*
M8211/0	*Tubular adenoma NOS*
M8211/3	*Tubular adenocarcinoma*
M8220/0	*Adenomatous polyposis coli*
M8220/3	*Adenocarcinoma in adenomatous polyposis coli*
M8221/0	*Multiple adenomatous polyps*
M8230/3	*Solid carcinoma NOS*
M8231/3	*Carcinoma simplex*
M8240/1	*Carcinoid tumor NOS*
M8240/3	*Carcinoid tumor, malignant*
M8241/1	*Carcinoid tumor, argentaffin NOS*
M8241/3	*Carcinoid tumor, argentaffin, malignant*
M8242/1	*Carcinoid tumor, nonargentaffin NOS*
M8242/3	*Carcinoid tumor, nonargentaffin, malignant*
M8243/3	*Mucocarcinoid tumor, malignant*
M8244/3	*Composite carcinoid*
M8250/1	*Pulmonary adenomatosis*
M8250/3	*Bronchiolo-alveolar adenocarcinoma*
M8251/0	*Alveolar adenoma*

M8251/3	*Alveolar adenocarcinoma*
M8260/0	*Papillary adenoma NOS*
M8260/3	*Papillary adenocarcinoma NOS*
M8261/1	*Villous adenoma NOS*
M8261/3	*Adenocarcinoma in villous adenoma*
M8262/3	*Villous adenocarcinoma*
M8263/0	*Tubulovillous adenoma*
M8270/0	*Chromophobe adenoma*
M8270/3	*Chromophobe carcinoma*
M8280/0	*Acidophil adenoma*
M8280/3	*Acidophil carcinoma*
M8281/0	*Mixed acidophil-basophil adenoma*
M8281/3	*Mixed acidophil-basophil carcinoma*
M8290/0	*Oxyphilic adenoma*
M8290/3	*Oxyphilic adenocarcinoma*
M8300/0	*Basophil adenoma*
M8300/3	*Basophil carcinoma*
M8310/0	*Clear cell adenoma*
M8310/3	*Clear cell adenocarcinoma NOS*
M8311/1	*Hypernephroid tumor*
M8312/3	*Renal cell carcinoma*
M8313/0	*Clear cell adenofibroma*
M8320/3	*Granular cell carcinoma*
M8321/0	*Chief cell adenoma*
M8322/0	*Water-clear cell adenoma*
M8322/3	*Water-clear cell adenocarcinoma*
M8323/0	*Mixed cell adenoma*
M8323/3	*Mixed cell adenocarcinoma*
M8324/0	*Lipoadenoma*
M8330/0	*Follicular adenoma*
M8330/3	*Follicular adenocarcinoma NOS*
M8331/3	*Follicular adenocarcinoma, well differentiated type*
M8332/3	*Follicular adenocarcinoma, trabecular type*
M8333/0	*Microfollicular adenoma*
M8334/0	*Macrofollicular adenoma*
M8340/3	*Papillary and follicular adenocarcinoma*
M8350/3	*Nonencapsulated sclerosing carcinoma*
M8360/1	*Multiple endocrine adenomas*
M8361/1	*Juxtaglomerular tumor*
M8370/0	*Adrenal cortical adenoma NOS*
M8370/3	*Adrenal cortical carcinoma*
M8371/0	*Adrenal cortical adenoma, compact cell type*
M8372/0	*Adrenal cortical adenoma, heavily pigmented variant*
M8373/0	*Adrenal cortical adenoma, clear cell type*
M8374/0	*Adrenal cortical adenoma, glomerulosa cell type*
M8375/0	*Adrenal cortical adenoma, mixed cell type*
M8380/0	*Endometrioid adenoma NOS*
M8380/1	*Endometrioid adenoma, borderline malignancy*
M8380/3	*Endometrioid carcinoma*
M8381/0	*Endometrioid adenofibroma NOS*
M8381/1	*Endometrioid adenofibroma, borderline malignancy*
M8381/3	*Endometrioid adenofibroma, malignant*

M839-M842 Adnexal and skin appendage neoplasms

M8390/0	*Skin appendage adenoma*
M8390/3	*Skin appendage carcinoma*
M8400/0	*Sweat gland adenoma*
M8400/1	*Sweat gland tumor NOS*
M8400/3	*Sweat gland adenocarcinoma*
M8401/0	*Apocrine adenoma*
M8401/3	*Apocrine adenocarcinoma*
M8402/0	*Eccrine acrospiroma*
M8403/0	*Eccrine spiradenoma*
M8404/0	*Hidrocystoma*
M8405/0	*Papillary hydradenoma*
M8406/0	*Papillary syringadenoma*
M8407/0	*Syringoma NOS*
M8410/0	*Sebaceous adenoma*
M8410/3	*Sebaceous adenocarcinoma*
M8420/0	*Ceruminous adenoma*
M8420/3	*Ceruminous adenocarcinoma*

M843 **Mucoepidermoid neoplasms**
M8430/1   *Mucoepidermoid tumor*
M8430/3   *Mucoepidermoid carcinoma*

M844-M849 **Cystic, mucinous, and serous neoplasms**
M8440/0   *Cystadenoma NOS*
M8440/3   *Cystadenocarcinoma NOS*
M8441/0   *Serous cystadenoma NOS*
M8441/1   *Serous cystadenoma, borderline malignancy*
M8441/3   *Serous cystadenocarcinoma NOS*
M8450/0   *Papillary cystadenoma NOS*
M8450/1   *Papillary cystadenoma, borderline malignancy*
M8450/3   *Papillary cystadenocarcinoma NOS*
M8460/0   *Papillary serous cystadenoma NOS*
M8460/1   *Papillary serous cystadenoma, borderline malignancy*
M8460/3   *Papillary serous cystadenocarcinoma*
M8461/0   *Serous surface papilloma NOS*
M8461/1   *Serous surface papilloma, borderline malignancy*
M8461/3   *Serous surface papillary carcinoma*
M8470/0   *Mucinous cystadenoma NOS*
M8470/1   *Mucinous cystadenoma, borderline malignancy*
M8470/3   *Mucinous cystadenocarcinoma NOS*
M8471/0   *Papillary mucinous cystadenoma NOS*
M8471/1   *Papillary mucinous cystadenoma, borderline malignancy*
M8471/3   *Papillary mucinous cystadenocarcinoma*
M8480/0   *Mucinous adenoma*
M8480/3   *Mucinous adenocarcinoma*
M8480/6   *Pseudomyxoma peritonei*
M8481/3   *Mucin-producing adenocarcinoma*
M8490/3   *Signet ring cell carcinoma*
M8490/6   *Metastatic signet ring cell carcinoma*

M850-M854 **Ductal, lobular, and medullary neoplasms**
M8500/2   *Intraductal carcinoma, noninfiltrating NOS*
M8500/3   *Infiltrating duct carcinoma*
M8501/2   *Comedocarcinoma, noninfiltrating*
M8501/3   *Comedocarcinoma NOS*
M8502/3   *Juvenile carcinoma of the breast*
M8503/0   *Intraductal papilloma*
M8503/2   *Noninfiltrating intraductal papillary adenocarcinoma*
M8504/0   *Intracystic papillary adenoma*
M8504/2   *Noninfiltrating intracystic carcinoma*
M8505/0   *Intraductal papillomatosis NOS*
M8506/0   *Subareolar duct papillomatosis*
M8510/3   *Medullary carcinoma NOS*
M8511/3   *Medullary carcinoma with amyloid stroma*
M8512/3   *Medullary carcinoma with lymphoid stroma*
M8520/2   *Lobular carcinoma in situ*
M8520/3   *Lobular carcinoma NOS*
M8521/3   *Infiltrating ductular carcinoma*
M8530/3   *Inflammatory carcinoma*
M8540/3   *Paget's disease, mammary*
M8541/3   *Paget's disease and infiltrating duct carcinoma of breast*
M8542/3   *Paget's disease, extramammary (except Paget's disease of bone)*

M855 **Acinar cell neoplasms**
M8550/0   *Acinar cell adenoma*
M8550/1   *Acinar cell tumor*
M8550/3   *Acinar cell carcinoma*

M856-M858 **Complex epithelial neoplasms**
M8560/3   *Adenosquamous carcinoma*
M8561/0   *Adenolymphoma*
M8570/3   *Adenocarcinoma with squamous metaplasia*
M8571/3   *Adenocarcinoma with cartilaginous and osseous metaplasia*
M8572/3   *Adenocarcinoma with spindle cell metaplasia*
M8573/3   *Adenocarcinoma with apocrine metaplasia*
M8580/0   *Thymoma, benign*
M8580/3   *Thymoma, malignant*

M859-M867 **Specialized gonadal neoplasms**
M8590/1   *Sex cord-stromal tumor*
M8600/0   *Thecoma NOS*
M8600/3   *Theca cell carcinoma*

M8610/0	*Luteoma NOS*
M8620/1	*Granulosa cell tumor NOS*
M8620/3	*Granulosa cell tumor, malignant*
M8621/1	*Granulosa cell-theca cell tumor*
M8630/0	*Androblastoma, benign*
M8630/1	*Androblastoma NOS*
M8630/3	*Androblastoma, malignant*
M8631/0	*Sertoli-Leydig cell tumor*
M8632/1	*Gynandroblastoma*
M8640/0	*Tubular androblastoma NOS*
M8640/3	*Sertoli cell carcinoma*
M8641/0	*Tubular androblastoma with lipid storage*
M8650/0	*Leydig cell tumor, benign*
M8650/1	*Leydig cell tumor NOS*
M8650/3	*Leydig cell tumor, malignant*
M8660/0	*Hilar cell tumor*
M8670/0	*Lipid cell tumor of ovary*
M8671/0	*Adrenal rest tumor*

M868-M871 Paragangliomas and glomus tumors

M8680/1	*Paraganglioma NOS*
M8680/3	*Paraganglioma, malignant*
M8681/1	*Sympathetic paraganglioma*
M8682/1	*Parasympathetic paraganglioma*
M8690/1	*Glomus jugulare tumor*
M8691/1	*Aortic body tumor*
M8692/1	*Carotid body tumor*
M8693/1	*Extra-adrenal paraganglioma NOS*
M8693/3	*Extra-adrenal paraganglioma, malignant*
M8700/0	*Pheochromocytoma NOS*
M8700/3	*Pheochromocytoma, malignant*
M8710/3	*Glomangiosarcoma*
M8711/0	*Glomus tumor*
M8712/0	*Glomangioma*

M872-M879 Nevi and melanomas

M8720/0	*Pigmented nevus NOS*
M8720/3	*Malignant melanoma NOS*
M8721/3	*Nodular melanoma*
M8722/0	*Balloon cell nevus*
M8722/3	*Balloon cell melanoma*
M8723/0	*Halo nevus*
M8724/0	*Fibrous papule of the nose*
M8725/0	*Neuronevus*
M8726/0	*Magnocellular nevus*
M8730/0	*Nonpigmented nevus*
M8730/3	*Amelanotic melanoma*
M8740/0	*Junctional nevus*
M8740/3	*Malignant melanoma in junctional nevus*
M8741/2	*Precancerous melanosis NOS*
M8741/3	*Malignant melanoma in precancerous melanosis*
M8742/2	*Hutchinson's melanotic freckle*
M8742/3	*Malignant melanoma in Hutchinson's melanotic freckle*
M8743/3	*Superficial spreading melanoma*
M8750/0	*Intradermal nevus*
M8760/0	*Compound nevus*
M8761/1	*Giant pigmented nevus*
M8761/3	*Malignant melanoma in giant pigmented nevus*
M8770/0	*Epithelioid and spindle cell nevus*
M8771/3	*Epithelioid cell melanoma*
M8772/3	*Spindle cell melanoma NOS*
M8773/3	*Spindle cell melanoma, type A*
M8774/3	*Spindle cell melanoma, type B*
M8775/3	*Mixed epithelioid and spindle cell melanoma*
M8780/0	*Blue nevus NOS*
M8780/3	*Blue nevus, malignant*
M8790/0	*Cellular blue nevus*

M880 Soft tissue tumors and sarcomas NOS

M8800/0	*Soft tissue tumor, benign*
M8800/3	*Sarcoma NOS*
M8800/9	*Sarcomatosis NOS*
M8801/3	*Spindle cell sarcoma*

M8802/3	*Giant cell sarcoma (except of bone M9250/3)*
M8803/3	*Small cell sarcoma*
M8804/3	*Epithelioid cell sarcoma*

M881-M883 Fibromatous neoplasms

M8810/0	*Fibroma NOS*
M8810/3	*Fibrosarcoma NOS*
M8811/0	*Fibromyxoma*
M8811/3	*Fibromyxosarcoma*
M8812/0	*Periosteal fibroma*
M8812/3	*Periosteal fibrosarcoma*
M8813/0	*Fascial fibroma*
M8813/3	*Fascial fibrosarcoma*
M8814/3	*Infantile fibrosarcoma*
M8820/0	*Elastofibroma*
M8821/1	*Aggressive fibromatosis*
M8822/1	*Abdominal fibromatosis*
M8823/1	*Desmoplastic fibroma*
M8830/0	*Fibrous histiocytoma NOS*
M8830/1	*Atypical fibrous histiocytoma*
M8830/3	*Fibrous histiocytoma, malignant*
M8831/0	*Fibroxanthoma NOS*
M8831/1	*Atypical fibroxanthoma*
M8831/3	*Fibroxanthoma, malignant*
M8832/0	*Dermatofibroma NOS*
M8832/1	*Dermatofibroma protuberans*
M8832/3	*Dermatofibrosarcoma NOS*

M884 Myxomatous neoplasms

| M8840/0 | *Myxoma NOS* |
| M8840/3 | *Myxosarcoma* |

M885-M888 Lipomatous neoplasms

M8850/0	*Lipoma NOS*
M8850/3	*Liposarcoma NOS*
M8851/0	*Fibrolipoma*
M8851/3	*Liposarcoma, well differentiated type*
M8852/0	*Fibromyxolipoma*
M8852/3	*Myxoid liposarcoma*
M8853/3	*Round cell liposarcoma*
M8854/3	*Pleomorphic liposarcoma*
M8855/3	*Mixed type liposarcoma*
M8856/0	*Intramuscular lipoma*
M8857/0	*Spindle cell lipoma*
M8860/0	*Angiomyolipoma*
M8860/3	*Angiomyoliposarcoma*
M8861/0	*Angiolipoma NOS*
M8861/1	*Angiolipoma, infiltrating*
M8870/0	*Myelolipoma*
M8880/0	*Hibernoma*
M8881/0	*Lipoblastomatosis*

M889-M892 Myomatous neoplasms

M8890/0	*Leiomyoma NOS*
M8890/1	*Intravascular leiomyomatosis*
M8890/3	*Leiomyosarcoma NOS*
M8891/1	*Epithelioid leiomyoma*
M8891/3	*Epithelioid leiomyosarcoma*
M8892/1	*Cellular leiomyoma*
M8893/0	*Bizarre leiomyoma*
M8894/0	*Angiomyoma*
M8894/3	*Angiomyosarcoma*
M8895/0	*Myoma*
M8895/3	*Myosarcoma*
M8900/0	*Rhabdomyoma NOS*
M8900/3	*Rhabdomyosarcoma NOS*
M8901/3	*Pleomorphic rhabdomyosarcoma*
M8902/3	*Mixed type rhabdomyosarcoma*
M8903/0	*Fetal rhabdomyoma*
M8904/0	*Adult rhabdomyoma*
M8910/3	*Embryonal rhabdomyosarcoma*
M8920/3	*Alveolar rhabdomyosarcoma*

M893-M899 Complex mixed and stromal neoplasms

M8930/3	*Endometrial stromal sarcoma*
M8931/1	*Endolymphatic stromal myosis*
M8932/0	*Adenomyoma*
M8940/0	*Pleomorphic adenoma*
M8940/3	*Mixed tumor, malignant NOS*
M8950/3	*Mullerian mixed tumor*
M8951/3	*Mesodermal mixed tumor*
M8960/1	*Mesoblastic nephroma*
M8960/3	*Nephroblastoma NOS*
M8961/3	*Epithelial nephroblastoma*
M8962/3	*Mesenchymal nephroblastoma*
M8970/3	*Hepatoblastoma*
M8980/3	*Carcinosarcoma NOS*
M8981/3	*Carcinosarcoma, embryonal type*
M8982/0	*Myoepithelioma*
M8990/0	*Mesenchymoma, benign*
M8990/1	*Mesenchymoma, NOS*
M8990/3	*Mesenchymoma, malignant*
M8991/3	*Embryonal sarcoma*

M900-M903 Fibroepithelial neoplasms

M9000/0	*Brenner tumor NOS*
M9000/1	*Brenner tumor, borderline malignancy*
M9000/3	*Brenner tumor, malignant*
M9010/0	*Fibroadenoma NOS*
M9011/0	*Intracanalicular fibroadenoma NOS*
M9012/0	*Pericanalicular fibroadenoma*
M9013/0	*Adenofibroma NOS*
M9014/0	*Serous adenofibroma*
M9015/0	*Mucinous adenofibroma*
M9020/0	*Cellular intracanalicular fibroadenoma*
M9020/1	*Cystosarcoma phyllodes NOS*
M9020/3	*Cystosarcoma phyllodes, malignant*
M9030/0	*Juvenile fibroadenoma*

M904 Synovial neoplasms

M9040/0	*Synovioma, benign*
M9040/3	*Synovial sarcoma NOS*
M9041/3	*Synovial sarcoma, spindle cell type*
M9042/3	*Synovial sarcoma, epithelioid cell type*
M9043/3	*Synovial sarcoma, biphasic type*
M9044/3	*Clear cell sarcoma of tendons and aponeuroses*

M905 Mesothelial neoplasms

M9050/0	*Mesothelioma, benign*
M9050/3	*Mesothelioma, malignant*
M9051/0	*Fibrous mesothelioma, benign*
M9051/3	*Fibrous mesothelioma, malignant*
M9052/0	*Epithelioid mesothelioma, benign*
M9052/3	*Epithelioid mesothelioma, malignant*
M9053/0	*Mesothelioma, biphasic type, benign*
M9053/3	*Mesothelioma, biphasic type, malignant*
M9054/0	*Adenomatoid tumor NOS*

M906-M909 Germ cell neoplasms

M9060/3	*Dysgerminoma*
M9061/3	*Seminoma NOS*
M9062/3	*Seminoma, anaplastic type*
M9063/3	*Spermatocytic seminoma*
M9064/3	*Germinoma*
M9070/3	*Embryonal carcinoma NOS*
M9071/3	*Endodermal sinus tumor*
M9072/3	*Polyembryoma*
M9073/1	*Gonadoblastoma*
M9080/0	*Teratoma, benign*
M9080/1	*Teratoma NOS*
M9080/3	*Teratoma, malignant NOS*
M9081/3	*Teratocarcinoma*
M9082/3	*Malignant teratoma, undifferentiated type*
M9083/3	*Malignant teratoma, intermediate type*
M9084/0	*Dermoid cyst*
M9084/3	*Dermoid cyst with malignant transformation*

M9090/0	*Struma ovarii NOS*
M9090/3	*Struma ovarii, malignant*
M9091/1	*Strumal carcinoid*

M910   **Trophoblastic neoplasms**
M9100/0	*Hydatidiform mole NOS*
M9100/1	*Invasive hydatidiform mole*
M9100/3	*Choriocarcinoma*
M9101/3	*Choriocarcinoma combined with teratoma*
M9102/3	*Malignant teratoma, trophoblastic*

M911   **Mesonephromas**
M9110/0	*Mesonephroma, benign*
M9110/1	*Mesonephric tumor*
M9110/3	*Mesonephroma, malignant*
M9111/1	*Endosalpingioma*

M912-M916   **Blood vessel tumors**
M9120/0	*Hemangioma NOS*
M9120/3	*Hemangiosarcoma*
M9121/0	*Cavernous hemangioma*
M9122/0	*Venous hemangioma*
M9123/0	*Racemose hemangioma*
M9124/3	*Kupffer cell sarcoma*
M9130/0	*Hemangioendothelioma, benign*
M9130/1	*Hemangioendothelioma NOS*
M9130/3	*Hemangioendothelioma, malignant*
M9131/0	*Capillary hemangioma*
M9132/0	*Intramuscular hemangioma*
M9140/3	*Kaposi's sarcoma*
M9141/0	*Angiokeratoma*
M9142/0	*Verrucous keratotic hemangioma*
M9150/0	*Hemangiopericytoma, benign*
M9150/1	*Hemangiopericytoma NOS*
M9150/3	*Hemangiopericytoma, malignant*
M9160/0	*Angiofibroma NOS*
M9161/1	*Hemangioblastoma*

M917   **Lymphatic vessel tumors**
M9170/0	*Lymphangioma NOS*
M9170/3	*Lymphangiosarcoma*
M9171/0	*Capillary lymphangioma*
M9172/0	*Cavernous lymphangioma*
M9173/0	*Cystic lymphangioma*
M9174/0	*Lymphangiomyoma*
M9174/1	*Lymphangiomyomatosis*
M9175/0	*Hemolymphangioma*

M918-M920   **Osteomas and osteosarcomas**
M9180/0	*Osteoma NOS*
M9180/3	*Osteosarcoma NOS*
M9181/3	*Chondroblastic osteosarcoma*
M9182/3	*Fibroblastic osteosarcoma*
M9183/3	*Telangiectatic osteosarcoma*
M9184/3	*Osteosarcoma in Paget's disease of bone*
M9190/3	*Juxtacortical osteosarcoma*
M9191/0	*Osteoid osteoma NOS*
M9200/0	*Osteoblastoma*

M921-M924   **Chondromatous neoplasms**
M9210/0	*Osteochondroma*
M9210/1	*Osteochondromatosis NOS*
M9220/0	*Chondroma NOS*
M9220/1	*Chondromatosis NOS*
M9220/3	*Chondrosarcoma NOS*
M9221/0	*Juxtacortical chondroma*
M9221/3	*Juxtacortical chondrosarcoma*
M9230/0	*Chondroblastoma NOS*
M9230/3	*Chondroblastoma, malignant*
M9240/3	*Mesenchymal chondrosarcoma*
M9241/0	*Chondromyxoid fibroma*

M925   **Giant cell tumors**
M9250/1	*Giant cell tumor of bone NOS*
M9250/3	*Giant cell tumor of bone, malignant*

M9251/1	Giant cell tumor of soft parts NOS
M9251/3	Malignant giant cell tumor of soft parts

M926   **Miscellaneous bone tumors**

M9260/3	Ewing's sarcoma
M9261/3	Adamantinoma of long bones
M9262/0	Ossifying fibroma

M927-M934 Odontogenic tumors

M9270/0	Odontogenic tumor, benign
M9270/1	Odontogenic tumor NOS
M9270/3	Odontogenic tumor, malignant
M9271/0	Dentinoma
M9272/0	Cementoma NOS
M9273/0	Cementoblastoma, benign
M9274/0	Cementifying fibroma
M9275/0	Gigantiform cementoma
M9280/0	Odontoma NOS
M9281/0	Compound odontoma
M9282/0	Complex odontoma
M9290/0	Ameloblastic fibro-odontoma
M9290/3	Ameloblastic odontosarcoma
M9300/0	Adenomatoid odontogenic tumor
M9301/0	Calcifying odontogenic cyst
M9310/0	Ameloblastoma NOS
M9310/3	Ameloblastoma, malignant
M9311/0	Odontoameloblastoma
M9312/0	Squamous odontogenic tumor
M9320/0	Odontogenic myxoma
M9321/0	Odontogenic fibroma NOS
M9330/0	Ameloblastic fibroma
M9330/3	Ameloblastic fibrosarcoma
M9340/0	Calcifying epithelial odontogenic tumor

M935-M937 Miscellaneous tumors

M9350/1	Craniopharyngioma
M9360/1	Pinealoma
M9361/1	Pineocytoma
M9362/3	Pineoblastoma
M9363/0	Melanotic neuroectodermal tumor
M9370/3	Chordoma

M938-M948 Gliomas

M9380/3	Glioma, malignant
M9381/3	Gliomatosis cerebri
M9382/3	Mixed glioma
M9383/1	Subependymal glioma
M9384/1	Subependymal giant cell astrocytoma
M9390/0	Choroid plexus papilloma NOS
M9390/3	Choroid plexus papilloma, malignant
M9391/3	Ependymoma NOS
M9392/3	Ependymoma, anaplastic type
M9393/1	Papillary ependymoma
M9394/1	Myxopapillary ependymoma
M9400/3	Astrocytoma NOS
M9401/3	Astrocytoma, anaplastic type
M9410/3	Protoplasmic astrocytoma
M9411/3	Gemistocytic astrocytoma
M9420/3	Fibrillary astrocytoma
M9421/3	Pilocytic astrocytoma
M9422/3	Spongioblastoma NOS
M9423/3	Spongioblastoma polare
M9430/3	Astroblastoma
M9440/3	Glioblastoma NOS
M9441/3	Giant cell glioblastoma
M9442/3	Glioblastoma with sarcomatous component
M9443/3	Primitive polar spongioblastoma
M9450/3	Oligodendroglioma NOS
M9451/3	Oligodendroglioma, anaplastic type
M9460/3	Oligodendroblastoma
M9470/3	Medulloblastoma NOS
M9471/3	Desmoplastic medulloblastoma
M9472/3	Medullomyoblastoma

| M9480/3 | *Cerebellar sarcoma NOS* |
| M9481/3 | *Monstrocellular sarcoma* |

M949-M952 Neuroepitheliomatous neoplasms

M9490/0	*Ganglioneuroma*
M9490/3	*Ganglioneuroblastoma*
M9491/0	*Ganglioneuromatosis*
M9500/3	*Neuroblastoma NOS*
M9501/3	*Medulloepithelioma NOS*
M9502/3	*Teratoid medulloepithelioma*
M9503/3	*Neuroepithelioma NOS*
M9504/3	*Spongioneuroblastoma*
M9505/1	*Ganglioglioma*
M9506/0	*Neurocytoma*
M9507/0	*Pacinian tumor*
M9510/3	*Retinoblastoma NOS*
M9511/3	*Retinoblastoma, differentiated type*
M9512/3	*Retinoblastoma, undifferentiated type*
M9520/3	*Olfactory neurogenic tumor*
M9521/3	*Esthesioneurocytoma*
M9522/3	*Esthesioneuroblastoma*
M9523/3	*Esthesioneuroepithelioma*

M953 Meningiomas

M9530/0	*Meningioma NOS*
M9530/1	*Meningiomatosis NOS*
M9530/3	*Meningioma, malignant*
M9531/0	*Meningotheliomatous meningioma*
M9532/0	*Fibrous meningioma*
M9533/0	*Psammomatous meningioma*
M9534/0	*Angiomatous meningioma*
M9535/0	*Hemangioblastic meningioma*
M9536/0	*Hemangiopericytic meningioma*
M9537/0	*Transitional meningioma*
M9538/1	*Papillary meningioma*
M9539/3	*Meningeal sarcomatosis*

M954-M957 Nerve sheath tumor

M9540/0	*Neurofibroma NOS*
M9540/1	*Neurofibromatosis NOS*
M9540/3	*Neurofibrosarcoma*
M9541/0	*Melanotic neurofibroma*
M9550/0	*Plexiform neurofibroma*
M9560/0	*Neurilemmoma NOS*
M9560/1	*Neurinomatosis*
M9560/3	*Neurilemmoma, malignant*
M9570/0	*Neuroma NOS*

M958 Granular cell tumors and alveolar soft part sarcoma

M9580/0	*Granular cell tumor NOS*
M9580/3	*Granular cell tumor, malignant*
M9581/3	*Alveolar soft part sarcoma*

M959-M963 Lymphomas, NOS or diffuse

M9590/0	*Lymphomatous tumor, benign*
M9590/3	*Malignant lymphoma NOS*
M9591/3	*Malignant lymphoma, non Hodgkin's type*
M9600/3	*Malignant lymphoma, undifferentiated cell type NOS*
M9601/3	*Malignant lymphoma, stem cell type*
M9602/3	*Malignant lymphoma, convoluted cell type NOS*
M9610/3	*Lymphosarcoma NOS*
M9611/3	*Malignant lymphoma, lymphoplasmacytoid type*
M9612/3	*Malignant lymphoma, immunoblastic type*
M9613/3	*Malignant lymphoma, mixed lymphocytic-histiocytic NOS*
M9614/3	*Malignant lymphoma, centroblastic-centrocytic, diffuse*
M9615/3	*Malignant lymphoma, follicular center cell NOS*
M9620/3	*Malignant lymphoma, lymphocytic, well differentiated NOS*
M9621/3	*Malignant lymphoma, lymphocytic, intermediate differentiation NOS*
M9622/3	*Malignant lymphoma, centrocytic*
M9623/3	*Malignant lymphoma, follicular center cell, cleaved NOS*
M9630/3	*Malignant lymphoma, lymphocytic, poorly differentiated NOS*
M9631/3	*Prolymphocytic lymphosarcoma*
M9632/3	*Malignant lymphoma, centroblastic type NOS*
M9633/3	*Malignant lymphoma, follicular center cell, noncleaved NOS*

M964	**Reticulosarcomas**
M9640/3	*Reticulosarcoma NOS*
M9641/3	*Reticulosarcoma, pleomorphic cell type*
M9642/3	*Reticulosarcoma, nodular*

M965-M966	**Hodgkin's disease**
M9650/3	*Hodgkin's disease NOS*
M9651/3	*Hodgkin's disease, lymphocytic predominance*
M9652/3	*Hodgkin's disease, mixed cellularity*
M9653/3	*Hodgkin's disease, lymphocytic depletion NOS*
M9654/3	*Hodgkin's disease, lymphocytic depletion, diffuse fibrosis*
M9655/3	*Hodgkin's disease, lymphocytic depletion, reticular type*
M9656/3	*Hodgkin's disease, nodular sclerosis NOS*
M9657/3	*Hodgkin's disease, nodular sclerosis, cellular phase*
M9660/3	*Hodgkin's paragranuloma*
M9661/3	*Hodgkin's granuloma*
M9662/3	*Hodgkin's sarcoma*

M969	**Lymphomas, nodular or follicular**
M9690/3	*Malignant lymphoma, nodular NOS*
M9691/3	*Malignant lymphoma, mixed lymphocytic-histiocytic, nodular*
M9692/3	*Malignant lymphoma, centroblastic-centrocytic, follicular*
M9693/3	*Malignant lymphoma, lymphocytic, well differentiated, nodular*
M9694/3	*Malignant lymphoma, lymphocytic, intermediate differentiation, nodular*
M9695/3	*Malignant lymphoma, follicular center cell, cleaved, follicular*
M9696/3	*Malignant lymphoma, lymphocytic, poorly differentiated, nodular*
M9697/3	*Malignant lymphoma, centroblastic type, follicular*
M9698/3	*Malignant lymphoma, follicular center cell, noncleaved, follicular*

M970	**Mycosis fungoides**
M9700/3	*Mycosis fungoides*
M9701/3	*Sezary's disease*

M971-M972	**Miscellaneous reticuloendothelial neoplasms**
M9710/3	*Microglioma*
M9720/3	*Malignant histiocytosis*
M9721/3	*Histiocytic medullary reticulosis*
M9722/3	*Letterer-Siwe's disease*

M973	**Plasma cell tumors**
M9730/3	*Plasma cell myeloma*
M9731/0	*Plasma cell tumor, benign*
M9731/1	*Plasmacytoma NOS*
M9731/3	*Plasma cell tumor, malignant*

M974	**Mast cell tumors**
M9740/1	*Mastocytoma NOS*
M9740/3	*Mast cell sarcoma*
M9741/3	*Malignant mastocytosis*

M975	**Burkitt's tumor**
M9750/3	*Burkitt's tumor*

M980-M994	**Leukemias**

M980	**Leukemias NOS**
M9800/3	*Leukemia NOS*
M9801/3	*Acute leukemia NOS*
M9802/3	*Subacute leukemia NOS*
M9803/3	*Chronic leukemia NOS*
M9804/3	*Aleukemic leukemia NOS*

M981	**Compound leukemias**
M9810/3	*Compound leukemia*

M982	**Lymphoid leukemias**
M9820/3	*Lymphoid leukemia NOS*
M9821/3	*Acute lymphoid leukemia*
M9822/3	*Subacute lymphoid leukemia*
M9823/3	*Chronic lymphoid leukemia*
M9824/3	*Aleukemic lymphoid leukemia*
M9825/3	*Prolymphocytic leukemia*

M983	**Plasma cell leukemias**
M9830/3	*Plasma cell leukemia*

M984	**Erythroleukemias**
M9840/3	*Erythroleukemia*
M9841/3	*Acute erythremia*

M9842/3	*Chronic erythremia*

M985	**Lymphosarcoma cell leukemias**
M9850/3	*Lymphosarcoma cell leukemia*

M986	**Myeloid leukemias**
M9860/3	*Myeloid leukemia NOS*
M9861/3	*Acute myeloid leukemia*
M9862/3	*Subacute myeloid leukemia*
M9863/3	*Chronic myeloid leukemia*
M9864/3	*Aleukemic myeloid leukemia*
M9865/3	*Neutrophilic leukemia*
M9866/3	*Acute promyelocytic leukemia*

M987	**Basophilic leukemias**
M9870/3	*Basophilic leukemia*

M988	**Eosinophilic leukemias**
M9880/3	*Eosinophilic leukemia*

M989	**Monocytic leukemias**
M9890/3	*Monocytic leukemia NOS*
M9891/3	*Acute monocytic leukemia*
M9892/3	*Subacute monocytic leukemia*
M9893/3	*Chronic monocytic leukemia*
M9894/3	*Aleukemic monocytic leukemia*

M990-M994	**Miscellaneous leukemias**
M9900/3	*Mast cell leukemia*
M9910/3	*Megakaryocytic leukemia*
M9920/3	*Megakaryocytic myelosis*
M9930/3	*Myeloid sarcoma*
M9940/3	*Hairy cell leukemia*

M995-M997	**Miscellaneous myeloproliferative and lymphoproliferative disorders**
M9950/1	*Polycythemia vera*
M9951/1	*Acute panmyelosis*
M9960/1	*Chronic myeloproliferative disease*
M9961/1	*Myelosclerosis with myeloid metaplasia*
M9962/1	*Idiopathic thrombocythemia*
M9970/1	*Chronic lymphoproliferative disease*

APPENDIX B:
GLOSSARY OF MENTAL DISORDERS

Note: *Appendix B Glossary of Mental Disorders* has been removed from the official ICD-9-CM CD-Rom effective with the FY2005 update.

APPENDIX C:
CLASSIFICATION OF DRUGS BY AMERICAN HOSPITAL FORMULARY SERVICE LIST NUMBER AND THEIR ICD-9-CM EQUIVALENTS

The coding of adverse effects of drugs is keyed to the continually revised Hospital Formulary of the American Hospital Formulary Service (AHFS) published under the direction of the American Society of Hospital Pharmacists.

AHFS*LIST		ICD-9-CM Diagnosis Code

The following section gives the ICD-9-CM diagnosis code for each AHFS list.

4:00	**ANTIHISTAMINE DRUGS**	963.0
8:00	**ANTI-INFECTIVE AGENTS**	
8:04	Amebacides	961.5
	hydroxyquinoline derivatives	961.3
	arsenical anti-infectives	961.1
8:08	Anthelmintics	961.6
	quinoline derivatives	961.3
8:12.04	Antifungal Antibiotics	960.1
	nonantibiotics	961.9
8:12.06	Cephalosporins	960.5
8:12.08	Chloramphenicol	960.2
8:12.12	The Erythromycins	960.3
8:12.16	The Penicillins	960.0
8:12.20	The Streptomycins	960.6
8:12.24	The Tetracyclines	960.4
8:12.28	Other Antibiotics	960.8
	antimycobacterial antibiotics	960.6
	macrolides	960.3
8:16	Antituberculars	961.8
	antibiotics	960.6
8:18	Antivirals	961.7
8:20	Plasmodicides (antimalarials)	961.4
8:24	Sulfonamides	961.0
8:26	The Sulfones	961.8
8:28	Treponemicides	961.2
8:32	Trichomonacides	961.5
	hydroxyquinoline derivatives	961.3
	nitrofuran derivatives	961.9
8:36	Urinary Germicides	961.9
	quinoline derivatives	961.3
8:40	Other Anti-Infectives	961.9
10:00	**ANTINEOPLASTIC AGENTS**	963.1
	antibiotics	960.7
	progestogens	962.2
12:00	**AUTONOMIC DRUGS**	
12:04	Parasympathomimetic (Cholinergic) Agents	971.0
12:08	Parasympatholytic (Cholinergic Blocking) Agents	971.1
12:12	Sympathomimetic (Adrenergic) Agents	971.2
12:16	Sympatholytic (Adrenergic Blocking) Agents	971.3

	AHFS*LIST	ICD-9-CM Diagnosis Code
12:20	Skeletal Muscle Relaxants	975.2
	central nervous system muscle-tone depressants	968.0
16:00	**BLOOD DERIVATIVES**	964.7
20:00	**BLOOD FORMATION AND COAGULATION**	
20:04	Antianemia Drugs	964.1
20:04.04	Iron Preparations	964.0
20:04.08	Liver and Stomach Preparations	964.1
20:12.04	Anticoagulants	964.2
20:12.08	Antiheparin agents	964.5
20:12.12	Coagulants	964.5
20:12.16	Hemostatics	964.5
	capillary-active drugs	972.8
	fibrinolysis-affecting agents	964.4
	natural products	964.7
24:00	**CARDIOVASCULAR DRUGS**	
24:04	Cardiac Drugs	972.9
	cardiotonic agents	972.1
	rhythm regulators	972.0
24:06	Antilipemic Agents	972.2
	thyroid derivatives	962.7
24:08	Hypotensive Agents	972.6
	adrenergic blocking agents	971.3
	ganglion-blocking agents	972.3
	vasodilators	972.5
24:12	Vasodilating Agents	972.5
	coronary	972.4
	nicotinic acid derivatives	972.2
24:16	Sclerosing Agents	972.7
28:00	**CENTRAL NERVOUS SYSTEM DRUGS**	
28:04	General Anesthetics	968.4
	gaseous anesthetics	968.2
	halothane	968.1
	intravenous anesthetics	968.3
28:08	Analgesics and Antipyretics	965.9
	antirheumatics	965.6
	aromatic analgesics	965.4
	non-narcotics NEC	965.7
	opium alkaloids	965.00
	heroin	965.01
	methadone	965.02
	specified type NEC	965.09
	pyrazole derivatives	965.5
	salicylates	965.1
	specified type NEC	965.8
28:10	Narcotic Antagonists	970.1
28:12	Anticonvulsants	966.3
	barbiturates	967.0
	benzodiazepine-based tranquilizers	969.4
	bromides	967.3
	hydantoin derivatives	966.1
	oxazolidine derivative	966.0
	succinimides	966.2
28:16.04	Antidepressants	969.0

AHFS*LIST	ICD-9-CM Diagnosis Code

28:16.08	Tranquilizers	969.5
	benzodiazepine-based	969.4
	butyrophenone-based	969.2
	major NEC	969.3
	phenothiazine-based	969.1
28:16.12	Other Psychotherapeutic Agents	969.8
28:20	Respiratory and Cerebral Stimulants	970.9
	analeptics	970.0
	anorexigenic agents	977.0
	psychostimulants	969.7
	specified type NEC	970.8
28:24	Sedatives and Hypnotics	967.9
	barbiturates	967.0
	benzodiazepine-based tranquilizers	969.4
	chloral hydrate group	967.1
	glutethamide group	967.5
	intravenous anesthetics	968.3
	methaqualone	967.4
	paraldehyde	967.2
	phenothiazine-based tranquilizers	969.1
	specified type NEC	967.8
	thiobarbiturates	968.3
	tranquilizer NEC	969.5
36:00	**DIAGNOSTIC AGENTS**	977.8
40:00	**ELECTROLYTE, CALORIC, AND WATER BALANCE AGENTS NEC**	974.5
40:04	Acidifying Agents	963.2
40:08	Alkalinizing Agents	963.3
40:10	Ammonia Detoxicants	974.5
40:12	Replacement Solutions NEC	974.5
	plasma volume expanders	964.8
40:16	Sodium-Removing Resins	974.5
40:18	Potassium-Removing Resins	974.5
40:20	Caloric Agents	974.5
40:24	Salt and Sugar Substitutes	974.5
40:28	Diuretics NEC	974.4
	carbonic acid anhydrase inhibitors	974.2
	mercurials	974.0
	purine derivatives	974.1
	saluretics	974.3
40:36	Irrigating Solutions	974.5
40:40	Uricosuric Agents	974.7
44:00	**ENZYMES NEC**	963.4
	fibrinolysis-affecting agents	964.4
	gastric agents	973.4
48:00	**EXPECTORANTS AND COUGH PREPARATIONS**	
	antihistamine agents	963.0
	antitussives	975.4
	codeine derivatives	965.09
	expectorants	975.5
	narcotic agents NEC	965.09

AHFS*LIST	ICD-9-CM Diagnosis Code

52:00 **EYE, EAR, NOSE, AND THROAT PREPARATIONS**

52:04	Anti-Infectives	
	ENT	976.6
	ophthalmic	976.5
52:04.04	Antibiotics	
	ENT	976.6
	ophthalmic	976.5
52:04.06	Antivirals	
	ENT	976.6
	ophthalmic	976.5
52:04.08	Sulfonamides	
	ENT	976.6
	ophthalmic	976.5
52:04.12	Miscellaneous Anti-Infectives	
	ENT	976.6
	ophthalmic	976.5
52:08	Anti-Inflammatory Agents	
	ENT	976.6
	ophthalmic	976.5
52:10	Carbonic Anhydrase Inhibitors	974.2
52:12	Contact Lens Solutions	976.5
52:16	Local Anesthetics	968.5
52:20	Miotics	971.0
52:24	Mydriatics	
	adrenergics	971.2
	anticholinergics	971.1
	antimuscarinics	971.1
	parasympatholytics	971.1
	spasmolytics	971.1
	sympathomimetics	971.2
52:28	Mouth Washes and Gargles	976.6
52:32	Vasoconstrictors	971.2
52:36	Unclassified Agents	
	ENT	976.6
	ophthalmic	976.5

56:00 **GASTROINTESTINAL DRUGS**

56:04	Antacids and Absorbants	973.0
56:08	Anti-Diarrhea Agents	973.5
56:10	Antiflatulents	973.8
56:12	Cathartics NEC	973.3
	emollients	973.2
	irritants	973.1
56:16	Digestants	973.4
56:20	Emetics and Antiemetics	
	antiemetics	963.0
	emetics	973.6
56:24	Lipotropic Agents	977.1

60:00 **GOLD COMPOUNDS** 965.6

64:00 **HEAVY METAL ANTAGONISTS** 963.8

68:00 **HORMONES AND SYNTHETIC SUBSTITUTES**

| 68:04 | Adrenals | 962.0 |
| 68:08 | Androgens | 962.1 |

*American Hospital Formulary Service

AHFS*LIST		ICD-9-CM Diagnosis Code
68:12	Contraceptives	962.2
68:16	Estrogens	962.2
68:18	Gonadotropins	962.4
68:20	Insulins and Antidiabetic Agents	962.3
68:20.08	Insulins	962.3
68:24	Parathyroid	962.6
68:28	Pituitary	
	anterior	962.4
	posterior	962.5
68:32	Progestogens	962.2
68:34	Other Corpus Luteum Hormones	962.2
68:36	Thyroid and Antithyroid	
	antithyroid	962.8
	thyroid	962.7
72:00	**LOCAL ANESTHETICS NEC**	968.9
	topical (surface) agents	968.5
	infiltrating agents (intradermal) (subcutaneous) (submucosal)	968.5
	nerve blocking agents (peripheral) (plexus)(regional)	968.6
	spinal	968.7
76:00	**OXYTOCICS**	975.0
78:00	**RADIOACTIVE AGENTS**	990
80:00	**SERUMS, TOXOIDS, AND VACCINES**	
80:04	Serums	979.9
	immune globulin (gamma) (human)	964.6
80:08	Toxoids NEC	978.8
	diphtheria	978.5
	and tetanus	978.9
	with pertussis component	978.6
	tetanus	978.4
	and diphtheria	978.9
	with pertussis component	978.6
80:12	Vaccines NEC	979.9
	bacterial NEC	978.8
	with	
	other bacterial component	978.9
	pertussis component	978.6
	viral and rickettsial component	979.7
	rickettsial NEC	979.6
	with	
	bacterial component	979.7
	pertussis component	978.6
	viral component	979.7
	viral NEC	979.6
	with	
	bacterial component	979.7
	pertussis component	978.6
	rickettsial component	979.7
84:00	**SKIN AND MUCOUS MEMBRANE PREPARATIONS**	
84:04	Anti-Infectives	976.0
84:04.04	Antibiotics	976.0
84:04.08	Fungicides	976.0
84:04.12	Scabicides and Pediculicides	976.0
84:04.16	Miscellaneous Local Anti-Infectives	976.0

	AHFS*LIST	ICD-9-CM Diagnosis Code
84:06	Anti-Inflammatory Agents	976.0
84:08	Antipruritics and Local Anesthetics	
	antipruritics	976.1
	local anesthetics	968.5
84:12	Astringents	976.2
84:16	Cell Stimulants and Proliferants	976.8
84:20	Detergents	976.2
84:24	Emollients, Demulcents, and Protectants	976.3
84:28	Keratolytic Agents	976.4
84:32	Keratoplastic Agents	976.4
84:36	Miscellaneous Agents	976.8
86:00	**SPASMOLYTIC AGENTS**	975.1
	antiasthmatics	975.7
	papaverine	972.5
	theophyllin	974.1
88:00	**VITAMINS**	
88:04	Vitamin A	963.5
88:08	Vitamin B Complex	963.5
	hematopoietic vitamin	964.1
	nicotinic acid derivatives	972.2
88:12	Vitamin C	963.5
88:16	Vitamin D	963.5
88:20	Vitamin E	963.5
88:24	Vitamin K Activity	964.3
88:28	Multivitamin Preparations	963.5
92:00	**UNCLASSIFIED THERAPEUTIC AGENTS**	

APPENDIX D:
CLASSIFICATION OF INDUSTRIAL ACCIDENTS
ACCORDING TO AGENCY

Annex B to the Resolution concerning Statistics of Employment Injuries adopted by the Tenth International Conference of Labor Statisticians on 12 October 1962

1 MACHINES

11   Prime-Movers, except Electrical Motors
111   Steam engines
112   Internal combustion engines
119   Others

12   Transmission Machinery
121   Transmission shafts
122   Transmission belts, cables, pulleys, pinions, chains, gears
129   Others

13   Metalworking Machines
131   Power presses
132   Lathes
133   Milling machines
134   Abrasive wheels
135   Mechanical shears
136   Forging machines
137   Rolling-mills
139   Others

14   Wood and Assimilated Machines
141   Circular saws
142   Other saws
143   Molding machines
144   Overhand planes
149   Others

15   Agricultural Machines
151   Reapers (including combine reapers)
152   Threshers
159   Others

16   Mining Machinery
161   Under-cutters
169   Others

19   Other Machines Not Elsewhere Classified
191   Earth-moving machines, excavating and scraping machines, except means of transport
192   Spinning, weaving and other textile machines
193   Machines for the manufacture of foodstuffs and beverages
194   Machines for the manufacture of paper
195   Printing machines
199   Others

2 MEANS OF TRANSPORT AND LIFTING EQUIPMENT

21   Lifting Machines and Appliances
211   Cranes
212   Lifts and elevators
213   Winches
214   Pulley blocks
219   Others

22   Means of Rail Transport
221   Inter-urban railways
222   Rail transport in mines, tunnels, quarries, industrial establishments, docks, etc.
229   Others

23   Other Wheeled Means of Transport, Excluding Rail Transport
231   Tractors
232   Lorries

2 MEANS OF TRANSPORT AND LIFTING EQUIPMENT *continued*

    233 Trucks
    234 Motor vehicles, not elsewhere classified
    235 Animal-drawn vehicles
    236 Hand-drawn vehicles
    239 Others

24 Means of Air Transport

25 Means of Water Transport
251 Motorized means of water transport
252 Non-motorized means of water transport

26 Other Means of Transport
261 Cable-cars
262 Mechanical conveyors, except cable-cars
269 Others

3 OTHER EQUIPMENT

31 Pressure Vessels
311 Boilers
312 Pressurized containers
313 Pressurized piping and accessories
314 Gas cylinders
315 Caissons, diving equipment
319 Others

32 Furnaces, Ovens, Kilns
321 Blast furnaces
322 Refining furnaces
323 Other furnaces
324 Kilns
325 Ovens

33 Refrigerating Plants

34 Electrical Installations, Including Electric Motors, but Excluding Electric Hand Tools
341 Rotating machines
342 Conductors
343 Transformers
344 Control apparatus
349 Others

35 Electric Hand Tools

36 Tools, Implements, and Appliances, Except Electric Hand Tools
361 Power-driven hand tools, except electric hand tools
362 Hand tools, not power-driven
369 Others

37 Ladders, Mobile Ramps

38 Scaffolding

39 Other Equipment, Not Elsewhere Classified

4 MATERIALS, SUBSTANCES AND RADIATIONS

41 Explosives

42 Dusts, Gases, Liquids and Chemicals, Excluding Explosives
421 Dusts
422 Gases, vapors, fumes
423 Liquids, not elsewhere classified
424 Chemicals, not elsewhere classified

43 Flying Fragments

44 Radiations
441 Ionizing radiations
449 Others

49 Other Materials and Substances Not Elsewhere Classified

5 WORKING ENVIRONMENT

51 Outdoor
511 Weather
512 Traffic and working surfaces
513 Water
519 Others

52 Indoor
521 Floors
522 Confined quarters
523 Stairs
524 Other traffic and working surfaces
525 Floor openings and wall openings
526 Environmental factors (lighting, ventilation, temperature, noise, etc.)
529 Others

53 Underground
531 Roofs and faces of mine roads and tunnels, etc.
532 Floors of mine roads and tunnels, etc.
533 Working-faces of mines, tunnels, etc.
534 Mine shafts
535 Fire
536 Water
539 Others

6 OTHER AGENCIES, NOT ELSEWHERE CLASSIFIED

61 Animals
611 Live animals
612 Animals products

69 Other Agencies, Not Elsewhere Classified

7 AGENCIES NOT CLASSIFIED FOR LACK OF SUFFICIENT DATA

APPENDIX E:
LIST OF THREE-DIGIT CATEGORIES

1. INFECTIOUS AND PARASITIC DISEASES

Intestinal infectious diseases (001-009)

- 001 Cholera
- 002 Typhoid and paratyphoid fevers
- 003 Other salmonella infections
- 004 Shigellosis
- 005 Other food poisoning (bacterial)
- 006 Amebiasis
- 007 Other protozoal intestinal diseases
- 008 Intestinal infections due to other organisms
- 009 Ill-defined intestinal infections

Tuberculosis (010-018)

- 010 Primary tuberculous infection
- 011 Pulmonary tuberculosis
- 012 Other respiratory tuberculosis
- 013 Tuberculosis of meninges and central nervous system
- 014 Tuberculosis of intestines, peritoneum, and mesenteric glands
- 015 Tuberculosis of bones and joints
- 016 Tuberculosis of genitourinary system
- 017 Tuberculosis of other organs
- 018 Miliary tuberculosis

Zoonotic bacterial diseases (020-027)

- 020 Plague
- 021 Tularemia
- 022 Anthrax
- 023 Brucellosis
- 024 Glanders
- 025 Melioidosis
- 026 Rat-bite fever
- 027 Other zoonotic bacterial diseases

Other bacterial diseases (030-041)

- 030 Leprosy
- 031 Diseases due to other mycobacteria
- 032 Diphtheria
- 033 Whooping cough
- 034 Streptococcal sore throat and scarlet fever
- 035 Erysipelas
- 036 Meningococcal infection
- 037 Tetanus
- 038 Septicemia
- 039 Actinomycotic infections
- 040 Other bacterial diseases
- 041 Bacterial infection in conditions classified elsewhere and of unspecified site

Human immunodeficiency virus (HIV) infection (042)

- 042 Human immunodeficiency virus [HIV] disease

Poliomyelitis and other non-arthropod-borne viral diseases of central nervous system (045-049)

- 045 Acute poliomyelitis
- 046 Slow virus infections and prion diseases of central nervous system
- 047 Meningitis due to enterovirus
- 048 Other enterovirus diseases of central nervous system
- 049 Other non-arthropod-borne viral diseases of central nervous system

Viral diseases generally accompanied by exanthem (050-059)

- 050 Smallpox
- 051 Cowpox and paravaccinia
- 052 Chickenpox
- 053 Herpes zoster
- 054 Herpes simplex
- 055 Measles
- 056 Rubella

1. INFECTIOUS AND PARASITIC DISEASES *continued*

    057   Other viral exanthemata
    058   Other human herpesviruses
    059   Other poxvirus infections

Arthropod-borne viral diseases (060-066)
    060   Yellow fever
    061   Dengue
    062   Mosquito-borne viral encephalitis
    063   Tick-borne viral encephalitis
    064   Viral encephalitis transmitted by other and unspecified arthropods
    065   Arthropod-borne hemorrhagic fever
    066   Other arthropod-borne viral diseases

Other diseases due to viruses and Chlamydiae (070-079)
    070   Viral hepatitis
    071   Rabies
    072   Mumps
    073   Ornithosis
    074   Specific diseases due to Coxsackie virus
    075   Infectious mononucleosis
    076   Trachoma
    077   Other diseases of conjunctiva due to viruses and Chlamydiae
    078   Other diseases due to viruses and Chlamydiae
    079   Viral and Chlamydial infection in conditions classified elsewhere and of unspecified site

Rickettsioses and other arthropod-borne diseases (080-088)
    080   Louse-borne [epidemic] typhus
    081   Other typhus
    082   Tick-borne rickettsioses
    083   Other rickettsioses
    084   Malaria
    085   Leishmaniasis
    086   Trypanosomiasis
    087   Relapsing fever
    088   Other arthropod-borne diseases

Syphilis and other venereal diseases (090-099)
    090   Congenital syphilis
    091   Early syphilis, symptomatic
    092   Early syphilis, latent
    093   Cardiovascular syphilis
    094   Neurosyphilis
    095   Other forms of late syphilis, with symptoms
    096   Late syphilis, latent
    097   Other and unspecified syphilis
    098   Gonococcal infections
    099   Other venereal diseases

Other spirochetal diseases (100-104)
    100   Leptospirosis
    101   Vincent's angina
    102   Yaws
    103   Pinta
    104   Other spirochetal infection

Mycoses (110-118)
    110   Dermatophytosis
    111   Dermatomycosis, other and unspecified
    112   Candidiasis
    114   Coccidioidomycosis
    115   Histoplasmosis
    116   Blastomycotic infection
    117   Other mycoses
    118   Opportunistic mycoses

Helminthiases (120-129)
    120   Schistosomiasis [bilharziasis]
    121   Other trematode infections

1. INFECTIOUS AND PARASITIC DISEASES *continued*

122 Echinococcosis
123 Other cestode infection
124 Trichinosis
125 Filarial infection and dracontiasis
126 Ancylostomiasis and necatoriasis
127 Other intestinal helminthiases
128 Other and unspecified helminthiases
129 Intestinal parasitism, unspecified

Other infectious and parasitic diseases (130-136)

130 Toxoplasmosis
131 Trichomoniasis
132 Pediculosis and phthirus infestation
133 Acariasis
134 Other infestation
135 Sarcoidosis
136 Other and unspecified infectious and parasitic diseases

Late effects of infectious and parasitic diseases (137-139)

137 Late effects of tuberculosis
138 Late effects of acute poliomyelitis
139 Late effects of other infectious and parasitic diseases

2. NEOPLASMS

Malignant neoplasm of lip, oral cavity, and pharynx (140-149)

140 Malignant neoplasm of lip
141 Malignant neoplasm of tongue
142 Malignant neoplasm of major salivary glands
143 Malignant neoplasm of gum
144 Malignant neoplasm of floor of mouth
145 Malignant neoplasm of other and unspecified parts of mouth
146 Malignant neoplasm of oropharynx
147 Malignant neoplasm of nasopharynx
148 Malignant neoplasm of hypopharynx
149 Malignant neoplasm of other and ill-defined sites within the lip, oral cavity, and pharynx

Malignant neoplasm of digestive organs and peritoneum (150-159)

150 Malignant neoplasm of esophagus
151 Malignant neoplasm of stomach
152 Malignant neoplasm of small intestine, including duodenum
153 Malignant neoplasm of colon
154 Malignant neoplasm of rectum, rectosigmoid junction, and anus
155 Malignant neoplasm of liver and intrahepatic bile ducts
156 Malignant neoplasm of gallbladder and extrahepatic bile ducts
157 Malignant neoplasm of pancreas
158 Malignant neoplasm of retroperitoneum and peritoneum
159 Malignant neoplasm of other and ill-defined sites within the digestive organs and peritoneum

Malignant neoplasm of respiratory and intrathoracic organs (160-165)

160 Malignant neoplasm of nasal cavities, middle ear, and accessory sinuses
161 Malignant neoplasm of larynx
162 Malignant neoplasm of trachea, bronchus, and lung
163 Malignant neoplasm of pleura
164 Malignant neoplasm of thymus, heart, and mediastinum
165 Malignant neoplasm of other and ill-defined sites within the respiratory system and intrathoracic organs

Malignant neoplasm of bone, connective tissue, skin, and breast (170-176)

170 Malignant neoplasm of bone and articular cartilage
171 Malignant neoplasm of connective and other soft tissue
172 Malignant melanoma of skin
173 Other malignant neoplasm of skin
174 Malignant neoplasm of female breast
175 Malignant neoplasm of male breast
176 Kaposi's sarcoma

2. NEOPLASMS *continued*

Malignant neoplasm of genitourinary organs (179-189)
179 Malignant neoplasm of uterus, part unspecified
180 Malignant neoplasm of cervix uteri
181 Malignant neoplasm of placenta
182 Malignant neoplasm of body of uterus
183 Malignant neoplasm of ovary and other uterine adnexa
184 Malignant neoplasm of other and unspecified female genital organs
185 Malignant neoplasm of prostate
186 Malignant neoplasm of testis
187 Malignant neoplasm of penis and other male genital organs
188 Malignant neoplasm of bladder
189 Malignant neoplasm of kidney and other and unspecified urinary organs

Malignant neoplasm of other and unspecified sites (190-199)
190 Malignant neoplasm of eye
191 Malignant neoplasm of brain
192 Malignant neoplasm of other and unspecified parts of nervous system
193 Malignant neoplasm of thyroid gland
194 Malignant neoplasm of other endocrine glands and related structures
195 Malignant neoplasm of other and ill-defined sites
196 Secondary and unspecified malignant neoplasm of lymph nodes
197 Secondary malignant neoplasm of respiratory and digestive systems
198 Secondary malignant neoplasm of other specified sites
199 Malignant neoplasm without specification of site

Malignant neoplasm of lymphatic and hematopoietic tissue (200-208)
200 Lymphosarcoma and reticulosarcoma and other specified malignant tumors of lymphatic tissue
201 Hodgkin's disease
202 Other malignant neoplasm of lymphoid and histiocytic tissue
203 Multiple myeloma and immunoproliferative neoplasms
204 Lymphoid leukemia
205 Myeloid leukemia
206 Monocytic leukemia
207 Other specified leukemia
208 Leukemia of unspecified cell type

Neuroendocrine tumors (209)
209 Neuroendocrine tumors

Benign neoplasms (210-229)
210 Benign neoplasm of lip, oral cavity, and pharynx
211 Benign neoplasm of other parts of digestive system
212 Benign neoplasm of respiratory and intrathoracic organs
213 Benign neoplasm of bone and articular cartilage
214 Lipoma
215 Other benign neoplasm of connective and other soft tissue
216 Benign neoplasm of skin
217 Benign neoplasm of breast
218 Uterine leiomyoma
219 Other benign neoplasm of uterus
220 Benign neoplasm of ovary
221 Benign neoplasm of other female genital organs
222 Benign neoplasm of male genital organs
223 Benign neoplasm of kidney and other urinary organs
224 Benign neoplasm of eye
225 Benign neoplasm of brain and other parts of nervous system
226 Benign neoplasm of thyroid gland
227 Benign neoplasm of other endocrine glands and related structures
228 Hemangioma and lymphangioma, any site
229 Benign neoplasm of other and unspecified sites

Carcinoma in situ (230-234)
230 Carcinoma in situ of digestive organs
231 Carcinoma in situ of respiratory system
232 Carcinoma in situ of skin
233 Carcinoma in situ of breast and genitourinary system
234 Carcinoma in situ of other and unspecified sites

2. NEOPLASMS *continued*

Neoplasms of uncertain behavior (235-238)

235 Neoplasm of uncertain behavior of digestive and respiratory systems
236 Neoplasm of uncertain behavior of genitourinary organs
237 Neoplasm of uncertain behavior of endocrine glands and nervous system
238 Neoplasm of uncertain behavior of other and unspecified sites and tissues

Neoplasm of unspecified nature (239)

239 Neoplasm of unspecified nature

3. ENDOCRINE, NUTRITIONAL AND METABOLIC DISEASES, AND IMMUNITY DISORDERS

Disorders of thyroid gland (240-246)

240 Simple and unspecified goiter
241 Nontoxic nodular goiter
242 Thyrotoxicosis with or without goiter
243 Congenital hypothyroidism
244 Acquired hypothyroidism
245 Thyroiditis
246 Other disorders of thyroid

Diseases of other endocrine glands (249-259)

249 Secondary diabetes mellitus
250 Diabetes mellitus
251 Other disorders of pancreatic internal secretion
252 Disorders of parathyroid gland
253 Disorders of the pituitary gland and its hypothalamic control
254 Diseases of thymus gland
255 Disorders of adrenal glands
256 Ovarian dysfunction
257 Testicular dysfunction
258 Polyglandular dysfunction and related disorders
259 Other endocrine disorders

Nutritional deficiencies (260-269)

260 Kwashiorkor
261 Nutritional marasmus
262 Other severe protein-calorie malnutrition
263 Other and unspecified protein-calorie malnutrition
264 Vitamin A deficiency
265 Thiamine and niacin deficiency states
266 Deficiency of B-complex components
267 Ascorbic acid deficiency
268 Vitamin D deficiency
269 Other nutritional deficiencies

Other metabolic and immunity disorders (270-279)

270 Disorders of amino-acid transport and metabolism
271 Disorders of carbohydrate transport and metabolism
272 Disorders of lipoid metabolism
273 Disorders of plasma protein metabolism
274 Gout
275 Disorders of mineral metabolism
276 Disorders of fluid, electrolyte, and acid-base balance
277 Other and unspecified disorders of metabolism
278 Overweight, obesity and other hyperalimentation
279 Disorders involving the immune mechanism

4. DISEASES OF THE BLOOD AND BLOOD-FORMING ORGANS

Diseases of blood and blood-forming organs (280-289)

280 Iron deficiency anemias
281 Other deficiency anemias
282 Hereditary hemolytic anemias
283 Acquired hemolytic anemias
284 Aplastic anemia and other bone marrow failure syndromes
285 Other and unspecified anemias
286 Coagulation defects
287 Purpura and other hemorrhagic conditions

5. MENTAL DISORDERS
288   Diseases of white blood cells
289   Other diseases of blood and blood-forming organs

Organic psychotic conditions (290-294)
290   Dementias
291   Alcohol-induced mental disorders
292   Drug-induced mental disorders
293   Transient mental disorders due to conditions classified elsewhere
294   Persistent mental disorders due to conditions classified elsewhere

Other psychoses (295-299)
295   Schizophrenic disorders
296   Episodic mood disorders
297   Delusional disorders
298   Other nonorganic psychoses
299   Pervasive developmental disorders

Neurotic disorders, personality disorders, and other nonpsychotic mental disorders (300-316)
300   Anxiety, dissociative and somatoform disorders
301   Personality disorders
302   Sexual and gender identity disorders
303   Alcohol dependence syndrome
304   Drug dependence
305   Nondependent abuse of drugs
306   Physiological malfunction arising from mental factors
307   Special symptoms or syndromes, not elsewhere classified
308   Acute reaction to stress
309   Adjustment reaction
310   Specific nonpsychotic mental disorders due to brain damage
311   Depressive disorder, not elsewhere classified
312   Disturbance of conduct, not elsewhere classified
313   Disturbance of emotions specific to childhood and adolescence
314   Hyperkinetic syndrome of childhood
315   Specific delays in development
316   Psychic factors associated with diseases classified elsewhere

Mental retardation (317-319)
317   Mild mental retardation
318   Other specified mental retardation
319   Unspecified mental retardation

6. DISEASES OF THE NERVOUS SYSTEM AND SENSE ORGANS

Inflammatory diseases of the central nervous system (320-326)
320   Bacterial meningitis
321   Meningitis due to other organisms
322   Meningitis of unspecified cause
323   Encephalitis, myelitis, and encephalomyelitis
324   Intracranial and intraspinal abscess
325   Phlebitis and thrombophlebitis of intracranial venous sinuses
326   Late effects of intracranial abscess or pyogenic infection

Organic sleep disorders (327)
327   Organic sleep disorders

Hereditary and degenerative diseases of the central nervous system (330-337)
330   Cerebral degenerations usually manifest in childhood
331   Other cerebral degenerations
332   Parkinson's disease
333   Other extrapyramidal disease and abnormal movement disorders
334   Spinocerebellar disease
335   Anterior horn cell disease
336   Other diseases of spinal cord
337   Disorders of the autonomic nervous system

Pain (338)
338   Pain, not elsewhere classified

Other headache syndromes (339)
339   Other headache syndromes

6. DISEASES OF THE NERVOUS SYSTEM AND SENSE ORGANS *continued*

Other disorders of the central nervous system (340-349)
- 340 Multiple sclerosis
- 341 Other demyelinating diseases of central nervous system
- 342 Hemiplegia and hemiparesis
- 343 Infantile cerebral palsy
- 344 Other paralytic syndromes
- 345 Epilepsy and recurrent seizures
- 346 Migraine
- 347 Cataplexy and narcolepsy
- 348 Other conditions of brain
- 349 Other and unspecified disorders of the nervous system

Disorders of the peripheral nervous system (350-359)
- 350 Trigeminal nerve disorders
- 351 Facial nerve disorders
- 352 Disorders of other cranial nerves
- 353 Nerve root and plexus disorders
- 354 Mononeuritis of upper limb and mononeuritis multiplex
- 355 Mononeuritis of lower limb and unspecified site
- 356 Hereditary and idiopathic peripheral neuropathy
- 357 Inflammatory and toxic neuropathy
- 358 Myoneural disorders
- 359 Muscular dystrophies and other myopathies

Disorders of the eye and adnexa (360-379)
- 360 Disorders of the globe
- 361 Retinal detachments and defects
- 362 Other retinal disorders
- 363 Chorioretinal inflammations, scars and other disorders of choroid
- 364 Disorders of iris and ciliary body
- 365 Glaucoma
- 366 Cataract
- 367 Disorders of refraction and accommodation
- 368 Visual disturbances
- 369 Blindness and low vision
- 370 Keratitis
- 371 Corneal opacity and other disorders of cornea
- 372 Disorders of conjunctiva
- 373 Inflammation of eyelids
- 374 Other disorders of eyelids
- 375 Disorders of lacrimal system
- 376 Disorders of the orbit
- 377 Disorders of optic nerve and visual pathways
- 378 Strabismus and other disorders of binocular eye movements
- 379 Other disorders of eye

Diseases of the ear and mastoid process (380-389)
- 380 Disorders of external ear
- 381 Nonsuppurative otitis media and Eustachian tube disorders
- 382 Suppurative and unspecified otitis media
- 383 Mastoiditis and related conditions
- 384 Other disorders of tympanic membrane
- 385 Other disorders of middle ear and mastoid
- 386 Vertiginous syndromes and other disorders of vestibular system
- 387 Otosclerosis
- 388 Other disorders of ear
- 389 Hearing loss

7. DISEASES OF THE CIRCULATORY SYSTEM

Acute rheumatic fever (390-392)
- 390 Rheumatic fever without mention of heart involvement
- 391 Rheumatic fever with heart involvement
- 392 Rheumatic chorea

Chronic rheumatic heart disease (393-398)
- 393 Chronic rheumatic pericarditis
- 394 Diseases of mitral valve

7. DISEASES OF THE CIRCULATORY SYSTEM *continued*

395 Diseases of aortic valve
396 Diseases of mitral and aortic valves
397 Diseases of other endocardial structures
398 Other rheumatic heart disease

Hypertensive disease (401-405)
401 Essential hypertension
402 Hypertensive heart disease
403 Hypertensive chronic kidney disease
404 Hypertensive heart and chronic kidney disease
405 Secondary hypertension

Ischemic heart disease (410-414)
410 Acute myocardial infarction
411 Other acute and subacute form of ischemic heart disease
412 Old myocardial infarction
413 Angina pectoris
414 Other forms of chronic ischemic heart disease

Diseases of pulmonary circulation (415-417)
415 Acute pulmonary heart disease
416 Chronic pulmonary heart disease
417 Other diseases of pulmonary circulation

Other forms of heart disease (420-429)
420 Acute pericarditis
421 Acute and subacute endocarditis
422 Acute myocarditis
423 Other diseases of pericardium
424 Other diseases of endocardium
425 Cardiomyopathy
426 Conduction disorders
427 Cardiac dysrhythmias
428 Heart failure
429 Ill-defined descriptions and complications of heart disease

Cerebrovascular disease (430-438)
430 Subarachnoid hemorrhage
431 Intracerebral hemorrhage
432 Other and unspecified intracranial hemorrhage
433 Occlusion and stenosis of precerebral arteries
434 Occlusion of cerebral arteries
435 Transient cerebral ischemia
436 Acute but ill-defined cerebrovascular disease
437 Other and ill-defined cerebrovascular disease
438 Late effects of cerebrovascular disease

Diseases of arteries, arterioles, and capillaries (440-449)
440 Atherosclerosis
441 Aortic aneurysm and dissection
442 Other aneurysm
443 Other peripheral vascular disease
444 Arterial embolism and thrombosis
445 Atheroembolism
446 Polyarteritis nodosa and allied conditions
447 Other disorders of arteries and arterioles
448 Diseases of capillaries
449 Septic arterial embolism

Diseases of veins and lymphatics, and other diseases of circulatory system (451-459)
451 Phlebitis and thrombophlebitis
452 Portal vein thrombosis
453 Other venous embolism and thrombosis
454 Varicose veins of lower extremities
455 Hemorrhoids
456 Varicose veins of other sites
457 Noninfective disorders of lymphatic channels
458 Hypotension
459 Other disorders of circulatory system

8. DISEASES OF THE RESPIRATORY SYSTEM

Acute respiratory infections (460-466)
- 460 Acute nasopharyngitis [common cold]
- 461 Acute sinusitis
- 462 Acute pharyngitis
- 463 Acute tonsillitis
- 464 Acute laryngitis and tracheitis
- 465 Acute upper respiratory infections of multiple or unspecified sites
- 466 Acute bronchitis and bronchiolitis

Other diseases of upper respiratory tract (470-478)
- 470 Deviated nasal septum
- 471 Nasal polyps
- 472 Chronic pharyngitis and nasopharyngitis
- 473 Chronic sinusitis
- 474 Chronic disease of tonsils and adenoids
- 475 Peritonsillar abscess
- 476 Chronic laryngitis and laryngotracheitis
- 477 Allergic rhinitis
- 478 Other diseases of upper respiratory tract

Pneumonia and influenza (480-488)
- 480 Viral pneumonia
- 481 Pneumococcal pneumonia [*Streptococcus pneumoniae* pneumonia]
- 482 Other bacterial pneumonia
- 483 Pneumonia due to other specified organism
- 484 Pneumonia in infectious diseases classified elsewhere
- 485 Bronchopneumonia, organism unspecified
- 486 Pneumonia, organism unspecified
- 487 Influenza
- 488 Influenza due to certain identified influenza viruses

Chronic obstructive pulmonary disease and allied conditions (490-496)
- 490 Bronchitis, not specified as acute or chronic
- 491 Chronic bronchitis
- 492 Emphysema
- 493 Asthma
- 494 Bronchiectasis
- 495 Extrinsic allergic alveolitis
- 496 Chronic airway obstruction, not elsewhere classified

Pneumoconioses and other lung diseases due to external agents (500-508)
- 500 Coal workers' pneumoconiosis
- 501 Asbestosis
- 502 Pneumoconiosis due to other silica or silicates
- 503 Pneumoconiosis due to other inorganic dust
- 504 Pneumopathy due to inhalation of other dust
- 505 Pneumoconiosis, unspecified
- 506 Respiratory conditions due to chemical fumes and vapors
- 507 Pneumonitis due to solids and liquids
- 508 Respiratory conditions due to other and unspecified external agents

Other diseases of respiratory system (510-519)
- 510 Empyema
- 511 Pleurisy
- 512 Pneumothorax
- 513 Abscess of lung and mediastinum
- 514 Pulmonary congestion and hypostasis
- 515 Postinflammatory pulmonary fibrosis
- 516 Other alveolar and parietoalveolar pneumopathy
- 517 Lung involvement in conditions classified elsewhere
- 518 Other diseases of lung
- 519 Other diseases of respiratory system

9. DISEASES OF THE DIGESTIVE SYSTEM

Diseases of oral cavity, salivary glands, and jaws (520-529)
- 520 Disorders of tooth development and eruption
- 521 Diseases of hard tissues of teeth
- 522 Diseases of pulp and periapical tissues

9. DISEASES OF THE DIGESTIVE SYSTEM *continued*

    523   Gingival and periodontal diseases
    524   Dentofacial anomalies, including malocclusion
    525   Other diseases and conditions of the teeth and supporting structures
    526   Diseases of the jaws
    527   Diseases of the salivary glands
    528   Diseases of the oral soft tissues, excluding lesions specific for gingiva and tongue
    529   Diseases and other conditions of the tongue

Diseases of esophagus, stomach, and duodenum (530-538)

    530   Diseases of esophagus
    531   Gastric ulcer
    532   Duodenal ulcer
    533   Peptic ulcer, site unspecified
    534   Gastrojejunal ulcer
    535   Gastritis and duodenitis
    536   Disorders of function of stomach
    537   Other disorders of stomach and duodenum
    538   Gastrointestinal mucositis (ulcerative)

Appendicitis (540-543)

    540   Acute appendicitis
    541   Appendicitis, unqualified
    542   Other appendicitis
    543   Other diseases of appendix

Hernia of abdominal cavity (550-553)

    550   Inguinal hernia
    551   Other hernia of abdominal cavity, with gangrene
    552   Other hernia of abdominal cavity, with obstruction, but without mention of gangrene
    553   Other hernia of abdominal cavity without mention of obstruction or gangrene

Noninfectious enteritis and colitis (555-558)

    555   Regional enteritis
    556   Ulcerative colitis
    557   Vascular insufficiency of intestine
    558   Other and unspecified noninfectious gastroenteritis and colitis

Other diseases of intestines and peritoneum (560-569)

    560   Intestinal obstruction without mention of hernia
    562   Diverticula of intestine
    564   Functional digestive disorders, not elsewhere classified
    565   Anal fissure and fistula
    566   Abscess of anal and rectal regions
    567   Peritonitis and retroperitoneal infections
    568   Other disorders of peritoneum
    569   Other disorders of intestine

Other diseases of digestive system (570-579)

    570   Acute and subacute necrosis of liver
    571   Chronic liver disease and cirrhosis
    572   Liver abscess and sequelae of chronic liver disease
    573   Other disorders of liver
    574   Cholelithiasis
    575   Other disorders of gallbladder
    576   Other disorders of biliary tract
    577   Diseases of pancreas
    578   Gastrointestinal hemorrhage
    579   Intestinal malabsorption

10. DISEASES OF THE GENITOURINARY SYSTEM

Nephritis, nephrotic syndrome, and nephrosis (580-589)

    580   Acute glomerulonephritis
    581   Nephrotic syndrome
    582   Chronic glomerulonephritis
    583   Nephritis and nephropathy, not specified as acute or chronic
    584   Acute kidney failure
    585   Chronic kidney disease (CKD)

10. DISEASES OF THE GENITOURINARY SYSTEM *continued*

- 586 Renal failure, unspecified
- 587 Renal sclerosis, unspecified
- 588 Disorders resulting from impaired renal function
- 589 Small kidney of unknown cause

Other diseases of urinary system (590-599)

- 590 Infections of kidney
- 591 Hydronephrosis
- 592 Calculus of kidney and ureter
- 593 Other disorders of kidney and ureter
- 594 Calculus of lower urinary tract
- 595 Cystitis
- 596 Other disorders of bladder
- 597 Urethritis, not sexually transmitted, and urethral syndrome
- 598 Urethral stricture
- 599 Other disorders of urethra and urinary tract

Diseases of male genital organs (600-608)

- 600 Hyperplasia of prostate
- 601 Inflammatory diseases of prostate
- 602 Other disorders of prostate
- 603 Hydrocele
- 604 Orchitis and epididymitis
- 605 Redundant prepuce and phimosis
- 606 Infertility, male
- 607 Disorders of penis
- 608 Other disorders of male genital organs

Disorders of breast (610-612)

- 610 Benign mammary dysplasias
- 611 Other disorders of breast
- 612 Deformity and disproportion of reconstructed breast

Inflammatory disease of female pelvic organs (614-616)

- 614 Inflammatory disease of ovary, fallopian tube, pelvic cellular tissue, and peritoneum
- 615 Inflammatory diseases of uterus, except cervix
- 616 Inflammatory disease of cervix, vagina, and vulva

Other disorders of female genital tract (617-629)

- 617 Endometriosis
- 618 Genital prolapse
- 619 Fistula involving female genital tract
- 620 Noninflammatory disorders of ovary, fallopian tube, and broad ligament
- 621 Disorders of uterus, not elsewhere classified
- 622 Noninflammatory disorders of cervix
- 623 Noninflammatory disorders of vagina
- 624 Noninflammatory disorders of vulva and perineum
- 625 Pain and other symptoms associated with female genital organs
- 626 Disorders of menstruation and other abnormal bleeding from female genital tract
- 627 Menopausal and postmenopausal disorders
- 628 Infertility, female
- 629 Other disorders of female genital organs

11. COMPLICATIONS OF PREGNANCY, CHILDBIRTH AND THE PUERPERIUM

Ectopic and molar pregnancy (630-633)

- 630 Hydatidiform mole
- 631 Other abnormal product of conception
- 632 Missed abortion
- 633 Ectopic pregnancy

Other pregnancy with abortive outcome (634-639)

- 634 Abortion
- 635 Legally induced abortion
- 636 Illegally induced abortion
- 637 Unspecified abortion
- 638 Failed attempted abortion
- 639 Complications following abortion and ectopic and molar pregnancies

11. COMPLICATIONS OF PREGNANCY, CHILDBIRTH AND THE PUERPERIUM *continued*

Complications mainly related to pregnancy (640-649)
- 640 Hemorrhage in early pregnancy
- 641 Antepartum hemorrhage, abruptio placentae, and placenta previa
- 642 Hypertension complicating pregnancy, childbirth, and the puerperium
- 643 Excessive vomiting in pregnancy
- 644 Early or threatened labor
- 645 Late pregnancy
- 646 Other complications of pregnancy, not elsewhere classified
- 647 Infectious and parasitic conditions in the mother classifiable elsewhere but complicating pregnancy, childbirth, and the puerperium
- 648 Other current conditions in the mother classifiable elsewhere but complicating pregnancy, childbirth, and the puerperium
- 649 Other conditions or status of the mother complicating pregnancy, childbirth or the puerperium

Normal delivery, and other indications for care in pregnancy, labor, and delivery (650-659)
- 650 Normal delivery
- 651 Multiple gestation
- 652 Malposition and malpresentation of fetus
- 653 Disproportion
- 654 Abnormality of organs and soft tissues of pelvis
- 655 Known or suspected fetal abnormality affecting management of mother
- 656 Other known or suspected fetal and placental problems affecting management of mother
- 657 Polyhydramnios
- 658 Other problems associated with amniotic cavity and membranes
- 659 Other indications for care or intervention related to labor and delivery and not elsewhere classified

Complications occurring mainly in the course of labor and delivery (660-669)
- 660 Obstructed labor
- 661 Abnormality of forces of labor
- 662 Long labor
- 663 Umbilical cord complications
- 664 Trauma to perineum and vulva during delivery
- 665 Other obstetrical trauma
- 666 Postpartum hemorrhage
- 667 Retained placenta or membranes, without hemorrhage
- 668 Complications of the administration of anesthetic or other sedation in labor and delivery
- 669 Other complications of labor and delivery, not elsewhere classified

Complications of the puerperium (670-677)
- 670 Major puerperal infection
- 671 Venous complications in pregnancy and the puerperium
- 672 Pyrexia of unknown origin during the puerperium
- 673 Obstetrical pulmonary embolism
- 674 Other and unspecified complications of the puerperium, not elsewhere classified
- 675 Infections of the breast and nipple associated with childbirth
- 676 Other disorders of the breast associated with childbirth, and disorders of lactation
- 677 Late effect of complication of pregnancy, childbirth, and the puerperium

Other maternal and fetal complications (678-679)
- 678 Other fetal conditions
- 679 Complications of in utero procedures

12. DISEASES OF THE SKIN AND SUBCUTANEOUS TISSUE

Infections of skin and subcutaneous tissue (680-686)
- 680 Carbuncle and furuncle
- 681 Cellulitis and abscess of finger and toe
- 682 Other cellulitis and abscess
- 683 Acute lymphadenitis
- 684 Impetigo
- 685 Pilonidal cyst
- 686 Other local infections of skin and subcutaneous tissue

Other inflammatory conditions of skin and subcutaneous tissue (690-698)
- 690 Erythematosquamous dermatosis
- 691 Atopic dermatitis and related conditions

12. DISEASES OF THE SKIN AND SUBCUTANEOUS TISSUE *continued*

692   Contact dermatitis and other eczema
693   Dermatitis due to substances taken internally
694   Bullous dermatoses
695   Erythematous conditions
696   Psoriasis and similar disorders
697   Lichen
698   Pruritus and related conditions

Other diseases of skin and subcutaneous tissue (700-709)

700   Corns and callosities
701   Other hypertrophic and atrophic conditions of skin
702   Other dermatoses
703   Diseases of nail
704   Diseases of hair and hair follicles
705   Disorders of sweat glands
706   Diseases of sebaceous glands
707   Chronic ulcer of skin
708   Urticaria
709   Other disorders of skin and subcutaneous tissue

13. DISEASES OF THE MUSCULOSKELETAL SYSTEM AND CONNECTIVE TISSUE

Arthropathies and related disorders (710-719)

710   Diffuse diseases of connective tissue
711   Arthropathy associated with infections
712   Crystal arthropathies
713   Arthropathy associated with other disorders classified elsewhere
714   Rheumatoid arthritis and other inflammatory polyarthropathies
715   Osteoarthrosis and allied disorders
716   Other and unspecified arthropathies
717   Internal derangement of knee
718   Other derangement of joint
719   Other and unspecified disorder of joint

Dorsopathies (720-724)

720   Ankylosing spondylitis and other inflammatory spondylopathies
721   Spondylosis and allied disorders
722   Intervertebral disc disorders
723   Other disorders of cervical region
724   Other and unspecified disorders of back

Rheumatism, excluding the back (725-729)

725   Polymyalgia rheumatica
726   Peripheral enthesopathies and allied syndromes
727   Other disorders of synovium, tendon, and bursa
728   Disorders of muscle, ligament, and fascia
729   Other disorders of soft tissues

Osteopathies, chondropathies, and acquired musculoskeletal deformities (730-739)

730   Osteomyelitis, periostitis, and other infections involving bone
731   Osteitis deformans and osteopathies associated with other disorders classified elsewhere
732   Osteochondropathies
733   Other disorders of bone and cartilage
734   Flat foot
735   Acquired deformities of toe
736   Other acquired deformities of limbs
737   Curvature of spine
738   Other acquired deformity
739   Nonallopathic lesions, not elsewhere classified

14. CONGENITAL ANOMALIES

740   Anencephalus and similar anomalies
741   Spina bifida
742   Other congenital anomalies of nervous system
743   Congenital anomalies of eye
744   Congenital anomalies of ear, face, and neck
745   Bulbus cordis anomalies and anomalies of cardiac septal closure

14. CONGENITAL ANOMALIES *continued*

746 Other congenital anomalies of heart
747 Other congenital anomalies of circulatory system
748 Congenital anomalies of respiratory system
749 Cleft palate and cleft lip
750 Other congenital anomalies of upper alimentary tract
751 Other congenital anomalies of digestive system
752 Congenital anomalies of genital organs
753 Congenital anomalies of urinary system
754 Certain congenital musculoskeletal deformities
755 Other congenital anomalies of limbs
756 Other congenital musculoskeletal anomalies
757 Congenital anomalies of the integument
758 Chromosomal anomalies
759 Other and unspecified congenital anomalies

15. CERTAIN CONDITIONS ORIGINATING IN THE PERINATAL PERIOD

Maternal causes of perinatal morbidity and mortality (760-763)

760 Fetus or newborn affected by maternal conditions which may be unrelated to present pregnancy
761 Fetus or newborn affected by maternal complications of pregnancy
762 Fetus or newborn affected by complications of placenta, cord, and membranes
763 Fetus or newborn affected by other complications of labor and delivery

Other conditions originating in the perinatal period (764-779)

764 Slow fetal growth and fetal malnutrition
765 Disorders relating to short gestation and low birthweight
766 Disorders relating to long gestation and high birthweight
767 Birth trauma
768 Intrauterine hypoxia and birth asphyxia
769 Respiratory distress syndrome
770 Other respiratory conditions of fetus and newborn
771 Infections specific to the perinatal period
772 Fetal and neonatal hemorrhage
773 Hemolytic disease of fetus or newborn, due to isoimmunization
774 Other perinatal jaundice
775 Endocrine and metabolic disturbances specific to the fetus and newborn
776 Hematological disorders of newborn
777 Perinatal disorders of digestive system
778 Conditions involving the integument and temperature regulation of fetus and newborn
779 Other and ill-defined conditions originating in the perinatal period

16. SYMPTOMS, SIGNS, AND ILL-DEFINED CONDITIONS

Symptoms (780-789)

780 General symptoms
781 Symptoms involving nervous and musculoskeletal systems
782 Symptoms involving skin and other integumentary tissue
783 Symptoms concerning nutrition, metabolism, and development
784 Symptoms involving head and neck
785 Symptoms involving cardiovascular system
786 Symptoms involving respiratory system and other chest symptoms
787 Symptoms involving digestive system
788 Symptoms involving urinary system
789 Other symptoms involving abdomen and pelvis

Nonspecific abnormal findings (790-796)

790 Nonspecific findings on examination of blood
791 Nonspecific findings on examination of urine
792 Nonspecific abnormal findings in other body substances
793 Nonspecific (abnormal) findings on radiological and other examination of body structure
794 Nonspecific abnormal results of function studies
795 Other and nonspecific abnormal cytological, histological, immunological and DNA test findings
796 Other nonspecific abnormal findings

Ill-defined and unknown causes of morbidity and mortality (797-799)

797 Senility without mention of psychosis

16. SYMPTOMS, SIGNS, AND ILL-DEFINED CONDITIONS *continued*

798   Sudden death, cause unknown
799   Other ill-defined and unknown causes of morbidity and mortality

17. INJURY AND POISONING

Fracture of skull (800-804)

800   Fracture of vault of skull
801   Fracture of base of skull
802   Fracture of face bones
803   Other and unqualified skull fractures
804   Multiple fractures involving skull or face with other bones

Fracture of neck and trunk (805-809)

805   Fracture of vertebral column without mention of spinal cord injury
806   Fracture of vertebral column with spinal cord injury
807   Fracture of rib(s), sternum, larynx, and trachea
808   Fracture of pelvis
809   Ill-defined fractures of bones of trunk

Fracture of upper limb (810-819)

810   Fracture of clavicle
811   Fracture of scapula
812   Fracture of humerus
813   Fracture of radius and ulna
814   Fracture of carpal bone(s)
815   Fracture of metacarpal bone(s)
816   Fracture of one or more phalanges of hand
817   Multiple fractures of hand bones
818   Ill-defined fractures of upper limb
819   Multiple fractures involving both upper limbs, and upper limb with rib(s) and sternum

Fracture of lower limb (820-829)

820   Fracture of neck of femur
821   Fracture of other and unspecified parts of femur
822   Fracture of patella
823   Fracture of tibia and fibula
824   Fracture of ankle
825   Fracture of one or more tarsal and metatarsal bones
826   Fracture of one or more phalanges of foot
827   Other, multiple, and ill-defined fractures of lower limb
828   Multiple fractures involving both lower limbs, lower with upper limb, and lower limb(s) with rib(s) and sternum
829   Fracture of unspecified bones

Dislocation (830-839)

830   Dislocation of jaw
831   Dislocation of shoulder
832   Dislocation of elbow
833   Dislocation of wrist
834   Dislocation of finger
835   Dislocation of hip
836   Dislocation of knee
837   Dislocation of ankle
838   Dislocation of foot
839   Other, multiple, and ill-defined dislocations

Sprains and strains of joints and adjacent muscles (840-848)

840   Sprains and strains of shoulder and upper arm
841   Sprains and strains of elbow and forearm
842   Sprains and strains of wrist and hand
843   Sprains and strains of hip and thigh
844   Sprains and strains of knee and leg
845   Sprains and strains of ankle and foot
846   Sprains and strains of sacroiliac region
847   Sprains and strains of other and unspecified parts of back
848   Other and ill-defined sprains and strains

Intracranial injury, excluding those with skull fracture (850-854)

850   Concussion
851   Cerebral laceration and contusion

17. INJURY AND POISONING *continued*

852 Subarachnoid, subdural, and extradural hemorrhage, following injury
853 Other and unspecified intracranial hemorrhage following injury
854 Intracranial injury of other and unspecified nature

Internal injury of thorax, abdomen, and pelvis (860-869)
860 Traumatic pneumothorax and hemothorax
861 Injury to heart and lung
862 Injury to other and unspecified intrathoracic organs
863 Injury to gastrointestinal tract
864 Injury to liver
865 Injury to spleen
866 Injury to kidney
867 Injury to pelvic organs
868 Injury to other intra-abdominal organs
869 Internal injury to unspecified or ill-defined organs

Open wound of head, neck, and trunk (870-879)
870 Open wound of ocular adnexa
871 Open wound of eyeball
872 Open wound of ear
873 Other open wound of head
874 Open wound of neck
875 Open wound of chest (wall)
876 Open wound of back
877 Open wound of buttock
878 Open wound of genital organs (external), including traumatic amputation
879 Open wound of other and unspecified sites, except limbs

Open wound of upper limb (880-887)
880 Open wound of shoulder and upper arm
881 Open wound of elbow, forearm, and wrist
882 Open wound of hand except finger(s) alone
883 Open wound of finger(s)
884 Multiple and unspecified open wound of upper limb
885 Traumatic amputation of thumb (complete) (partial)
886 Traumatic amputation of other finger(s) (complete) (partial)
887 Traumatic amputation of arm and hand (complete) (partial)

Open wound of lower limb (890-897)
890 Open wound of hip and thigh
891 Open wound of knee, leg [except thigh], and ankle
892 Open wound of foot except toe(s) alone
893 Open wound of toe(s)
894 Multiple and unspecified open wound of lower limb
895 Traumatic amputation of toe(s) (complete) (partial)
896 Traumatic amputation of foot (complete) (partial)
897 Traumatic amputation of leg(s) (complete) (partial)

Injury to blood vessels (900-904)
900 Injury to blood vessels of head and neck
901 Injury to blood vessels of thorax
902 Injury to blood vessels of abdomen and pelvis
903 Injury to blood vessels of upper extremity
904 Injury to blood vessels of lower extremity and unspecified sites

Late effects of injuries, poisonings, toxic effects, and other external causes (905-909)
905 Late effects of musculoskeletal and connective tissue injuries
906 Late effects of injuries to skin and subcutaneous tissues
907 Late effects of injuries to the nervous system
908 Late effects of other and unspecified injuries
909 Late effects of other and unspecified external causes

Superficial injury (910-919)
910 Superficial injury of face, neck, and scalp except eye
911 Superficial injury of trunk
912 Superficial injury of shoulder and upper arm
913 Superficial injury of elbow, forearm, and wrist
914 Superficial injury of hand(s) except finger(s) alone
915 Superficial injury of finger(s)

17. INJURY AND POISONING *continued*

916   Superficial injury of hip, thigh, leg, and ankle
917   Superficial injury of foot and toe(s)
918   Superficial injury of eye and adnexa
919   Superficial injury of other, multiple, and unspecified sites

Contusion with intact skin surface (920-924)

920   Contusion of face, scalp, and neck except eye(s)
921   Contusion of eye and adnexa
922   Contusion of trunk
923   Contusion of upper limb
924   Contusion of lower limb and of other and unspecified sites

Crushing injury (925-929)

925   Crushing injury of face, scalp, and neck
926   Crushing injury of trunk
927   Crushing injury of upper limb
928   Crushing injury of lower limb
929   Crushing injury of multiple and unspecified sites

Effects of foreign body entering through orifice (930-939)

930   Foreign body on external eye
931   Foreign body in ear
932   Foreign body in nose
933   Foreign body in pharynx and larynx
934   Foreign body in trachea, bronchus, and lung
935   Foreign body in mouth, esophagus, and stomach
936   Foreign body in intestine and colon
937   Foreign body in anus and rectum
938   Foreign body in digestive system, unspecified
939   Foreign body in genitourinary tract

Burns (940-949)

940   Burn confined to eye and adnexa
941   Burn of face, head, and neck
942   Burn of trunk
943   Burn of upper limb, except wrist and hand
944   Burn of wrist(s) and hand(s)
945   Burn of lower limb(s)
946   Burns of multiple specified sites
947   Burn of internal organs
948   Burns classified according to extent of body surface involved
949   Burn, unspecified

Injury to nerves and spinal cord (950-957)

950   Injury to optic nerve and pathways
951   Injury to other cranial nerve(s)
952   Spinal cord injury without evidence of spinal bone injury
953   Injury to nerve roots and spinal plexus
954   Injury to other nerve(s) of trunk excluding shoulder and pelvic girdles
955   Injury to peripheral nerve(s) of shoulder girdle and upper limb
956   Injury to peripheral nerve(s) of pelvic girdle and lower limb
957   Injury to other and unspecified nerves

Certain traumatic complications and unspecified injuries (958-959)

958   Certain early complications of trauma
959   Injury, other and unspecified

Poisoning by drugs, medicinal and biological substances (960-979)

960   Poisoning by antibiotics
961   Poisoning by other anti-infectives
962   Poisoning by hormones and synthetic substitutes
963   Poisoning by primarily systemic agents
964   Poisoning by agents primarily affecting blood constituents
965   Poisoning by analgesics, antipyretics, and antirheumatics
966   Poisoning by anticonvulsants and anti-Parkinsonism drugs
967   Poisoning by sedatives and hypnotics
968   Poisoning by other central nervous system depressants and anesthetics
969   Poisoning by psychotropic agents
970   Poisoning by central nervous system stimulants

17. INJURY AND POISONING *continued*

971 Poisoning by drugs primarily affecting the autonomic nervous system
972 Poisoning by agents primarily affecting the cardiovascular system
973 Poisoning by agents primarily affecting the gastrointestinal system
974 Poisoning by water, mineral, and uric acid metabolism drugs
975 Poisoning by agents primarily acting on the smooth and skeletal muscles and respiratory system
976 Poisoning by agents primarily affecting skin and mucous membrane, ophthalmological, otorhinolaryngological, and dental drugs
977 Poisoning by other and unspecified drugs and medicinals
978 Poisoning by bacterial vaccines
979 Poisoning by other vaccines and biological substances

Toxic effects of substances chiefly nonmedicinal as to source (980-989)

980 Toxic effect of alcohol
981 Toxic effect of petroleum products
982 Toxic effect of solvents other than petroleum-based
983 Toxic effect of corrosive aromatics, acids, and caustic alkalis
984 Toxic effect of lead and its compounds (including fumes)
985 Toxic effect of other metals
986 Toxic effect of carbon monoxide
987 Toxic effect of other gases, fumes, or vapors
988 Toxic effect of noxious substances eaten as food
989 Toxic effect of other substances, chiefly nonmedicinal as to source

Other and unspecified effects of external causes (990-995)

990 Effects of radiation, unspecified
991 Effects of reduced temperature
992 Effects of heat and light
993 Effects of air pressure
994 Effects of other external causes
995 Certain adverse effects, not elsewhere classified

Complications of surgical and medical care, not elsewhere classified (996-999)

996 Complications peculiar to certain specified procedures
997 Complications affecting specified body systems, not elsewhere classified
998 Other complications of procedures, not elsewhere classified
999 Complications of medical care, not elsewhere classified

SUPPLEMENTARY CLASSIFICATION OF FACTORS INFLUENCING HEALTH STATUS AND CONTACT WITH HEALTH SERVICES

Persons with potential health hazards related to communicable diseases (V01-V06)

V01 Contact with or exposure to communicable diseases
V02 Carrier or suspected carrier of infectious diseases
V03 Need for prophylactic vaccination and inoculation against bacterial diseases
V04 Need for prophylactic vaccination and inoculation against certain viral diseases
V05 Need for other prophylactic vaccination and inoculation against single diseases
V06 Need for prophylactic vaccination and inoculation against combinations of diseases

Persons with need for isolation, other potential health hazards and prophylactic measures (V07-V09)

V07 Need for isolation and other prophylactic measures
V08 Asymptomatic human immunodeficiency virus (HIV) infection status
V09 Infection with drug-resistant microorganisms

Persons with potential health hazards related to personal and family history (V10-V19)

V10 Personal history of malignant neoplasm
V11 Personal history of mental disorder
V12 Personal history of certain other diseases
V13 Personal history of other diseases
V14 Personal history of allergy to medicinal agents
V15 Other personal history presenting hazards to health
V16 Family history of malignant neoplasm
V17 Family history of certain chronic disabling diseases
V18 Family history of certain other specific conditions
V19 Family history of other conditions

Persons encountering health services in circumstances related to reproduction and development (V20-V29)

V20 Health supervision of infant or child
V21 Constitutional states in development

SUPPLEMENTARY CLASSIFICATION...HEALTH STATUS/HEALTH SERVICES *continued*

V22   Normal pregnancy
V23   Supervision of high-risk pregnancy
V24   Postpartum care and examination
V25   Encounter for contraceptive management
V26   Procreative management
V27   Outcome of delivery
V28   Encounter for antenatal screening of mother
V29   Observation and evaluation of newborns and infants for suspected condition not found

Liveborn infants according to type of birth (V30-V39)

V30   Single liveborn
V31   Twin, mate liveborn
V32   Twin, mate stillborn
V33   Twin, unspecified
V34   Other multiple, mates all liveborn
V35   Other multiple, mates all stillborn
V36   Other multiple, mates live- and stillborn
V37   Other multiple, unspecified
V39   Unspecified

Persons with a condition influencing their health status (V40-V49)

V40   Mental and behavioral problems
V41   Problems with special senses and other special functions
V42   Organ or tissue replaced by transplant
V43   Organ or tissue replaced by other means
V44   Artificial opening status
V45   Other postprocedural states
V46   Other dependence on machines and devices
V47   Other problems with internal organs
V48   Problems with head, neck, and trunk
V49   Other conditions influencing health status

Persons encountering health services for specific procedures and aftercare (V50-V59)

V50   Elective surgery for purposes other than remedying health states
V51   Aftercare involving the use of plastic surgery
V52   Fitting and adjustment of prosthetic device and implant
V53   Fitting and adjustment of other device
V54   Other orthopedic aftercare
V55   Attention to artificial openings
V56   Encounter for dialysis and dialysis catheter care
V57   Care involving use of rehabilitation procedures
V58   Encounter for other and unspecified procedures and aftercare
V59   Donors

Persons encountering health services in other circumstances (V60-V69)

V60   Housing, household, and economic circumstances
V61   Other family circumstances
V62   Other psychosocial circumstances
V63   Unavailability of other medical facilities for care
V64   Persons encountering health services for specific procedures, not carried out
V65   Other persons seeking consultation
V66   Convalescence and palliative care
V67   Follow-up examination
V68   Encounters for administrative purposes
V69   Problems related to lifestyle

Persons without reported diagnosis encountered during examination and investigation of individuals and populations (V70-V86)

V70   General medical examination
V71   Observation and evaluation for suspected conditions not found
V72   Special investigations and examinations
V73   Special screening examination for viral and chlamydial diseases
V74   Special screening examination for bacterial and spirochetal diseases
V75   Special screening examination for other infectious diseases
V76   Special screening for malignant neoplasms
V77   Special screening for endocrine, nutritional, metabolic, and immunity disorders
V78   Special screening for disorders of blood and blood-forming organs

SUPPLEMENTARY CLASSIFICATION...HEALTH STATUS/HEALTH SERVICES *continued*

  V79 Special screening for mental disorders and developmental handicaps
  V80 Special screening for neurological, eye, and ear diseases
  V81 Special screening for cardiovascular, respiratory, and genitourinary diseases
  V82 Special screening for other conditions
  V83 Genetic carrier status
  V84 Genetic susceptibility to disease
  V85 Body mass index
  V86 Estrogen receptor status
  V87 Other specified personal exposures and history presenting hazards to health
  V88 Acquired absence of other organs and tissue
  V89 Other suspected conditions not found

SUPPLEMENTARY CLASSIFICATION OF EXTERNAL CAUSES OF INJURY AND POISONING

External cause status (E000)

  E000 External cause status

Activity (E001-E030)

  E001 Activities involving walking and running
  E002 Activities involving water and water craft
  E003 Activities involving ice and snow
  E004 Activities involving climbing, rappelling and jumping off
  E005 Activities involving dancing and other rhythmic movement
  E006 Activities involving other sports and athletics played individually
  E007 Activities involving other sports and athletics played as a team or group
  E008 Activities involving other specified sports and athletics
  E009 Activities involving other cardiorespiratory exercise
  E010 Activities involving other muscle strengthening exercises
  E011 Activities involving computer technology and electronic devices
  E012 Activities involving arts and handcrafts
  E013 Activities involving personal hygiene and household maintenance
  E014 Activities involving person providing caregiving
  E015 Activities involving food preparation, cooking and grilling
  E016 Activities involving property and land maintenance, building and construction
  E017 Activities involving roller coasters and other types of external motion
  E018 Activities involving playing musical instruments
  E019 Activities involving animal care
  E029 Other activity
  E030 Unspecified activity

Railway accidents (E800-E807)

  E800 Railway accident involving collision with rolling stock
  E801 Railway accident involving collision with other object
  E802 Railway accident involving derailment without antecedent collision
  E803 Railway accident involving explosion, fire, or burning
  E804 Fall in, on, or from railway train
  E805 Hit by rolling stock
  E806 Other specified railway accident
  E807 Railway accident of unspecified nature

Motor vehicle traffic accidents (E810-E819)

  E810 Motor vehicle traffic accident involving collision with train
  E811 Motor vehicle traffic accident involving re-entrant collision with another motor vehicle
  E812 Other motor vehicle traffic accident involving collision with another motor vehicle
  E813 Motor vehicle traffic accident involving collision with other vehicle
  E814 Motor vehicle traffic accident involving collision with pedestrian
  E815 Other motor vehicle traffic accident involving collision on the highway
  E816 Motor vehicle traffic accident due to loss of control, without collision on the highway
  E817 Noncollision motor vehicle traffic accident while boarding or alighting
  E818 Other noncollision motor vehicle traffic accident
  E819 Motor vehicle traffic accident of unspecified nature

Motor vehicle nontraffic accidents (E820-E825)

  E820 Nontraffic accident involving motor-driven snow vehicle
  E821 Nontraffic accident involving other off-road motor vehicle
  E822 Other motor vehicle nontraffic accident involving collision with moving object
  E823 Other motor vehicle nontraffic accident involving collision with stationary object

SUPPLEMENTARY CLASSIFICATION...INJURY AND POISONING *continued*

E824 Other motor vehicle nontraffic accident while boarding and alighting

E825 Other motor vehicle nontraffic accident of other and unspecified nature

Other road vehicle accidents (E826-E829)

E826 Pedal cycle accident

E827 Animal-drawn vehicle accident

E828 Accident involving animal being ridden

E829 Other road vehicle accidents

Water transport accidents (E830-E838)

E830 Accident to watercraft causing submersion

E831 Accident to watercraft causing other injury

E832 Other accidental submersion or drowning in water transport accident

E833 Fall on stairs or ladders in water transport

E834 Other fall from one level to another in water transport

E835 Other and unspecified fall in water transport

E836 Machinery accident in water transport

E837 Explosion, fire, or burning in watercraft

E838 Other and unspecified water transport accident

Air and space transport accidents (E840-E845)

E840 Accident to powered aircraft at takeoff or landing

E841 Accident to powered aircraft, other and unspecified

E842 Accident to unpowered aircraft

E843 Fall in, on, or from aircraft

E844 Other specified air transport accidents

E845 Accident involving spacecraft

Vehicle accidents, not elsewhere classifiable (E846-E849)

E846 Accidents involving powered vehicles used solely within the buildings and premises of an industrial or commercial establishment

E847 Accidents involving cable cars not running on rails

E848 Accidents involving other vehicles, not elsewhere classifiable

E849 Place of occurrence

Accidental poisoning by drugs, medicinal substances, and biologicals (E850-E858)

E850 Accidental poisoning by analgesics, antipyretics, and antirheumatics

E851 Accidental poisoning by barbiturates

E852 Accidental poisoning by other sedatives and hypnotics

E853 Accidental poisoning by tranquilizers

E854 Accidental poisoning by other psychotropic agents

E855 Accidental poisoning by other drugs acting on central and autonomic nervous systems

E856 Accidental poisoning by antibiotics

E857 Accidental poisoning by other anti-infectives

E858 Accidental poisoning by other drugs

Accidental poisoning by other solid and liquid substances, gases, and vapors (E860-E869)

E860 Accidental poisoning by alcohol, not elsewhere classified

E861 Accidental poisoning by cleansing and polishing agents, disinfectants, paints, and varnishes

E862 Accidental poisoning by petroleum products, other solvents and their vapors, not elsewhere classified

E863 Accidental poisoning by agricultural and horticultural chemical and pharmaceutical preparations other than plant foods and fertilizers

E864 Accidental poisoning by corrosives and caustics, not elsewhere classified

E865 Accidental poisoning from poisonous foodstuffs and poisonous plants

E866 Accidental poisoning by other and unspecified solid and liquid substances

E867 Accidental poisoning by gas distributed by pipeline

E868 Accidental poisoning by other utility gas and other carbon monoxide

E869 Accidental poisoning by other gases and vapors

Misadventures to patients during surgical and medical care (E870-E876)

E870 Accidental cut, puncture, perforation, or hemorrhage during medical care

E871 Foreign object left in body during procedure

E872 Failure of sterile precautions during procedure

E873 Failure in dosage

E874 Mechanical failure of instrument or apparatus during procedure

E875 Contaminated or infected blood, other fluid, drug, or biological substance

E876 Other and unspecified misadventures during medical care

SUPPLEMENTARY CLASSIFICATION...INJURY AND POISONING *continued*

Surgical and medical procedures as the cause of abnormal reaction of patient or later complication, without mention of misadventure at the time of procedure (E878-E879)

E878 Surgical operation and other surgical procedures as the cause of abnormal reaction of patient, or of later complication, without mention of misadventure at the time of operation

E879 Other procedures, without mention of misadventure at the time of procedure, as the cause of abnormal reaction of patient, or of later complication

Accidental falls (E880-E888)

E880 Fall on or from stairs or steps

E881 Fall on or from ladders or scaffolding

E882 Fall from or out of building or other structure

E883 Fall into hole or other opening in surface

E884 Other fall from one level to another

E885 Fall on same level from slipping, tripping, or stumbling

E886 Fall on same level from collision, pushing or shoving, by or with other person

E887 Fracture, cause unspecified

E888 Other and unspecified fall

Accidents caused by fire and flames (E890-E899)

E890 Conflagration in private dwelling

E891 Conflagration in other and unspecified building or structure

E892 Conflagration not in building or structure

E893 Accident caused by ignition of clothing

E894 Ignition of highly inflammable material

E895 Accident caused by controlled fire in private dwelling

E896 Accident caused by controlled fire in other and unspecified building or structure

E897 Accident caused by controlled fire not in building or structure

E898 Accident caused by other specified fire and flames

E899 Accident caused by unspecified fire

Accidents due to natural and environmental factors (E900-E909)

E900 Excessive heat

E901 Excessive cold

E902 High and low air pressure and changes in air pressure

E903 Travel and motion

E904 Hunger, thirst, exposure, and neglect

E905 Venomous animals and plants as the cause of poisoning and toxic reactions

E906 Other injury caused by animals

E907 Lightning

E908 Cataclysmic storms, and floods resulting from storms

E909 Cataclysmic earth surface movements and eruptions

Accidents caused by submersion, suffocation, and foreign bodies (E910-E915)

E910 Accidental drowning and submersion

E911 Inhalation and ingestion of food causing obstruction of respiratory tract or suffocation

E912 Inhalation and ingestion of other object causing obstruction of respiratory tract or suffocation

E913 Accidental mechanical suffocation

E914 Foreign body accidentally entering eye and adnexa

E915 Foreign body accidentally entering other orifice

Other accidents (E916-E928)

E916 Struck accidentally by falling object

E917 Striking against or struck accidentally by objects or persons

E918 Caught accidentally in or between objects

E919 Accidents caused by machinery

E920 Accidents caused by cutting and piercing instruments or objects

E921 Accident caused by explosion of pressure vessel

E922 Accident caused by firearm and air gun missile

E923 Accident caused by explosive material

E924 Accident caused by hot substance or object, caustic or corrosive material, and steam

E925 Accident caused by electric current

E926 Exposure to radiation

E927 Overexertion and strenuous and repetitive movements or loads

E928 Other and unspecified environmental and accidental causes

SUPPLEMENTARY CLASSIFICATION...INJURY AND POISONING *continued*

Late effects of accidental injury (E929)
E929 Late effects of accidental injury

Drugs, medicinal and biological substances causing adverse effects in therapeutic use (E930-E949)
E930 Antibiotics
E931 Other anti-infectives
E932 Hormones and synthetic substitutes
E933 Primarily systemic agents
E934 Agents primarily affecting blood constituents
E935 Analgesics, antipyretics, and antirheumatics
E936 Anticonvulsants and anti-Parkinsonism drugs
E937 Sedatives and hypnotics
E938 Other central nervous system depressants and anesthetics
E939 Psychotropic agents
E940 Central nervous system stimulants
E941 Drugs primarily affecting the autonomic nervous system
E942 Agents primarily affecting the cardiovascular system
E943 Agents primarily affecting gastrointestinal system
E944 Water, mineral, and uric acid metabolism drugs
E945 Agents primarily acting on the smooth and skeletal muscles and respiratory system
E946 Agents primarily affecting skin and mucous membrane, ophthalmological, otorhinolaryngological, and dental drugs
E947 Other and unspecified drugs and medicinal substances
E948 Bacterial vaccines
E949 Other vaccines and biological substances

Suicide and self-inflicted injury (E950-E959)
E950 Suicide and self-inflicted poisoning by solid or liquid substances
E951 Suicide and self-inflicted poisoning by gases in domestic use
E952 Suicide and self-inflicted poisoning by other gases and vapors
E953 Suicide and self-inflicted injury by hanging, strangulation, and suffocation
E954 Suicide and self-inflicted injury by submersion [drowning]
E955 Suicide and self-inflicted injury by firearms, air guns and explosives
E956 Suicide and self-inflicted injury by cutting and piercing instruments
E957 Suicide and self-inflicted injuries by jumping from high place
E958 Suicide and self-inflicted injury by other and unspecified means
E959 Late effects of self-inflicted injury

Homicide and injury purposely inflicted by other persons (E960-E969)
E960 Fight, brawl, and rape
E961 Assault by corrosive or caustic substance, except poisoning
E962 Assault by poisoning
E963 Assault by hanging and strangulation
E964 Assault by submersion [drowning]
E965 Assault by firearms and explosives
E966 Assault by cutting and piercing instrument
E967 Perpetrator of child and adult abuse
E968 Assault by other and unspecified means
E969 Late effects of injury purposely inflicted by other person

Legal intervention (E970-E978)
E970 Injury due to legal intervention by firearms
E971 Injury due to legal intervention by explosives
E972 Injury due to legal intervention by gas
E973 Injury due to legal intervention by blunt object
E974 Injury due to legal intervention by cutting and piercing instruments
E975 Injury due to legal intervention by other specified means
E976 Injury due to legal intervention by unspecified means
E977 Late effects of injuries due to legal intervention
E978 Legal execution
E979 Terrorism

Injury undetermined whether accidentally or purposely inflicted (E980-E989)
E980 Poisoning by solid or liquid substances, undetermined whether accidentally or purposely inflicted
E981 Poisoning by gases in domestic use, undetermined whether accidentally or purposely inflicted

APPENDIX E

SUPPLEMENTARY CLASSIFICATION...INJURY AND POISONING *continued*

E982 Poisoning by other gases, undetermined whether accidentally or purposely inflicted
E983 Hanging, strangulation, or suffocation, undetermined whether accidentally or purposely inflicted
E984 Submersion [drowning], undetermined whether accidentally or purposely inflicted
E985 Injury by firearms, air guns and explosives, undetermined whether accidentally or purposely inflicted
E986 Injury by cutting and piercing instruments, undetermined whether accidentally or purposely inflicted
E987 Falling from high place, undetermined whether accidentally or purposely inflicted
E988 Injury by other and unspecified means, undetermined whether accidentally or purposely inflicted
E989 Late effects of injury, undetermined whether accidentally or purposely inflicted

Injury resulting from operations of war (E990-E999)

E990 Injury due to war operations by fires and conflagrations
E991 Injury due to war operations by bullets and fragments
E992 Injury due to war operations by explosion of marine weapons
E993 Injury due to war operations by other explosion
E994 Injury due to war operations by destruction of aircraft
E995 Injury due to war operations by other and unspecified forms of conventional warfare
E996 Injury due to war operations by nuclear weapons
E997 Injury due to war operations by other forms of unconventional warfare
E998 Injury due to war operations but occurring after cessation of hostilities
E999 Late effects of injury due to war operations and terrorism

DISEASES: ALPHABETIC INDEX

VOLUME 2

A

AAT (alpha-1 antitrypsin) deficiency 273.4
AAV (disease) (illness) (infection)—*see* Human
immunodeficiency virus (disease) (illness)
(infection)
Abactio —*see* Abortion, induced
Abactus venter —*see* Abortion, induced
Abarognosis 781.99
Abasia (-astasia) 307.9
  atactica 781.3
  choreic 781.3
  hysterical 300.11
  paroxysmal trepidant 781.3
  spastic 781.3
  trembling 781.3
  trepidans 781.3
Abderhalden-Kaufmann-Lignac syndrome
  (cystinosis) 270.0
Abdomen, abdominal —*see also* condition
  accordion 306.4
  acute 789.0
  angina 557.1
  burst 868.00
  convulsive equivalent (*see also* Epilepsy) 345.5
  heart 746.87
  muscle deficiency syndrome 756.79
  obstipum 756.79
Abdominalgia 789.0
  periodic 277.31
Abduction contracture, hip or other joint —*see*
  Contraction, joint
Abercrombie's syndrome (amyloid
  degeneration) 277.39
Aberrant (congenital)—*see also* Malposition,
  congenital
  adrenal gland 759.1
  blood vessel NEC 747.60
    arteriovenous NEC 747.60
    cerebrovascular 747.81
    gastrointestinal 747.61
    lower limb 747.64
    renal 747.62
    spinal 747.82
    upper limb 747.63
  breast 757.6
  endocrine gland NEC 759.2
  gastrointestinal vessel (peripheral) 747.61
  hepatic duct 751.69
  lower limb vessel (peripheral) 747.64
  pancreas 751.7
  parathyroid gland 759.2
  peripheral vascular vessel NEC 747.60
  pituitary gland (pharyngeal) 759.2
  renal blood vessel 747.62
  sebaceous glands, mucous membrane, mouth
    750.26
  spinal vessel 747.82
  spleen 759.0
  testis (descent) 752.51
  thymus gland 759.2
  thyroid gland 759.2
  upper limb vessel (peripheral) 747.63
Aberratio
  lactis 757.6
  testis 752.51
Aberration —*see also* Anomaly
  chromosome—*see* Anomaly, chromosome(s)
  distantial 368.9

Aberration—*continued*
  mental (*see also* Disorder, mental,
    nonpsychotic) 300.9
Abetalipoproteinemia 272.5
Abionarce 780.79
Abiotrophy 799.89
Ablatio
  placentae—*see* Placenta, ablatio
  retinae (*see also* Detachment, retina) 361.9
Ablation
  pituitary (gland) (with hypofunction) 253.7
  placenta—*see* Placenta, ablatio
  uterus 621.8
Ablepharia, ablepharon, ablephary 743.62
Ablepsia —*see* Blindness
Ablepsy —*see* Blindness
Ablutomania 300.3
Abnormal, abnormality, abnormalities —*see*
    also Anomaly
  acid-base balance 276.4
    fetus or newborn—*see* Distress, fetal
  adaptation curve, dark 368.63
  alveolar ridge 525.9
  amnion 658.9
    affecting fetus or newborn 762.9
  anatomical relationship NEC 759.9
  apertures, congenital, diaphragm 756.6
  auditory perception NEC 388.40
  autosomes NEC 758.5
    13 758.1
    18 758.2
    21 or 22 758.0
    D₁ 758.1
    E₃ 758.2
    G 758.0
  ballistocardiogram 794.39
  basal metabolic rate (BMR) 794.7
  biosynthesis, testicular androgen 257.2
  blood level (of)
    cobalt 790.6
    copper 790.6
    iron 790.6
    lead 790.6
    lithium 790.6
    magnesium 790.6
    mineral 790.6
    zinc 790.6
  blood pressure
    elevated (without diagnosis of hypertension)
      796.2
    low (*see also* Hypotension) 458.9
      reading (incidental) (isolated) (nonspecific)
        796.3
  blood sugar 790.29
  bowel sounds 787.5
  breathing behavior—*see* Respiration
  caloric test 794.19
  cervix (acquired) NEC 622.9
    congenital 752.40
    in pregnancy or childbirth 654.6
      causing obstructed labor 660.2
        affecting fetus or newborn 763.1
  chemistry, blood NEC 790.6
  chest sounds 786.7
  chorion 658.9
    affecting fetus or newborn 762.9
  chromosomal NEC 758.89
    analysis, nonspecific result 795.2

Abnormal, abnormality—*continued*
  autosomes (*see also* Abnormal, autosomes
    NEC) 758.5
  fetal, (suspected) affecting management of
    pregnancy 655.1
  sex 758.81
  clinical findings NEC 796.4
  communication—*see* Fistula
  configuration of pupils 379.49
  coronary
    artery 746.85
    vein 746.9
  cortisol-binding globulin 255.8
  course, Eustachian tube 744.24
  creatinine clearance 794.4
  dentofacial NEC 524.9
    functional 524.50
    specified type NEC 524.89
  development, developmental NEC 759.9
    bone 756.9
    central nervous system 742.9
  direction, teeth 524.30
  Dynia (*see also* Defect, coagulation) 286.9
  Ebstein 746.2
  echocardiogram 793.2
  echoencephalogram 794.01
  echogram NEC—*see* Findings, abnormal,
    structure
  electrocardiogram (ECG) (EKG) 794.31
  electroencephalogram (EEG) 794.02
  electromyogram (EMG) 794.17
    ocular 794.14
  electro-oculogram (EOG) 794.12
  electroretinogram (ERG) 794.11
  erythrocytes 289.9
    congenital, with perinatal jaundice 282.9
      [774.0]
  Eustachian valve 746.9
  excitability under minor stress 301.9
  fat distribution 782.9
  feces 787.7
  fetal heart rate—*see* Distress, fetal
  fetus NEC
    affecting management of pregnancy—*see*
      Pregnancy, management affected by, fetal
    causing disproportion 653.7
      affecting fetus or newborn 763.1
      causing obstructed labor 660.1
        affecting fetus or newborn 763.1
  findings without manifest disease—*see*
    Findings, abnormal
  fluid
    amniotic 792.3
    cerebrospinal 792.0
    peritoneal 792.9
    pleural 792.9
    synovial 792.9
    vaginal 792.9
  forces of labor NEC 661.9
    affecting fetus or newborn 763.7
  form, teeth 520.2
  function studies
    auditory 794.15
    bladder 794.9
    brain 794.00
    cardiovascular 794.30
    endocrine NEC 794.6
    kidney 794.4
    liver 794.8
    nervous system
      central 794.00

Abnormal, abnormality—*continued*
    peripheral 794.19
    oculomotor 794.14
    pancreas 794.9
    placenta 794.9
    pulmonary 794.2
    retina 794.11
    special senses 794.19
    spleen 794.9
    thyroid 794.5
    vestibular 794.16
  gait 781.2
    hysterical 300.11
  gastrin secretion 251.5
  globulin
    cortisol-binding 255.8
    thyroid-binding 246.8
  glucagon secretion 251.4
  glucose 790.29
    in pregnancy, childbirth, or puerperium 648.8
      fetus or newborn 775.0
    non-fasting 790.29
  gravitational (G) forces or states 994.9
  hair NEC 704.2
  hard tissue formation in pulp 522.3
  head movement 781.0
  heart
    rate
      fetus, affecting liveborn infant
        before the onset of labor 763.81
        during labor 763.82
        unspecified as to time of onset 763.83
      intrauterine
        before the onset of labor 763.81
        during labor 763.82
        unspecified as to time of onset 763.83
      newborn
        before the onset of labor 763.81
        during labor 763.82
        unspecified as to time of onset 763.83
    shadow 793.2
    sounds NEC 785.3
  hemoglobin (*see also* Disease, hemoglobin)
    282.7
    trait—*see* Trait, hemoglobin, abnormal
  hemorrhage, uterus—*see* Hemorrhage, uterus
  histology NEC 795.4
  increase in
    appetite 783.6
    development 783.9
  involuntary movement 781.0
  jaw closure 524.51
  karyotype 795.2
  knee jerk 796.1
  labor NEC 661.9
    affecting fetus or newborn 763.7
  laboratory findings—*see* Findings, abnormal
  length, organ or site, congenital—*see* Distortion
  liver function test 790.6
  loss of height 781.91
  loss of weight 783.21
  lung shadow 793.1
  mammogram 793.80
    calcification 793.89
    calculus 793.89
    microcalcification 793.81
  Mantoux test 795.5
  membranes (fetal)
    affecting fetus or newborn 762.9
    complicating pregnancy 658.8
  menstruation—*see* Menstruation

Abnormal, abnormality —*continued*
metabolism (*see also* condition) 783.9
movement 781.0
  disorder, NEC 333.90
    sleep related, unspecified 780.58
    specified, NEC 333.99
  head 781.0
  involuntary 781.0
  specified type NEC 333.99
muscle contraction, localized 728.85
myoglobin (Aberdeen) (Annapolis) 289.9
narrowness, eyelid 743.62
optokinetic response 379.57
organs or tissues of pelvis NEC
  in pregnancy or childbirth 654.9
    affecting fetus or newborn 763.89
    causing obstructed labor 660.2
      affecting fetus or newborn 763.1
origin—*see* Malposition, congenital
palmar creases 757.2
Papanicolaou (smear)
  anus 796.70
    with
      atypical squamous cells
        cannot exclude high grade squamous
          intraepithelial lesion (ASC-H)
          796.72
        of undetermined significance (ASC-US)
          796.71
      cytologic evidence of malignancy 796.76
      high grade squamous intraepithelial lesion
        (HGSIL) 796.74
      low grade squamous intraepithelial lesion
        (LGSIL) 796.73
    glandular 796.70
    specified finding NEC 796.79
  cervix 795.00
    with
      atypical squamous cell
        cannot exclude high grade squamous
          intraepithelial lesion (ASC-H)
          795.02
        of undetermined significance (ASC-US)
          795.01
      cytologic evidence of malignancy 795.06
      favor benign (ASCUS favor benign)
        795.01
      favor dysplasia (ASCUS favor dysplasia)
        795.02
      high grade squamous intraepithelial lesion
        (HGSIL) 795.04
      low grade squamous intraepithelial lesion
        (LGSIL) 795.03
    nonspecific finding NEC 795.09
    other site 796.9
  vagina 795.10
    with
      atypical squamous cells
        cannot exclude high grade squamous
          intraepithelial lesion (ASC-H)
          795.12
        of undetermined significance (ASC-US)
          795.11
      cytologic evidence of malignancy 795.16
      high grade squamous intraepithelial lesion
        (HGSIL) 795.14
      low grade squamous intraepithelial lesion
        (LGSIL) 795.13
    glandular 795.10
    specified finding NEC 795.19

Abnormal, abnormality —*continued*
parturition
  affecting fetus or newborn 763.9
  mother—*see* Delivery, complicated
pelvis (bony)—*see* Deformity, pelvis
percussion, chest 786.7
periods (grossly) (*see also* Menstruation) 626.9
phonocardiogram 794.39
placenta—*see* Placenta, abnormal
plantar reflex 796.1
plasma protein—*see* Deficiency, plasma, protein
pleural folds 748.8
position—*see also* Malposition
  gravid uterus 654.4
    causing obstructed labor 660.2
      affecting fetus or newborn 763.1
posture NEC 781.92
presentation (fetus)—*see* Presentation, fetus,
  abnormal
product of conception NEC 631
puberty—*see* Puberty
pulmonary
  artery 747.3
  function, newborn 770.89
  test results 794.2
  ventilation, newborn 770.89
    hyperventilation 786.01
pulsations in neck 785.1
pupil reflexes 379.40
quality of milk 676.8
radiological examination 793.99
  abdomen NEC 793.6
  biliary tract 793.3
  breast 793.89
    mammogram NOS 793.80
    mammographic
      calcification 793.89
      calculus 793.89
      microcalcification 793.81
  gastrointestinal tract 793.4
  genitourinary organs 793.5
  head 793.0
  image test inconclusive due to excess body fat
    793.91
  intrathoracic organ NEC 793.2
  lung (field) 793.1
  musculoskeletal system 793.7
  retroperitoneum 793.6
  skin and subcutaneous tissue 793.99
  skull 793.0
red blood cells 790.09
  morphology 790.09
  volume 790.09
reflex NEC 796.1
renal function test 794.4
respiration signs—*see* Respiration
response to nerve stimulation 794.10
retinal correspondence 368.34
rhythm, heart—*see also* Arrhythmia fetus—*see*
  Distress, fetal
saliva 792.4
scan
  brain 794.09
  kidney 794.4
  liver 794.8
  lung 794.2
  thyroid 794.5
secretion
  gastrin 251.5
  glucagon 251.4
semen 792.2

Abnormal, abnormality —*continued*
serum level (of)
acid phosphatase 790.5
alkaline phosphatase 790.5
amylase 790.5
enzymes NEC 790.5
lipase 790.5
shape
cornea 743.41
gallbladder 751.69
gravid uterus 654.4
affecting fetus or newborn 763.89
causing obstructed labor 660.2
affecting fetus or newborn 763.1
head (*see also* Anomaly, skull) 756.0
organ or site, congenital NEC—*see* Distortion
sinus venosus 747.40
size
fetus, complicating delivery 653.5
causing obstructed labor 660.1
gallbladder 751.69
head (*see also* Anomaly, skull) 756.0
organ or site, congenital NEC—*see* Distortion
teeth 520.2
skin and appendages, congenital NEC 757.9
soft parts of pelvis—*see* Abnormal, organs or
tissues of pelvis
spermatozoa 792.2
sputum (amount) (color) (excessive) (odor)
(purulent) 786.4
stool NEC 787.7
bloody 578.1
occult 792.1
bulky 787.7
color (dark) (light) 792.1
content (fat) (mucus) (pus) 792.1
occult blood 792.1
synchondrosis 756.9
test results without manifest disease—*see*
Findings, abnormal
thebesian valve 746.9
thermography—*see* Findings, abnormal,
structure
threshold, cones or rods (eye) 368.63
thyroid-binding globulin 246.8
thyroid product 246.8
toxicology (findings) NEC 796.0
tracheal cartilage (congenital) 748.3
transport protein 273.8
ultrasound results—*see* Findings, abnormal,
structure
umbilical cord
affecting fetus or newborn 762.6
complicating delivery 663.9
specified NEC 663.8
union
cricoid cartilage and thyroid cartilage 748.3
larynx and trachea 748.3
thyroid cartilage and hyoid bone 748.3
urination NEC 788.69
psychogenic 306.53
stream
intermittent 788.61
slowing 788.62
splitting 788.61
weak 788.62
urgency 788.63
urine (constituents) NEC 791.9

Abnormal, abnormality —*continued*
uterine hemorrhage (*see also* Hemorrhage,
uterus) 626.9
climacteric 627.0
postmenopausal 627.1
vagina (acquired) (congenital)
in pregnancy or childbirth 654.7
affecting fetus or newborn 763.89
causing obstructed labor 660.2
affecting fetus or newborn 763.1
vascular sounds 785.9
vectorcardiogram 794.39
visually evoked potential (VEP) 794.13
vulva (acquired) (congenital)
in pregnancy or childbirth 654.8
affecting fetus or newborn 763.89
causing obstructed labor 660.2
affecting fetus or newborn 763.1
weight
gain 783.1
of pregnancy 646.1
with hypertension—*see* Toxemia, of
pregnancy
loss 783.21
x-ray examination—*see* Abnormal, radiological
examination
Abnormally formed uterus —*see* Anomaly,
uterus
Abnormity (any organ or part)—*see* Anomaly
ABO
hemolytic disease 773.1
incompatibility reaction 999.6
Abocclusion 524.20
Abolition, language 784.69
Aborter, habitual or recurrent NEC
without current pregnancy 629.81
current abortion (*see also* Abortion,
spontaneous) 634.9
affecting fetus or newborn 761.8
observation in current pregnancy 646.3
Abortion (complete) (incomplete) (inevitable)
(with retained products of conception) 637.9

> Note—Use the following fifth-digit
> subclassification with categories 634-637:
>
> 0   unspecifhed
> 1   incomplete
> 2   complete

with
complication(s) (any) following previous
abortion—*see* category 639
damage to pelvic organ (laceration) (rupture)
(tear) 637.2
embolism (air) (amniotic fluid) (blood clot)
(pulmonary) (pyemic) (septic) (soap)
637.6
genital tract and pelvic infection 637.0
hemorrhage, delayed or excessive 637.1
metabolic disorder 637.4
renal failure (acute) 637.3
sepsis (genital tract) (pelvic organ) 637.0
urinary tract 637.7
shock (postoperative) (septic) 637.5
specified complication NEC 637.7
toxemia 637.3
unspecified complication(s) 637.8
urinary tract infection 637.7
accidental—*see* Abortion, spontaneous
artificial—*see* Abortion, induced
attempted (failed)—*see* Abortion, failed

Abortion—*continued*
  criminal—*see* Abortion, illegal
  early—*see* Abortion, spontaneous
  elective—*see* Abortion, legal
  failed (legal) 638.9
    with
      damage to pelvic organ (laceration) (rupture)
        (tear) 638.2
      embolism (air) (amniotic fluid) (blood clot)
        (pulmonary) (pyemic) (septic) (soap)
        638.6
      genital tract and pelvic infection 638.0
      hemorrhage, delayed or excessive 638.1
      metabolic disorder 638.4
      renal failure (acute) 638.3
      sepsis (genital tract) (pelvic organ) 638.0
        urinary tract 638.7
      shock (postoperative) (septic) 638.5
      specified complication NEC 638.7
      toxemia 638.3
      unspecified complication(s) 638.8
      urinary tract infection 638.7
  fetal indication—*see* Abortion, legal
  fetus 779.6
  following threatened abortion—*see* Abortion, by
    type
  habitual or recurrent (care during pregnancy)
    646.3
    with current abortion (*see also* Abortion,
      spontaneous) 634.9
      affecting fetus or newborn 761.8
    without current pregnancy 629.81
  homicidal—*see* Abortion, illegal
  illegal 636.9
    with
      damage to pelvic organ (laceration) (rupture)
        (tear) 636.2
      embolism (air) (amniotic fluid) (blood clot)
        (pulmonary) (pyemic) (septic) (soap)
        636.6
      genital tract and pelvic infection 636.0
      hemorrhage, delayed or excessive 636.1
      metabolic disorder 636.4
      renal failure 636.3
      sepsis (genital tract) (pelvic organ) 636.0
        urinary tract 636.7
      shock (postoperative) (septic) 636.5
      specified complication NEC 636.7
      toxemia 636.3
      unspecified complication(s) 636.8
      urinary tract infection 636.7
    fetus 779.6
  induced 637.9
    illegal—*see* Abortion, illegal
    legal indications—*see* Abortion, legal
    medical indications—*see* Abortion, legal
    therapeutic—*see* Abortion, legal
  late—*see* Abortion, spontaneous
  legal (legal indication) (medical indication)
    (under medical supervision) 635.9
    with
      damage to pelvic organ (laceration) (rupture)
        (tear) 635.2
      embolism (air) (amniotic fluid) (blood clot)
        (pulmonary) (pyemic) (septic) (soap) 635.6
      genital tract and pelvic infection 635.0
      hemorrhage, delayed or excessive 635.1
      metabolic disorder 635.4
      renal failure (acute) 635.3
      sepsis (genital tract) (pelvic organ) 635.0
        urinary tract 635.7

Abortion—*continued*
    shock (postoperative) (septic) 635.5
    specified complication NEC 635.7
    toxemia 635.3
    unspecified complication(s) 635.8
    urinary tract infection 635.7
  fetus 779.6
  medical indication—*see* Abortion, legal
  mental hygiene problem—*see* Abortion, legal
  missed 632
  operative—*see* Abortion, legal
  psychiatric indication—*see* Abortion, legal
  recurrent—*see* Abortion, spontaneous
  self-induced—*see* Abortion, illegal
  septic—*see* Abortion, by type, with sepsis
  spontaneous 634.9
    with
      damage to pelvic organ (laceration) (rupture)
        (tear) 634.2
      embolism (air) (amniotic fluid) (blood clot)
        (pulmonary) (pyemic) (septic) (soap)
        634.6
      genital tract and pelvic infection 634.0
      hemorrhage, delayed or excessive 634.1
      metabolic disorder 634.4
      renal failure 634.3
      sepsis (genital tract) (pelvic organ) 634.0
        urinary tract 634.7
      shock (postoperative) (septic) 634.5
      specified complication NEC 634.7
      toxemia 634.3
      unspecified complication(s) 634.8
      urinary tract infection 634.7
    fetus 761.8
    threatened 640.0
      affecting fetus or newborn 762.1
  surgical—*see* Abortion, legal
  therapeutic—*see* Abortion, legal
  threatened 640.0
    affecting fetus or newborn 762.1
  tubal—*see* Pregnancy, tubal
  voluntary—*see* Abortion, legal
Abortus fever 023.9
Aboulomania 301.6
Abrachia 755.20
Abrachiatism 755.20
Abrachiocephalia 759.89
Abrachiocephalus 759.89
Abrami's disease (acquired hemolytic jaundice)
    283.9
Abramov-Fiedler myocarditis (acute isolated
    myocarditis) 422.91
Abrasion —*see also* Injury, superficial, by site
  cornea 918.1
  dental 521.20
    extending into
      dentine 521.22
      pulp 521.23
    generalized 521.25
    limited to enamel 521.21
    localized 521.24
  teeth, tooth (dentifrice) (habitual) (hard tissues)
    (occupational) (ritual) (traditional) (wedge
    defect) (*see also* Abrasion, dental) 521.20
Abrikossov's tumor (M9580/0)—*see also*
    Neoplasm, connective tissue, benign
  malignant (M9580/3)—*see* Neoplasm,
    connective tissue, malignant
Abrism 988.8
Abruption, placenta —*see* Placenta, abruptio
Abruptio placentae —*see* Placenta, abruptio

Abscess (acute) (chronic) (infectional)
(lymphangitic) (metastatic) (multiple)
(pyogenic) (septic) (with lymphangitis) (*see
also* Cellulitis) 682.9
  abdomen, abdominal
    cavity 567.22
    wall 682.2
  abdominopelvic 567.22
  accessory sinus (chronic) (*see also* Sinusitis)
    473.9
  adrenal (capsule) (gland) 255.8
  alveolar 522.5
    with sinus 522.7
  amebic 006.3
    bladder 006.8
    brain (with liver or lung abscess) 006.5
    liver (without mention of brain or lung
      abscess) 006.3
      with
        brain abscess (and lung abscess) 006.5
        lung abscess 006.4
    lung (with liver abscess) 006.4
      with brain abscess 006.5
    seminal vesicle 006.8
    specified site NEC 006.8
    spleen 006.8
  anaerobic 040.0
  ankle 682.6
  anorectal 566
  antecubital space 682.3
  antrum (chronic) (Highmore) (*see also* Sinusitis,
    maxillary) 473.0
  anus 566
  apical (tooth) 522.5
    with sinus (alveolar) 522.7
  appendix 540.1
  areola (acute) (chronic) (nonpuerperal) 611.0
    puerperal, postpartum 675.1
  arm (any part, above wrist) 682.3
  artery (wall) 447.2
  atheromatous 447.2
  auditory canal (external) 380.10
  auricle (ear) (staphylococcal) (streptococcal)
    380.10
  axilla, axillary (region) 682.3
    lymph gland or node 683
  back (any part) 682.2
  Bartholin's gland 616.3
    with
      abortion—*see* Abortion, by type, with sepsis
      ectopic pregnancy (*see also* categories
        633.0-633.9) 639.0
      molar pregnancy (*see also* categories
        630-632) 639.0
    complicating pregnancy or puerperium 646.6
    following
      abortion 639.0
      ectopic or molar pregnancy 639.0
  bartholinian 616.3
  Bezold's 383.01
  bile, biliary, duct or tract (*see also* Cholecystitis)
    576.8
  bilharziasis 120.1
  bladder (wall) 595.89
    amebic 006.8
  bone (subperiosteal) (*see also* Osteomyelitis)
    730.0
    accessory sinus (chronic) (*see also* Sinusitis)
      473.9
    acute 730.0
    chronic or old 730.1

Abscess—*continued*
  jaw (lower) (upper) 526.4
  mastoid—*see* Mastoiditis, acute
  petrous (*see also* Petrositis) 383.20
  spinal (tuberculous) (*see also* Tuberculosis)
    015.0 *[730.88]*
    nontuberculous 730.08
  bowel 569.5
  brain (any part) 324.0
    amebic (with liver or lung abscess) 006.5
    cystic 324.0
    late effect—*see* category 326
    otogenic 324.0
    tuberculous (*see also* Tuberculosis) 013.3
  breast (acute) (chronic) (nonpuerperal) 611.0
    newborn 771.5
    puerperal, postpartum 675.1
    tuberculous (*see also* Tuberculosis) 017.9
  broad ligament (chronic) (*see also* Disease,
    pelvis, inflammatory) 614.4
    acute 614.3
  Brodie's (chronic) (localized) (*see also*
    Osteomyelitis) 730.1
  bronchus 519.19
  buccal cavity 528.3
  bulbourethral gland 597.0
  bursa 727.89
    pharyngeal 478.29
  buttock 682.5
  canaliculus, breast 611.0
  canthus 372.20
  cartilage 733.99
  cecum 569.5
    with appendicitis 540.1
  cerebellum, cerebellar 324.0
    late effect—*see* category 326
  cerebral (embolic) 324.0
    late effect—*see* category 326
  cervical (neck region) 682.1
    lymph gland or node 683
    stump (*see also* Cervicitis) 616.0
  cervix (stump) (uteri) (*see also* Cervicitis) 616.0
  cheek, external 682.0
    inner 528.3
  chest 510.9
    with fistula 510.0
    wall 682.2
  chin 682.0
  choroid 363.00
  ciliary body 364.3
  circumtonsillar 475
  cold (tuberculous)—*see also* Tuberculosis,
    abscess
    articular—*see* Tuberculosis, joint
  colon (wall) 569.5
  colostomy or enterostomy 569.6
  conjunctiva 372.00
  connective tissue NEC 682.9
  cornea 370.55
    with ulcer 370.00
  corpus
    cavernosum 607.2
    luteum (*see also* Salpingo-oophoritis) 614.2
  Cowper's gland 597.0
  cranium 324.0
  cul-de-sac (Douglas') (posterior) (*see also*
    Disease, pelvis, inflammatory) 614.4
    acute 614.3
  dental 522.5
    with sinus (alveolar) 522.7
  dentoalveolar 522.5

Abscess—*continued*
  with sinus (alveolar) 522.7
  diaphragm, diaphragmatic 567.22
  digit NEC 681.9
  Douglas' cul-de-sac or pouch (*see also* Disease,
    pelvis, inflammatory) 614.4
    acute 614.3
  Dubois' 090.5
  ductless gland 259.8
  ear
    acute 382.00
    external 380.10
    inner 386.30
    middle—*see* Otitis media
  elbow 682.3
  endamebic—*see* Abscess, amebic
  entamebic—*see* Abscess, amebic
  enterostomy 569.6
  epididymis 604.0
  epidural 324.9
    brain 324.0
    late effect—*see* category 326
    spinal cord 324.1
  epiglottis 478.79
  epiploon, epiploic 567.22
  erysipelatous (*see also* Erysipelas) 035
  esophagostomy 530.86
  esophagus 530.19
  ethmoid (bone) (chronic) (sinus) (*see also*
    Sinusitis, ethmoidal) 473.2
  external auditory canal 380.10
  extradural 324.9
    brain 324.0
    late effect—*see* category 326
    spinal cord 324.1
  extraperitoneal—*see* Abscess, peritoneum
  eye 360.00
  eyelid 373.13
  face (any part, except eye) 682.0
  fallopian tube (*see also* Salpingo-oophoritis)
    614.2
  fascia 728.89
  fauces 478.29
  fecal 569.5
  femoral (region) 682.6
  filaria, filarial (*see also* Infestation, filarial)
    125.9
  finger (any) (intrathecal) (periosteal)
    (subcutaneous) (subcuticular) 681.00
  fistulous NEC 682.9
  flank 682.2
  foot (except toe) 682.7
  forearm 682.3
  forehead 682.0
  frontal (sinus) (chronic) (*see also* Sinusitis,
    frontal) 473.1
  gallbladder (*see also* Cholecystitis, acute) 575.0
  gastric 535.0
  genital organ or tract NEC
    female 616.9
      with
        abortion—*see* Abortion, by type, with
          sepsis
        ectopic pregnancy (*see also* categories
          633.0-633.9) 639.0
        molar pregnancy (*see also* categories
          630-632) 639.0
      following
        abortion 639.0
        ectopic or molar pregnancy 639.0
      puerperal, postpartum, childbirth 670.8

Abscess—*continued*
  male 608.4
  genitourinary system, tuberculous (*see also*
    Tuberculosis) 016.9
  gingival 523.30
  gland, glandular (lymph) (acute) NEC 683
  glottis 478.79
  gluteal (region) 682.5
  gonorrheal NEC (*see also* Gonococcus) 098.0
  groin 682.2
  gum 523.30
  hand (except finger or thumb) 682.4
  head (except face) 682.8
  heart 429.89
  heel 682.7
  helminthic (*see also* Infestation, by specific
    parasite) 128.9
  hepatic 572.0
    amebic (*see also* Abscess, liver, amebic) 006.3
    duct 576.8
  hip 682.6
    tuberculous (active) (*see also* Tuberculosis)
      015.1
  ileocecal 540.1
  ileostomy (bud) 569.6
  iliac (region) 682.2
    fossa 540.1
  iliopsoas 567.31
    tuberculous (see also Tuberculosis) 015.0
      [730.88]
  infraclavicular (fossa) 682.3
  inguinal (region) 682.2
    lymph gland or node 683
  intersphincteric (anus) 566
  intestine, intestinal 569.5
    rectal 566
  intra-abdominal (*see also* Abscess, peritoneum)
    567.22
    postoperative 998.59
  intracranial 324.0
    late effect—*see* category 326
  intramammary—*see* Abscess, breast
  intramastoid (*see also* Mastoiditis, acute) 383.00
  intraorbital 376.01
  intraperitoneal 567.22
  intraspinal 324.1
    late effect—*see* category 326
  intratonsillar 475
  iris 364.3
  ischiorectal 566
  jaw (bone) (lower) (upper) 526.4
    skin 682.0
  joint (*see also* Arthritis, pyogenic) 711.0
    vertebral (tuberculous) (*see also* Tuberculosis)
      015.0 *[730.88]*
      nontuberculous 724.8
  kidney 590.2
    with
      abortion—*see* Abortion, by type, with
        urinary tract infection
      calculus 592.0
      ectopic pregnancy (*see also* categories
        633.0-633.9) 639.8
      molar pregnancy (*see also* categories
        630-632) 639.8
    complicating pregnancy or puerperium 646.6
      affecting fetus or newborn 760.1
    following
      abortion 639.8
      ectopic or molar pregnancy 639.8

Abscess—*continued*
  knee 682.6
    joint 711.06
    tuberculous (active) (*see also* Tuberculosis)
        015.2
  labium (majus) (minus) 616.4
    complicating pregnancy, childbirth, or
        puerperium 646.6
  lacrimal (passages) (sac) (*see also*
        Dacryocystitis) 375.30
    caruncle 375.30
    gland (*see also* Dacryoadenitis) 375.00
  lacunar 597.0
  larynx 478.79
  lateral (alveolar) 522.5
    with sinus 522.7
  leg, except foot 682.6
  lens 360.00
  lid 373.13
  lingual 529.0
    tonsil 475
  lip 528.5
  Littre's gland 597.0
  liver 572.0
    amebic 006.3
      with
        brain abscess (and lung abscess) 006.5
        lung abscess 006.4
      due to Entamoeba histolytica 006.3
    dysenteric (*see also* Abscess, liver, amebic)
        006.3
    pyogenic 572.0
    tropical (*see also* Abscess, liver, amebic)
        006.3
  loin (region) 682.2
  lumbar (tuberculous) (*see also* Tuberculosis)
        015.0 *[730.88]*
    nontuberculous 682.2
  lung (miliary) (putrid) 513.0
    amebic (with liver abscess) 006.4
      with brain abscess 006.5
  lymph, lymphatic, gland or node (acute) 683
    any site, except mesenteric 683
    mesentery 289.2
  lymphangitic, acute—*see* Cellulitis
  malar 526.4
  mammary gland—*see* Abscess, breast
  marginal (anus) 566
  mastoid (process) (*see also* Mastoiditis, acute)
        383.00
    subperiosteal 383.01
  maxilla, maxillary 526.4
    molar (tooth) 522.5
      with sinus 522.7
    premolar 522.5
    sinus (chronic) (*see also* Sinusitis, maxillary)
        473.0
  mediastinum 513.1
  meibomian gland 373.12
  meninges (*see also* Meningitis) 320.9
  mesentery, mesenteric 567.22
  mesosalpinx (*see also* Salpingo-oophoritis)
        614.2
  milk 675.1
  Monro's (psoriasis) 696.1
  mons pubis 682.2
  mouth (floor) 528.3
  multiple sites NEC 682.9
  mural 682.2
  muscle 728.89
    psoas 567.31

Abscess—*continued*
  myocardium 422.92
  nabothian (follicle) (*see also* Cervicitis) 616.0
  nail (chronic) (with lymphangitis) 681.9
    finger 681.02
    toe 681.11
  nasal (fossa) (septum) 478.19
    sinus (chronic) (*see also* Sinusitis) 473.9
  nasopharyngeal 478.29
  nates 682.5
  navel 682.2
    newborn NEC 771.4
  neck (region) 682.1
    lymph gland or node 683
  nephritic (*see also* Abscess, kidney) 590.2
  nipple 611.0
    puerperal, postpartum 675.0
  nose (septum) 478.19
    external 682.0
  omentum 567.22
  operative wound 998.59
  orbit, orbital 376.01
  ossifluent—*see* Abscess, bone
  ovary, ovarian (corpus luteum) (*see also*
        Salpingo-oophoritis) 614.2
  oviduct (*see also* Salpingo-oophoritis) 614.2
  palate (soft) 528.3
    hard 526.4
  palmar (space) 682.4
  pancreas (duct) 577.0
  paradontal 523.30
  parafrenal 607.2
  parametric, parametrium (chronic) (*see also*
        Disease, pelvis, inflammatory) 614.4
    acute 614.3
  paranephric 590.2
  parapancreatic 577.0
  parapharyngeal 478.22
  pararectal 566
  parasinus (*see also* Sinusitis) 473.9
  parauterine (*see also* Disease, pelvis,
        inflammatory) 614.4
    acute 614.3
  paravaginal (*see also* Vaginitis) 616.10
  parietal region 682.8
  parodontal 523.30
  parotid (duct) (gland) 527.3
    region 528.3
  parumbilical 682.2
    newborn 771.4
  pectoral (region) 682.2
  pelvirectal 567.22
  pelvis, pelvic
    female (chronic) (*see also* Disease, pelvis,
        inflammatory) 614.4
      acute 614.3
    male, peritoneal (cellular tissue)—*see*
        Abscess, peritoneum
    tuberculous (*see also* Tuberculosis) 016.9
  penis 607.2
    gonococcal (acute) 098.0
      chronic or duration of 2 months or over
        098.2
  perianal 566
  periapical 522.5
    with sinus (alveolar) 522.7
  periappendiceal 540.1
  pericardial 420.99
  pericecal 540.1
  pericemental 523.30

Abscess—*continued*
pericholecystic (*see also* Cholecystitis, acute)
575.0
pericoronal 523.30
peridental 523.30
perigastric 535.0
perimetric (*see also* Disease, pelvis,
inflammatory) 614.4
acute 614.3
perinephric, perinephritic (*see also* Abscess,
kidney) 590.2
perineum, perineal (superficial) 682.2
deep (with urethral involvement) 597.0
urethra 597.0
periodontal (parietal) 523.31
apical 522.5
periosteum, periosteal (*see also* Periostitis)
730.3
with osteomyelitis (*see also* Osteomyelitis)
730.2
acute or subacute 730.0
chrŏnic or old 730.1
peripleuritic 510.9
with fistula 510.0
periproctic 566
periprostatic 601.2
perirectal (staphylococcal) 566
perirenal (tissue) (*see also* Abscess, kidney)
590.2
perisinuous (nose) (*see also* Sinusitis) 473.9
peritoneum, peritoneal (perforated) (ruptured)
567.22
with
abortion—*see* Abortion, by type, with sepsis
appendicitis 540.1
ectopic pregnancy (*see also* categories
633.0-633.9) 639.0
molar pregnancy (*see also* categories
630-632) 639.0
following
abortion 639.0
ectopic or molar pregnancy 639.0
pelvic, female (*see also* Disease, pelvis,
inflammatory) 614.4
acute 614.3
postoperative 998.59
puerperal, postpartum, childbirth 670.8
tuberculous (*see also* Tuberculosis) 014.0
peritonsillar 475
perityphlic 540.1
periureteral 593.89
periurethral 597.0
gonococcal (acute) 098.0
chronic or duration of 2 months or over
098.2
periuterine (*see also* Disease, pelvis,
inflammatory) 614.4
acute 614.3
perivesical 595.89
pernicious NEC 682.9
petrous bone—*see* Petrositis
phagedenic NEC 682.9
chancroid 099.0
pharynx, pharyngeal (lateral) 478.29
phlegmonous NEC 682.9
pilonidal 685.0
pituitary (gland) 253.8
pleura 510.9
with fistula 510.0
popliteal 682.6
postanal 566

Abscess—*continued*
postcecal 540.1
postlaryngeal 478.79
postnasal 478.19
postpharyngeal 478.24
posttonsillar 475
posttyphoid 002.0
Pott's (*see also* Tuberculosis) 015.0 *[730.88]*
pouch of Douglas (chronic) (*see also* Disease,
pelvis, inflammatory) 614.4
premammary—*see* Abscess, breast
prepatellar 682.6
prostate (*see also* Prostatitis) 601.2
gonococcal (acute) 098.12
chronic or duration of 2 months or over 098.32
psoas 567.31
tuberculous (*see also* Tuberculosis) 015.0
[730.88]
pterygopalatine fossa 682.8
pubis 682.2
puerperal—Puerperal, abscess, by site
pulmonary—*see* Abscess, lung
pulp, pulpal (dental) 522.0
finger 681.01
toe 681.10
pyemic—*see* Septicemia
pyloric valve 535.0
rectovaginal septum 569.5
rectovesical 595.89
rectum 566
regional NEC 682.9
renal (*see also* Abscess, kidney) 590.2
retina 363.00
retrobulbar 376.01
retrocecal 567.22
retrolaryngeal 478.79
retromammary—*see* Abscess, breast
retroperineal 682.2
retroperitoneal 567.38
postprocedural 998.59
retropharyngeal 478.24
tuberculous (*see also* Tuberculosis) 012.8
retrorectal 566
retrouterine (*see also* Disease, pelvis,
inflammatory) 614.4
acute 614.3
retrovesical 595.89
root, tooth 522.5
with sinus (alveolar) 522.7
round ligament (*see also* Disease, pelvis,
inflammatory) 614.4
acute 614.3
rupture (spontaneous) NEC 682.9
sacrum (tuberculous) (*see also* Tuberculosis)
015.0 *[730.88]*
nontuberculous 730.08
salivary duct or gland 527.3
scalp (any part) 682.8
scapular 730.01
sclera 379.09
scrofulous (*see also* Tuberculosis) 017.2
scrotum 608.4
seminal vesicle 608.0
amebic 006.8
septal, dental 522.5
with sinus (alveolar) 522.7
septum (nasal) 478.19
serous (*see also* Periostitis) 730.3
shoulder 682.3
side 682.2
sigmoid 569.5

Abscess—*continued*
 sinus (accessory) (chronic) (nasal) (*see also*
  Sinusitis) 473.9
  intracranial venous (any) 324.0
  late effect—*see* category 326
 Skene's duct or gland 597.0
 skin NEC 682.9
  tuberculous (primary) (*see also* Tuberculosis)
   017.0
 sloughing NEC 682.9
 specified site NEC 682.8
  amebic 006.8
 spermatic cord 608.4
 sphenoidal (sinus) (*see also* Sinusitis,
   sphenoidal) 473.3
 spinal
  cord (any part) (staphylococcal) 324.1
   tuberculous (*see also* Tuberculosis) 013.5
  epidural 324.1
 spine (column) (tuberculous) (*see also*
   Tuberculosis) 015.0 *[730.88]*
  nontuberculous 730.08
 spleen 289.59
  amebic 006.8
 staphylococcal NEC 682.9
 stitch 998.59
 stomach (wall) 535.0
 strumous (tuberculous) (*see also* Tuberculosis)
   017.2
 subarachnoid 324.9
  brain 324.0
  cerebral 324.0
  late effect—*see* category 326
  spinal cord 324.1
 subareolar—*see also* Abscess, breast
  puerperal, postpartum 675.1
 subcecal 540.1
 subcutaneous NEC 682.9
 subdiaphragmatic 567.22
 subdorsal 682.2
 subdural 324.9
  brain 324.0
  late effect—*see* category 326
  spinal cord 324.1
 subgaleal 682.8
 subhepatic 567.22
 sublingual 528.3
  gland 527.3
 submammary—*see* Abscess, breast
 submandibular (region) (space) (triangle) 682.0
  gland 527.3
 submaxillary (region) 682.0
  gland 527.3
 submental (pyogenic) 682.0
  gland 527.3
 subpectoral 682.2
 subperiosteal—*see* Abscess, bone
 subperitoneal 567.22
 subphrenic—*see also* Abscess, peritoneum
   567.22
  postoperative 998.59
 subscapular 682.2
 subungual 681.9
 suburethral 597.0
 sudoriparous 705.89
 suppurative NEC 682.9
 supraclavicular (fossa) 682.3
 suprahepatic 567.22
 suprapelvic (*see also* Disease, pelvis,
   inflammatory) 614.4
  acute 614.3

Abscess—*continued*
 suprapubic 682.2
 suprarenal (capsule) (gland) 255.8
 sweat gland 705.89
 syphilitic 095.8
 teeth, tooth (root) 522.5
  with sinus (alveolar) 522.7
  supporting structures NEC 523.30
 temple 682.0
 temporal region 682.0
 temporosphenoidal 324.0
  late effect—*see* category 326
 tendon (sheath) 727.89
 testicle—*see* Orchitis
 thecal 728.89
 thigh (acquired) 682.6
 thorax 510.9
  with fistula 510.0
 throat 478.29
 thumb (intrathecal) (periosteal) (subcutaneous)
   (subcuticular) 681.00
 thymus (gland) 254.1
 thyroid (gland) 245.0
 toe (any) (intrathecal) (periosteal)
   (subcutaneous) (subcuticular) 681.10
 tongue (staphylococcal) 529.0
 tonsil(s) (lingual) 475
 tonsillopharyngeal 475
 tooth, teeth (root) 522.5
  with sinus (alveolar) 522.7
  supporting structure NEC 523.30
 trachea 478.9
 trunk 682.2
 tubal (*see also* Salpingo-oophoritis) 614.2
 tuberculous—*see* Tuberculosis, abscess
 tubo-ovarian (*see also* Salpingo-oophoritis)
   614.2
 tunica vaginalis 608.4
 umbilicus NEC 682.2
  newborn 771.4
 upper arm 682.3
 upper respiratory 478.9
 urachus 682.2
 urethra (gland) 597.0
 urinary 597.0
 uterus, uterine (wall) (*see also* Endometritis)
   615.9
  ligament (*see also* Disease, pelvis,
    inflammatory) 614.4
   acute 614.3
  neck (*see also* Cervicitis) 616.0
 uvula 528.3
 vagina (wall) (*see also* Vaginitis) 616.10
 vaginorectal (*see also* Vaginitis) 616.10
 vas deferens 608.4
 vermiform appendix 540.1
 vertebra (column) (tuberculous) (*see also*
   Tuberculosis) 015.0 *[730.88]*
  nontuberculous 730.0
 vesical 595.89
 vesicouterine pouch (*see also* Disease, pelvis,
   inflammatory) 614.4
 vitreous (humor) (pneumococcal) 360.04
 vocal cord 478.5
 von Bezold's 383.01
 vulva 616.4
  complicating pregnancy, childbirth, or
   puerperium 646.6
 vulvovaginal gland (*see also* Vaginitis) 616.3
 web-space 682.4
 wrist 682.4

Absence (organ or part) (complete or partial)
  acoustic nerve 742.8
  adrenal (gland) (congenital) 759.1
    acquired V45.79
  albumin (blood) 273.8
  alimentary tract (complete) (congenital) (partial)
    751.8
    lower 751.5
    upper 750.8
  alpha-fucosidase 271.8
  alveolar process (acquired) 525.8
    congenital 750.26
  anus, anal (canal) (congenital) 751.2
  aorta (congenital) 747.22
  aortic valve (congenital) 746.89
  appendix, congenital 751.2
  arm (acquired) V49.60
    above elbow V49.66
    below elbow V49.65
    congenital (*see also* Deformity, reduction,
      upper limb) 755.20
      lower—*see* Absence, forearm, congenital
      upper (complete) (partial) (with absence of
        distal elements, incomplete) 755.24
        with
          complete absence of distal elements
            755.21
          forearm (incomplete) 755.23
  artery (congenital) (peripheral) NEC (*see also*
    Anomaly, peripheral vascular system)
    747.60
    brain 747.81
    cerebral 747.81
    coronary 746.85
    pulmonary 747.3
    umbilical 747.5
  atrial septum 745.69
  auditory canal (congenital) (external) 744.01
  auricle (ear) (with stenosis or atresia of auditory
    canal), congenital 744.01
  bile, biliary duct (common) or passage
    (congenital) 751.61
    bladder (acquired) V45.74
    congenital 753.8
  bone (congenital) NEC 756.9
    marrow 284.9
      acquired (secondary) 284.89
      congenital 284.09
      hereditary 284.09
      idiopathic 284.9
    skull 756.0
  bowel sounds 787.5
  brain 740.0
    specified part 742.2
  breast(s) (acquired) V45.71
    congenital 757.6
  broad ligament (congenital) 752.19
  bronchus (congenital) 748.3
  calvarium, calvaria (skull) 756.0
  canaliculus lacrimalis, congenital 743.65
  carpal(s) (congenital) (complete) (partial) (with
    absence of distal elements, incomplete) (*see*
    also Deformity, reduction, upper limb)
    755.28
    with complete absence of distal elements
      755.21
  cartilage 756.9
  caudal spine 756.13
  cecum (acquired) (postoperative)
    (posttraumatic) V45.72
    congenital 751.2

Absence— *continued*
  cementum 520.4
  cerebellum (congenital) (vermis) 742.2
  cervix (acquired) (uteri) V88.01
    with remaining uterus V88.03
    and uterus V88.01
    congenital 752.49
  chin, congenital 744.89
  cilia (congenital) 743.63
    acquired 374.89
  circulatory system, part NEC 747.89
  clavicle 755.51
  clitoris (congenital) 752.49
  coccyx, congenital 756.13
  cold sense (*see also* Disturbance, sensation)
    782.0
  colon (acquired) (postoperative) V45.72
    congenital 751.2
  congenital
    lumen—*see* Atresia
    organ or site NEC—*see* Agenesis
    septum—*see* Imperfect, closure
  corpus callosum (congenital) 742.2
  cricoid cartilage 748.3
  diaphragm (congenital) (with hernia) 756.6
    with obstruction 756.6
  digestive organ(s) or tract, congenital (complete)
    (partial) 751.8
    acquired V45.79
    lower 751.5
    upper 750.8
  ductus arteriosus 747.89
  duodenum (acquired) (postoperative) V45.72
    congenital 751.1
  ear, congenital 744.09
    acquired V45.79
    auricle 744.01
    external 744.01
    inner 744.05
    lobe, lobule 744.21
    middle, except ossicles 744.03
      ossicles 744.04
    ossicles 744.04
  ejaculatory duct (congenital) 752.89
  endocrine gland NEC (congenital) 759.2
  epididymis (congenital) 752.89
    acquired V45.77
  epiglottis, congenital 748.3
  epileptic (atonic) (typical) (*see also* Epilepsy)
    345.0
  erythrocyte 284.9
  erythropoiesis 284.9
    congenital 284.01
  esophagus (congenital) 750.3
  Eustachian tube (congenital) 744.24
  extremity (acquired)
    congenital (*see also* Deformity, reduction)
      755.4
    lower V49.70
    upper V49.60
  extrinsic muscle, eye 743.69
  eye (acquired) V45.78
    adnexa (congenital) 743.69
    congenital 743.00
    muscle (congenital) 743.69
  eyelid (fold), congenital 743.62
    acquired 374.89
  face
    bones NEC 756.0
    specified part NEC 744.89

Absence—*continued*
  lip 750.26
  liver (congenital) (lobe) 751.69
  lumbar (congenital) (vertebra) 756.13
    isthmus 756.11
    pars articularis 756.11
  lumen—*see* Atresia
  lung (bilateral) (congenital) (fissure) (lobe)
    (unilateral) 748.5
    acquired (any part) V45.76
  mandible (congenital) 524.09
  maxilla (congenital) 524.09
  menstruation 626.0
  metacarpal(s), congenital (complete) (partial)
    (with absence of distal elements,
    incomplete) (*see also* Deformity, reduction,
    upper limb) 755.28
    with all fingers, complete 755.21
  metatarsal(s), congenital (complete) (partial)
    (with absence of distal elements,
    incomplete) (*see also* Deformity, reduction,
    lower limb) 755.38
    with complete absence of distal elements
     755.31
  muscle (congenital) (pectoral) 756.81
    ocular 743.69
  musculoskeletal system (congenital) NEC 756.9
  nail(s) (congenital) 757.5
  neck, part 744.89
  nerve 742.8
  nervous system, part NEC 742.8
  neutrophil 288.00
  nipple (congenital) 757.6
    acquired V45.71
  nose (congenital) 748.1
    acquired 738.0
  nuclear 742.8
  ocular muscle (congenital) 743.69
  organ
    of Corti (congenital) 744.05
    or site
      acquired V45.79
      congenital NEC 759.89
  osseous meatus (ear) 744.03
  ovary (acquired) V45.77
    congenital 752.0
  oviduct (acquired) V45.77
    congenital 752.19
  pancreas (congenital) 751.7
    acquired (postoperative) (posttraumatic)
     V45.79
  parathyroid gland (congenital) 759.2
  parotid gland(s) (congenital) 750.21
  patella, congenital 755.64
  pelvic girdle (congenital) 755.69
  penis (congenital) 752.69
    acquired V45.77
  pericardium (congenital) 746.89
  perineal body (congenital) 756.81
  phalange(s), congenital 755.4
    lower limb (complete) (intercalary) (partial)
     (terminal) (*see also* Deformity, reduction,
     lower limb) 755.39
     meaning all toes (complete) (partial) 755.31
     transverse 755.31
    upper limb (complete) (intercalary) (partial)
     (terminal) (*see also* Deformity, reduction,
     upper limb) 755.29
     meaning all digits (complete) (partial)
      755.21
     transverse 755.21

Absence—*continued*
  pituitary gland (congenital) 759.2
  postoperative—*see* Absence, by site, acquired
  prostate (congenital) 752.89
    acquired V45.77
  pulmonary
    artery 747.3
    trunk 747.3
    valve (congenital) 746.01
    vein 747.49
  punctum lacrimale (congenital) 743.65
  radius, congenital (complete) (partial) (with
    absence of distal elements, incomplete)
    755.26
    with
     complete absence of distal elements 755.21
     ulna 755.25
      with
       complete absence of distal elements
        755.21
       humerus (incomplete) 755.23
  ray, congenital 755.4
    lower limb (complete) (partial) (*see also*
     Deformity, reduction, lower limb) 755.38
     meaning all rays 755.31
     transverse 755.31
    upper limb (complete) (partial) (*see also*
     Deformity, reduction, upper limb) 755.28
     meaning all rays 755.21
     transverse 755.21
  rectum (congenital) 751.2
    acquired V45.79
  red cell 284.9
    acquired (secondary) 284.81
    congenital 284.01
    hereditary 284.01
    idiopathic 284.9
  respiratory organ (congenital) NEC 748.9
  rib (acquired) 738.3
    congenital 756.3
  roof of orbit (congenital) 742.0
  round ligament (congenital) 752.89
  sacrum, congenital 756.13
  salivary gland(s) (congenital) 750.21
  scapula 755.59
  scrotum, congenital 752.89
  seminal tract or duct (congenital) 752.89
    acquired V45.77
  septum (congenital)—*see also* Imperfect,
    closure, septum
    atrial 745.69
    and ventricular 745.7
    between aorta and pulmonary artery 745.0
    ventricular 745.3
    and atrial 745.7
  sex chromosomes 758.81
  shoulder girdle, congenital (complete) (partial)
    755.59
  skin (congenital) 757.39
  skull bone 756.0
    with
     anencephalus 740.0
     encephalocele 742.0
     hydrocephalus 742.3
      with spina bifida (*see also* Spina bifida)
       741.0
     microcephalus 742.1
  spermatic cord (congenital) 752.89
  spinal cord 742.59
  spine, congenital 756.13

Absence—*continued*
  spleen (congenital) 759.0
    acquired V45.79
  sternum, congenital 756.3
  stomach (acquired) (partial) (postoperative)
      V45.75
    congenital 750.7
    with postgastric surgery syndrome 564.2
  submaxillary gland(s) (congenital) 750.21
  superior vena cava (congenital) 747.49
  tarsal(s), congenital (complete) (partial) (with
      absence of distal elements, incomplete) (*see
      also* Deformity, reduction, lower limb)
      755.38
  teeth, tooth (congenital) 520.0
    with abnormal spacing 524.30
    acquired 525.10
      due to
        caries 525.13
        extraction 525.10
        periodontal disease 525.12
        trauma 525.11
      with malocclusion 524.30
  tendon (congenital) 756.81
  testis (congenital) 752.89
    acquired V45.77
  thigh (acquired) 736.89
  thumb (acquired) V49.61
    congenital 755.29
  thymus gland (congenital) 759.2
  thyroid (gland) (surgical) 246.8
    with hypothyroidism 244.0
    cartilage, congenital 748.3
    congenital 243
  tibia, congenital (complete) (partial) (with absence
      of distal elements, incomplete) (*see also*
      Deformity, reduction, lower limb) 755.36
    with
      complete absence of distal elements 755.31
      fibula 755.35
        with
          complete absence of distal elements
              755.31
        femur (incomplete) 755.33
          with complete absence of distal
              elements 755.31
  toe (acquired) V49.72
    congenital (complete) (partial) 755.39
      meaning all toes 755.31
      transverse 755.31
    great V49.71
  tongue (congenital) 750.11
  tooth, teeth, (congenital) 520.0
    with abnormal spacing 524.30
    acquired 525.10
      due to
        caries 525.13
        extraction 525.10
        periodontal disease 525.12
        trauma 525.11
      with malocclusion 524.30
  trachea (cartilage) (congenital) (rings) 748.3
  transverse aortic arch (congenital) 747.21
  tricuspid valve 746.1

Absence—*continued*
  ulna, congenital (complete) (partial) (with
      absence of distal elements, incomplete) (*see
      also* Deformity, reduction, upper limb)
      755.27
    with
      complete absence of distal elements 755.21
      radius 755.25
        with
          complete absence of distal elements
              755.21
          humerus (incomplete) 755.23
  umbilical artery (congenital) 747.5
  ureter (congenital) 753.4
    acquired V45.74
  urethra, congenital 753.8
    acquired V45.74
  urinary system, part NEC, congenital 753.8
    acquired V45.74
  uterus (acquired) V88.01
    with remaining cervical stump V88.02
    and cervix V88.01
    congenital 752.3
  uvula (congenital) 750.26
  vagina, congenital 752.49
    acquired V45.77
  vas deferens (congenital) 752.89
    acquired V45.77
  vein (congenital) (peripheral) NEC (*see also*
      Anomaly, peripheral vascular system)
      747.60
    brain 747.81
    great 747.49
    portal 747.49
    pulmonary 747.49
  vena cava (congenital) (inferior) (superior)
      747.49
  ventral horn cell 742.59
  ventricular septum 745.3
  vermis of cerebellum 742.2
  vertebra, congenital 756.13
  vulva, congenital 752.49
Absentia epileptica (*see also* Epilepsy) 345.0
Absinthemia (*see also* Dependence) 304.6
Absinthism (*see also* Dependence) 304.6
Absorbent system disease 459.89
Absorption
  alcohol, through placenta or breast milk 760.71
  antibiotics, through placenta or breast milk
      760.74
  anticonvulsants, through placenta or breast milk
      760.77
  antifungals, through placenta or breast milk
      760.74
  anti-infective, through placenta or breast milk
      760.74
  antimetabolics, through placenta or breast milk
      760.78
  chemical NEC 989.9
    specified chemical or substance—*see* Table of
        drugs and chemicals
    through placenta or breast milk (fetus or
        newborn) 760.70
      alcohol 760.71
      anticonvulsants 760.77
      antifungals 760.74
      anti-infective agents 760.74
      antimetabolics 760.78
      cocaine 760.75
      "crack" 760.75

Absorption—*continued*
diethylstilbestrol *[DES] 760.76*
hallucinogenic agents 760.73
medicinal agents NEC 760.79
narcotics 760.72
obstetric anesthetic or analgesic drug 763.5
specified agent NEC 760.79
suspected, affecting management of
pregnancy 655.5
cocaine, through placenta or breast milk 760.75
drug NEC (*see also* Reaction, drug)
through placenta or breast milk (fetus or
newborn) 760.70
alcohol 760.71
anticonvulsants 760.77
antifungals 760.74
anti-infective agents 760.74
antimetabolics 760.78
cocaine 760.75
"crack" 760.75
diethylstilbestrol (DES) 760.76
hallucinogenic agents 760.73
medicinal agents NEC 760.79
narcotics 760.72
obstetric anesthetic or analgesic drug 763.5
specified agent NEC 760.79
suspected, affecting management of
pregnancy 655.5
fat, disturbance 579.8
hallucinogenic agents, through placenta or
breast milk 760.73
immune sera, through placenta or breast milk
760.79
lactose defect 271.3
medicinal agents NEC, through placenta or
breast milk 760.79
narcotics, through placenta or breast milk
760.72
noxious substance,—*see* Absorption, chemical
protein, disturbance 579.8
pus or septic, general—*see* Septicemia
quinine, through placenta or breast milk 760.74
toxic substance—*see* Absorption, chemical
uremic—*see* Uremia
Abstinence symptoms or syndrome
alcohol 291.81
drug 292.0
neonatal 779.5
Abt-Letterer-Siwe syndrome (acute
histiocytosis X) (M9722/3) 202.5
Abulia 799.89
Abulomania 301.6
Abuse
adult 995.80
emotional 995.82
multiple forms 995.85
neglect (nutritional) 995.84
physical 995.81
psychological 995.82
sexual 995.83
alcohol (*see also* Alcoholism) 305.0
dependent 303.9
non-dependent 305.0
child 995.50
counseling
perpetrator
non-parent V62.83
parent V61.22
victim V61.21
emotional 995.51
multiple forms 995.59
neglect (nutritional) 995.52

Abuse—*continued*
physical 995.54
shaken infant syndrome 995.55
psychological 995.51
sexual 995.53
drugs, nondependent 305.9

*Note—Use the following fifth-digit
subclassification with the following codes:
305.0, 305.2-305.9:*

0   *unspecifidd*
1   *continuous*
2   *episodic*
3   *in remission*

amphetamine type 305.7
antidepressants 305.8
anxiolytic 305.4
barbiturates 305.4
caffeine 305.9
cannabis 305.2
cocaine type 305.6
hallucinogens 305.3
hashish 305.2
hypnotic 305.4
inhalant 305.9
LSD 305.3
marijuana 305.2
mixed 305.9
morphine type 305.5
opioid type 305.5
phencyclidine (PCP) 305.9
sedative 305.4
specified NEC 305.9
tranquilizers 305.4
spouse 995.80
tobacco 305.1
Acalcerosis 275.40
Acalcicosis 275.40
Acalculia 784.69
developmental 315.1
Acanthocheilonemiasis 125.4
Acanthocytosis 272.5
Acanthokeratodermia 701.1
Acantholysis 701.8
bullosa 757.39
Acanthoma (benign) (M8070/0)—*see also*
Neoplasm, by site, benign
malignant (M8070/3)—*see* Neoplasm, by site,
malignant
Acanthosis (acquired) (nigricans) 701.2
adult 701.2
benign (congenital) 757.39
congenital 757.39
glycogenic
esophagus 530.8
juvenile 701.2
tongue 529.8
Acanthrocytosis 272.5
Acapnia 276.3
Acarbia 276.2
Acardia 759.89
Acardiacus amorphus 759.89
Acardiotrophia 429.1
Acardius 759.89
Acariasis 133.9
sarcoptic 133.0
Acaridiasis 133.9
Acarinosis 133.9
Acariosis 133.9

Acarodermatitis 133.9
   urticarioides 133.9
Acarophobia 300.29
Acatalasemia 277.89
Acatalasia 277.89
Acatamathesia 784.69
Acataphasia 784.59
Acathisia 781.0
   due to drugs 333.99
Acceleration, accelerated
   atrioventricular conduction 426.7
   idioventricular rhythm 427.89
Accessory (congenital)
   adrenal gland 759.1
   anus 751.5
   appendix 751.5
   atrioventricular conduction 426.7
   auditory ossicles 744.04
   auricle (ear) 744.1
   autosome(s) NEC 758.5
      21 or 22 758.0
   biliary duct or passage 751.69
   bladder 753.8
   blood vessels (peripheral) (congenital) NEC (*see
      also* Anomaly, peripheral vascular system)
      747.60
      cerebral 747.81
      coronary 746.85
   bone NEC 756.9
      foot 755.67
   breast tissue, axilla 757.6
   carpal bones 755.56
   cecum 751.5
   cervix 752.49
   chromosome(s) NEC 758.5
      13-15 758.1
      16-18 758.2
      21 or 22 758.0
      autosome(s) NEC 758.5
      D₁ 758.1
      E₃ 758.2
      G 758.0
      sex 758.81
   coronary artery 746.85
   cusp(s), heart valve NEC 746.89
      pulmonary 746.09
   cystic duct 751.69
   digits 755.00
   ear (auricle) (lobe) 744.1
   endocrine gland NEC 759.2
   external os 752.49
   eyelid 743.62
   eye muscle 743.69
   face bone(s) 756.0
   fallopian tube (fimbria) (ostium) 752.19
   fingers 755.01
   foreskin 605
   frontonasal process 756.0
   gallbladder 751.69
   genital organ(s)
      female 752.89
         external 752.49
         internal NEC 752.89
      male NEC 752.89
         penis 752.69
   genitourinary organs NEC 752.89
   heart 746.89
      valve NEC 746.89
         pulmonary 746.09
   hepatic ducts 751.69
   hymen 752.49

Accessory—*continued*
   intestine (large) (small) 751.5
   kidney 753.3
   lacrimal canal 743.65
   leaflet, heart valve NEC 746.89
      pulmonary 746.09
   ligament, broad 752.19
   liver (duct) 751.69
   lobule (ear) 744.1
   lung (lobe) 748.69
   muscle 756.82
   navicular of carpus 755.56
   nervous system, part NEC 742.8
   nipple 757.6
   nose 748.1
   organ or site NEC—*see* Anomaly, specified type NEC
   ovary 752.0
   oviduct 752.19
   pancreas 751.7
   parathyroid gland 759.2
   parotid gland (and duct) 750.22
   pituitary gland 759.2
   placental lobe—*see* Placenta, abnormal
   preauricular appendage 744.1
   prepuce 605
   renal arteries (multiple) 747.62
   rib 756.3
      cervical 756.2
   roots (teeth) 520.2
   salivary gland 750.22
   sesamoids 755.8
   sinus—*see* condition
   skin tags 757.39
   spleen 759.0
   sternum 756.3
   submaxillary gland 750.22
   tarsal bones 755.67
   teeth, tooth 520.1
      causing crowding 524.31
   tendon 756.89
   thumb 755.01
   thymus gland 759.2
   thyroid gland 759.2
   toes 755.02
   tongue 750.13
   tragus 744.1
   ureter 753.4
   urethra 753.8
   urinary organ or tract NEC 753.8
   uterus 752.2
   vagina 752.49
   valve, heart NEC 746.89
      pulmonary 746.09
   vertebra 756.19
   vocal cords 748.3
   vulva 752.49
Accident, accidental —*see also* condition
   birth NEC 767.9
   cardiovascular (*see also* Disease,
      cardiovascular) 429.2
   cerebral (*see also* Disease, cerebrovascular,
      acute) 434.91
   cerebrovascular (current) (CVA) (*see also*
      Disease, cerebrovascular, acute) 434.91
      aborted 434.91
      embolic 434.11
      healed or old V12.54
      hemorrhagic—*see* Hemorrhage, brain
      impending 435.9
      ischemic 434.91

Accident, accidental—*continued*
late effect—*see* Late effect(s) (of)
cerebrovascular disease
postoperative 997.02
thrombotic 434.01
coronary (*see also* Infarct, myocardium) 410.9
craniovascular (*see also* Disease,
cerebrovascular, acute) 436
during pregnancy, to mother
affecting fetus or newborn 760.5
heart, cardiac (*see also* Infarct, myocardium)
410.9
intrauterine 779.89
vascular—*see* Disease, cerebrovascular, acute
Accommodation
disorder of 367.51
drug-induced 367.89
toxic 367.89
insufficiency of 367.4
paralysis of 367.51
hysterical 300.11
spasm of 367.53
Accouchement —*see* Delivery
Accreta placenta (without hemorrhage) 667.0
with hemorrhage 666.0
Accretio cordis (nonrheumatic) 423.1
Accretions on teeth 523.6
Accumulation secretion, prostate 602.8
Acephalia, acephalism, acephaly 740.0
Acephalic monster 740.0
Acephalobrachia monster 759.89
Acephalocardia 759.89
Acephalocardius 759.89
Acephalochiria 759.89
Acephalochirus monster 759.89
Acephalogaster 759.89
Acephalostomus monster 759.89
Acephalothorax 759.89
Acephalus 740.0
Acetonemia 790.6
diabetic 250.1
due to secondary diabetes 249.1
Acetonglycosuria 982.8
Acetonuria 791.6
Achalasia 530.0
cardia 530.0
digestive organs congenital NEC 751.8
esophagus 530.0
pelvirectal 751.3
psychogenic 306.4
pylorus 750.5
sphincteral NEC 564.89
Achard-Thiers syndrome (adrenogenital) 255.2
Ache (s)—*see* Pain
Acheilia 750.26
Acheiria 755.21
Achilloburistis 726.71
Achillodynia 726.71
Achlorhydria, achlorhydric 536.0
anemia 280.9
diarrhea 536.0
neurogenic 536.0
postvagotomy 564.2
psychogenic 306.4
secondary to vagotomy 564.2
Achloroblepsia 368.52
Achloropsia 368.52
Acholia 575.8
Acholuric jaundice (familial) (splenomegalic)
(*see also* Spherocytosis) 282.0
acquired 283.9

Achondroplasia 756.4
Achrestic anemia 281.8
Achroacytosis, lacrimal gland 375.00
tuberculous (*see also* Tuberculosis) 017.3
Achroma, cutis 709.00
Achromate (congenital) 368.54
Achromatopia 368.54
Achromatopsia (congenital) 368.54
Achromia
congenital 270.2
parasitica 111.0
unguium 703.8
Achylia
gastrica 536.8
neurogenic 536.3
psychogenic 306.4
pancreatica 577.1
Achylosis 536.8
Acid
burn—*see also* Burn, by site
from swallowing acid—*see* Burn, internal
organs
deficiency
amide nicotinic 265.2
amino 270.9
ascorbic 267
folic 266.2
nicotinic (amide) 265.2
pantothenic 266.2
intoxication 276.2
peptic disease 536.8
stomach 536.8
psychogenic 306.4
Acidemia 276.2
arginsuccinic 270.6
fetal
affecting management of pregnancy 656.3
before onset of labor, in liveborn infant 768.2
during labor and delivery, in liveborn infant
768.3
intrauterine—*see* Distress, fetal 656.3
unspecified as to time of onset, in liveborn
infant 768.4
newborn 775.81
pipecolic 270.7
Acidity, gastric (high) (low) 536.8
psychogenic 306.4
Acidocytopenia 288.59
Acidocytosis 288.3
Acidopenia 288.59
Acidosis 276.2
diabetic 250.1
due to secondary diabetes 249.1
fetal, affecting management of pregnancy 656.8
fetal, affecting newborn 775.81
kidney tubular 588.89
lactic 276.2
metabolic NEC 276.2
with respiratory acidosis 276.4
of newborn 775.81
late, of newborn 775.7
newborn 775.81
renal
hyperchloremic 588.89
tubular (distal) (proximal) 588.89
respiratory 276.2
complicated by
metabolic acidosis 276.4
of newborn 775.81
metabolic alkalosis 276.4

Aciduria 791.9
  arginosuccinic 270.6
  beta-aminoisobutyric (BAIB) 277.2
  glutaric
    type I 270.7
    type II (type IIA, IIB, IIC) 277.85
    type III 277.86
  glycolic 271.8
  methylmalonic 270.3
    with glycinemia 270.7
  organic 270.9
  orotic (congenital) (hereditary) (pyrimidine
    deficiency) 281.4
Acladiosis 111.8
  skin 111.8
Aclasis
  diaphyseal 756.4
  tarsoepiphyseal 756.59
Acleistocardia 745.5
Aclusion 524.4
Acmesthesia 782.0
Acne (pustular) (vulgaris) 706.1
  agminata (*see also* Tuberculosis) 017.0
  artificialis 706.1
  atrophica 706.0
  cachecticorum (Hebra) 706.1
  conglobata 706.1
  conjunctiva 706.1
  cystic 706.1
  decalvans 704.09
  erythematosa 695.3
  eyelid 706.1
  frontalis 706.0
  indurata 706.1
  keloid 706.1
  lupoid 706.0
  necrotic, necrotica 706.0
    miliaris 704.8
  neonatal 706.1
  nodular 706.1
  occupational 706.1
  papulosa 706.1
  rodens 706.0
  rosacea 695.3
  scorbutica 267
  scrofulosorum (Bazin) (*see also* Tuberculosis)
    017.0
  summer 692.72
  tropical 706.1
  varioliformis 706.0
Acneiform drug eruptions 692.3
Acnitis (primary) (*see also* Tuberculosis) 017.0
Acomia 704.00
Acontractile bladder 344.61
Aconuresis (*see also* Incontinence) 788.30
Acosta's disease 993.2
Acousma 780.1
Acoustic —*see* condition
Acousticophobia 300.29
Acquired —*see* condition
Acquired immunodeficiency syndrome —*see*
  Human immunodeficiency virus (disease)
  (illness) (infection)
Acragnosis 781.99
Acrania (monster) 740.0
Acroagnosis 781.99
Acroasphyxia, chronic 443.89
Acrobrachycephaly 756.0
Acrobystiolith 608.89
Acrobystitis 607.2
Acrocephalopolysyndactyly 755.55

Acrocephalosyndactyly 755.55
Acrocephaly 756.0
Acrochondrohyperplasia 759.82
Acrocyanosis 443.89
  newborn 770.83
Acrodermatitis 686.8
  atrophicans (chronica) 701.8
  continua (Hallopeau) 696.1
  enteropathica 686.8
  Hallopeau's 696.1
  perstans 696.1
  pustulosa continua 696.1
  recalcitrant pustular 696.1
Acrodynia 985.0
Acrodysplasia 755.55
Acrohyperhidrosis (*see also* Hyperhidrosis)
  780.8
Acrokeratosis verruciformis 757.39
Acromastitis 611.0
Acromegaly, acromegalia (skin) 253.0
Acromelalgia 443.82
Acromicria, acromikria 756.59
Acronyx 703.0
Acropachy, thyroid (*see also* Thyrotoxicosis)
  242.9
Acropachyderma 757.39
Acroparesthesia 443.89
  simple (Schultz's type) 443.89
  vasomotor (Nothnagel's type) 443.89
Acropathy thyroid (*see also* Thyrotoxicosis) 242.9
Acrophobia 300.29
Acroposthitis 607.2
Acroscleriasis (*see also* Scleroderma) 710.1
Acroscleroderma (*see also* Scleroderma) 710.1
Acrosclerosis (*see also* Scleroderma) 710.1
Acrosphacelus 785.4
Acrosphenosyndactylia 755.55
Acrospiroma, eccrine (M8402/0)—*see*
  Neoplasm, skin, benign
Acrostealgia 732.9
Acrosyndactyly (*see also* Syndactylism) 755.10
Acrotrophodynia 991.4
Actinic —*see also* condition
  cheilitis (due to sun) 692.72
    chronic NEC 692.74
    due to radiation, except from sun 692.82
  conjunctivitis 370.24
  dermatitis (due to sun) (*see also* Dermatitis,
    actinic) 692.70
  due to
    roentgen rays or radioactive substance
      692.82
    ultraviolet radiation, except from sun 692.82
    sun NEC 692.70
  elastosis solare 692.74
  granuloma 692.73
  keratitis 370.24
  ophthalmia 370.24
  reticuloid 692.73
Actinobacillosis, general 027.8
Actinobacillus
  lignieresii 027.8
  mallei 024
  muris 026.1
Actinocutitis NEC (*see also* Dermatitis, actinic)
  692.70
Actinodermatitis NEC (*see also* Dermatitis,
  actinic) 692.70
Actinomyces
  israelii (infection)—*see* Actinomycosis
  muris-ratti (infection) 026.1

Actinomycosis actinomycotic 039.9
  with
    pneumonia 039.1
  abdominal 039.2
  cervicofacial 039.3
  cutaneous 039.0
  pulmonary 039.1
  specified site NEC 039.8
  thoracic 039.1
Actinoneuritis 357.89
Action, heart
  disorder 427.9
    postoperative 997.1
  irregular 427.9
    postoperative 997.1
    psychogenic 306.2
Active —*see* condition
Activity decrease, functional 780.99
Acute —*see also* condition
  abdomen NEC 789.0
  gallbladder (*see also* Cholecystitis, acute) 575.0
Acyanoblepsia 368.53
Acyanopsia 368.53
Acystia 753.8
Acystinervia —*see* Neurogenic, bladder
Acystineuria —*see* Neurogenic, bladder
Adactylia, adactyly (congenital) 755.4
  lower limb (complete) (intercalary) (partial)
    (terminal) (*see also* Deformity, reduction,
    lower limb) 755.39
    meaning all digits (complete) (partial) 755.31
    transverse (complete) (partial) 755.31
  upper limb (complete) (intercalary) (partial)
    (terminal) (*see also* Deformity, reduction,
    upper limb) 755.29
    meaning all digits (complete) (partial) 755.21
    transverse (complete) (partial) 755.21
Adair-Dighton syndrome (brittle bones and blue
  sclera, deafness) 756.51
Adamantinoblastoma (M9310/0)—*see*
  Ameloblastoma
Adamantinoma (M9310/0)—*see* Ameloblastoma
Adamantoblastoma (M9310/0)—*see*
  Ameloblastoma
Adams-Stokes (-Morgagni) disease or syndrome
  (syncope with heart block) 426.9
Adaptation reaction (*see also* Reaction,
  adjustment) 309.9
Addiction —*see also* Dependence
  absinthe 304.6
  alcoholic (ethyl) (methyl) (wood) 303.9
    complicating pregnancy, childbirth, or
      puerperium 648.4
      affecting fetus or newborn 760.71
    suspected damage to fetus affecting
      management of pregnancy 655.4
  drug (*see also* Dependence) 304.9
  ethyl alcohol 303.9
  heroin 304.0
  hospital 301.51
  methyl alcohol 303.9
  methylated spirit 303.9
  morphine (-like substances) 304.0
  nicotine 305.1
  opium 304.0
  tobacco 305.1
  wine 303.9

Addison's
  anemia (pernicious) 281.0
  disease (bronze) (primary adrenal insufficiency)
    255.41
    tuberculous (*see also* Tuberculosis) 017.6
  keloid (morphea) 701.0
  melanoderma (adrenal cortical hypofunction)
    255.41
Addison-Biermer anemia (pernicious) 281.0
Addison-Gull disease —*see* Xanthoma
Addisonian crisis or melanosis (acute
  adrenocortical insufficiency) 255.41
Additional —*see also* Accessory
  chromosome(s) 758.5
    13-15 758.1
    16-18 758.2
    21 758.0
    autosome(s) NEC 758.5
    sex 758.81
Adduction contracture, hip or other joint —*see*
  Contraction, joint
ADEM (acute disseminated encephalomyelitis)
  (postinfectious) 136.9 *[323.61]*
  infectious 136.9 *[323.61]*
  noninfectious 323.81
Adenasthenia gastrica 536.0
Aden fever 061
Adenitis (*see also* Lymphadenitis) 289.3
  acute, unspecified site 683
    epidemic infectious 075
  axillary 289.3
    acute 683
    chronic or subacute 289.1
  Bartholin's gland 616.89
  bulbourethral gland (*see also* Urethritis) 597.89
  cervical 289.3
    acute 683
    chronic or subacute 289.1
  chancroid (Ducrey's bacillus) 099.0
  chronic (any lymph node, except mesenteric)
    289.1
    mesenteric 289.2
  Cowper's gland (*see also* Urethritis) 597.89
  epidemic, acute 075
  gangrenous 683
  gonorrheal NEC 098.89
  groin 289.3
    acute 683
    chronic or subacute 289.1
  infectious 075
  inguinal (region) 289.3
    acute 683
    chronic or subacute 289.1
  lymph gland or node, except mesenteric 289.3
    acute 683
    chronic or subacute 289.1
    mesenteric (acute) (chronic) (nonspecific)
      (subacute) 289.2
  mesenteric (acute) (chronic) (nonspecific)
    (subacute) 289.2
    due to Pasteurella multocida (P. septica) 027.2
  parotid gland (suppurative) 527.2
  phlegmonous 683
  salivary duct or gland (any) (recurring)
    (suppurative) 527.2
  scrofulous (*see also* Tuberculosis) 017.2
  septic 289.3
  Skene's duct or gland (*see also* Urethritis)
    597.89
  strumous, tuberculous (*see also* Tuberculosis)
    017.2

Adenitis—*continued*
  subacute, unspecified site 289.1
  sublingual gland (suppurative) 527.2
  submandibular gland (suppurative) 527.2
  submaxillary gland (suppurative) 527.2
  suppurative 683
  tuberculous—*see* Tuberculosis, lymph gland
  urethral gland (*see also* Urethritis) 597.89
  venereal NEC 099.8
  Wharton's duct (suppurative) 527.2
Adenoacanthoma (M8570/3)—*see* Neoplasm, by
  site, malignant
Adenoameloblastoma (M9300/0) 213.1
  upper jaw (bone) 213.0
Adenocarcinoma (M8140/3)—*see also*
  Neoplasm, by site, malignant

---

*Note—The list of adjectival modifiers below is
not exhaustive. A description of
adenocarcinoma that does not appear in this list
should be coded in the same manner as
carcinoma with that description. Thus, "mixed
acidophil-basophil adenocarcinoma," should be
coded in the same manner as "mixed
acidophil-basophil carcinoma," which appears
in the list under "Carcinoma."*

*Except where otherwise indicated, the
morphological varieties of adenocarcinoma in
the list below should be coded by site as for
"Neoplasm, malignant."*

---

  with
    apocrine metaplasia (M8573/3)
    cartilaginous (and osseous) metaplasia
      (M8571/3)
    osseous (and cartilaginous) metaplasia
      (M8571/3)
    spindle cell metaplasia (M8572/3)
    squamous metaplasia (M8570/3)
  acidophil (M8280/3)
    specified site—*see* Neoplasm, by site,
      malignant
    unspecified site 194.3
  acinar (M8550/3)
  acinic cell (M8550/3)
  adrenal cortical (M8370/3) 194.0
  alveolar (M8251/3)
  and
    epidermoid carcinoma, mixed (M8560/3)
    squamous cell carcinoma, mixed (M8560/3)
  apocrine (M8401/3)
    breast—*see* Neoplasm, breast, malignant
    specified site NEC—*see* Neoplasm, skin,
      malignant
    unspecified site 173.9
  basophil (M8300/3)
    specified site—*see* Neoplasm, by site,
      malignant
    unspecified site 194.3
  bile duct type (M8160/3)
    sliver 155.1
    specified site NEC—*see* Neoplasm, by site,
      malignant
    unspecified site 155.1
  bronchiolar (M8250/3)—*see* Neoplasm, lung,
    malignant
  ceruminous (M8420/3) 173.2
  chromophobe (M8270/3)
    specified site—*see* Neoplasm, by site,
      malignant
    unspecified site 194.3

Adenocarcinoma—*continued*
  clear cell (mesonephroid type) (M8310/3)
  colloid (M8480/3)
  cylindroid type (M8200/3)
  diffuse type (M8145/3)
    pecified site—*see* Neoplasm, by site,
      malignant
    unspecified site 151.9
  duct (infiltrating) (M8500/3)
    with Paget's disease (M8541/3)—*see*
      Neoplasm, breast, malignant
    specified site—*see* Neoplasm, by site,
      malignant
    unspecified site 174.9
  embryonal (M9070/3)
  endometrioid (M8380/3)—*see* Neoplasm, by
    site, malignant
  eosinophil (M8280/3)
    specified site—*see* Neoplasm, by site,
      malignant
    unspecified site 194.3
  follicular (M8330/3)
    and papillary (M8340/3) 193
    moderately differentiated type (M8332/3) 193
    pure follicle type (M8331/3) 193
    specified site—*see* Neoplasm, by site,
      malignant
    trabecular type (M8332/3) 193
    unspecified type 193
    well differentiated type (M8331/3) 193
  gelatinous (M8480/3)
  granular cell (M8320/3)
  Hürthle cell (M8290/3) 193
  in
    adenomatous
      polyp (M8210/3)
      polyposis coli (M8220/3) 153.9
    polypoid adenoma (M8210/3)
    tubular adenoma (M8210/3)
    villous adenoma (M8261/3)
  infiltrating duct (M8500/3)
    with Paget's disease (M8541/3)—*see*
      Neoplasm, breast, malignant
    specified site—*see* Neoplasm, by site,
      malignant
    unspecified site 174.9
  inflammatory (M8530/3)
    specified site—*see* Neoplasm, by site,
      malignant
    unspecified site 174.9
  in situ (M8140/2)—*see* Neoplasm, by site, in
    situ
  intestinal type (M8144/3)
    specified site—*see* Neoplasm, by site,
      malignant
    unspecified site 151.9
  intraductal (noninfiltrating) (M8500/2)
    papillary (M8503/2)
      specified site—*see* Neoplasm, by site, in situ
      unspecified site 233.0
    specified site—*see* Neoplasm, by site, in situ
    unspecified site 233.0
  islet cell (M8150/3)
    and exocrine, mixed (M8154/3)
      specified site—*see* Neoplasm, by site,
        malignant
      unspecified site 157.9
    pancreas 157.4
    specified site NEC—*see* Neoplasm, by site,
      malignant
    unspecified site 157.4

Adenocarcinoma—*continued*
lobular (M8520/3)
  specified site—*see* Neoplasm, by site,
    malignant
  unspecified site 174.9
medullary (M8510/3)
mesonephric (M9110/3)
mixed cell (M8323/3)
mucinous (M8480/3)
mucin-producing (M8481/3)
mucoid (M8480/3)—*see also* Neoplasm, by site,
    malignant
  cell (M8300/3)
    specified site—*see* Neoplasm, by site,
      malignant
    unspecified site 194.3
nonencapsulated sclerosing (M8350/3) 193
oncocytic (M8290/3)
oxyphilic (M8290/3)
papillary (M8260/3)
  and follicular (M8340/3) 193
  intraductal (noninfiltrating) (M8503/2)
    specified site—*see* Neoplasm, by site, in situ
    unspecified site 233.0
  serous (M8460/3)
    specified site—*see* Neoplasm, by site,
      malignant
    unspecified site 183.0
papillocystic (M8450/3)
  specified site—*see* Neoplasm, by site,
    malignant
  unspecified site 183.0
pseudomucinous (M8470/3)
  specified site—*see* Neoplasm, by site,
    malignant
  unspecified site 183.0
renal cell (M8312/3) 189.0
sebaceous (M8410/3)
serous (M8441/3)—*see also* Neoplasm, by site,
    malignant
  papillary
    specified site—*see* Neoplasm, by site,
      malignant
    unspecified site 183.0
signet ring cell (M8490/3)
superficial spreading (M8143/3)
sweat gland (M8400/3)—*see* Neoplasm, skin,
    malignant
trabecular (M8190/3)
tubular (M8211/3)
villous (M8262/3)
water-clear cell (M8322/3) 194.1
Adenofibroma (M9013/0)
clear cell (M8313/0)—*see* Neoplasm, by site,
    benign
endometrioid (M8381/0) 220
  borderline malignancy (M8381/1) 236.2
  malignant (M8381/3) 183.0
mucinous (M9015/0)
  specified site—*see* Neoplasm, by site, benign
  unspecified site 220
prostate 600.20
  with other lower urinary tract symptoms
    (LUTS) 600.21
  with urinary
    obstruction 600.21
    retention 600.21
serous (M9014/0)
  specified site—*see* Neoplasm, by site, benign
  unspecified site 220
specified site—*see* Neoplasm, by site, benign
unspecified site 220

Adenofibrosis
breast 610.2
endometrioid 617.0
Adenoiditis 474.01
acute 463
chronic 474.01
  with chronic tonsillitis 474.02
Adenoids (congenital) (of nasal fossa) 474.9
hypertrophy 474.12
vegetations 474.2
Adenolipomatosis (symmetrical) 272.8
Adenolymphoma (M8561/0)
specified site—*see* Neoplasm, by site, benign
unspecified 210.2
Adenoma (sessile) (M8140/0)—*see also*
  Neoplasm, by site, benign

> *Note—Except where otherwise indicated, the
> morphological varieties of adenoma in the list
> below should be coded by site as for
> "Neoplasm, benign."*

acidophil (M8280/0)
  specified site—*see* Neoplasm, by site, benign
  unspecified site 227.3
acinar (cell) (M8550/0)
acinic cell (M8550/0)
adrenal (cortex) (cortical) (functioning)
    (M8370/0) 227.0
  clear cell type (M8373/0) 227.0
  compact cell type (M8371/0) 227.0
  glomerulosa cell type (M8374/0) 227.0
  heavily pigmented variant (M8372/0) 227.0
  mixed cell type (M8375/0) 227.0
alpha cell (M8152/0)
  pancreas 211.7
  specified site NEC—*see* Neoplasm, by site,
    benign
  unspecified site 211.7
alveolar (M8251/0)
apocrine (M8401/0)
  breast 217
  specified site NEC—*see* Neoplasm, skin,
    benign
  unspecified site 216.9
basal cell (M8147/0)
basophil (M8300/0)
  specified site—*see* Neoplasm, by site, benign
  unspecified site 227.3
beta cell (M8151/0)
  pancreas 211.7
  specified site NEC—*see* Neoplasm, by site,
    benign
  unspecified site 211.7
bile duct (M8160/0) 211.5
black (M8372/0) 227.0
bronchial (M8140/1) 235.7
  carcinoid type (M8240/3)—*see* Neoplasm,
    lung, malignant
  cylindroid type (M8200/3)—*see* Neoplasm,
    lung, malignant
ceruminous (M8420/0) 216.2
chief cell (M8321/0) 227.1
  chromophobe (M8270/0)
    (specified site—*see* Neoplasm, by site, benign
    unspecified site 227.3
clear cell (M8310/0)
colloid (M8334/0)
  specified site—*see* Neoplasm, by site, benign
  unspecified site 226
cylindroid type, bronchus (M8200/3)—*see*
  Neoplasm, lung, malignant

Adenoma—*continued*
  duct (M8503/0)
  embryonal (M8191/0)
  endocrine, multiple (M8360/1)
    single specified site—*see* Neoplasm, by site,
      uncertain behavior
    two or more specified sites 237.4
    unspecified site 237.4
  endometrioid (M8380/0)—*see also* Neoplasm,
      by site, benign
    borderline malignancy (M8380/1)—*see*
      Neoplasm, by site, uncertain behavior
  eosinophil (M8280/0)
    specified site—*see* Neoplasm, by site, benign
    unspecified site 227.3
  fetal (M8333/0)
    specified site—*see* Neoplasm, by site, benign
    unspecified site 226
  follicular (M8330/0)
    specified site—*see* Neoplasm, by site, benign
    unspecified site 226
  hepatocellular (M8170/0) 211.5
  Hürthle cell (M8290/0) 226
  intracystic papillary (M8504/0)
  islet cell (functioning) (M8150/0)
    pancreas 211.7
    specified site NEC—*see* Neoplasm, by site,
      benign
    unspecified site 211.7
  liver cell (M8170/0) 211.5
  macrofollicular (M8334/0)
    specified site NEC—*see* Neoplasm, by site,
      benign
    unspecified site 226
  malignant, malignum (M8140/3)—*see*
      Neoplasm, by site, malignant
  mesonephric (M9110/0)
  microfollicular (M8333/0)
    specified site—*see* Neoplasm, by site, benign
    unspecified site 226
  mixed cell (M8323/0)
  monomorphic (M8146/0)
  mucinous (M8480/0)
  mucoid cell (M8300/0)
    specified site—*see* Neoplasm, by site, benign
    unspecified site 227.3
  multiple endocrine (M8360/1)
    single specified site—*see* Neoplasm, by site,
      uncertain behavior
    two or more specified sites 237.4
    unspecified site 237.4
  nipple (M8506/0) 217
  oncocytic (M8290/0)
  oxyphilic (M8290/0)
  papillary (M8260/0)—*see also* Neoplasm, by
      site, benign
    intracystic (M8504/0)
  papillotubular (M8263/0)
  Pick's tubular (M8640/0)
    specified site—*see* Neoplasm, by site, benign
    unspecified site
      female 220
      male 222.0
  pleomorphic (M8940/0)
  polypoid (M8210/0)

Adenoma—*continued*
  prostate (benign) 600.20
    with
      other lower urinary tract symptoms (LUTS)
        600.21
      urinary
        obstruction 600.21
        retention 600.21
  rete cell 222.0
  sebaceous, sebaceum (gland) (senile)
      (M8410/0)—*see also* Neoplasm, skin,
      benign
    disseminata 759.5
  Sertoli cell (M8640/0)
    specified site—*see* Neoplasm, by site, benign
    unspecified site
      female 220
      male 222.0
  skin appendage (M8390/0)—*see* Neoplasm,
      skin, benign
  sudoriferous gland (M8400/0)—*see* Neoplasm,
      skin, benign
  sweat gland or duct (M8400/0)—*see* Neoplasm,
      skin, benign
  testicular (M8640/0)
    specified site—*see* Neoplasm, by site, benign
    unspecified site
      female 220
      male 222.0
  thyroid 226
  trabecular (M8190/0)
  tubular (M8211/0)—*see also* Neoplasm, by site,
      benign
    papillary (M8460/3)
    Pick's (M8640/0)
      specified site—*see* Neoplasm, by site, benign
      unspecified site
        female 220
        male 222.0
  tubulovillous (M8263/0)
  villoglandular (M8263/0)
  villous (M8261/1)—*see* Neoplasm, by site,
      uncertain behavior
  water-clear cell (M8322/0) 227.1
  wolffian duct (M9110/0)
Adenomatosis (M8220/0)
  endocrine (multiple) (M8360/1)
    single specified site—*see* Neoplasm, by site,
      uncertain behavior
    two or more specified sites 237.4
    unspecified site 237.4
  erosive of nipple (M8506/0) 217
  pluriendocrine—*see* Adenomatosis, endocrine
  pulmonary (M8250/1) 235.7
    malignant (M8250/3)—*see* Neoplasm, lung,
      malignant
  specified site—*see* Neoplasm, by site, benign
  unspecified site 211.3
Adenomatous
  cyst, thyroid (gland)—*see* Goiter, nodular
  goiter (nontoxic) (*see also* Goiter, nodular)
      241.9
    toxic or with hyperthyroidism 242.3
Adenomyoma (M8932/0)—*see also* Neoplasm,
    by site, benign
  prostate 600.20
    with
      other lower urinary tract symptoms (LUTS)
        600.21
      urinary
        obstruction 600.21
        retention 600.21

Adenomyometritis 617.0
Adenomyosis (uterus) (internal) 617.0
Adenopathy (lymph gland) 785.6
  inguinal 785.6
  mediastinal 785.6
  mesentery 785.6
  syphilitic (secondary) 091.4
    tracheobronchial 785.6
  tuberculous (*see also* Tuberculosis) 012.1
    primary, progressive 010.8
  tuberculous (*see also* Tuberculosis, lymph
    gland) 017.2
    tracheobronchial 012.1
      primary, progressive 010.8
Adenopharyngitis 462
Adenophlegmon 683
Adenosalpingitis 614.1
Adenosarcoma (M8960/3) 189.0
Adenosclerosis 289.3
Adenosis
  breast (sclerosing) 610.2
  vagina, congenital 752.49
Adentia (complete) (partial) (*see also* Absence,
  teeth) 520.0
Adherent
  labium (minus) 624.4
  pericardium (nonrheumatic) 423.1
    rheumatic 393
  placenta 667.0
    with hemorrhage 666.0
  prepuce 605
  scar (skin) NEC 709.2
  tendon in scar 709.2
**Adhesion(s), adhesive (postinfectional)(postop-
erative)**
  abdominal (wall) (*see also* Adhesions,
    peritoneum) 568.0
  amnion to fetus 658.8
    affecting fetus or newborn 762.8
  appendix 543.9
  arachnoiditis—*see* Meningitis
  auditory tube (Eustachian) 381.89
  bands—*see also* Adhesions, peritoneum
    cervix 622.3
    uterus 621.5
  bile duct (any) 576.8
  bladder (sphincter) 596.8
  bowel (*see also* Adhesions, peritoneum) 568.0
  cardiac 423.1
    rheumatic 398.99
  cecum (*see also* Adhesions, peritoneum) 568.0
  cervicovaginal 622.3
    congenital 752.49
    postpartal 674.8
      old 622.3
  cervix 622.3
  clitoris 624.4
  colon (*see also* Adhesions, peritoneum) 568.0
  common duct 576.8
  congenital—*see also* Anomaly, specified type
    NEC
    fingers (*see also* Syndactylism, fingers)
      755.11
    labium (majus) (minus) 752.49
    omental, anomalous 751.4
    ovary 752.0
    peritoneal 751.4
    toes (*see also* Syndactylism, toes) 755.13
    tongue (to gum or roof of mouth) 750.12

Adhesion(s)—*continued*
  conjunctiva (acquired) (localized) 372.62
    congenital 743.63
    extensive 372.63
  cornea—*see* Opacity, cornea
  cystic duct 575.8
  diaphragm (*see also* Adhesions, peritoneum)
    568.0
  due to foreign body—*see* Foreign body
  duodenum (*see also* Adhesions, peritoneum)
    568.0
    with obstruction 537.3
  ear, middle—*see* Adhesions, middle ear
  epididymis 608.89
  epidural—*see* Adhesions, meninges
  epiglottis 478.79
  Eustachian tube 381.89
  eyelid 374.46
    postoperative 997.99
      surgically created V45.69
  gallbladder (*see also* Disease, gallbladder) 575.8
  globe 360.89
  heart 423.1
    rheumatic 398.99
  ileocecal (coil) (*see also* Adhesions,
    peritoneum) 568.0
  ileum (*see also* Adhesions, peritoneum) 568.0
  intestine (postoperative) (*see also* Adhesions,
    peritoneum) 568.0
    with obstruction 560.81
      with hernia—*see also* Hernia, by site, with
        obstruction
        gangrenous—*see* Hernia, by site, with
          gangrene
  intra-abdominal (*see also* Adhesions,
    peritoneum) 568.0
  iris 364.70
    to corneal graft 996.79
  joint (*see also* Ankylosis) 718.5
  kidney 593.89
  labium (majus) (minus), congenital 752.49
  liver 572.8
  lung 511.0
  mediastinum 519.3
  meninges 349.2
    cerebral (any) 349.2
      congenital 742.4
    congenital 742.8
    spinal (any) 349.2
      congenital 742.59
    tuberculous (cerebral) (spinal) (*see also*
      Tuberculosis, meninges) 013.0
  mesenteric (*see also* Adhesions, peritoneum)
    568.0
  middle ear (fibrous) 385.10
    drum head 385.19
      to
        incus 385.11
        promontorium 385.13
        stapes 385.12
    specified NEC 385.19
  nasal (septum) (to turbinates) 478.19
  nerve NEC 355.9
    spinal 355.9
      root 724.9
        cervical NEC 723.4
        lumbar NEC 724.4
        lumbosacral 724.4
        thoracic 724.4
  ocular muscle 378.60

Adhesion(s)—*continued*
  omentum (*see also* Adhesions, peritoneum)
    568.0
  organ or site, congenital NEC—*see* Anomaly,
    specified type NEC
  ovary 614.6
    congenital (to cecum, kidney, or omentum)
      752.0
  parauterine 614.6
  parovarian 614.6
  pelvic (peritoneal)
    female 614.6
    male (*see also* Adhesions, peritoneum) 568.0
    postpartal (old) 614.6
    tuberculous (*see also* Tuberculosis) 016.9
  penis to scrotum (congenital) 752.69
  periappendiceal (*see also* Adhesions,
    peritoneum) 568.0
  pericardium (nonrheumatic) 423.1
    rheumatic 393
    tuberculous (*see also* Tuberculosis) 017.9
      [420.0]
  pericholecystic 575.8
  perigastric (*see also* Adhesions, peritoneum)
    568.0
  periovarian 614.6
  periprostatic 602.8
  perirectal (*see also* Adhesions, peritoneum)
    568.0
  perirenal 593.89
  peritoneum, peritoneal (fibrous) (postoperative)
    568.0
    with obstruction (intestinal) 560.81
      with hernia—*see also* Hernia, by site, with
        obstruction
        gangrenous—*see* Hernia, by site, with
          gangrene
      duodenum 537.3
    congenital 751.4
    female, (postoperative) (postinfective) 614.6
    pelvic, female 614.6
    pelvic, male 568.0
    postpartal, pelvic 614.6
    to uterus 614.6
  peritubal 614.6
  periureteral 593.89
  periuterine 621.5
  perivesical 596.8
  perivesicular (seminal vesicle) 608.89
  pleura, pleuritic 511.0
    tuberculous (*see also* Tuberculosis, pleura)
      012.0
  pleuropericardial 511.0
  postoperative (gastrointestinal tract) (*See also*
    Adhesions, peritoneum) 568.0
    eyelid 997.99
      surgically created V45.69
    urethra 598.2
  postpartal, old 624.4
  preputial, prepuce 605
  pulmonary 511.0
  pylorus (*see also* Adhesions, peritoneum) 568.0
  Rosenmüller's fossa 478.29
  sciatic nerve 355.0
  seminal vesicle 608.89
  shoulder (joint) 726.0
  sigmoid flexure (*see also* Adhesions,
    peritoneum) 568.0
  spermatic cord (acquired) 608.89
    congenital 752.89

Adhesion(s)—*continued*
  spinal canal 349.2
    nerve 355.9
      root 724.9
        cervical NEC 723.4
        lumbar NEC 724.4
        lumbosacral 724.4
        thoracic 724.4
  stomach (*see also* Adhesions, peritoneum) 568.0
  subscapular 726.2
  tendonitis 726.90
    shoulder 726.0
  testicle 608.89
  tongue (congenital) (to gum or roof of mouth)
    750.12
    acquired 529.8
  trachea 519.19
  tubo-ovarian 614.6
  tunica vaginalis 608.89
  ureter 593.89
  uterus 621.5
    to abdominal wall 614.6
      in pregnancy or childbirth 654.4
        affecting fetus or newborn 763.89
  vagina (chronic) (postoperative) (postradiation)
    623.2
  vaginitis (congenital) 752.49
  vesical 596.8
  vitreous 379.29
Adie (-Holmes) syndrome (tonic pupillary
  reaction) 379.46
Adiponecrosis neonatorum 778.1
Adiposa dolorosa 272.8
Adiposalgia 272.8
Adiposis 278.0
  cerebralis 253.8
  dolorosa 272.8
  tuberosa simplex 272.8
Adiposity 278.02
  heart (*see also* Degeneration, myocardial) 429.1
  localized 278.1
Adiposogenital dystrophy 253.8
Adjustment
  prosthesis or other device—*see* Fitting of
  reaction—*see* Reaction, adjustment
Administration, prophylactic
  antibiotics V07.39
  antitoxin, any V07.2
  antivenin V07.2
  chemotherapeutic agent NEC V07.39
  chemotherapy NEC V07.39
  diphtheria antitoxin V07.2
  fluoride V07.31
  gamma globulin V07.2
  immune sera (gamma globulin) V07.2
  passive immunization agent V07.2
  RhoGAM V07.2
Admission (encounter)
  as organ donor—*see* Donor
  by mistake V68.9
  for
    adequacy testing (for)
      hemodialysis V56.31
      peritoneal dialysis V56.32
    adjustment (of)
      artificial
        arm (complete) (partial) V52.0
        eye V52.2
        leg (complete) (partial) V52.1
      brain neuropacemaker V53.02

Admission—*continued*
  for —*continued*
    adjustment (of)—*continued*
      breast
        implant V52.4
          exchange (different material) (different
            size) V52.4
        prosthesis V52.4
      cardiac device V53.39
        defibrillator, automatic implantable
          V53.32
        pacemaker V53.31
          carotid sinus V53.39
      catheter
        non-vascular V58.82
        vascular V58.81
      cerebral ventricle (communicating) shunt
        V53.01
      colostomy belt V53.5
      contact lenses V53.1
      cystostomy device V53.6
      dental prosthesis V52.3
      device, unspecified type V53.90
        abdominal V53.59
        cardiac V53.39
          defibrillator, automatic implantable
            V53.32
          pacemaker V53.31
            carotid sinus V53.39
        cerebral ventricle (communicating) shunt
          V53.01
        gastrointestinal NEC V53.59
        insulin pump V53.91
        intestinal V53.50
        intrauterine contraceptive V25.1
        nervous system V53.09
        orthodontic V53.4
        other device V53.99
        prosthetic V52.9
          breast V52.4
          dental V52.3
          eye V52.2
          specified type NEC V52.8
        special senses V53.09
        substitution
          auditory V53.09
          nervous system V53.09
          visual V53.09
        urinary V53.6
      dialysis catheter
        extracorporeal V56.1
        peritoneal V56.2
      diaphragm (contraceptive) V25.02
      gastric lap band V53.51
      gastrointestinal applicance and device NEC
        V53.59
      growth rod V54.02
      hearing aid V53.2
      ileostomy device V53.5
      intestinal appliance and device V53.50
      intrauterine contraceptive device V25.1
      neuropacemaker (brain) (peripheral nerve)
        (spinal cord) V53.02
      orthodontic device V53.4
      orthopedic (device) V53.7
        brace V53.7
        cast V53.7
        shoes V53.7

Admission—*continued*
  for —*continued*
    adjustment (of)—*continued*
      pacemaker
        brain V53.02
        cardiac V53.31
        carotid sinus V53.39
        peripheral nerve V53.02
        spinal cord V53.02
      prosthesis V52.9
        arm (complete) (partial) V52.0
        breast V52.4
        dental V52.3
        eye V52.2
        leg (complete) (partial) V52.1
        specified type NEC V52.8
      spectacles V53.1
      wheelchair V53.8
    adoption referral or proceedings V68.89
    aftercare (*see also* Aftercare) V58.9
      cardiac pacemaker V53.31
      chemotherapy (oral) (intravenous) V58.11
      dialysis
        extracorporeal (renal) V56.0
        peritoneal V56.8
        renal V56.0
      fracture (*see also* Aftercare, fracture) V54.9
      medical NEC V58.89
      organ transplant V58.44
      orthopedic V54.9
        specified type NEC V54.89
      pacemaker device
        brain V53.02
        cardiac V53.31
        carotid sinus V53.39
        nervous system V53.02
        spinal cord V53.02
      postoperative NEC V58.49
        wound closure, planned V58.41
      postpartum
        immediately after delivery V24.0
        routine follow-up V24.2
      postradiation V58.0
      radiation therapy V58.0
      removal of
        non-vascular catheter V58.82
        vascular catheter V58.81
        specified NEC V58.89
          removal of vascular catheter V58.81
        surgical NEC V58.49
          wound closure, planned V58.41
    antineoplastic
      chemotherapy (oral) (intravenous) V58.11
      immunotherapy V58.12
    assisted reproductive fertility procedure cycle
      V26.81
    artificial insemination V26.1
    attention to artificial opening (of) V55.9
      artificial vagina V55.7
      colostomy V55.3
      cystostomy V55.5
      enterostomy V55.4
      gastrostomy V55.1
      ileostomy V55.2
      jejunostomy V55.4
      nephrostomy V55.6
      specified site NEC V55.8
        intestinal tract V55.4
        urinary tract V55.6
      tracheostomy V55.0
      ureterostomy V55.6
      urethrostomy V55.6

Admission—*continued*
  for —*continued*
    battery replacement
      cardiac pacemaker V53.31
    blood typing V72.86
      Rh typing V72.86
    boarding V65.0
    breast
      augmentation or reduction V50.1
      implant exchange (different material)
          (different size) V52.4
      reconstruction following mastectomy V51.0
      removal
        prophylactic V50.41
        tissue expander without synchronous
            insertion of permanent implant V52.4
    change of
      cardiac pacemaker (battery) V53.31
      carotid sinus pacemaker V53.39
      catheter in artificial opening—*see* Attention
          to, artificial, opening
      drains V58.49
      dressing
        wound V58.30
          nonsurgical V58.30
          surgical V58.31
      fixation device
        external V54.89
        internal V54.01
      Kirschner wire V54.89
      neuropacemaker device (brain) (peripheral
          nerve) (spinal cord) V53.02
      nonsurgical wound dressing V58.30
      pacemaker device
        brain V53.02
        cardiac V53.31
        carotid sinus V53.39
        nervous system V53.02
      plaster cast V54.89
      splint, external V54.89
      Steinmann pin V54.89
      surgical wound dressing V58.31
      traction device V54.89
      wound packing V58.30
        nonsurgical V58.30
        surgical V58.31
    checkup only V70.0
    chemotherapy, (oral) (intravenous)
        antineoplastic V58.11
    circumcision, ritual or routine (in absence of
        medical indication) V50.2
    clinical research investigation (control)
        (normal comparison) (participant) V70.7
    closure of artificial opening—*see* Attention to,
        artificial, opening
    contraceptive
      counseling V25.09
        emergency V25.03
        postcoital V25.03
      management V25.9
        specified type NEC V25.8
    convalescence following V66.9
      chemotherapy V66.2
      psychotherapy V66.3
      radiotherapy V66.1
      surgery V66.0
      treatment (for) V66.5
        combined V66.6
        fracture V66.4
        mental disorder NEC V66.3
        specified condition NEC V66.5

Admission—*continued*
  for —*continued*
    cosmetic surgery NEC V50.1
      breast reconstruction following mastectomy
          V51.0
      following healed injury or operation V51.8
    counseling (*see also* Counseling) V65.40
      without complaint or sickness V65.49
      contraceptive management V25.09
        emergency V25.03
        postcoital V25.03
      dietary V65.3
      exercise V65.41
      fertility preservation (prior to cancer
          therapy) (prior to surgical removal of
          gonads) V26.42
      for
        nonattending third party V65.19
        pediatric
          pre-adoption visit for adoptive parent(s)
              V65.11
          pre-birth visit for expectant parent(s)
              V65.11
        victim of abuse
          child V61.21
          partner or spouse V61.11
      genetic V26.33
      gonorrhea V65.45
      HIV V65.44
      human immunodeficiency virus V65.44
      injury prevention V65.43
      insulin pump training V65.46
      natural family planning
        procreative V26.41
        to avoid pregnancy V25.04
      procreative management V26.49
        using natural family planning V26.41
      sexually transmitted disease NEC V65.45
        HIV V65.44
      specified reason NEC V65.49
      substance use and abuse V65.42
      syphilis V65.45
      victim of abuse
        child V61.21
        partner or spouse V61.11
    desensitization to allergens V07.1
    dialysis V56.0
      catheter
        fitting and adjustment
          extracorporeal V56.1
          peritoneal V56.2
        removal or replacement
          extracorporeal V56.1
          peritoneal V56.2
      extracorporeal (renal) V56.0
      peritoneal V56.8
      renal V56.0
    dietary surveillance and counseling V65.3
    drug monitoring, therapeutic V58.83
    ear piercing V50.3
    elective surgery V50.9
      breast
        augmentation or reduction V50.1
        removal, prophylactic V50.41
        reconstruction following mastectomy
            V51.0
      circumcision, ritual or routine (in absence of
          medical indication) V50.2

Admission—*continued*
for —*continued*
  elective surgery—*continued*
    cosmetic NEC V50.1
      breast reconstruction following mastecomy
        V51.0
      following healed injury or operation V51.8
    ear piercing V50.3
    face-lift V50.1
    hair transplant V50.0
    plastic
      breast reconstruction following mastecomy
        V51.0
      cosmetic NEC V50.1
      following healed injury or operation V51.8
    prophylactic organ removal V50.49
      breast V50.41
      ovary V50.42
    repair of scarred tissue (following healed
      injury or operation) V51.8
    specified type NEC V50.8
  end-of-life care V66.7
  examination (*see also* Examination) V70.9
    administrative purpose NEC V70.3
    adoption V70.3
    allergy V72.7
    antibody response V72.61
    at health care facility V70.0
    athletic team V70.3
    camp V70.3
    cardiovascular, preoperative V72.81
    clinical research investigation (control)
      (participant) V70.7
    dental V72.2
    developmental testing (child) (infant) V20.2
    donor (potential) V70.8
    driver's license V70.3
    ear V72.19
    employment V70.5
    eye V72.0
    follow-up (routine)—*see* Examination,
      follow-up
    for admission to
      old age home V70.3
      school V70.3
    general V70.9
      specified reason NEC V70.8
    gynecological V72.31
    health supervision
      child (over 28 days old) V20.2
      infant (over 28 days old) V20.2
      newborn
        8 to 28 days old V20.32
        under 8 days old V20.31
    hearing V72.19
      following failed hearing screening V72.11
    immigration V70.3
    infant
      8 to 28 days old V20.32
      over 28 days old, routine V20.2
      under 8 days old V20.31
    insurance certification V70.3
    laboratory V72.60
      ordered as part of a routine general
        medical examination V72.62
      pre-operative V72.63
      pre-procedural V72.63
      specified NEC V72.69
    marriage license V70.3
    medical (general) (*see also* Examination,
      medical) V70.9

Admission—*continued*
for —*continued*
  examination—*continued*
    medicolegal reasons V70.4
    naturalization V70.3
    pelvic (annual) (periodic) V72.31
    postpartum checkup V24.2
    pregnancy (possible) (unconfirmed) V72.40
      negative result V72.41
      positive result V72.42
    preoperative V72.84
      cardiovascular V72.81
      respiratory V72.82
      specified NEC V72.83
    preprocedural V72.84
      cardiovascular V72.81
      general physical V72.83
      respiratory V72.82
      specified NEC V72.83
    prior to chemotherapy V72.83
    prison V70.3
    psychiatric (general) V70.2
      requested by authority V70.1
    radiological NEC V72.5
    respiratory, preoperative V72.82
    school V70.3
    screening—*see* Screening
    skin hypersensitivity V72.7
    specified type NEC V72.85
    sport competition V70.3
    vision V72.0
    well baby and child care V20.2
  exercise therapy V57.1
  face-lift, cosmetic reason V50.1
  fertility preservation (prior to cancer therapy)
    (prior to surgical removal of gonads)
    V26.82
  fitting (of)
    artificial
      arm (complete) (partial) V52.0
      eye V52.2
      leg (complete) (partial) V52.1
    biliary drainage tube V58.82
    brain neuropacemaker V53.02
    breast V52.4
      implant V50.1
      prosthesis V52.4
    cardiac pacemaker V53.31
    catheter
      non-vascular V58.82
      vascular V58.81
    cerebral ventricle (communicating) shunt
      V53.01
    chest tube V58.82
    colostomy belt V53.5
    contact lenses V53.1
    cystostomy device V53.6
    dental prosthesis V52.3
    device, unspecified type V53.90
      abdominal V53.59
      cerebral ventricle (communicating) shunt
        V53.01
      gastrointestinal NEC V53.59
      insulin pump V53.91
      intestinal V53.50
      intrauterine contraceptive V25.1
      nervous system V53.09
      orthodontic V53.4
      other device V53.99

Admission—*continued*
for —*continued*
fitting (of)—*continued*
device—*continued*
prosthetic V52.9
breast V52.4
dental V52.3
eye V52.2
special senses V53.09
substitution
auditory V53.09
nervous system V53.09
visual V53.09
diaphragm (contraceptive) V25.02
fistula (sinus tract) drainage tube V58.82
gastric lap band V53.51
gastrointestinal appliance and device NEC
V53.59
growth rod V54.02
hearing aid V53.2
ileostomy device V53.5
intestinal appliance and device V53.50
intrauterine contraceptive device V25.1
neuropacemaker (brain) (peripheral nerve)
(spinal cord) V53.02
orthodontic device V53.4
orthopedic (device) V53.7
brace V53.7
cast V53.7
shoes V53.7
pacemaker
brain V53.02
cardiac V53.31
carotid sinus V53.39
spinal cord V53.02
pleural drainage tube V58.82
portacath V58.81
prosthesis V52.9
arm (complete) (partial) V52.0
breast V52.4
dental V52.3
eye V52.2
leg (complete) (partial) V52.1
specified type NEC V52.8
spectacles V53.1
wheelchair V53.8
follow-up examination (routine) (following)
V67.9
cancer chemotherapy V67.2
chemotherapy V67.2
high-risk medication NEC V67.51
injury NEC V67.59
psychiatric V67.3
psychotherapy V67.3
radiotherapy V67.1
specified surgery NEC V67.09
surgery V67.00
treatment (for) V67.9
combined V67.6
fracture V67.4
involving high-risk medication NEC
V67.51
mental disorder V67.3
specified NEC V67.59
vaginal pap smear V67.01
hair transplant, for cosmetic reason V50.0
health advice, education, or instruction V65.4
hearing conservation and treatment V72.12
hormone replacement therapy
(postmenopausal) V07.4
hospice care V66.7

Admission—*continued*
for —*continued*
immunizations (childhood) appropriate for age
V20.2
immunotherapy, antineoplastic V58.12
in vitro fertilization cycle V26.81
insertion (of)
subdermal implantable contraceptive V25.5
insulin pump titration V53.91
insulin pump training V65.46
intrauterine device
insertion V25.1
management V25.42
investigation to determine further disposition
V63.8
isolation V07.0
issue of
disability examination certificate V68.01
medical certificate NEC V68.09
repeat prescription NEC V68.1
contraceptive device NEC V25.49
kidney dialysis V56.0
lengthening of growth rod V54.02
mental health evaluation V70.2
requested by authority V70.1
natural family planning counseling and advice
procreative V26.41
to avoid pregnancy V25.04
nonmedical reason NEC V68.89
nursing care evaluation V63.8
observation (without need for further medical
care) (*see also* Observation) V71.9
accident V71.4
alleged rape or seduction V71.5
criminal assault V71.6
following accident V71.4
at work V71.3
foreign body ingestion V71.89
growth and development variations,
childhood V21.0
inflicted injury NEC V71.6
ingestion of deleterious agent or foreign
body V71.89
injury V71.6
malignant neoplasm V71.1
mental disorder V71.09
newborn—*see* Observation, suspected
condition, newborn
rape V71.5
specified NEC V71.89
suspected
abuse V71.81
accident V71.4
at work V71.3
benign neoplasm V71.89
cardiovascular V71.7
disorder V71.9
exposure
anthrax V71.82
biological agent NEC V71.83
SARS V71.83
heart V71.7
inflicted injury NEC V71.6
malignant neoplasm V71.1

Admission—*continued*
  for —*continued*
    observation—*continued*
      maternal and fetal problem not found
        amniotic cavity and membrane V89.01
        cervical shortening V89.05
        fetal anomaly V89.03
        fetal growth V89.04
        oligohydramnios V89.01
        other specified NEC V89.09
        placenta V89.02
        polyhydramnios V89.01
      mental NEC V71.09
      neglect V71.81
      specified condition NEC V71.89
      tuberculosis V71.2
     tuberculosis V71.2
    occupational therapy V57.21
    organ transplant, donor—*see* Donor
    ovary, ovarian removal, prophylactic V50.42
    palliative care V66.7
    Papanicolaou smear
     cervix V76.2
      for suspected malignant neoplasm V76.2
        no disease found V71.1
      routine, as part of gynecological
        examination V72.31
      to confirm findings of recent normal smear
        following initial abnormal smear
        V72.32
     vaginal V76.47
      following hysterectomy for malignant
        condition V67.01
    passage of sounds or bougie in artificial
      opening—*see* Attention to, artificial, opening
    paternity testing V70.4
    peritoneal dialysis V56.8
    physical therapy NEC V57.1
    plastic surgery
     breast reconstruction following mastectomy
      V51.0
     cosmetic NEC V50.1
     following healed injury or operation V51.8
    postmenopausal hormone replacement therapy
      V07.4
    postpartum observation
     immediately after delivery V24.0
     routine follow-up V24.2
    poststerilization (for restoration) V26.0
    procreative management V26.9
     assisted reproductive fertility procedure
      cycle V26.81
     in vitro fertilization cycle V26.81
     specified type NEC V26.89
    prophylactic
     administration of
      antibiotics V07.39
      antitoxin, any V07.2
      antivenin V07.2
      chemotherapeutic agent NEC V07.39
      chemotherapy NEC V07.39
      diphtheria antitoxin V07.2
      fluoride V07.31
      gamma globulin V07.2
      immune sera (gamma globulin) V07.2
      RhoGAM V07.2
      tetanus antitoxin V07.2
     breathing exercises V57.0
     chemotherapy NEC V07.39
     fluoride V07.31

Admission—*continued*
  for —*continued*
    prophylactic—*continued*
     measure V07.9
      specified type NEC V07.8
     organ removal V50.49
      breast V50.41
      ovary V50.42
    psychiatric examination (general) V70.2
     requested by authority V70.1
    radiation management V58.0
    radiotherapy V58.0
    reconstruction following mastectomy V51.0
    reforming of artificial opening—*see* Attention
      to, artificial, opening
    rehabilitation V57.9
     multiple types V57.89
     occupational V57.21
     orthoptic V57.4
     orthotic V57.81
     physical NEC V57.1
     specified type NEC V57.89
     speech (-language) V57.3
     vocational V57.22
    removal of
     breast tissue expander without synchronous
      insertion of permanent implant V52.4
     cardiac pacemaker V53.31
     cast (plaster) V54.89
     catheter from artificial opening—*see*
      Attention to, artificial, opening
     cerebral ventricle (communicating) shunt
      V53.01
     cystostomy catheter V55.5
     device
      cerebral ventricle (communicating) shunt
       V53.01
      fixation
       external V54.89
       internal V54.01
      intrauterine contraceptive V25.42
      traction, external V54.89
     drains V58.49
     dressing
      wound V58.30
       nonsurgical V58.30
       surgical V58.31
     fixation device
      external V54.89
      internal V54.01
     intrauterine contraceptive device V25.42
     Kirschner wire V54.89
     neuropacemaker (brain) (peripheral nerve)
      (spinal cord) V53.02
     nonsurgical wound dressing V58.30
     orthopedic fixation device
      external V54.89
      internal V54.01
     pacemaker device
      brain V53.02
      cardiac V53.31
      carotid sinus V53.39
      nervous system V53.02
     plaster cast V54.89
     plate (fracture) V54.01
     rod V54.01
     screw (fracture) V54.01
     splint, traction V54.89
     staples V58.32
     Steinmann pin V54.89
     subdermal implantable contraceptive V25.43

Admission—*continued*
  for —*continued*
    vaccination—*continued*
      smallpox V04.1
      specified type NEC V05.8
      Streptococcus pneumoniae
        [pneumococcus] V03.82
        with
          influenza V06.6
      tetanus toxoid alone V03.7
        with diphtheria [Td] [DT] V06.5
          and pertussis (DTP) (DTaP) V06.1
      tuberculosis (BCG) V03.2
      tularemia V03.4
      typhoid alone V03.1
        with diphtheria-tetanus-pertussis (TAB +
          DTP) V06.2
      typhoid-paratyphoid alone (TAB) V03.1
      typhus V05.8
      varicella V05.4
      viral encephalitis, arthropod-borne V05.0
      viral hepatitis V05.3
      yellow fever V04.4
    vasectomy V25.2
    vasoplasty for previous sterilization V26.0
    vision examination V72.0
    vocational therapy V57.22
    waiting period for admission to other facility
      V63.2
      undergoing social agency investigation
        V63.8
    well baby and child care V20.2
    x-ray of chest
      for suspected tuberculosis V71.2
      routine V72.5
Adnexitis (suppurative) (*see also*
  Salpingo-oophoritis) 614.2
Adolescence NEC V21.2
Adoption
  agency referral V68.89
  examination V70.3
  held for V68.89
Adrenal gland —*see* condition
Adrenalism 255.9
  tuberculous (*see also* Tuberculosis) 017.6
Adrenalitis, adrenitis 255.8
  meningococcal hemorrhagic 036.3
Adrenarche, precocious 259.1
Adrenocortical syndrome 255.2
Adrenogenital syndrome (acquired) (congenital)
  255.2
  iatrogenic, fetus or newborn 760.79
Adrenoleukodystrophy 277.86
  neonatal 277.86
  x-linked 277.86
Adrenomyeloneuropathy 277.86
Adventitious bursa —*see* Bursitis
Adynamia (episodica) (hereditary) (periodic)
  359.3
Adynamic
  ileus or intestine (*see also* ileus) 560.1
  ureter 753.22
Aeration lung imperfect, newborn 770.5
Aerobullosis 993.3
Aerocele —*see* Embolism, air
Aerodermectasia
  subcutaneous (traumatic) 958.7
    surgical 998.81
  surgical 998.81

Aerodontalgia 993.2
Aeroembolism 993.3
Aerogenes capsulatus infection (*see also*
  Gangrene, gas) 040.0
Aero-otitis media 993.0
Aerophagy, aerophagia 306.4
  psychogenic 306.4
Aerosinusitis 993.1
Aerotitis 993.0
Affection, affections —*see also* Disease
  sacroiliac (joint), old 724.6
  shoulder region NEC 726.2
Afibrinogenemia 286.3
  acquired 286.6
  congenital 286.3
  postpartum 666.3
African
  sleeping sickness 086.5
  tick fever 087.1
  trypanosomiasis 086.5
    Gambian 086.3
    Rhodesian 086.4
Aftercare V58.9
  amputation stump V54.89
  artificial openings—*see* Attention to, artificial,
    opening
  blood transfusion without reported diagnosis
    V58.2
  breathing exercise V57.0
  cardiac device V53.39
    defibrillator, automatic implantable V53.32
    pacemaker V53.31
      carotid sinus V53.39
  carotid sinus pacemaker V53.39
  cerebral ventricle (communicating) shunt
    V53.01
  chemotherapy (oral) (intravenous) session
    (adjunctive) (maintenance) V58.11
  defibrillator, automatic implantable cardiac
    V53.32
  exercise (remedial) (therapeutic) V57.1
    breathing V57.0
  extracorporeal dialysis (intermittent) (treatment)
    V56.0
  following surgery NEC V58.49
    wound closure, planned V58.41
    for
      injury V58.43
      neoplasm V58.42
      organ transplant V58.44
      trauma V58.43
    joint replacement V54.81
    of
      circulatory system V58.73
      digestive system V58.75
      genital organs V58.76
      genitourinary system V58.76
      musculoskeletal system V58.78
      nervous system V58.72
      oral cavity V58.75
      respiratory system V58.74
      sense organs V58.71
      skin V58.77
      subcutaneous tissue V58.77
      teeth V58.75
      urinary system V58.76
    spinal —*see* Aftercare, following surgery, of,
      specified body system

Agenesis —*see also* Absence, by site, congenital
  acoustic nerve 742.8
  adrenal (gland) 759.1
  alimentary tract (complete) (partial) NEC 751.8
    lower 751.2
    upper 750.8
  anus, anal (canal) 751.2
  aorta 747.22
  appendix 751.2
  arm (complete) (partial) (*see also* Deformity,
    reduction, upper limb) 755.20
  artery (peripheral) NEC (*see also* Anomaly,
    peripheral vascular system) 747.60
    brain 747.81
    coronary 746.85
    pulmonary 747.3
    umbilical 747.5
  auditory (canal) (external) 744.01
  auricle (ear) 744.01
  bile, biliary duct or passage 751.61
  bone NEC 756.9
  brain 740.0
    specified part 742.2
  breast 757.6
  bronchus 748.3
  canaliculus lacrimalis 743.65
  carpus NEC (*see also* Deformity, reduction,
    upper limb) 755.28
  cartilage 756.9
  cecum 751.2
  cerebellum 742.2
  cervix 752.49
  chin 744.89
  cilia 743.63
  circulatory system, part NEC 747.89
  clavicle 755.51
  clitoris 752.49
  coccyx 756.13
  colon 751.2
  corpus callosum 742.2
  cricoid cartilage 748.3
  diaphragm (with hernia) 756.6
  digestive organ(s) or tract (complete) (partial)
    NEC 751.8
    lower 751.2
    upper 750.8
  ductus arteriosus 747.89
  duodenum 751.1
  ear NEC 744.09
    auricle 744.01
    lobe 744.21
  ejaculatory duct 752.89
  endocrine (gland) NEC 759.2
  epiglottis 748.3
  esophagus 750.3
  Eustachian tube 744.24
  extrinsic muscle, eye 743.69
  eye 743.00
    adnexa 743.69
  eyelid (fold) 743.62
  face
    bones NEC 756.0
    specified part NEC 744.89
  fallopian tube 752.19
  femur NEC (*see also* Absence, femur,
    congenital) 755.34
  fibula NEC (*see also* Absence, fibula,
    congenital) 755.37
  finger NEC (*see also* Absence, finger,
    congenital) 755.29

Agenesis—*continued*
  foot (complete) (*see also* Deformity, reduction,
    lower limb) 755.31
  gallbladder 751.69
  gastric 750.8
  genitalia, genital (organ)
    female 752.89
      external 752.49
      internal NEC 752.89
    male 752.89
      penis 752.69
  glottis 748.3
  gonadal 758.6
  hair 757.4
  hand (complete) (*see also* Deformity, reduction,
    upper limb) 755.21
  heart 746.89
    valve NEC 746.89
      aortic 746.89
      mitral 746.89
      pulmonary 746.01
  hepatic 751.69
  humerus NEC (*see also* Absence, humerus,
    congenital) 755.24
  hymen 752.49
  ileum 751.1
  incus 744.04
  intestine (small) 751.1
    large 751.2
  iris (dilator fibers) 743.45
  jaw 524.09
  jejunum 751.1
  kidney(s) (partial) (unilateral) 753.0
  labium (majus) (minus) 752.49
  labyrinth, membranous 744.05
  lacrimal apparatus (congenital) 743.65
  larynx 748.3
  leg NEC (*see also* Deformity, reduction, lower
    limb) 755.30
  lens 743.35
  limb (complete) (partial) (*see also* Deformity,
    reduction) 755.4
    lower NEC 755.30
    upper 755.20
  lip 750.26
  liver 751.69
  lung (bilateral) (fissures) (lobe) (unilateral)
    748.5
  mandible 524.09
  maxilla 524.09
  metacarpus NEC 755.28
  metatarsus NEC 755.38
  muscle (any) 756.81
  musculoskeletal system NEC 756.9
  nail(s) 757.5
  neck, part 744.89
  nerve 742.8
  nervous system, part NEC 742.8
  nipple 757.6
  nose 748.1
  nuclear 742.8
  organ
    of Corti 744.05
    or site not listed—*see* Anomaly, specified type
      NEC
  osseous meatus (ear) 744.03
  ovary 752.0
  oviduct 752.19
  pancreas 751.7
  parathyroid (gland) 759.2
  patella 755.64

Agenesis—*continued*
pelvic girdle (complete) (partial) 755.69
penis 752.69
pericardium 746.89
perineal body 756.81
pituitary (gland) 759.2
prostate 752.89
pulmonary
    artery 747.3
    trunk 747.3
    vein 747.49
punctum lacrimale 743.65
radioulnar NEC (*see also* Absence, forearm,
    congenital) 755.25
radius NEC (*see also* Absence, radius,
    congenital) 755.26
rectum 751.2
renal 753.0
respiratory organ NEC 748.9
rib 756.3
roof of orbit 742.0
round ligament 752.89
sacrum 756.13
salivary gland 750.21
scapula 755.59
scrotum 752.89
seminal duct or tract 752.89
septum
    atrial 745.69
    between aorta and pulmonary artery 745.0
    ventricular 745.3
shoulder girdle (complete) (partial) 755.59
skull (bone) 756.0
    with
        anencephalus 740.0
        encephalocele 742.0
        hydrocephalus 742.3
            with spina bifida (*see also* Spina bifida)
                741.0
        microcephalus 742.1
spermatic cord 752.89
spinal cord 742.59
spine 756.13
    lumbar 756.13
        isthmus 756.11
        pars articularis 756.11
spleen 759.0
sternum 756.3
stomach 750.7
tarsus NEC 755.38
tendon 756.81
testicular 752.89
testis 752.89
thymus (gland) 759.2
thyroid (gland) 243
    cartilage 748.3
tibia NEC (*see also* Absence, tibia, congenital)
    755.36
tibiofibular NEC 755.35
toe (complete) (partial) (*see also* Absence, toe,
    congenital) 755.39
tongue 750.11
trachea (cartilage) 748.3
ulna NEC (*see also* Absence, ulna, congenital)
    755.27
ureter 753.4
urethra 753.8
urinary tract NEC 753.8
uterus 752.3
uvula 750.26
vagina 752.49

Agenesis—*continued*
vas deferens 752.89
vein(s) (peripheral) NEC (*see also* Anomaly,
    peripheral vascular system) 747.60
    brain 747.81
    great 747.49
    portal 747.49
    pulmonary 747.49
vena cava (inferior) (superior) 747.49
vermis of cerebellum 742.2
vertebra 756.13
    lumbar 756.13
        isthmus 756.11
        pars articularis 756.11
vulva 752.49
Ageusia (*see also* Disturbance, sensation) 781.1
Aggressiveness 301.3
Aggressive outburst (*see also* Disturbance,
    conduct) 312.0
    in children or adolescents 313.9
Aging skin 701.8
Agitated —*see* condition
Agitation 307.9
    catatonic (*see also* Schizophrenia) 295.2
Aglossia (congenital) 750.11
Aglycogenosis 271.0
Agnail (finger) (with lymphangitis) 681.02
Agnosia (body image) (tactile) 784.69
    verbal 784.69
        auditory 784.69
        developmental 315.8
        secondary to organic lesion 784.69
    visual 368.16
        object 368.16
Agoraphobia 300.22
    with panic disorder 300.21
Agrammatism 784.69
Agranulocytopenia (see also Agranulocytosis)
    288.09
Agranulocytosis (see also Neutropenia) 288.09
    chronic 288.09
    cyclical 288.02
    due to infection 288.04
    genetic 288.01
    infantile 288.01
    periodic 288.02
    pernicious 288.09
Agraphia (absolute) 784.69
    with alexia 784.61
    developmental 315.39
Agrypnia (*see also* Insomnia) 780.52
Ague (*see also* Malaria) 084.6
    brass-founders' 985.8
    dumb 084.6
    tertian 084.1
Agyria 742.2
Ahumada-del Castillo syndrome (nonpuerperal
    galactorrhea and amenorrhea) 253.1
AIDS 042
AIDS-associated retrovirus (disease) (illness) 042
    infection—*see* Human immunodeficiency virus,
        infection
AIDS-associated virus (disease) (illness) 042
    infection—*see* Human immunodeficiency virus,
        infection
AIDS-like disease (illness) (syndrome) 042
AIDS-related complex 042
AIDS-related conditions 042
AIDS-related virus (disease) (illness) 042
    infection—*see* Human immunodeficiency virus,
        infection

AIDS virus (disease) (illness) 042
  infection—*see* Human immunodeficiency virus,
    infection
Ailment, heart —*see* Disease, heart
Ailurophobia 300.29
AIN I [anal intraepithelial neoplasia I]
  (histologically confirmed) 569.44
AIN II [anal intraepithelial neoplasia II]
  (histologically confirmed) 569.44
AIN III [anal intraepithelial neoplasia III]
  230.6
  anal canal 230.5
Ainhum (disease) 136.0
Air
  anterior mediastinum 518.1
  compressed, disease 993.3
  embolism (any site) (artery) (cerebral) 958.0
    with
      abortion—*see* Abortion, by type, with
        embolism
      ectopic pregnancy (*see also* categories
        633.0-633.9) 639.6
      molar pregnancy (*see also* categories
        630-632) 639.6
    due to implanted device—*see* Complications,
      due to (presence of) any device, implant,
      or graft classified to 996.0-996.5 NEC
    following
      abortion 639.6
      ectopic or molar pregnancy 639.6
      infusion, perfusion, or transfusion 999.1
    in pregnancy, childbirth, or puerperium 673.0
    traumatic 958.0
  hunger 786.09
    psychogenic 306.1
  leak (lung) (pulmonary) (thorax) 512.8
    iatrogenic 512.1
    postoperative 512.1
  rarefied, effects of—*see* Effect, adverse, high altitude
  sickness 994.6
Airplane sickness 994.6
Akathisia, acathisia 781.0
  due to drugs 333.99
  neuroleptic-induced acute 333.99
Akinesia algeria 352.6
Akiyami 100.89
Akureyri disease (epidemic neuromyasthenia) 049.8
Alacrima (congenital) 743.65
Alactasia (hereditary) 271.3
Alagille syndrome 759.89
Alalia 784.3
  developmental 315.31
    receptive-expressive 315.32
  secondary to organic lesion 784.3
Alaninemia 270.8
Alastrim 050.1
Albarrán's disease (colibacilluria) 791.9
Albers-Schönberg's disease (marble bones)
  756.52
Albert's disease 726.71
Albinism, albino (choroid) (cutaneous) (eye)
  (generalized) (isolated) (ocular)
  (oculocutaneous) (partial) 270.2
Albinismus 270.2
Albright (-Martin) (-Bantam) disease
  (pseudohypoparathyroidism) 275.49
Albright (-McCune) (-Sternberg) syndrome
  (osteitis fibrosa disseminata) 756.59
Albuminous —*see* condition

Albuminuria, albuminuric (acute) (chronic)
  (subacute) 791.0
  Bence-Jones 791.0
  cardiac 785.9
  complicating pregnancy, childbirth, or
    puerperium 646.2
    with hypertension—*see* Toxemia, of
      pregnancy
    affecting fetus or newborn 760.1
  cyclic 593.6
  gestational 646.2
  gravidarum 646.2
    with hypertension—*see* Toxemia, of
      pregnancy
    affecting fetus or newborn 760.1
  heart 785.9
  idiopathic 593.6
  orthostatic 593.6
  postural 593.6
  pre-eclamptic (mild) 642.4
    affecting fetus or newborn 760.0
    severe 642.5
      affecting fetus or newborn 760.0
  recurrent physiologic 593.6
  scarlatinal 034.1
Albumosuria 791.0
  Bence-Jones 791.0
  myelopathic (M9730/3) 203.0
Alcaptonuria 270.2
Alcohol, alcoholic
  abstinance 291.81
  acute intoxication 305.0
    with dependence 303.0
  addiction (*see also* Alcoholism) 303.9
    maternal
      with suspected fetal damage affecting
        management of pregnancy 655.4
      affecting fetus or newborn 760.71
  amnestic disorder, persisting 291.1
  anxiety 291.89
  brain syndrome, chronic 291.2
  cardiopathy 425.5
  chronic (*see also* Alcoholism) 303.9
  cirrhosis (liver) 571.2
  delirium 291.0
    acute 291.0
    chronic 291.1
    tremens 291.0
    withdrawal 291.0
  dementia NEC 291.2
  deterioration 291.2
  drunkenness (simple) 305.0
  hallucinosis (acute) 291.3
  induced
    circadian rhythm sleep disorder 291.82
    hypersomnia 291.82
    insomnia 291.82
    mental disorder 291.9
      anxiety 291.89
      mood 291.89
      sexual 291.89
      sleep 291.82
      specified type 291.89
    parasomnia 291.82
    persisting
      amnestic disorder 291.1
      dementia 291.2
    psychotic disorder
      with
        delusions 291.5
        hallucinations 291.3
    sleep disorder 291.82

Alcohol, alcoholic—*continued*
insanity 291.9
intoxication (acute) 305.0
  with dependence 303.0
  pathological 291.4
jealousy 291.5
Korsakoff's, Korsakov's, Korsakow's 291.1
liver NEC 571.3
  acute 571.1
  chronic 571.2
mania (acute) (chronic) 291.9
mood 291.89
paranoia 291.5
paranoid (type) psychosis 291.5
pellagra 265.2
poisoning, accidental (acute) NEC 980.9
  specified type of alcohol—*see* Table of drugs
    and chemicals
psychosis (*see also* Psychosis, alcoholic) 291.9
  Korsakoff's, Korsakov's, Korsakow's 291.1
  polyneuritic 291.1
  with
    delusions 291.5
    hallucinations 291.3
related disorder 291.9
withdrawal symptoms, syndrome NEC 291.81
  delirium 291.0
  hallucinosis 291.3
Alcoholism 303.9

*Note—Use the following fifth-digit
subclassification with category 303:*

0 *unspecifhed*
1 *continuous*
2 *episodic*
3 *in remission*

with psychosis (*see also* Psychosis, alcoholic)
    291.9
acute 303.0
chronic 303.9
  with psychosis 291.9
complicating pregnancy, childbirth, or
    puerperium 648.4
affecting fetus or newborn 760.71
history V11.3
Korsakoff's, Korsakov's, Korsakow's 291.1
suspected damage to fetus affecting
    management of pregnancy 655.4
Alder's anomaly or syndrome (leukocyte
    granulation anomaly) 288.2
Alder-Reilly anomaly (leukocyte granulation) 288.2
Aldosteronism (primary) 255.10
  congenital 255.10
  familial type I 255.11
  glucocorticoid-remediable 255.11
  secondary 255.14
Aldosteronoma (M8370/1) 237.2
Aldrich (-Wiskott) syndrome
    (eczema-thrombocytopenia) 279.12
Aleppo boil 085.1
Aleukemic —*see* condition
Aleukia
  congenital 288.09
  hemorrhagica 284.9
    acquired (secondary) 284.89
    congenital 284.09
    idiopathic 284.9
  splenica 289.4
Alexia (congenital) (developmental) 315.01
  secondary to organic lesion 784.61

Algoneurodystrophy 733.7
Algophobia 300.29
Alibert's disease (mycosis fungoides) (M9700/3)
    202.1
Alibert-Bazin disease (M9700/3) 202.1
Alice in Wonderland syndrome 293.89
Alienation, mental (*see also* Psychosis) 298.9
Alkalemia 276.3
Alkalosis 276.3
  metabolic 276.3
    with respiratory acidosis 276.4
  respiratory 276.3
Alkaptonuria 270.2
Allen-Masters syndrome 620.6
Allergic bronchopulmonary aspergillosis 518.6
Allergy, allergic (reaction) 995.3
  air-borne substance (*see also* Fever, hay) 477.9
    specified allergen NEC 477.8
  alveolitis (extrinsic) 495.9
    due to
      Aspergillus clavatus 495.4
      cryptostroma corticale 495.6
      organisms (fungal, thermophilic
        actinomycete, other) growing in
        ventilation (air conditioning systems)
        495.7
    specified type NEC 495.8
  anaphylactic shock 999.4
    due to
      food—*see* Anaphylactic shock, due to, food
  angioneurotic edema 995.1
  animal (cat) (dog) (epidermal) 477.8
    dander 477.2
    hair 477.2
  arthritis (*see also* Arthritis, allergic) 716.2
  asthma—*see* Asthma
  bee sting (anaphylactic shock) 989.5
  biological—*see* Allergy, drug
  bronchial asthma—*see* Asthma
  conjunctivitis (eczematous) 372.14
  dander, animal (cat) (dog) 477.2
  dandruff 477.8
  dermatitis (venenata)—*see* Dermatitis
  diathesis V15.09
  drug, medicinal substance, and biological (any)
    (correct medicinal substance properly
    administered) (external) (internal) 995.27
    wrong substance given or taken NEC 977.9
      specified drug or substance—*see* Table of
        drugs and chemicals
  dust (house) (stock) 477.8
  eczema—*see* Eczema
  endophthalmitis 360.19
  epidermal (animal) 477.8
  existing dental restorative material 525.66
  feathers 477.8
  food (any) (ingested) 693.1
    atopic 691.8
    in contact with skin 692.5
  gastritis 535.4
  gastroenteritis 558.3
  gastrointestinal 558.3
  grain 477.0
  grass (pollen) 477.0
    asthma (*see also* Asthma) 493.0
    hay fever 477.0
  hair, animal (cat) (dog) 477.2
  hay fever (grass) (pollen) (ragweed) (tree) (*see
    also* Fever, hay) 477.9

Allergy, allergic—*continued*
history (of) V15.09
to
    arachnid bite V15.06
    eggs V15.03
    food additives V15.05
    insect bite V15.06
    latex V15.07
    milk products V15.02
    nuts V15.05
      peanuts V15.01
    radiographic dye V15.08
    seafood V15.04
    specified food NEC V15.05
    spider bite V15.06
horse serum—*see* Allergy, serum
inhalant 477.9
    dust 477.8
    pollen 477.0
    specified allergen other than pollen 477.8
kapok 477.8
medicine—*see* Allergy, drug
migraine 339.00
milk protein 558.3
pannus 370.62
pneumonia 518.3
pollen (any) (hay fever) 477.0
    asthma (*see also* Asthma) 493.0
primrose 477.0
primula 477.0
purpura 287.0
ragweed (pollen) (Senecio jacobae) 477.0
    asthma (*see also* Asthma) 493.0
    hay fever 477.0
respiratory (*see also* Allergy, inhalant) 477.9
    due to
      drug—*see* Allergy, drug
      food—*see* Allergy, food
rhinitis (*see also* Fever, hay) 477.9
    due to food 477.1
rose 477.0
Senecio jacobae 477.0
serum (prophylactic) (therapeutic) 999.5
    anaphylactic shock 999.4
shock (anaphylactic)
    due to
      adverse effect of correct medicinal substance
        properly administered 995.0
      food—*see* Anaphylactic shock, due to, food
    from serum or immunization 999.5
      anaphylactic 999.4
sinusitis (*see also* Fever, hay) 477.9
skin reaction 692.9
    specified substance—*see* Dermatitis, due to
tree (any) (hay fever) (pollen) 477.0
    asthma (*see also* Asthma) 493.0
upper respiratory (*see also* Fever, hay) 477.9
urethritis 597.89
urticaria 708.0
vaccine—*see* Allergy, serum
Allescheriosis 117.6
Alligator skin disease (ichthyosis congenita)
    757.1
    acquired 701.1
Allocheiria, allochiria (*see also* Disturbance,
    sensation) 782.0
Almeida's disease (Brazilian blastomycosis) 116.1
Alopecia (atrophicans) (pregnancy) (premature)
    (senile) 704.00
    adnata 757.4
    areata 704.01

Alopecia—*continued*
    celsi 704.01
    cicatrisata 704.09
    circumscripta 704.01
    congenital, congenitalis 757.4
    disseminata 704.01
    effluvium (telogen) 704.02
    febrile 704.09
    generalisata 704.09
    hereditaria 704.09
    marginalis 704.01
    mucinosa 704.09
    postinfectional 704.09
    seborrheica 704.09
    specific 091.82
    syphilitic (secondary) 091.82
    telogen effluvium 704.02
    totalis 704.09
    toxica 704.09
    universalis 704.09
    x-ray 704.09
Alper's disease 330.8
Alpha-lipoproteinemia 272.4
Alpha thalassemia 282.49
Alphos 696.1
Alpine sickness 993.2
Alport's syndrome (hereditary
    hematuria-nephropathy-deafness) 759.89
**ALPS (autoimmune lymphoproliferative
    syndrome)** 279.41
ALTE (apparent life threatening event) in
    newborn and infant 799.82
Alteration (of), altered
    awareness 780.09
      transient 780.02
    consciousness 780.09
      persistent vegetative state 780.03
      transient 780.02
    mental status 780.97
      amnesia (retrograde) 780.93
      memory loss 780.93
Alternaria (infection) 118
Alternating —*see* condition
Altitude, high (effects)—*see* Effect, adverse,
    high altitude
Aluminosis (of lung) 503
Alvarez syndrome (transient cerebral ischemia)
    435.9
Alveolar capillary block syndrome 516.3
Alveolitis
    allergic (extrinsic) 495.9
      due to organisms (fungal, thermophilic
        actinomycete, other) growing in
        ventilation (air conditioning systems)
        495.7
      specified type NEC 495.8
    due to
      Aspergillus clavatus 495.4
      Cryptostroma corticale 495.6
    fibrosing (chronic) (cryptogenic) (lung) 516.3
      idiopathic 516.3
      rheumatoid 714.81
    jaw 526.5
    sicca dolorosa 526.5
Alveolus, alveolar —*see* condition
Alymphocytosis (pure) 279.2
Alymphoplasia, thymic 279.2
Alzheimer's
    dementia (senile)
      with behavioral disturbance 331.0 *[294.11]*
      without behavioral disturbance 331.0 *[294.10]*

Alzheimer's—*continued*
  disease or sclerosis 331.0
    with dementia—*see* Alzheimer's, dementia
Amastia (*see also* Absence, breast) 611.89
Amaurosis (acquired) (congenital) (*see also*
  Blindness) 369.00
  fugax 362.34
  hysterical 300.11
  Leber's (congenital) 362.76
  tobacco 377.34
  uremic—*see* Uremia
Amaurotic familial idiocy (infantile) (juvenile)
  (late) 330.1
Ambisexual 752.7
Amblyopia (acquired) (congenital) (partial) 368.00
  color 368.59
  acquired 368.55
  deprivation 368.02
  ex anopsia 368.00
  hysterical 300.11
  nocturnal 368.60
    vitamin A deficiency 264.5
  refractive 368.03
  strabismic 368.01
  suppression 368.01
  tobacco 377.34
  toxic NEC 377.34
  uremic—*see* Uremia
Ameba, amebic (histolytica)–*see also* Amebiasis
  abscess 006.3
    bladder 006.8
    brain (with liver and lung abscess) 006.5
    liver 006.3
      with
        brain abscess (and lung abscess) 006.5
        lung abscess 006.4
    lung (with liver abscess) 006.4
      with brain abscess 006.5
    seminal vesicle 006.8
    spleen 006.8
  carrier (suspected of) V02.2
  meningoencephalitis
    due to Naegleria (gruberi) 136.29
    primary 136.29
Amebiasis NEC 006.9
  with
    brain abscess (with liver or lung abscess) 006.5
    liver abscess (without mention of brain or lung
      abscess) 006.3
    lung abscess (with liver abscess) 006.4
      with brain abscess 006.5
  acute 006.0
  bladder 006.8
  chronic 006.1
  cutaneous 006.6
  cutis 006.6
  due to organism other than Entamoeba
    histolytica 007.8
  hepatic (*see also* Abscess, liver, amebic) 006.3
  nondysenteric 006.2
  seminal vesicle 006.8
  specified
    organism NEC 007.8
    site NEC 006.8
Ameboma 006.8
Amelia 755.4
  lower limb 755.31
  upper limb 755.21

Ameloblastoma (M9310/0) 213.1
  jaw (bone) (lower) 213.1
    upper 213.0
  long bones (M9261/3)—*see* Neoplasm, bone,
    malignant
  malignant (M9310/3) 170.1
    jaw (bone) (lower) 170.1
      upper 170.0
  mandible 213.1
  tibial (M9261/3) 170.7
Amelogenesis imperfecta 520.5
  nonhereditaria (segmentalis) 520.4
Amenorrhea (primary) (secondary) 626.0
  due to ovarian dysfunction 256.8
  hyperhormonal 256.8
Amentia (*see also* Retardation, mental) 319
  Meynert's (nonalcoholic) 294.0
    alcoholic 291.1
  nevoid 759.6
American
  leishmaniasis 085.5
  mountain tick fever 066.1
  trypanosomiasis—*see* Trypanosomiasis,
    American
Ametropia (*see also* Disorder, accommodation) 367.9
Amianthosis 501
Amimia 784.69
Amino acid
  deficiency 270.9
    anemia 281.4
  metabolic disorder (*see also* Disorder, amino
    acid) 270.9
Aminoaciduria 270.9
  imidazole 270.5
Amnesia (retrograde) 780.93
  auditory 784.69
    developmental 315.31
    secondary to organic lesion 784.69
  dissociative 300.12
  hysterical or dissociative type 300.12
  psychogenic 300.12
  transient global 437.7
Amnestic (confabulatory) syndrome 294.0
  alcohol-induced persisting 291.1
  drug-induced persisting 292.83
  posttraumatic 294.0
Amniocentesis screening (for) V28.2
  alphafetoprotein level, raised V28.1
  chromosomal anomalies V28.0
Amnion, amniotic —*see also* condition
  nodosum 658.8
Amnionitis (complicating pregnancy) 658.4
  affecting fetus or newborn 762.7
Amoral trends 301.7
Amotio retinae (*see also* Detachment, retina) 361.9
Ampulla
  lower esophagus 530.89
  phrenic 530.89
Amputation
  any part of fetus, to facilitate delivery 763.89
  cervix (supravaginal) (uteri) 622.8
    in pregnancy or childbirth 654.6
      affecting fetus or newborn 763.89
  clitoris—*see* Wound, open, clitoris
  congenital
    lower limb 755.31
    upper limb 755.21
  neuroma (traumatic)—*see also* Injury, nerve, by
    site
    surgical complications (late) 997.61
  penis—*see* Amputation, traumatic, penis

Amputation—*continued*
status (without complication)—*see* Absence, by
   site, acquired
stump (surgical)(posttraumatic)
   abnormal, painful, or with complication (late)
      997.60
   healed or old NEC —*see also* Absence, by
      site, acquired
      lower V49.70
      upper V49.60
traumatic (complete) (partial)

> *Note*—*"Complicated" includes traumatic
> amputation with delayed healing, delayed
> treatment, foreign body, or infection.*

arm 887.4
   at or above elbow 887.2
      complicated 887.3
   below elbow 887.0
      complicated 887.1
   both (bilateral) (any level(s)) 887.6
      complicated 887.7
   complicated 887.5
   finger(s) (one or both hands) 886.0
      with thumb(s) 885.0
         complicated 885.1
      complicated 886.1
foot (except toe(s) only) 896.0
   and other leg 897.6
      complicated 897.7
   both (bilateral) 896.2
      complicated 896.3
   complicated 896.1
   toe(s) only (one or both feet) 895.0
      complicated 895.1
genital organ(s) (external) NEC 878.8
   complicated 878.9
hand (except finger(s) only) 887.0
   and other arm 887.6
      complicated 887.7
   both (bilateral) 887.6
      complicated 887.7
   complicated 887.1
   finger(s) (one or both hands) 886.0
      with thumb(s) 885.0
         complicated 885.1
      complicated 886.1
   thumb(s) (with fingers of either hand) 885.0
      complicated 885.1
head 874.9
late effect—*see* Late, effects (of), amputation
leg 897.4
   and other foot 897.6
      complicated 897.7
   at or above knee 897.2
      complicated 897.3
   below knee 897.0
      complicated 897.1
   both (bilateral) 897.6
      complicated 897.7
   complicated 897.5
lower limb(s) except toe(s)—*see* Amputation,
   traumatic, leg
nose—*see* Wound, open, nose
penis 878.0
   complicated 878.1
sites other than limbs—*see* Wound, open, by site
thumb(s) (with finger(s) of either hand) 885.0
   complicated 885.1
toe(s) (one or both feet) 895.0
   complicated 895.1
upper limb(s)—*see* Amputation, traumatic, arm

Amputee (bilateral) (old) —*see also* Absence, by
   site, acquired V49.70
Amusia 784.69
   developmental 315.39
   secondary to organic lesion 784.69
Amyelencephalus 740.0
Amyelia 742.59
Amygdalitis— *see* Tonsillitis
Amygdalolith 474.8
Amyloid disease or degeneration 277.30
   heart 277.39 *[425.7]*
Amyloidosis (familial) (general) (generalized)
   (genetic) (primary) 277.30
   with lung involvement 277.39 *[517.8]*
   cardiac, hereditary 277.39
   heart 277.39 *[425.7]*
   nephropathic 277.39 *[583.81]*
   neuropathic (Portuguese) (Swiss) 277.39
      [357.4]
   pulmonary 277.39 *[517.8]*
   secondary 277.39
   systemic, inherited 277.39
Amylopectinosis (brancher enzyme deficiency)
   271.0
Amylophagia 307.52
Amyoplasia, congenita 756.89
Amyotonia 728.2
   congenita 358.8
Amyotrophia, amyotrophy, amyotrophic 728.2
   congenita 756.89
   diabetic 250.6 *[353.5]*
      due to secondary diabetes 249.6 *[353.5]*
   lateral sclerosis (syndrome) 335.20
   neuralgic 353.5
   sclerosis (lateral) 335.20
   spinal progressive 335.21
Anacidity
   gastric 536.0
   psychogenic 306.4
Anaerosis of newborn 770.88
Analbuminemia 273.8
Analgesia (*see also* Anesthesia) 782.0
Analphalipoproteinemia 272.5
Anaphylactic shock or reaction (correct
   substance properly administered) 995.0
   due to
      food 995.60
         additives 995.66
         crustaceans 995.62
         eggs 995.68
         fish 995.65
         fruits 995.63
         milk products 995.67
         nuts (tree) 995.64
         peanuts 995.61
         *see*ds 995.64
         specified NEC 995.69
         tree nuts 995.64
         vegetables 995.63
      immunization 999.4
      overdose or wrong substance given or taken
         977.9
      specified drug—*see* Table of drugs and
         chemicals
   following sting(s) 989.5
   purpura 287.0
   serum 999.4
Anaphylactoid shock or reaction —*see*
   Anaphylactic shock
Anaphylaxis —*see* Anaphylactic shock
Anaplasia, cervix 622.10

Anarthria 784.51
Anarthritic rheumatoid disease 446.5
Anasarca 782.3
  cardiac (see also Failure, heart) 428.0
  fetus or newborn 778.0
  lung 514
  nutritional 262
  pulmonary 514
  renal (see also Nephrosis) 581.9
Anaspadias 752.62
Anastomosis
  aneurysmal—see Aneurysm
  arteriovenous, congenital NEC (see also
      Anomaly, arteriovenous) 747.60
    ruptured, of brain (see also Hemorrhage,
        subarachnoid) 430
  intestinal 569.89
    complicated NEC 997.4
      involving urinary tract 997.5
  retinal and choroidal vessels 743.58
    acquired 362.17
Anatomical narrow angle (glaucoma) 365.02
Ancylostoma (infection) (infestation) 126.9
  americanus 126.1
  braziliense 126.2
  caninum 126.8
  ceylanicum 126.3
  duodenale 126.0
  Necator americanus 126.1
Ancylostomiasis (intestinal) 126.9
  Ancylostoma
    americanus 126.1
    caninum 126.8
    ceylanicum 126.3
    duodenale 126.0
  braziliense 126.2
  Necator americanus 126.1
Anders' disease or syndrome (adiposis tuberosa
    simplex) 272.8
Andersen's glycogen storage disease 271.0
Anderson's disease 272.7
Andes disease 993.2
Andrews' disease (bacterid) 686.8
Androblastoma (M8630/1)
  benign (M8630/0)
    specified site—see Neoplasm, by site, benign
    unspecified site
      female 220
      male 222.0
  malignant (M8630/3)
    specified site—see Neoplasm, by site,
        malignant
    unspecified site
      female 183.0
      male 186.9
  specified site—see Neoplasm, by site, uncertain
      behavior
  tubular (M8640/0)
    with lipid storage (M8641/0)
      specified site—see Neoplasm, by site,
          benign
      unspecified site
        female 220
        male 222.0
    specified site—see Neoplasm, by site, benign
    unspecified site
      female 220
      male 222.0
  unspecified site
    female 236.2
    male 236.4

Android pelvis 755.69
  with disproportion (fetopelvic) 653.3
    affecting fetus or newborn 763.1
    causing obstructed labor 660.1
      affecting fetus or newborn 763.1
Anectasis, pulmonary (newborn or fetus) 770.5
Anemia 285.9
  in
    chronic illness NEC 285.29
    chronic kidney disease 285.21
    end-stage renal disease 285.21
    neoplastic disease 285.22
  with
    disorder of
      anaerobic glycolysis 282.3
      pentose phosphate pathway 282.2
    koilonychia 280.9
  6-phosphogluconic dehydrogenase deficiency
      282.2
  achlorhydric 280.9
  achrestic 281.8
  Addison's (pernicious) 281.0
  Addison-Biermer (pernicious) 281.0
  agranulocytic 288.09
  amino acid deficiency 281.4
  antineoplastic chemotherapy induced 285.3
  aplastic 284.9
    acquired (secondary) 284.89
    congenital 284.01
    constitutional 284.01
    due to
      antineoplastic chemotherapy 284.89
      chronic systemic disease 284.89
      drugs 284.89
      infection 284.89
      radiation 284.89
    idiopathic 284.9
    myxedema 244.9
    of or complicating pregnancy 648.2
    red cell (acquired) (adult) (with thymoma)
        284.81
      congenital 284.01
      pure 284.01
    specified type NEC 284.89
    toxic (paralytic) 284.89
  aregenerative 284.9
    congenital 284.01
  asiderotic 280.9
  atypical (primary) 285.9
  autohemolysis of Selwyn and Dacie (type I)
      282.2
  autoimmune hemolytic 283.0
  Baghdad Spring 282.2
  Balantidium coli 007.0
  Biermer's (pernicious) 281.0
  blood loss (chronic) 280.0
    acute 285.1
  bothriocephalus 123.4
  brickmakers' (see also Ancylostomiasis) 126.9
  cerebral 437.8
  childhood 282.9
  chlorotic 280.9
  chronica congenita aregenerativa 284.01
  chronic simple 281.9
  combined system disease NEC 281.0 [336.2]
    due to dietary deficiency 281.1 [336.2]
  complicating pregnancy or childbirth 648.2

Anemia—*continued*
  congenital (following fetal blood loss) 776.5
    aplastic 284.01
    due to isoimmunization NEC 773.2
    Heinz-body 282.7
    hereditary hemolytic NEC 282.9
    nonspherocytic
      Type I 282.2
      Type II 282.3
    pernicious 281.0
    spherocytic (*see also* Spherocytosis) 282.0
  Cooley's (erythroblastic) 282.49
  crescent—*see* Disease, sickle-cell
  cytogenic 281.0
  Dacie's (nonspherocytic)
    Type I 282.2
    Type II 282.3
  Davidson's (refractory) 284.9
  deficiency 281.9
    2, 3 diphosphoglycurate mutase 282.3
    2, 3 PG 282.3
    6-PGD 282.2
    6-phosphogluronic dehydrogenase 282.2
    amino acid 281.4
    combined B_{12} and folate 281.3
    enzyme, drug-induced (hemolytic) 282.2
    erythrocytic glutathione 282.2
    folate 281.2
      dietary 281.2
      drug-induced 281.2
    folic acid 281.2
      dietary 281.2
      drug-induced 281.2
    G-6-PD 282.2
    GGS-R 282.2
    glucose-6-phosphate dehydrogenase (G-6-PD) 282.2
    glucose-phosphate isomerase 282.3
    glutathione peroxidase 282.2
    glutathione reductase 282.2
    glyceraldehyde phosphate dehydrogenase 282.3
    GPI 282.3
    G SH 282.2
    hexokinase 282.3
    iron (Fe) 280.9
      specified NEC 280.8
    nutritional 281.9
      with
        poor iron absorption 280.9
        specified deficiency NEC 281.8
      due to inadequate dietary iron intake 280.1
      specified type NEC 281.8
    of or complicating pregnancy 648.2
    pentose phosphate pathway 282.2
    PFK 282.3
    phosphofructo-aldolase 282.3
    phosphofructokinase 282.3
    phosphoglycerate kinase 282.3
    PK 282.3
    protein 281.4
    pyruvate kinase (PK) 282.3
      TPI 282.3
    triosephosphate isomerase 282.3
    vitamin B_{12} NEC 281.1
      dietary 281.1
      pernicious 281.0
  Diamond-Blackfan (congenital hypoplastic) 284.01
  dibothriocephalus 123.4
  dimorphic 281.9

Anemia—*continued*
  diphasic 281.8
  diphtheritic 032.89
  Diphyllobothrium 123.4
  drepanocytic (*see also* Disease, sickle-cell) 282.60
  due to
    antineoplastic chemotherapy 285.3
    blood loss (chronic) 280.0
      acute 285.1
    chemotherapy, antineoplastic 285.3
    defect of Embden-Meyerhof pathway glycolysis 282.3
    disorder of glutathione metabolism 282.2
    drug - see Anemia, by type (see also Table of Drugs and Chemicals)
      chemotherapy, antineoplastic 285.3
    fetal blood loss 776.5
    fish tapeworm (D. latum) infestation 123.4
    glutathione metabolism disorder 282.2
    hemorrhage (chronic) 280.0
      acute 285.1
    hexose monophosphate (HMP) shunt deficiency 282.2
    impaired absorption 280.9
    loss of blood (chronic) 280.0
      acute 285.1
    myxedema 244.9
    Necator americanus 126.1
    prematurity 776.6
    selective vitamin B_{12} malabsorption with proteinuria 281.1
  Dyke-Young type (secondary) (symptomatic) 283.9
  dyserythropoietic (congenital) (types I, II, III) 285.8
  dyshemopoietic (congenital) 285.8
  Egypt (*see also* Ancylostomiasis) 126.9
  elliptocytosis (*see also* Elliptocytosis) 282.1
  enzyme deficiency, drug-induced 282.2
  epidemic (*see also* Ancylostomiasis) 126.9
  EPO resistant 285.21
  erythroblastic
    familial 282.49
    fetus or newborn (*see also* Disease, hemolytic) 773.2
    late 773.5
  erythrocytic glutathione deficiency 282.2
  erythropoietin-resistant (EPO resistant anemia) 285.21
  essential 285.9
  Faber's (achlorhydric anemia) 280.9
  factitious (self-induced blood letting) 280.0
  familial erythroblastic (microcytic) 282.49
  Fanconi's (congenital pancytopenia) 284.09
  favism 282.2
  fetal 678.0
    following blood loss, affecting newborn 776.5
  fetus or newborn
    due to
      ABO
        antibodies 773.1
        incompatibility, maternal/fetal 773.1
        isoimmunization 773.1
      Rh
        antibodies 773.0
        incompatibility, maternal/fetal 773.0
        isoimmunization 773.0
    following fetal blood loss 776.5
  fish tapeworm (D. latum) infestation 123.4

Anemia—*continued*
folate (folic acid) deficiency 281.2
    dietary 281.2
    drug-induced 281.2
folate malabsorption, congenital 281.2
folic acid deficiency 281.2
    dietary 281.2
    drug-induced 281.2
G-6-PD 282.2
general 285.9
glucose-6-phosphate dehydrogenase deficiency
        282.2
glutathione-reductase deficiency 282.2
goat's milk 281.2
granulocytic 288.09
Heinz-body, congenital 282.7
hemoglobin deficiency 285.9
hemolytic 283.9
    acquired 283.9
        with hemoglobinuria NEC 283.2
        autoimmune (cold type) (idiopathic)
            (primary) (secondary) (symptomatic)
            (warm type) 283.0
        due to
            cold reactive antibodies 283.0
            drug exposure 283.0
            warm reactive antibodies 283.0
        fragmentation 283.19
        idiopathic (chronic) 283.9
        infectious 283.19
            autoimmune 283.0
        non-autoimmune NEC 283.10
        toxic 283.19
        traumatic cardiac 283.19
    acute 283.9
        due to enzyme deficiency NEC 282.3
        fetus or newborn (*see also* Disease,
            hemolytic) 773.2
            late 773.5
        Lederer's (acquired infectious hemolytic
            anemia) 283.19
    autoimmune (acquired) 283.0
    chronic 282.9
        idiopathic 283.9
    cold type (secondary) (symptomatic) 283.0
    congenital (spherocytic) (*see also*
        Spherocytosis) 282.0
    nonspherocytic—*see* Anemia, hemolytic,
        nonspherocytic, congenital
    drug-induced 283.0
        enzyme deficiency 282.2
    due to
        cardiac conditions 283.19
        drugs 283.0
        enzyme deficiency NEC 282.3
            drug-induced 282.2
        presence of shunt or other internal prosthetic
            device 283.19
        thrombotic thrombocytopenic purpura 446.6
    elliptocytotic (*see also* Elliptocytosis) 282.1
    familial 282.9
    hereditary 282.9
        due to enzyme deficiency NEC 282.3
        specified NEC 282.8
    idiopathic (chronic) 283.9
    infectious (acquired) 283.19
    mechanical 283.19
    microangiopathic 283.19
    non-autoimmune NEC 283.10

Anemia—*continued*
hemolytic—*continued*
    nonspherocytic
        congenital or hereditary NEC 282.3
            glucose-6-phosphate dehydrogenase
                deficiency 282.2
            pyruvate kinase (PK) deficiency 282.3
            type I 282.2
            type II 282.3
            type I 282.2
            type II 282.3
    of or complicating pregnancy 648.2
    resulting from presence of shunt or other
        internal prosthetic device 283.19
    secondary 283.19
        autoimmune 283.0
    sickle-cell—*see* Disease, sickle-cell
    Stransky-Regala type (Hb-E) (*see also*
        Disease, hemoglobin) 282.7
    symptomatic 283.19
        autoimmune 283.0
    toxic (acquired) 283.19
    uremic (adult) (child) 283.11
    warm type (secondary) (symptomatic) 283.0
hemorrhagic (chronic) 280.0
    acute 285.1
HEMPAS 285.8
hereditary erythroblast multinuclearity- positive
        acidified serum test 285.8
Herrick's (hemoglobin S disease) 282.61
hexokinase deficiency 282.3
high A₂ 282.49
hookworm (*see also* Ancylostomiasis) 126.9
hypochromic (idiopathic) (microcytic)
        (normoblastic) 280.9
    with iron loading 285.0
    due to blood loss (chronic) 280.0
        acute 285.1
    familial sex linked 285.0
    pyridoxine-responsive 285.0
hypoplasia, red blood cells 284.81
    congenital or familial 284.01
hypoplastic (idiopathic) 284.9
    congenital 284.01
    familial 284.01
    of childhood 284.09
idiopathic 285.9
    hemolytic, chronic 283.9
infantile 285.9
infective, infectional 285.9
intertropical (*see also* Ancylostomiasis) 126.9
iron (Fe) deficiency 280.9
    due to blood loss (chronic) 280.0
        acute 285.1
    of or complicating pregnancy 648.2
    specified NEC 280.8
Jaksch's (pseudoleukemia infantum) 285.8
Joseph-Diamond-Blackfan (congenital
        hypoplastic) 284.01
labyrinth 386.50
Lederer's (acquired infectious hemolytic
        anemia) 283.19
leptocytosis (hereditary) 282.49
leukoerythroblastic 284.2
macrocytic 281.9
    nutritional 281.2
    of or complicating pregnancy 648.2
    tropical 281.2
malabsorption (familial), selective B₁₂ with
        proteinuria 281.1
malarial (*see also* Malaria) 084.6

Anemia—*continued*
  malignant (progressive) 281.0
  malnutrition 281.9
  marsh (*see also* Malaria) 084.6
  Mediterranean (with hemoglobinopathy) 282.49
  megaloblastic 281.9
    combined B_{12} and folate deficiency 281.3
    nutritional (of infancy) 281.2
    of infancy 281.2
    of or complicating pregnancy 648.2
    refractory 281.3
    specified NEC 281.3
  megalocytic 281.9
  microangiopathic hemolytic 283.19
  microcytic (hypochromic) 280.9
    due to blood loss (chronic) 280.0
      acute 285.1
    familial 282.49
    hypochromic 280.9
  microdrepanocytosis 282.49
  miners' (*see also* Ancylostomiasis) 126.9
  myelopathic 285.8
  myelophthisic (normocytic) 284.2
  newborn (*see also* Disease, hemolytic) 773.2
    due to isoimmunization (*see also* Disease,
      hemolytic) 773.2
    late, due to isoimmunization 773.5
    posthemorrhagic 776.5
  nonregenerative 284.9
  nonspherocytic hemolytic—*see* Anemia,
    hemolytic, nonspherocytic
  normocytic (infectional) (not due to blood loss)
    285.9
    due to blood loss (chronic) 280.0
      acute 285.1
    myelophthisic 284.2
  nutritional (deficiency) 281.9
    with
      poor iron absorption 280.9
      specified deficiency NEC 281.8
    due to inadequate dietary iron intake 280.1
    megaloblastic (of infancy) 281.2
  of childhood 282.9
  of chronic
    disease NEC 285.29
    illness NEC 285.29
  of or complicating pregnancy 648.2
    affecting fetus or newborn 760.8
  of prematurity 776.6
  orotic aciduric (congenital) (hereditary) 281.4
  osteosclerotic 289.89
  ovalocytosis (hereditary) (*see also*
    Elliptocytosis) 282.1
  paludal (*see also* Malaria) 084.6
  pentose phosphate pathway deficiency 282.2
  pernicious (combined system disease)
    (congenital) (dorsolateral spinal
    degeneration) (juvenile) (myelopathy)
    (neuropathy) (posterior sclerosis) (primary)
    (progressive) (spleen) 281.0
    of or complicating pregnancy 648.2
  pleochromic 285.9
    of sprue 281.8
  portal 285.8
  posthemorrhagic (chronic) 280.0
    acute 285.1
    newborn 776.5
  postoperative
    due to (acute) blood loss 285.1
      chronic blood loss 280.0
    other 285.9

Anemia—*continued*
  postpartum 648.2
  pressure 285.9
  primary 285.9
  profound 285.9
  progressive 285.9
    malignant 281.0
    pernicious 281.0
  protein-deficiency 281.4
  pseudoleukemica infantum 285.8
  puerperal 648.2
  pure red cell 284.81
    congenital 284.01
  pyridoxine-responsive (hypochromic) 285.0
  pyruvate kinase (PK) deficiency 282.3
  refractoria sideroblastica 238.72
  refractory (primary) 238.72
    with
      excess
        blasts-1 (RAEB-1) 238.72
        blasts-2 (RAEB-2) 238.73
      hemochromatosis 238.72
      ringed sideroblasts (RARS) 238.72
    due to
      drug 285.0
      myelodysplastic syndrome 238.72
      toxin 285.0
    hereditary 285.0
    idiopathic 238.72
    megaloblastic 281.3
    sideroblastic 238.72
      hereditary 285.0
      sideropenic 280.9
  Rietti-Greppi-Micheli (thalassemia minor)
    282.49
  scorbutic 281.8
  secondary (to) 285.9
    blood loss (chronic) 280.0
      acute 285.1
    hemorrhage 280.0
      acute 285.1
    inadequate dietary iron intake 280.1
  semiplastic 284.9
  septic 285.9
  sickle-cell (*see also* Disease, sickle-cell) 282.60
  sideroachrestic 285.0
  sideroblastic (acquired) (any type) (congenital)
    (drug-induced) (due to disease) (hereditary)
    (primary) (secondary) (sex-linked
    hypochromic) (vitamin B_6 responsive) 285.0
    refractory 238.72
      congenital 285.0
      drug-induced 285.0
      hereditary 285.0
      sex-linked hypochromic 285.0
      vitamin B_6-responsive 285.0
  sideropenic (refractory) 280.9
    due to blood loss (chronic) 280.0
      acute 285.1
  simple chronic 281.9
  specified type NEC 285.8
  spherocytic (hereditary) (*see also* Spherocytosis)
    282.0
  splenic 285.8
    familial (Gaucher's) 272.7
  splenomegalic 285.8
  stomatocytosis 282.8
  syphilitic 095.8
  target cell (oval) 282.49
  thalassemia 282.49

Anemia—*continued*
  thrombocytopenic (*see also* Thrombocytopenia)
      287.5
  toxic 284.89
  triosephosphate isomerase deficiency 282.3
  tropical, macrocytic 281.2
  tuberculous (*see also* Tuberculosis) 017.9
  vegan's 281.1
  vitamin
      B$_6$-responsive 285.0
      B$_{12}$ deficiency (dietary) 281.1
          pernicious 281.0
  von Jaksch's (pseudoleukemia infantum) 285.8
  Witts' (achlorhydric anemia) 280.9
  Zuelzer (-Ogden) (nutritional megaloblastic
      anemia) 281.2
Anencephalus, anencephaly 740.0
  fetal, affecting management of pregnancy 655.0
Anergasia (*see also* Psychosis, organic) 294.9
  senile 290.0
Anesthesia, anesthetic 782.0
  complication or reaction NEC 995.22
      due to
          correct substance properly administered
              995.22
          overdose or wrong substance given 968.4
          specified anesthetic—*see* Table of drugs
              and chemicals
  cornea 371.81
  death from
      correct substance properly administered 995.4
      during delivery 668.9
      overdose or wrong substance given 968.4
          specified anesthetic—*see* Table of drugs and
              chemicals
  eye 371.81
  functional 300.11
  hyperesthetic, thalamic 338.0
  hysterical 300.11
  local skin lesion 782.0
  olfactory 781.1
  sexual (psychogenic) 302.72
  shock
      due to
          correct substance properly administered 995.4
          overdose or wrong substance given 968.4
          specified anesthetic—*see* Table of drugs and
              chemicals
  skin 782.0
  tactile 782.0
  testicular 608.9
  thermal 782.0
Anetoderma (maculosum) 701.3
Aneuploidy NEC 758.5
Aneurin deficiency 265.1
Aneurysm (anastomotic) (artery) (cirsoid)
      (diffuse) (false) (fusiform) (multiple)
      (ruptured) (saccular) (varicose) 442.9
  abdominal (aorta) 441.4
      ruptured 441.3
      syphilitic 093.0
  aorta, aortic (nonsyphilitic) 441.9
      abdominal 441.4
          dissecting 441.02
          ruptured 441.3
          syphilitic 093.0
      arch 441.2
          ruptured 441.1
      arteriosclerotic NEC 441.9
          ruptured 441.5
      ascending 441.2
          ruptured 441.1

Aneurysm—*continued*
  aorta—*continued*
      congenital 747.29
      descending 441.9
          abdominal 441.4
              ruptured 441.3
          ruptured 441.5
          thoracic 441.2
              ruptured 441.1
      dissecting 441.00
          abdominal 441.02
          thoracic 441.01
          thoracoabdominal 441.03
      due to coarctation (aorta) 747.10
      ruptured 441.5
      sinus, right 747.29
      syphilitic 093.0
      thoracoabdominal 441.7
          ruptured 441.6
      thorax, thoracic (arch) (nonsyphilitic) 441.2
          dissecting 441.01
          ruptured 441.1
          syphilitic 093.0
      transverse 441.2
          ruptured 441.1
      valve (heart) (*see also* Endocarditis, aortic)
          424.1
  arteriosclerotic NEC 442.9
      cerebral 437.3
          ruptured (*see also* Hemorrhage,
              subarachnoid) 430
  arteriovenous (congenital) (peripheral) NEC
      (*see also* Anomaly, arteriovenous) 747.60
      acquired NEC 447.0
          brain 437.3
              ruptured (*see also* Hemorrhage,
                  subarachnoid) 430
          coronary 414.11
          pulmonary 417.0
      brain (cerebral) 747.81
          ruptured (*see also* Hemorrhage,
              subarachnoid) 430
      coronary 746.85
      pulmonary 747.3
      retina 743.58
      specified site NEC 747.89
          acquired 447.0
      traumatic (*see also* Injury, blood vessel, by
          site) 904.9
  basal—*see* Aneurysm, brain
  berry (congenital) (ruptured) (*see also*
      Hemorrhage, subarachnoid) 430
  brain 437.3
      arteriosclerotic 437.3
          ruptured (*see also* Hemorrhage,
              subarachnoid) 430
      arteriovenous 747.81
          acquired 437.3
              ruptured (*see also* Hemorrhage,
                  subarachnoid) 430
          ruptured (*see also* Hemorrhage,
              subarachnoid) 430
      berry (congenital) (ruptured) (*see also*
          Hemorrhage, subarachnoid) 430
      congenital 747.81
          ruptured (*see also* Hemorrhage,
              subarachnoid) 430
      meninges 437.3
          ruptured (*see also* Hemorrhage,
              subarachnoid) 430
      miliary (congenital) (ruptured) (*see also*
          Hemorrhage, subarachnoid) 430

Aneurysm—*continued*
  brain—*continued*
    mycotic 421.0
      ruptured (*see also* Hemorrhage,
        subarachnoid) 430
      nonruptured 437.3
    ruptured (*see also* Hemorrhage, subarachnoid)
      430
    syphilitic 094.87
    syphilitic (hemorrhage) 094.87
    traumatic—*see* Injury, intracranial
  cardiac (false) (*see also* Aneurysm, heart)
    414.10
  carotid artery (common) (external) 442.81
    internal (intracranial portion) 437.3
      extracranial portion 442.81
      ruptured into brain (*see also* Hemorrhage,
        subarachnoid) 430
    syphilitic 093.89
    intracranial 094.87
  cavernous sinus (*see also* Aneurysm, brain)
    437.3
    arteriovenous 747.81
      ruptured (*see also* Hemorrhage,
        subarachnoid) 430
    congenital 747.81
      ruptured (*see also* Hemorrhage,
        subarachnoid) 430
  celiac 442.84
  central nervous system, syphilitic 094.89
  cerebral—*see* Aneurysm, brain
  chest—*see* Aneurysm, thorax
  circle of Willis (*see also* Aneurysm, brain)
    437.3
    congenital 747.81
      ruptured (*see also* Hemorrhage,
        subarachnoid) 430
    ruptured (*see also* Hemorrhage, subarachnoid)
      430
  common iliac artery 442.2
  congenital (peripheral) NEC 747.60
    brain 747.81
      ruptured (*see also* Hemorrhage,
        subarachnoid) 430
    cerebral—*see* Aneurysm, brain, congenital
    coronary 746.85
    gastrointestinal 747.61
    lower limb 747.64
    pulmonary 747.3
    renal 747.62
    retina 743.58
    specified site NEC 747.89
    spinal 747.82
    upper limb 747.63
  conjunctiva 372.74
  conus arteriosus (*see also* Aneurysm, heart) 414.10
  coronary (arteriosclerotic) (artery) (vein) (*see
    also* Aneurysm, heart) 414.11
    arteriovenous 746.85
    congenital 746.85
    syphilitic 093.89
  cylindrical 441.9
    ruptured 441.5
    syphilitic 093.9
  dissecting 442.9
    aorta 441.00
      abdominal 441.02
      thoracic 441.01
      thoracoabdominal 441.03
    syphilitic 093.9
  ductus arteriosus 747.0

Aneurysm—*continued*
  embolic—*see* Embolism, artery
  endocardial, infective (any valve) 421.0
  femoral 442.3
  gastroduodenal 442.84
  gastroepiploic 442.84
  heart (chronic or with a stated duration of over 8
    weeks) (infectional) (wall) 414.10
    acute or with a stated duration of 8 weeks or
      less (*see also* Infarct, myocardium) 410.9
    congenital 746.89
    valve—*see* Endocarditis
  hepatic 442.84
  iliac (common) 442.2
  infective (any valve) 421.0
  innominate (nonsyphilitic) 442.89
    syphilitic 093.89
  interauricular septum (*see also* Aneurysm, heart)
    414.10
  interventricular septum (*see also* Aneurysm,
    heart) 414.10
  intracranial—*see* Aneurysm, brain
  intrathoracic (nonsyphilitic) 441.2
    ruptured 441.1
    syphilitic 093.0
  jugular vein 453.89
  lower extremity 442.3
  lung (pulmonary artery) 417.1
  malignant 093.9
  mediastinal (nonsyphilitic) 442.89
    syphilitic 093.89
  miliary (congenital) (ruptured) (*see also*
    Hemorrhage, subarachnoid) 430
  mitral (heart) (valve) 424.0
  mural (arteriovenous) (heart) (*see also*
    Aneurysm, heart) 414.10
  mycotic, any site 421.0
    ruptured, brain (*see also* Hemorrhage,
      subarachnoid) 430
    without endocarditis —*see* Aneurysm, by site
  myocardium (*see also* Aneurysm, heart) 414.10
  neck 442.81
  pancreaticoduodenal 442.84
  patent ductus arteriosus 747.0
  peripheral NEC 442.89
    congenital NEC (*see also* Aneurysm,
      congenital) 747.60
  popliteal 442.3
  pulmonary 417.1
    arteriovenous 747.3
      acquired 417.0
    syphilitic 093.89
    valve (heart) (*see also* Endocarditis,
      pulmonary) 424.3
  racemose 442.9
    congenital (peripheral) NEC 747.60
  radial 442.0
  Rasmussen's (*see also* Tuberculosis) 011.2
  renal 442.1
  retinal (acquired) 362.17
    congenital 743.58
    diabetic 250.5 *[362.01]*
      due to secondary diabetes 249.5 *[362.01]*
  sinus, aortic (of Valsalva) 747.29
  specified site NEC 442.89
  spinal (cord) 442.89
    congenital 747.82
    syphilitic (hemorrhage) 094.89
  spleen, splenic 442.83
  subclavian 442.82
    syphilitic 093.89

Aneurysm—*continued*
  superior mesenteric 442.84
  syphilitic 093.9
    aorta 093.0
    central nervous system 094.89
    congenital 090.5
    spine, spinal 094.89
  thoracoabdominal 441.7
    ruptured 441.6
  thorax, thoracic (arch) (nonsyphilitic) 441.2
    dissecting 441.01
    ruptured 441.1
    syphilitic 093.0
  traumatic (complication) (early)—*see* Injury,
    blood vessel, by site
  tricuspid (heart) (valve)—*see* Endocarditis,
    tricuspid
  ulnar 442.0
  upper extremity 442.0
  valve, valvular—*see* Endocarditis
  venous 456.8
  congenital NEC (*see also* Aneurysm,
    congenital) 747.60
  ventricle (arteriovenous) (*see also* Aneurysm,
    heart) 414.10
  visceral artery NEC 442.84
Angiectasis 459.89
Angiectopia 459.9
Angiitis 447.6
  allergic granulomatous 446.4
  hypersensitivity 446.20
    Goodpasture's syndrome 446.21
    specified NEC 446.29
  necrotizing 446.0
  Wegener's (necrotizing respiratory
    granulomatosis) 446.4
Angina (attack) (cardiac) (chest) (effort) (heart)
    (pectoris) (syndrome) (vasomotor) 413.9
  abdominal 557.1
  accelerated 411.1
  agranulocytic 288.03
  aphthous 074.0
  catarrhal 462
  crescendo 411.1
  croupous 464.4
  cruris 443.9
    due to atherosclerosis NEC (*see also*
      Arteriosclerosis, extremities) 440.20
  decubitus 413.0
  diphtheritic (membranous) 032.0
  equivalent 413.9
  erysipelatous 034.0
  erythematous 462
  exudative, chronic 476.0
  faucium 478.29
  gangrenous 462
    diphtheritic 032.0
  infectious 462
  initial 411.1
  intestinal 557.1
  ludovici 528.3
  Ludwig's 528.3
  malignant 462
    diphtheritic 032.0
  membranous 464.4
    diphtheritic 032.0
  mesenteric 557.1
  monocytic 075
  nocturnal 413.0
  phlegmonous 475
    diphtheritic 032.0

Angina—*continued*
  preinfarctional 411.1
  Prinzmetal's 413.1
  progressive 411.1
  pseudomembranous 101
  psychogenic 306.2
  pultaceous, diphtheritic 032.0
  scarlatinal 034.1
  septic 034.0
  simple 462
  stable NEC 413.9
  staphylococcal 462
  streptococcal 034.0
  stridulous, diphtheritic 032.3
  syphilitic 093.9
    congenital 090.5
  tonsil 475
  trachealis 464.4
  unstable 411.1
  variant 413.1
  Vincent's 101
Angioblastoma (M9161/1)—*see* Neoplasm,
  connective tissue, uncertain behavior
Angiocholecystitis (*see also* Cholecystitis, acute)
  575.0
Angiocholitis (*see also* Cholecystitis, acute) 576.1
Angiodysgensis spinalis 336.1
Angiodysplasia (intestinalis) (intestine) 569.84
  with hemorrhage 569.85
  duodenum 537.82
    with hemorrhage 537.83
  stomach 537.82
    with hemorrhage 537.83
Angioedema (allergic) (any site) (with urticaria)
  995.1
  hereditary 277.6
Angioendothelioma (M9130/1)—*see also*
  Neoplasm, by site, uncertain behavior
  benign (M9130/0) (*see also* Hemangioma, by
    site) 228.00
  bone (M9260/3)—*see* Neoplasm, bone,
    malignant
  Ewing's (M9260/3)—*see* Neoplasm, bone,
    malignant
  nervous system (M9130/0) 228.09
Angiofibroma (M9160/0)—*see also* Neoplasm,
  by site, benign
  juvenile (M9160/0) 210.7
    specified site—*see* Neoplasm, by site, benign
    unspecified site 210.7
Angiohemophilia (A) (B) 286.4
Angioid streaks (choroid) (retina) 363.43
Angiokeratoma (M9141/0)—*see also* Neoplasm,
  skin, benign
  corporis diffusum 272.7
Angiokeratosis
  diffuse 272.7
Angioleiomyoma (M8894/0)—*see* Neoplasm,
  connective tissue, benign
Angioleucitis 683
Angiolipoma (M8861/0) (*see also* Lipoma, by
  site) 214.9
  infiltrating (M8861/1)—*see* Neoplasm,
    connective tissue, uncertain behavior
Angioma (M9120/0) (*see also* Hemangioma, by
  site) 228.00
  capillary 448.1
  hemorrhagicum hereditaria 448.0
  malignant (M9120/3)—*see* Neoplasm,
    connective tissue, malignant
  pigmentosum et atrophicum 757.33

Angioma—*continued*
placenta—*see* Placenta, abnormal
plexiform (M9131/0)—*see* Hemangioma, by
  site
senile 448.1
serpiginosum 709.1
spider 448.1
stellate 448.1
Angiomatosis 757.32
bacillary 083.8
corporis diffusum universale 272.7
cutaneocerebral 759.6
encephalocutaneous 759.6
encephalofacial 759.6
encephalotrigeminal 759.6
hemorrhagic familial 448.0
hereditary familial 448.0
heredofamilial 448.0
meningo-oculofacial 759.6
multiple sites 228.09
neuro-oculocutaneous 759.6
retina (Hippel's disease) 759.6
retinocerebellosa 759.6
retinocerebral 759.6
systemic 228.09
Angiomyolipoma (M8860/0)
specified site—*see* Neoplasm, connective tissue,
  benign
unspecified site 223.0
Angiomyoliposarcoma (M8860/3)—*see*
  Neoplasm, connective tissue, malignant
Angiomyoma (M8894/0)—*see* Neoplasm,
  connective tissue, benign
Angiomyosarcoma (M8894/3)—*see* Neoplasm,
  connective tissue, malignant
Angioneurosis 306.2
Angioneurotic edema (allergic) (any site) (with
  urticaria) 995.1
hereditary 277.6
Angiopathia, angiopathy 459.9
diabetic (peripheral) 250.7 *[443.81]*
  due to secondary diabetes 249.7 [443.81]
peripheral 443.9
  diabetic 250.7 *[443.81]*
    due to secondary diabetes 249.7 [443.81]
  specified type NEC 443.89
retinae syphilitica 093.89
retinalis (juvenilis) 362.18
  background 362.10
  diabetic 250.5 *[362.01]*
    due to secondary diabetes 249.5 [362.01]
  proliferative 362.29
  tuberculous (*see also* Tuberculosis) 017.3 *[362.18]*
Angiosarcoma (M9120/3)—*see* Neoplasm,
  connective tissue, malignant
Angiosclerosis —*see* Arteriosclerosis
Angioscotoma, enlarged 368.42
Angiospasm 443.9
brachial plexus 353.0
cerebral 435.9
cervical plexus 353.2
nerve
  arm 354.9
    axillary 353.0
    median 354.1
    ulnar 354.2
  autonomic (*see also* Neuropathy, peripheral,
    autonomic) 337.9
  axillary 353.0
  leg 355.8
    plantar 355.6

Angiospasm—*continued*
nerve—*continued*
  lower extremity—*see* Angiospasm, nerve, leg
  median 354.1
  peripheral NEC 355.9
  spinal NEC 355.9
  sympathetic (*see also* Neuropathy, peripheral,
    autonomic) 337.9
  ulnar 354.2
  upper extremity—*see* Angiospasm, nerve, arm
peripheral NEC 443.9
traumatic 443.9
  foot 443.9
  leg 443.9
  vessel 443.9
Angiospastic disease or edema 443.9
Angle's
class I 524.21
class II 524.22
class III 524.23
Anguillulosis 127.2
Angulation
cecum (*see also* Obstruction, intestine) 560.9
coccyx (acquired) 738.6
  congenital 756.19
femur (acquired) 736.39
  congenital 755.69
intestine (large) (small) (*see also* Obstruction,
  intestine) 560.9
sacrum (acquired) 738.5
  congenital 756.19
sigmoid (flexure) (*see also* Obstruction,
  intestine) 560.9
spine (*see also* Curvature, spine) 737.9
tibia (acquired) 736.89
  congenital 755.69
ureter 593.3
wrist (acquired) 736.09
  congenital 755.59
Angulus infectiosus 686.8
Anhedonia 780.99
Anhidrosis (lid) (neurogenic) (thermogenic)
  705.0
Anhydration 276.51
with
  hypernatremia 276.0
  hyponatremia 276.1
Anhydremia 276.52
with
  hypernatremia 276.0
  hyponatremia 276.1
Anidrosis 705.0
Aniridia (congenital) 743.45
Anisakiasis (infection) (infestation) 127.1
Anisakis larva infestation 127.1
Aniseikonia 367.32
Anisocoria (pupil) 379.41
  congenital 743.46
Anisocytosis 790.09
Anisometropia (congenital) 367.31
Ankle —*see* condition
Ankyloblepharon (acquired) (eyelid) 374.46
  filiforme (adnatum) (congenital) 743.62
  total 743.62
Ankylodactly (*see also* Syndactylism) 755.10
Ankyloglossia 750.0
Ankylosis (fibrous) (osseous) 718.50
ankle 718.57
any joint, produced by surgical fusion V45.4
cricoarytenoid (cartilage) (joint) (larynx) 478.79
dental 521.6

Ankylosis—*continued*
 ear ossicle NEC 385.22
  malleus 385.21
 elbow 718.52
 finger 718.54
 hip 718.55
 incostapedial joint (infectional) 385.22
 joint, produced by surgical fusion NEC V45.4
 knee 718.56
 lumbosacral (joint) 724.6
 malleus 385.21
 multiple sites 718.59
 postoperative (status) V45.4
 sacroiliac (joint) 724.6
 shoulder 718.51
 specified site NEC 718.58
 spine NEC 724.9
 surgical V45.4
 teeth, tooth (hard tissues) 521.6
 temporomandibular joint 524.61
 wrist 718.53
Ankylostoma —*see* Ancylostoma
Ankylostomiasis (intestinal)—*see*
 Ancylostomiasis
Ankylurethria (*see also* Stricture, urethra) 598.9
Annular —*see also* condition
 detachment, cervix 622.8
 organ or site, congenital NEC—*see* Distortion
 pancreas (congenital) 751.7
Anodontia (complete) (partial) (vera) 520.0
 with abnormal spacing 524.30
 acquired 525.10
  causing malocclusion 524.30
  due to
   caries 525.13
   extraction 525.10
   periodontal disease 525.12
   trauma 525.11
Anomaly, anomalous (congenital) (unspecified
  type) 759.9
 abdomen 759.9
 abdominal wall 756.70
 acoustic nerve 742.9
 adrenal (gland) 759.1
 Alder (-Reilly) (leukocyte granulation) 288.2
 alimentary tract 751.9
  lower 751.5
  specified type NEC 751.8
  upper (any part, except tongue) 750.9
   tongue 750.10
    specified type NEC 750.19
 alveolar 524.70
  ridge (process) 525.8
  specified NEC 524.79
 ankle (joint) 755.69
 anus, anal (canal) 751.5
 aorta, aortic 747.20
  arch 747.21
  coarctation (postductal) (preductal) 747.10
  cusp or valve NEC 746.9
  septum 745.0
  specified type NEC 747.29
 aorticopulmonary septum 745.0
 apertures, diaphragm 756.6
 appendix 751.5
 aqueduct of Sylvius 742.3
  with spina bifida (*see also* Spina bifida) 741.0
 arm 755.50
  reduction (*see also* Deformity, reduction,
   upper limb) 755.20

Anomaly, anomalous—*continued*
 arteriovenous (congenital) (peripheral) NEC
   747.60
  brain 747.81
  cerebral 747.81
  coronary 746.85
  gastrointestinal 747.61
   acquired—*see* Angiodysplasia
  lower limb 747.64
  renal 747.62
  specified site NEC 747.69
  spinal 747.82
  upper limb 747.63
 artery (*see also* Anomaly, peripheral vascular
   system) NEC 747.60
  brain 747.81
  cerebral 747.81
  coronary 746.85
  eye 743.9
  pulmonary 747.3
  renal 747.62
  retina 743.9
  umbilical 747.5
 arytenoepiglottic folds 748.3
 atrial
  bands 746.9
  folds 746.9
  septa 745.5
 atrioventricular
  canal 745.69
  common 745.69
  conduction 426.7
  excitation 426.7
  septum 745.4
 atrium—*see* Anomaly, atrial
 auditory canal 744.3
  specified type NEC 744.29
   with hearing impairment 744.02
 auricle
  ear 744.3
   causing impairment of hearing 744.02
  heart 746.9
  septum 745.5
 autosomes, autosomal NEC 758.5
 Axenfeld's 743.44
 back 759.9
 band
  atrial 746.9
  heart 746.9
  ventricular 746.9
 Bartholin's duct 750.9
 biliary duct or passage 751.60
  atresia 751.61
 bladder (neck) (sphincter) (trigone) 753.9
  specified type NEC 753.8
 blood vessel 747.9
  artery—*see* Anomaly, artery
  peripheral vascular—*see* Anomaly, peripheral
   vascular system
  vein—*see* Anomaly, vein
 bone NEC 756.9
  ankle 755.69
  arm 755.50
  chest 756.3
  cranium 756.0
  face 756.0
  finger 755.50
  foot 755.67
  forearm 755.50
  frontal 756.0
  head 756.0

Anomaly, anomalous—*continued*
  bone—*continued*
    hip 755.63
    leg 755.60
    lumbosacral 756.10
    nose 748.1
    pelvic girdle 755.60
    rachitic 756.4
    rib 756.3
    shoulder girdle 755.50
    skull 756.0
      with
        anencephalus 740.0
        encephalocele 742.0
        hydrocephalus 742.3
          with spina bifida (*see also* Spina bifida)
            741.0
        microcephalus 742.1
    toe 755.66
  brain 742.9
    multiple 742.4
    reduction 742.2
    specified type NEC 742.4
    vessel 747.81
  branchial cleft NEC 744.49
    cyst 744.42
    fistula 744.41
    persistent 744.41
    sinus (external) (internal) 744.41
  breast 757.6
  broad ligament 752.10
    specified type NEC 752.19
  bronchus 748.3
  bulbar septum 745.0
  bulbus cordis 745.9
    persistent (in left ventricle) 745.8
  bursa 756.9
  canal of Nuck 752.9
  canthus 743.9
  capillary NEC (*see also* Anomaly, peripheral
    vascular system) 747.60
  cardiac 746.9
    septal closure 745.9
      acquired 429.71
    valve NEC 746.9
      pulmonary 746.00
      specified type NEC 746.89
  cardiovascular system 746.9
    complicating pregnancy, childbirth, or
      puerperium 648.5
  carpus 755.50
  cartilage, trachea 748.3
  cartilaginous 756.9
  caruncle, lacrimal, lachrymal 743.9
  cascade stomach 750.7
  cauda equina 742.59
  cecum 751.5
  cerebral—*see also* Anomaly, brain
    vessels 747.81
  cerebrovascular system 747.81
  cervix (uterus) 752.40
    with doubling of vagina and uterus 752.2
    in pregnancy or childbirth 654.6
      affecting fetus or newborn 763.89
      causing obstructed labor 660.2
        affecting fetus or newborn 763.1
  Chédiak-Higashi (-Steinbrinck) (congenital
    gigantism of peroxidase granules) 288.2
  cheek 744.9
  chest (wall) 756.3

Anomaly, anomalous—*continued*
  chin 744.9
    specified type NEC 744.89
  chordae tendineae 746.9
  choroid 743.9
    plexus 742.9
  chromosomes, chromosomal 758.9
    13 (13-15) 758.1
    18 (16-l8) 758.2
    21 or 22 758.0
    autosomes NEC (*see also* Abnormality,
      autosomes) 758.5
    deletion 758.39
      Christchurch 758.39
      D_1 758.1
      E_3 758.2
      G 758.0
    mitochondrial 758.9
    mosaics 758.89
    sex 758.81
      complement, XO 758.6
      complement, XXX 758.81
      complement, XYY 758.81
      gonadal dysgenesis 758.6
      Klinefelter's 758.7
      Turner's 758.6
    trisomy 21 758.0
  cilia 743.9
  circulatory system 747.9
    specified type NEC 747.89
  clavicle 755.51
  clitoris 752.40
  coccyx 756.10
  colon 751.5
  common duct 751.60
  communication
    coronary artery 746.85
    left ventricle with right atrium 745.4
  concha (ear) 744.3
  connection
    renal vessels with kidney 747.62
    total pulmonary venous 747.41
  connective tissue 756.9
    specified type NEC 756.89
  cornea 743.9
    shape 743.41
    size 743.41
    specified type NEC 743.49
  coronary
    artery 746.85
    vein 746.89
  cranium—*see* Anomaly, skull
  cricoid cartilage 748.3
  cushion, endocardial 745.60
    specified type NEC 745.69
  cystic duct 751.60
  dental arch 524.20
    specified NEC 524.29
  dental arch relationship 524.20
    angle's class I 524.21
    angle's class II 524.22
    angle's class III 524.23
    articulation
      anterior 524.27
      posterior 524.27
      reverse 524.27
    disto-occlusion 524.22
      division I 524.22
      division II 524.22
    excessive horizontal overlap 524.26
    interarch distance (excessive) (inadequate)
      524.28

Anomaly, anomalous—*continued*
  dental arch relationship—*continued*
    mesio-occlusion 524.23
    neutro-occlusion 524.21
    open
      anterior occlusal relationship 524.24
      posterior occlusal relationship 524.25
    specified NEC 524.29
  dentition 520.6
  dentofacial NEC 524.9
    functional 524.50
    specified type NEC 524.89
  dermatoglyphic 757.2
  Descemet's membrane 743.9
    specified type NEC 743.49
  development
    cervix 752.40
    vagina 752.40
    vulva 752.40
  diaphragm, diaphragmatic (apertures) NEC
    756.6
  digestive organ(s) or system 751.9
    lower 751.5
    specified type NEC 751.8
    upper 750.9
  distribution, coronary artery 746.85
  ductus
    arteriosus 747.0
    Botalli 747.0
  duodenum 751.5
  dura 742.9
    brain 742.4
    spinal cord 742.59
  ear 744.3
    causing impairment of hearing 744.00
      specified type NEC 744.09
    external 744.3
      causing impairment of hearing 744.02
      specified type NEC 744.29
    inner (causing impairment of hearing) 744.05
    middle, except ossicles (causing impairment
      of hearing) 744.03
      ossicles 744.04
    ossicles 744.04
    prominent auricle 744.29
    specified type NEC 744.29
      with hearing impairment 744.09
  Ebstein's (heart) 746.2
    tricuspid valve 746.2
  ectodermal 757.9
  Eisenmenger's (ventricular septal defect) 745.4
  ejaculatory duct 752.9
    specified type NEC 752.89
  elbow (joint) 755.50
  endocardial cushion 745.60
    specified type NEC 745.69
  endocrine gland NEC 759.2
  epididymis 752.9
  epiglottis 748.3
  esophagus 750.9
    specified type NEC 750.4
  Eustachian tube 744.3
    specified type NEC 744.24
  eye (any part) 743.9
    adnexa 743.9
      specified type NEC 743.69
    anophthalmos 743.00

Anomaly, anomalous—*continued*
  eye—*continued*
    anterior
      chamber and related structures 743.9
        angle 743.9
          specified type NEC 743.44
        specified type NEC 743.44
      segment 743.9
        combined 743.48
        multiple 743.48
        specified type NEC 743.49
    cataract (*see also* Cataract) 743.30
    glaucoma (*see also* Buphthalmia) 743.20
    lid 743.9
      specified type NEC 743.63
    microphthalmos (*see also* Microphthalmos) 743.10
    posterior segment 743.9
      specified type NEC 743.59
      vascular 743.58
      vitreous 743.9
        specified type NEC 743.51
    ptosis (eyelid) 743.61
    retina 743.9
      specified type NEC 743.59
    sclera 743.9
      specified type NEC 743.47
    specified type NEC 743.8
  eyebrow 744.89
  eyelid 743.9
    specified type NEC 743.63
  face (any part) 744.9
    bone(s) 756.0
    specified type NEC 744.89
  fallopian tube 752.10
    specified type NEC 752.19
  fascia 756.9
    specified type NEC 756.89
  femur 755.60
  fibula 755.60
  finger 755.50
    supernumerary 755.01
    webbed (*see also* Syndactylism, fingers) 755.11
  fixation, intestine 751.4
  flexion (joint) 755.9
    hip or thigh (*see also* Dislocation, hip,
      congenital) 754.30
  folds, heart 746.9
  foot 755.67
  foramen
    Botalli 745.5
    ovale 745.5
  forearm 755.50
  forehead (*see also* Anomaly, skull) 756.0
  form, teeth 520.2
  fovea centralis 743.9
  frontal bone (*see also* Anomaly, skull) 756.0
  gallbladder 751.60
  Gartner's duct 752.41
  gastrointestinal tract 751.9
    specified type NEC 751.8
    vessel 747.61
  genitalia, genital organ(s) or system
    female 752.9
      external 752.40
        specified type NEC 752.49
      internal NEC 752.9

Anomaly, anomalous—*continued*
  genitalia—*continued*
    male (external and internal) 752.9
      epispadias 752.62
      hidden penis 752.65
      hydrocele, congenital 778.6
      hypospadias 752.61
      micropenis 752.64
      testis, undescended 752.51
        retractile 752.52
      specified type NEC 752.89
  genitourinary NEC 752.9
  Gerbode 745.4
  globe (eye) 743.9
  glottis 748.3
  granulation or granulocyte, genetic 288.2
    constitutional 288.2
    leukocyte 288.2
  gum 750.9
  gyri 742.9
  hair 757.9
    specified type NEC 757.4
  hand 755.50
  hard tissue formation in pulp 522.3
  head (*see also* Anomaly, skull) 756.0
  heart 746.9
    auricle 746.9
    bands 746.9
    fibroelastosis cordis 425.3
    folds 746.9
    malposition 746.87
    maternal, affecting fetus or newborn 760.3
    obstructive NEC 746.84
    patent ductus arteriosus (Botalli) 747.0
    septum 745.9
      acquired 429.71
      aortic 745.0
      aorticopulmonary 745.0
      atrial 745.5
      auricular 745.5
      between aorta and pulmonary artery 745.0
      endocardial cushion type 745.60
        specified type NEC 745.69
      interatrial 745.5
      interventricular 745.4
        with pulmonary stenosis or atresia,
          dextraposition of aorta, and
          hypertrophy of right ventricle 745.2
        acquired 429.71
      specified type NEC 745.8
      ventricular 745.4
        with pulmonary stenosis or atresia,
          dextraposition of aorta, and
          hypertrophy of right ventricle 745.2
        acquired 429.71
    specified type NEC 746.89
    tetralogy of Fallot 745.2
    valve NEC 746.9
      aortic 746.9
        atresia 746.89
        bicuspid valve 746.4
        insufficiency 746.4
        specified type NEC 746.89
        stenosis 746.3
          subaortic 746.81
          supravalvular 747.22
      mitral 746.9
        atresia 746.89
        insufficiency 746.6
        specified type NEC 746.89
        stenosis 746.5

Anomaly, anomalous—*continued*
  heart—*continued*
    valve—*continued*
      pulmonary 746.00
        atresia 746.01
        insufficiency 746.09
        stenosis 746.02
          infundibular 746.83
          subvalvular 746.83
      tricuspid 746.9
        atresia 746.1
        stenosis 746.1
    ventricle 746.9
  heel 755.67
  Hegglin's 288.2
  hemianencephaly 740.0
  hemicephaly 740.0
  hemicrania 740.0
  hepatic duct 751.60
  hip (joint) 755.63
  hourglass
    bladder 753.8
    gallbladder 751.69
    stomach 750.7
  humerus 755.50
  hymen 752.40
  hypersegmentation of neutrophils, hereditary
    288.2
  hypophyseal 759.2
  ileocecal (coil) (valve) 751.5
  ileum (intestine) 751.5
  ilium 755.60
  integument 757.9
    specified type NEC 757.8
  interarch distance (excessive) (inadequate)
    524.28
  intervertebral cartilage or disc 756.10
  intestine (large) (small) 751.5
    fixational type 751.4
  iris 743.9
    specified type NEC 743.46
  ischium 755.60
  jaw NEC 524.9
    closure 524.51
    size NEC 524.00
    specified type NEC 524.89
  jaw-cranial base relationship 524.10
    specified NEC 524.19
  jejunum 751.5
  joint 755.9
    hip
      dislocation (*see also* Dislocation, hip,
        congenital) 754.30
      predislocation (*see also* Subluxation,
        congenital, hip) 754.32
      preluxation (*see also* Subluxation,
        congenital, hip) 754.32
      subluxation (*see also* Subluxation,
        congenital, hip) 754.32
    lumbosacral 756.10
      spondylolisthesis 756.12
      spondylosis 756.11
    multiple arthrogryposis 754.89
    sacroiliac 755.69
  Jordan's 288.2
  kidney(s) (calyx) (pelvis) 753.9
    vessel 747.62
  Klippel-Feil (brevicollis) 756.16

Anomaly, anomalous—*continued*
  knee (joint) 755.64
  labium (majus) (minus) 752.40
  labyrinth, membranous (causing impairment of
    hearing) 744.05
  lacrimal
    apparatus, duct or passage 743.9
      specified type NEC 743.65
    gland 743.9
      specified type NEC 743.64
  Langdon Down (mongolism) 758.0
  larynx, laryngeal (muscle) 748.3
    web, webbed 748.2
  leg (lower) (upper) 755.60
    reduction NEC (*see also* Deformity, reduction,
      lower limb) 755.30
  lens 743.9
    shape 743.36
    specified type NEC 743.39
  leukocytes, genetic 288.2
    granulation (constitutional) 288.2
  lid (fold) 743.9
  ligament 756.9
    broad 752.10
    round 752.9
  limb, except reduction deformity 755.9
    lower 755.60
      reduction deformity (*see also* Deformity,
        reduction, lower limb) 755.30
      specified type NEC 755.69
    upper 755.50
      reduction deformity (*see also* Deformity,
        reduction, upper limb) 755.20
      specified type NEC 755.59
  lip 750.9
    harelip (*see also* Cleft, lip) 749.10
    specified type NEC 750.26
  liver (duct) 751.60
    atresia 751.69
  lower extremity 755.60
    vessel 747.64
  lumbosacral (joint) (region) 756.10
  lung (fissure) (lobe) NEC 748.60
    agenesis 748.5
    specified type NEC 748.69
  lymphatic system 759.9
  Madelung's (radius) 755.54
  mandible 524.9
    size NEC 524.00
  maxilla 524.9
    size NEC 524.00
  May (-Hegglin) 288.2
  meatus urinarius 753.9
    specified type NEC 753.8
  meningeal bands or folds, constriction of 742.8
  meninges 742.9
    brain 742.4
    spinal 742.59
  meningocele (*see also* Spina bifida) 741.9
  mesentery 751.9
  metacarpus 755.50
  metatarsus 755.67
  middle ear, except ossicles (causing impairment
    of hearing) 744.03
    ossicles 744.04
  mitral (leaflets) (valve) 746.9
    atresia 746.89
    insufficiency 746.6
    specified type NEC 746.89
    stenosis 746.5

Anomaly, anomalous—*continued*
  mouth 750.9
    specified type NEC 750.26
  multiple NEC 759.7
    specified type NEC 759.89
  muscle 756.9
    eye 743.9
      specified type NEC 743.69
    specified type NEC 756.89
  musculoskeletal system, except limbs 756.9
    specified type NEC 756.9
  nail 757.9
    specified type NEC 757.5
  narrowness, eyelid 743.62
  nasal sinus or septum 748.1
  neck (any part) 744.9
    specified type NEC 744.89
  nerve 742.9
    acoustic 742.9
      specified type NEC 742.8
    optic 742.9
    specified type NEC 742.8
    specified type NEC 742.8
  nervous system NEC 742.9
    brain 742.9
      specified type NEC 742.4
    specified type NEC 742.8
  neurological 742.9
  nipple 757.6
  nonteratogenic NEC 754.89
  nose, nasal (bone) (cartilage) (septum) (sinus)
    748.1
  ocular muscle 743.9
  omphalomesenteric duct 751.0
  opening, pulmonary veins 747.49
  optic
    disc 743.9
      specified type NEC 743.57
    nerve 742.9
  opticociliary vessels 743.9
  orbit (eye) 743.9
    specified type NEC 743.66
  organ
    of Corti (causing impairment of hearing)
      744.05
    or site 759.9
      specified type NEC 759.89
  origin
    both great arteries from same ventricle 745.11
    coronary artery 746.85
    innominate artery 747.69
    left coronary artery from pulmonary artery
      746.85
    pulmonary artery 747.3
    renal vessels 747.62
    subclavian artery (left) (right) 747.21
  osseous meatus (ear) 744.03
  ovary 752.0
  oviduct 752.10
  palate (hard) (soft) 750.9
    cleft (*see also* Cleft, palate) 749.00
  pancreas (duct) 751.7
  papillary muscles 746.9
  parathyroid gland 759.2
  paraurethral ducts 753.9
  parotid (gland) 750.9
  patella 755.64
  Pelger-Huët (hereditary hyposegmentation)
    288.2
  pelvic girdle 755.60
    specified type NEC 755.69

Anomaly, anomalous—*continued*
  pelvis (bony) 755.60
    complicating delivery 653.0
      rachitic 268.1
        fetal 756.4
  penis (glans) 752.69
  pericardium 746.89
  peripheral vascular system NEC 747.60
    gastrointestinal 747.61
    lower limb 747.64
    renal 747.62
    specified site NEC 747.69
    spinal 747.82
    upper limb 747.63
  Peter's 743.44
  pharynx 750.9
    branchial cleft 744.41
    specified type NEC 750.29
  Pierre Robin 756.0
  pigmentation NEC 709.00
    congenital 757.33
  pituitary (gland) 759.2
  pleural folds 748.8
  portal vein 747.40
  position tooth, teeth 524.30
    crowding 524.31
    displacement 524.30
      horizontal 524.33
      vertical 524.34
    distance
      interocclusal
        excessive 524.37
        insufficient 524.36
      excessive spacing 524.32
      rotation 524.35
      specified NEC 524.39
  preauricular sinus 744.46
  prepuce 752.9
  prostate 752.9
  pulmonary 748.60
    artery 747.3
    circulation 747.3
    specified type NEC 748.69
    valve 746.00
      atresia 746.01
      insufficiency 746.09
      specified type NEC 746.09
      stenosis 746.02
        infundibular 746.83
        subvalvular 746.83
    vein 747.40
    venous
      connection 747.49
        partial 747.42
        total 747.41
      return 747.49
        partial 747.42
        total (TAPVR) (complete)
          (subdiaphragmatic)
          (supradiaphragmatic) 747.41
  pupil 743.9
  pylorus 750.9
    hypertrophy 750.5
    stenosis 750.5
  rachitic, fetal 756.4
  radius 755.50
  rectovaginal (septum) 752.40
  rectum 751.5
  refraction 367.9
  renal 753.9
    vessel 747.62

Anomaly, anomalous—*continued*
  respiratory system 748.9
    specified type NEC 748.8
  rib 756.3
    cervical 756.2
  Rieger's 743.44
  rings, trachea 748.3
  rotation—*see also* Malrotation
    hip or thigh (*see also* Subluxation, congenital,
      hip) 754.32
  round ligament 752.9
  sacroiliac (joint) 755.69
  sacrum 756.10
  saddle
    back 754.2
    nose 754.0
      syphilitic 090.5
  salivary gland or duct 750.9
    specified type NEC 750.26
  scapula 755.50
  sclera 743.9
    specified type NEC 743.47
  scrotum 752.9
  sebaceous gland 757.9
  seminal duct or tract 752.9
  sense organs 742.9
    specified type NEC 742.8
  septum
    heart—*see* Anomaly, heart, septum
    nasal 748.1
  sex chromosomes NEC (*see also* Anomaly,
    chromosomes) 758.81
  shoulder (girdle) (joint) 755.50
    specified type NEC 755.59
  sigmoid (flexure) 751.5
  sinus of Valsalva 747.29
  site NEC 759.9
  skeleton generalized NEC 756.50
  skin (appendage) 757.9
    specified type NEC 757.39
  skull (bone) 756.0
    with
      anencephalus 740.0
      encephalocele 742.0
      hydrocephalus 742.3
        with spina bifida (*see also* Spina bifida)
          741.0
      microcephalus 742.1
  specified type NEC
    adrenal (gland) 759.1
    alimentary tract (complete) (partial) 751.8
      lower 751.5
      upper 750.8
    ankle 755.69
    anus, anal (canal) 751.5
    aorta, aortic 747.29
      arch 747.21
    appendix 751.5
    arm 755.59
    artery (peripheral) NEC (*see also* Anomaly,
      peripheral vascular system) 747.60
      brain 747.81
      coronary 746.85
      eye 743.58
      pulmonary 747.3
      retinal 743.58
      umbilical 747.5
    auditory canal 744.29
      causing impairment of hearing 744.02
    bile duct or passage 751.69
    bladder 753.8
      neck 753.8

Anomaly, anomalous—*continued*
  specified type NEC—*continued*
    bone(s) 756.9
      arm 755.59
      face 756.0
      leg 755.69
      pelvic girdle 755.69
      shoulder girdle 755.59
      skull 756.0
        with
          anencephalus 740.0
          encephalocele 742.0
          hydrocephalus 742.3
            with spina bifida (*see also* Spina
              bifida) 741.0
          microcephalus 742.1
    brain 742.4
    breast 757.6
    broad ligament 752.19
    bronchus 748.3
    canal of Nuck 752.89
    cardiac septal closure 745.8
    carpus 755.59
    cartilaginous 756.9
    cecum 751.5
    cervix 752.49
    chest (wall) 756.3
    chin 744.89
    ciliary body 743.46
    circulatory system 747.89
    clavicle 755.51
    clitoris 752.49
    coccyx 756.19
    colon 751.5
    common duct 751.69
    connective tissue 756.89
    cricoid cartilage 748.3
    cystic duct 751.69
    diaphragm 756.6
    digestive organ(s) or tract 751.8
      lower 751.5
      upper 750.8
    duodenum 751.5
    ear 744.29
      auricle 744.29
        causing impairment of hearing 744.02
      causing impairment of hearing 744.09
      inner (causing impairment of hearing)
        744.05
      middle, except ossicles 744.03
        ossicles 744.04
    ejaculatory duct 752.89
    endocrine 759.2
    epiglottis 748.3
    esophagus 750.4
    Eustachian tube 744.24
    eye 743.8
      lid 743.63
      muscle 743.69
    face 744.89
      bone(s) 756.0
    fallopian tube 752.19
    fascia 756.89
    femur 755.69
    fibula 755.69
    finger 755.59
    foot 755.67
    fovea centralis 743.55
    gallbladder 751.69
    Gartner's duct 752.89
    gastrointestinal tract 751.8

Anomaly, anomalous—*continued*
  specified type NEC—*continued*
    genitalia, genital organ(s)
      female 752.89
        external 752.49
        internal NEC 752.89
      male 752.89
        penis 752.69
        scrotal transposition 752.81
    genitourinary tract NEC 752.89
    glottis 748.3
    hair 757.4
    hand 755.59
    heart 746.89
      valve NEC 746.89
        pulmonary 746.09
    hepatic duct 751.69
    hydatid of Morgagni 752.89
    hymen 752.49
    integument 757.8
    intestine (large) (small) 751.5
      fixational type 751.4
    iris 743.46
    jejunum 751.5
    joint 755.8
    kidney 753.3
    knee 755.64
    labium (majus) (minus) 752.49
    labyrinth, membranous 744.05
    larynx 748.3
    leg 755.69
    lens 743.39
    limb, except reduction deformity 755.8
      lower 755.69
        reduction deformity (*see also* Deformity,
          reduction, lower limb) 755.30
      upper 755.59
        reduction deformity (*see also* Deformity,
          reduction, upper limb) 755.20
    lip 750.26
    liver 751.69
    lung (fissure) (lobe) 748.69
    meatus urinarius 753.8
    metacarpus 755.59
    mouth 750.26
    muscle 756.89
      eye 743.69
    musculoskeletal system, except limbs 756.9
    nail 757.5
    neck 744.89
    nerve 742.8
      acoustic 742.8
      optic 742.8
    nervous system 742.8
    nipple 757.6
    nose 748.1
    organ NEC 759.89
      of Corti 744.05
    osseous meatus (ear) 744.03
    ovary 752.0
    oviduct 752.19
    pancreas 751.7
    parathyroid 759.2
    patella 755.64
    pelvic girdle 755.69
    penis 752.69
    pericardium 746.89
    peripheral vascular system NEC (*see also*
      Anomaly, peripheral vascular system)
      747.60
    pharynx 750.29

Anomaly, anomalous—*continued*
  specified type NEC—*continued*
    pituitary 759.2
    prostate 752.89
    radius 755.59
    rectum 751.5
    respiratory system 748.8
    rib 756.3
    round ligament 752.89
    sacrum 756.19
    salivary duct or gland 750.26
    scapula 755.59
    sclera 743.47
    scrotum 752.89
      transposition 752.81
    seminal duct or tract 752.89
    shoulder girdle 755.59
    site NEC 759.89
    skin 757.39
    skull (bone(s)) 756.0
      with
        anencephalus 740.0
        encephalocele 742.0
        hydrocephalus 742.3
          with spina bifida (*see also* Spina bifida)
            741.0
        microcephalus 742.1
    specified organ or site NEC 759.89
    spermatic cord 752.89
    spinal cord 742.59
    spine 756.19
    spleen 759.0
    sternum 756.3
    stomach 750.7
    tarsus 755.67
    tendon 756.89
    testis 752.89
    thorax (wall) 756.3
    thymus 759.2
    thyroid (gland) 759.2
      cartilage 748.3
    tibia 755.69
    toe 755.66
    tongue 750.19
    trachea (cartilage) 748.3
    ulna 755.59
    urachus 753.7
    ureter 753.4
      obstructive 753.29
    urethra 753.8
      obstructive 753.6
    urinary tract 753.8
    uterus 752.3
    uvula 750.26
    vagina 752.49
    vascular NEC (*see also* Anomaly, peripheral
      vascular system) 747.60
      brain 747.81
    vas deferens 752.89
    vein(s) (peripheral) NEC (*see also* Anomaly,
      peripheral vascular system) 747.60
      brain 747.81
      great 747.49
      portal 747.49
      pulmonary 747.49
    vena cava (inferior) (superior) 747.49
    vertebra 756.19
    vulva 752.49
  spermatic cord 752.9

Anomaly, anomalous—*continued*
  spine, spinal 756.10
    column 756.10
    cord 742.9
      meningocele (*see also* Spina bifida) 741.9
      specified type NEC 742.59
      spina bifida (*see also* Spina bifida) 741.9
      vessel 747.82
    meninges 742.59
    nerve root 742.9
  spleen 759.0
  Sprengel's 755.52
  sternum 756.3
  stomach 750.9
    specified type NEC 750.7
  submaxillary gland 750.9
  superior vena cava 747.40
  talipes—*see* Talipes
  tarsus 755.67
    with complete absence of distal elements
      755.31
  teeth, tooth NEC 520.9
    position 524.30
      crowding 524.31
      displacement 524.30
        horizontal 524.33
        vertical 524.34
      distance
        interocclusal
          excessive 524.37
          insufficient 524.36
        excessive spacing 524.32
      rotation 524.35
      specified NEC 524.39
    spacing 524.30
  tendon 756.9
    specified type NEC 756.89
  termination
    coronary artery 746.85
  testis 752.9
  thebesian valve 746.9
  thigh 755.60
    flexion (*see also* Subluxation, congenital, hip)
      754.32
  thorax (wall) 756.3
  throat 750.9
  thumb 755.50
    supernumerary 755.01
  thymus gland 759.2
  thyroid (gland) 759.2
    cartilage 748.3
  tibia 755.60
    saber 090.5
  toe 755.66
    supernumerary 755.02
    webbed (*see also* Syndactylism, toes) 755.13
  tongue 750.10
    specified type NEC 750.19
  trachea, tracheal 748.3
    cartilage 748.3
    rings 748.3
  tragus 744.3
  transverse aortic arch 747.21
  trichromata 368.59
  trichromatopsia 368.59
  tricuspid (leaflet) (valve) 746.9
    atresia 746.1
    Ebstein's 746.2
    specified type NEC 746.89
    stenosis 746.1

Anomaly, anomalous—*continued*
trunk 759.9
Uhl's (hypoplasia of myocardium, right
    ventricle) 746.84
ulna 755.50
umbilicus 759.9
    artery 747.5
union, trachea with larynx 748.3
unspecified site 759.9
upper extremity 755.50
    vessel 747.63
urachus 753.7
    specified type NEC 753.7
ureter 753.9
    obstructive 753.20
    specified type NEC 753.4
        obstructive 753.29
urethra (valve) 753.9
    obstructive 753.6
    specified type NEC 753.8
urinary tract or system (any part, except
    urachus) 753.9
    specified type NEC 753.8
    urachus 753.7
uterus 752.3
    with only one functioning horn 752.3
    in pregnancy or childbirth 654.0
        affecting fetus or newborn 763.89
        causing obstructed labor 660.2
            affecting fetus or newborn 763.1
uvula 750.9
vagina 752.40
valleculae 748.3
valve (heart) NEC 746.9
    formation, ureter 753.29
    pulmonary 746.00
    specified type NEC 746.89
vascular NEC (*see also* Anomaly, peripheral
    vascular system) 747.60
    ring 747.21
vas deferens 752.9
vein(s) (peripheral) NEC (*see also* Anomaly,
    peripheral vascular system) 747.60
    brain 747.81
    cerebral 747.81
    coronary 746.89
    great 747.40
        specified type NEC 747.49
    portal 747.40
    pulmonary 747.40
    retina 743.9
vena cava (inferior) (superior) 747.40
venous—*see* Anomaly, vein
venous return (pulmonary) 747.49
    partial 747.42
    total 747.41
ventricle, ventricular (heart) 746.9
    bands 746.9
    folds 746.9
    septa 745.4
vertebra 756.10
vesicourethral orifice 753.9
vessels NEC (*see also* Anomaly, peripheral
    vascular system) 747.60
    optic papilla 743.9
vitelline duct 751.0
vitreous humor 743.9
    specified type NEC 743.51
vulva 752.40
wrist (joint) 755.50
Anomia 784.69

Anonychia 757.5
    acquired 703.8
Anophthalmos, anophthalmus (clinical)
    (congenital) (globe) 743.00
    acquired V45.78
Anopsia (altitudinal) (quadrant) 368.46
Anorchia 752.89
Anorchism, anorchidism 752.89
Anorexia 783.0
    hysterical 300.11
    nervosa 307.1
Anosmia (*see also* Disturbance, sensation) 781.1
    hysterical 300.11
    postinfectional 478.9
    psychogenic 306.7
    traumatic 951.8
Anosognosia 780.99
Anosphrasia 781.1
Anosteoplasia 756.50
Anotia 744.09
Anovulatory cycle 628.0
Anoxemia 799.02
    newborn 770.88
Anoxia 799.02
    altitude 993.2
    cerebral 348.1
        with
            abortion—*see* Abortion, by type,
                with specified complication NEC
            ectopic pregnancy (*see also* categories
                633.0-633.9) 639.8
            molar pregnancy (*see also* categories
                630-632) 639.8
        complicating
            delivery (cesarean) (instrumental) 669.4
            ectopic or molar pregnancy 639.8
            obstetric anesthesia or sedation 668.2
        during or resulting from a procedure 997.01
        following
            abortion 639.8
            ectopic or molar pregnancy 639.8
        newborn (*see also* Distress, fetal, liveborn
            infant) 770.88
    due to drowning 994.1
    fetal, affecting newborn 770.88
    heart—*see* Insufficiency, coronary
    high altitude 993.2
    intrauterine
        fetal death (before onset of labor) 768.0
            during labor 768.1
        liveborn infant—*see* Distress, fetal, liveborn
            infant
    myocardial—*see* Insufficiency, coronary
    newborn 768.9
        mild or moderate 768.6
        severe 768.5
    pathological 799.02
Anteflexion —*see* Anteversion
Antenatal
    care, normal pregnancy V22.1
        first V22.0
    sampling
        chorionic villus V28.89
    screening of mother (for) V28.9
        based on amniocentesis NEC V28.2
            chromosomal anomalies V28.0
            raised alphafetoprotein levels V28.1
        chromosomal anomalies V28.0
        fetal growth retardation using ultrasonics
            V28.4
        genomic V28.89

Antenatal—*continued*
  screening of mother—*continued*
    isoimmunization V28.5
    malformations using ultrasonics V28.3
    proteomic V28.89
    raised alphafetoprotein levels in amniotic fluid V28.1
    risk
      pre-term labor V28.82
      specified condition NEC V28.89
    Streptococcus B V28.6
    survey
      fetal anatomic V28.81
    testing
      nuchal translucency V28.89
Antepartum —*see* condition
Anterior —*see also* condition
  spinal artery compression syndrome 721.1
Antero-occlusion 524.24
Anteversion
  cervix (—*see* Anteversion, uterus)
  femur (neck), congenital 755.63
  uterus, uterine (cervix) (postinfectional) (postpartal, old) 621.6
    congenital 752.3
    in pregnancy or childbirth 654.4
      affecting fetus or newborn 763.89
      causing obstructed labor 660.2
        affecting fetus or newborn 763.1
Anthracosilicosis (occupational) 500
Anthracosis (lung) (occupational) 500
  lingua 529.3
Anthrax 022.9
  with pneumonia 022.1 *[484.5]*
  colitis 022.2
  cutaneous 022.0
  gastrointestinal 022.2
  intestinal 022.2
  pulmonary 022.1
  respiratory 022.1
  septicemia 022.3
  specified manifestation NEC 022.8
Anthropoid pelvis 755.69
  with disproportion (fetopelvic) 653.2
    affecting fetus or newborn 763.1
    causing obstructed labor 660.1
      affecting fetus or newborn 763.1
Anthropophobia 300.29
Antibioma, breast 611.0
Antibodies
  maternal (blood group) (*see also* Incompatibility) 656.2
    anti-D, cord blood 656.1
    fetus or newborn 773.0
Antibody deficiency syndrome
  agammaglobulinemic 279.00
    congenital 279.04
  hypogammaglobulinemic 279.00
Anticoagulant, intrinsic, circulating, causing hemorrhagic disorder (*see also* Circulating anticoagulants) 286.5
Antimongolism syndrome 758.39
Antimonial cholera 985.4
Antisocial personality 301.7
Antithrombinemia (*see also* Circulating anticoagulants) 286.5
Antithromboplastinemia (*see also* Circulating anticoagulants) 286.5
Antithromboplastinogenemia (*see also* Circulating anticoagulants) 286.5

Antitoxin complication or reaction —*see* Complications, vaccination
Anton (-Babinski) syndrome (hemiasomatognosia) 307.9
Antritis (chronic) 473.0
  maxilla 473.0
    acute 461.0
  stomach 535.4
Antrum, antral —*see* condition
Anuria 788.5
  with
    abortion—*see* Abortion, by type, with renal failure
    ectopic pregnancy (*see also* categories 633.0-633.9) 639.3
    molar pregnancy (*see also* categories 630-632) 639.3
  calculus (impacted) (recurrent) 592.9
    kidney 592.0
    ureter 592.1
  congenital 753.3
  due to a procedure 997.5
  following
    abortion 639.3
    ectopic or molar pregnancy 639.3
  newborn 753.3
  postrenal 593.4
  puerperal, postpartum, childbirth 669.3
  specified as due to a procedure 997.5
  sulfonamide
    correct substance properly administered 788.5
    overdose or wrong substance given or taken 961.0
  traumatic (following crushing) 958.5
Anus, anal —*see also* condition
  high risk human papillomavirus (HPV) DNA test positive 796.75
  low risk human papillomavirus (HPV) DNA test positive 796.79
Anusitis 569.49
Anxiety (neurosis) (reaction) (state) 300.00
  alcohol-induced 291.89
  depression 300.4
  drug-induced 292.89
  due to or associated with physical condition 293.84
  generalized 300.02
  hysteria 300.20
  in
    acute stress reaction 308.0
    transient adjustment reaction 309.24
  panic type 300.01
  separation, abnormal 309.21
  syndrome (organic) (transient) 293.84
Aorta, aortic —*see* condition
Aortectasia 441.9
Aortitis (nonsyphilitic) 447.6
  arteriosclerotic 440.0
  calcific 447.6
  Döhle-Heller 093.1
  luetic 093.1
  rheumatic (*see also* Endocarditis, acute, rheumatic) 391.1
  rheumatoid—*see* Arthritis, rheumatoid
  specific 093.1
  syphilitic 093.1
    congenital 090.5
Apathetic 799.25
  thyroid storm (*see also* Thyrotoxicosis) 242.9
Apathy 799.25

Apepsia 536.8
  achlorhydric 536.0
  psychogenic 306.4
Aperistalsis, esophagus 530.0
Apert's syndrome (acrocephalosyndactyly) 755.55
Apert-Gallais syndrome (adrenogenital) 255.2
Apertognathia 524.20
Aphagia 787.20
  psychogenic 307.1
Aphakia (acquired) (bilateral) (postoperative) (unilateral) 379.31
  congenital 743.35
Aphalangia (congenital) 755.4
  lower limb (complete) (intercalary) (partial) (terminal) 755.39
    meaning all digits (complete) (partial) 755.31
    transverse 755.31
  upper limb (complete) (intercalary) (partial) (terminal) 755.29
    meaning all digits (complete) (partial) 755.21
    transverse 755.21
Aphasia (amnestic) (ataxic) (auditory) (Broca's) (choreatic) (classic) (expressive) (global) (ideational) (ideokinetic) (ideomotor) (jargon) (motor) (nominal) (receptive) (semantic) (sensory) (syntactic) (verbal) (visual) (Wernicke's) 784.3
  developmental 315.31
  syphilis, tertiary 094.89
  uremic—*see* Uremia
Aphemia 784.3
  uremic—*see* Uremia
Aphonia 784.41
  clericorum 784.49
  hysterical 300.11
  organic 784.41
  psychogenic 306.1
Aphthae, aphthous —*see also* condition
  Bednar's 528.2
  cachectic 529.0
  epizootic 078.4
  fever 078.4
  oral 528.2
  stomatitis 528.2
  thrush 112.0
  ulcer (oral) (recurrent) 528.2
    genital organ(s) NEC
      female 616.50
      male 608.89
    larynx 478.79
Apical —*see* condition
Apical ballooning syndrome 429.83
Aplasia —*see also* Agenesis
  alveolar process (acquired) 525.8
    congenital 750.26
  aorta (congenital) 747.22
  aortic valve (congenital) 746.89
  axialis extracorticalis (congenital) 330.0
  bone marrow (myeloid) 284.9
    acquired (secondary) 284.89
    congenital 284.01
    idiopathic 284.9
  brain 740.0
    specified part 742.2
  breast 757.6
  bronchus 748.3
  cementum 520.4
  cerebellar 742.2
  congenital (pure) red cell 284.01
  corpus callosum 742.2

Aplasia—*continued*
  erythrocyte 284.81
    congenital 284.01
  extracortical axial 330.0
  eye (congenital) 743.00
  fovea centralis (congenital) 743.55
  germinal (cell) 606.0
  iris 743.45
  labyrinth, membranous 744.05
  limb (congenital) 755.4
    lower NEC 755.30
    upper NEC 755.20
  lung (bilateral) (congenital) (unilateral) 748.5
  nervous system NEC 742.8
  nuclear 742.8
  ovary 752.0
  Pelizaeus-Merzbacher 330.0
  prostate (congenital) 752.89
  red cell (with thymoma) (adult) 284.81
    acquired (secondary) 284.81
    congenital 284.01
    hereditary 284.01
    of infants 284.01
    primary 284.01
    pure 284.01
  round ligament (congenital) 752.89
  salivary gland 750.21
  skin (congenital) 757.39
  spinal cord 742.59
  spleen 759.0
  testis (congenital) 752.89
  thymic, with immunodeficiency 279.2
  thyroid 243
  uterus 752.3
  ventral horn cell 742.59
Apleuria 756.3
Apnea, apneic (spells) 786.03
  newborn, neonatorum 770.81
    essential 770.81
    obstructive 770.82
    primary 770.81
    sleep 770.81
    specified NEC 770.82
  psychogenic 306.1
  sleep, unspecified 780.57
    with
      hypersomnia, unspecified 780.53
      hyposomnia, unspecified 780.51
      insomnia, unspecified 780.51
      sleep disturbance 780.57
    central, in conditions classified elsewhere 327.27
    obstructive (adult) (pediatric) 327.23
    organic 327.20
    other 327.29
    primary central 327.21
Apneumatosis newborn 770.4
Apodia 755.31
Apophysitis (bone) (*see also* Osteochondrosis) 732.9
  calcaneus 732.5
  juvenile 732.6
Apoplectiform convulsions (*see also* Disease, cerebrovascular, acute) 436
Apoplexia, apoplexy, apoplectic (*see also* Disease, cerebrovascular, acute) 436
  abdominal 569.89
  adrenal 036.3
  attack 436
  basilar (*see also* Disease, cerebrovascular, acute) 436

Apoplexia, apoplexy, apoplectic—*continued*
  brain (*see also* Disease, cerebrovascular, acute)
    436
  bulbar (*see also* Disease, cerebrovascular, acute)
    436
  capillary (*see also* Disease, cerebrovascular,
    acute) 436
  cardiac (*see also* Infarct, myocardium) 410.9
  cerebral (*see also* Disease, cerebrovascular,
    acute) 436
  chorea (*see also* Disease, cerebrovascular,
    acute) 436
  congestive (*see also* Disease, cerebrovascular,
    acute) 436
    newborn 767.4
  embolic (*see also* Embolism, brain) 434.1
  fetus 767.0
  fit (*see also* Disease, cerebrovascular, acute) 436
  healed or old V12.54
  heart (auricle) (ventricle) (*see also* Infarct,
    myocardium) 410.9
  heat 992.0
  hemiplegia (*see also* Disease, cerebrovascular,
    acute) 436
  hemorrhagic (stroke) (*see also* Hemorrhage,
    brain) 432.9
  ingravescent (*see also* Disease, cerebrovascular,
    acute) 436
  late effect—*see* Late effect(s) (of)
    cerebrovascular disease
  lung—*see* Embolism, pulmonary
  meninges, hemorrhagic (*see also* Hemorrhage,
    subarachnoid) 430
  neonatorum 767.0
  newborn 767.0
  pancreatitis 577.0
  placenta 641.2
  progressive (*see also* Disease, cerebrovascular,
    acute) 436
  pulmonary (artery) (vein)—*see* Embolism,
    pulmonary
  sanguineous (*see also* Disease, cerebrovascular,
    acute) 436
  seizure (*see also* Disease, cerebrovascular,
    acute) 436
  serous (*see also* Disease, cerebrovascular, acute)
    436
  spleen 289.59
  stroke (*see also* Disease, cerebrovascular, acute)
    436
  thrombotic (*see also* Thrombosis, brain) 434.0
  uremic—*see* Uremia
  uteroplacental 641.2
Appendage
  fallopian tube (cyst of Morgagni) 752.11
  intestine (epiploic) 751.5
  preauricular 744.1
  testicular (organ of Morgagni) 752.89
Appendicitis 541
  with
    perforation, peritonitis (generalized), or
      rupture 540.0
      with peritoneal abscess 540.1
    peritoneal abscess 540.1
  acute (catarrhal) (fulminating) (gangrenous)
    (inflammatory) (obstructive) (retrocecal)
    (suppurative) 540.9
    with
      perforation, peritonitis, or rupture 540.0
        with peritoneal abscess 540.1
      peritoneal abscess 540.1

Apendicitis—*continued*
  amebic 006.8
  chronic (recurrent) 542
  exacerbation—*see* Appendicitis, acute
  fulminating—*see* Appendicitis, acute
  gangrenous—*see* Appendicitis, acute
  healed (obliterative) 542
  interval 542
  neurogenic 542
  obstructive 542
  pneumococcal 541
  recurrent 542
  relapsing 542
  retrocecal 541
  subacute (adhesive) 542
  subsiding 542
  suppurative—*see* Appendicitis, acute
  tuberculous (*see also* Tuberculosis) 014.8
Appendiclausis 543.9
Appendicolithiasis 543.9
Appendicopathia oxyurica 127.4
Appendix, appendicular —*see also* condition
  Morgagni (male) 752.89
    fallopian tube 752.11
Appetite
  depraved 307.52
  excessive 783.6
    psychogenic 307.51
  lack or loss (*see also* Anorexia) 783.0
    nonorganic origin 307.59
  perverted 307.52
    hysterical 300.11
Apprehension, apprehensiveness (abnormal)
    (state) 300.00
  specified type NEC 300.09
Approximal wear 521.10
Apraxia (classic) (ideational) (ideokinetic)
    (ideomotor) (motor) 784.69
  oculomotor, congenital 379.51
  verbal 784.69
Aptyalism 527.7
Aqueous misdirection 365.83
Arabicum elephantiasis (*see also* Infestation,
    filarial) 125.9
Arachnidism 989.5
Arachnitis —*see* Meningitis
Arachnodactyly 759.82
Arachnoidism 989.5
Arachnoiditis (acute) (adhesive) (basic) (brain)
    (cerebrospinal) (chiasmal) (chronic) (spinal)
    (*see also* Meningitis) 322.9
  meningococcal (chronic) 036.0
  syphilitic 094.2
  tuberculous (*see also* Tuberculosis, meninges)
    013.0
Araneism 989.5
Arboencephalitis, Australian 062.4
Arborization block (heart) 426.6
Arbor virus, arbovirus (infection) NEC 066.9
ARC 042
Arches —*see* condition
Arcuatus uterus 752.3
Arcus (cornea)
  juvenilis 743.43
    interfering with vision 743.42
  senilis 371.41
Arc-welders' lung 503
Arc-welders' syndrome (photokeratitis) 370.24
Areflexia 796.1
Areola —*see* condition

Argentaffinoma (M8241/1)—*see also* Neoplasm, by site, uncertain behavior
benign (M8241/0)—*see* Neoplasm, by site, benign
malignant (M8241/3)—*see* Neoplasm, by site, malignant
syndrome 259.2
Argentinian hemorrhagic fever 078.7
Arginosuccinicaciduria 270.6
Argonz-Del Castillo syndrome (nonpuerperal galactorrhea and amenorrhea) 253.1
Argyll-Robertson phenomenon pupil, or syndrome (syphilitic) 094.89
atypical 379.45
nonluetic 379.45
nonsyphilitic 379.45
reversed 379.45
Argyria, argyriasis NEC 985.8
conjunctiva 372.55
cornea 371.16
from drug or medicinal agent
correct substance properly administered 709.09
overdose or wrong substance given or taken 961.2
Arhinencephaly 742.2
Arias-Stella phenomenon 621.30
Ariboflavinosis 266.0
Arizona enteritis 008.1
Arm —*see* condition
Armenian disease 277.31
Arnold-Chiari obstruction or syndrome (*see also* Spina bifida) 741.0
type I 348.4
type II (*see also* Spina bifida) 741.0
type III 742.0
type IV 742.2
Arousals
confusional 327.41
Arrest, arrested
active phase of labor 661.1
affecting fetus or newborn 763.7
any plane in pelvis
complicating delivery 660.1
affecting fetus or newborn 763.1
bone marrow (*see also* Anemia, aplastic) 284.9
cardiac 427.5
with
abortion—*see* Abortion, by type, with specified complication NEC
ectopic pregnancy (*see also* categories 633.0-633.9) 639.8
molar pregnancy (*see also* categories 630-632) 639.8
complicating
anesthesia
correct substance properly administered 427.5
obstetric 668.1
overdose or wrong substance given 968.4
specified anesthetic—*see* Table of drugs and chemicals
delivery (cesarean) (instrumental) 669.4
ectopic or molar pregnancy 639.8
surgery (nontherapeutic) (therapeutic) 997.1
fetus or newborn 779.85
following
abortion 639.8
ectopic or molar pregnancy 639.8
personal history, successfully rescucitated V12.53
postoperative (immediate) 997.1
long-term effect of cardiac surgery 429.4

Arrest, arrested—*continued*
cardiorespiratory (*see also* Arrest, cardiac) 427.5
deep transverse 660.3
affecting fetus or newborn 763.1
development or growth
bone 733.91
child 783.40
fetus 764.9
affecting management of pregnancy 656.5
tracheal rings 748.3
epiphyseal 733.91
granulopoiesis 288.09
heart—*see* Arrest, cardiac
respiratory 799.1
newborn 770.87
sinus 426.6
transverse (deep) 660.3
affecting fetus or newborn 763.1
Arrhenoblastoma (M8630.1)
benign (M8630/0)
specified site—*see* Neoplasm, by site, benign
unspecified site
female 220
male 222.0
malignant (M8630/3)
specified site— *see* Neoplasm, by site, malignant
unspecified site
female 183.0
male 186.9
specified site—*see* Neoplasm, by site, uncertain behavior
unspecified site
female 236.2
male 236.4
Arrhinencephaly 742.2
due to
trisomy 13 (13-15) 758.1
trisomy 18 (16-18) 758.2
Arrhythmia (auricle) (cardiac) (cordis) (gallop rhythm) (juvenile) (nodal) (reflex) (sinus) (supraventricular) (transitory) (ventricle) 427.9
bigeminal rhythm 427.89
block 426.9
bradycardia 427.89
contractions, premature 427.60
coronary sinus 427.89
ectopic 427.89
extrasystolic 427.60
postoperative 997.1
psychogenic 306.2
vagal 780.2
Arrillaga-Ayerza syndrome (pulmonary artery sclerosis with pulmonary hypertension) 416.0
Arsenical
dermatitis 692.4
keratosis 692.4
pigmentation 985.1
from drug or medicinal agent
correct substance properly administered 709.09
overdose or wrong substance given or taken 961.1
Arsenism 985.1
from drug or medicinal agent
correct substance properly administered 692.4
overdose or wrong substance given or taken 961.1
Arterial —*see* condition
Arteriectasis 447.8
Arteriofibrosis —*see* Arteriosclerosis
Arteriolar sclerosis —*see* Arteriosclerosis

Arteriolith —*see* Arteriosclerosis
Arteriolitis 447.6
  necrotizing, kidney 447.5
  renal—*see* Hypertension, kidney
Arteriolosclerosis —*see* Arteriosclerosis
Arterionephrosclerosis (*see also* Hypertension, kidney) 403.90
Arteriopathy 447.9
Arteriosclerosis, arteriosclerotic (artery) (deformans) (diffuse) (disease) (endarteritis) (general) (obliterans) (obliterative) (occlusive) (senile) (with calcification) 440.9
  with
    gangrene 440.24
    psychosis (*see also* Psychosis, arteriosclerotic) 290.40
    ulceration 440.23
  aorta 440.0
  arteries of extremities NEC — *see* Arteriosclerosis, extremities
  basilar (artery) (*see also* Occlusion, artery, basilar) 433.0
  brain 437.0
  bypass graft
    coronary artery 414.05
      autologous artery (gastroepiploic) (internal mammary) 414.04
      autologous vein 414.02
      nonautologous biological 414.03
      of transplanted heart 414.07
    extremity 440.30
      autologous vein 440.31
      nonautologous biological 440.32
  cardiac — *see* Arteriosclerosis, coronary
  cardiopathy — *see* Arteriosclerosis, coronary
  cardiorenal (*see also* Hypertension, cardiorenal) 404.90
  cardiovascular (*see also* Disease, cardiovascular) 429.2
  carotid (artery) (common) (internal) (*see also* Occlusion, artery, carotid) 433.1
  central nervous system 437.0
  cerebral 437.0
    late effect—*see* Late effect(s) (of) cerebrovascular disease
  cerebrospinal 437.0
  cerebrovascular 437.0
  coronary (artery) 414.00
    due to lipid rich plaque 414.3
    graft—*see* Arteriosclerosis, bypass graft
    native artery 414.01
    of transplanted heart 414.06
    of transplanted heart 414.06
  extremities (native artery) 440.20
    bypass graft 440.30
      autologous vein 440.31
      nonautologous biological 440.32
    claudication (intermittent) 440.21
    and
      gangrene 440.24
      rest pain 440.22
      and
        gangrene 440.24
        ulceration 440.23
          and gangrene 440.24
      ulceration 440.23
        and gangrene 440.24
    gangrene 440.24
    rest pain 440.22
      and gangrene 440.24
      and ulceration 440.23
        and gangrene 440.24

Arteriosclerosis, arteriosclerotic—*continued*
  extremities—*continued*
    specified site NEC 440.29
    ulceration 440.23
      and gangrene 440.24
  heart (disease) — *see also* Arteriosclerosis, coronary
    valve 424.99
      aortic 424.1
      mitral 424.0
      pulmonary 424.3
      tricuspid 424.2
  kidney (*see also* Hypertension, kidney) 403.90
  labyrinth, labyrinthine 388.00
  medial NEC 440.20
  mesentery (artery) 557.1
  Mönckeberg's 440.20
  myocarditis 429.0
  nephrosclerosis (*see also* Hypertension, kidney) 403.90
  peripheral (of extremities) *see* Arteriosclerosis, extremities
  precerebral 433.9
    specified artery NEC 433.8
  pulmonary (idiopathic) 416.0
  renal (*see also* Hypertension, kidney) 403.90
    arterioles (*see also* Hypertension, kidney) 403.90
    artery 440.1
  retinal (vascular) 440.8 *[362.13]*
  specified artery NEC 440.8
    with gangrene 440.8 *[785.4]*
  spinal (cord) 437.0
  vertebral (artery) (*see also* Occlusion, artery, vertebral) 433.2
Arteriospasm 443.9
Arteriovenous —*see* condition
Arteritis 447.6
  allergic (*see also* Angiitis, hypersensitivity) 446.20
  aorta (nonsyphilitic) 447.6
    syphilitic 093.1
  aortic arch 446.7
  brachiocephalica 446.7
  brain 437.4
    syphilitic 094.89
  branchial 446.7
  cerebral 437.4
    late effect—*see* Late effect(s) (of) cerebrovascular disease
    syphilitic 094.89
  coronary (artery) —*see also* Arteriosclerosis, coronary
    rheumatic 391.9
      chronic 398.99
    syphilitic 093.89
  cranial (left) (right) 446.5
  deformans—*see* Arteriosclerosis
  giant cell 446.5
  necrosing or necrotizing 446.0
  nodosa 446.0
  obliterans—*see also* Arteriosclerosis
    subclaviocarotica 446.7
  pulmonary 417.8
  retina 362.18
  rheumatic—*see* Fever, rheumatic
  senile—*see* Arteriosclerosis
  suppurative 447.2
  syphilitic (general) 093.89
    brain 094.89
    coronary 093.89
    spinal 094.89

Arteritis—*continued*
  temporal 446.5
  young female, syndrome 446.7
Artery, arterial —*see* condition
Arthralgia (*see also* Pain, joint) 719.4
  allergic (*see also* Pain, joint) 719.4
  in caisson disease 993.3
  psychogenic 307.89
  rubella 056.71
  Salmonella 003.23
  temporomandibular joint 524.62
Arthritis, arthritic (acute) (chronic) (subacute)
  716.9

---

*Note—Use the following fifth-digit
subclassification with categories 711-712,
715-716:*

0 *site unspecified*
1 *shoulder region*
2 *upper arm*
3 *forearm*
4 *hand*
5 *pelvic region and thigh*
6 *lower leg*
7 *ankle and foot*
8 *other specified sites*
9 *multiple sites*

---

  allergic 716.2
  ankylosing (crippling) (spine) 720.0
    sites other than spine 716.9
  atrophic 714.0
    spine 720.9
  back (*see also* Arthritis, spine) 721.90
  Bechterew's (ankylosing spondylitis) 720.0
  blennorrhagic 098.50
  cervical, cervicodorsal (*see also* Spondylosis,
    cervical) 721.0
  Charcot's 094.0 *[713.5]*
    diabetic 250.6 *[713.5]*
      due to secondary diabetes 249.6 *[713.5]*
    syringomyelic 336.0 *[713.5]*
    tabetic 094.0 *[713.5]*
  chylous (*see also* Filariasis) 125.9 *[711.7]*
  climacteric NEC 716.3
  coccyx 721.8
  cricoarytenoid 478.79
  crystal (-induced)—*see* Arthritis, due to crystals
  deformans (*see also* Osteoarthrosis) 715.9
    spine 721.90
      with myelopathy 721.91
  degenerative (*see also* Osteoarthrosis) 715.9
    idiopathic 715.09
    polyarticular 715.09
    spine 721.90
      with myelopathy 721.91
  dermatoarthritis, lipoid 272.8 *[713.0]*
  due to or associated with
    acromegaly 253.0 *[713.0]*
    actinomycosis 039.8 *[711.4]*
    amyloidosis 277.39 *[713.7]*
    bacterial disease NEC 040.89 *[711.4]*
    Behçet's syndrome 136.1 *[711.2]*
    blastomycosis 116.0 *[711.6]*
    brucellosis (*see also* Brucellosis) 023.9
      [711.4]
    caisson disease 993.3
    coccidioidomycosis 114.3 *[711.6]*
    coliform (Escherichia coli) 711.0
    colitis, ulcerative (*see also* Colitis, ulcerative)
      556.9 *[713.1]*

Arthritis, arthritic—*continued*
  due to or associated with—*continued*
    cowpox 051.01 *[711.5]*
    crystals (*see also* Gout)
      dicalcium phosphate 275.49 *[712.1]*
      pyrophosphate 275.49 *[712.2]*
      specified NEC 275.49 *[712.8]*
    dermatoarthritis, lipoid 272.8 *[713.0]*
    dermatological disorder NEC 709.9 *[713.3]*
    diabetes 250.6 *[713.0]*
      due to secondary diabetes 249.6 *[713.5]*
    diphtheria 032.89 *[711.4]*
    dracontiasis 125.7 *[711.7]*
    dysentery 009.0 *[711.3]*
    endocrine disorder NEC 259.9 *[713.0]*
    enteritis NEC 009.1 *[711.3]*
      infectious (*see also* Enteritis, infectious)
        009.0 *[711.3]*
        specified organism NEC 008.8 *[711.3]*
      regional (*see also* Enteritis, regional) 555.9
        [713.1]
      specified organism NEC 008.8 *[711.3]*
    epiphyseal slip, nontraumatic (old) 716.8
    erysipelas 035 *[711.4]*
    erythema
      epidemic 026.1
      multiforme 695.10 *[713.3]*
      nodosum 695.2 *[713.3]*
    Escherichia coli 711.0
    filariasis NEC 125.9 *[711.7]*
    gastrointestinal condition NEC 569.9 *[713.1]*
    glanders 024 *[711.4]*
    Gonococcus 098.50
    gout 274.00
    H. influenzae 711.0
    helminthiasis NEC 128.9 *[711.7]*
    hematological disorder NEC 289.9 *[713.2]*
    hemochromatosis 275.0 *[713.0]*
    hemoglobinopathy NEC (*see also* Disease,
      hemoglobin) 282.7 *[713.2]*
    hemophilia (*see also* Hemophilia) 286.0
      [713.2]
    Hemophilus influenzae (H. influenzae) 711.0
    Henoch (-Schönlein) purpura 287.0 *[713.6]*
    histoplasmosis NEC (*see also* Histoplasmosis)
      115.99 *[711.6]*
    human parvovirus 079.83 *[711.5]*
    hyperparathyroidism 252.00 *[713.0]*
    hypersensitivity reaction NEC 995.3 *[713.6]*
    hypogammaglobulinemia (*see also*
      Hypogammaglobulinemia) 279.00 *[713.0]*
    hypothyroidism NEC 244.9 *[713.0]*
    infection (*see also* Arthritis, infectious) 711.9
    infectious disease NEC 136.9 *[711.8]*
    leprosy (*see also* Leprosy) 030.9 *[711.4]*
    leukemia NEC (M9800/3) 208.9 *[713.2]*
    lipoid dermatoarthritis 272.8 *[713.0]*
    Lyme disease 088.81 *[711.8]*
    meaning Osteoarthritis—*see* Osteoarthrosis
    Mediterranean fever, familial 277.31 *[713.7]*
    meningococcal infection 036.82
    metabolic disorder NEC 277.9 *[713.0]*
    multiple myelomatosis (M9730/3) 203.0
      [713.2]
    mumps 072.79 *[711.5]*
    mycobacteria 031.8 *[711.4]*
    mycosis NEC 117.9 *[711.6]*
    neurological disorder NEC 349.9 *[713.5]*
    ochronosis 270.2 *[713.0]*
    O'Nyong Nyong 066.3 *[711.5]*
    parasitic disease NEC 136.9 *[711.8]*

Arthritis, arthritic—*continued*
  thoracic (*see also* Spondylosis, thoracic) 721.2
  toxic of menopause 716.3
  transient 716.4
  traumatic (chronic) (old) (post) 716.1
    current injury—*see* nature of injury
  tuberculous (*see also* Tuberculosis, arthritis)
    015.9 *[711.4]*
  urethritica 099.3 *[711.1]*
  urica, uratic 274.00
  venereal 099.3 *[711.1]*
  vertebral (*see also* Arthritis, spine) 721.90
  villous 716.8
  von Bechterew's 720.0
Arthrocele (*see also* Effusion, joint) 719.0
Arthrochondritis —*see* Arthritis
Arthrodesis status V45.4
Arthrodynia (*see also* Pain, joint) 719.4
  psychogenic 307.89
Arthrodysplasia 755.9
Arthrofibrosis, joint (*see also* Ankylosis) 718.5
Arthrogryposis 728.3
  multiplex, congenita 754.89
Arthrokatadysis 715.35
Arthrolithiasis 274.00
Arthro-onychodysplasia 756.89
Arthro-osteo-onychodysplasia 756.89
Arthropathy (*see also* Arthritis) 716.9

Note—Use the following fifth-digit
subclassification with categories 711-712, 716:

0 site unspecified
1 shoulder region
2 upper arm
3 forearm
4 hand
5 pelvic region and thigh
6 lower leg
7 ankle and foot
8 other specified sites
9 multiple sites

  Behçet's 136.1 *[711.2]*
  Charcot's 094.0 *[713.5]*
    diabetic 250.6 *[713.5]*
      due to secondary diabetes 249.6 *[713.5]*
    syringomyelic 336.0 *[713.5]*
    tabetic 094.0 *[713.5]*
  crystal (-induced)—*see* Arthritis, due to crystals
  gouty 274.00
    acute 274.01
    chronic (without mention of tophus (tophi))
      274.02
      with tophus (tophi) 274.03
  neurogenic, neuropathic (Charcot's) (tabetic)
    094.0 *[713.5]*
    diabetic 250.6 *[713.5]*
      due to secondary diabetes 249.6 *[713.5]*
    nonsyphilitic NEC 349.9 *[713.5]*
    syringomyelic 336.0 *[713.5]*
  postdysenteric NEC 009.0 *[711.3]*
  postrheumatic, chronic (Jaccoud's) 714.4
  psoriatic 696.0
  pulmonary 731.2
  specified NEC 716.8
  syringomyelia 336.0 *[713.5]*
  tabes dorsalis 094.0 *[713.5]*
  tabetic 094.0 *[713.5]*
  transient 716.4
  traumatic 716.1
  uric acid 274.00

Arthrophyte (*see also* Loose, body, joint) 718.1
Arthrophytis 719.80
  ankle 719.87
  elbow 719.82
  foot 719.87
  hand 719.84
  hip 719.85
  knee 719.86
  multiple sites 719.89
  pelvic region 719.85
  shoulder (region) 719.81
  specified site NEC 719.88
  wrist 719.83
Arthropyosis (*see also* Arthritis, pyogenic) 711.0
Arthroscopic surgical procedure converted to
  open procedure V64.43
Arthrosis (deformans) (degenerative) (*see also*
  Osteoarthrosis) 715.9
  Charcot's 094.0 *[713.5]*
  polyarticular 715.09
  spine (*see also* Spondylosis) 721.90
Arthus' phenomenon 995.21
  due to
    correct substance properly administered
      995.21
    overdose or wrong substance given or taken
      977.9
    specified drug—*see* Table of drugs and
      chemicals
  serum 999.5
Articular —*see also* condition
  disc disorder (reducing or non-reducing) 524.63
  spondylolisthesis 756.12
Articulation
  anterior 524.27
  posterior 524.27
  reverse 524.27
Artificial
  device (prosthetic)—*see* Fitting, device
  insemination V26.1
  menopause (states) (symptoms) (syndrome)
    627.4
  opening status (functioning) (without
    complication) V44.9
    anus (colostomy) V44.3
    colostomy V44.3
    cystostomy V44.50
      appendico-vesicostomy V44.52
      cutaneous-vesicostomy V44.51
      specified type NEC V44.59
    enterostomy V44.4
    gastrostomy V44.1
    ileostomy V44.2
    intestinal tract NEC V44.4
    jejunostomy V44.4
    nephrostomy V44.6
    specified site NEC V44.8
    tracheostomy V44.0
    ureterostomy V44.6
    urethrostomy V44.6
    urinary tract NEC V44.6
    vagina V44.7
  vagina status V44.7
ARV (disease) (illness) (infection)—*see* Human
  immunodeficiency virus (disease) (illness)
  (infection)
Arytenoid —*see* condition
Asbestosis (occupational) 501
Asboe-Hansen's disease (incontinentia pigmenti)
  757.33
Ascariasis (intestinal) (lung) 127.0
Ascaridiasis 127.0

Ascaridosis 127.0
Ascaris 127.0
  lumbricoides (infestation) 127.0
  pneumonia 127.0
Ascending —*see* condition
ASC-H (atypical squamous cells cannot exclude
  high grade squamous intraepithelial lesion)
  anus 796.72
  cervix 795.02
  vagina 795.12
Aschoff's bodies (*see also* Myocarditis,
  rheumatic) 398.0
Ascites 789.59
  abdominal NEC 789.59
  cancerous (M8000/6) 789.51
  cardiac 428.0
  chylous (nonfilarial) 457.8
    filarial (*see also* Infestation, filarial) 125.9
  congenital 778.0
  due to S. japonicum 120.2
  fetal, causing fetopelvic disproportion 653.7
  heart 428.0
  joint (*see also* Effusion, joint) 719.0
  malignant (M8000/6) 789.51
  pseudochylous 789.59
  syphilitic 095.2
  tuberculous (*see also* Tuberculosis) 014.0
Ascorbic acid (vitamin C) deficiency (scurvy)
  267
ASC-US (atypical squamous cells of
  undetermined significance)
  anus 796.71
  cervix 795.01
  vagina 795.11
ASCVD (arteriosclerotic cardiovascular disease)
  429.2
Aseptic —*see* condition
Asherman's syndrome 621.5
Asialia 527.7
Asiatic cholera (*see also* Cholera) 001.9
Asocial personality or trends 301.7
Asomatognosia 781.8
Aspergillosis 117.3
  with pneumonia 117.3 *[484.6]*
  allergic bronchopulmonary 518.6
  nonsyphilitic NEC 117.3
Aspergillus (flavus) (fumigatus) (infection)
  (terreus) 117.3
Aspermatogenesis 606.0
Aspermia (testis) 606.0
Asphyxia, asphyxiation (by) 799.01
  antenatal—*see* Distress, fetal
  bedclothes 994.7
  birth (*see also* Asphyxia, newborn) 768.9
  bunny bag 994.7
  carbon monoxide 986
  caul (*see also* Asphyxia, newborn) 768.9
  cave-in 994.7
    crushing—*see* Injury, internal, intrathoracic
      organs
  constriction 994.7
  crushing—*see* Injury, internal, intrathoracic
    organs
  drowning 994.1
  fetal, affecting newborn 768.9

Asphyxia, asphyxiation—*continued*
  food or foreign body (in larynx) 933.1
    bronchioles 934.8
    bronchus (main) 934.1
    lung 934.8
    nasopharynx 933.0
    nose, nasal passages 932
    pharynx 933.0
    respiratory tract 934.9
      specified part NEC 934.8
    throat 933.0
    trachea 934.0
  gas, fumes, or vapor NEC 987.9
    specified—*see* Table of drugs and chemicals
  gravitational changes 994.7
  hanging 994.7
  inhalation—*see* Inhalation
  intrauterine
    fetal death (before onset of labor) 768.0
      during labor 768.1
    liveborn infant—*see* Distress, fetal, liveborn
      infant
  local 443.0
  mechanical 994.7
    during birth (*see also* Distress, fetal) 768.9
  mucus 933.1
    bronchus (main) 934.1
    larynx 933.1
    lung 934.8
    nasal passages 932
    newborn 770.18
    pharynx 933.0
    respiratory tract 934.9
      specified part NEC 934.8
    throat 933.0
    trachea 934.0
    vaginal (fetus or newborn) 770.18
  newborn 768.9
    blue 768.6
    livida 768.6
    mild or moderate 768.6
    pallida 768.5
    severe 768.5
    white 768.5
    with neurologic involvement 768.5
  pathological 799.01
  plastic bag 994.7
  postnatal (*see also* Asphyxia, newborn) 768.9
    mechanical 994.7
  pressure 994.7
  reticularis 782.61
  strangulation 994.7
  submersion 994.1
  traumatic NEC—*see* Injury, internal,
    intrathoracic organs
  vomiting, vomitus—*see* Asphyxia, food or
    foreign body
Aspiration
  acid pulmonary (syndrome) 997.39
    obstetric 668.0
  amniotic fluid 770.13
    with respiratory symptoms 770.14
  bronchitis 507.0
  clear amniotic fluid 770.13
    with
      pneumonia 770.14
      pneumonitis 770.14
      respiratory symptoms 770.14
  contents of birth canal 770.17
    with respiratory symptoms 770.18

Aspiration—*continued*
  fetal 770.10
    blood 770.15
      with
        pneumonia 770.16
        pneumonitis 770.16
      pneumonitis 770.18
    food, foreign body, or gasoline (with
      asphyxiation)—*see* Asphyxia, food or
      foreign body
    meconium 770.11
      with
        pneumonia 770.12
        pneumonitis 770.12
        respiratory symptoms 770.12
      below vocal cords 770.11
        with respiratory symptoms 770.12
  mucus 933.1
    into
      bronchus (main) 934.1
      lung 934.8
      respiratory tract 934.9
        specified part NEC 934.8
      trachea 934.0
    newborn 770.17
    vaginal (fetus or newborn) 770.17
  newborn 770.10
    with respiratory symptoms 770.18
    blood 770.15
      with
        pneumonia 770.16
        pneumonitis 770.16
        respiratory symptoms 770.16
    pneumonia 507.0
      fetus or newborn 770.18
        meconium 770.12
    pneumonitis 507.0
      fetus or newborn 770.18
        meconium 770.12
      obstetric 668.0
    postnatal stomach contents 770.85
      with
        pneumonia 770.86
        pneumonitis 770.86
        respiratory symptoms 770.86
    syndrome of newborn (massive) 770.18
      meconium 770.12
    vernix caseosa 770.17
Asplenia 759.0
  with mesocardia 746.87
Assam fever 085.0
Assimilation, pelvis
  with disproportion 653.2
    affecting fetus or newborn 763.1
    causing obstructed labor 660.1
      affecting fetus or newborn 763.1
Assmann's focus (*see also* Tuberculosis) 011.0
Astasia (-abasia) 307.9
  hysterical 300.11
Asteatosis 706.8
  cutis 706.8
Astereognosis 780.99
Asterixis 781.3
  in liver disease 572.8
Asteroid hyalitis 379.22
Asthenia, asthenic 780.79
  cardiac (*see also* Failure, heart) 428.9
    psychogenic 306.2
  cardiovascular (*see also* Failure, heart) 428.9
    psychogenic 306.2

Asthenia—*continued*
  heart (*see also* Failure, heart) 428.9
    psychogenic 306.2
  hysterical 300.11
  myocardial (*see also* Failure, heart) 428.9
    psychogenic 306.2
  nervous 300.5
  neurocirculatory 306.2
  neurotic 300.5
  psychogenic 300.5
  psychoneurotic 300.5
  psychophysiologic 300.5
  reaction, psychoneurotic 300.5
  senile 797
  Stiller's 780.79
  tropical anhidrotic 705.1
Asthenopia 368.13
  accommodative 367.4
  hysterical (muscular) 300.11
  psychogenic 306.7
Asthenospermia 792.2
Asthma, asthmatic (bronchial) (catarrh)
  (spasmodic) 493.9

Note—The following fifth digit
subclassification is for use with codes
493.0-493.2, 493.9:

0 unspecified
1 with status asthmaticus
2 with (acute) exacerbation

---

  with
    chronic obstructive pulmonary disease
      (COPD) 493.2
    hay fever 493.0
    rhinitis, allergic 493.0
  allergic 493.9
    stated cause (external allergen) 493.0
  atopic 493.0
  cardiac (*see also* Failure, ventricular, left) 428.1
  cardiobronchial (*see also* Failure, ventricular,
    left) 428.1
  cardiorenal (*see also* Hypertension, cardiorenal)
    404.90
  childhood 493.0
  colliers' 500
  cough variant 493.82
  croup 493.9
  detergent 507.8
  due to
    detergent 507.8
    inhalation of fumes 506.3
    internal immunological process 493.0
  endogenous (intrinsic) 493.1
  eosinophilic 518.3
  exercise induced bronchospasm 493.81
  exogenous (cosmetics) (dander or dust) (drugs)
    (dust) (feathers) (food) (hay) (platinum)
    (pollen) 493.0
  extrinsic 493.0
  grinders' 502
  hay 493.0
  heart (*see also* Failure, ventricular, left) 428.1
  IgE 493.0
  infective 493.1
  intrinsic 493.1
  Kopp's 254.8
  late-onset 493.1
  meat-wrappers' 506.9
  Millar's (laryngismus stridulus) 478.75
  millstone makers' 502

Asthma—*continued*
  miners' 500
  Monday morning 504
  New Orleans (epidemic) 493.0
  platinum 493.0
  pneumoconiotic (occupational) NEC 505
  potters' 502
  psychogenic 316 *[493.9]*
  pulmonary eosinophilic 518.3
  red cedar 495.8
  Rostan's (*see also* Failure, ventricular, left) 428.1
  sandblasters' 502
  sequoiosis 495.8
  stonemasons' 502
  thymic 254.8
  tuberculous (*see also* Tuberculosis, pulmonary) 011.9
  Wichmann's (laryngismus stridulus) 478.75
  wood 495.8
Astigmatism (compound) (congenital) 367.20
  irregular 367.22
  regular 367.21
Astroblastoma (M9430/3)
  nose 748.1
  specified site—*see* Neoplasm, by site,
    malignant
  unspecified site 191.9
Astrocytoma (cystic) (M9400/3)
  anaplastic type (M9401/3)
    specified site—*see* Neoplasm, by site,
      malignant
    unspecified site 191.9
  fibrillary (M9420/3)
    specified site—*see* Neoplasm, by site,
      malignant
    unspecified site 191.9
  fibrous (M9420/3)
    specified site—*see* Neoplasm, by site,
      malignant
    unspecified site 191.9
  gemistocytic (M9411/3)
    specified site—*see* Neoplasm, by site,
      malignant
    unspecified site 191.9
  juvenile (M9421/3)
    specified site—*see* Neoplasm, by site,
      malignant
    unspecified site 191.9
  nose 748.1
  pilocytic (M9421/3)
    specified site—*see* Neoplasm, by site,
      malignant
    unspecified site 191.9
  piloid (M9421/3)
    specified site—*see* Neoplasm, by site, malignant
    unspecified site 191.9
  protoplasmic (M9410/3)
    specified site—*see* Neoplasm, by site,
      malignant
    unspecified site 191.9
  specified site—*see* Neoplasm, by site, malignant
  subependymal (M9383/1) 237.5
    giant cell (M9384/1) 237.5
  unspecified site 191.9
Astroglioma (M9400/3)
  nose 748.1
  specified site—*see* Neoplasm, by site, malignant
  unspecified site 191.9
Asymbolia 784.60
Asymmetrical breathing 786.09

Asymmetry —*see also* Distortion
  breast, between native and reconstructed 612.1
  chest 786.9
  face 754.0
  jaw NEC 524.12
    maxillary 524.11
  pelvis with disproportion 653.0
    affecting fetus or newborn 763.1
    causing obstructed labor 660.1
      affecting fetus or newborn 763.1
Asynergia 781.3
Asynergy 781.3
  ventricular 429.89
Asystole (heart) (*see also* Arrest, cardiac) 427.5
At risk for falling V15.88
Ataxia, ataxy, ataxic 781.3
  acute 781.3
  brain 331.89
  cerebellar 334.3
    hereditary (Marie's) 334.2
    in
      alcoholism 303.9 *[334.4]*
      myxedema (*see also* Myxedema) 244.9
        [334.4]
      neoplastic disease NEC 239.9 *[334.4]*
  cerebral 331.89
  family, familial 334.2
    cerebral (Marie's) 334.2
    spinal (Friedreich's) 334.0
  Friedreich's (heredofamilial) (spinal) 334.0
  frontal lobe 781.3
  gait 781.2
    hysterical 300.11
  general 781.3
  hereditary NEC 334.2
    cerebellar 334.2
    spastic 334.1
    spinal 334.0
  heredofamilial (Marie's) 334.2
  hysterical 300.11
  locomotor (progressive) 094.0
    diabetic 250.6 *[337.1]*
      due to secondary diabetes 249.6 *[337.1]*
  Marie's (cerebellar) (heredofamilial) 334.2
  nonorganic origin 307.9
  partial 094.0
  postchickenpox 052.7
  progressive locomotor 094.0
  psychogenic 307.9
  Sanger-Brown's 334.2
  spastic 094.0
    hereditary 334.1
    syphilitic 094.0
  spinal
    hereditary 334.0
    progressive locomotor 094.0
  telangiectasia 334.8
Ataxia-telangiectasia 334.8
Atelectasis (absorption collapse) (complete)
    (compression) (massive) (partial)
    (postinfective) (pressure collapse)
    (pulmonary) (relaxation) 518.0
  newborn (congenital) (partial) 770.5
    primary 770.4
  primary 770.4
  tuberculous (*see also* Tuberculosis, pulmonary)
    011.9
Ateleiosis, ateliosis 253.3
Atelia —*see* Distortion
Ateliosis 253.3
Atelocardia 746.9
Atelomyelia 742.59

Athelia 757.6
Atheroembolism
extremity
lower 445.02
upper 445.01
kidney 445.81
specified site NEC 445.89
Atheroma, atheromatous (*see also*
Arteriosclerosis) 440.9
aorta, aortic 440.0
valve (*see also* Endocarditis, aortic) 424.1
artery—*see* Arteriosclerosis
basilar, (artery) (*see also* Occlusion, artery,
basilar) 433.0
carotid (artery) (common) (internal) (*see also*
Occlusion, artery, carotid) 433.1
cerebral (arteries) 437.0
coronary (artery)—*see* Arteriosclerosis, coronary
degeneration—*see* Arteriosclerosis
heart, cardiac —*see* Arteriosclerosis, coronary
mitral (valve) 424.0
myocardium, myocardial —*see* Arteriosclerosis,
coronary
pulmonary valve (heart) (*see also* Endocarditis,
pulmonary) 424.3
skin 706.2
tricuspid (heart) (valve) 424.2
valve, valvular—*see* Endocarditis
vertebral (artery) (*see also* Occlusion, artery,
vertebral) 433.2
Atheromatosis —*see also* Arteriosclerosis
arterial, congenital 272.8
Atherosclerosis —*see* Arteriosclerosis
Athetosis (acquired) 781.0
bilateral 333.79
congenital (bilateral) 333.6
double 333.71
unilateral 781.0
Athlete's
foot 110.4
heart 429.3
Athletic team examination V70.3
Athrepsia 261
Athyrea (acquired) (*see also* Hypothyroidism) 244.9
congenital 243
Athyreosis (congenital) 243
acquired—*see* Hypothyroidism
Athyroidism (acquired) (*see also*
Hypothyroidism) 244.9
congenital 243
Atmospheric pyrexia 992.0
Atonia, atony, atonic
abdominal wall 728.2
bladder (sphincter) 596.4
neurogenic NEC 596.54
with cauda equina syndrome 344.61
capillary 448.9
cecum 564.89
psychogenic 306.4
colon 564.89
psychogenic 306.4
congenital 779.89
dyspepsia 536.3
psychogenic 306.4
intestine 564.89
psychogenic 306.4
stomach 536.3
neurotic or psychogenic 306.4
psychogenic 306.4

Atonia, atony, atonic—*continued*
uterus 661.2
affecting fetus or newborn 763.7
with hemorrhage (postpartum) 666.1
without hemorrhage
intrapartum 661.2
postpartum 669.8
vesical 596.4
Atopy NEC V15.09
Atransferrinemia, congenital 273.8
Atresia, atretic (congenital) 759.89
alimentary organ or tract NEC 751.8
lower 751.2
upper 750.8
ani, anus, anal (canal) 751.2
aorta 747.22
with hypoplasia of ascending aorta and
defective development of left ventricle
(with mitral valve atresia) 746.7
arch 747.11
ring 747.21
aortic (orifice) (valve) 746.89
arch 747.11
aqueduct of Sylvius 742.3
with spina bifida (*see also* Spina bifida) 741.0
artery NEC (*see also* Atresia, blood vessel)
747.60
cerebral 747.81
coronary 746.85
eye 743.58
pulmonary 747.3
umbilical 747.5
auditory canal (external) 744.02
bile, biliary duct (common) or passage 751.61
acquired (*see also* Obstruction, biliary) 576.2
bladder (neck) 753.6
blood vessel (peripheral) NEC 747.60
cerebral 747.81
gastrointestinal 747.61
lower limb 747.64
pulmonary artery 747.3
renal 747.62
spinal 747.82
upper limb 747.63
bronchus 748.3
canal, ear 744.02
cardiac
valve 746.89
aortic 746.89
mitral 746.89
pulmonary 746.01
tricuspid 746.1
cecum 751.2
cervix (acquired) 622.4
congenital 752.49
in pregnancy or childbirth 654.6
affecting fetus or newborn 763.89
causing obstructed labor 660.2
affecting fetus or newborn 763.1
choana 748.0
colon 751.2
cystic duct 751.61
acquired 575.8
with obstruction (*see also* Obstruction,
gallbladder) 575.2
digestive organs NEC 751.8
duodenum 751.1
ear canal 744.02
ejaculatory duct 752.89
epiglottis 748.3
esophagus 750.3

Atresia, atretic—*continued*
Eustachian tube 744.24
fallopian tube (acquired) 628.2
  congenital 752.19
follicular cyst 620.0
foramen of
  Luschka 742.3
    with spina bifida (*see also* Spina bifida) 741.0
  Magendie 742.3
    with spina bifida (*see also* Spina bifida)
      741.0
gallbladder 751.69
genital organ
  external
    female 752.49
    male NEC 752.89
      penis 752.69
  internal
    female 752.89
    male 752.89
glottis 748.3
gullet 750.3
heart
  valve NEC 746.89
    aortic 746.89
    mitral 746.89
    pulmonary 746.01
    tricuspid 746.1
hymen 752.42
  acquired 623.3
  postinfective 623.3
ileum 751.1
intestine (small) 751.1
  large 751.2
iris, filtration angle (*see also* Buphthalmia)
  743.20
jejunum 751.1
kidney 753.3
lacrimal, apparatus 743.65
  acquired—*see* Stenosis, lacrimal
larynx 748.3
ligament, broad 752.19
lung 748.5
meatus urinarius 753.6
mitral valve 746.89
  with atresia or hypoplasia of aortic orifice or
    valve, with hypoplasia of ascending aorta
    and defective development of left ventricle
    746.7
nares (anterior) (posterior) 748.0
nasolacrimal duct 743.65
nasopharynx 748.8
nose, nostril 748.0
  acquired 738.0
organ or site NEC—*see* Anomaly, specified
  type NEC
osseous meatus (ear) 744.03
oviduct (acquired) 628.2
  congenital 752.19
parotid duct 750.23
  acquired 527.8
pulmonary (artery) 747.3
  valve 746.01
  vein 747.49
pulmonic 746.01
pupil 743.46
rectum 751.2
salivary duct or gland 750.23
  acquired 527.8
sublingual duct 750.23
  acquired 527.8

Atresia, atretic—*continued*
submaxillary duct or gland 750.23
  acquired 527.8
trachea 748.3
tricuspid valve 746.1
ureter 753.29
ureteropelvic junction 753.21
ureterovesical orifice 753.22
urethra (valvular) 753.6
urinary tract NEC 753.29
uterus 752.3
  acquired 621.8
vagina (acquired) 623.2
  congenital 752.49
  postgonococcal (old) 098.2
  postinfectional 623.2
  senile 623.2
vascular NEC (*see also* Atresia, blood vessel)
  747.60
  cerebral 747.81
vas deferens 752.89
vein NEC (*see also* Atresia, blood vessel)
  747.60
  cardiac 746.89
  great 747.49
  portal 747.49
  pulmonary 747.49
vena cava (inferior) (superior) 747.49
vesicourethral orifice 753.6
vulva 752.49
  acquired 624.8
Atrichia, atrichosis 704.00
congenital (universal) 757.4
Atrioventricularis commune 745.69
Atrophia —*see also* Atrophy
alba 709.09
cutis 701.8
  idiopathica progressiva 701.8
  senilis 701.8
dermatological, diffuse (idiopathic) 701.8
flava hepatis (acuta) (subacuta) (*see also*
  Necrosis, liver) 570
gyrata of choroid and retina (central) 363.54
  generalized 363.57
senilis 797
  dermatological 701.8
unguium 703.8
  congenita 757.5
Atrophoderma, atrophodermia 701.9
diffusum (idiopathic) 701.8
maculatum 701.3
  et striatum 701.3
    due to syphilis 095.8
  syphilitic 091.3
neuriticum 701.8
pigmentosum 757.33
reticulatum symmetricum faciei 701.8
senile 701.8
symmetrical 701.8
vermiculata 701.8
Atrophy, atrophic
adrenal (autoimmune) (capsule) (cortex) (gland) 255.41
  with hypofunction 255.41
alveolar process or ridge (edentulous) 525.20
  mandible 525.20
    minimal 525.21
    moderate 525.22
    severe 525.23
  maxilla 525.20
    minimal 525.24
    moderate 525.25
    severe 525.26

Atrophy, atrophic—*continued*
appendix 543.9
Aran-Duchenne muscular 335.21
arm 728.2
arteriosclerotic—*see* Arteriosclerosis
arthritis 714.0
spine 720.9
bile duct (any) 576.8
bladder 596.8
blanche (of Milian) 701.3
bone (senile) 733.99
due to
disuse 733.7
infection 733.99
tabes dorsalis (neurogenic) 094.0
posttraumatic 733.99
brain (cortex) (progressive) 331.9
with dementia 290.10
Alzheimer's 331.0
with dementia—*see* Alzheimer's dementia
circumscribed (Pick's) 331.11
with dementia
with behavioral disturbance 331.11
[294.11]
without behavioral disturbance 331.11
[294.10]
congenital 742.4
hereditary 331.9
senile 331.2
breast 611.4
puerperal, postpartum 676.3
buccal cavity 528.9
cardiac (brown) (senile) (*see also* Degeneration, myocardial) 429.1
cartilage (infectional) (joint) 733.99
cast, plaster of Paris 728.2
cerebellar—*see* Atrophy, brain
cerebral—*see* Atrophy, brain
cervix (endometrium) (mucosa) (myometrium) (senile) (uteri) 622.8
menopausal 627.8
Charcot-Marie-Tooth 356.1
choroid 363.40
diffuse secondary 363.42
hereditary (*see also* Dystrophy, choroid) 363.50
gyrate
central 363.54
diffuse 363.57
generalized 363.57
senile 363.41
ciliary body 364.57
colloid, degenerative 701.3
conjunctiva (senile) 372.89
corpus cavernosum 607.89
cortical (*see also* Atrophy, brain) 331.9
Cruveilhier's 335.21
cystic duct 576.8
dacryosialadenopathy 710.2
degenerative
colloid 701.3
senile 701.3
Déjérine-Thomas 333.0
diffuse idiopathic, dermatological 701.8
disuse
bone 733.7
muscle 728.2
pelvic muscles and anal sphincter 618.83

Atrophy, atrophic—*continued*
Duchenne-Aran 335.21
ear 388.9
edentulous alveolar ridge 525.20
mandible 525.20
minimal 525.21
moderate 525.22
severe 525.23
maxilla 525.20
minimal 525.24
moderate 525.25
severe 525.26
emphysema, lung 492.8
endometrium (senile) 621.8
cervix 622.8
enteric 569.89
epididymis 608.3
eyeball, cause unknown 360.41
eyelid (senile) 374.50
facial (skin) 701.9
facioscapulohumeral (Landouzy-Déjérine) 359.1
fallopian tube (senile), acquired 620.3
fatty, thymus (gland) 254.8
gallbladder 575.8
gastric 537.89
gastritis (chronic) 535.1
gastrointestinal 569.89
genital organ, male 608.89
glandular 289.3
globe (phthisis bulbi) 360.41
gum (*see also* Recession, gingival) 523.20
hair 704.2
heart (brown) (senile) (*see also* Degeneration, myocardial) 429.1
hemifacial 754.0
Romberg 349.89
hydronephrosis 591
infantile 261
paralysis, acute (*see also* Poliomyelitis, with paralysis) 045.1
intestine 569.89
iris (generalized) (postinfectional) (sector shaped) 364.59
essential 364.51
progressive 364.51
sphincter 364.54
kidney (senile) (*see also* Sclerosis, renal) 587
with hypertension (*see also* Hypertension, kidney) 403.90
congenital 753.0
hydronephrotic 591
infantile 753.0
lacrimal apparatus (primary) 375.13
secondary 375.14
Landouzy-Déjérine 359.1
laryngitis, infection 476.0
larynx 478.79
Leber's optic 377.16
lip 528.5
liver (acute) (subacute) (*see also* Necrosis, liver) 570
chronic (yellow) 571.8

Atrophy, atrophic—*continued*
 liver—*continued*
  yellow (congenital) 570
   with
    abortion—*see* Abortion, by type, with
     specified complication NEC
    ectopic pregnancy (*see also* categories
     633.0-633.9) 639.8
    molar pregnancy (*see also* categories
     630-632) 639.8
   chronic 571.8
   complicating pregnancy 646.7
   following
    abortion 639.8
    ectopic or molar pregnancy 639.8
   from injection, inoculation or transfusion
    (onset within 8 months after
    administration)—*see* Hepatitis, viral
   healed 571.5
   obstetric 646.7
   postabortal 639.8
   postimmunization—*see* Hepatitis, viral
   posttransfusion—*see* Hepatitis, viral
   puerperal, postpartum 674.8
 lung (senile) 518.89
  congenital 748.69
 macular (dermatological) 701.3
  syphilitic, skin 091.3
   striated 095.8
 muscle, muscular 728.2
  disuse 728.2
  Duchenne-Aran 335.21
  extremity (lower) (upper) 728.2
  familial spinal 335.11
  general 728.2
  idiopathic 728.2
  infantile spinal 335.0
  myelopathic (progressive) 335.10
  myotonic 359.21
  neuritic 356.1
  neuropathic (peroneal) (progressive) 356.1
  peroneal 356.1
  primary (idiopathic) 728.2
  progressive (familial) (hereditary) (pure)
   335.21
   adult (spinal) 335.19
   infantile (spinal) 335.0
   juvenile (spinal) 335.11
   spinal 335.10
    adult 335.19
    hereditary or familial 335.11
    infantile 335.0
  pseudohypertrophic 359.1
   spinal (progressive) 335.10
   adult 335.19
   Aran-Duchenne 335.21
   familial 335.11
   hereditary 335.11
   infantile 335.0
   juvenile 335.11
  syphilitic 095.6
 myocardium (*see also* Degeneration,
  myocardial) 429.1
 myometrium (senile) 621.8
  cervix 622.8
 myotatic 728.2
 myotonia 359.21
 nail 703.8
  congenital 757.5
 nasopharynx 472.2

Atrophy, atrophic—*continued*
 nerve—*see also* Disorder, nerve
  abducens 378.54
  accessory 352.4
  acoustic or auditory 388.5
  cranial 352.9
   first (olfactory) 352.0
   second (optic) (*see also* Atrophy, optic
    nerve) 377.10
   third (oculomotor) (partial) 378.51
    total 378.52
   fourth (trochlear) 378.53
   fifth (trigeminal) 350.8
   sixth (abducens) 378.54
   seventh (facial) 351.8
   eighth (auditory) 388.5
   ninth (glossopharyngeal) 352.2
   tenth (pneumogastric) (vagus) 352.3
   eleventh (accessory) 352.4
   twelfth (hypoglossal) 352.5
  facial 351.8
  glossopharyngeal 352.2
  hypoglossal 352.5
  oculomotor (partial) 378.51
   total 378.52
  olfactory 352.0
  peripheral 355.9
  pneumogastric 352.3
  trigeminal 350.8
  trochlear 378.53
  vagus (pneumogastric) 352.3
 nervous system, congenital 742.8
 neuritic (*see also* Disorder, nerve) 355.9
 neurogenic NEC 355.9
  bone
   tabetic 094.0
 nutritional 261
 old age 797
 olivopontocerebellar 333.0
 optic nerve (ascending) (descending)
   (infectional) (nonfamilial) (papillomacular
   bundle) (postretinal) (secondary NEC)
   (simple) 377.10
  associated with retinal dystrophy 377.13
  dominant hereditary 377.16
  glaucomatous 377.14
  hereditary (dominant) (Leber's) 377.16
  Leber's (hereditary) 377.16
  partial 377.15
  postinflammatory 377.12
  primary 377.11
  syphilitic 094.84
   congenital 090.49
   tabes dorsalis 094.0
 orbit 376.45
 ovary (senile), acquired 620.3
 oviduct (senile), acquired 620.3
 palsy, diffuse 335.20
 pancreas (duct) (senile) 577.8
 papillary muscle 429.81
 paralysis 355.9
 parotid gland 527.0
 patches skin 701.3
  senile 701.8
 penis 607.89
 pharyngitis 472.1
 pharynx 478.29
 pluriglandular 258.8
 polyarthritis 714.0
 prostate 602.2
 pseudohypertrophic 359.1

Atrophy, atrophic—*continued*
renal (*see also* Sclerosis, renal) 587
reticulata 701.8
retina (*see also* Degeneration, retina) 362.60
  hereditary (*see also* Dystrophy, retina) 362.70
rhinitis 472.0
salivary duct or gland 527.0
scar NEC 709.2
sclerosis, lobar (of brain) 331.0
  with dementia
    with behavioral disturbance 331.0 *[294.11]*
    without behavioral disturbance 331.0
      [294.10]
scrotum 608.89
seminal vesicle 608.89
senile 797
  degenerative, of skin 701.3
skin (patches) (senile) 701.8
spermatic cord 608.89
spinal (cord) 336.8
  acute 336.8
  muscular (chronic) 335.10
    adult 335.19
    familial 335.11
    juvenile 335.10
  paralysis 335.10
    acute (*see also* Poliomyelitis, with paralysis)
      045.1
spine (column) 733.99
spleen (senile) 289.59
spots (skin) 701.3
  senile 701.8
stomach 537.89
striate and macular 701.3
  syphilitic 095.8
subcutaneous 701.9
  due to injection 999.9
sublingual gland 527.0
submaxillary gland 527.0
Sudeck's 733.7
suprarenal (autoimmune) (capsule) (gland)
  255.41
  with hypofunction 255.41
tarso-orbital fascia, congenital 743.66
testis 608.3
thenar, partial 354.0
throat 478.29
thymus (fat) 254.8
thyroid (gland) 246.8
  with
    cretinism 243
    myxedema 244.9
  congenital 243
tongue (senile) 529.8
  papillae 529.4
  smooth 529.4
trachea 519.19
tunica vaginalis 608.89
turbinate 733.99
tympanic membrane (nonflaccid) 384.82
  flaccid 384.81
ulcer (*see also* Ulcer, skin) 707.9
upper respiratory tract 478.9
uterus, uterine (acquired) (senile) 621.8
  cervix 622.8
  due to radiation (intended effect) 621.8
vagina (senile) 627.3
vascular 459.89
vas deferens 608.89
vertebra (senile) 733.99
vulva (primary) (senile) 624.1

Atrophy, atrophic—*continued*
  Werdnig-Hoffmann 335.0
  yellow (acute) (congenital) (liver) (subacute)
    (*see also* Necrosis, liver) 570
    chronic 571.8
    resulting from administration of blood,
      plasma, serum, or other biological
      substance (within 8 months of
      administration)—*see* Hepatitis, viral
Attack
  akinetic (*see also* Epilepsy) 345.0
  angina—*see* Angina
  apoplectic (*see also* Disease, cerebrovascular,
    acute) 436
  benign shuddering 333.93
  bilious—*see* Vomiting
  cataleptic 300.11
  cerebral (*see also* Disease, cerebrovascular,
    acute) 436
  coronary (*see also* Infarct, myocardium) 410.9
  cyanotic, newborn 770.83
  epileptic (*see also* Epilepsy) 345.9
  epileptiform 780.39
  heart (*see also* Infarct, myocardium) 410.9
  hemiplegia (*see also* Disease, cerebrovascular,
    acute) 436
  hysterical 300.11
  jacksonian (*see also* Epilepsy) 345.5
  myocardium, myocardial (*see also* Infarct,
    myocardium) 410.9
  myoclonic (*see also* Epilepsy) 345.1
  panic 300.01
  paralysis (*see also* Disease, cerebrovascular,
    acute) 436
  paroxysmal 780.39
  psychomotor (*see also* Epilepsy) 345.4
  salaam (*see also* Epilepsy) 345.6
  schizophreniform (*see also* Schizophrenia)
    295.4
  sensory and motor 780.39
  syncope 780.2
  toxic, cerebral 780.39
  transient ischemic (TIA) 435.9
  unconsciousness 780.2
    hysterical 300.11
  vasomotor 780.2
  vasovagal (idiopathic) (paroxysmal) 780.2
Attention to
  artificial
    opening (of) V55.9
      digestive tract NEC V55.4
      specified site NEC V55.8
      urinary tract NEC V55.6
      vagina V55.7
  colostomy V55.3
  cystostomy V55.5
  dressing
    wound V58.30
      nonsurgical V58.30
      surgical V58.31
  gastrostomy V55.1
  ileostomy V55.2
  jejunostomy V55.4
  nephrostomy V55.6
  surgical dressings V58.31
  sutures V58.32
  tracheostomy V55.0
  ureterostomy V55.6
  urethrostomy V55.6

Attrition
gum (*see also* Recession, gingival) 523.20
teeth (hard tissues) 521.10
  excessive 521.10
    extending into
      dentine 521.12
      pulp 521.13
    generalized 521.15
    limited to enamel 521.11
    localized 521.14
Atypical —*see also* condition
cells
  endocervical 795.00
  endometrial 795.00
  glandular
    anus 796.70
    cervical 795.00
    vaginal 795.10
distribution, vessel (congenital) (peripheral)
  NEC 747.60
endometrium 621.9
kidney 593.89
Atypism, cervix 622.10
Audible tinnitus (*see also* Tinnitus) 388.30
Auditory —*see* condition
Audry's syndrome (acropachyderma) 757.39
Aujeszky's disease 078.89
Aura
jacksonian (*see also* Epilepsy) 345.5
persistent migraine 346.5
  with cerebral infarction 346.6
  without cerebral infarction 346.5
Aurantiasis, cutis 278.3
Auricle, auricular —*see* condition
Auriculotemporal syndrome 350.8
Australian
Q fever 083.0
X disease 062.4
Autism, autistic (child) (infantile) 299.0
Autodigestion 799.89
Autoerythrocyte sensitization 287.2
Autographism 708.3
Autoimmune
cold sensitivity 283.0
disease NEC 279.49
hemolytic anemia 283.0
lymphoproliferative syndrome (ALPS) 279.41
thyroiditis 245.2
Autoinfection, septic —*see* Septicemia
Autointoxication 799.89
Automatism 348.89
epileptic (*see also* Epilepsy) 345.4
paroxysmal, idiopathic (*see also* Epilepsy) 345.4
Autonomic, autonomous
bladder 596.54
  neurogenic 596.54
    with cauda equine 344.61
dysreflexia 337.3
faciocephalalgia (*see also* Neuropathy,
  peripheral, autonomic) 337.9
hysterical seizure 300.11
imbalance (*see also* Neuropathy, peripheral,
  autonomic) 337.9
Autophony 388.40
Autosensitivity, erythrocyte 287.2
Autotopagnosia 780.99
Autotoxemia 799.89
Autumn —*see* condition
Avellis' syndrome 344.89

Aviators
disease or sickness (*see also* Effect, adverse,
  high altitude) 993.2
ear 993.0
effort syndrome 306.2
Avitaminosis (multiple NEC) (*see also*
  Deficiency, vitamin) 269.2
A 264.9
B 266.9
  with
    beriberi 265.0
    pellagra 265.2
B_1 265.1
B_2 266.0
B_6 266.1
B_{12} 266.2
C (with scurvy) 267
D 268.9
  with
    osteomalacia 268.2
    rickets 268.0
E 269.1
G 266.0
H 269.1
K 269.0
multiple 269.2
nicotinic acid 265.2
P 269.1
Avulsion (traumatic) 879.8
blood vessel—*see* Injury, blood vessel, by site
cartilage—*see also* Dislocation, by site
  knee, current (*see also* Tear, meniscus) 836.2
  symphyseal (inner), complicating delivery 665.6
complicated 879.9
diaphragm—*see* Injury, internal, diaphragm
ear—*see* Wound, open, ear
epiphysis of bone—*see* Fracture, by site
external site other than limb—*see* Wound, open,
  by site
eye 871.3
fingernail—*see* Wound, open, finger
fracture—*see* Fracture, by site
genital organs, external—*see* Wound, open,
  genital organs
head (intracranial) NEC—*see also* Injury,
  intracranial, with open intracranial wound
  complete 874.9
  external site NEC 873.8
  complicated 873.9
internal organ or site—*see* Injury, internal, by site
joint—*see also* Dislocation, by site
  capsule—*see* Sprain, by site
ligament—*see* Sprain, by site
limb—*see also* Amputation, traumatic, by site
  skin and subcutaneous tissue—*see* Wound,
    open, by site
muscle—*see* Sprain, by site
nerve (root)—*see* Injury, nerve, by site
scalp—*see* Wound, open, scalp
skin and subcutaneous tissue—*see* Wound,
  open, by site
symphyseal cartilage (inner), complicating
  delivery 665.6
tendon—*see also* Sprain, by site
  with open wound—*see* Wound, open, by site
toenail—*see* Wound, open, toe(s)
tooth 873.63
  complicated 873.73
Awaiting organ transplant status V49.83
Awareness of heart beat 785.1
Axe grinders' disease 502
Axenfeld's anomaly or syndrome 743.44

Axilla, axillary —*see also* condition
  breast 757.6
Axonotmesis —*see* Injury, nerve, by site
Ayala's disease 756.89
Ayerza's disease or syndrome (pulmonary
  artery sclerosis with pulmonary hypertension)
  416.0
Azoospermia 606.0
Azorean disease (of the nervous system) 334.8
Azotemia 790.6
  meaning uremia (*see also* Uremia) 586
Aztec ear 744.29
Azygos lobe, lung (fissure) 748.69

B

Baader's syndrome (erythema multiforme exudativum) 695.19
Baastrup's syndrome 721.5
Babesiasis 088.82
Babesiosis 088.82
Babington's disease (familial hemorrhagic telangiectasia) 448.0
Babinski's syndrome (cardiovascular syphilis) 093.89
Babinski-Fröhlich syndrome (adiposogenital dystrophy) 253.8
Babinski-Nageotte syndrome 344.89
Bacillary —*see* condition
Bacilluria 791.9
  asymptomatic, in pregnancy or puerperium 646.5
  tuberculous (*see also* Tuberculosis) 016.9
Bacillus —*see also* Infection, bacillus
  abortus infection 023.1
  anthracis infection 022.9
  coli
    infection 041.4
      generalized 038.42
      intestinal 008.00
      pyemia 038.42
      septicemia 038.42
  Flexner's 004.1
  fusiformis infestation 101
  mallei infection 024
  Shiga's 004.0
  suipestifer infection (*see also* Infection, Salmonella) 003.9
Back —*see* condition
Backache (postural) 724.5
  psychogenic 307.89
  sacroiliac 724.6
Backflow (pyelovenous) (*see also* Disease, renal) 593.9
Backknee (*see also* Genu, recurvatum) 736.5
Bacteremia (*see also* Infection, bacillus) 790.7
  newborn 771.83
Bacteria
  in blood (*see also* Bacteremia) 790.7
  in urine (*see also* Bacteriuria) 599.0
Bacterial —*see* condition
Bactericholia (*see also* Cholecystitis, acute) 575.0
Bacterid, bacteride (Andrews' pustular) 686.8
Bacteriuria, bacteruria 791.9
  with
    urinary tract infection 599.0
  asymptomatic 791.9
    in pregnancy or puerperium 646.5
      affecting fetus or newborn 760.1
Bad
  breath 784.99
  heart—*see* Disease, heart
  trip (*see also* Abuse, drugs, nondependent) 305.3
Baehr-Schiffrin disease (thrombotic thrombocytopenic purpura) 446.6
Baelz's disease (cheilitis glandularis apostematosa) 528.5
Baerensprung's disease (eczema marginatum) 110.3
Bagassosis (occupational) 495.1
Baghdad boil 085.1

Bagratuni's syndrome (temporal arteritis) 446.5
Baker's
  cyst (knee) 727.51
    tuberculous (*see also* Tuberculosis) 015.2
  itch 692.89
Bakwin-Krida syndrome (craniometaphyseal dysplasia) 756.89
Balanitis (circinata) (gangraenosa) (infectious) (vulgaris) 607.1
  amebic 006.8
  candidal 112.2
  chlamydial 099.53
  due to Ducrey's bacillus 099.0
  erosiva circinata et gangraenosa 607.1
  gangrenous 607.1
  gonococcal (acute) 098.0
    chronic or duration of 2 months or over 098.2
  nongonococcal 607.1
  phagedenic 607.1
  venereal NEC 099.8
  xerotica obliterans 607.81
Balanoposthitis 607.1
  chlamydial 099.53
  gonococcal (acute) 098.0
    chronic or duration of 2 months or over 098.2
  ulcerative NEC 099.8
Balanorrhagia —*see* Balanitis
Balantidiasis 007.0
Balantidiosis 007.0
Balbuties, balbutio 307.0
Bald
  patches on scalp 704.00
  tongue 529.4
Baldness (*see also* Alopecia) 704.00
Balfour's disease (chloroma) 205.3
Balint's syndrome (psychic paralysis of visual fixation) 368.16
Balkan grippe 083.0
Ball
  food 938
  hair 938
Ballantyne (-Runge) syndrome (postmaturity) 766.22
Balloon disease (*see also* Effect, adverse, high altitude) 993.2
Ballooning posterior leaflet syndrome 424.0
Baló's disease or concentric sclerosis 341.1
Bamberger's disease (hypertrophic pulmonary osteoarthropathy) 731.2
Bamberger-Marie disease (hypertrophic pulmonary osteoarthropathy) 731.2
Bamboo spine 720.0
Bancroft's filariasis 125.0
Band(s)
  adhesive (*see also* Adhesions, peritoneum) 568.0
  amniotic 658.8
    affecting fetus or newborn 762.8
  anomalous or congenital—*see also* Anomaly, specified type NEC
    atrial 746.9
    heart 746.9
    intestine 751.4
    omentum 751.4
    ventricular 746.9
  cervix 622.3
  gallbladder (congenital) 751.69

Band(s)—*continued*
  intestinal (adhesive) (*see also* Adhesions,
    peritoneum) 568.0
    congenital 751.4
  obstructive (*see also* Obstruction, intestine)
    560.81
  periappendiceal (congenital) 751.4
  peritoneal (adhesive) (*see also* Adhesions,
    peritoneum) 568.0
    with intestinal obstruction 560.81
    congenital 751.4
  uterus 621.5
  vagina 623.2
Bandemia (without diagnosis of specific
  infection) 288.66
Bandl's ring (contraction)
  complicating delivery 661.4
  affecting fetus or newborn 763.7
Bang's disease (Brucella abortus) 023.1
Bangkok hemorrhagic fever 065.4
Bannister's disease 995.1
Bantam-Albright-Martin disease
  (pseudohypoparathyroidism) 275.49
Banti's disease or syndrome (with cirrhosis)
  (with portal hypertension)—*see* Cirrhosis, liver
Bar
  calcaneocuboid 755.67
  calcaneonavicular 755.67
  cubonavicular 755.67
  prostate 600.90
    with
      other lower urinary tract symptoms (LUTS)
        600.91
      urinary
        obstruction 600.91
        retention 600.91
  talocalcaneal 755.67
Baragnosis 780.99
Barasheh, barashek 266.2
Barcoo disease or rot (*see also* Ulcer, skin) 707.9
Bard-Pic syndrome (carcinoma, head of
  pancreas) 157.0
Bärensprung's disease (eczema marginatum)
  110.3
Baritosis 503
Barium lung disease 503
Barlow's syndrome (meaning mitral valve
  prolapse) 424.0
Barlow (-Möller) disease or syndrome (meaning
  infantile scurvy) 267
Barodontalgia 993.2
Baron Münchausen syndrome 301.51
Barosinusitis 993.1
Barotitis 993.0
Barotrauma 993.2
  odontalgia 993.2
  otitic 993.0
  sinus 993.1
Barraquer's disease or syndrome (progressive
  lipodystrophy) 272.6
Barré-Guillain syndrome 357.0
Barré-Liéou syndrome (posterior cervical
  sympathetic) 723.2
Barrel chest 738.3
Barrett's esophagus 530.85
Barrett's syndrome or ulcer (chronic peptic
  ulcer of esophagus) 530.85
Bársony-Polgár syndrome (corkscrew
  esophagus) 530.5
Bársony-Teschendorf syndrome (corkscrew
  esophagus) 530.5

Barth syndrome 759.89
Bartholin's
  adenitis (*see also* Bartholinitis) 616.89
  gland—*see* condition
Bartholinitis (suppurating) 616.89
  gonococcal (acute) 098.0
  chronic or duration of 2 months or over 098.2
Bartonellosis 088.0
Bartter's syndrome (secondary
  hyperaldosteronism with juxtaglomerular
  hyperplasia) 255.13
Basal—*see* **condition**
Basan's (hidrotic) ectodermal dysplasia 757.31
Baseball finger 842.13
Basedow's disease or syndrome (exophthalmic
  goiter) 242.0
Basic —*see* condition
Basilar —*see* condition
Bason's (hidrotic) ectodermal dysplasia 757.31
Basopenia 288.59
Basophilia 288.65
Basophilism (corticoadrenal) (Cushing's)
  (pituitary) (thymic) 255.0
Bassen-Kornzweig syndrome
  (abetalipoproteinemia) 272.5
Bat ear 744.29
Bateman's
  disease 078.0
  purpura (senile) 287.2
Bathing cramp 994.1
Bathophobia 300.23
Batten's disease, retina 330.1 *[362.71]*
Batten-Mayou disease 330.1 *[362.71]*
Batten-Steinert syndrome 359.21
Battered
  adult (syndrome) 995.81
  baby or child (syndrome) 995.54
  spouse (syndrome) 995.81
Battey mycobacterium infection 031.0
Battledore placenta —*see* Placenta, abnormal
Battle exhaustion (*see also* Reaction, stress,
  acute) 308.9
Baumgarten-Cruveilhier (cirrhosis) disease, or
  syndrome 571.5
Bauxite
  fibrosis (of lung) 503
  workers' disease 503
Bayle's disease (dementia paralytica) 094.1
Bazin's disease (primary) (*see also* Tuberculosis)
  017.1
Beach ear 380.12
Beaded hair (congenital) 757.4
Beals syndrome 759.82
Beard's disease (neurasthenia) 300.5
Bearn-Kunkel (-Slater) syndrome (lupoid
  hepatitis) 571.49
Beat
  elbow 727.2
  hand 727.2
  knee 727.2
Beats
  ectopic 427.60
  escaped, heart 427.60
    postoperative 997.1
  premature (nodal) 427.60
    atrial 427.61
    auricular 427.61
    postoperative 997.1
    specified type NEC 427.69
    supraventricular 427.61
    ventricular 427.69

Beau's
disease or syndrome (*see also* Degeneration, myocardial) 429.1
lines (transverse furrows on fingernails) 703.8
Bechterew's disease (ankylosing spondylitis) 720.0
Bechterew-Strümpell-Marie syndrome (ankylosing spondylitis) 720.0
Beck's syndrome (anterior spinal artery occlusion) 433.8
Becker's
disease
idiopathic mural endomyocardial disease 425.2
myotonia congenita, recessive form 359.22
dystrophy 359.22
Beckwith (-Wiedemann) syndrome 759.89
Bedbugs bite(s) —*see* Injury, superfiical, by site
Bed confinement status V49.84
Bedclothes, asphyxiation or suffocation by 994.7
Bednar's aphthae 528.2
Bedsore (*see also* Ulcer, pressure) 707.00
with gangrene 707.00 *[785.4]*
Bedwetting (*see also* Enuresis) 788.36
Beer-drinkers' heart (disease) 425.5
Bee sting (with allergic or anaphylactic shock) 989.5
Begbie's disease (exophthalmic goiter) 242.0
Behavior disorder, disturbance —*see also* Disturbance, conduct
antisocial, without manifest psychiatric disorder
adolescent V71.02
adult V71.01
child V71.02
dyssocial, without manifest psychiatric disorder
adolescent V71.02
adult V71.01
child V71.02
high-risk—*see* Problem
Behçet's syndrome 136.1
Behr's disease 362.50
Beigel's disease or morbus (white piedra) 111.2
Bejel 104.0
Bekhterev's disease (ankylosing spondylitis) 720.0
Bekhterev-Strümpell-Marie syndrome (ankylosing spondylitis) 720.0
Belching (*see also* Eructation) 787.3
Bell's
disease (*see also* Psychosis, affective) 296.0
mania (*see also* Psychosis, affective) 296.0
palsy, paralysis 351.0
infant 767.5
newborn 767.5
syphilitic 094.89
spasm 351.0
Bence-Jones albuminuria, albuminosuria, or proteinuria 791.0
Bends 993.3
Benedikt's syndrome (paralysis) 344.89
Benign —*see also* condition
cellular changes, cervix 795.09
prostate
hyperplasia 600.20
with urinary retention 600.21
neoplasm 222.2
with
other lower urinary tract symptoms (LUTS) 600.21
urinary
obstruction 600.21
retention 600.21

Bennett's
disease (leukemia) 208.9
fracture (closed) 815.01
open 815.11
Benson's disease 379.22
Bent
back (hysterical) 300.11
nose 738.0
congenital 754.0
Bereavement V62.82
as adjustment reaction 309.0
Berger's paresthesia (lower limb) 782.0
Bergeron's disease (hysteroepilepsy) 300.11
Beriberi (acute) (atrophic) (chronic) (dry) (subacute) (wet) 265.0
with polyneuropathy 265.0 *[357.4]*
heart (disease) 265.0 *[425.7]*
leprosy 030.1
neuritis 265.0 *[357.4]*
Berlin's disease or edema (traumatic) 921.3
Berloque dermatitis 692.72
Bernard-Horner syndrome (*see also* Neuropathy, peripheral, autonomic) 337.9
Bernard-Sergent syndrome (acute adrenocortical insufficiency) 255.41
Bernard-Soulier disease or thrombopathy 287.1
Bernhardt's disease or paresthesia 355.1
Bernhardt-Roth disease or syndrome (paresthesia) 355.1
Bernheim's syndrome (*see also* Failure, heart) 428.0
Bertielliasis 123.8
Bertolotti's syndrome (sacralization of fifth lumbar vertebra) 756.15
Berylliosis (acute) (chronic) (lung) (occupational) 503
Besnier's
lupus pernio 135
prurigo (atopic dermatitis) (infantile eczema) 691.8
Besnier-Boeck disease or sarcoid 135
Besnier-Boeck-Schaumann disease (sarcoidosis) 135
Best's disease 362.76
Bestiality 302.1
Beta-adrenergic hyperdynamic circulatory state 429.82
Beta-aminoisobutyric aciduria 277.2
Beta-mercaptolactate-cysteine disulfiduria 270.0
Beta thalassemia (major) (minor) (mixed) 282.49
Beurmann's disease (sporotrichosis) 117.1
Bezoar 938
intestine 936
stomach 935.2
Bezold's abscess (*see also* Mastoiditis) 383.01
Bianchi's syndrome (aphasia-apraxia-alexia) 784.69
Bicornuate or bicornis uterus 752.3
in pregnancy or childbirth 654.0
with obstructed labor 660.2
affecting fetus or newborn 763.1
affecting fetus or newborn 763.89
Bicuspid aortic valve 746.4
Biedl-Bardet syndrome 759.89
Bielschowsky's disease 330.1
Bielschowsky-Jansky
amaurotic familial idiocy 330.1
disease 330.1
Biemond's syndrome (obesity, polydactyly, and mental retardation) 759.89

Biermer's anemia or disease (pernicious anemia) 281.0
Biett's disease 695.4
Bifid (congenital)—*see also* Imperfect, closure
  apex, heart 746.89
  clitoris 752.49
  epiglottis 748.3
  kidney 753.3
  nose 748.1
  patella 755.64
  scrotum 752.89
  toe 755.66
  tongue 750.13
  ureter 753.4
  uterus 752.3
  uvula 749.02
  with cleft lip (*see also* Cleft, palate, with cleft lip) 749.20
Biforis uterus (suprasimplex) 752.3
Bifurcation (congenital)—*see also* Imperfect, closure
  gallbladder 751.69
  kidney pelvis 753.3
  renal pelvis 753.3
  rib 756.3
  tongue 750.13
  trachea 748.3
  ureter 753.4
  urethra 753.8
  uvula 749.02
  with cleft lip (*see also* Cleft, palate, with cleft lip) 749.20
  vertebra 756.19
Bigeminal pulse 427.89
Bigeminy 427.89
Big spleen syndrome 289.4
Bilateral —*see* condition
Bile duct —*see* condition
Bile pigments in urine 791.4
Bilharziasis (*see also* Schistosomiasis) 120.9
  chyluria 120.0
  cutaneous 120.3
  galacturia 120.0
  hematochyluria 120.0
  intestinal 120.1
  lipemia 120.9
  lipuria 120.0
  Oriental 120.2
  piarhemia 120.9
  pulmonary 120.2
  tropical hematuria 120.0
  vesical 120.0
Biliary —*see* condition
Bilious (attack)—*see also* Vomiting
  fever, hemoglobinuric 084.8
Bilirubinuria 791.4
Biliuria 791.4
Billroth's disease
  meningocele (*see also* Spina bifida) 741.9
Bilobate placenta —*see* Placenta, abnormal
Bilocular
  heart 745.7
  stomach 536.8
Bing-Horton syndrome (histamine cephalgia) 339.00
Binswanger's disease or dementia 290.12
Biörck (-Thorson) syndrome (malignant carcinoid) 259.2

Biparta, bipartite —*see also* Imperfect, closure
  carpal scaphoid 755.59
  patella 755.64
  placenta—*see* Placenta, abnormal
  vagina 752.49
Bird
  face 756.0
  fanciers' lung or disease 495.2
  flu 488.0
Bird's disease (oxaluria) 271.8
Birth
  abnormal fetus or newborn 763.9
  accident, fetus or newborn—*see* Birth, injury
  complications in mother—*see* Delivery, complicated
  compression during NEC 767.9
  defect—*see* Anomaly
  delayed, fetus 763.9
  difficult NEC, affecting fetus or newborn 763.9
  dry, affecting fetus or newborn 761.1
  forced, NEC, affecting fetus or newborn 763.89
  forceps, affecting fetus or newborn 763.2
  hematoma of sternomastoid 767.8
  immature 765.1
    extremely 765.0
  inattention, after or at 995.52
  induced, affecting fetus or newborn 763.89
  infant—*see* Newborn
  injury NEC 767.9
    adrenal gland 767.8
    basal ganglia 767.0
    brachial plexus (paralysis) 767.6
    brain (compression) (pressure) 767.0
    cerebellum 767.0
    cerebral hemorrhage 767.0
    conjunctiva 767.8
    eye 767.8
    fracture
      bone, any except clavicle or spine 767.3
      clavicle 767.2
      femur 767.3
      humerus 767.3
      long bone 767.3
      radius and ulna 767.3
      skeleton NEC 767.3
      skull 767.3
      spine 767.4
      tibia and fibula 767.3
    hematoma 767.8
      liver (subcapsular) 767.8
      mastoid 767.8
      skull 767.19
      sternomastoid 767.8
      testes 767.8
      vulva 767.8
    intracranial (edema) 767.0
    laceration
      brain 767.0
      by scalpel 767.8
      peripheral nerve 767.7
      liver 767.8
    meninges
      brain 767.0
      spinal cord 767.4
    nerves (cranial, peripheral) 767.7
      brachial plexus 767.6
      facial 767.5
    paralysis 767.7
      brachial plexus 767.6
      Erb (-Duchenne) 767.6
      facial nerve 767.5
      Klumpke (-Déjérine) 767.6

Birth—*continued*
    radial nerve 767.6
    spinal (cord) (hemorrhage) (laceration)
        (rupture) 767.4
    rupture
        intracranial 767.0
        liver 767.8
        spinal cord 767.4
        spleen 767.8
        viscera 767.8
    scalp 767.19
    scalpel wound 767.8
    skeleton NEC 767.3
    specified NEC 767.8
    spinal cord 767.4
    spleen 767.8
    subdural hemorrhage 767.0
    tentorial, tear 767.0
    testes 767.8
    vulva 767.8
    instrumental, NEC, affecting fetus or newborn
        763.2
    lack of care, after or at 995.52
    multiple
        affected by maternal complications of
            pregnancy 761.5
        healthy liveborn—*see* Newborn, multiple
    neglect, after or at 995.52
    newborn—*see* Newborn
    palsy or paralysis NEC 767.7
    precipitate, fetus or newborn 763.6
    premature (infant) 765.1
    prolonged, affecting fetus or newborn 763.9
    retarded, fetus or newborn 763.9
    shock, newborn 779.89
    strangulation or suffocation
        due to aspiration of clear amniotic fluid 770.13
            with respiratory symptoms 770.14
        mechanical 767.8
    trauma NEC 767.9
    triplet
        affected by maternal complications of
            pregnancy 761.5
        healthy liveborn—*see* Newborn, multiple
    twin
        affected by maternal complications of
            pregnancy 761.5
        healthy liveborn—*see* Newborn, twin
    ventouse, affecting fetus or newborn 763.3
Birt-Hogg-Dube syndrome 759.89
Birthmark 757.32
Bisalbuminemia 273.8
Biskra button 085.1
Bite(s)
    with intact skin surface—*see* Contusion
    animal—*see* Wound, open, by site
        intact skin surface—*see* Contusion
    bedbug—*see* Injury, superficial, by site
    centipede 989.5
    chigger 133.8
    fire ant 989.5
    flea—*see* Injury, superficial, by site
    human (open wound)—*see also* Wound, open,
        by site
        intact skin surface—*see* Contusion
    insect
        nonvenomous—*see* Injury, superficial, by site
        venomous 989.5
    mad dog (death from) 071
    open
        anterior 524.24
        posterior 524.25

Bite(s)—*continued*
    poisonous 989.5
    red bug 133.8
    reptile 989.5
        nonvenomous—*see* Wound, open, by site
    snake 989.5
        nonvenomous—*see* Wound, open, by site
    spider (venomous) 989.5
        nonvenomous—*see* Injury, superficial, by site
    venomous 989.5
Biting
    cheek or lip 528.9
    nail 307.9
Black
    death 020.9
    eye NEC 921.0
    hairy tongue 529.3
    heel 924.20
    lung disease 500
    palm 923.20
Blackfan-Diamond anemia or syndrome
    (congenital hypoplastic anemia) 284.01
Blackhead 706.1
Blackout 780.2
Blackwater fever 084.8
Bladder —*see* Condition
Blast
    blindness 921.3
    concussion—*see* Blast, injury
    injury 869.0
        with open wound into cavity 869.1
        abdomen or thorax—*see* Injury, internal, by
            site
        brain (*see also* Concussion, brain) 850.9
            with skull fracture—*see* Fracture, skull
        ear (acoustic nerve trauma) 951.5
            with perforation, tympanic membrane—*see*
                Wound, open, ear, drum
        lung (*see also* Injury, internal, lung) 861.20
        otitic (explosive) 388.11
Blastomycosis, blastomycotic (chronic)
    (cutaneous) (disseminated) (lung) (pulmonary)
    (systemic) 116.0
    Brazilian 116.1
    European 117.5
    keloidal 116.2
    North American 116.0
    primary pulmonary 116.0
    South American 116.1
Bleb(s) 709.8
    emphysematous (bullous) (diffuse) (lung)
        (ruptured) (solitary) 492.0
    filtering, eye (postglaucoma) (status) V45.69
        with complication 997.99
        postcataract extraction (complication) 997.99
    lung (ruptured) 492.0
        congenital 770.5
    subpleural (emphysematous) 492.0
Bleeder (familial) (hereditary) (*see also* Defect,
    coagulation) 286.9
    nonfamilial 286.9
Bleeding (*see also* Hemorrhage) 459.0
    anal 569.3
    anovulatory 628.0
    atonic, following delivery 666.1
    capillary 448.9
    due to subinvolution 621.1
        puerperal 666.2
    ear 388.69
    excessive, associated with menopausal onset
        627.0
    familial (*see also* Defect, coagulation) 286.9

Bleeding—*continued*
  following intercourse 626.7
  gastrointestinal 578.9
  gums 523.8
  hemorrhoids—*see* Hemorrhoids, bleeding
  intermenstrual
    irregular 626.6
    regular 626.5
  intraoperative 998.11
  irregular NEC 626.4
  menopausal 627.0
  mouth 528.9
  nipple 611.79
  nose 784.7
  ovulation 626.5
  postclimacteric 627.1
  postcoital 626.7
  postmenopausal 627.1
    following induced menopause 627.4
  postoperative 998.11
  preclimacteric 627.0
  puberty 626.3
    excessive, with onset of menstrual periods
      626.3
  rectum, rectal 569.3
  tendencies (*see also* Defect, coagulation) 286.9
  throat 784.8
  umbilical stump 772.3
  umbilicus 789.9
  unrelated to menstrual cycle 626.6
  uterus, uterine 626.9
    climacteric 627.0
    dysfunctional 626.8
    functional 626.8
    unrelated to menstrual cycle 626.6
  vagina, vaginal 623.8
    functional 626.8
  vicarious 625.8
Blennorrhagia, blennorrhagic —*see*
  Blennorrhea
Blennorrhea (acute) 098.0
  adultorum 098.40
  alveolaris 523.40
  chronic or duration of 2 months or over 098.2
  gonococcal (neonatorum) 098.40
  inclusion (neonatal) (newborn) 771.6
  neonatorum 098.40
Blepharelosis (*see also* Entropion) 374.00
Blepharitis (eyelid) 373.00
  angularis 373.01
  ciliaris 373.00
    with ulcer 373.01
  marginal 373.00
    with ulcer 373.01
  scrofulous (*see also* Tuberculosis) 017.3
    [373.00]
  squamous 373.02
  ulcerative 373.01
Blepharochalasis 374.34
  congenital 743.62
Blepharoclonus 333.81
Blepharoconjunctivitis (*see also* Conjunctivitis)
  372.20
  angular 372.21
  contact 372.22
Blepharophimosis (eyelid) 374.46
  congenital 743.62
Blepharoplegia 374.89
Blepharoptosis 374.30
  congenital 743.61
Blepharopyorrhea 098.49

Blepharospasm 333.81
  due to drugs 333.85
Blessig's cyst 362.62
Blighted ovum 631
Blind
  bronchus (congenital) 748.3
  eye—*see also* Blindness
    hypertensive 360.42
    hypotensive 360.41
  loop syndrome (postoperative) 579.2
  sac, fallopian tube (congenital) 752.19
  spot, enlarged 368.42
  tract or tube (congenital) NEC—*see* Atresia
Blindness (acquired) (congenital) (both eyes) 369.00
  with deafness V49.85
  blast 921.3
    with nerve injury—*see* Injury, nerve, optic
  Bright's—*see* Uremia
  color (congenital) 368.59
    acquired 368.55
    blue 368.53
    green 368.52
    red 368.51
    total 368.54
  concussion 950.9
  cortical 377.75
  day 368.10
    acquired 368.10
    congenital 368.10
    hereditary 368.10
    specified type NEC 368.10
  due to
    injury NEC 950.9
    refractive error—*see* Error, refractive
  eclipse (total) 363.31
  emotional 300.11
  face 368.16
  hysterical 300.11
  legal (both eyes) (USA definition) 369.4
    with impairment of better (less impaired) eye
      near-total 369.02
        with
          lesser eye impairment 369.02
            near-total 369.04
            total 369.03
        profound 369.05
          with
            lesser eye impairment 369.05
              near-total 369.07
              profound 369.08
              total 369.06
        severe 369.21
          with
            lesser eye impairment 369.21
              blind 369.11
              near-total 369.13
              profound 369.14
              severe 369.22
              total 369.12
        total
          with lesser eye impairment total 369.01
  mind 784.69
  moderate
    both eyes 369.25
      with impairment of lesser eye (specified as)
        blind, not further specified 369.15
        low vision, not further specified 369.23
        near-total 369.17
        profound 369.18
        severe 369.24
        total 369.16

Blindness—*continued*
  one eye 369.74
    with vision of other eye (specified as)
      near-normal 369.75
      normal 369.76
  near-total
    both eyes 369.04
      with impairment of lesser eye (specified as)
        blind, not further specified 369.02
        total 369.03
    one eye 369.64
      with vision of other eye (specified as)
        near-normal 369.65
        normal 369.66
  night 368.60
    acquired 368.62
    congenital (Japanese) 368.61
    hereditary 368.61
    specified type NEC 368.69
    vitamin A deficiency 264.5
  nocturnal—*see* Blindness, night
  one eye 369.60
    with low vision of other eye 369.10
  profound
    both eyes 369.08
      with impairment of lesser eye (specified as)
        blind, not further specified 369.05
        near-total 369.07
        total 369.06
    one eye 369.67
      with vision of other eye (specified as)
        near-normal 369.68
        normal 369.69
  psychic 784.69
  severe
    both eyes 369.22
      with impairment of lesser eye (specified as)
        blind, not further specified 369.11
        low vision, not further specified 369.21
        near-total 369.13
        profound 369.14
        total 369.12
    one eye 369.71
      with vision of other eye (specified as)
        near-normal 369.72
        normal 369.73
  snow 370.24
  sun 363.31
  temporary 368.12
  total
    both eyes 369.01
    one eye 369.61
      with vision of other eye (specified as)
        near-normal 369.62
        normal 369.63
  transient 368.12
  traumatic NEC 950.9
  word (developmental) 315.01
    acquired 784.61
    secondary to organic lesion 784.61
Blister —*see also* Injury, superficial, by site
  beetle dermatitis 692.89
  due to burn—*see* Burn, by site, second degree
  fever 054.9
  multiple, skin, nontraumatic 709.8
Bloating 787.3
Bloch-Siemens syndrome (incontinentia pigmenti) 757.33
Bloch-Stauffer dyshormonal dermatosis 757.33
Bloch-Sulzberger disease or syndrome
  (incontinentia pigmenti) (melanoblastosis) 757.33

Block
  alveolar capillary 516.3
  arborization (heart) 426.6
  arrhythmic 426.9
  atrioventricular (AV) (incomplete) (partial) 426.10
    with
      2:1 atrioventricular response block 426.13
      atrioventricular dissociation 426.0
      first degree (incomplete) 426.11
      second degree (Mobitz type I) 426.13
        Mobitz (type) II 426.12
      third degree 426.0
    complete 426.0
      congenital 746.86
    congenital 746.86
    Mobitz (incomplete)
      type I (Wenckebach's) 426.13
      type II 426.12
    partial 426.13
  auriculoventricular (*see also* Block, atrioventricular) 426.10
    complete 426.0
      congenital 746.86
    congenital 746.86
  bifascicular (cardiac) 426.53
  bundle branch (complete) (false) (incomplete) 426.50
    bilateral 426.53
    left (complete) (main stem) 426.3
      with right bundle branch block 426.53
      anterior fascicular 426.2
        with
          posterior fascicular block 426.3
          right bundle branch block 426.52
      hemiblock 426.2
      incomplete 426.2
        with right bundle branch block 426.53
      posterior fascicular 426.2
        with
          anterior fascicular block 426.3
          right bundle branch block 426.51
    right 426.4
      with
        left bundle branch block (incomplete) (main stem) 426.53
        left fascicular block 426.53
          anterior 426.52
          posterior 426.51
    Wilson's type 426.4
  cardiac 426.9
  conduction 426.9
    complete 426.0
  Eustachian tube (*see also* Obstruction, Eustachian tube) 381.60
  fascicular (left anterior) (left posterior) 426.2
  foramen Magendie (acquired) 331.3
    congenital 742.3
      with spina bifida (*see also* Spina bifida) 741.0
  heart 426.9
    first degree (atrioventricular) 426.11
    second degree (atrioventricular) 426.13
    third degree (atrioventricular) 426.0
    bundle branch (complete) (false) (incomplete) 426.50
      bilateral 426.53
      left (*see also* Block, bundle branch, left) 426.3
      right (*see also* Block, bundle branch, right) 426.4

Block—*continued*
   complete (atrioventricular) 426.0
      congenital 746.86
   incomplete 426.13
   intra-atrial 426.6
   intraventricular NEC 426.6
   sinoatrial 426.6
   specified type NEC 426.6
   hepatic vein 453.0
   intraventricular (diffuse) (myofibrillar) 426.6
      bundle branch (complete) (false) (incomplete)
         426.50
         bilateral 426.53
         left (*see also* Block, bundle branch, left)
            426.3
         right (*see also* Block, bundle branch, right)
            426.4
   kidney (*see also* Disease, renal) 593.9
      postcystoscopic 997.5
   myocardial (*see also* Block, heart) 426.9
   nodal 426.10
   optic nerve 377.49
   organ or site (congenital) NEC—*see* Atresia
   parietal 426.6
   peri-infarction 426.6
   portal (vein) 452
   sinoatrial 426.6
   sinoauricular 426.6
   spinal cord 336.9
   trifascicular 426.54
   tubal 628.2
   vein NEC 453.9
Blocq's disease or syndrome (astasia-abasia)
   307.9
Blood
   constituents, abnormal NEC 790.6
   disease 289.9
      specified NEC 289.89
   donor V59.01
      other blood components V59.09
      stem cells V59.02
      whole blood V59.01
   dyscrasia 289.9
      with
         abortion—*see* Abortion, by type, with
            hemorrhage, delayed or excessive
         ectopic pregnancy (*see also* categories
            633.0-633.9) 639.1
         molar pregnancy (*see also* categories
            630-632) 639.1
         following
            abortion 639.1
            ectopic or molar pregnancy 639.1
         newborn NEC 776.9
         puerperal, postpartum 666.3
   flukes NEC (*see also* Infestation, Schistosoma)
      120.9
   in
      feces (*see also* Melena) 578.1
         occult 792.1
      urine (*see also* Hematuria) 599.70
   mole 631
   occult 792.1
   poisoning (*see also* Septicemia) 038.9
   pressure
      decreased, due to shock following injury 958.4
      fluctuating 796.4
      high (*see also* Hypertension) 401.9
         incidental reading (isolated) (nonspecific),
            without diagnosis of hypertension 796.2
      low (*see also* Hypotension) 458.9

Blood—*continued*
      incidental reading (isolated) (nonspecific),
         without diagnosis of hypotension 796.3
   spitting (*see also* Hemoptysis) 786.3
   staining cornea 371.12
   transfusion
      without reported diagnosis V58.2
      donor V59.01
         stem cells V59.02
      reaction or complication—*see* Complications,
         transfusion
   tumor—*see* Hematoma
   vessel rupture—*see* Hemorrhage
   vomiting (*see also* Hematemesis) 578.0
Blood-forming organ disease 289.9
Bloodgood's disease 610.1
Bloodshot eye 379.93
Bloom (-Machacek) (-Torre) syndrome 757.39
Blotch, palpebral 372.55
Blount's disease (tibia vara) 732.4
Blount-Barber syndrome (tibia vara) 732.4
Blue
   baby 746.9
   bloater 491.20
      with acute bronchitis 491.22
      with exacerbation (acute) 491.21
   diaper syndrome 270.0
   disease 746.9
   dome cyst 610.0
   drum syndrome 381.02
   sclera 743.47
      with fragility of bone and deafness 756.51
   toe syndrome 445.02
Blueness (cyanosis) 782.5
Blurred vision 368.8
Blushing (abnormal) (excessive) 782.62
BMI (body mass index)
   adult
      25.0-25.9 V85.21
      26.0-26.9 V85.22
      27.0-27.9 V85.23
      28.0-28.9 V85.24
      29.0-29.9 V85.25
      30.0-30.9 V85.30
      31.0-31.9 V85.31
      32.0-32.9 V85.32
      33.0-33.9 V85.33
      34.0-34.9 V85.34
      35.0-35.9 V85.35
      36.0-36.9 V85.36
      37.0-37.9 V85.37
      38.0-38.9 V85.38
      39.0-39.9 V85.39
      40 and over V85.4
      between 19-24 V85.1
      less than 19 V85.0
   pediatric
      5th percentile to less than 85th percentile for
         age V85.52
      85th percentile to less than 95th percentile for
         age V85.53
      greater than or equal to 95th percentile for age
         V85.54
      less than 5th percentile for age V85.51
Boarder, hospital V65.0
   infant V65.0
Bockhart's impetigo (superficial folliculitis) 704.8
Bodechtel-Guttmann disease (subacute
   sclerosing panencephalitis) 046.2
Boder-Sedgwick syndrome (ataxia-
   telangiectasia) 334.8

Bony block of joint—*continued*
multiple sites 718.89
pelvic region 718.85
shoulder (region) 718.81
specified site NEC 718.88
wrist 718.83
BOOP (bronchiolitis obliterans organized penumonia) 516.8
Borderline
intellectual functioning V62.89
osteopenia 733.90
pelvis 653.1
with obstruction during labor 660.1
affecting fetus or newborn 763.1
psychosis (*see also* Schizophrenia) 295.5
of childhood (*see also* Psychosis, childhood) 299.8
schizophrenia (*see also* Schizophrenia) 295.5
Borna disease 062.9
Bornholm disease (epidemic pleurodynia) 074.1
Borrelia vincentii (mouth) (pharynx) (tonsils) 101
Bostock's catarrh (*see also* Fever, hay) 477.9
Boston exanthem 048
Botalli, ductus (patent) (persistent) 747.0
Bothriocephalus latus infestation 123.4
Botulism 005.1
food poisoning 005.1
infant 040.41
non-foodborne 040.42
wound 040.42
Bouba (*see also* Yaws) 102.9
Bouffée délirante 298.3
Bouillaud's disease or syndrome (rheumatic heart disease) 391.9
Bourneville's disease (tuberous sclerosis) 759.5
Boutonneuse fever 082.1
Boutonniere
deformity (finger) 736.21
hand (intrinsic) 736.21
Bouveret (-Hoffmann) disease or syndrome (paroxysmal tachycardia) 427.2
Bovine heart —*see* Hypertrophy, cardiac
Bowel —*see* condition
Bowen's
dermatosis (precancerous) (M8081/2)—*see* Neoplasm, skin, in situ
disease (M8081/2)—*see* Neoplasm, skin, in situ
epithelioma (M8081/2)—*see* Neoplasm, skin, in situ
type
epidermoid carcinoma in situ (M8081/2)—*see* Neoplasm, skin, in situ
intraepidermal squamous cell carcinoma (M8081/2)–*see* Neoplasm, skin, in situ
Bowing
femur 736.89
congenital 754.42
fibula 736.89
congenital 754.43
forearm 736.09
away from midline (cubitus valgus) 736.01
toward midline (cubitus varus) 736.02
leg(s), long bones, congenital 754.44
radius 736.09
away from midline (cubitus valgus) 736.01
toward midline (cubitus varus) 736.02
tibia 736.89
congenital 754.43
Bowleg (s) 736.42
congenital 754.44
rachitic 268.1

Boyd's dysentery 004.2
Brachial —*see* condition
Brachman-de Lange syndrome (Amsterdam dwarf, mental retardation, and brachycephaly) 759.89
Brachycardia 427.89
Brachycephaly 756.0
Brachymorphism and ectopia lentis 759.89
Bradley's disease (epidemic vomiting) 078.82
Bradycardia 427.89
chronic (sinus) 427.81
newborn 779.81
nodal 427.89
postoperative 997.1
reflex 337.09
sinoatrial 427.89
with paroxysmal tachyarrhythmia or tachycardia 427.81
chronic 427.81
sinus 427.89
with paroxysmal tachyarrhythmia or tachycardia 427.81
chronic 427.81
persistent 427.81
severe 427.81
tachycardia syndrome 427.81
vagal 427.89
Bradykinesia 781.0
Bradypnea 786.09
Brailsford's disease 732.3
radial head 732.3
tarsal scaphoid 732.5
Brailsford-Morquio disease or syndrome (mucopolysaccharidosis IV) 277.5
Brain —*see also* condition
death 348.89
syndrome (acute) (chronic) (nonpsychotic) (organic) (with neurotic reaction) (with behavioral reaction) (*see also* Syndrome, brain) 310.9
with
presenile brain disease 290.10
psychosis, psychotic reaction (*see also* Psychosis, organic) 294.9
congenital (*see also* Retardation, mental) 319
Branched-chain amino-acid disease 270.3
Branchial —*see* condition
Brandt's syndrome (acrodermatitis enteropathica) 686.8
Brash (water) 787.1
Brass-founders' ague 985.8
Bravais-Jacksonian epilepsy (*see also* Epilepsy) 345.5
Braxton Hicks contractions 644.1
Braziers' disease 985.8
Brazilian
blastomycosis 116.1
leishmaniasis 085.5
BRBPR (bright red blood per rectum) 569.3
Break
cardiorenal—*see* Hypertension, cardiorenal
retina (*see also* Defect, retina) 361.30
Breakbone fever 061
Breakdown
device, implant, or graft—*see* Complications, mechanical
nervous (*see also* Disorder, mental, nonpsychotic) 300.9
perineum 674.2

Breast —*see also* condition
  buds 259.1
    in newborn 779.89
  dense 793.82
  nodule 793.89
Breast feeding difficulties 676.8
Breath
  foul 784.99
  holder, child 312.81
  holding spells 786.9
  shortness 786.05
Breathing
  asymmetrical 786.09
  bronchial 786.09
  exercises V57.0
  labored 786.09
  mouth 784.99
    causing malocclusion 524.59
  periodic 786.09
    high altitude 327.22
  tic 307.20
Breathlessness 786.09
Breda's disease (*see also* Yaws) 102.9
Breech
  delivery, affecting fetus or newborn 763.0
  extraction, affecting fetus or newborn 763.0
  presentation (buttocks) (complete) (frank) 652.2
    with successful version 652.1
    before labor, affecting fetus or newborn 761.7
    during labor, affecting fetus or newborn 763.0
Breisky's disease (kraurosis vulvae) 624.09
Brennemann's syndrome (acute mesenteric
  lymphadenitis) 289.2
Brenner's
  tumor (benign) (M9000/0) 220
    borderline malignancy (M9000/1) 236.2
    malignant (M9000/3) 183.0
    proliferating (M9000/1) 236.2
Bretonneau's disease (diphtheritic malignant
  angina) 032.0
Breus' mole 631
Brevicollis 756.16
Bricklayers' itch 692.89
Brickmakers' anemia 126.9
Bridge
  myocardial 746.85
Bright's
  blindness—*see* Uremia
  disease (*see also* Nephritis) 583.9
    arteriosclerotic (*see also* Hypertension,
      kidney) 403.90
Bright red blood per rectum (BRBPR) 569.3
Brill's disease (recrudescent typhus) 081.1
  flea-borne 081.0
  louse-borne 081.1
Brill-Symmers disease (follicular lymphoma)
  (M9690/3) 202.0
Brill-Zinsser disease (recrudescent typhus) 081.1
Brinton's disease (linitis plastica) (M8142/3)
  151.9
Brion-Kayser disease (*see also* Fever,
  paratyphoid) 002.9
Briquet's disorder or syndrome 300.81
Brissaud's
  infantilism (infantile myxedema) 244.9
  motor-verbal tic 307.23
Brissaud-Meige syndrome (infantile myxedema)
  244.9

Brittle
  bones (congenital) 756.51
  nails 703.8
    congenital 757.5
Broad —*see also* condition
  beta disease 272.2
  ligament laceration syndrome 620.6
Brock's syndrome (atelectasis due to enlarged
  lymph nodes) 518.0
Brocq's disease 691.8
  atopic (diffuse) neurodermatitis 691.8
  lichen simplex chronicus 698.3
  parakeratosis psoriasiformis 696.2
  parapsoriasis 696.2
Brocq-Duhring disease (dermatitis
  herpetiformis) 694.0
Brodie's
  abscess (localized) (chronic) (*see also*
    Osteomyelitis) 730.1
  disease (joint) (*see also* Osteomyelitis) 730.1
Broken
  arches 734
    congenital 755.67
  back—*see* Fracture, vertebra, by site
  bone—*see* Fracture, by site
  compensation—*see* Disease, heart
  heart syndrome 429.83
  implant or internal device—*see* listing under
    Complications, mechanical
  neck—*see* Fracture, vertebra, cervical
  nose 802.0
    open 802.1
  tooth, teeth 873.63
    complicated 873.73
Bromhidrosis 705.89
Bromidism, bromism
  acute 967.3
    correct substance properly administered
      349.82
    overdose or wrong substance given or taken
      967.3
  chronic (*see also* Dependence) 304.1
Bromidrosiphobia 300.23
Bromidrosis 705.89
Bronchi, bronchial —*see* condition
Bronchiectasis (cylindrical) (diffuse) (fusiform)
  (localized) (moniliform) (postinfectious)
  (recurrent) (saccular) 494.0
  with acute exacerbation 494.1
  congenital 748.61
  tuberculosis (*see also* Tuberculosis) 011.5
Bronchiolectasis —*see* Bronchiectasis
Bronchiolitis (acute) (infectious) (subacute)
  466.19
  with
    bronchospasm or obstruction 466.19
    influenza, flu, or grippe 487.1
  catarrhal (acute) (subacute) 466.19
  chemical 506.0
    chronic 506.4
  chronic (obliterative) 491.8
  due to external agent—*see* Bronchitis, acute,
    due to
  fibrosa obliterans 491.8
  influenzal 487.1
  obliterans 491.8
    status post lung transplant 996.84
    with organizing pneumonia (BOOP) 516.8
  obliterative (chronic) (diffuse) (subacute) 491.8
    due to fumes or vapors 506.4
  respiratory syncytial virus 466.11
  vesicular—*see* Pneumonia, broncho-

Bronchospasm 519.11
  with
    asthma—*see* Asthma
    bronchiolitis, acute 466.19
      due to respiratory syncytial virus 466.11
    bronchitis—*see* Bronchitis
    chronic obstructive pulmonary disease
      (COPD) 496
    emphysema—*see* Emphysema
    due to external agent—*see* Condition,
      respiratory, acture, due to
  acute 519.11
    due to external agent—*see* Condition,
      respiratory, acute, due to
  exercise induced 493.81
Bronchospirochetosis 104.8
Bronchostenosis 519.19
Bronchus —*see* condition
Bronze, bronzed
  diabetes 275.0
  disease (Addison's) (skin) 255.41
  tuberculous (*see also* Tuberculosis) 017.6
Brooke's disease or tumor (M8100/0)—*see*
  Neoplasm, skin, benign
Brow presentation complicating delivery 652.4
Brown's tendon sheath syndrome 378.61
Brown enamel of teeth (hereditary) 520.5
Brown-Séquard's paralysis (syndrome) 344.89
Brucella, brucellosis (infection) 023.9
  abortus 023.1
  canis 023.3
  dermatitis, skin 023.9
  melitensis 023.0
  mixed 023.8
  suis 023.2
Bruck's disease 733.99
Bruck-de Lange disease or syndrome
  (Amsterdam dwarf, mental retardation, and
  brachycephaly) 759.89
Brugada syndrome 746.89
Brug's filariasis 125.1
Brugsch's syndrome (acropachyderma) 757.39
Bruhl's disease (splenic anemia with fever) 285.8
Bruise (skin surface intact)—*see also* Contusion
  with
    fracture—*see* Fracture, by site
    open wound—*see* Wound, open, by site
  internal organ (abdomen, chest, or pelvis)—*see*
    Injury, internal, by site
  umbilical cord 663.6
    affecting fetus or newborn 762.6
Bruit 785.9
  arterial (abdominal) (carotid) 785.9
  supraclavicular 785.9
Brushburn —*see* Injury, superficial, by site
Bruton's X-linked agammaglobulinemia 279.04
Bruxism 306.8
  sleep related 327.53
Bubbly lung syndrome 770.7
Bubo 289.3
  blennorrhagic 098.89
  chancroidal 099.0
  climatic 099.1
  due to Hemophilus ducreyi 099.0
  gonococcal 098.89
  indolent NEC 099.8
  inguinal NEC 099.8
    chancroidal 099.0
    climatic 099.1
    due to H. ducreyi 099.0

Bubo—*continued*
  scrofulous (*see also* Tuberculosis) 017.2
  soft chancre 099.0
  suppurating 683
  syphilitic 091.0
    congenital 090.0
  tropical 099.1
  venereal NEC 099.8
  virulent 099.0
Bubonic plague 020.0
Bubonocele —*see* Hernia, inguinal
Buccal —*see* condition
Buchanan's disease (juvenile osteochondrosis of
  iliac crest) 732.1
Buchem's syndrome (hyperostosis corticalis)
  733.3
Buchman's disease (osteochondrosis, juvenile)
  732.1
Bucket handle fracture (semilunar cartilage)
  (*see also* Tear, meniscus) 836.2
Budd-Chiari syndrome (hepatic vein
  thrombosis) 453.0
Budgerigar-fanciers' disease or lung 495.2
Büdinger-Ludloff-Läwen disease 717.89
Buds
  breast 259.1
  in newborn 779.89
Buerger's disease (thromboangiitis obliterans)
  443.1
Bulbar —*see* condition
Bulbus cordis 745.9
  persistent (in left ventricle) 745.8
Bulging fontanels (congenital) 756.0
Bulimia 783.6
  nervosa 307.51
  nonorganic origin 307.51
Bulky uterus 621.2
Bulla(e) 709.8
  lung (emphysematous) (solitary) 492.0
Bullet wound —*see also* Wound, open, by site
  fracture—*see* Fracture, by site, open
  internal organ (abdomen, chest, or pelvis)—*see*
    Injury, internal, by site, with open wound
  intracranial—*see* Laceration, brain, with open
    wound
Bullis fever 082.8
Bullying (*see also* Disturbance, conduct) 312.0
Bundle
  branch block (complete) (false) (incomplete)
    426.50
    bilateral 426.53
    left (*see also* Block, bundle branch, left) 426.3
      hemiblock 426.2
    right (*see also* Block, bundle branch, right)
      426.4
  of His—*see* condition
  of Kent syndrome (anomalous atrioventricular
    excitation) 426.7
Bungpagga 040.81
Bunion 727.1
Bunionette 727.1
Bunyamwera fever 066.3
Buphthalmia, buphthalmos (congenital) 743.20
  associated with
    keratoglobus, congenital 743.22
    megalocornea 743.22
    ocular anomalies NEC 743.22
  isolated 743.21
  simple 743.21
Bürger-Grütz disease or syndrome (essential
  familial hyperlipemia) 272.3

Buried roots 525.3
Burke's syndrome 577.8
Burkitt's
tumor (M9750/3) 200.2
type malignant, lymphoma, lymphoblastic, or
undifferentiated (M9750/3) 200.2
Burn (acid) (cathode ray) (caustic) (chemical)
(electric heating appliance) (electricity) (fire)
(flame) (hot liquid or object) (irradiation)
(lime) (radiation) (steam) (thermal) (x-ray)
949.0

---

*Note—Use the following fifth-digit
subclassification with category 948 to indicate
the percent of body surface with third degree
burn:*

0 less than 10% or unspecified
1 10-19%
2 20-29%
3 30-39%
4 40-49%
5 50-59%
6 60-69%
7 70-79%
8 80-89%
9 90% or more of body surface

---

with
  blisters—*see* Burn, by site, second degree
  erythema—*see* Burn, by site, first degree
  skin loss (epidermal)—*see also* Burn, by site,
    second degree
    full thickness—*see also* Burn, by site, third
     degree
     with necrosis of underlying tissues—*see*
      Burn, by site, third degree, deep
first degree—*see* Burn, by site, first degree
second degree—*see* Burn, by site, second degree
third degree—*see also* Burn, by site, third degree
  deep—*see* Burn, by site, third degree, deep
abdomen, abdominal (muscle) (wall) 942.03
  with
    trunk—*see* Burn, trunk, multiple sites
  first degree 942.13
  second degree 942.23
  third degree 942.33
    deep 942.43
     with loss of body part 942.53
ankle 945.03
  with
    lower limb(s)–*see* Burn, leg, multiple sites
  first degree 945.13
  second degree 945.23
  third degree 945.33
    deep 945.43
     with loss of body part 945.53
anus—*see* Burn, trunk, specified site NEC
arm(s) 943.00
  first degree 943.10
  second degree 943.20
  third degree 943.30
    deep 943.40
     with loss of body part 943.50
  lower—*see* Burn, forearm(s)
  multiple sites, except hand(s) or wrist(s) 943.09
    first degree 943.19
    second degree 943.29
    third degree 943.39
     deep 943.49
      with loss of body part 943.59

Burn—*continued*
  arm(s)—*continued*
    upper 943.03
     first degree 943.13
     second degree 943.23
     third degree 943.33
      deep 943.43
       with loss of body part 943.53
  auditory canal (external)—*see* Burn, ear
  auricle (ear)—*see* Burn, ear
  axilla 943.04
    with
     upper limb(s) except hand(s) or wrist(s)—*see*
      Burn, arm(s), multiple sites
    first degree 943.14
    second degree 943.24
    third degree 943.34
     deep 943.44
      with loss of body part 943.54
  back 942.04
    with
     trunk—*see* Burn, trunk, multiple sites
    first degree 942.14
    second degree 942.24
    third degree 942.34
     deep 942.44
      with loss of body part 942.54
  biceps
    brachii—*see* Burn, arm(s), upper
    femoris—*see* Burn, thigh
  breast(s) 942.01
    with
     trunk—*see* Burn, trunk, multiple sites
    first degree 942.11
    second degree 942.21
    third degree 942.31
     deep 942.41
      with loss of body part 942.51
  brow—*see* Burn, forehead
  buttock(s)—*see* Burn, back
  canthus (eye) 940.1
    chemical 940.0
  cervix (uteri) 947.4
  cheek (cutaneous) 941.07
    with
     face or head—*see* Burn, head, multiple sites
    first degree 941.17
    second degree 941.27
    third degree 941.37
     deep 941.47
      with loss of body part 941.57
  chest wall (anterior) 942.02
    with
     trunk—*see* Burn, trunk, multiple sites
    first degree 942.12
    second degree 942.22
    third degree 942.32
     deep 942.42
      with loss of body part 942.52
  chin 941.04
    with
     face or head—*see* Burn, head, multiple sites
    first degree 941.14
    second degree 941.24
    third degree 941.34
     deep 941.44
      with loss of body part 941.54
  clitoris—*see* Burn, genitourinary organs,
    external
  colon 947.3

Burn—*continued*
conjunctiva (and cornea) 940.4
  chemical
    acid 940.3
    alkaline 940.2
cornea (and conjunctiva) 940.4
  chemical
    acid 940.3
    alkaline 940.2
costal region—*see* Burn, chest wall
due to ingested chemical agent—*see* Burn,
  internal organs
ear (auricle) (canal) (drum) (external) 941.01
  with
    face or head—*see* Burn, head, multiple sites
  first degree 941.11
  second degree 941.21
  third degree 941.31
    deep 941.41
      with loss of a body part 941.51
elbow 943.02
  with
    hand(s) and wrist(s)—*see* Burn, multiple
      specified sites
    upper limb(s) except hand(s) or
      wrist(s)—*see also* Burn, arm(s), multiple
      sites
  first degree 943.12
  second degree 943.22
  third degree 943.32
    deep 943.42
      with loss of body part 943.52
electricity, electric current—*see* Burn, by site
entire body—*see* Burn, multiple, specified sites
epididymis—*see* Burn, genitourinary organs,
  external
epigastric region—*see* Burn, abdomen
epiglottis 947.1
esophagus 947.2
extent (percent of body surface)
  less than 10 percent 948.0
  10-19 percent 948.1
  20-29 percent 948.2
  30-39 percent 948.3
  40-49 percent 948.4
  50-59 percent 948.5
  60-69 percent 948.6
  70-79 percent 948.7
  80-89 percent 948.8
  90 percent or more 948.9
extremity
  lower—*see* Burn, leg
  upper—*see* Burn, arm(s)
eye(s) (and adnexa) (only) 940.9
  with
    face, head, or neck 941.02
      first degree 941.12
      second degree 941.22
      third degree 941.32
        deep 941.42
          with loss of body part 941.52
    other sites (classifiable to more than one
      category in 940-945)—*see* Burn,
      multiple, specified sites
    resulting rupture and destruction of eyeball
      940.5
  specified part—*see* Burn, by site
eyeball—*see also* Burn, eye
  with resulting rupture and destruction of
    eyeball 940.5

Burn—*continued*
eyelid(s) 940.1
  chemical 940.0
face—*see* Burn, head
finger (nail) (subungual) 944.01
  with
    hand(s)—*see* Burn, hand(s), multiple sites
    other sites—*see* Burn, multiple, specified
      sites
    thumb 944.04
      first degree 944.14
      second degree 944.24
      third degree 944.34
        deep 944.44
          with loss of body part 944.54
  first degree 944.11
  second degree 944.21
  third degree 944.31
    deep 944.41
      with loss of body part 944.51
  multiple (digits) 944.03
    with thumb—*see* Burn, finger, with thumb
    first degree 944.13
    second degree 944.23
    third degree 944.33
      deep 944.43
        with loss of body part 944.53
flank—*see* Burn, abdomen
foot 945.02
  with
    lower limb(s)—*see* Burn, leg, multiple sites
  first degree 945.12
  second degree 945.22
  third degree 945.32
    deep 945.42
      with loss of body part 945.52
forearm(s) 943.01
  with
    upper limb(s) except hand(s) or
      wrist(s)—*see* Burn, arm(s), multiple sites
  first degree 943.11
  second degree 943.21
  third degree 943.31
    deep 943.41
      with loss of body part 943.51
forehead 941.07
  with
    face or head—*see* Burn, head, multiple sites
  first degree 941.17
  second degree 941.27
  third degree 941.37
    deep 941.47
      with loss of body part 941.57
fourth degree—*see* Burn, by site, third degree,
  deep
friction—*see* Injury, superficial, by site
from swallowing caustic or corrosive substance
  NEC—*see* Burn, internal organs
full thickness—*see* Burn, by site, third degree
gastrointestinal tract 947.3
genitourinary organs
  external 942.05
    with
      trunk—*see* Burn, trunk, multiple sites
    first degree 942.15
    second degree 942.25
    third degree 942.35
      deep 942.45
        with loss of body part 942.55
  internal 947.8
globe (eye)—*see* Burn, eyeball

Burn—*continued*
  groin—*see* Burn, abdomen
  gum 947.0
  hand(s) (phalanges) (and wrist) 944.00
    first degree 944.10
    second degree 944.20
    third degree 944.30
      deep 944.40
        with loss of body part 944.50
    back (dorsal surface) 944.06
      first degree 944.16
      second degree 944.26
      third degree 944.36
        deep 944.46
          with loss of body part 944.56
    multiple sites 944.08
      first degree 944.18
      second degree 944.28
      third degree 944.38
        deep 944.48
          with loss of body part 944.58
  head (and face) 941.00
    eye(s) only 940.9
      specified part—*see* Burn, by site
    first degree 941.10
    second degree 941.20
    third degree 941.30
      deep 941.40
        with loss of body part 941.50
    multiple sites 941.09
      with eyes—*see* Burn, eyes, with face, head,
        or neck
      first degree 941.19
      second degree 941.29
      third degree 941.39
        deep 941.49
          with loss of body part 941.59
  heel—*see* Burn, foot
  hip—*see* Burn, trunk, specified site NEC
  iliac region—*see* Burn, trunk, specified site
    NEC
  infected 958.3
  inhalation (*see also* Burn, internal organs) 947.9
  internal organs 947.9
    from caustic or corrosive substance
      (swallowing) NEC 947.9
    specified NEC (*see also* Burn, by site) 947.8
  interscapular region—*see* Burn, back
  intestine (large) (small) 947.3
  iris—*see* Burn, eyeball
  knee 945.05
    with
      lower limb(s)—*see* Burn, leg, multiple sites
    first degree 945.15
    second degree 945.25
    third degree 945.35
      deep 945.45
        with loss of body part 945.55
  labium (majus) (minus)—*see* Burn,
    genitourinary organs, external
  lacrimal apparatus, duct, gland, or sac 940.1
    chemical 940.0
  larynx 947.1
  late effect—*see* Late, effects (of), burn
  leg 945.00
    first degree 945.10
    second degree 945.20
    third degree 945.30
      deep 945.40
        with loss of body part 945.50

Burn—*continued*
  leg —*continued*
    lower 945.04
      with other part(s) of lower limb(s)—*see*
        Burn, leg, multiple sites
      first degree 945.14
      second degree 945.24
      third degree 945.34
        deep 945.44
          with loss of body part 945.54
    multiple sites 945.09
      first degree 945.19
      second degree 945.29
      third degree 945.39
        deep 945.49
          with loss of body part 945.59
    upper—*see* Burn, thigh
  lightning—*see* Burn, by site
  limb(s)
    lower (including foot or toe(s))—*see* Burn, leg
    upper (except wrist and hand)—*see* Burn,
      arm(s)
  lip(s) 941.03
    with
      face or head—*see* Burn, head, multiple sites
      first degree 941.13
      second degree 941.23
      third degree 941.33
        deep 941.43
          with loss of body part 941.53
  lumbar region—*see* Burn, back
  lung 947.1
  malar region—*see* Burn, cheek
  mastoid region—*see* Burn, scalp
  membrane, tympanic—*see* Burn, ear
  midthoracic region—*see* Burn, chest wall
  mouth 947.0
  multiple (*see also* Burn, unspecified) 949.0
    specified sites (classifiable to more than one
      category in 940-945) 946.0
      first degree 946.1
      second degree 946.2
      third degree 946.3
        deep 946.4
          with loss of body part 946.5
  muscle, abdominal—*see* Burn, abdomen
  nasal (septum)—*see* Burn, nose
  neck 941.08
    with
      face or head—*see* Burn, head, multiple sites
      first degree 941.18
      second degree 941.28
      third degree 941.38
        deep 941.48
          with loss of body part 941.58
  nose (septum) 941.05
    with
      face or head—*see* Burn, head, multiple sites
      first degree 941.15
      second degree 941.25
      third degree 941.35
        deep 941.45
          with loss of body part 941.55
  occipital region—*see* Burn, scalp
  orbit region 940.1
    chemical 940.0
  oronasopharynx 947.0
  palate 947.0

Burn—*continued*
palm(s) 944.05
  with
    hand(s) and wrist(s)—*see* Burn, hand(s),
      multiple sites
    first degree 944.15
    second degree 944.25
    third degree 944.35
      deep 944.45
        with loss of a body part 944.55
parietal region—*see* Burn, scalp
penis—*see* Burn, genitourinary organs, external
perineum—*see* Burn, genitourinary organs,
  external
periocular area 940.1
  chemical 940.0
pharynx 947.0
pleura 947.1
popliteal space—*see* Burn, knee
prepuce—*see* Burn, genitourinary organs,
  external
pubic region—*see* Burn, genitourinary organs,
  external
pudenda—*see* Burn, genitourinary organs,
  external
rectum 947.3
sac, lacrimal 940.1
  chemical 940.0
sacral region—*see* Burn, back
salivary (ducts) (glands) 947.0
scalp 941.06
  with
    face or neck—*see* Burn, head, multiple sites
    first degree 941.16
    second degree 941.26
    third degree 941.36
      deep 941.46
        with loss of body part 941.56
scapular region 943.06
  with
    upper limb(s), except hand(s) or
      wrist(s)—*see* Burn, arm(s), multiple sites
    first degree 943.16
    second degree 943.26
    third degree 943.36
      deep 943.46
        with loss of body part 943.56
sclera—*see* Burn, eyeball
scrotum—*see* Burn, genitourinary organs,
  external
septum, nasal—*see* Burn, nose
shoulder(s) 943.05
  with
    hand(s) and wrist(s)—*see* Burn, multiple,
      specified sites
    upper limb(s), except hand(s) or
      wrist(s)—*see* Burn, arm(s), multiple sites
    first degree 943.15
    second degree 943.25
    third degree 943.35
      deep 943.45
        with loss of body part 943.55
skin NEC (*see also* Burn, unspecified) 949.0
skull—*see* Burn, head
small intestine 947.3
sternal region—*see* Burn, chest wall
stomach 947.3
subconjunctival—*see* Burn, conjunctiva
subcutaneous—*see* Burn, by site, third degree
submaxillary region—*see* Burn, head
submental region—*see* Burn, chin

Burn—*continued*
sun—*see* Sunburn
supraclavicular fossa—*see* Burn, neck
supraorbital—*see* Burn, forehead
temple—*see* Burn, scalp
temporal region—*see* Burn, scalp
testicle—*see* Burn, genitourinary organs,
  external
testis—*see* Burn, genitourinary organs, external
thigh 945.06
  with
    lower limb(s)—*see* Burn, leg, multiple sites
    first degree 945.16
    second degree 945.26
    third degree 945.36
      deep 945.46
        with loss of body part 945.56
thorax (external)—*see* Burn, chest wall
throat 947.0
thumb(s) (nail) (subungual) 944.02
  with
    finger(s)—*see* Burn, finger, with other sites,
      thumb
    hand(s) and wrist(s)—*see* Burn, hand(s),
      multiple sites
    first degree 944.12
    second degree 944.22
    third degree 944.32
      deep 944.42
        with loss of body part 944.52
toe (nail) (subungual) 945.01
  with
    lower limb(s)—*see* Burn, leg, multiple sites
    first degree 945.11
    second degree 945.21
    third degree 945.31
      deep 945.41
        with loss of body part 945.51
tongue 947.0
tonsil 947.0
trachea 947.1
trunk 942.00
  first degree 942.10
  second degree 942.20
  third degree 942.30
    deep 942.40
      with loss of body part 942.50
  multiple sites 942.09
    first degree 942.19
    second degree 942.29
    third degree 942.39
      deep 942.49
        with loss of body part 942.59
  specified site NEC 942.09
    first degree 942.19
    second degree 942.29
    third degree 942.39
      deep 942.49
        with loss of body part 942.59
tunica vaginalis—*see* Burn, genitourinary
  organs, external
tympanic membrane—*see* Burn, ear
tympanum—*see* Burn, ear
ultraviolet 692.82

Burn—*continued*
  unspecified site (multiple) 949.0
    with extent of body surface involved specified
      less than 10 percent 948.0
      10-19 percent 948.1
      20-29 percent 948.2
      30-39 percent 948.3
      40-49 percent 948.4
      50-59 percent 948.5
      60-69 percent 948.6
      70-79 percent 948.7
      80-89 percent 948.8
      90 percent or more 948.9
    first degree 949.1
    second degree 949.2
    third degree 949.3
      deep 949.4
        with loss of body part 949.5
  uterus 947.4
  uvula 947.0
  vagina 947.4
  vulva—*see* Burn, genitourinary organs, external
  wrist(s) 944.07
    with
      hand(s)—*see* Burn, hand(s), multiple sites
    first degree 944.17
    second degree 944.27
    third degree 944.37
      deep 944.47
        with loss of body part 944.57
Burnett's syndrome (milk-alkali) 275.42
Burnier's syndrome (hypophyseal dwarfism)
    253.3
Burning
  feet syndrome 266.2
  sensation (*see also* Disturbance, sensation)
    782.0
  tongue 529.6
Burns' disease (osteochondrosis, lower ulna)
    732.3
Bursa —*see also* condition
  pharynx 478.29
Bursitis NEC 727.3
  Achilles tendon 726.71
  adhesive 726.90
    shoulder 726.0
  ankle 726.79
  buttock 726.5
  calcaneal 726.79
  collateral ligament
    fibular 726.63
    tibial 726.62
  Duplay's 726.2
  elbow 726.33
  finger 726.8
  foot 726.79
  gonococcal 098.52
  hand 726.4
  hip 726.5
  infrapatellar 726.69
  ischiogluteal 726.5
  knee 726.60
  occupational NEC 727.2
  olecranon 726.33
  pes anserinus 726.61
  pharyngeal 478.29
  popliteal 727.51
  prepatellar 726.65
  radiohumeral 727.3
  scapulohumeral 726.19
    adhesive 726.0

Bursitis—*continued*
  shoulder 726.10
    adhesive 726.0
  subacromial 726.19
    adhesive 726.0
  subcoracoid 726.19
  subdeltoid 726.19
    adhesive 726.0
  subpatellar 726.69
  syphilitic 095.7
  Thornwaldt's, Tornwaldt's (pharyngeal) 478.29
  toe 726.79
  trochanteric area 726.5
  wrist 726.4
Burst stitches or sutures (complication of
    surgery) (external) (*see also* Dehiscence)
    998.32
  internal 998.31
Buruli ulcer 031.1
Bury's disease (erythema elevatum diutinum)
    695.89
Buschke's disease or scleredema (adultorum)
    710.1
Busquet's disease (osteoperiostitis) (*see also*
    Osteomyelitis) 730.1
Busse-Buschke disease (cryptococcosis) 117.5
Buttock —*see* condition
Button
  Biskra 085.1
  Delhi 085.1
  oriental 085.1
Buttonhole hand (intrinsic) 736.21
Bwamba fever (encephalitis) 066.3
Byssinosis (occupational) 504
Bywaters' syndrome 958.5

C

Cacergasia 300.9
Cachexia 799.4
cancerous —*see also* Neoplasm, by site,
    malignant 799.4
cardiac—*see* Disease, heart
dehydration 276.51
    with
        hypernatremia 276.0
        hyponatremia 276.1
    due to malnutrition 799.4
    exophthalmic 242.0
    heart—*see* Disease, heart
    hypophyseal 253.2
    hypopituitary 253.2
    lead 984.9
        specified type of lead—*see* Table of drugs and
            chemicals
    malaria 084.9
    malignant —*see also* Neoplasm, by site,
        malignant 799.4
    marsh 084.9
    nervous 300.5
    old age 797
    pachydermic—*see* Hypothyroidism
    paludal 084.9
    pituitary (postpartum) 253.2
    renal (*see also* Disease, renal) 593.9
    saturnine 984.9
        specified type of lead—*see* Table of drugs and
            chemicals
    senile 797
    Simmonds' (pituitary cachexia) 253.2
    splenica 289.59
    strumipriva (*see also* Hypothyroidism) 244.9
    tuberculous NEC (*see also* Tuberculosis) 011.9
café au lait spots 709.09
Caffey's disease or syndrome (infantile cortical
    hyperostosis) 756.59
Caisson disease 993.3
Caked breast (puerperal, postpartum) 676.2
Cake kidney 753.3
Calabar swelling 125.2
Calcaneal spur 726.73
Calcaneoapophysitis 732.5
Calcaneonavicular bar 755.67
Calcareous —*see* condition
Calcicosis (occupational) 502
Calciferol (vitamin D) deficiency 268.9
    with
        osteomalacia 268.2
        rickets (*see also* Rickets) 268.0
Calcification
    adrenal (capsule) (gland) 255.41
        tuberculous (*see also* Tuberculosis) 017.6
    aorta 440.0
    artery (annular)—*see* Arteriosclerosis
    auricle (ear) 380.89
    bladder 596.8
        due to S. hematobium 120.0
    brain (cortex)—*see* Calcification, cerebral
    bronchus 519.19
    bursa 727.82
    cardiac (*see also* Degeneration, myocardial) 429.1
    cartilage (postinfectional) 733.99
    cerebral (cortex) 348.89
        artery 437.0
    cervix (uteri) 622.8

Calcification—*continued*
    choroid plexus 349.2
    conjunctiva 372.54
    corpora cavernosa (penis) 607.89
    cortex (brain)—*see* Calcification, cerebral
    dental pulp (nodular) 522.2
    dentinal papilla 520.4
    disc, intervertebral 722.90
        cervical, cervicothoracic 722.91
        lumbar, lumbosacral 722.93
        thoracic, thoracolumbar 722.92
    fallopian tube 620.8
    falx cerebri—*see* Calcification, cerebral
    fascia 728.89
    gallbladder 575.8
    general 275.40
    heart (*see also* Degeneration, myocardial) 429.1
        valve—*see* Endocarditis
    intervertebral cartilage or disc (postinfectional)
        722.90
        cervical, cervicothoracic 722.91
        lumbar, lumbosacral 722.93
        thoracic, thoracolumbar 722.92
    intracranial—*see* Calcification, cerebral
    intraspinal ligament 728.89
    joint 719.80
        ankle 719.87
        elbow 719.82
        foot 719.87
        hand 719.84
        hip 719.85
        knee 719.86
        multiple sites 719.89
        pelvic region 719.85
        shoulder (region) 719.81
        specified site NEC 719.88
        wrist 719.83
    kidney 593.89
        tuberculous (*see also* Tuberculosis) 016.0
    larynx (senile) 478.79
    lens 366.8
    ligament 728.89
        intraspinal 728.89
        knee (medial collateral) 717.89
    lung 518.89
        active 518.89
        postinfectional 518.89
        tuberculous (*see also* Tuberculosis,
            pulmonary) 011.9
    lymph gland or node (postinfectional) 289.3
        tuberculous (*see also* Tuberculosis, lymph
            gland) 017.2
    mammographic 793.89
    massive (paraplegic) 728.10
    medial NEC (*see also* Arteriosclerosis,
        extremities) 440.20
    meninges (cerebral) 349.2
    metastatic 275.40
    Mönckeberg's—*see* Arteriosclerosis
    muscle 728.10
        heterotopic, postoperative 728.13
    myocardium, myocardial (*see also*
        Degeneration, myocardial) 429.1
    ovary 620.8
    pancreas 577.8
    penis 607.99
    periarticular 728.89
    pericardium (*see also* Pericarditis) 423.8

Calcification—*continued*
  pineal gland 259.8
  pleura 511.0
    postinfectional 518.89
    tuberculous (*see also* Tuberculosis, pleura)
      012.0
  pulp (dental) (nodular) 522.2
  renal 593.89
  rider's bone 733.99
  sclera 379.16
  semilunar cartilage 717.89
  spleen 289.59
  subcutaneous 709.3
  suprarenal (capsule) (gland) 255.41
  tendon (sheath) 727.82
    with bursitis, synovitis or tenosynovitis 727.82
  trachea 519.19
  ureter 593.89
  uterus 621.8
  vitreous 379.29
Calcified —*see also* Calcification
  hematoma NEC 959.9
Calcinosis (generalized) (interstitial) (tumoral)
    (universalis) 275.49
  circumscripta 709.3
  cutis 709.3
  intervertebralis 275.49 *[722.90]*
  Raynaud's
    phenomenonsclerodactylytelangiectasis
      (CRST) 710.1
Calciphylaxis (*see also* Calcification, by site)
    275.49
Calcium
  blood
    high (*see also* Hypercalcemia) 275.42
    low (*see also* Hypocalcemia) 275.41
  deposits—*see also* Calcification, by site
    in bursa 727.82
    in tendon (sheath) 727.82
      with bursitis, synovitis or tenosynovitis
        727.82
  salts or soaps in vitreous 379.22
Calciuria 791.9
Calculi —*see* Calculus
Calculosis, intrahepatic —*see*
    Choledocholithiasis
Calculus, calculi, calculous 592.9
  ampulla of Vater—*see* Choledocholithiasis
  anuria (impacted) (recurrent) 592.0
  appendix 543.9
  bile duct (any)—*see* Choledocholithiasis
  biliary—*see* Cholelithiasis
  bilirubin, multiple—*see* Cholelithiasis
  bladder (encysted) (impacted) (urinary) 594.1
    diverticulum 594.0
  bronchus 518.89
  calyx (kidney) (renal) 592.0
    congenital 753.3
  cholesterol (pure) (solitary)—*see* Cholelithiasis
  common duct (bile)—*see* Choledocholithiasis
  conjunctiva 372.54
  cystic 594.1
    duct—*see* Cholelithiasis
  dental 523.6
    subgingival 523.6
    supragingival 523.6
  epididymis 608.89

Calculus, calculi, calculous—*continued*
  gallbladder—*see also* Cholelithiasis
    congenital 751.69
  hepatic (duct)—*see* Choledocholithiasis
  intestine (impaction) (obstruction) 560.39
  kidney (impacted) (multiple) (pelvis) (recurrent)
      (staghorn) 592.0
    congenital 753.3
  lacrimal (passages) 375.57
  liver (impacted)—*see* Choledocholithiasis
  lung 518.89
  mammographic 793.89
  nephritic (impacted) (recurrent) 592.0
  nose 478.19
  pancreas (duct) 577.8
  parotid gland 527.5
  pelvis, encysted 592.0
  prostate 602.0
  pulmonary 518.89
  renal (impacted) (recurrent) 592.0
    congenital 753.3
  salivary (duct) (gland) 527.5
  seminal vesicle 608.89
  staghorn 592.0
  Stensen's duct 527.5
  sublingual duct or gland 527.5
    congenital 750.26
  submaxillary duct, gland, or region 527.5
  suburethral 594.8
  tonsil 474.8
  tooth, teeth 523.6
  tunica vaginalis 608.89
  ureter (impacted) (recurrent) 592.1
  urethra (impacted) 594.2
  urinary (duct) (impacted) (passage) (tract) 592.9
    lower tract NEC 594.9
      specified site 594.8
  vagina 623.8
  vesical (impacted) 594.1
  Wharton's duct 527.5
Caliectasis 593.89
California
  disease 114.0
  encephalitis 062.5
Caligo cornea 371.03
Callositas, callosity (infected) 700
Callus (infected) 700
  bone 726.91
  excessive, following fracture—*see also* Late,
    effect (of), fracture
Calvé (-Perthes) disease (osteochondrosis,
    femoral capital) 732.1
Calvities (*see also* Alopecia) 704.00
Cameroon fever (*see also* Malaria) 084.6
Camptocormia 300.11
Camptodactyly (congenital) 755.59
Camurati-Engelmann disease (diaphyseal
    sclerosis) 756.59
Canal —*see* condition
Canaliculitis (lacrimal) (acute) 375.31
  Actinomyces 039.8
  chronic 375.41
Canavan's disease 330.0

Cancer (M8000/3)—*see also* Neoplasm, by site, malignant

> *Note—The term "cancer" when modified by an adjective or adjectival phrase indicating a morphological type should be coded in the same manner as "carcinoma" with that adjective or phrase. Thus, "squamous-cell cancer" should be coded in the same manner as "squamous-cell carcinoma," which appears in the list under "Carcinoma."*

  bile duct type (M8160/3), liver 155.1
  hepatocellular (M8170/3) 155.0
Cancerous (M8000/3)—*see* Neoplasm, by site, malignant
Cancerphobia 300.29
Cancrum oris 528.1
Candidiasis, candidal 112.9
  with pneumonia 112.4
  balanitis 112.2
  congenital 771.7
  disseminated 112.5
  endocarditis 112.81
  esophagus 112.84
  intertrigo 112.3
  intestine 112.85
  lung 112.4
  meningitis 112.83
  mouth 112.0
  nails 112.3
  neonatal 771.7
  onychia 112.3
  otitis externa 112.82
  otomycosis 112.82
  paronychia 112.3
  perionyxis 112.3
  pneumonia 112.4
  pneumonitis 112.4
  skin 112.3
  specified site NEC 112.89
  systemic 112.5
  urogenital site NEC 112.2
  vagina 112.1
  vulva 112.1
  vulvovaginitis 112.1
Candidiosis —*see* Candidiasis
Candiru infection or infestation 136.8
Canities (premature) 704.3
  congenital 757.4
Canker (mouth) (sore) 528.2
  rash 034.1
Cannabinosis 504
Canton fever 081.9
Cap
  cradle 690.11
Capillariasis 127.5
Capillary —*see* condition
Caplan's syndrome 714.81
Caplan-Colinet syndrome 714.81
Capsule —*see* condition
Capsulitis (joint) 726.90
  adhesive (shoulder) 726.0
  hip 726.5
  knee 726.60
  labyrinthine 387.8
  thyroid 245.9
  wrist 726.4
Caput
  crepitus 756.0
  medusae 456.8
  succedaneum 767.19

Carapata disease 087.1
Carate —*see* Pinta
Carbohydrate-deficient glycoprotein syndrome (CDGS) 271.8
Carboxyhemoglobinemia 986
Carbuncle 680.9
  abdominal wall 680.2
  ankle 680.6
  anus 680.5
  arm (any part, above wrist) 680.3
  auditory canal, external 680.0
  axilla 680.3
  back (any part) 680.2
  breast 680.2
  buttock 680.5
  chest wall 680.2
  corpus cavernosum 607.2
  ear (any part) (external) 680.0
  eyelid 373.13
  face (any part, except eye) 680.0
  finger (any) 680.4
  flank 680.2
  foot (any part) 680.7
  forearm 680.3
  genital organ (male) 608.4
  gluteal (region) 680.5
  groin 680.2
  hand (any part) 680.4
  head (any part, except face) 680.8
  heel 680.7
  hip 680.6
  kidney (*see also* Abscess, kidney) 590.2
  knee 680.6
  labia 616.4
  lacrimal
    gland (*see also* Dacryoadenitis) 375.00
    passages (duct) (sac) (*see also* Dacryocystitis) 375.30
  leg, any part except foot 680.6
  lower extremity, any part except foot 680.6
  malignant 022.0
  multiple sites 680.9
  neck 680.1
  nose (external) (septum) 680.0
  orbit, orbital 376.01
  partes posteriores 680.5
  pectoral region 680.2
  penis 607.2
  perineum 680.2
  pinna 680.0
  scalp (any part) 680.8
  scrotum 608.4
  seminal vesicle 608.0
  shoulder 680.3
  skin NEC 680.9
  specified site NEC 680.8
  spermatic cord 608.4
  temple (region) 680.0
  testis 608.4
  thigh 680.6
  thumb 680.4
  toe (any) 680.7
  trunk 680.2
  tunica vaginalis 608.4
  umbilicus 680.2
  upper arm 680.3
  urethra 597.0
  vas deferens 608.4
  vulva 616.4
  wrist 680.4
Carbunculus (*see also* Carbuncle) 680.9

Carcinoid (tumor) (M8240/1)—see Tumor,
carcinoid
Carcinoidosis 259.2
Carcinoma (M8010/3)—*see also* Neoplasm, by
site, malignant

*Note—Except where otherwise indicated, the
morphological varieties of carcinoma in the list
below should be coded by site as for
"Neoplasm, malignant."*

with
apocrine metaplasia (M8573/3)
cartilaginous (and osseous) metaplasia
(M8571/3)
osseous (and cartilaginous) metaplasia
(M8571/3)
productive fibrosis (M8141/3)
spindle cell metaplasia (M8572/3)
squamous metaplasia (M8570/3)
acidophil (M8280/3)
specified site—*see* Neoplasm, by site,
malignant
unspecified site 194.3
acidophil-basophil, mixed (M8281/3)
specified site—*see* Neoplasm, by site,
malignant
unspecified site 194.3
acinar (cell) (M8550/3)
acinic cell (M8550/3)
adenocystic (M8200/3)
adenoid
cystic (M8200/3)
squamous cell (M8075/3)
adenosquamous (M8560/3)
adnexal (skin) (M8390/3)—*see* Neoplasm, skin,
malignant
adrenal cortical (M8370/3) 194.0
alveolar (M8251/3)
cell (M8250/3)—*see* Neoplasm, lung,
malignant
anaplastic type (M8021/3)
apocrine (M8401/3)
breast—*see* Neoplasm, breast, malignant
specified site NEC—*see* Neoplasm, skin,
malignant
unspecified site 173.9
basal cell (pigmented) (M8090/3)—*see also*
Neoplasm, skin, malignant
fibro-epithelial type (M8093/3)—*see*
Neoplasm, skin, malignant
morphea type (M8092/3)—*see* Neoplasm,
skin, malignant
multicentric (M8091/3)—*see* Neoplasm, skin,
malignant
basaloid (M8123/3)
basal-squamous cell, mixed (M8094/3)—*see*
Neoplasm, skin, malignant
basophil (M8300/3)
specified site—*see* Neoplasm, by site,
malignant
unspecified site 194.3
basophil-acidophil, mixed (M8281/3)
specified site—*see* Neoplasm, by site,
malignant
unspecified site 194.3
basosquamous (M8094/3)—*see* Neoplasm, skin,
malignant

Carcinoma—*continued*
bile duct type (M8160/3)
and hepatocellular, mixed (M8180/3) 155.0
liver 155.1
specified site NEC—*see* Neoplasm, by site,
malignant
unspecified site 155.1
branchial or branchiogenic 146.8
bronchial or bronchogenic—*see* Neoplasm,
lung, malignant
bronchiolar (terminal) (M8250/3)—*see*
Neoplasm, lung, malignant
bronchiolo-alveolar (M8250/3)—*see* Neoplasm,
lung, malignant
bronchogenic (epidermoid) 162.9
C cell (M8510/3)
specified site—*see* Neoplasm, by site,
malignant
unspecified site 193
ceruminous (M8420/3) 173.2
chorionic (M9100/3)
specified site—*see* Neoplasm, by site,
malignant
unspecified site
female 181
male 186.9
chromophobe (M8270/3)
specified site—*see* Neoplasm, by site,
malignant
unspecified site 194.3
clear cell (mesonephroid type) (M8310/3)
cloacogenic (M8124/3)
specified site—*see* Neoplasm, by site,
malignant
unspecified site 154.8
colloid (M8480/3)
cribriform (M8201/3)
cylindroid type (M8200/3)
diffuse type (M8145/3)
specified site—*see* Neoplasm, by site,
malignant
unspecified site 151.9
duct (cell) (M8500/3)
with Paget's disease (M8541/3)—*see*
Neoplasm, breast, malignant
infiltrating (M8500/3)
specified site—*see* Neoplasm, by site,
malignant
unspecified site 174.9
ductal (M8500/3)
ductular, infiltrating (M8521/3)
embryonal (M9070/3)
and teratoma, mixed (M9081/3)
combined with choriocarcinoma
(M9101/3)—*see* Neoplasm, by site,
malignant
infantile type (M9071/3)
liver 155.0
polyembryonal type (M9072/3)
endometrioid (M8380/3)
eosinophil (M8280/3)
specified site—*see* Neoplasm, by site,
malignant
unspecified site 194.3
epidermoid (M8070/3)—*see also* Carcinoma,
squamous cell
and adenocarcinoma, mixed (M8560/3)
in situ, Bowen's type (M8081/2)—*see*
Neoplasm, skin, in situ
intradermal—*see* Neoplasm, skin, in situ

Carcinoma—*continued*
fibroepithelial type basal cell (M8093/3)—*see*
　　Neoplasm, skin, malignant
follicular (M8330/3)
　and papillary (mixed) (M8340/3) 193
　moderately differentiated type (M8332/3) 193
　pure follicle type (M8331/3) 193
　specified site—*see* Neoplasm, by site,
　　malignant
　trabecular type (M8332/3) 193
　unspecified site 193
　well differentiated type (M8331/3) 193
gelatinous (M8480/3)
giant cell (M8031/3)
　and spindle cell (M8030/3)
granular cell (M8320/3)
granulosa cell (M8620/3) 183.0
hepatic cell (M8170/3) 155.0
hepatocellular (M8170/3) 155.0
　and bile duct, mixed (M8180/3)
　　155.0
hepatocholangiolitic (M8180/3) 155.0
Hurthle cell (thyroid) 193
hypernephroid (M8311/3)
in
　adenomatous
　　polyp (M8210/3)
　　polyposis coli (M8220/3) 153.9
　pleomorphic adenoma (M8940/3)
　polypoid adenoma (M8210/3)
　situ (M8010/3)—*see* Carcinoma,
　　in situ
　tubular adenoma (M8210/3)
　villous adenoma (M8261/3)
infiltrating duct (M8500/3)
　with Paget's disease (M8541/3)—*see*
　　Neoplasm, breast, malignant
　specified site—*see* Neoplasm, by site,
　　malignant
　unspecified site 174.9
inflammatory (M8530/3)
　specified site—*see* Neoplasm, by site,
　　malignant
　unspecified site 174.9
in situ (M8010/2)—*see also* Neoplasm, by site,
　in situ
　epidermoid (M8070/2)—*see also* Neoplasm,
　　by site, in situ
　　with questionable stromal invasion
　　　(M8076/2)
　　specified site—*see* Neoplasm, by site, in
　　　situ
　　unspecified site 233.1
　　Bowen's type (M8081/2)—*see* Neoplasm,
　　　skin, in situ
　intraductal (M8500/2)
　　specified site—*see* Neoplasm, by site, in situ
　　unspecified site 233.0
　lobular (M8520/2)
　　specified site—*see* Neoplasm, by site, in situ
　　unspecified site 233.0
　papillary (M8050/2)—*see* Neoplasm, by site,
　　in situ
　squamous cell (M8070/2)—*see also*
　　Neoplasm, by site, in situ
　　with questionable stromal invasion
　　　(M8076/2)
　specified site—*see* Neoplasm, by site, in situ
　　unspecified site 233.1
　transitional cell (M8120/2)—*see* Neoplasm,
　　by site, in situ

Carcinoma—*continued*
intestinal type (M8144/3)
　specified site—*see* Neoplasm, by site,
　　malignant
　unspecified site 151.9
intraductal (noninfiltrating) (M8500/2)
　papillary (M8503/2)
　　specified site—*see* Neoplasm, by site, in situ
　　unspecified site 233.0
　specified site—*see* Neoplasm, by site, in situ
　unspecified site 233.0
intraepidermal (M8070/2)—*see also* Neoplasm,
　skin, in situ
　squamous cell, Bowen's type (M8081/2)—*see*
　　Neoplasm, skin, in situ
intraepithelial (M8010/2)—*see also* Neoplasm,
　by site, in situ
　squamous cell (M8072/2)—*see* Neoplasm, by
　　site, in situ
intraosseous (M9270/3) 170.1
　upper jaw (bone) 170.0
islet cell (M8150/3)
　and exocrine, mixed (M8154/3)
　　specified site—*see* Neoplasm, by site,
　　　malignant
　　unspecified site 157.9
　pancreas 157.4
　specified site NEC—*see* Neoplasm, by site,
　　malignant
　unspecified site 157.4
juvenile, breast (M8502/3)—*see* Neoplasm,
　breast, malignant
Kulchitsky's cell (carcinoid tumor of intestine)
　259.2
large cell (M8012/3)
　squamous cell, nonkeratinizing type
　　(M8072/3)
Leydig cell (testis) (M8650/3)
　specified site—*see* Neoplasm, by site,
　　malignant
　unspecified site 186.9
　　female 183.0
　　male 186.9
liver cell (M8170/3) 155.0
lobular (infiltrating) (M8520/3)
　non-infiltrating (M8520/3)
　　specified site—*see* Neoplasm, by site, in situ
　　unspecified site 233.0
　specified site—*see* Neoplasm, by site,
　　malignant
　unspecified site 174.9
lymphoepithelial (M8082/3)
medullary (M8510/3)
　with
　　amyloid stroma (M8511/3)
　　　specified site—*see* Neoplasm, by site,
　　　　malignant
　　　unspecified site 193
　　lymphoid stroma (M8512/3)
　　　specified site—*see* Neoplasm, by site,
　　　　malignant
　　　unspecified site 174.9

Carcinoma—*continued*
  Merkel cell 209.36
    buttock 209.36
    ear 209.31
    eyelid, including canthus 209.31
    face 209.31
    genitals 209.36
    lip 209.31
    lower limb 209.34
    neck 209.32
    nodal presentation 209.75
    scalp 209.32
    secondary (any site) 209.75
    specified site NEC 209.36
    trunk 209.35
    unknown primary site 209.75
    upper limb 209.33
    visceral metastatic presentation 209.75
  mesometanephric (M9110/3)
  mesonephric (M9110/3)
  metastatic (M8010/6)—*see* Metastasis, cancer
  metatypical (M8095/3)—*see* Neoplasm, skin,
    malignant
  morphea type basal cell (M8092/3)—*see*
    Neoplasm, skin, malignant
  mucinous (M8480/3)
  mucin-producing (M8481/3)
  mucin-secreting (M8481/3)
  mucoepidermoid (M8430/3)
  mucoid (M8480/3)
    cell (M8300/3)
      specified site—*see* Neoplasm, by site,
        malignant
      unspecified site 194.3
  mucous (M8480/3)
  neuroendocrine
    high grade (M8240/3) 209.30
    malignant poorly differentiated (M8240/3)
      209.30
  nonencapsulated sclerosing (M8350/3) 193
  noninfiltrating
    intracystic (M8504/2)—*see* Neoplasm, by site,
      in situ
    intraductal (M8500/2)
      papillary (M8503/2)
        specified site—*see* Neoplasm, by site, in
          situ
        unspecified site 233.0
      specified site—*see* Neoplasm, by site, in situ
      unspecified site 233.0
    lobular (M8520/2)
      specified site—*see* Neoplasm, by site, in situ
      unspecified site 233.0
  oat cell (M8042/3)
    specified site—*see* Neoplasm, by site,
      malignant
    unspecified site 162.9
  odontogenic (M9270/3) 170.1
    upper jaw (bone) 170.0
  onocytic (M8290/3)
  oxyphilic (M8290/3)
  papillary (M8050/3)
    and follicular (mixed) (M8340/3) 193
    epidermoid (M8052/3)
    intraductal (noninfiltrating) (M8503/2)
      specified site—*see* Neoplasm, by site, in situ
      unspecified site 233.0

Carcinoma—*continued*
  papillary—*continued*
    serous (M8460/3)
      specified site—*see* Neoplasm, by site,
        malignant
      surface (M8461/3)
        specified site—*see* Neoplasm, by site,
          malignant
        unspecified site 183.0
      unspecified site 183.0
    squamous cell (M8052/3)
    transitional cell (M8130/3)
  papillocystic (M8450/3)
    specified site—*see* Neoplasm, by site,
      malignant
    unspecified site 183.0
  parafollicular cell (M8510/3)
    specified site—*see* Neoplasm, by site,
      malignant
    unspecified site 193
  pleomorphic (M8022/3)
  polygonal cell (M8034/3)
  prickle cell (M8070/3)
  pseudoglandular, squamous cell (M8075/3)
  pseudomucinous (M8470/3)
    specified site—*see* Neoplasm, by site,
      malignant
    unspecified site 183.0
  pseudosarcomatous (M8033/3)
  regaud type (M8082/3)—*see* Neoplasm,
    nasopharynx, malignant
  renal cell (M8312/3) 189.0
  reserve cell (M8041/3)
  round cell (M8041/3)
  Schmincke (M8082/3)—*see* Neoplasm,
    nasopharynx, malignant
  Schneiderian (M8121/3)
    specified site—*see* Neoplasm, by site,
      malignant
    unspecified site 160.0
  scirrhous (M8141/3)
  sebaceous (M8410/3)—*see* Neoplasm, skin,
    malignant
  secondary (M8010/6)—*see* Neoplasm, by site,
    malignant, secondary
  secretory, breast (M8502/3)—*see* Neoplasm,
    breast, malignant
  serous (M8441/3)
    papillary (M8460/3)
      specified site—*see* Neoplasm, by site,
        malignant
      unspecified site 183.0
    surface, papillary (M8461/3)
      specified site—*see* Neoplasm, by site,
        malignant
      unspecified site 183.0
  Sertoli cell (M8640/3)
    specified site—*see* Neoplasm, by site,
      malignant
    unspecified site 186.9
  signet ring cell (M8490/3)
    metastatic (M8490/6)—*see* Neoplasm, by site,
      secondary
  simplex (M8231/3)
  skin appendage (M8390/3)—*see* Neoplasm,
    skin, malignant
  small cell (M8041/3)
    fusiform cell type (M8043/3)
    squamous cell, non-keratinizing type
      (M8073/3)

Carcinoma—*continued*
  solid (M8230/3)
    with amyloid stroma (M8511/3)
      specified site—*see* Neoplasm, by site,
        malignant
      unspecified site 193
  spheroidal cell (M8035/3)
  spindle cell (M8032/3)
    and giant cell (M8030/3)
  spinous cell (M8070/3)
  squamous (cell) (M8070/3)
    adenoid type (M8075/3)
    and adenocarcinoma, mixed (M8560/3)
    intraepidermal, Bowen's type—*see* Neoplasm,
      skin, in situ
    keratinizing type (large cell) (M8071/3)
    large cell, non-keratinizing type (M8072/3)
    microinvasive (M8076/3)
      specified site—*see* Neoplasm, by site,
        malignant
      unspecified site 180.9
    non-keratinizing type (M8072/3)
    papillary (M8052/3)
    pseudoglandular (M8075/3)
    small cell, non-keratinizing type (M8073/3)
    spindle cell type (M8074/3)
    verrucous (M8051/3)
  superficial spreading (M8143/3)
  sweat gland (M8400/3)—*see* Neoplasm, skin,
    malignant
  theca cell (M8600/3) 183.0
  thymic (M8580/3) 164.0
  trabecular (M8190/3)
  transitional (cell) (M8120/3)
    papillary (M8130/3)
    spindle cell type (M8122/3)
  tubular (M8211/3)
  undifferentiated type (M8020/3)
  urothelial (M8120/3)
  ventriculi 151.9
  verrucous (epidermoid) (squamous cell)
    (M8051/3)
  villous (M8262/3)
  water-clear cell (M8322/3) 194.1
  wolffian duct (M9110/3)
Carcinomaphobia 300.29
Carcinomatosis
  peritonei (M8010/6) 197.6
  specified site NEC (M8010/3)—*see* Neoplasm,
    by site, malignant
  unspecified site (M8010/6) 199.0
Carcinosarcoma (M8980/3)—*see also*
  Neoplasm, by site, malignant
  embryonal type (M8981/3)—*see* Neoplasm, by
    site, malignant
Cardia, cardial —*see* condition
Cardiac —*see also* condition
  death—*see* Disease, heart
  device
    defibrillator, automatic implantable V45.02
    in situ NEC V45.00
    pacemaker
      cardiac
        fitting or adjustment V53.3
        in situ V45.01
      carotid sinus
        fitting or adjustment V53.3
        in situ V45.09
    pacemaker—*see* Cardiac, device, pacemaker
    tamponade 423.3
Cardialgia (*see also* Pain, precordial) 786.51
Cardiectasis —*see* Hypertrophy, cardiac

Cardiochalasia 530.81
Cardiomalacia (*see also* Degeneration,
  myocardial) 429.1
Cardiomegalia glycogenica diffusa 271.0
Cardiomegaly (*see also* Hypertrophy, cardiac)
  429.3
  congenital 746.89
  glycogen 271.0
  hypertensive (*see also* Hypertension, heart)
    402.90
  idiopathic 429.3
Cardiomyoliposis (*see also* Degeneration,
  myocardial) 429.1
Cardiomyopathy (congestive) (constrictive)
  (familial) (infiltrative) (obstructive)
  (restrictive) (sporadic) 425.4
  alcoholic 425.5
  amyloid 277.39 *[425.7]*
  beriberi 265.0 *[425.7]*
  cobalt-beer 425.5
  congenital 425.3
  due to
    amyloidosis 277.39 *[425.7]*
    beriberi 265.0 *[425.7]*
    cardiac glycogenesis 271.0 *[425.7]*
    Chagas' disease 086.0
    Friedreich's ataxia 334.0 *[425.8]*
    mucopolysaccharidosis 277.5 *[425.7]*
    myotonia atrophica 359.21 *[425.8]*
    progressive muscular dystrophy 359.1 *[425.8]*
    sarcoidosis 135 *[425.8]*
  glycogen storage 271.0 *[425.7]*
  hypertensive—*see* Hypertension, with, heart
    involvement
  hypertrophic
    nonobstructive 425.4
    obstructive 425.1
      congenital 746.84
  idiopathic (concentric) 425.4
  in
    Chagas' disease 086.0
    sarcoidosis 135 *[425.8]*
  ischemic 414.8
  metabolic NEC 277.9 *[425.7]*
    amyloid 277.39 *[425.7]*
    thyrotoxic (*see also* Thyrotoxicosis) 242.9
      [425.7]
    thyrotoxicosis (*see also* Thyrotoxicosis) 242.9
      [425.7]
  newborn 425.4
    congenital 425.3
  nutritional 269.9 *[425.7]*
    beriberi 265.0 *[425.7]*
  obscure of Africa 425.2
  peripartum 674.5
  postpartum 674.5
  primary 425.4
  secondary 425.9
  stress induced 429.83
  takotsubo 429.83
  thyrotoxic (*see also* Thyrotoxicosis) 242.9 *[425.7]*
  toxic NEC 425.9
  tuberculous (*see also* Tuberculosis) 017.9 *[425.8]*
Cardionephritis —*see* Hypertension, cardiorenal
Cardionephropathy —*see* Hypertension,
  cardiorenal
Cardionephrosis —*see* Hypertension,
  cardiorenal
Cardioneurosis 306.2
Cardiopathia nigra 416.0

Cardiopathy (*see also* Disease, heart) 429.9
  hypertensive (*see also* Hypertension, heart) 402.90
  idiopathic 425.4
  mucopolysaccharidosis 277.5 *[425.7]*
Cardiopericarditis (*see also* Pericarditis) 423.9
Cardiophobia 300.29
Cardioptosis 746.87
Cardiorenal —*see* condition
Cardiorrhexis (*see also* Infarct, myocardium) 410.9
Cardiosclerosis —*see* Arteriosclerosis, coronary
Cardiosis —*see* Disease, heart
Cardiospasm (esophagus) (reflex) (stomach) 530.0
  congenital 750.7
Cardiostenosis —*see* Disease, heart
Cardiosymphysis 423.1
Cardiothyrotoxicosis —*see* Hyperthyroidism
Cardiovascular —*see* condition
Carditis (acute) (bacterial) (chronic) (subacute) 429.89
  Coxsackie 074.20
  hypertensive (*see also* Hypertension, heart) 402.90
  meningococcal 036.40
  rheumatic—*see* Disease, heart, rheumatic
  rheumatoid 714.2
Care (of)
  child (routine) V20.1
  convalescent following V66.9
    chemotherapy V66.2
    medical NEC V66.5
    psychotherapy V66.3
    radiotherapy V66.1
    surgery V66.0
    surgical NEC V66.0
    treatment (for) V66.5
      combined V66.6
      fracture V66.4
      mental disorder NEC V66.3
      specified type NEC V66.5
  end-of-life care V66.7
  family member (handicapped) (sick)
    creating problem for family V61.49
    provided away from home for holiday relief V60.5
    unavailable, due to
      absence (person rendering care) (sufferer) V60.4
      inability (any reason) of person rendering care V60.4
  holiday relief V60.5
  hospice V66.7
  lack of (at or after birth) (infant) (child) 995.52
    adult 995.84
  lactation of mother V24.1
  palliative V66.7
  postpartum
    immediately after delivery V24.0
    routine follow-up V24.2
  prenatal V22.1
    first pregnancy V22.0
    high risk pregnancy V23.9
      specified problem NEC V23.8
  terminal V66.7
  unavailable, due to
    absence of person rendering care V60.4
    inability (any reason) of person rendering care V60.4
  well baby V20.1

Caries (bone) (*see also* Tuberculosis, bone) 015.9 *[730.8]*
  arrested 521.04
  cementum 521.03
  cerebrospinal (tuberculous) 015.0 *[730.88]*
  dental (acute) (chronic) (incipient) (infected) 521.00
    with pulp exposure 521.03
    extending to
      dentine 521.02
      pulp 521.03
    other specified NEC 521.09
    pit and fissure 521.06
    primary
      pit and fissure origin 521.06
      root surface 521.08
      smooth surface origin 521.07
    root surface 521.08
    smooth surface 521.07
  dentin (acute) (chronic) 521.02
  enamel (acute) (chronic) (incipient) 521.01
  external meatus 380.89
  hip (*see also* Tuberculosis) 015.1 *[730.85]*
  initial 521.01
  knee 015.2 *[730.86]*
  labyrinth 386.8
  limb NEC 015.7 *[730.88]*
  mastoid (chronic) (process) 383.1
  middle ear 385.89
  nose 015.7 *[730.88]*
  orbit 015.7 *[730.88]*
  ossicle 385.24
  petrous bone 383.20
  sacrum (tuberculous) 015.0 *[730.88]*
  spine, spinal (column) (tuberculous) 015.0 *[730.88]*
  syphilitic 095.5
    congenital 090.0 *[730.8]*
  teeth (internal) 521.00
    initial 521.01
  vertebra (column) (tuberculous) 015.0 *[730.88]*
Carini's syndrome (ichthyosis congenita) 757.1
Carious teeth 521.00
Carneous mole 631
Carnosinemia 270.5
Carotid body or sinus syndrome 337.01
Carotidynia 337.01
Carotinemia (dietary) 278.3
Carotinosis (cutis) (skin) 278.3
Carpal tunnel syndrome 354.0
Carpenter's syndrome 759.89
Carpopedal spasm (*see also* Tetany) 781.7
Carpoptosis 736.05
Carrier (suspected) of
  amebiasis V02.2
  bacterial disease (meningococcal, staphylococcal, streptococcal) NEC V02.59
  cholera V02.0
  cystic fibrosis gene V83.81
  defective gene V83.89
  diphtheria V02.4
  dysentery (bacillary) V02.3
    amebic V02.2
  Endamoeba histolytica V02.2
  gastrointestinal pathogens NEC V02.3
  genetic defect V83.89
  gonorrhea V02.7
  group B streptococcus V02.51
  HAA (hepatitis Australian-antigen) V02.61
  hemophilia A (asymptomatic) V83.01
    symptomatic V83.02

Carrier—*continued*
  hepatitis V02.60
    Australian-antigen (HAA) V02.61
    B V02.61
    C V02.62
    serum V02.61
    specified type NEC V02.69
    viral V02.60
  infective organism NEC V02.9
  malaria V02.9
  paratyphoid V02.3
  Salmonella V02.3
    typhosa V02.1
  serum hepatitis V02.61
  Shigella V02.3
  Staphylococcus NEC V02.59
    methicillin
      resistant Staphylococcus aureus V02.54
      susceptible Staphylococcus aureus V02.53
  Streptococcus NEC V02.52
    group B V02.51
  typhoid V02.1
  venereal disease NEC V02.8
Carrión's disease (Bartonellosis) 088.0
Car sickness 994.6
Carter's
  relapsing fever (Asiatic) 087.0
Cartilage —*see* condition
Caruncle (inflamed)
  abscess, lacrimal (*see also* Dacryocystitis) 375.30
  conjunctiva 372.00
    acute 372.00
  eyelid 373.00
  labium (majus) (minus) 616.89
  lacrimal 375.30
  urethra (benign) 599.3
  vagina (wall) 616.89
Cascade stomach 537.6
Caseation lymphatic gland (*see also*
  Tuberculosis) 017.2
Caseous
  bronchitis—*see* Tuberculosis, pulmonary
  meningitis 013.0
  pneumonia—*see* Tuberculosis, pulmonary
Cassidy (-Scholte) syndrome (malignant
  carcinoid) 259.2
Castellani's bronchitis 104.8
Castleman's tumor or lymphoma (mediastinal
  lymph node hyperplasia) 785.6
Castration, traumatic 878.2
  complicated 878.3
Casts in urine 791.7
Cat's ear 744.29
Catalepsy 300.11
  catatonic (acute) (*see also* Schizophrenia) 295.2
  hysterical 300.11
  schizophrenic (*see also* Schizophrenia) 295.2
Cataphasia 307.0
Cataplexy (idiopathic) *see also* Narcolepsy
Cataract (anterior cortical) (anterior polar)
  (black) (capsular) (central) (cortical)
  (hypermature) (immature) (incipient) (mature)
  366.9
  anterior
    and posterior axial embryonal 743.33
    pyramidal 743.31
    subcapsular polar
      infantile, juvenile, or presenile 366.01
      senile 366.13

Cataract—*continued*
  associated with
    calcinosis 275.40 *[366.42]*
    craniofacial dysostosis 756.0 *[366.44]*
    galactosemia 271.1 *[366.44]*
    hypoparathyroidism 252.1 *[366.42]*
    myotonic disorders 359.21 *[366.43]*
    neovascularization 366.33
  blue dot 743.39
  cerulean 743.39
  complicated NEC 366.30
  congenital 743.30
    capsular or subcapsular 743.31
    cortical 743.32
    nuclear 743.33
    specified type NEC 743.39
    total or subtotal 743.34
    zonular 743.32
  coronary (congenital) 743.39
    acquired 366.12
  cupuliform 366.14
  diabetic 250.5 *[366.41]*
    due to secondary diabetes 249.5 *[366.41]*
  drug-induced 366.45
  due to
    chalcosis 360.24 *[366.34]*
    chronic choroiditis (*see also* Choroiditis)
      363.20 *[366.32]*
    degenerative myopia 360.21 *[366.34]*
    glaucoma (*see also* Glaucoma) 365.9 *[366.31]*
    infection, intraocular NEC 366.32
    inflammatory ocular disorder NEC 366.32
    iridocyclitis, chronic 364.10 *[366.33]*
    pigmentary retinal dystrophy 362.74 *[366.34]*
    radiation 366.46
  electric 366.46
  glassblowers' 366.46
  heat ray 366.46
  heterochromic 366.33
  in eye disease NEC 366.30
  infantile (*see also* Cataract, juvenile) 366.00
  intumescent 366.12
  irradiational 366.46
  juvenile 366.00
    anterior subcapsular polar 366.01
    combined forms 366.09
    cortical 366.03
    lamellar 366.03
    nuclear 366.04
    posterior subcapsular polar 366.02
    specified NEC 366.09
    zonular 366.03
  lamellar 743.32
    infantile, juvenile, or presenile 366.03
  morgagnian 366.18
  myotonic 359.21 *[366.43]*
  myxedema 244.9 *[366.44]*
  nuclear 366.16
  posterior, polar (capsular) 743.31
    infantile, juvenile, or presenile 366.02
    senile 366.14
  presenile (*see also* Cataract, juvenile) 366.00
  punctate
    acquired 366.12
    congenital 743.39
  secondary (membrane) 366.50
    obscuring vision 366.53
    specified type, not obscuring vision 366.52

Cataract—*continued*
  senile 366.10
    anterior subcapsular polar 366.13
    combined forms 366.19
    cortical 366.15
    hypermature 366.18
    immature 366.12
    incipient 366.12
    mature 366.17
    nuclear 366.16
    posterior subcapsular polar 366.14
    specified NEC 366.19
    total or subtotal 366.17
  snowflake 250.5 *[366.41]*
    due to secondary diabetes 249.5 *[366.41]*
  specified NEC 366.8
  subtotal (senile) 366.17
    congenital 743.34
  sunflower 360.24 *[366.34]*
  tetanic NEC 252.1 *[366.42]*
  total (mature) (senile) 366.17
    congenital 743.34
    localized 366.21
    traumatic 366.22
  toxic 366.45
  traumatic 366.20
    partially resolved 366.23
    total 366.22
  zonular (perinuclear) 743.32
    infantile, juvenile, or presenile 366.03
Cataracta 366.10
  brunescens 366.16
  cerulea 743.39
  complicata 366.30
  congenita 743.30
  coralliformis 743.39
  coronaria (congenital) 743.39
    acquired 366.12
  diabetic 250.5 *[366.41]*
    due to secondary diabetes 249.5 *[366.41]*
  floriformis 360.24 *[366.34]*
  membranacea
    accreta 366.50
    congenita 743.39
  nigra 366.16
Catarrh, catarrhal (inflammation) (*see also*
    condition) 460
  acute 460
  asthma, asthmatic (*see also* Asthma) 493.9
  Bostock's (*see also* Fever, hay) 477.9
  bowel—*see* Enteritis
  bronchial 490
    acute 466.0
    chronic 491.0
    subacute 466.0
  cervix, cervical (canal) (uteri)—*see* Cervicitis
  chest (*see also* Bronchitis) 490
  chronic 472.0
  congestion 472.0
  conjunctivitis 372.03
  due to syphilis 095.9
    congenital 090.0
  enteric—*see* Enteritis
  epidemic 487.1
  Eustachian 381.50
  eye (acute) (vernal) 372.03
  fauces (*see also* Pharyngitis) 462
  febrile 460
  fibrinous acute 466.0
  gastroenteric—*see* Enteritis
  gastrointestinal—*see* Enteritis

Catarrh, catarrhal—*continued*
  gingivitis 523.00
  hay (*see also* Fever, hay) 477.9
  infectious 460
  intestinal—*see* Enteritis
  larynx (*see also* Laryngitis, chronic) 476.0
  liver 070.1
    with hepatic coma 070.0
  lung (*see also* Bronchitis) 490
    acute 466.0
    chronic 491.0
  middle ear (chronic)—*see* Otitis media, chronic
  mouth 528.00
  nasal (chronic) (*see also* Rhinitis) 472.0
    acute 460
  nasobronchial 472.2
  nasopharyngeal (chronic) 472.2
    acute 460
  nose—*see* Catarrh, nasal
  ophthalmia 372.03
  pneumococcal, acute 466.0
  pulmonary (*see also* Bronchitis) 490
    acute 466.0
    chronic 491.0
  spring (eye) 372.13
  suffocating (*see also* Asthma) 493.9
  summer (hay) (*see also* Fever, hay) 477.9
  throat 472.1
  tracheitis 464.10
    with obstruction 464.11
  tubotympanal 381.4
    acute (*see also* Otitis media, acute,
      nonsuppurative) 381.00
    chronic 381.10
  vasomotor (*see also* Fever, hay) 477.9
  vesical (bladder)—*see* Cystitis
Catarrhus aestivus (*see also* Fever, hay) 477.9
Catastrophe, cerebral (*see also* Disease,
    cerebrovascular, acute) 436
Catatonia, catatonic (acute) 781.99
  agitation 295.2
  dementia (praecox) 295.2
  due to or associated with physical condition 293.89
  excitation 295.2
  excited type 295.2
  in conditions classified elsewhere 293.89
  schizophrenia 295.2
  stupor 295.2
  with
    affective psychosis —*see* Psychosis, affective
Cat-scratch —*see also* Injury, superficial
  disease or fever 078.3
Cauda equina —*see also* condition syndrome
    344.60
Cauliflower ear 738.7
Caul over face 768.9
Causalgia 355.9
  lower limb 355.71
  upper limb 354.4
Cause
  external, general effects NEC 994.9
  not stated 799.9
  unknown 799.9
Caustic burn —*see also* Burn, by site
  from swallowing caustic or corrosive
    substance—*see* Burn, internal organs
Cavare's disease (familial periodic paralysis) 359.3
Cave-in, injury
  crushing (severe) (*see also* Crush, by site) 869.1
  suffocation 994.7
Cavernitis (penis) 607.2
  lymph vessel—*see* Lymphangioma

Cavernositis 607.2
Cavernous —*see* condition
Cavitation of lung (*see also* Tuberculosis) 011.2
  nontuberculous 518.89
  primary, progressive 010.8
Cavity
  lung—*see* Cavitation of lung
  optic papilla 743.57
  pulmonary—*see* Cavitation of lung
  teeth 521.00
  vitreous (humor) 379.21
Cavovarus foot, congenital 754.59
Cavus foot (congenital) 754.71
  acquired 736.73
Cazenave's
  disease (pemphigus) NEC 694.4
  lupus (erythematosus) 695.4
CDGS (carbohydrate-deficient glycoprotein syndrome) 271.8
Cecitis —*see* Appendicitis
Cecocele —*see* Hernia
Cecum —*see* condition
Celiac
  artery compression syndrome 447.4
  disease 579.0
  infantilism 579.0
Cell, cellular —*see also* condition
  anterior chamber (eye) (positive aqueous ray) 364.04
Cellulitis (diffuse) (with lymphangitis) (*see also* Abscess) 682.9
  abdominal wall 682.2
  anaerobic (*see also* Gas gangrene) 040.0
  ankle 682.6
  anus 566
  areola 611.0
  arm (any part, above wrist) 682.3
  auditory canal (external) 380.10
  axilla 682.3
  back (any part) 682.2
  breast 611.0
    postpartum 675.1
  broad ligament (*see also* Disease, pelvis, inflammatory) 614.4
    acute 614.3
  buttock 682.5
  cervical (neck region) 682.1
  cervix (uteri) (*see also* Cervicitis) 616.0
  cheek, external 682.0
    internal 528.3
  chest wall 682.2
  chronic NEC 682.9
  colostomy 569.61
  corpus cavernosum 607.2
  digit 681.9
  Douglas' cul-de-sac or pouch (chronic) (*see also* Disease, pelvis, inflammatory) 614.4
    acute 614.3
  drainage site (following operation) 998.59
  ear, external 380.10
  enterostomy 569.61
  erysipelar (*see also* Erysipelas) 035
  esophagostomy 530.86
  eyelid 373.13
  face (any part, except eye) 682.0
  finger (intrathecal) (periosteal) (subcutaneous) (subcuticular) 681.00
  flank 682.2
  foot (except toe) 682.7
  forearm 682.3
  gangrenous (*see also* Gangrene) 785.4

Cellulitis—*continued*
  genital organ NEC
    female—*see* Abscess, genital organ, female
    male 608.4
  glottis 478.71
  gluteal (region) 682.5
  gonococcal NEC 098.0
  groin 682.2
  hand (except finger or thumb) 682.4
  head (except face) NEC 682.8
  heel 682.7
  hip 682.6
  jaw (region) 682.0
  knee 682.6
  labium (majus) (minus) (*see also* Vulvitis) 616.10
  larynx 478.71
  leg, except foot 682.6
  lip 528.5
  mammary gland 611.0
  mouth (floor) 528.3
  multiple sites NEC 682.9
  nasopharynx 478.21
  navel 682.2
    newborn NEC 771.4
  neck (region) 682.1
  nipple 611.0
  nose 478.19
    external 682.0
  orbit, orbital 376.01
  palate (soft) 528.3
  pectoral (region) 682.2
  pelvis, pelvic
    with
      abortion—*see* Abortion, by type, with sepsis
      ectopic pregnancy (*see also* categories 633.0-633.9) 639.0
      molar pregnancy (*see also* categories 630-632) 639.0
    female (*see also* Disease, pelvis, inflammatory) 614.4
      acute 614.3
    following
      abortion 639.0
      ectopic or molar pregnancy 639.0
    male 567.21
    puerperal, postpartum, childbirth 670.8
  penis 607.2
  perineal, perineum 682.2
  perirectal 566
  peritonsillar 475
  periurethral 597.0
  periuterine (*see also* Disease, pelvis, inflammatory) 614.4
    acute 614.3
  pharynx 478.21
  phlegmonous NEC 682.9
  rectum 566
  retromammary 611.0
  retroperitoneal (*see also* Peritonitis) 567.238
  round ligament (*see also* Disease, pelvis, inflammatory) 614.4
    acute 614.3
  scalp (any part) 682.8
    dissecting 704.8
  scrotum 608.4
  seminal vesicle 608.0
  septic NEC 682.9
  shoulder 682.3
  specified sites NEC 682.8
  spermatic cord 608.4

Cellulitis—*continued*
submandibular (region) (space) (triangle) 682.0
gland 527.3
submaxillary 528.3
gland 527.3
submental (pyogenic) 682.0
gland 527.3
suppurative NEC 682.9
testis 608.4
thigh 682.6
thumb (intrathecal) (periosteal) (subcutaneous)
(subcuticular) 681.00
toe (intrathecal) (periosteal) (subcutaneous)
(subcuticular) 681.10
tonsil 475
trunk 682.2
tuberculous (primary) (*see also* Tuberculosis)
017.0
tunica vaginalis 608.4
umbilical 682.2
newborn NEC 771.4
vaccinal 999.39
vagina—*see* Vaginitis
vas deferens 608.4
vocal cords 478.5
vulva (*see also* Vulvitis) 616.10
wrist 682.4
Cementoblastoma, benign (M9273/0) 213.1
upper jaw (bone) 213.0
Cementoma (M9273/0) 213.1
gigantiform (M9276/0) 213.1
upper jaw (bone) 213.0
upper jaw (bone) 213.0
Cementoperiostitis 523.40
acute 523.33
apical 523.40
Cephalgia, cephalalgia (*see also* Headache) 784.0
histamine 339.00
nonorganic origin 307.81
other trigeminal autonomic (TACS) 339.09
psychogenic 307.81
tension 307.81
Cephalhematocele, cephalematocele
due to birth injury 767.19
fetus or newborn 767.19
traumatic (*see also* Contusion, head) 920
Cephalhematoma, cephalematoma (calcified)
due to birth injury 767.19
fetus or newborn 767.19
traumatic (*see also* Contusion, head) 920
Cephalic —*see* condition
Cephalitis —*see* Encephalitis
Cephalocele 742.0
Cephaloma —*see* Neoplasm, by site,
malignant
Cephalomenia 625.8
Cephalopelvic —*see* condition
Cercomoniasis 007.3
Cerebellitis —*see* Encephalitis
Cerebellum (cerebellar)—*see* condition
Cerebral —*see* condition
Cerebritis —*see* Encephalitis
Cerebrohepatorenal syndrome 759.89
Cerebromacular degeneration 330.1
Cerebromalacia (*see also* Softening, brain) 434.9
Cerebrosidosis 272.7
Cerebrospasticity —*see* Palsy, cerebral
Cerebrospinal —*see* condition
Cerebrum —*see* condition
Ceroid storage disease 272.7
Cerumen (accumulation) (impacted) 380.4

Cervical —*see also* condition
auricle 744.43
high risk human papillomavirus (HPV) DNA
test positive 795.05
intraepithelial glandular neoplasia 233.1
low rish human papillomavirus (Hpv) DNA test
positive 795.09
rib 756.2
shortening —*see* Short, cervical
Cervicalgia 723.1
Cervicitis (acute) (chronic) (nonvenereal)
(subacute) (with erosion or ectropion) 616.0
with
abortion—*see* Abortion, by type, with sepsis
ectopic pregnancy (*see also* categories
633.0-633.9) 639.0
molar pregnancy (*see also* categories 630-632)
639.0
ulceration 616.0
chlamydial 099.53
complicating pregnancy or puerperium 646.6
affecting fetus or newborn 760.8
following
abortion 639.0
ectopic or molar pregnancy 639.0
gonococcal (acute) 098.15
chronic or duration of 2 months or more 098.35
senile (atrophic) 616.0
syphilitic 095.8
trichomonal 131.09
tuberculous (*see also* Tuberculosis) 016.7
Cervicoaural fistula 744.49
Cervicocolpitis (emphysematosa) (*see also*
Cervicitis) 616.0
Cervix —*see* condition
Cesarean delivery, operation or section NEC
669.7
affecting fetus or newborn 763.4
post mortem, affecting fetus or newborn 761.6
previous, affecting management of pregnancy
654.2
Céstan's syndrome 344.89
Céstan-Chenais paralysis 344.89
Céstan-Raymond syndrome 433.8
Cestode infestation NEC 123.9
specified type NEC 123.8
Cestodiasis 123.9
CGF (congenital generalized fibromatosis) 759.89
Chaberts' disease 022.9
Chacaleh 266.2
Chafing 709.8
Chagas' disease (*see also* Trypanosomiasis,
American) 086.2
with heart involvement 086.0
Chagres fever 084.0
Chalasia (cardiac sphincter) 530.81
Chalazion 373.2
Chalazoderma 757.39
Chalcosis 360.24
cornea 371.15
crystalline lens 360.24 *[366.34]*
retina 360.24
Chalicosis (occupational) (pulmonum) 502
Chancre (any genital site) (hard) (indurated)
(infecting) (primary) (recurrent) 091.0
congenital 090.0
conjunctiva 091.2
Ducrey's 099.0
extragenital 091.2
eyelid 091.2
Hunterian 091.0

Chancre—*continued*
  lip (syphilis) 091.2
  mixed 099.8
  nipple 091.2
  Nisbet's 099.0
  of
    carate 103.0
    pinta 103.0
    yaws 102.0
  palate, soft 091.2
  phagedenic 099.0
  Ricord's 091.0
  Rollet's (syphilitic) 091.0
  seronegative 091.0
  seropositive 091.0
  simple 099.0
  soft 099.0
    bubo 099.0
  urethra 091.0
  yaws 102.0
Chancriform syndrome 114.1
Chancroid 099.0
  anus 099.0
  penis (Ducrey's bacillus) 099.0
  perineum 099.0
  rectum 099.0
  scrotum 099.0
  urethra 099.0
  vulva 099.0
Chandipura fever 066.8
Chandler's disease (osteochondritis dissecans, hip) 732.7
Change(s) (of)—*see also* Removal of
  arteriosclerotic—*see* Arteriosclerosis
  battery
    cardiac pacemaker V53.31
  bone 733.90
    diabetic 250.8 *[731.8]*
    due to secondary diabetes 249.8 [731.8]
  in disease, unknown cause 733.90
  bowel habits 787.99
  cardiorenal (vascular) (*see also* Hypertension, cardiorenal) 404.90
  cardiovascular—*see* Disease, cardiovascular
  circulatory 459.9
  cognitive or personality change of other type, nonpsychotic 310.1
  color, teeth, tooth
    during formation 520.8
    extrinsic 523.6
    intrinsic posteruptive 521.7
  contraceptive device V25.42
  cornea, corneal
    degenerative NEC 371.40
    membrane NEC 371.30
    senile 371.41
  coronary (*see also* Ischemia, heart) 414.9
  degenerative
    chamber angle (anterior) (iris) 364.56
    ciliary body 364.57
    spine or vertebra (*see also* Spondylosis) 721.90
  dental pulp, regressive 522.2
  drains V58.49
  dressing
    wound V58.30
      nonsurgical V58.30
      surgical V58.31
  fixation device V54.89
    external V54.89
    internal V54.01

Change(s) (of)—*continued*
  heart—*see also* Disease, heart
  hip joint 718.95
  hyperplastic larynx 478.79
  hypertrophic
    nasal sinus (*see also* Sinusitis) 473.9
    turbinate, nasal 478.0
    upper respiratory tract 478.9
  inflammatory—*see* Inflammation
  joint (*see also* Derangement, joint) 718.90
    sacroiliac 724.6
  Kirschner wire V54.89
  knee 717.9
  macular, congenital 743.55
  malignant (M——/3)—*see also* Neoplasm, by site, malignant

Note—for malignant change occurring in a neoplasm, use the appropriate M code with behavior digit /3 e.g., malignant change in uterine fibroid—M8890/3. For malignant change occurring in a nonneoplastic condition (e.g., gastric ulcer) use the M code M8000/3.

  mental (status) NEC 780.97
    due to or associated with physical condition—*see* Syndrome, brain
  myocardium, myocardial—*see* Degeneration, myocardial
  of life (*see also* Menopause) 627.2
  pacemaker battery (cardiac) V53.31
  peripheral nerve 355.9
  personality (nonpsychotic) NEC 310.1
  plaster cast V54.89
  refractive, transient 367.81
  regressive, dental pulp 522.2
  retina 362.9
    myopic (degenerative) (malignant) 360.21
    vascular appearance 362.13
  sacroiliac joint 724.6
  scleral 379.19
    degenerative 379.16
  senile (*see also* Senility) 797
  sensory (*see also* Disturbance, sensation) 782.0
  skin texture 782.8
  spinal cord 336.9
  splint, external V54.89
  subdermal implantable contraceptive V25.5
  suture V58.32
  traction device V54.89
  trophic 355.9
    arm NEC 354.9
    leg NEC 355.8
    lower extremity NEC 355.8
    upper extremity NEC 354.9
  vascular 459.9
  vasomotor 443.9
  voice 784.49
    psychogenic 306.1
  wound packing V58.30
    nonsurgical V58.30
    surgical V58.31
Changing sleep-work schedule, affecting sleep 327.36
Changuinola fever 066.0
Chapping skin 709.8
Character
  depressive 301.12
Charcot's
  arthropathy 094.0 *[713.5]*
  cirrhosis—*see* Cirrhosis, biliary
  disease 094.0
    spinal cord 094.0

Charcot's—*continued*
  fever (biliary) (hepatic) (intermittent)—*see*
    Choledocholithiasis
  joint (disease) 094.0 *[713.5]*
    diabetic 250.6 *[713.5]*
      due to secondary diabetes 249.6 [713.5]
    syringomyelic 336.0 *[713.5]*
  syndrome (intermittent claudication) 443.9
    due to atherosclerosis 440.21
Charcot-Marie-Tooth disease paralysis, or
  syndrome 356.1
CHARGE association (syndrome) 759.89
Charleyhorse (quadriceps) 843.8
  muscle, except quadriceps—*see* Sprain, by site
Charlouis' disease (*see also* Yaws) 102.9
Chauffeur's fracture —*see* Fracture, ulna, lower
  end
Cheadle (-Möller) (-Barlow) disease or syndrome
  (infantile scurvy) 267
Checking (of)
  contraceptive device (intrauterine) V25.42
  device
    fixation V54.89
      external V54.89
      internal V54.09
      traction V54.89
    Kirschner wire V54.89
    plaster cast V54.89
    splint, external V54.89
Checkup
  following treatment—*see* Examination
  health V70.0
  infant (over 28 days old) (not sick) V20.2
  newborn, routine
    8 to 28 days old V20.32
    over 28 days old, routine V20.2
    under 8 days old V20.31
    weight V20.32
  pregnancy (normal) V22.1
    first V22.0
    high risk pregnancy V23.9
      specified problem NEC V23.8
Chédiak-Higashi (-Steinbrinck) anomaly,
  disease, or syndrome (congenital gigantism of
  peroxidase granules) 288.2
Cheek —*see also* condition
  biting 528.9
Cheese itch 133.8
Cheese washers' lung 495.8
Cheilitis 528.5
  actinic (due to sun) 692.72
    chronic NEC 692.74
      due to radiation, except from sun 692.82
    due to radiation, except from sun 692.82
  acute 528.5
  angular 528.5
  catarrhal 528.5
  chronic 528.5
  exfoliative 528.5
  gangrenous 528.5
  glandularis apostematosa 528.5
  granulomatosa 351.8
  infectional 528.5
  membranous 528.5
  Miescher's 351.8
  suppurative 528.5
  ulcerative 528.5
  vesicular 528.5
Cheilodynia 528.5
Cheilopalatoschisis (*see also* Cleft, palate, with
  cleft lip) 749.20
Cheilophagia 528.9

Cheiloschisis (*see also* Cleft, lip) 749.10
Cheilosis 528.5
  with pellagra 265.2
  angular 528.5
  due to
    dietary deficiency 266.0
    vitamin deficiency 266.0
Cheiromegaly 729.89
Cheiropompholyx 705.81
Cheloid (*see also* Keloid) 701.4
Chemical burn —*see also* Burn, by site
  from swallowing chemical—*see* Burn, internal
  organs
Chemodectoma (M8693/1)—*see* Paraganglioma,
  nonchromaffin
Chemoprophylaxis NEC V07.39
Chemosis, conjunctiva 372.73
Chemotherapy
  convalescence V66.2
  encounter (for) (oral) (intravenous) V58.11
  maintenance (oral) (intravenous) V58.11
  prophylactic NEC V07.39
    fluoride V07.31
Cherubism 526.89
Chest —*see* condition
Cheyne-Stokes respiration (periodic) 786.04
Chiari's
  disease or syndrome (hepatic vein thrombosis)
    453.0
  malformation
    type I 348.4
    type II (*see also* Spina bifida) 741.0
    type III 742.0
    type IV 742.2
  network 746.89
Chiari-Frommel syndrome 676.6
Chicago disease (North American blastomycosis)
  116.0
Chickenpox (*see also* Varicella) 052.9
  exposure to V01.71
  vaccination and inoculation (prophylactic) V05.4
Chiclero ulcer 085.4
Chiggers 133.8
Chignon 111.2
  fetus or newborn (from vacuum extraction)
    767.19
Chigoe disease 134.1
Chikungunya fever 066.3
Chilaiditi's syndrome (subphrenic displacement,
  colon) 751.4
Chilblains 991.5
  lupus 991.5
Child
  behavior causing concern V61.20
    adopted child V61.24
    biological child V61.23
    foster child V61.25
Childbed fever 670.8
Childbirth —*see also* Delivery
  puerperal complications—*see* Puerperal
Childhood, period of rapid growth V21.0
Chill (s) 780.64
  with fever 780.60
  without fever 780.64
  congestive 780.99
    in malarial regions 084.6
  septic—*see* Septicemia
  urethral 599.84
Chilomastigiasis 007.8
Chin —*see* condition
Chinese dysentery 004.9

Chiropractic dislocation (*see also* Lesion,
  nonallopathic, by site) 739.9
Chitral fever 066.0
Chlamydia, chlamydial -*see* condition
Chloasma 709.09
  cachecticorum 709.09
  eyelid 374.52
    congenital 757.33
    hyperthyroid 242.0
  gravidarum 646.8
  idiopathic 709.09
  skin 709.09
  symptomatic 709.09
Chloroma (M9930/3) 205.3
Chlorosis 280.9
  Egyptian (*see also* Ancylostomiasis) 126.9
  miners' (*see also* Ancylostomiasis) 126.9
Chlorotic anemia 280.9
Chocolate cyst (ovary) 617.1
Choked
  disk or disc—*see* Papilledema
  on food, phlegm, or vomitus NEC (*see also*
    Asphyxia, food) 933.1
  phlegm 933.1
  while vomiting NEC (*see also* Asphyxia, food)
    933.1
Chokes (resulting from bends) 993.3
Choking sensation 784.99
Cholangiectasis (*see also* Disease, gallbladder)
  575.8
Cholangiocarcinoma (M8160/3)
  and hepatocellular carcinoma, combined
    (M8180/3) 155.0
  liver 155.1
  specified site NEC—*see* Neoplasm, by site,
    malignant
  unspecified site 155.1
Cholangiohepatitis 575.8
  due to fluke infestation 121.1
Cholangiohepatoma (M8180/3) 155.0
Cholangiolitis (acute) (chronic) (extrahepatic)
  (gangrenous) 576.1
  intrahepatic 575.8
  paratyphoidal (*see also* Fever, paratyphoid) 002.9
  typhoidal 002.0
Cholangioma (M8160/0) 211.5
  malignant—*see* Cholangiocarcinoma
Cholangitis (acute) (ascending) (catarrhal)
  (chronic) (infective) (malignant) (primary)
  (recurrent) (sclerosing) (secondary)
  (stenosing) (suppurative) 576.1
  chronic nonsuppurative destructive 571.6
  nonsuppurative destructive (chronic) 571.6
Cholecystdocholithiasis —*see*
  Choledocholithiasis
Cholecystitis 575.10
  with
    calculus, stones in
      bile duct (common) (hepatic)—*see*
        Choledocholithiasis
      gallbladder—*see* Cholelithiasis
  acute and chronic 575.12
  chronic 575.11
  emphysematous (acute) (*see also* Cholecystitis,
    acute) 575.0
  gangrenous (*see also* Cholecystitis, acute) 575.0
  paratyphoidal, current (*see also* Fever,
    paratyphoid) 002.9
  suppurative (*see also* Cholecystitis, acute) 575.0
  typhoidal 002.0

Choledochitis (suppurative) 576.1
Choledocholith —*see* Choledocholithiasis
Choledocholithiasis 574.5

> *Note—Use the following fifth-digit*
> *subclassification with category 574:*
>
> *0 without mention of obstruction*
> *1 with obstruction*

  with
    cholecystitis 574.4
      acute 574.3
      chronic 574.4
    cholelithiasis 574.9
      with
        cholecystitis 574.7
          acute 574.6
            and chronic 574.8
          chronic 574.7
Cholelithiasis (impacted) (multiple) 574.2

> *Note—Use the following fifth-digit*
> *subclassification with category 574:*
>
> *0 without mention of obstruction*
> *1 with obstruction*

  with
    cholecystitis 574.1
      acute 574.0
      chronic 574.1
    choledocholithiasis 574.9
      with
        cholecystitis 574.7
          acute 574.6
            and chronic 574.8
          chronic cholecystitis 574.7
Cholemia (*see also* Jaundice) 782.4
  familial 277.4
  Gilbert's (familial nonhemolytic) 277.4
Cholemic gallstone —*see* Cholelithiasis
Choleperitoneum, choleperitonitis (*see also*
  Disease, gallbladder) 567.81
Cholera (algid) (Asiatic) (asphyctic) (epidemic)
  (gravis) (Indian) (malignant) (morbus)
  (pestilential) (spasmodic) 001.9
  antimonial 985.4
  carrier (suspected) of V02.0
  classical 001.0
  contact V01.0
  due to
    Vibrio
      cholerae (Inaba, Ogawa, Hikojima
        serotypes) 001.0
      El Tor 001.1
  El Tor 001.1
  exposure to V01.0
  vaccination, prophylactic (against) V03.0
Cholerine (*see also* Cholera) 001.9
Cholestasis 576.8
  due to total parenteral nutrition (TPN) 573.8
Cholesteatoma (ear) 385.30
  attic (primary) 385.31
  diffuse 385.35
  external ear (canal) 380.21
  marginal (middle ear) 385.32
    with involvement of mastoid cavity 385.33
    secondary (with middle ear involvement) 385.33
  mastoid cavity 385.30

Cholesteatoma—*continued*
  middle ear (secondary) 385.32
    with involvement of mastoid cavity 385.33—
    postmastoidectomy cavity (recurrent) 383.32
    primary 385.31
    recurrent, postmastoidectomy cavity 383.32
    secondary (middle ear) 385.32
    with involvement of mastoid cavity 385.33
Cholesteatosis (middle ear) (*see also*
  Cholesteatoma) 385.30
  diffuse 385.35
Cholesteremia 272.0
Cholesterin
  granuloma, middle ear 385.82
  in vitreous 379.22
Cholesterol
  deposit
    retina 362.82
    vitreous 379.22
  elevated (high) 272.0
    with elevated (high) triglycerides 272.2
  imbibition of gallbladder (*see also* Disease,
    gallbladder) 575.6
Cholesterolemia 272.0
  essential 272.0
  familial 272.0
  hereditary 272.0
Cholesterosis, cholesterolosis (gallbladder) 575.6
  middle ear (*see also* Cholesteatoma) 385.30
  with
    cholecystitis—*see* Cholecystitis
    cholelithiasis—*see* Cholelithiasis
Cholocolic fistula (*see also* Fistula, gallbladder)
  575.5
Choluria 791.4
Chondritis (purulent) 733.99
  auricle 380.03
  costal 733.6
    Tietze's 733.6
  patella, posttraumatic 717.7
  pinna 380.03
  posttraumatica patellae 717.7
  tuberculous (active) (*see also* Tuberculosis) 015.9
    intervertebral 015.0 *[730.88]*
Chondroangiopathia calcarea seu punctate
  756.59
Chondroblastoma (M9230/0)—*see also*
  Neoplasm, bone, benign
  malignant (M9230/3)—*see* Neoplasm, bone,
    malignant
Chondrocalcinosis (articular) (crystal deposition)
  (dihydrate) (*see also* Arthritis, due to, crystals)
  275.49 *[712.3]*
  due to
    calcium pyrophosphate 275.49 *[712.2]*
    dicalcium phosphate crystals 275.49 *[712.1]*
    pyrophosphate crystals 275.4 *[712.2]*
Chondrodermatitis nodularis helicis 380.00
Chondrodysplasia 756.4
  angiomatose 756.4
  calcificans congenita 756.59
  epiphysialis punctata 756.59
  hereditary deforming 756.4
  rhizomelic punctata 277.86
Chondrodystrophia (fetalis) 756.4
  calcarea 756.4
  calcificans congenita 756.59
  fetalis hypoplastica 756.59
  hypoplastica calcinosa 756.59
  punctata 756.59
  tarda 277.5

Chondrodystrophy (familial) (hypoplastic) 756.4
  myotonic (congenital) 359.23
Chondroectodermal dysplasia 756.55
Chondrolysis 733.99
Chondroma (M9220/0)—*see also* Neoplasm
  cartilage, benign
  juxtacortical (M9221/0)—*see* Neoplasm, bone,
    benign
  periosteal (M9221/0)—*see* Neoplasm, bone,
    benign
Chondromalacia 733.92
  epiglottis (congenital) 748.3
  generalized 733.92
  knee 717.7
  larynx (congenital) 748.3
  localized, except patella 733.92
  patella, patellae 717.7
  systemic 733.92
  tibial plateau 733.92
  trachea (congenital) 748.3
Chondromatosis (M9220/1)—*see* Neoplasm,
  cartilage, uncertain behavior
Chondromyxosarcoma (M9220/3)—*see*
  Neoplasm, cartilage, malignant
Chondro-osteodysplasia (Morquio-Brailsford
  type) 277.5
Chondro-osteodystrophy 277.5
Chondro-osteodystrophy 277.5
Chondro-osteoma (M9210/0)—*see* Neoplasm,
  bone, benign
Chondropathia tuberosa 733.6
Chondrosarcoma (M9220/3)—*see also*
  Neoplasm, cartilage, malignant
  juxtacortical (M9221/3)—*see* Neoplasm, bone,
    malignant
  mesenchymal (M9240/3)—*see* Neoplasm,
    connective tissue, malignant
Chordae tendineae rupture (chronic) 429.5
Chordee (nonvenereal) 607.89
  congenital 752.63
  gonococcal 098.2
Chorditis (fibrinous) (nodosa) (tuberosa) 478.5
Chordoma (M9370/3)—*see* Neoplasm, by site,
  malignant
Chorea (gravis) (minor) (spasmodic) 333.5
  with
    heart involvement—*see* Chorea with
      rheumatic heart disease
    rheumatic heart disease (chronic, inactive, or
      quiescent) (conditions classifiable to
      393-398)—*see also* Rheumatic heart
      condition involved
      active or acute (conditions classifiable to
        391) 392.0
  acute—*see* Chorea, Sydenham's
  apoplectic (*see also* Disease, cerebrovascular,
    acute) 436
  chronic 333.4
  electric 049.8
  gravidarum—*see* Eclampsia, pregnancy
  habit 307.22
  hereditary 333.4
  Huntington's 333.4
  posthemiplegic 344.89
  pregnancy—*see* Eclampsia, pregnancy
  progressive 333.4
    chronic 333.4
    hereditary 333.4
  rheumatic (chronic) 392.9
    with heart disease or involvement—*see*
      Chorea, with rheumatic heart disease

Chorea—*continued*
  senile 333.5
  Sydenham's 392.9
    with heart involvement—*see* Chorea, with
      rheumatic heart disease
    nonrheumatic 333.5
  variabilis 307.23
Choreoathetosis (paroxysmal) 333.5
Chorioadenoma (destruens) (M9100/1) 236.1
Chorioamnionitis 658.4
  affecting fetus or newborn 762.7
Chorioangioma (M9120/0) 219.8
Choriocarcinoma (M9100/3)
  combined with
    embryonal carcinoma (M9101/3)—*see*
      Neoplasm, by site, malignant
    teratoma (M9101/3)—*see* Neoplasm, by site,
      malignant
  specified site—*see* Neoplasm, by site, malignant
  unspecified site
    female 181
    male 186.9
Chorioencephalitis, lymphocytic (acute)
    (serous) 049.0
Chorioepithelioma (M9100/3)—*see*
  Choriocarcinoma
Choriomeningitis (acute) (benign) (lymphocytic)
    (serous) 049.0
Chorionepithelioma (M9100/3)—*see*
  Choriocarcinoma
Chorionitis (*see also* Scleroderma) 710.1
Chorioretinitis 363.20
  disseminated 363.10
    generalized 363.13
    in
      neurosyphilis 094.83
      secondary syphilis 091.51
    peripheral 363.12
    posterior pole 363.11
    tuberculous (*see also* Tuberculosis) 017.3
      [363.13]
  due to
    histoplasmosis (*see also* Histoplasmosis) 115.92
    toxoplasmosis (acquired) 130.2
      congenital (active) 771.2
  focal 363.00
    juxtapapillary 363.01
    peripheral 363.04
    posterior pole NEC 363.03
  juxtapapillaris, juxtapapillary 363.01
  progressive myopia (degeneration) 360.21
  syphilitic (secondary) 091.51
    congenital (early) 090.0 *[363.13]*
      late 090.5 *[363.13]*
    late 095.8 *[363.13]*
  tuberculous (*see also* Tuberculosis) 017.3 *[363.13]*
Choristoma —*see* Neoplasm, by site, benign
Choroid —*see* condition
Choroideremia, choroidermia (initial stage)
    (late stage) (partial or total atrophy) 363.55
Choroiditis (*see also* Chorioretinitis) 363.20
  leprous 030.9 *[363.13]*
  senile guttate 363.41
  sympathetic 360.11
  syphilitic (secondary) 091.51
    congenital (early) 090.0 *[363.13]*
      late 090.5 *[363.13]*
    late 095.8 *[363.13]*
  Tay's 363.41
  tuberculous (*see also* Tuberculosis) 017.3
    [363.13]

Choroidopathy NEC 363.9
  degenerative (*see also* Degeneration, choroid)
    363.40
  hereditary (*see also* Dystrophy, choroid) 363.50
  specified type NEC 363.8
Choroidoretinitis —*see* Chorioretinitis
Choroidosis, central serous 362.41
Choroidretinopathy, serous 362.41
Christian's syndrome (chronic histiocytosis X)
    277.89
Christian-Weber disease (nodular
    nonsuppurative panniculitis) 729.30
Christmas disease 286.1
Chromaffinoma (M8700/0)—*see also*
    Neoplasm, by site, benign
  malignant (M8700/3)—*see* Neoplasm, by site,
    malignant
Chromatopsia 368.59
Chromhidrosis, chromidrosis 705.89
Chromoblastomycosis 117.2
Chromomycosis 117.2
Chromophytosis 111.0
Chromotrichomycosis 111.8
Chronic —*see* condition
Churg-Strauss syndrome 446.4
Chyle cyst, mesentery 457.8
Chylocele (nonfilarial) 457.8
  filarial (*see also* Infestation, filarial) 125.9
  tunica vaginalis (nonfilarial) 608.84
    filarial (*see also* Infestation, filarial) 125.9
Chylomicronemia (fasting) (with
    hyperprebetalipoproteinemia) 272.3
Chylopericardium (acute) 420.90
Chylothorax (nonfilarial) 457.8
  filarial (*see also* Infestation, filarial) 125.9
Chylous
  ascites 457.8
  cyst of peritoneum 457.8
  hydrocele 603.9
  hydrothorax (nonfilarial) 457.8
    filarial (*see also* Infestation, filarial) 125.9
Chyluria 791.1
  bilharziasis 120.0
  due to
    Brugia (malayi) 125.1
    Wuchereria (bancrofti) 125.0
      malayi 125.1
  filarial (*see also* Infestation, filarial) 125.9
  filariasis (*see also* Infestation, filarial) 125.9
  nonfilarial 791.1
Cicatricial (deformity)—*see* Cicatrix
Cicatrix (adherent) (contracted) (painful)
    (vicious) 709.2
  adenoid 474.8
  alveolar process 525.8
  anus 569.49
  auricle 380.89
  bile duct (*see also* Disease, biliary) 576.8
  bladder 596.8
  bone 733.99
  brain 348.89
  cervix (postoperative) (postpartal) 622.3
    in pregnancy or childbirth 654.6
      causing obstructed labor 660.2
  chorioretinal 363.30
    disseminated 363.35
    macular 363.32
    peripheral 363.34
    posterior pole NEC 363.33
  choroid—*see* Cicatrix, chorioretinal

Cicatrix—*continued*
 common duct (*see also* Disease, biliary) 576.8
 congenital 757.39
 conjunctiva 372.64
 cornea 371.00
  tuberculous (*see also* Tuberculosis) 017.3 *[371.05]*
 duodenum (bulb) 537.3
 esophagus 530.3
 eyelid 374.46
  with
   ectropion—*see* Ectropion
   entropion—*see* Entropion
 hypopharynx 478.29
 knee, semilunar cartilage 717.5
 lacrimal
  canaliculi 375.53
  duct
   acquired 375.56
   neonatal 375.55
  punctum 375.52
  sac 375.54
 larynx 478.79
 limbus (cystoid) 372.64
 lung 518.89
 macular 363.32
  disseminated 363.35
  peripheral 363.34
 middle ear 385.89
 mouth 528.9
 muscle 728.89
 nasolacrimal duct
  acquired 375.56
  neonatal 375.55
 nasopharynx 478.29
 palate (soft) 528.9
 penis 607.89
 prostate 602.8
 rectum 569.49
 retina 363.30
  disseminated 363.35
  macular 363.32
  peripheral 363.34
  posterior pole NEC 363.33
 semilunar cartilage—*see* Derangement,
  meniscus
 seminal vesicle 608.89
 skin 709.2
  infected 686.8
  postinfectional 709.2
  tuberculous (*see also* Tuberculosis) 017.0
 specified site NEC 709.2
 throat 478.29
 tongue 529.8
 tonsil (and adenoid) 474.8
 trachea 478.9
 tuberculous NEC (*see also* Tuberculosis) 011.9
 ureter 593.89
 urethra 599.84
 uterus 621.8
 vagina 623.4
  in pregnancy or childbirth 654.7
   causing obstructed labor 660.2
 vocal cord 478.5
 wrist, constricting (annular) 709.2
**CIDP (chronic inflammatory demyelinating
  polyneuropathy)** 357.81
CIN I [cervical intraepithelial neoplasia I] 622.11
CIN II [cervical intraepithelial neoplasia II] 622.12
CIN III [cervical intraepithelial neoplasia III] 233.1

Cinchonism
 correct substance properly administered 386.9
 overdose or wrong substance given or taken
  961.4
Circine herpes 110.5
Circle of Willis —*see* condition
Circular —*see also* condition
 hymen 752.49
**Circulating, intrinsic anticoagulants causing
  hemorrhagic disorder** 286.5
 following childbirth 666.3
 postpartum 666.3
Circulation
 collateral (venous), any site 459.89
 defective 459.9
  congenital 747.9
  lower extremity 459.89
 embryonic 747.9
 failure 799.89
  fetus or newborn 779.89
  peripheral 785.59
 fetal, persistent 747.83
 heart, incomplete 747.9
Circulatory system —*see* condition
Circulus senilis 371.41
Circumcision
 in absence of medical indication V50.2
 ritual V50.2
 routine V50.2
Circumscribed —*see* condition
Circumvallata placenta —*see* Placenta,
  abnormal
Cirrhosis, cirrhotic 571.5
 with alcoholism 571.2
 alcoholic (liver) 571.2
 atrophic (of liver)—*see* Cirrhosis, portal
 Baumgarten-Cruveilhier 571.5
 biliary (cholangiolitic) (cholangitic)
   (cholestatic) (extrahepatic) (hypertrophic)
   (intrahepatic) (nonobstructive) (obstructive)
   (pericholangiolitic) (posthepatic) (primary)
   (secondary) (xanthomatous) 571.6
  due to
   clonorchiasis 121.1
   flukes 121.3
 brain 331.9
 capsular—*see* Cirrhosis, portal
 cardiac 571.5
  alcoholic 571.2
 central (liver)—*see* Cirrhosis, liver
 Charcot's 571.6
 cholangiolitic—*see* Cirrhosis, biliary
 cholangitic—*see* Cirrhosis, biliary
 cholestatic—*see* Cirrhosis, biliary
 clitoris (hypertrophic) 624.2
 coarsely nodular 571.5
 congestive (liver)—*see* Cirrhosis, cardiac
 Cruveilhier-Baumgarten 571.5
 cryptogenic (of liver) 571.5
  alcoholic 571.2
 dietary (*see also* Cirrhosis, portal) 571.5
 due to
  bronzed diabetes 275.0
  congestive hepatomegaly—*see* Cirrhosis,
   cardiac
  cystic fibrosis 277.00
  hemochromatosis 275.0
  hepatolenticular degeneration 275.1
  passive congestion (chronic)—*see* Cirrhosis,
   cardiac
  Wilson's disease 275.1
  xanthomatosis 272.2

Cirrhosis, cirrhotic—*continued*
  extrahepatic (obstructive)—*see* Cirrhosis, biliary
  fatty 571.8
    alcoholic 571.0
    florid 571.2
  Glisson's—*see* Cirrhosis, portal
  Hanot's (hypertrophic)—*see* Cirrhosis, biliary
  hepatic—*see* Cirrhosis, liver
  hepatolienal—*see* Cirrhosis, liver
  hobnail—*see* Cirrhosis, portal
  hypertrophic—*see also* Cirrhosis, liver
    biliary—*see* Cirrhosis, biliary
    Hanot's—*see* Cirrhosis, biliary
  infectious NEC—*see* Cirrhosis, portal
  insular—*see* Cirrhosis, portal
  intrahepatic (obstructive) (primary)
    (secondary)—*see* Cirrhosis, biliary
  juvenile (*see also* Cirrhosis, portal) 571.5
  kidney (*see also* Sclerosis, renal) 587
  Laennec's (of liver) 571.2
    nonalcoholic 571.5
  liver (chronic) (hepatolienal) (hypertrophic)
    (nodular) (splenomegalic) (unilobar) 571.5
    with alcoholism 571.2
    alcoholic 571.2
    congenital (due to failure of obliteration of
      umbilical vein) 777.8
    cryptogenic 571.5
      alcoholic 571.2
    fatty 571.8
      alcoholic 571.0
    macronodular 571.5
      alcoholic 571.2
    micronodular 571.5
      alcoholic 571.2
    nodular, diffuse 571.5
      alcoholic 571.2
    pigmentary 275.0
    portal 571.5
      alcoholic 571.2
    postnecrotic 571.5
      alcoholic 571.2
    syphilitic 095.3
  lung (chronic) (*see also* Fibrosis, lung) 515
  macronodular (of liver) 571.5
    alcoholic 571.2
  malarial 084.9
  metabolic NEC 571.5
  micronodular (of liver) 571.5
    alcoholic 571.2
  monolobular—*see* Cirrhosis, portal
  multilobular—*see* Cirrhosis, portal
  nephritis (*see also* Sclerosis, renal) 587
  nodular—*see* Cirrhosis, liver
  nutritional (fatty) 571.5
  obstructive (biliary) (extrahepatic)
    (intrahepatic)—*see* Cirrhosis, biliary
  ovarian 620.8
  paludal 084.9
  pancreas (duct) 577.8
  pericholangiolitic—*see* Cirrhosis, biliary
  periportal—*see* Cirrhosis, portal
  pigment, pigmentary (of liver) 275.0
  portal (of liver) 571.5
    alcoholic 571.2
  posthepatitic (*see also* Cirrhosis, postnecrotic) 571.5
  postnecrotic (of liver) 571.5
    alcoholic 571.2
  primary (intrahepatic)—*see* Cirrhosis, biliary
  pulmonary (*see also* Fibrosis, lung) 515
  renal (*see also* Sclerosis, renal) 587

Cirrhosis, cirrhotic—*continued*
  septal (*see also* Cirrhosis, postnecrotic) 571.5
  spleen 289.51
  splenomegalic (of liver)—*see* Cirrhosis, liver
  stasis (liver)—*see* Cirrhosis, liver
  stomach 535.4
  Todd's (*see also* Cirrhosis, biliary) 571.6
  toxic (nodular)—*see* Cirrhosis, postnecrotic
  trabecular—*see* Cirrhosis, postnecrotic
  unilobar—*see* Cirrhosis, liver
  vascular (of liver)—*see* Cirrhosis, liver
  xanthomatous (biliary) (*see also* Cirrhosis,
    biliary) 571.6
    due to xanthomatosis (familial) (metabolic)
      (primary) 272.2
Cistern, subarachnoid 793.0
Citrullinemia 270.6
Citrullinuria 270.6
Ciuffini-Pancoast tumor (M8010/3) (carcinoma,
  pulmonary apex) 162.3
Civatte's disease or poikiloderma 709.09
CJD (Creutzfeldt-Jakob disease) 046.19
  variant (vCJD) 046.11
Clam diggers' itch 120.3
Clap —*see* Gonorrhea
Clark's paralysis 343.9
Clarke-Hadfield syndrome (pancreatic
  infantilism) 577.8
Clastothrix 704.2
Claude's syndrome 352.6
Claude Bernard-Horner syndrome (*see also*
  Neuropathy, peripheral, autonomic) 337.9
Claudication, intermittent 443.9
  cerebral (artery) (*see also* Ischemia, cerebral,
    transient) 435.9
  due to atherosclerosis 440.21
  spinal cord (arteriosclerotic) 435.1
    syphilitic 094.89
  spinalis 435.1
  venous (axillary) 453.89
Claudicatio venosa intermittens 453.89
Claustrophobia 300.29
Clavus (infected) 700
Claw foot (congenital) 754.71
  acquired 736.74
Claw hand (acquired) 736.06
  congenital 755.59
Clawtoe (congenital) 754.71
  acquired 735.5
Clay eating 307.52
Clay shovelers' fracture —*see* Fracture,
  vertebra, cervical
Cleansing of artificial opening (*see also*
  Attention to artificial opening) V55.9
Cleft (congenital)—*see also* Imperfect, closure
  alveolar process 525.8
  branchial (persistent) 744.41
    cyst 744.42
  clitoris 752.49
  cricoid cartilage, posterior 748.3
  facial (*see also* Cleft, lip) 749.10
  lip 749.10
    with cleft palate 749.20
      bilateral (lip and palate) 749.24
        with unilateral lip or palate 749.25
        complete 749.23
        incomplete 749.24
      unilateral (lip and palate) 749.22
        with bilateral lip or palate 749.25
        complete 749.21
        incomplete 749.22

Cleft—*continued*
lip —*continued*
  bilateral 749.14
    with cleft palate, unilateral 749.25
    complete 749.13
    incomplete 749.14
  unilateral 749.12
    with cleft palate, bilateral 749.25
    complete 749.11
    incomplete 749.12
  nose 748.1
  palate 749.00
    with cleft lip 749.20
      bilateral (lip and palate) 749.24
        with unilateral lip or palate 749.25
        complete 749.23
        incomplete 749.24
      unilateral (lip and palate) 749.22
        with bilateral lip or palate 749.25
        complete 749.21
        incomplete 749.22
    bilateral 749.04
      with cleft lip, unilateral 749.25
      complete 749.03
      incomplete 749.04
    unilateral 749.02
      with cleft lip, bilateral 749.25
      complete 749.01
      incomplete 749.02
  penis 752.69
  posterior, cricoid cartilage 748.3
  scrotum 752.89
  sternum (congenital) 756.3
  thyroid cartilage (congenital) 748.3
  tongue 750.13
  uvula 749.02
    with cleft lip (*see also* Cleft, lip, with cleft
      palate) 749.20
  water 366.12
Cleft hand (congenital) 755.58
Cleidocranial dysostosis 755.59
Cleidotomy, fetal 763.89
Cleptomania 312.32
Clérambault's syndrome 297.8
  erotomania 302.89
Clergyman's sore throat 784.49
Click, clicking
  systolic syndrome 785.2
Clifford's syndrome (postmaturity) 766.22
Climacteric (*see also* Menopause) 627.2
  arthritis NEC (*see also* Arthritis, climacteric)
    716.3
  depression (*see also* Psychosis, affective) 296.2
  disease 627.2
    recurrent episode 296.3
    single episode 296.2
  female (symptoms) 627.2
  male (symptoms) (syndrome) 608.89
  melancholia (*see also* Psychosis, affective) 296.2
    recurrent episode 296.3
    single episode 296.2
  paranoid state 297.2
  paraphrenia 297.2
  polyarthritis NEC 716.39
    male 608.89
  symptoms (female) 627.2
Clinical research investigation (control)
  (participant) V70.7
Clinodactyly 755.59
Clitoris —*see* condition
Cloaca, persistent 751.5
Clonorchiasis 121.1

Clonorchiosis 121.1
Clonorchis infection, liver 121.1
Clonus 781.0
Closed bite 524.20
Closed surgical procedure converted to open
  procedure
  arthroscopic V64.43
  laparoscopic V64.41
  thoracoscopic V64.42
Closure
  artificial opening (*see also* Attention to artificial
    opening) V55.9
  congenital, nose 748.0
  cranial sutures, premature 756.0
  defective or imperfect NEC—*see* Imperfect,
    closure
  fistula, delayed—*see* Fistula
  fontanelle, delayed 756.0
  foramen ovale, imperfect 745.5
  hymen 623.3
  interauricular septum, defective 745.5
  interventricular septum, defective 745.4
  lacrimal duct 375.56
    congenital 743.65
    neonatal 375.55
  nose (congenital) 748.0
    acquired 738.0
  vagina 623.2
  valve—*see* Endocarditis
  vulva 624.8
Clot (blood)
  artery (obstruction) (occlusion) (*see also*
    Embolism) 444.9
  atrial appendage 429.89
  bladder 596.7
  brain (extradural or intradural) (*see also*
    Thrombosis, brain) 434.0
    late effect—*see* Late effect(s) (of)
      cerebrovascular disease
  circulation 444.9
  heart (*see also* Infarct, myocardium) 410.9
    without myocardial infarction 429.89
  vein (*see also* Thrombosis) 453.9
Clotting defect NEC (*see also* Defect,
  coagulation) 286.9
Clouded state 780.09
  epileptic (*see also* Epilepsy) 345.9
  paroxysmal (idiopathic) (*see also* Epilepsy) 345.9
Clouding
  corneal graft 996.51
Cloudy
  antrum, antra 473.0
  dialysis effluent 792.5
Clouston's (hidrotic) ectodermal dysplasia 757.31
Clubbing of fingers 781.5
Clubfinger 736.29
  acquired 736.29
  congenital 754.89
Clubfoot (congenital) 754.70
  acquired 736.71
  equinovarus 754.51
  paralytic 736.71
Club hand (congenital) 754.89
  acquired 736.07
Clubnail (acquired) 703.8
  congenital 757.5
Clump kidney 753.3
Clumsiness 781.3
  syndrome 315.4
Cluttering 307.0
Clutton's joints 090.5

Coagulation, intravascular (diffuse)
  (disseminated) (*see also* Fibrinolysis) 286.6
  newborn 776.2
Coagulopathy (*see also* Defect, coagulation) 286.9
  consumption 286.6
  intravascular (disseminated) NEC 286.6
    newborn 776.2
Coalition
  calcaneoscaphoid 755.67
  calcaneus 755.67
  tarsal 755.67
Coal miners'
  elbow 727.2
  lung 500
Coal workers' lung or pneumoconiosis 500
Coarctation
  aorta (postductal) (preductal) 747.10
  pulmonary artery 747.3
Coated tongue 529.3
Coats' disease 362.12
Cocainism (*see also* Dependence) 304.2
Coccidioidal granuloma 114.3
Coccidioidomycosis 114.9
  with pneumonia 114.0
  cutaneous (primary) 114.1
  disseminated 114.3
  extrapulmonary (primary) 114.1
  lung 114.5
    acute 114.0
    chronic 114.4
    primary 114.0
  meninges 114.2
  primary (pulmonary) 114.0
    acute 114.0
  prostate 114.3
  pulmonary 114.5
    acute 114.0
    chronic 114.4
    primary 114.0
  specified site NEC 114.3
Coccidioidosis 114.9
  lung 114.5
    acute 114.0
    chronic 114.4
    primary 114.0
  meninges 114.2
Coccidiosis (colitis) (diarrhea) (dysentery) 007.2
Cocciuria 791.9
Coccus in urine 791.9
Coccydynia 724.79
Coccygodynia 724.79
Coccyx —*see* condition
Cochin-China
  diarrhea 579.1
    anguilluliasis 127.2
  ulcer 085.1
Cock's peculiar tumor 706.2
Cockayne's disease or syndrome (microcephaly
  and dwarfism) 759.89
Cockayne-Weber syndrome (epidermolysis
  bullosa) 757.39
Cocked-up toe 735.2
Codman's tumor (benign chondroblastoma)
  (M9230/0)—*see* Neoplasm, bone, benign
Coenurosis 123.8
Coffee workers' lung 495.8
Cogan's syndrome 370.52
  congenital oculomotor apraxia 379.51
  nonsyphilitic interstitial keratitis 370.52
Coiling, umbilical cord —*see* Complications,
  umbilical cord

Coitus, painful (female) 625.0
  male 608.89
  psychogenic 302.76
Cold 460
  with influenza, flu, or grippe 487.1
  abscess—*see also* Tuberculosis, abscess
    articular—*see* Tuberculosis, joint
  agglutinin
    disease (chronic) or syndrome 283.0
    hemoglobinuria 283.0
      paroxysmal (cold) (nocturnal) 283.2
  allergic (*see also* Fever, hay) 477.9
  bronchus or chest—*see* Bronchitis
    with grippe or influenza 487.1
  common (head) 460
    vaccination, prophylactic (against) V04.7
  deep 464.10
  effects of 991.9
    specified effect NEC 991.8
  excessive 991.9
    specified effect NEC 991.8
  exhaustion from 991.8
  exposure to 991.9
    specified effect NEC 991.8
  grippy 487.1
  head 460
  injury syndrome (newborn) 778.2
  intolerance 780.99
  on lung—*see* Bronchitis
  rose 477.0
  sensitivity, autoimmune 283.0
  virus 460
Coldsore (*see also* Herpes, simplex) 054.9
Colibacillosis 041.4
  generalized 038.42
Colibacilluria 791.9
Colic (recurrent) 789.7
  abdomen 789.7
    (recurrent)psychogenic 307.89
  appendicular 543.9
  appendix 543.9
  bile duct—*see* Choledocholithiasis
  biliary—*see* Cholelithiasis
  bilious—*see* Cholelithiasis
  common duct—*see* Choledocholithiasis
  Devonshire NEC 984.9
    specified type of lead—*see* Table of drugs and
      chemicals
  flatulent 787.3
  gallbladder or gallstone—*see* Cholelithiasis
  gastric 536.8
  hepatic (duct)—*see* Choledocholithiasis
  hysterical 300.11
  in
    adult 789.0
    child over 12 months old 789.0
    infant 789.7
  infantile 789.7
  intestinal 789.7
  kidney 788.0
  lead NEC 984.9
    specified type of lead—*see* Table of drugs and
      chemicals
  liver (duct)—*see* Choledocholithiasis
  mucous 564.9
    psychogenic 316 *[564.9]*
  nephritic 788.0
  painter's NEC 984.9
  pancreas 577.8
  psychogenic 306.4
  renal 788.0

Colic—*continued*
  saturnine NEC 984.9
    specified type of lead—*see* Table of drugs and chemicals
  spasmodic 789.7
  ureter 788.0
  urethral 599.84
    due to calculus 594.2
  uterus 625.8
    menstrual 625.3
  vermicular 543.9
  virus 460
  worm NEC 128.9
Colicystitis (*see also* Cystitis) 595.9
Colitis (acute) (catarrhal) (croupous) (cystica superficialis) (exudative) (hemorrhagic) (noninfectious) (phlegmonous) (presumed noninfectious) 558.9
  adaptive 564.9
  allergic 558.3
  amebic (*see also* Amebiasis) 006.9
    nondysenteric 006.2
  anthrax 022.2
  bacillary (*see also* Infection, Shigella) 004.9
  balantidial 007.0
  chronic 558.9
    ulcerative (*see also* Colitis, ulcerative) 556.9
  coccidial 007.2
  dietetic 558.9
  due to radiation 558.1
  eosinophilic 558.42
  functional 558.9
  gangrenous 009.0
  giardial 007.1
  granulomatous 555.1
  gravis (*see also* Colitis, ulcerative) 556.9
  infectious (*see also* Enteritis, due to, specific organism) 009.0
    presumed 009.1
  ischemic 557.9
    acute 557.0
    chronic 557.1
    due to mesenteric artery insufficiency 557.1
  membranous 564.9
    psychogenic 316 *[564.9]*
  mucous 564.9
    psychogenic 316 *[564.9]*
  necrotic 009.0
  polyposa (*see also* Colitis, ulcerative) 556.9
  protozoal NEC 007.9
  pseudomembranous 008.45
  pseudomucinous 564.9
  regional 555.1
  segmental 555.1
  septic (*see also* Enteritis, due to, specific organism) 009.0
  spastic 564.9
    psychogenic 316 *[564.9]*
  staphylococcus 008.41
    food 005.0
  thromboulcerative 557.0
  toxic 558.2
  transmural 555.1
  trichomonal 007.3
  tuberculous (ulcerative) 014.8

Colitis—*continued*
  ulcerative (chronic) (idiopathic) (nonspecific) 556.9
    entero- 556.0
    fulminant 557.0
    ileo- 556.1
    left-sided 556.5
    procto- 556.2
    proctosigmoid 556.3
    psychogenic 316 *[556]*
    specified NEC 556.8
    universal 556.6
Collagen disease NEC 710.9
  nonvascular 710.9
  vascular (allergic) (*see also* Angiitis, hypersensitivity) 446.20
Collagenosis (*see also* Collagen disease) 710.9
  cardiovascular 425.4
  mediastinal 519.3
Collapse 780.2
  adrenal 255.8
  cardiorenal (*see also* Hypertension, cardiorenal) 404.90
  cardiorespiratory 785.51
    fetus or newborn 779.85
  cardiovascular (*see also* Disease, heart) 785.51
    fetus or newborn 779.85
  circulatory (peripheral) 785.59
    with
      abortion—*see* Abortion, by type, with shock
      ectopic pregnancy (*see also* categories 633.0-633.9) 639.5
      molar pregnancy (*see also* categories 630-632) 639.5
    during or after labor and delivery 669.1
    fetus or newborn 779.85
    following
      abortion 639.5
      ectopic or molar pregnancy 639.5
    during or after labor and delivery 669.1
    fetus or newborn 779.89
  external ear canal 380.50
    secondary to
      inflammation 380.53
      surgery 380.52
      trauma 380.51
  general 780.2
  heart—*see* Disease, heart
  heat 992.1
  hysterical 300.11
  labyrinth, membranous (congenital) 744.05
  lung (massive) (*see also* Atelectasis) 518.0
    pressure, during labor 668.0
  myocardial—*see* Disease, heart
  nervous (*see also* Disorder, mental, nonpsychotic) 300.9
  neurocirculatory 306.2
  nose 738.0
  postoperative (cardiovascular) 998.0
  pulmonary (*see also* Atelectasis) 518.0
    fetus or newborn 770.5
      partial 770.5
      primary 770.4
  thorax 512.8
    iatrogenic 512.1
    postoperative 512.1
  trachea 519.19
  valvular—*see* Endocarditis

Collapse—*continued*
  vascular (peripheral) 785.59
    with
      abortion—*see* Abortion, by type, with shock
      ectopic pregnancy (*see also* categories
        633.0-633.9) 639.5
      molar pregnancy (*see also* categories
        630-632) 639.5
    cerebral (*see also* Disease, cerebrovascular,
      acute) 436
    during or after labor and delivery 669.1
    fetus or newborn 779.89
    following
      abortion 639.5
      ectopic or molar pregnancy 639.5
    vasomotor 785.59
    vertebra 733.13
Collateral —*see also* condition
  circulation (venous) 459.89
  dilation, veins 459.89
Colles' fracture (closed) (reversed) (separation)
  813.41
  open 813.51
Collet's syndrome 352.6
Collet-Sicard syndrome 352.6
Colliculitis urethralis (*see also* Urethritis) 597.89
Colliers'
  asthma 500
  lung 500
  phthisis (*see also* Tuberculosis) 011.4
Collodion baby (ichthyosis congenita) 757.1
Colloid milium 709.3
Coloboma NEC 743.49
  choroid 743.59
  fundus 743.52
  iris 743.46
  lens 743.36
  lids 743.62
  optic disc (congenital) 743.57
    acquired 377.23
  retina 743.56
  sclera 743.47
Coloenteritis —*see* Enteritis
Colon —*see* condition
Colonization
  MRSA (methicillin resistant Staphylococcus
    aureus) V02.54
  MSSA (methicillin susceptible Staphylococcus
    aureus) V02.53
Coloptosis 569.89
Color
  amblyopia NEC 368.59
    acquired 368.55
  blindness NEC (congenital) 368.59
    acquired 368.55
Colostomy
  attention to V55.3
  fitting or adjustment V53.5
  malfunctioning 569.62
  status V44.3
Colpitis (*see also* Vaginitis) 616.10
Colpocele 618.6
Colpocystitis (*see also* Vaginitis) 616.10
Colporrhexis 665.4
Colpospasm 625.1
Column, spinal, vertebral —*see* condition
Coma 780.01
  apoplectic (*see also* Disease, cerebrovascular,
    acute) 436

Coma—*continued*
  diabetic (with ketoacidosis) 250.3
    due to secondary diabetes 249.3
  hyperosmolar 250.2
    due to secondary diabetes 249.2
  eclamptic (*see also* Eclampsia) 780.39
  epileptic 345.3
  hepatic 572.2
  hyperglycemic 250.2
    due to secondary diabetes 249.2
  hyperosmolar (diabetic) (nonketotic) 250.2
    due to secondary diabetes 249.2
  hypoglycemic 251.0
    diabetic 250.3
      due to secondary diabetes 249.3
  insulin 250.3
    due to secondary diabetes 249.3
    hyperosmolar 250.2
      due to secondary diabetes 249.2
    non-diabetic 251.0
    organic hyperinsulinism 251.0
  Kussmaul's (diabetic) 250.3
    due to secondary diabetes 249.3
  liver 572.2
  newborn 779.2
  prediabetic 250.2
    due to secondary diabetes 249.2
  uremic—*see* Uremia
Combat fatigue (*see also* Reaction, stress, acute)
  308.9
Combined —*see* condition
Comedo 706.1
Comedocarcinoma (M8501/3)—*see also*
  Neoplasm, breast, malignant
  noninfiltrating (M8501/2)
    specified site—*see* Neoplasm, by site, in situ
    unspecified site 233.0
Comedomastitis 610.4
Comedones 706.1
  lanugo 757.4
Comma bacillus, carrier (suspected) of V02.3
Comminuted fracture —*see* Fracture, by site
Common
  aortopulmonary trunk 745.0
  atrioventricular canal (defect) 745.69
  atrium 745.69
  cold (head) 460
    vaccination, prophylactic (against) V04.7
  truncus (arteriosus) 745.0
  ventricle 745.3
Commotio (current)
  cerebri (*see also* Concussion, brain) 850.9
    with skull fracture—*see* Fracture, skull, by site
  retinae 921.3
  spinalis—*see* Injury, spinal, by site
Commotion (current)
  brain (without skull fracture) (*see also*
    Concussion, brain) 850.9
    with skull fracture—*see* Fracture, skull, by site
  spinal cord—*see* Injury, spinal, by site
Communication
  abnormal—*see also* Fistula
    between
      base of aorta and pulmonary artery 745.0
      left ventricle and right atrium 745.4
      pericardial sac and pleural sac 748.8
      pulmonary artery and pulmonary vein 747.3
    congenital, between uterus and anterior
      abdominal wall 752.3
      bladder 752.3
      intestine 752.3
      rectum 752.3

Communication—*continued*
　left ventricular-right atrial 745.4
　pulmonary artery-pulmonary vein 747.3
Compartment syndrome —*see* Syndrome,
　compartment
Compensation
　broken—*see* Failure, heart
　failure—*see* Failure, heart
　neurosis, psychoneurosis 300.11
Complaint —*see also* Disease
　bowel, functional 564.9
　　psychogenic 306.4
　intestine, functional 564.9
　　psychogenic 306.4
　kidney (*see also* Disease, renal) 593.9
　liver 573.9
　miners' 500
Complete —*see* condition
Complex
　cardiorenal (*see also* Hypertension, cardiorenal)
　　404.90
　castration 300.9
　Costen's 524.60
　ego-dystonic homosexuality 302.0
　Eisenmenger's (ventricular septal defect) 745.4
　homosexual, ego-dystonic 302.0
　hypersexual 302.89
　inferiority 301.9
　jumped process
　　spine—*see* Dislocation, vertebra
　primary, tuberculosis (*see also* Tuberculosis) 010.0
　regional pain syndrome 355.9
　type I 337.20
　　lower limb 337.22
　　specified site NEC 337.29
　　upper limb 337.21
　type II
　　lower limb 355.71
　　upper limb 354.4
　Taussig-Bing (transposition, aorta and
　　overriding pulmonary artery) 745.11
Complications
　abortion NEC—*see* categories 634-639
　accidental puncture or laceration during a
　　procedure 998.2
　amniocentesis, fetal 679.1
　amputation stump (late) (surgical) 997.60
　　traumatic—*see* Amputation, traumatic
　anastomosis (and bypass)—*see also*
　　Complications, due to (presence of) any
　　device, implant, or graft classified to
　　996.0-996.5 NEC
　　hemorrhage NEC 998.11
　　intestinal (internal) NEC 997.4
　　　involving urinary tract 997.5
　　mechanical—*see* Complications, mechanical,
　　　graft
　　urinary tract (involving intestinal tract) 997.5
　anesthesia, anesthetic NEC (*see also* Anesthesia,
　　complication) 995.22
　　in labor and delivery 668.9
　　　affecting fetus or newborn 763.5
　　　cardiac 668.1
　　　central nervous system 668.2
　　　pulmonary 668.0
　　　specified type NEC 668.8
　aortocoronary (bypass) graft 996.03
　　atherosclerosis —*see* Arteriosclerosis,
　　　coronary
　　embolism 996.72
　　occlusion NEC 996.72
　　thrombus 996.72

Complications—*continued*
　arthroplasty (*see also* Complications, prosthetic
　　joint) 996.49
　artificial opening
　　cecostomy 569.60
　　colostomy 569.6
　　cystostomy 997.5
　　enterostomy 569.60
　　esophagostomy 530.87
　　　infection 530.86
　　　mechanical 530.87
　　gastrostomy 536.40
　　ileostomy 569.60
　　jejunostomy 569.60
　　nephrostomy 997.5
　　tracheostomy 519.00
　　ureterostomy 997.5
　　urethrostomy 997.5
　bariatric surgery 997.4
　bile duct implant (prosthetic) NEC 996.79
　　infection or inflammation 996.69
　　mechanical 996.59
　bleeding (intraoperative) (postoperative) 998.11
　blood vessel graft 996.1
　　aortocoronary 996.03
　　　atherosclerosis —*see* Arteriosclerosis,
　　　　coronary
　　　embolism 996.72
　　　occlusion NEC 996.72
　　　thrombus 996.72
　　atherosclerosis —*see* Arteriosclerosis,
　　　extremities
　　　embolism 996.74
　　　occlusion NEC 996.74
　　　thrombus 996.74
　bone growth stimulator NEC 996.78
　　infection or inflammation 996.67
　bone marrow transplant 996.85
　breast implant (prosthetic) NEC 996.79
　　infection or inflammation 996.69
　　mechanical 996.54
　bypass—*see also* Complications, anastomosis
　　aortocoronary 996.03
　　　atherosclerosis —*see* Arteriosclerosis,
　　　　coronary
　　　embolism 996.72
　　　occlusion NEC 996.72
　　　thrombus 996.72
　　carotid artery 996.1
　　　atherosclerosis —*see* Arteriosclerosis,
　　　　extremities
　　　embolism 996.74
　　　occlusion NEC 996.74
　　　thrombus 996.74
　cardiac (*see also* Disease, heart) 429.9
　　device, implant, or graft NEC 996.72
　　　infection or inflammation 996.61
　　　long-term effect 429.4
　　　mechanical (*see also* Complications,
　　　　mechanical, by type) 996.00
　　　valve prosthesis 996.71
　　　　infection or inflammation 996.61
　　postoperative NEC 997.1
　　　long-term effect 429.4
　　cardiorenal (*see also* Hypertension, cardiorenal)
　　　404.90
　carotid artery bypass graft 996.1
　　atherosclerosis —*see* Arteriosclerosis,
　　　extremities
　　embolism 996.74
　　occlusion NEC 996.74
　　thrombus 996.74

Complications—*continued*
  cataract fragments in eye 998.82
  catheter device—*see also* Complications, due to
    (presence of) any device, implant, or graft
    classified to 996.0-996.5 NEC
    mechanical—*see* Complications, mechanical,
      catheter
  cecostomy 569.60
  cesarean section wound 674.3
  chemotherapy (antineoplastic) 995.29
  chin implant (prosthetic) NEC 996.79
    infection or inflammation 996.69
    mechanical 996.59
  colostomy (enterostomy) 569.60
    specified type NEC 569.69
  contraceptive device, intrauterine NEC 996.76
    infection 996.65
    inflammation 996.65
    mechanical 996.32
  cord (umbilical)—*see* Complications, umbilical cord
  cornea
    due to contact lens 371.82
  coronary (artery) bypass (graft) NEC 996.03
    atherosclerosis —*see* Arteriosclerosis, coronary
    embolism 996.72
    infection or inflammation 996.61
    mechanical 996.03
    occlusion NEC 996.72
    specified type NEC 996.72
    thrombus 996.72
  cystostomy 997.5
  delivery 669.9
    procedure (instrumental) (manual) (surgical) 669.4
    specified type NEC 669.8
  dialysis (hemodialysis) (peritoneal) (renal) NEC 999.9
    catheter NEC—*see also* Complications, due to
      (presence of) any device, implant or graft
      classified to 996.0-996.5 NEC
    infection or inflammation 996.62
      peritoneal 996.68
    mechanical 996.1
      peritoneal 996.56
  drug NEC 995.29
  due to (presence of) any device, implant, or graft
    classified to 996.0-996.5 NEC 996.70
    with infection or inflammation—*see*
      Complications, infection or inflammation,
      due to (presence of) any device, implant,
      or graft classified to 996.0-996.5 NEC
    arterial NEC 996.74
      coronary NEC 996.03
        atherosclerosis —*see* Arteriosclerosis, coronary
      embolism 996.72
      occlusion NEC 996.72
      specified type NEC 996.72
      thrombus 996.72
      renal dialysis 996.73
    arteriovenous fistula or shunt NEC 996.74
    bone growth stimulator 996.78
    breast NEC 996.79
    cardiac NEC 996.72
      defibrillator 996.72
      pacemaker 996.72
      valve prosthesis 996.71
    catheter NEC 996.79
      spinal 996.75
      urinary, indwelling 996.76
      vascular NEC 996.74
        renal dialysis 996.73
      ventricular shunt 996.75

Complications—*continued*
  due to—*continued*
    coronary (artery) bypass (graft) NEC 996.03
      atherosclerosis —*see* Arteriosclerosis, coronary
      embolism 996.72
      occlusion NEC 996.72
      thrombus 996.72
    electrodes
      brain 996.75
      heart 996.72
    esophagostomy 530.87
    gastrointestinal NEC 996.79
    genitourinary NEC 996.76
    heart valve prosthesis NEC 996.71
    infusion pump 996.74
    insulin pump 996.57
    internal
      joint prosthesis 996.77
      orthopedic NEC 996.78
      specified type NEC 996.79
    intrauterine contraceptive device NEC 996.76
    joint prosthesis, internal NEC 996.77
    mechanical—*see* Complications, mechanical
    nervous system NEC 996.75
    ocular lens NEC 996.79
    orbital NEC 996.79
    orthopedic NEC 996.78
      joint, internal 996.77
    renal dialysis 996.73
    specified type NEC 996.79
    urinary catheter, indwelling 996.76
    vascular NEC 996.74
    ventricular shunt 996.75
  during dialysis NEC 999.9
  ectopic or molar pregnancy NEC 639.9
  electroshock therapy NEC 999.9
  enterostomy 569.60
    specified type NEC 569.69
  esophagostomy 530.87
    infection 530.86
    mechanical 530.87
  external (fixation) device with internal
    component(s) NEC 996.78
    infection or inflammation 996.67
    mechanical 996.49
  extracorporeal circulation NEC 999.9
  eye implant (prosthetic) NEC 996.79
    infection or inflammation 996.69
    mechanical
      ocular lens 996.53
      orbital globe 996.59
  fetal, from amniocentesis 679.1
  gastrointestinal, postoperative NEC (*see also*
    Complications, surgical procedures) 997.4
  gastrostomy 536.40
    specified type NEC 536.49
  genitourinary device, implant or graft NEC 996.76
    infection or inflammation 996.65
      urinary catheter, indwelling 996.64
    mechanical (*see also* Complications,
      mechanical, by type) 996.30
      specified NEC 996.39
  graft (bypass) (patch)—*see also* Complications,
    due to (presence of) any device, implant, or
    graft classified to 996.0-996.5 NEC
    bone marrow 996.85
    corneal NEC 996.79
      infection or inflammation 996.69
      rejection or reaction 996.51

Complications—*continued*
  graft—*continued*
    mechanical—*see* Complications, mechanical,
      graft
    organ (immune or nonimmune cause) (partial)
      (total) 996.80
      bone marrow 996.85
      heart 996.83
      intestines 996.87
      kidney 996.81
      liver 996.82
      lung 996.84
      pancreas 996.86
      specified NEC 996.89
    skin NEC 996.79
      infection or inflammation 996.69
      rejection 996.52
        artificial 996.55
      decellularized allodermis 996.55
  heart—*see also* Disease, heart
    transplant (immune or nonimmune cause)
      996.83
  hematoma (intraoperative) (postoperative)
    998.12
  hemorrhage (intraoperative) (postoperative)
    998.11
  hyperalimentation therapy NEC 999.9
  immunization (procedure)—*see* Complications,
    vaccination
  implant—*see also* Complications, due to
    (presence of) any device, implant, or graft
    classified to 996.0-996.5 NEC
    dental placement, hemorrhagic 525.71
    mechanical—*see* Complications, mechanical,
      implant
  infection and inflammation
    due to (presence of) any device, implant, or
      graft classified to 996.0-996.5 NEC 996.60
    arterial NEC 996.62
      coronary 996.61
      renal dialysis 996.62
    arteriovenous fistula or shunt 996.62
    artificial heart 996.61
    bone growth stimulator 996.67
    breast 996.69
    cardiac 996.61
    catheter NEC 996.69
      central venous 999.31
      Hickman 999.31
      peripherally inserted central (PICC) 999.31
      peritoneal 996.68
      portacath (port-a-cath) 999.31
      spinal 996.63
      triple lumen 999.31
      umbilical venous 999.31
      urinary, indwelling 996.64
      vascular (arterial) (dialysis) (peripheral
        venous) NEC 996.62
      ventricular shunt 996.63
    central venous catheter 999.31
    coronary artery bypass 996.61
    electrodes
      brain 996.63
      heart 996.61
    gastrointestinal NEC 996.69
    genitourinary NEC 996.65
      indwelling urinary catheter 996.64
    heart assist device 996.61
    heart valve 996.61
    Hickman catheter 999.31
    infusion pump 996.62

Complications—*continued*
  infection and inflammation—*continued*
    due to—*continued*
      insulin pump 996.69
      intrauterine contraceptive device 996.65
      joint prosthesis, internal 996.66
      ocular lens 996.69
      orbital (implant) 996.69
      orthopedic NEC 996.67
        joint, internal 996.66
      peripherally inserted central catheter (PICC)
        999.31
      portacath (port-a-cath) 999.31
      specified type NEC 996.69
      triple lumen catheter 999.31
      umbilical venous catheter 999.31
      urinary catheter, indwelling 996.64
      ventricular shunt 996.63
  infusion (procedure) 999.88
    blood—*see* Complications, transfusion
    infection NEC 999.39
    sepsis NEC 999.39
  inhalation therapy NEC 999.9
  injection (procedure) 999.9
    drug reaction (*see also* Reaction, drug) 995.27
    infection NEC 999.39
    sepsis NEC 999.39
    serum (prophylactic) (therapeutic)—*see*
      Complications, vaccination
    vaccine (any)—*see* Complications,
      vaccination
  inoculation (any)—*see* Complications, vaccination
  insulin pump 996.57
  internal device (catheter) (electronic) (fixation)
    (prosthetic) NEC—*see also* Complications,
    due to (presence of) any device, implant, or
    graft classified to 996.0-996.5 NEC
    mechanical—*see* Complications, mechanical
  intestinal pouch, specified NEC 569.79
  intestinal transplant (immune or nonimmune
    cause) 996.87
  intraoperative bleeding or hemorrhage 998.11
  intrauterine contraceptive device (*see also*
    Complications, contraceptive device) 996.76
    infection or inflammation 996.65
    with fetal damage affecting management of
      pregnancy 655.8
  in utero procedure
    fetal 679.1
    maternal 679.0
  jejunostomy 569.60
  kidney transplant (immune or nonimmune
    cause) 996.81
  labor 669.9
    specified condition NEC 669.8
  liver transplant (immune or nonimmune cause)
    996.82
  lumbar puncture 349.0
  mechanical
    anastomosis—*see* Complications, mechanical,
      graft
    artificial heart 996.09
    bypass—*see* Complications, mechanical, graft
    catheter NEC 996.59
      cardiac 996.09
      cystostomy 996.39
      dialysis (hemodialysis) 996.1
        peritoneal 996.56
      during a procedure 998.2
      urethral, indwelling 996.31
    colostomy 569.62

Complications—*continued*
mechanical—*continued*
  device NEC 996.59
    balloon (counterpulsation), intra-aortic 996.1
    cardiac 996.00
      automatic implantable defibrillator 996.04
      long-term effect 429.4
      specified NEC 996.09
    contraceptive, intrauterine 996.32
    counterpulsation, intra-aortic 996.1
    fixation, external, with internal components 996.49
    fixation, internal (nail, rod, plate) 996.40
    genitourinary 996.30
      specified NEC 996.39
    insulin pump 996.57
    nervous system 996.2
    orthopedic, internal 996.40
      prosthetic joint (*see also* Complications, mechanical device, orthopedic, prosthetic, joint) 996.47
    prosthetic NEC 996.59
      joint 996.47
        articular bearing surface wear 996.46
        aseptic loosening 996.41
        breakage 996.43
        dislocation 996.42
        failure 996.47
        fracture 996.43
          around prosthetic 996.44
          peri-prosthetic 996.44
        instability 996.42
        loosening 996.41
        peri-prosthetic osteolysis 996.45
        subluxation 996.42
        wear 996.46
    umbrella, vena cava 996.1
    vascular 996.1
  dorsal column stimulator 996.2
  electrode NEC 996.59
    brain 996.2
    cardiac 996.01
    spinal column 996.2
  enterostomy 569.62
  esophagostomy 530.87
  fistula, arteriovenous, surgically created 996.1
  gastrostomy 536.42
  graft NEC 996.52
    aortic (bifurcation) 996.1
    aortocoronary bypass 996.03
    blood vessel NEC 996.1
    bone 996.49
    cardiac 996.00
    carotid artery bypass 996.1
    cartilage 996.49
    corneal 996.51
    coronary bypass 996.03
    decellularized allodermis 996.55
    genitourinary 996.30
      specified NEC 996.39
    muscle 996.49
    nervous system 996.2
    organ (immune or nonimmune cause) 996.80
      heart 996.83
      intestines 996.87
      kidney 996.81
      liver 996.82
      lung 996.84
      pancreas 996.86
      specified NEC 996.89
    orthopedic, internal 996.49

Complications—*continued*
mechanical—*continued*
  graft—*continued*
    peripheral nerve 996.2
    prosthetic NEC 996.59
    skin 996.52
      artificial 996.55
    specified NEC 996.59
    tendon 996.49
    tissue NEC 996.52
    tooth 996.59
    ureter, without mention of resection 996.39
    vascular 996.1
  heart valve prosthesis 996.02
    long-term effect 429.4
  implant NEC 996.59
    cardiac 996.00
      automatic implantable defibrillator 996.04
      long-term effect 429.4
      specified NEC 996.09
    electrode NEC 996.59
      brain 996.2
      cardiac 996.01
      spinal column 996.2
    genitourinary 996.30
    nervous system 996.2
    orthopedic, internal 996.49
    prosthetic NEC 996.59
      in
        bile duct 996.59
        breast 996.54
        chin 996.59
        eye
          ocular lens 996.53
          orbital globe 996.59
        vascular 996.1
  insulin pump 996.57
  nonabsorbable surgical material 996.59
  pacemaker NEC 996.59
    brain 996.2
    cardiac 996.01
    nerve (phrenic) 996.2
  patch—*see* Complications, mechanical, graft
  prosthesis NEC 996.59
    bile duct 996.59
    breast 996.54
    chin 996.59
    ocular lens 996.53
    reconstruction, vas deferens 996.39
  reimplant NEC 996.59
    extremity (*see also* Complications, reattached, extremity) 996.90
    organ (*see also* Complications, transplant, organ, by site) 996.80
  repair—*see* Complications, mechanical, graft
  respirator (ventilator) V46.14
  shunt NEC 996.59
    arteriovenous, surgically created 996.1
    ventricular (communicating) 996.2
  stent NEC 996.59
  tracheostomy 519.02
  vas deferens reconstruction 996.39
  ventilator (respirator) V46.14
medical care NEC 999.9
  cardiac NEC 997.1
  gastrointestinal NEC 997.4
  nervous system NEC 997.00
  peripheral vascular NEC 997.2
  respiratory NEC 997.39
  urinary NEC 997.5

Complications—*continued*
 medical care—*continued*
  vascular
   mesenteric artery 997.71
   other vessels 997.79
   peripheral vessels 997.2
   renal artery 997.72
  nephrostomy 997.5
  nervous system
   device, implant, or graft NEC 349.1
    mechanical 996.2
   postoperative NEC 997.00
  obstetric 669.9
   procedure (instrumental) (manual) (surgical)
    669.4
   specified NEC 669.8
   surgical wound 674.3
  ocular lens implant NEC 996.79
   infection or inflammation 996.69
   mechanical 996.53
  organ transplant—*see* Complications, transplant,
   organ, by site
  orthopedic device, implant, or graft
   internal (fixation) (nail) (plate) (rod) NEC
    996.78
    infection or inflammation 996.67
   joint prosthesis 996.77
    infection or inflammation 996.66
    mechanical 996.40
   pacemaker (cardiac) 996.72
    infection or inflammation 996.61
    mechanical 996.01
  pancreas transplant (immune or nonimmune
   cause) 996.86
  perfusion NEC 999.9
  perineal repair (obstetrical) 674.3
   disruption 674.2
  pessary (uterus) (vagina)—*see* Complications,
   contraceptive device
  phototherapy 990
  postcystoscopic 997.5
  postmastoidectomy NEC 383.30
  postoperative—*see* Complications, surgical
   procedures
  pregnancy NEC 646.9
   affecting fetus or newborn 761.9
  prosthetic device, internal—*see also*
   Complications, due to (presence of) any
   device, implant, or graft classified to
   996.0-996.5 NEC
   mechanical NEC (*see also* Complications,
    mechanical) 996.59
  puerperium NEC (*see also* Puerperal) 674.9
  puncture, spinal 349.0
  pyelogram 997.5
  radiation 990
  radiotherapy 990
  reattached
   body part, except extremity 996.99
   extremity (infection) (rejection) 996.90
    arm(s) 996.94
    digit(s) (hand) 996.93
     foot 996.95
    finger(s) 996.93
    foot 996.95
    forearm 996.91
    hand 996.92
    leg 996.96
    lower NEC 996.96
    toe(s) 996.95
    upper NEC 996.94

Complications—*continued*
 reimplant—*see also* Complications, due to
  (presence of) any device, implant, or graft
  classified to 996.0-996.5 NEC
  bone marrow 996.85
  extremity (*see also* Complications, reattached,
   extremity) 996.90
   due to infection 996.90
  mechanical—*see* Complications, mechanical,
   reimplant
  organ (immune or nonimmune cause) (partial)
   (total) (*see also* Complications, transplant,
   organ, by site) 996.80
 renal allograft 996.81
 renal dialysis—*see* Complications, dialysis
 respirator (ventilator), mechanical V46.14
 respiratory 519.9
  device, implant or graft NEC 996.79
   infection or inflammation 996.69
   mechanical 996.59
  distress syndrome, adult, following trauma or
   surgery 518.5
  insufficiency, acute, postoperative 518.5
  postoperative NEC 997.39
  therapy NEC 999.9
 sedation during labor and delivery 668.9
  affecting fetus or newborn 763.5
  cardiac 668.1
  central nervous system 668.2
  pulmonary 668.0
  specified type NEC 668.8
 seroma (intraoperative) (postoperative)
  (noninfected) 998.13
  infected 998.51
 shunt—*see also* Complications, due to (presence
  of) any device, implant, or graft classified to
  996.0-996.5 NEC
  mechanical—*see* Complications, mechanical,
   shunt
 specified body system NEC
  device, implant, or graft—*see* Complications,
   due to (presence of) any device, implant,
   or graft classified to 996.0-996.5 NEC
  postoperative NEC 997.99
 spinal puncture or tap 349.0
 stoma, external
  gastrointestinal tract
   colostomy 569.60
   enterostomy 569.60
   esophagostomy 530.87
    infection 530.86
    mechanical 530.87
   gastrostomy 536.40
  urinary tract 997.5
 stomach banding 997.4
 stomach stapling 997.4
 surgical procedures 998.9
  accidental puncture or laceration 998.2
  amputation stump (late) 997.60
  anastomosis—*see* Complications, anastomosis
  burst stitches or sutures (external) (*see also*
   Dehiscence) 998.32
   internal 998.31
  cardiac 997.1
   long-term effect following cardiac surgery
    429.4
  cataract fragments in eye 998.82
  catheter device—*see* Complications, catheter
   device
  cecostomy malfunction 569.62
  colostomy malfunction 569.62

Complications—*continued*
surgical procedures—*continued*
  cystostomy malfunction 997.5
  dehiscence (of incision) (external) (*see also*
    Dehiscence) 998.32
    internal 998.31
  dialysis NEC (*see also* Complications,
    dialysis) 999.9
  disruption (*see also* Dehiscence)
    anastomosis (internal)—*see* Complications,
      mechanical, graft
    internal suture (line) 998.31
    wound (external) 998.32
      internal 998.31
  dumping syndrome (postgastrectomy) 564.2
  elephantiasis or lymphedema 997.99
    postmastectomy 457.0
  emphysema (surgical) 998.81
  enterostomy malfunction 569.62
  esophagostomy malfunction 530.87
  evisceration 998.32
  fistula (persistent postoperative) 998.6
  foreign body inadvertently left in wound
    (sponge) (suture) (swab) 998.4
  from nonabsorbable surgical material
    (Dacron) (mesh) (permanent suture)
    (reinforcing) (Teflon)—*see* Complications,
    due to (presence of) any device, implant,
    or graft classified to 996.0-996.5 NEC
  gastrointestinal NEC 997.4
  gastrostomy malfunction 536.42
  hematoma 998.12
  hemorrhage 998.11
  ileostomy malfunction 569.62
  internal prosthetic device NEC (*see also*
    Complications, internal device) 996.70
    hemolytic anemia 283.19
    infection or inflammation 996.60
    malfunction—*see* Complications,
      mechanical
    mechanical complication—*see*
      Complications, mechanical
    thrombus 996.70
  jejunostomy malfunction 569.62
  nervous system NEC 997.00
  obstruction, internal anastomosis—*see*
    Complications, mechanical, graft
  other body system NEC 997.99
  peripheral vascular NEC 997.2
  postcardiotomy syndrome 429.4
  postcholecystectomy syndrome 576.0
  postcommissurotomy syndrome 429.4
  postgastrectomy dumping syndrome 564.2
  postmastectomy lymphedema syndrome 457.0
  postmastoidectomy 383.30
    cholesteatoma, recurrent 383.32
    cyst, mucosal 383.31
    granulation 383.33
    inflammation, chronic 383.33
  postvagotomy syndrome 564.2
  postvalvulotomy syndrome 429.4
  reattached extremity (infection) (rejection)
    (*see also* Complications, reattached,
    extremity) 996.90
  respiratory NEC 997.39
  seroma 998.13
  shock (endotoxic) (hypovolemic) (septic)
    998.0

Complications—*continued*
surgical procedures—*continued*
  shunt, prosthetic (thrombus)—*see also*
    Complications, due to (presence of) any
    device, implant, or graft classified to
    996.0-996.5 NEC
    hemolytic anemia 283.19
  specified complication NEC 998.89
  stitch abscess 998.59
  transplant—*see* Complications, graft
  ureterostomy malfunction 997.5
  urethrostomy malfunction 997.5
  urinary NEC 997.5
  vascular
    mesenteric artery 997.71
    other vessels 997.79
    peripheral vessels 997.2
    renal artery 997.72
  wound infection 998.59
therapeutic misadventure NEC 999.9
  surgical treatment 998.9
tracheostomy 519.00
transfusion (blood) (lymphocytes) (plasma)
  NEC 999.89
  acute lung injury (TRALI) 518.7
  atrophy, liver, yellow, subacute (within 8
    months of administration)—*see* Hepatitis,
    viral
  bone marrow 996.85
  embolism
    air 999.1
    thrombus 999.2
  hemolysis NEC 999.89
    bone marrow 996.85
  hepatitis (serum) (type B) (within 8 months
    after administration) *see* Hepatitis, viral
  incompatibility reaction
    ABO 999.6
    minor blood group 999.89
    Rh (factor) 999.7
  infection 999.39
  jaundice (serum) (within 8 months after
    administration) *see* Hepatitis, viral
  sepsis 999.39
  shock or reaction NEC 999.89
    bone marrow 996.85
  subacute yellow atrophy of liver (within 8
    months after administration) *see* Hepatitis,
    viral
  thromboembolism 999.2
transplant—*see also* Complications, due to
  (presence of) any device, implant, or graft
  classified to 996.0-996.5 NEC
  bone marrow 996.85
  organ (immune or nonimmune cause) (partial)
    (total) 996.80
    bone marrow 996.85
    heart 996.83
    intestines 996.87
    kidney 996.81
    liver 996.82
    lung 996.84
    pancreas 996.86
    specified NEC 996.89
trauma NEC (early) 958.8
ultrasound therapy NEC 999.9
umbilical cord
  affecting fetus or newborn 762.6
  complicating delivery 663.9
    affecting fetus or newborn 762.6
    specified type NEC 663.8

Complications—*continued*
  urethral catheter NEC 996.76
    infection or inflammation 996.64
    mechanical 996.31
  urinary, postoperative NEC 997.5
  vaccination 999.9
    anaphylaxis NEC 999.4
    cellulitis 999.39
    encephalitis or encephalomyelitis 323.51
    hepatitis (serum) (type B) (within 8 months
      after administration) *see* Hepatitis, viral
    infection (general) (local) NEC 999.39
    jaundice (serum) (within 8 months after
      administration) *see* Hepatitis, viral
    meningitis 997.09 *[321.8]*
    myelitis 323.52
    protein sickness 999.5
    reaction (allergic) 999.5
      Herxheimer's 995.0
      serum 999.5
    sepsis 999.39
    serum intoxication, sickness, rash, or other
      serum reaction NEC 999.5
    shock (allergic) (anaphylactic) 999.4
    subacute yellow atrophy of liver (within 8
      months after administration) *see* Hepatitis,
      viral
    vaccinia (generalized) 999.0
    localized 999.39
  vascular
    device, implant, or graft NEC 996.74
      infection or inflammation 996.62
      mechanical NEC 996.1
        cardiac (*see also* Complications,
          mechanical, by type) 996.00
    following infusion, perfusion, or transfusion
      999.2
    postoperative NEC 997.2
      mesenteric artery 997.71
      other vessels 997.79
      peripheral vessels 997.2
      renal artery 997.72
  ventilation therapy NEC 999.9
  ventilator (respirator), mechanical V46.14
Compound presentation complicating delivery
  652.8
  causing obstructed labor 660.0
Compressed air disease 993.3
Compression
  with injury—*see* specific injury
  arm NEC 354.9
  artery 447.1
    celiac, syndrome 447.4
  brachial plexus 353.0
  brain (stem) 348.4
    due to
      contusion, brain—*see* Contusion, brain
      injury NEC—*see also* Hemorrhage, brain,
        traumatic
        birth—*see* Birth, injury, brain
      laceration, brain—*see* Laceration, brain
    osteopathic 739.0
  bronchus 519.19
  by cicatrix—*see* Cicatrix
  cardiac 423.9
  cauda equina 344.60
    with neurogenic bladder 344.61
  celiac (artery) (axis) 447.4
  cerebral—*see* Compression, brain
  cervical plexus 353.2

Compression—*continued*
  cord (umbilical)—*see* Compression, umbilical
    cord
  cranial nerve 352.9
    second 377.49
    third (partial) 378.51
      total 378.52
    fourth 378.53
    fifth 350.8
    sixth 378.54
    seventh 351.8
  divers' squeeze 993.3
  duodenum (external) (*see also* Obstruction,
    duodenum) 537.3
  during birth 767.9
  esophagus 530.3
    congenital, external 750.3
  Eustachian tube 381.63
  facies (congenital) 754.0
  fracture—*see* Fracture, by site
  heart—*see* Disease, heart
  intestine (*see also* Obstruction, intestine) 560.9
    with hernia—*see* Hernia, by site, with
      obstruction
  laryngeal nerve, recurrent 478.79
  leg NEC 355.8
  lower extremity NEC 355.8
  lumbosacral plexus 353.1
  lung 518.89
  lymphatic vessel 457.1
  medulla—*see* Compression, brain
  nerve NEC—*see also* Disorder, nerve
    arm NEC 354.9
    autonomic nervous system (*see also*
      Neuropathy, peripheral, autonomic) 337.9
    axillary 353.0
    cranial NEC 352.9
    due to displacement of intervertebral disc
      722.2
      with myelopathy 722.70
      cervical 722.0
        with myelopathy 722.71
      lumbar, lumbosacral 722.10
        with myelopathy 722.73
      thoracic, thoracolumbar 722.11
        with myelopathy 722.72
    iliohypogastric 355.79
    ilioinguinal 355.79
    leg NEC 355.8
    lower extremity NEC 355.8
  nerve—*continued*
    median (in carpal tunnel) 354.0
    obturator 355.79
    optic 377.49
    plantar 355.6
    posterior tibial (in tarsal tunnel) 355.5
    root (by scar tissue) NEC 724.9
      cervical NEC 723.4
      lumbar NEC 724.4
      lumbosacral 724.4
      thoracic 724.4
    saphenous 355.79
    sciatic (acute) 355.0
    sympathetic 337.9
    traumatic—*see* Injury, nerve
    ulnar 354.2
    upper extremity NEC 354.9
  peripheral—*see* Compression, nerve

Compression—*continued*
  spinal (cord) (old or nontraumatic) 336.9
    by displacement of intervertebral disc—*see*
      Displacement, intervertebral disc
    nerve
      root NEC 724.9
        postoperative 722.80
          cervical region 722.81
          lumbar region 722.83
          thoracic region 722.82
        traumatic—*see* Injury, nerve, spinal
      traumatic—*see* Injury, nerve, spinal
    spondylogenic 721.91
      cervical 721.1
      lumbar, lumbosacral 721.42
      thoracic 721.41
    traumatic—*see also* Injury, spinal, by site
      with fracture, vertebra—*see* Fracture,
        vertebra, by site, with spinal cord injury
    spondylogenic—*see* Compression, spinal cord,
      spondylogenic
  subcostal nerve (syndrome) 354.8
  sympathetic nerve NEC 337.9
  syndrome 958.5
  thorax 512.8
    iatrogenic 512.1
    postoperative 512.1
  trachea 519.19
    congenital 748.3
  ulnar nerve (by scar tissue) 354.2
  umbilical cord
    affecting fetus or newborn 762.5
      cord prolapsed 762.4
    complicating delivery 663.2
      cord around neck 663.1
      cord prolapsed 663.0
  upper extremity NEC 354.9
  ureter 593.3
  urethra—*see* Stricture, urethra
  vein 459.2
  vena cava (inferior) (superior) 459.2
  vertebral NEC—*see* Compression, spinal (cord)
Compulsion, compulsive
  eating 307.51
  neurosis (obsessive) 300.3
  personality 301.4
  states (mixed) 300.3
  swearing 300.3
    in Gilles de la Tourette's syndrome 307.23
  tics and spasms 307.22
  water drinking NEC (syndrome) 307.9
Concato's disease (pericardial polyserositis) 423.2
  peritoneal 568.82
  pleural—*see* Pleurisy
Concavity, chest wall 738.3
Concealed
  hemorrhage NEC 459.0
  penis 752.65
Concentric fading 368.12
Concern (normal) about sick person in family
  V61.49
Concrescence (teeth) 520.2
Concretio cordis 423.1
  rheumatic 393
Concretion —*see also* Calculus
  appendicular 543.9
  canaliculus 375.57
  clitoris 624.8
  conjunctiva 372.54
  eyelid 374.56
  intestine (impaction) (obstruction) 560.39

Concretion—*continued*
  lacrimal (passages) 375.57
  prepuce (male) 605
    female (clitoris) 624.8
  salivary gland (any) 527.5
  seminal vesicle 608.89
  stomach 537.89
  tonsil 474.8
Concussion (current) 850.9
  with
    loss of consciousness 850.5
      brief (less than one hour)
        30 minutes or less 850.11
        31-59 minutes 850.12
      moderate (1-24 hours) 850.2
      prolonged (more than 24 hours) (with
        complete recovery) (with return to
        pre-existing conscious level) 850.3
      without return to pre-existing conscious
        level 850.4
    mental confusion or disorientation (without
      loss of consciousness) 850.0
      with loss of consciousness—*see* Concussion,
        with, loss of consciousness
  without loss of consciousness 850.0
  blast (air) (hydraulic) (immersion) (underwater)
    869.0
    with open wound into cavity 869.1
    abdomen or thorax—*see* Injury, internal, by site
    brain—*see* Concussion, brain
    ear (acoustic nerve trauma) 951.5
      with perforation, tympanic membrane—*see*
        Wound, open, ear drum
    thorax—*see* Injury, internal, intrathoracic
      organs NEC
  brain or cerebral (without skull fracture) 850.9
    with
      loss of consciousness 850.5
        brief (less than one hour)
          30 minutes or less 850.11
          31-59 minutes 850.12
        moderate (1-24 hours) 850.2
        prolonged (more than 24 hours) (with
          complete recovery) (with return to
          pre-existing conscious level) 850.3
        without return to pre-existing conscious
          level 850.4
      mental confusion or disorientation (without
        loss of consciousness) 850.0
      with loss of consciousness—*see*
        Concussion, brain, with, loss of
        consciousness
    skull fracture—*see* Fracture, skull, by site
    without loss of consciousness 850.0
  cauda equina 952.4
  cerebral—*see* Concussion, brain
  conus medullaris (spine) 952.4
  hydraulic—*see* Concussion, blast
  internal organs—*see* Injury, internal, by site
  labyrinth—*see* Injury, intracranial
  ocular 921.3
  osseous labyrinth—*see* Injury, intracranial
  spinal (cord)—*see also* Injury, spinal, by site
    due to
      broken
        back—*see* Fracture, vertebra, by site, with
          spinal cord injury
        neck—*see* Fracture, vertebra, cervical,
          with spinal cord injury

Concussion—*continued*
  spinal (cord)—*continued*
    fracture, fracture dislocation, or compression
      fracture of spine or vertebra—*see*
      Fracture, vertebra, by site, with spinal
      cord injury
  syndrome 310.2
  underwater blast—*see* Concussion, blast
Condition —*see also* Disease
  fetal hematologic 678.0
  psychiatric 298.9
  respiratory NEC 519.9
    acute or subacute NEC 519.9
      due to
        external agent 508.9
          specified type NEC 508.8
          fumes or vapors (chemical) (inhalation) 506.3
          radiation 508.0
    chronic NEC 519.9
      due to
        external agent 508.9
          specified type NEC 508.8
          fumes or vapors (chemical) (inhalation) 506.4
          radiation 508.1
      due to
        external agent 508.9
          specified type NEC 508.8
          fumes or vapors (chemical) (inhalation)
           506.9
Conduct disturbance (*see also* Disturbance,
  conduct) 312.9
  adjustment reaction 309.3
  hyperkinetic 314.2
Condyloma NEC 078.11
  acuminatum 078.11
  gonorrheal 098.0
  latum 091.3
  syphilitic 091.3
    congenital 090.0
  venereal, syphilitic 091.3
Confinement —*see* Delivery
Conflagration —*see also* Burn, by site
  asphyxia (by inhalation of smoke, gases, fumes,
    or vapors) 987.9
    specified agent—*see* Table of drugs and
      chemicals
Conflict
  family V61.9
    specified circumstance NEC V61.8
  interpersonal NEC V62.81
  marital V61.10
    involving
      divorce V61.03
      estrangement V61.09
  parent(guardian)-child V61.20
    adopted child V61.24
    biological child V61.23
    foster child V61.25
  partner V61.10
Confluent —*see* condition
Confusion, confused (mental) (state) (*see also*
  State, confusional) 298.9
  acute 293.0
  epileptic 293.0
  postoperative 293.9
  psychogenic 298.2
  reactive (from emotional stress, psychological
    trauma) 298.2
  subacute 293.1
Confusional arousals 327.41
Congelation 991.9

Congenital —*see also* condition
  aortic septum 747.29
  generalized fibromatosis (CGF) 759.89
  intrinsic factor deficiency 281.0
  malformation—*see* Anomaly
Congestion, congestive
  asphyxia, newborn 768.9
  bladder 596.8
  bowel 569.89
  brain (*see also* Disease, cerebrovascular NEC)
    437.8
    malarial 084.9
  breast 611.79
  bronchi 519.19
  bronchial tube 519.19
  catarrhal 472.0
  cerebral—*see* Congestion, brain
  cerebrospinal—*see* Congestion, brain
  chest 786.9
  chill 780.99
    malarial (*see also* Malaria) 084.6
  circulatory NEC 459.9
  conjunctiva 372.71
  due to disturbance of circulation 459.9
  duodenum 537.3
  enteritis—*see* Enteritis
  eye 372.71
  fibrosis syndrome (pelvic) 625.5
  gastroenteritis—*see* Enteritis
  general 799.89
  glottis 476.0
  heart (*see also* Failure, heart) 428.0
  hepatic 573.0
  hypostatic (lung) 514
  intestine 569.89
  intracranial—*see* Congestion, brain
  kidney 593.89
  labyrinth 386.50
  larynx 476.0
  liver 573.0
  lung 786.9
    active or acute (*see also* Pneumonia) 486
      congenital 770.0
    chronic 514
    hypostatic 514
    idiopathic, acute 518.5
    passive 514
  malaria, malarial (brain) (fever) (*see also*
    Malaria) 084.6
  medulla—*see* Congestion, brain
  nasal 478.19
  nose 478.19
  orbit, orbital 376.33
    inflammatory (chronic) 376.10
      acute 376.00
  ovary 620.8
  pancreas 577.8
  pelvic, female 625.5
  pleural 511.0
  prostate (active) 602.1
  pulmonary—*see* Congestion, lung
  renal 593.89
  retina 362.89
  seminal vesicle 608.89
  spinal cord 336.1
  spleen 289.51
    chronic 289.51
  stomach 537.89
  trachea 464.11
  urethra 599.84

Congestion, congestive—*continued*
uterus 625.5
with subinvolution 621.1
viscera 799.89
Congestive —*see* Congestion
Conical
cervix 622.6
cornea 371.60
teeth 520.2
Conjoined twins 759.4
causing disproportion (fetopelvic) 678.1
fetal 678.1
Conjugal maladjustment V61.10
involving
divorce V61.03
estrangement V61.09
Conjunctiva —*see* condition
Conjunctivitis (exposure) (infectious)
(nondiphtheritic) (pneumococcal) (pustular)
(staphylococcal) (streptococcal) NEC 372.30
actinic 370.24
acute 372.00
atopic 372.05
chemical 372.06
contagious 372.03
follicular 372.02
hemorrhagic (viral) 077.4
toxic 372.06
adenoviral (acute) 077.3
allergic (chronic) 372.14
with hay fever 372.05
anaphylactic 372.05
angular 372.03
Apollo (viral) 077.4
atopic 372.05
blennorrhagic (neonatorum) 098.40
catarrhal 372.03
chemical 372.06
allergic 372.05
meaning corrosion, *see* Burn, conjunctiva
chlamydial 077.98
due to
Chlamydial trachomatis—*see* Trachoma
paratrachoma 077.0
chronic 372.10
allergic 372.14
follicular 372.12
simple 372.11
specified type NEC 372.14
vernal 372.13
diphtheritic 032.81
due to
dust 372.05
enterovirus type 70 077.4
erythema multiforme 695.10 *[372.33]*
filariasis (*see also* Filariasis) 125.9 *[372.15]*
mucocutaneous
disease NEC 372.33
leishmaniasis 085.5 *[372.15]*
Reiter's disease 099.3 *[372.33]*
syphilis 095.8 *[372.10]*
toxoplasmosis (acquired) 130.1
congenital (active) 771.2
trachoma—*see* Trachoma
dust 372.05
eczematous 370.31
epidemic 077.1
hemorrhagic 077.4
follicular (acute) 372.02
adenoviral (acute) 077.3
chronic 372.12

Conjunctivitis— *continued*
glare 370.24
gonococcal (neonatorum) 098.40
granular (trachomatous) 076.1
late effect 139.1
hemorrhagic (acute) (epidemic) 077.4
herpetic (simplex) 054.43
zoster 053.21
inclusion 077.0
infantile 771.6
influenzal 372.03
Koch-Weeks 372.03
light 372.05
medicamentosa 372.05
membranous 372.04
meningococcic 036.89
Morax-Axenfeld 372.02
mucopurulent NEC 372.03
neonatal 771.6
gonococcal 098.40
Newcastle's 077.8
nodosa 360.14
of Beal 077.3
parasitic 372.15
filariasis (*see also* Filariasis) 125.9 *[372.15]*
mucocutaneous leishmaniasis 085.5 *[372.15]*
Parinaud's 372.02
petrificans 372.39
phlyctenular 370.31
pseudomembranous 372.04
diphtheritic 032.81
purulent 372.03
Reiter's 099.3 *[372.33]*
rosacea 695.3 *[372.31]*
serous 372.01
viral 077.99
simple chronic 372.11
specified NEC 372.39
sunlamp 372.04
swimming pool 077.0
toxic 372.06
trachomatous (follicular) 076.1
acute 076.0
late effect 139.1
traumatic NEC 372.39
tuberculous (*see also* Tuberculosis) 017.3 *[370.31]*
tularemic 021.3
tularensis 021.3
vernal 372.13
limbar 372.13 *[370.32]*
viral 077.99
acute hemorrhagic 077.4
specified NEC 077.8
Conjunctivochalasis 372.81
Conjunctoblepharitis —*see* Conjunctivitis
Conn (-Louis) syndrome (primary aldosteronism)
255.12
Connective tissue —*see* condition
Conradi (-Hünermann) syndrome or disease
(chondrodysplasia calcificans congenita)
756.59
Consanguinity V19.7
Consecutive —*see* condition
Consolidated lung (base)—*see* Pneumonia, lobar
Constipation 564.00
atonic 564.09
drug induced
correct substance properly administered 564.09
overdose or wrong substance given or taken 977.9
specified drug—*see* Table of drugs and
chemicals

Constipation—*continued*
  neurogenic 564.09
  other specified NEC 564.09
  outlet dysfunction 564.02
  psychogenic 306.4
  simple 564.00
  slow transit 564.01
  spastic 564.09
Constitutional —*see also* condition
  arterial hypotension (*see also* Hypotension) 458.9
  obesity 278.00
    morbid 278.01
  psychopathic state 301.9
  short stature in childhood 783.43
  state, developmental V21.9
    specified development NEC V21.8
  substandard 301.6
Constitutionally substandard 301.6
Constriction
  anomalous, meningeal bands or folds 742.8
  aortic arch (congenital) 747.10
  asphyxiation or suffocation by 994.7
  bronchus 519.19
  canal, ear (*see also* Stricture, ear canal,
    acquired) 380.50
  duodenum 537.3
  gallbladder (*see also* Obstruction, gallbladder) 575.2
    congenital 751.69
  intestine (*see also* Obstruction, intestine) 560.9
  larynx 478.74
    congenital 748.3
  meningeal bands or folds, anomalous 742.8
  organ or site, congenital NEC—*see* Atresia
  prepuce (congenital) 605
  pylorus 537.0
    adult hypertrophic 537.0
    congenital or infantile 750.5
    newborn 750.5
  ring (uterus) 661.4
    affecting fetus or newborn 763.7
  spastic—*see also* Spasm
    ureter 593.3
    urethra—*see* Stricture, urethra
  stomach 537.89
  ureter 593.3
  urethra—*see* Stricture, urethra
  visual field (functional) (peripheral) 368.45
Constrictive —*see* condition
Consultation V65.9
  medical—*see also* Counseling, medical
  specified reason NEC V65.8
  without complaint or sickness V65.9
    feared complaint unfounded V65.5
    specified reason NEC V65.8
Consumption —*see* Tuberculosis
Contact
  with
    AIDS virus V01.79
    anthrax V01.81
    asbestos V15.84
    cholera V01.0
    communicable disease V01.9
      specified type NEC V01.89
      viral NEC V01.79
    Escherichia coli (E. coli) V01.83
    German measles V01.4
    gonorrhea V01.6
    HIV V01.79
    human immunodeficiency virus V01.79
    lead V15.86
    meningococcus V01.84

Contact—*continued*
  with—*continued*
    parasitic disease NEC V01.89
    poliomyelitis V01.2
    potentially hazardous body fluids V15.85
    rabies V01.5
    rubella V01.4
    SARS-associated coronavirus V01.82
    smallpox V01.3
    syphilis V01.6
    tuberculosis V01.1
    varicella V01.71
    venereal disease V01.6
    viral disease NEC V01.79
  dermatitis—*see* Dermatitis
Contamination, food (*see also* Poisoning, food) 005.9
Contraception, contraceptive
  advice NEC V25.09
    family planning V25.09
    fitting of diaphragm V25.02
    prescribing or use of
      oral contraceptive agent V25.01
      specified agent NEC V25.02
  counseling NEC V25.09
    emergency V25.03
    family planning V25.09
    fitting of diaphragm V25.02
    prescribing or use of
      oral contraceptive agent V25.01
        emergency V25.03
        postcoital V25.03
      specified agent NEC V25.02
  device (in situ) V45.59
    causing menorrhagia 996.76
    checking V25.42
    complications 996.32
    insertion V25.1
    intrauterine V45.51
    reinsertion V25.42
    removal V25.42
    subdermal V45.52
  fitting of diaphragm V25.02
  insertion
    intrauterine contraceptive device V25.1
    subdermal implantable V25.5
  maintenance V25.40
    examination V25.40
      intrauterine device V25.42
      oral contraceptive V25.41
      specified method NEC V25.49
      subdermal implantable V25.43
    intrauterine device V25.42
    oral contraceptive V25.41
    specified method NEC V25.49
    subdermal implantable V25.43
  management NEC V25.49
  prescription
    oral contraceptive agent V25.01
      emergency V25.03
      postcoital V25.03
      repeat V25.41
    specified agent NEC V25.02
      repeat V25.49
  sterilization V25.2
  surveillance V25.40
    intrauterine device V25.42
    oral contraceptive agent V25.41
    specified method NEC V25.49
    subdermal implantable V25.43

Contraction, contracture, contracted
Achilles tendon (*see also* Short, tendon, Achilles) 727.81
anus 564.89
axilla 729.90
bile duct (*see also* Disease, biliary) 576.8
bladder 596.8
  neck or sphincter 596.0
bowel (*see also* Obstruction, intestine) 560.9
Braxton Hicks 644.1
breast implant, capsular 611.83
bronchus 519.19
burn (old)—*see* Cicatrix
capsular, of breast implant 611.83
cecum (*see also* Obstruction, intestine) 560.9
cervix (*see also* Stricture, cervix) 622.4
  congenital 752.49
cicatricial—*see* Cicatrix
colon (*see also* Obstruction, intestine) 560.9
conjunctiva trachomatous, active 076.1
  late effect 139.1
Dupuytren's 728.6
eyelid 374.41
eye socket (after enucleation) 372.64
face 729.90
fascia (lata) (postural) 728.89
  Dupuytren's 728.6
  palmar 728.6
  plantar 728.71
finger NEC 736.29
  congenital 755.59
  joint (*see also* Contraction, joint) 718.44
flaccid, paralytic
  joint (*see also* Contraction, joint) 718.4
  muscle 728.85
    ocular 378.50
gallbladder (*see also* Obstruction, gallbladder) 575.2
hamstring 728.89
  tendon 727.81
heart valve—*see* Endocarditis
Hicks' 644.1
hip (*see also* Contraction, joint) 718.4
hourglass
  bladder 596.8
    congenital 753.8
  gallbladder (*see also* Obstruction, gallbladder) 575.2
    congenital 751.69
  stomach 536.8
    congenital 750.7
    psychogenic 306.4
  uterus 661.4
    affecting fetus or newborn 763.7
hysterical 300.11
infantile (*see also* Epilepsy) 345.6
internal os (*see also* Stricture, cervix) 622.4
intestine (*see also* Obstruction, intestine) 560.9
joint (abduction) (acquired) (adduction) (flexion) (rotation) 718.40
  ankle 718.47
  congenital NEC 755.8
    generalized or multiple 754.89
      lower limb joints 754.89
    hip (*see also* Subluxation, congenital, hip) 754.32
    lower limb (including pelvic girdle) not involving hip 754.89
    upper limb (including shoulder girdle) 755.59
  elbow 718.42

Contraction—*continued*
joint—*continued*
  foot 718.47
  hand 718.44
  hip 718.45
  hysterical 300.11
  knee 718.46
  multiple sites 718.49
  pelvic region 718.45
  shoulder (region) 718.41
  specified site NEC 718.48
  wrist 718.43
kidney (granular) (secondary) (*see also* Sclerosis, renal) 587
  congenital 753.3
  hydronephritic 591
  pyelonephritic (*see also* Pyelitis, chronic) 590.00
  tuberculous (*see also* Tuberculosis) 016.0
ligament 728.89
  congenital 756.89
liver—*see* Cirrhosis, liver
muscle (postinfectional) (postural) NEC 728.85
  congenital 756.89
    sternocleidomastoid 754.1
  extraocular 378.60
  eye (extrinsic) (*see also* Strabismus) 378.9
    paralytic (*see also* Strabismus, paralytic) 378.50
  flaccid 728.85
  hysterical 300.11
  ischemic (Volkmann's) 958.6
  paralytic 728.85
  posttraumatic 958.6
  psychogenic 306.0
    specified as conversion reaction 300.11
myotonic 728.85
neck (*see also* Torticollis) 723.5
  congenital 754.1
  psychogenic 306.0
ocular muscle (*see also* Strabismus) 378.9
  paralytic (*see also* Strabismus, paralytic) 378.50
organ or site, congenital NEC—*see* Atresia
outlet (pelvis)—*see* Contraction, pelvis
palmar fascia 728.6
paralytic
  joint (*see also* Contraction, joint) 718.4
  muscle 728.85
    ocular (*see also* Strabismus, paralytic) 378.50
pelvis (acquired) (general) 738.6
  affecting fetus or newborn 763.1
  complicating delivery 653.1
    causing obstructed labor 660.1
  generally contracted 653.1
    causing obstructed labor 660.1
  inlet 653.2
    causing obstructed labor 660.1
  midpelvic 653.8
    causing obstructed labor 660.1
  midplane 653.8
    causing obstructed labor 660.1
  outlet 653.3
    causing obstructed labor 660.1
plantar fascia 728.71
premature
  atrial 427.61
  auricular 427.61
  auriculoventricular 427.61
  heart (junctional) (nodal) 427.60
  supraventricular 427.61
  ventricular 427.69

Contraction—*continued*
prostate 602.8
pylorus (*see also* Pylorospasm) 537.81
rectosigmoid (*see also* Obstruction, intestine) 560.9
rectum, rectal (sphincter) 564.89
    psychogenic 306.4
ring (Bandl's) 661.4
    affecting fetus or newborn 763.7
scar—*see* Cicatrix
sigmoid (*see also* Obstruction, intestine) 560.9
socket, eye 372.64
spine (*see also* Curvature, spine) 737.9
stomach 536.8
    hourglass 536.8
        congenital 750.7
        psychogenic 306.4
    psychogenic 306.4
tendon (sheath) (*see also* Short, tendon) 727.81
toe 735.8
ureterovesical orifice (postinfectional) 593.3
urethra 599.84
uterus 621.8
    abnormal 661.9
        affecting fetus or newborn 763.7
    clonic, hourglass or tetanic 661.4
        affecting fetus or newborn 763.7
    dyscoordinate 661.4
        affecting fetus or newborn 763.7
    hourglass 661.4
        affecting fetus or newborn 763.7
    hypotonic NEC 661.2
        affecting fetus or newborn 763.7
    incoordinate 661.4
        affecting fetus or newborn 763.7
    inefficient or poor 661.2
        affecting fetus or newborn 763.7
    irregular 661.2
        affecting fetus or newborn 763.7
    tetanic 661.4
        affecting fetus or newborn 763.7
vagina (outlet) 623.2
vesical 596.8
    neck or urethral orifice 596.0
visual field, generalized 368.45
Volkmann's (ischemic) 958.6
Contusion (skin surface intact) 924.9
with
    crush injury—*see* Crush
    dislocation—*see* Dislocation, by site
    fracture—*see* Fracture, by site
    internal injury—*see also* Injury, internal, by
        site
        heart—*see* Contusion, cardiac
        kidney—*see* Contusion, kidney
        liver—*see* Contusion, liver
        lung—*see* Contusion, lung
        spleen—*see* Contusion, spleen
    intracranial injury—*see* Injury, intracranial
    nerve injury—*see* Injury, nerve
    open wound—*see* Wound, open, by site
abdomen, abdominal (muscle) (wall) 922.2
    organ(s) NEC 868.00
adnexa, eye NEC 921.9
ankle 924.21
    with other parts of foot 924.20
arm 923.9
    lower (with elbow) 923.10
    upper 923.03
        with shoulder or axillary region 923.09

Contusion—*continued*
auditory canal (external) (meatus) (and other
    part(s) of neck, scalp, or face, except eye)
    920
auricle, ear (and other part(s) of neck, scalp, or
    face except eye) 920
axilla 923.02
    with shoulder or upper arm 923.09
back 922.31
bone NEC 924.9
brain (cerebral) (membrane) (with hemorrhage)
    851.8

*Note—Use the following fifth-digit
subclassification with categories 851-854:*

0 unspecified state of consciousness
1 with no loss of consciousness
*2 with brief [less than one hour] loss
    of consciousness*
*3 with moderate [1-24 hours] loss of
    consciousness*
*4 with prolonged [more than 24 hours] loss of
    consciousness and return to pre-existing
    conscious level*
*5 with prolonged [more than 24 hours] loss of
    consciousness, without return to pre-existing
    conscious level*
*Use fifth-digit 5 to designate when a patient is
unconscious and dies before regaining
conciousness, regardless of the duration of the
loss of conciousness*
*6 with loss of consciousness of unspecified
    duration*
9 with concussion, unspecified

with
    open intracranial wound 851.9
    skull fracture—*see* Fracture, skull, by site
cerebellum 851.4
    with open intracranial wound 851.5
cortex 851.0
    with open intracranial wound 851.1
occipital lobe 851.4
    with open intracranial wound 851.5
stem 851.4
    with open intracranial wound 851.5
breast 922.0
brow (and other part(s) of neck, scalp, or face,
    except eye) 920
buttock 922.32
canthus 921.1
cardiac 861.01
    with open wound into thorax 861.11
cauda equina (spine) 952.4
cerebellum—*see* Contusion, brain, cerebellum
cerebral—*see* Contusion, brain
cheek(s) (and other part(s) of neck, scalp, or
    face, except eye) 920
chest (wall) 922.1
chin (and other part(s) of neck, scalp, or face,
    except eye) 920
clitoris 922.4
conjunctiva 921.1
conus medullaris (spine) 952.4
cornea 921.3
corpus cavernosum 922.4
cortex (brain) (cerebral)—*see* Contusion, brain,
    cortex
costal region 922.1
ear (and other part(s) of neck, scalp, or face
    except eye) 920

Contusion—*continued*
  elbow 923.11
    with forearm 923.10
  epididymis 922.4
  epigastric region 922.2
  eye NEC 921.9
  eyeball 921.3
  eyelid(s) (and periocular area) 921.1
  face (and neck, or scalp any part, except eye) 920
  femoral triangle 922.2
  fetus or newborn 772.6
  finger(s) (nail) (subungual) 923.3
  flank 922.2
  foot (with ankle) (excluding toe(s)) 924.20
  forearm (and elbow) 923.10
  forehead (and other part(s) of neck, scalp, or face, except eye) 920
  genital organs, external 922.4
  globe (eye) 921.3
  groin 922.2
  gum(s) (and other part(s) of neck, scalp, or face, except eye) 920
  hand(s) (except fingers alone) 923.20
  head (any part, except eye) (and face) (and neck) 920
  heart—*see* Contusion, cardiac
  heel 924.20
  hip 924.01
    with thigh 924.00
  iliac region 922.2
  inguinal region 922.2
  internal organs (abdomen, chest, or pelvis) NEC—*see* Injury, internal, by site
  interscapular region 922.33
  iris (eye) 921.3
  kidney 866.01
    with open wound into cavity 866.11
  knee 924.11
    with lower leg 924.10
  labium (majus) (minus) 922.4
  lacrimal apparatus, gland, or sac 921.1
  larynx (and other part(s) of neck, scalp, or face, except eye) 920
  late effect—*see* Late, effects (of), contusion
  leg 924.5
    lower (with knee) 924.10
  lens 921.3
  lingual (and other part(s) of neck, scalp, or face, except eye) 920
  lip(s) (and other part(s) of neck, scalp, or face, except eye) 920
  liver 864.01
    with
      laceration—*see* Laceration, liver
      open wound into cavity 864.11
  lower extremity 924.5
    multiple sites 924.4
  lumbar region 922.31
  lung 861.21
    with open wound into thorax 861.31
  malar region (and other part(s) of neck, scalp, or face, except eye) 920
  mandibular joint (and other part(s) of neck, scalp, or face, except eye) 920
  mastoid region (and other part(s) of neck, scalp, or face, except eye) 920
  membrane, brain—*see* Contusion, brain
  midthoracic region 922.1
  mouth (and other part(s) of neck, scalp, or face, except eye) 920

Contusion—*continued*
  multiple sites (not classifiable to same three-digit category) 924.8
    lower limb 924.4
    trunk 922.8
    upper limb 923.8
  muscle NEC 924.9
  myocardium—*see* Contusion, cardiac
  nasal (septum) (and other part(s) of neck, scalp, or face, except eye) 920
  neck (and scalp, or face any part, except eye) 920
  nerve—*see* Injury, nerve, by site
  nose (and other part(s) of neck, scalp, or face, except eye) 920
  occipital region (scalp) (and neck or face, except eye) 920
    lobe—*see* Contusion, brain, occipital lobe
  orbit (region) (tissues) 921.2
  palate (soft) (and other part(s) of neck, scalp, or face, except eye) 920
  parietal region (scalp) (and neck, or face, except eye) 920
    lobe—*see* Contusion, brain
  penis 922.4
  pericardium—*see* Contusion, cardiac
  perineum 922.4
  periocular area 921.1
  pharynx (and other part(s) of neck, scalp, or face, except eye) 920
  popliteal space (*see also* Contusion, knee) 924.11
  prepuce 922.4
  pubic region 922.4
  pudenda 922.4
  pulmonary—*see* Contusion, lung
  quadriceps femoralis 924.00
  rib cage 922.1
  sacral region 922.32
  salivary ducts or glands (and other part(s) of neck, scalp, or face, except eye) 920
  scalp (and neck, or face any part, except eye) 920
  scapular region 923.01
    with shoulder or upper arm 923.09
  sclera (eye) 921.3
  scrotum 922.4
  shoulder 923.00
    with upper arm or axillar regions 923.09
  skin NEC 924.9
  skull 920
  spermatic cord 922.4
  spinal cord—*see also* Injury, spinal, by site
    cauda equina 952.4
    conus medullaris 952.4
  spleen 865.01
    with open wound into cavity 865.11
  sternal region 922.1
  stomach—*see* Injury, internal, stomach
  subconjunctival 921.1
  subcutaneous NEC 924.9
  submaxillary region (and other part(s) of neck, scalp, or face, except eye) 920
  submental region (and other part(s) of neck, scalp, or face, except eye) 920
  subperiosteal NEC 924.9
  supraclavicular fossa (and other part(s) of neck, scalp, or face, except eye) 920
  supraorbital (and other part(s) of neck, scalp, or face, except eye) 920
  temple (region) (and other part(s) of neck, scalp, or face, except eye) 920

Cord's angiopathy (*see also* Tuberculosis) 017.3
  [362.18]
Cordis ectopia 746.87
Corditis (spermatic) 608.4
Corectopia 743.46
Cori type glycogen storage disease —*see*
  Disease, glycogen storage
Cork-handlers' disease or lung 495.3
Corkscrew esophagus 530.5
Corlett's pyosis (impetigo) 684
Corn (infected) 700
Cornea—*see also* condition
  donor V59.5
  guttata (dystrophy) 371.57
  plana 743.41
Cornelia de Lange's syndrome (Amsterdam
  dwarf, mental retardation, and brachycephaly)
  759.89
Cornual gestation or pregnancy —*see*
  Pregnancy, cornual
Cornu cutaneum 702.8
Coronary (artery)—*see also* condition
  arising from aorta or pulmonary trunk 746.85
Corpora —*see also* condition
  amylacea (prostate) 602.8
  cavernosa—*see* condition
Corpulence (*see also* Obesity) 278.0
Corpus —*see* condition
Corrigan's disease —*see* Insufficiency, aortic
Corrosive burn —*see* Burn, by site
Corsican fever (*see also* Malaria) 084.6
Cortical —*see also* condition
  blindness 377.75
  necrosis, kidney (bilateral) 583.6
Corticoadrenal —*see* condition
Corticosexual syndrome 255.2
Coryza (acute) 460
  with grippe or influenza 487.1
  syphilitic 095.8
    congenital (chronic) 090.0
Costen's syndrome or complex 524.60
Costiveness (*see also* Constipation) 564.00
Costochondritis 733.6
Cotard's syndrome (paranoia) 297.1
Cot death 798.0
Cotia virus 059.8
Cotungo's disease 724.3
Cough 786.2
  with hemorrhage (*see also* Hemoptysis) 786.3
  affected 786.2
  bronchial 786.2
    with grippe or influenza 487.1
  chronic 786.2
  epidemic 786.2
  functional 306.1
  hemorrhagic 786.3
  hysterical 300.11
  laryngeal, spasmodic 786.2
  nervous 786.2
  psychogenic 306.1
  smokers' 491.0
  tea tasters' 112.89
Counseling NEC V65.40
  without complaint or sickness V65.49
  abuse victim NEC V62.89
    child V61.21
    partner V61.11
    spouse V61.11
  child abuse, maltreatment, or neglect V61.21

Counseling—*continued*
  contraceptive NEC V25.09
    device (intrauterine) V25.02
    maintenance V25.40
      intrauterine contraceptive device V25.42
      oral contraceptive (pill) V25.41
      specified type NEC V25.49
      subdermal implantable V25.43
    management NEC V25.9
      oral contraceptive (pill) V25.01
        emergency V25.03
        postcoital V25.03
    prescription NEC V25.02
      oral contraceptive (pill) V25.01
        emergency V25.03
        postcoital V25.03
      repeat prescription V25.41
    repeat prescription V25.40
    subdermal implantable V25.43
    surveillance V25.40
  dietary V65.3
  exercise V65.41
  expectant parents(s)
    pediatric pre-adoption visit V65.11
    pediatric pre-birth visit V65.11
  explanation of
    investigation finding NEC V65.49
    medication NEC V65.49
  family planning V25.09
    natural
      procreative V26.41
      to avoid pregnancy V25.04
  for nonattending third party V65.19
  genetic V26.33
  gonorrhea V65.45
  health (advice) (education) (instruction) NEC
    V65.49
  HIV V65.44
  human immunodeficiency virus V65.44
  injury prevention V65.43
  insulin pump training V65.46
  marital V61.10
  medical (for) V65.9
    boarding school resident V60.6
    condition not demonstrated V65.5
    feared complaint and no disease found V65.5
    institutional resident V60.6
    on behalf of another V65.19
    person living alone V60.3
  natural family planning
    procreative V26.41
    to avoid pregnancy V25.04
  parent(guardian)-child conflict V61.20
    adopted child V61.24
    biological child V61.23
    foster child V61.25
    specified problem NEC V61.29
  partner abuse
    perpetrator V61.12
    victim V61.11
  pediatric
    pre-adoption visit for adoptive parent(s)
      V65.11
    pre-birth visit for expectant parent(s) V65.11
  perpetrator of
    child abuse V62.83
      parental V61.22
    partner abuse V61.12
    spouse abuse V61.12
  procreative V65.49

Counseling—*continued*
  sex NEC V65.49
    transmitted disease NEC V65.45
      HIV V65.44
  specified reason NEC V65.49
  spousal abuse
    perpetrator V61.12
    victim V61.11
  substance use and abuse V65.42
  syphilis V65.45
  victim (of)
    abuse NEC V62.89
    child abuse V61.21
    partner abuse V61.11
    spousal abuse V61.11
Coupled rhythm 427.89
Couvelaire uterus (complicating delivery)—*see*
  Placenta, separation
Cowper's gland —*see* condition
Cowperitis (*see also* Urethritis) 597.89
  gonorrheal (acute) 098.0
    chronic or duration of 2 months or over 098.2
Cowpox (abortive) 051.01
  due to vaccination 999.0
  eyelid 051.01 *[373.5]*
    postvaccination 999.0 *[373.5]*
Coxa
  plana 732.1
  valga (acquired) 736.31
    congenital 755.61
    late effect of rickets 268.1
  vara (acquired) 736.32
    congenital 755.62
    late effect of rickets 268.1
Coxae malum senilis 715.25
Coxalgia (nontuberculous) 719.45
  tuberculous (*see also* Tuberculosis) 015.1 *[730.85]*
Coxalgic pelvis 736.30
Coxitis 716.65
Coxsackie (infection) (virus) 079.2
  central nervous system NEC 048
  endocarditis 074.22
  enteritis 008.67
  meningitis (aseptic) 047.0
  myocarditis 074.23
  pericarditis 074.21
  pharyngitis 074.0
  pleurodynia 074.1
  specific disease NEC 074.8
Crabs, meaning pubic lice 132.2
Crack baby 760.75
Cracked
  nipple 611.2
    puerperal, postpartum 676.1
  puerperal, postpartum 676.1
  tooth 521.81
Cradle cap 690.11
Craft neurosis 300.89
Craigiasis 007.8
Cramp(s) 729.82
  abdominal 789.0
  bathing 994.1
  colic 789.7
    infantile 789.7
    psychogenic 306.4
  due to immersion 994.1
  extremity (lower) (upper) NEC 729.82
  fireman 992.2
  heat 992.2
  hysterical 300.11
  immersion 994.1

Cramp(s)—*continued*
  intestinal 789.0
    psychogenic 306.4
  linotypist's 300.89
    organic 333.84
  muscle (extremity) (general) 729.82
    due to immersion 994.1
    hysterical 300.11
  occupational (hand) 300.89
    organic 333.84
  psychogenic 307.89
  salt depletion 276.1
  sleep related leg 327.52
  stoker 992.2
  stomach 789.0
  telegraphers' 300.89
    organic 333.84
  typists' 300.89
    organic 333.84
  uterus 625.8
    menstrual 625.3
  writers' 333.84
    organic 333.84
    psychogenic 300.89
Cranial —*see* condition
Cranioclasis, fetal 763.89
Craniocleidodysostosis 755.59
Craniofenestria (skull) 756.0
Craniolacunia (skull) 756.0
Craniopagus 759.4
Craniopathy, metabolic 733.3
Craniopharyngeal —*see* condition
Craniopharyngioma (M9350/1) 237.0
Craniorachischisis (totalis) 740.1
Cranioschisis 756.0
Craniostenosis 756.0
Craniosynostosis 756.0
Craniotabes (cause unknown) 733.3
  rachitic 268.1
  syphilitic 090.5
Craniotomy, fetal 763.89
Cranium —*see* condition
Craw-craw 125.3
CRBSI (catheter-related bloodstream infec-
  tion) 999.31
Creaking joint 719.60
  ankle 719.67
  elbow 719.62
  foot 719.67
  hand 719.64
  hip 719.65
  knee 719.66
  multiple sites 719.69
  pelvic region 719.65
  shoulder (region) 719.61
  specified site NEC 719.68
  wrist 719.63
Creeping
  eruption 126.9
  palsy 335.21
  paralysis 335.21
Crenated tongue 529.8
Creotoxism 005.9
Crepitus
  caput 756.0
  joint 719.60
    ankle 719.67
    elbow 719.62
    foot 719.67
    hand 719.64
    hip 719.65

Crepitus—*continued*
  joint—*continued*
    knee 719.66
    multiple sites 719.69
    pelvic region 719.65
    shoulder (region) 719.61
    specified site NEC 719.68
    wrist 719.63
Crescent or conus choroid, congenital 743.57
Cretin, cretinism (athyrotic) (congenital)
  (endemic) (metabolic) (nongoitrous)
  (sporadic) 243
  goitrous (sporadic) 246.1
  pelvis (dwarf type) (male type) 243
    with disproportion (fetopelvic) 653.1
      affecting fetus or newborn 763.1
      causing obstructed labor 660.1
        affecting fetus or newborn 763.1
  pituitary 253.3
Cretinoid degeneration 243
Creutzfeldt-Jakob disease (CJD) (syndrome)
  046.19
  with dementia
    with behavioral disturbance 046.19 *[294.11]*
    without behavioral disturbance 046.19
      [294.10]
  familial 046.19
  iatrogenic 046.19
  specified NEC 046.19
  sporadic 046.19
  variant (vCJD) 046.11
    with dementia
      with behavioral disturbance 046.11 *[294.11]*
      without behavioral disturbance 046.11
        [294.10]
Crib death 798.0
Cribriform hymen 752.49
Cri-du-chat syndrome 758.31
Crigler-Najjar disease or syndrome (congenital
  hyperbilirubinemia) 277.4
Crimean hemorrhagic fever 065.0
Criminalism 301.7
Crisis
  abdomen 789.0
  addisonian (acute adrenocortical insufficiency)
    255.41
  adrenal (cortical) 255.41
  asthmatic—*see* Asthma
  brain, cerebral (*see also* Disease,
    cerebrovascular, acute) 436
  celiac 579.0
  Dietl's 593.4
  emotional NEC 309.29
    acute reaction to stress 308.0
    adjustment reaction 309.9
    specific to childhood or adolescence 313.9
  gastric (tabetic) 094.0
  glaucomatocyclitic 364.22
  heart (*see also* Failure, heart) 428.9
  hypertensive—*see* Hypertension
  nitritoid
    correct substance properly administered
      458.29
    overdose or wrong substance given or taken
      961.1
  oculogyric 378.87
    psychogenic 306.7
  Pel's 094.0
  psychosexual identity 302.6
  rectum 094.0
  renal 593.81

Crisis—*continued*
  sickle cell 282.62
  stomach (tabetic) 094.0
  tabetic 094.0
  thyroid (*see also* Thyrotoxicosis) 242.9
  thyrotoxic (*see also* Thyrotoxicosis) 242.9
  vascular—*see* Disease, cerebrovascular, acute
Crocq's disease (acrocyanosis) 443.89
Crohn's disease (*see also* Enteritis, regional) 555.9
Cronkhite-Canada syndrome 211.3
Crooked septum, nasal 470
Cross
  birth (of fetus) complicating delivery 652.3
    with successful version 652.1
    causing obstructed labor 660.0
  bite, anterior or posterior 524.27
  eye (*see also* Esotropia) 378.00
Crossed ectopia of kidney 753.3
Crossfoot 754.50
Croup, croupus (acute) (angina) (catarrhal)
  (infective) (inflammatory) (laryngeal)
  (membranous) (nondiphtheritic)
  (pseudomembranous) 464.4
  asthmatic (*see also* Asthma) 493.9
  bronchial 466.0
  diphtheritic (membranous) 032.3
  false 478.75
  spasmodic 478.75
    diphtheritic 032.3
  stridulous 478.75
    diphtheritic 032.3
Crouzon's disease (craniofacial dysostosis)
  756.0
Crowding, teeth 524.31
CRST syndrome (cutaneous systemic sclerosis)
  710.1
Cruchet's disease (encephalitis lethargica) 049.8
Cruelty in children (*see also* Disturbance,
  conduct) 312.9
Crural ulcer (*see also* Ulcer, lower extremity)
  707.10
Crush, crushed, crushing (injury) 929.9
  abdomen 926.19
    internal—*see* Injury, internal, abdomen
  ankle 928.21
    with other parts of foot 928.20
  arm 927.9
    lower (and elbow) 927.10
    upper 927.03
      with shoulder or axillary region 927.09
  axilla 927.02
    with shoulder or upper arm 927.09
  back 926.11
  breast 926.19
  buttock 926.12
  cheek 925.1
  chest—*see* Injury, internal, chest
  ear 925.1
  elbow 927.11
    with forearm 927.10
  face 925.1
  finger(s) 927.3
    with hand(s) 927.20
    and wrist(s) 927.21
  flank 926.19
  foot, excluding toe(s) alone (with ankle) 928.20
  forearm (and elbow) 927.10
  genitalia, external (female) (male) 926.0
    internal—*see* Injury, internal, genital organ NEC
  hand, except finger(s) alone (and wrist) 927.20
  head—*see* Fracture, skull, by site

Crush, crushed, crushing—*continued*
  heel 928.20
  hip 928.01
    with thigh 928.00
  internal organ (abdomen, chest, or pelvis)—*see*
    Injury, internal, by site
  knee 928.11
    with leg, lower 928.10
  labium (majus) (minus) 926.0
  larynx 925.2
  late effect—*see* Late, effects (of), crushing
  leg 928.9
    lower 928.10
      and knee 928.11
    upper 928.00
  limb
    lower 928.9
      multiple sites 928.8
    upper 927.9
      multiple sites 927.8
  multiple sites NEC 929.0
  neck 925.2
  nerve—*see* Injury, nerve, by site
  nose 802.0
    open 802.1
  penis 926.0
  pharynx 925.2
  scalp 925.2
  scapular region 927.01
    with shoulder or upper arm 927.09
  scrotum 926.0
  shoulder 927.00
    with upper arm or axillary region 927.09
  skull or cranium—*see* Fracture, skull, by site
  spinal cord—*see* Injury, spinal, by site
  syndrome (complication of trauma) 958.5
  testis 926.0
  thigh (with hip) 928.00
  throat 925.2
  thumb(s) (and fingers) 927.3
  toe(s) 928.3
    with foot 928.20
      and ankle 928.21
  tonsil 925.2
  trunk 926.9
    chest—*see* Injury, internal, intrathoracic
      organs NEC
    internal organ—*see* Injury, internal, by site
    multiple sites 926.8
    specified site NEC 926.19
  vulva 926.0
  wrist 927.21
    with hand(s), except fingers alone 927.20
Crusta lactea 690.11
Crusts 782.8
Crutch paralysis 953.4
Cruveilhier's disease 335.21
Cruveilhier-Baumgarten cirrhosis, disease, or
  syndrome 571.5
Cruz-Chagas disease (*see also* Trypanosomiasis)
  086.2
Crying
  constant, continuous
    adolescent 780.95
    adult 780.95
    baby 780.92
    child 780.95
    infant 780.92
    newborn 780.92

Crying—*continued*
  excessive
    adolescent 780.95
    adult 780.95
    baby 780.92
    child 780.95
    infant 780.92
    newborn 780.92
Cryofibrinogenemia 273.2
Cryoglobulinemia (mixed) 273.2
Crypt (anal) (rectal) 569.49
Cryptitis (anal) (rectal) 569.49
Cryptococcosis (European) (pulmonary)
  (systemic) 117.5
Cryptococcus 117.5
  epidermicus 117.5
  neoformans, infection by 117.5
Cryptopapillitis (anus) 569.49
Cryptophthalmos (eyelid) 743.06
Cryptorchid, cryptorchism, cryptorchidism
  752.51
Cryptosporidiosis 007.4
  hepatobiliary 136.8
  respiratory 136.8
Cryptotia 744.29
Crystallopathy
  calcium pyrophosphate (*see also* Arthritis)
    275.49 *[712.2]*
  dicalcium phosphate (*see also* Arthritis) 275.49
    [712.1]
  gouty 274.00
  pyrophosphate NEC (*see also* Arthritis) 275.49
    [712.2]
  uric acid 274.00
Crystalluria 791.9
Csillag's disease (lichen sclerosus et atrophicus)
  701.0
Cuban itch 050.1
Cubitus
  valgus (acquired) 736.01
    congenital 755.59
    late effect of rickets 268.1
  varus (acquired) 736.02
    congenital 755.59
    late effect of rickets 268.1
Cultural deprivation V62.4
Cupping of optic disc 377.14
Curling's ulcer —*see* Ulcer, duodenum
Curling esophagus 530.5
Curschmann (-Batten) (-Steinert) disease or
  syndrome 359.21
Curvature
  organ or site, congenital NEC—*see* Distortion
  penis (lateral) 752.69
  Pott's (spinal) (*see also* Tuberculosis) 015.0
    [737.43]
  radius, idiopathic, progressive (congenital)
    755.54
  spine (acquired) (angular) (idiopathic)
    (incorrect) (postural) 737.9
    congenital 754.2
    due to or associated with
      Charcot-Marie-Tooth disease 356.1 *[737.40]*
      mucopolysaccharidosis 277.5 *[737.40]*
      neurofibromatosis 237.71 *[737.40]*
      osteitis
        deformans 731.0 *[737.40]*
        fibrosa cystica 252.01 *[737.40]*
      osteoporosis (*see also* Osteoporosis) 733.00
        [737.40]

Curvature—*continued*
  spine—*continued*
    due to—*continued*
      poliomyelitis (*see also* Poliomyelitis) 138
        [737.40]
      tuberculosis (Pott's curvature) (*see also*
        Tuberculosis) 015.0 *[737.43]*
      kyphoscoliotic (*see also* Kyphoscoliosis)
        737.30
      kyphotic (*see also* Kyphosis) 737.10
      late effect of rickets 268.1 *[737.40]*
      Pott's 015.0 *[737.40]*
      scoliotic (*see also* Scoliosis) 737.30
      specified NEC 737.8
      tuberculous 015.0 *[737.40]*
Cushing's
  basophilism, disease, or syndrome (iatrogenic)
    (idiopathic) (pituitary basophilism) (pituitary
    dependent) 255.0
  ulcer—*see* Ulcer, peptic
Cushingoid due to steroid therapy
  correct substance properly administered 255.0
  overdose or wrong substance given or taken
    962.0
Cut (external)—*see* Wound, open, by site
Cutaneous —*see also* condition
  hemorrhage 782.7
  horn (cheek) (eyelid) (mouth) 702.8
  larva migrans 126.9
Cutis —*see also* condition
  hyperelastic 756.83
    acquired 701.8
  laxa 756.83
    senilis 701.8
  marmorata 782.61
  osteosis 709.3
  pendula 756.83
    acquired 701.8
  rhomboidalis nuchae 701.8
  verticis gyrata 757.39
    acquired 701.8
Cyanopathy, newborn 770.83
Cyanosis 782.5
  autotoxic 289.7
  common atrioventricular canal 745.69
  congenital 770.83
  conjunctiva 372.71
  due to
    endocardial cushion defect 745.60
    nonclosure, foramen botalli 745.5
    patent foramen botalli 745.5
    persistent foramen ovale 745.5
  enterogenous 289.7
  fetus or newborn 770.83
  ostium primum defect 745.61
  paroxysmal digital 443.0
  retina, retinal 362.10
Cycle
  anovulatory 628.0
  menstrual, irregular 626.4
Cyclencephaly 759.89
Cyclical vomiting 536.2
  associated with migraine 346.2
  psychogenic 306.4
Cyclitic membrane 364.74
Cyclitis (*see also* Iridocyclitis) 364.3
  acute 364.00
    primary 364.01
    recurrent 364.02

Cyclitis—*continued*
  chronic 364.10
  in
    sarcoidosis 135 *[364.11]*
    tuberculosis (*see also* Tuberculosis) 017.3
      [364.11]
  Fuchs' heterochromic 364.21
  granulomatous 364.10
  lens induced 364.23
  nongranulomatous 364.00
  posterior 363.21
  primary 364.01
  recurrent 364.02
  secondary (noninfectious) 364.04
    infectious 364.03
  subacute 364.00
    primary 364.01
    recurrent 364.02
Cyclokeratitis —*see* Keratitis
Cyclophoria 378.44
Cyclopia, cyclops 759.89
Cycloplegia 367.51
Cyclospasm 367.53
Cyclosporiasis 007.5
Cyclothymia 301.13
Cyclothymic personality 301.13
Cyclotropia 378.33
Cyesis —*see* Pregnancy
Cylindroma (M8200/3)—*see also* Neoplasm, by
  site, malignant
  eccrine dermal (M8200/0)—*see* Neoplasm, skin, benign
  skin (M8200/0)—*see* Neoplasm, skin, benign
Cylindruria 791.7
Cyllosoma 759.89
Cynanche
  diphtheritic 032.3
  tonsillaris 475
Cynorexia 783.6
Cyphosis —*see* Kyphosis
Cyprus fever (*see also* Brucellosis) 023.9
Cyriax's syndrome (slipping rib) 733.99
Cyst (mucus) (retention) (serous) (simple)

> *Note*—In general, cysts are not neoplastic and
> are classified to the appropriate category for
> disease of the specified anatomical site. This
> generalization does not apply to certain types of
> cysts which are neoplastic in nature, for
> example, dermoid, nor does it apply to cysts of
> certain structures, for example, branchial cleft,
> which are classified as developmental
> anomalies. The following listing includes some
> of the most frequently reported sites of cysts as
> well as qualifiers which indicate the type of cyst.
> The latter qualifiers usually are not repeated
> under the anatomical sites. Since the code
> assignment for a given site may vary depending
> upon the type of cyst, the coder should refer to
> the listings under the specified type of cyst
> before consideration is given to the site.

  accessory, fallopian tube 752.11
  adenoid (infected) 474.8
  adrenal gland 255.8
    congenital 759.1
  air, lung 518.89
  allantoic 753.7
  alveolar process (jaw bone) 526.2
  amnion, amniotic 658.8

Cyst —*continued*
anterior chamber (eye) 364.60
  exudative 364.62
  implantation (surgical) (traumatic) 364.61
  parasitic 360.13
anterior nasopalatine 526.1
antrum 478.19
anus 569.49
apical (periodontal) (tooth) 522.8
appendix 543.9
arachnoid, brain 348.0
arytenoid 478.79
auricle 706.2
Baker's (knee) 727.51
  tuberculous (*see also* Tuberculosis) 015.2
Bartholin's gland or duct 616.2
bile duct (*see also* Disease, biliary) 576.8
bladder (multiple) (trigone) 596.8
Blessig's 362.62
blood, endocardial (*see also* Endocarditis)
  424.90
blue dome 610.0
bone (local) 733.20
  aneurysmal 733.22
  jaw 526.2
    developmental (odontogenic) 526.0
    fissural 526.1
    latent 526.89
  solitary 733.21
  unicameral 733.21
brain 348.0
  congenital 742.4
  hydatid (*see also* Echinococcus) 122.9
  third ventricle (colloid) 742.4
branchial (cleft) 744.42
branchiogenic 744.42
breast (benign) (blue dome) (pedunculated)
  (solitary) (traumatic) 610.0
  involution 610.4
  sebaceous 610.8
broad ligament (benign) 620.8
  embryonic 752.11
bronchogenic (mediastinal) (sequestration)
  518.89
  congenital 748.4
buccal 528.4
bulbourethral gland (Cowper's) 599.89
bursa, bursal 727.49
  pharyngeal 478.26
calcifying odontogenic (M9301/0) 213.1
  upper jaw (bone) 213.0
canal of Nuck (acquired) (serous) 629.1
  congenital 752.41
canthus 372.75
carcinomatous (M8010/3)—*see* Neoplasm, by
  site, malignant
cartilage (joint)—*see* Derangement, joint
cauda equina 336.8
cavum septi pellucidi NEC 348.0
celomic (pericardium) 746.89
cerebellopontine (angle)—*see* Cyst, brain
cerebellum—*see* Cyst, brain
cerebral—*see* Cyst, brain
cervical lateral 744.42
cervix 622.8
  embryonal 752.41
  nabothian (gland) 616.0
chamber, anterior (eye) 364.60
  exudative 364.62
  implantation (surgical) (traumatic) 364.61
  parasitic 360.13

Cyst —*continued*
chiasmal, optic NEC (*see also* Lesion, chiasmal)
  377.54
chocolate (ovary) 617.1
choledochal (congenital) 751.69
  acquired 576.8
choledochus 751.69
chorion 658.8
choroid plexus 348.0
chyle, mesentery 457.8
ciliary body 364.60
  exudative 364.64
  implantation 364.61
  primary 364.63
clitoris 624.8
coccyx (*see also* Cyst, bone) 733.20
colloid
  third ventricle (brain) 742.4
  thyroid gland—*see* Goiter
colon 569.89
common (bile) duct (*see also* Disease, biliary)
  576.8
congenital NEC 759.89
  adrenal glands 759.1
  epiglottis 748.3
  esophagus 750.4
  fallopian tube 752.11
  kidney 753.10
    multiple 753.19
    single 753.11
  larynx 748.3
  liver 751.62
  lung 748.4
  mediastinum 748.8
  ovary 752.0
  oviduct 752.11
  pancreas 751.7
  periurethral (tissue) 753.8
  prepuce NEC 752.69
    penis 752.69
  sublingual 750.26
  submaxillary gland 750.26
  thymus (gland) 759.2
  tongue 750.19
  ureterovesical orifice 753.4
  vulva 752.41
conjunctiva 372.75
cornea 371.23
corpora quadrigemina 348.0
corpus
  albicans (ovary) 620.2
  luteum (ruptured) 620.1
Cowper's gland (benign) (infected) 599.89
cranial meninges 348.0
craniobuccal pouch 253.8
craniopharyngeal pouch 253.8
cystic duct (*see also* Disease, gallbladder) 575.8
Cysticercus (any site) 123.1
Dandy-Walker 742.3
  with spina bifida (*see also* Spina bifida) 741.0
dental 522.8
  developmental 526.0
  eruption 526.0
  lateral periodontal 526.0
  primordial (keratocyst) 526.0
  root 522.8
dentigerous 526.0
  mandible 526.0
  maxilla 526.0

Cyst —*continued*
dermoid (M9084/0)—*see also* Neoplasm, by
site, benign
with malignant transformation (M9084/3)
183.0
implantation
external area or site (skin) NEC 709.8
iris 364.61
skin 709.8
vagina 623.8
vulva 624.8
mouth 528.4
oral soft tissue 528.4
sacrococcygeal 685.1
with abscess 685.0
developmental of ovary, ovarian 752.0
dura (cerebral) 348.0
spinal 349.2
ear (external) 706.2
echinococcal (*see also* Echinococcus) 122.9
embryonal
cervix uteri 752.41
genitalia, female external 752.41
uterus 752.3
vagina 752.41
endometrial 621.8
ectopic 617.9
endometrium (uterus) 621.8
ectopic—*see* Endometriosis
enteric 751.5
enterogenous 751.5
epidermal (inclusion) (*see also* Cyst, skin) 706.2
epidermoid (inclusion) (*see also* Cyst, skin)
706.2
mouth 528.4
not of skin—*see* Cyst, by site
oral soft tissue 528.4
epididymis 608.89
epiglottis 478.79
epiphysis cerebri 259.8
epithelial (inclusion) (*see also* Cyst, skin) 706.2
epoophoron 752.11
eruption 526.0
esophagus 530.89
ethmoid sinus 478.19
eye (retention) 379.8
congenital 743.03
posterior segment, congenital 743.54
eyebrow 706.2
eyelid (sebaceous) 374.84
infected 373.13
sweat glands or ducts 374.84
falciform ligament (inflammatory) 573.8
fallopian tube 620.8
congenital 752.11
female genital organs NEC 629.89
fimbrial (congenital) 752.11
fissural (oral region) 526.1
follicle (atretic) (graafian) (ovarian) 620.0
nabothian (gland) 616.0
follicular (atretic) (ovarian) 620.0
dentigerous 526.0
frontal sinus 478.19
gallbladder or duct 575.8
ganglion 727.43
Gartner's duct 752.41
gas, of mesentery 568.89
gingiva 523.8
gland of moll 374.84
globulomaxillary 526.1
graafian follicle 620.0

Cyst —*continued*
granulosal lutein 620.2
hemangiomatous (M9121/0) (*see also*
Hemangioma) 228.00
hydatid (*see also* Echinococcus) 122.9
fallopian tube (Morgagni) 752.11
liver NEC 122.8
lung NEC 122.9
Morgagni 752.89
fallopian tube 752.11
specified site NEC 122.9
hymen 623.8
embryonal 752.41
hypopharynx 478.26
hypophysis, hypophyseal (duct) (recurrent)
253.8
cerebri 253.8
implantation (dermoid)
anterior chamber (eye) 364.61
external area or site (skin) NEC 709.8
iris 364.61
vagina 623.8
vulva 624.8
incisor, incisive canal 526.1
inclusion (epidermal) (epithelial) (epidermoid)
(mucous) (squamous) (*see also* Cyst, skin)
706.2
not of skin—*see* Neoplasm, by site, benign
intestine (large) (small) 569.89
intracranial—*see* Cyst, brain
intraligamentous 728.89
knee 717.89
intrasellar 253.8
iris (idiopathic) 364.60
exudative 364.62
implantation (surgical) (traumatic) 364.61
miotic pupillary 364.55
parasitic 360.13
Iwanoff's 362.62
jaw (bone) (aneurysmal) (extravasation)
(hemorrhagic) (traumatic) 526.2
developmental (odontogenic) 526.0
fissural 526.1
keratin 706.2
kidney (congenital) 753.10
acquired 593.2
calyceal (*see also* Hydronephrosis) 591
multiple 753.19
pyelogenic (*see also* Hydronephrosis) 591
simple 593.2
single 753.11
solitary (not congenital) 593.2
labium (majus) (minus) 624.8
sebaceous 624.8
lacrimal
apparatus 375.43
gland or sac 375.12
larynx 478.79
lens 379.39
congenital 743.39
lip (gland) 528.5
liver 573.8
congenital 751.62
hydatid (*see also* Echinococcus) 122.8
granulosis 122.0
multilocularis 122.5
lung 518.89
congenital 748.4
giant bullous 492.0
lutein 620.1
lymphangiomatous (M9173/0) 228.1

Cyst —*continued*
lymphoepithelial
  mouth 528.4
  oral soft tissue 528.4
macula 362.54
malignant (M8000/3)—*see* Neoplasm, by site,
  malignant
mammary gland (sweat gland) (*see also* Cyst,
  breast) 610.0
mandible 526.2
  dentigerous 526.0
  radicular 522.8
maxilla 526.2
  dentigerous 526.0
  radicular 522.8
median
  anterior maxillary 526.1
  palatal 526.1
mediastinum (congenital) 748.8
meibomian (gland) (retention) 373.2
  infected 373.12
membrane, brain 348.0
meninges (cerebral) 348.0
  spinal 349.2
meniscus knee 717.5
mesentery, mesenteric (gas) 568.89
  chyle 457.8
  gas 568.89
mesonephric duct 752.89
mesothelial
  peritoneum 568.89
  pleura (peritoneal) 568.89
milk 611.5
miotic pupillary (iris) 364.55
Morgagni (hydatid) 752.89
  fallopian tube 752.11
mouth 528.4
Müllerian duct 752.89
  appendix testis 608.89
  cervix (embryonal) 752.41
  fallopian tube 752.11
  prostatic utricle 599.89
  vagina (embryonal) 752.41
multilocular (ovary) (M8000/1) 239.5
myometrium 621.8
nabothian (follicle) (ruptured) 616.0
nasal sinus 478.19
nasoalveolar 528.4
nasolabial 528.4
nasopalatine (duct) 526.1
  anterior 526.1
nasopharynx 478.26
neoplastic (M8000/1)—*see also* Neoplasm, by
  site, unspecified nature
  benign (M8000/0)—*see* Neoplasm, by site, benign
  uterus 621.8
nervous system—*see* Cyst, brain
neuroenteric 742.59
neuroepithelial ventricle 348.0
nipple 610.0
nose 478.19
  skin of 706.2
odontogenic, developmental 526.0
omentum (lesser) 568.89
  congenital 751.8
oral soft tissue (dermoid) (epidermoid)
  (lymphoepithelial) 528.4
ora serrata 361.19
orbit 376.81

Cyst —*continued*
ovary, ovarian (twisted) 620.2
  adherent 620.2
  chocolate 617.1
  corpus
    albicans 620.2
    luteum 620.1
  dermoid (M9084/0) 220
  developmental 752.0
  due to failure of involution NEC 620.2
  endometrial 617.1
  follicular (atretic) (graafian) (hemorrhagic)
    620.0
  hemorrhagic 620.2
  in pregnancy or childbirth 654.4
    affecting fetus or newborn 763.89
    causing obstructed labor 660.2
      affecting fetus or newborn 763.1
  multilocular (M8000/1) 239.5
  pseudomucinous (M8470/0) 220
  retention 620.2
  serous 620.2
  theca lutein 620.2
  tuberculous (*see also* Tuberculosis) 016.6
  unspecified 620.2
oviduct 620.8
palatal papilla (jaw) 526.1
palate 526.1
  fissural 526.1
  median (fissural) 526.1
palatine, of papilla 526.1
pancreas, pancreatic 577.2
  congenital 751.7
  false 577.2
  hemorrhagic 577.2
  true 577.2
paralabral
  hip 718.85
  shoulder 840.7
paramesonephric duct - see Cyst, Müllerian duct
paranephric 593.2
para ovarian 752.11
paraphysis, cerebri 742.4
parasitic NEC 136.9
parathyroid (gland) 252.8
paratubal (fallopian) 620.8
paraurethral duct 599.89
paroophoron 752.11
parotid gland 527.6
  mucous extravasation or retention 527.6
parovarian 752.11
pars planus 364.60
  exudative 364.64
  primary 364.63
pelvis, female
  in pregnancy or childbirth 654.4
    affecting fetus or newborn 763.89
    causing obstructed labor 660.2
      affecting fetus or newborn 763.1
penis (sebaceous) 607.89
periapical 522.8
pericardial (congenital) 746.89
  acquired (secondary) 423.8
pericoronal 526.0
perineural (Tarlov's) 355.9
periodontal 522.8
  lateral 526.0
peripancreatic 577.2
peripelvic (lymphatic) 593.2
peritoneum 568.89
  chylous 457.8

Cyst —*continued*
pharynx (wall) 478.26
pilonidal (infected) (rectum) 685.1
  with abscess 685.0
  malignant (M9084/3) 173.5
pituitary (duct) (gland) 253.8
placenta (amniotic)—*see* Placenta, abnormal
pleura 519.8
popliteal 727.51
porencephalic 742.4
  acquired 348.0
postanal (infected) 685.1
  with abscess 685.0
posterior segment of eye, congenital 743.54
postmastoidectomy cavity 383.31
preauricular 744.47
prepuce 607.89
  congenital 752.69
primordial (jaw) 526.0
prostate 600.3
pseudomucinous (ovary) (M8470/0) 220
pudenda (sweat glands) 624.8
pupillary, miotic 364.55
  sebaceous 624.8
radicular (residual) 522.8
radiculodental 522.8
ranular 527.6
Rathke's pouch 253.8
rectum (epithelium) (mucous) 569.49
renal—*see* Cyst, kidney
residual (radicular) 522.8
retention (ovary) 620.2
retina 361.19
  macular 362.54
  parasitic 360.13
  primary 361.13
  secondary 361.14
retroperitoneal 568.89
sacrococcygeal (dermoid) 685.1
  with abscess 685.0
salivary gland or duct 527.6
  mucous extravasation or retention 527.6
Sampson's 617.1
sclera 379.19
scrotum (sebaceous) 706.2
  sweat glands 706.2
sebaceous (duct) (gland) 706.2
  breast 610.8
  eyelid 374.84
  genital organ NEC
    female 629.89
    male 608.89
  scrotum 706.2
semilunar cartilage (knee) (multiple) 717.5
seminal vesicle 608.89
serous (ovary) 620.2
sinus (antral) (ethmoidal) (frontal) (maxillary)
    (nasal) (sphenoidal) 478.19
Skene's gland 599.89
skin (epidermal) (epidermoid, inclusion)
    (epithelial) (inclusion) (retention)
    (sebaceous) 706.2
  breast 610.8
  eyelid 374.84
  genital organ NEC
    female 629.89
    male 608.89
  neoplastic 216.3
  scrotum 706.2
  sweat gland or duct 705.89

Cyst —*continued*
solitary
  bone 733.21
  kidney 593.2
spermatic cord 608.89
sphenoid sinus 478.19
spinal meninges 349.2
spine (*see also* Cyst, bone) 733.20
spleen NEC 289.59
  congenital 759.0
  hydatid (*see also* Echinococcus) 122.9
spring water (pericardium) 746.89
subarachnoid 348.0
  intrasellar 793.0
subdural (cerebral) 348.0
  spinal cord 349.2
sublingual gland 527.6
  mucous extravasation or retention 527.6
submaxillary gland 527.6
  mucous extravasation or retention 527.6
suburethral 599.89
suprarenal gland 255.8
suprasellar—*see* Cyst, brain
sweat gland or duct 705.89
sympathetic nervous system 337.9
synovial 727.40
  popliteal space 727.51
Tarlov's 355.9
tarsal 373.2
tendon (sheath) 727.42
testis 608.89
theca-lutein (ovary) 620.2
Thornwaldt's, Tornwaldt's 478.26
thymus (gland) 254.8
thyroglossal (duct) (infected) (persistent) 759.2
thyroid (gland) 246.2
  adenomatous—*see* Goiter, nodular
  colloid (*see also* Goiter) 240.9
thyrolingual duct (infected) (persistent) 759.2
tongue (mucous) 529.8
tonsil 474.8
tooth (dental root) 522.8
tubo-ovarian 620.8
  inflammatory 614.1
tunica vaginalis 608.89
turbinate (nose) (*see also* Cyst, bone) 733.20
Tyson's gland (benign) (infected) 607.89
umbilicus 759.89
urachus 753.7
ureter 593.89
ureterovesical orifice 593.89
  congenital 753.4
urethra 599.84
urethral gland (Cowper's) 599.89
uterine
  ligament 620.8
    embryonic 752.11
  tube 620.8
uterus (body) (corpus) (recurrent) 621.8
  embryonal 752.3
utricle (ear) 386.8
  prostatic 599.89
utriculus masculinus 599.89
vagina, vaginal (squamous cell) (wall) 623.8
  embryonal 752.41
  implantation 623.8
  inclusion 623.8
vallecula, vallecular 478.79
ventricle, neuroepithelial 348.0
verumontanum 599.89
vesical (orifice) 596.8

Cyst —*continued*
 vitreous humor 379.29
 vulva (sweat glands) 624.8
  congenital 752.41
  implantation 624.8
  inclusion 624.8
  sebaceous gland 624.8
  vulvovaginal gland 624.8
  wolffian 752.89
Cystadenocarcinoma (M8440/3)—*see also*
  Neoplasm, by site, malignant
 bile duct type (M8161/3) 155.1
 endometrioid (M8380/3)—*see* Neoplasm, by
  site, malignant
 mucinous (M8470/3)
  papillary (M8471/3)
   specified site—*see* Neoplasm, by site,
    malignant
   unspecified site 183.0
  specified site—*see* Neoplasm, by site,
   malignant
  unspecified site 183.0
 papillary (M8450/3)
  mucinous (M8471/3)
   specified site—*see* Neoplasm, by site,
    malignant
   unspecified site 183.0
  pseudomucinous (M8471/3)
   specified site—*see* Neoplasm, by site,
    malignant
   unspecified site 183.0
  serous (M8460/3)
   specified site—*see* Neoplasm, by site,
    malignant
   unspecified site 183.0
  specified site—*see* Neoplasm, by site,
   malignant
  unspecified 183.0
 pseudomucinous (M8470/3)
  papillary (M8471/3)
   specified site—*see* Neoplasm, by site,
    malignant
   unspecified site 183.0
  specified site—*see* Neoplasm, by site,
   malignant
  unspecified site 183.0
 serous (M8441/3)
  papillary (M8460/3)
   specified site—*see* Neoplasm, by site,
    malignant
   unspecified site 183.0
  specified site—*see* Neoplasm, by site,
   malignant
  unspecified site 183.0
Cystadenofibroma (M9013/0)
 clear cell (M8313/0)—*see* Neoplasm, by site,
  benign
 endometrioid (M8381/0) 220
  borderline malignancy (M8381/1) 236.2
  malignant (M8381/3) 183.0
 mucinous (M9015/0)
  specified site—*see* Neoplasm, by site, benign
  unspecified site 220
 serous (M9014/0)
  specified site—*see* Neoplasm, by site, benign
  unspecified site 220
 specified site—*see* Neoplasm, by site, benign
 unspecified site 220

Cystadenoma (M8440/0)—*see also* Neoplasm,
  by site, benign
 bile duct (M8161/0) 211.5
 endometrioid (M8380/0)—*see also* Neoplasm,
  by site, benign
  borderline malignancy (M8380/1)—*see*
   Neoplasm, by site, uncertain behavior
 malignant (M8440/3)—*see* Neoplasm, by site,
  malignant
 mucinous (M8470/0)
  borderline malignancy (M8470/1)
   specified site—*see* Neoplasm, uncertain
    behavior
   unspecified site 236.2
  papillary (M8471/0)
   borderline malignancy (M8471/1)
    specified site—*see* Neoplasm, by site,
     uncertain behavior
    unspecified site 236.2
   specified site—*see* Neoplasm, by site,
    benign
   unspecified site 220
  specified site—*see* Neoplasm, by site, benign
  unspecified site 220
 papillary (M8450/0)
  borderline malignancy (M8450/1)
   specified site—*see* Neoplasm, by site,
    uncertain behavior
   unspecified site 236.2
  lymphomatosum (M8561/0) 210.2
  mucinous (M8471/0)
   borderline malignancy (M8471/1)
    specified site—*see* Neoplasm, by site,
     uncertain behavior
    unspecified site 236.2
   specified site—*see* Neoplasm, by site,
    benign
   unspecified site 220
  pseudomucinous (M8471/0)
   borderline malignancy (M8471/1)
    specified site—*see* Neoplasm, by site,
     uncertain behavior
    unspecified site 236.2
   specified site—*see* Neoplasm, by site,
    benign
   unspecified site 220
  serous (M8460/0)
   borderline malignancy (M8460/1)
    specified site—*see* Neoplasm, by site,
     uncertain behavior
    unspecified site 236.2
   specified site—*see* Neoplasm, by site,
    benign
   unspecified site 220
  specified site—*see* Neoplasm, by site, benign
  unspecified site 220
 pseudomucinous (M8470/0)
  borderline malignancy (M8470/1)
   specified site—*see* Neoplasm, by site,
    uncertain behavior
   unspecified site 236.2
  papillary (M8471/0)
   borderline malignancy (M8471/1)
    specified site—*see* Neoplasm, by site,
     uncertain behavior
    unspecified site 236.2
   specified site—*see* Neoplasm, by site,
    benign
   unspecified site 220
  specified site—*see* Neoplasm, by site, benign
  unspecified site 220

Cystadenoma—*continued*
serous (M8441/0)
  borderline malignancy (M8441/1)
    specified site—*see* Neoplasm, by site,
      uncertain behavior
    unspecified site 236.2
  papillary (M8460/0)
    borderline malignancy (M8460/1)
      specified site—*see* Neoplasm, by site,
        uncertain behavior
      unspecified site 236.2
    specified site—*see* Neoplasm, by site,
      benign
    unspecified site 220
  specified site—*see* Neoplasm, by site, benign
  unspecified site 220
  thyroid 226
Cystathioninemia 270.4
Cystathioninuria 270.4
Cystic —*see also* condition
  breast, chronic 610.1
  corpora lutea 620.1
  degeneration, congenital
    brain 742.4
    kidney (*see also* Cystic, disease, kidney)
      753.10
  disease
    breast, chronic 610.1
    kidney, congenital 753.10
      medullary 753.16
      multiple 753.19
      polycystic—*see* Polycystic, kidney
      single 753.11
      specified NEC 753.19
    liver, congenital 751.62
    lung 518.89
      congenital 748.4
    pancreas, congenital 751.7
    semilunar cartilage 717.5
  duct—*see* condition
  eyeball, congenital 743.03
  fibrosis (pancreas) 277.00
    with
      manifestations
        gastrointestinal 277.03
        pulmonary 277.02
        specified NEC 277.09
      meconium ileus 277.01
      pulmonary exacerbation 277.02
  hygroma (M9173/0) 228.1
  kidney, congenital 753.10
    medullary 753.16
    multiple 753.19
    polycystic—*see* Polycystic, kidney
    single 753.11
    specified NEC 753.19
  liver, congenital 751.62
  lung 518.89
    congenital 748.4
  mass—*see* Cyst
  mastitis, chronic 610.1
  ovary 620.2
  pancreas, congenital 751.7
Cysticerciasis 123.1
Cysticercosis (mammary) (subretinal) 123.1
Cysticercus 123.1
  cellulosae infestation 123.1
Cystinosis (malignant) 270.0
Cystinuria 270.0

Cystitis (bacillary) (colli) (diffuse) (exudative)
(hemorrhagic) (purulent) (recurrent) (septic)
(suppurative) (ulcerative) 595.9
  with
    abortion—*see* Abortion, by type, with urinary
      tract infection
    ectopic pregnancy (*see also* categories
      633.0-633.9) 639.8
    fibrosis 595.1
    leukoplakia 595.1
    malakoplakia 595.1
    metaplasia 595.1
    molar pregnancy (*see also* categories 630-632)
      639.8
  actinomycotic 039.8 *[595.4]*
  acute 595.0
    of trigone 595.3
  allergic 595.89
  amebic 006.8 *[595.4]*
  bilharzial 120.9 *[595.4]*
  blennorrhagic (acute) 098.11
    chronic or duration of 2 months or more
      098.31
  bullous 595.89
  calculous 594.1
  chlamydial 099.53
  chronic 595.2
    interstitial 595.1
    of trigone 595.3
  complicating pregnancy, childbirth, or
    puerperium 646.6
    affecting fetus or newborn 760.1
  cystic(a) 595.81
  diphtheritic 032.84
  echinococcal
    granulosus 122.3 *[595.4]*
    multilocularis 122.6 *[595.4]*
  emphysematous 595.89
  encysted 595.81
  follicular 595.3
  following
    abortion 639.8
    ectopic or molar pregnancy 639.8
  gangrenous 595.89
  glandularis 595.89
  gonococcal (acute) 098.11
    chronic or duration of 2 months or more
      098.31
  incrusted 595.89
  interstitial 595.1
  irradiation 595.82
  irritation 595.89
  malignant 595.89
  monilial 112.2
  of trigone 595.3
  panmural 595.1
  polyposa 595.89
  prostatic 601.3
  radiation 595.82
  Reiter's (abacterial) 099.3
  specified NEC 595.89
  subacute 595.2
  submucous 595.1
  syphilitic 095.8
  trichomoniasis 131.09
  tuberculous (*see also* Tuberculosis) 016.1
  ulcerative 595.1

Cystocele
  female (without uterine prolapse) 618.01
    with uterine prolapse 618.4
      complete 618.3
      incomplete 618.2
    lateral 618.02
    midline 618.01
    paravaginal 618.02
  in pregnancy or childbirth 654.4
    affecting fetus or newborn 763.89
    causing obstructed labor 660.2
      affecting fetus or newborn 763.1
  male 596.8
Cystoid
  cicatrix limbus 372.64
  degeneration macula 362.53
Cystolithiasis 594.1
Cystoma (M8440/0)—*see also* Neoplasm, by
    site, benign
  endometrial, ovary 617.1
  mucinous (M8470/0)
    specified site—*see* Neoplasm, by site, benign
    unspecified site 220
  serous (M8441/0)
    specified site—*see* Neoplasm, by site, benign
    unspecified site 220
  simple (ovary) 620.2
Cystoplegia 596.53
Cystoptosis 596.8
Cystopyelitis (*see also* Pyelitis) 590.80
Cystorrhagia 596.8
Cystosarcoma phyllodes (M9020/1) 238.3
  benign (M9020/0) 217
  malignant (M9020/3)—*see* Neoplasm, breast,
    malignant
Cystostomy status V44.50
  appendico-vesicostomy V44.52
  cutaneous-vesicostomy V44.51
  specified type NEC V44.59
  with complication 997.5
Cystourethritis (*see also* Urethritis) 597.89
Cystourethrocele (*see also* Cystocele)
  female (without uterine prolapse) 618.09
    with uterine prolapse 618.4
      complete 618.3
      incomplete 618.2
  male 596.8
Cytomegalic inclusion disease 078.5
  congenital 771.1
Cytomycosis, reticuloendothelial (*see also*
    Histoplasmosis, American) 115.00
Cytopenia 289.9
  refractory
    with
      multilineage dysplasia (RCMD) 238.72
        and ringed sideroblasts (RCMD-RS)
          238.72

D

Daae (-Finsen) disease (epidemic pleurodynia) 074.1
Dabney's grip 074.1
Da Costa's syndrome (neurocirculatory asthenia) 306.2
Dacryoadenitis, dacryadenitis 375.00
  acute 375.01
  chronic 375.02
Dacryocystitis 375.30
  acute 375.32
  chronic 375.42
  neonatal 771.6
  phlegmonous 375.33
  syphilitic 095.8
    congenital 090.0
  trachomatous, active 076.1
    late effect 139.1
  tuberculous (*see also* Tuberculosis) 017.3
Dacryocystoblennorrhea 375.42
Dacryocystocele 375.43
Dacryolith, dacryolithiasis 375.57
Dacryoma 375.43
Dacryopericystitis (acute) (subacute) 375.32
  chronic 375.42
Dacryops 375.11
Dacryosialadenopathy, atrophic 710.2
Dacryostenosis 375.56
  congenital 743.65
Dactylitis
  bone (*see also* Osteomyelitis) 730.2
  sickle-cell 282.62
    Hb-C 282.64
    Hb-SS 282.62
    specified NEC 282.69
  syphilitic 095.5
  tuberculous (*see also* Tuberculosis) 015.5
Dactylolysis spontanea 136.0
Dactylosymphysis (*see also* Syndactylism) 755.10
Damage
  arteriosclerotic—*see* Arteriosclerosis
  brain 348.9
    anoxic, hypoxic 348.1
      during or resulting from a procedure 997.01
      ischemic, in newborn 768.70
        mild 768.71
        moderate 768.72
        severe 768.73
    child NEC 343.9
    due to birth injury 767.0
    minimal (child) (*see also* Hyperkinesia) 314.9
    newborn 767.0
  cardiac—*see also* Disease, heart
  cardiorenal (vascular) (*see also* Hypertension, cardiorenal) 404.90
  central nervous system—*see* Damage, brain
  cerebral NEC—*see* Damage, brain
  coccyx, complicating delivery 665.6
  coronary (*see also* Ischemia, heart) 414.9
  eye, birth injury 767.8
  heart—*see also* Disease, heart
    valve—*see* Endocarditis
  hypothalamus NEC 348.9
  liver 571.9
    alcoholic 571.3
  medication 995.20

Damage—*continued*
  myocardium (*see also* Degeneration, myocardial) 429.1
  pelvic
    joint or ligament, during delivery 665.6
    organ NEC
      with
        abortion—*see* Abortion, by type, with damage to pelvic organs
        ectopic pregnancy (*see also* categories 633.0-633.9) 639.2
        molar pregnancy (*see also* categories 630-632) 639.2
      during delivery 665.5
      following
        abortion 639.2
        ectopic or molar pregnancy 639.2
  renal (*see also* Disease, renal) 593.9
  skin, solar 692.79
    acute 692.72
    chronic 692.74
  subendocardium, subendocardial (*see also* Degeneration, myocardial) 429.1
  vascular 459.9
Dameshek's syndrome (erythroblastic anemia) 282.49
Dana-Putnam syndrome (subacute combined sclerosis with pernicious anemia) 281.0 *[336.2]*
Danbolt (-Closs) syndrome (acrodermatitis enteropathica) 686.8
Dandruff 690.18
Dandy fever 061
Dandy-Walker deformity or syndrome (atresia, foramen of Magendie) 742.3
  with spina bifida (*see also* Spina bifida) 741.0
Dangle foot 736.79
Danielssen's disease (anesthetic leprosy) 030.1
Danlos' syndrome 756.83
Darier's disease (congenital) (keratosis follicularis) 757.39
  due to vitamin A deficiency 264.8
  meaning erythema annulare centrifugum 695.0
Darier-Roussy sarcoid 135
Dark area on retina 239.81
Darling's
  disease (*see also* Histoplasmosis, American) 115.00
  histoplasmosis (*see also* Histoplasmosis, American) 115.00
Dartre 054.9
Darwin's tubercle 744.29
Davidson's anemia (refractory) 284.9
Davies' disease 425.0
Davies-Colley syndrome (slipping rib) 733.99
Dawson's encephalitis 046.2
Day blindness (*see also* Blindness, day) 368.60
Dead
  fetus
    retained (in utero) 656.4
      early pregnancy (death before 22 completed weeks gestation) 632
      late (death after 22 completed weeks gestation) 656.4
    syndrome 641.3
  labyrinth 386.50
  ovum, retained 631

Deaf and dumb NEC 389.7
Deaf mutism (acquired) (congenital) NEC 389.7
  endemic 243
  hysterical 300.11
  syphilitic, congenital 090.0
Deafness (acquired) (complete) (congenital)
  (hereditary) (middle ear) (partial) 389.9
  with
    blindness V49.85
    blue sclera and fragility of bone 756.51
  auditory fatigue 389.9
  aviation 993.0
    nerve injury 951.5
  boilermakers' 951.5
  central 389.14
    with conductive hearing loss 389.20
      bilateral 389.22
      unilateral 389.21
  conductive (air) 389.00
    with sensorineural hearing loss 389.20
      bilateral 389.22
      unilateral 389.21
    bilateral 389.06
    combined types 389.08
    external ear 389.01
    inner ear 389.04
    middle ear 389.03
    multiple types 389.08
    tympanic membrane 389.02
    unilateral 389.05
  emotional (complete) 300.11
  functional (complete) 300.11
  high frequency 389.8
  hysterical (complete) 300.11
  injury 951.5
  low frequency 389.8
  mental 784.69
  mixed conductive and sensorineural 389.20
    bilateral 389.22
    unilateral 389.21
  nerve
    with conductive hearing loss 389.20
      bilateral 389.22
      unilateral 389.21
    bilateral 389.12
    unilateral 389.13
  neural
    with conductive hearing loss 389.20
      bilateral 389.22
      unilateral 389.21
    bilateral 389.12
    unilateral 389.13
  noise-induced 388.12
    nerve injury 951.5
  nonspeaking 389.7
  perceptive 389.10
    with conductive hearing loss 389.20
      bilateral 389.22
      unilateral 389.21
    central 389.14
    neural
      bilateral 389.12
      unilateral 389.13
    sensorineural 389.10
      asymmetrical 389.16
      bilateral 389.18
      unilateral 389.15
    sensory
      bilateral 389.11
      unilateral 389.17
  psychogenic (complete) 306.7

Deafness—*continued*
  sensorineural (*see also* Deafness, perceptive)
    389.10
    asymmetrical 389.16
    bilateral 389.18
    unilateral 389.15
  sensory
    with conductive hearing loss 389.20
      bilateral 389.22
      unilateral 389.21
    bilateral 389.11
    unilateral 389.17
  specified type NEC 389.8
  sudden NEC 388.2
  syphilitic 094.89
  transient ischemic 388.02
  transmission—*see* Deafness, conductive
  traumatic 951.5
  word (secondary to organic lesion) 784.69
    developmental 315.31
Death
  after delivery (cause not stated) (sudden) 674.9
  anesthetic
    due to
      correct substance properly administered
        995.4
      overdose or wrong substance given 968.4
        specified anesthetic—*see* Table of drugs
          and chemicals
    during delivery 668.9
  brain 348.89
  cardiac (sudden) (SCD)—code to underlying
    condition
    family history of V17.41
    personal history of, successfully resuscitated
      V12.53
  cause unknown 798.2
  cot (infant) 798.0
  crib (infant) 798.0
  fetus, fetal (cause not stated) (intrauterine) 779.9
    early, with retention (before 22 completed
      weeks gestation) 632
    from asphyxia or anoxia (before labor) 768.0
      during labor 768.1
    late, affecting management of pregnancy (after
      22 completed weeks gestation) 656.4
  from pregnancy NEC 646.9
  instantaneous 798.1
  intrauterine (*see also* Death, fetus) 779.9
    complicating pregnancy 656.4
  maternal, affecting fetus or newborn 761.6
  neonatal NEC 779.9
  sudden (cause unknown) 798.1
    cardiac (SCD)
      family history of V17.41
      personal history of, successfully resuscitated
        V12.53
    during delivery 669.9
    under anesthesia NEC 668.9
    infant, syndrome (SIDS) 798.0
    puerperal, during puerperium 674.9
  unattended (cause unknown) 798.9
  under anesthesia NEC
    due to
      correct substance properly administered
        995.4
      overdose or wrong substance given 968.4
        specified anesthetic—*see* Table of drugs
          and chemicals
    during delivery 668.9
  violent 798.1

de Beurmann-Gougerot disease (sporotrichosis) 117.1
Debility (general) (infantile) (postinfectional) 799.3
  with nutritional difficulty 269.9
  congenital or neonatal NEC 779.9
  nervous 300.5
  old age 797
  senile 797
Débove's disease (splenomegaly) 789.2
Decalcification
  bone (*see also* Osteoporosis) 733.00
  teeth 521.89
Decapitation 874.9
  fetal (to facilitate delivery) 763.89
Decapsulation, kidney 593.89
Decay
  dental 521.00
  senile 797
  tooth, teeth 521.00
Decensus, uterus —*see* Prolapse, uterus
Deciduitis (acute)
  with
    abortion—*see* Abortion, by type, with sepsis
    ectopic pregnancy (*see also* categories 633.0-633.9) 639.0
    molar pregnancy (*see also* categories 630-632) 639.0
  affecting fetus or newborn 760.8
  following
    abortion 639.0
    ectopic or molar pregnancy 639.0
  in pregnancy 646.6
  puerperal, postpartum 670.1
Deciduoma malignum (M9100/3) 181
Deciduous tooth (retained) 520.6
Decline (general) (*see also* Debility) 799.3
Decompensation
  cardiac (acute) (chronic) (*see also* Disease, heart) 429.9
    failure—*see* Failure, heart
  cardiorenal (*see also* Hypertension, cardiorenal) 404.90
  cardiovascular (*see also* Disease, cardiovascular) 429.2
  heart (*see also* Disease, heart) 429.9
    failure—*see* Failure, heart
  hepatic 572.2
  myocardial (acute) (chronic) (*see also* Disease, heart) 429.9
    failure—*see* Failure, heart
  respiratory 519.9
Decompression sickness 993.3
Decrease, decreased
  blood
    platelets (*see also* Thrombocytopenia) 287.5
    pressure 796.3
      due to shock following
        injury 958.4
        operation 998.0
    white cell count 288.50
      specified NEC 288.59
  cardiac reserve—*see* Disease, heart
  estrogen 256.39
    postablative 256.2
  fetal movements 655.7
  fragility of erythrocytes 289.89
  function
    adrenal (cortex) 255.41
      medulla 255.5
    ovary in hypopituitarism 253.4

Decrease, decreased—*continued*
    parenchyma of pancreas 577.8
    pituitary (gland) (lobe) (anterior) 253.2
      posterior (lobe) 253.8
    functional activity 780.99
  glucose 790.29
  haptoglobin (serum) NEC 273.8
  leukocytes 288.50
  libido 799.81
  lymphocytes 288.51
  platelets (*see also* Thrombocytopenia) 287.5
  pulse pressure 785.9
  respiration due to shock following injury 958.4
  sexual desire 799.81
  tear secretion NEC 375.15
  tolerance
    fat 579.8
    salt and water 276.9
  vision NEC 369.9
  white blood cell count 288.50
Decubital gangrene (*see also* Ulcer, pressure) 707.00 *[785.4]*
Decubiti (*see also* Ulcer, pressure) 707.00
Decubitus (ulcer) (*see also* Ulcer, pressure) 707.00
  with gangrene 707.00 *[785.4]*
  ankle 707.06
  back
    lower 707.03
    upper 707.02
  buttock 707.05
  coccyx 707.03
  elbow 707.01
  head 707.09
  heel 707.07
  hip 707.04
  other site 707.09
  sacrum 707.03
  shoulder blades 707.02
Deepening acetabulum 718.85
Defect, defective 759.9
  3-beta-hydroxysteroid dehydrogenase 255.2
  11-hydroxylase 255.2
  21-hydroxylase 255.2
  abdominal wall, congenital 756.70
  aorticopulmonary septum 745.0
  aortic septal 745.0
  atrial septal (ostium secundum type) 745.5
    acquired 429.71
    ostium primum type 745.61
    sinus venosus 745.8
  atrioventricular
    canal 745.69
    septum 745.4
      acquired 429.71
  atrium secundum 745.5
    acquired 429.71
  auricular septal 745.5
    acquired 429.71
  bilirubin excretion 277.4
  biosynthesis, testicular androgen 257.2
  bridge 525.60
  bulbar septum 745.0
  butanol-insoluble iodide 246.1
  chromosome—*see* Anomaly, chromosome
  circulation (acquired) 459.9
    congenital 747.9
    newborn 747.9
  clotting NEC (*see also* Defect, coagulation) 286.9

Defect, defective—*continued*
  coagulation (factor) (*see also* Deficiency,
    coagulation factor) 286.9
    with
      abortion—*see* Abortion, by type, with
        hemorrhage
      ectopic pregnancy (*see also* categories
        634-638) 639.1
      molar pregnancy (*see also* categories
        630-632) 639.1
    acquired (any) 286.7
    antepartum or intrapartum 641.3
      affecting fetus or newborn 762.1
    causing hemorrhage of pregnancy or delivery
      641.3
    complicating pregnancy, childbirth, or the
      puerperium 649.3
    due to
      liver disease 286.7
      vitamin K deficiency 286.7
    newborn, transient 776.3
    postpartum 666.3
    specified type NEC 286.9
  conduction (heart) 426.9
    bone (*see also* Deafness, conductive) 389.00
  congenital, organ or site NEC—*see also*
    Anomaly
  circulation 747.9
  Descemet's membrane 743.9
    specified type NEC 743.49
  diaphragm 756.6
  ectodermal 757.9
  esophagus 750.9
  pulmonic cusps—*see* Anomaly, heart valve
  respiratory system 748.9
    specified type NEC 748.8
  crown 525.60
  cushion endocardial 745.60
  dental restoration 525.60
  dentin (hereditary) 520.5
  Descemet's membrane (congenital) 743.9
    acquired 371.30
    specific type NEC 743.49
  deutan 368.52
  developmental—*see also* Anomaly, by site
    cauda equina 742.59
    left ventricle 746.9
      with atresia or hypoplasia of aortic orifice or
        valve, with hypoplasia of ascending
        aorta 746.7
      in hypoplastic left heart syndrome 746.7
    testis 752.9
    vessel 747.9
  diaphragm
    with elevation, eventration, or hernia—*see*
      Hernia, diaphragm
    congenital 756.6
      with elevation, eventration, or hernia 756.6
      gross (with elevation, eventration, or hernia)
        756.6
  ectodermal, congenital 757.9
  Eisenmenger's (ventricular septal defect) 745.4
  endocardial cushion 745.60
    specified type NEC 745.69
  esophagus, congenital 750.9
  extensor retinaculum 728.9
  fibrin polymerization (*see also* Defect,
    coagulation) 286.3

Defect, defective—*continued*
  filling
    biliary tract 793.3
    bladder 793.5
    dental 525.60
    gallbladder 793.3
    kidney 793.5
    stomach 793.4
    ureter 793.5
  fossa ovalis 745.5
  gene, carrier (suspected) of V83.89
  Gerbode 745.4
  glaucomatous, without elevated tension 365.89
  Hageman (factor) (*see also* Defect, coagulation)
    286.3
  hearing (*see also* Deafness) 389.9
  high grade 317
  homogentisic acid 270.2
  interatrial septal 745.5
    acquired 429.71
  interauricular septal 745.5
    acquired 429.71
  interventricular septal 745.4
    with pulmonary stenosis or atresia,
      dextroposition of aorta, and hypertrophy of
      right ventricle 745.2
    acquired 429.71
    in tetralogy of Fallot 745.2
  iodide trapping 246.1
  iodotyrosine dehalogenase 246.1
  kynureninase 270.2
  learning, specific 315.2
  major osseous 731.3
  mental (*see also* Retardation, mental) 319
  osseous, major 731.3
  osteochondral NEC 738.8
  ostium
    primum 745.61
    secundum 745.5
  pericardium 746.89
  peroxidase-binding 246.1
  placental blood supply—*see* Placenta,
    insufficiency
  platelet (qualitative) 287.1
    constitutional 286.4
  postural, spine 737.9
  protan 368.51
  pulmonic cusps, congenital 746.00
  renal pelvis 753.9
    obstructive 753.29
    specified type NEC 753.3
  respiratory system, congenital 748.9
    specified type NEC 748.8
  retina, retinal 361.30
    with detachment (*see also* Detachment, retina,
      with retinal defect) 361.00
    multiple 361.33
      with detachment 361.02
    nerve fiber bundle 362.85
    single 361.30
      with detachment 361.01
  septal (closure) (heart) NEC 745.9
    acquired 429.71
    atrial 745.5
    specified type NEC 745.8
  speech NEC 784.59
    developmental 315.39
    late effect of cerebrovascular disease — *see*
      Late effect(s) (of) cerebrovascular disease,
      speech and language deficit
    secondary to organic lesion 784.59

Defect, defective—*continued*
  Taussig-Bing (transposition, aorta and
     overriding pulmonary artery) 745.11
  teeth, wedge 521.20
  thyroid hormone synthesis 246.1
  tritan 368.53
  ureter 753.9
    obstructive 753.29
  vascular (acquired) (local) 459.9
    congenital (peripheral) NEC 747.60
      gastrointestinal 747.61
      lower limb 747.64
      renal 747.62
      specified NEC 747.69
      spinal 747.82
      upper limb 747.63
  ventricular septal 745.4
    with pulmonary stenosis or atresia,
      dextraposition of aorta, and hypertrophy of
      right ventricle 745.2
    acquired 429.71
    atrioventricular canal type 745.69
    between infundibulum and anterior portion
      745.4
    in tetralogy of Fallot 745.2
    isolated anterior 745.4
  vision NEC 369.9
  visual field 368.40
    arcuate 368.43
    heteronymous, bilateral 368.47
    homonymous, bilateral 368.46
    localized NEC 368.44
    nasal step 368.44
    peripheral 368.44
    sector 368.43
  voice and resonance 784.40
  wedge, teeth (abrasion) 521.20
Defeminization syndrome 255.2
Deferentitis 608.4
  gonorrheal (acute) 098.14
    chronic or duration of 2 months or over 098.34
Defibrination syndrome (*see also* Fibrinolysis)
  286.6
Deficiency, deficient
  3-beta-hydroxysteroid dehydrogenase 255.2
  6-phosphogluconic dehydrogenase (anemia)
    282.2
  11-beta-hydroxylase 255.2
  17-alpha-hydroxylase 255.2
  18-hydroxysteroid dehydrogenase 255.2
  20-alpha-hydroxylase 255.2
  21-hydroxylase 255.2
  AAT (alpha-1 antitrypsin) 273.4
  abdominal muscle syndrome 756.79
  accelerator globulin (Ac G) (blood) (*see also*
    Defect, coagulation) 286.3
  AC globulin (congenital) (*see also* Defect,
    coagulation) 286.3
    acquired 286.7
  activating factor (blood) (*see also* Defect,
    coagulation) 286.3
  adenohypophyseal 253.2
  adenosine deaminase 277.2
  aldolase (hereditary) 271.2
  alpha-1-antitrypsin 273.4
  alpha-1-trypsin inhibitor 273.4
  alpha-fucosidase 271.8
  alpha-lipoprotein 272.5
  alpha-mannosidase 271.8
  amino acid 270.9
  anemia—*see* Anemia, deficiency

Deficiency, deficient—*continued*
  aneurin 265.1
    with beriberi 265.0
  antibody NEC 279.00
  antidiuretic hormone 253.5
  antihemophilic
    factor (A) 286.0
      B 286.1
      C 286.2
    globulin (AHG) NEC 286.0
  antithrombin III 289.81
  antitrypsin 273.4
  argininosuccinate synthetase or lyase 270.6
  ascorbic acid (with scurvy) 267
  autoprothrombin
    I (*see also* Defect, coagulation) 286.3
    II 286.1
    C (*see also* Defect, coagulation) 286.3
  bile salt 579.8
  biotin 266.2
  biotinidase 277.6
  bradykinase-1 277.6
  brancher enzyme (amylopectinosis) 271.0
  calciferol 268.9
    with
      osteomalacia 268.2
      rickets (*see also* Rickets) 268.0
  calcium 275.40
    dietary 269.3
  calorie, severe 261
  carbamyl phosphate synthetase 270.6
  cardiac (*see also* Insufficiency, myocardial)
    428.0
  carnitine 277.81
    due to
      hemodialysis 277.83
      inborn errors of metabolism 277.82
      valproic acid therapy 277.83
    iatrogenic 277.83
    palmitoyltransferase (CPT1, CPT2) 277.85
    palmityl transferase (CPT1, CPT2) 277.85
    primary 277.81
    secondary 277.84
  carotene 264.9
  Carr factor (*see also* Defect, coagulation) 286.9
  central nervous system 349.9
  ceruloplasmin 275.1
  cevitamic acid (with scurvy) 267
  choline 266.2
  Christmas factor 286.1
  chromium 269.3
  citrin 269.1
  clotting (blood) (*see also* Defect, coagulation)
    286.9
  coagulation factor NEC 286.9
    with
      abortion—*see* Abortion, by type, with
        hemorrhage
      ectopic pregnancy (*see also* categories
        634-638) 639.1
      molar pregnancy (*see also* categories
        630-632) 639.1
    acquired (any) 286.7
    antepartum or intrapartum 641.3
      affecting fetus or newborn 762.1
    complicating pregnancy, childbirth, or the
      puerperium 649.3
    due to
      liver disease 286.7
      vitamin K deficiency 286.7
    newborn, transient 776.3

Deficiency, deficient—*continued*
  coagulation factor —*continued*
    postpartum 666.3
    specified type NEC 286.3
  color vision (congenital) 368.59
    acquired 368.55
  combined glucocorticoid and mineralocorticoid
    255.41
  combined, two or more coagulation factors (*see
    also* Defect, coagulation) 286.9
  complement factor NEC 279.8
  contact factor (*see also* Defect, coagulation)
    286.3
  copper NEC 275.1
  corticoadrenal 255.41
  craniofacial axis 756.0
  cyanocobalamin (vitamin B$_{12}$) 266.2
  debrancher enzyme (limit dextrinosis) 271.0
  desmolase 255.2
  diet 269.9
  dihydrofolate reductase 281.2
  dihydropteridine reductase 270.1
  disaccharidase (intestinal) 271.3
  disease NEC 269.9
  ear(s) V48.8
  edema 262
  endocrine 259.9
  enzymes, circulating NEC (*see also* Deficiency,
    by specific enzyme) 277.6
  ergosterol 268.9
    with
      osteomalacia 268.2
      rickets (*see also* Rickets) 268.0
  erythrocytic glutathione (anemia) 282.2
  eyelid(s) V48.8
  factor (*see also* Defect, coagulation) 286.9
    I (congenital) (fibrinogen) 286.3
      antepartum or intrapartum 641.3
        affecting fetus or newborn 762.1
      newborn, transient 776.3
      postpartum 666.3
    II (congenital) (prothrombin) 286.3
    V (congenital) (labile) 286.3
    VII (congenital) (stable) 286.3
    VIII (congenital) (functional) 286.0
      with
        functional defect 286.0
        vascular defect 286.4
    IX (Christmas) (congenital) (functional) 286.1
    X (congenital) (Stuart-Prower) 286.3
    XI (congenital) (plasma thromboplastin
      antecedent) 286.2
    XII (congenital) (Hageman) 286.3
    XIII (congenital) (fibrin stabilizing) 286.3
    Hageman 286.3
    multiple (congenital) 286.9
      acquired 286.7
  fibrinase (*see also* Defect, coagulation) 286.3
  fibrinogen (congenital) (*see also* Defect,
    coagulation) 286.3
    acquired 286.6
  fibrin stabilizing factor (congenital) (*see also*
    Defect, coagulation) 286.3
    acquired 286.7
  finger—*see* Absence, finger
  Fletcher factor (*see also* Defect, coagulation)
    286.9
  fluorine 269.3
  folate, anemia 281.2
  folic acid (vitamin B$_c$) 266.2
    anemia 281.2

Deficiency, deficient—*continued*
  follicle-stimulating hormone (FSH) 253.4
  fructokinase 271.2
  fructose-1, 6-diphosphate 271.2
  fructose-1-phosphate aldolase 271.2
  FSH (follicle-stimulating hormone) 253.4
  fucosidase 271.8
  galactokinase 271.1
  galactose-1-phosphate uridyl transferase 271.1
  gamma globulin in blood 279.00
  glass factor (*see also* Defect, coagulation) 286.3
  glucocorticoid 255.41
  glucose-6-phosphatase 271.0
  glucose-6-phosphate dehydrogenase anemia 282.2
  glucuronyl transferase 277.4
  glutathione-reductase (anemia) 282.2
  glycogen synthetase 271.0
  growth hormone 253.3
  Hageman factor (congenital) (*see also* Defect,
    coagulation) 286.3
  head V48.0
  hemoglobin (*see also* Anemia) 285.9
  hepatophosphorylase 271.0
  hexose monophosphate (HMP) shunt 282.2
  HGH (human growth hormone) 253.3
  HG-PRT 277.2
  homogentisic acid oxidase 270.2
  hormone—*see also* Deficiency, by specific
    hormone
    anterior pituitary (isolated) (partial) NEC
      253.4
      growth (human) 253.3
    follicle-stimulating 253.4
    growth (human) (isolated) 253.3
    human growth 253.3
    interstitial cell-stimulating 253.4
    luteinizing 253.4
    melanocyte-stimulating 253.4
    testicular 257.2
  human growth hormone 253.3
  humoral 279.00
    with
      hyper-IgM 279.05
        autosomal recessive 279.05
        X-linked 279.05
      increased IgM 279.05
    congenital hypogammaglobulinemia 279.04
    non-sex-linked 279.06
    selective immunoglobulin NEC 279.03
      IgA 279.01
      IgG 279.03
      IgM 279.02
        increased 279.05
    specified NEC 279.09
  hydroxylase 255.2
  hypoxanthine-guanine
    phosphoribosyltransferase (HG-PRT) 277.2
  ICSH (interstitial cell-stimulating hormone)
    253.4
  immunity NEC 279.3
    cell-mediated 279.10
      with
        hyperimmunoglobulinemia 279.2
        thrombocytopenia and eczema 279.12
      specified NEC 279.19
    combined (severe) 279.2
      syndrome 279.2
    common variable 279.06
    humoral NEC 279.00
    IgA (secretory) 279.01
    IgG 279.03
    IgM 279.02

Deficiency, deficient—*continued*
  psychobiological 301.6
  PTA 286.2
  PTC 286.1
  purine nucleoside phosphorylase 277.2
  pyracin (alpha) (beta) 266.1
  pyridoxal 266.1
  pyridoxamine 266.1
  pyridoxine (derivatives) 266.1
  pyruvate carboxylase 271.8
  pyruvate dehydrogenase 271.8
  pyruvate kinase (PK) 282.3
  riboflavin (vitamin B₂) 266.0
  saccadic eye movements 379.57
  salivation 527.7
  salt 276.1
  secretion
    ovary 256.39
    salivary gland (any) 527.7
    urine 788.5
  selenium 269.3
  serum
    antitrypsin, familial 273.4
    protein (congenital) 273.8
  short chain acyl CoA dehydrogenase (SCAD)
      277.85
  short stature homeobox gene (SHOX)
    with
      dyschondrosteosis 756.89
      short stature (idiopathic) 783.43
      Turner's syndrome 758.6
  smooth pursuit movements (eye) 379.58
  sodium (Na) 276.1
  SPCA (*see also* Defect, coagulation) 286.3
  specified NEC 269.8
  stable factor (congenital) (*see also* Defect,
      coagulation) 286.3
    acquired 286.7
  Stuart (-Prower) factor (*see also* Defect,
      coagulation) 286.3
  sucrase 271.3
  sucrase-isomaltase 271.3
  sulfite oxidase 270.0
  syndrome, multiple 260
  thiamine, thiaminic (chloride) 265.1
  thrombokinase (*see also* Defect, coagulation) 286.3
    newborn 776.0
  thrombopoieten 287.39
  thymolymphatic 279.2
  thyroid (gland) 244.9
  tocopherol 269.1
  toe—*see* Absence, toe
  tooth bud (*see also* Anodontia) 520.0
  trunk V48.1
  UDPG-glycogen transferase 271.0
  upper limb V49.0
    congenital 755.20
      with complete absence of distal elements
          755.21
      longitudinal (complete) (partial) (with distal
          deficiencies, incomplete) 755.22
        carpal(s) 755.28
        combined humeral, radial, ulnar
            (incomplete) 755.23
        humeral 755.24
        metacarpal(s) 755.28
        phalange(s) 755.29
          meaning all digits 755.21
        radial 755.26
        radioulnar 755.25
        ulnar 755.27
      transverse (complete) (partial) 755.21

Deficiency, deficient—*continued*
  vascular 459.9
  vasopressin 253.5
  viosterol (*see also* Deficiency, calciferol) 268.9
  vitamin (multiple) NEC 269.2
    A 264.9
      with
        Bitôt's spot 264.1
          corneal 264.2
            with corneal ulceration 264.3
        keratomalacia 264.4
        keratosis, follicular 264.8
        night blindness 264.5
        scar of cornea, xerophthalmic 264.6
        specified manifestation NEC 264.8
          ocular 264.7
        xeroderma 264.8
        xerophthalmia 264.7
        xerosis
          conjunctival 264.0
            with Bitôt's spot 264.1
          corneal 264.2
            with corneal ulceration 264.3
    B (complex) NEC 266.9
      with
        beriberi 265.0
        pellagra 265.2
        specified type NEC 266.2
    B₁ NEC 265.1
      beriberi 265.0
    B₂ 266.0
    B₆ 266.1
    B₁₂ 266.2
    Bₑ (folic acid) 266.2
    C (ascorbic acid) (with scurvy) 267
    D (calciferol) (ergosterol) 268.9
      with
        osteomalacia 268.2
        rickets (*see also* Rickets) 268.0
    E 269.1
    folic acid 266.2
    G 266.0
    H 266.2
    K 269.0
      of newborn 776.0
    nicotinic acid 265.2
    P 269.1
    PP 265.2
    specified NEC 269.1
    zinc 269.3
Deficient —*see also* Deficiency
  blink reflex 374.45
  craniofacial axis 756.0
  number of teeth (*see also* Anodontia) 520.0
  secretion of urine 788.5
Deficit
  neurologic NEC 781.99
    due to
      cerebrovascular lesion (*see also* Disease,
          cerebrovascular, acute) 436
      late effect—*see* Late effect(s) (of)
          cerebrovascular disease
      transient ischemic attack 435.9
    ischemic
      reversible (RIND) 434.91
        history of (personal) V12.54
      prolonged (PRIND) 434.91
        history of (personal) V12.54
  oxygen 799.02

Deflection
  radius 736.09
  septum (acquired) (nasal) (nose) 470
  spine—*see* Curvature, spine
  turbinate (nose) 470
Defluvium
  capillorum (*see also* Alopecia) 704.00
  ciliorum 374.55
  unguium 703.8
Deformity 738.9
  abdomen, congenital 759.9
  abdominal wall
    acquired 738.8
    congenital 756.70
    muscle deficiency syndrome 756.79
  acquired (unspecified site) 738.9
    specified site NEC 738.8
  adrenal gland (congenital) 759.1
  alimentary tract, congenital 751.9
    lower 751.5
    specified type NEC 751.8
    upper (any part, except tongue) 750.9
      specified type NEC 750.8
      tongue 750.10
        specified type NEC 750.19
  ankle (joint) (acquired) 736.70
    abduction 718.47
    congenital 755.69
    contraction 718.47
    specified NEC 736.79
  anus (congenital) 751.5
    acquired 569.49
  aorta (congenital) 747.20
    acquired 447.8
    arch 747.21
      acquired 447.8
    coarctation 747.10
  aortic
    arch 747.21
      acquired 447.8
    cusp or valve (congenital) 746.9
      acquired (*see also* Endocarditis, aortic) 424.1
    ring 747.21
  appendix 751.5
  arm (acquired) 736.89
    congenital 755.50
  arteriovenous (congenital) (peripheral) NEC 747.60
    gastrointestinal 747.61
    lower limb 747.64
    renal 747.62
    specified NEC 747.69
    spinal 747.82
    upper limb 747.63
  artery (congenital) (peripheral) NEC (*see also* Deformity, vascular) 747.60
    acquired 447.8
    cerebral 747.81
    coronary (congenital) 746.85
      acquired (*see also* Ischemia, heart) 414.9
    retinal 743.9
    umbilical 747.5
  atrial septal (congenital) (heart) 745.5
  auditory canal (congenital) (external) (*see also* Deformity, ear) 744.3
    acquired 380.50
  auricle
    ear (congenital) (*see also* Deformity, ear) 744.3
      acquired 380.32
    heart (congenital) 746.9

Deformity—*continued*
  back (acquired)—*see* Deformity, spine
  Bartholin's duct (congenital) 750.9
  bile duct (congenital) 751.60
    acquired 576.8
    with calculus, choledocholithiasis, or stones—*see* Choledocholithiasis
  biliary duct or passage (congenital) 751.60
    acquired 576.8
    with calculus, choledocholithiasis, or stones—*see* Choledocholithiasis
  bladder (neck) (sphincter) (trigone) (acquired) 596.8
    congenital 753.9
  bone (acquired) NEC 738.9
    congenital 756.9
    turbinate 738.0
  boutonniere (finger) 736.21
  brain (congenital) 742.9
    acquired 348.89
    multiple 742.4
    reduction 742.2
    vessel (congenital) 747.81
  breast (acquired) 611.89
    congenital 757.6
    reconstructed 612.0
  bronchus (congenital) 748.3
    acquired 519.19
  bursa, congenital 756.9
  canal of Nuck 752.9
  canthus (congenital) 743.9
    acquired 374.89
  capillary (acquired) 448.9
    congenital NEC (*see also* Deformity, vascular) 747.60
  cardiac—*see* Deformity, heart
  cardiovascular system (congenital) 746.9
  caruncle, lacrimal (congenital) 743.9
    acquired 375.69
  cascade, stomach 537.6
  cecum (congenital) 751.5
    acquired 569.89
  cerebral (congenital) 742.9
    acquired 348.89
  cervix (acquired) (uterus) 622.8
    congenital 752.40
  cheek (acquired) 738.19
    congenital 744.9
  chest (wall) (acquired) 738.3
    congenital 754.89
    late effect of rickets 268.1
  chin (acquired) 738.19
    congenital 744.9
  choroid (congenital) 743.9
    acquired 363.8
    plexus (congenital) 742.9
      acquired 349.2
  cicatricial—*see* Cicatrix
  cilia (congenital) 743.9
    acquired 374.89
  circulatory system (congenital) 747.9
  clavicle (acquired) 738.8
    congenital 755.51
  clitoris (congenital) 752.40
    acquired 624.8
  clubfoot—*see* Clubfoot
  coccyx (acquired) 738.6
    congenital 756.10
  colon (congenital) 751.5
    acquired 569.89

Deformity—*continued*
  concha (ear) (congenital) (*see also* Deformity,
    ear) 744.3
    acquired 380.32
  congenital, organ or site not listed (*see also*
    Anomaly) 759.9
  cornea (congenital) 743.9
    acquired 371.70
  coronary artery (congenital) 746.85
    acquired (*see also* Ischemia, heart) 414.9
  cranium (acquired) 738.19
    congenital (*see also* Deformity, skull,
      congenital) 756.0
  cricoid cartilage (congenital) 748.3
    acquired 478.79
  cystic duct (congenital) 751.60
    acquired 575.8
  Dandy-Walker 742.3
    with spina bifida (*see also* Spina bifida) 741.0
  diaphragm (congenital) 756.6
    acquired 738.8
  digestive organ(s) or system (congenital) NEC
    751.9
    specified type NEC 751.8
  ductus arteriosus 747.0
  duodenal bulb 537.89
  duodenum (congenital) 751.5
    acquired 537.89
  dura (congenital) 742.9
    brain 742.4
      acquired 349.2
    spinal 742.59
      acquired 349.2
  ear (congenital) 744.3
    acquired 380.32
    auricle 744.3
      causing impairment of hearing 744.02
    causing impairment of hearing 744.00
    external 744.3
      causing impairment of hearing 744.02
    internal 744.05
    lobule 744.3
    middle 744.03
      ossicles 744.04
    ossicles 744.04
  ectodermal (congenital) NEC 757.9
    specified type NEC 757.8
  ejaculatory duct (congenital) 752.9
    acquired 608.89
  elbow (joint) (acquired) 736.00
    congenital 755.50
    contraction 718.42
  endocrine gland NEC 759.2
  epididymis (congenital) 752.9
    acquired 608.89
    torsion 608.24
  epiglottis (congenital) 748.3
    acquired 478.79
  esophagus (congenital) 750.9
    acquired 530.89
  Eustachian tube (congenital) NEC 744.3
    specified type NEC 744.24
  extremity (acquired) 736.9
    congenital, except reduction deformity 755.9
      lower 755.60
      upper 755.50
    reduction—*see* Deformity, reduction
  eye (congenital) 743.9
    acquired 379.8
    muscle 743.9
  eyebrow (congenital) 744.89

Deformity—*continued*
  eyelid (congenital) 743.9
    acquired 374.89
    specified type NEC 743.62
  face (acquired) 738.19
    congenital (any part) 744.9
    due to intrauterine malposition and pressure 754.0
  fallopian tube (congenital) 752.10
    acquired 620.8
  femur (acquired) 736.89
    congenital 755.60
  fetal
    with fetopelvic disproportion 653.7
      affecting fetus or newborn 763.1
    causing obstructed labor 660.1
      affecting fetus or newborn 763.1
    known or suspected, affecting management of
      pregnancy 655.9
  finger (acquired) 736.20
    boutonniere type 736.21
    congenital 755.50
    flexion contracture 718.44
    swan neck 736.22
  flexion (joint) (acquired) 736.9
    congenital NEC 755.9
    hip or thigh (acquired) 736.39
      congenital (*see also* Subluxation, congenital,
        hip) 754.32
  foot (acquired) 736.70
    cavovarus 736.75
      congenital 754.59
    congenital NEC 754.70
      specified type NEC 754.79
    valgus (acquired) 736.79
      congenital 754.60
        specified type NEC 754.69
    varus (acquired) 736.79
      congenital 754.50
        specified type NEC 754.59
  forearm (acquired) 736.00
    congenital 755.50
  forehead (acquired) 738.19
    congenital (*see also* Deformity, skull,
      congenital) 756.0
  frontal bone (acquired) 738.19
    congenital (*see also* Deformity, skull,
      congenital) 756.0
  gallbladder (congenital) 751.60
    acquired 575.8
  gastrointestinal tract (congenital) NEC 751.9
    acquired 569.89
    specified type NEC 751.8
  genitalia, genital organ(s) or system NEC
    congenital 752.9
    female (congenital) 752.9
      acquired 629.89
      external 752.40
      internal 752.9
    male (congenital) 752.9
      acquired 608.89
  globe (eye) (congenital) 743.9
    acquired 360.89
  gum (congenital) 750.9
    acquired 523.9
  gunstock 736.02
  hand (acquired) 736.00
    claw 736.06
    congenital 755.50
    minus (and plus) (intrinsic) 736.09
    pill roller (intrinsic) 736.09
    plus (and minus) (intrinsic) 736.09
    swan neck (intrinsic) 736.09

Deformity—*continued*
  head (acquired) 738.10
    congenital (*see also* Deformity, skull,
        congenital) 756.0
    specified NEC 738.19
  heart (congenital) 746.9
    auricle (congenital) 746.9
    septum 745.9
      auricular 745.5
      specified type NEC 745.8
      ventricular 745.4
    valve (congenital) NEC 746.9
      acquired—*see* Endocarditis
      pulmonary (congenital) 746.00
      specified type NEC 746.89
    ventricle (congenital) 746.9
  heel (acquired) 736.76
    congenital 755.67
  hepatic duct (congenital) 751.60
    acquired 576.8
      with calculus, choledocholithiasis, or
          stones—*see* Choledocholithiasis
  hip (joint) (acquired) 736.30
    congenital NEC 755.63
    flexion 718.45
      congenital (*see also* Subluxation, congenital,
          hip) 754.32
  hourglass—*see* Contraction, hourglass
  humerus (acquired) 736.89
    congenital 755.50
  hymen (congenital) 752.40
  hypophyseal (congenital) 759.2
  ileocecal (coil) (valve) (congenital) 751.5
    acquired 569.89
  ileum (intestine) (congenital) 751.5
    acquired 569.89
  ilium (acquired) 738.6
    congenital 755.60
  integument (congenital) 757.9
  intervertebral cartilage or disc (acquired)—*see
      also* Displacement, intervertebral disc
    congenital 756.10
  intestine (large) (small) (congenital) 751.5
    acquired 569.89
  iris (acquired) 364.75
    congenital 743.9
    prolapse 364.89
  ischium (acquired) 738.6
    congenital 755.60
  jaw (acquired) (congenital) NEC 524.9
    due to intrauterine malposition and pressure
        754.0
  joint (acquired) NEC 738.8
    congenital 755.9
    contraction (abduction) (adduction) (extension)
        (flexion)—*see* Contraction, joint
  kidney(s) (calyx) (pelvis) (congenital) 753.9
    acquired 593.89
    vessel 747.62
      acquired 459.9
  Klippel-Feil (brevicollis) 756.16
  knee (acquired) NEC 736.6
    congenital 755.64
  labium (majus) (minus) (congenital) 752.40
    acquired 624.8
  lacrimal apparatus or duct (congenital) 743.9
    acquired 375.69
  larynx (muscle) (congenital) 748.3
    acquired 478.79
    web (glottic) (subglottic) 748.2

Deformity—*continued*
  leg (lower) (upper) (acquired) NEC 736.89
    congenital 755.60
    reduction—*see* Deformity, reduction, lower limb
  lens (congenital) 743.9
    acquired 379.39
  lid (fold) (congenital) 743.9
    acquired 374.89
  ligament (acquired) 728.9
    congenital 756.9
  limb (acquired) 736.9
    congenital, except reduction deformity 755.9
      lower 755.60
        reduction (*see also* Deformity, reduction,
            lower limb) 755.30
      upper 755.50
        reduction (*see also* Deformity, reduction,
            lower limb) 755.20
    specified NEC 736.89
  lip (congenital) NEC 750.9
    acquired 528.5
    specified type NEC 750.26
  liver (congenital) 751.60
    acquired 573.8
    duct (congenital) 751.60
      acquired 576.8
        with calculus, choledocholithiasis, or
            stones—*see* Choledocholithiasis
  lower extremity—*see* Deformity, leg
  lumbosacral (joint) (region) (congenital) 756.10
    acquired 738.5
  lung (congenital) 748.60
    acquired 518.89
    specified type NEC 748.69
  lymphatic system, congenital 759.9
  Madelung's (radius) 755.54
  maxilla (acquired) (congenital) 524.9
  meninges or membrane (congenital) 742.9
    brain 742.4
      acquired 349.2
    spinal (cord) 742.59
      acquired 349.2
  mesentery (congenital) 751.9
    acquired 568.89
  metacarpus (acquired) 736.00
    congenital 755.50
  metatarsus (acquired) 736.70
    congenital 754.70
  middle ear, except ossicles (congenital) 744.03
    ossicles 744.04
  mitral (leaflets) (valve) (congenital) 746.9
    acquired—*see* Endocarditis, mitral
    Ebstein's 746.89
    parachute 746.5
    specified type NEC 746.89
    stenosis, congenital 746.5
  mouth (acquired) 528.9
    congenital NEC 750.9
      specified type NEC 750.26
  multiple, congenital NEC 759.7
    specified type NEC 759.89
  muscle (acquired) 728.9
    congenital 756.9
      specified type NEC 756.89
      sternocleidomastoid (due to intrauterine
          malposition and pressure) 754.1
  musculoskeletal system, congenital NEC 756.9
    specified type NEC 756.9
  nail (acquired) 703.9
    congenital 757.9
  nasal—*see* Deformity, nose

Deformity—*continued*
neck (acquired) NEC 738.2
  congenital (any part) 744.9
    sternocleidomastoid 754.1
nervous system (congenital) 742.9
nipple (congenital) 757.6
  acquired 611.89
nose, nasal (cartilage) (acquired) 738.0
  bone (turbinate) 738.0
  congenital 748.1
    bent 754.0
    squashed 754.0
  saddle 738.0
    syphilitic 090.5
  septum 470
    congenital 748.1
  sinus (wall) (congenital) 748.1
    acquired 738.0
  syphilitic (congenital) 090.5
    late 095.8
ocular muscle (congenital) 743.9
  acquired 378.60
opticociliary vessels (congenital) 743.9
orbit (congenital) (eye) 743.9
  acquired NEC 376.40
    associated with craniofacial deformities 376.44
    due to
      bone disease 376.43
      surgery 376.47
      trauma 376.47
organ of Corti (congenital) 744.05
ovary (congenital) 752.0
  acquired 620.8
oviduct (congenital) 752.10
  acquired 620.8
palate (congenital) 750.9
  acquired 526.89
  cleft (congenital) (*see also* Cleft, palate) 749.00
  hard, acquired 526.89
  soft, acquired 528.9
pancreas (congenital) 751.7
  acquired 577.8
parachute, mitral valve 746.5
parathyroid (gland) 759.2
parotid (gland) (congenital) 750.9
  acquired 527.8
patella (acquired) 736.6
  congenital 755.64
pelvis, pelvic (acquired) (bony) 738.6
  with disproportion (fetopelvic) 653.0
    affecting fetus or newborn 763.1
    causing obstructed labor 660.1
      affecting fetus or newborn 763.1
  congenital 755.60
  rachitic (late effect) 268.1
penis (glans) (congenital) 752.9
  acquired 607.89
pericardium (congenital) 746.9
  acquired—*see* Pericarditis
pharynx (congenital) 750.9
  acquired 478.29
Pierre Robin (congenital) 756.0
pinna (acquired) 380.32
  congenital 744.3
pituitary (congenital) 759.2
pleural folds (congenital) 748.8
portal vein (congenital) 747.40
posture—*see* Curvature, spine
prepuce (congenital) 752.9
  acquired 607.89
prostate (congenital) 752.9
  acquired 602.8

Deformity—*continued*
pulmonary valve—*see* Endocarditis, pulmonary
pupil (congenital) 743.9
  acquired 364.75
pylorus (congenital) 750.9
  acquired 537.89
rachitic (acquired), healed or old 268.1
radius (acquired) 736.00
  congenital 755.50
    reduction—*see* Deformity, reduction, upper
      limb
rectovaginal septum (congenital) 752.40
  acquired 623.8
rectum (congenital) 751.5
  acquired 569.49
reduction (extremity) (limb) 755.4
  brain 742.2
  lower limb 755.30
    with complete absence of distal elements
      755.31
    longitudinal (complete) (partial) (with distal
      deficiencies, incomplete) 755.32
      with complete absence of distal elements
        755.31
      combined femoral, tibial, fibular
        (incomplete) 755.33
      femoral 755.34
      fibular 755.37
      metatarsal(s) 755.38
      phalange(s) 755.39
        meaning all digits 755.31
      tarsal(s) 755.38
      tibia 755.36
      tibiofibular 755.35
      transverse 755.31
  upper limb 755.20
    with complete absence of distal elements 755.21
    longitudinal (complete) (partial) (with distal
      deficiencies, incomplete) 755.22
      with complete absence of distal elements
        755.21
      carpal(s) 755.28
      combined humeral, radial, ulnar
        (incomplete) 755.23
      humeral 755.24
      metacarpal(s) 755.28
      phalange(s) 755.29
        meaning all digits 755.21
      radial 755.26
      radioulnar 755.25
      ulnar 755.27
    transverse (complete) (partial) 755.21
  renal—*see* Deformity, kidney
respiratory system (congenital) 748.9
  specified type NEC 748.8
rib (acquired) 738.3
  congenital 756.3
    cervical 756.2
rotation (joint) (acquired) 736.9
  congenital 755.9
  hip or thigh 736.39
    congenital (*see also* Subluxation, congenital,
      hip) 754.32
sacroiliac joint (congenital) 755.69
  acquired 738.5
sacrum (acquired) 738.5
  congenital 756.10
saddle
  back 737.8
  nose 738.0
    syphilitic 090.5

Deformity—*continued*
  salivary gland or duct (congenital) 750.9
    acquired 527.8
  scapula (acquired) 736.89
    congenital 755.50
  scrotum (congenital) 752.9
    acquired 608.89
  sebaceous gland, acquired 706.8
  seminal tract or duct (congenital) 752.9
    acquired 608.89
  septum (nasal) (acquired) 470
    congenital 748.1
  shoulder (joint) (acquired) 736.89
    congenital 755.50
      specified type NEC 755.59
    contraction 718.41
  sigmoid (flexure) (congenital) 751.5
    acquired 569.89
  sinus of Valsalva 747.29
  skin (congenital) 757.9
    acquired NEC 709.8
  skull (acquired) 738.19
    congenital 756.0
      with
        anencephalus 740.0
        encephalocele 742.0
        hydrocephalus 742.3
          with spina bifida (*see also* Spina bifida)
            741.0
        microcephalus 742.1
      due to intrauterine malposition and pressure
        754.0
  soft parts, organs or tissues (of pelvis)
    in pregnancy or childbirth NEC 654.9
      affecting fetus or newborn 763.89
      causing obstructed labor 660.2
        affecting fetus or newborn 763.1
  spermatic cord (congenital) 752.9
    acquired 608.89
    torsion 608.22
      extravaginal 608.21
      intravaginal 608.22
  spinal
    column—*see* Deformity, spine
    cord (congenital) 742.9
      acquired 336.8
      vessel (congenital) 747.82
    nerve root (congenital) 742.9
      acquired 724.9
    vessel 747.82
  spine (acquired) NEC 738.5
    congenital 756.10
      due to intrauterine malposition and pressure
        754.2
    kyphoscoliotic (*see also* Kyphoscoliosis)
      737.30
    kyphotic (*see also* Kyphosis) 737.10
    lordotic (*see also* Lordosis) 737.20
    rachitic 268.1
    scoliotic (*see also* Scoliosis) 737.30
  spleen
    acquired 289.59
    congenital 759.0
  Sprengel's (congenital) 755.52
  sternum (acquired) 738.3
    congenital 756.3
  stomach (congenital) 750.9
    acquired 537.89
  submaxillary gland (congenital) 750.9
    acquired 527.8

Deformity—*continued*
  swan neck (acquired)
    finger 736.22
    hand 736.09
  talipes—*see* Talipes
  teeth, tooth NEC 520.9
  testis (congenital) 752.9
    acquired 608.89
    torsion 608.20
  thigh (acquired) 736.89
    congenital 755.60
  thorax (acquired) (wall) 738.3
    congenital 754.89
    late effect of rickets 268.1
  thumb (acquired) 736.20
    congenital 755.50
  thymus (tissue) (congenital) 759.2
  thyroid (gland) (congenital) 759.2
    cartilage 748.3
      acquired 478.79
  tibia (acquired) 736.89
    congenital 755.60
    saber 090.5
  toe (acquired) 735.9
    congenital 755.66
    specified NEC 735.8
  tongue (congenital) 750.10
    acquired 529.8
  tooth, teeth NEC 520.9
  trachea (rings) (congenital) 748.3
    acquired 519.19
  transverse aortic arch (congenital) 747.21
  tricuspid (leaflets) (valve) (congenital) 746.9
    acquired—*see* Endocarditis, tricuspid
    atresia or stenosis 746.1
    specified type NEC 746.89
  trunk (acquired) 738.3
    congenital 759.9
  ulna (acquired) 736.00
    congenital 755.50
  upper extremity—*see* Deformity, arm
  urachus (congenital) 753.7
  ureter (opening) (congenital) 753.9
    acquired 593.89
  urethra (valve) (congenital) 753.9
    acquired 599.84
  urinary tract or system (congenital) 753.9
    urachus 753.7
  uterus (congenital) 752.3
    acquired 621.8
  uvula (congenital) 750.9
    acquired 528.9
  vagina (congenital) 752.40
    acquired 623.8
  valve, valvular (heart) (congenital) 746.9
    acquired—*see* Endocarditis
    pulmonary 746.00
    specified type NEC 746.89
  vascular (congenital) (peripheral) NEC 747.60
    acquired 459.9
    gastrointestinal 747.61
    lower limb 747.64
    renal 747.62
    specified site NEC 747.69
    spinal 747.82
    upper limb 747.63
  vas deferens (congenital) 752.9
    acquired 608.89

Deformity—*continued*
  vein (congenital) NEC (*see also* Deformity,
    vascular) 747.60
    brain 747.81
    coronary 746.9
    great 747.40
  vena cava (inferior) (superior) (congenital)
    747.40
  vertebra—*see* Deformity, spine
  vesicourethral orifice (acquired) 596.8
    congenital NEC 753.9
      specified type NEC 753.8
  vessels of optic papilla (congenital) 743.9
  visual field (contraction) 368.45
  vitreous humor (congenital) 743.9
    acquired 379.29
  vulva (congenital) 752.40
    acquired 624.8
  wrist (joint) (acquired) 736.00
    congenital 755.50
    contraction 718.43
    valgus 736.03
      congenital 755.59
    varus 736.04
      congenital 755.59

Degeneration, degenerative
  adrenal (capsule) (gland) 255.8
    with hypofunction 255.41
    fatty 255.8
    hyaline 255.8
    infectional 255.8
    lardaceous 277.39
  amyloid (any site) (general) 277.39
  anterior cornua, spinal cord 336.8
  anterior labral 840.8
  aorta, aortic 440.0
    fatty 447.8
    valve (heart) (*see also* Endocarditis, aortic)
      424.1
  arteriovascular—*see* Arteriosclerosis
  artery, arterial (atheromatous) (calcareous)—*see
    also* Arteriosclerosis
    amyloid 277.39
    lardaceous 277.39
    medial NEC (*see also* Arteriosclerosis,
      extremities) 440.20
  articular cartilage NEC (*see also* Disorder,
    cartilage, articular) 718.0
    elbow 718.02
    knee 717.5
    patella 717.7
    shoulder 718.01
    spine (*see also* Spondylosis) 721.90
  atheromatous—*see* Arteriosclerosis
  bacony (any site) 277.39
  basal nuclei or ganglia NEC 333.0
  bone 733.90
  brachial plexus 353.0
  brain (cortical) (progressive) 331.9
    arteriosclerotic 437.0
    childhood 330.9
      specified type NEC 330.8
    congenital 742.4
    cystic 348.0
      congenital 742.4
    familial NEC 331.89
    grey matter 330.8
    heredofamilial NEC 331.89

Degeneration, degenerative—*continued*
  brain—*continued*
    in
      alcoholism 303.9 *[331.7]*
      beriberi 265.0 *[331.7]*
      cerebrovascular disease 437.9 *[331.7]*
      congenital hydrocephalus 742.3 *[331.7]*
        with spina bifida (*see also* Spina bifida)
          741.0 *[331.7]*
      Fabry's disease 272.7 *[330.2]*
      Gaucher's disease 272.7 *[330.2]*
      Hunter's disease or syndrome 277.5 *[330.3]*
      lipidosis
        cerebral 330.1
        generalized 272.7 *[330.2]*
      mucopolysaccharidosis 277.5 *[330.3]*
      myxedema (*see also* Myxedema) 244.9
        [331.7]
      neoplastic disease NEC (M8000/1) 239.9
        [331.7]
      Niemann-Pick disease 272.7 *[330.2]*
      sphingolipidosis 272.7 *[330.2]*
      vitamin B_{12} deficiency 266.2 *[331.7]*
    motor centers 331.89
    senile 331.2
    specified type NEC 331.89
  breast—*see* Disease, breast
  Bruch's membrane 363.40
  bundle of His 426.50
    left 426.3
    right 426.4
  calcareous NEC 275.49
  capillaries 448.9
    amyloid 277.39
    fatty 448.9
    lardaceous 277.39
  cardiac (brown) (calcareous) (fatty) (fibrous)
    (hyaline) (mural) (muscular) (pigmentary)
    (senile) (with arteriosclerosis) (*see also*
    Degeneration, myocardial) 429.1
    valve, valvular—*see* Endocarditis
  cardiorenal (*see also* Hypertension, cardiorenal)
    404.90
  cardiovascular (*see also* Disease, cardiovascular)
    429.2
    renal (*see also* Hypertension, cardiorenal) 404.90
  cartilage (joint)—*see* Derangement, joint
  cerebellar NEC 334.9
    primary (hereditary) (sporadic) 334.2
  cerebral—*see* Degeneration, brain
  cerebromacular 330.1
  cerebrovascular 437.1
    due to hypertension 437.2
    late effect—*see* Late effect(s) (of)
      cerebrovascular disease
  cervical plexus 353.2
  cervix 622.8
    due to radiation (intended effect) 622.8
      adverse effect or misadventure 622.8
  changes, spine or vertebra (*see also*
    Spondylosis) 721.90
  chitinous 277.39
  chorioretinal 363.40
    congenital 743.53
    hereditary 363.50
  choroid (colloid) (drusen) 363.40
    hereditary 363.50
    senile 363.41
      diffuse secondary 363.42
  cochlear 386.8

Degeneration, degenerative—*continued*
  collateral ligament (knee) (medial) 717.82
    lateral 717.81
  combined (spinal cord) (subacute) 266.2 *[336.2]*
    with anemia (pernicious) 281.0 *[336.2]*
      due to dietary deficiency 281.1 *[336.2]*
      due to vitamin B$_{12}$ deficiency anemia (dietary) 281.1 *[336.2]*
  conjunctiva 372.50
    amyloid 277.39 *[372.50]*
  cornea 371.40
    calcerous 371.44
    familial (hereditary) (*see also* Dystrophy, cornea) 371.50
      macular 371.55
      reticular 371.54
    hyaline (of old scars) 371.41
    marginal (Terrien's) 371.48
    mosaic (shagreen) 371.41
    nodular 371.46
    peripheral 371.48
    senile 371.41
  cortical (cerebellar) (parenchymatous) 334.2
    alcoholic 303.9 *[334.4]*
    diffuse, due to arteriopathy 437.0
  corticostriatal-spinal 334.8
  cretinoid 243
  cruciate ligament (knee) (posterior) 717.84
    anterior 717.83
  cutis 709.3
    amyloid 277.39
  dental pulp 522.2
  disc disease—*see* Degeneration, intervertebral disc
  dorsolateral (spinal cord)—*see* Degeneration, combined
  endocardial 424.90
  extrapyramidal NEC 333.90
  eye NEC 360.40
    macular (*see also* Degeneration, macula) 362.50
      congenital 362.75
      hereditary 362.76
  fatty (diffuse) (general) 272.8
    liver 571.8
      alcoholic 571.0
    localized site—*see* Degeneration, by site, fatty
    placenta—*see* Placenta, abnormal
  globe (eye) NEC 360.40
    macular—*see* Degeneration, macula
  grey matter 330.8
  heart (brown) (calcareous) (fatty) (fibrous)
      (hyaline) (mural) (muscular) (pigmentary)
      (senile) (with arteriosclerosis) (*see also*
      Degeneration, myocardial) 429.1
    amyloid 277.39 *[425.7]*
    atheromatous —*see* Arteriosclerosis, coronary
    gouty 274.82
    hypertensive (*see also* Hypertension, heart) 402.90
    ischemic 414.9
    valve, valvular—*see* Endocarditis
  hepatolenticular (Wilson's) 275.1
  hepatorenal 572.4
  heredofamilial
    brain NEC 331.89
    spinal cord NEC 336.8
  hyaline (diffuse) (generalized) 728.9
    localized—*see also* Degeneration, by site
      cornea 371.41
      keratitis 371.41
  hypertensive vascular—*see* Hypertension
  infrapatellar fat pad 729.31

Degeneration, degenerative—*continued*
  internal semilunar cartilage 717.3
  intervertebral disc 722.6
    with myelopathy 722.70
    cervical, cervicothoracic 722.4
      with myelopathy 722.71
    lumbar, lumbosacral 722.52
      with myelopathy 722.73
    thoracic, thoracolumbar 722.51
      with myelopathy 722.72
  intestine 569.89
    amyloid 277.39
    lardaceous 277.39
  iris (generalized) (*see also* Atrophy, iris) 364.59
    pigmentary 364.53
    pupillary margin 364.54
  ischemic—*see* Ischemia
  joint disease (*see also* Osteoarthrosis) 715.9
    multiple sites 715.09
    spine (*see also* Spondylosis) 721.90
  kidney (*see also* Sclerosis, renal) 587
    amyloid 277.39 *[583.81]*
    cyst, cystic (multiple) (solitary) 593.2
      congenital (*see also* Cystic, disease, kidney) 753.10
    fatty 593.89
    fibrocystic (congenital) 753.19
    lardaceous 277.39 *[583.81]*
    polycystic (congenital) 753.12
      adult type (APKD) 753.13
      autosomal dominant 753.13
      autosomal recessive 753.14
      childhood type (CPKD) 753.14
      infantile type 753.14
    waxy 277.39 *[583.81]*
  Kuhnt-Junius (retina) 362.52
  labyrinth, osseous 386.8
  lacrimal passages, cystic 375.12
  lardaceous (any site) 277.39
  lateral column (posterior), spinal cord (*see also*
      Degeneration, combined) 266.2 *[336.2]*
  lattice 362.63
  lens 366.9
    infantile, juvenile, or presenile 366.00
    senile 366.10
  lenticular (familial) (progressive) (Wilson's)
      (with cirrhosis of liver) 275.1
    striate artery 437.0
  lethal ball, prosthetic heart valve 996.02
  ligament
    collateral (knee) (medial) 717.82
      lateral 717.81
    cruciate (knee) (posterior) 717.84
      anterior 717.83
  liver (diffuse) 572.8
    amyloid 277.39
    congenital (cystic) 751.62
    cystic 572.8
      congenital 751.62
    fatty 571.8
      alcoholic 571.0
    hypertrophic 572.8
    lardaceous 277.39
    parenchymatous, acute or subacute (*see also*
        Necrosis, liver) 570
    pigmentary 572.8
    toxic (acute) 573.8
    waxy 277.39
  lung 518.8
  lymph gland 289.3
    hyaline 289.3
    lardaceous 277.39

Degeneration, degenerative— *continued*
  senile— *continued*
    retina, cystic 362.50
    vascular— *see* Arteriosclerosis
  silicone rubber poppet (prosthetic valve) 996.02
  sinus (cystic) (*see also* Sinusitis) 473.9
    polypoid 471.1
  skin 709.3
    amyloid 277.39
    colloid 709.3
  spinal (cord) 336.8
    amyloid 277.39
    column 733.90
    combined (subacute) (*see also* Degeneration,
        combined) 266.2 *[336.2]*
      with anemia (pernicious) 281.0 *[336.2]*
    dorsolateral (*see also* Degeneration,
        combined) 266.2 *[336.2]*
    familial NEC 336.8
    fatty 336.8
    funicular (*see also* Degeneration, combined)
        266.2 *[336.2]*
    heredofamilial NEC 336.8
    posterolateral (*see also* Degeneration,
        combined) 266.2 *[336.2]*
    subacute combined— *see* Degeneration,
        combined
    tuberculous (*see also* Tuberculosis) 013.8
  spine 733.90
  spleen 289.59
    amyloid 277.39
    lardaceous 277.39
  stomach 537.89
    lardaceous 277.39
  strionigral 333.0
  sudoriparous (cystic) 705.89
  suprarenal (capsule) (gland) 255.8
    with hypofunction 255.41
  sweat gland 705.89
  synovial membrane (pulpy) 727.9
  tapetoretinal 362.74
    adult or presenile form 362.50
  testis (postinfectional) 608.89
  thymus (gland) 254.8
    fatty 254.8
    lardaceous 277.39
  thyroid (gland) 246.8
  tricuspid (heart) (valve)— *see* Endocarditis,
      tricuspid
  tuberculous NEC (*see also* Tuberculosis) 011.9
  turbinate 733.90
  uterus 621.8
    cystic 621.8
  vascular (senile)— *see also* Arteriosclerosis
    hypertensive— *see* Hypertension
  vitreoretinal (primary) 362.73
    secondary 362.66
  vitreous humor (with infiltration) 379.21
  wallerian NEC— *see* Disorder, nerve
  waxy (any site) 277.39
  Wilson's hepatolenticular 275.1
Deglutition
  paralysis 784.99
    hysterical 300.11
  pneumonia 507.0
Degos' disease or syndrome 447.8
**Degradation disorder, branched-chain
    amino-acid** 270.3
Dehiscence
  anastomosis— *see* Complications, anastomosis
  cesarean wound 674.1

Dehiscence— *continued*
  closure of
    cornea 998.32
    fascia, superficial or muscular 998.31
    internal organ 998.31
    mucosa 998.32
    muscle or muscle flap 998.31
    ribs or rib cage 998.31
    skin 998.32
    skull or craniotomy 998.31
    sternum or sternotomy 998.31
    subcutaneous tissue 998.32
    tendon or ligament 998.31
    traumatic laceration (external) (internal)
        998.33
  episiotomy 674.2
  operation wound 998.32
    deep 998.31
    external 998.32
    internal 998.31
    superficial 998.32
  perineal wound (postpartum) 674.2
  postoperative 998.32
    abdomen 998.32
      internal 998.31
    internal 998.31
  traumatic injury wound repair 998.33
  uterine wound 674.1
Dehydration (cachexia) 276.51
  newborn 775.5
  with
    hypernatremia 276.0
    hyponatremia 276.1
Deiters' nucleus syndrome 386.19
Déjérine's disease 356.0
Déjérine-Klumpke paralysis 767.6
Déjérine-Roussy syndrome 338.0
Déjérine-Sottas disease or neuropathy
    (hypertrophic) 356.0
Déjérine-Thomas atrophy or syndrome 333.0
de Lange's syndrome (Amsterdam dwarf, mental
    retardation, and brachycephaly) 759.89
Delay, delayed
  adaptation, cones or rods 368.63
  any plane in pelvis
    affecting fetus or newborn 763.1
    complicating delivery 660.1
  birth or delivery NEC 662.1
    affecting fetus or newborn 763.9
    second twin, triplet, or multiple mate 662.3
  closure— *see also* Fistula
    cranial suture 756.0
    fontanel 756.0
  coagulation NEC 790.92
  conduction (cardiac) (ventricular) 426.9
  delivery NEC 662.1
    second twin, triplet, etc. 662.3
      affecting fetus or newborn 763.89
  development
    in childhood 783.40
      physiological 783.40
    intellectual NEC 315.9
    learning NEC 315.2
    reading 315.00
    sexual 259.0
    speech 315.39
      and language due to hearing loss 315.34
      associated with hyperkinesis 314.1
    spelling 315.09
  gastric emptying 536.8

Delay, delayed—*continued*
  menarche 256.39
    due to pituitary hypofunction 253.4
  menstruation (cause unknown) 626.8
  milestone in childhood 783.42
  motility—*see* Hypomotility
  passage of meconium (newborn) 777.1
  primary respiration 768.9
  puberty 259.0
  separation of umbilical cord 779.83
  sexual maturation, female 259.0
  vaccination V64.00
Del Castillo's syndrome (germinal aplasia) 606.0
Deleage's disease 359.89
Deletion syndrome
  5p 758.31
  22q11.2 758.32
  autosomal NEC 758.39
  constitutional 5q deletion 758.39
Delhi (boil) (button) (sore) 085.1
Delinquency (juvenile) 312.9
  group (*see also* Disturbance, conduct) 312.2
  neurotic 312.4
Delirium, delirious 780.09
  acute (psychotic) 293.0
  alcoholic 291.0
    acute 291.0
    chronic 291.1
  alcoholicum 291.0
  chronic (*see also* Psychosis) 293.89
    due to or associated with physical
      condition—*see* Psychosis, organic
  due to conditions classified elsewhere 293.0
  drug-induced 292.81
  eclamptic (*see also* Eclampsia) 780.39
  exhaustion (*see also* Reaction, stress, acute)
    308.9
  hysterical 300.11
  in
    presenile dementia 290.11
    senile dementia 290.3
  induced by drug 292.81
  manic, maniacal (acute) (*see also* Psychosis,
    affective) 296.0
    recurrent episode 296.1
    single episode 296.0
  puerperal 293.9
  senile 290.3
  subacute (psychotic) 293.1
  thyroid (*see also* Thyrotoxicosis) 242.9
  traumatic—*see also* Injury, intracranial
    with
      lesion, spinal cord—*see* Injury, spinal, by
        site
      shock, spinal—*see* Injury, spinal, by site
  tremens (impending) 291.0
  uremic—*see* Uremia
  withdrawal
    alcoholic (acute) 291.0
      chronic 291.1
    drug 292.0

Delivery

Note—Use the following fifth-digit
subclassification with categories
640-649, 651-676:

0 unspecified as to episode of care
1 delivered, with or without mention of
   antepartum condition
2 delivered, with mention of
   postpartum complication
3 antepartum condition or complication
4 postpartum condition or
   complication

  breech (assisted) (spontaneous) 652.2
    affecting fetus or newborn 763.0
    extraction NEC 669.6
  cesarean (for) 669.7
    abnormal
      cervix 654.6
      pelvic organs or tissues 654.9
      pelvis (bony) (major) NEC 653.0
      presentation or position 652.9
        in multiple gestation 652.6
      size, fetus 653.5
      soft parts (of pelvis) 654.9
      uterus, congenital 654.0
      vagina 654.7
      vulva 654.8
    abruptio placentae 641.2
    acromion presentation 652.8
    affecting fetus or newborn 763.4
    anteversion, cervix or uterus 654.4
    atony, uterus 661.2
      with hemorrhage 666.1
    bicornis or bicornuate uterus 654.0
    breech presentation 652.2
    brow presentation 652.4
    cephalopelvic disproportion (normally formed
      fetus) 653.4
    chin presentation 652.4
    cicatrix of cervix 654.6
    contracted pelvis (general) 653.1
      inlet 653.2
      outlet 653.3
    cord presentation or prolapse 663.0
    cystocele 654.4
    deformity (acquired) (congenital)
      pelvic organs or tissues NEC 654.9
      pelvis (bony) NEC 653.0
    displacement, uterus NEC 654.4
    disproportion NEC 653.9
    distress
      fetal 656.8
      maternal 669.0
    eclampsia 642.6
    face presentation 652.4
    failed
      forceps 660.7
      trial of labor NEC 660.6
      vacuum extraction 660.7
      ventouse 660.7
    fetal deformity 653.7
    fetal-maternal hemorrhage 656.0
    fetus, fetal
      distress 656.8
      prematurity 656.8
    fibroid (tumor) (uterus) 654.1
    footling 652.8
      with successful version 652.1

Delivery—*continued*
cesarean—*continued*
  hemorrhage (antepartum) (intrapartum) NEC
      641.9
  hydrocephalic fetus 653.6
  incarceration of uterus 654.3
  incoordinate uterine action 661.4
  inertia, uterus 661.2
    primary 661.0
    secondary 661.1
  lateroversion, uterus or cervix 654.4
  mal lie 652.9
  malposition
    fetus 652.9
      in multiple gestation 652.6
    pelvic organs or tissues NEC 654.9
    uterus NEC or cervix 654.4
  malpresentation NEC 652.9
    in multiple gestation 652.6
  maternal
    diabetes mellitus (conditions classifiable to
        249 and 250) 648.0
    heart disease NEC 648.6
  meconium in liquor 656.8
    staining only 792.3
  oblique presentation 652.3
  oversize fetus 653.5
  pelvic tumor NEC 654.9
  placental insufficiency 656.5
  placenta previa 641.0
    with hemorrhage 641.1
  poor dilation, cervix 661.0
  pre-eclampsia 642.4
    severe 642.5
  previous
    cesarean delivery 654.2
    surgery (to)
      cervix 654.6
      gynecological NEC 654.9
      rectum 654.8
      uterus NEC 654.9
        from previous cesarean delivery 654.2
      vagina 654.7
  prolapse
    arm or hand 652.7
    uterus 654.4
  prolonged labor 662.1
  rectocele 654.4
  retroversion, uterus or cervix 654.3
  rigid
    cervix 654.6
    pelvic floor 654.4
    perineum 654.8
    vagina 654.7
    vulva 654.8
  sacculation, pregnant uterus 654.4
  scar(s)
    cervix 654.6
    cesarean delivery 654.2
    uterus NEC 654.9
      due to previous cesarean delivery 654.2
  Shirodkar suture in situ 654.5
  shoulder presentation 652.8
  stenosis or stricture, cervix 654.6
  transverse presentation or lie 652.3
  tumor, pelvic organs or tissues NEC 654.4
  umbilical cord presentation or prolapse 663.0
  completely normal case—*see* category 650

Delivery—*continued*
complicated (by) NEC 669.9
  abdominal tumor, fetal 653.7
    causing obstructed labor 660.1
  abnormal, abnormality of
    cervix 654.6
      causing obstructed labor 660.2
    forces of labor 661.9
    formation of uterus 654.0
    pelvic organs or tissues 654.9
      causing obstructed labor 660.2
    pelvis (bony) (major) NEC 653.0
      causing obstructed labor 660.1
    presentation or position NEC 652.9
      causing obstructed labor 660.0
    size, fetus 653.5
      causing obstructed labor 660.1
    soft parts (of pelvis) 654.9
      causing obstructed labor 660.2
    uterine contractions NEC 661.9
    uterus (formation) 654.0
      causing obstructed labor 660.2
    vagina 654.7
      causing obstructed labor 660.2
  abnormally formed uterus (any type)
      (congenital) 654.0
    causing obstructed labor 660.2
  acromion presentation 652.8
    causing obstructed labor 660.0
  adherent placenta 667.0
    with hemorrhage 666.0
  adhesions, uterus (to abdominal wall) 654.4
  advanced maternal age NEC 659.6
    multigravida 659.6
    primigravida 659.5
  air embolism 673.0
  amnionitis 658.4
  amniotic fluid embolism 673.1
  anesthetic death 668.9
  annular detachment, cervix 665.3
  antepartum hemorrhage—*see* Delivery,
      complicated, hemorrhage
  anteversion, cervix or uterus 654.4
    causing obstructed labor 660.2
  apoplexy 674.0
    placenta 641.2
  arrested active phase 661.1
  asymmetrical pelvis bone 653.0
    causing obstructed labor 660.1
  atony, uterus with hemorrhage (hypotonic)
      (inertia) 666.1
    hypertonic 661.4
  Bandl's ring 661.4
  battledore placenta—*see* Placenta, abnormal
  bicornis or bicornuate uterus 654.0
    causing obstructed labor 660.2
  birth injury to mother NEC 665.9
  bleeding (*see also* Delivery, complicated,
      hemorrhage) 641.9
  breech presentation (assisted) (buttocks)
      (complete) (frank) (spontaneous) 652.2
    with successful version 652.1
  brow presentation 652.4
  cephalopelvic disproportion (normally formed
      fetus) 653.4
    causing obstructed labor 660.1
  cerebral hemorrhage 674.0
  cervical dystocia 661.2
  chin presentation 652.4
    causing obstructed labor 660.0

Delivery—*continued*
  complicated by—*continued*
    cicatrix
      cervix 654.6
        causing obstructed labor 660.2
      vagina 654.7
        causing obstructed labor 660.2
    coagulation defect 649.3
    colporrhexis 665.4
      with perineal laceration 664.0
    compound presentation 652.8
      causing obstructed labor 660.0
    compression of cord (umbilical) 663.2
      around neck 663.1
      cord prolapsed 663.0
    contraction, contracted pelvis 653.1
      causing obstructed labor 660.1
      general 653.1
        causing obstructed labor 660.1
      inlet 653.2
        causing obstructed labor 660.1
      midpelvic 653.8
        causing obstructed labor 660.1
      midplane 653.8
        causing obstructed labor 660.1
      outlet 653.3
        causing obstructed labor 660.1
    contraction ring 661.4
    cord (umbilical) 663.9
      around neck, tightly or with compression 663.1
        without compression 663.3
      bruising 663.6
      complication NEC 663.9
        specified type NEC 663.8
      compression NEC 663.2
      entanglement NEC 663.3
        with compression 663.2
      forelying 663.0
      hematoma 663.6
      marginal attachment 663.8
      presentation 663.0
      prolapse (complete) (occult) (partial) 663.0
      short 663.4
      specified complication NEC 663.8
      thrombosis (vessels) 663.6
      vascular lesion 663.6
      velamentous insertion 663.8
    Couvelaire uterus 641.2
    cretin pelvis (dwarf type) (male type) 653.1
      causing obstructed labor 660.1
    crossbirth 652.3
      with successful version 652.1
      causing obstructed labor 660.0
    cyst (Gartner's duct) 654.7
    cystocele 654.4
      causing obstructed labor 660.2
    death of fetus (near term) 656.4
      early (before 22 completed weeks'
        gestation) 632
    deformity (acquired) (congenital)
      fetus 653.7
        causing obstructed labor 660.1
      pelvic organs or tissues NEC 654.9
        causing obstructed labor 660.2
      pelvis (bony) NEC 653.0
        causing obstructed labor 660.1
    delay, delayed
      delivery in multiple pregnancy 662.3
      due to locked mates 660.5
      following rupture of membranes
        (spontaneous) 658.2
        artificial 658.3

Delivery—*continued*
  complicated by—*continued*
    depressed fetal heart tones 659.7
    diastasis recti 665.8
    dilatation
      bladder 654.4
        causing obstructed labor 660.2
      cervix, incomplete, poor or slow 661.0
    diseased placenta 656.7
    displacement uterus NEC 654.4
      causing obstructed labor 660.2
    disproportion NEC 653.9
      causing obstructed labor 660.1
    disruptio uteri—*see* Delivery, complicated,
      rupture, uterus
    distress
      fetal 656.8
      maternal 669.0
    double uterus (congenital) 654.0
      causing obstructed labor 660.2
    dropsy amnion 657
    dysfunction, uterus 661.9
      hypertonic 661.4
      hypotonic 661.2
        primary 661.0
        secondary 661.1
      incoordinate 661.4
    dystocia
      cervical 661.2
      fetal—*see* Delivery, complicated, abnormal,
        presentation
      maternal—*see* Delivery, complicated,
        prolonged labor
      pelvic—*see* Delivery, complicated,
        contraction pelvis
      positional 652.8
      shoulder girdle 660.4
    eclampsia 642.6
    ectopic kidney 654.4
      causing obstructed labor 660.2
    edema, cervix 654.6
      causing obstructed labor 660.2
    effusion, amniotic fluid 658.1
    elderly multigravida 659.6
    elderly primigravida 659.5
    embolism (pulmonary) 673.2
      air 673.0
      amniotic fluid 673.1
      blood-clot 673.2
      cerebral 674.0
      fat 673.8
      pyemic 673.3
      septic 673.3
    entanglement, umbilical cord 663.3
      with compression 663.2
      around neck (with compression) 663.1
    eversion, cervix or uterus 665.2
    excessive
      fetal growth 653.5
        causing obstructed labor 660.1
      size of fetus 653.5
        causing obstructed labor 660.1
    face presentation 652.4
      causing obstructed labor 660.0
      to pubes 660.3
    failure, fetal head to enter pelvic brim 652.5
      causing obstructed labor 660.0
    female genital mutilation 660.8

Delivery—*continued*
  complicated by—*continued*
    fetal
      acid-base balance 656.8
      death (near term) NEC 656.4
        early (before 22 completed weeks'
          gestation) 632
      deformity 653.7
        causing obstructed labor 660.1
      distress 656.8
      heart rate or rhythm 659.7
      reduction of multiple fetuses reduced to
        single fetus 651.7
    fetopelvic disproportion 653.4
      causing obstructed labor 660.1
    fever during labor 659.2
    fibroid (tumor) (uterus) 654.1
      causing obstructed labor 660.2
    fibromyomata 654.1
      causing obstructed labor 660.2
    forelying umbilical cord 663.0
    fracture of coccyx 665.6
    hematoma 664.5
      broad ligament 665.7
      ischial spine 665.7
      pelvic 665.7
      perineum 664.5
      soft tissues 665.7
      subdural 674.0
      umbilical cord 663.6
      vagina 665.7
      vulva or perineum 664.5
    hemorrhage (uterine) (antepartum)
      (intrapartum) (pregnancy) 641.9
    accidental 641.2
    associated with
      afibrinogenemia 641.3
      coagulation defect 641.3
        hyperfibrinolysis 641.3
        hypofibrinogenemia 641.3
    cerebral 674.0
    due to
      low-lying placenta 641.1
      placenta previa 641.1
      premature separation of placenta (normally
        implanted) 641.2
      retained placenta 666.0
      trauma 641.8
      uterine leiomyoma 641.8
    marginal sinus rupture 641.2
    placenta NEC 641.9
    postpartum (atonic) (immediate) (within 24
      hours) 666.1
      with retained or trapped placenta 666.0
      third stage 666.0
      delayed 666.2
      secondary 666.2
  hourglass contraction, uterus 661.4
  hydramnios 657
  hydrocephalic fetus 653.6
    causing obstructed labor 660.1
  hydrops fetalis 653.7
    causing obstructed labor 660.1
  hypertension—*see* Hypertension, complicating
    pregnancy
  hypertonic uterine dysfunction 661.4
  hypotonic uterine dysfunction 661.2
  impacted shoulders 660.4
  incarceration, uterus 654.3
    causing obstructed labor 660.2
  incomplete dilation (cervix) 661.0
  incoordinate uterus 661.4

Delivery—*continued*
  complicated by—*continued*
    indication NEC 659.9
      specified type NEC 659.8
    inertia, uterus 661.2
      hypertonic 661.4
      hypotonic 661.2
      primary 661.0
      secondary 661.1
    infantile
      genitalia 654.4
        causing obstructed labor 660.2
      uterus (os) 654.4
        causing obstructed labor 660.2
    injury (to mother) NEC 665.9
    intrauterine fetal death (near term) NEC 656.4
      early (before 22 completed weeks'
        gestation) 632
    inversion, uterus 665.2
    kidney, ectopic 654.4
      causing obstructed labor 660.2
    knot (true), umbilical cord 663.2
    labor, premature (before 37 completed weeks
      gestation) 644.2
    laceration 664.9
      anus (sphincter) (healed) (old) 654.8
        not associated with third-degree perineal
          laceration 664.6
        with mucosa 664.3
      bladder (urinary) 665.5
      bowel 665.5
      central 664.4
      cervix (uteri) 665.3
      fourchette 664.0
      hymen 664.0
      labia (majora) (minora) 664.0
      pelvic
        floor 664.1
        organ NEC 665.5
      perineum, perineal 664.4
        first degree 664.0
        second degree 664.1
        third degree 664.2
        fourth degree 664.3
        central 664.4
        extensive NEC 664.4
        muscles 664.1
        skin 664.0
        slight 664.0
      peritoneum 665.5
      periurethral tissue 664.8
      rectovaginal (septum) (without perineal
        laceration) 665.4
        with perineum 664.2
        with anal or rectal mucosa 664.3
      skin (perineum) 664.0
      specified site or type NEC 664.8
      sphincter ani (healed) (old) 654.8
        not associated with third-degree perineal
          laceration 664.6
        with mucosa 664.3
      urethra 665.5
      uterus 665.1
        before labor 665.0
      vagina, vaginal (deep) (high) (sulcus) (wall)
        (without perineal laceration) 665.4
        with perineum 664.0
        muscles, with perineum 664.1
      vulva 664.0
    lateroversion, uterus or cervix 654.4
      causing obstructed labor 660.2
    locked mates 660.5

Delivery—*continued*
  complicated by—*continued*
    low implantation of placenta—*see* Delivery,
      complicated, placenta, previa
    mal lie 652.9
    malposition
      fetus NEC 652.9
        causing obstructed labor 660.0
      pelvic organs or tissues NEC 654.9
        causing obstructed labor 660.2
      placenta 641.1
        without hemorrhage 641.0
      uterus NEC or cervix 654.4
        causing obstructed labor 660.2
    malpresentation 652.9
      causing obstructed labor 660.0
    marginal sinus (bleeding) (rupture) 641.2
    maternal hypotension syndrome 669.2
    meconium in liquor 656.8
    membranes, retained—*see* Delivery,
      complicated, placenta, retained
    mentum presentation 652.4
      causing obstructed labor 660.0
    metrorrhagia (myopathia)—*see* Delivery,
      complicated, hemorrhage
    metrorrhexis—*see* Delivery, complicated,
      rupture, uterus
    multiparity (grand) 659.4
    myelomeningocele, fetus 653.7
      causing obstructed labor 660.1
    Nägele's pelvis 653.0
      causing obstructed labor 660.1
    nonengagement, fetal head 652.5
      causing obstructed labor 660.0
    oblique presentation 652.3
      causing obstructed labor 660.0
    obstetric
      shock 669.1
      trauma NEC 665.9
    obstructed labor 660.9
      due to
        abnormality pelvic organs or tissues
          (conditions classifiable to 654.0-654.9)
          660.2
        deep transverse arrest 660.3
        impacted shoulders 660.4
        locked twins 660.5
        malposition and malpresentation of fetus
          (conditions classifiable to 652.0-652.9)
          660.0
        persistent occipitoposterior 660.3
        shoulder dystocia 660.4
    occult prolapse of umbilical cord 663.0
    oversize fetus 653.5
      causing obstructed labor 660.1
    pathological retraction ring, uterus 661.4
    pelvic
      arrest (deep) (high) (of fetal head)
        (transverse) 660.3
      deformity (bone)—*see also* Deformity,
        pelvis, with disproportion
      soft tissue 654.9
        causing obstructed labor 660.2
      tumor NEC 654.9
        causing obstructed labor 660.2
    penetration, pregnant uterus by instrument
      665.1
    perforation—*see* Delivery, complicated,
      laceration

Delivery—*continued*
  complicated by—*continued*
    persistent
      hymen 654.8
        causing obstructed labor 660.2
      occipitoposterior 660.3
    placenta, placental
      ablatio 641.2
      abnormality 656.7
        with hemorrhage 641.2
      abruptio 641.2
      accreta 667.0
        with hemorrhage 666.0
      adherent (without hemorrhage) 667.0
        with hemorrhage 666.0
      apoplexy 641.2
      battledore 663.8
      detachment (premature) 641.2
      disease 656.7
      hemorrhage NEC 641.9
      increta (without hemorrhage) 667.0
        with hemorrhage 666.0
      low (implantation) 641.1
        without hemorrhage 641.0
      malformation 656.7
        with hemorrhage 641.2
      malposition 641.1
        without hemorrhage 641.0
      marginal sinus rupture 641.2
      percreta 667.0
        with hemorrhage 666.0
      premature separation 641.2
      previa (central) (lateral) (marginal) (partial)
        641.1
        without hemorrhage 641.0
      retained (with hemorrhage) 666.0
        without hemorrhage 667.0
      rupture of marginal sinus 641.2
      separation (premature) 641.2
      trapped 666.0
        without hemorrhage 667.0
      vicious insertion 641.1
    polyhydramnios 657
    polyp, cervix 654.6
      causing obstructed labor 660.2
    precipitate labor 661.3
    premature
      labor (before 37 completed weeks gestation)
        644.2
      rupture, membranes 658.1
        delayed delivery following 658.2
    presenting umbilical cord 663.0
    previous
      cesarean delivery 654.2
      surgery
        cervix 654.6
          causing obstructed labor 660.2
        gynecological NEC 654.9
          causing obstructed labor 660.2
        perineum 654.8
        rectum 654.8
        uterus NEC 654.9
          due to previous cesarean delivery 654.2
        vagina 654.7
          causing obstructed labor 660.2
        vulva 654.8
    primary uterine inertia 661.0
    primipara, elderly or old 659.5

Delivery—*continued*
  complicated by—*continued*
  prolapse
    arm or hand 652.7
      causing obstructed labor 660.0
    cord (umbilical) 663.0
    fetal extremity 652.8
    foot or leg 652.8
      causing obstructed labor 660.0
    umbilical cord (complete) (occult) (partial)
      663.0
    uterus 654.4
      causing obstructed labor 660.2
  prolonged labor 662.1
    active phase 661.2
    due to
      cervical dystocia 661.2
      contraction ring 661.4
      tetanic uterus 661.4
      uterine inertia 661.2
        primary 661.0
        secondary 661.1
    first stage 662.0
    latent phase 661.0
    second stage 662.2
  pyrexia during labor 659.2
  rachitic pelvis 653.2
    causing obstructed labor 660.1
  rectocele 654.4
    causing obstructed labor 660.2
  retained membranes or portions of placenta
    666.2
    without hemorrhage 667.1
  retarded (prolonged) birth 662.1
  retention secundines (with hemorrhage) 666.2
    without hemorrhage 667.1
  retroversion, uterus or cervix 654.3
    causing obstructed labor 660.2
  rigid
    cervix 654.6
      causing obstructed labor 660.2
    pelvic floor 654.4
      causing obstructed labor 660.2
    perineum or vulva 654.8
      causing obstructed labor 660.2
    vagina 654.7
      causing obstructed labor 660.2
  Robert's pelvis 653.0
    causing obstructed labor 660.1
  rupture—*see also* Delivery, complicated,
    laceration
    bladder (urinary) 665.5
    cervix 665.3
    marginal sinus 641.2
    membranes, premature 658.1
    pelvic organ NEC 665.5
    perineum (without mention of other
      laceration)—*see* Delivery, complicated,
      laceration, perineum
    peritoneum 665.5
    urethra 665.5
    uterus (during labor) 665.1
      before labor 665.0
  sacculation, pregnant uterus 654.4
  sacral teratomas, fetal 653.7
    causing obstructed labor 660.1

Delivery—*continued*
  complicated by—*continued*
  scar(s)
    cervix 654.6
      causing obstructed labor 660.2
    cesarean delivery 654.2
      causing obstructed labor 660.2
    perineum 654.8
      causing obstructed labor 660.2
    uterus NEC 654.9
      causing obstructed labor 660.2
      due to previous cesarean delivery 654.2
    vagina 654.7
      causing obstructed labor 660.2
    vulva 654.8
      causing obstructed labor 660.2
  scoliotic pelvis 653.0
    causing obstructed labor 660.1
  secondary uterine inertia 661.1
  secundines, retained—*see* Delivery,
    complicated, placenta, retained
  separation
    placenta (premature) 641.2
    pubic bone 665.6
    symphysis pubis 665.6
  septate vagina 654.7
    causing obstructed labor 660.2
  shock (birth) (obstetric) (puerperal) 669.1
  short cord syndrome 663.4
  shoulder
    girdle dystocia 660.4
    presentation 652.8
      causing obstructed labor 660.0
  Siamese twins 678.1
  slow slope active phase 661.2
  spasm
    cervix 661.4
    uterus 661.4
  spondylolisthesis, pelvis 653.3
    causing obstructed labor 660.1
  spondylolysis (lumbosacral) 653.3
    causing obstructed labor 660.1
  spondylosis 653.0
    causing obstructed labor 660.1
  stenosis or stricture
    cervix 654.6
      causing obstructed labor 660.2
    vagina 654.7
      causing obstructed labor 660.2
  sudden death, unknown cause 669.9
  tear (pelvic organ) (*see also* Delivery,
    complicated, laceration) 664.9
    anal sphincter (healed) (old) 654.8
      not associated with third-degree perineal
        laceration 664.6
  teratomas, sacral, fetal 653.7
    causing obstructed labor 660.1
  tetanic uterus 661.4
  tipping pelvis 653.0
    causing obstructed labor 660.1
  transverse
    arrest (deep) 660.3
    presentation or lie 652.3
      with successful version 652.1
      causing obstructed labor 660.0
  trauma (obstetrical) NEC 665.9

Delivery—*continued*
complicated by—*continued*
tumor
abdominal, fetal 653.7
causing obstructed labor 660.1
pelvic organs or tissues NEC 654.9
causing obstructed labor 660.2
umbilical cord (*see also* Delivery,
complicated, cord) 663.9
around neck tightly, or with compression
663.1
entanglement NEC 663.3
with compression 663.2
prolapse (complete) (occult) (partial) 663.0
unstable lie 652.0
causing obstructed labor 660.0
uterine
inertia (*see also* Delivery, complicated,
inertia, uterus) 661.2
spasm 661.4
vasa previa 663.5
velamentous insertion of cord 663.8
young maternal age 659.8
delayed NEC 662.1
following rupture of membranes (spontaneous)
658.2
artificial 658.3
second twin, triplet, etc. 662.3
difficult NEC 669.9
previous, affecting management of pregnancy
or childbirth V23.49
specified type NEC 669.8
early onset (spontaneous) 644.2
forceps NEC 669.5
affecting fetus or newborn 763.2
footling 652.8
with successful version 652.1
missed (at or near term) 656.4
multiple gestation NEC 651.9
with fetal loss and retention of one or more
fetus(es) 651.6
following (elective) fetal reduction 651.7
specified type NEC 651.8
with fetal loss and retention of one or more
fetus(es) 651.6
following (elective) fetal reduction 651.7
nonviable infant 656.4
normal—*see* category 650
precipitate 661.3
affecting fetus or newborn 763.6
premature NEC (before 37 completed weeks
gestation) 644.2
previous, affecting management of pregnancy
V23.41
quadruplet NEC 651.2
with fetal loss and retention of one or more
fetus(es) 651.5
following (elective) fetal reduction 651.7
quintuplet NEC 651.8
with fetal loss and retention of one or more
fetus(es) 651.6
following (elective) fetal reduction 651.7
sextuplet NEC 651.8
with fetal loss and retention of one or more
fetus(es) 651.6
following (elective) fetal reduction 651.7
specified complication NEC 669.8
stillbirth (near term) NEC 656.4
early (before 22 completed weeks' gestation)
632

Delivery—*continued*
term pregnancy (live birth) NEC—*see* category
650
stillbirth NEC 656.4
threatened premature 644.2
triplets NEC 651.1
with fetal loss and retention of one or more
fetus(es) 651.4
delayed delivery (one or more mates) 662.3
following (elective) fetal reduction 651.7
locked mates 660.5
twins NEC 651.0
with fetal loss and retention of one or more
fetus(es) 651.3
delayed delivery (one or more mates) 662.3
following (elective) fetal reduction 651.7
locked mates 660.5
uncomplicated—*see* category 650
vacuum extractor NEC 669.5
affecting fetus or newborn 763.3
ventouse NEC 669.5
affecting fetus or newborn 763.3
Dellen, cornea 371.41
Delusions (paranoid) 297.9
grandiose 297.1
parasitosis 300.29
systematized 297.1
Dementia 294.8
alcohol-induced persisting (*see also* Psychosis,
alcoholic) 291.2
Alzheimer's—*see* Alzheimer's dementia
arteriosclerotic (simple type) (uncomplicated)
290.40
with
acute confusional state 290.41
delirium 290.41
delusions 290.42
depressed mood 290.43
depressed type 290.43
paranoid type 290.42
Binswanger's 290.12
catatonic (acute) (*see also* Schizophrenia) 295.2
congenital (*see also* Retardation, mental) 319
degenerative 290.9
presenile-onset—*see* Dementia, presenile
senile-onset—*see* Dementia, senile
developmental (*see also* Schizophrenia) 295.9
dialysis 294.8
transient 293.9
drug-induced persisting (*see also* Psychosis,
drug) 292.82
due to or associated with condition(s) classified
elsewhere
Alzheimer's
with behavioral disturbance 331.0 [294.11]
without behavioral disturbance 331.0
[294.10]
cerebral lipidoses
with behavioral disturbance 330.1 [294.11]
without behavioral disturbance 330.1
[294.10]
epilepsy
with behavioral disturbance 345.9 [294.11]
without behavioral disturbance 345.9
[294.10]
hepatolenticular degeneration
with behavioral disturbance 275.1 [294.11]
without behavioral disturbance 275.1
[294.10]
HIV
with behavioral disturbance 042 [294.11]
without behavioral disturbance 042 [294.10]

Dementia—*continued*
  due to or associated with—*continued*
  Huntington's chorea
    with behavioral disturbance 333.4 *[294.11]*
    without behavioral disturbance 333.4
      [294.10]
  Jakob-Creutzfeldt disease (CJD)
    with behavioral disturbance 046.19 *[294.11]*
    without behavioral disturbance 046.19
      [294.10]
    variant (vCJD) 046.11
      with dementia
        with behavioral disturbance 046.11
          [294.11]
        without behavioral disturbance 046.11
          [294.10]
  Lewy bodies
    with behavioral disturbance 331.82 *[294.11]*
    without behavioral disturbance 331.82
      [294.10]
  multiple sclerosis
    with behavioral disturbance 340 *[294.11]*
    without behavioral disturbance 340 *[294.10]*
  neurosyphilis
    with behavioral disturbance 094.9 *[294.11]*
    without behavioral disturbance 094.9
      [294.10]
  Parkinsonism
    with behavioral disturbance 331.82 *[294.11]*
    without behavioral disturbance 331.82
      [294.10]
  Pelizaeus-Merzbacher disease
    with behavioral disturbance 333.0 *[294.11]*
    without behavioral disturbance 333.0
      [294.10]
  Pick's disease
    with behavioral disturbance 331.11 *[294.11]*
    without behavioral disturbance 331.11
      [294.10]
  polyarteritis nodosa
    with behavioral disturbance 446.0 *[294.11]*
    without behavioral disturbance 446.0
      [294.10]
  syphilis
    with behavioral disturbance 094.1 *[294.11]*
    without behavioral disturbance 094.1
      [294.10]
  Wilson's disease
    with behavioral disturbance 275.1 *[294.11]*
    without behavioral disturbance 275.1
      [294.10]
  frontal 331.19
    with behavioral disturbance 331.19 *[294.11]*
    without behavioral disturbance 331.19
      [294.10]
  frontotemporal 331.19
    with behavioral disturbance 331.19 *[294.11]*
    without behavioral disturbance 331.19
      [294.10]
  hebephrenic (acute) 295.1
  Heller's (infantile psychosis) (*see also*
    Psychosis, childhood) 299.1
  idiopathic 290.9
    presenile-onset—*see* Dementia, presenile
    senile-onset—*see* Dementia, senile
  in
    arteriosclerotic brain disease 290.40
    senility 290.0
  induced by drug 292.82
  infantile, infantilia (*see also* Psychosis,
    childhood) 299.0

Dementia—*continued*
  Lewy body 331.82
    with behavioral disturbance 331.82 *[294.11]*
    without behavioral disturbance 331.82 *[294.10]*
  multi-infarct (cerebrovascular) (*see also*
    Dementia, arteriosclerotic) 290.40
  old age 290.0
  paralytica, paralytic 094.1
    juvenilis 090.40
    syphilitic 094.1
      congenital 090.40
    tabetic form 094.1
  paranoid (*see also* Schizophrenia) 295.3
  paraphrenic (*see also* Schizophrenia) 295.3
  paretic 094.1
  praecox (*see also* Schizophrenia) 295.9
  presenile 290.10
    with
      acute confusional state 290.11
      delirium 290.11
      delusional features 290.12
      depressive features 290.13
    depressed type 290.13
    paranoid type 290.12
    simple type 290.10
    uncomplicated 290.10
  primary (acute) (*see also* Schizophrenia) 295.0
  progressive, syphilitic 094.1
  puerperal—*see* Psychosis, puerperal
  schizophrenic (*see also* Schizophrenia) 295.9
  senile 290.0
    with
      acute confusional state 290.3
      delirium 290.3
      delusional features 290.20
      depressive features 290.21
    depressed type 290.21
    exhaustion 290.0
    paranoid type 290.20
  simple type (acute) (*see also* Schizophrenia) 295.0
  simplex (acute) (*see also* Schizophrenia) 295.0
  syphilitic 094.1
  uremic—*see* Uremia
  vascular 290.40
    with
      delirium 290.41
      delusions 290.42
      depressed mood 290.43
Demerol dependence (*see also* Dependence)
  304.0
Demineralization, ankle (*see also* Osteoporosis)
  733.00
Demodex folliculorum (infestation) 133.8
Demoralization 799.25
de Morgan's spots (senile angiomas) 448.1
Demyelinating
  polyneuritis, chronic inflammatory 357.81
Demyelination, demyelinization
  central nervous system 341.9
    specified NEC 341.8
  corpus callosum (central) 341.8
  global 340
Dengue (fever) 061
  sandfly 061
  vaccination, prophylactic (against) V05.1
  virus hemorrhagic fever 065.4
Dens
  evaginatus 520.2
  in dente 520.2
  invaginatus 520.2
Dense breast(s) —*omit code*

Density
  increased, bone (disseminated) (generalized)
    (spotted) 733.99
  lung (nodular) 518.89
Dental —*see also* condition
  examination only V72.2
Dentia praecox 520.6
Denticles (in pulp) 522.2
Dentigerous cyst 526.0
Dentin
  irregular (in pulp) 522.3
  opalescent 520.5
  secondary (in pulp) 522.3
  sensitive 521.89
Dentinogenesis imperfecta 520.5
Dentinoma (M9271/0) 213.1
  upper jaw (bone) 213.0
Dentition 520.7
  abnormal 520.6
  anomaly 520.6
  delayed 520.6
  difficult 520.7
  disorder of 520.6
  precocious 520.6
  retarded 520.6
Denture sore (mouth) 528.9
Dependence

Note—Use the following fifth-digit
subclassification with category 304:

0 unspecified
1 continuous
2 episodic
3 in remission

---

  with
    withdrawal symptoms
      alcohol 291.81
      drug 292.0
  14-hydroxy-dihydromorphinone 304.0
  absinthe 304.6
  acemorphan 304.0
  acetanilid(e) 304.6
  acetophenetidin 304.6
  acetorphine 304.0
  acetyldihydrocodeine 304.0
  acetyldihydrocodeinone 304.0
  Adalin 304.1
  Afghanistan black 304.3
  agrypnal 304.1
  alcohol, alcoholic (ethyl) (methyl) (wood) 303.9
    maternal, with suspected fetal damage
      affecting management of pregnancy 655.4
  allobarbitone 304.1
  allonal 304.1
  allylisopropylacetylurea 304.1
  alphaprodine (hydrochloride) 304.0
  Alurate 304.1
  Alvodine 304.0
  amethocaine 304.6
  amidone 304.0
  amidopyrine 304.6
  aminopyrine 304.6
  amobarbital 304.1
  amphetamine(s) (type) (drugs classifiable to
    969.7) 304.4
  amylene hydrate 304.6
  amylobarbitone 304.1
  amylocaine 304.6

Dependence—*continued*
  Amytal (sodium) 304.1
  analgesic (drug) NEC 304.6
    synthetic with morphine-like effect 304.0
  anesthetic (agent) (drug) (gas) (general) (local)
    NEC 304.6
  Angel dust 304.6
  anileridine 304.0
  antipyrine 304.6
  anxiolytic 304.1
  aprobarbital 304.1
  aprobarbitone 304.1
  atropine 304.6
  Avertin (bromide) 304.6
  barbenyl 304.1
  barbital(s) 304.1
  barbitone 304.1
  barbiturate(s) (compounds) (drugs classifiable to
    967.0) 304.1
  barbituric acid (and compounds) 304.1
  benzedrine 304.4
  benzylmorphine 304.0
  Beta-chlor 304.1
  bhang 304.3
  blue velvet 304.0
  Brevital 304.1
  bromal (hydrate) 304.1
  bromide(s) NEC 304.1
  bromine compounds NEC 304.1
  bromisovalum 304.1
  bromoform 304.1
  Bromo-seltzer 304.1
  bromural 304.1
  butabarbital (sodium) 304.1
  butabarpal 304.1
  butallylonal 304.1
  butethal 304.1
  buthalitone (sodium) 304.1
  Butisol 304.1
  butobarbitone 304.1
  butyl chloral (hydrate) 304.1
  caffeine 304.4
  cannabis (indica) (sativa) (resin) (derivatives)
    (type) 304.3
  carbamazepine 304.6
  Carbrital 304.1
  carbromal 304.1
  carisoprodol 304.6
  Catha (edulis) 304.4
  chloral (betaine) (hydrate) 304.1
  chloralamide 304.1
  chloralformamide 304.1
  chloralose 304.1
  chlordiazepoxide 304.1
  Chloretone 304.1
  chlorobutanol 304.1
  chlorodyne 304.1
  chloroform 304.6
  Cliradon 304.0
  coca (leaf) and derivatives 304.2
  cocaine 304.2
    hydrochloride 304.2
    salt (any) 304.2
  codeine 304.0
  combination of drugs (excluding morphine or
    opioid type drug) NEC 304.8
    morphine or opioid type drug with any other
      drug 304.7

Dependence—*continued*
croton-chloral 304.1
cyclobarbital 304.1
cyclobarbitone 304.1
dagga 304.3
Delvinal 304.1
Demerol 304.0
desocodeine 304.0
desomorphine 304.0
desoxyephedrine 304.4
DET 304.5
dexamphetamine 304.4
dexedrine 304.4
dextromethorphan 304.0
dextromoramide 304.0
dextronorpseudophedrine 304.4
dextrorphan 304.0
diacetylmorphine 304.0
Dial 304.1
diallylbarbituric acid 304.1
diamorphine 304.0
diazepam 304.1
dibucaine 304.6
dichloroethane 304.6
diethyl barbituric acid 304.1
diethylsulfone-diethylmethane 304.1
difencloxazine 304.0
dihydrocodeine 304.0
dihydrocodeinone 304.0
dihydrohydroxycodeinone 304.0
dihydroisocodeine 304.0
dihydromorphine 304.0
dihydromorphinone 304.0
dihydroxcodeinone 304.0
Dilaudid 304.0
dimenhydrinate 304.6
dimethylmeperidine 304.0
dimethyltriptamine 304.5
Dionin 304.0
diphenoxylate 304.6
dipipanone 304.0
d-lysergic acid diethylamide 304.5
DMT 304.5
Dolophine 304.0
DOM 304.2
Doriden 304.1
dormiral 304.1
Dormison 304.1
Dromoran 304.0
drug NEC 304.9
 analgesic NEC 304.6
 combination (excluding morphine or opioid
  type drug) NEC 304.8
   morphine or opioid type drug with any other
    drug 304.7
 complicating pregnancy, childbirth, or
  puerperium 648.3
  affecting fetus or newborn 779.5
 hallucinogenic 304.5
 hypnotic NEC 304.1
 narcotic NEC 304.9
 psychostimulant NEC 304.4
 sedative 304.1
 soporific NEC 304.1
 specified type NEC 304.6
 suspected damage to fetus affecting
  management of pregnancy 655.5
 synthetic, with morphine-like effect 304.0
 tranquilizing 304.1
duboisine 304.6

Dependence—*continued*
ectylurea 304.1
Endocaine 304.6
Equanil 304.1
Eskabarb 304.1
ethchlorvynol 304.1
ether (ethyl) (liquid) (vapor) (vinyl) 304.6
ethidene 304.6
ethinamate 304.1
ethoheptazine 304.6
ethyl
 alcohol 303.9
 bromide 304.6
 carbamate 304.6
 chloride 304.6
 morphine 304.0
ethylene (gas) 304.6
 dichloride 304.6
ethylidene chloride 304.6
etilfen 304.1
etorphine 304.0
etoval 304.1
eucodal 304.0
euneryl 304.1
Evipal 304.1
Evipan 304.1
fentanyl 304.0
ganja 304.3
gardenal 304.1
gardenpanyl 304.1
gelsemine 304.6
Gelsemium 304.6
Gemonil 304.1
glucochloral 304.1
glue (airplane) (sniffing) 304.6
glutethimide 304.1
hallucinogenics 304.5
hashish 304.3
headache powder NEC 304.6
Heavenly Blue 304.5
hedonal 304.1
hemp 304.3
heptabarbital 304.1
Heptalgin 304.0
heptobarbitone 304.1
heroin 304.0
 salt (any) 304.0
hexethal (sodium) 304.1
hexobarbital 304.1
Hycodan 304.0
hydrocodone 304.0
hydromorphinol 304.0
hydromorphinone 304.0
hydromorphone 304.0
hydroxycodeine 304.0
hypnotic NEC 304.1
Indian hemp 304.3
inhalant 304.6
intranarcon 304.1
Kemithal 304.1
ketobemidone 304.0
khat 304.4
kif 304.3
Lactuca (virosa) extract 304.1
lactucarium 304.1
laudanum 304.0
Lebanese red 304.3
Leritine 304.0

Dependence—*continued*
  lettuce opium 304.1
  Levanil 304.1
  Levo-Dromoran 304.0
  levo-iso-methadone 304.0
  levorphanol 304.0
  Librium 304.1
  Lomotil 304.6
  Lotusate 304.1
  LSD (-25) (and derivatives) 304.5
  Luminal 304.1
  lysergic acid 304.5
    amide 304.5
  maconha 304.3
  magic mushroom 304.5
  marihuana 304.3
  MDA (methylene dioxyamphetamine) 304.4
  Mebaral 304.1
  Medinal 304.1
  Medomin 304.1
  megahallucinogenics 304.5
  meperidine 304.0
  mephobarbital 304.1
  meprobamate 304.1
  mescaline 304.5
  methadone 304.0
  methamphetamine(s) 304.4
  methaqualone 304.1
  metharbital 304.1
  methitural 304.1
  methobarbitone 304.1
  methohexital 304.1
  methopholine 304.6
  methyl
    alcohol 303.9
    bromide 304.6
    morphine 304.0
    sulfonal 304.1
  methylated spirit 303.9
  methylbutinol 304.6
  methyldihydromorphinone 304.0
  methylene
    chloride 304.6
    dichloride 304.6
    dioxyamphetamine (MDA) 304.4
  methylparafynol 304.1
  methylphenidate 304.4
  methyprylone 304.1
  metopon 304.0
  Miltown 304.1
  morning glory *seeds* 304.5
  morphinan(s) 304.0
  morphine (sulfate) (sulfite) (type) (drugs
      classifiable to 965.00-965.09) 304.0
  morphine or opioid type drug (drugs classifiable
      to 965.00-965.09) with any other drug 304.7
  morphinol(s) 304.0
  morphinon 304.0
  morpholinylethylmorphine 304.0
  mylomide 304.1
  myristicin 304.5
  narcotic (drug) NEC 304.9
  nealbarbital 304.1
  nealbarbitone 304.1
  Nembutal 304.1
  Neonal 304.1
  Neraval 304.1
  Neravan 304.1
  neurobarb 304.1
  nicotine 305.1
  Nisentil 304.0

Dependence—*continued*
  nitrous oxide 304.6
  Noctec 304.1
  Noludar 304.1
  nonbarbiturate sedatives and tranquilizers with
      similar effect 304.1
  noptil 304.1
  normorphine 304.0
  noscapine 304.0
  Novocaine 304.6
  Numorphan 304.0
  nunol 304.1
  Nupercaine 304.6
  Oblivon 304.1
  on
    aspirator V46.0
    hemodialysis V45.11
    hyperbaric chamber V46.8
    iron lung V46.11
    machine (enabling) V46.9
      specified type NEC V46.8
    peritoneal dialysis V45.11
    Possum (Patient-Operated-Selector-
        Mechanism) V46.8
    renal dialysis machine V45.11
    respirator (ventilator) V46.11
      encounter
        during
          mechanical failure V46.14
          power failure V46.12
        for weaning V46.13
    supplemental oxygen V46.2
    wheelchair V46.3
  opiate 304.0
  opioids 304.0
  opioid type drug 304.0
    with any other drug 304.7
  opium (alkaloids) (derivatives) (tincture) 304.0
  ortal 304.1
  Oxazepam 304.1
  oxycodone 304.0
  oxymorphone 304.0
  Palfium 304.0
  Panadol 304.6
  pantopium 304.0
  pantopon 304.0
  papaverine 304.0
  paracetamol 304.6
  paracodin 304.0
  paraldehyde 304.1
  paregoric 304.0
  Parzone 304.7
  PCP (phencyclidine) 304.6
  Pearly Gates 304.5
  pentazocine 304.0
  pentobarbital 304.1
  pentobarbitone (sodium) 304.1
  Pentothal 304.1
  Percaine 304.6
  Percodan 304.0
  Perichlor 304.1
  Pernocton 304.1
  Pernoston 304.1
  peronine 304.0
  pethidine (hydrochloride) 304.0
  petrichloral 304.1
  peyote 304.5
  Phanodorn 304.1
  phenacetin 304.6
  phenadoxone 304.0
  phenaglycodol 304.1
  phenazocine 304.0

Dependence—*continued*
phencyclidine 304.6
phenmetrazine 304.4
phenobal 304.1
phenobarbital 304.1
phenobarbitone 304.1
phenomorphan 304.0
phenonyl 304.1
phenoperidine 304.0
pholcodine 304.0
piminodine 304.0
Pipadone 304.0
Pitkin's solution 304.6
Placidyl 304.1
polysubstance 304.8
Pontocaine 304.6
pot 304.3
potassium bromide 304.1
Preludin 304.4
Prinadol 304.0
probarbital 304.1
procaine 304.6
propanal 304.1
propoxyphene 304.6
psilocibin 304.5
psilocin 304.5
psilocybin 304.5
psilocyline 304.5
psilocyn 304.5
psychedelic agents 304.5
psychostimulant NEC 304.4
psychotomimetic agents 304.5
pyrahexyl 304.3
Pyramidon 304.6
quinalbarbitone 304.1
racemoramide 304.0
racemorphan 304.0
Rela 304.6
scopolamine 304.6
secobarbital 304.1
Seconal 304.1
sedative NEC 304.1
　nonbarbiturate with barbiturate effect 304.1
Sedormid 304.1
sernyl 304.1
sodium bromide 304.1
Soma 304.6
Somnal 304.1
Somnos 304.1
Soneryl 304.1
soporific (drug) NEC 304.1
specified drug NEC 304.6
speed 304.4
spinocaine 304.6
Stovaine 304.6
STP 304.5
stramonium 304.6
Sulfonal 304.1
sulfonethylmethane 304.1
sulfonmethane 304.1
Surital 304.1
synthetic drug with morphine-like effect 304.0
talbutal 304.1
tetracaine 304.6
tetrahydrocannabinol 304.3
tetronal 304.1
THC 304.3
thebacon 304.0
thebaine 304.0
thiamil 304.1
thiamylal 304.1

Dependence—*continued*
thiopental 304.1
tobacco 305.1
toluene, toluol 304.6
tranquilizer NEC 304.1
　nonbarbiturate with barbiturate effect 304.1
tribromacetaldehyde 304.6
tribromethanol 304.6
tribromomethane 304.6
trichloroethanol 304.6
trichoroethyl phosphate 304.1
triclofos 304.1
Trional 304.1
Tuinal 304.1
Turkish Green 304.3
urethan(e) 304.6
Valium 304.1
Valmid 304.1
veganin 304.0
veramon 304.1
Veronal 304.1
versidyne 304.6
vinbarbital 304.1
vinbarbitone 304.1
vinyl bitone 304.1
vitamin B_6 266.1
wine 303.9
Zactane 304.6
Dependency
passive 301.6
reactions 301.6
Depersonalization (episode, in neurotic state) (neurotic) (syndrome) 300.6
Depletion
carbohydrates 271.9
complement factor 279.8
extracellular fluid 276.52
plasma 276.52
potassium 276.8
　nephropathy 588.89
salt or sodium 276.1
　causing heat exhaustion or prostration 992.4
　nephropathy 593.9
volume 276.50
　extracellular fluid 276.52
　plasma 276.52
Deployment (military)
personal history of V62.22
returned from V62.22
status V62.21
Deposit
argentous, cornea 371.16
bone, in Boeck's sarcoid 135
calcareous, calcium—*see* Calcification
cholesterol
　retina 362.82
　skin 709.3
　vitreous (humor) 379.22
conjunctival 372.56
cornea, corneal NEC 371.10
　argentous 371.16
　in
　　cystinosis 270.0 *[371.15]*
　　mucopolysaccharidosis 277.5 *[371.15]*
crystalline, vitreous (humor) 379.22
hemosiderin, in old scars of cornea 371.11
metallic, in lens 366.45
skin 709.3
teeth, tooth (betel) (black) (green) (materia alba) (orange) (soft) (tobacco) 523.6
urate, in kidney (*see also* Disease, renal) 593.9
Depraved appetite 307.52

Depression 311
  acute (*see also* Psychosis, affective) 296.2
    recurrent episode 296.3
    single episode 296.2
  agitated (*see also* Psychosis, affective) 296.2
    recurrent episode 296.3
    single episode 296.2
  anaclitic 309.21
  anxiety 300.4
  arches 734
    congenital 754.61
  autogenous (*see also* Psychosis, affective) 296.2
    recurrent episode 296.3
    single episode 296.2
  basal metabolic rate (BMR) 794.7
  bone marrow 289.9
  central nervous system 799.1
    newborn 779.2
  cerebral 331.9
    newborn 779.2
  cerebrovascular 437.8
    newborn 779.2
  chest wall 738.3
  endogenous (*see also* Psychosis, affective) 296.2
    recurrent episode 296.3
    single episode 296.2
  functional activity 780.99
  hysterical 300.11
  involutional, climacteric, or menopausal (*see also* Psychosis, affective) 296.2
    recurrent episode 296.3
    single episode 296.2
  manic (*see also* Psychosis, affective) 296.80
  medullary 348.89
    newborn 779.2
  mental 300.4
  metatarsal heads—*see* Depression, arches
  metatarsus—*see* Depression, arches
  monopolar (*see also* Psychosis, affective) 296.2
    recurrent episode 296.3
    single episode 296.2
  nervous 300.4
  neurotic 300.4
  nose 738.0
  postpartum 648.4
  psychogenic 300.4
    reactive 298.0
  psychoneurotic 300.4
  psychotic (*see also* Psychosis, affective) 296.2
    reactive 298.0
    recurrent episode 296.3
    single episode 296.2
  reactive 300.4
    neurotic 300.4
    psychogenic 298.0
    psychoneurotic 300.4
    psychotic 298.0
  recurrent 296.3
  respiratory center 348.89
    newborn 770.89
  scapula 736.89
  senile 290.21
  situational (acute) (brief) 309.0
    prolonged 309.1
  skull 754.0
  sternum 738.3
  visual field 368.40
Depressive reaction —*see also* Reaction, depressive
  acute (transient) 309.0
    with anxiety 309.28

Depressive reaction—*continued*
    prolonged 309.1
  situational (acute) 309.0
    prolonged 309.1
Deprivation
  cultural V62.4
  emotional V62.89
    affecting
      adult 995.82
      infant or child 995.51
  food 994.2
    specific substance NEC 269.8
  protein (familial) (kwashiorkor) 260
  sleep V69.4
  social V62.4
    affecting
      adult 995.82
      infant or child 995.51
  symptoms, syndrome
    alcohol 291.81
    drug 292.0
  vitamins (*see also* Deficiency, vitamin) 269.2
  water 994.3
de Quervain's
  disease (tendon sheath) 727.04
  thyroiditis (subacute granulomatous thyroiditis) 245.1
  syndrome 259.51
Derangement
  ankle (internal) 718.97
    current injury (*see also* Dislocation, ankle) 837.0
    recurrent 718.37
  cartilage (articular) NEC (*see also* Disorder, cartilage, articular) 718.0
    knee 717.9
      recurrent 718.36
    recurrent 718.3
  collateral ligament (knee) (medial) (tibial) 717.82
    current injury 844.1
      lateral (fibular) 844.0
    lateral (fibular) 717.81
      current injury 844.0
  cruciate ligament (knee) (posterior) 717.84
    anterior 717.83
      current injury 844.2
    current injury 844.2
  elbow (internal) 718.92
    current injury (*see also* Dislocation, elbow) 832.00
    recurrent 718.32
  gastrointestinal 536.9
  heart—*see* Disease, heart
  hip (joint) (internal) (old) 718.95
    current injury (*see also* Dislocation, hip) 835.00
    recurrent 718.35
  intervertebral disc—*see* Displacement, intervertebral disc
  joint (internal) 718.90
    ankle 718.97
    current injury—*see also* Dislocation, by site
      knee, meniscus or cartilage (*see also* Tear, meniscus) 836.2
    elbow 718.92
    foot 718.97
    hand 718.94
    hip 718.95
    knee 717.9
    multiple sites 718.99

Derangement—*continued*
  joint—*continued*
    pelvic region 718.95
    recurrent 718.30
      ankle 718.37
      elbow 718.32
      foot 718.37
      hand 718.34
      hip 718.35
      knee 718.36
      multiple sites 718.39
      pelvic region 718.35
      shoulder (region) 718.31
      specified site NEC 718.38
      temporomandibular (old) 524.69
      wrist 718.33
    shoulder (region) 718.91
    specified site NEC 718.98
    spine NEC 724.9
    temporomandibular 524.69
    wrist 718.93
  knee (cartilage) (internal) 717.9
    current injury (*see also* Tear, meniscus) 836.2
    ligament 717.89
      capsular 717.85
      collateral—*see* Derangement, collateral
        ligament
      cruciate—*see* Derangement, cruciate
        ligament
      specified NEC 717.85
    recurrent 718.36
  low back NEC 724.9
  meniscus NEC (knee) 717.5
    current injury (*see also* Tear, meniscus) 836.2
    lateral 717.40
      anterior horn 717.42
      posterior horn 717.43
      specified NEC 717.49
    medial 717.3
      anterior horn 717.1
      posterior horn 717.2
    recurrent 718.3
    site other than knee—*see* Disorder, cartilage,
      articular
  mental (*see also* Psychosis) 298.9
  rotator cuff (recurrent) (tear) 726.10
    current 840.4
  sacroiliac (old) 724.6
    current—*see* Dislocation, sacroiliac
  semilunar cartilage (knee) 717.5
    current injury 836.2
      lateral 836.1
      medial 836.0
    recurrent 718.3
  shoulder (internal) 718.91
    current injury (*see also* Dislocation, shoulder)
      831.00
    recurrent 718.31
  spine (recurrent) NEC 724.9
    current—*see* Dislocation, spine
  temporomandibular (internal) (joint) (old)
    524.69
    current—*see* Dislocation, jaw
Dercum's disease or syndrome (adiposis
    dolorosa) 272.8
Derealization (neurotic) 300.6
Dermal —*see* condition
Dermaphytid —*see* Dermatophytosis
Dermatergosis —*see* Dermatitis

Dermatitis (allergic) (contact) (occupational)
    (venenata) 692.9
  ab igne 692.82
  acneiform 692.9
  actinic (due to sun) 692.70
    acute 692.72
    chronic NEC 692.74
    other than from sun NEC 692.82
  ambustionis
    due to
      burn or scald—*see* Burn, by site
      sunburn (*see also* Sunburn) 692.71
  amebic 006.6
  ammonia 691.0
  anaphylactoid NEC 692.9
  arsenical 692.4
  artefacta 698.4
    psychogenic 316 [698.4]
  asthmatic 691.8
  atopic (allergic) (intrinsic) 691.8
    psychogenic 316 [691.8]
  atrophicans 701.8
    diffusa 701.8
    maculosa 701.3
  autoimmune progesterone 279.49
  berlock, berloque 692.72
  blastomycetic 116.0
  blister beetle 692.89
  Brucella NEC 023.9
  bullosa 694.9
    striata pratensis 692.6
  bullous 694.9
    mucosynechial, atrophic 694.60
      with ocular involvement 694.61
    seasonal 694.8
  calorica
    due to
      burn or scald—*see* Burn, by site
      cold 692.89
      sunburn (*see also* Sunburn) 692.71
  caterpillar 692.89
  cercarial 120.3
  combustionis
    due to
      burn or scald—*see* Burn, by site
      sunburn (*see also* Sunburn) 692.71
  congelationis 991.5
  contusiformis 695.2
  diabetic 250.8
  diaper 691.0
  diphtheritica 032.85
  due to
    acetone 692.2
    acids 692.4
    adhesive plaster 692.4
    alcohol (skin contact) (substances classifiable
      to 980.0-980.9) 692.4
      taken internally 693.8
    alkalis 692.4
    allergy NEC 692.9
    ammonia (household) (liquid) 692.4
    animal
      dander (cat) (dog) 692.84
      hair (cat) (dog) 692.84
    arnica 692.3
    arsenic 692.4
      taken internally 693.8
    blister beetle 692.89
    cantharides 692.3
    carbon disulphide 692.2
    caterpillar 692.89

Dermatitis—*continued*
　due to—*continued*
　　caustics 692.4
　　cereal (ingested) 693.1
　　　contact with skin 692.5
　　chemical(s) NEC 692.4
　　　internal 693.8
　　　irritant NEC 692.4
　　　taken internally 693.8
　　chlorocompounds 692.2
　　coffee (ingested) 693.1
　　　contact with skin 692.5
　　cold weather 692.89
　　cosmetics 692.81
　　cyclohexanes 692.2
　　dander, animal (cat) (dog) 692.84
　　deodorant 692.81
　　detergents 692.0
　　dichromate 692.4
　　drugs and medicinals (correct substance
　　　　properly administered) (internal use) 693.0
　　　external (in contact with skin) 692.3
　　　　wrong substance given or taken 976.9
　　　　　specified substance—*see* Table of drugs
　　　　　　and chemicals
　　　wrong substance given or taken 977.9
　　　　specified substance—*see* Table of drugs
　　　　　and chemicals
　　dyes 692.89
　　　hair 692.89
　　epidermophytosis—*see* Dermatophytosis
　　esters 692.2
　　external irritant NEC 692.9
　　　specified agent NEC 692.89
　　eye shadow 692.81
　　fish (ingested) 693.1
　　　contact with skin 692.5
　　flour (ingested) 693.1
　　　contact with skin 692.5
　　food (ingested) 693.1
　　　in contact with skin 692.5
　　fruit (ingested) 693.1
　　　contact with skin 692.5
　　fungicides 692.3
　　furs 692.84
　　glycols 692.2
　　greases NEC 692.1
　　hair, animal (cat) (dog) 692.84
　　hair dyes 692.89
　　hot
　　　objects and materials—*see* Burn, by site
　　　weather or places 692.89
　　hydrocarbons 692.2
　　infrared rays, except from sun 692.82
　　　solar NEC (*see also* Dermatitis, due to, sun)
　　　　692.70
　　ingested substance 693.9
　　　drugs and medicinals (*see also* Dermatitis,
　　　　due to, drugs and medicinals) 693.0
　　　food 693.1
　　　specified substance NEC 693.8
　　ingestion or injection of
　　　chemical 693.8
　　　drug (correct substance properly
　　　　administered) 693.0
　　　　wrong substance given or taken 977.9
　　　　　specified substance—*see* Table of drugs
　　　　　　and chemicals
　　insecticides 692.4

Dermatitis—*continued*
　due to—*continued*
　　internal agent 693.9
　　　drugs and medicinals (*see also* Dermatitis,
　　　　due to, drugs and medicinals) 693.0
　　　food (ingested) 693.1
　　　　in contact with skin 692.5
　　　specified agent NEC 693.8
　　iodine 692.3
　　iodoform 692.3
　　irradiation 692.82
　　jewelry 692.83
　　keratolytics 692.3
　　ketones 692.2
　　lacquer tree (Rhus verniciflua) 692.6
　　light (sun) NEC (*see also* Dermatitis, due to,
　　　　sun) 692.70
　　　other 692.82
　　low temperature 692.89
　　mascara 692.81
　　meat (ingested) 693.1
　　　contact with skin 692.5
　　mercury, mercurials 692.3
　　metals 692.83
　　milk (ingested) 693.1
　　　contact with skin 692.5
　　Neomycin 692.3
　　nylon 692.4
　　oils NEC 692.1
　　paint solvent 692.2
　　pediculocides 692.3
　　petroleum products (substances classifiable to
　　　　981) 692.4
　　phenol 692.3
　　photosensitiveness, photosensitivity (sun)
　　　　692.72
　　　other light 692.82
　　plants NEC 692.6
　　plasters, medicated (any) 692.3
　　plastic 692.4
　　poison
　　　ivy (Rhus toxicodendron) 692.6
　　　oak (Rhus diversiloba) 692.6
　　　plant or vine 692.6
　　　sumac (Rhus venenata) 692.6
　　　vine (Rhus radicans) 692.6
　　preservatives 692.89
　　primrose (primula) 692.6
　　primula 692.6
　　radiation 692.82
　　　sun NEC (*see also* Dermatitis, due to, sun)
　　　　692.70
　　　tanning bed 692.82
　　radioactive substance 692.82
　　radium 692.82
　　ragweed (Senecio jacobae) 692.6
　　Rhus (diversiloba) (radicans) (toxicodendron)
　　　　(venenata) (verniciflua) 692.6
　　rubber 692.4
　　scabicides 692.3
　　Senecio jacobae 692.6
　　solar radiation—*see* Dermatitis, due to, sun
　　solvents (any) (substances classifiable to
　　　　982.0-982.8) 692.2
　　　chlorocompound group 692.2
　　　cyclohexane group 692.2
　　　ester group 692.2
　　　glycol group 692.2
　　　hydrocarbon group 692.2
　　　ketone group 692.2
　　　paint 692.2

Dermatitis—*continued*
due to—*continued*
  specified agent NEC 692.89
  sun 692.70
    acute 692.72
    chronic NEC 692.74
    specified NEC 692.79
  sunburn (*see also* Sunburn) 692.71
  sunshine NEC (*see also* Dermatitis, due to, sun) 692.70
  tanning bed 692.82
  tetrachlorethylene 692.2
  toluene 692.2
  topical medications 692.3
  turpentine 692.2
  ultraviolet rays, except from sun 692.82
    sun NEC (*see also* Dermatitis, due to, sun) 692.70
  x-rays 692.82
  vaccine or vaccination (correct substance properly administered) 693.0
    wrong substance given or taken
      bacterial vaccine 978.8
        specified—*see* Table of drugs and chemicals
      other vaccines NEC 979.9
        specified—*see* Table of drugs and chemicals
  varicose veins (*see also* Varicose, vein, inflamed or infected) 454.1
  x-rays 692.82
dyshydrotic 705.81
dysmenorrheica 625.8
eczematoid NEC 692.9
  infectious 690.8
eczematous NEC 692.9
epidemica 695.89
erysipelatosa 695.81
escharotica—*see* Burn, by site
exfoliativa, exfoliative 695.89
  generalized 695.89
  infantum 695.81
  neonatorum 695.81
eyelid 373.31
  allergic 373.32
  contact 373.32
  eczematous 373.31
  herpes (zoster) 053.20
    simplex 054.41
  infective 373.5
    due to
      actinomycosis 039.3 *[373.5]*
      herpes
        simplex 054.41
        zoster 053.20
      impetigo 684 *[373.5]*
      leprosy (*see also* Leprosy) 030.0 *[373.4]*
      lupus vulgaris (tuberculous) (*see also* Tuberculosis) 017.0 *[373.4]*
      mycotic dermatitis (*see also* Dermatomycosis) 111.9 *[373.5]*
      vaccinia 051.02 *[373.5]*
        postvaccination 999.0 *[373.5]*
      yaws (*see also* Yaws) 102.9 *[373.4]*
facta, factitia 698.4
  psychogenic 316 *[698.4]*
ficta 698.4
  psychogenic 316 *[698.4]*
flexural 691.8
follicularis 704.8
friction 709.8

Dermatitis—*continued*
fungus 111.9
  specified type NEC 111.8
gangrenosa, gangrenous (infantum) (*see also* Gangrene) 785.4
gestationis 646.8
gonococcal 098.89
gouty 274.89
harvest mite 133.8
heat 692.89
herpetiformis (bullous) (erythematous) (pustular) (vesicular) 694.0
  juvenile 694.2
  senile 694.5
hiemalis 692.89
hypostatic, hypostatica 454.1
  with ulcer 454.2
impetiginous 684
infantile (acute) (chronic) (intertriginous) (intrinsic) (seborrheic) 690.12
infectiosa eczematoides 690.8
infectious (staphylococcal) (streptococcal) 686.9
  eczematoid 690.8
infective eczematoid 690.8
Jacquet's (diaper dermatitis) 691.0
leptus 133.8
lichenified NEC 692.9
lichenoid, chronic 701.0
lichenoides purpurica pigmentosa 709.1
meadow 692.6
medicamentosa (correct substance properly administered) (internal use) (*see also* Dermatitis, due to, drugs or medicinals) 693.0
  due to contact with skin 692.3
mite 133.8
multiformis 694.0
  juvenile 694.2
  senile 694.5
napkin 691.0
neuro 698.3
neurotica 694.0
nummular NEC 692.9
osteatosis, osteatotic 706.8
papillaris capillitii 706.1
pellagrous 265.2
perioral 695.3
perstans 696.1
photosensitivity (sun) 692.72
  other light 692.82
pigmented purpuric lichenoid 709.1
polymorpha dolorosa 694.0
primary irritant 692.9
pruriginosa 694.0
pruritic NEC 692.9
psoriasiform nodularis 696.2
psychogenic 316
purulent 686.00
pustular contagious 051.2
pyococcal 686.00
pyocyaneus 686.09
pyogenica 686.00
radiation 692.82
repens 696.1
Ritter's (exfoliativa) 695.81
Schamberg's (progressive pigmentary dermatosis) 709.09
schistosome 120.3
seasonal bullous 694.8
seborrheic 690.10
  infantile 690.12

Dermatitis—*continued*
 sensitization NEC 692.9
 septic (*see also* Septicemia) 686.00
   gonococcal 098.89
 solar, solare NEC (*see also* Dermatitis, due to,
   sun) 692.70
 stasis 454.1
   due to
     postphlebitic syndrome 459.12
       with ulcer 459.13
     varicose veins—*see* Varicose
   ulcerated or with ulcer (varicose) 454.2
 sunburn (*see also* Sunburn) 692.71
 suppurative 686.00
 traumatic NEC 709.8
 trophoneurotica 694.0
 ultraviolet, except from sun 692.82
   due to sun NEC (*see also* Dermatitis, due to,
     sun) 692.70
 varicose 454.1
   with ulcer 454.2
 vegetans 686.8
 verrucosa 117.2
 xerotic 706.8
Dermatoarthritis, lipoid 272.8 *[713.0]*
Dermatochalasia, dermatochalasis 374.87
Dermatofibroma (lenticulare) (M8832/0)—*see*
   also Neoplasm, skin, benign
 protuberans (M8832/1)—*see* Neoplasm, skin,
   uncertain behavior
Dermatofibrosarcoma (protuberans) (M8832/3)
   see Neoplasm, skin, malignant
Dermatographia 708.3
Dermatolysis (congenital) (exfoliativa) 757.39
 acquired 701.8
 eyelids 374.34
 palpebrarum 374.34
 senile 701.8
Dermatomegaly NEC 701.8
Dermatomucomyositis 710.3
Dermatomycosis 111.9
 furfuracea 111.0
 specified type NEC 111.8
Dermatomyositis (acute) (chronic) 710.3
Dermatoneuritis of children 985.0
Dermatophiliasis 134.1
Dermatophytide —*see* Dermatophytosis
Dermatophytosis (Epidermophyton) (infection)
   (microsporum) (tinea) (Trichophyton) 110.9
 beard 110.0
 body 110.5
 deep seated 110.6
 fingernails 110.1
 foot 110.4
 groin 110.3
 hand 110.2
 nail 110.1
 perianal (area) 110.3
 scalp 110.0
 scrotal 110.8
 specified site NEC 110.8
 toenails 110.1
 vulva 110.8
Dermatopolyneuritis 985.0
Dermatorrhexis 756.83
 acquired 701.8
Dermatosclerosis (*see also* Scleroderma) 710.1
 localized 701.0
Dermatosis 709.9
 Andrews' 686.8
 atopic 691.8

Dermatosis—*continued*
 Bowen's (M8081/2)—*see* Neoplasm, skin, in situ
 bullous 694.9
   specified type NEC 694.8
 erythematosquamous 690.8
 exfoliativa 695.89
 factitial 698.4
 gonococcal 098.89
 herpetiformis 694.0
   juvenile 694.2
   senile 694.5
 hysterical 300.11
 linear IgA 694.8
 menstrual NEC 709.8
 neutrophilic, acute febrile 695.89
 occupational (*see also* Dermatitis) 692.9
 papulosa nigra 709.8
 pigmentary NEC 709.00
   progressive 709.09
   Schamberg's 709.09
   Siemens-Bloch 757.33
 progressive pigmentary 709.09
 psychogenic 316
 pustular subcorneal 694.1
 Schamberg's (progressive pigmentary) 709.09
 senile NEC 709.3
 Unna's (seborrheic dermatitis) 690.10
Dermographia 708.3
Dermographism 708.3
Dermoid (cyst) (M9084/0)—*see also* Neoplasm,
   by site, benign
 with malignant transformation (M9084/3) 183.0
Dermopathy
 infiltrative, with thyrotoxicosis 242.0
 nephrogenic fibrosing 701.8
 senile NEC 709.3
Dermophytosis —*see* Dermatophytosis
Descemet's membrane —*see* condition
Descemetocele 371.72
Descending —*see* condition
Descensus uteri (complete) (incomplete) (partial)
   (without vaginal wall prolapse) 618.1
   with mention of vaginal wall prolapse—*see*
     Prolapse, uterovaginal
Desensitization to allergens V07.1
Desert
 rheumatism 114.0
 sore (*see also* Ulcer, skin) 707.9
Desertion (child) (newborn) 995.52
 adult 995.84
Desmoid (extra-abdominal) (tumor) (M8821/1)—*see*
   also Neoplasm, connective tissue, uncertain behavior
 abdominal (M8822/1)—*see* Neoplasm,
   connective tissue, uncertain behavior
Despondency 300.4
Desquamative dermatitis NEC 695.89
Destruction
 articular facet (*see also* Derangement, joint) 718.9
   vertebra 724.9
 bone 733.90
   syphilitic 095.5
 joint (*see also* Derangement, joint) 718.9
   sacroiliac 724.6
 kidney 593.89
 live fetus to facilitate birth NEC 763.89
 ossicles (ear) 385.24
 rectal sphincter 569.49
 septum (nasal) 478.19
 tuberculous NEC (*see also* Tuberculosis) 011.9
 tympanic membrane 384.82
 tympanum 385.89
 vertebral disc—*see* Degeneration, intervertebral disc

Destructiveness (*see also* Disturbance, conduct)
  312.9
  adjustment reaction 309.3
Detachment
  cartilage—*see also* Sprain, by site
    knee—*see* Tear, meniscus
  cervix, annular 622.8
    complicating delivery 665.3
  choroid (old) (postinfectional) (simple)
      (spontaneous) 363.70
    hemorrhagic 363.72
    serous 363.71
  knee, medial meniscus (old) 717.3
    current injury 836.0
  ligament—*see* Sprain, by site
  placenta (premature)—*see* Placenta, separation
  retina (recent) 361.9
    with retinal defect (rhegmatogenous) 361.00
      giant tear 361.03
      multiple 361.02
      partial
        with
          giant tear 361.03
          multiple defects 361.02
          retinal dialysis (juvenile) 361.04
          single defect 361.01
        retinal dialysis (juvenile) 361.04
        single 361.01
        subtotal 361.05
        total 361.05
    delimited (old) (partial) 361.06
    old
      delimited 361.06
      partial 361.06
      total or subtotal 361.07
    pigment epithelium (RPE) (serous) 362.42
      exudative 362.42
      hemorrhagic 362.43
    rhegmatogenous (*see also* Detachment, retina,
        with retinal defect) 361.00
    serous (without retinal defect) 361.2
    specified type NEC 361.89
    traction (with vitreoretinal organization)
        361.81
  vitreous humor 379.21
Detergent asthma 507.8
Deterioration
  epileptic
    with behavioral disturbance 345.9 *[294.11]*
    without behavioral disturbance 345.9 *[294.10]*
  heart, cardiac (*see also* Degeneration,
      myocardial) 429.1
  mental (*see also* Psychosis) 298.9
  myocardium, myocardial (*see also*
      Degeneration, myocardial) 429.1
  senile (simple) 797
  transplanted organ—*see* Complications,
      transplant, organ, by site
de Toni-Fanconi syndrome (cystinosis) 270.0
Deuteranomaly 368.52
Deuteranopia (anomalous trichromat) (complete)
  (incomplete) 368.52
Deutschländer's disease —*see* Fracture, foot
Development
  abnormal, bone 756.9
  arrested 783.40
    bone 733.91
    child 783.40
    due to malnutrition (protein-calorie) 263.2
    fetus or newborn 764.9
    tracheal rings (congenital) 748.3

Development—*continued*
  defective, congenital—*see also* Anomaly
    cauda equina 742.59
    left ventricle 746.9
      with atresia or hypoplasia of aortic orifice or
        valve with hypoplasia of ascending aorta
        746.7
      in hypoplastic left heart syndrome 746.7
  delayed (*see also* Delay, development) 783.40
    arithmetical skills 315.1
    language (skills) 315.31
      and speech due to hearing loss 315.34
      expressive 315.31
      mixed receptive-expressive 315.32
    learning skill, specified NEC 315.2
    mixed skills 315.5
    motor coordination 315.4
    reading 315.00
    specified
      learning skill NEC 315.2
      type NEC, except learning 315.8
    speech 315.39
      and language due to hearing loss 315.34
      associated with hyperkinesia 314.1
      phonological 315.39
    spelling 315.09
    written expression 315.2
  imperfect, congenital—*see also* Anomaly
    heart 746.9
    lungs 748.60
  improper (fetus or newborn) 764.9
  incomplete (fetus or newborn) 764.9
    affecting management of pregnancy 656.5
    bronchial tree 748.3
    organ or site not listed—*see* Hypoplasia
    respiratory system 748.9
  sexual, precocious NEC 259.1
  tardy, mental (*see also* Retardation, mental) 319
Developmental —*see* condition
Devergie's disease (pityriasis rubra pilaris) 696.4
Deviation
  conjugate (eye) 378.87
    palsy 378.81
    spasm, spastic 378.82
  esophagus 530.89
  eye, skew 378.87
  mandible, opening and closing 524.53
  midline (jaw) (teeth) 524.29
    specified site NEC—*see* Malposition
  occlusal plane 524.76
  organ or site, congenital NEC—*see* Malposition,
      congenital
  septum (acquired) (nasal) 470
    congenital 754.0
  sexual 302.9
    bestiality 302.1
    coprophilia 302.89
    ego-dystonic
      homosexuality 302.0
      lesbianism 302.0
    erotomania 302.89
      Clérambault's 297.8
    exhibitionism (sexual) 302.4
    fetishism 302.81
      transvestic 302.3
    frotteurism 302.89
    homosexuality, ego-dystonic 302.0
      pedophilic 302.2
    lesbianism, ego-dystonic 302.0
    masochism 302.83
    narcissism 302.89

Deviation—*continued*
  sexual—*continued*
    necrophilia 302.89
    nymphomania 302.89
    pederosis 302.2
    pedophilia 302.2
    sadism 302.84
    sadomasochism 302.84
    satyriasis 302.89
    specified type NEC 302.89
    transvestic fetishism 302.3
    transvestism 302.3
    voyeurism 302.82
    zoophilia (erotica) 302.1
  teeth, midline 524.29
  trachea 519.19
  ureter (congenital) 753.4
Devic's disease 341.0
Device
  cerebral ventricle (communicating) in situ V45.2
  contraceptive—*see* Contraceptive, device
  drainage, cerebrospinal fluid V45.2
Devil's
  grip 074.1
  pinches (purpura simplex) 287.2
Devitalized tooth 522.9
Devonshire colic 984.9
  specified type of lead—*see* Table of drugs and chemicals
Dextraposition, aorta 747.21
  with ventricular septal defect, pulmonary stenosis or atresia, and hypertrophy of right ventricle 745.2
  in tetralogy of Fallot 745.2
Dextratransposition, aorta 745.11
Dextrinosis, limit (debrancher enzyme deficiency) 271.0
Dextrocardia (corrected) (false) (isolated) (secondary) (true) 746.87
  with
    complete transposition of viscera 759.3
    situs inversus 759.3
Dextroversion, kidney (left) 753.3
Dhobie itch 110.3
Diabetes, diabetic (brittle) (congenital) (familial) (mellitus) (severe) (slight) (without complication) 250.0

Note—Use the following fifth-digit subclassification with category 250:

0 type II or unspecified type, not stated as uncontrolled
  Fifth-digit 0 is for use for type II patients, even if the patient requires insulin
1 type I [juvenile type], not stated as uncontrolled
2 type II or unspecified type, uncontrolled
  Fifth-digit 2 is for use for type II patients, even if the paiten requires insulin
3 type I [juvenile type], uncontrolled

---

  with
    coma (with ketoacidosis) 250.3
      due to secondary diabetes 249.3
    hyperosmolar (nonketotic) 250.2
      due to secondary diabetes 249.2
    complication NEC 250.9
      due to secondary diabetes 249.9
    specified NEC 250.8
      due to secondary diabetes 249.8

Diabetes, diabetic—*continued*
  with—*continued*
    gangrene 250.7 *[785.4]*
      due to secondary diabetes 249.7 *[785.4]*
    hyperglycemia — code to Diabetes, by type, with 5th digit for not stated as uncontrolled
    hyperosmolarity 250.2
      due to secondary diabetes 249.2
    ketosis, ketoacidosis 250.1
      due to secondary diabetes 249.1
    osteomyelitis 250.8 *[731.8]*
      due to secondary diabetes 249.8 *[731.8]*
    specified manifestations NEC 250.8
      due to secondary diabetes 249.8
  acetonemia 250.1
    due to secondary diabetes 249.1
  acidosis 250.1
    due to secondary diabetes 249.1
  amyotrophy 250.6 *[353.5]*
    due to secondary diabetes 249.6 *[353.5]*
  angiopathy, peripheral 250.7 *[443.81]*
    due to secondary diabetes 249.7 *[443.81]*
  asymptomatic 790.29
  autonomic neuropathy (peripheral) 250.6 *[337.1]*
    due to secondary diabetes 249.6 *[337.1]*
  bone change 250.8 *[731.8]*
    due to secondary diabetes 249.8 *[731.8]*
  bronze, bronzed 275.0
  cataract 250.5 *[366.41]*
    due to secondary diabetes 249.5 *[366.41]*
  chemical induced—see Diabetes, secondary
  complicating pregnancy, childbirth, or puerperium 648.0
  coma (with ketoacidosis) 250.3
    due to secondary diabetes 249.3
    hyperglycemic 250.3
      due to secondary diabetes 249.3
    hyperosmolar (nonketotic) 250.2
      due to secondary diabetes 249.2
    hypoglycemic 250.3
      due to secondary diabetes 249.3
    insulin 250.3
      due to secondary diabetes 249.3
  complicating pregnancy, childbirth, or puerperium (maternal) (conditions classifiable to 249 and 250) 648.0
    affecting fetus or newborn 775.0
  complication NEC 250.9
    due to secondary diabetes 249.9
    specified NEC 250.8
      due to secondary diabetes 249.8
  dorsal sclerosis 250.6 *[340]*
    due to secondary diabetes 249.6 *[340]*
  drug induced—*see also* Diabetes, secondary
    overdose or wrong substance given or taken — *see* Table of Drugs and Chemicals
  due to
    cystic fibrosis — *see* Diabetes, secondary
    infection — *see* Diabetes, secondary
  dwarfism-obesity syndrome 258.1
  gangrene 250.7 *[785.4]*
    due to secondary diabetes 249.7 *[785.4]*
  gastroparesis 250.6 *[536.3]*
    due to secondary diabetes 249.6 *[536.3]*
  gestational 648.8
    complicating pregnancy, childbirth, or puerperium 648.8
  glaucoma 250.5 *[365.44]*
    due to secondary diabetes 249.5 *[365.44]*
  glomerulosclerosis (intercapillary) 250.4 *[581.81]*
    due to secondary diabetes 249.4 *[581.81]*

Diabetes, diabetic—*continued*
glycogenosis, secondary 250.8 *[259.8]*
  due to secondary diabetes 249.8 *[259.8]*
hemochromatosis 275.0
hyperosmolar coma 250.2
  due to secondary diabetes 249.2
hyperosmolarity 250.2
  due to secondary diabetes 249.2
hypertension-nephrosis syndrome 250.4 *[581.81]*
  due to secondary diabetes 249.4 *[581.81]*
hypoglycemia 250.8
  due to secondary diabetes 249.8
hypoglycemic shock 250.8
  due to secondary diabetes 249.8
inadequately controlled—code to Diabetes, by
  type, with 5th digit for not stated as
  uncontrolled
insipidus 253.5
  nephrogenic 588.1
  pituitary 253.5
  vasopressin-resistant 588.1
intercapillary glomerulosclerosis 250.4 *[581.81]*
  due to secondary diabetes 249.4 *[581.81]*
iritis 250.5 *[364.42]*
  due to secondary diabetes 249.5 *[364.42]*
ketosis, ketoacidosis 250.1
  due to secondary diabetes 249.1
Kimmelstiel (-Wilson) disease or syndrome
  (intercapillary glomerulosclerosis) 250.4
  [581.81]
  due to secondary diabetes 249.4 *[581.81]*
Lancereaux's (diabetes mellitus with marked
  emaciation) 250.8 *[261]*
  due to secondary diabetes 249.8 *[261]*
latent (chemical)—*see* Diabetes, secondary
complicating pregnancy, childbirth, or
  puerperium 648.0
lipoidosis 250.8 *[272.7]*
  due to secondary diabetes 249.8 *[272.7]*
macular edema 250.5 *[362.07]*
  due to secondary diabetes 249.5 *[362.07]*
maternal
  with manifest disease in the infant 775.1
  affecting fetus or newborn 775.0
microaneurysms, retinal 250.5 *[362.01]*
  due to secondary diabetes 249.5 *[362.01]*
mononeuropathy 250.6 *[355.9]*
  due to secondary diabetes 249.6 *[355.9]*
neonatal, transient 775.1
nephropathy 250.4 *[583.81]*
  due to secondary diabetes 249.4 *[583.81]*
nephrosis (syndrome) 250.4 *[581.81]*
  due to secondary diabetes 249.4 *[581.81]*
neuralgia 250.6 *[357.2]*
  due to secondary diabetes 249.6 *[357.2]*
neuritis 250.6 *[357.2]*
  due to secondary diabetes 249.6 *[357.2]*
neurogenic arthropathy 250.6 *[713.5]*
  due to secondary diabetes 249.6 *[713.5]*
neuropathy 250.6 *[357.2]*
  autonomic (peripheral) 250.6 *[337.1]*
    due to secondary diabetes 249.6 *[337.1]*
  due to secondary diabetes 249.6 *[357.2]*
nonclinical 790.29
osteomyelitis 250.8 *[731.8]*
  due to secondary diabetes 249.8 *[731.8]*
out of control—code to Diabetes, by type, with
  5th digit for uncontrolled
peripheral autonomic neuropathy 250.6 *[337.1]*
  due to secondary diabetes 249.6 *[337.1]*
phosphate 275.3

Diabetes, diabetic—*continued*
polyneuropathy 250.6 *[357.2]*
  due to secondary diabetes 249.6 *[357.2]*
poorly controlled—code to Diabetes, by type,
  with 5th digit for not stated as uncontrolled
renal (true) 271.4
retinal
  edema 250.5 *[362.07]*
    due to secondary diabetes 249.5 *[362.07]*
  hemorrhage 250.5 *[362.01]*
    due to secondary diabetes 249.5 *[362.01]*
  microaneurysms 250.5 *[362.01]*
    due to secondary diabetes 249.5 *[362.01]*
retinitis 250.5 *[362.01]*
  due to secondary diabetes 249.5 *[362.01]*
retinopathy 250.5 *[362.01]*
  due to secondary diabetes 249.5 *[362.01]*
  background 250.5 *[362.01]*
    due to secondary diabetes 249.5 *[362.01]*
  nonproliferative 250.5 *[362.03]*
    due to secondary diabetes 249.5 *[362.03]*
    mild 250.5 *[362.04]*
      due to secondary diabetes 249.5 *[362.04]*
    moderate 250.5 *[362.05]*
      due to secondary diabetes 249.5 *[362.05]*
    severe 250.5 *[362.06]*
      due to secondary diabetes 249.5 *[362.06]*
  proliferative 250.5 *[362.02]*
    due to secondary diabetes 249.5 *[362.02]*
secondary (chemical-induced) (due to chronic
  condition) (due to infection) (drug-induced)
  249.0
  with
    coma (with ketoacidosis) 249.3
      hyperosmolar (nonketotic) 249.2
    complication NEC 249.9
      specified NEC 249.8
    gangrene 249.7 *[785.4]*
    hyperosmolarity 249.2
    ketosis, ketoacidosis 249.1
    osteomyelitis 249.8 *[731.8]*
    specified manifestations NEC 249.8
  acetonemia 249.1
  acidosis 249.1
  amyotrophy 249.6 *[353.5]*
  angiopathy, peripheral 249.7 *[443.81]*
  autonomic neuropathy (peripheral) 249.6
    [337.1]
  bone change 249.8 *[731.8]*
  cataract 249.5 *[366.41]*
  coma (with ketoacidosis) 249.3
    hyperglycemic 249.3
    hyperosmolar (nonketotic) 249.2
    hypoglycemic 249.3
    insulin 249.3
  complicating pregnancy, childbirth, or
    puerperium (maternal) 648.0
    affecting fetus or newborn 775.0
  complication NEC 249.9
    specified NEC 249.8
  dorsal sclerosis 249.6 *[340]*
  due to overdose or wrong substance given or
    taken — *see* Table of Drugs and
    Chemicals
  gangrene 249.7 *[785.4]*
  gastroparesis 249.6 *[536.3]*
  glaucoma 249.5 *[365.44]*
  glomerulosclerosis (intercapillary) 249.4
    [581.81]
  glycogenosis, secondary 249.8 *[259.8]*
  hyperosmolar coma 249.2

Diabetes, diabetic—*continued*
  secondary—*continued*
    hyperosmolarity 249.2
    hypertension-nephrosis syndrome 249.4 *[581.81]*
    hypoglycemia 249.8
    hypoglycemic shock 249.8
    intercapillary glomerulosclerosis 249.4 *[581.81]*
    iritis 249.5 *[364.42]*
    ketosis, ketoacidosis 249.1
    Kimmelstiel (-Wilson) disease or syndrome
      (intercapillary glomerulosclerosis) 249.4
      [581.81]
    Lancereaux's (diabetes mellitus with marked
      emaciation) 249.8 *[261]*
    lipoidosis 249.8 *[272.7]*
    macular edema 249.5 *[362.07]*
    maternal
      with manifest disease in the infant 775.1
      affecting fetus or newborn 775.0
    microaneurysms, retinal 249.5 *[362.01]*
    mononeuropathy 249.6 *[355.9]*
    nephropathy 249.4 *[583.81]*
    nephrosis (syndrome) 249.4 *[581.81]*
    neuralgia 249.6 *[357.2]*
    neuritis 249.6 *[357.2]*
    neurogenic arthropathy 249.6 *[713.5]*
    neuropathy 249.6 *[357.2]*
      autonomic (peripheral) 249.6 *[337.1]*
    osteomyelitis 249.8 *[731.8]*
    peripheral autonomic neuropathy 249.6 *[337.1]*
    polyneuropathy 249.6 *[357.2]*
    retinal
      edema 249.5 *[362.07]*
      hemorrhage 249.5 *[362.01]*
      microaneurysms 249.5 *[362.01]*
    retinitis 249.5 *[362.01]*
    retinopathy 249.5 *[362.01]*
      background 249.5 *[362.01]*
      nonproliferative 249.5 *[362.03]*
        mild 249.5 *[362.04]*
        moderate 249.5 *[362.05]*
        severe 249.5 *[362.06]*
      proliferative 249.5 *[362.02]*
    ulcer (skin) 249.8 *[707.9]*
      lower extremity 249.8 *[707.10]*
        ankle 249.8 *[707.13]*
        calf 249.8 *[707.12]*
        foot 249.8 *[707.15]*
        heel 249.8 *[707.14]*
        knee 249.8 *[707.19]*
        specified site NEC 249.8 *[707.19]*
        thigh 249.8 *[707.11]*
        toes 249.8 *[707.15]*
      specified site NEC 249.8 *[707.8]*
    xanthoma 249.8 *[272.2]*
  steroid induced—*see also* Diabetes, secondary
    overdose or wrong substance given or taken
    962.0
  stress 790.29
  subclinical 790.29
  subliminal 790.29
  sugar 250.0
  ulcer (skin) 250.8 *[707.9]*
    due to secondary diabetes 249.8 *[707.9]*
    lower extremity 250.8 *[707.10]*
      due to secondary diabetes 249.8 *[707.10]*
      ankle 250.8 *[707.13]*
        due to secondary diabetes 249.8 *[707.13]*
      calf 250.8 *[707.12]*
        due to secondary diabetes 249.8 *[707.12]*

Diabetes, diabetic—*continued*
  ulcer—*continued*
    lower extremity—*continued*
      foot 250.8 *[707.15]*
        due to secondary diabetes 249.8 *[707.15]*
      heel 250.8 *[707.14]*
        due to secondary diabetes 249.8 *[707.14]*
      knee 250.8 *[707.19]*
        due to secondary diabetes 249.8 *[707.19]*
      specified site NEC 250.8 *[707.19]*
        due to secondary diabetes 249.8 *[707.19]*
      thigh 250.8 *[707.11]*
        due to secondary diabetes 249.8 *[707.11]*
      toes 250.8 *[707.15]*
        due to secondary diabetes 249.8 *[707.15]*
    specified site NEC 250.8 *[707.8]*
      due to secondary diabetes 249.8 *[707.8]*
    xanthoma 250.8 *[272.2]*
      due to secondary diabetes 249.8 *[272.2]*
Diacyclothrombopathia 287.1
Diagnosis deferred 799.9
Dialysis (intermittent) (treatment)
  anterior retinal (juvenile) (with detachment)
    361.04
  extracorporeal V56.0
  hemodialysis V56.0
    status only V45.11
  peritoneal V56.8
    status only V45.11
  renal V56.0
    status only V45.11
  specified type NEC V56.8
Diamond-Blackfan anemia or syndrome
  (congenital hypoplastic anemia) 284.01
Diamond-Gardener syndrome (autoerythrocyte
  sensitization) 287.2
Diaper rash 691.0
Diaphoresis (excessive) NEC (*see also*
  Hyperhidrosis) 780.8
Diaphragm —*see* condition
Diaphragmalgia 786.52
Diaphragmitis 519.4
Diaphyseal aclasis 756.4
Diaphysitis 733.99
Diarrhea, diarrheal (acute) (autumn) (bilious)
  (bloody) (catarrhal) (choleraic) (chronic)
  (gravis) (green) (infantile) (lienteric)
  (noninfectious) (presumed noninfectious)
  (putrefactive) (secondary) (sporadic)
  (summer) (symptomatic) (thermic) 787.91
  achlorhydric 536.0
  allergic 558.3
  amebic (*see also* Amebiasis) 006.9
    with abscess—*see* Abscess, amebic
    acute 006.0
    chronic 006.1
    nondysenteric 006.2
  bacillary—*see* Dysentery, bacillary
  bacterial NEC 008.5
  balantidial 007.0
  bile salt-induced 579.8
  cachectic NEC 787.91
  chilomastix 007.8
  choleriformis 001.1
  coccidial 007.2
  Cochin-China 579.1
    anguilluliasis 127.2
    psilosis 579.1
  Dientamoeba 007.8
  dietetic 787.91

Diarrhea, diarrheal—*continued*
due to
  achylia gastrica 536.8
  Aerobacter aerogenes 008.2
  Bacillus coli—*see* Enteritis, E. coli
  bacteria NEC 008.5
  bile salts 579.8
  Capillaria
    hepatica 128.8
    philippinensis 127.5
  Clostridium perfringens (C) (F) 008.46
  Enterobacter aerogenes 008.2
  enterococci 008.49
  Escherichia coli—*see* Enteritis, E. coli
  Giardia lamblia 007.1
  Heterophyes heterophyes 121.6
  irritating foods 787.91
  Metagonimus yokogawai 121.5
  Necator americanus 126.1
  Paracolobactrum arizonae 008.1
  Paracolon bacillus NEC 008.47
    Arizona 008.1
  Proteus (bacillus) (mirabilis) (Morganii) 008.3
  Pseudomonas aeruginosa 008.42
  S. japonicum 120.2
  specified organism NEC 008.8
    bacterial 008.49
    viral NEC 008.69
  Staphylococcus 008.41
  Streptococcus 008.49
    anaerobic 008.46
  Strongyloides stercoralis 127.2
  Trichuris trichiuria 127.3
  virus NEC (*see also* Enteritis, viral) 008.69
dysenteric 009.2
  due to specified organism NEC 008.8
dyspeptic 787.91
endemic 009.3
epidemic 009.3
fermentative 787.91
flagellate 007.9
Flexner's (ulcerative) 004.1
functional 564.5
  following gastrointestinal surgery 564.4
  psychogenic 306.4
giardial 007.1
Giardia lamblia 007.1
hill 579.1
hyperperistalsis (nervous) 306.4
infectious 009.2
  presumed 009.3
inflammatory 787.91
  due to specified organism NEC 008.8
malarial (*see also* Malaria) 084.6
mite 133.8
mycotic 117.9
nervous 306.4
neurogenic 564.5
parenteral NEC 009.2
postgastrectomy 564.4
postvagotomy 564.4
prostaglandin induced 579.8
protozoal NEC 007.9
psychogenic 306.4
septic 009.2
  due to specified organism NEC 008.8
specified organism NEC 008.8
  bacterial 008.49
  viral NEC 008.69
Staphylococcus 008.41

Diarrhea, diarrheal—*continued*
Streptococcus 008.49
  anaerobic 088.46
toxic 558.2
travelers' 009.2
  due to specified organism NEC 008.8
trichomonal 007.3
tropical 579.1
tuberculous 014.8
ulcerative (chronic) (*see also* Colitis, ulcerative)
  556.9
viral (*see also* Enteritis, viral) 008.8
zymotic NEC 009.2
Diastasis
cranial bones 733.99
  congenital 756.0
joint (traumatic)—*see* Dislocation, by site
muscle 728.84
  congenital 756.89
recti (abdomen) 728.84
  complicating delivery 665.8
  congenital 756.79
Diastema, teeth, tooth 524.30
Diastematomyelia 742.51
Diataxia, cerebral, infantile 343.0
Diathesis
allergic V15.09
bleeding (familial) 287.9
cystine (familial) 270.0
gouty 274.9
hemorrhagic (familial) 287.9
  newborn NEC 776.0
oxalic 271.8
scrofulous (*see also* Tuberculosis) 017.2
spasmophilic (*see also* Tetany) 781.7
ulcer 536.9
uric acid 274.9
Diaz's disease or osteochondrosis 732.5
Dibothriocephaliasis 123.4
  larval 123.5
Dibothriocephalus (infection) (infestation)
  (latus) 123.4
  larval 123.5
Dicephalus 759.4
Dichotomy, teeth 520.2
Dichromat, dichromata (congenital) 368.59
Dichromatopsia (congenital) 368.59
Dichuchwa 104.0
Dicroceliasis 121.8
Didelphys, didelphic (*see also* Double uterus)
  752.2
Didymitis (*see also* Epididymitis) 604.90
Died —*see also* Death
without
  medical attention (cause unknown) 798.9
  sign of disease 798.2
Dientamoeba diarrhea 007.8
Dietary
inadequacy or deficiency 269.9
surveillance and counseling V65.3
Dietl's crisis 593.4
Dieulafoy lesion (hemorrhagic) of
duodenum 537.84
esophagus 530.82
intestine 569.86
stomach 537.84
Dieulafoy's ulcer —*see* Ulcer, stomach
Difficult
birth, affecting fetus or newborn 763.9
delivery NEC 669.9

Difficulty
  feeding 783.3
    adult 783.3
    breast 676.8
    child 783.3
    elderly 783.3
    infant 783.3
    newborn 779.31
  nonorganic (infant) NEC 307.59
  mechanical, gastroduodenal stoma 537.89
  reading 315.00
  specific, spelling 315.09
  swallowing (*see also* Dysphagia) 787.20
  walking 719.7
Diffuse —*see* condition
Diffused ganglion 727.42
DiGeorge's syndrome (thymic hypoplasia)
    279.11
Digestive —*see* condition
Di Guglielmo's disease or syndrome (M9841/3)
    207.0
Diktyoma (M9051/3)—*see* Neoplasm, by site,
    malignant
Dilaceration, tooth 520.4
Dilatation
  anus 564.89
    venule—*see* Hemorrhoids
  aorta (focal) (general) (*see also* Aneurysm,
      aorta) 441.9
    congenital 747.29
    infectional 093.0
    ruptured 441.5
    syphilitic 093.0
  appendix (cystic) 543.9
  artery 447.8
  bile duct (common) (cystic) (congenital) 751.69
    acquired 576.8
  bladder (sphincter) 596.8
    congenital 753.8
    in pregnancy or childbirth 654.4
      causing obstructed labor 660.2
        affecting fetus or newborn 763.1
  blood vessel 459.89
  bronchus, bronchi 494.0
    with acute exacerbation 494.1
  calyx (due to obstruction) 593.89
  capillaries 448.9
  cardiac (acute) (chronic) (*see also* Hypertrophy,
      cardiac) 429.3
    congenital 746.89
    valve NEC 746.89
      pulmonary 746.09
    hypertensive (*see also* Hypertension, heart)
        402.90
  cavum septi pellucidi 742.4
  cecum 564.89
    psychogenic 306.4
  cervix (uteri)—*see also* Incompetency, cervix
    incomplete, poor, slow
      affecting fetus or newborn 763.7
      complicating delivery 661.0
        affecting fetus or newborn 763.7
  colon 564.7
    congenital 751.3
    due to mechanical obstruction 560.89
    psychogenic 306.4
  common bile duct (congenital) 751.69
    acquired 576.8
      with calculus, choledocholithiasis, or
        stones—*see* Choledocholithiasis

Dilatation—*continued*
  cystic duct 751.69
    acquired (any bile duct) 575.8
  duct, mammary 610.4
  duodenum 564.89
  esophagus 530.89
    congenital 750.4
    due to
      achalasia 530.0
      cardiospasm 530.0
  Eustachian tube, congenital 744.24
  fontanel 756.0
  gallbladder 575.8
    congenital 751.69
  gastric 536.8
    acute 536.1
    psychogenic 306.4
  heart (acute) (chronic) (*see also* Hypertrophy,
      cardiac) 429.3
    congenital 746.89
    hypertensive (*see also* Hypertension, heart)
        402.90
    valve—*see also* Endocarditis
      congenital 746.89
  ileum 564.89
    psychogenic 306.4
  inguinal rings—*see* Hernia, inguinal
  jejunum 564.89
    psychogenic 306.4
  kidney (calyx) (collecting structures) (cystic)
      (parenchyma) (pelvis) 593.89
  lacrimal passages 375.69
  lymphatic vessel 457.1
  mammary duct 610.4
  Meckel's diverticulum (congenital) 751.0
  meningeal vessels, congenital 742.8
  myocardium (acute) (chronic) (*see also*
      Hypertrophy, cardiac) 429.3
  organ or site, congenital NEC—*see* Distortion
  pancreatic duct 577.8
  pelvis, kidney 593.89
  pericardium—*see* Pericarditis
  pharynx 478.29
  prostate 602.8
  pulmonary
    artery (idiopathic) 417.8
      congenital 747.3
    valve, congenital 746.09
  pupil 379.43
  rectum 564.89
  renal 593.89
  saccule vestibularis, congenital 744.05
  salivary gland (duct) 527.8
  sphincter ani 564.89
  stomach 536.8
    acute 536.1
    psychogenic 306.4
  submaxillary duct 527.8
  trachea, congenital 748.3
  ureter (idiopathic) 593.89
    congenital 753.20
    due to obstruction 593.5
  urethra (acquired) 599.84
  vasomotor 443.9
  vein 459.89
  ventricular, ventricle (acute) (chronic) (*see also*
      Hypertrophy, cardiac) 429.3
    cerebral, congenital 742.4
    hypertensive (*see also* Hypertension, heart) 402.90
  venule 459.89
    anus—*see* Hemorrhoids
  vesical orifice 596.8

Dilated, dilation —*see* Dilatation
Diminished
  hearing (acuity) (*see also* Deafness) 389.9
  pulse pressure 785.9
  vision NEC 369.9
  vital capacity 794.2
Diminuta taenia 123.6
Diminution, sense or sensation (cold) (heat)
  (tactile) (vibratory) (*see also* Disturbance,
  sensation) 782.0
Dimitri-Sturge-Weber disease
  (encephalocutaneous angiomatosis) 759.6
Dimple
  parasacral 685.1
    with abscess 685.0
  pilonidal 685.1
    with abscess 685.0
  postanal 685.1
    with abscess 685.0
Dioctophyma renale (infection) (infestation) 128.8
Dipetalonemiasis 125.4
Diphallus 752.69
Diphtheria, diphtheritic (gangrenous)
  (hemorrhagic) 032.9
  carrier (suspected) of V02.4
  cutaneous 032.85
  cystitis 032.84
  faucial 032.0
  infection of wound 032.85
  inoculation (anti) (not sick) V03.5
  laryngeal 032.3
  myocarditis 032.82
  nasal anterior 032.2
  nasopharyngeal 032.1
  neurological complication 032.89
  peritonitis 032.83
  specified site NEC 032.89
Diphyllobothriasis (intestine) 123.4
  larval 123.5
Diplacusis 388.41
Diplegia (upper limbs) 344.2
  brain or cerebral 437.8
  congenital 343.0
  facial 351.0
    congenital 352.6
  infantile or congenital (cerebral) (spastic)
    (spinal) 343.0
  lower limbs 344.1
  syphilitic, congenital 090.49
Diplococcus, diplococcal —*see* condition
Diplomyelia 742.59
Diplopia 368.2
  refractive 368.15
Dipsomania (*see also* Alcoholism) 303.9
  with psychosis (*see also* Psychosis, alcoholic)
    291.9
Dipylidiasis 123.8
  intestine 123.8
Direction, teeth, abnormal 524.30
Dirt-eating child 307.52
Disability
  heart—*see* Disease, heart
  learning NEC 315.2
  special spelling 315.09
Disarticulation (*see also* Derangement, joint)
  718.9
  meaning
    amputation
      status—*see* Absence, by site
      traumatic —*see* Amputation, traumatic
    dislocation, traumatic or congenital—*see*
      Dislocation

Disaster, cerebrovascular (*see also* Disease,
  cerebrovascular, acute) 436
Discharge
  anal NEC 787.99
  breast (female) (male) 611.79
  conjunctiva 372.89
  continued locomotor idiopathic (*see also*
    Epilepsy) 345.5
  diencephalic autonomic idiopathic (*see also*
    Epilepsy) 345.5
  ear 388.60
    blood 388.69
    cerebrospinal fluid 388.61
  excessive urine 788.42
  eye 379.93
  nasal 478.19
  nipple 611.79
  patterned motor idiopathic (*see also* Epilepsy)
    345.5
  penile 788.7
  postnasal—*see* Sinusitis
  sinus, from mediastinum 510.0
  umbilicus 789.9
  urethral 788.7
    bloody 599.84
  vaginal 623.5
Discitis 722.90
  cervical, cervicothoracic 722.91
  lumbar, lumbosacral 722.93
  thoracic, thoracolumbar 722.92
Discogenic syndrome —*see* Displacement,
  intervertebral disc
Discoid
  kidney 753.3
  meniscus, congenital 717.5
  semilunar cartilage 717.5
Discoloration
  mouth 528.9
  nails 703.8
  teeth 521.7
    due to
      drugs 521.7
      metals (copper) (silver) 521.7
      pulpal bleeding 521.7
    during formation 520.8
    extrinsic 523.6
    intrinsic posteruptive 521.7
Discomfort
  chest 786.59
  visual 368.13
Discomycosis —*see* Actinomycosis
Discontinuity, ossicles, ossicular chain 385.23
Discrepancy
  centric occlusion
    maximum intercuspation 524.55
    of teeth 524.55
  leg length (acquired) 736.81
    congenital 755.30
  uterine size-date 649.6
Discrimination
  political V62.4
  racial V62.4
  religious V62.4
  sex V62.4
Disease, diseased —*see also* Syndrome
  Abrami's (acquired hemolytic jaundice) 283.9
  absorbent system 459.89
  accumulation—*see* Thesaurismosis
  acid-peptic 536.8
  Acosta's 993.2
  Adams-Stokes (-Morgagni) (syncope with heart
    block) 426.9

Disease, diseased—*continued*
  Addison's (bronze) (primary adrenal
      insufficiency) 255.41
    anemia (pernicious) 281.0
    tuberculous (*see also* Tuberculosis) 017.6
  Addison-Gull—*see* Xanthoma
  adenoids (and tonsils) (chronic) 474.9
  adrenal (gland) (capsule) (cortex) 255.9
    hyperfunction 255.3
    hypofunction 255.41
    specified type NEC 255.8
  ainhum (dactylolysis spontanea) 136.0
  akamushi (scrub typhus) 081.2
  Akureyri (epidemic neuromyasthenia) 049.8
  Albarrán's (colibacilluria) 791.9
  Albers-Schönberg's (marble bones) 756.52
  Albert's 726.71
  Albright (-Martin) (-Bantam) 275.49
  Alibert's (mycosis fungoides) (M9700/3) 202.1
  Alibert-Bazin (M9700/3) 202.1
  alimentary canal 569.9
  alligator skin (ichthyosis congenital) 757.1
    acquired 701.1
  Almeida's (Brazilian blastomycosis) 116.1
  Alpers' 330.8
  alpine 993.2
  altitude 993.2
  alveoli, teeth 525.9
  Alzheimer's—*see* Alzheimer's
  amyloid (any site) 277.30
  anarthritic rheumatoid 446.5
  Anders' (adiposis tuberosa simplex) 272.8
  Andersen's (glycogenosis IV) 271.0
  Anderson's (angiokeratoma corporis diffusum)
      272.7
  Andes 993.2
  Andrews' (bacterid) 686.8
  angiospastic, angiospasmodic 443.9
    cerebral 435.9
      with transient neurologic deficit 435.9
    vein 459.89
  anterior
    chamber 364.9
    horn cell 335.9
      specified type NEC 335.8
  antral (chronic) 473.0
    acute 461.0
  anus NEC 569.49
  aorta (nonsyphilitic) 447.9
    syphilitic NEC 093.89
  aortic (heart) (valve) (*see also* Endocarditis,
      aortic) 424.1
  apollo 077.4
  aponeurosis 726.90
  appendix 543.9
  aqueous (chamber) 364.9
  arc-welders' lung 503
  Armenian 277.31
  Arnold-Chiari (*see also* Spina bifida) 741.0
  arterial 447.9
    occlusive (*see also* Occlusion, by site) 444.22
      with embolus or thrombus—*see* Occlusion,
          by site
    due to stricture or stenosis 447.1
    specified type NEC 447.8
  arteriocardiorenal (*see also* Hypertension,
      cardiorenal) 404.90
  arteriolar (generalized) (obliterative) 447.9
    specified type NEC 447.8
  arteriorenal—*see* Hypertension, kidney

Disease, diseased—*continued*
  arteriosclerotic—*see also* Arteriosclerosis
    cardiovascular 429.2
    coronary —*see* Arteriosclerosis, coronary
    heart —*see* Arteriosclerosis, coronary
  artery 447.9
    cerebral 437.9
    coronary —*see* Arteriosclerosis, coronary
    specified type NEC 447.8
  arthropod-borne NEC 088.9
    specified type NEC 088.89
  Asboe-Hansen's (incontinentia pigmenti) 757.33
  atticoantral, chronic (with posterior or superior
      marginal perforation of ear drum) 382.2
  auditory canal, ear 380.9
  Aujeszky's 078.89
  auricle, ear NEC 380.30
  Australian X 062.4
  autoimmune NEC 279.49
    hemolytic (cold type) (warm type) 283.0
    parathyroid 252.1
    thyroid 245.2
  aviators' (*see also* Effect, adverse, high altitude)
      993.2
  ax(e)-grinders' 502
  Ayala's 756.89
  Ayerza's (pulmonary artery sclerosis with
      pulmonary hypertension) 416.0
  Azorean (of the nervous system) 334.8
  Babington's (familial hemorrhagic
      telangiectasia) 448.0
  back bone NEC 733.90
  bacterial NEC 040.89
    zoonotic NEC 027.9
    specified type NEC 027.8
  Baehr-Schiffrin (thrombotic thrombocytopenic
      purpura) 446.6
  Baelz's (cheilitis glandularis apostematosa)
      528.5
  Baerensprung's (eczema marginatum) 110.3
  Balfour's (chloroma) 205.3
  balloon (*see also* Effect, adverse, high altitude)
      993.2
  Baló's 341.1
  Bamberger (-Marie) (hypertrophic pulmonary
      osteoarthropathy) 731.2
  Bang's (Brucella abortus) 023.1
  Bannister's 995.1
  Banti's (with cirrhosis) (with portal
      hypertension)—*see* Cirrhosis, liver
  Barcoo (*see also* Ulcer, skin) 707.9
  barium lung 503
  Barlow (-Möller) (infantile scurvy) 267
  barometer makers' 985.0
  Barraquer (-Simons) (progressive lipodystrophy)
      272.6
  basal ganglia 333.90
    degenerative NEC 333.0
    specified NEC 333.89
  Basedow's (exophthalmic goiter) 242.0
  basement membrane NEC 583.89
    with
      pulmonary hemorrhage (Goodpasture's
          syndrome) 446.21 *[583.81]*
  Bateman's 078.0
    purpura (senile) 287.2
  Batten's 330.1 *[362.71]*
  Batten-Mayou (retina) 330.1 *[362.71]*
  Batten-Steinert 359.21
  Battey 031.0
  Baumgarten-Cruveilhier (cirrhosis of liver) 571.5
  bauxite-workers' 503

Disease, diseased—*continued*
Bayle's (dementia paralytica) 094.1
Bazin's (primary) (*see also* Tuberculosis) 017.1
Beard's (neurasthenia) 300.5
Beau's (*see also* Degeneration, myocardial) 429.1
Bechterew's (ankylosing spondylitis) 720.0
Becker's
  idiopathic mural endomyocardial disease 425.2
  myotonia congenita, recessive form 359.22
Begbie's (exophthalmic goiter) 242.0
Behr's 362.50
Beigel's (white piedra) 111.2
Bekhterev's (ankylosing spondylitis) 720.0
Bell's (*see also* Psychosis, affective) 296.0
Bennett's (leukemia) 208.9
Benson's 379.22
Bergeron's (hysteroepilepsy) 300.11
Berlin's 921.3
Bernard-Soulier (thrombopathy) 287.1
Bernhardt (-Roth) 355.1
beryllium 503
Besnier-Boeck (-Schaumann) (sarcoidosis) 135
Best's 362.76
Beurmann's (sporotrichosis) 117.1
Bielschowsky (-Jansky) 330.1
Biermer's (pernicious anemia) 281.0
Biett's (discoid lupus erythematosus) 695.4
bile duct (*see also* Disease, biliary) 576.9
biliary (duct) (tract) 576.9
  with calculus, choledocholithiasis, or
    stones—*see* Choledocholithiasis
Billroth's (meningocele) (*see also* Spina bifida)
  741.9
Binswanger's 290.12
Bird's (oxaluria) 271.8
bird fanciers' 495.2
black lung 500
bladder 596.9
  specified NEC 596.8
bleeder's 286.0
Bloch-Sulzberger (incontinentia pigmenti) 757.33
Blocq's (astasia-abasia) 307.9
blood (-forming organs) 289.9
  specified NEC 289.89
  vessel 459.9
Bloodgood's 610.1
Blount's (tibia vara) 732.4
blue 746.9
Bodechtel-Guttmann (subacute sclerosing
  panencephalitis) 046.2
Boeck's (sarcoidosis) 135
bone 733.90
  fibrocystic NEC 733.29
    jaw 526.2
  marrow 289.9
  Paget's (osteitis deformans) 731.0
  specified type NEC 733.99
  von Recklinghausen's (osteitis fibrosa cystica)
    252.01
Bonfils'—*see* Disease, Hodgkin's
Borna 062.9
Bornholm (epidemic pleurodynia) 074.1
Bostock's (*see also* Fever, hay) 477.9
Bouchard's (myopathic dilatation of the
  stomach) 536.1
Bouillaud's (rheumatic heart disease) 391.9
Bourneville (-Brissaud) (tuberous sclerosis) 759.5
Bouveret (-Hoffmann) (paroxysmal tachycardia)
  427.2
bowel 569.9
  functional 564.9
    psychogenic 306.4

Disease, diseased—*continued*
Bowen's (M8081/2)—*see* Neoplasm, skin, in situ
Bozzolo's (multiple myeloma) (M9730/3) 203.0
Bradley's (epidemic vomiting) 078.82
Brailsford's 732.3
  radius, head 732.3
  tarsal, scaphoid 732.5
Brailsford-Morquio (mucopolysaccharidosis IV)
  277.5
brain 348.9
  Alzheimer's 331.0
    with dementia—*see* Alzheimer's, dementia
  arterial, artery 437.9
  arteriosclerotic 437.0
  congenital 742.9
  degenerative—*see* Degeneration, brain
  inflammatory—*see also* Encephalitis
  late effect—*see* category 326
  organic 348.9
    arteriosclerotic 437.0
  parasitic NEC 123.9
  Pick's 331.11
    with dementia
      with behavioral disturbance 331.11
        [294.11]
      without behavioral disturbance 331.11
        [294.10]
  senile 331.2
braziers' 985.8
breast 611.9
  cystic (chronic) 610.1
  fibrocystic 610.1
  inflammatory 611.0
  Paget's (M8540/3) 174.0
  puerperal, postpartum NEC 676.3
  specified NEC 611.89
Breda's (*see also* Yaws) 102.9
Breisky's (kraurosis vulvae) 624.09
Bretonneau's (diphtheritic malignant angina)
  032.0
Bright's (*see also* Nephritis) 583.9
  arteriosclerotic (*see also* Hypertension,
    kidney) 403.90
Brill's (recrudescent typhus) 081.1
  flea-borne 081.0
  louse-borne 081.1
Brill-Symmers (follicular lymphoma)
  (M9690/3) 202.0
Brill-Zinsser (recrudescent typhus) 081.1
Brinton's (leather bottle stomach) (M8142/3)
  151.9
Brion-Kayser (*see also* Fever, paratyphoid)
  002.9
broad
  beta 272.2
  ligament, noninflammatory 620.9
    specified NEC 620.8
Brocq's 691.8
  meaning
    atopic (diffuse) neurodermatitis 691.8
    dermatitis herpetiformis 694.0
    lichen simplex chronicus 698.3
    parapsoriasis 696.2
    prurigo 698.2
Brocq-Duhring (dermatitis herpetiformis) 694.0
Brodie's (joint) (*see also* Osteomyelitis) 730.1
bronchi 519.19
bronchopulmonary 519.19
bronze (Addison's) 255.41
  tuberculous (*see also* Tuberculosis) 017.6
Brown-Séquard 344.89
Bruck's 733.99

Disease, diseased—*continued*
Bruck-de Lange (Amsterdam dwarf, mental retardation, and brachycephaly) 759.89
Bruhl's (splenic anemia with fever) 285.8
Bruton's (X-linked agammaglobulinemia) 279.04
buccal cavity 528.9
Buchanan's (juvenile osteochondrosis, iliac crest) 732.1
Buchman's (osteochondrosis juvenile) 732.1
Budgerigar-fanciers' 495.2
Büdinger-Ludloff-Läwen 717.89
Buerger's (thromboangiitis obliterans) 443.1
Bürger-Grütz (essential familial hyperlipemia) 272.3
Burns' (lower ulna) 732.3
bursa 727.9
Bury's (erythema elevatum diutinum) 695.89
Buschke's 710.1
Busquet's (*see also* Osteomyelitis) 730.1
Busse-Buschke (cryptococcosis) 117.5
C₂ (*see also* Alcoholism) 303.9
Caffey's (infantile cortical hyperostosis) 756.59
caisson 993.3
calculous 592.9
California 114.0
Calvé (-Perthes) (osteochondrosis, femoral capital) 732.1
Camurati-Engelmann (diaphyseal sclerosis) 756.59
Canavan's 330.0
capillaries 448.9
Carapata 087.1
cardiac-*see* Disease, heart
cardiopulmonary, chronic 416.9
cardiorenal (arteriosclerotic) (hepatic) (hypertensive) (vascular) (*see also* Hypertension, cardiorenal) 404.90
cardiovascular (arteriosclerotic) 429.2
  congenital 746.9
  hypertensive (*see also* Hypertension, heart) 402.90
    benign 402.10
    malignant 402.00
  renal (*see also* Hypertension, cardiorenal) 404.90
  syphilitic (asymptomatic) 093.9
carotid gland 259.8
Carrión's (Bartonellosis) 088.0
cartilage NEC 733.90
  specified NEC 733.99
Castellani's 104.8
cat-scratch 078.3
Cavare's (familial periodic paralysis) 359.3
Cazenave's (pemphigus) 694.4
cecum 569.9
celiac (adult) 579.0
  infantile 579.0
cellular tissue NEC 709.9
central core 359.0
cerebellar, cerebellum—*see* Disease, brain
cerebral (*see also* Disease, brain) 348.9
  arterial, artery 437.9
  degenerative—*see* Degeneration, brain
cerebrospinal 349.9

C_2

Disease, diseased—*continued*
cerebrovascular NEC 437.9
  acute 436
    embolic—*see* Embolism, brain
    late effect—*see* Late effect(s) (of) cerebrovascular disease
    puerperal, postpartum, childbirth 674.0
    thrombotic—*see* Thrombosis, brain
  arteriosclerotic 437.0
    embolic—*see* Embolism, brain
    ischemic, generalized NEC 437.1
    late effect—*see* Late effect(s) (of) cerebrovascular disease
    occlusive 437.1
    puerperal, postpartum, childbirth 674.0
    specified type NEC 437.8
    thrombotic—*see* Thrombosis, brain
ceroid storage 272.7
cervix (uteri)
  inflammatory 616.0
  noninflammatory 622.9
    specified NEC 622.8
Chabert's 022.9
Chagas' (*see also* Trypanosomiasis, American) 086.2
Chandler's (osteochondritis dissecans, hip) 732.7
Charcot's (joint) 094.0 *[713.5]*
  spinal cord 094.0
Charcot-Marie-Tooth 356.1
Charlouis' (*see also* Yaws) 102.9
Cheadle (-Möller) (-Barlow) (infantile scurvy) 267
Chédiak-Steinbrinck (-Higashi) (congenital gigantism of peroxidase granules) 288.2
cheek, inner 528.9
chest 519.9
Chiari's (hepatic vein thrombosis) 453.0
Chicago (North American blastomycosis) 116.0
chignon (white piedra) 111.2
chigoe, chigo (jigger) 134.1
childhood granulomatous 288.1
Chinese liver fluke 121.1
chlamydial NEC 078.88
cholecystic (*see also* Disease, gallbladder) 575.9
choroid 363.9
  degenerative (*see also* Degeneration, choroid) 363.40
  hereditary (*see also* Dystrophy, choroid) 363.50
  specified type NEC 363.8
Christian's (chronic histiocytosis X) 277.89
Christian-Weber (nodular nonsuppurative panniculitis) 729.30
Christmas 286.1
ciliary body 364.9
  specified NEC 364.89
circulatory (system) NEC 459.9
  chronic, maternal, affecting fetus or newborn 760.3
  specified NEC 459.89
  syphilitic 093.9
    congenital 090.5
Civatte's (poikiloderma) 709.09
climacteric 627.2
  male 608.89
coagulation factor deficiency (congenital) (*see also* Defect, coagulation) 286.9
Coats' 362.12

Disease, diseased—*continued*
coccidioidal pulmonary 114.5
  acute 114.0
  chronic 114.4
  primary 114.0
  residual 114.4
Cockayne's (microcephaly and dwarfism) 759.89
Cogan's 370.52
cold
  agglutinin 283.0
    or hemoglobinuria 283.0
      paroxysmal (cold) (nocturnal) 283.2
  hemagglutinin (chronic) 283.0
collagen NEC 710.9
  nonvascular 710.9
  specified NEC 710.8
  vascular (allergic) (*see also* Angiitis, hypersensitivity) 446.20
colon 569.9
  functional 564.9
    congenital 751.3
  ischemic 557.0
combined system (of spinal cord) 266.2 *[336.2]*
  with anemia (pernicious) 281.0 *[336.2]*
compressed air 993.3
Concato's (pericardial polyserositis) 423.2
  peritoneal 568.82
  pleural—*see* Pleurisy
congenital NEC 799.89
conjunctiva 372.9
  chlamydial 077.98
    specified NEC 077.8
  specified type NEC 372.89
  viral 077.99
    specified NEC 077.8
connective tissue, diffuse (*see also* Disease, collagen) 710.9
Conor and Bruch's (boutonneuse fever) 082.1
Conradi (-Hünermann) 756.59
Cooley's (erythroblastic anemia) 282.49
Cooper's 610.1
Corbus' 607.1
cork-handlers' 495.3
cornea (*see also* Keratopathy) 371.9
coronary (*see also* Ischemia, heart) 414.9
  congenital 746.85
  ostial, syphilitic 093.20
    aortic 093.22
    mitral 093.21
    pulmonary 093.24
    tricuspid 093.23
Corrigan's—*see* Insufficiency, aortic
Cotugno's 724.3
Coxsackie (virus) NEC 074.8
cranial nerve NEC 352.9
Creutzfeldt-Jakob (CJD) 046.19
  with dementia
    with behavioral disturbance 046.19 *[294.11]*
    without behavioral disturbance 046.19 *[294.10]*
  familial 046.19
  iatrogenic 046.19
  specified NEC 046.19
  sporadic 046.19
  variant (vCJD) 046.11
    with dementia
      with behavioral disturbance 046.11 *[294.11]*
      without behavioral disturbance 046.11 *[294.10]*

Disease, diseased—*continued*
Crigler-Najjar (congenital hyperbilirubinemia) 277.4
Crocq's (acrocyanosis) 443.89
Crohn's (intestine) (*see also* Enteritis, regional) 555.9
Crouzon's (craniofacial dysostosis) 756.0
Cruchet's (encephalitis lethargica) 049.8
Cruveilhier's 335.21
Cruz-Chagas (*see also* Trypanosomiasis, American) 086.2
crystal deposition (*see also* Arthritis, due to, crystals) 712.9
Csillag's (lichen sclerosus et atrophicus) 701.0
Curschmann's 359.21
Cushing's (pituitary basophilism) 255.0
cystic
  breast (chronic) 610.1
  kidney, congenital (*see also* Cystic, disease, kidney) 753.10
  liver, congenital 751.62
  lung 518.89
    congenital 748.4
  pancreas 577.2
    congenital 751.7
  renal, congenital (*see also* Cystic, disease, kidney) 753.10
  semilunar cartilage 717.5
cysticercus 123.1
cystine storage (with renal sclerosis) 270.0
cytomegalic inclusion (generalized) 078.5
  with
    pneumonia 078.5 *[484.1]*
  congenital 771.1
Daae (-Finsen) (epidemic pleurodynia) 074.1
dancing 297.8
Danielssen's (anesthetic leprosy) 030.1
Darier's (congenital) (keratosis follicularis) 757.39
  erythema annulare centrifugum 695.0
  vitamin A deficiency 264.8
Darling's (histoplasmosis) (*see also* Histoplasmosis, American) 115.00
Davies' 425.0
de Beurmann-Gougerot (sporotrichosis) 117.1
Débove's (splenomegaly) 789.2
deer fly (*see also* Tularemia) 021.9
deficiency 269.9
degenerative—*see also* Degeneration
  disc—*see* Degeneration, intervertebral disc
Degos' 447.8
Déjérine (-Sottas) 356.0
Deleage's 359.89
demyelinating, demyelinizating (brain stem) (central nervous system) 341.9
  multiple sclerosis 340
  specified NEC 341.8
de Quervain's (tendon sheath) 727.04
  thyroid (subacute granulomatous thyroiditis) 245.1
Dercum's (adiposis dolorosa) 272.8
Deutschländer's—*see* Fracture, foot
Devergie's (pityriasis rubra pilaris) 696.4
Devic's 341.0
diaphorase deficiency 289.7
diaphragm 519.4
diarrheal, infectious 009.2
diatomaceous earth 502
Diaz's (osteochondrosis astragalus) 732.5
digestive system 569.9

Disease, diseased—*continued*

Di Guglielmo's (erythemic myelosis) (M9841/3) 207.0

Dimitri-Sturge-Weber (encephalocutaneous angiomatosis) 759.6

disc, degenerative—*see* Degeneration, intervertebral disc

discogenic (*see also* Disease, intervertebral disc) 722.90

diverticular—*see* Diverticula

Down's (mongolism) 758.0

Dubini's (electric chorea) 049.8

Dubois' (thymus gland) 090.5

Duchenne's 094.0
  locomotor ataxia 094.0
  muscular dystrophy 359.1
  paralysis 335.22
  pseudohypertrophy, muscles 359.1

Duchenne-Griesinger 359.1

ductless glands 259.9

Duhring's (dermatitis herpetiformis) 694.0

Dukes (-Filatov) 057.8

duodenum NEC 537.9
  specified NEC 537.89

Duplay's 726.2

Dupré's (meningism) 781.6

Dupuytren's (muscle contracture) 728.6

Durand-Nicolas-Favre (climatic bubo) 099.1

Duroziez's (congenital mitral stenosis) 746.5

Dutton's (trypanosomiasis) 086.9

Eales' 362.18

ear (chronic) (inner) NEC 388.9
  middle 385.9
    adhesive (*see also* Adhesions, middle ear) 385.10
    specified NEC 385.89

Eberth's (typhoid fever) 002.0

Ebstein's
  heart 746.2
  meaning diabetes 250.4 *[581.81]*
    due to secondary diabetes 249.4 *[581.81]*

Echinococcus (*see also* Echinococcus) 122.9

ECHO virus NEC 078.89

Economo's (encephalitis lethargica) 049.8

Eddowes' (brittle bones and blue sclera) 756.51

Edsall's 992.2

Eichstedt's (pityriasis versicolor) 111.0

Ellis-van Creveld (chondroectodermal dysplasia) 756.55

endocardium—*see* Endocarditis

endocrine glands or system NEC 259.9
  specified NEC 259.8

endomyocardial, idiopathic mural 425.2

Engel-von Recklinghausen (osteitis fibrosa cystica) 252.01

Engelmann's (diaphyseal sclerosis) 756.59

English (rickets) 268.0

Engman's (infectious eczematoid dermatitis) 690.8

enteroviral, enterovirus NEC 078.89
  central nervous system NEC 048

epidemic NEC 136.9

epididymis 608.9

epigastric, functional 536.9
  psychogenic 306.4

Erb (-Landouzy) 359.1

Erb-Goldflam 358.00

Erdheim-Chester (ECD) 277.89

Erichsen's (railway spine) 300.16

esophagus 530.9
  functional 530.5
  psychogenic 306.4

Disease, diseased—*continued*

Eulenburg's (congenital paramyotonia) 359.29

Eustachian tube 381.9

Evans' (thrombocytopenic purpura) 287.32

external auditory canal 380.9

extrapyramidal NEC 333.90

eye 379.90
  anterior chamber 364.9
  inflammatory NEC 364.3
  muscle 378.9

eyeball 360.9

eyelid 374.9

eyeworm of Africa 125.2

Fabry's (angiokeratoma corporis diffusum) 272.7

facial nerve (seventh) 351.9
  newborn 767.5

Fahr-Volhard (malignant nephrosclerosis) 403.00

fallopian tube, noninflammatory 620.9
  specified NEC 620.8

familial periodic 277.31
  paralysis 359.3

Fanconi's (congenital pancytopenia) 284.09

Farber's (disseminated lipogranulomatosis) 272.8

fascia 728.9
  inflammatory 728.9

Fauchard's (periodontitis) 523.40

Favre-Durand-Nicolas (climatic bubo) 099.1

Favre-Racouchot (elastoidosis cutanea nodularis) 701.8

Fede's 529.0

Feer's 985.0

Felix's (juvenile osteochondrosis, hip) 732.1

Fenwick's (gastric atrophy) 537.89

Fernels' (aortic aneurysm) 441.9

fibrocaseous, of lung (*see also* Tuberculosis, pulmonary) 011.9

fibrocystic—*see also* Fibrocystic, disease
  newborn 277.01

Fiedler's (leptospiral jaundice) 100.0

fifth 057.0

Filatoff's (infectious mononucleosis) 075

Filatov's (infectious mononucleosis) 075

file-cutters' 984.9
  specified type of lead—*see* Table of drugs and chemicals

filterable virus NEC 078.89

fish skin 757.1
  acquired 701.1

Flajani (-Basedow) (exophthalmic goiter) 242.0

Flatau-Schilder 341.1

flax-dressers' 504

Fleischner's 732.3

flint 502

fluke—*see* Infestation, fluke

Følling's (phenylketonuria) 270.1

foot and mouth 078.4

foot process 581.3

Forbes' (glycogenosis III) 271.0

Fordyce's (ectopic sebaceous glands) (mouth) 750.26

Fordyce-Fox (apocrine miliaria) 705.82

Fothergill's
  meaning scarlatina anginosa 034.1
  neuralgia (*see also* Neuralgia, trigeminal) 350.1

Fournier's 608.83

fourth 057.8

Fox (-Fordyce) (apocrine miliaria) 705.82

Francis' (*see also* Tularemia) 021.9

Disease, diseased—*continued*
  Franklin's (heavy chain) 273.2
  Frei's (climatic bubo) 099.1
  Freiberg's (flattening metatarsal) 732.5
  Friedländer's (endarteritis obliterans)—*see*
      Arteriosclerosis
  Friedreich's
    combined systemic or ataxia 334.0
    facial hemihypertrophy 756.0
    myoclonia 333.2
  Fröhlich's (adiposogenital dystrophy) 253.8
  Frommel's 676.6
  frontal sinus (chronic) 473.1
    acute 461.1
  Fuller's earth 502
  fungus, fungous NEC 117.9
  Gaisböck's (polycythemia hypertonica) 289.0
  gallbladder 575.9
    congenital 751.60
  Gamna's (siderotic splenomegaly) 289.51
  Gamstorp's (adynamia episodica hereditaria)
      359.3
  Gandy-Nanta (siderotic splenomegaly) 289.51
  gannister (occupational) 502
  Garré's (*see also* Osteomyelitis) 730.1
  gastric (*see also* Disease, stomach) 537.9
  gastroesophageal reflux (GERD) 530.81
  gastrointestinal (tract) 569.9
    amyloid 277.39
    functional 536.9
      psychogenic 306.4
  Gaucher's (adult) (cerebroside lipidosis)
      (infantile) 272.7
  Gayet's (superior hemorrhagic
      polioencephalitis) 265.1
  Gee (-Herter) (-Heubner) (-Thaysen)
      (nontropical sprue) 579.0
  generalized neoplastic (M8000/6) 199.0
  genital organs NEC
    female 629.9
      specified NEC 629.89
    male 608.9
  Gerhardt's (erythromelalgia) 443.82
  Gerlier's (epidemic vertigo) 078.81
  Gibert's (pityriasis rosea) 696.3
  Gibney's (perispondylitis) 720.9
  Gierke's (glycogenosis I) 271.0
  Gilbert's (familial nonhemolytic jaundice) 277.4
  Gilchrist's (North American blastomycosis)
      116.0
  Gilford (-Hutchinson) (progeria) 259.8
  Gilles de la Tourette's (motor-verbal tic) 307.23
  Giovannini's 117.9
  gland (lymph) 289.9
  Glanzmann's (hereditary hemorrhagic
      thrombasthenia) 287.1
  glassblowers' 527.1
  Glénard's (enteroptosis) 569.89
  Glisson's (*see also* Rickets) 268.0
  glomerular
    membranous, idiopathic 581.1
    minimal change 581.3
  glycogen storage (Andersen's) (Cori types 1-7)
      (Forbes') (McArdle-Schmid-Pearson)
      (Pompe's) (types I-VII) 271.0
    cardiac 271.0 *[425.7]*
    generalized 271.0
    glucose-6-phosphatase deficiency 271.0
    heart 271.0 *[425.7]*
    hepatorenal 271.0
    liver and kidneys 271.0
    myocardium 271.0 *[425.7]*

Disease, diseased—*continued*
  von Gierke's (glycogenosis I) 271.0
  Goldflam-Erb 358.00
  Goldscheider's (epidermolysis bullosa) 757.39
  Goldstein's (familial hemorrhagic
      telangiectasia) 448.0
  gonococcal NEC 098.0
  Goodall's (epidemic vomiting) 078.82
  Gordon's (exudative enteropathy) 579.8
  Gougerot's (trisymptomatic) 709.1
  Gougerot-Carteaud (confluent reticulate
      papillomatosis) 701.8
  Gougerot-Hailey-Hailey (benign familial
      chronic pemphigus) 757.39
  graft-versus-host 279.50
    acute 279.51
      on chronic 279.53
    chronic 279.52
  grain-handlers' 495.8
  Grancher's (splenopneumonia)—*see* Pneumonia
  granulomatous (childhood) (chronic) 288.1
  graphite lung 503
  Graves' (exophthalmic goiter) 242.0
  Greenfield's 330.0
  green monkey 078.89
  Griesinger's (*see also* Ancylostomiasis) 126.9
  grinders' 502
  Grisel's 723.5
  Gruby's (tinea tonsurans) 110.0
  Guertin's (electric chorea) 049.8
  Guillain-Barré 357.0
  Guinon's (motor-verbal tic) 307.23
  Gull's (thyroid atrophy with myxedema) 244.8
  Gull and Sutton's—*see* Hypertension, kidney
  gum NEC 523.9
  Günther's (congenital erythropoietic porphyria)
      277.1
  gynecological 629.9
    specified NEC 629.89
  H 270.0
  Haas' 732.3
  Habermann's (acute parapsoriasis varioliformis)
      696.2
  Haff 985.1
  Hageman (congenital factor XII deficiency) (*see
      also* Defect, congenital) 286.3
  Haglund's (osteochondrosis os tibiale externum)
      732.5
  Hagner's (hypertrophic pulmonary
      osteoarthropathy) 731.2
  Hailey-Hailey (benign familial chronic
      pemphigus) 757.39
  hair (follicles) NEC 704.9
    specified type NEC 704.8
  Hallervorden-Spatz 333.0
  Hallopeau's (lichen sclerosus et atrophicus)
      701.0
  Hamman's (spontaneous mediastinal
      emphysema) 518.1
  hand, foot, and mouth 074.3
  Hand-Schüller-Christian (chronic histiocytosis
      X) 277.89
  Hanot's—*see* Cirrhosis, biliary
  Hansen's (leprosy) 030.9
    benign form 030.1
    malignant form 030.0
  Harada's 363.22
  Harley's (intermittent hemoglobinuria) 283.2
  Hart's (pellagra-cerebellar ataxia renal
      aminoaciduria) 270.0
  Hartnup (pellagra-cerebellar ataxia-renal
      aminoaciduria) 270.0

Disease, diseased—*continued*
  Hashimoto's (struma lymphomatosa) 245.2
  Hb—*see* Disease, hemoglobin
  heart (organic) 429.9
    with
      acute pulmonary edema (*see also* Failure,
        ventricular, left) 428.1
      hypertensive 402.91
        with renal failure 404.92
        benign 402.11
          with renal failure 404.12
        malignant 402.01
          with renal failure 404.02
      kidney disease—*see* Hypertension,
        cardiorenal
      rheumatic fever (conditions classifiable to
        390)
        active 391.9
          with chorea 392.0
        inactive or quiescent (with chorea) 398.90
    amyloid 277.39 *[425.7]*
    aortic (valve) (*see also* Endocarditis, aortic)
      424.1
    arteriosclerotic or sclerotic (minimal)
      (senile)—*see* Arteriosclerosis, coronary
    artery, arterial —*see* Arteriosclerosis,
      coronary
    atherosclerotic —*see* Arteriosclerosis,
      coronary
    beer drinkers' 425.5
    beriberi 265.0 *[425.7]*
    black 416.0
    congenital NEC 746.9
      cyanotic 746.9
      maternal, affecting fetus or newborn 760.3
      specified type NEC 746.89
    congestive (*see also* Failure, heart) 428.0
    coronary 414.9
    cryptogenic 429.9
    due to
      amyloidosis 277.39 *[425.7]*
      beriberi 265.0 *[425.7]*
      cardiac glycogenosis 271.0 *[425.7]*
      Friedreich's ataxia 334.0 *[425.8]*
      gout 274.82
      mucopolysaccharidosis 277.5 *[425.7]*
      myotonia atrophica 359.21 *[425.8]*
      progressive muscular dystrophy 359.1
        [425.8]
      sarcoidosis 135 *[425.8]*
    fetal 746.9
      inflammatory 746.89
    fibroid (*see also* Myocarditis) 429.0
    functional 427.9
      postoperative 997.1
      psychogenic 306.2
    glycogen storage 271.0 *[425.7]*
    gonococcal NEC 098.85
    gouty 274.82
    hypertensive (*see also* Hypertension, heart)
      402.90
      benign 402.10
      malignant 402.00
    hyperthyroid (*see also* Hyperthyroidism)
      242.9 *[425.7]*
    incompletely diagnosed—*see* Disease, heart

Disease, diseased—*continued*
  heart—*continued*
    ischemic (chronic) (*see also* Ischemia, heart)
      414.9
      acute (*see also* Infarct, myocardium) 410.9
        without myocardial infarction 411.89
          with coronary (artery) occlusion 411.81
      asymptomatic 412
      diagnosed on ECG or other special
        investigation but currently presenting no
        symptoms 412
    kyphoscoliotic 416.1
    mitral (*see also* Endocarditis, mitral) 394.9
    muscular (*see also* Degeneration, myocardial)
      429.1
    postpartum 674.8
    psychogenic (functional) 306.2
    pulmonary (chronic) 416.9
      acute 415.0
      specified NEC 416.8
    rheumatic (chronic) (inactive) (old)
      (quiescent) (with chorea) 398.90
      active or acute 391.9
        with chorea (active) (rheumatic)
          (Sydenham's) 392.0
        specified type NEC 391.8
      maternal, affecting fetus or newborn 760.3
    rheumatoid—*see* Arthritis, rheumatoid
    sclerotic —*see* Arteriosclerosis, coronary
    senile (*see also* Myocarditis) 429.0
    specified type NEC 429.89
    syphilitic 093.89
      aortic 093.1
        aneurysm 093.0
      asymptomatic 093.89
      congenital 090.5
    thyroid (gland) (*see also* Hyperthyroidism)
      242.9 *[425.7]*
    thyrotoxic (*see also* Thyrotoxicosis) 242.9
      [425.7]
    tuberculous (*see also* Tuberculosis) 017.9
      [425.8]
    valve, valvular (obstructive)
      (regurgitant)—*see also* Endocarditis
      congenital NEC (*see also* Anomaly, heart,
        valve) 746.9
      pulmonary 746.00
      specified type NEC 746.89
    vascular—*see* Disease, cardiovascular
  heavy-chain (gamma G) 273.2
  Heberden's 715.04
  Hebra's
    dermatitis exfoliativa 695.89
    erythema multiforme exudativum 695.19
    pityriasis
      maculata et circinata 696.3
      rubra 695.89
      pilaris 696.4
    prurigo 698.2
  Heerfordt's (uveoparotitis) 135
  Heidenhain's 290.10
    with dementia 290.10
  Heilmeyer-Schöner (M9842/3) 207.1
  Heine-Medin (*see also* Poliomyelitis) 045.9
  Heller's (*see also* Psychosis, childhood) 299.1
  Heller-Döhle (syphilitic aortitis) 093.1
  hematopoietic organs 289.9

Disease, diseased—*continued*
  hemoglobin (Hb) 282.7
    with thalassemia 282.49
    abnormal (mixed) NEC 282.7
      with thalassemia 282.49
    AS genotype 282.5
    Bart's 282.49
    C (Hb-C) 282.7
      with other abnormal hemoglobin NEC 282.7
      elliptocytosis 282.7
      Hb-S (without crisis) 282.63
        with
          crisis 282.64
          vaso-occlusive pain 282.64
        sickle-cell (without crisis) 282.63
        with
          crisis 282.64
          vaso-occlusive pain 282.64
      thalassemia 282.49
    constant spring 282.7
    D (Hb-D) 282.7
      with other abnormal hemoglobin NEC 282.7
      Hb-S (without crisis) 282.68
        with crisis 282.69
      sickle-cell (without crisis) 282.68
        with crisis 282.69
      thalassemia 282.49
    E (Hb-E) 282.7
      with other abnormal hemoglobin NEC 282.7
      Hb-S (without crisis) 282.68
        with crisis 282.69
      sickle-cell (without crisis) 282.68
        with crisis 282.69
      thalassemia 282.49
    elliptocytosis 282.7
    F (Hb-F) 282.7
    G (Hb-G) 282.7
    H (Hb-H) 282.49
    hereditary persistence, fetal (HPFH) ("Swiss
      variety") 282.7
    high fetal gene 282.7
    I thalassemia 282.49
    M 289.7
    S—*see also* Disease, sickle-cell, Hb-S
      thalassemia (without crisis) 282.41
        with
          crisis 282.42
          vaso-occlusive pain 282.42
    spherocytosis 282.7
    unstable, hemolytic 282.7
    Zurich (Hb-Zurich) 282.7
  hemolytic (fetus) (newborn) 773.2
    autoimmune (cold type) (warm type) 283.0
    due to or with
      incompatibility
        ABO (blood group) 773.1
        blood (group) (Duffy) (Kell) (Kidd)
          (Lewis) (M) (S) NEC 773.2
        Rh (blood group) (factor) 773.0
        Rh negative mother 773.0
    unstable hemoglobin 282.7
  hemorrhagic 287.9
    newborn 776.0
  Henoch (-Schönlein) (purpura nervosa) 287.0
  hepatic—*see* Disease, liver
  hepatolenticular 275.1
  heredodegenerative NEC
    brain 331.89
    spinal cord 336.8
  Hers' (glycogenosis VI) 271.0
  Herter (-Gee) (-Heubner) (nontropical sprue) 579.0

Disease, diseased—*continued*
  Herxheimer's (diffuse idiopathic cutaneous
    atrophy) 701.8
  Heubner's 094.89
  Heubner-Herter (nontropical sprue) 579.0
  high fetal gene or hemoglobin thalassemia 282.49
  Hildenbrand's (typhus) 081.9
  hip (joint) NEC 719.95
    congenital 755.63
    suppurative 711.05
    tuberculous (*see also* Tuberculosis) 015.1
      [730.85]
  Hippel's (retinocerebral angiomatosis) 759.6
  Hirschfeld's (acute diabetes mellitus) (*see also*
    Diabetes) 250.0
    due to secondary diabetes 249.0
  Hirschsprung's (congenital megacolon) 751.3
  His (-Werner) (trench fever) 083.1
  HIV 042
  Hodgkin's (M9650/3) 201.9

> *Note—Use the following fifth-digit
> subclassification with categories 201:*
>
> 0 *unspecified site*
> 1 *lymph nodes of head, face, and neck*
> 2 *intrathoracic lymph nodes*
> 3 *intra-abdominal lymph nodes*
> 4 *lymph nodes of axilla and upper limb*
> 5 *lymph nodes of inguinal region and
>   lower limb*
> 6 *intrapelvic lymph nodes*
> 7 *spleen*
> 8 *lymph nodes of multiple sites*

    lymphocytic
      depletion (M9653/3) 201.7
        diffuse fibrosis (M9654/3) 201.7
        reticular type (M9655/3) 201.7
      predominance (M9651/3) 201.4
    lymphocytic-histiocytic predominance
      (M9651/3) 201.4
    mixed cellularity (M9652/3) 201.6
    nodular sclerosis (M9656/3) 201.5
      cellular phase (M9657/3) 201.5
  Hodgson's 441.9
    ruptured 441.5
  Hoffa (-Kastert) (liposynovitis prepatellaris)
    272.8
  Holla (*see also* Spherocytosis) 282.0
  homozygous-Hb-S 282.61
  hoof and mouth 078.4
  hookworm (*see also* Ancylostomiasis) 126.9
  Horton's (temporal arteritis) 446.5
  host-versus-graft (immune or nonimmune cause)
    279.50
  HPFH (hereditary persistence of fetal
    hemoglobin) ("Swiss variety") 282.7
  Huchard's (continued arterial hypertension)
    401.9
  Huguier's (uterine fibroma) 218.9
  human immunodeficiency (virus) 042
  hunger 251.1
  Hunt's
    dyssynergia cerebellaris myoclonica 334.2
    herpetic geniculate ganglionitis 053.11
  Huntington's 333.4
  Huppert's (multiple myeloma) (M9730/3) 203.0
  Hurler's (mucopolysaccharidosis I) 277.5
  Hutchinson's, meaning
    angioma serpiginosum 709.1
    cheiropompholyx 705.81
    prurigo estivalis 692.72

Disease, diseased—*continued*
Hutchinson-Boeck (sarcoidosis) 135
Hutchinson-Gilford (progeria) 259.8
hyaline (diffuse) (generalized) 728.9
  membrane (lung) (newborn) 769
hydatid (*see also* Echinococcus) 122.9
Hyde's (prurigo nodularis) 698.3
hyperkinetic (*see also* Hyperkinesia) 314.9
  heart 429.82
hypertensive (*see also* Hypertension) 401.9
hypophysis 253.9
  hyperfunction 253.1
  hypofunction 253.2
Iceland (epidemic neuromyasthenia) 049.8
I cell 272.7
ill-defined 799.89
immunologic NEC 279.9
immunoproliferative 203.8
inclusion 078.5
  salivary gland 078.5
infancy, early NEC 779.9
infective NEC 136.9
inguinal gland 289.9
internal semilunar cartilage, cystic 717.5
intervertebral disc 722.90
  with myelopathy 722.70
  cervical, cervicothoracic 722.91
    with myelopathy 722.71
  lumbar, lumbosacral 722.93
    with myelopathy 722.73
  thoracic, thoracolumbar 722.92
    with myelopathy 722.72
intestine 569.9
  functional 564.9
    congenital 751.3
    psychogenic 306.4
  lardaceous 277.39
  organic 569.9
  protozoal NEC 007.9
iris 364.9
  specified NEC 364.89
iron
  metabolism 275.0
  storage 275.0
Isambert's (*see also* Tuberculosis, larynx) 012.3
Iselin's (osteochondrosis, fifth metatarsal) 732.5
Island (scrub typhus) 081.2
itai-itai 985.5
Jadassohn's (maculopapular erythroderma) 696.2
Jadassohn-Pellizari's (anetoderma) 701.3
Jakob-Creutzfeldt (CJD) 046.19
  with dementia
    with behavioral disturbance 046.19 *[294.11]*
    without behavioral disturbance 046.19
      [294.10]
  familial 046.19
  iatrogenic 046.19
  specified NEC 046.19
  sporadic 046.19
  variant (vCJD) 046.11
    with dementia
      with behavioral disturbance 046.11 *[294.11]*
      without behavioral disturbance 046.11
        [294.10]
Jaksch (-Luzet) (pseudoleukemia infantum) 285.8
Janet's 300.89
Jansky-Bielschowsky 330.1
jaw NEC 526.9
  fibrocystic 526.2
Jensen's 363.05
Jeune's (asphyxiating thoracic dystrophy) 756.4
jigger 134.1

Disease, diseased—*continued*
Johnson-Stevens (erythema multiforme
  exudativum) 695.13
joint NEC 719.9
  ankle 719.97
  Charcot 094.0 *[713.5]*
  degenerative (*see also* Osteoarthrosis) 715.9
    multiple 715.09
    spine (*see also* Spondylosis) 721.90
  elbow 719.92
  foot 719.97
  hand 719.94
  hip 719.95
  hypertrophic (chronic) (degenerative) (*see also*
    Osteoarthrosis) 715.9
    spine (*see also* Spondylosis) 721.90
  knee 719.96
  Luschka 721.90
  multiple sites 719.99
  pelvic region 719.95
  sacroiliac 724.6
  shoulder (region) 719.91
  specified site NEC 719.98
  spine NEC 724.9
    pseudarthrosis following fusion 733.82
    sacroiliac 724.6
  wrist 719.93
Jourdain's (acute gingivitis) 523.00
Jüngling's (sarcoidosis) 135
Kahler (-Bozzolo) (multiple myeloma)
  (M9730/3) 203.0
Kalischer's 759.6
Kaposi's 757.33
  lichen ruber 697.8
    acuminatus 696.4
    moniliformis 697.8
  xeroderma pigmentosum 757.33
Kaschin-Beck (endemic polyarthritis) 716.00
  ankle 716.07
  arm 716.02
    lower (and wrist) 716.03
    upper (and elbow) 716.02
  foot (and ankle) 716.07
  forearm (and wrist) 716.03
  hand 716.04
  leg 716.06
    lower 716.06
    upper 716.05
  multiple sites 716.09
  pelvic region (hip) (thigh) 716.05
  shoulder region 716.01
  specified site NEC 716.08
Katayama 120.2
Kawasaki 446.1
Kedani (scrub typhus) 081.2
kidney (functional) (pelvis) (*see also* Disease,
  renal) 593.9
  chronic 585.9
    requiring chronic dialysis 585.6
    stage
      I 585.1
      II (mild) 585.2
      III (moderate) 585.3
      IV (severe) 585.4
      V 585.5
  cystic (congenital) 753.10
    multiple 753.19
    single 753.11
    specified NEC 753.19
  fibrocystic (congenital) 753.19
  in gout 274.10

Disease, diseased—*continued*
kidney—*continued*
  polycystic (congenital) 753.12
    adult type (APKD) 753.13
    autosomal dominant 753.13
    autosomal recessive 753.14
    childhood type (CPKD) 753.14
    infantile type 753.14
  Kienböck's (carpal lunate) (wrist) 732.3
  Kimmelstiel (-Wilson) (intercapillary
    glomerulosclerosis) 250.4 *[581.81]*
  due to secondary diabetes 249.4 *[581.81]*
  Kinnier Wilson's (hepatolenticular
    degeneration) 275.1
  kissing 075
  Kleb's (*see also* Nephritis) 583.9
  Klinger's 446.4
  Klippel's 723.8
  Klippel-Feil (brevicollis) 756.16
  knight's 911.1
  Köbner's (epidermolysis bullosa) 757.39
  Koenig-Wichmann (pemphigus) 694.4
  Köhler's
    first (osteoarthrosis juvenilis) 732.5
    second (Freiberg's infraction, metatarsal head)
      732.5
    patellar 732.4
    tarsal navicular (bone) (osteoarthrosis
      juvenilis) 732.5
  Köhler-Freiberg (infraction, metatarsal head) 732.5
  Köhler-Mouchet (osteoarthrosis juvenilis) 732.5
  Köhler-Pellegrini-Stieda (calcification, knee
    joint) 726.62
  Kok 759.89
  König's (osteochondritis dissecans) 732.7
  Korsakoff's (nonalcoholic) 294.0
    alcoholic 291.1
  Kostmann's (infantile genetic agranulocytosis)
    288.01
  Krabbe's 330.0
  Kraepelin-Morel (*see also* Schizophrenia) 295.9
  Kraft-Weber-Dimitri 759.6
  Kufs' 330.1
  Kugelberg-Welander 335.11
  Kuhnt-Junius 362.52
  Kümmell's (-Verneuil) (spondylitis) 721.7
  Kundrat's (lymphosarcoma) 200.1
  kuru 046.0
  Kussmaul (-Meier) (polyarteritis nodosa) 446.0
  Kyasanur Forest 065.2
  Kyrle's (hyperkeratosis follicularis in cutem
    penetrans) 701.1
  labia
    inflammatory 616.10
    noninflammatory 624.9
      specified NEC 624.8
  labyrinth, ear 386.8
  lacrimal system (apparatus) (passages) 375.9
    gland 375.00
    specified NEC 375.89
  Lafora's 333.2
  Lagleyze-von Hippel (retinocerebral
    angiomatosis) 759.6
  Lancereaux-Mathieu (leptospiral jaundice) 100.0
  Landry's 357.0
  Lane's 569.89
  lardaceous (any site) 277.39
  Larrey-Weil (leptospiral jaundice) 100.0
  Larsen (-Johansson) (juvenile osteopathia
    patellae) 732.4
  larynx 478.70
  Lasègue's (persecution mania) 297.9

Disease, diseased—*continued*
Leber's 377.16
Lederer's (acquired infectious hemolytic
  anemia) 283.19
Legg's (capital femoral osteochondrosis) 732.1
Legg-Calvé-Perthes (capital femoral
  osteochondrosis) 732.1
Legg-Calvé-Waldenström (femoral capital
  osteochondrosis) 732.1
Legg-Perthes (femoral capital osteochondrosis)
  732.1
Legionnaires' 482.84
Leigh's 330.8
Leiner's (exfoliative dermatitis) 695.89
Leloir's (lupus erythematosus) 695.4
Lenegre's 426.0
lens (eye) 379.39
Leriche's (osteoporosis, posttraumatic) 733.7
Letterer-Siwe (acute histiocytosis X) (M9722/3)
  202.5
Lev's (acquired complete heart block) 426.0
Lewandowski's (*see also* Tuberculosis) 017.0
Lewandowski-Lutz (epidermodysplasia
  verruciformis) 078.19
Lewy body 331.82
  with dementia
    with behavioral disturbance 331.82 *[294.11]*
    without behavioral disturbance 331.82
      [294.10]
Leyden's (periodic vomiting) 536.2
Libman-Sacks (verrucous endocarditis) 710.0
  [424.91]
Lichtheim's (subacute combined sclerosis with
  pernicious anemia) 281.0 *[336.2]*
ligament 728.9
light chain 203.0
Lightwood's (renal tubular acidosis) 588.89
Lignac's (cystinosis) 270.0
Lindau's (retinocerebral angiomatosis) 759.6
Lindau-von Hippel (angiomatosis
  retinocerebellosa) 759.6
lip NEC 528.5
lipidosis 272.7
lipoid storage NEC 272.7
Lipschütz's 616.50
Little's—*see* Palsy, cerebral
liver 573.9
  alcoholic 571.3
    acute 571.1
    chronic 571.3
  chronic 571.9
    alcoholic 571.3
  cystic, congenital 751.62
  drug-induced 573.3
  due to
    chemicals 573.3
    fluorinated agents 573.3
    hypersensitivity drugs 573.3
    isoniazids 573.3
  end stage NEC 572.8
    due to hepatitis —*see* Hepatitis
  fibrocystic (congenital) 751.62
  glycogen storage 271.0
  organic 573.9
  polycystic (congenital) 751.62
Lobo's (keloid blastomycosis) 116.2
Lobstein's (brittle bones and blue sclera) 756.61
locomotor system 334.9
Lorain's (pituitary dwarfism) 253.3
Lou Gehrig's 335.20
Lucas-Championnière (fibrinous bronchitis) 466.0
Ludwig's (submaxillary cellulitis) 528.3

Disease, diseased—*continued*
luetic—*see* Syphilis
lumbosacral region 724.6
lung NEC 518.89
  black 500
  congenital 748.60
  cystic 518.89
    congenital 748.4
  fibroid (chronic) (*see also* Fibrosis, lung) 515
  fluke 121.2
    Oriental 121.2
  in
    amyloidosis 277.39 *[517.8]*
    polymyositis 710.4 *[517.8]*
    sarcoidosis 135 *[517.8]*
    Sjögren's syndrome 710.2 *[517.8]*
    syphilis 095.1
    systemic lupus erythematosus 710.0 *[517.8]*
    systemic sclerosis 710.1 *[517.2]*
  interstitial (chronic) 515
    acute 136.3
  nonspecific, chronic 496
  obstructive (chronic) (COPD) 496
    with
      acute
        bronchitis 491.22
        exacerbation NEC 491.21
    alveolitis, allergic (*see also* Alveolitis,
      allergic) 495.9
    asthma (chronic) (obstructive) 493.2
    bronchiectasis 494.0
      with exacerbation (acute) 494.1
    bronchitis (chronic) 491.20
      with
        acute bronchitis 491.22
        exacerbation (acute) 491.21
      decompensated 491.21
        with exacerbation 491.21
    emphysema NEC 492.8
    diffuse (with fibrosis) 496
  polycystic 518.89
    asthma (chronic) (obstructive) 493.2
    congenital 748.4
  purulent (cavitary) 513.0
  restrictive 518.89
  rheumatoid 714.81
    diffuse interstitial 714.81
  specified NEC 518.89
Lutembacher's (atrial septal defect with mitral
  stenosis) 745.5
Lutz-Miescher (elastosis perforans serpiginosa)
  701.1
Lutz-Splendore-de Almeida (Brazilian
  blastomycosis) 116.1
Lyell's (toxic epidermal necrolysis) 695.15
  due to drug
    correct substance properly administered
      695.15
    overdose or wrong substance given or taken
      977.9
    specific drug—*see* Table of drugs and
      chemicals
Lyme 088.81
lymphatic (gland) (system) 289.9
  channel (noninfective) 457.9
  vessel (noninfective) 457.9
  specified NEC 457.8
lymphoproliferative (chronic) (M9970/1) 238.79
Machado-Joseph 334.8
Madelung's (lipomatosis) 272.8

Disease, diseased—*continued*
Madura (actinomycotic) 039.9
  mycotic 117.4
Magitot's 526.4
Majocchi's (purpura annularis telangiectodes)
  709.1
malarial (*see also* Malaria) 084.6
Malassez's (cystic) 608.89
Malibu 919.8
  infected 919.9
malignant (M8000/3)—*see also* Neoplasm, by
  site, malignant
  previous, affecting management of pregnancy
    V23.8
Manson's 120.1
maple bark 495.6
maple syrup (urine) 270.3
Marburg (virus) 078.89
Marchiafava (-Bignami) 341.8
Marfan's 090.49
  congenital syphilis 090.49
  meaning Marfan's syndrome 759.82
Marie-Bamberger (hypertrophic pulmonary
  osteoarthropathy) (secondary) 731.2
  primary or idiopathic (acropachyderma)
    757.39
  pulmonary (hypertrophic osteoarthropathy)
    731.2
Marie-Strümpell (ankylosing spondylitis) 720.0
Marion's (bladder neck obstruction) 596.0
Marsh's (exophthalmic goiter) 242.0
Martin's 715.27
mast cell 757.33
  systemic (M9741/3) 202.6
mastoid (*see also* Mastoiditis) 383.9
  process 385.9
maternal, unrelated to pregnancy NEC, affecting
  fetus or newborn 760.9
Mathieu's (leptospiral jaundice) 100.0
Mauclaire's 732.3
Mauriac's (erythema nodosum syphiliticum)
  091.3
Maxcy's 081.0
McArdle (-Schmid-Pearson) (glycogenosis V)
  271.0
mediastinum NEC 519.3
Medin's (*see also* Poliomyelitis) 045.9
Mediterranean (with hemoglobinopathy) 282.49
medullary center (idiopathic) (respiratory)
  348.89
Meige's (chronic hereditary edema) 757.0
Meleda 757.39
Ménétrier's (hypertrophic gastritis) 535.2
Ménière's (active) 386.00
  cochlear 386.02
  cochleovestibular 386.01
  inactive 386.04
  in remission 386.04
  vestibular 386.03
  meningeal—*see* Meningitis
mental (*see also* Psychosis) 298.9
Merzbacher-Pelizaeus 330.0
mesenchymal 710.9
mesenteric embolic 557.0
metabolic NEC 277.9
metal polishers' 502
metastatic—*see* Metastasis
Mibelli's 757.39
microdrepanocytic 282.49
microvascular —*code to condition*
Miescher's 709.3

Disease, diseased—*continued*
Mikulicz's (dryness of mouth, absent or
  decreased lacrimation) 527.1
Milkman (-Looser) (osteomalacia with
  pseudofractures) 268.2
Miller's (osteomalacia) 268.2
Mills' 335.29
Milroy's (chronic hereditary edema) 757.0
Minamata 985.0
Minor's 336.1
Minot's (hemorrhagic disease, newborn) 776.0
Minot-von Willebrand-Jürgens
  (angiohemophilia) 286.4
Mitchell's (erythromelalgia) 443.82
mitral—*see* Endocarditis, mitral
Mljet (mal de Meleda) 757.39
Möbius', Moebius' 346.2
Moeller's 267
Möller (-Barlow) (infantile scurvy) 267
Mönckeberg's (*see also* arteriosclerosis,
  extremities) 440.20
Mondor's (thrombophlebitis of breast) 451.89
Monge's 993.2
Morel-Kraepelin (*see also* Schizophrenia) 295.9
Morgagni's (syndrome) (hyperostosis frontalis
  interna) 733.3
Morgagni-Adams-Stokes (syncope with heart
  block) 426.9
Morquio (-Brailsford) (-Ullrich)
  (mucopolysaccharidosis IV) 277.5
Morton's (with metatarsalgia) 355.6
Morvan's 336.0
motor neuron (bulbar) (mixed type) 335.20
Mouchet's (juvenile osteochondrosis, foot)
  732.5
mouth 528.9
Moyamoya 437.5
Mucha's (acute parapsoriasis varioliformis)
  696.2
mu-chain 273.2
mucolipidosis (I) (II) (III) 272.7
Münchmeyer's (exostosis luxurians) 728.11
Murri's (intermittent hemoglobinuria) 283.2
muscle 359.9
  inflammatory 728.9
  ocular 378.9
musculoskeletal system 729.90
mushroom workers' 495.5
Myà's (congenital dilation, colon) 751.3
mycotic 117.9
myeloproliferative (chronic) (M9960/1) 238.79
myocardium, myocardial (*see also*
  Degeneration, myocardial) 429.1
hypertensive (*see also* Hypertension, heart)
  402.90
primary (idiopathic) 425.4
myoneural 358.9
Naegeli's 287.1
nail 703.9
  specified type NEC 703.8
Nairobi sheep 066.1
nasal 478.19
  cavity NEC 478.19
  sinus (chronic)—*see* Sinusitis
navel (newborn) NEC 779.89
  delayed separation of umbilical cord 779.83
nemaline body 359.0
neoplastic, generalized (M8000/6) 199.0
nerve—*see* Disorder, nerve

Disease, diseased—*continued*
nervous system (central) 349.9
  autonomic, peripheral (*see also* Neuropathy,
    peripheral, autonomic) 337.9
  congenital 742.9
  inflammatory—*see* Encephalitis
  parasympathetic (*see also* Neuropathy,
    peripheral, autonomic) 337.9
  peripheral NEC 355.9
  prion NEC 046.79
  specified NEC 349.89
  sympathetic (*see also* Neuropathy, peripheral,
    autonomic) 337.9
  vegetative (*see also* Neuropathy, peripheral,
    autonomic) 337.9
Nettleship's (urticaria pigmentosa) 757.33
Neumann's (pemphigus vegetans) 694.4
neurologic (central) NEC (*see also* Disease,
  nervous system) 349.9
  peripheral NEC 355.9
neuromuscular system NEC 358.9
Newcastle 077.8
Nicolas (-Durand) -Favre (climatic bubo) 099.1
Niemann-Pick (lipid histiocytosis) 272.7
nipple 611.9
  Paget's (M8540/3) 174.0
Nishimoto (-Takeuchi) 437.5
nonarthropod-borne NEC 078.89
  central nervous system NEC 049.9
  enterovirus NEC 078.89
non-autoimmune hemolytic NEC 283.10
Nonne-Milroy-Meige (chronic hereditary
  edema) 757.0
Norrie's (congenital progressive
  oculoacousticocerebral degeneration) 743.8
nose 478.19
nucleus pulposus—*see* Disease, intervertebral
  disc
nutritional 269.9
  maternal, affecting fetus or newborn 760.4
oasthouse, urine 270.2
obliterative vascular 447.1
Odelberg's (juvenile osteochondrosis) 732.1
Oguchi's (retina) 368.61
Ohara's (*see also* Tularemia) 021.9
Ollier's (chondrodysplasia) 756.4
Opitz's (congestive splenomegaly) 289.51
Oppenheim's 358.8
Oppenheim-Urbach (necrobiosis lipoidica
  diabeticorum) 250.8 *[709.3]*
  due to secondary diabetes 249.8 *[709.3]*
optic nerve NEC 377.49
orbit 376.9
  specified NEC 376.89
Oriental liver fluke 121.1
Oriental lung fluke 121.2
Ormond's 593.4
Osgood's tibia (tubercle) 732.4
Osgood-Schlatter 732.4
Osler (-Vaquez) (polycythemia vera) (M9950/1)
  238.4
Osler-Rendu (familial hemorrhagic
  telangiectasia) 448.0
osteofibrocystic 252.01
Otto's 715.35
outer ear 380.9
ovary (noninflammatory) NEC 620.9
  cystic 620.2
  polycystic 256.4
  specified NEC 620.8
Owren's (congenital) (*see also* Defect,
  coagulation) 286.3

Disease, diseased—*continued*
Paas' 756.59
Paget's (osteitis deformans) 731.0
  with infiltrating duct carcinoma of the breast
    (M8541/3)—*see* Neoplasm, breast, malignant
  bone 731.0
    osteosarcoma in (M9184/3)—*see* Neoplasm,
      bone, malignant
  breast (M8540/3) 174.0
  extramammary (M8542/3)—*see also*
    Neoplasm, skin, malignant
    anus 154.3
    skin 173.5
  malignant (M8540/3)
    breast 174.0
    specified site NEC (M8542/3)—*see*
      Neoplasm, skin, malignant
    unspecified site 174.0
  mammary (M8540/3) 174.0
  nipple (M8540/3) 174.0
  palate (soft) 528.9
Paltauf-Sternberg 201.9
pancreas 577.9
  cystic 577.2
    congenital 751.7
  fibrocystic 277.00
Panner's 732.3
  capitellum humeri 732.3
  head of humerus 732.3
  tarsal navicular (bone) (osteochondrosis) 732.5
panvalvular—*see* Endocarditis, mitral
parametrium 629.9
parasitic NEC 136.9
  cerebral NEC 123.9
  intestinal NEC 129
  mouth 112.0
  skin NEC 134.9
  specified type—*see* Infestation
  tongue 112.0
parathyroid (gland) 252.9
  specified NEC 252.8
Parkinson's 332.0
parodontal 523.9
Parrot's (syphilitic osteochondritis) 090.0
Parry's (exophthalmic goiter) 242.0
Parson's (exophthalmic goiter) 242.0
Pavy's 593.6
Paxton's (white piedra) 111.2
Payr's (splenic flexure syndrome) 569.89
pearl-workers' (chronic osteomyelitis) (*see also*
  Osteomyelitis) 730.1
Pel-Ebstein—*see* Disease, Hodgkin's
Pelizaeus-Merzbacher 330.0
  with dementia
    with behavioral disturbance 330.0 *[294.11]*
    without behavioral disturbance 330.0
      [294.10]
Pellegrini-Stieda (calcification, knee joint) 726.62
pelvis, pelvic
  female NEC 629.9
    specified NEC 629.89
  gonococcal (acute) 098.19
    chronic or duration of 2 months or over 098.39
  infection (*see also* Disease, pelvis, inflammatory)
    614.9

Disease, diseased—*continued*
pelvic—*continued*
  inflammatory (female) (PID) 614.9
    with
      abortion—*see* Abortion, by type, with sepsis
      ectopic pregnancy (*see also* categories
        633.0-633.9) 639.0
      molar pregnancy (*see also* categories
        630-632) 639.0
    acute 614.3
    chronic 614.4
    complicating pregnancy 646.6
      affecting fetus or newborn 760.8
    following
      abortion 639.0
      ectopic or molar pregnancy 639.0
    peritonitis (acute) 614.5
      chronic NEC 614.7
    puerperal, postpartum, childbirth 670.8
    specified NEC 614.8
  organ, female NEC 629.9
    specified NEC 629.89
  peritoneum, female NEC 629.9
    specified NEC 629.89
penis 607.9
  inflammatory 607.2
peptic NEC 536.9
  acid 536.8
periapical tissues NEC 522.9
pericardium 423.9
  specified type NEC 423.8
perineum
  female
    inflammatory 616.9
      specified NEC 616.89
    noninflammatory 624.9
      specified NEC 624.8
  male (inflammatory) 682.2
periodic (familial) (Reimann's) NEC 277.31
  paralysis 359.3
periodontal NEC 523.9
  specified NEC 523.8
periosteum 733.90
peripheral
  arterial 443.9
  autonomic nervous system (*see also*
    Neuropathy, autonomic) 337.9
  nerve NEC (*see also* Neuropathy) 356.9
    multiple—*see* Polyneuropathy
  vascular 443.9
    specified type NEC 443.89
peritoneum 568.9
  pelvic, female 629.9
    specified NEC 629.89
Perrin-Ferraton (snapping hip) 719.65
persistent mucosal (middle ear) (with posterior
  or superior marginal perforation of ear
  drum) 382.2
Perthes' (capital femoral osteochondrosis) 732.1
Petit's (*see also* Hernia, lumbar) 553.8
Peutz-Jeghers 759.6
Peyronie's 607.85
Pfeiffer's (infectious mononucleosis) 075
pharynx 478.20
Phocas' 610.1
photochromogenic (acid-fast bacilli)
  (pulmonary) 031.0
  nonpulmonary 031.9

Disease, diseased—*continued*
  Pick's
    brain 331.11
      with dementia
        with behavioral disturbance 331.11
          [294.11]
        without behavioral disturbance 331.11
          [294.10]
      cerebral atrophy 331.11
        with dementia
          with behavioral disturbance 331.11
            [294.11]
          without behavioral disturbance 331.11
            [294.10]
      lipid histiocytosis 272.7
      liver (pericardial pseudocirrhosis of liver) 423.2
      pericardium (pericardial pseudocirrhosis of
        liver) 423.2
      polyserositis (pericardial pseudocirrhosis of
        liver) 423.2
  Pierson's (osteochondrosis) 732.1
  pigeon fancier's or breeders' 495.2
  pineal gland 259.8
  pink 985.0
  Pinkus' (lichen nitidus) 697.1
  pinworm 127.4
  pituitary (gland) 253.9
    hyperfunction 253.1
    hypofunction 253.2
  pituitary snuff-takers' 495.8
  placenta
    affecting fetus or newborn 762.2
    complicating pregnancy or childbirth 656.7
  pleura (cavity) (*see also* Pleurisy) 511.0
  Plummer's (toxic nodular goiter) 242.3
  pneumatic
    drill 994.9
    hammer 994.9
  policeman's 729.2
  Pollitzer's (hidradenitis suppurativa) 705.83
  polycystic (congenital) 759.89
    kidney or renal 753.12
      adult type (APKD) 753.13
      autosomal dominant 753.13
      autosomal recessive 753.14
      childhood type (CPKD) 753.14
      infantile type 753.14
    liver or hepatic 751.62
    lung or pulmonary 518.89
      congenital 748.4
    ovary, ovaries 256.4
    spleen 759.0
  Pompe's (glycogenosis II) 271.0
  Poncet's (tuberculous rheumatism) (*see also*
    Tuberculosis) 015.9
  Posada-Wernicke 114.9
  Potain's (pulmonary edema) 514
  Pott's (*see also* Tuberculosis) 015.0 *[730.88]*
    osteomyelitis 015.0 *[730.88]*
    paraplegia 015.0 *[730.88]*
    spinal curvature 015.0 *[737.43]*
    spondylitis 015.0 *[720.81]*
  Potter's 753.0
  Poulet's 714.2
  pregnancy NEC (*see also* Pregnancy) 646.9
  Preiser's (osteoporosis) 733.09
  Pringle's (tuberous sclerosis) 759.5
  Profichet's 729.90
  prostate 602.9
    specified type NEC 602.8
  protozoal NEC 136.8
    intestine, intestinal NEC 007.9

Disease, diseased—*continued*
  pseudo-Hurler's (mucolipidosis III) 272.7
  psychiatric (*see also* Psychosis) 298.9
  psychotic (*see also* Psychosis) 298.9
  Puente's (simple glandular cheilitis) 528.5
  puerperal NEC (*see also* Puerperal) 674.9
  pulmonary—*see also* Disease, lung
    amyloid 277.39 *[517.8]*
    artery 417.9
    circulation, circulatory 417.9
      specified NEC 417.8
    diffuse obstructive (chronic) 496
      with
        acute bronchitis 491.22
        asthma (chronic) (obstructive) 493.2
        bronchitis (chronic) 491.20
          with exacerbation (acute) 491.21
          exacerbation NEC (acute) 491.21
    heart (chronic) 416.9
      specified NEC 416.8
    hypertensive (vascular) 416.0
      cardiovascular 416.0
    obstructive diffuse (chronic) 496
      decompensated 491.21
        with exacerbation 491.21
      with
        acute bronchitis 491.22
        asthma (chronic) (obstructive) 493.2
        bronchitis (chronic) 491.20
          with
            exacerbation (acute) 491.21
            acute 491.22
          exacerbation NEC (acute) 491.21
    valve (*see also* Endocarditis, pulmonary) 424.3
  pulp (dental) NEC 522.9
  pulseless 446.7
  Putnam's (subacute combined sclerosis with
    pernicious anemia) 281.0 *[336.2]*
  Pyle (-Cohn) (craniometaphyseal dysplasia) 756.89
  pyramidal tract 333.90
  Quervain's
    tendon sheath 727.04
    thyroid (subacute granulomatous thyroiditis)
      245.1
  Quincke's—*see* Edema, angioneurotic
  Quinquaud (acne decalvans) 704.09
  rag sorters' 022.1
  Raynaud's (Paroxysmal digital cyanosis) 443.0
  reactive airway—*see* Asthma
  Recklinghausen's (M9540/1) 237.71
    bone (osteitis fibrosa cystica) 252.01
  Recklinghausen-Applebaum (hemochromatosis)
    275.0
  Reclus' (cystic) 610.1
  rectum NEC 569.49
  Refsum's (heredopathia atactica
    polyneuritiformis) 356.3
  Reichmann's (gastrosuccorrhea) 536.8
  Reimann's (periodic) 277.31
  Reiter's 099.3
  renal (functional) (pelvis) (*see also* Disease,
    kidney) 593.9
    with
      edema (*see also* Nephrosis) 581.9
      exudative nephritis 583.89
      lesion of interstitial nephritis 583.89
      stated generalized cause—*see* Nephritis
    acute 593.9
    basement membrane NEC 583.89
      with
        pulmonary hemorrhage (Goodpasture's
          syndrome) 446.21 *[583.81]*

Disease, diseased—*continued*
　renal—*continued*
　　chronic (*see also* Disease, kidney, chronic)
　　　585.9
　　complicating pregnancy or puerperium NEC
　　　646.2
　　　with hypertension—*see* Toxemia, of
　　　　pregnancy
　　　affecting fetus or newborn 760.1
　　cystic, congenital (*see also* Cystic, disease,
　　　kidney) 753.10
　　diabetic 250.4 *[583.81]*
　　　due to secondary diabetes 249.4 *[581.81]*
　　due to
　　　amyloidosis 277.39 *[583.81]*
　　　diabetes mellitus 250.4 *[583.81]*
　　　　due to secondary diabetes 249.4 *[581.81]*
　　　systemic lupus erythematosis 710.0 *[583.81]*
　　end-stage 585.6
　　exudative 583.89
　　fibrocystic (congenital) 753.19
　　gonococcal 098.19 *[583.81]*
　　gouty 274.10
　　hypertensive (*see also* Hypertension, kidney)
　　　403.90
　　immune complex NEC 583.89
　　interstitial (diffuse) (focal) 583.89
　　lupus 710.0 *[583.81]*
　　maternal, affecting fetus or newborn 760.1
　　　hypertensive 760.0
　　phosphate-losing (tubular) 588.0
　　polycystic (congenital) 753.12
　　　adult type (APKD) 753.13
　　　autosomal dominant 753.13
　　　autosomal recessive 753.14
　　　childhood type (CPKD) 753.14
　　　infantile type 753.14
　　specified lesion or cause NEC (*see also*
　　　Glomerulonephritis) 583.89
　　subacute 581.9
　　syphilitic 095.4
　　tuberculous (*see also* Tuberculosis) 016.0
　　　[583.81]
　　tubular (*see also* Nephrosis, tubular) 584.5
　Rendu-Olser-Weber (familial hemorrhagic
　　telangiectasia) 448.0
　renovascular (arteriosclerotic) (*see also*
　　Hypertension, kidney) 403.90
　respiratory (tract) 519.9
　　acute or subacute (upper) NEC 465.9
　　　due to fumes or vapors 506.3
　　　multiple sites NEC 465.8
　　　noninfectious 478.9
　　　streptococcal 034.0
　　chronic 519.9
　　　arising in the perinatal period 770.7
　　　due to fumes or vapors 506.4
　　due to
　　　aspiration of liquids or solids 508.9
　　　external agents NEC 508.9
　　　　specified NEC 508.8
　　　fumes or vapors 506.9
　　　　acute or subacute NEC 506.3
　　　　chronic 506.4
　　fetus or newborn NEC 770.9
　　obstructive 496
　　specified type NEC 519.8
　　upper (acute) (infectious) NEC 465.9
　　　multiple sites NEC 465.8
　　　noninfectious NEC 478.9
　　　streptococcal 034.0

Disease, diseased—*continued*
　retina, retinal NEC 362.9
　　Batten's or Batten-Mayou 330.1 *[362.71]*
　　degeneration 362.89
　　vascular lesion 362.17
　rheumatic (*see also* Arthritis) 716.8
　　heart—*see* Disease, heart, rheumatic
　rheumatoid (heart)—*see* Arthritis, rheumatoid
　rickettsial NEC 083.9
　　specified type NEC 083.8
　Riedel's (ligneous thyroiditis) 245.3
　Riga (-Fede) (cachectic aphthae) 529.0
　Riggs' (compound periodontitis) 523.40
　Ritter's 695.81
　Rivalta's (cervicofacial actinomycosis) 039.3
　Robles' (onchocerciasis) 125.3 *[360.13]*
　Roger's (congenital interventricular septal
　　defect) 745.4
　Rokitansky's (*see also* Necrosis, liver) 570
　Romberg's 349.89
　Rosenthal's (factor XI deficiency) 286.2
　Rossbach's (hyperchlorhydria) 536.8
　　psychogenic 306.4
　Roth (-Bernhardt) 355.1
　Runeberg's (progressive pernicious anemia)
　　281.0
　Rust's (tuberculous spondylitis) (*see also*
　　Tuberculosis) 015.0 *[720.81]*
　Rustitskii's (multiple myeloma) (M9730/3)
　　203.0
　Ruysch's (Hirschsprung's disease) 751.3
　Sachs (-Tay) 330.1
　sacroiliac NEC 724.6
　salivary gland or duct NEC 527.9
　　inclusion 078.5
　　streptococcal 034.0
　　virus 078.5
　Sander's (paranoia) 297.1
　Sandhoff's 330.1
　sandworm 126.9
　Savill's (epidemic exfoliative dermatitis) 695.89
　Schamberg's (progressive pigmentary
　　dermatosis) 709.09
　Schaumann's (sarcoidosis) 135
　Schenck's (sporotrichosis) 117.1
　Scheuermann's (osteochondrosis) 732.0
　Schilder (-Flatau) 341.1
　Schimmelbusch's 610.1
　Schlatter's tibia (tubercle) 732.4
　Schlatter-Osgood 732.4
　Schmorl's 722.30
　　cervical 722.39
　　lumbar, lumbosacral 722.32
　　specified region NEC 722.39
　　thoracic, thoracolumbar 722.31
　Scholz's 330.0
　Schönlein (-Henoch) (purpura rheumatica) 287.0
　Schottmüller's (*see also* Fever, paratyphoid)
　　002.9
　Schüller-Christian (chronic histiocytosis X)
　　277.89
　Schultz's (agranulocytosis) 288.09
　Schwalbe-Ziehen-Oppenheimer 333.6
　Schwartz-Jampel 359.23
　Schweninger-Buzzi (macular atrophy) 701.3
　sclera 379.19
　scrofulous (*see also* Tuberculosis) 017.2
　scrotum 608.9
　sebaceous glands NEC 706.9
　Secretan's (posttraumatic edema) 782.3

Disease, diseased—*continued*
  semilunar cartilage, cystic 717.5
  seminal vesicle 608.9
  Senear-Usher (pemphigus erythematosus) 694.4
  serum NEC 999.5
  Sever's (osteochondrosis calcaneum) 732.5
  sexually transmitted —*see* Disease, venereal
  Sézary's (reticulosis) (M9701/3) 202.2
  Shaver's (bauxite pneumoconiosis) 503
  Sheehan's (postpartum pituitary necrosis) 253.2
  shimamushi (scrub typhus) 081.2
  shipyard 077.1
  sickle-cell 282.60
    with
      crisis 282.62
      Hb-S disease 282.61
      other abnormal hemoglobin (Hb-D) (Hb-E)
        (Hb-G) (Hb-J) (Hb-K) (Hb-O) (Hb-P)
        (high fetal gene) (without crisis) 282.68
        with crisis 282.69
    elliptocytosis 282.60
    Hb-C (without crisis) 282.63
      with
        crisis 282.64
        vaso-occlusive pain 282.64
    Hb-S 282.61
      with
        crisis 282.62
        Hb-C (without crisis) 282.63
          with
            crisis 282.64
            vaso-occlusive pain 282.64
        other abnormal hemoglobin (Hb-D) (Hb-E)
          (Hb-G) (Hb-J) (Hb-K) (Hb-O) (Hb-P)
          (high fetal gene) (without crisis) 282.68
          with crisis 282.69
    spherocytosis 282.60
    thalassemia (without crisis) 282.41
      with
        crisis 282.42
        vaso-occlusive pain 282.42
  Siegal-Cattan-Mamou (periodic) 277.31
  silo fillers' 506.9
  Simian B 054.3
  Simmonds' (pituitary cachexia) 253.2
  Simons' (progressive lipodystrophy) 272.6
  Sinding-Larsen (juvenile osteopathia patellae)
    732.4
  sinus—*see also* Sinusitis
    brain 437.9
    specified NEC 478.19
  Sirkari's 085.0
  sixth (*see also* Exanthem subitum) 058.10
  Sjögren (-Gougerot) 710.2
    with lung involvement 710.2 *[517.8]*
  Skevas-Zerfus 989.5
  skin NEC 709.9
    due to metabolic disorder 277.9
    specified type NEC 709.8
  sleeping (*see also* Narcolepsy) 347.00
    meaning sleeping sickness (*see also*
      Trypanosomiasis) 086.5
  small vessel 443.9
  Smith-Strang (oasthouse urine) 270.2
  Sneddon-Wilkinson (subcorneal pustular
    dermatosis) 694.1
  South African creeping 133.8
  Spencer's (epidemic vomiting) 078.82
  Spielmeyer-Stock 330.1
  Spielmeyer-Vogt 330.1

Disease, diseased—*continued*
  spine, spinal 733.90
    combined system (*see also* Degeneration,
      combined) 266.2 *[336.2]*
      with pernicious anemia 281.0 *[336.2]*
    cord NEC 336.9
    congenital 742.9
    demyelinating NEC 341.8
    joint (*see also* Disease, joint, spine) 724.9
    tuberculous 015.0 *[730.8]*
  spinocerebellar 334.9
    specified NEC 334.8
  spleen (organic) (postinfectional) 289.50
    amyloid 277.39
    lardaceous 277.39
    polycystic 759.0
    specified NEC 289.59
  sponge divers' 989.5
  Stanton's (melioidosis) 025
  Stargardt's 362.75
  Startle 759.89
  Steinert's 359.21
  Sternberg's—*see* Disease, Hodgkin's
  Stevens-Johnson (erythema multiforme
    exudativum) 695.13
  Sticker's (erythema infectiosum) 057.0
  Stieda's (calcification, knee joint) 726.62
  Still's (juvenile rheumatoid arthritis) 714.30
    adult onset 714.2
  Stiller's (asthenia) 780.79
  Stokes' (exophthalmic goiter) 242.0
  Stokes-Adams (syncope with heart block) 426.9
  Stokvis (-Talma) (enterogenous cyanosis) 289.7
  stomach NEC (organic) 537.9
    functional 536.9
      psychogenic 306.4
    lardaceous 277.39
  stonemasons' 502
  storage
    glycogen (*see also* Disease, glycogen storage)
      271.0
    lipid 272.7
    mucopolysaccharide 277.5
  striatopallidal system 333.90
    specified NEC 333.89
  Strümpell-Marie (ankylosing spondylitis) 720.0
  Stuart's (congenital factor X deficiency) (*see
    also* Defect, coagulation) 286.3
  Stuart-Prower (congenital factor X deficiency)
    (*see also* Defect, coagulation) 286.3
  Sturge (-Weber) (-Dimitri) (encephalocutaneous
    angiomatosis) 759.6
  Stuttgart 100.89
  Sudeck's 733.7
  supporting structures of teeth NEC 525.9
  suprarenal (gland) (capsule) 255.9
    hyperfunction 255.3
    hypofunction 255.41
  Sutton's 709.09
  Sutton and Gull's—*see* Hypertension, kidney
  sweat glands NEC 705.9
    specified type NEC 705.89
  sweating 078.2
  Sweeley-Klionsky 272.4
  Swift (-Feer) 985.0
  swimming pool (bacillus) 031.1
  swineherd's 100.89
  Sylvest's (epidemic pleurodynia) 074.1
  Symmers (follicular lymphoma) (M9690/3)
    202.0

Disease, diseased—*continued*
  sympathetic nervous system (*see also*
    Neuropathy, peripheral, autonomic) 337.9
  synovium 727.9
  syphilitic—*see* Syphilis
  systemic tissue mast cell (M9741/3) 202.6
  Taenzer's 757.4
  Takayasu's (pulseless) 446.7
  Talma's 728.85
  Tangier (familial high-density lipoprotein
    deficiency) 272.5
  Tarral-Besnier (pityriasis rubra pilaris) 696.4
  Tay-Sachs 330.1
  Taylor's 701.8
  tear duct 375.69
  teeth, tooth 525.9
    hard tissues 521.9
      specified NEC 521.89
    pulp NEC 522.9
  tendon 727.9
    inflammatory NEC 727.9
  terminal vessel 443.9
  testis 608.9
  Thaysen-Gee (nontropical sprue) 579.0
  Thomsen's 359.22
  Thomson's (congenital poikiloderma) 757.33
  Thornwaldt's, Tornwaldt's (pharyngeal bursitis)
    478.29
  throat 478.20
    septic 034.0
  thromboembolic (*see also* Embolism) 444.9
  thymus (gland) 254.9
    specified NEC 254.8
  thyroid (gland) NEC 246.9
    heart (*see also* Hyperthyroidism) 242.9
      [425.7]
    lardaceous 277.39
    specified NEC 246.8
  Tietze's 733.6
  Tommaselli's
    correct substance properly administered
      599.70
    overdose or wrong substance given or taken
      961.4
  tongue 529.9
  tonsils, tonsillar (and adenoids) (chronic) 474.9
    specified NEC 474.8
  tooth, teeth 525.9
    hard tissues 521.9
      specified NEC 521.89
    pulp NEC 522.9
  Tornwaldt's (pharyngeal bursitis) 478.29
  Tourette's 307.23
  trachea 519.19
  tricuspid—*see* Endocarditis, tricuspid
  triglyceride-storage, type I, II, III 272.7
  triple vessel (coronary arteries) —*see*
    Arteriosclerosis, coronary
  trisymptomatic, Gougerot's 709.1
  trophoblastic (*see also* Hydatidiform mole) 630
    previous, affecting management of pregnancy
      V23.1
  tsutsugamushi (scrub typhus) 081.2
  tube (fallopian), noninflammatory 620.9
    specified NEC 620.8
  tuberculous NEC (*see also* Tuberculosis) 011.9
  tubo-ovarian
    inflammatory (*see also* Salpingo-oophoritis)
      614.2
    noninflammatory 620.9
      specified NEC 620.8

Disease, diseased—*continued*
  tubotympanic, chronic (with anterior perforation
    of ear drum) 382.1
  tympanum 385.9
  Uhl's 746.84
  umbilicus (newborn) NEC 779.89
    delayed separation 779.83
  Underwood's (sclerema neonatorum) 778.1
  undiagnosed 799.9
  Unna's (seborrheic dermatitis) 690.18
  unstable hemoglobin hemolytic 282.7
  Unverricht (-Lundborg) 345.1
  Urbach-Oppenheim (necrobiosis lipoidica
    diabeticorum) 250.8 *[709.3]*
    due to secondary diabetes 249.8 *[709.3]*
  Urbach-Wiethe (lipoid proteinosis) 272.8
  ureter 593.9
  urethra 599.9
    specified type NEC 599.84
  urinary (tract) 599.9
    bladder 596.9
      specified NEC 596.8
    maternal, affecting fetus or newborn 760.1
  Usher-Senear (pemphigus erythematosus) 694.4
  uterus (organic) 621.9
    infective (*see also* Endometritis) 615.9
    inflammatory (*see also* Endometritis) 615.9
    noninflammatory 621.9
      specified type NEC 621.8
  uveal tract
    anterior 364.9
    posterior 363.9
  vagabonds' 132.1
  vagina, vaginal
    inflammatory 616.10
    noninflammatory 623.9
      specified NEC 623.8
  Valsuani's (progressive pernicious anemia,
    puerperal) 648.2
    complicating pregnancy or puerperium 648.2
  valve, valvular—*see also* Endocarditis
    congenital NEC (*see also* Anomaly, heart,
      valve) 746.9
    pulmonary 746.00
      specified type NEC 746.89
  van Bogaert-Nijssen (-Peiffer) 330.0
  van Creveld-von Gierke (glycogenosis I) 271.0
  van den Bergh's (enterogenous cyanosis) 289.7
  van Neck's (juvenile osteochondrosis) 732.1
  Vaquez (-Osler) (polycythemia vera) (M9950/1)
    238.4
  vascular 459.9
    arteriosclerotic—*see* Arteriosclerosis
    hypertensive—*see* Hypertension
    obliterative 447.1
      peripheral 443.9
    occlusive 459.9
    peripheral (occlusive) 443.9
      in (due to) (with) diabetes mellitus 250.7
        [443.81]
      in (due to) (with) secondary diabetes 249.7
        [443.81]
    specified type NEC 443.89
  vas deferens 608.9
  vasomotor 443.9
  vasospastic 443.9
  vein 459.9

Disease, diseased—*continued*
venereal 099.9
fifth 099.1
sixth 099.1
chlamydial NEC 099.50
anus 099.52
bladder 099.53
cervix 099.53
epididymis 099.54
genitourinary NEC 099.55
lower 099.53
specified NEC 099.54
pelvic inflammatory disease 099.54
perihepatic 099.56
peritoneum 099.56
pharynx 099.51
rectum 099.52
specified site NEC 099.59
testis 099.54
vagina 099.53
vulva 099.53
complicating pregnancy, childbirth, or
puerperium 647.2
specified nature or type NEC 099.8
chlamydial—*see* Disease, venereal,
chlamydial
Verneuil's (syphilitic bursitis) 095.7
Verse's (calcinosis intervertebralis) 275.49
[722.90]
vertebra, vertebral NEC 733.90
disc—*see* Disease, Intervertebral disc
vibration NEC 994.9
Vidal's (lichen simplex chronicus) 698.3
Vincent's (trench mouth) 101
Virchow's 733.99
virus (filterable) NEC 078.89
arbovirus NEC 066.9
arthropod-borne NEC 066.9
central nervous system NEC 049.9
specified type NEC 049.8
complicating pregnancy, childbirth, or
puerperium 647.6
contact (with) V01.79
varicella V01.71
exposure to V01.79
varicella V01.71
Marburg 078.89
maternal
with fetal damage affecting management of
pregnancy 655.3
nonarthropod-borne NEC 078.89
central nervous system NEC 049.9
specified NEC 049.8
vaccination, prophylactic (against) V04.89
vitreous 379.29
vocal cords NEC 478.5
Vogt's (Cecile) 333.71
Vogt-Spielmeyer 330.1
Volhard-Fahr (malignant nephrosclerosis)
403.00
Volkmann's
acquired 958.6
von Bechterew's (ankylosing spondylitis) 720.0
von Economo's (encephalitis lethargica) 049.8
von Eulenburg's (congenital paramyotonia)
359.29
von Gierke's (glycogenosis I) 271.0
von Graefe's 378.72
von Hippel's (retinocerebral angiomatosis)
759.6
von Hippel-Lindau (angiomatosis
retinocerebellosa) 759.6

Disease, diseased—*continued*
von Jaksch's (pseudoleukemia infantum) 285.8
von Recklinghausen's (M9540/1) 237.71
bone (osteitis fibrosa cystica) 252.01
von Recklinghausen-Applebaum
(hemochromatosis) 275.0
von Willebrand (-Jürgens) (angiohemophilia)
286.4
von Zambusch's (lichen sclerosus et atrophicus)
701.0
Voorhoeve's (dyschondroplasia) 756.4
Vrolik's (osteogenesis imperfecta) 756.51
vulva
inflammatory 616.10
noninflammatory 624.9
specified NEC 624.8
Wagner's (colloid milium) 709.3
Waldenström's (osteochondrosis capital
femoral) 732.1
Wallgren's (obstruction of splenic vein with
collateral circulation) 459.89
Wardrop's (with lymphangitis) 681.9
finger 681.02
toe 681.11
Wassilieff's (leptospiral jaundice) 100.0
wasting NEC 799.4
due to malnutrition 261
paralysis 335.21
Waterhouse-Friderichsen 036.3
waxy (any site) 277.39
Weber-Christian (nodular nonsuppurative
panniculitis) 729.30
Wegner's (syphilitic osteochondritis) 090.0
Weil's (leptospiral jaundice) 100.0
of lung 100.0
Weir Mitchell's (erythromelalgia) 443.82
Werdnig-Hoffmann 335.0
Werlhof's (*see also* Purpura, thrombocytopenic)
287.39
Wermer's 258.01
Werner's (progeria adultorum) 259.8
Werner-His (trench fever) 083.1
Werner-Schultz (agranulocytosis) 288.09
Wernicke's (superior hemorrhagic
polioencephalitis) 265.1
Wernicke-Posadas 114.9
Whipple's (intestinal lipodystrophy) 040.2
whipworm 127.3
white
blood cell 288.9
specified NEC 288.8
spot 701.0
White's (congenital) (keratosis follicularis)
757.39
Whitmore's (melioidosis) 025
Widal-Abrami (acquired hemolytic jaundice)
283.9
Wilkie's 557.1
Wilkinson-Sneddon (subcorneal pustular
dermatosis) 694.1
Willis' (diabetes mellitus) (*see also* Diabetes)
250.0
due to secondary diabetes 249.0
Wilson's (hepatolenticular degeneration) 275.1
Wilson-Brocq (dermatitis exfoliativa) 695.89
winter vomiting 078.82
Wise's 696.2
Wohlfart-Kugelberg-Welander 335.11
Woillez's (acute idiopathic pulmonary
congestion) 518.5
Wolman's (primary familial xanthomatosis)
272.7

Disease, diseased—*continued*
  wool-sorters' 022.1
  Zagari's (xerostomia) 527.7
  Zahorsky's (exanthem subitum) 058.10
  Ziehen-Oppenheim 333.6
  zoonotic, bacterial NEC 027.9
    specified type NEC 027.8
Disfigurement (due to scar) 709.2
  head V48.6
  limb V49.4
  neck V48.7
  trunk V48.7
Disgerminoma —*see* Dysgerminoma
Disinsertion, retina 361.04
Disintegration, complete, of the body 799.89
  traumatic 869.1
Disk kidney 753.3
Dislocatable hip, congenita l (*see also*
  Dislocation, hip, congenital) 754.30
Dislocation (articulation) (closed) (displacement)
  (simple) (subluxation) 839.8

> *Note—"Closed" includes simple, complete,
> partial, uncomplicated, and unspecified
> dislocation. "Open" includes dislocation
> specified as infected or compound and
> dislocation with foreign body. "Chronic,"
> "habitual," "old," or "recurrent" dislocations
> should be coded as indicated under the entry
> "Dislocation, recurrent"; and "pathological"
> as indicated under the entry "Dislocation,
> pathological." For late effect of dislocation see
> Late, effect, dislocation.*

  with fracture—*see* Fracture, by site
  acromioclavicular (joint) (closed) 831.04
    open 831.14
  anatomical site (closed)
    specified NEC 839.69
      open 839.79
    unspecified or ill-defined 839.8
      open 839.9
  ankle (scaphoid bone) (closed) 837.0
    open 837.1
  arm (closed) 839.8
    open 839.9
  astragalus (closed) 837.0
    open 837.1
  atlanto-axial (closed) 839.01
    open 839.11
  atlas (closed) 839.01
    open 839.11
  axis (closed) 839.02
    open 839.12
  back (closed) 839.8
    open 839.9
  Bell-Daly 723.8
  breast bone (closed) 839.61
    open 839.71
  capsule, joint—*see* Dislocation, by site
  carpal (bone)—*see* Dislocation, wrist
  carpometacarpal (joint) (closed) 833.04
    open 833.14
  cartilage (joint)—*see also* Dislocation, by site
    knee—*see* Tear, meniscus
  cervical, cervicodorsal, or cervicothoracic
    (spine) (vertebra)—*see* Dislocation,
    vertebra, cervical
  chiropractic (*see also* Lesion, nonallopathic)
    739.9
  chondrocostal—*see* Dislocation, costochondral
  chronic—*see* Dislocation, recurrent

Dislocation—*continued*
  clavicle (closed) 831.04
    open 831.14
  coccyx (closed) 839.41
    open 839.51
  collar bone (closed) 831.04
    open 831.14
  compound (open) NEC 839.9
  congenital NEC 755.8
    hip (*see also* Dislocation, hip, congenital)
      754.30
    lens 743.37
    rib 756.3
    sacroiliac 755.69
    spine NEC 756.19
    vertebra 756.19
  coracoid (closed) 831.09
    open 831.19
  costal cartilage (closed) 839.69
    open 839.79
  costochondral (closed) 839.69
    open 839.79
  cricoarytenoid articulation (closed) 839.69
    open 839.79
  cricothyroid (cartilage) articulation (closed)
    839.69
    open 839.79
  dorsal vertebrae (closed) 839.21
    open 839.31
  ear ossicle 385.23
  elbow (closed) 832.00
    anterior (closed) 832.01
      open 832.11
    congenital 754.89
    divergent (closed) 832.09
      open 832.19
    lateral (closed) 832.04
      open 832.14
    medial (closed) 832.03
      open 832.13
    open 832.10
    posterior (closed) 832.02
      open 832.12
    recurrent 718.32
    specified type NEC 832.09
      open 832.19
  eye 360.81
    lateral 376.36
  eyeball 360.81
    lateral 376.36
  femur
    distal end (closed) 836.50
      anterior 836.52
        open 836.62
      lateral 836.54
        open 836.64
      medial 836.53
        open 836.63
      open 836.60
      posterior 836.51
        open 836.61
    proximal end (closed) 835.00
      anterior (pubic) 835.03
        open 835.13
      obturator 835.02
        open 835.12
      open 835.10
      posterior 835.01
        open 835.11

Dislocation—*continued*
  fibula
    distal end (closed) 837.0
      open 837.1
    proximal end (closed) 836.59
      open 836.69
  finger(s) (phalanx) (thumb) (closed) 834.00
    interphalangeal (joint) 834.02
      open 834.12
    metacarpal (bone), distal end 834.01
      open 834.11
    metacarpophalangeal (joint) 834.01
      open 834.11
    open 834.10
    recurrent 718.34
  foot (closed) 838.00
    open 838.10
    recurrent 718.37
  forearm (closed) 839.8
    open 839.9
  fracture—*see* Fracture, by site
  glenoid (closed) 831.09
    open 831.19
  habitual—*see* Dislocation, recurrent
  hand (closed) 839.8
    open 839.9
  hip (closed) 835.00
    anterior 835.03
      obturator 835.02
        open 835.12
      open 835.13
    congenital (unilateral) 754.30
      with subluxation of other hip 754.35
      bilateral 754.31
    developmental 718.75
    open 835.10
    posterior 835.01
      open 835.11
    recurrent 718.35
  humerus (closed) 831.00
    distal end (*see also* Dislocation, elbow) 832.00
    open 831.10
    proximal end (closed) 831.00
      anterior (subclavicular) (subcoracoid)
        (subglenoid) (closed) 831.01
        open 831.11
      inferior (closed) 831.03
        open 831.13
      open 831.10
      posterior (closed) 831.02
        open 831.12
  implant—*see* Complications, mechanical
  incus 385.23
  infracoracoid (closed) 831.01
    open 831.11
  innominate (pubic junction) (sacral junction)
    (closed) 839.69
    acetabulum (*see also* Dislocation, hip) 835.00
    open 839.79
  interphalangeal (joint)
    finger or hand (closed) 834.02
      open 834.12
    foot or toe (closed) 838.06
      open 838.16
  jaw (cartilage) (meniscus) (closed) 830.0
    open 830.1
    recurrent 524.69
  joint NEC (closed) 839.8
    developmental 718.7
    open 839.9
    pathological—*see* Dislocation, pathological
    recurrent—*see* Dislocation, recurrent

Dislocation—*continued*
  knee (closed) 836.50
    anterior 836.51
      open 836.61
    congenital (with genu recurvatum) 754.41
    habitual 718.36
    lateral 836.54
      open 836.64
    medial 836.53
      open 836.63
    old 718.36
    open 836.60
    posterior 836.52
      open 836.62
    recurrent 718.36
    rotatory 836.59
      open 836.69
  lacrimal gland 375.16
  leg (closed) 839.8
    open 839.9
  lens (crystalline) (complete) (partial) 379.32
    anterior 379.33
    congenital 743.37
    ocular implant 996.53
    posterior 379.34
    traumatic 921.3
  ligament—*see* Dislocation, by site
  lumbar (vertebrae) (closed) 839.20
    open 839.30
  lumbosacral (vertebrae) (closed) 839.20
    congenital 756.19
    open 839.30
  mandible (closed) 830.0
    open 830.1
  maxilla (inferior) (closed) 830.0
    open 830.1
  meniscus (knee)—*see also* Tear, meniscus
    other sites—*see* Dislocation, by site
  metacarpal (bone)
    distal end (closed) 834.01
      open 834.11
    proximal end (closed) 833.05
      open 833.15
  metacarpophalangeal (joint) (closed) 834.01
    open 834.11
  metatarsal (bone) (closed) 838.04
    open 838.14
  metatarsophalangeal (joint) (closed) 838.05
    open 838.15
  midcarpal (joint) (closed) 833.03
    open 833.13
  midtarsal (joint) (closed) 838.02
    open 838.12
  Monteggia's—*see* Dislocation, hip
  multiple locations (except fingers only or toes
    only) (closed) 839.8
    open 839.9
  navicular (bone) foot (closed) 837.0
    open 837.1
  neck (*see also* Dislocation, vertebra, cervical)
    839.00
  Nélaton's—*see* Dislocation, ankle
  nontraumatic (joint)—*see* Dislocation,
    pathological
  nose (closed) 839.69
    open 839.79
  not recurrent, not current injury—*see*
    Dislocation, pathological
  occiput from atlas (closed) 839.01
    open 839.11
  old—*see* Dislocation, recurrent
    open (compound) NEC 839.9

Dislocation—*continued*
ossicle, ear 385.23
paralytic (flaccid) (spastic)—*see* Dislocation,
  pathological
patella (closed) 836.3
  congenital 755.64
  open 836.4
pathological NEC 718.20
  ankle 718.27
  elbow 718.22
  foot 718.27
  hand 718.24
  hip 718.25
  knee 718.26
  lumbosacral joint 724.6
  multiple sites 718.29
  pelvic region 718.25
  sacroiliac 724.6
  shoulder (region) 718.21
  specified site NEC 718.28
  spine 724.8
    sacroiliac 724.6
  wrist 718.23
pelvis (closed) 839.69
  acetabulum (*see also* Dislocation, hip) 835.00
  open 839.79
phalanx
  foot or toe (closed) 838.09
    open 838.19
  hand or finger (*see also* Dislocation, finger)
    834.00
postpoliomyelitic—*see* Dislocation,
  pathological
prosthesis, internal—*see* Complications,
  mechanical
radiocarpal (joint) (closed) 833.02
  open 833.12
radioulnar (joint)
  distal end (closed) 833.01
    open 833.11
  proximal end (*see also* Dislocation, elbow)
    832.00
radius
  distal end (closed) 833.00
    open 833.10
  proximal end (closed) 832.01
    open 832.11
recurrent (*see also* Derangement, joint,
  recurrent) 718.3
  elbow 718.32
  hip 718.35
  joint NEC 718.38
  knee 718.36
  lumbosacral (joint) 724.6
  patella 718.36
  sacroiliac 724.6
  shoulder 718.31
  temporomandibular 524.69
rib (cartilage) (closed) 839.69
  congenital 756.3
  open 839.79
sacrococcygeal (closed) 839.42
  open 839.52
sacroiliac (joint) (ligament) (closed) 839.42
  congenital 755.69
  open 839.52
  recurrent 724.6
sacrum (closed) 839.42
  open 839.52

Dislocation—*continued*
scaphoid (bone)
  ankle or foot (closed) 837.0
    open 837.1
  wrist (closed) (*see also* Dislocation, wrist)
    833.0
    open 833.10
scapula (closed) 831.09
  open 831.19
semilunar cartilage, knee—*see* Tear, meniscus
septal cartilage (nose) (closed) 839.69
  open 839.79
septum (nasal) (old) 470
sesamoid bone—*see* Dislocation, by site
shoulder (blade) (ligament) (closed) 831.00
  anterior (subclavicular) (subcoracoid)
    (subglenoid) (closed) 831.01
    open 831.11
  chronic 718.31
  inferior 831.03
    open 831.13
  open 831.10
  posterior (closed) 831.02
    open 831.12
  recurrent 718.31
skull—*see* Injury, intracranial
Smith's—*see* Dislocation, foot
spine (articular process) (*see also* Dislocation,
  vertebra) (closed) 839.40
  atlanto-axial (closed) 839.01
    open 839.11
    recurrent 723.8
  cervical, cervicodorsal, cervicothoracic
    (closed) (*see also* Dislocation, vertebrae,
    cervical) 839.00
    open 839.10
    recurrent 723.8
  coccyx 839.41
    open 839.51
  congenital 756.19
  due to birth trauma 767.4
  open 839.50
  recurrent 724.9
  sacroiliac 839.42
    recurrent 724.6
  sacrum (sacrococcygeal) (sacroiliac) 839.42
    open 839.52
spontaneous—*see* Dislocation, pathological
sternoclavicular (joint) (closed) 839.61
  open 839.71
sternum (closed) 839.61
  open 839.71
subastragalar—*see* Dislocation, foot
subglenoid (closed) 831.01
  open 831.11
symphysis
  jaw (closed) 830.0
    open 830.1
  mandibular (closed) 830.0
    open 830.1
  pubis (closed) 839.69
    open 839.79
tarsal (bone) (joint) 838.01
  open 838.11
tarsometatarsal (joint) 838.03
  open 838.13
temporomandibular (joint) (closed) 830.0
  open 830.1
  recurrent 524.69

Dislocation—*continued*
  thigh
    distal end (*see also* Dislocation, femur, distal
        end) 836.50
    proximal end (*see also* Dislocation, hip) 835.00
  thoracic (vertebrae) (closed) 839.21
    open 839.31
  thumb(s) (*see also* Dislocation, finger) 834.00
  thyroid cartilage (closed) 839.69
    open 839.79
  tibia
    distal end (closed) 837.0
      open 837.1
    proximal end (closed) 836.50
      anterior 836.51
        open 836.61
      lateral 836.54
        open 836.64
      medial 836.53
        open 836.63
      open 836.60
      posterior 836.52
        open 836.62
      rotatory 836.59
        open 836.69
  tibiofibular
    distal (closed) 837.0
      open 837.1
    superior (closed) 836.59
      open 836.69
  toe(s) (closed) 838.09
    open 838.19
  trachea (closed) 839.69
    open 839.79
  ulna
    distal end (closed) 833.09
      open 833.19
    proximal end—*see* Dislocation, elbow
  vertebra (articular process) (body) (closed)
      (traumatic) 839.40
    cervical, cervicodorsal or cervicothoracic
        (closed) 839.00
      first (atlas) 839.01
        open 839.11
      second (axis) 839.02
        open 839.12
      third 839.03
        open 839.13
      fourth 839.04
        open 839.14
      fifth 839.05
        open 839.15
      sixth 839.06
        open 839.16
      seventh 839.07
        open 839.17
      congenital 756.19
      multiple sites 839.08
        open 839.18
      open 839.10
    congenital 756.19
    dorsal 839.21
      open 839.31
      recurrent 724.9
    lumbar, lumbosacral 839.20
      open 839.30
    non-traumatic —*see* Displacement,
        intervertebral disc
    open NEC 839.50
    recurrent 724.9
    specified region NEC 839.49
      open 839.59

Dislocation—*continued*
  vertebra—*continued*
    thoracic 839.21
      open 839.31
  wrist (carpal bone) (scaphoid) (semilunar)
      (closed) 833.00
    carpometacarpal (joint) 833.04
      open 833.14
    metacarpal bone, proximal end 833.05
      open 833.15
    midcarpal (joint) 833.03
      open 833.13
    open 833.10
    radiocarpal (joint) 833.02
      open 833.12
    radioulnar (joint) 833.01
      open 833.11
    recurrent 718.33
    specified site NEC 833.09
      open 833.19
  xiphoid cartilage (closed) 839.61
    open 839.71
Dislodgement
  artificial skin graft 996.55
  decellularized allodermis graft 996.55
Disobedience, hostile (covert) (overt) (*see also*
    Disturbance, conduct) 312.0
Disorder —*see also* Disease
  academic underachievement, childhood and
      adolescence 313.83
  accommodation 367.51
    drug-induced 367.89
    toxic 367.89
  adjustment (*see also* Reaction, adjustment) 309.9
    with
      anxiety 309.24
      anxiety and depressed mood 309.28
      depressed mood 309.0
      disturbance of conduct 309.3
      disturbance of emotions and conduct 309.4
  adrenal (capsule) (cortex) (gland) 255.9
    specified type NEC 255.8
  adrenogenital 255.2
  affective (*see also* Psychosis, affective) 296.90
    atypical 296.81
  aggressive, unsocialized (*see also* Disturbance,
      conduct) 312.0
  alcohol, alcoholic (*see also* Alcohol) 291.9
  allergic—*see* Allergy
  amino acid (metabolic) (*see also* Disturbance,
      metabolism, amino acid) 270.9
    albinism 270.2
    alkaptonuria 270.2
    argininosuccinicaciduria 270.6
    beta-amino-isobutyricaciduria 277.2
    cystathioninuria 270.4
    cystinosis 270.0
    cystinuria 270.0
    glycinuria 270.0
    homocystinuria 270.4
    imidazole 270.5
    maple syrup (urine) disease 270.3
    neonatal, transitory 775.89
    oasthouse urine disease 270.2
    ochronosis 270.2
    phenylketonuria 270.1
    phenylpyruvic oligophrenia 270.1
    purine NEC 277.2
    pyrimidine NEC 277.2
    renal transport NEC 270.0
    specified type NEC 270.8

Disorder—*continued*
amino acid—*continued*
transport NEC 270.0
renal 270.0
xanthinuria 277.2
amnestic (*see also* Amnestic syndrome) 294.08
alcohol-induced persisting 291.1
drug-induced persisting 292.83
in conditions classified elsewhere 294.0
anaerobic glycolysis with anemia 282.3
anxiety (*see also* Anxiety) 300.00
due to or associated with physical condition 293.84
arteriole 447.9
specified type NEC 447.8
artery 447.9
specified type NEC 447.8
articulation—*see* Disorder, joint
Asperger's 299.8
attachment of infancy or early childhood 313.89
attention deficit 314.00
with hyperactivity 314.01
predominantly
combined hyperactive/inattentive 314.01
hyperactive/impulsive 314.01
inattentive 314.00
residual type 314.8
auditory processing disorder 388.45
acquired 388.45
developmental 315.32
autistic 299.0
autoimmune NEC 279.49
hemolytic (cold type) (warm type) 283.0
parathyroid 252.1
thyroid 245.2
avoidant, childhood or adolescence 313.21
balance
acid-base 276.9
mixed (with hypercapnia) 276.4
electrolyte 276.9
fluid 276.9
behavior NEC (*see also* Disturbance, conduct) 312.9
disruptive 312.9
bilirubin excretion 277.4
bipolar (affective) (alternating) 296.80

Note—Use the following fifth-digit subclassification with categories 296.0-296.6:

0   *unspecified*
1   *mild*
2   *moderate*
3   *severe, without mention of psychotic behavior*
4   *severe, specified as with psychotic behavior*
5   *in partial or unspecified remission*
6   *in full remission*

atypical 296.7
currently
depressed 296.5
hypomanic 296.4
manic 296.4
mixed 296.6
specified type NEC 296.89

Disorder—*continued*
bipolar—*continued*
type I 296.7
most recent episode (or current)
depressed 296.5
hypomanic 296.4
manic 296.4
mixed 296.6
unspecified 296.7
single manic episode 296.0
type II (recurrent major depressive episodes with hypomania) 296.89
bladder 596.9
functional NEC 596.59
specified NEC 596.8
bleeding 286.9
bone NEC 733.90
specified NEC 733.99
brachial plexus 353.0
branched-chain amino-acid degradation 270.3
breast 611.9
puerperal, postpartum 676.3
specified NEC 611.89
Briquet's 300.81
bursa 727.9
shoulder region 726.10
carbohydrate metabolism, congenital 271.9
cardiac, functional 427.9
postoperative 997.1
psychogenic 306.2
cardiovascular, psychogenic 306.2
cartilage NEC 733.90
articular 718.00
ankle 718.07
elbow 718.02
foot 718.07
hand 718.04
hip 718.05
knee 717.9
multiple sites 718.09
pelvic region 718.05
shoulder region 718.01
specified
site NEC 718.08
type NEC 733.99
wrist 718.03
catatonic—*see* Catatonia
central auditory processing 315.32
acquired 388.45
developmental 315.32
cervical region NEC 723.9
cervical root (nerve) NEC 353.2
character NEC (*see also* Disorder, personality) 301.9
ciliary body 364.9
specified NEC 364.89
coagulation (factor) (*see also* Defect, coagulation) 286.9
factor VIII (congenital) (functional) 286.0
factor IX (congenital) (functional) 286.1
neonatal, transitory 776.3
coccyx 724.70
specified NEC 724.79
cognitive 294.9
colon 569.9
functional 564.9
congenital 751.3
communication 307.9

Disorder—*continued*
  conduct (*see also* Disturbance, conduct) 312.9
    adjustment reaction 309.3
    adolescent onset type 312.82
    childhood onset type 312.81
    compulsive 312.30
      specified type NEC 312.39
    hyperkinetic 314.2
    onset unspecified 312.89
    socialized (type) 312.20
      aggressive 312.23
      unaggressive 312.21
    specified NEC 312.89
  conduction, heart 426.9
    specified NEC 426.89
  conflict
    sexual orientation 302.0
  congenital
    glycosylation (CDG) 271.8
  convulsive (secondary) (*see also* Convulsions)
    780.39
    due to injury at birth 767.0
    idiopathic 780.39
  coordination 781.3
  cornea NEC 371.89
    due to contact lens 371.82
  corticosteroid metabolism NEC 255.2
  cranial nerve—*see* Disorder, nerve, cranial
  cyclothymic 301.13
  degradation, branched-chain amino acid 270.3
  delusional 297.1
  dentition 520.6
  depersonalization 300.6
  depressive NEC 311
    atypical 296.82
    major (*see also* Psychosis, affective) 296.2
      recurrent episode 296.3
      single episode 296.2
  development, specific 315.9
    associated with hyperkinesia 314.1
    coordination 315.4
    language 315.31
      and speech due to hearing loss 315.34
    learning 315.2
      arithmetical 315.1
      reading 315.00
    mixed 315.5
    motor coordination 315.4
    specified type NEC 315.8
    speech 315.39
      and language due to hearing loss 315.34
  diaphragm 519.4
  digestive 536.9
    fetus or newborn 777.9
      specified NEC 777.8
    psychogenic 306.4
  disintegrative, childhood 299.1
  dissociative 300.15
    identity 300.14
    nocturnal 307.47
  drug-related 292.9
  dysmorphic body 300.7
  dysthymic 300.4
  ear 388.9
    degenerative NEC 388.00
    external 380.9
      specified 380.89
    pinna 380.30
    specified type NEC 388.8
    vascular NEC 388.00
  eating NEC 307.50

Disorder—*continued*
  electrolyte NEC 276.9
    with
      abortion—*see* Abortion, by type, with
        metabolic disorder
      ectopic pregnancy (*see also* categories
        633.0-633.9) 639.4
      molar pregnancy (*see also* categories
        630-632) 639.4
    acidosis 276.2
      metabolic 276.2
      respiratory 276.2
    alkalosis 276.3
      metabolic 276.3
      respiratory 276.3
    following
      abortion 639.4
      ectopic or molar pregnancy 639.4
    neonatal, transitory NEC 775.5
  emancipation as adjustment reaction 309.22
  emotional (*see also* Disorder, mental,
    nonpsychotic) V40.9
  endocrine 259.9
    specified type NEC 259.8
  esophagus 530.9
    functional 530.5
    psychogenic 306.4
  explosive
    intermittent 312.34
    isolated 312.35
  expressive language 315.31
  eye 379.90
    globe—*see* Disorder, globe
    ill-defined NEC 379.99
    limited duction NEC 378.63
    specified NEC 379.8
  eyelid 374.9
    degenerative 374.50
    sensory 374.44
    specified type NEC 374.89
    vascular 374.85
  factitious (with combined psychological and
    physical signs and symptoms) (with
    predominantly physical signs and
    symptoms) 300.19
    with predominantly psychological signs and
      symptoms 300.16
  factor, coagulation (*see also* Defect, coagulation)
    286.9
    VIII (congenital) (functional) 286.0
    IX (congenital) (functional) 286.1
  fascia 728.9
  fatty acid oxidation 277.85
  feeding —*see* Feeding
  female sexual arousal 302.72
  fluid NEC 276.9
  gastric (functional) 536.9
    motility 536.8
    psychogenic 306.4
    secretion 536.8
  gastrointestinal (functional) NEC 536.9
    newborn (neonatal) 777.9
      specified NEC 777.8
    psychogenic 306.4
  gender (child) 302.6
    adult 302.85
  gender identity (childhood) 302.6
    adolescents 302.85
    adults (-life) 302.85
  genitourinary system, psychogenic 306.50

Disorder—*continued*
globe 360.9
degenerative 360.20
specified NEC 360.29
specified type NEC 360.89
hearing—*see also* Deafness
conductive type (air) (*see also* Deafness,
conductive) 389.00
mixed conductive and sensorineural 389.20
bilateral 389.22
unilateral 389.21
nerve
bilateral 389.12
unilateral 389.13
perceptive (*see also* Deafness, perceptive)
389.10
sensorineural type NEC (*see also* Deafness,
sensorineural) 389.10
heart action 427.9
postoperative 997.1
hematological, transient neonatal 776.9
specified type NEC 776.8
hematopoietic organs 289.9
hemorrhagic NEC 287.9
due to intrinsic circulating anticoagulants
286.5
specified type NEC 287.8
hemostasis (*see also* Defect, coagulation) 286.9
homosexual conflict 302.0
hypomanic (chronic) 301.11
identity
childhood and adolescence 313.82
gender 302.6
gender 302.6
immune mechanism (immunity) 279.9
single complement (C_1-C_9) 279.8
specified type NEC 279.8
impulse control (*see also* Disturbance, conduct,
compulsive) 312.30
infant sialic acid storage 271.8
integument, fetus or newborn 778.9
specified type NEC 778.8
interactional psychotic (childhood) (*see also*
Psychosis, childhood) 299.1
intermittent explosive 312.34
intervertebral disc 722.90
cervical, cervicothoracic 722.91
lumbar, lumbosacral 722.93
thoracic, thoracolumbar 722.92
intestinal 569.9
functional NEC 564.9
congenital 751.3
postoperative 564.4
psychogenic 306.4
introverted, of childhood and adolescence
313.22
involuntary emotional expression (IEED) 310.8
iris 364.9
specified NEC 364.89
iron, metabolism 275.0
isolated explosive 312.35
joint NEC 719.90
ankle 719.97
elbow 719.92
foot 719.97
hand 719.94
hip 719.95
knee 719.96
multiple sites 719.99
pelvic region 719.95
psychogenic 306.0

Disorder—*continued*
joint—*continued*
shoulder (region) 719.91
specified site NEC 719.98
temporomandibular 524.60
sounds on opening or closing 524.64
specified NEC 524.69
wrist 719.93
kidney 593.9
functional 588.9
specified NEC 588.89
labyrinth, labyrinthine 386.9
specified type NEC 386.8
lactation 676.9
language (developmental) (expressive) 315.31
mixed receptive-expressive 315.32
learning 315.9
ligament 728.9
ligamentous attachments, peripheral—*see also*
Enthesopathy
spine 720.1
limb NEC 729.90
psychogenic 306.0
lipid
metabolism, congenital 272.9
storage 272.7
lipoprotein deficiency (familial) 272.5
low back NEC 724.9
psychogenic 306.0
lumbosacral
plexus 353.1
root (nerve) NEC 353.4
lymphoproliferative (chronic) NEC (M9970/1)
238.79
post-transplant (PTLD) 238.77
major depressive (*see also* Psychosis, affective)
296.2
recurrent episode 296.3
single episode 296.2
male erectile 607.84
nonorganic origin 302.72
manic (*see also* Psychosis, affective) 296.0
atypical 296.81
mathematics 315.1
meniscus NEC (*see also* Disorder, cartilage,
articular) 718.0
menopausal 627.9
specified NEC 627.8
menstrual 626.9
psychogenic 306.52
specified NEC 626.8
mental (nonpsychotic) 300.9
affecting management of pregnancy,
childbirth, or puerperium 648.4
drug-induced 292.9
hallucinogen persistent perception 292.89
specified type NEC 292.89
due to or associated with
alcoholism 291.9
drug consumption NEC 292.9
specified type NEC 292.89
physical condition NEC 293.9
induced by drug 292.9
specified type NEC 292.89
neurotic (*see also* Neurosis) 300.9
of infancy, childhood or adolescence 313.9
persistent
other
due to conditions classified elsewhere 294.8
unspecified
due to conditions classified elsewhere 294.9

Disorder—*continued*
  mental—*continued*
    presenile 310.1
      psychotic NEC 290.10
    previous, affecting management of pregnancy
      V23.8
    psychoneurotic (*see also* Neurosis) 300.9
    psychotic (*see also* Psychosis) 298.9
      brief 298.8
      senile 290.20
    specific, following organic brain damage 310.9
      cognitive or personality change of other type
        310.1
      frontal lobe syndrome 310.0
      postconcussional syndrome 310.2
      specified type NEC 310.8
    transient
      in conditions classified elsewhere 293.9
  metabolism NEC 277.9
    with
      abortion—*see* Abortion, by type, with
        metabolic disorder
      ectopic pregnancy (*see also* categories
        633.0-633.9) 639.4
      molar pregnancy (*see also* categories
        630-632) 639.4
    alkaptonuria 270.2
    amino acid (*see also* Disorder, amino acid)
      270.9
      specified type NEC 270.8
    ammonia 270.6
    arginine 270.6
    argininosuccinic acid 270.6
    basal 794.7
    bilirubin 277.4
    calcium 275.40
    carbohydrate 271.9
      specified type NEC 271.8
    cholesterol 272.9
    citrulline 270.6
    copper 275.1
    corticosteroid 255.2
    cystine storage 270.0
    cystinuria 270.0
    fat 272.9
    fatty acid oxidation 277.85
    following
      abortion 639.4
      ectopic or molar pregnancy 639.4
    fructosemia 271.2
    fructosuria 271.2
    fucosidosis 271.8
    due to conditions classified elsewhere 294.8
    galactose-1-phosphate uridyl transferase 271.1
    glutamine 270.7
    glycine 270.7
    glycogen storage NEC 271.0
      hepatorenal 271.0
    hemochromatosis 275.0
    in labor and delivery 669.0
    iron 275.0
    lactose 271.3
    lipid 272.9
      specified type NEC 272.8
      storage 272.7
    lipoprotein—*see also* Hyperlipemia deficiency
      (familial) 272.5
    lysine 270.7
    magnesium 275.2
    mannosidosis 271.8
    mineral 275.9
      specified type NEC 275.8

Disorder—*continued*
  metabolism—*continued*
    mitochondrial 277.87
    mucopolysaccharide 277.5
    nitrogen 270.9
    ornithine 270.6
    oxalosis 271.8
    pentosuria 271.8
    phenylketonuria 270.1
    phosphate 275.3
    phosphorus 275.3
    plasma protein 273.9
      specified type NEC 273.8
    porphyrin 277.1
    purine 277.2
    pyrimidine 277.2
    serine 270.7
    sodium 276.9
    specified type NEC 277.89
    steroid 255.2
    threonine 270.7
    urea cycle 270.6
    xylose 271.8
  micturition NEC 788.69
    psychogenic 306.53
  misery and unhappiness, of childhood and
    adolescence 313.1
  mitochondrial metabolism 277.87
  mitral valve 424.0
  mood (*see also* Disorder, bipolar) 296.90
    episodic 296.90
      specified NEC 296.99
    in conditions classified elsewhere 293.83
  motor tic 307.20
    chronic 307.22
    transient (childhood) 307.21
  movement NEC 333.90
    hysterical 300.11
    medication-induced 333.90
    periodic limb 327.51
    sleep related, unspecified 780.58
      other organic 327.59
    specified type NEC 333.99
    stereotypic 307.3
  mucopolysaccharide 277.5
  muscle 728.9
    psychogenic 306.0
    specified type NEC 728.3
  muscular attachments, peripheral—*see also*
    Enthesopathy
    spine 720.1
  musculoskeletal system NEC 729.90
    psychogenic 306.0
  myeloproliferative (chronic) NEC (M9960/1)
    238.79
  myoneural 358.9
    due to lead 358.2
    specified type NEC 358.8
    toxic 358.2
  myotonic 359.29
  neck region NEC 723.9
  nerve 349.9
    abducens NEC 378.54
    accessory 352.4
    acoustic 388.5
    auditory 388.5
    auriculotemporal 350.8
    axillary 353.0
    cerebral—*see* Disorder, nerve, cranial

Disorder—*continued*
nerve—*continued*
  cranial 352.9
    first 352.0
    second 377.49
    third
      partial 378.51
      total 378.52
    fourth 378.53
    fifth 350.9
    sixth 378.54
    seventh NEC 351.9
    eighth 388.5
    ninth 352.2
    tenth 352.3
    eleventh 352.4
    twelfth 352.5
    multiple 352.6
  entrapment—*see* Neuropathy, entrapment
  facial 351.9
    specified NEC 351.8
  femoral 355.2
  glossopharyngeal NEC 352.2
  hypoglossal 352.5
  iliohypogastric 355.79
  ilioinguinal 355.79
  intercostal 353.8
  lateral
    cutaneous of thigh 355.1
    popliteal 355.3
  lower limb NEC 355.8
  medial, popliteal 355.4
  median NEC 354.1
  obturator 355.79
  oculomotor
    partial 378.51
    total 378.52
  olfactory 352.0
  optic 377.49
    hypoplasia 377.43
    ischemic 377.41
    nutritional 377.33
    toxic 377.34
  peroneal 355.3
  phrenic 354.8
  plantar 355.6
  pneumogastric 352.3
  posterior tibial 355.5
  radial 354.3
  recurrent laryngeal 352.3
  root 353.9
    specified NEC 353.8
  saphenous 355.79
  sciatic NEC 355.0
  specified NEC 355.9
    lower limb 355.79
    upper limb 354.8
  spinal 355.9
  sympathetic NEC 337.9
  trigeminal 350.9
    specified NEC 350.8
  trochlear 378.53
  ulnar 354.2
  upper limb NEC 354.9
  vagus 352.3

Disorder—*continued*
  nervous system NEC 349.9
    autonomic (peripheral) (*see also* Neuropathy, peripheral, autonomic) 337.9
    cranial 352.9
    parasympathetic (*see also* Neuropathy, peripheral, autonomic) 337.9
    specified type NEC 349.89
    sympathetic (*see also* Neuropathy, peripheral, autonomic) 337.9
    vegetative (*see also* Neuropathy, peripheral, autonomic) 337.9
  neurohypophysis NEC 253.6
  neurological NEC 781.99
    peripheral NEC 355.9
  neuromuscular NEC 358.9
    hereditary NEC 359.1
    specified NEC 358.8
    toxic 358.2
  neurotic 300.9
    specified type NEC 300.89
  neutrophil, polymorphonuclear (functional) 288.1
  nightmare 307.47
  night terror 307.46
  obsessive-compulsive 300.3
  oppositional defiant, childhood and adolescence 313.81
  optic
    chiasm 377.54
      associated with
        inflammatory disorders 377.54
        neoplasm NEC 377.52
          pituitary 377.51
        pituitary disorders 377.51
        vascular disorders 377.53
    nerve 377.49
    radiations 377.63
    tracts 377.63
  orbit 376.9
    specified NEC 376.89
  orgasmic
    female 302.73
    male 302.74
  overanxious, of childhood and adolescence 313.0
  oxidation, fatty acid 277.85
  pancreas, internal secretion (other than diabetes mellitus) 251.9
    specified type NEC 251.8
  panic 300.01
    with agoraphobia 300.21
  papillary muscle NEC 429.81
  paranoid 297.9
    induced 297.3
    shared 297.3
  parathyroid 252.9
    specified type NEC 252.8
  paroxysmal, mixed 780.39
  pentose phosphate pathway with anemia 282.2
  periodic limb movement 327.51
  peroxisomal 277.86
  personality 301.9
    affective 301.10
    aggressive 301.3
    amoral 301.7
    anancastic, anankastic 301.4
    antisocial 301.7
    asocial 301.7
    asthenic 301.6

Disorder—*continued*
  personality—*continued*
    avoidant 301.82
    borderline 301.83
    compulsive 301.4
    cyclothymic 301.13
    dependent-passive 301.6
    dyssocial 301.7
    emotional instability 301.59
    epileptoid 301.3
    explosive 301.3
    following organic brain damage 310.1
    histrionic 301.50
    hyperthymic 301.11
    hypomanic (chronic) 301.11
    hypothymic 301.12
    hysterical 301.50
    immature 301.89
    inadequate 301.6
    introverted 301.21
    labile 301.59
    moral deficiency 301.7
    narcissistic 301.81
    obsessional 301.4
    obsessive-compulsive 301.4
    overconscientious 301.4
    paranoid 301.0
    passive (-dependent) 301.6
    passive-aggressive 301.84
    pathological NEC 301.9
    pseudosocial 301.7
    psychopathic 301.9
    schizoid 301.20
      introverted 301.21
      schizotypal 301.22
    schizotypal 301.22
    seductive 301.59
    type A 301.4
    unstable 301.59
  pervasive developmental 299.9
    childhood-onset 299.8
    specified NEC 299.8
  phonological 315.39
  pigmentation, choroid (congenital) 743.53
  pinna 380.30
    specified type NEC 380.39
  pituitary, thalamic 253.9
    anterior NEC 253.4
    iatrogenic 253.7
    postablative 253.7
    specified NEC 253.8
  pityriasis-like NEC 696.8
  platelets (blood) 287.1
  polymorphonuclear neutrophils (functional) 288.1
  porphyrin metabolism 277.1
  postmenopausal 627.9
    specified type NEC 627.8
  post-transplant lymphoproliferative (PTLD) 238.77
  post-traumatic stress (PTSD) 309.81
    acute 309.81
    brief 309.81
    chronic 309.81
  premenstrual dysphoric (PMDD) 625.4
  psoriatic-like NEC 696.8
  psychic, with diseases classified elsewhere 316

Disorder—*continued*
  psychogenic NEC (*see also* condition) 300.9
    allergic NEC
      respiratory 306.1
    anxiety 300.00
      atypical 300.00
      generalized 300.02
    appetite 307.59
    articulation, joint 306.0
    asthenic 300.5
    blood 306.8
    cardiovascular (system) 306.2
    compulsive 300.3
    cutaneous 306.3
    depressive 300.4
    digestive (system) 306.4
    dysmenorrheic 306.52
    dyspneic 306.1
    eczematous 306.3
    endocrine (system) 306.6
    eye 306.7
    feeding 307.59
    functional NEC 306.9
    gastric 306.4
    gastrointestinal (system) 306.4
    genitourinary (system) 306.50
    heart (function) (rhythm) 306.2
    hemic 306.8
    hyperventilatory 306.1
    hypochondriacal 300.7
    hysterical 300.10
    intestinal 306.4
    joint 306.0
    learning 315.2
    limb 306.0
    lymphatic (system) 306.8
    menstrual 306.52
    micturition 306.53
    monoplegic NEC 306.0
    motor 307.9
    muscle 306.0
    musculoskeletal 306.0
    neurocirculatory 306.2
    obsessive 300.3
    occupational 300.89
    organ or part of body NEC 306.9
    organs of special sense 306.7
    paralytic NEC 306.0
    phobic 300.20
    physical NEC 306.9
    pruritic 306.3
    rectal 306.4
    respiratory (system) 306.1
    rheumatic 306.0
    sexual (function) 302.70
      specified type NEC 302.79
    sexual orientation conflict 302.0
    skin (allergic) (eczematous) (pruritic) 306.3
    sleep 307.40
      initiation or maintenance 307.41
        persistent 307.42
        transient 307.41
      movement 780.58
      sleep terror 307.46
      specified type NEC 307.49
    specified part of body NEC 306.8
    stomach 306.4
  psychomotor NEC 307.9
    hysterical 300.11

Disorder—*continued*
  psychoneurotic (*see also* Neurosis) 300.9
    mixed NEC 300.89
  psychophysiologic (*see also* Disorder,
    psychosomatic) 306.9
  psychosexual identity (childhood) 302.6
    adult-life 302.85
  psychosomatic NEC 306.9
    allergic NEC
      respiratory 306.1
    articulation, joint 306.0
    cardiovascular (system) 306.2
    cutaneous 306.3
    digestive (system) 306.4
    dysmenorrheic 306.52
    dyspneic 306.1
    endocrine (system) 306.6
    eye 306.7
    gastric 306.4
    gastrointestinal (system) 306.4
    genitourinary (system) 306.50
    heart (functional) (rhythm) 306.2
    hyperventilatory 306.1
    intestinal 306.4
    joint 306.0
    limb 306.0
    lymphatic (system) 306.8
    menstrual 306.52
    micturition 306.53
    monoplegic NEC 306.0
    muscle 306.0
    musculoskeletal 306.0
    neurocirculatory 306.2
    organs of special sense 306.7
    paralytic NEC 306.0
    pruritic 306.3
    rectal 306.4
    respiratory (system) 306.1
    rheumatic 306.0
    sexual (function) 302.70
      specified type NEC 302.79
    skin 306.3
    specified part of body NEC 306.8
    stomach 306.4
  psychotic (*see also* Psychosis) 298.9
    brief 298.8
  PTSD (post-traumatic stress disorder) 309.81
  purine metabolism NEC 277.2
  pyrimidine metabolism NEC 277.2
  reactive attachment of infancy or early
    childhood 313.89
  reading, developmental 315.00
  reflex 796.1
  REM sleep behavior 327.42
  renal function, impaired 588.9
    specified type NEC 588.89
  renal transport NEC 588.89
  respiration, respiratory NEC 519.9
    due to
      aspiration of liquids or solids 508.9
      inhalation of fumes or vapors 506.9
    psychogenic 306.1
  retina 362.9
    specified type NEC 362.89
  rumination 307.53
  sacroiliac joint NEC 724.6
  sacrum 724.6
  schizo-affective (*see also* Schizophrenia) 295.7
  schizoid, childhood or adolescence 313.22
  schizophreniform 295.4
  schizotypal personality 301.22

Disorder—*continued*
  secretion, thyrocalcitonin 246.0
  seizure 345.9
    recurrent 345.9
      epileptic—*see* Epilepsy
  semantic pragmatic 315.39
    with autism 299.0
  sense of smell 781.1
    psychogenic 306.7
  separation anxiety 309.21
  sexual (*see also* Deviation, sexual) 302.9
    aversion 302.79
    desire, hypoactive 302.71
    function, psychogenic 302.70
  shyness, of childhood and adolescence 313.21
  single complement (C_1-C_9) 279.8
  skin NEC 709.9
    fetus or newborn 778.9
      specified type 778.8
    psychogenic (allergic) (eczematous) (pruritic)
      306.3
    specified type NEC 709.8
    vascular 709.1
  sleep 780.50
    alcohol induced 291.82
    arousal 307.46
      confusional 327.41
    circadian rhythm 327.30
      advanced sleep phase type 327.32
      alcohol induced 291.82
      delayed sleep phase type 327.31
      drug induced 292.85
      free running type 327.34
      in conditions classified elsewhere 327.37
      irregular sleep-wake type 327.33
      jet lag type 327.35
      other 327.39
      shift work type 327.36
    drug induced 292.85
    initiation or maintenance (*see also* Insomnia)
      780.52
      nonorganic origin (transient) 307.41
        persistent 307.42
    nonorganic origin 307.40
      specified type NEC 307.49
    organic specified type NEC 327.8
    periodic limb movement 327.51
    specified NEC 780.59
    wake
      cycle—*see* Disorder, sleep, circadian rhythm
      schedule—*see* Disorder, sleep, circadian rhythm
    with apnea—*see* Apnea, sleep
  social, of childhood and adolescence 313.22
  soft tissue 729.90
    specified type NEC 729.99
  somatization 300.81
  somatoform (atypical) (undifferentiated) 300.82
    severe 300.81
    specified type NEC 300.89
  speech NEC 784.59
    nonorganic origin 307.9
  spine NEC 724.9
    ligamentous or muscular attachments,
      peripheral 720.1
  steroid metabolism NEC 255.2
  stomach (functional) (*see also* Disorder, gastric) 536.9
    psychogenic 306.4
  storage, iron 275.0

Disorder—*continued*
  stress (*see also* Reaction, stress, acute) 308.3
    posttraumatic
      acute 309.81
      brief 309.81
      chronic 309.81
    substitution 300.11
  suspected—*see* Observation
  synovium 727.9
  temperature regulation, fetus or newborn 778.4
  temporomandibular joint NEC 524.60
    sounds on opening or closing 524.64
    specified NEC 524.69
  tendon 727.9
    shoulder region 726.10
  thoracic root (nerve) NEC 353.3
  thyrocalcitonin secretion 246.0
  thyroid (gland) NEC 246.9
    specified type NEC 246.8
  tic 307.20
    chronic (motor or vocal) 307.22
    motor-verbal 307.23
    organic origin 333.1
    transient (of childhood) 307.21
  tooth NEC 525.9
    development NEC 520.9
      specified type NEC 520.8
    eruption 520.6
    specified type NEC 525.8
  Tourette's 307.23
  transport, carbohydrate 271.9
    specified type NEC 271.8
  tubular, phosphate-losing 588.0
  tympanic membrane 384.9
  unaggressive, unsocialized (*see also*
    Disturbance, conduct) 312.1
  undersocialized, unsocialized—*see also*
    Disturbance, conduct
    aggressive (type) 312.0
    unaggressive (type) 312.1
  vision, visual NEC 368.9
    binocular NEC 368.30
    cortex 377.73
      associated with
        inflammatory disorders 377.73
        neoplasms 377.71
        vascular disorders 377.72
    pathway NEC 377.63
      associated with
        inflammatory disorders 377.63
        neoplasms 377.61
        vascular disorders 377.62
  vocal tic
    chronic 307.22
  wakefulness (*see also* Hypersomnia) 780.54
    nonorganic origin (transient) 307.43
    persistent 307.44
  written expression 315.2
Disorganized globe 360.29
Displacement, displaced

> *Note—For acquired displacement of bones,
> cartilage, joints, tendons, due to injury, see also
> Dislocation. Displacements at ages under one
> year should be considered congenital, provided
> there is no indication the condition was
> acquired after birth.*

  acquired traumatic of bond, cartilage, joint,
    tendon NEC (without fracture) (*see also*
    Dislocation) 839.8
    with fracture—*see* Fracture, by site

Displacement, displaced—*continued*
  adrenal gland (congenital) 759.1
  alveolus and teeth, vertical 524.75
  appendix, retrocecal (congenital) 751.5
  auricle (congenital) 744.29
  bladder (acquired) 596.8
    congenital 753.8
  brachial plexus (congenital) 742.8
  brain stem, caudal 742.4
  canaliculus lacrimalis 743.65
  cardia, through esophageal hiatus 750.6
  cerebellum, caudal 742.4
  cervix —*see* Displacement, uterus
  colon (congenital) 751.4
  device, implant, or graft—*see* Complications,
    mechanical
  epithelium
    columnar of cervix 622.10
    cuboidal, beyond limits of external os (uterus)
      752.49
  esophageal mucosa into cardia of stomach,
    congenital 750.4
  esophagus (acquired) 530.89
    congenital 750.4
  eyeball (acquired) (old) 376.36
    congenital 743.8
    current injury 871.3
    lateral 376.36
  fallopian tube (acquired) 620.4
    congenital 752.19
    opening (congenital) 752.19
  gallbladder (congenital) 751.69
  gastric mucosa 750.7
    into
      duodenum 750.7
      esophagus 750.7
      Meckel's diverticulum, congenital 750.7
  globe (acquired) (lateral) (old) 376.36
    current injury 871.3
  graft
    artificial skin graft 996.55
    decellularized allodermis graft 996.55
  heart (congenital) 746.87
    acquired 429.89
  hymen (congenital) (upward) 752.49
  internal prosthesis NEC—*see* Complications,
    mechanical
  intervertebral disc (with neuritis, radiculitis,
    sciatica, or other pain) 722.2
    with myelopathy 722.70
    cervical, cervicodorsal, cervicothoracic 722.0
      with myelopathy 722.71
      due to major trauma—*see* Dislocation,
        vertebra, cervical
    due to trauma—*see* Dislocation, vertebra
    lumbar, lumbosacral 722.10
      with myelopathy 722.73
      due to major trauma—*see* Dislocation,
        vertebra, lumbar
    thoracic, thoracolumbar 722.11
      with myelopathy 722.72
      due to major trauma—*see* Dislocation,
        vertebra, thoracic
  intrauterine device 996.32
  kidney (acquired) 593.0
    congenital 753.3
  lacrimal apparatus or duct (congenital) 743.65
  macula (congenital) 743.55
  Meckel's diverticulum (congenital) 751.0
  nail (congenital) 757.5
    acquired 703.8

Displacement, displaced—*continued*
  opening of Wharton's duct in mouth 750.26
  organ or site, congenital NEC—*see* Malposition,
    congenital
  ovary (acquired) 620.4
    congenital 752.0
    free in peritoneal cavity (congenital) 752.0
    into hernial sac 620.4
  oviduct (acquired) 620.4
    congenital 752.19
  parathyroid (gland) 252.8
  parotid gland (congenital) 750.26
  punctum lacrimale (congenital) 743.65
  sacroiliac (congenital) (joint) 755.69
    current injury—*see* Dislocation, sacroiliac
    old 724.6
  spine (congenital) 756.19
  spleen, congenital 759.0
  stomach (congenital) 750.7
    acquired 537.89
  subglenoid (closed) 831.01
  sublingual duct (congenital) 750.26
  teeth, tooth 524.30
    horizontal 524.33
    vertical 524.34
  tongue (congenital) (downward) 750.19
  trachea (congenital) 748.3
  ureter or ureteric opening or orifice (congenital)
    753.4
  uterine opening of oviducts or fallopian tubes
    752.19
  uterus, uterine (*see also* Malposition, uterus) 621.6
    congenital 752.3
  ventricular septum 746.89
    with rudimentary ventricle 746.89
  xyphoid bone (process) 738.3
Disproportion 653.9
  affecting fetus or newborn 763.1
  breast, reconstructed 612.1
    between native and reconstructed 612.1
  caused by
    conjoined twins 678.1
    contraction, pelvis (general) 653.1
      inlet 653.2
      midpelvic 653.8
      midplane 653.8
      outlet 653.3
    fetal
      ascites 653.7
      hydrocephalus 653.6
      hydrops 653.7
      meningomyelocele 653.7
      sacral teratoma 653.7
      tumor 653.7
    hydrocephalic fetus 653.6
    pelvis, pelvic, abnormality (bony) NEC 653.0
    unusually large fetus 653.5
  causing obstructed labor 660.1
  cephalopelvic, normally formed fetus 653.4
    causing obstructed labor 660.1
  fetal NEC 653.5
    causing obstructed labor 660.1
  fetopelvic, normally formed fetus 653.4
    causing obstructed labor 660.1
  mixed maternal and fetal origin, normally
    formed fetus 653.4
  pelvis, pelvic (bony) NEC 653.1
    causing obstructed labor 660.1
  specified type NEC 653.8

Disruption
  cesarean wound 674.1
  family V61.09
    due to
      child in
        care of non-parental family member
          V61.06
        foster care V61.06
        welfare custody V61.05
      death of family member V61.07
      divorce V61.03
      estrangement V61.09
        parent-child V61.04
      extended absence of family member NEC
        V61.08
      family member
        on military deployment V61.01
        return from military deployment V61.02
      legal separation V61.03
  gastrointestinal anastomosis 997.4
  ligament(s)—*see also* Sprain
    knee
      current injury—*see* Dislocation, knee
      old 717.89
        capsular 717.85
        collateral (medial) 717.82
          lateral 717.81
        cruciate (posterior) 717.84
          anterior 717.83
        specified site NEC 717.85
  marital V61.10
    involving
      divorce V61.03
      estrangement V61.09
  operation wound (external) (*see also*
    Dehiscence) 998.32
    internal 998.31
  organ transplant, anastomosis site—*see*
    Complications, transplant, organ, by site
  ossicles, ossicular chain 385.23
    traumatic—*see* Fracture, skull, base
  parenchyma
    liver (hepatic)—*see* Laceration, liver, major
    spleen—*see* Laceration, spleen, parenchyma,
      massive
  phase-shift, of 24 hour sleep wake cycle,
    unspecified 780.55
    nonorganic origin 307.45
  sleep wake cycle (24 hour), unspecified 780.55
    circadian rhythm 327.33
    nonorganic origin 307.45
  suture line (external) (*see also* Dehiscence)
    998.32
    internal 998.31
  wound 998.30
    cesarean operation 674.1
    episiotomy 674.2
    operation (surgical) 998.32
      cesarean 674.1
      internal 998.31
    perineal (obstetric) 674.2
    uterine 674.1
Disruptio uteri —*see also* Rupture, uterus
  complicating delivery—*see* Delivery,
    complicated, rupture, uterus
Dissatisfaction with
  employment V62.29
  school environment V62.3
Dissecting —*see* condition

Dissection
  aorta 441.00
    abdominal 441.02
    thoracic 441.01
    thoracoabdominal 441.03
  artery, arterial
    carotid 443.21
    coronary 414.12
    iliac 443.22
    renal 443.23
    specified NEC 443.29
    vertebral 443.24
  vascular 459.9
  wound—*see* Wound, open, by site
Disseminated —*see* condition
Dissociated personality NEC 300.15
Dissociation
  auriculoventricular or atrioventricular (any
    degree) (AV) 426.89
    with heart block 426.0
  interference 426.89
  isorhythmic 426.89
  rhythm
    atrioventricular (AV) 426.89
    interference 426.89
Dissociative
  identity disorder 300.14
  reaction NEC 300.15
Dissolution, vertebra (*see also* Osteoporosis)
  733.00
Distention
  abdomen (gaseous) 787.3
  bladder 596.8
  cecum 569.89
  colon 569.89
  gallbladder 575.8
  gaseous (abdomen) 787.3
  intestine 569.89
  kidney 593.89
  liver 573.9
  seminal vesicle 608.89
  stomach 536.8
    acute 536.1
    psychogenic 306.4
  ureter 593.5
  uterus 621.8
Distichia, distichiasis (eyelid) 743.63
Distoma hepaticum infestation 121.3
Distomiasis 121.9
  bile passages 121.3
    due to Clonorchis sinensis 121.1
  hemic 120.9
  hepatic (liver) 121.3
    due to Clonorchis sinensis (clonorchiasis) 121.1
  intestinal 121.4
  liver 121.3
    due to Clonorchis sinensis 121.1
  lung 121.2
  pulmonary 121.2
Distomolar (fourth molar) 520.1
  causing crowding 524.31
Disto-occlusion (division I) (division II) 524.22
Distortion (congenital)
  adrenal (gland) 759.1
  ankle (joint) 755.69
  anus 751.5
  aorta 747.29
  appendix 751.5
  arm 755.59
  artery (peripheral) NEC (*see also* Distortion,
    peripheral vascular system) 747.60

Distortion—*continued*
  artery—*continued*
    cerebral 747.81
    coronary 746.85
    pulmonary 747.3
    retinal 743.58
    umbilical 747.5
  auditory canal 744.29
    causing impairment of hearing 744.02
  bile duct or passage 751.69
  bladder 753.8
  brain 742.4
  bronchus 748.3
  cecum 751.5
  cervix (uteri) 752.49
  chest (wall) 756.3
  clavicle 755.51
  clitoris 752.49
  coccyx 756.19
  colon 751.5
  common duct 751.69
  cornea 743.41
  cricoid cartilage 748.3
  cystic duct 751.69
  duodenum 751.5
  ear 744.29
    auricle 744.29
      causing impairment of hearing 744.02
    causing impairment of hearing 744.09
    external 744.29
      causing impairment of hearing 744.02
    inner 744.05
    middle, except ossicles 744.03
      ossicles 744.04
    ossicles 744.04
  endocrine (gland) NEC 759.2
  epiglottis 748.3
  Eustachian tube 744.24
  eye 743.8
    adnexa 743.69
  face bone(s) 756.0
  fallopian tube 752.19
  femur 755.69
  fibula 755.69
  finger(s) 755.59
  foot 755.67
  gallbladder 751.69
  genitalia, genital organ(s)
    female 752.89
      external 752.49
      internal NEC 752.89
    male 752.89
      penis 752.69
  glottis 748.3
  gyri 742.4
  hand bone(s) 755.59
  heart (auricle) (ventricle) 746.89
    valve (cusp) 746.89
  hepatic duct 751.69
  humerus 755.59
  hymen 752.49
  ileum 751.5
  intestine (large) (small) 751.5
    with anomalous adhesions, fixation or
      malrotation 751.4
  jaw NEC 524.89
  jejunum 751.5
  kidney 753.3
  knee (joint) 755.64
  labium (majus) (minus) 752.49
  larynx 748.3
  leg 755.69

Distortion—*continued*
  lens 743.36
  liver 751.69
  lumbar spine 756.19
    with disproportion (fetopelvic) 653.0
      affecting fetus or newborn 763.1
      causing obstructed labor 660.1
  lumbosacral (joint) (region) 756.19
  lung (fissures) (lobe) 748.69
  nerve 742.8
  nose 748.1
  organ
    of Corti 744.05
    or site not listed—*see* Anomaly, specified type NEC
  ossicles, ear 744.04
  ovary 752.0
  oviduct 752.19
  pancreas 751.7
  parathyroid (gland) 759.2
  patella 755.64
  peripheral vascular system NEC 747.60
    gastrointestinal 747.61
    lower limb 747.64
    renal 747.62
    spinal 747.82
    upper limb 747.63
  pituitary (gland) 759.2
  radius 755.59
  rectum 751.5
  rib 756.3
  sacroiliac joint 755.69
  sacrum 756.19
  scapula 755.59
  shoulder girdle 755.59
  site not listed—*see* Anomaly, specified type NEC
  skull bone(s) 756.0
    with
      anencephalus 740.0
      encephalocele 742.0
      hydrocephalus 742.3
        with spina bifida (*see also* Spina bifida) 741.0
      microcephalus 742.1
  spinal cord 742.59
  spine 756.19
  spleen 759.0
  sternum 756.3
  thorax (wall) 756.3
  thymus (gland) 759.2
  thyroid (gland) 759.2
    cartilage 748.3
  tibia 755.69
  toe(s) 755.66
  tongue 750.19
  trachea (cartilage) 748.3
  ulna 755.59
  ureter 753.4
    causing obstruction 753.20
  urethra 753.8
    causing obstruction 753.6
  uterus 752.3
  vagina 752.49
  vein (peripheral) NEC (*see also* Distortion,
    peripheral vascular system) 747.60
    great 747.49
    portal 747.49
    pulmonary 747.49
  vena cava (inferior) (superior) 747.49
  vertebra 756.19
  visual NEC 368.15
    shape or size 368.14
  vulva 752.49
  wrist (bones) (joint) 755.59

Distress
  abdomen 789.0
  colon 789.0
  emotional V40.9
  epigastric 789.0
  fetal (syndrome) 768.4
    affecting management of pregnancy or
      childbirth 656.8
    liveborn infant 768.4
      first noted
        before onset of labor 768.2
        during labor and delivery 768.3
      stillborn infant (death before onset of labor)
        768.0
        death during labor 768.1
  gastrointestinal (functional) 536.9
    psychogenic 306.4
  intestinal (functional) NEC 564.9
    psychogenic 306.4
  intrauterine (*see* Distress, fetal)
  leg 729.5
  maternal 669.0
  mental V40.9
  respiratory 786.09
    acute (adult) 518.82
    adult syndrome (following shock, surgery, or
      trauma) 518.5
      specified NEC 518.82
    fetus or newborn 770.89
    syndrome (idiopathic) (newborn) 769
  stomach 536.9
    psychogenic 306.4
Distribution vessel, atypical NEC 747.60
  coronary artery 746.85
  spinal 747.82
Districhiasis 704.2
Disturbance —*see also* Disease
  absorption NEC 579.9
    calcium 269.3
    carbohydrate 579.8
    fat 579.8
    protein 579.8
    specified type NEC 579.8
    vitamin (*see also* Deficiency, vitamin) 269.2
  acid-base equilibrium 276.9
  activity and attention, simple, with hyperkinesis
    314.01
  amino acid (metabolic) (*see also* Disorder,
    amino acid) 270.9
    imidazole 270.5
    maple syrup (urine) disease 270.3
    transport 270.0
  assimilation, food 579.9
  attention, simple 314.00
    with hyperactivity 314.01
  auditory, nerve, except deafness 388.5
  behavior (*see also* Disturbance, conduct) 312.9
  blood clotting (hypoproteinemia) (mechanism)
    (*see also* Defect, coagulation) 286.9
  central nervous system NEC 349.9
  cerebral nerve NEC 352.9
  circulatory 459.9

Disturbance—*continued*
conduct 312.9

---

*Note—Use the following fifth-digit
subclassification with categories 312.0-312.2:*

0   *unspecified*
1   *mild*
2   *moderate*
3   *severe*

---

adjustment reaction 309.3
adolescent onset type 312.82
childhood onset type 312.81
compulsive 312.30
intermittent explosive disorder 312.34
isolated explosive disorder 312.35
kleptomania 312.32
pathological gambling 312.31
pyromania 312.33
hyperkinetic 314.2
intermittent explosive 312.34
isolated explosive 312.35
memory (*see also* Amnesia) 780.99
mixed with emotions 312.4
socialized (type) 312.20
aggressive 312.23
unaggressive 312.21
specified type NEC 312.89
undersocialized, unsocialized
aggressive (type) 312.0
unaggressive (type) 312.1
coordination 781.3
cranial nerve NEC 352.9
deep sensibility—*see* Disturbance, sensation
digestive 536.9
psychogenic 306.4
electrolyte—*see* Imbalance, electrolyte
emotions specific to childhood or adolescence
313.9
with
academic underachievement 313.83
anxiety and fearfulness 313.0
elective mutism 313.23
identity disorder 313.82
jealousy 313.3
misery and unhappiness 313.1
oppositional defiant disorder 313.81
overanxiousness 313.0
sensitivity 313.21
shyness 313.21
social withdrawal 313.22
withdrawal reaction 313.22
involving relationship problems 313.3
mixed 313.89
specified type NEC 313.89
endocrine (gland) 259.9
neonatal, transitory 775.9
specified NEC 775.89
equilibrium 780.4
feeding (elderly) (infant) 783.3
newborn 779.31
nonorganic origin NEC 307.59
psychogenic NEC 307.59
fructose metabolism 271.2
gait 781.2
hysterical 300.11
gastric (functional) 536.9
motility 536.8
psychogenic 306.4
secretion 536.8

Disturbance—*continued*
gastrointestinal (functional) 536.9
psychogenic 306.4
habit, child 307.9
hearing, except deafness 388.40
heart, functional (conditions classifiable to 426,
427, 428)
due to presence of (cardiac) prosthesis 429.4
postoperative (immediate) 997.1
long-term effect of cardiac surgery 429.4
psychogenic 306.2
hormone 259.9
innervation uterus, sympathetic,
parasympathetic 621.8
keratinization NEC
gingiva 523.10
lip 528.5
oral (mucosa) (soft tissue) 528.79
residual ridge mucosa
excessive 528.72
minimal 528.71
tongue 528.79
labyrinth, labyrinthine (vestibule) 386.9
learning, specific NEC 315.2
memory (*see also* Amnesia) 780.93
mild, following organic brain damage 310.8
mental (*see also* Disorder, mental) 300.9
associated with diseases classified elsewhere
316
metabolism (acquired) (congenital) (*see also*
Disorder, metabolism) 277.9
with
abortion—*see* Abortion, by type, with
metabolic disorder
ectopic pregnancy (*see also* categories
633.0-633.9) 639.4
molar pregnancy (*see also* categories
630-632) 639.4
amino acid (*see also* Disorder, amino acid)
270.9
aromatic NEC 270.2
branched-chain 270.3
specified type NEC 270.8
straight-chain NEC 270.7
sulfur-bearing 270.4
transport 270.0
ammonia 270.6
arginine 270.6
argininosuccinic acid 270.6
carbohydrate NEC 271.9
cholesterol 272.9
citrulline 270.6
cystathionine 270.4
fat 272.9
following
abortion 639.4
ectopic or molar pregnancy 639.4
general 277.9
carbohydrate 271.9
iron 275.0
phosphate 275.3
sodium 276.9
glutamine 270.7
glycine 270.7
histidine 270.5
homocystine 270.4
in labor or delivery 669.0
iron 275.0
isoleucine 270.3
leucine 270.3

Disturbance—*continued*
  metabolism—*continued*
    lipoid 272.9
      specified type NEC 272.8
    lysine 270.7
    methionine 270.4
    neonatal, transitory 775.9
      specified type NEC 775.89
    nitrogen 788.99
    ornithine 270.6
    phosphate 275.3
    phosphatides 272.7
    serine 270.7
    sodium NEC 276.9
    threonine 270.7
    tryptophan 270.2
    tyrosine 270.2
    urea cycle 270.6
    valine 270.3
  motor 796.1
  nervous functional 799.21
  neuromuscular mechanism (eye) due to syphilis
    094.84
  nutritional 269.9
    nail 703.8
  ocular motion 378.87
    psychogenic 306.7
  oculogyric 378.87
    psychogenic 306.7
  oculomotor NEC 378.87
    psychogenic 306.7
  olfactory nerve 781.1
  optic nerve NEC 377.49
  oral epithelium, including tongue 528.79
    residual ridge mucosa
      excessive 528.72
      minimal 528.71
  personality (pattern) (trait) (*see also* Disorder,
    personality) 301.9
    following organic brain damage 310.1
  polyglandular 258.9
  psychomotor 307.9
  pupillary 379.49
  reflex 796.1
  rhythm, heart 427.9
    postoperative (immediate) 997.1
      long-term effect of cardiac surgery 429.4
    psychogenic 306.2
  salivary secretion 527.7
  sensation (cold) (heat) (localization) (tactile
    discrimination localization) (texture)
    (vibratory) NEC 782.0
    hysterical 300.11
    skin 782.0
    smell 781.1
    taste 781.1
  sensory (*see also* Disturbance, sensation) 782.0
    innervation 782.0
  situational (transient) (*see also* Reaction,
    adjustment) 309.9
    acute 308.3
  sleep 780.50
    initiation or maintenance (*see also* Insomnia)
      780.52
      nonorganic origin 307.41
    nonorganic origin 307.40
      specified type NEC 307.49
    specified NEC 780.59
      nonorganic origin 307.49
    wakefulness (*see also* Hypersomnia) 780.54
      nonorganic origin 307.43
    with apnea—*see* Apnea, sleep

Disturbance—*continued*
  sociopathic 301.7
  speech NEC 784.59
    developmental 315.39
      associated with hyperkinesis 314.1
    secondary to organic lesion 784.59
  stomach (functional) (*see also* Disturbance,
    gastric) 536.9
  sympathetic (nerve) (*see also* Neuropathy,
    peripheral, autonomic) 337.9
  temperature sense 782.0
    hysterical 300.11
  tooth
    eruption 520.6
    formation 520.4
    structure, hereditary NEC 520.5
  touch (*see also* Disturbance, sensation) 782.0
  vascular 459.9
    arteriosclerotic—*see* Arteriosclerosis
  vasomotor 443.9
  vasospastic 443.9
  vestibular labyrinth 386.9
  vision, visual NEC 368.9
    psychophysical 368.16
    specified NEC 368.8
    subjective 368.10
  voice and resonance 784.40
  wakefulness (initiation or maintenance) (*see
    also* Hypersomnia) 780.54
    nonorganic origin 307.43
Disulfiduria, beta-mercaptolactate-cysteine 270.0
Disuse atrophy, bone 733.7
Ditthomska syndrome 307.81
Diuresis 788.42
Divers'
  palsy or paralysis 993.3
  squeeze 993.3
Diverticula, diverticulosis, diverticulum (acute)
    (multiple) (perforated) (ruptured) 562.10
  with diverticulitis 562.11
  aorta (Kommerell's) 747.21
  appendix (noninflammatory) 543.9
  bladder (acquired) (sphincter) 596.3
    congenital 753.8
  broad ligament 620.8
  bronchus (congenital) 748.3
    acquired 494.0
      with acute exacerbation 494.1
  calyx, calyceal (kidney) 593.89
  cardia (stomach) 537.1
  cecum 562.10
    with
      diverticulitis 562.11
        with hemorrhage 562.13
      hemorrhage 562.12
    congenital 751.5
  colon (acquired) 562.10
    with
      diverticulitis 562.11
        with hemorrhage 562.13
      hemorrhage 562.12
    congenital 751.5
  duodenum 562.00
    with
      diverticulitis 562.01
        with hemorrhage 562.03
      hemorrhage 562.02
    congenital 751.5
  epiphrenic (esophagus) 530.6

Diverticula, diverticulosis—*continued*
  esophagus (congenital) 750.4
    acquired 530.6
    epiphrenic 530.6
    pulsion 530.6
    traction 530.6
    Zenker's 530.6
  Eustachian tube 381.89
  fallopian tube 620.8
  gallbladder (congenital) 751.69
  gastric 537.1
  heart (congenital) 746.89
  ileum 562.00
    with
      diverticulitis 562.01
        with hemorrhage 562.03
      hemorrhage 562.02
  intestine (large) 562.10
    with
      diverticulitis 562.11
        with hemorrhage 562.13
      hemorrhage 562.12
    congenital 751.5
    small 562.00
      with
        diverticulitis 562.01
          with hemorrhage 562.03
        hemorrhage 562.02
      congenital 751.5
  jejunum 562.00
    with
      diverticulitis 562.01
        with hemorrhage 562.03
      hemorrhage 562.02
  kidney (calyx) (pelvis) 593.89
    with calculus 592.0
  Kommerell's 747.21
  laryngeal ventricle (congenital) 748.3
  Meckel's (displaced) (hypertrophic) 751.0
  midthoracic 530.6
  organ or site, congenital NEC—*see* Distortion
  pericardium (congenital) (cyst) 746.89
    acquired (true) 423.8
  pharyngoesophageal (pulsion) 530.6
  pharynx (congenital) 750.27
  pulsion (esophagus) 530.6
  rectosigmoid 562.10
    with
      diverticulitis 562.11
        with hemorrhage 562.13
      hemorrhage 562.12
    congenital 751.5
  rectum 562.10
    with
      diverticulitis 562.11
        with hemorrhage 562.13
      hemorrhage 562.12
  renal (calyces) (pelvis) 593.89
    with calculus 592.0
  Rokitansky's 530.6
  seminal vesicle 608.0
  sigmoid 562.10
    with
      diverticulitis 562.11
        with hemorrhage 562.13
      hemorrhage 562.12
    congenital 751.5
  small intestine 562.00
    with
      diverticulitis 562.01
        with hemorrhage 562.03
      hemorrhage 562.02

Diverticula, diverticulosis—*continued*
  stomach (cardia) (juxtacardia) (juxtapyloric)
    (acquired) 537.1
    congenital 750.7
  subdiaphragmatic 530.6
  trachea (congenital) 748.3
    acquired 519.19
  traction (esophagus) 530.6
  ureter (acquired) 593.89
    congenital 753.4
  ureterovesical orifice 593.89
  urethra (acquired) 599.2
    congenital 753.8
  ventricle, left (congenital) 746.89
  vesical (urinary) 596.3
    congenital 753.8
  Zenker's (esophagus) 530.6
Diverticulitis (acute) (*see also* Diverticula) 562.11
  with hemorrhage 562.13
  bladder (urinary) 596.3
  cecum (perforated) 562.11
    with hemorrhage 562.13
  colon (perforated) 562.11
    with hemorrhage 562.13
  duodenum 562.01
    with hemorrhage 562.03
  esophagus 530.6
  ileum (perforated) 562.01
    with hemorrhage 562.03
  intestine (large) (perforated) 562.11
    with hemorrhage 562.13
    small 562.01
      with hemorrhage 562.03
  jejunum (perforated) 562.01
    with hemorrhage 562.03
  Meckel's (perforated) 751.0
  pharyngoesophageal 530.6
  rectosigmoid (perforated) 562.11
    with hemorrhage 562.13
  rectum 562.11
    with hemorrhage 562.13
  sigmoid (old) (perforated) 562.11
    with hemorrhage 562.13
  small intestine (perforated) 562.01
    with hemorrhage 562.03
  vesical (urinary) 596.3
Diverticulosis —*see* Diverticula
Division
  cervix uteri 622.8
    external os into two openings by frenum 752.49
  external (cervical) into two openings by frenum
    752.49
  glans penis 752.69
  hymen 752.49
  labia minora (congenital) 752.49
  ligament (partial or complete) (current)—*see*
    also Sprain, by site
    with open wound—*see* Wound, open, by site
  muscle (partial or complete) (current)—*see also*
    Sprain, by site
    with open wound—*see* Wound, open, by site
  nerve—*see* Injury, nerve, by site
  penis glans 752.69
  spinal cord—*see* Injury, spinal, by site
  vein 459.9
    traumatic—*see* Injury, vascular, by site
Divorce V61.03
Dix-Hallpike neurolabyrinthitis 386.12
Dizziness 780.4
  hysterical 300.11
  psychogenic 306.9

Doan-Wiseman syndrome (primary splenic
neutropenia) 289.53
Dog bite —*see* Wound, open, by site
Döhle-Heller aortitis 093.1
Döhle body-panmyelopathic syndrome 288.2
Dolichocephaly, dolichocephalus 754.0
Dolichocolon 751.5
Dolichostenomelia 759.82
Donohue's syndrome (leprechaunism) 259.8
Donor
  blood V59.01
    other blood components V59.09
    stem cells V59.02
    whole blood V59.01
  bone V59.2
    marrow V59.3
  cornea V59.5
  egg (oocyte) (ovum) V59.70
    age 35 and over V59.73
      anonymous recipient V59.73
      designated recipient V59.74
    under age 35 V59.71
      anonymous recipient V59.71
      designated recipient V59.72
  heart V59.8
  kidney V59.4
  liver V59.6
  lung V59.8
  lymphocyte V59.8
  organ V59.9
    specified NEC V59.8
  potential, examination of V70.8
  skin V59.1
  specified organ or tissue NEC V59.8
  sperm V59.8
  stem cells V59.02
  tissue V59.9
    specified type NEC V59.8
Donovanosis (granuloma venereum) 099.2
DOPS (diffuse obstructive pulmonary syndrome) 496
Double
  albumin 273.8
  aortic arch 747.21
  auditory canal 744.29
  auricle (heart) 746.82
  bladder 753.8
  external (cervical) os 752.49
  kidney with double pelvis (renal) 753.3
  larynx 748.3
  meatus urinarius 753.8
  organ or site NEC—*see* Accessory
  orifice
    heart valve NEC 746.89
      pulmonary 746.09
  outlet, right ventricle 745.11
  pelvis (renal) with double ureter 753.4
  penis 752.69
  tongue 750.13
  ureter (one or both sides) 753.4
    with double pelvis (renal) 753.4
  urethra 753.8
  urinary meatus 753.8
  uterus (any degree) 752.2
    with doubling of cervix and vagina 752.2
    in pregnancy or childbirth 654.0
      affecting fetus or newborn 763.89
  vagina 752.49
    with doubling of cervix and uterus 752.2
  vision 368.2
  vocal cords 748.3
  vulva 752.49
  whammy (syndrome) 360.81

Douglas' pouch, cul-de-sac —*see* condition
Down's disease or syndrome (mongolism) 758.0
Down-growth, epithelial (anterior chamber)
364.61
Dracontiasis 125.7
Dracunculiasis 125.7
Dracunculosis 125.7
Drainage
  abscess (spontaneous)—*see* Abscess
  anomalous pulmonary veins to hepatic veins or
    right atrium 747.41
  stump (amputation) (surgical) 997.62
  suprapubic, bladder 596.8
Dream state, hysterical 300.13
Drepanocytic anemia (*see also* Disease, sickle
cell) 282.60
Dresbach's syndrome (elliptocytosis) 282.1
Dreschlera (infection) 118
  hawaiiensis 117.8
Dressler's syndrome (postmyocardial infarction)
411.0
Dribbling (post-void) 788.35
Drift, ulnar 736.09
Drinking (alcohol)—*see also* Alcoholism
  excessive, to excess NEC (*see also* Abuse,
    drugs, nondependent) 305.0
    bouts, periodic 305.0
    continual 303.9
    episodic 305.0
    habitual 303.9
    periodic 305.0
Drip, postnasal (chronic) 784.91
  due to
    allergic rhinitis —*see* Rhinitis, allergic
    common cold 460
    gastroesophageal reflux —*see* Reflux,
      gastroesophageal
    nasopharyngitis —*see* Nasopharyngitis
    other known condition —*code to condition*
    sinusitis —*see* Sinusitis
Drivers' license examination V70.3
Droop
  Cooper's 611.81
  facial 781.94
Drop
  finger 736.29
  foot 736.79
  hematocrit (precipitous) 790.01
  hemoglobin 790.01
  toe 735.8
  wrist 736.05
Dropped
  dead 798.1
  heart beats 426.6
Dropsy, dropsical (*see also* Edema) 782.3
  abdomen 789.59
  amnion (*see also* Hydramnios) 657
  brain—*see* Hydrocephalus
  cardiac (*see also* Failure, heart) 428.0
  cardiorenal (*see also* Hypertension, cardiorenal)
    404.90
  chest 511.9
  fetus or newborn 778.0
    due to isoimmunization 773.3
  gangrenous (*see also* Gangrene) 785.4
  heart (*see also* Failure, heart) 428.0
  hepatic—*see* Cirrhosis, liver
  infantile—*see* Hydrops, fetalis
  kidney (*see also* Nephrosis) 581.9
  liver—*see* Cirrhosis, liver
  lung 514

Dropsy, dropsical—*continued*
  malarial (*see also* Malaria) 084.9
  neonatorum—*see* Hydrops, fetalis
  nephritic 581.9
  newborn—*see* Hydrops, fetalis
  nutritional 269.9
  ovary 620.8
  pericardium (*see also* Pericarditis) 423.9
  renal (*see also* Nephrosis) 581.9
  uremic—*see* Uremia
Drowned, drowning (near) 994.1
  lung 518.5
Drowsiness 780.09
Drug —*see also* condition
  addiction (*see also* listing under Dependence)
    304.9
  adverse effect NEC, correct substance properly
    administered 995.20
  allergy 995.27
  dependence (*see also* listing under Dependence)
    304.9
  habit (*see also* listing under Dependence) 304.9
  hypersensitivity 995.27
  induced
    circadian rhythm sleep disorder 292.85
    hypersomnia 292.85
    insomnia 292.85
    mental disorder 292.9
      anxiety 292.89
      mood 292.84
      sexual 292.89
      sleep 292.85
      specified type 292.89
    parasomnia 292.85
    persisting
      amnestic disorder 292.83
      dementia 292.82
    psychotic disorder
      with
        delusions 292.11
        hallucinations 292.12
    sleep disorder 292.85
  intoxication 292.89
  overdose—*see* Table of drugs and chemicals
  poisoning—*see* Table of drugs and chemicals
  therapy (maintenance) status NEC
    chemotherapy, antineoplastic V58.11
    immunotherapy, antineoplastic V58.12
    long-term (current) use V58.69
      antibiotics V58.62
      anticoagulants V58.61
      anti-inflammatories, non-steroidal (NSAID)
        V58.64
      antiplatelets V58.63
      antithrombotics V58.63
      aspirin V58.66
      high-risk medications NEC V58.69
      insulin V58.67
      methadone V58.69
      opiate analgesic V58.69
      steroids V58.65
  wrong substance given or taken in error—*see*
    Table of drugs and chemicals
Drunkenness (*see also* Abuse, drugs,
  nondependent) 305.0
  acute in alcoholism (*see also* Alcoholism) 303.0
  chronic (*see also* Alcoholism) 303.9
  pathologic 291.4
  simple (acute) 305.0
    in alcoholism 303.0
  sleep 307.47

Drusen
  optic disc or papilla 377.21
  retina (colloid) (hyaloid degeneration) 362.57
    hereditary 362.77
Drusenfieber 075
Dry, dryness —*see also* condition
  eye 375.15
    syndrome 375.15
  larynx 478.79
  mouth 527.7
  nose 478.19
  skin syndrome 701.1
  socket (teeth) 526.5
  throat 478.29
DSAP (disseminated superficial actinic
  porokeratosis) 692.75
Duane's retraction syndrome 378.71
Duane-Stilling-Turk syndrome (ocular
  retraction syndrome) 378.71
Dubin-Johnson disease or syndrome 277.4
Dubini's disease (electric chorea) 049.8
Dubois' abscess or disease 090.5
Duchenne's
  disease 094.0
    locomotor ataxia 094.0
    muscular dystrophy 359.1
    pseudohypertrophy, muscles 359.1
  paralysis 335.22
  syndrome 335.22
Duchenne-Aran myelopathic muscular atrophy
  (nonprogressive) (progressive) 335.21
Duchenne-Griesinger disease 359.1
Ducrey's
  bacillus 099.0
  chancre 099.0
  disease (chancroid) 099.0
Duct, ductus —*see* condition
Duengero 061
Duhring's disease (dermatitis herpetiformis) 694.0
Dukes (-Filatov) disease 057.8
Dullness
  cardiac (decreased) (increased) 785.3
Dumb ague (*see also* Malaria) 084.6
Dumbness (*see also* Aphasia) 784.3
Dumdum fever 085.0
Dumping syndrome (postgastrectomy) 564.2
  nonsurgical 536.8
Duodenitis (nonspecific) (peptic) 535.60
  due to
    Strongyloides stercoralis 127.2
  with hemorrhage 535.61
Duodenocholangitis 575.8
Duodenum, duodenal —*see* condition
Duplay's disease, periarthritis, or syndrome
  726.2
Duplex —*see also* Accessory
  kidney 753.3
  placenta—*see* Placenta, abnormal
  uterus 752.2
Duplication —*see also* Accessory
  anus 751.5
  aortic arch 747.21
  appendix 751.5
  biliary duct (any) 751.69
  bladder 753.8
  cecum 751.5
    and appendix 751.5
  clitoris 752.49
  cystic duct 751.69
  digestive organs 751.8

Duplication—*continued*
  duodenum 751.5
  esophagus 750.4
  fallopian tube 752.19
  frontonasal process 756.0
  gallbladder 751.69
  ileum 751.5
  intestine (large) (small) 751.5
  jejunum 751.5
  kidney 753.3
  liver 751.69
  nose 748.1
  pancreas 751.7
  penis 752.69
  respiratory organs NEC 748.9
  salivary duct 750.22
  spinal cord (incomplete) 742.51
  stomach 750.7
  ureter 753.4
  vagina 752.49
  vas deferens 752.89
  vocal cords 748.3
Dupré's disease or syndrome (meningism) 781.6
Dupuytren's
  contraction 728.6
  disease (muscle contracture) 728.6
  fracture (closed) 824.4
    ankle (closed) 824.4
      open 824.5
    fibula (closed) 824.4
      open 824.5
      open 824.5
    radius (closed) 813.42
      open 813.52
  muscle contracture 728.6
Durand-Nicolas-Favre disease (climatic bubo) 099.1
Durotomy incidental (inadvertent) (*see also* Tear, dural) 349.31
Duroziez's disease (congenital mitral stenosis) 746.5
Dust
  conjunctivitis 372.05
  reticulation (occupational) 504
Dutton's
  disease (trypanosomiasis) 086.9
  relapsing fever (West African) 087.1
Dwarf, dwarfism 259.4
  with infantilism (hypophyseal) 253.3
  achondroplastic 756.4
  Amsterdam 759.89
  bird-headed 759.89
  congenital 259.4
  constitutional 259.4
  hypophyseal 253.3
  infantile 259.4
  Levi type 253.3
  Lorain-Levi (pituitary) 253.3
  Lorain type (pituitary) 253.3
  metatropic 756.4
  nephrotic-glycosuric, with hypophosphatemic rickets 270.0
  nutritional 263.2
  ovarian 758.6
  pancreatic 577.8
  pituitary 253.3
  polydystrophic 277.5
  primordial 253.3
  psychosocial 259.4

Dwarf, dwarfism—*continued*
  renal 588.0
  with hypertension—*see* Hypertension, kidney
  Russell's (uterine dwarfism and craniofacial dysostosis) 759.89
Dyke-Young anemia or syndrome (acquired macrocytic hemolytic anemia) (secondary) (symptomatic) 283.9
Dynia abnormality (*see also* Defect, coagulation) 286.9
Dysacousis 388.40
Dysadrenocortism 255.9
  hyperfunction 255.3
  hypofunction 255.41
Dysarthria 784.51
  due to late effect of cerebrovascular disease (*see also* Late effect(s) (of) cerebrovascular disease) 438.13
Dysautonomia (*see also* Neuropathy, peripheral, autonomic) 337.9
  familial 742.8
Dysbarism 993.3
Dysbasia 719.7
  angiosclerotica intermittens 443.9
    due to atherosclerosis 440.21
  hysterical 300.11
  lordotica (progressiva) 333.6
  nonorganic origin 307.9
  psychogenic 307.9
Dysbetalipoproteinemia (familial) 272.2
Dyscalculia 315.1
Dyschezia (*see also* Constipation) 564.00
Dyschondroplasia (with hemangiomata) 756.4
  Voorhoeve's 756.4
Dyschondrosteosis 756.59
Dyschromia 709.00
Dyscollagenosis 710.9
Dyscoria 743.41
Dyscraniopyophalangy 759.89
Dyscrasia
  blood 289.9
    with antepartum hemorrhage 641.3
    hemorrhage, subungual 287.8
    puerperal, postpartum 666.3
  ovary 256.8
  plasma cell 273.9
  pluriglandular 258.9
  polyglandular 258.9
Dysdiadochokinesia 781.3
Dysectasia, vesical neck 596.8
Dysendocrinism 259.9
Dysentery, dysenteric (bilious) (catarrhal) (diarrhea) (epidemic) (gangrenous) (hemorrhagic) (infectious) (sporadic) (tropical) (ulcerative) 009.0
  abscess, liver (*see also* Abscess, amebic) 006.3
  amebic (*see also* Amebiasis) 006.9
    with abscess—*see* Abscess, amebic
    acute 006.0
    carrier (suspected) of V02.2
    chronic 006.1
  arthritis (*see also* Arthritis, due to, dysentery) 009.0 *[711.3]*
    bacillary 004.9 *[711.3]*
  asylum 004.9
  bacillary 004.9
    arthritis 004.9 *[711.3]*
    Boyd 004.2
    Flexner 004.1
    Schmitz (-Stutzer) 004.0
    Shiga 004.0

Dysentery, dysenteric—*continued*
  bacillary—*continued*
    Shigella 004.9
      group A 004.0
      group B 004.1
      group C 004.2
      group D 004.3
      specified type NEC 004.8
    Sonne 004.3
    specified type NEC 004.8
  bacterium 004.9
  balantidial 007.0
  Balantidium coli 007.0
  Boyd's 004.2
  Chilomastix 007.8
  Chinese 004.9
  choleriform 001.1
  coccidial 007.2
  Dientamoeba fragilis 007.8
  due to specified organism NEC—*see* Enteritis,
      due to, by organism
  Embadomonas 007.8
  Endolimax nana—*see* Dysentery, amebic
  Entamoba, entamebic—*see* Dysentery, amebic
  Flexner's 004.1
  Flexner-Boyd 004.2
  giardial 007.1
  Giardia lamblia 007.1
  Hiss-Russell 004.1
  lamblia 007.1
  leishmanial 085.0
  malarial (*see also* Malaria) 084.6
  metazoal 127.9
  Monilia 112.89
  protozoal NEC 007.9
  Russell's 004.8
  salmonella 003.0
  schistosomal 120.1
  Schmitz (-Stutzer) 004.0
  Shiga 004.0
  Shigella NEC (*see also* Dysentery, bacillary)
      004.9
    boydii 004.2
    dysenteriae 004.0
      Schmitz 004.0
      Shiga 004.0
    flexneri 004.1
    Group A 004.0
    Group B 004.1
    Group C 004.2
    Group D 004.3
    Schmitz 004.0
    Shiga 004.0
    Sonnei 004.3
  Sonne 004.3
  strongyloidiasis 127.2
  trichomonal 007.3
  tuberculous (*see also* Tuberculosis) 014.8
  viral (*see also* Enteritis, viral) 008.8
Dysequilibrium 780.4
Dysesthesia 782.0
  hysterical 300.11
Dysfibrinogenemia (congenital) (*see also* Defect,
    coagulation) 286.3
Dysfunction
  adrenal (cortical) 255.9
    hyperfunction 255.3
    hypofunction 255.41
  associated with sleep stages or arousal from
      sleep 780.56
    nonorganic origin 307.47

Dysfunction—*continued*
  bladder NEC 596.59
  bleeding, uterus 626.8
  brain, minimal (*see also* Hyperkinesia) 314.9
  cerebral 348.30
  colon 564.9
    psychogenic 306.4
  colostomy or enterostomy 569.62
  cystic duct 575.8
  diastolic 429.9
    with heart failure—*see* Failure, heart
    due to
      cardiomyopathy—*see* Cardiomyopathy
      hypertension—*see* Hypertension, heart
  endocrine NEC 259.9
  endometrium 621.8
  enteric stoma 569.62
  enterostomy 569.62
  erectile 607.84
    nonorganic origin 302.72
  esophagostomy 530.87
  Eustachian tube 381.81
  gallbladder 575.8
  gastrointestinal 536.9
  gland, glandular NEC 259.9
  heart 427.9
    postoperative (immediate) 997.1
      long-term effect of cardiac surgery 429.4
  hemoglobin 289.89
  hepatic 573.9
  hepatocellular NEC 573.9
  hypophysis 253.9
    hyperfunction 253.1
    hypofunction 253.2
    posterior lobe 253.6
      hypofunction 253.5
  kidney (*see also* Disease, renal) 593.9
  labyrinthine 386.50
    specified NEC 386.58
  liver 573.9
    constitutional 277.4
  minimal brain (child) (*see also* Hyperkinesia)
      314.9
  ovary, ovarian 256.9
    hyperfunction 256.1
      estrogen 256.0
    hypofunction 256.39
      postablative 256.2
    postablative 256.2
    specified NEC 256.8
  papillary muscle 429.81
    with myocardial infarction 410.8
  parathyroid 252.8
    hyperfunction 252.00
    hypofunction 252.1
  pineal gland 259.8
  pituitary (gland) 253.9
    hyperfunction 253.1
    hypofunction 253.2
    posterior 253.6
      hypofunction 253.5
  placental—*see* Placenta, insufficiency
  platelets (blood) 287.1
  polyglandular 258.9
    specified NEC 258.8

Dysfunction—*continued*
  psychosexual 302.70
  with
    dyspareunia (functional) (psychogenic)
      302.76
    frigidity 302.72
    impotence 302.72
    inhibition
      orgasm
        female 302.73
        male 302.74
      sexual
        desire 302.71
        excitement 302.72
    premature ejaculation 302.75
    sexual aversion 302.79
    specified disorder NEC 302.79
    vaginismus 306.51
  pylorus 537.9
  rectum 564.9
    psychogenic 306.4
  segmental (*see also* Dysfunction, somatic) 739.9
  senile 797
  sexual 302.70
  sinoatrial node 427.81
  somatic 739.9
    abdomen 739.9
    acromioclavicular 739.7
    cervical 739.1
    cervicothoracic 739.1
    costochondral 739.8
    costovertebral 739.8
    extremities
      lower 739.6
      upper 739.7
    head 739.0
    hip 739.5
    umbar, lumbosacral 739.3
    occipitocervical 739.0
    pelvic 739.5
    pubic 739.5
    rib cage 739.8
    sacral 739.4
    sacrococcygeal 739.4
    sacroiliac 739.4
    specified site NEC 739.9
    sternochondral 739.8
    sternoclavicular 739.7
    temporomandibular 739.0
    thoracic, thoracolumbar 739.2
  stomach 536.9
    psychogenic 306.4
  suprarenal 255.9
    hyperfunction 255.3
    hypofunction 255.41
  symbolic NEC 784.60
    specified type NEC 784.69
  systolic 429.9
    with heart failure—*see* Failure, heart
  temporomandibular (joint)
    (joint-pain-syndrome) NEC 524.60
    sounds on opening or closing 524.64
    specified NEC 524.69
  testicular 257.9
    hyperfunction 257.0
    hypofunction 257.2
    specified type NEC 257.8
  thymus 254.9

Dysfunction—*continued*
  thyroid 246.9
    complicating pregnancy, childbirth, or
      puerperium 648.1
    hyperfunction—*see* Hyperthyroidism
    hypofunction—*see* Hypothyroidism
  uterus, complicating delivery 661.9
    affecting fetus or newborn 763.7
    hypertonic 661.4
    hypotonic 661.2
      primary 661.0
      secondary 661.1
  velopharyngeal (acquired) 528.9
    congenital 750.29
  ventricular 429.9
    with congestive heart failure (*see also* Failure,
      heart) 428.0
    due to
      cardiomyopathy—*see* Cardiomyopathy
      hypertension—*see* Hypertension, heart
    left, reversible following sudden emotional
      stress 429.83
  vesicourethral NEC 596.59
  vestibular 386.50
    specified type NEC 386.58
Dysgammaglobulinemia 279.06
Dysgenesis
  gonadal (due to chromosomal anomaly) 758.6
    pure 752.7
  kidney(s) 753.0
  ovarian 758.6
  renal 753.0
  reticular 279.2
  seminiferous tubules 758.6
  tidal platelet 287.31
Dysgerminoma (M9060/3)
  specified site—*see* Neoplasm, by site, malignant
  unspecified site
    female 183.0
    male 186.9
Dysgeusia 781.1
Dysgraphia 781.3
Dyshidrosis 705.81
Dysidrosis 705.81
Dysinsulinism 251.8
Dyskaryotic cervical smear 795.09
Dyskeratosis (*see also* Keratosis) 701.1
  bullosa hereditaria 757.39
  cervix 622.10
  congenital 757.39
  follicularis 757.39
    vitamin A deficiency 264.8
  gingiva 523.8
  oral soft tissue NEC 528.79
  tongue 528.79
  uterus NEC 621.8
Dyskinesia 781.3
  biliary 575.8
  esophagus 530.5
  hysterical 300.11
  intestinal 564.89
  neuroleptic-induced tardive 333.85
  nonorganic origin 307.9
  orofacial 333.82
    due to drugs 333.85
  psychogenic 307.9
  subacute, due to drugs 333.85
  tardive (oral) 333.85
Dyslalia 784.59
  developmental 315.39

Dyslexia 784.61
  developmental 315.02
  secondary to organic lesion 784.61
Dyslipidemia 272.4
Dysmaturity (*see also* Immaturity) 765.1
  lung 770.4
  pulmonary 770.4
Dysmenorrhea (essential) (exfoliative)
    (functional) (intrinsic) (membranous)
    (primary) (secondary) 625.3
  psychogenic 306.52
Dysmetabolic syndrome X 277.7
Dysmetria 781.3
Dysmorodystrophia mesodermalis congenita
    759.82
Dysnomia 784.3
Dysorexia 783.0
  hysterical 300.11
Dysostosis
  cleidocranial, cleidocranialis 755.59
  craniofacial 756.0
  Fairbank's (idiopathic familial generalized
    osteophytosis) 756.50
  mandibularis 756.0
  mandibulofacial, incomplete 756.0
  multiplex 277.5
  orodigitofacial 759.89
Dyspareunia (female) 625.0
  male 608.89
  psychogenic 302.76
Dyspepsia (allergic) (congenital) (fermentative)
    (flatulent) (functional) (gastric) (gastrointestinal)
    (neurogenic) (occupational) (reflex) 536.8
  acid 536.8
  atonic 536.3
    psychogenic 306.4
  diarrhea 787.91
    psychogenic 306.4
  intestinal 564.89
    psychogenic 306.4
  nervous 306.4
  neurotic 306.4
  psychogenic 306.4
Dysphagia 787.20
  cervical 787.29
  functional 300.11
  hysterical 300.11
  nervous 300.11
  neurogenic 787.29
  oral phase 787.21
  oropharyngeal phase 787.22
  pharyngeal phase 787.23
  pharyngoesophageal phase 787.24
  psychogenic 306.4
  sideropenic 280.8
  spastica 530.5
  specified NEC 787.29
Dysphagocytosis, congenital 288.1
Dysphasia 784.59
Dysphonia 784.42
  clericorum 784.49
  functional 300.11
  hysterical 300.11
  psychogenic 306.1
  spastica 478.79
Dyspigmentation —*see also* Pigmentation
  eyelid (acquired) 374.52
Dyspituitarism 253.9
  hyperfunction 253.1
  hypofunction 253.2
  posterior lobe 253.6

Dysplasia —*see also* Anomaly
  anus 569.44
    intraepithelial neoplasia I [AIN I]
      (histologically confirmed) 569.44
    intraepithelial neoplasia II [AIN II]
      (histologically confirmed) 569.44
    intraepithelial neoplasia III [AIN III] 230.6
      anal canal 230.5
    mild (histologically confirmed) 569.44
    moderate (histologically confirmed) 569.44
    severe 230.6
      anal canal 230.5
  artery
    fibromuscular NEC 447.8
      carotid 447.8
      renal 447.3
  bladder 596.8
  bone (fibrous) NEC 733.29
    diaphyseal, progressive 756.59
    jaw 526.89
    monostotic 733.29
    polyostotic 756.54
    solitary 733.29
  brain 742.9
  bronchopulmonary, fetus or newborn 770.7
  cervix (uteri) 622.10
    cervical intraepithelial neoplasia I [CIN 1]
      622.11
    cervical intraepithelial neoplasia II [CIN II]
      622.12
    cervical intraepithelial neoplasia III [CIN III]
      233.1
    CIN I 622.11
    CIN II 622.12
    CIN III 233.1
    mild 622.11
    moderate 622.12
    severe 233.1
  chondroectodermal 756.55
  chondromatose 756.4
  colon 211.3
  craniocarpotarsal 759.89
  craniometaphyseal 756.89
  dentinal 520.5
  diaphyseal, progressive 756.59
  ectodermal (anhidrotic) (Bason) (Clouston's)
      (congenital) (Feinmesser) (hereditary)
      (hidrotic) (Marshall) (Robinson's) 757.31
  epiphysealis 756.9
    multiplex 756.56
    punctata 756.59
  epiphysis 756.9
    multiple 756.56
  epithelial
    epiglottis 478.79
    uterine cervix 622.10
  erythroid NEC 289.89
  eye (*see also* Microphthalmos) 743.10
  familial metaphyseal 756.89
  fibromuscular, artery NEC 447.8
    carotid 447.8
    renal 447.3
  fibrous
    bone NEC 733.29
    diaphyseal, progressive 756.59
    jaw 526.89
    monostotic 733.29
    polyostotic 756.54
    solitary 733.29
  high grade, focal—*see* Neoplasm, by site,
      benign

Dysplasia—*continued*
 hip (congenital) 755.63
  with dislocation (*see also* Dislocation, hip,
    congenital) 754.30
 hypohidrotic ectodermal 757.31
 joint 755.8
 kidney 753.15
 leg 755.69
 linguofacialis 759.89
 lung 748.5
 macular 743.55
 mammary (benign) (gland) 610.9
  cystic 610.1
  specified type NEC 610.8
 metaphyseal 756.9
  familial 756.89
 monostotic fibrous 733.29
 muscle 756.89
 myeloid NEC 289.89
 nervous system (general) 742.9
 neuroectodermal 759.6
 oculoauriculovertebral 756.0
 oculodentodigital 759.89
 olfactogenital 253.4
 osteo-onycho-arthro (hereditary) 756.89
 periosteum 733.99
 polyostotic fibrous 756.54
 progressive diaphyseal 756.59
 prostate 602.3
  intraepithelial neoplasia I [PIN I] 602.3
  intraepithelial neoplasia II [PIN II] 602.3
  intraepithelial neoplasia III [PIN III] 233.4
 renal 753.15
 renofacialis 753.0
 retinal NEC 743.56
 retrolental (*see also* Retinopathy of prematurity)
    362.21
 skin 709.8
 spinal cord 742.9
 thymic, with immunodeficiency 279.2
 vagina 623.0
  mild 623.0
  moderate 623.0
  severe 233.31
 vocal cord 478.5
 vulva 624.8
  intraepithelial neoplasia I [VIN I] 624.01
  intraepithelial neoplasia II [VIN II] 624.02
  intraepithelial neoplasia III [VIN III] 233.32
  mild 624.01
  moderate 624.02
  severe 233.32
  VIN I 624.01
  VIN II 624.02
  VIN III 233.32
Dyspnea (nocturnal) (paroxysmal) 786.09
 asthmatic (bronchial) (*see also* Asthma) 493.9
  with bronchitis (*see also* Asthma) 493.9
   chronic 493.2
 cardiac (*see also* Failure, ventricular, left) 428.1
 cardiac (*see also* Failure, ventricular, left) 428.1
 functional 300.11
 hyperventilation 786.01
 hysterical 300.11
 Monday morning 504
 newborn 770.89
 psychogenic 306.1
 uremic—*see* Uremia
Dyspraxia 781.3
 syndrome 315.4

Dysproteinemia 273.8
 transient with copper deficiency 281.4
Dysprothrombinemia (constitutional) (*see also*
  Defect, coagulation) 286.3
Dysreflexia, autonomic 337.3
Dysrhythmia
 cardiac 427.9
  postoperative (immediate) 997.1
   long-term effect of cardiac surgery 429.4
  specified type NEC 427.89
 cerebral or cortical 348.30
Dyssecretosis, mucoserous 710.2
**Dyssocial reaction without manifest psychiatric
  disorder**
 adolescent V71.02
 adult V71.01
 child V71.02
Dyssomnia NEC 780.56
 nonorganic origin 307.47
Dyssplenism 289.4
Dyssynergia
 biliary (*see also* Disease, biliary) 576.8
 cerebellaris myoclonica 334.2
 detrusor sphincter (bladder) 596.55
 ventricular 429.89
Dystasia, hereditary areflexic 334.3
Dysthymia 300.4
Dysthymic disorder 300.4
Dysthyroidism 246.9
Dystocia 660.9
 affecting fetus or newborn 763.1
 cervical 661.2
  affecting fetus or newborn 763.7
 contraction ring 661.4
  affecting fetus or newborn 763.7
 fetal 660.9
  abnormal size 653.5
  affecting fetus or newborn 763.1
  deformity 653.7
 maternal 660.9
  affecting fetus or newborn 763.1
 positional 660.0
  affecting fetus or newborn 763.1
 shoulder (girdle) 660.4
  affecting fetus or newborn 763.1
 uterine NEC 661.4
  affecting fetus or newborn 763.7
Dystonia
 acute
  due to drugs 333.72
   neuroleptic-induced acute 333.72
 deformans progressiva 333.6
 lenticularis 333.6
 musculorum deformans 333.6
 torsion (idiopathic) 333.6
  acquired 333.79
  fragments (of) 333.89
  genetic 333.6
  symptomatic 333.79
Dystonic
 movements 781.0
Dystopia kidney 753.3
Dystrophy, dystrophia 783.9
 adiposogenital 253.8
 asphyxiating thoracic 756.4
 Becker's type 359.22
 brevicollis 756.16
 Bruch's membrane 362.77
 cervical (sympathetic) NEC 337.09
 chondro-osseus with punctate epiphyseal
    dysplasia 756.59

Dystrophy, dystrophia—*continued*
  choroid (hereditary) 363.50
    central (areolar) (partial) 363.53
      total (gyrate) 363.54
    circinate 363.53
    circumpapillary (partial) 363.51
      total 363.52
    diffuse
      partial 363.56
      total 363.57
    generalized
      partial 363.56
      total 363.57
    gyrate
      central 363.54
      generalized 363.57
    helicoid 363.52
    peripapillary—*see* Dystrophy, choroid,
      circumpapillary
    serpiginous 363.54
  cornea (hereditary) 371.50
    anterior NEC 371.52
    Cogan's 371.52
    combined 371.57
    crystalline 371.56
    endothelial (Fuchs') 371.57
    epithelial 371.50
      juvenile 371.51
      microscopic cystic 371.52
    granular 371.53
    lattice 371.54
    macular 371.55
    marginal (Terrien's) 371.48
    Meesman's 371.51
    microscopic cystic (epithelial) 371.52
    nodular, Salzmann's 371.46
    polymorphous 371.58
    posterior NEC 371.58
    ring-like 371.52
    Salzmann's nodular 371.46
    stromal NEC 371.56
  dermatochondrocorneal 371.50
  Duchenne's 359.1
  due to malnutrition 263.9
  Erb's 359.1
  familial
    hyperplastic periosteal 756.59
    osseous 277.5
  foveal 362.77
  Fuchs', cornea 371.57
  Gowers' muscular 359.1
  hair 704.2
  hereditary, progressive muscular 359.1
  hypogenital, with diabetic tendency 759.81
  Landouzy-Déjérine 359.1
  Leyden-Möbius 359.1
  mesodermalis congenita 759.82
  muscular 359.1
    congenital (hereditary) 359.0
      myotonic 359.22
    distal 359.1
    Duchenne's 359.1
    Erb's 359.1
    fascioscapulohumeral 359.1
    Gowers' 359.1
    hereditary (progressive) 359.1
    Landouzy-Déjérine 359.1
    limb-girdle 359.1
    myotonic 359.21
    progressive (hereditary) 359.1
      Charcot-Marie-Tooth 356.1
    pseudohypertrophic (infantile) 359.1

Dystrophy, dystrophia—*continued*
  myocardium, myocardial (*see also*
    Degeneration, myocardial) 429.1
  myotonic 359.21
  myotonica 359.21
  nail 703.8
    congenital 757.5
  neurovascular (traumatic) (*see also* Neuropathy,
    peripheral, autonomic) 337.9
  nutritional 263.9
  ocular 359.1
  oculocerebrorenal 270.8
  oculopharyngeal 359.1
  ovarian 620.8
  papillary (and pigmentary) 701.1
  pelvicrural atrophic 359.1
  pigmentary (*see also* Acanthosis) 701.2
  pituitary (gland) 253.8
  polyglandular 258.8
  posttraumatic sympathetic—*see* Dystrophy,
    sympathetic
  progressive ophthalmoplegic 359.1
  reflex neuromuscular—*see* Dystrophy,
    sympathetic
  retina, retinal (hereditary) 362.70
    albipunctate 362.74
    Bruch's membrane 362.77
    cone, progressive 362.75
    hyaline 362.77
    in
      Bassen-Kornzweig syndrome 272.5
        [362.72]
      cerebroretinal lipidosis 330.1 *[362.71]*
      Refsum's disease 356.3 *[362.72]*
      systemic lipidosis 272.7 *[362.71]*
    juvenile (Stargardt's) 362.75
    pigmentary 362.74
    pigment epithelium 362.76
    progressive cone (-rod) 362.75
    pseudoinflammatory foveal 362.77
    rod, progressive 362.75
    sensory 362.75
    vitelliform 362.76
  Salzmann's nodular 371.46
  scapuloperoneal 359.1
  skin NEC 709.9
  sympathetic (posttraumatic) (reflex) 337.20
    lower limb 337.22
    specified NEC 337.29
    upper limb 337.21
  tapetoretinal NEC 362.74
  thoracic asphyxiating 756.4
  unguium 703.8
    congenital 757.5
  vitreoretinal (primary) 362.73
    secondary 362.66
  vulva 624.09
Dysuria 788.1
  psychogenic 306.53

E

Eagle-Barrett syndrome 756.71
Eales' disease (syndrome) 362.18
Ear —*see also* condition
ache 388.70
  otogenic 388.71
  referred 388.72
lop 744.29
piercing V50.3
swimmers' acute 380.12
tank 380.12
tropical 111.8 *[380.15]*
wax 380.4
Earache 388.70
otogenic 388.71
referred 388.72
Early satiety 780.94
Eaton-Lambert syndrome (*see also* Neoplasm,
by site, malignant) 199.1 *[358.1]*
Eberth's disease (typhoid fever) 002.0
Ebstein's
anomaly or syndrome (downward displacement,
  tricuspid valve into right ventricle) 746.2
disease (diabetes) 250.4 *[581.81]*
  due to secondary diabetes 249.4 *[581.81]*
Eccentro-osteochondrodysplasia 277.5
Ecchondroma (M9210/0)—*see* Neoplasm, bone,
benign
Ecchondrosis (M9210/1) 238.0
Ecchordosis physaliphora 756.0
Ecchymosis (multiple) 459.89
conjunctiva 372.72
eye (traumatic) 921.0
eyelids (traumatic) 921.1
newborn 772.6
spontaneous 782.7
traumatic—*see* Contusion
ECD (Erdheim-Chester disease) 277.89
Echinococciasis —*see* Echinococcus
Echinococcosis —*see* Echinococcus
Echinococcus (infection) 122.9
granulosus 122.4
  liver 122.0
  lung 122.1
  orbit 122.3 *[376.13]*
  specified site NEC 122.3
  thyroid 122.2
liver NEC 122.8
  granulosus 122.0
  multilocularis 122.5
lung NEC 122.9
  granulosus 122.1
  multilocularis 122.6
multilocularis 122.7
  liver 122.5
  specified site NEC 122.6
orbit 122.9 *[376.13]*
  granulosus 122.3 *[376.13]*
  multilocularis 122.6 *[376.13]*
specified site NEC 122.9
  granulosus 122.3
  multilocularis 122.6 *[376.13]*
thyroid NEC 122.9
  granulosus 122.2
  multilocularis 122.6
Echinorhynchiasis 127.7
Echinostomiasis 121.8
Echolalia 784.69
ECHO virus infection NEC 079.1

Eclampsia, eclamptic (coma) (convulsions)
(delirium) 780.39
female, child-bearing age NEC—*see* Eclampsia,
  pregnancy
gravidarum—*see* Eclampsia, pregnancy
male 780.39
not associated with pregnancy or childbirth
  780.39
pregnancy, childbirth or puerperium 642.6
  with pre-existing hypertension 642.7
  affecting fetus or newborn 760.0
uremic 586
Eclipse blindness (total) 363.31
Economic circumstance affecting care V60.9
specified type NEC V60.89
Economo's disease (encephalitis lethargica)
049.8
Ectasia, ectasis
aorta (*see also* Aneurysm, aorta) 441.9
  ruptured 441.5
breast 610.4
capillary 448.9
cornea (marginal) (postinfectional) 371.71
duct (mammary) 610.4
gastric antral vascular (GAVE) 537.82
  with hemorrhage 537.83
  without hemorrhage 537.82
kidney 593.89
mammary duct (gland) 610.4
papillary 448.9
renal 593.89
salivary gland (duct) 527.8
scar, cornea 371.71
sclera 379.11
Ecthyma 686.8
contagiosum 051.2
gangrenosum 686.09
infectiosum 051.2
Ectocardia 746.87
Ectodermal dysplasia, congenital 757.31
Ectodermosis erosiva pluriorificialis 695.19
Ectopic, ectopia (congenital) 759.89
abdominal viscera 751.8
  due to defect in anterior abdominal wall
    756.79
ACTH syndrome 255.0
adrenal gland 759.1
anus 751.5
auricular beats 427.61
beats 427.60
bladder 753.5
bone and cartilage in lung 748.69
brain 742.4
breast tissue 757.6
cardiac 746.87
cerebral 742.4
cordis 746.87
endometrium 617.9
gallbladder 751.69
gastric mucosa 750.7
gestation—*see* Pregnancy, ectopic
heart 746.87
hormone secretion NEC 259.3
hyperparathyroidism 259.3
kidney (crossed) (intrathoracic) (pelvis) 753.3
  in pregnancy or childbirth 654.4
    causing obstructed labor 660.2

Ectopic, ectopia—*continued*
lens 743.37
lentis 743.37
mole—*see* Pregnancy, ectopic
organ or site NEC—*see* Malposition, congenital
ovary 752.0
pancreas, pancreatic tissue 751.7
pregnancy—*see* Pregnancy, ectopic
pupil 364.75
renal 753.3
sebaceous glands of mouth 750.26
secretion
  ACTH 255.0
  adrenal hormone 259.3
  adrenalin 259.3
  adrenocorticotropin 255.0
  antidiuretic hormone (ADH) 259.3
  epinephrine 259.3
  hormone NEC 259.3
  norepinephrine 259.3
  pituitary (posterior) 259.3
spleen 759.0
testis 752.51
thyroid 759.2
ureter 753.4
ventricular beats 427.69
vesicae 753.5
Ectrodactyly 755.4
finger (*see also* Absence, finger, congenital) 755.29
toe (*see also* Absence, toe, congenital) 755.39
Ectromelia 755.4
lower limb 755.30
upper limb 755.20
Ectropion 374.10
anus 569.49
cervix 622.0
  with mention of cervicitis 616.0
cicatricial 374.14
congenital 743.62
eyelid 374.10
  cicatricial 374.14
  congenital 743.62
  mechanical 374.12
  paralytic 374.12
  senile 374.11
  spastic 374.13
iris (pigment epithelium) 364.54
lip (congenital) 750.26
  acquired 528.5
mechanical 374.12
paralytic 374.12
rectum 569.49
senile 374.11
spastic 374.13
urethra 599.84
uvea 364.54
Eczema (acute) (allergic) (chronic)
  (erythematous) (fissum) (occupational)
  (rubrum) (squamous) 692.9
asteatotic 706.8
atopic 691.8
contact NEC 692.9
dermatitis NEC 692.9
due to specified cause—*see* Dermatitis, due to
dyshidrotic 705.81
external ear 380.22
flexural 691.8
gouty 274.89
herpeticum 054.0
hypertrophicum 701.8
hypostatic—*see* Varicose, vein
impetiginous 684

Eczema—*continued*
infantile (acute) (chronic) (due to any substance)
  (intertriginous) (seborrheic) 690.12
intertriginous NEC 692.9
  infantile 690.12
intrinsic 691.8
lichenified NEC 692.9
marginatum 110.3
nummular 692.9
pustular 686.8
seborrheic 690.18
  infantile 690.12
solare 692.72
stasis (lower extremity) 454.1
  ulcerated 454.2
vaccination, vaccinatum 999.0
varicose (lower extremity)—*see* Varicose, vein
verrucosum callosum 698.3
Eczematoid, exudative 691.8
Eddowes' syndrome (brittle bones and blue
  sclera) 756.51
Edema, edematous 782.3
with nephritis (*see also* Nephrosis) 581.9
allergic 995.1
angioneurotic (allergic) (any site) (with
  urticaria) 995.1
  hereditary 277.6
angiospastic 443.9
Berlin's (traumatic) 921.3
brain 348.5
  due to birth injury 767.8
  fetus or newborn 767.8
cardiac (*see also* Failure, heart) 428.0
cardiovascular (*see also* Failure, heart) 428.0
cerebral—*see* Edema, brain
cerebrospinal vessel—*see* Edema, brain
cervix (acute) (uteri) 622.8
  puerperal, postpartum 674.8
chronic hereditary 757.0
circumscribed, acute 995.1
  hereditary 277.6
complicating pregnancy (gestational) 646.1
  with hypertension—*see* Toxemia, of pregnancy
conjunctiva 372.73
connective tissue 782.3
cornea 371.20
  due to contact lenses 371.24
  idiopathic 371.21
  secondary 371.22
due to
  lymphatic obstruction—*see* Edema, lymphatic
  salt retention 276.0
epiglottis—*see* Edema, glottis
essential, acute 995.1
  hereditary 277.6
extremities, lower—*see* Edema, legs
eyelid NEC 374.82
familial, hereditary (legs) 757.0
famine 262
fetus or newborn 778.5
genital organs
  female 629.89
  male 608.86
gestational 646.1
  with hypertension—*see* Toxemia, of pregnancy
glottis, glottic, glottides (obstructive) (passive)
  478.6
  allergic 995.1
    hereditary 277.6
  due to external agent—*see* Condition,
    respiratory, acute, due to specified agent

Edema, edematous—*continued*
　heart (*see also* Failure, heart) 428.0
　　newborn 779.89
　heat 992.7
　hereditary (legs) 757.0
　inanition 262
　infectious 782.3
　intracranial 348.5
　　due to injury at birth 767.8
　iris 364.89
　joint (*see also* Effusion, joint) 719.0
　larynx (*see also* Edema, glottis) 478.6
　legs 782.3
　　due to venous obstruction 459.2
　　hereditary 757.0
　localized 782.3
　　due to venous obstruction 459.2
　　lower extremity 459.2
　lower extremities—*see* Edema, legs
　lungs 514
　　acute 518.4
　　　with heart disease or failure (*see also*
　　　　Failure, ventricular, left) 428.1
　　　　congestive 428.0
　　　chemical (due to fumes or vapors) 506.1
　　　due to
　　　　external agent(s) NEC 508.9
　　　　　specified NEC 508.8
　　　　fumes and vapors (chemical) (inhalation)
　　　　　506.1
　　　　radiation 508.0
　　chemical (acute) 506.1
　　　chronic 506.4
　　chronic 514
　　　chemical (due to fumes or vapors) 506.4
　　　due to
　　　　external agent(s) NEC 508.9
　　　　　specified NEC 508.8
　　　　fumes or vapors (chemical) (inhalation)
　　　　　506.4
　　　　radiation 508.1
　　due to
　　　external agent 508.9
　　　　specified NEC 508.8
　　　high altitude 993.2
　　　near drowning 994.1
　　postoperative 518.4
　　terminal 514
　lymphatic 457.1
　　due to mastectomy operation 457.0
　macula 362.83
　　cystoid 362.53
　　diabetic 250.5 *[362.07]*
　　　due to secondary diabetes 249.5 *[362.07]*
　malignant (*see also* Gangrene, gas) 040.0
　Milroy's 757.0
　nasopharynx 478.25
　neonatorum 778.5
　nutritional (newborn) 262
　　with dyspigmentation, skin and hair 260
　optic disc or nerve—*see* Papilledema
　orbit 376.33
　　circulatory 459.89
　palate (soft) (hard) 528.9
　pancreas 577.8
　penis 607.83
　periodic 995.1
　　hereditary 277.6
　pharynx 478.25
　pitting 782.3
　pulmonary—*see* Edema, lung

Edema, edematous—*continued*
　Quincke's 995.1
　　hereditary 277.6
　renal (*see also* Nephrosis) 581.9
　retina (localized) (macular) (peripheral) 362.83
　　cystoid 362.53
　　diabetic 250.5 *[362.07]*
　　　due to secondary diabetes 249.5 *[362.07]*
　salt 276.0
　scrotum 608.86
　seminal vesicle 608.86
　spermatic cord 608.86
　spinal cord 336.1
　starvation 262
　stasis (*see also* Hypertension, venous) 459.30
　subconjunctival 372.73
　subglottic (*see also* Edema, glottis) 478.6
　supraglottic (*see also* Edema, glottis) 478.6
　testis 608.86
　toxic NEC 782.3
　traumatic NEC 782.3
　tunica vaginalis 608.86
　vas deferens 608.86
　vocal cord—*see* Edema, glottis
　vulva (acute) 624.8
Edentia (complete) (partial) (*see also* Absence,
　tooth) 520.0
　acquired (*see also* Edentulism) 525.40
　　due to
　　　caries 525.13
　　　extraction 525.10
　　　periodontal disease 525.12
　　　specified NEC 525.19
　　　trauma 525.11
　　causing malocclusion 524.30
　congenital (deficiency of tooth buds) 520.0
Edentulism 525.40
　complete 525.40
　　class I 525.41
　　class II 525.42
　　class III 525.43
　　class IV 525.44
　partial 525.50
　　class I 525.51
　　class II 525.52
　　class III 525.53
　　class IV 525.54
Edsall's disease 992.2
Educational handicap V62.3
Edwards' syndrome 758.2
Effect, adverse NEC
　abnormal gravitational (G) forces or states 994.9
　air pressure—*see* Effect, adverse, atmospheric
　　pressure
　altitude (high)—*see* Effect, adverse, high altitude
　anesthetic
　　in labor and delivery NEC 668.9
　　　affecting fetus or newborn 763.5
　antitoxin—*see* Complications, vaccination
　atmospheric pressure 993.9
　　due to explosion 993.4
　　high 993.3
　　low—*see* Effect, adverse, high altitude
　　specified effect NEC 993.8
　biological, correct substance properly
　　administered (*see also* Effect, adverse, drug)
　　995.20
　blood (derivatives) (serum) (transfusion)—*see*
　　Complications, transfusion
　chemical substance NEC 989.9
　　specified—*see* Table of drugs and chemicals

Effect, adverse—*continued*
  cobalt, radioactive (*see also* Effect, adverse,
    radioactive substance) 990
  cold (temperature) (weather) 991.9
    chilblains 991.5
    frostbite—*see* Frostbite
    specified effect NEC 991.8
  drugs and medicinals 995.20
    correct substance properly administered
      995.20
    overdose or wrong substance given or taken
      977.9
      specified drug—*see* Table of drugs and
        chemicals
  electric current (shock) 994.8
    burn—*see* Burn, by site
  electricity (electrocution) (shock) 994.8
    burn—*see* Burn, by site
  exertion (excessive) 994.5
  exposure 994.9
    exhaustion 994.4
  external cause NEC 994.9
  fallout (radioactive) NEC 990
  fluoroscopy NEC 990
  foodstuffs
    allergic reaction (*see also* Allergy, food) 693.1
      anaphylactic shock due to food NEC 995.60
    noxious 988.9
      specified type NEC (*see also* Poisoning, by
        name of noxious foodstuff) 988.8
  gases, fumes, or vapors—*see* Table of drugs and
    chemicals
  glue (airplane) sniffing 304.6
  heat—*see* Heat
  high altitude NEC 993.2
    anoxia 993.2
    on
      fears 993.0
      sinuses 993.1
    polycythemia 289.0
  hot weather—*see* Heat
  hunger 994.2
  immersion, foot 991.4
  immunization—*see* Complications, vaccination
  immunological agents—*see* Complications,
    vaccination
  implantation (removable) of isotope or radium
    NEC 990
  infrared (radiation) (rays) NEC 990
    burn—*see* Burn, by site
    dermatitis or eczema 692.82
  infusion—*see* Complications, infusion
  ingestion or injection of isotope (therapeutic)
    NEC 990
  irradiation NEC (*see also* Effect, adverse,
    radiation) 990
  isotope (radioactive) NEC 990
  lack of care (child) (infant) (newborn) 995.52
    adult 995.84
  lightning 994.0
    burn—*see* Burn, by site
  Lirugin—*see* Complications, vaccination
  medicinal substance, correct, properly
    administered (*see also* Effect, adverse,
    drugs) 995.20
  mesothorium NEC 990
  motion 994.6
  noise, inner ear 388.10
  other drug, medicinal and biological substance
    995.29

Effect, adverse—*continued*
  overheated places—*see* Heat
  polonium NEC 990
  psychosocial, of work environment V62.1
  radiation (diagnostic) (fallout) (infrared) (natural
    source) (therapeutic) (tracer) (ultraviolet)
    (x-ray) NEC 990
    with pulmonary manifestations
      acute 508.0
      chronic 508.1
    dermatitis or eczema 692.82
      due to sun NEC (*see also* Dermatitis, due to,
        sun) 692.70
    fibrosis of lungs 508.1
    maternal with suspected damage to fetus
      affecting management of pregnancy 655.6
    pneumonitis 508.0
  radioactive substance NEC 990
    dermatitis or eczema 692.82
  radioactivity NEC 990
  radiotherapy NEC 990
    dermatitis or eczema 692.82
  radium NEC 990
  reduced temperature 991.9
    frostbite—*see* Frostbite
    immersion, foot (hand) 991.4
    specified effect NEC 991.8
  roentgenography NEC 990
  roentgenoscopy NEC 990
  roentgen rays NEC 990
  serum (prophylactic) (therapeutic) NEC 999.5
  specified NEC 995.89
    external cause NEC 994.9
  strangulation 994.7
  submersion 994.1
  teletherapy NEC 990
  thirst 994.3
  transfusion—*see* Complications, transfusion
  ultraviolet (radiation) (rays) NEC 990
    burn—*see also* Burn, by site
      from sun (*see also* Sunburn) 692.71
    dermatitis or eczema 692.82
      due to sun NEC (*see also* Dermatitis, due to,
        sun) 692.70
  uranium NEC 990
  vaccine (any)—*see* Complications, vaccination
  weightlessness 994.9
  whole blood—*see also* Complications,
    transfusion
    overdose or wrong substance given (*see also*
      Table of drugs and chemicals) 964.7
  working environment V62.1
  x-rays NEC 990
    dermatitis or eczema 692.82
Effect, remote
  of cancer —*see* condition
Effects, late —*see* Late, effect (of)
Effluvium, telogen 704.02
Effort
  intolerance 306.2
  syndrome (aviators) (psychogenic) 306.2
Effusion
  Amniotic fluid (*see also* Rupture, membranes,
    premature) 658.1
  brain (serous) 348.5
  bronchial (*see also* Bronchitis) 490
  cerebral 348.5
  cerebrospinal (*see also* Meningitis) 322.9
    vessel 348.5
  chest—*see* Effusion, pleura
  intracranial 348.5

Effusion—*continued*
  joint 719.00
    ankle 719.07
    elbow 719.02
    foot 719.07
    hand 719.04
    hip 719.05
    knee 719.06
    multiple sites 719.09
    pelvic region 719.05
    shoulder (region) 719.01
    specified site NEC 719.08
    wrist 719.03
  meninges (*see also* Meningitis) 322.9
  pericardium, pericardial (*see also* Pericarditis) 423.9
    acute 420.90
  peritoneal (chronic) 568.82
  pleura, pleurisy, pleuritic, pleuropericardial 511.9
    bacterial, nontuberculous 511.1
    fetus or newborn 511.9
    malignant 511.81
    nontuberculous 511.9
      bacterial 511.1
    pneumococcal 511.1
    staphylococcal 511.1
    streptococcal 511.1
    tuberculous (*see also* Tuberculosis, pleura) 012.0
      primary progressive 010.1
    traumatic 862.29
      with open wound 862.39
  pulmonary—*see* Effusion, pleura
  spinal (*see also* Meningitis) 322.9
  thorax, thoracic—*see* Effusion, pleura
Egg (oocyte) (ovum)
  donor V59.70
    age 35 and over V59.73
      anonymous recipient V59.73
      designated recipient V59.74
    under age 35 V59.71
      anonymous recipient V59.71
      designated recipient V59.72
Eggshell nails 703.8
  congenital 757.5
Ego-dystonic
  homosexuality 302.0
  lesbianism 302.0
  sexual orientation 302.0
Egyptian splenomegaly 120.1
Ehlers-Danlos syndrome 756.83
Ehrlichiosis 082.40
  chaffeensis 082.41
  specified type NEC 082.49
Eichstedt's disease (pityriasis versicolor) 111.0
EIN (endometrial intraepithelial neoplasia) 621.35
Eisenmenger's complex or syndrome
  (ventricular septal defect) 745.4
Ejaculation, semen
  painful 608.89
    psychogenic 306.59
  premature 302.75
  retrograde 608.87
Ekbom syndrome (restless legs) 333.94
Ekman's syndrome (brittle bones and blue
  sclera) 756.51
Elastic skin 756.83
  acquired 701.8
Elastofibroma (M8820/0)—*see* Neoplasm,
  connective tissue, benign
Elastoidosis
  cutanea nodularis 701.8
  cutis cystica et comedonica 701.8

Elastoma 757.39
  juvenile 757.39
  Miescher's (elastosis perforans serpiginosa) 701.1
Elastomyofibrosis 425.3
Elastosis 701.8
  atrophicans 701.8
  perforans serpiginosa 701.1
  reactive perforating 701.1
  senilis 701.8
  solar (actinic) 692.74
Elbow —*see* condition
Electric
  current, electricity, effects (concussion) (fatal)
    (nonfatal) (shock) 994.8
    burn—*see* Burn, by site
  feet (foot) syndrome 266.2
  shock from electroshock gun (taser) 994.8
Electrocution 994.8
Electrolyte imbalance 276.9
  with
    abortion—*see* Abortion, by type, with
      metabolic disorder
    ectopic pregnancy (*see also* categories
      633.0-633.9) 639.4
    hyperemesis gravidarum (before 22 completed
      weeks gestation) 643.1
    molar pregnancy (*see also* categories 630-632)
      639.4
  following
    abortion 639.4
    ectopic or molar pregnancy 639.4
Elephant man syndrome 237.71
Elephantiasis (nonfilarial) 457.1
  arabicum (*see also* Infestation, filarial) 125.9
  congenita hereditaria 757.0
  congenital (any site) 757.0
  due to
    Brugia (malayi) 125.1
    mastectomy operation 457.0
    Wuchereria (bancrofti) 125.0
      malayi 125.1
  eyelid 374.83
  filarial (*see also* Infestation, filarial) 125.9
  filariensis (*see also* Infestation, filarial) 125.9
  gingival 523.8
  glandular 457.1
  graecorum 030.9
  lymphangiectatic 457.1
  lymphatic vessel 457.1
    due to mastectomy operation 457.0
  neuromatosa 237.71
  postmastectomy 457.0
  scrotum 457.1
  streptococcal 457.1
  surgical 997.99
    postmastectomy 457.0
  telangiectodes 457.1
  vulva (nonfilarial) 624.8
Elevated —*see also* Elevation
  findings on laboratory examination — see
    Findings, abnormal, without diagnosis
    (examination) (laboratory test)
  GFR (glomerular filtration rate) — see Findings,
    abnormal, without diagnosis (examination)
    (laboratory test)
Elevation
  17-ketosteroids 791.9
  acid phosphatase 790.5
  alkaline phosphatase 790.5
  amylase 790.5
  antibody titers 795.79

Elevation—*continued*
  basal metabolic rate (BMR) 794.7
  blood pressure (*see also* Hypertension) 401.9
    reading (incidental) (isolated) (nonspecific),
      no diagnosis of hypertension 796.2
  blood sugar 790.29
  body temperature (of unknown origin) (*see also*
    Pyrexia) 780.60
  C-reactive protein (CRP) 790.95
  cancer antigen 125 [CA 125] 795.82
  carcinoembryonic antigen [CEA] 795.81
  cholesterol 272.0
    with high triglycerides 272.2
  conjugate, eye 378.81
  CRP (C-reactive protein) 790.95
  diaphragm, congenital 756.6
  GFR (glomerular filtration rate) — see Findings,
    abnormal, without diagnosis (examination)
    (laboratory test)
  glucose
    fasting 790.21
    tolerance test 790.22
  immunoglobulin level 795.79
  indolacetic acid 791.9
  lactic acid dehydrogenase (LDH) level 790.4
  leukocytes 288.60
  lipase 790.5
  lipoprotein a level 272.8
  liver function test (LFT) 790.6
    alkaline phosphatase 790.5
    aminotransferase 790.4
    bilirubin 782.4
    hepatic enzyme NEC 790.5
    lactate dehydrogenase 790.4
  lymphocytes 288.61
  prostate specific antigen (PSA) 790.93
  renin 790.99
    in hypertension (*see also* Hypertension,
      renovascular) 405.91
  Rh titer 999.7
  scapula, congenital 755.52
  sedimentation rate 790.1
  SGOT 790.4
  SGPT 790.4
  transaminase 790.4
  triglycerides 272.1
    with high cholesterol 272.2
  vanillylmandelic acid 791.9
  venous pressure 459.89
  VMA 791.9
  white blood cell count 288.60
    specified NEC 288.69
Elliptocytosis (congenital) (hereditary) 282.1
  Hb-C (disease) 282.7
  hemoglobin disease 282.7
  sickle-cell (disease) 282.60
    trait 282.5
Ellis-van Creveld disease or syndrome
  (chondroectodermal dysplasia) 756.55
Ellison-Zollinger syndrome (gastric
  hypersecretion with pancreatic islet cell
  tumor) 251.5
Elongation, elongated (congenital)—*see also*
  Distortion
  bone 756.9
  cervix (uteri) 752.49
    acquired 622.6
    hypertrophic 622.6
  colon 751.5
  common bile duct 751.69
  cystic duct 751.69

Elongation, elongated—*continued*
  frenulum, penis 752.69
  labia minora, acquired 624.8
  ligamentum patellae 756.89
  petiolus (epiglottidis) 748.3
  styloid bone (process) 733.99
  tooth, teeth 520.2
  uvula 750.26
    acquired 528.9
Elschnig bodies or pearls 366.51
El Tor cholera 001.1
Emaciation (due to malnutrition) 261
Emancipation disorder 309.22
Embadomoniasis 007.8
Embarrassment heart, cardiac —*see* Disease,
  heart
Embedded tooth, teeth 520.6
  root only 525.3
Embolic —*see* condition
Embolism 444.9
  with
    abortion—*see* Abortion, by type, with
      embolism
    ectopic pregnancy (*see also* categories
      633.0-633.9) 639.6
    molar pregnancy (*see also* categories 630-632)
      639.6
  air (any site) 958.0
    with
      abortion—*see* Abortion, by type, with
        embolism
      ectopic pregnancy (*see also* categories
        633.0-633.9) 639.6
      molar pregnancy (*see also* categories
        630-632) 639.6
    due to implanted device—*see* Complications,
      due to (presence of) any device, implant,
      or graft classified to 996.0-996.5 NEC
    following
      abortion 639.6
      ectopic or molar pregnancy 639.6
      infusion, perfusion, or transfusion 999.1
    in pregnancy, childbirth, or puerperium 673.0
    traumatic 958.0
  amniotic fluid (pulmonary) 673.1
    with
      abortion—*see* Abortion, by type, with
        embolism
      ectopic pregnancy (*see also* categories
        633.0-633.9) 639.6
      molar pregnancy (*see also* categories
        630-632) 639.6
    following
      abortion 639.6
      ectopic or molar pregnancy 639.6
  aorta, aortic 444.1
    abdominal 444.0
    bifurcation 444.0
    saddle 444.0
    thoracic 444.1
  artery 444.9
    auditory, internal 433.8
    basilar (*see also* Occlusion, artery, basilar)
      433.0
    bladder 444.89
    carotid (common) (internal) (*see also*
      Occlusion, artery, carotid) 433.1
    cerebellar (anterior inferior) (posterior
      inferior) (superior) 433.8
    cerebral (*see also* Embolism, brain) 434.1
    choroidal (anterior) 433.8

Embolism—*continued*
  artery—*continued*
    communicating posterior 433.8
    coronary (*see also* Infarct, myocardium) 410.9
      without myocardial infarction 411.81
    extremity 444.22
      lower 444.22
      upper 444.21
    hypophyseal 433.8
    mesenteric (with gangrene) 557.0
    ophthalmic (*see also* Occlusion, retina) 362.30
    peripheral 444.22
    pontine 433.8
    precerebral NEC—*see* Occlusion, artery,
      precerebral
    pulmonary—*see* Embolism, pulmonary
    pyemic 449
      pulmonary 415.12
    renal 593.81
    retinal (*see also* Occlusion, retina) 362.30
    septic 449
      pulmonary 415.12
    specified site NEC 444.89
    vertebral (*see also* Occlusion, artery,
      vertebral) 433.2
  auditory, internal 433.8
  basilar (artery) (*see also* Occlusion, artery,
    basilar) 433.0
  birth, mother—*see* Embolism, obstetrical
  blood-clot
    with
      abortion—*see* Abortion, by type, with embolism
      ectopic pregnancy (*see also* categories
        633.0-633.9) 639.6
      molar pregnancy (*see also* categories
        630-632) 639.6
    following
      abortion 639.6
      ectopic or molar pregnancy 639.6
    in pregnancy, childbirth, or puerperium 673.2
  brain 434.1
    with
      abortion—*see* Abortion, by type, with embolism
      ectopic pregnancy (*see also* categories
        633.0-633.9) 639.6
      molar pregnancy (*see also* categories
        630-632) 639.6
    following
      abortion 639.6
      ectopic or molar pregnancy 639.6
    late effect—*see* Late effect(s) (of)
      cerebrovascular disease
    puerperal, postpartum, childbirth 674.0
  capillary 448.9
  cardiac (*see also* Infarct, myocardium) 410.9
  carotid (artery) (common) (internal) (*see also*
    Occlusion, artery, carotid) 433.1
  cavernous sinus (venous)—*see* Embolism,
    intracranial venous sinus
  cerebral (*see also* Embolism, brain) 434.1
  cholesterol—*see* Atheroembolism
  choroidal (anterior) (artery) 433.8
  coronary (artery or vein) (systemic) (*see also*
    Infarct, myocardium) 410.9
    without myocardial infarction 411.81
  due to (presence of) any device, implant, or graft
    classifiable to 996.0-996.5 —*see*
    Complications, due to (presence of) any
    device, implant, or graft classified to
    996.0-996.5 NEC
  encephalomalacia (*see also* Embolism, brain) 434.1

Embolism—*continued*
  extremities 444.22
    lower 444.22
    upper 444.21
  eye 362.30
  fat (cerebral) (pulmonary) (systemic) 958.1
    with
      abortion—*see* Abortion, by type, with embolism
      ectopic pregnancy (*see also* categories
        633.0-633.9) 639.6
      molar pregnancy (*see also* categories
        630-632) 639.6
    complicating delivery or puerperium 673.8
    following
      abortion 639.6
      ectopic or molar pregnancy 639.6
    in pregnancy, childbirth, or the puerperium 673.8
  femoral (artery) 444.22
    vein 453.6
      deep 453.41
  following
    abortion 639.6
    ectopic or molar pregnancy 639.6
    infusion, perfusion, or transfusion
      air 999.1
      thrombus 999.2
  heart (fatty) (*see also* Infarct, myocardium) 410.9
  hepatic (vein) 453.0
  iliac (artery) 444.81
  iliofemoral 444.81
  in pregnancy, childbirth, or puerperium
    (pulmonary)—*see* Embolism, obstetrical
  intestine (artery) (vein) (with gangrene) 557.0
  intracranial (*see also* Embolism, brain) 434.1
    venous sinus (any) 325
      late effect—*see* category 326
      nonpyogenic 437.6
        in pregnancy or puerperium 671.5
  kidney (artery) 593.81
  lateral sinus (venous)—*see* Embolism,
    intracranial venous sinus
  longitudinal sinus (venous)—*see* Embolism,
    intracranial venous sinus
  lower extremity 444.22
  lung (massive)—*see* Embolism, pulmonary
  meninges (*see also* Embolism, brain) 434.1
  mesenteric (artery) (with gangrene) 557.0
  multiple NEC 444.9
  obstetrical (pulmonary) 673.2
    air 673.0
    amniotic fluid (pulmonary) 673.1
    blood-clot 673.2
    cardiac 674.8
    fat 673.8
    heart 674.8
    pyemic 673.3
    septic 673.3
    specified NEC 674.8
  ophthalmic (*see also* Occlusion, retina) 362.30
  paradoxical NEC 444.9
  penis 607.82
  peripheral arteries NEC 444.22
    lower 444.22
    upper 444.21
  pituitary 253.8
  popliteal (artery) 444.22
  portal (vein) 452

Embolism—*continued*
  postoperative NEC 997.2
    cerebral 997.02
    mesenteric artery 997.71
    other vessels 997.79
    peripheral vascular 997.2
    pulmonary 415.11
      septic 415.11
    renal artery 997.72
  precerebral artery (*see also* Occlusion, artery,
    precerebral) 433.9
  puerperal—*see* Embolism, obstetrical
  pulmonary (acute) (artery) (vein) 415.19
    with
      abortion—*see* Abortion, by type, with
        embolism
      ectopic pregnancy (*see also* categories
        633.0-633.9) 639.6
      molar pregnancy (*see also* categories
        630-632) 639.6
    chronic 416.2
    following
      abortion 639.6
      ectopic or molar pregnancy 639.6
    healed or old V12.51
    iatrogenic 415.11
    in pregnancy, childbirth, or puerperium—*see*
      Embolism, obstetrical
    personal history of V12.51
    postoperative 415.11
    septic 415.12
  pyemic (multiple) (*see also* Septicemia) 415.12
    with
      abortion—*see* Abortion, by type, with embolism
      ectopic pregnancy (*see also* categories
        633.0-633.9) 639.6
      molar pregnancy (*see also* categories
        630-632) 639.6
    Aerobacter aerogenes 415.12
    enteric gram-negative bacilli 415.12
    Enterobacter aerogenes 415.12
    Escherichia coli 415.12
    following
      abortion 639.6
      ectopic or molar pregnancy 639.6
    Hemophilus influenzae 415.12
    pneumococcal 415.12
    Proteus vulgaris 415.12
    Pseudomonas (aeruginosa) 415.12
    puerperal, postpartum, childbirth (any
      organism) 673.3
    Serratia 415.12
    specified organism NEC 415.12
    staphylococcal 415.12
      aureus 415.12
      specified organism NEC 415.12
    streptococcal 415.12
  renal (artery) 593.81
    vein 453.3
  retina, retinal (*see also* Occlusion, retina) 362.30
  saddle (aorta) 444.0
  septic 415.12
    arterial 449
  septicemic—*see* Embolism, pyemic
  sinus—*see* Embolism, intracranial venous sinus

Embolism—*continued*
  soap
    with
      abortion—*see* Abortion, by type, with embolism
      ectopic pregnancy (*see also* categories
        633.0-633.9) 639.6
      molar pregnancy (*see also* categories
        630-632) 639.6
    following
      abortion 639.6
      ectopic or molar pregnancy 639.6
  spinal cord (nonpyogenic) 336.1
    in pregnancy or puerperium 671.5
    pyogenic origin 324.1
      late effect—*see* category 326
  spleen, splenic (artery) 444.89
  thrombus (thromboembolism) following
    infusion, perfusion, or transfusion 999.2
  upper extremity 444.21
  vein 453.9
    with inflammation or phlebitis—*see*
      Thrombophlebitis
    antecubital
      acute 453.81
      chronic 453.71
    axillary
      acute 453.84
      chronic 453.74
    basilic
      acute 453.81
      chronic 453.71
    brachial
      acute 453.82
      chronic 453.72
    brachiocephalic (innominate)
      acute 453.87
      chronic 453.77
    cephalic
      acute 453.81
      chronic 453.71
    cerebral (*see also* Embolism, brain) 434.1
    coronary (*see also* Infarct, myocardium) 410.9
      without myocardial infarction 411.81
    hepatic 453.0
    internal jugular
      acute 453.86
      chronic 453.76
    lower extremity (superficial) 453.6
      deep 453.40
        acute 453.40
          calf 453.42
          distal (lower leg) 453.42
          femoral 453.41
          iliac 453.41
          lower leg 453.42
          peroneal 453.42
          popliteal 453.41
          proximal (upper leg) 453.41
          thigh 453.41
          tibial 453.42
        chronic 453.50
          calf 453.52
          distal (lower leg) 453.52
          femoral 453.51
          iliac 453.51
          lower leg 453.52
          peroneal 453.52
          popliteal 453.51
          proximal (upper leg) 453.51
          thigh 453.51
          tibial 453.52

Embolism—*continued*
vein—*continued*
lower extremity—*continued*
saphenous (greater) (lesser) 453.6
superficial 453.6
mesenteric (with gangrene) 557.0
portal 452
pulmonary—*see* Embolism, pulmonary
radial
acute 453.82
chronic 453.72
renal 453.3
saphenous (greater) (lesser) 453.6
specified NEC (acute) 453.89
chronic 453.79
with inflammation or phlebitis—*see*
Thrombophlebitis
subclavian
acute 453.85
chronic 453.75
superior vena cava
acute 453.87
chronic 453.77
thoracic
acute 453.87
chronic 453.77
ulnar
acute 453.82
chronic 453.72
upper extremity 453.83
acute 453.83
deep 453.82
superficial 453.81
chronic 453.73
deep 453.72
superficial 453.71
vena cava
inferior 453.2
superior
acute 453.87
chronic 453.77
vessels of brain (*see also* Embolism, brain)
434.1
Embolization —*see* Embolism
Embolus —*see* Embolism
Embryoma (M9080/1)—*see also* Neoplasm, by
site, uncertain behavior
benign (M9080/0)—*see* Neoplasm, by site, benign
kidney (M8960/3) 189.0
liver (M8970/3) 155.0
malignant (M9080/3)—*see also* Neoplasm, by
site, malignant
kidney (M8960/3) 189.0
liver (M8970/3) 155.0
testis (M9070/3) 186.9
undescended 186.0
testis (M9070/3) 186.9
undescended 186.0
Embryonic
circulation 747.9
heart 747.9
vas deferens 752.89
Embryopathia NEC 759.9
Embryotomy, fetal 763.89
Embryotoxon 743.43
interfering with vision 743.42
Emesis —*see also* Vomiting
bilious 787.04
gravidarum—*see* Hyperemesis, gravidarum
Emissions, nocturnal (semen) 608.89

Emotional
crisis—*see* Crisis, emotional
disorder (*see also* Disorder, mental) 300.9
instability (excessive) 301.3
lability 799.24
overlay—*see* Reaction, adjustment
upset 300.9
Emotionality, pathological 301.3
Emotogenic disease (*see also* Disorder,
psychogenic) 306.9
Emphysema (atrophic) (centriacinar)
(centrilobular) (chronic) (diffuse) (essential)
(hypertrophic) (interlobular) (lung)
(obstructive) (panlobular) (paracicatricial)
(paracinar) (postural) (pulmonary) (senile)
(subpleural) (traction) (unilateral) (unilobular)
(vesicular) 492.8
with bronchitis
chronic 491.20
with
acute bronchitis 491.22
exacerbation (acute) 491.21
bullous (giant) 492.0
cellular tissue 958.7
surgical 998.81
compensatory 518.2
congenital 770.2
conjunctiva 372.89
connective tissue 958.7
surgical 998.81
due to fumes or vapors 506.4
eye 376.89
eyelid 374.85
surgical 998.81
traumatic 958.7
fetus or newborn (interstitial) (mediastinal)
(unilobular) 770.2
heart 416.9
interstitial 518.1
congenital 770.2
fetus or newborn 770.2
laminated tissue 958.7
surgical 998.81
mediastinal 518.1
fetus or newborn 770.2
newborn (interstitial) (mediastinal) (unilobular)
770.2
obstructive diffuse with fibrosis 492.8
orbit 376.89
subcutaneous 958.7
due to trauma 958.7
nontraumatic 518.1
surgical 998.81
surgical 998.81
thymus (gland) (congenital) 254.8
traumatic 958.7
tuberculous (*see also* Tuberculosis, pulmonary)
011.9
Employment examination (certification) V70.5
Empty sella (turcica) syndrome 253.8
Empyema (chest) (diaphragmatic) (double)
(encapsulated) (general) (interlobar) (lung)
(medial) (necessitatis) (perforating chest wall)
(pleura) (pneumococcal) (residual) (sacculated)
(streptococcal) (supradiaphragmatic) 510.9
with fistula 510.0
accessory sinus (chronic) (*see also* Sinusitis) 473.9
acute 510.9
with fistula 510.0
antrum (chronic) (*see also* Sinusitis, maxillary)
473.0

Empyema—*continued*
  brain (any part) (*see also* Abscess, brain) 324.0
  ethmoidal (sinus) (chronic) (*see also* Sinusitis,
      ethmoidal) 473.2
  extradural (*see also* Abscess, extradural) 324.9
  frontal (sinus) (chronic) (*see also* Sinusitis,
      frontal) 473.1
  gallbladder (*see also* Cholecystitis, acute) 575.0
  mastoid (process) (acute) (*see also* Mastoiditis,
      acute) 383.00
  maxilla, maxillary 526.4
    sinus (chronic) (*see also* Sinusitis, maxillary)
      473.0
  nasal sinus (chronic) (*see also* Sinusitis) 473.9
  sinus (accessory) (nasal) (*see also* Sinusitis) 473.9
  sphenoidal (chronic) (sinus) (*see also* Sinusitis,
      sphenoidal) 473.3
  subarachnoid (*see also* Abscess, extradural) 324.9
  subdural (*see also* Abscess, extradural) 324.9
  tuberculous (*see also* Tuberculosis, pleura) 012.0
  ureter (*see also* Ureteritis) 593.89
  ventricular (*see also* Abscess, brain) 324.0
Enameloma 520.2
Encephalitis (bacterial) (chronic) (hemorrhagic)
      (idiopathic) (nonepidemic) (spurious)
      (subacute) 323.9
  acute—*see also* Encephalitis, viral
    disseminated (postinfectious) NEC 136.9 *[323.61]*
      postimmunization or postvaccination 323.51
    inclusional 049.8
    inclusion body 049.8
    necrotizing 049.8
  arboviral, arbovirus NEC 064
  arthropod-borne (*see also* Encephalitis, viral,
      arthropod-borne) 064
  Australian X 062.4
  Bwamba fever 066.3
  California (virus) 062.5
  Central European 063.2
  Czechoslovakian 063.2
  Dawson's (inclusion body) 046.2
  diffuse sclerosing 046.2
  due to
    actinomycosis 039.8 *[323.41]*
    cat-scratch disease 078.3 *[323.01]*
    human herpesvirus 6 058.21
    human herpesvirus 7 058.29
    human herpesvirus NEC 058.29
    infection classified elsewhere 136.9 *[323.41]*
    infectious mononucleosis 075 *[323.01]*
    malaria (*see also* Malaria) 084.6 *[323.2]*
    Negishi virus 064
    ornithosis 073.7 *[323.01]*
    prophylactic inoculation against smallpox 323.51
    rickettsiosis (*see also* Rickettsiosis) 083.9
      [323.1]
    rubella 056.01
    toxoplasmosis (acquired) 130.0
      congenital (active) 771.2 *[323.41]*
    typhus (fever) (*see also* Typhus) 081.9 *[323.1]*
    vaccination (smallpox) 323.51
  Eastern equine 062.2
  endemic 049.8
  epidemic 049.8
  equine (acute) (infectious) (viral) 062.9
    Eastern 062.2
    Venezuelan 066.2
    Western 062.1
  Far Eastern 063.0
  following vaccination or other immunization
      procedure 323.51

Encephalitis—*continued*
  herpes 054.3
  human herpesvirus 6 058.21
  human herpesvirus 7 058.29
  human herpesvirus NEC 058.29
  Ilheus (virus) 062.8
  inclusion body 046.2
  infectious (acute) (virus) NEC 049.8
  influenza 487.8 *[323.41]*
    lethargic 049.8
  Japanese (B type) 062.0
  La Crosse 062.5
  Langat 063.8
  late effect—*see* Late, effect, encephalitis
  lead 984.9 *[323.71]*
  lethargic (acute) (infectious) (influenzal) 049.8
  lethargica 049.8
  louping ill 063.1
  lupus 710.0 *[323.81]*
  lymphatica 049.0
  Mengo 049.8
  meningococcal 036.1
  mumps 072.2
  Murray Valley 062.4
  myoclonic 049.8
  Negishi virus 064
  otitic NEC 382.4 *[323.41]*
  parasitic NEC 123.9 *[323.41]*
  periaxialis (concentrica) (diffusa) 341.1
  postchickenpox 052.0
  postexanthematous NEC 057.9 *[323.62]*
  postimmunization 323.51
  postinfectious NEC 136.9 *[323.62]*
  postmeasles 055.0
  posttraumatic 323.81
  postvaccinal (smallpox) 323.51
  postvaricella 052.0
  postviral NEC 079.99 *[323.62]*
    postexanthematous 057.9 *[323.62]*
      specified NEC 057.8 *[323.62]*
  Powassan 063.8
  progressive subcortical (Binswanger's) 290.12
  Rasmussen 323.81
  Rio Bravo 049.8
  rubella 056.01
  Russian
    autumnal 062.0
    spring-summer type (taiga) 063.0
  saturnine 984.9 *[323.71]*
  Semliki Forest 062.8
  serous 048
  slow-acting virus NEC 046.8
  specified cause NEC 323.81
  St. Louis type 062.3
  subacute sclerosing 046.2
  subcorticalis chronica 290.12
  summer 062.0
  suppurative 324.0
  syphilitic 094.81
    congenital 090.41
  tick-borne 063.9
  torula, torular 117.5 *[323.41]*
  toxic NEC 989.9 *[323.71]*
  toxoplasmic (acquired) 130.0
    congenital (active) 771.2 *[323.41]*
  trichinosis 124 *[323.41]*
  Trypanosomiasis (*see also* Trypanosomiasis)
      086.9 *[323.2]*
  tuberculous (*see also* Tuberculosis) 013.6
  type B (Japanese) 062.0
  type C 062.3
  van Bogaert's 046.2

Encephalitis—*continued*
  Venezuelan 066.2
  Vienna type 049.8
  viral, virus 049.9
    arthropod-borne NEC 064
      mosquito-borne 062.9
        Australian X disease 062.4
        California virus 062.5
        Eastern equine 062.2
        Ilheus virus 062.8
        Japanese (B type) 062.0
        Murray Valley 062.4
        specified type NEC 062.8
        St. Louis 062.3
        type B 062.0
        type C 062.3
        Western equine 062.1
      tick-borne 063.9
        biundulant 063.2
        Central European 063.2
        Czechoslovakian 063.2
        diphasic meningoencephalitis 063.2
        Far Eastern 063.0
        Langat 063.8
        louping ill 063.1
        Powassan 063.8
        Russian spring-summer (taiga) 063.0
        specified type NEC 063.8
        vector unknown 064
    slow acting NEC 046.8
    specified type NEC 049.8
    vaccination, prophylactic (against) V05.0
  von Economo's 049.8
  Western equine 062.1
  West Nile type 066.41
Encephalocele 742.0
  orbit 376.81
Encephalocystocele 742.0
Encephalomalacia (brain) (cerebellar) (cerebral)
  (cerebrospinal) (*see also* Softening, brain)
  434.9
  due to
    hemorrhage (*see also* Hemorrhage, brain) 431
    recurrent spasm of artery 435.9
  embolic (cerebral) (*see also* Embolism, brain)
    434.1
  subcorticalis chronicus arteriosclerotica 290.12
  thrombotic (*see also* Thrombosis, brain) 434.0
Encephalomeningitis —*see* Meningoencephalitis
Encephalomeningocele 742.0
Encephalomeningomyelitis —*see*
  Meningoencephalitis
Encephalomeningopathy (*see also*
  Meningoencephalitis) 349.9
Encephalomyelitis (chronic) (granulomatous)
  (myalgic, benign) (*see also* Encephalitis)
  323.9
  abortive disseminated 049.8
  acute disseminated (ADEM) (postinfectious)
    136.9 *[323.61]*
    infectious 136.9 *[323.61]*
    noninfectious 323.81
    postimmunization 323.51
  due to
    cat-scratch disease 078.3 *[323.01]*
    infectious mononucleosis 075 *[323.01]*
    ornithosis 073.7 *[323.01]*
    vaccination (any) 323.51
  equine (acute) (infectious) 062.9
    Eastern 062.2
    Venezuelan 066.2
    Western 062.1

Encephalomyelitis—*continued*
  funicularis infectiosa 049.8
  late effect—*see* Late, effect, encephalitis
  Munch-Peterson's 049.8
  postchickenpox 052.0
  postimmunization 323.51
  postmeasles 055.0
  postvaccinal (smallpox) 323.51
  rubella 056.01
  specified cause NEC 323.81
  syphilitic 094.81
  West Nile 066.41
Encephalomyelocele 742.0
Encephalomyelomeningitis —*see*
  Meningoencephalitis
Encephalomyeloneuropathy 349.9
Encephalomyelopathy 349.9
  subacute necrotizing (infantile) 330.8
Encephalomyeloradiculitis (acute) 357.0
Encephalomyeloradiculoneuritis (acute) 357.0
Encephalomyeloradiculopathy 349.9
Encephalomyocarditis 074.23
Encephalopathia hyperbilirubinemica
  newborn 774.7
  due to isoimmunization (conditions classifiable
    to 773.0-773.2) 773.4
Encephalopathy (acute) 348.30
  alcoholic 291.2
  anoxic—*see* Damage, brain, anoxic
  arteriosclerotic 437.0
    late effect—*see* Late effect(s) (of)
      cerebrovascular disease
  bilirubin, newborn 774.7
    due to isoimmunization 773.4
  congenital 742.9
  demyelinating (callosal) 341.8
  due to
    birth injury (intracranial) 767.8
    dialysis 294.8
      transient 293.9
    drugs (—see also Table of Drugs and
      Chemicals) 348.39
    hyperinsulinism—*see* Hyperinsulinism
    influenza (virus) 487.8
    lack of vitamin (*see also* Deficiency, vitamin)
      269.2
    nicotinic acid deficiency 291.2
    serum (nontherapeutic) (therapeutic) 999.5
    syphilis 094.81
    trauma (postconcussional) 310.2
      current (*see also* Concussion, brain) 850.9
        with skull fracture—*see* Fracture, skull, by
          site, with intracranial injury
    vaccination 323.51
  hepatic 572.2
  hyperbilirubinemic, newborn 774.7
    due to isoimmunization (conditions
      classifiable to 773.0-773.2) 773.4
  hypertensive 437.2
  hypoglycemic 251.2
  hypoxic—*see also* Damage, brain, anoxic
    ischemic (HIE) 768.70
      mild 768.71
      moderate 768.72
      severe 768.73
  infantile cystic necrotizing (congenital) 341.8
  lead 984.9 *[323.71]*
  leukopolio 330.0
  metabolic (*see also* Delirium) 348.31
    toxic 349.82

Encephalopathy—*continued*
  necrotizing
    hemorrhagic (acute) 323.61
    subacute 330.8
  other specified type NEC 348.39
  pellagrous 265.2
  portal-systemic 572.2
  postcontusional 310.2
  posttraumatic 310.2
  saturnine 984.9 *[323.71]*
  septic 348.31
  spongioform, subacute (viral) 046.19
  subacute
    necrotizing 330.8
    spongioform 046.19
    viral, spongioform 046.19
  subcortical progressive (Schilder) 341.1
    chronic (Binswanger's) 290.12
  toxic 349.82
    metabolic 349.82
  traumatic (postconcussional) 310.2
    current (*see also* Concussion, brain) 850.9
      with skull fracture—*see* Fracture, skull, by
        site, with intracranial injury
  vitamin B deficiency NEC 266.9
  Wernicke's (superior hemorrhagic
    polioencephalitis) 265.1
Enchephalorrhagia (*see also* Hemorrhage,
  brain) 432.9
  healed or old V12.54
  late effect—*see* Late effect(s) (of)
    cerebrovascular disease
Encephalosis, posttraumatic 310.2
Enchondroma (M9220/0)—*see also* Neoplasm,
  bone, benign
  multiple, congenital 756.4
Enchondromatosis (cartilaginous) (congenital)
  (multiple) 756.4
Enchondroses, multiple (cartilaginous)
  (congenital) 756.4
Encopresis (*see also* Incontinence, feces) 787.6
  nonorganic origin 307.7
Encounter for —*see also* Admission for
  administrative purpose only V68.9
    referral of patient without examination or
      treatment V68.81
    specified purpose NEC V68.89
  chemotherapy, (oral) (intravenous)
    antineoplastic V58.11
  disability examination V68.01
  end-of-life care V66.7
  hospice care V66.7
  immunizations (childhood) appropriate for age
    V20.2
  immunotherapy, antineoplastic V58.12
  palliative care V66.7
  radiotherapy V58.0
  respirator (ventilator) dependence
    during
      mechanical failure V46.14
      power failure V46.12
    for weaning V46.13
  routine infant and child vision and hearing
    testing V20.2
  school examination V70.3
    following surgery V67.09
  screening mammogram NEC V76.12
    for high-risk patient V76.11
  paternity testing V70.4
  terminal care V66.7
  weaning from respirator (ventilator) V46.13
Encystment —*see* Cyst

End-of-life care V66.7
Endamebiasis —*see* Amebiasis
Endamoeba —*see* Amebiasis
Endarteritis (bacterial, subacute) (infective)
  (septic) 447.6
  brain, cerebral or cerebrospinal 437.4
    late effect—*see* Late effect(s) (of)
      cerebrovascular disease
  coronary (artery) —*see* Arteriosclerosis,
    coronary
  deformans—*see* Arteriosclerosis
  embolic (*see also* Embolism) 444.9
  obliterans—*see also* Arteriosclerosis
    pulmonary 417.8
  pulmonary 417.8
  retina 362.18
  senile—*see* Arteriosclerosis
  syphilitic 093.89
    brain or cerebral 094.89
    congenital 090.5
    spinal 094.89
  tuberculous (*see also* Tuberculosis) 017.9
Endemic —*see* condition
Endocarditis (chronic) (indeterminate)
  (interstitial) (marantic) (nonbacterial
  thrombotic) (residual) (sclerotic) (sclerous)
  (senile) (valvular) 424.90
  with
    rheumatic fever (conditions classifiable to
      390)
      active—*see* Endocarditis, acute, rheumatic
      inactive or quiescent (with chorea) 397.9
  acute or subacute 421.9
    rheumatic (aortic) (mitral) (pulmonary)
      (tricuspid) 391.1
      with chorea (acute) (rheumatic)
        (Sydenham's) 392.0
  aortic (heart) (nonrheumatic) (valve) 424.1
    with
      mitral (valve) disease 396.9
        active or acute 391.1
          with chorea (acute) (rheumatic)
            (Sydenham's) 392.0
      rheumatic fever (conditions classifiable to
        390)
        active—*see* Endocarditis, acute, rheumatic
        inactive or quiescent (with chorea) 395.9
          with mitral disease 396.9
    acute or subacute 421.9
    arteriosclerotic 424.1
    congenital 746.89
    hypertensive 424.1
    rheumatic (chronic) (inactive) 395.9
      with mitral (valve) disease 396.9
        active or acute 391.1
          with chorea (acute) (rheumatic)
            (Sydenham's) 392.0
      active or acute 391.1
        with chorea (acute) (rheumatic)
          (Sydenham's) 392.0
    specified cause, except rheumatic 424.1
    syphilitic 093.22
  arteriosclerotic or due to arteriosclerosis 424.99
  atypical verrucous (Libman-Sacks) 710.0
    [424.91]
  bacterial (acute) (any valve) (chronic) (subacute)
    421.0
  blastomycotic 116.0 *[421.1]*
  candidal 112.81
  congenital 425.3
  constrictive 421.0

Endocarditis—*continued*
Coxsackie 074.22
due to
blastomycosis 116.0 *[421.1]*
candidiasis 112.81
Coxsackie (virus) 074.22
disseminated lupus erythematosus 710.0
[424.91]
histoplasmosis (*see also* Histoplasmosis) 115.94
hypertension (benign) 424.99
moniliasis 112.81
prosthetic cardiac valve 996.61
Q fever 083.0 *[421.1]*
serratia marcescens 421.0
typhoid (fever) 002.0 *[421.1]*
fetal 425.3
gonococcal 098.84
hypertensive 424.99
infectious or infective (acute) (any valve)
(chronic) (subacute) 421.0
lenta (acute) (any valve) (chronic) (subacute)
421.0
Libman-Sacks 710.0 *[424.91]*
Loeffler's (parietal fibroplastic) 421.0
malignant (acute) (any valve) (chronic)
(subacute) 421.0
meningococcal 036.42
mitral (chronic) (double) (fibroid) (heart)
(inactive) (valve) (with chorea) 394.9
with
aortic (valve) disease 396.9
active or acute 391.1
with chorea (acute) (rheumatic)
(Sydenham's) 392.0
rheumatic fever (conditions classifiable to
390)
active—*see* Endocarditis, acute, rheumatic
inactive or quiescent (with chorea) 394.9
with aortic valve disease 396.9
active or acute 391.1
bacterial 421.0
with chorea (acute) (rheumatic)
(Sydenham's) 392.0
arteriosclerotic 424.0
congenital 746.89
hypertensive 424.0
nonrheumatic 424.0
acute or subacute 421.9
syphilitic 093.21
monilial 112.81
mycotic (acute) (any valve) (chronic) (subacute)
421.0
pneumococcic (acute) (any valve) (chronic)
(subacute) 421.0
pulmonary (chronic) (heart) (valve) 424.3
with
rheumatic fever (conditions classifiable to
390)
active—*see* Endocarditis, acute, rheumatic
inactive or quiescent (with chorea) 397.1
acute or subacute 421.9
rheumatic 391.1
with chorea (acute) (rheumatic)
(Sydenham's) 392.0
arteriosclerotic or due to arteriosclerosis 424.3
congenital 746.09
hypertensive or due to hypertension (benign)
424.3

Endocarditis—*continued*
pulmonary—*continued*
rheumatic (chronic) (inactive) (with chorea)
397.1
active or acute 391.1
with chorea (acute) (rheumatic)
(Sydenham's) 392.0
syphilitic 093.24
purulent (acute) (any valve) (chronic) (subacute)
421.0
rheumatic (chronic) (inactive) (with chorea)
397.9
active or acute (aortic) (mitral) (pulmonary)
(tricuspid) 391.1
with chorea (acute) (rheumatic)
(Sydenham's) 392.0
septic (acute) (any valve) (chronic) (subacute)
421.0
specified cause, except rheumatic 424.99
streptococcal (acute) (any valve) (chronic)
(subacute) 421.0
subacute—*see* Endocarditis, acute
suppurative (any valve) (acute) (chronic)
(subacute) 421.0
syphilitic NEC 093.20
toxic (*see also* Endocarditis, acute) 421.9
tricuspid (chronic) (heart) (inactive) (rheumatic)
(valve) (with chorea) 397.0
with
rheumatic fever (conditions classifiable to
390)
active—*see* Endocarditis, acute, rheumatic
inactive or quiescent (with chorea) 397.0
active or acute 391.1
with chorea (acute) (rheumatic)
(Sydenham's) 392.0
arteriosclerotic 424.2
congenital 746.89
hypertensive 424.2
nonrheumatic 424.2
acute or subacute 421.9
specified cause, except rheumatic 424.2
syphilitic 093.23
tuberculous (*see also* Tuberculosis) 017.9
[424.91]
typhoid 002.0 *[421.1]*
ulcerative (acute) (any valve) (chronic)
(subacute) 421.0
vegetative (acute) (any valve) (chronic)
(subacute) 421.0
verrucous (acute) (any valve) (chronic)
(subacute) NEC 710.0 *[424.91]*
nonbacterial 710.0 *[424.91]*
nonrheumatic 710.0 *[424.91]*
Endocardium, endocardial —*see also* condition
cushion defect 745.60
specified type NEC 745.69
Endocervicitis (*see also* Cervicitis) 616.0
due to
intrauterine (contraceptive) device 996.65
gonorrheal (acute) 098.15
chronic or duration of 2 months or over 098.35
hyperplastic 616.0
syphilitic 095.8
trichomonal 131.09
tuberculous (*see also* Tuberculosis) 016.7
Endocrine —*see* condition
Endocrinopathy, pluriglandular 258.9
Endodontitis 522.0
Endomastoiditis (*see also* Mastoiditis) 383.9
Endometrioma 617.9

Enlargement, enlarged—*continued*
  sella turcica 793.0
  spleen (*see also* Splenomegaly) 789.2
    congenital 759.0
  thymus (congenital) (gland) 254.0
  thyroid (gland) (*see also* Goiter) 240.9
  tongue 529.8
  tonsils 474.11
    and adenoids 474.10
  uterus 621.2
Enophthalmos 376.50
  due to
    atrophy of orbital tissue 376.51
    surgery 376.52
    trauma 376.52
Enostosis 526.89
Entamebiasis —*see* Amebiasis
Entamebic —*see* Amebiasis
Entanglement, umbilical cord (s) 663.3
  with compression 663.2
  affecting fetus or newborn 762.5
  around neck with compression 663.1
  twins in monoamniotic sac 663.2
Enteralgia 789.0
Enteric —*see* condition
Enteritis (acute) (catarrhal) (choleraic) (chronic)
    (congestive) (diarrheal) (exudative) (follicular)
    (hemorrhagic) (infantile) (lienteric)
    (noninfectious) (perforative) (phlegmonous)
    (presumed noninfectious)
    (pseudomembranous) 558.9
  adaptive 564.9
  aertrycke infection 003.0
  allergic 558.3
  amebic (*see also* Amebiasis) 006.9
    with abscess—*see* Abscess, amebic
    acute 006.0
      with abscess—*see* Abscess, amebic
      nondysenteric 006.2
    chronic 006.1
      with abscess—*see* Abscess, amebic
      nondysenteric 006.2
    nondysenteric 006.2
  anaerobic (cocci) (gram-negative)
    (gram-positive) (mixed) NEC 008.46
  bacillary NEC 004.9
  bacterial NEC 008.5
    specified NEC 008.49
  Bacteroides (fragilis) (melaninogeniscus)
    (oralis) 008.46
  Butyrivibrio (fibriosolvens) 008.46
  Campylobacter 008.43
  Candida 112.85
  Chilomastix 007.8
  choleriformis 001.1
  chronic 558.9
    ulcerative (*see also* Colitis, ulcerative) 556.9
  cicatrizing (chronic) 555.0
  Clostridium
    botulinum 005.1
    difficile 008.45
    haemolyticum 008.46
    novyi 008.46
    perfringens (C) (F) 008.46
    specified type NEC 008.46
  coccidial 007.2
  dietetic 558.9

Enteritis—*continued*
  due to
    achylia gastrica 536.8
    adenovirus 008.62
    Aerobacter aerogenes 008.2
    anaerobes—*see* Enteritis, anaerobic 008.46
    Arizona (bacillus) 008.1
    astrovirus 008.66
    Bacillus coli—*see* Enteritis, E. coli 008.0
    bacteria NEC 008.5
      specified NEC 008.49
    Bacteroides 008.46
    Butyrivibrio (fibriosolvens) 008.46
    calicivirus 008.65
    Campylobacter 008.43
    Clostridium—*see* Enteritis, Clostridium
    Cockle agent 008.64
    Coxsackie (virus) 008.67
    Ditchling agent 008.64
    ECHO virus 008.67
    Enterobacter aerogenes 008.2
    enterococci 008.49
    enterovirus NEC 008.67
    Escherichia coli—*see* Enteritis, E. coli
    Eubacterium 008.46
    Fusobacterium (nucleatum) 008.46
    gram-negative bacteria NEC 008.47
      anaerobic NEC 008.46
    Hawaii agent 008.63
    irritating foods 558.9
    Klebsiella aerogenes 008.47
    Marin County agent 008.66
    Montgomery County agent 008.63
    norovirus 008.63
    Norwalk-like agent 008.63
    Norwalk virus 008.63
    Otofuke agent 008.63
    Paracolobactrum arizonae 008.1
    paracolon bacillus NEC 008.47
      Arizona 008.1
    Paramatta agent 008.64
    Peptococcus 008.46
    Peptostreptococcus 008.46
    Propionibacterium 008.46
    Proteus (bacillus) (mirabilis) (morganii) 008.3
    Pseudomonas aeruginosa 008.42
    radiation 558.1
    Rotavirus 008.61
    Sapporo agent 008.63
    small round virus (SRV) NEC 008.64
      featureless NEC 008.63
      structured NEC 008.63
    Snow Mountain (SM) agent 008.63
    specified
      bacteria NEC 008.49
      organism, nonbacterial NEC 008.8
      virus NEC 008.69
    Staphylococcus 008.41
    Streptococcus 008.49
      anaerobic 008.46
    Taunton agent 008.63
    Torovirus 008.69
    Treponema 008.46
    Veillonella 008.46
    virus 008.8
      specified type NEC 008.69
    Wollan (W) agent 008.64
    Yersinia enterocolitica 008.44
  dysentery—*see* Dysentery

Enteritis—*continued*
  E. coli 008.00
    enterohemorrhagic 008.04
    enteroinvasive 008.03
    enteropathogenic 008.01
    enterotoxigenic 008.02
    specified type NEC 008.09
  el tor 001.1
  embadomonial 007.8
  eosinophilic 558.41
  epidemic 009.0
  Eubacterium 008.46
  fermentative 558.9
  fulminant 557.0
  Fusobacterium (nucleatum) 008.46
  gangrenous (*see also* Enteritis, due to, by
    organism) 009.0
  giardial 007.1
  gram-negative bacteria NEC 008.47
    anaerobic NEC 008.46
  infectious NEC (*see also* Enteritis, due to, by
    organism) 009.0
    presumed 009.1
  influenzal 487.8
  ischemic 557.9
    acute 557.0
    chronic 557.1
    due to mesenteric artery insufficiency 557.1
  membranous 564.9
  mucous 564.9
  myxomembranous 564.9
  necrotic (*see also* Enteritis, due to, by organism) 009.0
  necroticans 005.2
  necrotizing of fetus or newborn (*see also*
    Enterocolitis, necrotizing, newborn) 777.50
  neurogenic 564.9
  newborn 777.8
    necrotizing (*see also* Enterocolitis,
      necrotizing, newborn) 777.50
  parasitic NEC 129
  paratyphoid (fever) (*see also* Fever,
    paratyphoid) 002.9
  Peptococcus 008.46
  Peptostreptococcus 008.46
  Propionibacterium 008.46
  protozoal NEC 007.9
  radiation 558.1
  regional (of) 555.9
    intestine
      large (bowel, colon, or rectum) 555.1
        with small intestine 555.2
      small (duodenum, ileum, or jejunum) 555.0
        with large intestine 555.2
  Salmonella infection 003.0
  salmonellosis 003.0
  segmental (*see also* Enteritis, regional) 555.9
  septic (*see also* Enteritis, due to, by organism)
    009.0
  Shigella 004.9
  simple 558.9
  spasmodic 564.9
  spastic 564.9
  staphylococcal 008.41
    due to food 005.0
  streptococcal 008.49
    anaerobic 008.46
  toxic 558.2
  Treponema (denticola) (macrodentium) 008.46
  trichomonal 007.3
  tuberculous (*see also* Tuberculosis) 014.8
  typhosa 002.0

Enteritis—*continued*
  ulcerative (chronic) (*see also* Colitis, ulcerative)
    556.9
  Veillonella 008.46
  viral 008.8
    adenovirus 008.62
    enterovirus 008.67
    specified virus NEC 008.69
  Yersinia enterocolitica 008.44
  zymotic 009.0
Enteroarticular syndrome 099.3
Enterobiasis 127.4
Enterobius vermicularis 127.4
Enterocele (*see also* Hernia) 553.9
  pelvis, pelvic (acquired) (congenital) 618.6
  vagina, vaginal (acquired) (congenital) 618.6
Enterocolitis —*see also* Enteritis
  fetus or newborn (*see also* Enterocolitis,
    necrotizing, newborn) 777.8
    necrotizing 777.50
  fulminant 557.0
  granulomatous 555.2
  hemorrhagic (acute) 557.0
    chronic 557.1
  necrotizing (acute) (membranous) 557.0
    newborn 777.50
      with
        perforation 777.53
        pneumatosis without perforation 777.52
        pneumatosis and perforation 777.53
      stage I 777.51
      stage II 777.52
      stage III 777.53
      without pneumatosis, without perforation
        777.51
  primary necrotizing (*see also* Enterocolitis,
    necrotizing, newborn) 777.50
  pseudomembranous 008.45
    newborn 008.45
  radiation 558.1
    newborn (*see also* Enterocolitis, necrotizing,
      newborn) 777.50
  ulcerative 556.0
Enterocystoma 751.5
Enterogastritis —*see* Enteritis
Enterogenous cyanosis 289.7
Enterolith, enterolithiasis (impaction) 560.39
  with hernia—*see also* Hernia, by site, with
    obstruction
  gangrenous—*see* Hernia, by site, with
    gangrene
Enteropathy 569.9
  exudative (of Gordon) 579.8
  gluten 579.0
  hemorrhagic, terminal 557.0
  protein-losing 579.8
Enteroperitonitis (*see also* Peritonitis) 567.9
Enteroptosis 569.89
Enterorrhagia 578.9
Enterospasm 564.9
  psychogenic 306.4
Enterostenosis (*see also* Obstruction, intestine)
  560.9
Enterostomy status V44.4
  with complication 569.60
Enthesopathy 726.39
  ankle and tarsus 726.70
  elbow region 726.30
    specified NEC 726.39
  hip 726.5

Enthesopathy—*continued*
  knee 726.60
  peripheral NEC 726.8
  shoulder region 726.10
    adhesive 726.0
  spinal 720.1
  wrist and carpus 726.4
Entrance, air into vein —*see* Embolism, air
Entrapment, nerve —*see* Neuropathy,
  entrapment
Entropion (eyelid) 374.00
  cicatricial 374.04
  congenital 743.62
  late effect of trachoma (healed) 139.1
  mechanical 374.02
  paralytic 374.02
  senile 374.01
  spastic 374.03
Enucleation of eye (current) (traumatic) 871.3
Enuresis 788.30
  habit disturbance 307.6
  nocturnal 788.36
    psychogenic 307.6
  nonorganic origin 307.6
  psychogenic 307.6
Enzymopathy 277.9
Eosinopenia 288.59
Eosinophilia 288.3
  allergic 288.3
  hereditary 288.3
  idiopathic 288.3
  infiltrative 518.3
  Loeffler's 518.3
  myalgia syndrome 710.5
  pulmonary (tropical) 518.3
  secondary 288.3
  tropical 518.3
Eosinophilic —*see also* condition
  fasciitis 728.89
  granuloma (bone) 277.89
  infiltration lung 518.3
Ependymitis (acute) (cerebral) (chronic)
  (granular) (*see also* Meningitis) 322.9
Ependymoblastoma (M9392/3)
  specified site—*see* Neoplasm, by site, malignant
  unspecified site 191.9
Ependymoma (epithelial) (malignant) (M9391/3)
  anaplastic type (M9392/3)
    specified site—*see* Neoplasm, by site, malignant
    unspecified site 191.9
  benign (M9391/0)
    specified site—*see* Neoplasm, by site, benign
    unspecified site 225.0
  myxopapillary (M9394/1) 237.5
  papillary (M9393/1) 237.5
  specified site—*see* Neoplasm, by site, malignant
  unspecified site 191.9
Ependymopathy 349.2
  spinal cord 349.2
Ephelides, ephelis 709.09
Ephemeral fever (*see also* Pyrexia) 780.60
Epiblepharon (congenital) 743.62
Epicanthus, epicanthic fold (congenital) (eyelid)
  743.63
Epicondylitis (elbow) (lateral) 726.32
  medial 726.31

Epicystitis (*see also* Cystitis) 595.9
Epidemic —*see* condition
Epidermidalization, cervix —*see* condition
Epidermidization, cervix —*see* condition
Epidermis, epidermal —*see* condition
Epidermization, cervix —*see* condition
Epidermodysplasia verruciformis 078.19
Epidermoid
  cholesteatoma—*see* Cholesteatoma
  inclusion (*see also* Cyst, skin) 706.2
Epidermolysis
  acuta (combustiformis) (toxica) 695.15
  bullosa 757.39
  necroticans combustiformis 695.15
    due to drug
      correct substance properly administered 695.15
      overdose or wrong substance given or taken
        977.9
      specified drug—*see* Table of drugs and
        chemicals
Epidermophytid —*see* Dermatophytosis
Epidermophytosis (infected)—*see*
  Dermatophytosis
Epidermosis, ear (middle) (*see also*
  Cholesteatoma) 385.30
Epididymis —*see* condition
Epididymitis (nonvenereal) 604.90
  with abscess 604.0
  acute 604.99
  blennorrhagic (acute) 098.0
    chronic or duration of 2 months or over 098.2
  caseous (*see also* Tuberculosis) 016.4
  chlamydial 099.54
  diphtheritic 032.89 *[604.91]*
  filarial 125.9 *[604.91]*
  gonococcal (acute) 098.0
    chronic or duration of 2 months or over 098.2
  recurrent 604.99
  residual 604.99
  syphilitic 095.8 *[604.91]*
  tuberculous (*see also* Tuberculosis) 016.4
Epididymo-orchitis (*see also* Epididymitis)
  604.90
  with abscess 604.0
  chlamydial 099.54
  gonococcal (acute) 098.13
    chronic or duration of 2 months or over 098.33
Epidural —*see* condition
Epigastritis (*see also* Gastritis) 535.5
Epigastrium, epigastric —*see* condition
Epigastrocele (*see also* Hernia, epigastric) 553.29
Epiglottiditis (acute) 464.30
  with obstruction 464.31
  chronic 476.1
  viral 464.30
    with obstruction 464.31
Epiglottis —*see* condition
Epiglottitis (acute) 464.30
  with obstruction 464.31
  chronic 476.1
  viral 464.30
    with obstruction 464.31
Epignathus 759.4
Epilepsia
  partialis continua (*see also* Epilepsy) 345.7
  procursiva (*see also* Epilepsy) 345.8

Epilepsy, epileptic (idiopathic) 345.9

> *Note—use the following fifth-digit*
> *subclassification with categories 345.0, 345.1,*
> *345.4-345.9*
>
> *0 without mention of intractable epilepsy*
> *1 with intractable epilepsy*
>   *pharmacoresistant (pharmacologically*
>   *resistant)*
>   *poorly controlled*
>   *refractory (medically)*
>   *treatment resistant*

abdominal 345.5
absence (attack) 345.0
akinetic 345.0
  psychomotor 345.4
automatism 345.4
autonomic diencephalic 345.5
brain 345.9
Bravais-Jacksonian 345.5
cerebral 345.9
climacteric 345.9
clonic 345.1
clouded state 345.9
coma 345.3
communicating 345.4
complicating pregnancy, childbirth or the
  puerperium 649.4
congenital 345.9
convulsions 345.9
cortical (focal) (motor) 345.5
cursive (running) 345.8
cysticercosis 123.1
deterioration
  with behavioral disturbance 345.9 *[294.11]*
  without behavioral disturbance 345.9 *[294.10]*
due to syphilis 094.89
equivalent 345.5
fit 345.9
focal (motor) 345.5
gelastic 345.8
generalized 345.9
  convulsive 345.1
  flexion 345.1
  nonconvulsive 345.0
grand mal (idiopathic) 345.1
Jacksonian (motor) (sensory) 345.5
Kojevnikoff's, Kojevnikov's, Kojewnikoff's
  345.7
laryngeal 786.2
limbic system 345.4
localization related (focal) (partial) and epileptic
  syndromes
  with
    complex partial seizures 345.4
    simple partial seizures 345.5
major (motor) 345.1
minor 345.0
mixed (type) 345.9
motor partial 345.5
musicogenic 345.1
myoclonus, myoclonic 345.1
  progressive (familial) 345.1
nonconvulsive, generalized 345.0
parasitic NEC 123.9

Epilepsy, epileptic—*continued*
partial (focalized) 345.5
  with
    impairment of consciousness 345.4
    memory and ideational disturbances 345.4
  abdominal type 345.5
  motor type 345.5
  psychomotor type 345.4
  psychosensory type 345.4
  secondarily generalized 345.4
  sensory type 345.5
  somatomotor type 345.5
  somatosensory type 345.5
  temporal lobe type 345.4
  visceral type 345.5
  visual type 345.5
  without impairment of consciousness 345.5
peripheral 345.9
petit mal 345.0
photokinetic 345.8
progressive myoclonic (familial) 345.1
psychic equivalent 345.5
psychomotor 345.4
psychosensory 345.4
reflex 345.1
seizure 345.9
senile 345.9
sensory-induced 345.5
sleep (*see also* Narcolepsy) 347.00
somatomotor type 345.5
somatosensory 345.5
specified type NEC 345.8
status (grand mal) 345.3
  focal motor 345.7
  petit mal 345.2
  psychomotor 345.7
  temporal lobe 345.7
symptomatic 345.9
temporal lobe 345.4
tonic (-clonic) 345.1
traumatic (injury unspecified) 907.0
  injury specified—*see* Late, effect (of)
    specified injury
twilight 293.0
uncinate (gyrus) 345.4
Unverricht (-Lundborg) (familial myoclonic)
  345.1
visceral 345.5
visual 345.5
Epileptiform
convulsions 780.39
seizure 780.39
Epiloia 759.5
Epimenorrhea 626.2
Epipharyngitis (*see also* Nasopharyngitis) 460
Epiphora 375.20
due to
  excess lacrimation 375.21
  insufficient drainage 375.22
Epiphyseal arrest 733.91
femoral head 732.2
Epiphyseolysis, epiphysiolysis (*see also*
  Osteochondrosis) 732.9
Epiphysitis (*see also* Osteochondrosis) 732.9
juvenile 732.6
marginal (Scheuermann's) 732.0
os calcis 732.5
syphilitic (congenital) 090.0
vertebral (Scheuermann's) 732.0
Epiplocele (*see also* Hernia) 553.9
Epiploitis (*see also* Peritonitis) 567.9

Epiplosarcomphalocele (*see also* Hernia, umbilicus) 553.1
Episcleritis 379.00
  gouty 274.89 *[379.09]*
  nodular 379.02
  periodica fugax 379.01
  angioneurotic—*see* Edema, angioneurotic
  specified NEC 379.09
  staphylococcal 379.00
  suppurative 379.00
  syphilitic 095.0
  tuberculous (*see also* Tuberculosis) 017.3 *[379.09]*
Episode
  brain (*see also* Disease, cerebrovascular, acute) 436
  cerebral (*see also* Disease, cerebrovascular, acute) 436
  depersonalization (in neurotic state) 300.6
  hyporesponsive 780.09
  psychotic (*see also* Psychosis) 298.9
    organic, transient 293.9
  schizophrenic (acute) NEC (*see also* Schizophrenia) 295.4
Epispadias
  female 753.8
  male 752.62
Episplenitis 289.59
Epistaxis (multiple) 784.7
  hereditary 448.0
  vicarious menstruation 625.8
Epithelioma (malignant) (M8011/3)—*see also* Neoplasm, by site, malignant
  adenoides cysticum (M8100/0)—*see* Neoplasm, skin, benign
  basal cell (M8090/3)—*see* Neoplasm, skin, malignant
  benign (M8011/0)—*see* Neoplasm, by site, benign
  Bowen's (M8081/2)—*see* Neoplasm, skin, in situ
  calcifying (benign) (Malherbe's) (M8110/0)—*see* Neoplasm, skin, benign
  external site—*see* Neoplasm, skin, malignant
  intraepidermal, Jadassohn (M8096/0)—*see* Neoplasm, skin, benign
  squamous cell (M8070/3)—*see* Neoplasm, by site, malignant
Epitheliopathy
  pigment, retina 363.15
  posterior multifocal placoid (acute) 363.15
Epithelium, epithelial —*see* condition
Epituberculosis (allergic) (with atelectasis) (*see also* Tuberculosis) 010.8
Eponychia 757.5
Epstein's
  nephrosis or syndrome (*see also* Nephrosis) 581.9
  pearl (mouth) 528.4
Epstein-Barr infection (viral) 075
  chronic 780.79 *[139.8]*
Epulis (giant cell) (gingiva) 523.8
Equinia 024
Equinovarus (congenital) 754.51
  acquired 736.71
Equivalent
  angina 413.9
  convulsive (abdominal) (*see also* Epilepsy) 345.5
  epileptic (psychic) (*see also* Epilepsy) 345.5

Erb's
  disease 359.1
  palsy, paralysis (birth) (brachial) (newborn) 767.6
    spinal (spastic) syphilitic 094.89
  pseudohypertrophic muscular dystrophy 359.1
Erb (-Duchenne) paralysis (birth injury) (newborn) 767.6
Erb-Goldflam disease or syndrome 358.00
Erdheim-Chester disease (ECD) 277.89
Erdheim's syndrome (acromegalic macrospondylitis) 253.0
Erection, painful (persistent) 607.3
Ergosterol deficiency (vitamin D) 268.9
  with
    osteomalacia 268.2
    rickets (*see also* Rickets) 268.0
Ergotism (ergotized grain) 988.2
  from ergot used as drug (migraine therapy)
    correct substance properly administered 349.82
    overdose or wrong substance given or taken 975.0
Erichsen's disease (railway spine) 300.16
Erlacher-Blount syndrome (tibia vara) 732.4
Erosio interdigitalis blastomycetica 112.3
Erosion
  arteriosclerotic plaque—*see* Arteriosclerosis, by site
  artery NEC 447.2
    without rupture 447.8
  bone 733.99
  bronchus 519.19
  cartilage (joint) 733.99
  cervix (uteri) (acquired) (chronic) (congenital) 622.0
    with mention of cervicitis 616.0
  cornea (recurrent) (*see also* Keratitis) 371.42
    traumatic 918.1
  dental (idiopathic) (occupational) 521.30
    extending into
      dentine 521.32
      pulp 521.33
    generalized 521.35
    limited to enamel 521.31
    localized 521.34
  duodenum, postpyloric—*see* Ulcer, duodenum
  esophagus 530.89
  gastric 535.4
  intestine 569.89
  lymphatic vessel 457.8
  pylorus, pyloric (ulcer) 535.4
  sclera 379.16
  spine, aneurysmal 094.89
  spleen 289.59
  stomach 535.4
  teeth (idiopathic) (occupational) (*see also* Erosion, dental) 521.30
    due to
      medicine 521.30
      persistent vomiting 521.30
  urethra 599.84
  uterus 621.8
  vertebra 733.99
Erotomania 302.89
  Clérambault's 297.8

Error
in diet 269.9
refractive 367.9
  astigmatism (*see also* Astigmatism) 367.20
  drug-induced 367.89
  hypermetropia 367.0
  hyperopia 367.0
  myopia 367.1
  presbyopia 367.4
  toxic 367.89
Eructation 787.3
nervous 306.4
psychogenic 306.4
Eruption
creeping 126.9
drug—*see* Dermatitis, due to, drug
Hutchinson, summer 692.72
Kaposi's varicelliform 054.0
napkin (psoriasiform) 691.0
polymorphous
  light (sun) 692.72
    other source 692.82
psoriasiform, napkin 691.0
recalcitrant pustular 694.8
ringed 695.89
skin (*see also* Dermatitis) 782.1
  creeping (meaning hookworm) 126.9
  due to
    chemical(s) NEC 692.4
      internal use 693.8
    drug—*see* Dermatitis, due to, drug
    prophylactic inoculation or vaccination
      against disease—*see* Dermatitis, due to,
      vaccine
    smallpox vaccination NEC—*see* Dermatitis,
      due to, vaccine
  erysipeloid 027.1
  feigned 698.4
  Hutchinson, summer 692.72
  Kaposi's, varicelliform 054.0
    vaccinia 999.0
  lichenoid, axilla 698.3
  polymorphous, due to light 692.72
  toxic NEC 695.0
  vesicular 709.8
teeth, tooth
  accelerated 520.6
  delayed 520.6
  difficult 520.6
  disturbance of 520.6
  in abnormal sequence 520.6
  incomplete 520.6
  late 520.6
  natal 520.6
  neonatal 520.6
  obstructed 520.6
  partial 520.6
  persistent primary 520.6
  premature 520.6
  prenatal 520.6
  vesicular 709.8
Erysipelas (gangrenous) (infantile) (newborn)
  (phlegmonous) (suppurative) 035
  external ear 035 *[380.13]*
  puerperal, postpartum, childbirth 670.8
Erysipelatoid (Rosenbach's) 027.1
Erysipeloid (Rosenbach's) 027.1

Erythema, erythematous (generalized) 695.9
ab igne—*see* Burn, by site, first degree
annulare (centrifugum) (rheumaticum) 695.0
arthriticum epidemicum 026.1
brucellum (*see also* Brucellosis) 023.9
bullosum 695.19
caloricum—*see* Burn, by site, first degree
chronicum migrans 088.81
  chronicum 088.81
circinatum 695.19
diaper 691.0
due to
  chemical (contact) NEC 692.4
    internal 693.8
  drug (internal use) 693.0
    contact 692.3
elevatum diutinum 695.89
endemic 265.2
epidemic, arthritic 026.1
figuratum perstans 695.0
gluteal 691.0
gyratum (perstans) (repens) 695.19
heat—*see* Burn, by site, first degree
ichthyosiforme congenitum 757.1
induratum (primary) (scrofulosorum) (*see also*
  Tuberculosis) 017.1
  nontuberculous 695.2
infantum febrile 057.8
infectional NEC 695.9
infectiosum 057.0
inflammation NEC 695.9
intertrigo 695.89
iris 695.10
lupus (discoid) (localized) (*see also* Lupus,
  erythematosus) 695.4
marginatum 695.0
  rheumaticum—*see* Fever, rheumatic
medicamentosum—*see* Dermatitis, due to, drug
migrans 529.1
multiforme 695.10
  bullosum 695.19
  conjunctiva 695.19
  exudativum (Hebra) 695.19
  major 695.12
  minor 695.11
  pemphigoides 694.5
napkin 691.0
neonatorum 778.8
nodosum 695.2
  tuberculous (*see also* Tuberculosis) 017.1
nummular, nummulare 695.19
palmar 695.0
palmaris hereditarium 695.0
pernio 991.5
perstans solare 692.72
rash, newborn 778.8
scarlatiniform (exfoliative) (recurrent) 695.0
simplex marginatum 057.8
solare (*see also* Sunburn) 692.71
streptogenes 696.5
toxic, toxicum NEC 695.0
  newborn 778.8
tuberculous (primary) (*see also* Tuberculosis)
  017.0
venenatum 695.0
Erythematosus —*see* condition
Erythematous —*see* condition
Erythermalgia (primary) 443.82
Erythralgia 443.82
Erythrasma 039.0

Erythredema 985.0
polyneuritica 985.0
polyneuropathy 985.0
Erythremia (acute) (M9841/3) 207.0
chronic (M9842/3) 207.1
secondary 289.0
Erythroblastopenia (acquired) 284.89
congenital 284.01
Erythroblastophthisis 284.01
Erythroblastosis (fetalis) (newborn) 773.2
due to
ABO
antibodies 773.1
incompatibility, maternal/fetal 773.1
isoimmunization 773.1
Rh
antibodies 773.0
incompatibility, maternal/fetal 773.0
isoimmunization 773.0
Erythrocyanosis (crurum) 443.89
Erythrocythemia —*see* Erythremia
Erythrocytopenia 285.9
Erythrocytosis (megalosplenic)
familial 289.6
oval, hereditary (*see also* Elliptocytosis) 282.1
secondary 289.0
stress 289.0
Erythroderma (*see also* Erythema) 695.9
desquamativa (in infants) 695.89
exfoliative 695.89
ichthyosiform, congenital 757.1
infantum 695.89
maculopapular 696.2
neonatorum 778.8
psoriaticum 696.1
secondary 695.9
Erythrodysesthesia, palmar plantar (PPE) 693.0
Erythrogenesis imperfecta 284.09
Erythroleukemia (M9840/3) 207.0
Erythromelalgia 443.82
Erythromelia 701.8
Erythropenia 285.9
Erythrophagocytosis 289.9
Erythrophobia 300.23
Erythroplakia
oral mucosa 528.79
tongue 528.79
Erythroplasia (Queyrat) (M8080/2)
specified site—*see* Neoplasm, skin, in situ
unspecified site 233.5
Erythropoiesis, idiopathic ineffective 285.0
Escaped beats, heart 427.60
postoperative 997.1
Esoenteritis —*see* Enteritis
Esophagalgia 530.89
Esophagectasis 530.89
due to cardiospasm 530.0
Esophagismus 530.5
Esophagitis (alkaline) (chemical) (chronic)
(infectional) (necrotic) (postoperative) 530.10
acute 530.12
candidal 112.84
eosinophilic 530.13
reflux 530.11
specified NEC 530.19
tuberculous (*see also* Tuberculosis) 017.8
ulcerative 530.19
Esophagocele 530.6
Esophagodynia 530.89

Esophagomalacia 530.89
Esophagoptosis 530.89
Esophagospasm 530.5
Esophagostenosis 530.3
Esophagostomiasis 127.7
Esophagostomy
complication 530.87
infection 530.86
malfunctioning 530.87
mechanical 530.87
Esophagotracheal —*see* condition
Esophagus —*see* condition
Esophoria 378.41
convergence, excess 378.84
divergence, insufficiency 378.85
Esotropia (nonaccommodative) 378.00
accommodative 378.35
alternating 378.05
with
A pattern 378.06
specified noncomitancy NEC 378.08
V pattern 378.07
X pattern 378.08
Y pattern 378.08
intermittent 378.22
intermittent 378.20
alternating 378.22
monocular 378.21
monocular 378.01
with
A pattern 378.02
specified noncomitancy NEC 378.04
V pattern 378.03
X pattern 378.04
Y pattern 378.04
intermittent 378.21
Espundia 085.5
Essential —*see* condition
Esterapenia 289.89
Esthesioneuroblastoma (M9522/3) 160.0
Esthesioneurocytoma (M9521/3) 160.0
Esthesioneuroepithelioma (M9523/3) 160.0
Esthiomene 099.1
Estivo-autumnal
fever 084.0
malaria 084.0
Estrangement V61.09
Estriasis 134.0
Ethanolaminuria 270.8
Ethanolism (*see also* Alcoholism) 303.9
Ether dependence, dependency (*see also*
Dependence) 304.6
Etherism (*see also* Dependence) 304.6
Ethmoid, ethmoidal —*see* condition
Ethmoiditis (chronic) (nonpurulent) (purulent)
(*see also* Sinusitis, ethmoidal) 473.2
influenzal 487.1
Woakes' 471.1
Ethylism (*see also* Alcoholism) 303.9
Eulenburg's disease (congenital paramyotonia)
359.29
Eunuchism 257.2
Eunuchoidism 257.2
hypogonadotropic 257.2
European blastomycosis 117.5
Eustachian —*see* condition
Euthyroid sick syndrome 790.94
Euthyroidism 244.9

Evaluation
fetal lung maturity 659.8
for suspected condition (*see also* Observation) V71.9
  abuse V71.81
  exposure
    antrax V71.82
    biologic agent NEC V71.83
    SARS V71.83
  neglect V71.81
  newborn—*see* Observation, suspected,
    condition, newborn
  specified condition NEC V71.89
mental health V70.2
  requested by authority V70.1
nursing care V63.8
social service V63.8
Evans' syndrome (thrombocytopenic purpura) 287.32
Event, apparent life threatening in newborn and infant (ALTE) 799.82
Eventration
colon into chest—*see* Hernia, diaphragm
diaphragm (congenital) 756.6
Eversion
bladder 596.8
cervix (uteri) 622.0
  with mention of cervicitis 616.0
foot NEC 736.79
  congenital 755.67
lacrimal punctum 375.51
punctum lacrimale (postinfectional) (senile) 375.51
ureter (meatus) 593.89
urethra (meatus) 599.84
uterus 618.1
  complicating delivery 665.2
    affecting fetus or newborn 763.89
  puerperal, postpartum 674.8
Evidence
of malignancy
  cytologic
    without histologic confirmation
      anus 796.76
      cervix 795.06
      vagina 795.16
Evisceration
birth injury 767.8
bowel (congenital)—*see* Hernia, ventral
congenital (*see also* Hernia, ventral) 553.29
operative wound 998.32
traumatic NEC 869.1
  eye 871.3
Evulsion —*see* Avulsion
Ewing's
angioendothelioma (M9260/3)—*see* Neoplasm, bone, malignant
sarcoma (M9260/3)—*see* Neoplasm, bone, malignant
tumor (M9260/3)—*see* Neoplasm, bone, malignant
Exaggerated lumbosacral angle (with impinging spine) 756.12
Examination (general) (routine) (of) (for) V70.9
allergy V72.7
annual V70.0
cardiovascular preoperative V72.81
cervical Papanicolaou smear V76.2
  as a part of routine gynecological examination V72.31
  to confirm findings of recent normal smear following initial abnormal smear V72.32
child care (routine) V20.2
clinical research investigation (normal control patient) (participant) V70.7

Examination—*continued*
dental V72.2
developmental testing (child) (infant) V20.2
donor (potential) V70.8
ear V72.19
eye V72.0
following
  accident (motor vehicle) V71.4
  alleged rape or seduction (victim or culprit) V71.5
  inflicted injury (victim or culprit) NEC V71.6
  rape or seduction, alleged (victim or culprit) V71.5
  treatment (for) V67.9
    combined V67.6
    fracture V67.4
    involving high-risk medication NEC V67.51
    mental disorder V67.3
    specified condition NEC V67.59
follow-up (routine) (following) V67.9
  cancer chemotherapy V67.2
  chemotherapy V67.2
  disease NEC V67.59
  high-risk medication NEC V67.51
  injury NEC V67.59
  population survey V70.6
  postpartum V24.2
  psychiatric V67.3
  psychotherapy V67.3
  radiotherapy V67.1
  specified surgery NEC V67.09
  surgery V67.00
    vaginal pap smear V67.01
gynecological V72.31
  for contraceptive maintenance V25.40
    intrauterine device V25.42
    pill V25.41
    specified method NEC V25.49
health (of)
  armed forces personnel V70.5
  checkup V70.0
  child, routine V20.2
  defined subpopulation NEC V70.5
  inhabitants of institutions V70.5
  occupational V70.5
  pre-employment screening V70.5
  preschool children V70.5
    for admission to school V70.3
  prisoners V70.5
    for entrance into prison V70.3
  prostitutes V70.5
  refugees V70.5
  school children V70.5
  students V70.5
hearing V72.19
  following failed hearing screening V72.11
infant
  8 to 28 days old V20.32
  over 28 days old, routine V20.2
  under 8 days old V20.31
laboratory V72.60
  ordered as part of a routine general medical examination V72.62
  pre-operative V72.63
  pre-procedural V72.63
  specified NEC V72.69
lactating mother V24.1
medical (for) (of) V70.9
  administrative purpose NEC V70.3
  admission to
    old age home V70.3
    prison V70.3
    school V70.3
  adoption V70.3

Examination—*continued*
  medical (for) (of)—*continued*
    armed forces personnel V70.5
    at health care facility V70.0
    camp V70.3
    child, routine V20.2
    clinical research investigation (control)
      (normal comparison) (participant) V70.7
    defined subpopulation NEC V70.5
    donor (potential) V70.8
    driving license V70.3
    general V70.9
      routine V70.0
      specified reason NEC V70.8
    immigration V70.3
    inhabitants of institutions V70.5
    insurance certification V70.3
    marriage V70.3
    medicolegal reasons V70.4
    naturalization V70.3
    occupational V70.5
    population survey V70.6
    pre-employment V70.5
    preschool children V70.5
      for admission to school V70.3
    prison V70.3
    prisoners V70.5
      for entrance into prison V70.3
    prostitutes V70.5
    refugees V70.5
    school children V70.5
    specified reason NEC V70.8
    sport competition V70.3
    students V70.5
  medicolegal reason V70.4
  pelvic (annual) (periodic) V72.31
  periodic (annual) (routine) V70.0
  postpartum
    immediately after delivery V24.0
    routine follow-up V24.2
  pregnancy (unconfirmed) (possible) V72.40
    negative result V72.41
    positive result V72.42
  prenatal V22.1
    first pregnancy V22.0
    high-risk pregnancy V23.9
      specified problem NEC V23.8
  preoperative V72.84
    cardiovascular V72.81
    respiratory V72.82
    specified NEC V72.83
  preprocedural V72.84
    cardiovascular V72.81
    general physical V72.83
    respiratory V72.82
    specified NEC V72.83
  prior to chemotherapy V72.83
  psychiatric V70.2
    follow-up not needing further care V67.3
    requested by authority V70.1
  radiological NEC V72.5
  respiratory preoperative V72.82
  screening—*see* Screening
  sensitization V72.7
  skin V72.7
    hypersensitivity V72.7
  special V72.9
  specified type or reason NEC V72.85
    preoperative V72.83
      specified NEC V72.83

Examination—*continued*
  teeth V72.2
  vaginal Papanicolaou smear V76.47
    following hysterectomy for malignant
      condition V67.01
  victim or culprit following
    alleged rape or seduction V71.5
    inflicted injury NEC V71.6
  vision V72.0
  well baby V20.2
Exanthem, exanthema (*see also* Rash) 782.1
  Boston 048
  epidemic, with meningitis 048
  lichenoid psoriasiform 696.2
  subitum 058.10
    due to
      human herpesvirus 6 058.11
      human herpesvirus 7 058.12
  viral, virus NEC 057.9
    specified type NEC 057.8
Excess, excessive, excessively
  alcohol level in blood 790.3
  carbohydrate tissue, localized 278.1
  carotene (dietary) 278.3
  cold 991.9
    specified effect NEC 991.8
  convergence 378.84
  crying 780.95
    of
      adolescent 780.95
      adult 780.95
      baby 780.92
      child 780.95
      infant (baby) 780.92
      newborn 780.92
  development, breast 611.1
  diaphoresis (*see also* Hyperhidrosis) 780.8
  distance, interarch 524.28
  divergence 378.85
  drinking (alcohol) NEC (*see also* Abuse, drugs,
    nondependent) 305.0
    continual (*see also* Alcoholism) 303.9
    habitual (*see also* Alcoholism) 303.9
  eating 783.6
  eyelid fold (congenital) 743.62
  fat 278.02
    in heart (*see also* Degeneration, myocardial) 429.1
    tissue, localized 278.1
  foreskin 605
  gas 787.3
  gastrin 251.5
  glucagon 251.4
  heat (*see also* Heat) 992.9
  horizontal
    overjet 524.26
    overlap 524.26
  interarch distance 524.28
  intermaxillary vertical dimension 524.37
  interocclusal distance of teeth 524.37
  large
    colon 564.7
      congenital 751.3
    fetus or infant 766.0
      with obstructed labor 660.1
      affecting management of pregnancy 656.6
      causing disproportion 653.5
    newborn (weight of 4500 grams or more) 766.0

Excess, excessive, excessively—*continued*
long
  colon 751.5
  organ or site, congenital NEC—*see* Anomaly,
    specified type NEC
  umbilical cord (entangled)
    affecting fetus or newborn 762.5
    in pregnancy or childbirth 663.3
      with compression 663.2
menstruation 626.2
number of teeth 520.1
  causing crowding 524.31
nutrients (dietary) NEC 783.6
potassium (K) 276.7
salivation (*see also* Ptyalism) 527.7
secretion—*see also* Hypersecretion
  milk 676.6
  sputum 786.4
  sweat (*see also* Hyperhidrosis) 780.8
short
  organ or site, congenital NEC—*see* Anomaly,
    specified type NEC
  umbilical cord
    affecting fetus or newborn 762.6
    in pregnancy or childbirth 663.4
skin NEC 701.9
  eyelid 743.62
    acquired 374.30
sodium (Na) 276.0
spacing of teeth 524.32
sputum 786.4
sweating (*see also* Hyperhidrosis) 780.8
tearing (ducts) (eye) (*see also* Epiphora) 375.20
thirst 783.5
  due to deprivation of water 994.3
tissue in reconstructed breast 612.0
tuberosity 524.07
vitamin
  A (dietary) 278.2
    administered as drug (chronic) (prolonged
      excessive intake) 278.2
    reaction to sudden overdose 963.5
  D (dietary) 278.4
    administered as drug (chronic) (prolonged
      excessive intake) 278.4
    reaction to sudden overdose 963.5
weight 278.02
  gain 783.1
    of pregnancy 646.1
  loss 783.21
Excitability, abnormal, under minor stress
  309.29
Excitation
catatonic (*see also* Schizophrenia) 295.2
psychogenic 298.1
reactive (from emotional stress, psychological
  trauma) 298.1
Excitement
manic (*see also* Psychosis, affective) 296.0
  recurrent episode 296.1
  single episode 296.0
mental, reactive (from emotional stress,
  psychological trauma) 298.1
state, reactive (from emotional stress,
  psychological trauma) 298.1
Excluded pupils 364.76
Excoriation (traumatic) (*see also* Injury,
  superficial, by site) 919.8
neurotic 698.4
Excyclophoria 378.44
Excyclotropia 378.33
Exencephalus, exencephaly 742.0

Exercise
breathing V57.0
remedial NEC V57.1
therapeutic NEC V57.1
Exfoliation
skin
  due to erythematous condition 695.50
    involving (percent of body surface)
      less than 10 percent 695.50
      10-19 percent 695.51
      20-29 percent 695.52
      30-39 percent 695.53
      40-49 percent 695.54
      50-59 percent 695.55
      60-69 percent 695.56
      70-79 percent 695.57
      80-89 percent 695.58
      90 percent or more 695.59
teeth
  due to systemic causes 525.0
Exfoliative —*see also* condition
dermatitis 695.89
Exhaustion, exhaustive (physical NEC) 780.79
battle (*see also* Reaction, stress, acute) 308.9
cardiac (*see also* Failure, heart) 428.9
delirium (*see also* Reaction, stress, acute) 308.9
due to
  cold 991.8
  excessive exertion 994.5
  exposure 994.4
  overexertion 994.5
fetus or newborn 779.89
heart (*see also* Failure, heart) 428.9
heat 992.5
  due to
    salt depletion 992.4
    water depletion 992.3
manic (*see also* Psychosis, affective) 296.0
  recurrent episode 296.1
  single episode 296.0
maternal, complicating delivery 669.8
  affecting fetus or newborn 763.89
mental 300.5
myocardium, myocardial (*see also* Failure,
  heart) 428.9
nervous 300.5
old age 797
postinfectional NEC 780.79
psychogenic 300.5
psychosis (*see also* Reaction, stress, acute)
  308.9
senile 797
  dementia 290.0
Exhibitionism (sexual) 302.4
Exomphalos 756.72
Exophoria 378.42
convergence, insufficiency 378.83
divergence, excess 378.85
Exophthalmic
cachexia 242.0
goiter 242.0
ophthalmoplegia 242.0 *[376.22]*
Exophthalmos 376.30
congenital 743.66
constant 376.31
endocrine NEC 259.9 *[376.22]*
hyperthyroidism 242.0 *[376.21]*
intermittent NEC 376.34
malignant 242.0 *[376.21]*
pulsating 376.35
  endocrine NEC 259.9 *[376.22]*
thyrotoxic 242.0 *[376.21]*

Exostosis 726.91
  cartilaginous (M9210/0)—*see* Neoplasm, bone, benign
  congenital 756.4
  ear canal, external 380.81
  gonococcal 098.89
  hip 726.5
  intracranial 733.3
  jaw (bone) 526.81
  luxurians 728.11
  multiple (cancellous) (congenital) (hereditary) 756.4
  nasal bones 726.91
  orbit, orbital 376.42
  osteocartilaginous (M9210/0)—*see* Neoplasm, bone, benign
  spine 721.8
    with spondylosis—*see* Spondylosis
  syphilitic 095.5
  wrist 726.4
Exotropia 378.10
  alternating 378.15
    with
      A pattern 378.16
      specified noncomitancy 378.18
      V pattern 378.17
      X pattern 378.18
      Y pattern 378.18
    intermittent 378.24
  intermittent 378.20
    alternating 378.24
    monocular 378.23
  monocular 378.11
    with
      A pattern 378.12
      specified noncomitancy NEC 378.14
      V pattern 378.13
      X pattern 378.14
      Y pattern 378.14
    intermittent 378.23
Explanation of
  investigation finding V65.4
  medication V65.4
Exposure (suspected) 994.9
  algae bloom V87.32
  cold 991.9
    specified effect NEC 991.8
  effects of 994.9
  exhaustion due to 994.4
  to
    AIDS virus V01.79
    anthrax V01.81
    aromatic
      amines V87.11
      dyes V87.19
    arsenic V87.01
    asbestos V15.84
    benzene V87.12
    body fluids (hazardous) V15.85
    cholera V01.0
    communicable disease V01.9
      specified type NEC V01.89
    chromium compounds V87.09
    dyes V87.2
      aromatic V87.19
    Escherichia coli (E. coli) V01.83
    German measles V01.4
    gonorrhea V01.6

Exposure—*continued*
  to —*continued*
    hazardous
      aromatic compounds NEC V87.19
      body fluids V15.85
      chemicals NEC V87.2
      metals V87.09
      substances V87.39
    HIV V01.79
    human immunodeficiency virus V01.79
    lead V15.86
    meningococcus V01.84
    mold V87.31
    nickel dust V87.09
    parasitic disease V01.89
    poliomyelitis V01.2
    polycyclic aromatic hydrocarbons V87.19
    potentially hazardous body fluids V15.85
    rabies V01.5
    rubella V01.4
    SARS-associated coronavirus V01.82
    smallpox V01.3
    syphilis V01.6
    tuberculosis V01.1
    varicella V01.71
    venereal disease V01.6
    viral disease NEC V01.79
      varicella V01.71
Exsanguination, fetal 772.0
Exstrophy
  abdominal content 751.8
  bladder (urinary) 753.5
Extensive —*see* condition
Extra —*see also* Accessory
  rib 756.3
    cervical 756.2
Extraction
  with hook 763.89
  breech NEC 669.6
    affecting fetus or newborn 763.0
  cataract postsurgical V45.61
  manual NEC 669.8
    affecting fetus or newborn 763.89
Extrasystole 427.60
  atrial 427.61
  postoperative 997.1
  ventricular 427.69
Extrauterine gestation or pregnancy —*see* Pregnancy, ectopic
Extravasation
  blood 459.0
    lower extremity 459.0
  chemotherapy, vesicant 999.81
  chyle into mesentery 457.8
  pelvicalyceal 593.4
  pyelosinus 593.4
  urine 788.8
    from ureter 788.8
  vesicant
    agent NEC 999.82
    chemotherapy 999.81
Extremity —*see* condition
Extrophy —*see* Exstrophy
Extroversion
  bladder 753.5
  uterus 618.1
    complicating delivery 665.2
      affecting fetus or newborn 763.89
    postpartal (old) 618.1

Extruded tooth 524.34
Extrusion
  alveolus and teeth 524.75
  breast implant (prosthetic) 996.54
  device, implant, or graft—*see* Complications,
       mechanical
  eye implant (ball) (globe) 996.59
  intervertebral disc—*see* Displacement,
       intervertebral disc
  lacrimal gland 375.43
  mesh (reinforcing) 996.59
  ocular lens implant 996.53
  prosthetic device NEC—*see* Complications,
       mechanical
  vitreous 379.26
Exudate, pleura —*see* Effusion, pleura
Exudates, retina 362.82
Exudative —*see* condition
Eye, eyeball, eyelid—*see* condition
Eyestrain 368.13
Eyeworm disease of Africa 125.2

F

Faber's anemia or syndrome (achlorhydric
    anemia) 280.9
Fabry's disease (angiokeratoma corporis
    diffusum) 272.7
Face, facial —see condition
Facet of cornea 371.44
Faciocephalalgia, autonomic (see also
    Neuropathy, peripheral, autonomic) 337.9
Facioscapulohumeral myopathy 359.1
Factitious disorder, illness —see Illness,
    factitious
Factor
    deficiency—see Deficiency, factor
    psychic, associated with diseases classified
        elsewhere 316
    risk—see Problem
Fahr-Volhard disease (malignant
    nephrosclerosis) 403.00
Failure, failed
    adenohypophyseal 253.2
    attempted abortion (legal) (see also Abortion,
        failed) 638.9
    bone marrow (anemia) 284.9
        acquired (secondary) 284.89
        congenital 284.09
        idiopathic 284.9
    cardiac (see also Failure, heart) 428.9
        newborn 779.89
    cardiorenal (chronic) 428.9
        hypertensive (see also Hypertension,
            cardiorenal) 404.93
    cardiorespiratory 799.1
        specified during or due to a procedure 997.1
            long-term effect of cardiac surgery 429.4
    cardiovascular (chronic) 428.9
    cerebrovascular 437.8
    cervical dilatation in labor 661.0
        affecting fetus or newborn 763.7
    circulation, circulatory 799.89
        fetus or newborn 779.89
        peripheral 785.50
    compensation—see Disease, heart
    conscious sedation, during procedure 995.24
    congestive (see also Failure, heart) 428.0
    coronary (see also Insufficiency, coronary) 411.89
    dental implant 525.79
        due to
            infection 525.71
            lack of attached gingiva 525.72
            occlusal trauma (caused by poor prosthetic
                design) 525.72
            parafunctional habits 525.72
            periodontal infection (peri-implantitis) 525.72
            poor oral hygiene 525.72
            unintentional loading 525.71
        endosseous NEC 525.79
        mechanical 525.73
        osseointegration 525.71
            due to
                complications of systemic disease 525.71
                poor bone quality 525.71
                premature loading 525.71
            iatrogenic 525.71
            prior to intentional prosthetic loading 525.71

Failure, failed—continued
    dental implant—continued
        post-osseointegration
            biological 525.72
            iatrogenic 525.72
            due to complications of systemic disease 525.72
            mechanical 525.73
        pre-integration 525.71
        pre-osseointegration 525.71
    dental prosthesis causing loss of dental implant
        525.73
    dental restoration
        marginal integrity 525.61
        periodontal anatomical integrity 525.65
    descent of head (at term) 652.5
        affecting fetus or newborn 763.1
        in labor 660.0
            affecting fetus or newborn 763.1
    device, implant, or graft—see Complications,
        mechanical
    engagement of head NEC 652.5
        in labor 660.0
    extrarenal 788.99
    fetal head to enter pelvic brim 652.5
        affecting fetus or newborn 763.1
        in labor 660.0
            affecting fetus or newborn 763.1
    forceps NEC 660.7
        affecting fetus or newborn 763.1
    fusion (joint) (spinal) 996.49
    growth in childhood 783.43
    heart (acute) (sudden) 428.9
        with
            abortion—see Abortion, by type, with
                specified complication NEC
            acute pulmonary edema (see also Failure,
                ventricular, left) 428.1
                with congestion (see also Failure, heart)
                    428.0
            decompensation (see also Failure, heart) 428.0
            dilation—see Disease, heart
            ectopic pregnancy (see also categories
                633.0-633.9) 639.8
            molar pregnancy (see also categories
                630-632) 639.8
        arteriosclerotic 440.9
        combined left-right sided 428.0
        combined systolic and diastolic 428.40
            acute 428.41
            acute on chronic 428.43
            chronic 428.42
        compensated (see also Failure, heart) 428.0
        complicating
            abortion—see Abortion, by type, with
                specified complication NEC
            delivery (cesarean) (instrumental) 669.4
            ectopic pregnancy (see also categories
                633.0-633.9) 639.8
            molar pregnancy (see also categories
                630-632) 639.8
            obstetric anesthesia or sedation 668.1
            surgery 997.1
        congestive (compensated) (decompensated)
            (see also Failure, heart) 428.0
            with rheumatic fever (conditions classifiable
                to 390)
                active 391.8
                inactive or quiescent (with chorea) 398.91

Failure, failed—*continued*
heart—*continued*
  congestive—*continued*
    fetus or newborn 779.89
    hypertensive (*see also* Hypertension, heart)
      402.91
      with renal disease (*see also* Hypertension,
        cardiorenal) 404.91
        with renal failure 404.93
      benign 402.11
      malignant 402.01
    rheumatic (chronic) (inactive) (with chorea)
      398.91
      active or acute 391.8
        with chorea (Sydenham's) 392.0
  decompensated (*see also* Failure, heart) 428.0
  degenerative (*see also* Degeneration,
    myocardial) 429.1
  diastolic 428.30
    acute 428.31
    acute or chronic 428.33
    chronic 428.32
  due to presence of (cardiac) prosthesis 429.4
  fetus or newborn 779.89
  following
    abortion 639.8
    cardiac surgery 429.4
    ectopic or molar pregnancy 639.8
  high output NEC 428.9
  hypertensive (*see also* Hypertension, heart) 402.91
    with renal disease (*see also* Hypertension,
      cardiorenal) 404.91
      with renal failure 404.93
    benign 402.11
    malignant 402.01
  left (ventricular) (*see also* Failure, ventricular,
    left) 428.1
    with right-sided failure (*see also* Failure,
      heart) 428.0
  low output (syndrome) NEC 428.9
  organic—*see* Disease, heart
  postoperative (immediate) 997.1
    long term effect of cardiac surgery 429.4
  rheumatic (chronic) (congestive) (inactive) 398.91
  right (secondary to left heart failure,
    conditions classifiable to 428.1)
    (ventricular) (*see also* Failure, heart) 428.0
  senile 797
  specified during or due to a procedure 997.1
    long-term effect of cardiac surgery 429.4
  systolic 428.20
    acute 428.21
    acute on chronic 428.23
    chronic 428.22
  thyrotoxic (*see also* Thyrotoxicosis) 242.9 *[425.7]*
  valvular—*see* Endocarditis
hepatic 572.8
  acute 570
  due to a procedure 997.4
hepatorenal 572.4
hypertensive heart (*see also* Hypertension,
  heart) 402.91
  benign 402.11
  malignant 402.01
induction (of labor) 659.1
  abortion (legal) (*see also* Abortion, failed)
    638.9
  affecting fetus or newborn 763.89
  by oxytocic drugs 659.1
  instrumental 659.0
  mechanical 659.0

Failure, failed—*continued*
induction (of labor)—*continued*
  medical 659.1
  surgical 659.0
initial alveolar expansion, newborn 770.4
involution, thymus (gland) 254.8
kidney—*see* Failure, renal
lactation 676.4
Leydig's cell, adult 257.2
liver 572.8
  acute 570
medullary 799.89
mitral—*see* Endocarditis, mitral
moderate sedation, during procedure 995.24
myocardium, myocardial (*see also* Failure,
  heart) 428.9
  chronic (*see also* Failure, heart) 428.0
  congestive (*see also* Failure, heart) 428.0
ovarian (primary) 256.39
  iatrogenic 256.2
  postablative 256.2
  postirradiation 256.2
  postsurgical 256.2
ovulation 628.0
prerenal 788.99
renal (kidney) 586
  with
    abortion—*see* Abortion, by type, with renal
      failure
    ectopic pregnancy (*see also* categories
      633.0-633.9) 639.3
    edema (*see also* Nephrosis) 581.9
    hypertension (*see also* Hypertension,
      kidney) 403.91
    hypertensive heart disease (conditions
      classifiable to 402) 404.92
      with heart failure 404.93
      benign 404.12
        with heart failure 404.13
      malignant 404.02
        with heart failure 404.03
    molar pregnancy (*see also* categories
      630-632) 639.3
    tubular necrosis (acute) 584.5
  acute 584.9
    with lesion of
      necrosis
        cortical (renal) 584.6
        medullary (renal) (papillary) 584.7
        tubular 584.5
      specified pathology NEC 584.8
  chronic 585.9
    hypertensive or with hypertension (*see also*
      Hypertension, kidney) 403.91
  due to a procedure 997.5
  following
    abortion 639.3
    crushing 958.5
    ectopic or molar pregnancy 639.3
    labor and delivery (acute) 669.3
  hypertensive (*see also* Hypertension, kidney)
    403.91
  puerperal, postpartum 669.3
respiration, respiratory 518.81
  acute 518.81
  acute and chronic 518.84
  center 348.89
    newborn 770.84
  chronic 518.83
  due to trauma, surgery or shock 518.5
  newborn 770.84

Failure, failed—*continued*
  rotation
    cecum 751.4
    colon 751.4
    intestine 751.4
    kidney 753.3
  sedation, during procedure
    conscious 995.24
    moderate 995.24
  segmentation—*see also* Fusion
    fingers (*see also* Syndactylism, fingers)
        755.11
    toes (*see also* Syndactylism, toes) 755.13
  seminiferous tubule, adult 257.2
  senile (general) 797
    with psychosis 290.20
  testis, primary (seminal) 257.2
  to progress 661.2
  to thrive
    adult 783.7
    child 783.41
    newborn 779.34
  transplant 996.80
    bone marrow 996.85
    organ (immune or nonimmune cause) 996.80
      bone marrow 996.85
      heart 996.83
      intestines 996.87
      kidney 996.81
      liver 996.82
      lung 996.84
      pancreas 996.86
      specified NEC 996.89
    skin 996.52
      artificial 996.55
      decellularized allodermis 996.55
      temporary allograft or pigskin graft—*omit code*
  trial of labor NEC 660.6
    affecting fetus or newborn 763.1
  tubal ligation 998.89
  urinary 586
  vacuum extraction
    abortion—*see* Abortion, failed
    delivery NEC 660.7
      affecting fetus or newborn 763.1
  vasectomy 998.89
  ventouse NEC 660.7
    affecting fetus or newborn 763.1
  ventricular (*see also* Failure, heart) 428.9
    left 428.1
      with rheumatic fever (conditions classifiable
          to 390)
        active 391.8
          with chorea 392.0
        inactive or quiescent (with chorea) 398.91
      hypertensive (*see also* Hypertension, heart)
          402.91
        benign 402.11
        malignant 402.01
      rheumatic (chronic) (inactive) (with chorea)
          398.91
        active or acute 391.8
          with chorea 392.0
    right (*see also* Failure, heart) 428.0
  vital centers, fetus or newborn 779.8
  weight gain in childhood 783.41
Fainting (fit) (spell) 780.2
Falciform hymen 752.49
Fall, maternal, affecting fetus or newborn 760.5
Fallen arches 734
Falling, any organ or part —*see* Prolapse

Fallopian
  insufflation
    fertility testing V26.21
    following sterilization reversal V26.22
  tube—*see* condition
Fallot's
  pentalogy 745.2
  tetrad or tetralogy 745.2
  triad or trilogy 746.09
Fallout, radioactive (adverse effect) NEC 990
False —*see also* condition
  bundle branch block 426.50
  bursa 727.89
  croup 478.75
  joint 733.82
  labor (pains) 644.1
  opening, urinary, male 752.69
  passage, urethra (prostatic) 599.4
  positive
    serological test for syphilis 795.6
    Wassermann reaction 795.6
  pregnancy 300.11
Family, familial —*see also* condition
  affected by
    family member
      currently on deployment (military) V61.01
      returned from deployment (military) (current
          or past conflict) V61.02
  disruption (*see also* Disruption, family) V61.09
  estrangement V61.09
  hemophagocytic
    lymphohistiocytosis 288.4
    reticulosis 288.4
  Li-fraumeni (syndrome) V84.01
  planning advice V25.09
    natural
      procreative V26.41
      to avoid pregnancy V25.04
  problem V61.9
    specified circumstance NEC V61.8
  retinoblastoma (syndrome) 190.5
Famine 994.2
  edema 262
Fanconi's anemia (congenital pancytopenia) 284.09
Fanconi (-de Toni) (-Debré) syndrome
    (cystinosis) 270.0
Farber (-Uzman) syndrome or disease
    (disseminated lipogranulomatosis) 272.8
Farcin 024
Farcy 024
Farmers'
  lung 495.0
  skin 692.74
Farsightedness 367.0
Fascia —*see* condition
Fasciculation 781.0
Fasciculitis optica 377.32
Fasciitis 729.4
  eosinophilic 728.89
  necrotizing 728.86
  nodular 728.79
  perirenal 593.4
  plantar 728.71
  pseudosarcomatous 728.79
  traumatic (old) NEC 728.79
    current—*see* Sprain, by site
Fasciola hepatica infestation 121.3
Fascioliasis 121.3
Fasciolopsiasis (small intestine) 121.4
Fasciolopsis (small intestine) 121.4
Fast pulse 785.0

Fat
  embolism (cerebral) (pulmonary) (systemic)
    958.1
    with
      abortion—*see* Abortion, by type, with
        embolism
      ectopic pregnancy (*see also* categories
        633.0-633.9) 639.6
      molar pregnancy (*see also* categories
        630-632) 639.6
    complicating delivery or puerperium 673.8
    following
      abortion 639.6
      ectopic or molar pregnancy 639.6
    in pregnancy, childbirth, or the puerperium
      673.8
  excessive 278.02
    in heart (*see also* Degeneration, myocardial)
      429.1
  general 278.02
  hernia, herniation 729.30
    eyelid 374.34
    knee 729.31
    orbit 374.34
    retro-orbital 374.34
    retropatellar 729.31
    specified site NEC 729.39
  indigestion 579.8
  in stool 792.1
  localized (pad) 278.1
    heart (*see also* Degeneration, myocardial) 429.1
    knee 729.31
    retropatellar 729.31
  necrosis—*see also* Fatty, degeneration
    breast (aseptic) (segmental) 611.3
    mesentery 567.82
    omentum 567.82
    peritoneum 567.82
    pad 278.1
Fatal familial insomnia (FFI) 046.72
Fatal syncope 798.1
Fatigue 780.79
  auditory deafness (*see also* Deafness) 389.9
  chronic, syndrome 780.71
  combat (*see also* Reaction, stress, acute) 308.9
  during pregnancy 646.8
  general 780.79
    psychogenic 300.5
  heat (transient) 992.6
  muscle 729.89
  myocardium (*see also* Failure, heart) 428.9
  nervous 300.5
  neurosis 300.5
  operational 300.89
  postural 729.89
  posture 729.89
  psychogenic (general) 300.5
  senile 797
  syndrome NEC 300.5
    chronic 780.71
  undue 780.79
  voice 784.49
Fatness 278.02
Fatty —*see also* condition
  apron 278.1
  degeneration (diffuse) (general) NEC 272.8
    localized—*see* Degeneration, by site, fatty
  placenta—*see* Placenta, abnormal
  heart (enlarged) (*see also* Degeneration,
    myocardial) 429.1

Fatty—*continued*
  infiltration (diffuse) (general) (*see also*
    Degeneration, by site, fatty) 272.8
    heart (enlarged) (*see also* Degeneration,
      myocardial) 429.1
  liver 571.8
    alcoholic 571.0
  necrosis—*see* Degeneration, fatty
  phanerosis 272.8
Fauces —*see* condition
Fauchard's disease (periodontitis) 523.40
Faucitis 478.29
Faulty —*see also* condition
  position of teeth 524.30
Favism (anemia) 282.2
Favre-Racouchot disease (elastoidosis cutanea
  nodularis) 701.8
Favus 110.9
  beard 110.0
  capitis 110.0
  corporis 110.5
  eyelid 110.8
  foot 110.4
  hand 110.2
  scalp 110.0
  specified site NEC 110.8
Fear, fearfulness (complex) (reaction) 300.20
  child 313.0
  of
    animals 300.29
    closed spaces 300.29
    crowds 300.29
    eating in public 300.23
    heights 300.29
    open spaces 300.22
      with panic attacks 300.21
    public speaking 300.23
    streets 300.22
      with panic attacks 300.21
    travel 300.22
      with panic attacks 300.21
    washing in public 300.23
  transient 308.0
Feared complaint unfounded V65.5
Febricula (continued) (simple) (*see also* Pyrexia)
  780.60
Febrile (*see also* Pyrexia) 780.60
  convulsion (simple) 780.31
    complex 780.32
  seizure (simple) 780.31
    atypical 780.32
    complex 780.32
    complicated 780.32
Febris (*see also* Fever) 780.60
  aestiva (*see also* Fever, hay) 477.9
  flava (*see also* Fever, yellow) 060.9
  melitensis 023.0
  pestis (*see also* Plague) 020.9
  puerperalis 672
  recurrens (*see also* Fever, relapsing) 087.9
    pediculo vestimenti 087.0
  rubra 034.1
  typhoidea 002.0
  typhosa 002.0
Fecal —*see* condition
Fecalith (impaction) 560.39
  with hernia—*see also* Hernia, by site, with
    obstruction
    gangrenous—*see* Hernia, by site, with gangrene
  appendix 543.9
  congenital 777.1

Fede's disease 529.0
Feeble-minded 317
Feeble rapid pulse due to shock following
    injury 958.4
Feeding
    faulty (elderly) (infant) 783.3
        newborn 779.31
    formula check V20.2
    improper (elderly) (infant) 783.3
        newborn 779.31
    problem (elderly) (infant) 783.3
        newborn 779.31
    nonorganic origin 307.59
Feeling of foreign body in throat 784.99
Feer's disease 985.0
Feet —see condition
Feigned illness V65.2
Feil-Klippel syndrome (brevicollis) 756.16
Feinmesser's (hidrotic) ectodermal dysplasia
    757.31
Felix's disease (juvenile osteochondrosis, hip)
    732.1
Felon (any digit) (with lymphangitis) 681.01
    herpetic 054.6
Felty's syndrome (rheumatoid arthritis with
    splenomegaly and leukopenia) 714.1
Feminism in boys 302.6
Feminization, testicular 259.51
    with pseudohermaphroditism, male 259.51
Femoral hernia —see Hernia, femoral
Femora vara 736.32
Femur, femoral —see condition
Fenestrata placenta —see Placenta, abnormal
Fenestration, fenestrated —see also Imperfect,
    closure
    aorta-pulmonary 745.0
    aorticopulmonary 745.0
    aortopulmonary 745.0
    cusps, heart valve NEC 746.89
        pulmonary 746.09
    hymen 752.49
    pulmonic cusps 746.09
Fenwick's disease 537.89
Fermentation (gastric) (gastrointestinal)
    (stomach) 536.8
    intestine 564.89
        psychogenic 306.4
    psychogenic 306.4
Fernell's disease (aortic aneurysm) 441.9
Fertile eunuch syndrome 257.2
Fertility, meaning multiparity—see Multiparity
Fetal
    alcohol syndrome 760.71
    anemia 678.0
    thrombocytopenia 678.0
    twin to twin transfusion 678.0
Fetalis uterus 752.3
Fetid
    breath 784.99
    sweat 705.89
Fetishism 302.81
    transvestic 302.3
Fetomaternal hemorrhage
    affecting management of pregnancy 656.0
    fetus or newborn 772.0
Fetus, fetal —see also condition
    papyraceous 779.89
    type lung tissue 770.4

Fever 780.60
    with chills 780.60
        in malarial regions (see also Malaria) 084.6
    abortus NEC 023.9
    Aden 061
    African tick-borne 087.1
    American
        mountain tick 066.1
        spotted 082.0
    and ague (see also Malaria) 084.6
    aphthous 078.4
    arbovirus hemorrhagic 065.9
    Assam 085.0
    Australian A or Q 083.0
    Bangkok hemorrhagic 065.4
    biliary, Charcot's intermittent—see
        Choledocholithiasis
    bilious, hemoglobinuric 084.8
    blackwater 084.8
    blister 054.9
    Bonvale Dam 780.79
    boutonneuse 082.1
    brain 323.9
        late effect—see category 326
    breakbone 061
    Bullis 082.8
    Bunyamwera 066.3
    Burdwan 085.0
    Bwamba (encephalitis) 066.3
    Cameroon (see also Malaria) 084.6
    Canton 081.9
    catarrhal (acute) 460
        chronic 472.0
    cat-scratch 078.3
    cerebral 323.9
        late effect—see category 326
    cerebrospinal (meningococcal) (see also
        Meningitis, cerebrospinal) 036.0
    Chagres 084.0
    Chandipura 066.8
    changuinola 066.0
    Charcot's (biliary) (hepatic) (intermittent)—see
        Choledocholithiasis
    Chikungunya (viral) 066.3
        hemorrhagic 065.4
    childbed 670.8
    Chitral 066.0
    Colombo (see also Fever, paratyphoid) 002.9
    Colorado tick (virus) 066.1
    congestive
        malarial (see also Malaria) 084.6
        remittent (see also Malaria) 084.6
    Congo virus 065.0
    continued 780.60
        malarial 084.0
    Corsican (see also Malaria) 084.6
    Crimean hemorrhagic 065.0
    Cyprus (see also Brucellosis) 023.9
    dandy 061
    deer fly (see also Tularemia) 021.9
    dehydration, newborn 778.4
    dengue (virus) 061
        hemorrhagic 065.4
    desert 114.0
    due to heat 992.0
    Dumdum 085.0
    enteric 002.0
    ephemeral (of unknown origin) (see also
        Pyrexia) 780.60
    epidemic, hemorrhagic of the Far East 065.0
    erysipelatous (see also Erysipelas) 035

Fever—*continued*
  estivo-autumnal (malarial) 084.0
  etiocholanolone 277.31
  famine—*see also* Fever, relapsing
    meaning typhus—*see* Typhus
  Far Eastern hemorrhagic 065.0
  five day 083.1
  Fort Bragg 100.89
  gastroenteric 002.0
  gastromalarial (*see also* Malaria) 084.6
  Gibraltar (*see also* Brucellosis) 023.9
  glandular 075
  Guama (viral) 066.3
  Haverhill 026.1
  hay (allergic) (with rhinitis) 477.9
    with
      asthma (bronchial) (*see also* Asthma) 493.0
    due to
      dander, animal (cat) (dog) 477.2
      dust 477.8
      fowl 477.8
      hair, animal (cat) (dog) 477.2
      pollen, any plant or tree 477.0
      specified allergen other than pollen 477.8
  heat (effects) 992.0
  hematuric, bilious 084.8
  hemoglobinuric (malarial) 084.8
    bilious 084.8
  hemorrhagic (arthropod-borne) NEC 065.9
    with renal syndrome 078.6
    arenaviral 078.7
    Argentine 078.7
    Bangkok 065.4
    Bolivian 078.7
    Central Asian 065.0
    chikungunya 065.4
    Crimean 065.0
    dengue (virus) 065.4
    Ebola 065.8
    epidemic 078.6
      of Far East 065.0
    Far Eastern 065.0
    Junin virus 078.7
    Korean 078.6
    Kyasanur forest 065.2
    Machupo virus 078.7
    mite-borne NEC 065.8
    mosquito-borne 065.4
    Omsk 065.1
    Philippine 065.4
    Russian (Yaroslav) 078.6
    Singapore 065.4
    Southeast Asia 065.4
    Thailand 065.4
    tick-borne NEC 065.3
  hepatic (*see also* Cholecystitis) 575.8
    intermittent (Charcot's)—*see*
      Choledocholithiasis
  herpetic (*see also* Herpes) 054.9
  Hyalomma tick 065.0
  icterohemorrhagic 100.0
  inanition 780.60
    newborn 778.4
  in conditions classified elsewhere 780.61
  infective NEC 136.9
  intermittent (bilious) (*see also* Malaria) 084.6
    hepatic (Charcot)—*see* Choledocholithiasis
    of unknown origin (*see also* Pyrexia) 780.60
  pernicious 084.0

Fever—*continued*
  iodide
    correct substance properly administered
      780.60
    overdose or wrong substance given or taken
      975.5
  Japanese river 081.2
  jungle yellow 060.0
  Junin virus, hemorrhagic 078.7
  Katayama 120.2
  Kedani 081.2
  Kenya 082.1
  Korean hemorrhagic 078.6
  Lassa 078.89
  Lone Star 082.8
  lung—*see* Pneumonia
  Machupo virus, hemorrhagic 078.7
  malaria, malarial (*see also* Malaria) 084.6
  Malta (*see also* Brucellosis) 023.9
  Marseilles 082.1
  marsh (*see also* Malaria) 084.6
  Mayaro (viral) 066.3
  Mediterranean (*see also* Brucellosis) 023.9
    familial 277.31
    tick 082.1
  meningeal—*see* Meningitis
  metal fumes NEC 985.8
  Meuse 083.1
  Mexican—*see* Typhus, Mexican
  Mianeh 087.1
  miasmatic (*see also* Malaria) 084.6
  miliary 078.2
  milk, female 672
  mill 504
  mite-borne hemorrhagic 065.8
  Monday 504
  mosquito-borne NEC 066.3
    hemorrhagic NEC 065.4
  mountain 066.1
    meaning
      Rocky Mountain spotted 082.0
      undulant fever (*see also* Brucellosis) 023.9
    tick (American) 066.1
  Mucambo (viral) 066.3
  mud 100.89
  Neapolitan (*see also* Brucellosis) 023.9
  neutropenic 288.00
  newborn (environmentally induced) 778.4
  nine-mile 083.0
  nonexanthematous tick 066.1
  North Asian tick-borne typhus 082.2
  Omsk hemorrhagic 065.1
  O'nyong-nyong (viral) 066.3
  Oropouche (viral) 066.3
  Oroya 088.0
  paludal (*see also* Malaria) 084.6
  Panama 084.0
  pappataci 066.0
  paratyphoid 002.9
    A 002.1
    B (Schottmüller's) 002.2
    C (Hirschfeld) 002.3
  parrot 073.9
  periodic 277.31
  pernicious, acute 084.0
  persistent (of unknown origin) (*see also*
    Pyrexia) 780.60
  petechial 036.0
  pharyngoconjunctival 077.2
    adenoviral type 3 077.2
  Philippine hemorrhagic 065.4

Fever—*continued*
  phlebotomus 066.0
  Piry 066.8
  Pixuna (viral) 066.3
  Plasmodium ovale 084.3
  pleural (*see also* Pleurisy) 511.0
  pneumonic—*see* Pneumonia
  polymer fume 987.8
  postimmunization 780.63
  postoperative 780.62
    due to infection 998.59
  postvaccination 780.63
  pretibial 100.89
  puerperal, postpartum 672
  putrid—*see* Septicemia
  pyemic—*see* Septicemia
  Q 083.0
    with pneumonia 083.0 *[484.8]*
  quadrilateral 083.0
  quartan (malaria) 084.2
  Queensland (coastal) 083.0
    seven-day 100.89
  Quintan (A) 083.1
  quotidian 084.0
  rabbit (*see also* Tularemia) 021.9
  rat-bite 026.9
    due to
      Spirillum minor or minus 026.0
      Spirochaeta morsus muris 026.0
      Streptobacillus moniliformis 026.1
  recurrent—*see* Fever, relapsing
  relapsing 087.9
    Carter's (Asiatic) 087.0
    Dutton's (West African) 087.1
    Koch's 087.9
    louse-borne (epidemic) 087.0
    Novy's (American) 087.1
    Obermeyer's (European) 087.0
    spirillum NEC 087.9
    tick-borne (endemic) 087.1
  remittent (bilious) (congestive) (gastric) (*see also* Malaria) 084.6
  rheumatic (active) (acute) (chronic) (subacute) 390
    with heart involvement 391.9
      carditis 391.9
      endocarditis (aortic) (mitral) (pulmonary) (tricuspid) 391.1
      multiple sites 391.8
      myocarditis 391.2
      pancarditis, acute 391.8
      pericarditis 391.0
      specified type NEC 391.8
      valvulitis 391.1
    inactive or quiescent with cardiac hypertrophy 398.99
      carditis 398.90
      endocarditis 397.9
        aortic (valve) 395.9
          with mitral (valve) disease 396.9
        mitral (valve) 394.9
          with aortic (valve) disease 396.9
        pulmonary (valve) 397.1
        tricuspid (valve) 397.0
      heart conditions (classifiable to 429.3, 429.6, 429.9) 398.99
        failure (congestive) (conditions classifiable to 428.0, 428.9) 398.91
        left ventricular failure (conditions classifiable to 428.1) 398.91
      myocardial degeneration (conditions classifiable to 429.1) 398.0

Fever—*continued*
  rheumatic—*continued*
    inactive—*continued*
      myocarditis (conditions classifiable to 429.0) 398.0
      pancarditis 398.99
      pericarditis 393
  Rift Valley (viral) 066.3
  Rocky Mountain spotted 082.0
  rose 477.0
  Ross river (viral) 066.3
  Russian hemorrhagic 078.6
  sandfly 066.0
  San Joaquin (valley) 114.0
  São Paulo 082.0
  scarlet 034.1
  septic—*see* Septicemia
  seven-day 061
    Japan 100.89
    Queensland 100.89
  shin bone 083.1
  Singapore hemorrhagic 065.4
  solar 061
  sore 054.9
  South African tick-bite 087.1
  Southeast Asia hemorrhagic 065.4
  spinal—*see* Meningitis
  spirillary 026.0
  splenic (*see also* Anthrax) 022.9
  spotted (Rocky Mountain) 082.0
    American 082.0
    Brazilian 082.0
    Colombian 082.0
    meaning
      cerebrospinal meningitis 036.0
      typhus 082.9
  spring 309.23
  steroid
    correct substance properly administered 780.60
    overdose or wrong substance given or taken 962.0
  streptobacillary 026.1
  subtertian 084.0
  Sumatran mite 081.2
  sun 061
  swamp 100.89
  sweating 078.2
  swine 003.8
  sylvatic yellow 060.0
  Tahyna 062.5
  tertian—*see* Malaria, tertian
  Thailand hemorrhagic 065.4
  thermic 992.0
  three day 066.0
    with Coxsackie exanthem 074.8
  tick
    American mountain 066.1
    Colorado 066.1
    Kemerovo 066.1
    Mediterranean 082.1
    mountain 066.1
    nonexanthematous 066.1
    Quaranfil 066.1
  tick-bite NEC 066.1
  tick-borne NEC 066.1
    hemorrhagic NEC 065.3
  transitory of newborn 778.4
  trench 083.1
  tsutsugamushi 081.2
  typhogastric 002.0

Fever—*continued*
  typhoid (abortive) (ambulant) (any site)
    (hemorrhagic) (infection) (intermittent)
    (malignant) (rheumatic) 002.0
  typhomalarial (*see also* Malaria) 084.6
  typhus—*see* Typhus
  undulant (*see also* Brucellosis) 023.9
  unknown origin (*see also* Pyrexia) 780.60
  uremic—*see* Uremia
  uveoparotid 135
  valley (Coccidioidomycosis) 114.0
  Venezuelan equine 066.2
  Volhynian 083.1
  Wesselsbron (viral) 066.3
  West
    African 084.8
    Nile (viral) 066.40
      with
        cranial nerve disorders 066.42
        encephalitis 066.41
        optic neuritis 066.42
        other complications 066.49
        other neurologic manifestations 066.42
        polyradiculitis 066.42
  Whitmore's 025
  Wolhynian 083.1
  worm 128.9
  Yaroslav hemorrhagic 078.6
  yellow 060.9
    jungle 060.0
    sylvatic 060.0
    urban 060.1
    vaccination, prophylactic (against) V04.4
  Zika (viral) 066.3
Fibrillation
  atrial (established) (paroxysmal) 427.31
  auricular (atrial) (established) 427.31
  cardiac (ventricular) 427.41
  coronary (*see also* Infarct, myocardium) 410.9
  heart (ventricular) 427.41
  muscular 728.9
  postoperative 997.1
  ventricular 427.41
Fibrin
  ball or bodies, pleural (sac) 511.0
  chamber, anterior (eye) (gelatinous exudate)
    364.04
Fibrinogenolysis (hemorrhagic)—*see*
  Fibrinolysis
Fibrinogenopenia (congenital) (hereditary) (*see*
  also Defect, coagulation) 286.3
  acquired 286.6
Fibrinolysis (acquired) (hemorrhagic)
  (pathologic) 286.6
  with
    abortion—*see* Abortion, by type, with
      hemorrhage, delayed or excessive
    ectopic pregnancy (*see also* categories
      633.0-633.9) 639.1
    molar pregnancy (*see also* categories 630-632)
      639.1
  antepartum or intrapartum 641.3
    affecting fetus or newborn 762.1
  following
    abortion 639.1
    ectopic or molar pregnancy 639.1
  newborn, transient 776.2
  postpartum 666.3
Fibrinopenia (hereditary) (*see also* Defect,
  coagulation) 286.3
  acquired 286.6
Fibrinopurulent —*see* condition

Fibrinous —*see* condition
Fibroadenoma (M9010/0)
  cellular intracanalicular (M9020/0) 217
  giant (intracanalicular) (M9020/0) 217
  intracanalicular (M9011/0)
    cellular (M9020/0) 217
    giant (M9020/0) 217
    specified site—*see* Neoplasm, by site, benign
    unspecified site 217
  juvenile (M9030/0) 217
  pericanalicular (M9012/0)
    specified site—*see* Neoplasm, by site, benign
    unspecified site 217
  phyllodes (M9020/0) 217
  prostate 600.20
    with
      other lower urinary tract symptoms (LUTS)
        600.21
      urinary
        obstruction 600.21
        retention 600.21
  specified site—*see* Neoplasm, by site, benign
  unspecified site 217
Fibroadenosis, breast (chronic) (cystic) (diffuse)
  (periodic) (segmental) 610.2
Fibroangioma (M9160/0)—*see also* Neoplasm,
  by site, benign
  juvenile (M9160/0)
    specified site—*see* Neoplasm, by site, benign
    unspecified site 210.7
Fibrocellulitis progressiva ossificans 728.11
Fibrochondrosarcoma (M9220/3)—*see*
  Neoplasm, cartilage, malignant
Fibrocystic
  disease 277.00
    bone NEC 733.29
    breast 610.1
    jaw 526.2
    kidney (congenital) 753.19
    liver 751.62
    lung 518.89
      congenital 748.4
    pancreas 277.00
  kidney (congenital) 753.19
Fibrodysplasia ossificans multiplex
  (progressiva) 728.11
Fibroelastosis (cordis) (endocardial)
  (endomyocardial) 425.3
Fibroid (tumor) (M8890/0)—*see also* Neoplasm,
  connective tissue, benign
  disease, lung (chronic) (*see also* Fibrosis, lung)
    515
  heart (disease) (*see also* Myocarditis) 429.0
  induration, lung (chronic) (*see also* Fibrosis,
    lung) 515
  in pregnancy or childbirth 654.1
    affecting fetus or newborn 763.89
    causing obstructed labor 660.2
      affecting fetus or newborn 763.1
  liver—*see* Cirrhosis, liver
  lung (*see also* Fibrosis, lung) 515
  pneumonia (chronic) (*see also* Fibrosis, lung)
    515
  uterus (M8890/0) (*see also* Leiomyoma, uterus)
    218.9
Fibrolipoma (M8851/0) (*see also* Lipoma, by
  site) 214.9
Fibroliposarcoma (M8850/3)—*see* Neoplasm,
  connective tissue, malignant

Fibroma (M8810/0)—*see also* Neoplasm,
   connective tissue, benign
  ameloblastic (M9330/0) 213.1
    upper jaw (bone) 213.0
  bone (nonossifying) 733.99
    ossifying (M9262/0)—*see* Neoplasm, bone,
     benign
  cementifying (M9274/0)—*see* Neoplasm, bone,
   benign
  chondromyxoid (M9241/0)—*see* Neoplasm,
   bone, benign
  desmoplastic (M8823/1)—*see* Neoplasm,
   connective tissue, uncertain behavior
  facial (M8813/0)—*see* Neoplasm, connective
   tissue, benign
  invasive (M8821/1)—*see* Neoplasm, connective
   tissue, uncertain behavior
  molle (M8851/0) (*see also* Lipoma, by site) 214.9
  myxoid (M8811/0)—*see* Neoplasm, connective
   tissue, benign
  nasopharynx, nasopharyngeal (juvenile)
   (M9160/0) 210.7
  nonosteogenic (nonossifying)—*see* Dysplasia,
   fibrous
  odontogenic (M9321/0) 213.1
   upper jaw (bone) 213.0
  ossifying (M9262/0)—*see* Neoplasm, bone,
   benign
  periosteal (M8812/0)—*see* Neoplasm, bone,
   benign
  prostate 600.20
   with
    other lower urinary tract symptoms (LUTS)
     600.21
    urinary
     obstruction 600.21
     retention 600.21
  soft (M8851/0) (*see also* Lipoma, by site) 214.9
Fibromatosis 728.79
  abdominal (M8822/1)—*see* Neoplasm,
   connective tissue, uncertain behavior
  aggressive (M8821/1)—*see* Neoplasm,
   connective tissue, uncertain behavior
  congenital generalized (CGF) 759.89
  Dupuytren's 728.6
  gingival 523.8
  plantar fascia 728.71
  proliferative 728.79
  pseudosarcomatous (proliferative)
   (subcutaneous) 728.79
  subcutaneous pseudosarcomatous (proliferative)
   728.79
Fibromyalgia 729.1
Fibromyoma (M8890/0)—*see also* Neoplasm,
  connective tissue, benign
  uterus (corpus) (*see also* Leiomyoma, uterus)
   218.9
   in pregnancy or childbirth 654.1
    affecting fetus or newborn 763.89
    causing obstructed labor 660.2
     affecting fetus or newborn 763.1
Fibromyositis (*see also* Myositis) 729.1
  scapulohumeral 726.2
Fibromyxolipoma (M8852/0) (*see also* Lipoma,
  by site) 214.9
Fibromyxoma (M8811/0)—*see* Neoplasm,
  connective tissue, benign
Fibromyxosarcoma (M8811/3)—*see* Neoplasm,
  connective tissue, malignant
Fibro-odontoma, ameloblastic (M9290/0) 213.1
  upper jaw (bone) 213.0

Fibro-osteoma (M9262/0)—*see* Neoplasm, bone,
  benign
Fibroplasia, retrolental (*see also* Retinopathy of
  prematurity) 362.21
Fibropurulent —*see* condition
Fibrosarcoma (M8810/3)—*see also* Neoplasm,
  connective tissue, malignant
  ameloblastic (M9330/3) 170.1
   upper jaw (bone) 170.0
  congenital (M8814/3)—*see* Neoplasm,
   connective tissue, malignant
  fascial (M8813/3)—*see* Neoplasm, connective
   tissue, malignant
  infantile (M8814/3)—*see* Neoplasm, connective
   tissue, malignant
  odontogenic (M9330/3) 170.1
   upper jaw (bone) 170.0
  periosteal (M8812/3)—*see* Neoplasm, bone,
   malignant
Fibrosclerosis
  breast 610.3
  corpora cavernosa (penis) 607.89
  familial multifocal NEC 710.8
  multifocal (idiopathic) NEC 710.8
  penis (corpora cavernosa) 607.89
Fibrosis, fibrotic
  adrenal (gland) 255.8
  alveolar (diffuse) 516.3
  amnion 658.8
  anal papillae 569.49
  anus 569.49
  appendix, appendiceal, noninflammatory 543.9
  arteriocapillary—*see* Arteriosclerosis
  bauxite (of lung) 503
  biliary 576.8
   due to Clonorchis sinensis 121.1
  bladder 596.8
   interstitial 595.1
   localized submucosal 595.1
   panmural 595.1
  bone, diffuse 756.59
  breast 610.3
  capillary—*see also* Arteriosclerosis
   lung (chronic) (*see also* Fibrosis, lung) 515
  cardiac (*see also* Myocarditis) 429.0
  cervix 622.8
  chorion 658.8
  corpus cavernosum 607.89
  cystic (of pancreas) 277.00
   with
    manifestations
     gastrointestinal 277.03
     pulmonary 277.02
     specified NEC 277.09
    meconium ileus 277.01
    pulmonary exacerbation 277.02
  due to (presence of) any device, implant, or
   graft—*see* Complications, due to (presence
   of) any device, implant, or graft classified to
   996.0-996.5 NEC
  ejaculatory duct 608.89
  endocardium (*see also* Endocarditis) 424.90
  endomyocardial (African) 425.0
  epididymis 608.89
  eye muscle 378.62
  graphite (of lung) 503
  heart (*see also* Myocarditis) 429.0
  hepatic—*see also* Cirrhosis, liver
   due to Clonorchis sinensis 121.1
  hepatolienal—*see* Cirrhosis, liver
  hepatosplenic—*see* Cirrhosis, liver

Fibrosis, fibrotic—*continued*
  infrapatellar fat pad 729.31
  interstitial pulmonary, newborn 770.7
  intrascrotal 608.89
  kidney (*see also* Sclerosis, renal) 587
  liver—*see* Cirrhosis, liver
  lung (atrophic) (capillary) (chronic) (confluent)
      (massive) (perialveolar) (peribronchial) 515
    with
      anthracosilicosis (occupational) 500
      anthracosis (occupational) 500
      asbestosis (occupational) 501
      bagassosis (occupational) 495.1
      bauxite 503
      berylliosis (occupational) 503
      byssinosis (occupational) 504
      calcicosis (occupational) 502
      chalicosis (occupational) 502
      dust reticulation (occupational) 504
      farmers' lung 495.0
      gannister disease (occupational) 502
      graphite 503
      pneumonoconiosis (occupational) 505
      pneumosiderosis (occupational) 503
      siderosis (occupational) 503
      silicosis (occupational) 502
      tuberculosis (*see also* Tuberculosis) 011.4
    diffuse (idiopathic) (interstitial) 516.3
    due to
      bauxite 503
      fumes or vapors (chemical) (inhalation) 506.4
      graphite 503
    following radiation 508.1
    postinflammatory 515
    silicotic (massive) (occupational) 502
    tuberculous (*see also* Tuberculosis) 011.4
  lymphatic gland 289.3
  median bar 600.90
    with
      other lower urinary tract symptoms (LUTS)
          600.91
      urinary
        obstruction 600.91
        retention 600.91
  mediastinum (idiopathic) 519.3
  meninges 349.2
  muscle NEC 728.2
    iatrogenic (from injection) 999.9
  myocardium, myocardial (*see also* Myocarditis)
      429.0
  oral submucous 528.8
  ovary 620.8
  oviduct 620.8
  pancreas 577.8
    cystic 277.00
      with
        manifestations
          gastrointestinal 277.03
          pulmonary 277.02
          specified NEC 277.09
        meconium ileus 277.01
        pulmonary exacerbation 277.02
  penis 607.89
  periappendiceal 543.9
  periarticular (*see also* Ankylosis) 718.5
  pericardium 423.1
  perineum, in pregnancy or childbirth 654.8
    affecting fetus or newborn 763.89
    causing obstructed labor 660.2
      affecting fetus or newborn 763.1

Fibrosis, fibrotic—*continued*
  perineural NEC 355.9
    foot 355.6
  periureteral 593.89
  placenta—*see* Placenta, abnormal
  pleura 511.0
  popliteal fat pad 729.31
  preretinal 362.56
  prostate (chronic) 600.90
    with
      other lower urinary tract symptoms (LUTS)
          600.91
      urinary
        obstruction 600.91
        retention 600.91
  pulmonary (chronic) (*see also* Fibrosis, lung)
      515
    alveolar capillary block 516.3
    interstitial
      diffuse (idiopathic) 516.3
      newborn 770.7
  radiation—*see* Effect, adverse, radiation
  rectal sphincter 569.49
  retroperitoneal, idiopathic 593.4
  sclerosing mesenteric (idiopathic) 567.82
  scrotum 608.89
  seminal vesicle 608.89
  senile 797
  skin NEC 709.2
  spermatic cord 608.89
  spleen 289.59
    bilharzial (*see also* Schistosomiasis) 120.9
  subepidermal nodular (M8832/0)—*see*
      Neoplasm, skin, benign
  submucous NEC 709.2
    oral 528.8
    tongue 528.8
  syncytium—*see* Placenta, abnormal
  testis 608.89
    chronic, due to syphilis 095.8
  thymus (gland) 254.8
  tunica vaginalis 608.89
  ureter 593.89
  urethra 599.84
  uterus (nonneoplastic) 621.8
    bilharzial (*see also* Schistosomiasis) 120.9
    neoplastic (*see also* Leiomyoma, uterus) 218.9
  vagina 623.8
  valve, heart (*see also* Endocarditis) 424.90
  vas deferens 608.89
  vein 459.89
    lower extremities 459.89
  vesical 595.1
Fibrositis (periarticular) (rheumatoid) 729.0
  humeroscapular region 726.2
  nodular, chronic
    Jaccoud's 714.4
    rheumatoid 714.4
  ossificans 728.11
  scapulohumeral 726.2
Fibrothorax 511.0
Fibrotic —*see* Fibrosis
Fibrous —*see* condition
Fibroxanthoma (M8831/0)—*see also* Neoplasm,
    connective tissue, benign
  atypical (M8831/1)—*see* Neoplasm, connective
      tissue, uncertain behavior
  malignant (M8831/3)—*see* Neoplasm,
      connective tissue, malignant
Fibroxanthosarcoma (M8831/3)—*see*
    Neoplasm, connective tissue, malignant

Fiedler's
  disease (leptospiral jaundice) 100.0
  myocarditis or syndrome (acute isolated
    myocarditis) 422.91
Fiessinger-Leroy (-Reiter) syndrome 099.3
Fiessinger-Rendu syndrome (erythema
  muliforme exudativum) 695.19
Fifth disease (eruptive) 057.0
  venereal 099.1
Filaria, filarial —*see* Infestation, filarial
Filariasis (*see also* Infestation, filarial) 125.9
  bancroftian 125.0
  Brug's 125.1
  due to
    bancrofti 125.0
    Brugia (Wuchereria) (malayi) 125.1
    Loa loa 125.2
    malayi 125.1
    organism NEC 125.6
    Wuchereria (bancrofti) 125.0
      malayi 125.1
  Malayan 125.1
  ozzardi 125.5
  specified type NEC 125.6
Filatoff's, Filatov's, Filatow's disease
  (infectious mononucleosis) 075
File-cutters' disease 984.9
  specified type of lead—*see* Table of drugs and
    chemicals
Filling defect
  biliary tract 793.3
  bladder 793.5
  duodenum 793.4
  gallbladder 793.3
  gastrointestinal tract 793.4
  intestine 793.4
  kidney 793.5
  stomach 793.4
  ureter 793.5
Filtering bleb, eye (postglaucoma) (status)
  V45.69
  with complication or rupture 997.99
  postcataract extraction (complication) 997.99
Fimbrial cyst (congenital) 752.11
Fimbriated hymen 752.49
Financial problem affecting care V60.2
Findings (abnormal), without diagnosis
  (examination) (laboratory test) 796.4
  17-ketosteroids, elevated 791.9
  acetonuria 791.6
  acid phosphatase 790.5
  albumin-globulin ratio 790.99
  albuminuria 791.0
  alcohol in blood 790.3
  alkaline phosphatase 790.5
  amniotic fluid 792.3
  amylase 790.5
  anisocytosis 790.09
  antenatal screening 796.5
  anthrax positive 795.31
  antibody titers, elevated 795.79
  anticardiolipin antibody 795.79
  antigen-antibody reaction 795.79
  antiphospholipid antibody 795.79
  bacteriuria 791.9
  ballistocardiogram 794.39
  bicarbonate 276.9
  bile in urine 791.4
  bilirubin 277.4
  bleeding time (prolonged) 790.92
  blood culture, positive 790.7
  blood gas level 790.91

Findings —*continued*
  blood sugar level 790.29
    high 790.29
      fasting glucose 790.21
      glucose tolerance test 790.22
    low 251.2
  C-reactive protein (CRP) 790.95
  calcium 275.40
  cancer antigen 125 [CA 125] 795.82
  carbonate 276.9
  carcinoembryonic antigen [CEA] 795.81
  casts, urine 791.7
  catecholamines 791.9
  cells, urine 791.7
  cerebrospinal fluid (color) (content) (pressure)
    792.0
  cervical
    high risk human papillomavirus (HPV) DNA
      test positive 795.05
    low risk human papillomavirus (HPV) DNA
      test positive 795.09
  chloride 276.9
  cholesterol 272.9
    high 272.0
      with high triglycerides 272.2
  chromosome analysis 795.2
  chyluria 791.1
  circulation time 794.39
  cloudy dialysis effluent 792.5
  cloudy urine 791.9
  coagulation study 790.92
  cobalt, blood 790.6
  color of urine (unusual) NEC 791.9
  copper, blood 790.6
  creatinine clearance 794.4
  crystals, urine 791.9
  culture, positive NEC 795.39
    blood 790.7
    HIV V08
    human immunodeficiency virus V08
    nose 795.39
      Staphylococcus — *see* Carrier (suspected)
        of, Staphylococcus
    skin lesion NEC 795.39
    spinal fluid 792.0
    sputum 795.39
    stool 792.1
    throat 795.39
    urine 791.9
    viral
      human immunodeficiency V08
    wound 795.39
  cytology specified site NEC 796.9
  echocardiogram 793.2
  echoencephalogram 794.01
  echogram NEC—*see* Findings, abnormal,
    structure
  electrocardiogram (ECG) (EKG) 794.31
  electroencephalogram (EEG) 794.02
  electrolyte level, urinary 791.9
  electromyogram (EMG) 794.17
    ocular 794.14
  electro-oculogram (EOG) 794.12
  electroretinogram (ERG) 794.11
  enzymes, serum NEC 790.5
  fibrinogen titer coagulation study 790.92
  filling defect—*see* Filling defect

Findings—*continued*
function study NEC 794.9
  auditory 794.15
  bladder 794.9
  brain 794.00
  cardiac 794.30
  endocrine NEC 794.6
    thyroid 794.5
  kidney 794.4
  liver 794.8
  nervous system
    central 794.00
    peripheral 794.19
  oculomotor 794.14
  pancreas 794.9
  placenta 794.9
  pulmonary 794.2
  retina 794.11
  special senses 794.19
  spleen 794.9
  vestibular 794.16
gallbladder, nonvisualization 793.3
glucose 790.29
  elevated
    fasting 790.21
    tolerance test 790.22
glycosuria 791.5
heart
  shadow 793.2
  sounds 785.3
hematinuria 791.2
hematocrit
  drop (precipitous) 790.01
  elevated 282.7
  low 285.9
hematologic NEC 790.99
hematuria 599.70
hemoglobin
  drop 790.01
  elevated 282.7
  low 285.9
hemoglobinuria 791.2
histological NEC 795.4
hormones 259.9
immunoglobulins, elevated 795.79
indolacetic acid, elevated 791.9
iron 790.6
karyotype 795.2
ketonuria 791.6
lactic acid dehydrogenase (LDH) 790.4
lead 790.6
lipase 790.5
lipids NEC 272.9
lithium, blood 790.6
liver function test 790.6
lung field (coin lesion) (shadow) 793.1
magnesium, blood 790.6
mammogram 793.80
  calcification 793.89
  caclulus 793.89
  dense breasts 793.82
  inconclusive 793.82
    due to dense breasts 793.82
  microcalcification 793.81
mediastinal shift 793.2
melanin, urine 791.9
microbiologic NEC 795.39
mineral, blood NEC 790.6
myoglobinuria 791.3
nasal swab, anthrax 795.31
neonatal screening 796.6
nitrogen derivatives, blood 790.6

Findings—*continued*
nonvisualization of gallbladder 793.3
nose culture, positive 795.39
odor of urine (unusual) NEC 791.9
oxygen saturation 790.91
Papanicolaou (smear) 796.9
  anus 796.70
    with
      atypical squamous cells
        cannot exclude high grade squamous
          intraepithelial lesion (ASC-H)
          796.72
        of undetermined significance (ASC-US)
          796.71
      cytologic evidence of malignancy 796.76
      high grade squamous intraepithelial lesion
        (HGSIL) 796.74
      low grade squamous intraepithelial lesion
        (LGSIL) 796.73
    glandular 796.70
    specified finding NEC 796.79
  cervix 795.00
    with
      atypical squamous cells
        cannot exclude high grade squamous
          intrepithelial lesion (ASC-H) 795.02
        of undetermined significance (ASC-US)
          795.01
      cytologic evidence of malignancy 795.06
      high grade squamous intraepithelial lesion
        (HGSIL) 795.04
      low grade squamous intraepithelial lesion
        (LGSIL) 795.03
    dyskaryotic 795.09
    nonspecific finding NEC 795.09
  other site 796.9
  vagina 795.10
    with
      atypical squamous cells
        cannot exclude high grade squamous
          intraepithelial lesion (ASC-H)
          795.12
        of undetermined significance (ASC-US)
          795.11
      cytologic evidence of malignancy 795.16
      high grade squamous intraepithelial lesion
        (HGSIL) 795.14
      low grade squamous intraepithelial lesion
        (LGSIL) 795.13
    glandular 795.10
    specified NEC 795.19
peritoneal fluid 792.9
phonocardiogram 794.39
phosphorus 275.3
pleural fluid 792.9
pneumoencephalogram 793.0
PO_2-oxygen ratio 790.91
poikilocytosis 790.09
potassium
  deficiency 276.8
  excess 276.7
PPD 795.5
prostate specific antigen (PSA) 790.93
protein, serum NEC 790.99
proteinuria 791.0
prothrombin time (partial) (prolonged) (PT)
  (PTT) 790.92
pyuria 791.9

Findings —*continued*
  radiologic (x-ray) 793.99
    abdomen 793.6
    biliary tract 793.3
    breast 793.89
      abnormal mammogram NOS 793.80
      mammographic
        calcification 793.89
        calculus 793.89
        microcalcification 793.81
    gastrointestinal tract 793.4
    genitourinary organs 793.5
    head 793.0
    image test inconclusive due to excess body fat
      793.91
    intrathoracic organs NEC 793.2
    lung 793.1
    musculoskeletal 793.7
    placenta 793.99
    retroperitoneum 793.6
    skin 793.99
    skull 793.0
    subcutaneous tissue 793.99
  red blood cell 790.09
    count 790.09
    morphology 790.09
    sickling 790.09
    volume 790.09
  saliva 792.4
  scan NEC 794.9
    bladder 794.9
    bone 794.9
    brain 794.09
    kidney 794.4
    liver 794.8
    lung 794.2
    pancreas 794.9
    placental 794.9
    spleen 794.9
    thyroid 794.5
  sedimentation rate, elevated 790.1
  semen 792.2
  serological (for)
    human immunodeficiency virus (HIV)
      inconclusive 795.71
      positive V08
    syphilis—*see* Findings, serology for syphilis
  serology for syphilis
    false positive 795.6
    positive 097.1
      false 795.6
      follow-up of latent syphilis—*see* Syphilis,
        latent
      only finding—*see* Syphilis, latent
  serum 790.99
    blood NEC 790.99
    enzymes NEC 790.5
    proteins 790.99
  SGOT 790.4
  SGPT 790.4
  sickling of red blood cells 790.09
  skin test, positive 795.79
    tuberculin (without active tuberculosis) 795.5
  sodium 790.6
    deficiency 276.1
    excess 276.0
  specified NEC 796.9
  spermatozoa 792.2
  spinal fluid 792.0
    culture, positive 792.0
  sputum culture, positive 795.39

Findings —*continued*
    for acid-fast bacilli 795.39
  stool NEC 792.1
    bloody 578.1
      occult 792.1
    color 792.1
    culture, positive 792.1
    occult blood 792.1
  stress test 794.39
  structure, body (echogram) (thermogram)
      (ultrasound) (x-ray) NEC 793.99
    abdomen 793.6
    breast 793.89
      abnormal mammogram 793.80
      mammographic
        calcification 793.89
        calculus 793.89
        microcalcification 793.81
    gastrointestinal tract 793.4
    genitourinary organs 793.5
    head 793.0
    echogram (ultrasound) 794.01
    intrathoracic organs NEC 793.2
    lung 793.1
    musculoskeletal 793.7
    placenta 793.99
    retroperitoneum 793.6
    skin 793.99
    subcutaneous tissue NEC 793.99
  synovial fluid 792.9
  thermogram—*see* Finding, abnormal, structure
  throat culture, positive 795.39
  thyroid (function) 794.5
    metabolism (rate) 794.5
    scan 794.5
    uptake 794.5
  total proteins 790.99
  toxicology (drugs) (heavy metals) 796.0
  transaminase (level) 790.4
  triglycerides 272.9
    high 272.1
      with high cholesterol 272.2
  tuberculin skin test (without active tuberculosis)
      795.5
  tumor markers NEC 795.89
  ultrasound—*see also* Finding, abnormal,
      structure
    cardiogram 793.2
  uric acid, blood 790.6
  urine, urinary constituents 791.9
    acetone 791.6
    albumin 791.0
    bacteria 791.9
    bile 791.4
    blood 599.70
    casts or cells 791.7
    chyle 791.1
    culture, positive 791.9
    glucose 791.5
    hemoglobin 791.2
    ketone 791.6
    protein 791.0
    pus 791.9
    sugar 791.5
  vaginal
    fluid 792.9
    high risk human papillomavirus (HPV) DNA
      test positive 795.15
    low risk human papillomavirus (HPV) DNA
      test positive 795.19
  vanillylmandelic acid, elevated 791.9

Fistula—*continued*
  carotid-cavernous
    congenital 747.81
      with hemorrhage 430
    traumatic 900.82
      with hemorrhage (*see also* Hemorrhage,
        brain, traumatic) 853.0
      late effect 908.3
  cecosigmoidal 569.81
  cecum 569.81
  cerebrospinal (fluid) 349.81
  cervical, lateral (congenital) 744.41
  cervicoaural (congenital) 744.49
  cervicosigmoidal 619.1
  cervicovesical 619.0
  cervix 619.8
  chest (wall) 510.0
  cholecystocolic (*see also* Fistula, gallbladder)
    575.5
  cholecystocolonic (*see also* Fistula, gallbladder)
    575.5
  cholecystoduodenal (*see also* Fistula,
    gallbladder) 575.5
  cholecystoenteric (*see also* Fistula, gallbladder)
    575.5
  cholecystogastric (*see also* Fistula, gallbladder)
    575.5
  cholecystointestinal (*see also* Fistula,
    gallbladder) 575.5
  choledochoduodenal 576.4
  cholocolic (*see also* Fistula, gallbladder) 575.5
  coccyx 685.1
    with abscess 685.0
  colon 569.81
  colostomy 569.69
  colovaginal (acquired) 619.1
  common duct (bile duct) 576.4
  congenital, NEC—*see* Anomaly, specified type
    NEC
  cornea, causing hypotony 360.32
  coronary, arteriovenous 414.19
    congenital 746.85
  costal region 510.0
  cul-de-sac, Douglas' 619.8
  cutaneous 686.9
  cystic duct (*see also* Fistula, gallbladder) 575.5
    congenital 751.69
  dental 522.7
  diaphragm 510.0
    bronchovisceral 510.0
    pleuroperitoneal 510.0
    pulmonoperitoneal 510.0
  duodenum 537.4
  ear (canal) (external) 380.89
  enterocolic 569.81
  enterocutaneous 569.81
  enteroenteric 569.81
  entero-uterine 619.1
    congenital 752.3
  enterovaginal 619.1
    congenital 752.49
  enterovesical 596.1
  epididymis 608.89
    tuberculous (*see also* Tuberculosis) 016.4
  esophagobronchial 530.89
    congenital 750.3
  esophagocutaneous 530.89
  esophagopleurocutaneous 530.89
  esophagotracheal 530.84
    congenital 750.3

Fistula—*continued*
  esophagus 530.89
    congenital 750.4
  ethmoid (*see also* Sinusitis, ethmoidal) 473.2
  eyeball (cornea) (sclera) 360.32
  eyelid 373.11
  fallopian tube (external) 619.2
  fecal 569.81
    congenital 751.5
  from periapical lesion 522.7
  frontal sinus (*see also* Sinusitis, frontal) 473.1
  gallbladder 575.5
    with calculus, cholelithiasis, stones (*see also*
      Cholelithiasis) 574.2
    congenital 751.69
  gastric 537.4
  gastrocolic 537.4
    congenital 750.7
    tuberculous (*see also* Tuberculosis) 014.8
  gastroenterocolic 537.4
  gastroesophageal 537.4
  gastrojejunal 537.4
  gastrojejunocolic 537.4
  genital
    organs
      female 619.9
        specified site NEC 619.8
      male 608.89
    tract-skin (female) 619.2
  hepatopleural 510.0
  hepatopulmonary 510.0
  horseshoe 565.1
  ileorectal 569.81
  ileosigmoidal 569.81
  ileostomy 569.69
  ileovesical 596.1
  ileum 569.81
  in ano 565.1
    tuberculous (*see also* Tuberculosis) 014.8
  inner ear (*see also* Fistula, labyrinth) 386.40
  intestine 569.81
  intestinocolonic (abdominal) 569.81
  intestinoureteral 593.82
  intestinouterine 619.1
  intestinovaginal 619.1
    congenital 752.49
  intestinovesical 596.1
  involving female genital tract 619.9
    digestive-genital 619.1
    genital tract-skin 619.2
    specified site NEC 619.8
    urinary-genital 619.0
  ischiorectal (fossa) 566
  jejunostomy 569.69
  jejunum 569.81
  joint 719.80
    ankle 719.87
    elbow 719.82
    foot 719.87
    hand 719.84
    hip 719.85
    knee 719.86
    multiple sites 719.89
    pelvic region 719.85
    shoulder (region) 719.81
    specified site NEC 719.88
    tuberculous—*see* Tuberculosis, joint
    wrist 719.83
  kidney 593.89
  labium (majus) (minus) 619.8

Fistula—*continued*
  labyrinth, labyrinthine NEC 386.40
    combined sites 386.48
    multiple sites 386.48
    oval window 386.42
    round window 386.41
  semicircular canal 386.43
  lacrimal, lachrymal (duct) (gland) (sac) 375.61
  lacrimonasal duct 375.61
  laryngotracheal 748.3
  larynx 478.79
  lip 528.5
    congenital 750.25
  lumbar, tuberculous (*see also* Tuberculosis)
    015.0 *[730.8]*
  lung 510.0
  lymphatic (node) (vessel) 457.8
  mamillary 611.0
  mammary (gland) 611.0
    puerperal, postpartum 675.1
  mastoid (process) (region) 383.1
  maxillary (*see also* Sinusitis, maxillary) 473.0
  mediastinal 510.0
  mediastinobronchial 510.0
  mediastinocutaneous 510.0
  middle ear 385.89
  mouth 528.3
  nasal 478.19
    sinus (*see also* Sinusitis) 473.9
  nasopharynx 478.29
  nipple—*see* Fistula, breast
  nose 478.19
  oral (cutaneous) 528.3
    maxillary (*see also* Sinusitis, maxillary) 473.0
    nasal (with cleft palate) (*see also* Cleft, palate)
      749.00
  orbit, orbital 376.10
  oro-antral (*see also* Sinusitis, maxillary) 473.0
  oval window (internal ear) 386.42
  oviduct (external) 619.2
  palate (hard) 526.89
    soft 528.9
  pancreatic 577.8
  pancreaticoduodenal 577.8
  parotid (gland) 527.4
    region 528.3
  pelvoabdominointestinal 569.81
  penis 607.89
  perianal 565.1
  pericardium (pleura) (sac) (*see also* Pericarditis)
    423.8
  pericecal 569.81
  perineal—*see* Fistula, perineum
  perineorectal 569.81
  perineosigmoidal 569.81
  perineo-urethroscrotal 608.89
  perineum, perineal (with urethral involvement)
    NEC 599.1
    tuberculous (*see also* Tuberculosis) 017.9
    ureter 593.82
  perirectal 565.1
    tuberculous (*see also* Tuberculosis) 014.8
  peritoneum (*see also* Peritonitis) 567.22
  periurethral 599.1
  pharyngo-esophageal 478.29
  pharynx 478.29
    branchial cleft (congenital) 744.41
  pilonidal (infected) (rectum) 685.1
    with abscess 685.0

Fistula—*continued*
  pleura, pleural, pleurocutaneous,
    pleuroperitoneal 510.0
    stomach 510.0
    tuberculous (*see also* Tuberculosis) 012.0
  pleuropericardial 423.8
  postauricular 383.81
  postoperative, persistent 998.6
  preauricular (congenital) 744.46
  prostate 602.8
  pulmonary 510.0
    arteriovenous 417.0
      congenital 747.3
    tuberculous (*see also* Tuberculosis,
      pulmonary) 011.9
  pulmonoperitoneal 510.0
  rectolabial 619.1
  rectosigmoid (intercommunicating) 569.81
  rectoureteral 593.82
  rectourethral 599.1
    congenital 753.8
  rectouterine 619.1
    congenital 752.3
  rectovaginal 619.1
    congenital 752.49
    old, postpartal 619.1
    tuberculous (*see also* Tuberculosis) 014.8
  rectovesical 596.1
    congenital 753.8
  rectovesicovaginal 619.1
  rectovulvar 619.1
    congenital 752.49
  rectum (to skin) 565.1
    tuberculous (*see also* Tuberculosis) 014.8
  renal 593.89
  retroauricular 383.81
  round window (internal ear) 386.41
  salivary duct or gland 527.4
    congenital 750.24
  sclera 360.32
  scrotum (urinary) 608.89
    tuberculous (*see also* Tuberculosis) 016.5
  semicircular canals (internal ear) 386.43
  sigmoid 569.81
    vesicoabdominal 596.1
  sigmoidovaginal 619.1
    congenital 752.49
  skin 686.9
    ureter 593.82
    vagina 619.2
  sphenoidal sinus (*see also* Sinusitis, sphenoidal)
    473.3
  splenocolic 289.59
  stercoral 569.81
  stomach 537.4
  sublingual gland 527.4
    congenital 750.24
  submaxillary
    gland 527.4
      congenital 750.24
    region 528.3
  thoracic 510.0
    duct 457.8
  thoracicoabdominal 510.0
  thoracicogastric 510.0
  thoracicointestinal 510.0
  thoracoabdominal 510.0
  thoracogastric 510.0
  thorax 510.0
  thyroglossal duct 759.2
  thyroid 246.8
  trachea (congenital) (external) (internal) 748.3

Fistula—*continued*
  tracheoesophageal 530.84
    congenital 750.3
    following tracheostomy 519.09
  traumatic
    arteriovenous (*see also* Injury, blood vessel,
      by site) 904.9
    brain—*see* Injury, intracranial
  tuberculous—*see* Tuberculosis, by site
  typhoid 002.0
  umbilical 759.89
  umbilico-urinary 753.8
  urachal, urachus 753.7
  ureter (persistent) 593.82
  ureteroabdominal 593.82
  ureterocervical 593.82
  ureterorectal 593.82
  ureterosigmoido-abdominal 593.82
  ureterovaginal 619.0
  ureterovesical 596.2
  urethra 599.1
    congenital 753.8
    tuberculous (*see also* Tuberculosis) 016.3
  urethroperineal 599.1
  urethroperineovesical 596.2
  urethrorectal 599.1
    congenital 753.8
  urethroscrotal 608.89
  urethrovaginal 619.0
  urethrovesical 596.2
  urethrovesicovaginal 619.0
  urinary (persistent) (recurrent) 599.1
  uteroabdominal (anterior wall) 619.2
    congenital 752.3
  uteroenteric 619.1
  uterofecal 619.1
  uterointestinal 619.1
    congenital 752.3
  uterorectal 619.1
    congenital 752.3
  uteroureteric 619.0
  uterovaginal 619.8
  uterovesical 619.0
    congenital 752.3
  uterus 619.8
  vagina (wall) 619.8
    postpartal, old 619.8
  vaginocutaneous (postpartal) 619.2
  vaginoileal (acquired) 619.1
  vaginoperineal 619.2
  vesical NEC 596.2
  vesicoabdominal 596.2
  vesicocervicovaginal 619.0
  vesicocolic 596.1
  vesicocutaneous 596.2
  vesicoenteric 596.1
  vesicointestinal 596.1
  vesicometrorectal 619.1
  vesicoperineal 596.2
  vesicorectal 596.1
    congenital 753.8
  vesicosigmoidal 596.1
  vesicosigmoidovaginal 619.1
  vesicoureteral 596.2
  vesicoureterovaginal 619.0
  vesicourethral 596.2
  vesicourethrorectal 596.1
  vesicouterine 619.0
    congenital 752.3
  vesicovaginal 619.0
  vulvorectal 619.1
    congenital 752.49

Fit 780.39
  apoplectic (*see also* Disease, cerebrovascular,
    acute) 436
    late effect—*see* Late effect(s) (of)
      cerebrovascular disease
  epileptic (*see also* Epilepsy) 345.9
  fainting 780.2
  hysterical 300.11
  newborn 779.0
Fitting (of)
  artificial
    arm (complete) (partial) V52.0
    breast V52.4
      implant exchange (different material)
        (different size) V52.4
    eye(s) V52.2
    leg(s) (complete) (partial) V52.1
  brain neuropacemaker V53.02
  cardiac pacemaker V53.31
  carotid sinus pacemaker V53.39
  cerebral ventricle (communicating) shunt
    V53.01
  colostomy belt V53.5
  contact lenses V53.1
  cystostomy device V53.6
  defibrillator, automatic implantable V53.32
  dentures V52.3
  device, unspecified type V53.90
    abdominal V53.5
    cardiac
      defibrillator, automatic implantable V53.32
      pacemaker V53.31
      specified NEC V53.39
    cerebral ventricle (communicating) shunt
      V53.01
    insulin pump V53.91
    intrauterine contraceptive V25.1
    nervous system V53.09
    orthodontic V53.4
    orthoptic V53.1
    other device V53.99
    prosthetic V52.9
      breast V52.4
      dental V52.3
      eye V52.2
      specified type NEC V52.8
    special senses V53.09
    substitution
      auditory V53.09
      nervous system V53.09
      visual V53.09
    urinary V53.6
  diaphragm (contraceptive) V25.02
  glasses (reading) V53.1
  growth rod V54.02
  hearing aid V53.2
  ileostomy device V53.5
  intestinal appliance or device NEC V53.5
  intrauterine contraceptive device V25.1
  neuropacemaker (brain) (peripheral nerve)
    (spinal cord) V53.02
  orthodontic device V53.4
  orthopedic (device) V53.7
    brace V53.7
    cast V53.7
    corset V53.7
    shoes V53.7
  pacemaker (cardiac) V53.31
    brain V53.02
    carotid sinus V53.39
    peripheral nerve V53.02
    spinal cord V53.02

Fitting—*continued*
  prosthesis V52.9
    arm (complete) (partial) V52.0
    breast V52.4
      implant exchange (different material)
        (different size) V52.4
    dental V52.3
    eye V52.2
    leg (complete) (partial) V52.1
    specified type NEC V52.8
  spectacles V53.1
  wheelchair V53.8
Fitz's syndrome (acute hemorrhagic pancreatitis) 577.0
Fitz-Hugh and Curtis syndrome 098.86
  due to
    Chlamydia trachomatis 099.56
    Neisseria gonorrhoeae (gonococcal peritonitis) 098.86
Fixation
  joint—*see* Ankylosis
  larynx 478.79
  pupil 364.76
  stapes 385.22
    deafness (*see also* Deafness, conductive) 389.04
  uterus (acquired)—*see* Malposition, uterus
  vocal cord 478.5
Flaccid —*see* condition
  foot 736.79
  forearm 736.09
  palate, congenital 750.26
Flail
  chest 807.4
    newborn 767.3
  joint (paralytic) 718.80
    ankle 718.87
    elbow 718.82
    foot 718.87
    hand 718.84
    hip 718.85
    knee 718.86
    multiple sites 718.89
    pelvic region 718.85
    shoulder (region) 718.81
    specified site NEC 718.88
    wrist 718.83
Flajani (-Basedow) syndrome or disease (exophthalmic goiter) 242.0
Flap, liver 572.8
Flare, anterior chamber (aqueous) (eye) 364.04
Flashback phenomena (drug) (hallucinogenic) 292.89
Flat
  chamber (anterior) (eye) 360.34
  chest, congenital 754.89
  electroencephalogram (EEG) 348.89
  foot (acquired) (fixed type) (painful) (postural) (spastic) 734
    congenital 754.61
      rocker bottom 754.61
      vertical talus 754.61
    rachitic 268.1
    rocker bottom (congenital) 754.61
    vertical talus, congenital 754.61
  organ or site, congenital NEC—*see* Anomaly, specified type NEC
  pelvis 738.6
    with disproportion (fetopelvic) 653.2
      affecting fetus or newborn 763.1
      causing obstructed labor 660.1
        affecting fetus or newborn 763.1
    congenital 755.69

Flatau-Schilder disease 341.1
Flattening
  head, femur 736.39
  hip 736.39
  lip (congenital) 744.89
  nose (congenital) 754.0
    acquired 738.0
Flatulence 787.3
Flatus 787.3
  vaginalis 629.89
Flax dressers' disease 504
Flea bite —*see* Injury, superficial, by site
Fleischer (-Kayser) ring (corneal pigmentation) 275.1 *[371.14]*
Fleischner's disease 732.3
Fleshy mole 631
Flexibilitas cerea (*see also* Catalepsy) 300.11
Flexion
  cervix —*see* Flexion, uterus
  contracture, joint (*see also* Contraction, joint) 718.4
  deformity, joint (*see also* Contraction, joint) 736.9
    hip, congenital (*see also* Subluxation, congenital, hip) 754.32
  uterus (*see also* Malposition, uterus) 621.6
Flexner's
  bacillus 004.1
  diarrhea (ulcerative) 004.1
  dysentery 004.1
Flexner-Boyd dysentery 004.2
Flexure —*see* condition
Floater, vitreous 379.24
Floating
  cartilage (joint) (*see also* Disorder, cartilage, articular) 718.0
    knee 717.6
  gallbladder (congenital) 751.69
  kidney 593.0
    congenital 753.3
  liver (congenital) 751.69
  rib 756.3
  spleen 289.59
Flooding 626.2
Floor —*see* condition
Floppy
  infant NEC 781.99
  iris syndrome 364.81
  valve syndrome (mitral) 424.0
Flu —*see also* Influenza
  bird 488.0
  gastric NEC 008.8
  swine 488.0
Fluctuating blood pressure 796.4
Fluid
  abdomen 789.59
  chest (*see also* Pleurisy, with effusion) 511.9
  heart (*see also* Failure, heart) 428.0
  joint (*see also* Effusion, joint) 719.0
  loss (acute) 276.50
    with
      hypernatremia 276.0
      hyponatremia 276.1
  lung—*see also* Edema, lung
    encysted 511.89
  peritoneal cavity 789.59
    malignant 789.51
  pleural cavity (*see also* Pleurisy, with effusion) 511.9
  retention 276.6
Flukes NEC (*see also* Infestation, fluke) 121.9
  blood NEC (*see also* Infestation, Schistosoma) 120.9
  liver 121.3

Fluor (albus) (vaginalis) 623.5
   trichomonal (Trichomonas vaginalis) 131.00
Fluorosis (dental) (chronic) 520.3
Flushing 782.62
   menopausal 627.2
Flush syndrome 259.2
Flutter
   atrial or auricular 427.32
   heart (ventricular) 427.42
      atrial 427.32
   impure 427.32
   postoperative 997.1
   ventricular 427.42
Flux (bloody) (serosanguineous) 009.0
Focal —*see* condition
Fochier's abscess —*see* Abscess, by site
Focus, Assmann's (*see also* Tuberculosis) 011.0
Fogo selvagem 694.4
Foix-Alajouanine syndrome 336.1
Folds, anomalous —*see also* Anomaly, specified
   type NEC
   Bowman's membrane 371.31
   Descemet's membrane 371.32
   epicanthic 743.63
   heart 746.89
   posterior segment of eye, congenital 743.54
Folie à deux 297.3
Follicle
   cervix (nabothian) (ruptured) 616.0
   graafian, ruptured, with hemorrhage 620.0
   nabothian 616.0
Folliclis (primary) (*see also* Tuberculosis) 017.0
Follicular —*see also* condition
   cyst (atretic) 620.0
Folliculitis 704.8
   abscedens et suffodiens 704.8
   decalvans 704.09
   gonorrheal (acute) 098.0
      chronic or duration of 2 months or more 098.2
   keloid, keloidalis 706.1
   pustular 704.8
   ulerythematosa reticulata 701.8
Folliculosis, conjunctival 372.02
Folling's disease (phenylketonuria) 270.1
Follow-up (examination) (routine) (following) V67.9
   cancer chemotherapy V67.2
   chemotherapy V67.2
   fracture V67.4
   high-risk medication V67.51
   injury NEC V67.59
   postpartum
      immediately after delivery V24.0
      routine V24.2
   psychiatric V67.3
   psychotherapy V67.3
   radiotherapy V67.1
   specified condition NEC V67.59
   specified surgery NEC V67.09
   surgery V67.00
      vaginal pap smear V67.01
   treatment V67.9
      combined NEC V67.6
      fracture V67.4
      involving high-risk medication NEC V67.51
      mental disorder V67.3
      specified NEC V67.59
Fong's syndrome (hereditary
   osteoonychodysplasia) 756.89

Food
   allergy 693.1
   anaphylactic shock—*see* Anaphylactic shock,
      due to, food
   asphyxia (from aspiration or inhalation) (*see*
      also Asphyxia, food) 933.1
   choked on (*see also* Asphyxia, food) 933.1
   deprivation 994.2
      specified kind of food NEC 269.8
   intoxication (*see also* Poisoning, food) 005.9
   lack of 994.2
   poisoning (*see also* Poisoning, food) 005.9
   refusal or rejection NEC 307.59
   strangulation or suffocation (*see also* Asphyxia,
      food) 933.1
   toxemia (*see also* Poisoning, food) 005.9
Foot —*see also* condition
   and mouth disease 078.4
   process disease 581.3
Foramen ovale (nonclosure) (patent) (persistent)
   745.5
Forbes' (glycogen storage) disease 271.0
Forbes-Albright syndrome (nonpuerperal
   amenorrhea and lactation associated with
   pituitary tumor) 253.1
Forced birth or delivery NEC 669.8
   affecting fetus or newborn NEC 763.89
Forceps
   delivery NEC 669.5
   affecting fetus or newborn 763.2
Fordyce's disease (ectopic sebaceous glands)
   (mouth) 750.26
Fordyce-Fox disease (apocrine miliaria) 705.82
Forearm —*see* condition
Foreign body

> *Note—For foreign body with open wound or
> other injury, see Wound, open, or the type of
> injury specified.*

   accidentally left during a procedure 998.4
   anterior chamber (eye) 871.6
      magnetic 871.5
         retained or old 360.51
      retained or old 360.61
   ciliary body (eye) 871.6
      magnetic 871.5
         retained or old 360.52
      retained or old 360.62
   entering through orifice (current) (old)
      accessory sinus 932
      air passage (upper) 933.0
         lower 934.8
      alimentary canal 938
      alveolar process 935.0
      antrum (Highmore) 932
      anus 937
      appendix 936
      asphyxia due to (*see also* Asphyxia, food)
         933.1
      auditory canal 931
      auricle 931
      bladder 939.0
      bronchioles 934.8
      bronchus (main) 934.1
      buccal cavity 935.0
      canthus (inner) 930.1
      cecum 936
      cervix (canal) uterine 939.1
      coil, ileocecal 936
      colon 936

Foreign body—*continued*
entering through—*continued*
conjunctiva 930.1
conjunctival sac 930.1
cornea 930.0
digestive organ or tract NEC 938
duodenum 936
ear (external) 931
esophagus 935.1
eye (external) 930.9
combined sites 930.8
intraocular—*see* Foreign body, by site
specified site NEC 930.8
eyeball 930.8
intraocular—*see* Foreign body, intraocular
eyelid 930.1
retained or old 374.86
frontal sinus 932
gastrointestinal tract 938
genitourinary tract 939.9
globe 930.8
penetrating 871.6
magnetic 871.5
retained or old 360.50
retained or old 360.60
gum 935.0
Highmore's antrum 932
hypopharynx 933.0
ileocecal coil 936
ileum 936
inspiration (of) 933.1
intestine (large) (small) 936
lacrimal apparatus, duct, gland, or sac 930.2
larynx 933.1
lung 934.8
maxillary sinus 932
mouth 935.0
nasal sinus 932
nasopharynx 933.0
nose (passage) 932
nostril 932
oral cavity 935.0
palate 935.0
penis 939.3
pharynx 933.0
pyriform sinus 933.0
rectosigmoid 937
junction 937
rectum 937
respiratory tract 934.9
specified part NEC 934.8
sclera 930.1
sinus 932
accessory 932
frontal 932
maxillary 932
nasal 932
pyriform 933.0
small intestine 936
stomach (hairball) 935.2
suffocation by (*see also* Asphyxia, food) 933.1
swallowed 938
tongue 933.0
tear ducts or glands 930.2
throat 933.0
tongue 935.0
swallowed 933.0
tonsil, tonsillar 933.0
fossa 933.0
trachea 934.0
ureter 939.0

Foreign body—*continued*
entering through—*continued*
urethra 939.0
uterus (any part) 939.1
vagina 939.2
vulva 939.2
wind pipe 934.0
feeling of, in throat 784.99
granuloma (old) 728.82
bone 733.99
in operative wound (inadvertently left) 998.4
due to surgical material intentionally
left—*see* Complications, due to
(presence of) any device, implant, or
graft classified to 996.0-996.5 NEC
muscle 728.82
skin 709.4
soft tissue 709.1
subcutaneous tissue 709.4
in
bone (residual) 733.99
open wound—*see* Wound, open, by site
complicated
soft tissue (residual) 729.6
inadvertently left in operation wound (causing
adhesions, obstruction, or perforation) 998.4
ingestion, ingested NEC 938
inhalation or inspiration (*see also* Asphyxia,
food) 933.1
internal organ, not entering through an
orifice—*see* Injury, internal, by site, with
open wound
intraocular (nonmagnetic) 871.6
combined sites 871.6
magnetic 871.5
retained or old 360.59
retained or old 360.69
magnetic 871.5
retained or old 360.50
retained or old 360.60
specified site NEC 871.6
magnetic 871.5
retained or old 360.59
retained or old 360.69
iris (nonmagnetic) 871.6
magnetic 871.5
retained or old 360.52
retained or old 360.62
lens (nonmagnetic) 871.6
magnetic 871.5
retained or old 360.53
retained or old 360.63
lid, eye 930.1
ocular muscle 870.4
retained or old 376.6
old or residual
bone 733.99
eyelid 374.86
middle ear 385.83
muscle 729.6
ocular 376.6
retrobulbar 376.6
skin 729.6
with granuloma 709.4
soft tissue 729.6
with granuloma 709.4
subcutaneous tissue 729.6
with granuloma 709.4
operation wound, left accidentally 998.4
orbit 870.4
retained or old 376.6

Foreign body—*continued*
  posterior wall, eye 871.6
    magnetic 871.5
      retained or old 360.55
    retained or old 360.65
  respiratory tree 934.9
    specified site NEC 934.8
  retained (old) (nonmagnetic) (in)
    anterior chamber (eye) 360.61
      magnetic 360.51
    ciliary body 360.62
      magnetic 360.52
    eyelid 374.86
    globe 360.60
      magnetic 360.50
    intraocular 360.60
      magnetic 360.50
      specified site NEC 360.69
        magnetic 360.59
    iris 360.62
      magnetic 360.52
    lens 360.63
      magnetic 360.53
    muscle 729.6
    orbit 376.6
    posterior wall of globe 360.65
      magnetic 360.55
    retina 360.65
      magnetic 360.55
    retrobulbar 376.6
    skin 729.6
      with granuloma 709.4
    soft tissue 729.6
      with granuloma 709.4
    subcutaneous tissue 729.6
      with granuloma 709.4
    vitreous 360.64
      magnetic 360.54
  retina 871.6
    magnetic 871.5
      retained or old 360.55
    retained or old 360.65
  superficial, without major open wound (*see also*
      Injury, superficial, by site) 919.6
  swallowed NEC 938
  throat, feeling of 784.99
  vitreous (humor) 871.6
    magnetic 871.5
      retained or old 360.54
    retained or old 360.64
Forking, aqueduct of Sylvius 742.3
  with spina bifida (*see also* Spina bifida) 741.0
Formation
  bone in scar tissue (skin) 709.3
  connective tissue in vitreous 379.25
  Elschnig pearls (postcataract extraction) 366.51
  hyaline in cornea 371.49
  sequestrum in bone (due to infection) (*see also*
      Osteomyelitis) 730.1
  valve
    colon, congenital 751.5
    ureter (congenital) 753.29
Formication 782.0
Fort Bragg fever 100.89
Fossa —*see also* condition
  pyriform—*see* condition
Foster care (status) V60.81
Foster-Kennedy syndrome 377.04
Fothergill's
  disease, meaning scarlatina anginosa 034.1
  neuralgia (*see also* Neuralgia, trigeminal) 350.1
Foul breath 784.99

Found dead (cause unknown) 798.9
Foundling V20.0
Fournier's disease (idiopathic gangrene) 608.83
Fourth
  cranial nerve—*see* condition
  disease 057.8
  molar 520.1
Foville's syndrome 344.89
Fox's
  disease (apocrine miliaria) 705.82
  impetigo (contagiosa) 684
Fox-Fordyce disease (apocrine miliaria) 705.82
Fracture (abduction) (adduction) (avulsion)
    (compression) (crush) (dislocation) (oblique)
    (separation) (closed) 829.0

---

*Note—For fracture of any of the following sites with
fracture of other bones—see Fracture, multiple.*

*"Closed" includes the following descriptions of
fractures, with or without delayed healing,
unless they are specified as open or compound:*

  comminuted
  depressed
  elevated
  fissured
  greenstick
  impacted
  linear
  simple
  slipped epiphysis
  spiral
  unspecified

*"Open" includes the following descriptions of
fractures, with or without delayed healing:*

  compound
  infected
  missile
  puncture
  with foreign body

*For late effect of fracture, see Late, effect,
fracture, by site.*

---

  with
    internal injuries in same region (conditions
        classifiable to 860-869)—*see also* Injury,
        internal, by site
    pelvic region—*see* Fracture, pelvis
  acetabulum (with visceral injury) (closed) 808.0
    open 808.1
  acromion (process) (closed) 811.01
    open 811.11
  alveolus (closed) 802.8
    open 802.9
  ankle (malleolus) (closed) 824.8
    bimalleolar (Dupuytren's) (Pott's) 824.4
      open 824.5
    bone 825.21
      open 825.31
    lateral malleolus only (fibular) 824.2
      open 824.3
    medial malleolus only (tibial) 824.0
      open 824.1
    open 824.9
    pathologic 733.16
    talus 825.21
      open 825.31
    trimalleolar 824.6
      open 824.7

Fracture—*continued*
antrum—*see* Fracture, skull, base
arm (closed) 818.0
  and leg(s) (any bones) 828.0
    open 828.1
  both (any bones) (with rib(s)) (with sternum)
    819.0
    open 819.1
  lower 813.80
    open 813.90
  open 818.1
  upper—*see* Fracture, humerus
astragalus (closed) 825.21
  open 825.31
atlas—*see* Fracture, vertebra, cervical, first
axis—*see* Fracture, vertebra, cervical, second
back—*see* Fracture, vertebra, by site
Barton's—*see* Fracture, radius, lower end
basal (skull)—*see* Fracture, skull, base
Bennett's (closed) 815.01
  open 815.11
bimalleolar (closed) 824.4
  open 824.5
bone (closed) NEC 829.0
  birth injury NEC 767.3
  open 829.1
  pathologic NEC (*see also* Fracture,
    pathologic) 733.10
  stress NEC (*see also* Fracture, stress) 733.95
boot top—*see* Fracture, fibula
boxers'—*see* Fracture, metacarpal bone(s)
breast bone—*see* Fracture, sternum
bucket handle (semilunar cartilage)—*see* Tear,
  meniscus
buckle — see Fracture, torus
burst—*see* Fracture, traumatic, by site
bursting—*see* Fracture, phalanx, hand, distal
calcaneus (closed) 825.0
  open 825.1
capitate (bone) (closed) 814.07
  open 814.17
capitellum (humerus) (closed) 812.49
  open 812.59
carpal bone(s) (wrist NEC) (closed) 814.00
  open 814.10
  specified site NEC 814.09
    open 814.19
cartilage, knee (semilunar)—*see* Tear, meniscus
cervical—*see* Fracture, vertebra, cervical
chauffeur's—*see* Fracture, ulna, lower end
chisel—*see* Fracture, radius, upper end
chronic — see Fracture, pathologic
clavicle (interligamentous part) (closed) 810.00
  acromial end 810.03
    open 810.13
  due to birth trauma 767.2
  open 810.10
  shaft (middle third) 810.02
    open 810.12
  sternal end 810.01
    open 810.11
clayshovelers'—*see* Fracture, vertebra, cervical
coccyx—*see also* Fracture, vertebra, coccyx
  complicating delivery 665.6
collar bone—*see* Fracture, clavicle
Colles' (reversed) (closed) 813.41
  open 813.51
comminuted—*see* Fracture, by site
compression—*see also* Fracture, by site
  nontraumatic—*see* Fracture, pathologic
congenital 756.9

Fracture—*continued*
coracoid process (closed) 811.02
  open 811.12
coronoid process (ulna) (closed) 813.02
  mandible (closed) 802.23
    open 802.33
  open 813.12
corpus cavernosum penis 959.13
costochondral junction—*see* Fracture, rib
costosternal junction—*see* Fracture, rib
cranium—*see* Fracture, skull, by site
cricoid cartilage (closed) 807.5
  open 807.6
cuboid (ankle) (closed) 825.23
  open 825.33
cuneiform
  foot (closed) 825.24
    open 825.34
  wrist (closed) 814.03
    open 814.13
dental implant 525.73
dental restorative material
  with loss of material 525.64
  without loss of material 525.63
due to
  birth injury—*see* Birth injury, fracture
  gunshot—*see* Fracture, by site, open
  neoplasm—*see* Fracture, pathologic
  osteoporosis—*see* Fracture, pathologic
Dupuytren's (ankle) (fibula) (closed) 824.4
  open 824.5
  radius 813.42
    open 813.52
Duverney's—*see* Fracture, ilium
elbow—*see also* Fracture, humerus, lower end
  olecranon (process) (closed) 813.01
    open 813.11
  supracondylar (closed) 812.41
    open 812.51
ethmoid (bone) (sinus)—*see* Fracture, skull,
  base
face bone(s) (closed) NEC 802.8
  with
    other bone(s)—*see also* Fracture, multiple,
      skull
    skull—*see also* Fracture, skull
      involving other bones—*see* Fracture,
        multiple, skull
  open 802.9
fatigue—*see* Fracture, march
femur, femoral (closed) 821.00
  cervicotrochanteric 820.03
    open 820.13
  condyles, epicondyles 821.21
    open 821.31
  distal end—*see* Fracture, femur, lower end
  epiphysis (separation)
    capital 820.01
      open 820.11
    head 820.01
      open 820.11
    lower 821.22
      open 821.32
    trochanteric 820.01
      open 820.11
    upper 820.01
      open 820.11
  head 820.09
    open 820.19

Fracture—*continued*
  femur—*continued*
    lower end or extremity (distal end) (closed) 821.20
      condyles, epicondyles 821.21
        open 821.31
      epiphysis (separation) 821.22
        open 821.32
      multiple sites 821.29
        open 821.39
      open 821.30
      specified site NEC 821.29
        open 821.39
      supracondylar 821.23
        open 821.33
      T-shaped 821.21
        open 821.31
    neck (closed) 820.8
      base (cervicotrochanteric) 820.03
      open 820.13
      extracapsular 820.20
      open 820.30
      intertrochanteric (section) 820.21
      open 820.31
      intracapsular 820.00
      open 820.10
      intratrochanteric 820.21
      open 821.31
      midcervical 820.02
      open 820.12
      open 820.9
      pathologic 733.14
        specified part NEC 733.15
      specified site NEC 820.09
      open 820.19
      transcervical 820.02
      open 820.12
      transtrochanteric 820.20
      open 820.30
    open 821.10
    pathologic 733.14
      specified part NEC 733.15
    peritrochanteric (section) 820.20
      open 820.30
    shaft (lower third) (middle third) (upper third) 821.01
      open 821.11
    subcapital 820.09
      open 820.19
    subtrochanteric (region) (section) 820.22
      open 820.32
    supracondylar 821.23
      open 821.33
    transepiphyseal 820.01
      open 820.11
    trochanter (greater) (lesser) (*see also* Fracture, femur, neck, by site) 820.20
      open 820.30
    T-shaped, into knee joint 821.21
      open 821.31
    upper end 820.8
      open 820.9
  fibula (closed) 823.81
    with tibia 823.82
      open 823.92
    distal end 824.8
      open 824.9
    epiphysis
      lower 824.8
        open 824.9
      upper—*see* Fracture, fibula, upper end

Fracture—*continued*
  fibula—*continued*
    head—*see* Fracture, fibula, upper end
    involving ankle 824.2
      open 824.3
    lower end or extremity 824.8
      open 824.9
    malleolus (external) (lateral) 824.2
      open 824.3
    open NEC 823.91
    pathologic 733.16
    proximal end—*see* Fracture, fibula, upper end
    shaft 823.21
      with tibia 823.22
        open 823.32
      open 823.31
    stress 733.93
    torus 853.41
      with tibia 823.42
    upper end or extremity (epiphysis) (head) (proximal end) (styloid) 823.01
      with tibia 823.02
        open 823.12
      open 823.11
  finger(s), of one hand (closed) (*see also* Fracture, phalanx, hand) 816.00
    with
      metacarpal bone(s), of same hand 817.0
        open 817.1
      thumb of same hand 816.03
        open 816.13
    open 816.10
  foot, except toe(s) alone (closed) 825.20
    open 825.30
  forearm (closed) NEC 813.80
    lower end (distal end) (lower epiphysis) 813.40
      open 813.50
    open 813.90
    shaft 813.20
      open 813.30
    upper end (proximal end) (upper epiphysis) 813.00
      open 813.10
  fossa, anterior, middle, or posterior—*see* Fracture, skull, base
  frontal (bone)—*see also* Fracture, skull, vault
    sinus—*see* Fracture, skull base
  Galeazzi's—*see* Fracture, radius, lower end
  glenoid (cavity) (fossa) (scapula) (closed) 811.03
    open 811.13
  Gosselin's—*see* Fracture, ankle
  greenstick—*see* Fracture, by site
  grenade-throwers'—*see* Fracture, humerus, shaft
  gutter—*see* Fracture, skull, vault
  hamate (closed) 814.08
    open 814.18
  hand, one (closed) 815.00
    carpals 814.00
      open 814.10
      specified site NEC 814.09
        open 814.19
    metacarpals 815.00
      open 815.10
    multiple, bones of one hand 817.0
      open 817.1
    open 815.10
    phalanges (*see also* Fracture, phalanx, hand) 816.00
      open 816.10

Fracture—*continued*
  healing
    aftercare (*see also* Aftercare, fracture) V54.89
    change of cast V54.89
    complications—*see* condition
    convalescence V66.4
    removal of
      cast V54.89
      fixation device
        external V54.89
        internal V54.01
  heel bone (closed) 825.0
    open 825.1
  Hill-Sachs 812.09
  hip (closed) (*see also* Fracture, femur, neck)
    820.8
    open 820.9
    pathologic 733.14
  humerus (closed) 812.20
    anatomical neck 812.02
      open 812.12
    articular process (*see also* Fracture, humerus,
      condyle(s)) 812.44
      open 812.54
    capitellum 812.49
      open 812.59
    condyle(s) 812.44
      lateral (external) 812.42
        open 812.52
      medial (internal epicondyle) 812.43
        open 812.53
      open 812.54
    distal end—*see* Fracture, humerus, lower end
    epiphysis
      lower (*see also* Fracture, humerus,
        condyle(s)) 812.44
        open 812.54
      upper 812.09
        open 812.19
    external condyle 812.42
      open 812.52
    great tuberosity 812.03
      open 812.13
    head 812.09
      open 812.19
    internal epicondyle 812.43
      open 812.53
    lesser tuberosity 812.09
      open 812.19
    lower end or extremity (distal end) (*see also*
      Fracture, humerus, by site) 812.40
    multiple sites NEC 812.49
      open 812.59
    open 812.50
    specified site NEC 812.49
      open 812.59
    neck 812.01
      open 812.11
    open 812.30
    pathologic 733.11
    proximal end—*see* Fracture, humerus, upper
      end
    shaft 812.21
      open 812.31
    supracondylar 812.41
      open 812.51
    surgical neck 812.01
      open 812.11
    trochlea 812.49
      open 812.59

Fracture—*continued*
  humerus—*continued*
    T-shaped 812.44
      open 812.54
    tuberosity—*see* Fracture, humerus, upper end
    upper end or extremity (proximal end) (*see*
      also Fracture, humerus, by site) 812.00
      open 812.10
      specified site NEC 812.09
        open 812.19
  hyoid bone (closed) 807.5
    open 807.6
  hyperextension—*see* Fracture, radius, lower end
  ilium (with visceral injury) (closed) 808.41
    open 808.51
  impaction, impacted—*see* Fracture, by site
  incus—*see* Fracture, skull, base
  innominate bone (with visceral injury) (closed)
    808.49
    open 808.59
  instep, of one foot (closed) 825.20
    with toe(s) of same foot 827.0
      open 827.1
    open 825.30
  insufficiency—*see* Fracture, pathologic, by site
  internal
    ear—*see* Fracture, skull, base
    semilunar cartilage, knee—*see* Tear,
      meniscus, medial
  intertrochanteric—*see* Fracture, femur, neck,
    intertrochanteric
  ischium (with visceral injury) (closed) 808.42
    open 808.52
  jaw (bone) (lower) (closed) (*see also* Fracture,
    mandible) 802.20
    angle 802.25
      open 802.35
    open 802.30
    upper—*see* Fracture, maxilla
  knee
    cap (closed) 822.0
      open 822.1
    cartilage (semilunar)—*see* Tear, meniscus
  labyrinth (osseous)—*see* Fracture, skull, base
  larynx (closed) 807.5
    open 807.6
  late effect—*see* Late, effects (of), fracture
  Le Fort's—*see* Fracture, maxilla
  leg (closed) 827.0
    with rib(s) or sternum 828.0
      open 828.1
    both (any bones) 828.0
      open 828.1
    lower—*see* Fracture, tibia
      open 827.1
    upper—*see* Fracture, femur
  limb
    lower (multiple) (closed) NEC 827.0
      open 827.1
    upper (multiple) (closed) NEC 818.0
      open 818.1
  long bones, due to birth trauma—*see* Birth
    injury, fracture
  lumbar—*see* Fracture, vertebra, lumbar
  lunate bone (closed) 814.02
    open 814.12
  malar bone (closed) 802.4
    open 802.5
  Malgaigne's (closed) 808.43
    open 808.53

Fracture—*continued*
malleolus (closed)0 824.8
  bimalleolar 824.4
    open 824.5
  lateral 824.2
    and medial—*see also* Fracture, malleolus,
      bimalleolar
      with lip of tibia—*see* Fracture, malleolus,
        trimalleolar
    open 824.3
  medial (closed) 824.0
    and lateral—*see also* Fracture, malleolus,
      bimalleolar
      with lip of tibia—*see* Fracture, malleolus,
        trimalleolar
    open 824.1
  open 824.9
  trimalleolar (closed) 824.6
    open 824.7
malleus—*see* Fracture, skull, base
malunion 733.81
mandible (closed) 802.20
  angle 802.25
    open 802.35
  body 802.28
    alveolar border 802.27
      open 802.37
    open 802.38
    symphysis 802.26
      open 802.36
  condylar process 802.21
    open 802.31
  coronoid process 802.23
    open 802.33
  multiple sites 802.29
    open 802.39
  open 802.30
  ramus NEC 802.24
    open 802.34
  subcondylar 802.22
    open 802.32
manubrium—*see* Fracture, sternum
march 733.95
  fibula 733.93
  metatarsals 733.94
  tibia 733.93
maxilla, maxillary (superior) (upper jaw)
  (closed) 802.4
  inferior—*see* Fracture, mandible
  open 802.5
meniscus, knee—*see* Tear, meniscus
metacarpus, metacarpal (bone(s)), of one hand
  (closed) 815.00
  with phalanx, phalanges, hand (finger(s))
    (thumb) of same hand 817.0
    open 817.1
  base 815.02
    first metacarpal 815.01
      open 815.11
    open 815.12
    thumb 815.01
      open 815.11
  multiple sites 815.09
    open 815.19
  neck 815.04
    open 815.14
  open 815.10
  shaft 815.03
    open 815.13

Fracture—*continued*
metatarsus, metatarsal (bone(s)), of one foot
  (closed) 825.25
  with tarsal bone(s) 825.29
    open 825.39
  open 825.35
Monteggia's (closed) 813.03
  open 813.13
Moore's—*see* Fracture, radius, lower end
multangular bone (closed)
  larger 814.05
    open 814.15
  smaller 814.06
    open 814.16
multiple (closed) 829.0

---

*Note—Multiple fractures of sites classifiable to
the same three- or four-digit category are coded
to that category, except for sites classifiable to
810-818 or 820-827 in different limbs.*

*Multiple fractures of sites classifiable to
different fourth-digit subdivisions within the
same three-digit category should be dealt with
according to coding rules.*

*Multiple fractures of sites classifiable to
different three-digit categories (identifiable
from the listing under "Fracture"), and of sites
classifiable to 810-818 or 820-827 in different
limbs should be coded according to the
following list, which should be referred to in the
following priority order: skull or face bones,
pelvis or vertebral column, legs, arms.*

---

  arm (multiple bones in same arm except in
    hand alone) (sites classifiable to 810-817
    with sites classifiable to a different
    three-digit category in 810-817 in same
    arm) (closed) 818.0
    open 818.1
  arms, both or arm(s) with rib(s) or sternum
    (sites classifiable to 810-818 with sites
    classifiable to same range of categories in
    other limb or to 807) (closed) 819.0
    open 819.1
  bones of trunk NEC (closed) 809.0
    open 809.1
  hand, metacarpal bone(s) with phalanx or
    phalanges of same hand (sites classifiable
    to 815 with sites classifiable to 816 in
    same hand) (closed) 817.0
    open 817.1
  leg (multiple bones in same leg) (sites
    classifiable to 820-826 with sites
    classifiable to a different three-digit
    category in that range in same leg) (closed)
    827.0
    open 827.1
  legs, both or leg(s) with arm(s), rib(s), or
    sternum (sites classifiable to 820-
    827 with sites classifiable to same range of
    categories in other leg or to 807 or
    810-819) (closed) 828.0
    open 828.1
  open 829.1
  pelvis with other bones except skull or face
    bones (sites classifiable to 808 with sites
    classifiable to 805-807 or 810-829)
    (closed) 809.0
    open 809.1

Fracture INDEX TO DISEASES

Fracture—*continued*
multiple—*continued*
  skull, specified or unspecified bones, or face
    bone(s) with any other bone(s) (sites
    classifiable to 800-803 with sites
    classifiable to 805-829) (closed) 804.0

*Note—Use the following fifth-digit
subclassification with categories 800, 801, 803,
and 804:*

0 unspecified state of consciousness
1 with no loss of consciousness
*2 with brief [less than one hour] loss of
    consciousness*
*3 with moderate [1-24 hours] loss of
    consciousness*
*4 with prolonged [more than 24 hours] loss of
    consciousness and return to pre-existing
    conscious level*
*5 with prolonged [more than 24 hours] loss of
    consciousness, without return to pre-existing
    conscious level*
*Use fifth-digit 5 to designate when a patient is
unconcious and dies before regaining
conciousness, regardless of the duration of the
loss of conciousness*
*6 with loss of consciousness of unspecified
    duration*
9 with concussion, unspecified

with
  contusion, cerebral 804.1
  epidural hemorrhage 804.2
  extradural hemorrhage 804.2
  hemorrhage (intracranial) NEC 804.3
  intracranial injury NEC 804.4
  laceration, cerebral 804.1
  subarachnoid hemorrhage 804.2
  subdural hemorrhage 804.2
open 804.5
  with
    contusion, cerebral 804.6
    epidural hemorrhage 804.7
    extradural hemorrhage 804.7
    hemorrhage (intracranial) NEC 804.8
    intracranial injury NEC 804.9
    laceration, cerebral 804.6
    subarachnoid hemorrhage 804.7
    subdural hemorrhage 804.7
  vertebral column with other bones, except
    skull or face bones (sites classifiable to
    805 or 806 with sites classifiable to
    807-808 or 810-829) (closed) 809.0
    open 809.1
nasal (bone(s)) (closed) 802.0
  open 802.1
sinus—Fracture, skull, base
navicular
  carpal (wrist) (closed) 814.01
    open 814.11
  tarsal (ankle) (closed) 825.22
    open 825.32
neck—*see* Fracture, vertebra, cervical
neural arch—*see* Fracture, vertebra, by site
nonunion 733.82
nose, nasal (bone) (septum) (closed) 802.0
  open 802.1
occiput—*see* Fracture, skull, base
odontoid process—*see* Fracture, vertebra,
  cervical

Fracture—*continued*
olecranon (process) (ulna) (closed) 813.01
  open 813.11
open 829.1
orbit, orbital (bone) (region) (closed) 802.8
  floor (blow-out) 802.6
    open 802.7
  open 802.9
  roof—*see* Fracture, skull, base
  specified part NEC 802.8
    open 802.9
os
  calcis (closed) 825.0
    open 825.1
  magnum (closed) 814.07
    open 814.17
  pubis (with visceral injury) (closed) 808.2
    open 808.3
  triquetrum (closed) 814.03
    open 814.13
osseous
  auditory meatus—*see* Fracture, skull, base
  labyrinth—*see* Fracture, skull, base
ossicles, auditory (incus) (malleus)
  (stapes)—*see* Fracture, skull, base
osteoporotic—*see* Fracture, pathologic
palate (closed) 802.8
  open 802.9
paratrooper—*see* Fracture, tibia, lower end
parietal bone—*see* Fracture, skull, vault
parry—*see* Fracture, Monteggia's
patella (closed) 822.0
  open 822.1
pathologic (cause unknown) 733.10
  ankle 733.16
  femur (neck) 733.14
    specified NEC 733.15
  fibula 733.16
  hip 733.14
  humerus 733.11
  radius 733.12
  specified site NEC 733.19
  tibia 733.16
  ulna 733.12
  vertebrae (collapse) 733.13
  wrist 733.12
pedicle (of vertebral arch)—*see* Fracture,
  vertebra, by site
pelvis, pelvic (bone(s)) (with visceral injury)
  (closed) 808.8
  multiple (with disruption of pelvic circle)
    808.43
    open 808.53
  open 808.9
  rim (closed) 808.49
    open 808.59
peritrochanteric (closed) 820.20
  open 820.30
phalanx, phalanges, of one
  foot (closed) 826.0
    with bone(s) of same lower limb 827.0
      open 827.1
    open 826.1
  hand (closed) 816.00
    with metacarpal bone(s) of same hand 817.0
      open 817.1
    distal 816.02
      open 816.12
    middle 816.01
      open 816.11

1102

Fracture—*continued*
phalanx, phalanges—*continued*
  hand—*continued*
    multiple sites NEC 816.03
      open 816.13
    open 816.10
    proximal 816.01
      open 816.11
  pisiform (closed) 814.04
    open 814.14
  pond—Fracture, skull, vault
  Pott's (closed) 824.4
    open 824.5
  prosthetic device, internal—*see* Complications,
    mechanical
  pubis (with visceral injury) (closed) 808.2
    open 808.3
  Quervain's (closed) 814.01
    open 814.11
  radius (alone) (closed) 813.81
    with ulna NEC 813.83
      open 813.93
    distal end—*see* Fracture, radius, lower end
    epiphysis
      lower—*see* Fracture, radius, lower end
      upper—*see* Fracture, radius, upper end
    head—*see* Fracture, radius, upper end
    lower end or extremity (distal end) (lower
      epiphysis) 813.42
      with ulna (lower end) 813.44
        open 813.54
      open 813.52
      torus 813.45
        with ulna 813.47
    neck—*see* Fracture, radius, upper end
    open NEC 813.91
    pathologic 733.12
    proximal end—*see* Fracture, radius, upper end
    shaft (closed) 813.21
      with ulna (shaft) 813.23
        open 813.33
      open 813.31
    upper end 813.07
      with ulna (upper end) 813.08
        open 813.18
      epiphysis 813.05
        open 813.15
      head 813.05
        open 813.15
      multiple sites 813.07
        open 813.17
      neck 813.06
        open 813.16
      open 813.17
      specified site NEC 813.07
        open 813.17
  ramus
    inferior or superior (with visceral injury)
      (closed) 808.2
      open 808.3
    ischium—*see* Fracture, ischium
    mandible 802.24
      open 802.34

Fracture—*continued*
  rib(s) (closed) 807.0

Note—Use the following fifth-digit
subclassification with categories 807.0-807.1:

0 rib(s), unspecified
1 one rib
2 two ribs
3 three ribs
4 four ribs
5 five ribs
6 six ribs
7 seven ribs
8 eight or more ribs
9 multiple ribs, unspecified

---

    with flail chest (open) 807.4
    open 807.1
  root, tooth 873.63
    complicated 873.73
  sacrum—*see* Fracture, vertebra, sacrum
  scaphoid
    ankle (closed) 825.22
      open 825.32
    wrist (closed) 814.01
      open 814.11
  scapula (closed) 811.00
    acromial, acromion (process) 811.01
      open 811.11
    body 811.09
      open 811.19
    coracoid process 811.02
      open 811.12
    glenoid (cavity) (fossa) 811.03
      open 811.13
    neck 811.03
      open 811.13
    open 811.10
  semilunar
    bone, wrist (closed) 814.02
      open 814.12
    cartilage (interior) (knee)—*see* Tear, meniscus
  sesamoid bone—*see* Fracture, by site
  Shepherd's (closed) 825.21
    open 825.31
  shoulder—*see also* Fracture, humerus, upper
    end
    blade—*see* Fracture, scapula
  silverfork—*see* Fracture, radius, lower end
  sinus (ethmoid) (frontal) (maxillary) (nasal)
    (sphenoidal)—*see* Fracture, skull, base
    maxillary—*see* Fracture, maxilla
  Skillern's—*see* Fracture, radius, shaft

Fracture—*continued*
  skull (multiple NEC) (with face bones) (closed)
    803.0

---

*Note—Use the following fifth-digit
subclassification with categories 800, 801, 803,
and 804:*

0 unspecified state of consciousness
1 with no loss of consciousness
*2 with brief [less than one hour] loss of
consciousness*
*3 with moderate [1-24 hours] loss of
consciousness*
*4 with prolonged [more than 24 hours] loss of
consciousness and return to pre-existing
conscious level*
*5 with prolonged [more than 24 hours] loss of
consciousness, without return to pre-existing
conscious level*
*Use fifth-digit 5 to designate when a patient is
unconscious and dies before regaining
consciousness, regardless of the duration of the
loss of consciousness*
*6 with loss of consciousness of unspecified
duration*
9 with concussion, unspecified

---

    with
      contusion, cerebral 803.1
      epidural hemorrhage 803.2
      extradural hemorrhage 803.2
      hemorrhage (intracranial) NEC 803.3
      intracranial injury NEC 803.4
      laceration, cerebral 803.1
      other bones—*see* Fracture, multiple, skull
      subarachnoid hemorrhage 803.2
      subdural hemorrhage 803.2
    base (antrum) (ethmoid bone) (fossa) (internal
      ear) (nasal sinus) (occiput) (sphenoid)
      (temporal bone) (closed) 801.0
    with
      contusion, cerebral 801.1
      epidural hemorrhage 801.2
      extradural hemorrhage 801.2
      hemorrhage (intracranial) NEC 801.3
      intracranial injury NEC 801.4
      laceration, cerebral 801.1
      subarachnoid hemorrhage 801.2
      subdural hemorrhage 801.2
    open 801.5
      with
        contusion, cerebral 801.6
        epidural hemorrhage 801.7
        extradural hemorrhage 801.7
        hemorrhage (intracranial) NEC 801.8
        intracranial injury NEC 801.9
        laceration, cerebral 801.6
        subarachnoid hemorrhage 801.7
        subdural hemorrhage 801.7
    birth injury 767.3
    face bones—*see* Fracture, face bones
    open 803.5
      with
        contusion, cerebral 803.6
        epidural hemorrhage 803.7
        extradural hemorrhage 803.7
        hemorrhage (intracranial) NEC 803.8
        intracranial injury NEC 803.9
        laceration, cerebral 803.6
        subarachnoid hemorrhage 803.7
        subdural hemorrhage 803.7

Fracture—*continued*
  skull—*continued*
    vault (frontal bone) (parietal bone) (vertex)
      (closed) 800.0
    with
      contusion, cerebral 800.1
      epidural hemorrhage 800.2
      extradural hemorrhage 800.2
      hemorrhage (intracranial) NEC 800.3
      intracranial injury NEC 800.4
      laceration, cerebral 800.1
      subarachnoid hemorrhage 800.2
      subdural hemorrhage 800.2
    open 800.5
      with
        contusion, cerebral 800.6
        epidural hemorrhage 800.7
        extradural hemorrhage 800.7
        hemorrhage (intracranial) NEC 800.8
        intracranial injury NEC 800.9
        laceration, cerebral 800.6
        subarachnoid hemorrhage 800.7
        subdural hemorrhage 800.7
  Smith's 813.41
    open 813.51
  sphenoid (bone) (sinus)—*see* Fracture, skull,
    base
  spine—*see also* Fracture, vertebra, by site
    due to birth trauma 767.4
  spinous process—*see* Fracture, vertebra, by site
  spontaneous—*see* Fracture, pathologic
  sprinters'—*see* Fracture, ilium
  stapes—*see* Fracture, skull, base
  stave—*see also* Fracture, metacarpus,
    metacarpal bone(s)
  spine—*see* Fracture, tibia, upper end
  sternum (closed) 807.2
    with flail chest (open) 807.4
    open 807.3
  Stieda's—*see* Fracture, femur, lower end
  stress 733.95
    fibula 733.93
    metatarsals 733.94
    specified site NEC 733.95
    tibia 733.93
  styloid process
    metacarpal (closed) 815.02
      open 815.12
    radius—*see* Fracture, radius, lower end
    temporal bone—*see* Fracture, skull, base
    ulna—*see* Fracture, ulna, lower end
  supracondylar, elbow 812.41
    open 812.51
  symphysis pubis (with visceral injury) (closed)
    808.2
    open 808.3
  talus (ankle bone) (closed) 825.21
    open 825.31
  tarsus, tarsal bone(s) (with metatarsus) of one
    foot (closed) NEC 825.29
    open 825.39
  temporal bone (styloid)—*see* Fracture, skull,
    base
  tendon—*see* Sprain, by site
  thigh—*see* Fracture, femur, shaft
  thumb (and finger(s)) of one hand (closed) (*see
    also* Fracture, phalanx, hand) 816.00
    with metacarpal bone(s) of same hand 817.0
      open 817.1
    metacarpal(s)—*see* Fracture, metacarpus
    open 816.10

Fracture—*continued*
thyroid cartilage (closed) 807.5
 open 807.6
tibia (closed) 823.80
 with fibula 823.82
  open 823.92
 condyles—*see* Fracture, tibia, upper end
 distal end 824.8
  open 824.9
 epiphysis
  lower 824.8
   open 824.9
  upper—*see* Fracture, tibia, upper end
 head (involving knee joint)—*see* Fracture,
  tibia, upper end
 intercondyloid eminence—*see* Fracture, tibia,
  upper end
 involving ankle 824.0
  open 824.1
 lower end or extremity (anterior lip) (posterior
  lip) 824.8
  open 824.9
 malleolus (internal) (medial) 824.0
  open 824.1
 open NEC 823.90
 pathologic 733.16
 proximal end—*see* Fracture, tibia, upper end
 shaft 823.20
  with fibula 823.22
   open 823.32
  open 823.30
 spine—*see* Fracture, tibia, upper end
 stress 733.93
 torus 823.40
  with tibia 823.42
 tuberosity—*see* Fracture, tibia, upper end
 upper end or extremity (condyle) (epiphysis)
  (head) (spine) (proximal end) (tuberosity)
  823.00
  with fibula 823.02
   open 823.12
  open 823.10
toe(s), of one foot (closed) 826.0
 with bone(s) of same lower limb 827.0
  open 827.1
 open 826.1
tooth (root) 873.63
 complicated 873.73
torus
 fibula 823.41
  with tibia 823.42
 humerus 812.49
 radius (alone) 813.45
  with ulna 813.47
 tibia 823.40
  with fibula 823.42
 ulna (alone) 813.46
  with radius 813.47
trachea (closed) 807.5
 open 807.6
transverse process—*see* Fracture, vertebra, by
 site
trapezium (closed) 814.05
 open 814.15
trapezoid bone (closed) 814.06
 open 814.16
trimalleolar (closed) 824.6
 open 824.7
triquetral (bone) (closed) 814.03
 open 814.13

Fracture—*continued*
trochanter (greater) (lesser) (closed) (*see also*
 Fracture, femur, neck, by site) 820.20
 open 820.30
trunk (bones) (closed) 809.0
 open 809.1
tuberosity (external)—*see* Fracture, by site
ulna (alone) (closed) 813.82
 with radius NEC 813.83
  open 813.93
 coronoid process (closed) 813.02
  open 813.12
 distal end—*see* Fracture, ulna, lower end
 epiphysis
  lower—*see* Fracture, ulna, lower end
  upper—*see* Fracture, ulna, upper, end
 head—*see* Fracture, ulna, lower end
 lower end (distal end) (head) (lower epiphysis)
  (styloid process) 813.43
  with radius (lower end) 813.44
   open 813.54
  open 813.53
 olecranon process (closed) 813.01
  open 813.11
 open NEC 813.92
 pathologic 733.12
 proximal end—*see* Fracture, ulna, upper end
 shaft 813.22
  with radius (shaft) 813.23
   open 813.33
  open 813.32
 styloid process—*see* Fracture, ulna, lower end
 torus 813.46
  with radius 813.47
 transverse—*see* Fracture, ulna, by site
 upper end (epiphysis) 813.04
  with radius (upper end) 813.08
   open 813.18
  multiple sites 813.04
   open 813.14
  open 813.14
  specified site NEC 813.04
   open 813.14
unciform (closed) 814.08
 open 814.18
vertebra, vertebral (back) (body) (column)
 (neural arch) (pedicle) (spine) (spinous
 process) (transverse process) (closed) 805.8
 with
  hematomyelia—*see* Fracture, vertebra, by
   site, with spinal cord injury
  injury to
   cauda equina—*see* Fracture, vertebra,
    sacrum, with spinal cord injury
   nerve—*see* Fracture, vertebra, by site, with
    spinal cord injury
  paralysis—*see* Fracture, vertebra, by site,
   with spinal cord injury
  paraplegia—*see* Fracture, vertebra, by site,
   with spinal cord injury
  quadriplegia—*see* Fracture, vertebra, by site,
   with spinal cord injury
  spinal concussion—*see* Fracture, vertebra,
   by site, with spinal cord injury

Fracture—*continued*
  vertebra—*continued*
    with—*continued*
      spinal cord injury (closed) NEC 806.8

Note—Use the following fifth-digit
subclassification with categories 806.0-806.3:

C_1-C_4 *or unspecified level and* D_1-D_6 *(T_1-T_6) or*
unspecified level with:

0 *unspecified spinal cord injury*
1 *complete lesion of cord*
2 *anterior cord syndrome*
3 *central cord syndrome*
4 *specified injury NEC*

C_5-C_7 *level and* D_7-D_{12} *level with:*

5 *unspecified spinal cord injury*
6 *complete lesion of cord*
7 *anterior cord syndrome*
8 *central cord syndrome*
9 *specified injury NEC*

      cervical 806.0
        open 806.1
      dorsal, dorsolumbar 806.2
        open 806.3
        open 806.9
      thoracic, thoracolumbar 806.2
        open 806.3
    atlanto-axial—*see* Fracture, vertebra, cervical
    cervical (hangman) (teardrop) (closed) 805.00
      with spinal cord injury—*see* Fracture,
        vertebra, with spinal cord injury, cervical
      first (atlas) 805.01
        open 805.11
      second (axis) 805.02
        open 805.12
      third 805.03
        open 805.13
      fourth 805.04
        open 805.14
      fifth 805.05
        open 805.15
      sixth 805.06
        open 805.16
      seventh 805.07
        open 805.17
      multiple sites 805.08
        open 805.18
      open 805.10
    chronic 733.13
    coccyx (closed) 805.6
      with spinal cord injury (closed) 806.60
        cauda equina injury 806.62
          complete lesion 806.61
            open 806.71
            open 806.72
          open 806.70
        specified type NEC 806.69
          open 806.79
        open 805.7
    collapsed 733.13
    compression, not due to trauma 733.13
    dorsal (closed) 805.2
      with spinal cord injury—*see* Fracture,
        vertebra, with spinal cord injury, dorsal
      open 805.3

Fracture—*continued*
  vertebra—*continued*
    dorsolumbar (closed) 805.2
      with spinal cord injury—*see* Fracture,
        vertebra, with spinal cord injury, dorsal
      open 805.3
    due to osteoporosis 733.13
    fetus or newborn 767.4
    lumbar (closed) 805.4
      with spinal cord injury (closed) 806.4
        open 806.5
      open 805.5
    nontraumatic 733.13
    open NEC 805.9
    pathologic 733.13
    sacrum (closed) 805.6
      with spinal cord injury 806.60
        cauda equina injury 806.62
          complete lesion 806.61
            open 806.71
          open 806.72
        open 806.70
        specified type NEC 806.69
          open 806.79
      open 805.7
    site unspecified (closed) 805.8
      with spinal cord injury (closed) 806.8
        open 806.9
      open 805.9
    stress (any site) 733.95
    thoracic (closed) 805.2
      with spinal cord injury—*see* Fracture,
        vertebra, with spinal cord injury,
        thoracic
      open 805.3
  vertex—*see* Fracture, skull, vault
  vomer (bone) 802.0
    open 802.1
  Wagstaffe's—*see* Fracture, ankle
  wrist (closed) 814.00
    open 814.10
    pathologic 733.12
  xiphoid (process)—*see* Fracture, sternum
  zygoma (zygomatic arch) (closed) 802.4
    open 802.5
Fragile X syndrome 759.83
Fragilitas
  crinium 704.2
  hair 704.2
  ossium 756.51
    with blue sclera 756.51
  unguium 703.8
    congenital 757.5
Fragility
  bone 756.51
    with deafness and blue sclera 756.51
  capillary (hereditary) 287.8
  hair 704.2
  nails 703.8
Fragmentation —*see* Fracture, by site
Frailty 797
Frambesia, frambesial (tropica) (*see also* Yaws)
  102.9
  initial lesion or ulcer 102.0
  primary 102.0
Frambeside
  gummatous 102.4
  of early yaws 102.2
Frambesioma 102.1
Franceschetti's syndrome (mandibulofacial
  dysostosis) 756.0
Francis' disease (*see also* Tularemia) 021.9

Frank's essential thrombocytopenia (*see also*
Purpura, thrombocytopenic) 287.39
Franklin's disease (heavy chain) 273.2
Fraser's syndrome 759.89
Freckle 709.09
malignant melanoma in (M8742/3)—*see*
Melanoma
melanotic (of Hutchinson) (M8742/2)—*see*
Neoplasm, skin, in situ
retinal 239.81
Freeman-Sheldon syndrome 759.89
Freezing 991.9
specified effect NEC 991.8
Frei's disease (climatic bubo) 099.1
Freiberg's
disease (osteochondrosis, second metatarsal) 732.5
infraction of metatarsal head 732.5
osteochondrosis 732.5
Fremitus, friction, cardiac 785.3
Frenulum lingua 750.0
Frenum
external os 752.49
tongue 750.0
Frequency (urinary) NEC 788.41
micturition 788.41
nocturnal 788.43
psychogenic 306.53
Frey's syndrome (auriculotemporal syndrome)
705.22
Friction
burn (*see also* Injury, superficial, by site) 919.0
fremitus, cardiac 785.3
precordial 785.3
sounds, chest 786.7
Friderichsen-Waterhouse syndrome or disease
036.3
Friedländer's
B (bacillus) NEC (*see also* condition) 041.3
sepsis or septicemia 038.49
disease (endarteritis obliterans)—*see*
Arteriosclerosis
Friedreich's
ataxia 334.0
combined systemic disease 334.0
disease 333.2
combined systemic 334.0
myoclonia 333.2
sclerosis (spinal cord) 334.0
Friedrich-Erb-Arnold syndrome
(acropachyderma) 757.39
Frigidity 302.72
psychic or psychogenic 302.72
Fröhlich's disease or syndrome (adiposogenital
dystrophy) 253.8
Froin's syndrome 336.8
Frommel's disease 676.6
Frommel-Chiari syndrome 676.6
Frontal —*see also* condition
lobe syndrome 310.0
Frostbite 991.3
face 991.0
foot 991.2
hand 991.1
specified site NEC 991.3
Frotteurism 302.89
Frozen 991.9
pelvis 620.8
shoulder 726.0
Fructosemia 271.2
Fructosuria (benign) (essential) 271.2

Fuchs'
black spot (myopic) 360.21
corneal dystrophy (endothelial) 371.57
heterochromic cyclitis 364.21
Fucosidosis 271.8
Fugue 780.99
dissociative 300.13
hysterical (dissociative) 300.13
reaction to exceptional stress (transient) 308.1
Fukuhara syndrome 277.87
Fuller Albright's syndrome (osteitis fibrosa
disseminata) 756.59
Fuller's earth disease 502
Fulminant, fulminating —*see* condition
Functional —*see* condition
Functioning
borderline intellectual V62.89
Fundus —*see also* condition
flavimaculatus 362.76
Fungemia 117.9
Fungus, fungous
cerebral 348.89
disease NEC 117.9
infection—*see* Infection, fungus
testis (*see also* Tuberculosis) 016.5 *[608.81]*
Funiculitis (acute) 608.4
chronic 608.4
endemic 608.4
gonococcal (acute) 098.14
chronic or duration of 2 months or over 098.34
tuberculous (*see also* Tuberculosis) 016.5
FUO (fever of unknown origin) (*see also* Pyrexia)
780.60
Funnel
breast (acquired) 738.3
congenital 754.81
late effect of rickets 268.1
chest (acquired) 738.3
congenital 754.81
late effect of rickets 268.1
pelvis (acquired) 738.6
with disproportion (fetopelvic) 653.3
affecting fetus or newborn 763.1
causing obstructed labor 660.1
affecting fetus or newborn 763.1
congenital 755.69
tuberculous (*see also* Tuberculosis) 016.9
Furfur 690.18
microsporon 111.0
Furor, paroxysmal (idiopathic) (*see also*
Epilepsy) 345.8
Furriers' lung 495.8
Furrowed tongue 529.5
congenital 750.13
Furrowing nail (s) (transverse) 703.8
congenital 757.5
Furuncle 680.9
abdominal wall 680.2
ankle 680.6
anus 680.5
arm (any part, above wrist) 680.3
auditory canal, external 680.0
axilla 680.3
back (any part) 680.2
breast 680.2
buttock 680.5
chest wall 680.2
corpus cavernosum 607.2
ear (any part) 680.0
eyelid 373.13

Furuncle—*continued*
  face (any part, except eye) 680.0
  finger (any) 680.4
  flank 680.2
  foot (any part) 680.7
  forearm 680.3
  gluteal (region) 680.5
  groin 680.2
  hand (any part) 680.4
  head (any part, except face) 680.8
  heel 680.7
  hip 680.6
  kidney (*see also* Abscess, kidney) 590.2
  knee 680.6
  labium (majus) (minus) 616.4
  lacrimal
    gland (*see also* Dacryoadenitis) 375.00
    passages (duct) (sac) (*see also* Dacryocystitis) 375.30
  leg, any part except foot 680.6
  malignant 022.0
  multiple sites 680.9
  neck 680.1
  nose (external) (septum) 680.0
  orbit 376.01
  partes posteriores 680.5
  pectoral region 680.2
  penis 607.2
  perineum 680.2
  pinna 680.0
  scalp (any part) 680.8
  scrotum 608.4
  seminal vesicle 608.0
  shoulder 680.3
  skin NEC 680.9
  specified site NEC 680.8
  spermatic cord 608.4
  temple (region) 680.0
  testis 604.90
  thigh 680.6
  thumb 680.4
  toe (any) 680.7
  trunk 680.2
  tunica vaginalis 608.4
  umbilicus 680.2
  upper arm 680.3
  vas deferens 608.4
  vulva 616.4
  wrist 680.4
Furunculosis (*see also* Furuncle) 680.9
  external auditory meatus 680.0 *[380.13]*
Fusarium (infection) 118
Fusion, fused (congenital)
  anal (with urogenital canal) 751.5
  aorta and pulmonary artery 745.0
  astragaloscaphoid 755.67
  atria 745.5
  atrium and ventricle 745.69
  auditory canal 744.02
  auricles, heart 745.5
  binocular, with defective stereopsis 368.33
  bone 756.9
  cervical spine—*see* Fusion, spine
  choanal 748.0
  commissure, mitral valve 746.5
  cranial sutures, premature 756.0
  cusps, heart valve NEC 746.89
    mitral 746.5
    tricuspid 746.89
  ear ossicles 744.04
  fingers (*see also* Syndactylism, fingers) 755.11

Fusion, fused—*continued*
  hymen 752.42
  hymeno-urethral 599.89
    causing obstructed labor 660.1
      affecting fetus or newborn 763.1
  joint (acquired)—*see also* Ankylosis
    congenital 755.8
  kidneys (incomplete) 753.3
  labium (majus) (minus) 752.49
  larynx and trachea 748.3
  limb 755.8
    lower 755.69
    upper 755.59
  lobe, lung 748.5
  lumbosacral (acquired) 724.6
    congenital 756.15
    surgical V45.4
  nares (anterior) (posterior) 748.0
  nose, nasal 748.0
  nostril(s) 748.0
  organ or site NEC—*see* Anomaly, specified type NEC
  ossicles 756.9
    auditory 744.04
  pulmonary valve segment 746.02
  pulmonic cusps 746.02
  ribs 756.3
  sacroiliac (acquired) (joint) 724.6
    congenital 755.69
    surgical V45.4
  skull, imperfect 756.0
  spine (acquired) 724.9
    arthrodesis status V45.4
    congenital (vertebra) 756.15
    postoperative status V45.4
  sublingual duct with submaxillary duct at opening in mouth 750.26
  talonavicular (bar) 755.67
  teeth, tooth 520.2
  testes 752.89
  toes (*see also* Syndactylism, toes) 755.13
  trachea and esophagus 750.3
  twins 759.4
  urethral-hymenal 599.89
  vagina 752.49
  valve cusps—*see* Fusion, cusps, heart valve
  ventricles, heart 745.4
  vertebra (arch)—*see* Fusion, spine
  vulva 752.49
Fusospirillosis (mouth) (tongue) (tonsil) 101
Fussy infant (baby) 780.91

G

Gafsa boil 085.1
Gain, weight (abnormal) (excessive) (see also
    Weight, gain) 783.1
Gaisböck's disease or syndrome (polycythemia
    hypertonica) 289.0
Gait
  abnormality 781.2
    hysterical 300.11
  ataxic 781.2
    hysterical 300.11
  disturbance 781.2
    hysterical 300.11
  paralytic 781.2
  scissor 781.2
  spastic 781.2
  staggering 781.2
    hysterical 300.11
Galactocele (breast) (infected) 611.5
  puerperal, postpartum 676.8
Galactophoritis 611.0
  puerperal, postpartum 675.2
Galactorrhea 676.6
  not associated with childbirth 611.6
Galactosemia (classic) (congenital) 271.1
Galactosuria 271.1
Galacturia 791.1
  bilharziasis 120.0
Galen's vein —*see* condition
Gallbladder —*see also* condition
  acute (*see also* Disease, gallbladder) 575.0
Gall duct —*see* condition
Gallop rhythm 427.89
Gallstone (cholemic) (colic) (impacted)—*see
    also* Cholelithiasis
  causing intestinal obstruction 560.31
Gambling, pathological 312.31
Gammaloidosis 277.39
Gammopathy 273.9
  macroglobulinemia 273.3
  monoclonal (benign) (essential) (idiopathic)
    (with lymphoplasmacytic dyscrasia) 273.1
Gamna's disease (siderotic splenomegaly)
    289.51
Gampsodactylia (congenital) 754.71
Gamstorp's disease (adynamia episodica
    hereditaria) 359.3
Gandy-Nanta disease (siderotic splenomegaly)
    289.51
**Gang activity without manifest psychiatric
    disorder** V71.09
  adolescent V71.02
  adult V71.01
  child V71.02
Gangliocytoma (M9490/0)—*see* Neoplasm,
    connective tissue, benign
Ganglioglioma (M9505/1)—*see* Neoplasm, by
    site, uncertain behavior
Ganglion 727.43
  joint 727.41
  of yaws (early) (late) 102.6
  periosteal (*see also* Periostitis) 730.3
  tendon sheath (compound) (diffuse) 727.42
  tuberculous (*see also* Tuberculosis) 015.9
Ganglioneuroblastoma (M9490/3)—*see*
    Neoplasm, connective tissue, malignant

Ganglioneuroma (M9490/0)—*see also*
    Neoplasm, connective tissue, benign
Ganglioneuroma—*continued*
  malignant (M9490/3)—*see* Neoplasm,
    connective tissue, malignant
Ganglioneuromatosis (M9491/0)—*see*
    Neoplasm, connective tissue, benign
Ganglionitis
  fifth nerve (*see also* Neuralgia, trigeminal)
    350.1
  gasserian 350.1
  geniculate 351.1
    herpetic 053.11
    newborn 767.5
  herpes zoster 053.11
  herpetic geniculate (Hunt's syndrome) 053.11
Gangliosidosis 330.1
Gangosa 102.5
Gangrene, gangrenous (anemia) (artery)
    (cellulitis) (dermatitis) (dry) (infective)
    (moist) (pemphigus) (septic) (skin) (stasis)
    (ulcer) 785.4
  with
    arteriosclerosis (native artery) 440.24
      bypass graft 440.30
        autologous vein 440.31
        nonautologous biological 440.32
    diabetes (mellitus) 250.7 *[785.4]*
      due to secondary diabetes 249.7 *[785.4]*
  abdomen (wall) 785.4
  adenitis 683
  alveolar 526.5
  angina 462
    diphtheritic 032.0
  anus 569.49
  appendices epiploicae—*see* Gangrene,
    mesentery
  appendix—*see* Appendicitis, acute
  arteriosclerotic —*see* Arteriosclerosis, with,
    gangrene
  auricle 785.4
  Bacillus welchii (*see also* Gangrene, gas) 040.0
  bile duct (*see also* Cholangitis) 576.8
  bladder 595.89
  bowel—*see* Gangrene, intestine
  cecum—*see* Gangrene, intestine
  Clostridium perfringens or welchii (*see also*
    Gangrene, gas) 040.0
  colon—*see* Gangrene, intestine
  connective tissue 785.4
  cornea 371.40
  corpora cavernosa (infective) 607.2
    noninfective 607.89
  cutaneous, spreading 785.4
  decubital (*see also* Ulcer, pressure) 707.00
    [785.4]
  diabetic (any site) 250.7 *[785.4]*
    due to secondary diabetes 249.7 *[785.4]*
  dropsical 785.4
  emphysematous (*see also* Gangrene, gas) 040.0
  epidemic (ergotized grain) 988.2
  epididymis (infectional) (*see also* Epididymitis)
    604.99
  erysipelas (*see also* Erysipelas) 035
  extremity (lower) (upper) 785.4
  gallbladder or duct (*see also* Cholecystitis,
    acute) 575.0

Gangrene, gangrenous—*continued*
  gas (bacillus) 040.0
    with
      abortion—*see* Abortion, by type, with sepsis
      ectopic pregnancy (*see also* categories
        633.0-633.9) 639.0
      molar pregnancy (*see also* categories
        630-632) 639.0
    following
      abortion 639.0
      ectopic or molar pregnancy 639.0
      puerperal, postpartum, childbirth 670.8
  glossitis 529.0
  gum 523.8
  hernia—*see* Hernia, by site, with gangrene
  hospital noma 528.1
  intestine, intestinal (acute) (hemorrhagic)
    (massive) 557.0
    with
      hernia—*see* Hernia, by site, with gangrene
      mesenteric embolism or infarction 557.0
      obstruction (*see also* Obstruction, intestine)
        560.9
  laryngitis 464.00
    with obstruction 464.01
  liver 573.8
  lung 513.0
    spirochetal 104.8
  lymphangitis 457.2
  Meleney's (cutaneous) 686.09
  mesentery 557.0
    with
      embolism or infarction 557.0
      intestinal obstruction (*see also* Obstruction,
        intestine) 560.9
  mouth 528.1
  noma 528.1
  orchitis 604.90
  ovary (*see also* Salpingo-oophoritis) 614.2
  pancreas 577.0
  penis (infectional) 607.2
    noninfective 607.89
  perineum 785.4
  pharynx 462
    septic 034.0
  pneumonia 513.0
  Pott's 440.24
  presenile 443.1
  pulmonary 513.0
  pulp, tooth 522.1
  quinsy 475
  Raynaud's (symmetric gangrene) 443.0 *[785.4]*
  rectum 569.49
  retropharyngeal 478.24
  rupture—*see* Hernia, by site, with gangrene
  scrotum 608.4
    noninfective 608.83
  senile 440.24
  sore throat 462
  spermatic cord 608.4
    noninfective 608.89
  spine 785.4
  spirochetal NEC 104.8
  spreading cutaneous 785.4
  stomach 537.89
  stomatitis 528.1
  symmetrical 443.0 *[785.4]*
  testis (infectional) (*see also* Orchitis) 604.99
    noninfective 608.89
  throat 462
    diphtheritic 032.0

Gangrene, gangrenous—*continued*
  thyroid (gland) 246.8
  tonsillitis (acute) 463
  tooth (pulp) 522.1
  tuberculous NEC (*see also* Tuberculosis) 011.9
  tunica vaginalis 608.4
    noninfective 608.89
  umbilicus 785.4
  uterus (*see also* Endometritis) 615.9
  uvulitis 528.3
  vas deferens 608.4
    noninfective 608.89
  vulva (*see also* Vulvitis) 616.10
Gannister disease (occupational) 502
  with tuberculosis—*see* Tuberculosis, pulmonary
Ganser's syndrome, hysterical 300.16
Gardner-Diamond syndrome (autoerythrocyte
  sensitization) 287.2
Gargoylism 277.5
Garré's
  disease (*see also* Osteomyelitis) 730.1
  osteitis (sclerosing) (*see also* Osteomyelitis)
    730.1
  osteomyelitis (*see also* Osteomyelitis) 730.1
Garrod's pads, knuckle 728.79
Gartner's duct
  cyst 752.41
  persistent 752.41
Gas 787.3
  asphyxia, asphyxiation, inhalation, poisoning,
    suffocation NEC 987.9
    specified gas—*see* Table of drugs and
      chemicals
  bacillus gangrene or infection—*see* Gas,
    gangrene
  cyst, mesentery 568.89
  excessive 787.3
  gangrene 040.0
    with
      abortion—*see* Abortion, by type, with sepsis
      ectopic pregnancy (*see also* categories
        633.0-633.9) 639.0
      molar pregnancy (*see also* categories
        630-632) 639.0
    following
      abortion 639.0
      ectopic or molar pregnancy 639.0
      puerperal, postpartum, childbirth 670.8
  on stomach 787.3
  pains 787.3
Gastradenitis 535.0
Gastralgia 536.8
  psychogenic 307.89
Gastrectasis, gastrectasia 536.1
  psychogenic 306.4
Gastric —*see* condition
Gastrinoma (M8153/1)
  malignant (M8153/3)
    pancreas 157.4
    specified site NEC—*see* Neoplasm, by site,
      malignant
    unspecified site 157.4
  specified site—*see* Neoplasm, by site,
    uncertain behavior
  unspecified site 235.5

Gastritis 535.5

> *Note—Use the following fifth-digit*
> *subclassification for category 535:*
>
> 0 *without mention of hemorrhage*
> 1 *with hemorrhage*

acute 535.0
alcoholic 535.3
allergic 535.4
antral 535.4
atrophic 535.1
atrophic-hyperplastic 535.1
bile-induced 535.4
catarrhal 535.0
chronic (atrophic) 535.1
cirrhotic 535.4
corrosive (acute) 535.4
dietetic 535.4
due to diet deficiency 269.9 *[535.4]*
eosinophilic 535.7
erosive 535.4
follicular 535.4
  chronic 535.1
giant hypertrophic 535.2
glandular 535.4
  chronic 535.1
hypertrophic (mucosa) 535.2
  chronic giant 211.1
irritant 535.4
nervous 306.4
phlegmonous 535.0
psychogenic 306.4
sclerotic 535.4
spastic 536.8
subacute 535.0
superficial 535.4
suppurative 535.0
toxic 535.4
tuberculous (*see also* Tuberculosis) 017.9
Gastrocarcinoma (M8010/3) 151.9
Gastrocolic —*see* condition
Gastrocolitis —*see* Enteritis
Gastrodisciasis 121.8
Gastroduodenitis (*see also* Gastritis) 535.5
catarrhal 535.0
infectional 535.0
virus, viral 008.8
  specified type NEC 008.69
Gastrodynia 536.8
Gastroenteritis (acute) (catarrhal) (congestive)
  (hemorrhagic) (noninfectious) (*see also*
  Enteritis) 558.9
aertrycke infection 003.0
allergic 558.3
chronic 558.9
  ulcerative (*see also* Colitis, ulcerative) 556.9
dietetic 558.9
due to
  antineoplastic chemotherapy 558.9
  food poisoning (*see also* Poisoning, food) 005.9
  radiation 558.1
eosinophilic 558.41
epidemic 009.0
functional 558.9
infectious (*see also* Enteritis, due to, by
  organism) 009.0
  presumed 009.1
salmonella 003.0
septic (*see also* Enteritis, due to, by organism)
  009.0

Gastroenteritis—*continued*
toxic 558.2
tuberculous (*see also* Tuberculosis) 014.8
ulcerative (*see also* Colitis, ulcerative) 556.9
viral NEC 008.8
  specified type NEC 008.69
zymotic 009.0
Gastroenterocolitis —*see* Enteritis
Gastroenteropathy, protein-losing 579.8
Gastroenteroptosis 569.89
Gastroesophageal laceration-hemorrhage
  syndrome 530.7
Gastroesophagitis 530.19
Gastrohepatitis (*see also* Gastritis) 535.5
Gastrointestinal —*see* condition
Gastrojejunal —*see* condition
Gastrojejunitis (*see also* Gastritis) 535.5
Gastrojejunocolic —*see* condition
Gastroliths 537.89
Gastromalacia 537.89
Gastroparalysis 536.3
diabetic 250.6 *[536.3]*
  due to secondary diabetes 249.6 *[536.3]*
Gastroparesis 536.3
diabetic 250.6 *[536.3]*
  due to secondary diabetes 249.6 *[536.3]*
Gastropathy 537.9
congestive portal 537.89
erythematous 535.5
exudative 579.8
portal hypertension 537.89
Gastroptosis 537.5
Gastrorrhagia 578.0
Gastrorrhea 536.8
psychogenic 306.4
Gastroschisis (congenital) 756.73
acquired 569.89
Gastrospasm (neurogenic) (reflex) 536.8
neurotic 306.4
psychogenic 306.4
Gastrostaxis 578.0
Gastrostenosis 537.89
Gastrostomy
attention to V55.1
complication 536.40
  specified type 536.49
infection 536.41
malfunctioning 536.42
status V44.1
Gastrosuccorrhea (continuous) (intermittent) 536.8
neurotic 306.4
psychogenic 306.4
Gaucher's
disease (adult) (cerebroside lipidosis) (infantile)
  272.7
hepatomegaly 272.7
splenomegaly (cerebroside lipidosis) 272.7
GAVE (gastric antral vascular ectasia) 537.82
with hemorrhage 537.83
without hemorrhage 537.82
Gayet's disease (superior hemorrhagic
  polioencephalitis) 265.1
Gayet-Wernicke's syndrome (superior
  hemorrhagic polioencephalitis) 265.1
Gee (-Herter) (-Heubner) (-Thaysen) disease or
  syndrome (nontropical sprue) 579.0
Gélineau's syndrome (*see also* Narcolepsy) 347.00
Gemination, teeth 520.2
Gemistocytoma (M9411/3)
specified site—*see* Neoplasm, by site, malignant
unspecified site 191.9

General, generalized —*see* condition
Genetic
  susceptibility to
    MEN (multiple endocrine neoplasia) V84.81
    neoplasia
      multiple endocrine [MEN] V84.81
    neoplasm
      malignant, of
        breast V84.01
        endometrium V84.04
        other V84.09
        ovary V84.02
        prostate V84.03
      specified disease NEC V84.89
Genital —*see* condition
  warts 078.11
Genito-anorectal syndrome 099.1
Genitourinary system —*see* condition
Genu
  congenital 755.64
  extrorsum (acquired) 736.42
    congenital 755.64
    late effects of rickets 268.1
  introrsum (acquired) 736.41
    congenital 755.64
    late effects of rickets 268.1
  rachitic (old) 268.1
  recurvatum (acquired) 736.5
    congenital 754.40
      with dislocation of knee 754.41
    late effects of rickets 268.1
  valgum (acquired) (knock-knee) 736.41
    congenital 755.64
    late effects of rickets 268.1
  varum (acquired) (bowleg) 736.42
    congenital 755.64
    late effects of rickets 268.1
Geographic tongue 529.1
Geophagia 307.52
Geotrichosis 117.9
  intestine 117.9
  lung 117.9
  mouth 117.9
Gephyrophobia 300.29
Gerbode defect 745.4
GERD (gastroesophageal reflux disease) 530.81
Gerhardt's
  disease (erythromelalgia) 443.82
  syndrome (vocal cord paralysis) 478.30
Gerlier's disease (epidemic vertigo) 078.81
German measles 056.9
  exposure to V01.4
Germinoblastoma (diffuse) (M9614/3) 202.8
  follicular (M9692/3) 202.0
Germinoma (M9064/3)—*see* Neoplasm, by site,
  malignant
Gerontoxon 371.41
Gerstmann's syndrome (finger agnosia) 784.69
Gerstmann-Sträussler-Scheinker syndrome
  (GSS) 046.71
Gestation (period)—*see also* Pregnancy
  ectopic NEC (*see also* Pregnancy, ectopic) 633.90
    with intrauterine pregnancy 633.91
Gestational proteinuria 646.2
  with hypertension—*see* Toxemia, of pregnancy
Ghon tubercle primary infection (*see also*
  Tuberculosis) 010.0
Ghost
  teeth 520.4
  vessels, cornea 370.64
Ghoul hand 102.3

Gianotti Crosti syndrome 057.8
  due to known virus—*see* Infection, virus
  due to unknown virus 057.8
Giant
  cell
    epulis 523.8
    peripheral (gingiva) 523.8
    tumor, tendon sheath 727.02
  colon (congenital) 751.3
  esophagus (congenital) 750.4
  kidney 753.3
  urticaria 995.1
    hereditary 277.6
Giardia lamblia infestation 007.1
Giardiasis 007.1
Gibert's disease (pityriasis rosea) 696.3
Gibraltar fever —*see* Brucellosis
Giddiness 780.4
  hysterical 300.11
  psychogenic 306.9
Gierke's disease (glycogenosis I) 271.0
Gigantism (cerebral) (hypophyseal) (pituitary)
  253.0
Gilbert's disease or cholemia (familial
  nonhemolytic jaundice) 277.4
Gilchrist's disease (North American
  blastomycosis) 116.0
Gilford (-Hutchinson) disease or syndrome
  (progeria) 259.8
Gilles de la Tourette's disease (motor-verbal tic)
  307.23
Gillespie's syndrome (dysplasia
  oculodentodigitalis) 759.89
Gingivitis 523.10
  acute 523.00
    necrotizing 101
    non-plaque induced 523.01
    plaque induced 523.00
  catarrhal 523.00
  chronic 523.10
    non-plaque induced 523.11
  desquamative 523.10
  expulsiva 523.40
  hyperplastic 523.10
  marginal, simple 523.10
  necrotizing, acute 101
  non-plaque induced 523.11
  pellagrous 265.2
  plaque induced 523.10
  ulcerative 523.10
    acute necrotizing 101
    Vincent's 101
Gingivoglossitis 529.0
Gingivopericementitis 523.40
Gingivosis 523.10
Gingivostomatitis 523.10
  herpetic 054.2
Giovannini's disease 117.9
GISA (glycopeptide intermediate staphylococcus
  aureus) V09.8
Gland, glandular —*see* condition
Glanders 024
Glanzmann (-Naegeli) disease or thrombasthenia
  287.1
Glassblowers' disease 527.1
Glaucoma (capsular) (inflammatory)
  (noninflammatory) (primary) 365.9
  with increased episcleral venous pressure 365.82
  absolute 360.42

Glaucoma—*continued*
  acute 365.22
    narrow angle 365.22
    secondary 365.60
  angle closure 365.20
    acute 365.22
    chronic 365.23
    intermittent 365.21
    interval 365.21
    residual stage 365.24
    subacute 365.21
  border line 365.00
  chronic 365.11
    noncongestive 365.11
    open angle 365.11
    simple 365.11
  closed angle—*see* Glaucoma, angle closure
  congenital 743.20
    associated with other eye anomalies 743.22
    simple 743.21
  congestive—*see* Glaucoma, narrow angle
  corticosteroid-induced (glaucomatous stage)
      365.31
    residual stage 365.32
  hemorrhagic 365.60
  hypersecretion 365.81
  in or with
    aniridia 365.42
    Axenfeld's anomaly 365.41
    congenital syndromes NEC 759.89 *[365.44]*
    disorder of lens NEC 365.59
    inflammation, ocular 365.62
    iris
      anomalies NEC 365.42
      atrophy, essential 365.42
      bombé 365.61
    microcornea 365.43
    neurofibromatosis 237.71 *[365.44]*
    ocular
      cysts NEC 365.64
      disorders NEC 365.60
      trauma 365.65
      tumors NEC 365.64
    pupillary block or seclusion 365.61
    Rieger's anomaly or syndrome 365.41
    seclusion of pupil 365.61
    Sturge-Weber (-Dimitri) syndrome 759.6
        [365.44]
    systemic syndrome NEC 365.44
    tumor of globe 365.64
    vascular disorders NEC 365.63
  infantile 365.14
    congenital 743.20
      associated with other eye anomalies 743.22
      simple 743.21
  juvenile 365.14
  low tension 365.12
  malignant 365.83
  narrow angle (primary) 365.20
    acute 365.22
    chronic 365.23
    intermittent 365.21
    interval 365.21
    residual stage 365.24
    subacute 365.21
  newborn 743.20
    associated with other eye anomalies 743.22
    simple 743.21
  noncongestive (chronic) 365.11
  nonobstructive (chronic) 365.11

Glaucoma—*continued*
  obstructive 365.60
    due to lens changes 365.59
  open angle 365.10
    with
      borderline intraocular pressure 365.01
      cupping of optic discs 365.01
    primary 365.11
    residual stage 365.15
  phacolytic 365.51
  pigmentary 365.13
  postinfectious 365.60
  pseudoexfoliation 365.52
      [365.52]
  secondary NEC 365.60
  simple (chronic) 365.11
  simplex 365.11
  steroid responders 365.03
  suspect 365.00
  syphilitic 095.8
  traumatic NEC 365.65
    newborn 767.8
  wide angle (*see also* Glaucoma, open angle)
      365.10
Glaucomatous flecks (subcapsular) 366.31
Glazed tongue 529.4
Gleet 098.2
Glénard's disease or syndrome (enteroptosis)
    569.89
Glinski-Simmonds syndrome (pituitary
    cachexia) 253.2
Glioblastoma (multiforme) (M9440/3)
  with sarcomatous component (M9442/3)
    specified site—*see* Neoplasm, by site,
      malignant
    unspecified site 191.9
  giant cell (M9441/3)
    specified site—*see* Neoplasm, by site, malignant
    unspecified site 191.9
  specified site—*see* Neoplasm, by site, malignant
  unspecified site 191.9
Glioma (malignant) (M9380/3)
  astrocytic (M9400/3)
    specified site—*see* Neoplasm, by site,
      malignant
    unspecified site 191.9
  mixed (M9382/3)
    specified site—*see* Neoplasm, by site,
      malignant
    unspecified site 191.9
  nose 748.1
  specified site NEC—*see* Neoplasm, by site,
      malignant
  subependymal (M9383/1) 237.5
  unspecified site 191.9
Gliomatosis cerebri (M9381/3) 191.0
Glioneuroma (M9505/1)—*see* Neoplasm, by
    site, uncertain behavior
Gliosarcoma (M9380/3)
  specified site—*see* Neoplasm, by site, malignant
  unspecified site 191.9
Gliosis (cerebral) 349.89
  spinal 336.0
Glisson's
  cirrhosis—*see* Cirrhosis, portal
  disease (*see also* Rickets) 268.0
Glissonitis 573.3
Globinuria 791.2
Globus 306.4
  hystericus 300.11

Glomangioma (M8712/0) (*see also* Hemangioma) 228.00
Glomangiosarcoma (M8710/3)—*see* Neoplasm, connective tissue, malignant
Glomerular nephritis (*see also* Nephritis) 583.9
Glomerulitis (*see also* Nephritis) 583.9
Glomerulonephritis (*see also* Nephritis) 583.9
  with
    edema (*see also* Nephrosis) 581.9
    lesion of
      exudative nephritis 583.89
      interstitial nephritis (diffuse) (focal) 583.89
      necrotizing glomerulitis 583.4
        acute 580.4
        chronic 582.4
      renal necrosis 583.9
        cortical 583.6
        medullary 583.7
      specified pathology NEC 583.89
        acute 580.89
        chronic 582.89
    necrosis, renal 583.9
      cortical 583.6
      medullary (papillary) 583.7
    specified pathology or lesion NEC 583.89
  acute 580.9
    with
      exudative nephritis 580.89
      interstitial nephritis (diffuse) (focal) 580.89
      necrotizing glomerulitis 580.4
    extracapillary with epithelial crescents 580.4
    poststreptococcal 580.0
    proliferative (diffuse) 580.0
    rapidly progressive 580.4
    specified pathology NEC 580.89
  arteriolar (*see also* Hypertension, kidney) 403.90
  arteriosclerotic (*see also* Hypertension, kidney) 403.90
  ascending (*see also* Pyelitis) 590.80
  basement membrane NEC 583.89
    with
      pulmonary hemorrhage (Goodpasture's syndrome) 446.21 *[583.81]*
  chronic 582.9
    with
      exudative nephritis 582.89
      interstitial nephritis (diffuse) (focal) 582.89
      necrotizing glomerulitis 582.4
      specified pathology or lesion NEC 582.89
    endothelial 582.2
    extracapillary with epithelial crescents 582.4
    hypocomplementemic persistent 582.2
    lobular 582.2
    membranoproliferative 582.2
    membranous 582.1
      and proliferative (mixed) 582.2
      sclerosing 582.1
    mesangiocapillary 582.2
    mixed membranous and proliferative 582.2
    proliferative (diffuse) 582.0
    rapidly progressive 582.4
    sclerosing 582.1
  cirrhotic—*see* Sclerosis, renal
  desquamative—*see* Nephrosis
  due to or associated with
    amyloidosis 277.39 *[583.81]*
      with nephrotic syndrome 277.39 *[581.81]*
      chronic 277.39 *[582.81]*

Glomerulonephritis—*continued*
    diabetes mellitus 250.4 *[583.81]*
      due to secondary diabetes 249.4 *[581.81]*
      with nephrotic syndrome 250.4 *[581.81]*
        due to secondary diabetes 249.4 *[581.81]*
    diphtheria 032.89 *[580.81]*
    gonococcal infection (acute) 098.19 *[583.81]*
      chronic or duration or 2 months or over 098.39 *[583.81]*
    infectious hepatitis 070.9 *[580.81]*
    malaria (with nephrotic syndrome) 084.9 *[581.81]*
    mumps 072.79 *[580.81]*
    polyarteritis (nodosa) (with nephrotic syndrome) 446.0 *[581.81]*
    specified pathology NEC 583.89
      acute 580.89
      chronic 582.89
    streptotrichosis 039.8 *[583.81]*
    subacute bacterial endocarditis 421.0 *[580.81]*
    syphilis (late) 095.4
      congenital 090.5 *[583.81]*
      early 091.69 *[583.81]*
    systemic lupus erythematosus 710.0 *[583.81]*
      with nephrotic syndrome 710.0 *[581.81]*
      chronic 710.0 *[582.81]*
    tuberculosis (*see also* Tuberculosis) 016.0 *[583.81]*
    typhoid fever 002.0 *[580.81]*
  extracapillary with epithelial crescents 583.4
    acute 580.4
    chronic 582.4
  exudative 583.89
    acute 580.89
    chronic 582.89
  focal (*see also* Nephritis) 583.9
    embolic 580.4
  granular 582.89
  granulomatous 582.89
  hydremic (*see also* Nephrosis) 581.9
  hypocomplementemic persistent 583.2
    with nephrotic syndrome 581.2
    chronic 582.2
  immune complex NEC 583.89
  infective (*see also* Pyelitis) 590.80
  interstitial (diffuse) (focal) 583.89
    with nephrotic syndrome 581.89
    acute 580.89
    chronic 582.89
  latent or quiescent 582.9
  lobular 583.2
    with nephrotic syndrome 581.2
    chronic 582.2
  membranoproliferative 583.2
    with nephrotic syndrome 581.2
    chronic 582.2
  membranous 583.1
    with nephrotic syndrome 581.1
    and proliferative (mixed) 583.2
      with nephrotic syndrome 581.2
      chronic 582.2
    chronic 582.1
    sclerosing 582.1
      with nephrotic syndrome 581.1
  mesangiocapillary 583.2
    with nephrotic syndrome 581.2
    chronic 582.2
  minimal change 581.3
  mixed membranous and proliferative 583.2
    with nephrotic syndrome 581.2
    chronic 582.2

Glomerulonephritis—*continued*
  necrotizing 583.4
    acute 580.4
    chronic 582.4
  nephrotic (*see also* Nephrosis) 581.9
  old—*see* Glomerulonephritis, chronic
  parenchymatous 581.89
  poststreptococcal 580.0
  proliferative (diffuse) 583.0
    with nephrotic syndrome 581.0
    acute 580.0
    chronic 582.0
  purulent (*see also* Pyelitis) 590.80
  quiescent—*see* Nephritis, chronic
  rapidly progressive 583.4
    acute 580.4
    chronic 582.4
  sclerosing membranous (chronic) 582.1
    with nephrotic syndrome 581.1
  septic (*see also* Pyelitis) 590.80
  specified pathology or lesion NEC 583.89
    with nephrotic syndrome 581.89
    acute 580.89
    chronic 582.89
  suppurative (acute) (disseminated) (*see also*
    Pyelitis) 590.80
  toxic—*see* Nephritis, acute
  tubal, tubular—*see* Nephrosis, tubular
  type II (Ellis)—*see* Nephrosis
  vascular—*see* Hypertension, kidney
Glomerulosclerosis (*see also* Sclerosis, renal) 587
  focal 582.1
    with nephrotic syndrome 581.1
  intercapillary (nodular) (with diabetes) 250.4
    [581.81]
    due to secondary diabetes 249.4 *[581.81]*
Glossagra 529.6
Glossalgia 529.6
Glossitis 529.0
  areata exfoliativa 529.1
  atrophic 529.4
  benign migratory 529.1
  gangrenous 529.0
  Hunter's 529.4
  median rhomboid 529.2
  Moeller's 529.4
  pellagrous 265.2
Glossocele 529.8
Glossodynia 529.6
  exfoliativa 529.4
Glossoncus 529.8
Glossophytia 529.3
Glossoplegia 529.8
Glossoptosis 529.8
Glossopyrosis 529.6
Glossotrichia 529.3
Glossy skin 701.9
Glottis —*see* condition
Glottitis —*see* Glossitis
Glucagonoma (M8152/0)
  malignant (M8152/3)
    pancreas 157.4
    specified site NEC—*see* Neoplasm, by site,
      malignant
    unspecified site 157.4
  pancreas 211.7
  specified site NEC—*see* Neoplasm, by site,
    benign
  unspecified site 211.7

Glucoglycinuria 270.7
Glue ear syndrome 381.20
Glue sniffing (airplane glue) (*see also*
  Dependence) 304.6
Glycinemia (with methylmalonic acidemia) 270.7
Glycinuria (renal) (with ketosis) 270.0
Glycogen
  infiltration (*see also* Disease, glycogen storage)
    271.0
  storage disease (*see also* Disease, glycogen
    storage) 271.0
Glycogenosis (*see also* Disease, glycogen
  storage) 271.0
  cardiac 271.0 *[425.7]*
  Cori, types I-VII 271.0
  diabetic, secondary 250.8 *[259.8]*
    due to secondary diabetes 249.8 *[259.8]*
  diffuse (with hepatic cirrhosis) 271.0
  generalized 271.0
  glucose-6-phosphatase deficiency 271.0
  hepatophosphorylase deficiency 271.0
  hepatorenal 271.0
  myophosphorylase deficiency 271.0
Glycopenia 251.2
Glycopeptide
  intermediate staphylococcus aureus (GISA)
    V09.8
  resistent
    enterococcus V09.8
    staphylococcus aureus (GRSA) V09.8
Glycoprolinuria 270.8
Glycosuria 791.5
  renal 271.4
Gnathostoma (spinigerum) (infection)
  (infestation) 128.1
  wandering swellings from 128.1
Gnathostomiasis 128.1
Goiter (adolescent) (colloid) (diffuse) (dipping)
  (due to iodine deficiency) (endemic)
  (euthyroid) (heart) (hyperplastic) (internal)
  (intrathoracic) (juvenile) (mixed type)
  (nonendemic) (parenchymatous) (plunging)
  (sporadic) (subclavicular) (substernal) 240.9
  with
    hyperthyroidism (recurrent) (*see also* Goiter,
      toxic) 242.0
    thyrotoxicosis (*see also* Goiter, toxic) 242.0
  adenomatous (*see also* Goiter, nodular) 241.9
  cancerous (M8000/3) 193
  complicating pregnancy, childbirth, or
    puerperium 648.1
  congenital 246.1
  cystic (*see also* Goiter, nodular) 241.9
  due to enzyme defect in synthesis of thyroid
    hormone (butane-insoluble iodine)
    (coupling) (deiodinase) (iodide trapping or
    organification) (iodotyrosine dehalogenase)
    (peroxidase) 246.1
  dyshormonogenic 246.1
  exophthalmic (*see also* Goiter, toxic) 242.0
  familial (with deaf-mutism) 243
  fibrous 245.3
  lingual 759.2
  lymphadenoid 245.2
  malignant (M8000/3) 193
  multinodular (nontoxic) 241.1
    toxic or with hyperthyroidism (*see also* Goiter,
      toxic) 242.2

Goiter—*continued*
nodular (nontoxic) 241.9
  with
    hyperthyroidism (*see also* Goiter, toxic)
      242.3
    thyrotoxicosis (*see also* Goiter, toxic) 242.3
  endemic 241.9
  exophthalmic (diffuse) (*see also* Goiter, toxic)
    242.0
  multinodular (nontoxic) 241.1
  sporadic 241.9
  toxic (*see also* Goiter, toxic) 242.3
  uninodular (nontoxic) 241.0
nontoxic (nodular) 241.9
  multinodular 241.1
  uninodular 241.0
pulsating (*see also* Goiter, toxic) 242.0
simple 240.0
toxic 242.0

*Note—Use the following fifth-digit
subclassification with category 242:*

*0 without mention of thyrotoxic crisis
   or storm*
1 with mention of thyrotoxic crisis or storm

  adenomatous 242.3
    multinodular 242.2
    uninodular 242.1
  multinodular 242.2
  nodular 242.3
    multinodular 242.2
    uninodular 242.1
  uninodular 242.1
  uninodular (nontoxic) 241.0
  toxic or with hyperthyroidism (*see also* Goiter,
    toxic) 242.1
Goldberg (-Maxwell) (-Morris) syndrome
  (testicular feminization) 259.51
Goldblatt's
  hypertension 440.1
  kidney 440.1
Goldenhar's syndrome (oculoauriculovertebral
  dysplasia) 756.0
Goldflam-Erb disease or syndrome 358.00
Goldscheider's disease (epidermolysis bullosa)
  757.39
Goldstein's disease (familial hemorrhagic
  telangiectasia) 448.0
Golfer's elbow 726.32
Goltz-Gorlin syndrome (dermal hypoplasia)
  757.39
Gonadoblastoma (M9073/1)
  specified site—*see* Neoplasm, by site uncertain
    behavior
  unspecified site
    female 236.2
    male 236.4
Gonecystitis (*see also* Vesiculitis) 608.0
Gongylonemiasis 125.6
  mouth 125.6
Goniosynechiae 364.73
Gonococcemia 098.89
Gonococcus, gonococcal (disease) (infection)
  (*see also* condition) 098.0
  anus 098.7
  bursa 098.52
  chronic NEC 098.2

Gonococcus, gonococcal—*continued*
  complicating pregnancy, childbirth, or
    puerperium 647.1
    affecting fetus or newborn 760.2
  conjunctiva, conjunctivitis (neonatorum) 098.40
  dermatosis 098.89
  endocardium 098.84
  epididymo-orchitis 098.13
    chronic or duration of 2 months or over 098.33
  eye (newborn) 098.40
  fallopian tube (chronic) 098.37
    acute 098.17
  genitourinary (acute) (organ) (system) (tract)
    (*see also* Gonorrhea) 098.0
    lower 098.0
      chronic 098.2
    upper 098.10
      chronic 098.30
  heart NEC 098.85
  joint 098.50
  keratoderma 098.81
  keratosis (blennorrhagica) 098.81
  lymphatic (gland) (node) 098.89
  meninges 098.82
  orchitis (acute) 098.13
    chronic or duration of 2 months or over 098.33
  pelvis (acute) 098.19
    chronic or duration of 2 months or over 098.39
  pericarditis 098.83
  peritonitis 098.86
  pharyngitis 098.6
  pharynx 098.6
  proctitis 098.7
  pyosalpinx (chronic) 098.37
    acute 098.17
  rectum 098.7
  septicemia 098.89
  skin 098.89
  specified site NEC 098.89
  synovitis 098.51
  tendon sheath 098.51
  throat 098.6
  urethra (acute) 098.0
    chronic or duration of 2 months or over 098.2
  vulva (acute) 098.0
    chronic or duration of 2 months or over 098.2
Gonocytoma (M9073/1)
  specified site—*see* Neoplasm, by site, uncertain
    behavior
  unspecified site
    female 236.2
    male 236.4
Gonorrhea 098.0
  acute 098.0
  Bartholin's gland (acute) 098.0
    chronic or duration of 2 months or over 098.2
  bladder (acute) 098.11
    chronic or duration of 2 months or over 098.31
  carrier (suspected of) V02.7
  cervix (acute) 098.15
    chronic or duration of 2 months or over 098.35
  chronic 098.2
  complicating pregnancy, childbirth, or
    puerperium 647.1
    affecting fetus or newborn 760.2
  conjunctiva, conjunctivitis (neonatorum) 098.40
  contact V01.6
  Cowper's gland (acute) 098.0
    chronic or duration of 2 months or over 098.2
  duration of two months or over 098.2

Gonorrhea—*continued*
  exposure to V01.6
  fallopian tube (chronic) 098.37
    acute 098.17
  genitourinary (acute) (organ) (system) (tract)
    098.0
    chronic 098.2
    duration of two months or over 098.2
  kidney (acute) 098.19
    chronic or duration of 2 months or over 098.39
  ovary (acute) 098.19
    chronic or duration of 2 months or over 098.39
  pelvis (acute) 098.19
    chronic or duration of 2 months or over 098.39
  penis (acute) 098.0
    chronic or duration of 2 months or over 098.2
  prostate (acute) 098.12
    chronic or duration of 2 months or over 098.32
  seminal vesicle (acute) 098.14
    chronic or duration of 2 months or over 098.34
  specified site NEC—*see* Gonococcus
  spermatic cord (acute) 098.14
    chronic or duration of 2 months or over 098.34
  urethra (acute) 098.0
    chronic or duration of 2 months or over 098.2
  vagina (acute) 098.0
    chronic or duration of 2 months or over 098.2
  vas deferens (acute) 098.14
    chronic or duration of 2 months or over 098.34
  vulva (acute) 098.0
    chronic or duration of 2 months or over 098.2
Goodpasture's syndrome (pneumorenal) 446.21
Good's syndrome 279.06
Gopalan's syndrome (burning feet) 266.2
Gordon's disease (exudative enteropathy) 579.8
Gorlin-Chaudhry-Moss syndrome 759.89
Gougerot's syndrome (trisymptomatic) 709.1
Gougerot-Blum syndrome (pigmented purpuric
  lichenoid dermatitis) 709.1
Gougerot-Carteaud disease or syndrome
  (confluent reticulate papillomatosis) 701.8
Gougerot-Hailey-Hailey disease (benign familial
  chronic pemphigus) 757.39
Gougerot (-Houwer) -Sjögren syndrome
  (keratoconjunctivitis sicca) 710.2
Gouley's syndrome (constrictive pericarditis)
  423.2
Goundou 102.6
Gout, gouty 274.9
  with
    specified manifestations NEC 274.89
    tophi (tophus) 274.03
  acute 274.01
  arthritis 274.00
    acute 274.01
  arthropathy 274.00
    acute 274.01
    chronic (without mention of tophus (tophi))
      274.02
      with tophus (tophi) 274.03
  attack 274.01
  chronic 274.02
    tophaceous 274.03
  degeneration, heart 274.82
  diathesis 274.9
  eczema 274.89
  episcleritis 274.89 *[379.09]*
  external ear (tophus) 274.81
  flare 274.01
  glomerulonephritis 274.10
  iritis 274.89 *[364.11]*

Gout, gouty—*continued*
  joint 274.00
  kidney 274.10
  lead 984.9
    specified type of lead—*see* Table of drugs and
      chemicals
  nephritis 274.10
  neuritis 274.89 *[357.4]*
  phlebitis 274.89 *[451.9]*
  rheumatic 714.0
  saturnine 984.9
    specified type of lead—*see* Table of drugs and
      chemicals
  spondylitis 274.00
  synovitis 274.00
  syphilitic 095.8
  tophi 274.03
    ear 274.81
    heart 274.82
    specified site NEC 274.82
Gowers'
  muscular dystrophy 359.1
  syndrome (vasovagal attack) 780.2
Gowers-Paton-Kennedy syndrome 377.04
Gradenigo's syndrome 383.02
Graft-versus-host disease 279.50
  due to organ transplant NEC—*see*
    Complications, transplant, organ
Graham Steell's murmur (pulmonic
  regurgitation) (*see also* Endocarditis,
  pulmonary) 424.3
Grain-handlers' disease or lung 495.8
Grain mite (itch) 133.8
Grand
  mal (idiopathic) (*see also* Epilepsy) 345.1
    hysteria of Charcot 300.11
    nonrecurrent or isolated 780.39
  multipara
    affecting management of labor and delivery
      659.4
    status only (not pregnant) V61.5
Granite workers' lung 502
Granular —*see also* condition
  inflammation, pharynx 472.1
  kidney (contracting) (*see also* Sclerosis, renal) 587
  liver—*see* Cirrhosis, liver
  nephritis—*see* Nephritis
Granulation tissue, abnormal —*see also*
    Granuloma
  abnormal or excessive 701.5
  postmastoidectomy cavity 383.33
  postoperative 701.5
  skin 701.5
Granulocytopenia, granulocytopenic (primary)
    288.00
  malignant 288.09
Granuloma NEC 686.1
  abdomen (wall) 568.89
    skin (pyogenicum) 686.1
      from residual foreign body 709.4
  annulare 695.89
  anus 569.49
  apical 522.6
  appendix 543.9
  aural 380.23
  beryllium (skin) 709.4
    lung 503
  bone (*see also* Osteomyelitis) 730.1
    eosinophilic 277.89
    from residual foreign body 733.99
  canaliculus lacrimalis 375.81

Granuloma—*continued*
  cerebral 348.89
  cholesterin, middle ear 385.82
  coccidioidal (progressive) 114.3
    lung 114.4
    meninges 114.2
    primary (lung) 114.0
  colon 569.89
  conjunctiva 372.61
  dental 522.6
  ear, middle (cholesterin) 385.82
    with otitis media—*see* Otitis media
  eosinophilic 277.89
    bone 277.89
    lung 277.89
    oral mucosa 528.9
  exuberant 701.5
  eyelid 374.89
  facial
    lethal midline 446.3
    malignant 446.3
  faciale 701.8
  fissuratum (gum) 523.8
  foot NEC 686.1
  foreign body (in soft tissue) NEC 728.82
    bone 733.99
    in operative wound 998.4
    muscle 728.82
    skin 709.4
    subcutaneous tissue 709.4
  fungoides 202.1
  gangraenescens 446.3
  giant cell (central) (jaw) (reparative) 526.3
    gingiva 523.8
    peripheral (gingiva) 523.8
  gland (lymph) 289.3
  Hodgkin's (M9661/3) 201.1
  ileum 569.89
  infectious NEC 136.9
  inguinale (Donovan) 099.2
    venereal 099.2
  intestine 569.89
  iridocyclitis 364.10
  jaw (bone) 526.3
    reparative giant cell 526.3
  kidney (*see also* Infection, kidney) 590.9
  lacrimal sac 375.81
  larynx 478.79
  lethal midline 446.3
  lipid 277.89
  lipoid 277.89
  liver 572.8
  lung (infectious) (*see also* Fibrosis, lung) 515
    coccidioidal 114.4
    eosinophilic 277.89
  lymph gland 289.3
  Majocchi's 110.6
  malignant, face 446.3
  mandible 526.3
  mediastinum 519.3
  midline 446.3
  monilial 112.3
  muscle 728.82
    from residual foreign body 728.82
  nasal sinus (*see also* Sinusitis) 473.9
  operation wound 998.59
    foreign body 998.4
    stitch (external) 998.89
      internal organ 998.89
    talc 998.7
  oral mucosa, eosinophilic or pyogenic 528.9

Granuloma—*continued*
  orbit, orbital 376.11
  paracoccidioidal 116.1
  penis, venereal 099.2
  periapical 522.6
  peritoneum 568.89
    due to ova of helminths NEC (*see also*
      Helminthiasis) 128.9
  postmastoidectomy cavity 383.33
  postoperative–*see* Granuloma, operation wound
  prostate 601.8
  pudendi (ulcerating) 099.2
  pudendorum (ulcerative) 099.2
  pulp, internal (tooth) 521.49
  pyogenic, pyogenicum (skin) 686.1
    maxillary alveolar ridge 522.6
    oral mucosa 528.9
  rectum 569.49
  reticulohistiocytic 277.89
  rubrum nasi 705.89
  sarcoid 135
  Schistosoma 120.9
  septic (skin) 686.1
  silica (skin) 709.4
  sinus (accessory) (infectional) (nasal) (*see also*
      Sinusitis) 473.9
  skin (pyogenicum) 686.1
    from foreign body or material 709.4
  sperm 608.89
  spine
    syphilitic (epidural) 094.89
    tuberculous (*see also* Tuberculosis) 015.0
      [730.88]
  stitch (postoperative) 998.89
    internal wound 998.89
  suppurative (skin) 686.1
  suture (postoperative) 998.89
    internal wound 998.89
  swimming pool 031.1
  talc 728.82
    in operation wound 998.7
  telangiectaticum (skin) 686.1
  tracheostomy 519.09
  trichophyticum 110.6
  tropicum 102.4
  umbilicus 686.1
    newborn 771.4
  urethra 599.84
  uveitis 364.10
  vagina 099.2
  venereum 099.2
  vocal cords 478.5
  Wegener's (necrotizing respiratory
      granulomatosis) 446.4
Granulomatosis NEC 686.1
  disciformis chronica et progressiva 709.3
  infantiseptica 771.2
  lipoid 277.89
  lipophagic, intestinal 040.2
  miliary 027.0
  necrotizing, respiratory 446.4
  progressive, septic 288.1
  Wegener's (necrotizing respiratory) 446.4
Granulomatous tissue —*see* Granuloma
Granulosis rubra nasi 705.89
Graphite fibrosis (of lung) 503
Graphospasm 300.89
  organic 333.84
Grating scapula 733.99
Gravel (urinary) (*see also* Calculus) 592.9
Graves' disease (exophthalmic goiter) (*see also*
      Goiter, toxic) 242.0

Gravis —*see* condition
Grawitz's tumor (hypernephroma) (M8312/3) 189.0
Grayness, hair (premature) 704.3
  congenital 757.4
Gray or grey syndrome (chloramphenicol) (newborn) 779.4
Greenfield's disease 330.0
Green sickness 280.9
Greenstick fracture —*see* Fracture, by site
Greig's syndrome (hypertelorism) 756.0
Grief 309.0
Griesinger's disease (*see also* Ancylostomiasis) 126.9
Grinder's
  asthma 502
  lung 502
  phthisis (*see also* Tuberculosis) 011.4
Grinding, teeth 306.8
Grip
  Dabney's 074.1
  devil's 074.1
Grippe, grippal —*see also* Influenza
  Balkan 083.0
  intestinal 487.8
  summer 074.8
Grippy cold 487.1
Grisel's disease 723.5
Groin —*see* condition
Grooved
  nails (transverse) 703.8
  tongue 529.5
    congenital 750.13
Ground itch 126.9
Growing pains, children 781.99
Growth (fungoid) (neoplastic) (new) (M8000/1)—*see also* Neoplasm, by site, unspecified nature
  adenoid (vegetative) 474.12
  benign (M8000/0)—*see* Neoplasm, by site, benign
  fetal, poor 764.9
    affecting management of pregnancy 656.5
  malignant (M8000/3)—*see* Neoplasm, by site malignant
  rapid, childhood V21.0
  secondary (M8000/6)—*see* Neoplasm, by site, malignant, secondary
GRSA (glycopeptide resistant staphylococcus aureus) V09.8
Gruber's hernia —*see* Hernia, Gruber's
Gruby's disease (tinea tonsurans) 110.0
GSS (Gerstmann-Straussler-Scheinker syndrome) 046.71
G-trisomy 758.0
Guama fever 066.3
Gubler (-Millard) paralysis or syndrome 344.89
Guérin-Stern syndrome (arthrogryposis multiplex congenita) 754.89
Guertin's disease (electric chorea) 049.8
Guillain-Barré disease or syndrome 357.0
Guinea worms (infection) (infestation) 125.7
Guinon's disease (motor-verbal tic) 307.23
Gull's disease (thyroid atrophy with myxedema) 244.8
Gull and Sutton's disease —*see* Hypertension, kidney
Gum —*see* condition
Gumboil 522.7

Gumma (syphilitic) 095.9
  artery 093.89
    cerebral or spinal 094.89
  bone 095.5
    of yaws (late) 102.6
  brain 094.89
  cauda equina 094.89
  central nervous system NEC 094.9
  ciliary body 095.8 *[364.11]*
  congenital 090.5
    testis 090.5
  eyelid 095.8 *[373.5]*
  heart 093.89
  intracranial 094.89
  iris 095.8 *[364.11]*
  kidney 095.4
  larynx 095.8
  leptomeninges 094.2
  liver 095.3
  meninges 094.2
  myocardium 093.82
  nasopharynx 095.8
  neurosyphilitic 094.9
  nose 095.8
  orbit 095.8
  palate (soft) 095.8
  penis 095.8
  pericardium 093.81
  pharynx 095.8
  pituitary 095.8
  scrofulous (*see also* Tuberculosis) 017.0
  skin 095.8
  specified site NEC 095.8
  spinal cord 094.89
  tongue 095.8
  tonsil 095.8
  trachea 095.8
  tuberculous (*see also* Tuberculosis) 017.0
  ulcerative due to yaws 102.4
  ureter 095.8
  yaws 102.4
    bone 102.6
Gunn's syndrome (jaw-winking syndrome) 742.8
Gunshot wound —*see also* Wound, open, by site
  fracture—*see* Fracture, by site, open
  internal organs (abdomen, chest, or pelvis)—*see* Injury, internal, by site, with open wound
  intracranial—*see* Laceration, brain, with open intracranial wound
Günther's disease or syndrome (congenital erythropoietic porphyria) 277.1
Gustatory hallucination 780.1
Gynandrism 752.7
Gynandroblastoma (M8632/1)
  specified site—*see* Neoplasm, by site, uncertain behavior
  unspecified site
    female 236.2
    male 236.4
Gynandromorphism 752.7
Gynatresia (congenital) 752.49
Gynecoid pelvis, male 738.6
Gynecological examination V72.31
  for contraceptive maintenance V25.40
Gynecomastia 611.1
Gynephobia 300.29
Gyrate scalp 757.39

H

Haas' disease (osteochondrosis head of humerus) 732.3
Habermann's disease (acute parapsoriasis varioliformis) 696.2
Habit, habituation
chorea 307.22
disturbance, child 307.9
drug (see also Dependence) 304.9
laxative (see also Abuse, drugs, nondependent) 305.9
spasm 307.20
chronic 307.22
transient (of childhood) 307.21
tic 307.20
chronic 307.22
transient (of childhood) 307.21
use of
nonprescribed drugs (see also Abuse, drugs, nondependent) 305.9
patent medicines (see also Abuse, drugs, nondependent) 305.9
vomiting 536.2
Hadfield-Clarke syndrome (pancreatic infantilism) 577.8
Haff disease 985.1
Hageman factor defect, deficiency, or disease (see also Defect, coagulation) 286.3
Haglund's disease (osteochondrosis os tibiale externum) 732.5
Haglund-Läwen-Fründ syndrome 717.89
Hagner's disease (hypertrophic pulmonary osteoarthropathy) 731.2
Hag teeth, tooth 524.39
Hailey-Hailey disease (benign familial chronic pemphigus) 757.39
Hair —see also condition
plucking 307.9
Hairball in stomach 935.2
Hairy black tongue 529.3
Half vertebra 756.14
Halitosis 784.99
Hallermann-Streiff syndrome 756.0
Hallervorden-Spatz disease or syndrome 333.0
Hallopeau's
acrodermatitis (continua) 696.1
disease (lichen sclerosis et atrophicus) 701.0
Hallucination (auditory) (gustatory) (olfactory) (tactile) 780.1
alcohol-induced 291.3
drug-induced 292.12
visual 368.16
Hallucinosis 298.9
alcohol-induced (acute) 291.3
drug-induced 292.12
Hallus —see Hallux
Hallux 735.9
limitus 735.8
malleus (acquired) 735.3
rigidus (acquired) 735.2
congenital 755.66
late effects of rickets 268.1
valgus (acquired) 735.0
congenital 755.66
varus (acquired) 735.1
congenital 755.66
Halo, visual 368.15
Hamartoblastoma 759.6

Hamartoma 759.6
epithelial (gingival), odontogenic, central, or peripheral (M9321/0) 213.1
upper jaw (bone) 213.0
vascular 757.32
Hamartosis, hamartoses NEC 759.6
Hamman's disease or syndrome (spontaneous mediastinal emphysema) 518.1
Hamman-Rich syndrome (diffuse interstitial pulmonary fibrosis) 516.3
Hammer toe (acquired) 735.4
congenital 755.66
late effects of rickets 268.1
Hand —see condition
Hand-Schüller-Christian disease or syndrome (chronic histiocytosis x) 277.89
Hand-foot syndrome 693.0
Hanging (asphyxia) (strangulation) (suffocation) 994.7
Hangnail (finger) (with lymphangitis) 681.02
Hangover (alcohol) (see also Abuse, drugs, nondependent) 305.0
Hanot's cirrhosis or disease —see Cirrhosis, biliary
Hanot-Chauffard (-Troisier) syndrome (bronze diabetes) 275.0
Hansen's disease (leprosy) 030.9
benign form 030.1
malignant form 030.0
Harada's disease or syndrome 363.22
Hard chancre 091.0
Hard firm prostate 600.10
with
urinary
obstruction 600.11
retention 600.11
Hardening
artery—see Arteriosclerosis
brain 348.89
liver 571.8
Hare's syndrome (M8010/3) (carcinoma, pulmonary apex) 162.3
Harelip (see also Cleft, lip) 749.10
Harkavy's syndrome 446.0
Harlequin (fetus) 757.1
color change syndrome 779.89
Harley's disease (intermittent hemoglobinuria) 283.2
Harris'
lines 733.91
syndrome (organic hyperinsulinism) 251.1
Hart's disease or syndrome (pellagra-cerebellar ataxia-renal aminoaciduria) 270.0
Hartmann's pouch (abnormal sacculation of gallbladder neck) 575.8
of intestine V44.3
attention to V55.3
Hartnup disease (pellagra-cerebellar ataxia-renal aminoaciduria) 270.0
Harvester lung 495.0
Hashimoto's disease or struma (struma lymphomatosa) 245.2
Hassall-Henle bodies (corneal warts) 371.41
Haut mal (see also Epilepsy) 345.1
Haverhill fever 026.1
Hawaiian wood rose dependence 304.5
Hawkins' keloid 701.4

Hay
asthma (*see also* Asthma) 493.0
  fever (allergic) (with rhinitis) 477.9with
    asthma (bronchial) (*see also* Asthma) 493.0
  allergic, due to grass, pollen, ragweed, or tree
    477.0
  conjunctivitis 372.05
  due to
    dander, animal (cat) (dog) 477.2
    dust 477.8
    fowl 477.8
    hair, animal (cat) (dog) 477.2
    pollen 477.0
    specified allergen other than pollen 477.8
Hayem-Faber syndrome (achlorhydric anemia)
  280.9
Hayem-Widal syndrome (acquired hemolytic
  jaundice) 283.9
Haygarth's nodosities 715.04
Hazard-Crile tumor (M8350/3) 193
Hb (abnormal)
  disease—*see* Disease, hemoglobin
  trait—*see* Trait
H disease 270.0
Head —*see also* condition
  banging 307.3
Headache 784.0
  allergic 339.00
  associated with sexual activity 339.82
  cluster 339.00
    chronic 339.02
    episodic 339.01
  daily
    chronic 784.0
    new persistent (NPDH) 339.42
  drug induced 339.3
  due to
    loss, spinal fluid 349.0
    lumbar puncture 349.0
    saddle block 349.0
  emotional 307.81
  histamine 339.00
  hypnic 339.81
  lumbar puncture 349.0
  medication overuse 339.3
  menopausal 627.2
  menstrual 346.4
  migraine 346.9
  nasal septum 784.0
  nonorganic origin 307.81
  orgasmic 339.82
  postspinal 349.0
  post-traumatic 339.20
    acute 339.21
    chronic 339.22
  premenstrual 346.4
  preorgasmic 339.82
  primary
    cough 339.83
    exertional 339.84
    stabbing 339.85
    thunderclap 339.43
  psychogenic 307.81
  psychophysiologic 307.81
  rebound 339.3
  short lasting unilateral neuralgiform with
    conjunctival injection and tearing (SUNCT)
    339.05
  sick 346.9

Headache—*continued*
  spinal 349.0
    complicating labor and delivery 668.8
    postpartum 668.8
  spinal fluid loss 349.0
  syndrome
    cluster 339.00
    complicated NEC 339.44
    periodic in child or adolescent 346.2
    specified NEC 339.89
  tension 307.81
    type 339.10
      chronic 339.12
      episodic 339.11
  vascular 784.0
    migraine type 346.9
  vasomotor 346.9
Health
  advice V65.4
  audit V70.0
  checkup V70.0
  education V65.4
  hazard (*see also* History of) V15.9
    falling V15.88
    specified cause NEC V15.89
  instruction V65.4
  services provided because (of)
    boarding school residence V60.6
    holiday relief for person providing home care
      V60.5
    inadequate
      housing V60.1
      resources V60.2
    lack of housing V60.0
    no care available in home V60.4
    person living alone V60.3
    poverty V60.3
    residence in institution V60.6
    specified cause NEC V60.89
    vacation relief for person providing home care
      V60.5
Healthy
  donor (*see also* Donor) V59.9
  infant or child
    accompanying sick mother V65.0
    receiving care V20.1
  person
    accompanying sick relative V65.0
    admitted for sterilization V25.2
    receiving prophylactic inoculation or
      vaccination (*see also* Vaccination,
      prophylactic) V05.9
Hearing
  conservation and treatment V72.12
  examination V72.19
    following failed hearing screening V72.11
Heart —*see* condition
Heartburn 787.1
  psychogenic 306.4
Heat (effects) 992.9
  apoplexy 992.0
  burn—*see also* Burn, by site
    from sun (*see also* Sunburn) 692.71
  collapse 992.1
  cramps 992.2
  dermatitis or eczema 692.89
  edema 992.7
  erythema—*see* Burn, by site
  excessive 992.9
    specified effect NEC 992.8

Heat —*continued*
exhaustion 992.5
  anhydrotic 992.3
  due to
    salt (and water) depletion 992.4
    water depletion 992.3
fatigue (transient) 992.6
fever 992.0
hyperpyrexia 992.0
prickly 705.1
prostration—*see* Heat, exhaustion
pyrexia 992.0
rash 705.1
specified effect NEC 992.8
stroke 992.0
sunburn (*see also* Sunburn) 692.71
syncope 992.1
Heavy-chain disease 273.2
Heavy-for-dates (fetus or infant) 766.1
4500 grams or more 766.0
exceptionally 766.0
Hebephrenia, hebephrenic (acute) (*see also* Schizophrenia) 295.1
dementia (praecox) (*see also* Schizophrenia) 295.1
schizophrenia (*see also* Schizophrenia) 295.1
Heberden's
disease or nodes 715.04
syndrome (angina pectoris) 413.9
Hebra's disease
dermatitis exfoliativa 695.89
erythema multiforme exudativum 695.19
pityriasis 695.89
  maculata et circinata 696.3
  rubra 695.89
    pilaris 696.4
prurigo 698.2
Hebra, nose 040.1
Hedinger's syndrome (malignant carcinoid) 259.2
Heel —*see* condition
Heerfordt's disease or syndrome (uveoparotitis) 135
Hegglin's anomaly or syndrome 288.2
Heidenhain's disease 290.10
with dementia 290.10
Heilmeyer-Schöner disease (M9842/3) 207.1
Heine-Medin disease (*see also* Poliomyelitis) 045.9
Heinz-body anemia, congenital 282.7
Heller's disease or syndrome (infantile psychosis) (*see also* Psychosis, childhood) 299.1
H.E.L.L.P. 642.5
Helminthiasis (*see also* Infestation, by specific parasite) 128.9
Ancylostoma (*see also* Ancylostoma) 126.9
intestinal 127.9
  mixed types (types classifiable to more than one of the titles 120.0-127.7) 127.8
  specified type 127.7
mixed types (intestinal) (types classifiable to more than one of the titles 120.0-127.7) 127.8
Necator americanus 126.1
specified type NEC 128.8
Trichinella 124
Heloma 700
Hemangioblastoma (M9161/1)—*see also* Neoplasm, connective tissue, uncertain behavior
malignant (M9161//3)—*see* Neoplasm, connective tissue, malignant

Hemangioblastomatosis, cerebelloretinal 759.6
Hemangioendothelioma (M9130/1)—*see also* Neoplasm, by site, uncertain behavior
benign (M9130/0) 228.00
bone (diffuse) (M9130/3)—*see* Neoplasm, bone, malignant
malignant (M9130/3)—*see* Neoplasm, connective tissue, malignant
nervous system (M9130/0) 228.09
Hemangioendotheliosarcoma (M9130/3)—*see* Neoplasm, connective tissue, malignant
Hemangiofibroma (M9160/0)—*see* Neoplasm, by site, benign
Hemangiolipoma (M8861/0)—*see* Lipoma
Hemangioma (M9120/0) 228.00
arteriovenous (M9123/0)—*see* Hemangioma, by site
brain 228.02
capillary (M9131/0)—*see* Hemangioma, by site
cavernous (M9121/0)—*see* Hemangioma, by site
central nervous system NEC 228.09
choroid 228.09
heart 228.09
infantile (M9131/0)—*see* Hemangioma, by site
intra-abdominal structures 228.04
intracranial structures 228.02
intramuscular (M9132/0)—*see* Hemangioma, by site
iris 228.09
juvenile (M9131/0)—*see* Hemangioma, by site
malignant (M9120/3)—*see* Neoplasm, connective tissue, malignant
meninges 228.09
  brain 228.02
  spinal cord 228.09
peritoneum 228.04
placenta—*see* Placenta, abnormal
plexiform (M9131/0)—*see* Hemangioma, by site
racemose (M9123/0)—*see* Hemangioma, by site
retina 228.03
retroperitoneal tissue 228.04
sclerosing (M8832/0)—*see* Neoplasm, skin, benign
simplex (M9131/0)—*see* Hemangioma, by site
skin and subcutaneous tissue 228.01
specified site NEC 228.09
spinal cord 228.09
venous (M9122/0)—*see* Hemangioma, by site
verrucous keratotic (M9142/0)—*see* Hemangioma, by site
Hemangiomatosis (systemic) 757.32
involving single site—*see* Hemangioma
Hemangiopericytoma (M9150/1)—*see also* Neoplasm, connective tissue, uncertain behavior
benign (M9150/0)—*see* Neoplasm, connective tissue, benign
malignant (M9150/3)—*see* Neoplasm, connective tissue, malignant
Hemangiosarcoma (M9120/3)—*see* Neoplasm, connective tissue, malignant
Hemarthrosis (nontraumatic) 719.0
ankle 719.17
elbow 719.12
foot 719.17
hand 719.14
hip 719.15
knee 719.16
multiple sites 719.19
pelvic region 719.15
shoulder (region) 719.11

Hemarthrosis—*continued*
  specified site NEC 719.18
  traumatic—*see* Sprain, by site
  wrist 719.13
Hematemesis 578.0
  with ulcer—*see* Ulcer, by site, with hemorrhage
  due to S. japonicum 120.2
  Goldstein's (familial hemorrhagic
    telangiectasia) 448.0
  newborn 772.4
    due to swallowed maternal blood 777.3
Hematidrosis 705.89
Hematinuria (*see also* Hemoglobinuria) 791.2
  malarial 084.8
  paroxysmal 283.2
Hematite miners' lung 503
Hematobilia 576.8
Hematocele (congenital) (diffuse) (idiopathic)
  608.83
  broad ligament 620.7
  canal of Nuck 629.0
  cord, male 608.83
  fallopian tube 620.8
  female NEC 629.0
  ischiorectal 569.89
  male NEC 608.83
  ovary 629.0
  pelvis, pelvic
    female 629.0
      with ectopic pregnancy (*see also* Pregnancy,
        ectopic) 633.90
      with intrauterine pregnancy 633.91
    male 608.83
  periuterine 629.0
  retrouterine 629.0
  scrotum 608.83
  spermatic cord (diffuse) 608.83
  testis 608.84
  traumatic—*see* Injury, internal, pelvis
  tunica vaginalis 608.83
  uterine ligament 629.0
  uterus 621.4
  vagina 623.6
  vulva 624.5
Hematocephalus 742.4
Hematochezia (*see also* Melena) 578.1
Hematochyluria (*see also* Infestation, filarial)
  125.9
Hematocolpos 626.8
Hematocornea 371.12
Hematogenous —*see* condition
Hematoma (skin surface intact) (traumatic)—*see*
  also Contusion

Note—*Hematomas are coded according to
origin and the nature and site of the hematoma
or the accompanying injury. Hematomas of
unspecified origin are coded as injuries of the
sites involved, except:*
(a) *hematomas of genital organs which are
coded as diseases of the organ involved
unless they complicate pregnancy or
delivery*
(b) *hematomas of the eye which are coded as
diseases of the eye.*

*For late effect of hematoma classifiable to
920-924 see Late, effect, contusion*

Hematoma—*continued*
  with
    crush injury—*see* Crush
    fracture—*see* Fracture, by site
    injury of internal organs—*see also* Injury,
      internal, by site
      kidney—*see* Hematoma, kidney, traumatic
      liver—*see* Hematoma, liver, traumatic
      spleen—*see* Hematoma, spleen
    nerve injury—*see* Injury, nerve
    open wound—*see* Wound, open, by site
    skin surface intact—*see* Contusion
  abdomen (wall)—*see* Contusion, abdomen
  amnion 658.8
  aorta, dissecting 441.00
    abdominal 441.02
    thoracic 441.01
    thoracoabdominal 441.03
  arterial (complicating trauma) 904.9
    specified site—*see* Injury, blood vessel, by
      site
  auricle (ear) 380.31
  birth injury 767.8
    skull 767.19
  brain (traumatic) 853.0

Note—*Use the following fifth-digit
subclassification with categories 851-854:*

0 *unspecified state of consciousness*
1 *with no loss of consciousness*
2 *with brief [less than one hour] loss of
   consciousness*
3 *with moderate [1-24 hours] loss of
   consciousness*
4 *with prolonged [more than 24 hours] loss of
   consciousness and return to pre-existing
   conscious level*
5 *with prolonged [more than 24 hours] loss of
   consciousness, without return to pre-existing
   conscious level*
*Use fifth-digit 5 to designate when a patient is
unconscious and dies before regaining
consciousness, regardless of the duration of the
loss of consciousness*
6 *with loss of consciousness of unspecified
   duration*
9 *with concussion, unspecified*

  with
    cerebral
      contusion—*see* Contusion, brain
      laceration—*see* Laceration, brain
    open intracranial wound 853.1
    skull fracture—*see* Fracture, skull, by site
  extradural or epidural 852.4
    with open intracranial wound 852.5
    fetus or newborn 767.0
    nontraumatic 432.0
  fetus or newborn NEC 767.0
  nontraumatic (*see also* Hemorrhage, brain)
    431
    epidural or extradural 432.0
    newborn NEC 772.8
    subarachnoid, arachnoid, or meningeal (*see
      also* Hemorrhage, subarachnoid) 430
    subdural (*see also* Hemorrhage, subdural)
      432.1
  subarachnoid, arachnoid, or meningeal 852.0
    with open intracranial wound 852.1
    fetus or newborn 772.2
    nontraumatic (*see also* Hemorrhage,
      subarachnoid) 430

Hematoma—*continued*
  brain—*continued*
    subdural 852.2
      with open intracranial wound 852.3
      fetus or newborn (localized) 767.0
      nontraumatic (*see also* Hemorrhage,
        subdural) 432.1
  breast (nontraumatic) 611.89
  broad ligament (nontraumatic) 620.7
    complicating delivery 665.7
    traumatic—*see* Injury, internal, broad
      ligament
  calcified NEC 959.9
  capitis 920
    due to birth injury 767.19
    newborn 767.19
  cerebral—*see* Hematoma, brain
  cesarean section wound 674.3
  chorion—*see* Placenta, abnormal
  complicating delivery (perineum) (vulva) 664.5
    pelvic 665.7
    vagina 665.7
  corpus
    cavernosum (nontraumatic) 607.82
    luteum (nontraumatic) (ruptured) 620.1
  dura (mater)—*see* Hematoma, brain, subdural
  epididymis (nontraumatic) 608.83
  epidural (traumatic)—*see also* Hematoma,
    brain, extradural
    spinal—*see* Injury, spinal, by site
  episiotomy 674.3
  external ear 380.31
  extradural—*see also* Hematoma, brain,
    extradural
    fetus or newborn 767.0
    nontraumatic 432.0
      fetus or newborn 767.0
  fallopian tube 620.8
  genital organ (nontraumatic)
    female NEC 629.89
    male NEC 608.83
    traumatic (external site) 922.4
      intern: '—*see* Injury, internal, genital organ
  graafian follicle (ruptured) 620.0
  internal organs (abdomen, chest, or pelvis)—*see
    also* Injury, internal, by site
    kidney—*see* Hematoma, kidney, traumatic
    liver—*see* Hematoma, liver, traumatic
    spleen—*see* Hematoma, spleen
  intracranial—*see* Hematoma, brain
  kidney, cystic 593.81
    traumatic 866.01
      with open wound into cavity 866.11
  labia (nontraumatic) 624.5
  lingual (and other parts of neck, scalp, or face,
    except eye) 920
  liver (subcapsular) 573.8
    birth injury 767.8
    fetus or newborn 767.8
    traumatic NEC 864.01
      with
        laceration—*see* Laceration, liver
        open wound into cavity 864.11
  mediastinum—*see* Injury, internal, mediastinum
  meninges, meningeal (brain)—*see also*
    Hematoma, brain, subarachnoid
    spinal—*see* Injury, spinal, by site
  mesosalpinx (nontraumatic) 620.8
    traumatic—*see* Injury, internal, pelvis
  muscle (traumatic)—*see* Contusion, by site
    nontraumatic 729.92

Hematoma—*continued*
  nasal (septum) (and other part(s) of neck, scalp,
    or face, except eye) 920
  obstetrical surgical wound 674.3
  orbit, orbital (nontraumatic) 376.32
    traumatic 921.2
  ovary (corpus luteum) (nontraumatic) 620.1
    traumatic—*see* Injury, internal, ovary
  pelvis (female) (nontraumatic) 629.89
    complicating delivery 665.7
    male 608.83
    traumatic—*see also* Injury, internal, pelvis
      specified organ NEC (*see also* Injury,
        internal, pelvis) 867.6
  penis (nontraumatic) 607.82
  pericranial (and neck, or face any part, except
    eye) 920
    due to injury at birth 767.19
  perineal wound (obstetrical) 674.3
    complicating delivery 664.5
  perirenal, cystic 593.81
  pinna 380.31
  placenta—*see* Placenta, abnormal
  postoperative 998.12
  retroperitoneal (nontraumatic) 568.81
    traumatic—*see* Injury, internal,
      retroperitoneum
  retropubic, male 568.81
  scalp (and neck, or face any part, except eye)
    920
    fetus or newborn 767.19
  scrotum (nontraumatic) 608.83
    traumatic 922.4
  seminal vesicle (nontraumatic) 608.83
    traumatic—*see* Injury, internal, seminal
      vesicle
  soft tissue 729.92
  spermatic cord—*see also* Injury, internal,
    spermatic cord
    nontraumatic 608.83
  spinal (cord) (meninges)—*see also* Injury,
    spinal, by site
    fetus or newborn 767.4
    nontraumatic 336.1
  spleen 865.01
    with
      laceration—*see* Laceration, spleen
      open wound into cavity 865.11
  sternocleidomastoid, birth injury 767.8
  sternomastoid, birth injury 767.8
  subarachnoid—*see also* Hematoma, brain,
    subarachnoid
    fetus or newborn 772.2
    nontraumatic (*see also* Hemorrhage,
      subarachnoid) 430
      newborn 772.2
  subdural—*see also* Hematoma, brain, subdural
    fetus or newborn (localized) 767.0
    nontraumatic (*see also* Hemorrhage, subdural)
      432.1
  subperiosteal (syndrome) 267
    traumatic—*see* Hematoma, by site
  superficial, fetus or newborn 772.6
  syncytium—*see* Placenta, abnormal
  testis (nontraumatic) 608.83
    birth injury 767.8
    traumatic 922.4
  tunica vaginalis (nontraumatic) 608.83
  umbilical cord 663.6
    affecting fetus or newborn 762.6
  uterine ligament (nontraumatic) 620.7
    traumatic—*see* Injury, internal, pelvis

Hematoma—*continued*
  uterus 621.4
    traumatic—*see* Injury, internal, pelvis
  vagina (nontraumatic) (ruptured) 623.6
    complicating delivery 665.7
    traumatic 922.4
  vas deferens (nontraumatic) 608.83
    traumatic—*see* Injury, internal, vas deferens
  vitreous 379.23
  vocal cord 920
  vulva (nontraumatic) 624.5
    complicating delivery 664.5
    fetus or newborn 767.8
    traumatic 922.4
Hematometra 621.4
Hematomyelia 336.1
  with fracture of vertebra (*see also* Fracture,
    vertebra, by site, with spinal cord injury)
    806.8
  fetus or newborn 767.4
Hematomyelitis 323.9
  late effect—*see* category 326
Hematoperitoneum (*see also* Hemoperitoneum)
  568.81
Hematopneumothorax (*see also* Hemothorax)
  511.89
Hematopoiesis, cyclic 288.02
Hematoporphyria (acquired) (congenital) 277.1
Hematoporphyrinuria (acquired) (congenital)
  277.1
Hematorachis, hematorrhachis 336.1
  fetus or newborn 767.4
Hematosalpinx 620.8
  with
    ectopic pregnancy (*see also* categories
      633.0-633.9) 639.2
    molar pregnancy (*see also* categories 630-632)
      639.2
  infectional (*see also* Salpingo-oophoritis) 614.2
Hematospermia 608.82
Hematothorax (*see also* Hemothorax) 511.89
Hematotympanum 381.03
Hematuria (benign) (essential) (idiopathic)
  599.70
  due to S. hematobium 120.0
  endemic 120.0
  gross 599.71
  intermittent 599.70
  malarial 084.8
  microscopic 599.72
  paroxysmal 599.70
  sulfonamide
    correct substance properly administered
      599.70
    overdose or wrong substance given or taken
      961.0
  tropical (bilharziasis) 120.0
  tuberculous (*see also* Tuberculosis) 016.9
Hematuric bilious fever 084.8
Hemeralopia 368.10
  acquired 286.5
Hemiabiotrophy 799.89
Hemi-akinesia 781.8
Hemianalgesia (*see also* Disturbance, sensation)
  782.0
Hemianencephaly 740.0
Hemianesthesia (*see also* Disturbance, sensation)
  782.0

Hemianopia, hemianopsia (altitudinal)
  (homonymous) 368.46
  binasal 368.47
  bitemporal 368.47
  heteronymous 368.47
  syphilitic 095.8
Hemiasomatognosia 307.9
Hemiathetosis 781.0
Hemiatrophy 799.89
  cerebellar 334.8
  face 349.89
    progressive 349.89
  fascia 728.9
  leg 728.2
  tongue 529.8
Hemiballism (us) 333.5
Hemiblock (cardiac) (heart) (left) 426.2
Hemicardia 746.89
Hemicephalus, hemicephaly 740.0
Hemichorea 333.5
Hemicrania 346.9
  congenital malformation 740.0
  continua 339.41
  paroxysmal 339.03
    chronic 339.04
    episodic 339.03
Hemidystrophy —*see* Hemiatrophy
Hemiectromelia 755.4
Hemihypalgesia (*see also* Disturbance,
  sensation) 782.0
Hemihypertrophy (congenital) 759.89
  cranial 756.0
Hemihypesthesia (*see also* Disturbance,
  sensation) 782.0
Hemi-inattention 781.8
Hemimelia 755.4
  lower limb 755.30
    paraxial (complete) (incomplete) (intercalary)
      (terminal) 755.32
      fibula 755.37
      tibia 755.36
    transverse (complete) (partial) 755.31
  upper limb 755.20
    paraxial (complete) (incomplete) (intercalary)
      (terminal) 755.22
      radial 755.26
      ulnar 755.27
    transverse (complete) (partial) 755.21
Hemiparalysis (*see also* Hemiplegia) 342.9
Hemiparesis (*see also* Hemiplegia) 342.9
Hemiparesthesia (*see also* Disturbance,
  sensation) 782.0
Hemiplegia 342.9
  acute (*see also* Disease, cerebrovascular, acute)
    436
  alternans facialis 344.89
  apoplectic (*see also* Disease, cerebrovascular,
    acute) 436
    late effect or residual
      affecting
        dominant side 438.21
        nondominant side 438.22
        unspecified side 438.20
  arteriosclerotic 437.0
    late effect or residual
      affecting
        dominant side 438.21
        nondominant side 438.22
        unspecified side 438.20
  ascending (spinal) NEC 344.89

Hemiplegia—*continued*
attack (*see also* Disease, cerebrovascular, acute)
436
brain, cerebral (current episode) 437.8
congenital 343.1
cerebral—*see* Hemiplegia, brain
congenital (cerebral) (spastic) (spinal) 343.1
conversion neurosis (hysterical) 300.11
cortical—*see* Hemiplegia, brain
due to
arteriosclerosis 437.0
late effect or residual
affecting
dominant side 438.21
nondominant side 438.22
unspecified side 438.20
cerebrovascular lesion (*see also* Disease,
cerebrovascular, acute) 436
late effect
affecting
dominant side 438.21
nondominant side 438.22
unspecified side 438.20
embolic (current) (*see also* Embolism, brain)
434.1
late effect
affecting
dominant side 438.21
nondominant side 438.22
unspecified side 438.20
flaccid 342.0
hypertensive (current episode) 437.8
infantile (postnatal) 343.4
late effect
birth injury, intracranial or spinal 343.4
cerebrovascular lesion—*see* Late effect(s) (of)
cerebrovascular disease
viral encephalitis 139.0
middle alternating NEC 344.89
newborn NEC 767.0
seizure (current episode) (*see also* Disease,
cerebrovascular, acute) 436
spastic 342.1
congenital or infantile 343.1
specified NEC 342.8
thrombotic (current) (*see also* Thrombosis,
brain) 434.0
late effect—*see* late effect(s) (of)
cerebrovascular disease
Hemisection, spinal cord —*see* Fracture,
vertebra, by site, with spinal cord injury
Hemispasm 781.0
facial 781.0
Hemispatial neglect 781.8
Hemisporosis 117.9
Hemitremor 781.0
Hemivertebra 756.14
Hemobilia 576.8
Hemocholecyst 575.8
Hemochromatosis (acquired) (diabetic)
(hereditary) (liver) (myocardium) (primary
idiopathic) (secondary) 275.0
with refractory anemia 238.72
Hemodialysis V56.0
Hemoglobin —*see also* condition
abnormal (disease)—*see* Disease, hemoglobin
AS genotype 282.5
fetal, hereditary persistence 282.7
high-oxygen-affinity 289.0
low NEC 285.9
S (Hb-S), heterozygous 282.5

Hemoglobinemia 283.2
due to blood transfusion NEC 999.89
bone marrow 996.85
paroxysmal 283.2
Hemoglobinopathy (mixed) (*see also* Disease,
hemoglobin) 282.7
with thalassemia 282.49
sickle-cell 282.60
with thalassemia (without crisis) 282.41
with
crisis 282.42
vaso-occlusive pain 282.42
Hemoglobinuria, hemoglobinuric 791.2
with anemia, hemolytic, acquired (chronic) NEC
283.2
cold (agglutinin) (paroxysmal) (with Raynaud's
syndrome) 283.2
due to
exertion 283.2
hemolysis (from external causes) NEC 283.2
exercise 283.2
fever (malaria) 084.8
infantile 791.2
intermittent 283.2
malarial 084.8
march 283.2
nocturnal (paroxysmal) 283.2
paroxysmal (cold) (nocturnal) 283.2
Hemolymphangioma (M9175/0) 228.1
Hemolysis
fetal—*see* Jaundice, fetus or newborn
intravascular (disseminated) NEC 286.6
with
abortion—*see* Abortion, by type, with
hemorrhage, delayed or excessive
ectopic pregnancy (*see also* categories
633.0-633.9) 639.1
hemorrhage of pregnancy 641.3
affecting fetus or newborn 762.1
molar pregnancy (*see also* categories
630-632) 639.1
acute 283.2
following
abortion 639.1
ectopic or molar pregnancy 639.1
neonatal—*see* Jaundice, fetus or newborn
transfusion NEC 999.89
bone marrow 996.85
Hemolytic —*see also* condition
anemia—*see* Anemia, hemolytic
uremic syndrome 283.11
Hemometra 621.4
Hemopericardium (with effusion) 423.0
newborn 772.8
traumatic (*see also* Hemothorax, traumatic) 860.2
with open wound into thorax 860.3
Hemoperitoneum 568.81
infectional (*see also* Peritonitis) 567.29
traumatic—*see* Injury, internal, peritoneum
Hemophagocytic syndrome 288.4
infection-associated 288.4
Hemophilia (familial) (hereditary) 286.0
A 286.0
carrier (asymptomatic) V83.01
symptomatic V83.02
B (Leyden) 286.1
C 286.2
calcipriva (*see also* Fibrinolysis) 286.7
classical 286.0
nonfamilial 286.7
secondary 286.5
vascular 286.4

Hemophilus influenzae NEC 041.5
  arachnoiditis (basic) (brain) (spinal) 320.0
    late effect—*see* category 326
  bronchopneumonia 482.2
  cerebral ventriculitis 320.0
    late effect—*see* category 326
  cerebrospinal inflammation 320.0
    late effect—*see* category 326
  infection NEC 041.5
  leptomeningitis 320.0
    late effect—*see* category 326
  meningitis (cerebral) (cerebrospinal) (spinal)
    320.0
    late effect—*see* category 326
  meningomyelitis 320.0
    late effect—*see* category 326
  pachymeningitis (adhesive) (fibrous)
    (hemorrhagic) (hypertrophic) (spinal) 320.0
    late effect—*see* category 326
  pneumonia (broncho-) 482.2
Hemophthalmos 360.43
Hemopneumothorax (*see also* Hemothorax)
  511.89
  traumatic 860.4
    with open wound into thorax 860.5
Hemoptysis 786.3
  due to Paragonimus (westermani) 121.2
  newborn 770.3
  tuberculous (*see also* Tuberculosis, pulmonary)
    011.9
Hemorrhage, hemorrhagic (nontraumatic) 459.0
  abdomen 459.0
  accidental (antepartum) 641.2
    affecting fetus or newborn 762.1
  adenoid 474.8
  adrenal (capsule) (gland) (medulla) 255.41
    newborn 772.5
  after labor—*see* Hemorrhage, postpartum
  alveolar
    lung, newborn 770.3
    process 525.8
  alveolus 525.8
  amputation stump (surgical) 998.11
    secondary, delayed 997.69
  anemia (chronic) 280.0
    acute 285.1
  antepartum—*see* Hemorrhage, pregnancy
  anus (sphincter) 569.3
  apoplexy (stroke) 432.9
  arachnoid—*see* Hemorrhage, subarachnoid
  artery NEC 459.0
    brain (*see also* Hemorrhage, brain) 431
    middle meningeal—*see* Hemorrhage,
      subarachnoid
  basilar (ganglion) (*see also* Hemorrhage, brain)
    431
  bladder 596.8
  blood dyscrasia 289.9
  bowel 578.9
    newborn 772.4
  brain (miliary) (nontraumatic) 431
    with
      birth injury 767.0
    arachnoid—*see* Hemorrhage, subarachnoid
    due to
      birth injury 767.0
      rupture of aneurysm (congenital) (*see also*
        Hemorrhage, subarachnoid) 430
        mycotic 431
      syphilis 094.89
    epidural or extradural—*see* Hemorrhage,
      extradural

Hemorrhage, hemorrhagic—*continued*
  brain—*continued*
    fetus or newborn (anoxic) (hypoxic) (due to
      birth trauma) (nontraumatic) 767.0
      intraventricular 772.10
        grade I 772.11
        grade II 772.12
        grade III 772.13
        grade IV 772.14
    iatrogenic 997.02
    postoperative 997.02
    puerperal, postpartum, childbirth 674.0
    stem 431
    subarachnoid, arachnoid or meningeal—*see*
      Hemorrhage, subarachnoid
    subdural—*see* Hemorrhage, subdural
    traumatic NEC 853.0

---

*Note—Use the following fifth-digit
subclassification with categories 851-854:*

*0 unspecified state of consciousness
1 with no loss of consciousness
2 with brief [less than one hour] loss of
consciousness
3 with moderate [1-24 hours] loss of
consciousness
4 with prolonged [more than 24 hours] loss of
consciousness and return to pre-existing
conscious level
5 with prolonged [more than 24 hours] loss of
consciousness, without return to pre-existing
conscious level
Use fifth-digit 5 to designate when a patient is
unconscious and dies before regaining
consciousness, regardless of the duration of the
loss of consciousness
6 with loss of consciousness of unspecified
duration
9 with concussion, unspecified*

---

    with
      cerebral
        contusion—*see* Contusion, brain
        laceration—*see* Laceration, brain
        open intracranial wound 853.1
        skull fracture—*see* Fracture, skull, by site
      extradural or epidural 852.4
        with open intracranial wound 852.5
      subarachnoid 852.0
        with open intracranial wound 852.1
      subdural 852.2
        with open intracranial wound 852.3
  breast 611.79
  bronchial tube—*see* Hemorrhage, lung
  bronchopulmonary—*see* Hemorrhage, lung
  bronchus (cause unknown) (*see also*
    Hemorrhage, lung) 786.3
  bulbar (*see also* Hemorrhage, brain) 431
  bursa 727.89
  capillary 448.9
    primary 287.8
  capsular—*see* Hemorrhage, brain
  cardiovascular 429.89
  cecum 578.9
  cephalic (*see also* Hemorrhage, brain) 431
  cerebellar (*see also* Hemorrhage, brain) 431
  cerebellum (*see also* Hemorrhage, brain) 431
  cerebral (*see also* Hemorrhage, brain) 431
    fetus or newborn (anoxic) (traumatic) 767.0
  cerebromeningeal (*see also* Hemorrhage, brain)
    431

Hemorrhage, hemorrhagic—*continued*
  cerebrospinal (*see also* Hemorrhage, brain) 431
  cerebrovascular accident—*see* Hemorrhage, brain
  cerebrum (*see also* Hemorrhage, brain) 431
  cervix (stump) (uteri) 622.8
  cesarean section wound 674.3
  chamber, anterior (eye) 364.41
  childbirth—*see* Hemorrhage, complicating, delivery
  choroid 363.61
    expulsive 363.62
  ciliary body 364.41
  cochlea 386.8
  colon—*see* Hemorrhage, intestine
  complicating
    delivery 641.9
      affecting fetus or newborn 762.1
      associated with
        afibrinogenemia 641.3
          affecting fetus or newborn 763.89
        coagulation defect 641.3
          affecting fetus or newborn 763.89
        hyperfibrinolysis 641.3
          affecting fetus or newborn 763.89
        hypofibrinogenemia 641.3
          affecting fetus or newborn 763.89
      due to
        low-lying placenta 641.1
          affecting fetus or newborn 762.0
        placenta previa 641.1
          affecting fetus or newborn 762.0
        premature separation of placenta 641.2
          affecting fetus or newborn 762.1
        retained
          placenta 666.0
          secundines 666.2
        trauma 641.8
          affecting fetus or newborn 763.89
        uterine leiomyoma 641.8
          affecting fetus or newborn 763.89
      surgical procedure 998.11
  complication(s)
    of dental implant placement 525.71
  concealed NEC 459.0
  congenital 772.9
  conjunctiva 372.72
    newborn 772.8
  cord, newborn 772.0
    slipped ligature 772.3
    stump 772.3
  corpus luteum (ruptured) 620.1
  cortical (*see also* Hemorrhage, brain) 431
  cranial 432.9
  cutaneous 782.7
    newborn 772.6
  cyst, pancreas 577.2
  cystitis—*see* Cystitis
  delayed
    with
      abortion—*see* Abortion, by type, with hemorrhage, delayed or excessive
      ectopic pregnancy (*see also* categories 633.0-633.9) 639.1
      molar pregnancy (*see also* categories 630-632) 639.1
    following
      abortion 639.1
      ectopic or molar pregnancy 639.1
    postpartum 666.2
  diathesis (familial) 287.9
    newborn 776.0

Hemorrhage, hemorrhagic—*continued*
  disease 287.9
    newborn 776.0
    specified type NEC 287.8
  disorder 287.9
    due to intrinsic circulating anticoagulants 286.5
    specified type NEC 287.8
  due to
    any device, implant, or graft (presence of) classifiable to 996.0-996.5—*see* Complications, due to (presence of) any device, implant, or graft classified to 996.0—996.5 NEC
    intrinsic circulating anticoagulant 286.5
  duodenum, duodenal 537.89
    ulcer—*see* Ulcer, duodenum, with hemorrhage
  dura mater—*see* Hemorrhage, subdural
  endotracheal—*see* Hemorrhage, lung
  epicranial subaponeurotic (massive) 767.11
  epidural—*see* Hemorrhage, extradural
  episiotomy 674.3
  esophagus 530.82
    varix (*see also* Varix, esophagus, bleeding) 456.0
  excessive
    with
      abortion—*see* Abortion, by type, with hemorrhage, delayed or excessive
      ectopic pregnancy (*see also* categories 633.0-633.9) 639.1
      molar pregnancy (*see also* categories 630-632) 639.1
    following
      abortion 639.1
      ectopic or molar pregnancy 639.1
  external 459.0
  extradural (traumatic)—*see also* Hemorrhage, brain, traumatic, extradural
    birth injury 767.0
    fetus or newborn (anoxic) (traumatic) 767.0
    nontraumatic 432.0
  eye 360.43
    chamber (anterior) (aqueous) 364.41
    fundus 362.81
  eyelid 374.81
  fallopian tube 620.8
  fetomaternal 772.0
    affecting management of pregnancy or puerperium 656.0
  fetus, fetal, affecting newborn 772.0
    from
      cut end of co-twin's cord 772.0
      placenta 772.0
      ruptured cord 772.0
      vasa previa 772.0
    into
      co-twin 772.0
      mother's circulation 772.0
        affecting management of pregnancy or puerperium 656.0
  fever (*see also* Fever, hemorrhagic) 065.9
    with renal syndrome 078.6
    arthropod-borne NEC 065.9
    Bangkok 065.4
    Crimean 065.0
    dengue virus 065.4
    epidemic 078.6
    Junin virus 078.7
    Korean 078.6
    Machupo virus 078.7
    mite-borne 065.8
    mosquito-borne 065.4

Hemorrhage, hemorrhagic—*continued*
  fever—*continued*
    Philippine 065.4
    Russian (Yaroslav) 078.6
    Singapore 065.4
    southeast Asia 065.4
    Thailand 065.4
    tick-borne NEC 065.3
  fibrinogenolysis (*see also* Fibrinolysis) 286.6
  fibrinolytic (acquired) (*see also* Fibrinolysis) 286.6
  fontanel 767.19
  from tracheostomy stoma 519.09
  fundus, eye 362.81
  funis
    affecting fetus or newborn 772.0
    complicating delivery 663.8
  gastric (*see also* Hemorrhage, stomach) 578.9
  gastroenteric 578.9
    newborn 772.4
  gastrointestinal (tract) 578.9
    newborn 772.4
  genitourinary (tract) NEC 599.89
  gingiva 523.8
  globe 360.43
  gravidarum—*see* Hemorrhage, pregnancy
  gum 523.8
  heart 429.89
  hypopharyngeal (throat) 784.8
  intermenstrual 626.6
    irregular 626.6
    regular 626.5
  internal (organs) 459.0
    capsule (*see also* Hemorrhage, brain) 431
    ear 386.8
    newborn 772.8
  intestine 578.9
    congenital 772.4
    newborn 772.4
  into
    bladder wall 596.7
    bursa 727.89
    corpus luysii (*see also* Hemorrhage, brain) 431
  intra-abdominal 459.0
    during or following surgery 998.11
  intra-alveolar, newborn (lung) 770.3
  intracerebral (*see also* Hemorrhage, brain) 431
  intracranial NEC 432.9
    puerperal, postpartum, childbirth 674.0
    traumatic—*see* Hemorrhage, brain, traumatic
  intramedullary NEC 336.1
  intraocular 360.43
  intraoperative 998.11
  intrapartum—*see* Hemorrhage, complicating, delivery
  intrapelvic
    female 629.89
    male 459.0
  intraperitoneal 459.0
  intrapontine (*see also* Hemorrhage, brain) 431
  intrauterine 621.4
    complicating delivery—*see* Hemorrhage, complicating, delivery
    in pregnancy or childbirth—*see* Hemorrhage, pregnancy
    postpartum (*see also* Hemorrhage, postpartum) 666.1

Hemorrhage, hemorrhagic—*continued*
  intraventricular (*see also* Hemorrhage, brain) 431
    fetus or newborn (anoxic) (traumatic) 772.10
    grade I 772.11
    grade II 772.12
    grade III 772.13
    grade IV 772.14
  intravesical 596.7
  iris (postinfectional) (postinflammatory) (toxic) 364.41
  joint (nontraumatic) 719.10
    ankle 719.17
    elbow 719.12
    foot 719.17
    forearm 719.13
    hand 719.14
    hip 719.15
    knee 719.16
    lower leg 719.16
    multiple sites 719.19
    pelvic region 719.15
    shoulder (region) 719.11
    specified site NEC 719.18
    thigh 719.15
    upper arm 719.12
    wrist 719.13
  kidney 593.81
  knee (joint) 719.16
  labyrinth 386.8
  leg NEC 459.0
  lenticular striate artery (*see also* Hemorrhage, brain) 431
  ligature, vessel 998.11
  liver 573.8
  lower extremity NEC 459.0
  lung 786.3
    newborn 770.3
    tuberculous (*see also* Tuberculosis, pulmonary) 011.9
  malaria 084.8
  marginal sinus 641.2
  massive subaponeurotic, birth injury 767.11
  maternal, affecting fetus or newborn 762.1
  mediastinum 786.3
  medulla (*see also* Hemorrhage, brain) 431
  membrane (brain) (*see also* Hemorrhage, subarachnoid) 430
    spinal cord—*see* Hemorrhage, spinal cord
  meninges, meningeal (brain) (middle) (*see also* Hemorrhage, subarachnoid) 430
    spinal cord—*see* Hemorrhage, spinal cord
  mesentery 568.81
  metritis 626.8
  midbrain (*see also* Hemorrhage, brain) 431
  mole 631
  mouth 528.9
  mucous membrane NEC 459.0
    newborn 772.8
  muscle 728.89
  nail (subungual) 703.8
  nasal turbinate 784.7
    newborn 772.8
  nasopharynx 478.29
  navel, newborn 772.3
  newborn 772.9
    adrenal 772.5
    alveolar (lung) 770.3
    brain (anoxic) (hypoxic) (due to birth trauma) 767.0
    cerebral (anoxic) (hypoxic) (due to birth trauma) 767.0

Hemorrhage, hemorrhagic—*continued*
  newborn—*continued*
    conjunctiva 772.8
    cutaneous 772.6
    diathesis 776.0
    due to vitamin K deficiency 776.0
    epicranial subaponeurotic (massive) 767.11
    gastrointestinal 772.4
    internal (organs) 772.8
    intestines 772.4
    intra-alveolar (lung) 770.3
    intracranial (from any perinatal cause) 767.0
    intraventricular (from any perinatal cause) 772.10
      grade I 772.11
      grade II 772.12
      grade III 772.13
      grade IV 772.14
    lung 770.3
    pulmonary (massive) 770.3
    spinal cord, traumatic 767.4
    stomach 772.4
    subaponeurotic (massive) 767.11
    subarachnoid (from any perinatal cause) 772.2
    subconjunctival 772.8
    subgaleal 767.11
    umbilicus 772.0
      slipped ligature 772.3
      vasa previa 772.0
  nipple 611.79
  nose 784.7
    newborn 772.8
  obstetrical surgical wound 674.3
  omentum 568.89
    newborn 772.4
  optic nerve (sheath) 377.42
  orbit 376.32
  ovary 620.1
  oviduct 620.8
  pancreas 577.8
  parathyroid (gland) (spontaneous) 252.8
  parturition—*see* Hemorrhage, complicating, delivery
  penis 607.82
  pericardium, pericarditis 423.0
  perineal wound (obstetrical) 674.3
  peritoneum, peritoneal 459.0
  peritonsillar tissue 474.8
    after operation on tonsils 998.11
    due to infection 475
  petechial 782.7
  pituitary (gland) 253.8
  placenta NEC 641.9
    affecting fetus or newborn 762.1
    from surgical or instrumental damage 641.8
      affecting fetus or newborn 762.1
    previa 641.1
      affecting fetus or newborn 762.0
  pleura—*see* Hemorrhage, lung
  polioencephalitis, superior 265.1
  polymyositis—*see* Polymyositis
  pons (*see also* Hemorrhage, brain) 431
  pontine (*see also* Hemorrhage, brain) 431
  popliteal 459.0
  postcoital 626.7
  postextraction (dental) 998.11
  postmenopausal 627.1
  postnasal 784.7
  postoperative 998.11

Hemorrhage, hemorrhagic—*continued*
  postpartum (atonic) (following delivery of placenta) 666.1
    delayed or secondary (after 24 hours) 666.2
    retained placenta 666.0
    third stage 666.0
  pregnancy (concealed) 641.9
    accidental 641.2
      affecting fetus or newborn 762.1
    affecting fetus or newborn 762.1
    before 22 completed weeks gestation 640.9
      affecting fetus or newborn 762.1
    due to
      abruptio placenta 641.2
        affecting fetus or newborn 762.1
      afibrinogenemia or other coagulation defect (conditions classifiable to 286.0-286.9) 641.3
        affecting fetus or newborn 762.1
      coagulation defect 641.3
        affecting fetus or newborn 762.1
      hyperfibrinolysis 641.3
        affecting fetus or newborn 762.1
      hypofibrinogenemia 641.3
        affecting fetus or newborn 762.1
      leiomyoma, uterus 641.8
        affecting fetus or newborn 762.1
      low-lying placenta 641.1
        affecting fetus or newborn 762.1
      marginal sinus (rupture) 641.2
        affecting fetus or newborn 762.1
      placenta previa 641.1
        affecting fetus or newborn 762.0
      premature separation of placenta (normally implanted) 641.2
        affecting fetus or newborn 762.1
      threatened abortion 640.0
        affecting fetus or newborn 762.1
      trauma 641.8
        affecting fetus or newborn 762.1
    early (before 22 completed weeks gestation) 640.9
      affecting fetus or newborn 762.1
    previous, affecting management of pregnancy or childbirth V23.49
    unavoidable—*see* Hemorrhage, pregnancy, due to placenta previa
  prepartum (mother)—*see* Hemorrhage, pregnancy
  preretinal, cause unspecified 362.81
  prostate 602.1
  puerperal (*see also* Hemorrhage, postpartum) 666.1
  pulmonary—*see also* Hemorrhage, lung
    newborn (massive) 770.3
    renal syndrome 446.21
  purpura (primary) (*see also* Purpura, thrombocytopenic) 287.39
  rectum (sphincter) 569.3
  recurring, following initial hemorrhage at time of injury 958.2
  renal 593.81
    pulmonary syndrome 446.21
  respiratory tract (*see also* Hemorrhage, lung) 786.3
  retina, retinal (deep) (superficial) (vessels) 362.81
    diabetic 250.5 *[362.01]*
      due to secondary diabetes 249.5 *[362.01]*
    due to birth injury 772.8
  retrobulbar 376.89

Hemosalpinx 620.8
Hemosiderosis 275.0
  dietary 275.0
  pulmonary (idiopathic) 275.0 *[516.1]*
  transfusion NEC 999.89
    bone marrow 996.85
Hemospermia 608.82
Hemothorax 511.89
  bacterial, nontuberculous 511.1
  newborn 772.8
  nontuberculous 511.89
    bacterial 511.1
  pneumococcal 511.1
  postoperative 998.11
  staphylococcal 511.1
  streptococcal 511.1
  traumatic 860.2
    with
      open wound into thorax 860.3
      pneumothorax 860.4
        with open wound into thorax 860.5
  tuberculous (*see also* Tuberculosis, pleura) 012.0
Hemotympanum 385.89
Hench-Rosenberg syndrome (palindromic
  arthritis) (*see also* Rheumatism, palindromic)
  719.3
Henle's warts 371.41
Henoch (-Schönlein)
  disease or syndrome (allergic purpura) 287.0
  purpura (allergic) 287.0
Henpue, henpuye 102.6
Heparitinuria 277.5
Hepar lobatum 095.3
Heparin-induced thrombocytopenia (HIT)
  289.84
Hepatalgia 573.8
Hepatic *—see also* condition
  flexure syndrome 569.89
Hepatitis 573.3
  acute (*see also* Necrosis, liver) 570
    alcoholic 571.1
    infective 070.1
      with hepatic coma 070.0
  alcoholic 571.1
  amebic—*see* Abscess, liver, amebic
  anicteric (acute)—*see* Hepatitis, viral
  antigen-associated (HAA) *see* Hepatitis, viral,
    type B
  Australian antigen (positive) *see* Hepatitis, viral,
    type B
  autoimmune 571.42
  catarrhal (acute) 070.1
    with hepatic coma 070.0
    chronic 571.40
    newborn 070.1
      with hepatic coma 070.0
  chemical 573.3
  cholangiolitic 573.8
  cholestatic 573.8
  chronic 571.40
    active 571.49
      viral—*see* Hepatitis, viral
    aggressive 571.49
    persistent 571.41
    viral—*see* Hepatitis, viral
  cytomegalic inclusion virus 078.5 *[573.1]*
  diffuse 573.3
  "dirty needle"—*see* Hepatitis, viral
    with hepatic coma 070.2
  drug-induced 573.3

Hepatitis—*continued*
  due to
    Coxsackie 074.8 *[573.1]*
    cytomegalic inclusion virus 078.5 *[573.1]*
    infectious mononucleosis 075 *[573.1]*
    malaria 084.9 *[573.2]*
    mumps 072.71
    secondary syphilis 091.62
    toxoplasmosis (acquired) 130.5
      congenital (active) 771.2
  epidemic—*see* Hepatitis, viral, type A
  fetus or newborn 774.4
  fibrous (chronic) 571.49
    acute 570
  from injection, inoculation, or transfusion
    (blood) (other substance) (plasma) (serum)
    (onset within 8 months after administration)
    see Hepatitis, viral
  fulminant (viral) (*see also* Hepatitis, viral) 070.9
    with hepatic coma 070.6
    type A 070.1
      with hepatic coma 070.0
    type B—*see* Hepatitis, viral, Type B
  giant cell (neonatal) 774.4
  hemorrhagic 573.8
  history of
    B V12.09
    C V12.09
  homologous serum—*see* Hepatitis, viral
  hypertrophic (chronic) 571.49
    acute 570
  nfectious, infective (acute) (chronic) (subacute)
    070.1
    with hepatic coma 070.0
  inoculation—*see* Hepatitis, viral
  interstitial (chronic) 571.49
    acute 570
  lupoid 571.49
  malarial 084.9 *[573.2]*
  malignant (*see also* Necrosis, liver) 570
  neonatal (toxic) 774.4
  newborn 774.4
  parenchymatous (acute) (*see also* Necrosis,
    liver) 570
  peliosis 573.3
  persistent, chronic 571.41
  plasma cell 571.49
  postimmunization—*see* Hepatitis, viral
  postnecrotic 571.49
  posttransfusion—*see* Hepatitis, viral
  recurrent 571.49
  septic 573.3
  serum—*see* Hepatitis, viral
    carrier (suspected) of V02.61
  subacute (*see also* Necrosis, liver) 570
  suppurative (diffuse) 572.0
  syphilitic (late) 095.3
    congenital (early) 090.0 *[573.2]*
      late 090.5 *[573.2]*
    secondary 091.62
  toxic (noninfectious) 573.3
    fetus or newborn 774.4
  tuberculous (*see also* Tuberculosis) 017.9

Hepatitis—*continued*
  viral (acute) (anicteric) (cholangiolitic)
    (cholestatic) (chronic) (subacute) 070.9
    with hepatic coma 070.6
    AU-SH type virus—*see* Hepatitis, viral, type
      B
    Australian antigen—*see* Hepatitis, viral, type
      B
    B-antigen—*see* Hepatitis, viral, type B
    Coxsackie 074.8 *[573.1]*
    cytomegalic inclusion 078.5 *[573.1]*
    IH (virus)—*see* Hepatitis, viral, type A
    infectious hepatitis virus—*see* Hepatitis, viral,
      type A
    serum hepatitis virus—*see* Hepatitis, viral,
      type B
    SH—*see* Hepatitis, viral, type B
    specified type NEC 070.59
      with hepatic coma 070.49
    type A 070.1
      with hepatic coma 070.0
    type B (acute) 070.30
      with
        hepatic coma 070.20
          with hepatitis delta 070.21
        hepatitis delta 070.31
          with hepatic coma 070.21
      carrier status V02.61
      chronic 070.32
        with
          hepatic coma 070.22
            with hepatitis delta 070.23
          hepatitis delta 070.33
            with hepatic coma 070.23
    type C
      with hepatic coma 070.41
      acute 070.51
        with hepatic coma 070.41
      carrier status V02.62
      chronic 070.54
        with hepatic coma 070.44
      in remission 070.54
      unspecified 070.70
        with hepatic coma 070.71
    type delta (with hepatitis B carrier state)
      070.52
      with
        active hepatitis B disease—*see* Hepatitis,
          viral, type B
        hepatic coma 070.42
    type E 070.53
      with hepatic coma 070.43
    vaccination and inoculation (prophylactic)
      V05.3
  Waldenström's (lupoid hepatitis) 571.49
Hepatization, lung (acute)—*see also* Pneumonia,
  lobar
  chronic (*see also* Fibrosis, lung) 515
Hepatoblastoma (M8970/3) 155.0
Hepatocarcinoma (M8170/3) 155.0
Hepatocholangiocarcinoma (M8180/3) 155.0
Hepatocholangioma, benign (M8180/0) 211.5
Hepatocholangitis 573.8
Hepatocystitis (*see also* Cholecystitis) 575.10
Hepatodystrophy 570
Hepatolenticular degeneration 275.1
Hepatolithiasis —*see* Choledocholithiasis
Hepatoma (malignant) (M8170/3) 155.0
  benign (M8170/0) 211.5
  congenital (M8970/3) 155.0
  embryonal (M8970/3) 155.0
Hepatomegalia glycogenica diffusa 271.0

Hepatomegaly (*see also* Hypertrophy, liver)
  789.1
  congenital 751.69
    syphilitic 090.0
  due to Clonorchis sinensis 121.1
  Gaucher's 272.7
  syphilitic (congenital) 090.0
Hepatoptosis 573.8
Hepatorrhexis 573.8
Hepatosis, toxic 573.8
Hepatosplenomegaly 571.8
  due to S. japonicum 120.2
  hyperlipemic (Burger-Grutz type) 272.3
Herald patch 696.3
Hereditary —*see* condition
Heredodegeneration 330.9
  macular 362.70
Heredopathia atactica polyneuritiformis 356.3
Heredosyphilis (*see also* Syphilis, congenital)
  090.9
Hermaphroditism (true) 752.7
  with specified chromosomal anomaly—*see*
    Anomaly, chromosomes, sex
Hernia, hernial (acquired) (recurrent) 553.9
  with
    gangrene (obstructed) NEC 551.9
    obstruction NEC 552.9
      and gangrene 551.9
  abdomen (wall)—*see* Hernia, ventral
  abdominal, specified site NEC 553.8
    with
      gangrene (obstructed) 551.8
      obstruction 552.8
        and gangrene 551.8
  appendix 553.8
    with
      gangrene (obstructed) 551.8
      obstruction 552.8
        and gangrene 551.8
  bilateral (inguinal)—*see* Hernia, inguinal
  bladder (sphincter)
    congenital (female) (male) 756.71
    female (*see also* Cystocele, female) 618.01
    male 596.8
  brain 348.4
    congenital 742.0
  broad ligament 553.8
  cartilage, vertebral—*see* Displacement,
    intervertebral disc
  cerebral 348.4
    congenital 742.0
    endaural 742.0
  ciliary body 364.89
    traumatic 871.1
  colic 553.9
    with
      gangrene (obstructed) 551.9
      obstruction 552.9
        and gangrene 551.9
  colon 553.9
    with
      gangrene (obstructed) 551.9
      obstruction 552.9
        and gangrene 551.9
  colostomy (stoma) 569.69
  Cooper's (retroperitoneal) 553.8
    with
      gangrene (obstructed) 551.8
      obstruction 552.8
        and gangrene 551.8
  crural—*see* Hernia, femoral

Hernia, hernial—*continued*
  diaphragm, diaphragmatic 553.3
    with
      gangrene (obstructed) 551.3
      obstruction 552.3
        and gangrene 551.3
    congenital 756.6
    due to gross defect of diaphragm 756.6
    traumatic 862.0
      with open wound into cavity 862.1
  direct (inguinal)—*see* Hernia, inguinal
  disc, intervertebral—*see* Displacement,
    intervertebral disc
  diverticulum, intestine 553.9
    with
      gangrene (obstructed) 551.9
      obstruction 552.9
        and gangrene 551.9
  double (inguinal)—*see* Hernia, inguinal
  due to adhesion with obstruction 560.81
  duodenojejunal 553.8
    with
      gangrene (obstructed) 551.8
      obstruction 552.8
        and gangrene 551.8
  en glissade—*see* Hernia, inguinal
  enterostomy (stoma) 569.69
  epigastric 553.29
    with
      gangrene (obstruction) 551.29
      obstruction 552.29
        and gangrene 551.29
    recurrent 553.21
      with
        gangrene (obstructed) 551.21
        obstruction 552.21
          and gangrene 551.21
  esophageal hiatus (sliding) 553.3
    with
      gangrene (obstructed) 551.3
      obstruction 552.3
        and gangrene 551.3
    congenital 750.6
  external (inguinal)—*see* Hernia, inguinal
  fallopian tube 620.4
  fascia 728.89
  fat 729.30
    eyelid 374.34
    orbital 374.34
    pad 729.30
      eye, eyelid 374.34
      knee 729.31
      orbit 374.34
      popliteal (space) 729.31
      specified site NEC 729.39
  femoral (unilateral) 553.00
    with
      gangrene (obstructed) 551.00
      obstruction 552.00
        with gangrene 551.00
    bilateral 553.02
      gangrenous (obstructed) 551.02
      obstructed 552.02
        with gangrene 551.02
      recurrent 553.03
        gangrenous (obstructed) 551.03
        obstructed 552.03
          with gangrene 551.03

Hernia, hernial—*continued*
  recurrent (unilateral) 553.01
    bilateral 553.03
      gangrenous (obstructed) 551.03
      obstructed 552.03
        with gangrene 551.03
    gangrenous (obstructed) 551.01
    obstructed 552.01
      with gangrene 551.01
  foramen
    Bochdalek 553.3
      with
        gangrene (obstructed) 551.3
        obstruction 552.3
          and gangrene 551.3
      congenital 756.6
    magnum 348.4
    Morgagni, morgagnian 553.3
      with
        gangrene 551.3
        obstruction 552.3
          and gangrene 551.3
      congenital 756.6
  funicular (umbilical) 553.1
    with
      gangrene (obstructed) 551.1
      obstruction 552.1
        and gangrene 551.1
    spermatic cord—*see* Hernia, inguinal
  gangrenous—*see* Hernia, by site, with gangrene
  gastrointestinal tract 553.9
    with
      gangrene (obstructed) 551.9
      obstruction 552.9
        and gangrene 551.9
  gluteal—*see* Hernia, femoral
  Gruber's (internal mesogastric) 553.8
    with
      gangrene (obstructed) 551.8
      obstruction 552.8
        and gangrene 551.8
  Hesselbach's 553.8
    with
      gangrene (obstructed) 551.8
      obstruction 552.8
        and gangrene 551.8
  hiatal (esophageal) (sliding) 553.3
    with
      gangrene (obstructed) 551.3
      obstruction 552.3
        and gangrene 551.3
    congenital 750.6
  incarcerated (*see also* Hernia, by site, with
    obstruction) 552.9
    gangrenous (*see also* Hernia, by site, with
    gangrene) 551.9
  incisional 553.21
    with
      gangrene (obstructed) 551.21
      obstruction 552.21
        and gangrene 551.21
    lumbar—*see* Hernia, lumbar
    recurrent 553.21
      with
        gangrene (obstructed) 551.21
        obstruction 552.21
          and gangrene 551.21
  indirect (inguinal)—*see* Hernia, inguinal
  infantile—*see* Hernia, inguinal

Hernia, hernial—*continued*
  infrapatellar fat pad 729.31
  inguinal (direct) (double) (encysted) (external)
    (funicular) (indirect) (infantile) (internal)
    (interstitial) (oblique) (scrotal) (sliding)
    550.9

Note—Use the following fifth-digit
subclassification with category 550:

0 unilateral or unspecified (not specified as
    recurrent)
1 unilateral or unspecified, recurrent
2 bilateral (not specified as recurrent)
3 bilateral, recurrent

---

    with
      gangrene (obstructed) 550.0
      obstruction 550.1
        and gangrene 550.0
  internal 553.8
    with
      gangrene (obstructed) 551.8
      obstruction 552.8
        and gangrene 551.8
    inguinal—*see* Hernia, inguinal
  interstitial 553.9
    with
      gangrene (obstructed) 551.9
      obstruction 552.9
        and gangrene 551.9
    inguinal—*see* Hernia, inguinal
  intervertebral cartilage or disc—*see*
    Displacement, intervertebral disc
  intestine, intestinal 553.9
    with
      gangrene (obstructed) 551.9
      obstruction 552.9
        and gangrene 551.9
  intra-abdominal 553.9
    with
      gangrene (obstructed) 551.9
      obstruction 552.9
        and gangrene 551.9
  intraparietal 553.9
    with
      gangrene (obstructed) 551.9
      obstruction 552.9
        and gangrene 551.9
  iris 364.89
    traumatic 871.1
  irreducible (*see also* Hernia, by site, with
    obstruction) 552.9
    gangrenous (with obstruction) (*see also*
      Hernia, by site, with gangrene) 551.9
  ischiatic 553.8
    with
      gangrene (obstructed) 551.8
      obstruction 552.8
        and gangrene 551.8
  ischiorectal 553.8
    with
      gangrene (obstructed) 551.8
      obstruction 552.8
        and gangrene 551.8
  lens 379.32
    traumatic 871.1
  linea
    alba—*see* Hernia, epigastric
    semilunaris—*see* Hernia, spigelian

Hernia, hernial—*continued*
  Littre's (diverticular) 553.9
    with
      gangrene (obstructed) 551.9
      obstruction 552.9
        and gangrene 551.9
  lumbar 553.8
    with
      gangrene (obstructed) 551.8
      obstruction 552.8
        and gangrene 551.8
    intervertebral disc 722.10
  lung (subcutaneous) 518.89
    congenital 748.69
  mediastinum 519.3
  mesenteric (internal) 553.8
    with
      gangrene (obstructed) 551.8
      obstruction 552.8
        and gangrene 551.8
  mesocolon 553.8
    with
      gangrene (obstructed) 551.8
      obstruction 552.8
        and gangrene 551.8
  muscle (sheath) 728.89
  nucleus pulposus—*see* Displacement,
    intervertebral disc
  oblique (inguinal)—*see* Hernia, inguinal
  obstructive (*see also* Hernia, by site, with
    obstruction) 552.9
    gangrenous (with obstruction) (*see also*
      Hernia, by site, with gangrene) 551.9
  obturator 553.8
    with
      gangrene (obstructed) 551.8
      obstruction 552.8
        and gangrene 551.8
  omental 553.8
    with
      gangrene (obstructed) 551.8
      obstruction 552.8
        and gangrene 551.8
  orbital fat (pad) 374.34
  ovary 620.4
  oviduct 620.4
  paracolostomy (stoma) 569.69
  paraduodenal 553.8
    with
      gangrene (obstructed) 551.8
      obstruction 552.8
        and gangrene 551.8
  paraesophageal 553.3
    with
      gangrene (obstructed) 551.3
      obstruction 552.3
        and gangrene 551.3
    congenital 750.6
  parahiatal 553.3
    with
      gangrene (obstructed) 551.3
      obstruction 552.3
        and gangrene 551.3
  paraumbilical 553.1
    with
      gangrene (obstructed) 551.1
      obstruction 552.1
        and gangrene 551.1

Hernia, hernial—*continued*
parietal 553.9
  with
    gangrene (obstructed) 551.9
    obstruction 552.9
    and gangrene 551.9
perineal 553.8
  with
    gangrene (obstructed) 551.8
    obstruction 552.8
    and gangrene 551.8
peritoneal sac, lesser 553.8
  with
    gangrene (obstructed) 551.8
    obstruction 552.8
    and gangrene 551.8
popliteal fat pad 729.31
postoperative 553.21
  with
    gangrene (obstructed) 551.21
    obstruction 552.21
    and gangrene 551.21
pregnant uterus 654.4
prevesical 596.8
properitoneal 553.8
  with
    gangrene (obstructed) 551.8
    obstruction 552.8
    and gangrene 551.8
pudendal 553.8
  with
    gangrene (obstructed) 551.8
    obstruction 552.8
    and gangrene 551.8
rectovaginal 618.6
retroperitoneal 553.8
  with
    gangrene (obstructed) 551.8
    obstruction 552.8
    and gangrene 551.8
Richter's (parietal) 553.9
  with
    gangrene (obstructed) 551.9
    obstruction 552.9
    and gangrene 551.9
Rieux's, Riex's (retrocecal) 553.8
  with
    gangrene (obstructed) 551.8
    obstruction 552.8
    and gangrene 551.8
sciatic 553.8
  with
    gangrene (obstructed) 551.8
    obstruction 552.8
    and gangrene 551.8
scrotum, scrotal—*see* Hernia, inguinal
sliding (inguinal)—*see also* Hernia, inguinal
hiatus—*see* Hernia, hiatal
spigelian 553.29
  with
    gangrene (obstructed) 551.29
    obstruction 552.29
    and gangrene 551.29
spinal (*see also* Spina bifida) 741.9
  with hydrocephalus 741.0
strangulated (*see also* Hernia, by site, with
  obstruction) 552.9
  gangrenous (with obstruction) (*see also*
    Hernia, by site, with gangrene) 551.9
supraumbilicus (linea alba)—*see* Hernia,
  epigastric

Hernia, hernial—*continued*
tendon 727.9
testis (nontraumatic) 550.9
  meaning
    scrotal hernia 550.9
    symptomatic late syphilis 095.8
Treitz's (fossa) 553.8
  with
    gangrene (obstructed) 551.8
    obstruction 552.8
    and gangrene 551.8
tunica
  albuginea 608.89
  vaginalis 752.89
umbilicus, umbilical 553.1
  with
    gangrene (obstructed) 551.1
    obstruction 552.1
    and gangrene 551.1
ureter 593.89
  with obstruction 593.4
uterus 621.8
  pregnant 654.4
vaginal (posterior) 618.6
Velpeau's (femoral) (*see also* Hernia, femoral)
  553.00
ventral 553.20
  with
    gangrene (obstructed) 551.20
    obstruction 552.20
    and gangrene 551.20
  recurrent 553.21
    with
      gangrene (obstructed) 551.21
      obstruction 552.21
      and gangrene 551.21
vesical
  congenital (female) (male) 756.71
  female (*see also* Cystocele, female) 618.01
  male 596.8
vitreous (into anterior chamber) 379.21
  traumatic 871.1
Herniation —*see also* Hernia
brain (stem) 348.4
cerebral 348.4
gastric mucosa (into duodenal bulb) 537.89
mediastinum 519.3
nucleus pulposus—*see* Displacement,
  intervertebral disc
Herpangina 074.0
Herpes, herpetic 054.9
auricularis (zoster) 053.71
  simplex 054.73
blepharitis (zoster) 053.20
  simplex 054.41
circinate 110.5
circinatus 110.5
  bullous 694.5
conjunctiva (simplex) 054.43
  zoster 053.21
cornea (simplex) 054.43
  disciform (simplex) 054.43
  zoster 053.21
encephalitis 054.3
eye (zoster) 053.29
  simplex 054.40
eyelid (zoster) 053.20
  simplex 054.41
febrilis 054.9
fever 054.9
geniculate ganglionitis 053.11

Herpes, herpetic—*continued*
  genital, genitalis 054.10
    specified site NEC 054.19
  gestationis 646.8
  gingivostomatitis 054.2
  iridocyclitis (simplex) 054.44
    zoster 053.22
  iris (any site) 695.10
  iritis (simplex) 054.44
  keratitis (simplex) 054.43
    dendritic 054.42
    disciform 054.43
    interstitial 054.43
      zoster 053.21
  keratoconjunctivitis (simplex) 054.43
    zoster 053.21
  labialis 054.9
    meningococcal 036.89
  lip 054.9
  meningitis (simplex) 054.72
    zoster 053.0
  ophthalmicus (zoster) 053.20
    simplex 054.40
  otitis externa (zoster) 053.71
    simplex 054.73
  penis 054.13
  perianal 054.10
  pharyngitis 054.79
  progenitalis 054.10
  scrotum 054.19
  septicemia 054.5
  simplex 054.9
    complicated 054.8
      ophthalmic 054.40
        specified NEC 054.49
      specified NEC 054.79
    congenital 771.2
    external ear 054.73
    keratitis 054.43
      dendritic 054.42
    meningitis 054.72
    myelitis 054.74
    neuritis 054.79
    specified complication NEC 054.79
      ophthalmic 054.49
    visceral 054.71
  stomatitis 054.2
  tonsurans 110.0
    maculosus (of Hebra) 696.3
  visceral 054.71
  vulva 054.12
  vulvovaginitis 054.11
  whitlow 054.6
  zoster 053.9
    auricularis 053.71
    complicated 053.8
      specified NEC 053.79
    conjunctiva 053.21
    cornea 053.21
    ear 053.71
    eye 053.29
    geniculate 053.11
    keratitis 053.21
      interstitial 053.21
    myelitis 053.14
    neuritis 053.10
    ophthalmicus(a) 053.20
    oticus 053.71
    otitis externa 053.71
    specified complication NEC 053.79
    specified site NEC 053.9
  zosteriform, intermediate type 053.9

Herrick's
  anemia (hemoglobin S disease) 282.61
  syndrome (hemoglobin S disease) 282.61
Hers' disease (glycogenosis VI) 271.0
Herter's infantilism (nontropical sprue) 579.0
Herter (-Gee) disease or syndrome (nontropical
    sprue) 579.0
Herxheimer's disease (diffuse idiopathic
    cutaneous atrophy) 701.8
Herxheimer's reaction 995.0
Hesitancy, urinary 788.64
Hesselbach's hernia —*see* Hernia, Hesselbach's
Heterochromia (congenital) 743.46
  acquired 364.53
  cataract 366.33
  cyclitis 364.21
  hair 704.3
  iritis 364.21
  retained metallic foreign body 360.62
    magnetic 360.52
  uveitis 364.21
Heterophoria 378.40
  alternating 378.45
  vertical 378.43
Heterophyes, small intestine 121.6
Heterophyiasis 121.6
Heteropsia 368.8
Heterotopia, heterotopic —*see also*
    Malposition, congenital
  cerebralis 742.4
  pancreas, pancreatic 751.7
  spinalis 742.59
Heterotropia 378.30
  intermittent 378.20
    vertical 378.31
  vertical (constant) (intermittent) 378.31
Heubner's disease 094.89
Heubner-Herter disease or syndrome
    (nontropical sprue) 579.0
Hexadactylism 755.00
Heyd's syndrome (hepatorenal) 572.4
HGSIL (high grade squamous intrepithelial
    lesion) (cytologic finding) (Pap smear finding)
  anus 796.74
  cervix 795.04
    biopsy finding —code to CIN II or CIN III
  vagina 795.14
Hibernoma (M8880/0)—*see* Lipoma
Hiccough 786.8
  epidemic 078.89
  psychogenic 306.1
Hiccup (*see also* Hiccough) 786.8
Hicks (-Braxton) contractures 644.1
Hidden penis 752.65
Hidradenitis (axillaris) (suppurative) 705.83
Hidradenoma (nodular) (M8400/0)—*see also*
    Neoplasm, skin, benign
  clear cell (M8402/0)—*see* Neoplasm, skin,
    benign
  papillary (M8405/0)—*see* Neoplasm, skin,
    benign
Hidrocystoma (M8404/0)—*see* Neoplasm, skin,
    benign
HIE (hypoxic-ischemic encephalopathy) 768.70
  mild 768.71
  moderate 768.72
  severe 768.73

High
  A₂ anemia 282.49
  altitude effects 993.2
    anoxia 993.2
    on
      ears 993.0
      sinuses 993.1
    polycythemia 289.0
  arch
    foot 755.67
    palate 750.26
  artery (arterial) tension (*see also* Hypertension)
      401.9
    without diagnosis of hypertension 796.2
  basal metabolic rate (BMR) 794.7
  blood pressure (*see also* Hypertension) 401.9
    incidental reading (isolated) (nonspecific), no
      diagnosis of hypertension 796.2
  cholesterol 272.0
    with high triglycerides 272.2
  compliance bladder 596.4
  diaphragm (congenital) 756.6
  frequency deafness (congenital) (regional) 389.8
  head at term 652.5
  output failure (cardiac) (*see also* Failure, heart)
      428.9
  oxygen-affinity hemoglobin 289.0
  palate 750.26
  risk
    behavior —*see* Problem
    family situation V61.9
      specified circumstance NEC V61.8
    human papillomavirus (HPV) DNA test
      positive
      anal 796.75
      cervical 795.05
      vaginal 795.15
    individual NEC V62.89
    infant NEC V20.1
    patient taking drugs (prescribed) V67.51
      nonprescribed (*see also* Abuse, drugs,
        nondependent) 305.9
    pregnancy V23.9
      inadequate prenatal care V23.7
      specified problem NEC V23.8
    temperature (of unknown origin) (*see also*
        Pyrexia) 780.60
    thoracic rib 756.3
    triglycerides 272.1
      with high cholesterol 272.2
Hildenbrand's disease (typhus) 081.9
Hilger's syndrome 337.09
Hill diarrhea 579.1
Hilliard's lupus (*see also* Tuberculosis) 017.0
Hilum —*see* condition
Hip —*see* condition
Hippel's disease (retinocerebral angiomatosis) 759.6
Hippus 379.49
Hirschfeld's disease (acute diabetes mellitus) (*see
  also* Diabetes) 250.0
  due to secondary diabetes 249.0
Hirschsprung's disease or megacolon
  (congenital) 751.3
Hirsuties (*see also* Hypertrichosis) 704.1
Hirsutism (*see also* Hypertrichosis) 704.1
Hirudiniasis (external) (internal) 134.2
His-Werner disease (trench fever) 083.1
Hiss-Russell dysentery 004.1
Histamine cephalgia 339.00
Histidinemia 270.5
Histidinuria 270.5

Histiocytic syndromes 288.4
Histiocytoma (M8832/0)—*see also* Neoplasm,
    skin, benign
  fibrous (M8830/0)—*see also* Neoplasm, skin,
    benign
    atypical (M8830/1)—*see* Neoplasm,
      connective tissue, uncertain behavior
    malignant (M8830/0)—*see* Neoplasm,
      connective tissue, malignant
Histiocytosis (acute) (chronic) (subacute) 277.89
  acute differentiated progressive (M9722/3) 202.5
  cholesterol 277.89
  essential 277.89
  lipid, lipoid (essential) 272.7
  lipochrome (familial) 288.1
  malignant (M9720/3) 202.3
  non-Langerhans cell 277.89
  polyostotic sclerosing 277.89
  X (chronic) 277.89
    acute (progressive) (M9722/3) 202.5
Histoplasmosis 115.90
  with
    endocarditis 115.94
    meningitis 115.91
    pericarditis 115.93
    pneumonia 115.95
    retinitis 115.92
    specified manifestation NEC 115.99
  African (due to Histoplasma duboisii) 115.10
    with
      endocarditis 115.14
      meningitis 115.11
      pericarditis 115.13
      pneumonia 115.15
      retinitis 115.12
      specified manifestation NEC 115.19
  American (due to Histoplasma capsulatum) 115.00
    with
      endocarditis 115.04
      meningitis 115.01
      pericarditis 115.03
      pneumonia 115.05
      retinitis 115.02
      specified manifestation NEC 115.09
  Darling's—*see* Histoplasmosis, American
  large form (*see also* Histoplasmosis, African) 115.10
  lung 115.05
  small form (*see also* Histoplasmosis, American)
    115.00
History (personal) of
  abuse
    emotional V15.42
    neglect V15.42
    physical V15.41
    sexual V15.41
  affective psychosis V11.1
  alcoholism V11.3
    specified as drinking problem (*see also* Abuse,
      drugs, nondependent) 305.0
  allergy to
    analgesic agent NEC V14.6
    anesthetic NEC V14.4
    antibiotic agent NEC V14.1
      penicillin V14.0
    anti-infective agent NEC V14.3
    arachnid bite V15.06
    diathesis V15.09
    drug V14.9
      specified type NEC V14.8
    eggs V15.03
    food additives V15.05

History—*continued*
  allergy to—*continued*
    insect bite V15.06
    latex V15.07
    medicinal agents V14.9
      specified type NEC V14.8
    milk products V15.02
    narcotic agent NEC V14.5
    nuts V15.05
      peanuts V15.01
    penicillin V14.0
    radiographic dye V15.08
    seafood V15.04
    serum V14.7
    specified food NEC V15.05
    specified nonmedicinal agents NEC V15.09
    spider bite V15.06
    sulfa V14.2
    sulfonamides V14.2
    therapeutic agent NEC V15.09
    vaccine V14.7
  anemia V12.3
  arrest, sudden cardiac V12.53
  arthritis V13.4
  attack, transient ischemic (TIA) V12.54
  benign neoplasm of brain V12.41
  blood disease V12.3
  calculi, urinary V13.01
  cardiovascular disease V12.50
    myocardial infarction 412
  chemotherapy, antineoplastic V87.41
  child abuse V15.41
  cigarette smoking V15.82
  circulatory system disease V12.50
    myocardial infarction 412
  congenital malformation V13.69
  contraception V15.7
  death, sudden, successfully resuscitated V12.53
  deficit
    prolonged reversible ischemic neurologic
      (PRIND) V12.54
    reversible ischemic neurologic (RIND) V12.54
  diathesis, allergic V15.09
  digestive system disease V12.70
    peptic ulcer V12.71
    polyps, colonic V12.72
    specified NEC V12.79
  disease (of) V13.9
    blood V12.3
    blood-forming organs V12.3
    cardiovascular system V12.50
    circulatory system V12.50
      specified NEC V12.59
    digestive system V12.70
      peptic ulcer V12.71
      polyps, colonic V12.72
      specified NEC V12.79
    infectious V12.00
      malaria V12.03
      methicillin resistant Staphylococcus aureus
        (MRSA) V12.04
      MRSA (methicillin resistant Staphylococcus
        aureus) V12.04
      poliomyelitis V12.02
      specified NEC V12.09
      tuberculosis V12.01
    parasitic V12.00
      specified NEC V12.09
    respiratory system V12.60
      pneumonia V12.61
      specified NEC V12.69

History—*continued*
  disease—*continued*
    skin V13.3
    specified site NEC V13.8
    subcutaneous tissue V13.3
    trophoblastic V13.1
      affecting management of pregnancy V23.1
  disorder (of) V13.9
    endocrine V12.2
    genital system V13.29
    hematological V12.3
    immunity V12.2
    mental V11.9
      affective type V11.1
      manic-depressive V11.1
      neurosis V11.2
      schizophrenia V11.0
      specified type NEC V11.8
    metabolic V12.2
    musculoskeletal NEC V13.59
    nervous system V12.40
      specified type NEC V12.49
    obstetric V13.29
      affecting management of current pregnancy
        V23.49
      pre-term labor V13.21
    sense organs V12.40
      specified type NEC V12.49
    specified site NEC V13.8
    urinary system V13.00
      calculi V13.01
      infection V13.02
      nephrotic syndrome V13.03
      specified NEC V13.09
  drug use
    nonprescribed (*see also* Abuse, drugs,
      nondependent) 305.9
    patent (*see also* Abuse, drugs, nondependent)
      305.9
  dysplasia
    cervical (conditions classifiable to 622.10-
      622.12) V13.22
  effect NEC of external cause V15.89
  embolism (pulmonary) V12.51
  emotional abuse V15.42
  encephalitis V12.42
  endocrine disorder V12.2
  estrogen therapy V87.43
  extracorporeal membrane oxygenation (ECMO)
    V15.87
  failed
    conscious sedation V15.80
    moderate sedation V15.80
  falling V15.88
  family
    allergy V19.6
    anemia V18.2
    arteriosclerosis V17.49
    arthritis V17.7
    asthma V17.5
    blindness V19.0
    blood disorder NEC V18.3
    cardiovascular disease V17.49
    carrier, genetic disease V18.9
    cerebrovascular disease V17.1
    chronic respiratory condition NEC V17.6
    colonic polyps V18.51
    congenital anomalies V19.5
    consanguinity V19.7
    coronary artery disease V17.3
    cystic fibrosis V18.19

History—*continued*
  family—*continued*
    deafness V19.2
    diabetes mellitus V18.0
    digestive disorders V18.59
    disease or disorder (of)
      allergic V19.6
      blood NEC V18.3
      cardiovascular NEC V17.49
      cerebrovascular V17.1
      colonic polyps V18.51
      coronary artery V17.3
      death, sudden cardiac (SCD) V17.41
      digestive V18.59
      ear NEC V19.3
      endocrine V18.19
        multiple neoplasia [MEN] syndrome
          V18.11
      eye NEC V19.1
      genitourinary NEC V18.7
      hypertensive V17.49
      infectious V18.8
      ischemic heart V17.3
      kidney V18.69
        polycystic V18.61
      mental V17.0
      metabolic V18.19
      musculoskeletal NEC V17.89
        osteoporosis V17.81
      neurological NEC V17.2
      parasitic V18.8
      psychiatric condition V17.0
      skin condition V19.4
    ear disorder NEC V19.3
    endocrine disease V18.19
      multiple neoplasia [MEN] syndrome V18.11
    epilepsy V17.2
    eye disorder NEC V19.1
    genetic disease carrier V18.9
    genitourinary disease NEC V18.7
    glomerulonephritis V18.69
    gout V18.19
    hay fever V17.6
    hearing loss V19.2
    hematopoietic neoplasia V16.7
    Hodgkin's disease V16.7
    Huntington's chorea V17.2
    hydrocephalus V19.5
    hypertension V17.49
    infarction, myocardial V17.3
    infectious disease V18.8
    ischemic heart disease V17.3
    kidney disease V18.69
      polycystic V18.61
    leukemia V16.6
    lymphatic malignant neoplasia NEC V16.7
    malignant neoplasm (of) NEC V16.9
      anorectal V16.0
      anus V16.0
      appendix V16.0
      bladder V16.52
      bone V16.8
      brain V16.8
      breast V16.3
        male V16.8
      bronchus V16.1
      cecum V16.0
      cervix V16.49
      colon V16.0
      duodenum V16.0
      esophagus V16.0

History—*continued*
  family—*continued*
    malignant neoplasm—*continued*
      eye V16.8
      gallbladder V16.0
      gastrointestinal tract V16.0
      genital organs V16.40
      hemopoietic NEC V16.7
      ileum V16.0
      ilium V16.8
      intestine V16.0
      intrathoracic organs NEC V16.2
      kidney V16.51
      larynx V16.2
      liver V16.0
      lung V16.1
      lymphatic NEC V16.7
      ovary V16.41
      oviduct V16.41
      pancreas V16.0
      penis V16.49
      prostate V16.42
      rectum V16.0
      respiratory organs NEC V16.2
      skin V16.8
      specified site NEC V16.8
      stomach V16.0
      testis V16.43
      trachea V16.1
      ureter V16.59
      urethra V16.59
      urinary organs V16.59
      uterus V16.49
      vagina V16.49
      vulva V16.49
    MEN (multiple endocrine neoplasia
      syndrome) V18.11
    mental retardation V18.4
    metabolic disease NEC V18.19
    mongolism V19.5
    multiple
      endocrine neoplasia [MEN] syndrome
        V18.11
      myeloma V16.7
    musculoskeletal disease NEC V17.89
      osteoporosis V17.81
    myocardial infarction V17.3
    nephritis V18.69
    nephrosis V18.69
    osteoporosis V17.81
    parasitic disease V18.8
    polycystic kidney disease V18.61
    psychiatric disorder V17.0
    psychosis V17.0
    retardation, mental V18.4
    retinitis pigmentosa V19.1
    schizophrenia V17.0
    skin conditions V19.4
    specified condition NEC V19.8
    stroke (cerebrovascular) V17.1
    sudden cardiac death (SCD) V17.41
    visual loss V19.0
  fracture, healed
    pathologic V13.51
    stress V13.52
    traumatic V15.51
  genital system disorder V13.29
    pre-term labor V13.21
  health hazard V15.9
    falling V15.88
    specified cause NEC V15.89

History—*continued*
  hepatitis
    B V12.09
    C V12.09
  Hodgkin's disease V10.72
  hypospadias V13.61
  immunity disorder V12.2
  immunosuppression therapy V87.46
  infarction, cerebral, without residual deficits
      V12.54
  infection
    central nervous system V12.42
    urinary (tract) V13.02
  infectious disease V12.00
    malaria V12.03
    methicillin resistant Staphylococcus aureus
        (MRSA) V12.04
    MRSA (methicillin resistant Staphylococcus
        aureus) V12.04
    poliomyelitis V12.02
    specified NEC V12.09
    tuberculosis V12.01
  injury NEC V15.59
    traumatic brain V15.52
  insufficient prenatal care V23.7
  in utero procedure
    during pregnancy V15.21
    while a fetus V15.22
  irradiation V15.3
  leukemia V10.60
    lymphoid V10.61
    monocytic V10.63
    myeloid V10.62
    specified type NEC V10.69
  little or no prenatal care V23.7
  low birth weight (*see also* Status, low birth
      weight) V21.30
  lymphosarcoma V10.71
  malaria V12.03
  malignant carcinoid tumor V10.91
  malignant neuroendocrine tumor V10.91
  malignant neoplasm (of) V10.90
    accessory sinus V10.22
    adrenal V10.88
    anus V10.06
    bile duct V10.09
    bladder V10.51
    bone V10.81
    brain V10.85
    breast V10.3
    bronchus V10.11
    cervix uteri V10.41
    colon V10.05
    connective tissue NEC V10.89
    corpus uteri V10.42
    digestive system V10.00
      specified part NEC V10.09
    duodenum V10.09
    endocrine gland NEC V10.88
    epididymis V10.48
    esophagus V10.03
    eye V10.84
    fallopian tube V10.44
    female genital organ V10.40
      specified site NEC V10.44
    gallbladder V10.09
    gastrointestinal tract V10.00
    gum V10.02
    hematopoietic NEC V10.79
    hypopharynx V10.02
    ileum V10.09

History—*continued*
  malignant neoplasm—*continued*
    intrathoracic organs NEC V10.20
    jejunum V10.09
    kidney V10.52
    large intestine V10.05
    larynx V10.21
    lip V10.02
    liver V10.07
    lung V10.11
    lymphatic NEC V10.79
    lymph glands or nodes NEC V10.79
    male genital organ V10.45
      specified site NEC V10.49
    mediastinum V10.29
    melanoma (of skin) V10.82
    middle ear V10.22
    mouth V10.02
      specified part NEC V10.02
    nasal cavities V10.22
    nasopharynx V10.02
    nervous system NEC V10.86
    nose V10.22
    oropharynx V10.02
    ovary V10.43
    pancreas V10.09
    parathyroid V10.88
    penis V10.49
    pharynx V10.02
    pineal V10.88
    pituitary V10.88
    placenta V10.44
    pleura V10.29
    prostate V10.46
    rectosigmoid junction V10.06
    rectum V10.06
    renal pelvis V10.53
    respiratory organs NEC V10.20
    salivary gland V10.02
    skin V10.83
      melanoma V10.82
    small intestine NEC V10.09
    soft tissue NEC V10.89
    specified site NEC V10.89
    stomach V10.04
    testis V10.47
    thymus V10.29
    thyroid V10.87
    tongue V10.01
    trachea V10.12
    ureter V10.59
    urethra V10.59
    urinary organ V10.50
    uterine adnexa V10.44
    uterus V10.42
    vagina V10.44
    vulva V10.44
  manic-depressive psychosis V11.1
  meningitis V12.42
  mental disorder V11.9
    affective type V11.1
    manic-depressive V11.1
    neurosis V11.2
    schizophrenia V11.0
    specified type NEC V11.8
  Merkel cell carcinoma V10.91
  metabolic disorder V12.2
  methicillin resistant Staphylococcus aureus
      (MRSA) V12.04
  MRSA (methicillin resistant Staphylococcus
      aureus) V12.04

History—*continued*
musculoskeletal disorder NEC V13.59
myocardial infarction 412
neglect (emotional) V15.42
nephrotic syndrome V13.03
nervous system disorder V12.40
    specified type NEC V12.49
neurosis V11.2
noncompliance with medical treatment V15.81
nutritional deficiency V12.1
obstetric disorder V13.29
    affecting management of current pregnancy
        V23.49
        pre-term labor V23.41
    pre-term labor V13.41
parasitic disease V12.00
    specified NEC V12.09
perinatal problems V13.7
    low birth weight (*see also* Status, low birth
        weight) V21.30
physical abuse V15.41
poisoning V15.6
poliomyelitis V12.02
polyps, colonic V12.72
poor obstetric V23.49
    affecting management of current pregnancy
        V23.49
        pre-term labor V23.41
    pre-term labor V13.41
prolonged reversible ischemic neurologic
    deficits (PRIND) V12.54
psychiatric disorder V11.9
    affective type V11.1
    manic-depressive V11.1
    neurosis V11.2
    schizophrenia V11.0
    specified type NEC V11.8
psychological trauma V15.49
    emotional abuse V15.42
    neglect V15.42
    physical abuse V15.41
    rape V15.41
psychoneurosis V11.2
radiation therapy V15.3
rape V15.41
respiratory system disease V12.60
    pneumonia V12.61
    specified NEC V12.69
reticulosarcoma V10.71
return from military deployment V62.22
reversible ischemic neurologic deficit (RIND)
    V12.54
schizophrenia V11.0
skin disease V13.3
smoking (tobacco) V15.82
steroid therapy V87.45
    inhaled V87.44
    systemic V87.45
stroke without residual deficits V12.54
subcutaneous tissue disease V13.3
sudden
    cardiac
        arrest V12.53
        death (successfully resuscitated) V12.53
surgery (to)
    great vessels V15.1
    heart V15.1
    in utero
        during pregnancy V15.21
        while a fetus V15.22
    organs NEC V15.29

History—*continued*
syndrome, nephrotic V13.03
therapy
    antineoplastic drug V87.41
    drug NEC V87.49
    estrogen V87.43
    immunosuppression V87.46
    monoclonal drug V87.42
    steroid V87.45
        inhaled V87.44
        systemic V87.45
thrombophlebitis V12.52
thrombosis V12.51
tobacco use V15.82
trophoblastic disease V13.1
    affecting management of pregnancy V23.1
tuberculosis V12.01
ulcer, peptic V12.71
urinary system disorder V13.00
    calculi V13.01
    infection V13.02
    nephrotic syndrome V13.03
    specified NEC V13.09
HIT (heparin-induced thrombocytopenia) 289.84
HIV infection (disease) (illness)—*see* Human
    immunodeficiency virus (disease) (illness)
    (infection)
Hives (bold) (*see also* Urticaria) 708.9
Hoarseness 784.42
Hobnail liver —*see* Cirrhosis, portal
Hobo, hoboism V60.0
Hodgkin's
disease (M9650/3) 201.9
    lymphocytic
        depletion (M9653/3) 201.7
            diffuse fibrosis (M9654/3) 201.7
            reticular type (M9655/3) 201.7
        predominance (M9651/3) 201.4
        lymphocytic-histiocytic predominance
            (M9651/3) 201.4
        mixed cellularity (M9652/3) 201.6
        nodular sclerosis (M9656/3) 201.5
            cellular phase (M9657/3) 201.5
    granuloma (M9661/3) 201.1
    lymphogranulomatosis (M9650/3) 201.9
    lymphoma (M9650/3) 201.9
    lymphosarcoma (M9650/3) 201.9
    paragranuloma (M9660/3) 201.0
    sarcoma (M9662/3) 201.2
Hodgson's disease (aneurysmal dilatation of
    aorta) 441.9
    ruptured 441.5
Hodi-potsy 111.0
Hoffa -(Kastert) disease or syndrome
    (liposynovitis prepatellaris) 272.8
Hoffmann's syndrome 244.9 *[359.5]*
Hoffmann-Bouveret syndrome (paroxysmal
    tachycardia) 427.2
Hole
macula 362.54
optic disc, crater-like 377.22
retina (macula) 362.54
    round 361.31
        with detachment 361.01
Holla disease (*see also* Spherocytosis) 282.0
Holländer-Simons syndrome (progressive
    lipodystrophy) 272.6
Hollow foot (congenital) 754.71
    acquired 736.73
Holmes' syndrome (visual disorientation) 368.16

Holoprosencephaly 742.2
due to
trisomy 13 758.1
trisomy 18 758.2
Holthouse's hernia —*see* Hernia, inguinal
Homesickness 309.89
Homocystinemia 270.4
Homocystinuria 270.4
Homologous serum jaundice (prophylactic)
(therapeutic)—*see* Hepatitis, viral
Homosexuality —*omit code*
ego-dystonic 302.0
pedophilic 302.2
problems with 302.0
Homozygous Hb-S disease 282.61
Honeycomb lung 518.89
congenital 748.4
Hong Kong ear 117.3
HOOD (hereditary osteo-onychodysplasia) 756.89
Hooded
clitoris 752.49
penis 752.69
Hookworm (anemia) (disease) (infestation)—*see*
Ancylostomiasis
Hoppe-Goldflam syndrome 358.00
Hordeolum (external) (eyelid) 373.11
internal 373.12
Horn
cutaneous 702.8
cheek 702.8
eyelid 702.8
penis 702.8
iliac 756.89
nail 703.8
congenital 757.5
papillary 700
Horner's
syndrome (*see also* Neuropathy, peripheral,
autonomic) 337.9
traumatic 954.0
teeth 520.4
Horseshoe kidney (congenital) 753.3
Horton's
disease (temporal arteritis) 446.5
headache or neuralgia 339.00
Hospice care V66.7
Hospitalism (in children) NEC 309.83
Hourglass contraction, contracture
bladder 596.8
gallbladder 575.2
congenital 751.69
stomach 536.8
congenital 750.7
psychogenic 306.4
uterus 661.4
affecting fetus or newborn 763.7
Household circumstance affecting care V60.9
specified type NEC V60.89
Housemaid's knee 727.2
Housing circumstance affecting care V60.9
specified type NEC V60.89
Huchard's disease (continued arterial
hypertension) 401.9
Hudson-Stähli lines 371.11
Huguier's disease (uterine fibroma) 218.9
Hum, venous —*omit code*
Human bite (open wound)—*see also* Wound,
open, by site
intact skin surface—*see* Contusion

Human immunodeficiency virus (disease)
(illness) 042
infection V08
with symptoms, symptomatic 042
Human immunodeficiency virus-2 infection
079.53
Human immunovirus (disease) (illness)
(infection)—*see* Human immunodeficiency
virus (disease) (illness) (infection)
Human papillomavirus 079.4
high risk, DNA test positive
anal 796.75
cervical 795.05
vaginal 795.15
low risk, DNA test positive
anal 796.79
cervical 795.09
vaginal 795.19
Human parovirus 079.83
Human T-cell lymphotrophic virus I infection
079.51
Human T-cell lymphotrophic virus II infection
079.52
Human T-cell lymphotropic virus-III (disease)
(illness) (infection)—*see* Human
immunodeficiency virus (disease) (illness)
(infection)
Hungry bone syndrome 275.5
HTLV-I infection 079.51
HTLV-II infection 079.52
HTLV-III (disease) (illness) (infection)—*see*
Human immunodeficiency virus (disease)
(illness) (infection)
HTLV-III/LAV
(disease) (illness) (infection)—*see* Human
immunodeficiency virus (disease) (illness)
(infection)
Humpback (acquired) 737.9
congenital 756.19
Hunchback (acquired) 737.9
congenital 756.19
Hunger 994.2
air, psychogenic 306.1
disease 251.1
Hunner's ulcer (*see also* Cystitis) 595.1
Hunt's
neuralgia 053.11
syndrome (herpetic geniculate ganglionitis)
053.11
dyssynergia cerebellaris myoclonica 334.2
Hunter's glossitis 529.4
Hunter (-Hurler) syndrome
(mucopolysaccharidosis II) 277.5
Hunterian chancre 091.0
Huntington's
chorea 333.4
disease 333.4
Huppert's disease (multiple myeloma)
(M9730/3) 203.0
Hurler (-Hunter) disease or syndrome
(mucopolysaccharidosis II) 277.5
Hürthle cell
adenocarcinoma (M8290/3) 193
adenoma (M8290/0) 226
carcinoma (M8290/3) 193
tumor (M8290/0) 226

Hutchinson's
 disease meaning
  angioma serpiginosum 709.1
  cheiropompholyx 705.81
  prurigo estivalis 692.72
  summer eruption, or summer prurigo 692.72
 incisors 090.5
 melanotic freckle (M8742/2)—*see also*
  Neoplasm, skin, in situ
  malignant melanoma in (M8742/3)—*see*
  Melanoma
 teeth or incisors (congenital syphilis) 090.5
Hutchinson-Boeck disease or syndrome
 (sarcoidosis) 135
Hutchinson-Gilford disease or syndrome
 (progeria) 259.8
Hyaline
 degeneration (diffuse) (generalized) 728.9
  localized—*see* Degeneration, by site
 membrane (disease) (lung) (newborn) 769
Hyalinosis cutis et mucosae 272.8
Hyalin plaque, sclera, senile 379.16
Hyalitis (asteroid) 379.22
 syphilitic 095.8
Hydatid
 cyst or tumor—*see also* Echinococcus
  fallopian tube 752.11
 mole—*see* Hydatidiform mole
 Morgagni (congenital) 752.89
  fallopian tube 752.11
Hydatidiform mole (benign) (complicating
 pregnancy) (delivered) (undelivered) 630
 invasive (M9100/1) 236.1
 malignant (M9100/1) 236.1
 previous, affecting management of pregnancy
  V23.1
Hydatidosis —*see* Echinococcus
Hyde's disease (prurigo nodularis) 698.3
Hydradenitis 705.83
Hydradenoma (M8400/0)—*see* Hidradenoma
Hydralazine lupus or syndrome
 correct substance properly administered 695.4
 overdose or wrong substance given or taken
  972.6
Hydramnios 657
 affecting fetus or newborn 761.3
Hydrancephaly 742.3
 with spina bifida (*see also* Spina bifida) 741.0
Hydranencephaly 742.3
 with spina bifida (*see also* Spina bifida) 741.0
Hydrargyrism NEC 985.0
Hydrarthrosis (*see also* Effusion, joint) 719.0
 gonococcal 098.50
 intermittent (*see also* Rheumatism, palindromic)
  719.3
 of yaws (early) (late) 102.6
 syphilitic 095.8
  congenital 090.5
Hydremia 285.9
Hydrencephalocele (congenital) 742.0
Hydrencephalomeningocele (congenital) 742.0
Hydroa 694.0
 aestivale 692.72
 gestationis 646.8
 herpetiformis 694.0
 pruriginosa 694.0
 vacciniforme 692.72
Hydroadenitis 705.83
Hydrocalycosis (*see also* Hydronephrosis) 591
 congenital 753.29
Hydrocalyx (*see also* Hydronephrosis) 591

Hydrocele (calcified) (chylous) (idiopathic)
 (infantile) (inguinal canal) (recurrent) (senile)
 (spermatic cord) (testis) (tunica vaginalis)
 603.9
 canal of Nuck (female) 629.1
  male 603.9
 congenital 778.6
 encysted 603.0
  congenital 778.6
 female NEC 629.89
 infected 603.1
 round ligament 629.89
 specified type NEC 603.8
  congenital 778.6
 spinalis (*see also* Spina bifida) 741.9
 vulva 624.8
Hydrocephalic fetus
 affecting management of pregnancy 655.0
 causing disproportion 653.6
  with obstructed labor 660.1
   affecting fetus or newborn 763.1
Hydrocephalus (acquired) (external) (internal)
 (malignant) (noncommunicating) (obstructive)
 (recurrent) 331.4
 aqueduct of Sylvius stricture 742.3
  with spina bifida (*see also* Spina bifida) 741.0
 chronic 742.3
  with spina bifida (*see also* Spina bifida) 741.0
 communicating 331.3
 congenital (external) (internal) 742.3
  with spina bifida (*see also* Spina bifida) 741.0
 due to
  stricture of aqueduct of Sylvius 742.3
   with spina bifida (*see also* Spina bifida)
    741.0
  toxoplasmosis (congenital) 771.2
 fetal affecting management of pregnancy 655.0
 foramen Magendie block (acquired) 331.3
  congenital 742.3
   with spina bifida (*see also* Spina bifida)
    741.0
 newborn 742.3
  with spina bifida (*see also* Spina bifida) 741.0
 normal pressure 331.5
  idiopathic (INPH) 331.5
  secondary 331.3
 otitic 348.2
 syphilitic, congenital 090.49
 tuberculous (*see also* Tuberculosis) 013.8
Hydrocolpos (congenital) 623.8
Hydrocystoma (M8404/0)—*see* Neoplasm, skin,
 benign
Hydroencephalocele (congenital) 742.0
Hydroencephalomeningocele (congenital) 742.0
Hydrohematopneumothorax (*see also*
 Hemothorax) 511.89
Hydromeningitis —*see* Meningitis
Hydromeningocele (spinal) (*see also* Spina
 bifida) 741.9
 cranial 742.0
Hydrometra 621.8
Hydrometrocolpos 623.8
Hydromicrocephaly 742.1
Hydromphalus (congenital) (since birth) 757.39
Hydromyelia 742.53
Hydromyelocele (*see also* Spina bifida) 741.9
Hydronephrosis 591
 atrophic 591
 congenital 753.29
 due to S. hematobium 120.0
 early 591

Hydronephrosis—*continued*
functionless (infected) 591
infected 591
intermittent 591
primary 591
secondary 591
tuberculous (*see also* Tuberculosis) 016.0
Hydropericarditis (*see also* Pericarditis) 423.9
Hydropericardium (*see also* Pericarditis) 423.9
Hydroperitoneum 789.59
Hydrophobia 071
Hydrophthalmos (*see also* Buphthalmia) 743.20
Hydropneumohemothorax (*see also* Hemothorax) 511.89
Hydropneumopericarditis (*see also* Pericarditis) 423.9
Hydropneumopericardium (*see also* Pericarditis) 423.9
Hydropneumothorax 511.89
nontuberculous 511.89
bacterial 511.1
pneumococcal 511.1
staphylococcal 511.1
streptococcal 511.1
traumatic 860.0
with open wound into thorax 860.1
tuberculous (*see also* Tuberculosis, pleural) 012.0
Hydrops 782.3
abdominis 789.59
amnii (complicating pregnancy) (*see also* Hydramnios) 657
articulorum intermittens (*see also* Rheumatism, palindromic) 719.3
cardiac (*see also* Failure, heart) 428.0
congenital—*see* Hydrops, fetalis
endolymphatic (*see also* Disease, Ménière's) 386.00
fetal(is) or newborn 778.0
due to isoimmunization 773.3
not due to isoimmunization 778.0
gallbladder 575.3
idiopathic (fetus or newborn) 778.0
joint (*see also* Effusion, joint) 719.0
labyrinth (*see also* Disease, Ménière's) 386.00
meningeal NEC 331.4
nutritional 262
pericardium—*see* Pericarditis
pleura (*see also* Hydrothorax) 511.89
renal (*see also* Nephrosis) 581.9
spermatic cord (*see also* Hydrocele) 603.9
Hydropyonephrosis (*see also* Pyelitis) 590.80
chronic 590.00
Hydrorachis 742.53
Hydrorrhea (nasal) 478.19
gravidarum 658.1
pregnancy 658.1
Hydrosadenitis 705.83
Hydrosalpinx (fallopian tube) (follicularis) 614.1
Hydrothorax (double) (pleural) 511.89
chylous (nonfilarial) 457.8
filaria (*see also* Infestation, filarial) 125.9
nontuberculous 511.89
bacterial 511.1
pneumococcal 511.1
staphylococcal 511.1
streptococcal 511.1
traumatic 862.29
with open wound into thorax 862.39
tuberculous (*see also* Tuberculosis, pleura) 012.0
Hydroureter 593.5
congenital 753.22

Hydroureteronephrosis (*see also* Hydronephrosis) 591
Hydrourethra 599.84
Hydroxykynureninuria 270.2
Hydroxyprolinemia 270.8
Hydroxyprolinuria 270.8
Hygroma (congenital) (cystic) (M9173/0) 228.1
prepatellar 727.3
subdural—*see* Hematoma, subdural
Hymen —*see* condition
Hymenolepiasis (diminuta) (infection) (infestation) (nana) 123.6
Hymenolepis (diminuta) (infection) (infestation) (nana) 123.6
Hypalgesia (*see also* Disturbance, sensation) 782.0
Hyperabduction syndrome 447.8
Hyperacidity, gastric 536.8
psychogenic 306.4
Hyperactive, hyperactivity 314.01
basal cell, uterine cervix 622.10
bladder 596.51
bowel (syndrome) 564.9
sounds 787.5
cervix epithelial (basal) 622.10
child 314.01
colon 564.9
gastrointestinal 536.8
psychogenic 306.4
intestine 564.9
labyrinth (unilateral) 386.51
with loss of labyrinthine reactivity 386.58
bilateral 386.52
nasal mucous membrane 478.19
stomach 536.8
thyroid (gland) (*see also* Thyrotoxicosis) 242.9
Hyperacusis 388.42
Hyperadrenalism (cortical) 255.3
medullary 255.6
Hyperadrenocorticism 255.3
congenital 255.2
iatrogenic
correct substance properly administered 255.3
overdose or wrong substance given or taken 962.0
Hyperaffectivity 301.11
Hyperaldosteronism (atypical) (hyperplastic) (normoaldosteronal) (normotensive) (primary) 255.10
secondary 255.14
Hyperalgesia (*see also* Disturbance, sensation) 782.0
Hyperalimentation 783.6
carotene 278.3
specified NEC 278.8
vitamin A 278.2
vitamin D 278.4
Hyperaminoaciduria 270.9
arginine 270.6
citrulline 270.6
cystine 270.0
glycine 270.0
lysine 270.7
ornithine 270.6
renal (types I, II, III) 270.0
Hyperammonemia (congenital) 270.6
Hyperamnesia 780.99
Hyperamylasemia 790.5
Hyperaphia 782.0
Hyperazotemia 791.9

Hyperbetalipoproteinemia (acquired) (essential) (familial) (hereditary) (primary) (secondary) 272.0
  with pre-betalipoproteinemia 272.2
Hyperbilirubinemia 782.4
  congenital 277.4
  constitutional 277.4
  neonatal (transient) (*see also* Jaundice, fetus or newborn) 774.6
  of prematurity 774.2
Hyperbilirubinemica encephalopathia, newborn 774.7
  due to isoimmunization 773.4
Hypercalcemia, hypercalcemic (idiopathic) 275.42
  nephropathy 588.89
Hypercalcinuria 275.40
Hypercapnia 786.09
  with mixed acid-base disorder 276.4
  fetal, affecting newborn 770.89
Hypercarotinemia 278.3
Hypercementosis 521.5
Hyperchloremia 276.9
Hyperchlorhydria 536.8
  neurotic 306.4
  psychogenic 306.4
Hypercholesterinemia —*see* Hypercholesterolemia
Hypercholesterolemia 272.0
  with hyperglyceridemia, endogenous 272.2
  essential 272.0
  familial 272.0
  hereditary 272.0
  primary 272.0
  pure 272.0
Hypercholesterolosis 272.0
Hyperchylia gastricsa 536.8
  psychogenic 306.4
Hyperchylomicronemia (familial) (with hyperbetalipoproteinemia) 272.3
Hypercoagulation syndrome (primary) 289.81
  secondary 289.82
Hypercorticosteronism
  correct substance properly administered 255.3
  overdose or wrong substance given or taken 962.0
Hypercortisonism
  correct substance properly administered 255.3
  overdose or wrong substance given or taken 962.0
Hyperdynamic beta-adrenergic state or syndrome (circulatory) 429.82
Hyperekplexia 759.89
Hyperelectrolytemia 276.9
Hyperemesis 536.2
  arising during pregnancy—*see* Hyperemesis, gravidarum
  gravidarum (mild) (before 22 completed weeks gestation) 643.0
  with
    carbohydrate depletion 643.1
    dehydration 643.1
    electrolyte imbalance 643.1
    metabolic disturbance 643.1
    affecting fetus or newborn 761.8
    severe (with metabolic disturbance) 643.1
  psychogenic 306.4

Hyperemia (acute) 780.99
  anal mucosa 569.49
  bladder 596.7
  cerebral 437.8
  conjunctiva 372.71
  ear, internal, acute 386.30
  enteric 564.89
  eye 372.71
  eyelid (active) (passive) 374.82
  intestine 564.89
  iris 364.41
  kidney 593.81
  labyrinth 386.30
  liver (active) (passive) 573.8
  lung 514
  ovary 620.8
  passive 780.99
  pulmonary 514
  renal 593.81
  retina 362.89
  spleen 289.59
  stomach 537.89
Hyperesthesia (body surface) (*see also* Disturbance, sensation) 782.0
  larynx (reflex) 478.79
    hysterical 300.11
  pharynx (reflex) 478.29
Hyperestrinism 256.0
Hyperestrogenism 256.0
Hyperestrogenosis 256.0
Hyperexplexia 759.89
Hyperextension, joint 718.80
  ankle 718.87
  elbow 718.82
  foot 718.87
  hand 718.84
  hip 718.85
  knee 718.86
  multiple sites 718.89
  pelvic region 718.85
  shoulder (region) 718.81
  specified site NEC 718.88
  wrist 718.83
Hyperfibrinolysis —*see* Fibrinolysis
Hyperfolliculinism 256.0
Hyperfructosemia 271.2
Hyperfunction
  adrenal (cortex) 255.3
    androgenic, acquired benign 255.3
    medulla 255.6
    virilism 255.2
  corticoadrenal NEC 255.3
  labyrinth—*see* Hyperactive, labyrinth
  medulloadrenal 255.6
  ovary 256.1
    estrogen 256.0
  pancreas 577.8
  parathyroid (gland) 252.00
  pituitary (anterior) (gland) (lobe) 253.1
  testicular 257.0
Hypergammaglobulinemia 289.89
  monoclonal, benign (BMH) 273.1
  polyclonal 273.0
  Waldenström's 273.0
Hyperglobulinemia 273.8
Hyperglycemia 790.29
  maternal
    affecting fetus or newborn 775.0
    manifest diabetes in infant 775.1
  postpancreatectomy (complete) (partial) 251.3

Hyperglyceridemia 272.1
  endogenous 272.1
  essential 272.1
  familial 272.1
  hereditary 272.1
  mixed 272.3
  pure 272.1
Hyperglycinemia 270.7
Hypergonadism
  ovarian 256.1
  testicular (infantile) (primary) 257.0
Hyperheparinemia (*see also* Circulating
  anticoagulants) 286.5
Hyperhidrosis, hyperidrosis 705.21
  axilla 705.21
  face 705.21
  focal (localized) 705.21
    primary 705.21
      axilla 705.21
      face 705.21
      palms 705.21
      soles 705.21
    secondary 705.22
      axilla 705.22
      face 705.22
      palms 705.22
      soles 705.22
  generalized 780.8
  palms 705.21
  psychogenic 306.3
  secondary 780.8
  soles 705.21
Hyperhistidinemia 270.5
Hyperinsulinism (ectopic) (functional) (organic)
  NEC 251.1
  iatrogenic 251.0
  reactive 251.2
  spontaneous 251.2
  therapeutic misadventure (from administration
    of insulin) 962.3
Hyperiodemia 276.9
Hyperirritability (cerebral), in newborn 779.1
Hyperkalemia 276.7
Hyperkeratosis (*see also* Keratosis) 701.1
  cervix 622.2
  congenital 757.39
  cornea 371.89
  due to yaws (early) (late) (palmar or plantar) 102.3
  eccentrica 757.39
  figurata centrifuga atrophica 757.39
  follicularis 757.39
    in cutem penetrans 701.1
  limbic (cornea) 371.89
  palmoplantaris climacterica 701.1
  pinta (carate) 103.1
  senile (with pruritus) 702.0
  tongue 528.79
  universalis congenita 757.1
  vagina 623.1
  vocal cord 478.5
  vulva 624.09
Hyperkinesia, hyperkinetic (disease) (reaction)
  (syndrome) 314.9
  with
    attention deficit —*see* Disorder, attention deficit
    conduct disorder 314.2
    developmental delay 314.1
    simple disturbance of activity and attention
      314.01
    specified manifestation NEC 314.8
  heart (disease) 429.82
  of childhood or adolescence NEC 314.9

Hyperlacrimation (*see also* Epiphora) 375.20
Hyperlipemia (*see also* Hyperlipidemia) 272.4
Hyperlipidemia 272.4
  carbohydrate-induced 272.1
  combined 272.2
  endogenous 272.1
  exogenous 272.3
  fat-induced 272.3
  group
    A 272.0
    B 272.1
    C 272.2
    D 272.3
  mixed 272.2
  specified type NEC 272.4
Hyperlipidosis 272.7
  hereditary 272.7
Hyperlipoproteinemia (acquired) (essential)
  (familial) (hereditary) (primary) (secondary)
  272.4
  Fredrickson type
    I 272.3
    IIa 272.0
    IIb 272.2
    III 272.2
    IV 272.1
    V 272.3
  low-density-lipoid-type (LDL) 272.0
  very-low-density-lipoid-type [VLDL] 272.1
Hyperlucent lung, unilateral 492.8
Hyperluteinization 256.1
Hyperlysinemia 270.7
Hypermagnesemia 275.2
  neonatal 775.5
Hypermaturity (fetus or newborn)
  post-term infant 766.21
  prolonged gestation infant 766.22
Hypermenorrhea 626.2
Hypermetabolism 794.7
Hypermethioninemia 270.4
Hypermetropia (congenital) 367.0
Hypermobility
  cecum 564.9
  coccyx 724.71
  colon 564.9
    psychogenic 306.4
  ileum 564.89
  joint (acquired) 718.80
    ankle 718.87
    elbow 718.82
    foot 718.87
    hand 718.84
    hip 718.85
    knee 718.86
    multiple sites 718.89
    pelvic region 718.85
    shoulder (region) 718.81
    specified site NEC 718.88
    wrist 718.83
  kidney, congenital 753.3
  meniscus (knee) 717.5
  scapula 718.81
  stomach 536.8
    psychogenic 306.4
  syndrome 728.5
  testis, congenital 752.52
  urethral 599.81
Hypermotility
  gastrointestinal 536.8
  intestine 564.9
    psychogenic 306.4
  stomach 536.8

Hypernasality 784.43
Hypernatremia 276.0
  with water depletion 276.0
Hypernephroma (M8312/3) 189.0
Hyperopia 367.0
Hyperorexia 783.6
Hyperornithinemia 270.6
Hyperosmia (*see also* Disturbance, sensation)
  781.1
Hyperosmolality 276.0
Hyperosteogenesis 733.99
Hyperostosis 733.99
  calvarial 733.3
  cortical 733.3
    infantile 756.59
  frontal, internal of skull 733.3
  interna frontalis 733.3
  monomelic 733.99
  skull 733.3
    congenital 756.0
  vertebral 721.8
    with spondylosis—*see* Spondylosis
    ankylosing 721.6
Hyperovarianism 256.1
Hyperovarism, hyperovaria 256.1
Hyperoxaluria (primary) 271.8
Hyperoxia 987.8
Hyperparathyroidism 252.00
  ectopic 259.3
  other 252.08
  primary 252.01
  secondary (of renal origin) 588.81
    non-renal 252.02
  tertiary 252.08
Hyperpathia (*see also* Disturbance, sensation)
  782.0
  psychogenic 307.80
Hyperperistalsis 787.4
  psychogenic 306.4
Hyperpermeability, capillary 448.9
Hyperphagia 783.6
Hyperphenylalaninemia 270.1
Hyperphoria 378.40
  alternating 378.45
Hyperphosphatemia 275.3
Hyperpiesia (*see also* Hypertension) 401.9
Hyperpiesis (*see also* Hypertension) 401.9
Hyperpigmentation —*see* Pigmentation
Hyperpinealism 259.8
Hyperpipecolatemia 270.7
Hyperpituitarism 253.1
Hyperplasia, hyperplastic
  adenoids (lymphoid tissue) 474.12
    and tonsils 474.10
  adrenal (capsule) (cortex) (gland) 255.8
    with
      sexual precocity (male) 255.2
      virilism, adrenal 255.2
      virilization (female) 255.2
    congenital 255.2
    due to excess ACTH (ectopic) (pituitary) 255.0
    medulla 255.8
  alpha cells (pancreatic)
    with
      gastrin excess 251.5
      glucagon excess 251.4
  appendix (lymphoid) 543.0
  artery, fibromuscular NEC 447.8
    carotid 447.8
    renal 447.3

Hyperplasia, hyperplastic—*continued*
  bone 733.99
    marrow 289.9
  breast (*see also* Hypertrophy, breast) 611.1
    ductal 610.8
      atypical 610.8
  carotid artery 447.8
  cementation, cementum (teeth) (tooth) 521.5
  cervical gland 785.6
  cervix (uteri) 622.10
    basal cell 622.10
    congenital 752.49
    endometrium 622.10
    polypoid 622.10
  chin 524.05
  clitoris, congenital 752.49
  dentin 521.5
  endocervicitis 616.0
  endometrium, endometrial (adenomatous)
    (atypical) (cystic) (glandular) (polypoid)
    (uterus) 621.30
    with atypia 621.33
    without atypia
      complex 621.32
      simple 621.31
    benign 621.34
    cervix 622.10
  epithelial 709.8
    focal, oral, including tongue 528.79
    mouth (focal) 528.79
    nipple 611.89
    skin 709.8
    tongue (focal) 528.79
    vaginal wall 623.0
  erythroid 289.9
  fascialis ossificans (progressiva) 728.11
  fibromuscular, artery NEC 447.8
    carotid 447.8
    renal 447.3
  genital
    female 629.89
    male 608.89
  gingiva 523.8
  glandularis
    cystica uteri 621.30
    endometrium (uterus) 621.30
    interstitialis uteri 621.30
  granulocytic 288.69
  gum 523.8
  hymen, congenital 752.49
  islands of Langerhans 251.1
  islet cell (pancreatic) 251.9
    alpha cells
      with excess
        gastrin 251.5
        glucagon 251.4
    beta cells 251.1
  juxtaglomerular (complex) (kidney) 593.89
  kidney (congenital) 753.3
  liver (congenital) 751.69
  lymph node (gland) 785.6
  lymphoid (diffuse) (nodular) 785.6
    appendix 543.0
    intestine 569.89
  mandibular 524.02
    alveolar 524.72
    unilateral condylar 526.89
  Marchand multiple nodular (liver)—*see*
    Cirrhosis, postnecrotic
  maxillary 524.01
    alveolar 524.71

Hyperplasia, hyperplastic—*continued*
  medulla, adrenal 255.8
  myometrium, myometrial 621.2
  nose (lymphoid) (polypoid) 478.19
  oral soft tissue (inflammatory) (irritative)
      (mucosa) NEC 528.9
    gingiva 523.8
    tongue 529.8
  organ or site, congenital NEC—*see* Anomaly,
      specified type NEC
  ovary 620.8
  palate, papillary 528.9
  pancreatic islet cells 251.9
    alpha
      with excess
        gastrin 251.5
        glucagon 251.4
    beta 251.1
  parathyroid (gland) 252.01
  persistent, vitreous (primary) 743.51
  pharynx (lymphoid) 478.29
  prostate 600.90
    with
      other lower urinary tract symptoms (LUTS)
          600.91
      urinary
        obstruction 600.91
        retention 600.91
    adenofibromatous 600.20
      with
        other lower urinary tract symptoms
            (LUTS) 600.21
        urinary
          obstruction 600.21
          retention 600.21
    nodular 600.10
      with
        urinary
          obstruction 600.11
          retention 600.11
  renal artery (fibromuscular) 447.3
  reticuloendothelial (cell) 289.9
  salivary gland (any) 527.1
  Schimmelbusch's 610.1
  suprarenal (capsule) (gland) 255.8
  thymus (gland) (persistent) 254.0
  thyroid (*see also* Goiter) 240.9
    primary 242.0
    secondary 242.2
  tonsil (lymphoid tissue) 474.11
    and adenoids 474.10
  urethrovaginal 599.89
  uterus, uterine (myometrium) 621.2
    endometrium (*see also* Hyperplasia,
        endometrium) 621.30
  vitreous (humor), primary persistent 743.51
  vulva 624.3
  zygoma 738.11
Hyperpnea (*see also* Hyperventilation) 786.01
Hyperpotassemia 276.7
Hyperprebetalipoproteinemia 272.1
  with chylomicronemia 272.3
  familial 272.1
Hyperprolactinemia 253.1
Hyperprolinemia 270.8
Hyperproteinemia 273.8
Hyperprothrombinemia 289.89
Hyperpselaphesia 782.0

Hyperpyrexia 780.60
  heat (effects of) 992.0
  malarial (*see also* Malaria) 084.6
  malignant, due to anesthetic 995.86
  rheumatic—*see* Fever, rheumatic
  unknown origin (*see also* Pyrexia) 780.60
Hyperreactor, vascular 780.2
Hyperreflexia 796.1
  bladder, autonomic 596.54
    with cauda equina 344.61
  detrusor 344.61
Hypersalivation (*see also* Ptyalism) 527.7
Hypersarcosinemia 270.8
Hypersecretion
  ACTH 255.3
  androgens (ovarian) 256.1
  calcitonin 246.0
  corticoadrenal 255.3
  cortisol 255.0
  estrogen 256.0
  gastric 536.8
    psychogenic 306.4
  gastrin 251.5
  glucagon 251.4
  hormone
    ACTH 255.3
    anterior pituitary 253.1
    growth NEC 253.0
    ovarian androgen 256.1
    testicular 257.0
    thyroid stimulating 242.8
  insulin—*see* Hyperinsulinism
  lacrimal glands (*see also* Epiphora) 375.20
  medulloadrenal 255.6
  milk 676.6
  ovarian androgens 256.1
  pituitary (anterior) 253.1
  salivary gland (any) 527.7
  testicular hormones 257.0
  thyrocalcitonin 246.0
  upper respiratory 478.9
Hypersegmentation, hereditary 288.2
  eosinophils 288.2
  neutrophil nuclei 288.2
Hypersensitive, hypersensitiveness,
    hypersensitivity —*see also* Allergy
  angiitis 446.20
    specified NEC 446.29
  carotid sinus 337.01
  colon 564.9
    psychogenic 306.4
  DNA (deoxyribonucleic acid) NEC 287.2
  drug (*see also* Allergy, drug) 995.27
  esophagus 530.89
  insect bites—*see* Injury, superficial, by site
  labyrinth 386.58
  pain (*see also* Disturbance, sensation) 782.0
  pneumonitis NEC 495.9
  reaction (*see also* Allergy) 995.3
    upper respiratory tract NEC 478.8
  stomach (allergic) (nonallergic) 536.8
    psychogenic 306.4
Hypersomatotropism (classic) 253.0
Hypersomnia, unspecified 780.54
  with sleep apnea, unspecified 780.53
  alcohol induced 291.82
  drug induced 291.85
  due to
    medical condition classified elsewhere 327.14
    mental disorder 327.15

Hypersomnia—*continued*
  idiopathic
    with long sleep time 327.11
    without long sleep time 327.12
  menstrual related 327.13
  nonorganic origin 307.43
    persistent (primary) 307.44
    transient 307.43
  organic 327.10
    other 327.19
  primary 307.44
  recurrent 327.13
Hypersplenia 289.4
Hypersplenism 289.4
Hypersteatosis 706.3
Hyperstimulation, ovarian 256.1
Hypersuprarenalism 255.3
Hypersusceptibility —*see* Allergy
Hyper-TBG-nemia 246.8
Hypertelorism 756.0
  orbit, orbital 376.41

*"H" listing resumes after
Hypertension table...*

Hypertension, hypertensive

	Malignant	Benign	Unspecified
(arterial) (arteriolar) (crisis) (degeneration) (disease) (essential) (fluctuating) (idiopathic) (intermittent) (labile) (low renin) (orthostatic) (paroxysmal) (primary) (systemic) (uncontrolled) (vascular)	401.0	401.1	401.9
with			
chronic kidney disease			
stage I through stage IV, or unspecified	403.00	403.10	403.90
stage V or end stage renal disease	403.01	403.11	403.91
heart involvement (conditions classifiable to 429.0-429.3, 429.8, 429.9 due to hypertension) (*see also* Hypertension, heart)	402.00	402.10	402.90
with kidney involvement—*see* Hypertension, cardiorenal			
renal (kidney) involvement (only conditions classifiable to 585) (excludes conditions classifiable to 584) (*see also* Hypertension, kidney).	403.00	403.10	403.90
with heart involvement—*see* Hypertension, cardiorenal			
failure (and sclerosis) (*see also* Hypertension, kidney) . .	403.01	403.11	403.91
sclerosis without failure (*see also* Hypertension, kidney) .	403.00	403.10	403.90
accelerated (*see also* Hypertension, by type, malignant)	401.0	—	—
antepartum—*see* Hypertension complicating pregnancy, childbirth, or the puerperium			
cardiorenal (disease)	404.00	404.10	404.90
with			
chronic kidney disease			
stage I through stage IV, or unspecified	404.00	404.10	404.90
and heart failure	404.01	404.11	404.91
stage V or end stage renal disease	404.02	404.12	404.92
and heart failure	404.03	404.13	404.93
heart failure	404.01	404.11	404.91
and chronic kidney disease	404.01	404.11	404.91
stage I through stage IV or unspecified	404.01	404.11	404.91
stage V or end stage renal disease	404.03	404.13	404.93
cardiovascular disease (arteriosclerotic) (sclerotic)	402.00	402.10	402.90
with			
heart failure	402.01	402.11	402.91
renal involvement (conditions classifiable to 403) (*see also* Hypertension, cardiorenal)	404.00	404.10	404.90
cardiovascular renal (disease) (sclerosis) (*see also* Hypertension cardiorenal)	404.00	404.10	404.90
cerebrovascular disease NEC	437.2	437.2	437.2
complicating pregnancy, childbirth, or the puerperium	642.2	642.0	642.9
with			
albuminuria (and edema) (mild)	—	—	642.4
severe	—	—	642.5
chronic kidney disease	642.2	642.2	642.2
and heart disease	642.2	642.2	642.2
edema (mild)	—	—	642.4
severe	—	—	642.5
heart disease	642.2	642.2	642.2
and chronic kidney disease	642.2	642.2	642.2
renal disease	642.2	642.2	642.2
and heart disease	642.2	642.2	642.2
chronic	642.2	642.0	642.0
with pre-eclampsia or eclampsia	642.7	642.7	642.7
fetus or newborn	760.0	760.0	760.0
essential	—	642.0	642.0
with pre-eclampsia or eclampsia	—	642.7	642.7
fetus or newborn	760.0	760.0	760.0
fetus or newborn	760.0	760.0	760.0
gestational	—	—	642.3
pre-existing	642.2	642.0	642.0
with pre-eclampsia or eclampsia	642.7	642.7	642.7
fetus or newborn	760.0	760.0	760.0
secondary to renal disease	642.1	642.1	642.1
with pre-eclampsia or eclampsia	642.7	642.7	642.7
fetus or newborn	760.0	760.0	760.0
transient	—	—	642.3
due to			
aldosteronism, primary	405.09	405.19	405.99
brain tumor	405.09	405.19	405.99
bulbar poliomyelitis	405.09	405.19	405.99
calculus			
kidney	405.09	405.19	405.99
ureter	405.09	405.19	405.99
coarctation, aorta	405.09	405.19	405.99
Cushing's disease	405.09	405.19	405.99
glomerulosclerosis (*see also* Hypertension, kidney)	403.00	403.10	403.90

	Malignant	Benign	Unspecified
periarteritis nodosa	405.09	405.19	405.99
pheochromocytoma	405.09	405.19	405.99
polycystic kidney(s)	405.09	405.19	405.99
polycythemia	405.09	405.19	405.99
porphyria	405.09	405.19	405.99
pyelonephritis	405.09	405.19	405.99
renal (artery)			
aneurysm	405.01	405.11	405.91
anomaly	405.01	405.11	405.91
embolism	405.01	405.11	405.91
fibromuscular hyperplasia	405.01	405.11	405.91
occlusion	405.01	405.11	405.91
stenosis	405.01	405.11	405.91
thrombosis	405.01	405.11	405.91
encephalopathy	437.2	437.2	437.2
gestational (transient) NEC	—	—	642.3
Goldblatt's	440.1	440.1	440.1
heart (disease) (conditions classifiable to 429.0-429.3, 429.8, 429.9 due to hypertension)	402.00	402.10	402.90
with			
heart failure	402.01	402.11	402.91
hypertensive kidney disease (conditions classifiable to 403) (*see also* Hypertension, cardiorenal)	404.00	404.10	404.90
renal sclerosis (*see also* Hypertension, cardiorenal)	404.00	404.10	404.90
intracranial, benign	—	348.2	—
intraocular	—	—	365.04
kidney	403.00	403.10	403.90
with			
chronic kidney disease			
stage I through stage IV, or unspecified	403.00	403.10	403.90
stage V or end stage renal disease	403.01	403.11	403.91
heart involvement (conditions classifiable to 429.0-429.3, 429.8, 429.9 due to hypertension) (*see also* Hypertension cardiorenal)	404.00	404.10	404.90
hypertensive heart (disease) (conditions classifiable to 402) (*see also* Hypertension, cardiorenal)	404.00	404.10	404.90
lesser circulation	—	—	416.0
necrotizing	401.0	—	—
ocular	—	—	365.04
pancreatic duct—code to underlying condition			
with chronic pancreatitis	—	—	577.1
portal (due to chronic liver disease)	—	—	572.3
postoperative	—	—	997.91
psychogenic	—	—	306.2
puerperal, postpartum—*see* Hypertension, complicating pregnancy, childbirth, or the puerperium			
pulmonary (artery)	—	—	416.8
idiopathic	—	—	416.0
primary	—	—	416.0
of newborn	—	—	747.83
with cor pulmonale (chronic)	—	—	416.8
acute	—	—	415.0
secondary	—	—	416.8
renal (disease) (*see also* Hypertension, kidney)	403.00	403.10	403.90
renovascular NEC	405.01	405.11	405.91
secondary NEC	405.09	405.19	405.99
due to			
aldosteronism, primary	405.09	405.19	405.99
brain tumor	405.09	405.19	405.99
bulbar poliomyelitis	405.09	405.19	405.99
calculus			
kidney	405.09	405.19	405.99
ureter	405.09	405.19	405.99
coarctation, aorta	405.09	405.19	405.99
Cushing's disease	405.09	405.19	405.99
glomerulosclerosis (*see also* Hypertension, kidney)	403.00	403.10	403.90
periarteritis nodosa	405.09	405.19	405.99
pheochromocytoma	405.09	405.19	405.99
polycystic kidney(s)	405.09	405.19	405.99
polycythemia	405.09	405.19	405.99
porphyria	405.09	405.19	405.99
pyelonephritis	405.09	405.19	405.99
renal (artery)			
aneurysm	405.01	405.11	405.91
anomaly	405.01	405.11	405.91
embolism	405.01	405.11	405.91
fibromuscular hyperplasia	405.01	405.11	405.91
occlusion	405.01	405.11	405.91
stenosis	405.01	405.11	405.91

	Malignant	Benign	Unspecified
thrombosis	405.01	405.11	405.91
transient	—	—	796.2
of pregnancy	—	—	642.3
venous, chronic (asymptomatic) (idiopathic)	—	—	459.30
with			
complication, NEC	—	—	459.39
due to			
deep vein thrombosis (*see also* Syndrome, postphlebetic) .	—	—	459.10
inflammation	—	—	459.32
with ulcer	—	—	459.33
ulcer	—	—	459.31
with inflammation	—	—	459.33

Hyperthecosis, ovary 256.8
Hyperthermia (of unknown origin) (*see also*
    Pyrexia) 780.60
    malignant (due to anesthesia) 995.86
    newborn 778.4
Hyperthymergasia (*see also* Psychosis,
    affective) 296.0
    reactive (from emotional stress, psychological
        trauma) 298.1
    recurrent episode 296.1
    single episode 296.0
Hyperthymism 254.8
Hyperthyroid (recurrent)—*see* Hyperthyroidism
Hyperthyroidism (latent) (preadult) (recurrent)
    (without goiter) 242.9

> *Note—Use the following fifth-digit*
> *subclassification with category 242:*
>
> *0 without mention of thyrotoxic crisis or storm*
> *1 with mention of thyrotoxic crisis or storm*

with
    goiter (diffuse) 242.0
        adenomatous 242.3
            multinodular 242.2
            uninodular 242.1
        nodular 242.3
            multinodular 242.2
            uninodular 242.1
        thyroid nodule 242.1
    complicating pregnancy, childbirth, or
        puerperium 648.1
    neonatal (transient) 775.3
Hypertonia —Hypertonicity
Hypertonicity
    bladder 596.51
    fetus or newborn 779.89
    gastrointestinal (tract) 536.8
    infancy 779.89
        due to electrolyte imbalance 779.89
    muscle 728.85
    stomach 536.8
        psychogenic 306.4
    uterus, uterine (contractions) 661.4
        affecting fetus or newborn 763.7
Hypertony —*see* Hypertonicity
Hypertransaminemia 790.4
Hypertrichosis 704.1
    congenital 757.4
    eyelid 374.54
    lanuginosa 757.4
        acquired 704.1
Hypertriglyceridemia, essential 272.1
Hypertrophy, hypertrophic
    adenoids (infectional) 474.12
        and tonsils (faucial) (infective) (lingual)
            (lymphoid) 474.10
    adrenal 255.8
    alveolar process or ridge 525.8
    anal papillae 569.49
    apocrine gland 705.82
    artery NEC 447.8
        carotid 447.8
        congenital (peripheral) NEC 747.60
        gastrointestinal 747.61
        lower limb 747.64
        renal 747.62
        specified NEC 747.69
        spinal 747.82
    arthritis (chronic) (*see also* Osteoarthrosis) 715.9
    spine (*see also* Spondylosis) 721.90

Hypertrophy, hypertrophic—*continued*
arytenoid 478.79
asymmetrical (heart) 429.9
auricular—*see* Hypertrophy, cardiac
Bartholin's gland 624.8
bile duct 576.8
bladder (sphincter) (trigone) 596.8
blind spot, visual field 368.42
bone 733.99
brain 348.89
breast 611.1
    cystic 610.1
    fetus or newborn 778.7
    fibrocystic 610.1
    massive pubertal 611.1
    puerperal, postpartum 676.3
    senile (parenchymatous) 611.1
cardiac (chronic) (idiopathic) 429.3
    with
        rheumatic fever (conditions classifiable to
            390)
            active 391.8
                with chorea 392.0
            inactive or quiescent (with chorea) 398.99
    congenital NEC 746.89
    fatty (*see also* Degeneration, myocardial)
        429.1
    hypertensive (*see also* Hypertension, heart)
        402.90
    rheumatic (with chorea) 398.99
        active or acute 391.8
            with chorea 392.0
    valve (*see also* Endocarditis) 424.90
        congenital NEC 746.89
cartilage 733.99
cecum 569.89
cervix (uteri) 622.6
    congenital 752.49
    elongation 622.6
clitoris (cirrhotic) 624.2
    congenital 752.49
colon 569.89
    congenital 751.3
conjunctiva, lymphoid 372.73
cornea 371.89
corpora cavernosa 607.89
duodenum 537.89
endometrium (uterus) (*see also* Hyperplasia,
    endometrium) 621.30
    cervix 622.6
epididymis 608.89
esophageal hiatus (congenital) 756.6
    with hernia—*see* Hernia, diaphragm
eyelid 374.30
falx, skull 733.99
fat pad 729.30
    infrapatellar 729.31
    knee 729.31
    orbital 374.34
    popliteal 729.31
    prepatellar 729.31
    retropatellar 729.31
    specified site NEC 729.39
foot (congenital) 755.67
frenum, frenulum (tongue) 529.8
    linguae 529.8
    lip 528.5
gallbladder or cystic duct 575.8
gastric mucosa 535.2
gingiva 523.8

Hypertrophy, hypertrophic—*continued*
gland, glandular (general) NEC 785.6
gum (mucous membrane) 523.8
heart (idiopathic)—*see also* Hypertrophy,
  cardiac
  valve—*see also* Endocarditis
    congenital NEC 746.89
hemifacial 754.0
hepatic—*see* Hypertrophy, liver
hiatus (esophageal) 756.6
hilus gland 785.6
hymen, congenital 752.49
ileum 569.89
infrapatellar fat pad 729.31
intestine 569.89
jejunum 569.89
kidney (compensatory) 593.1
  congenital 753.3
labial frenulum 528.5
labium (majus) (minus) 624.3
lacrimal gland, chronic 375.03
ligament 728.9
  spinal 724.8
linguae frenulum 529.8
lingual tonsil (infectional) 474.11
lip (frenum) 528.5
  congenital 744.81
liver 789.1
  acute 573.8
  cirrhotic—*see* Cirrhosis, liver
  congenital 751.69
  fatty—*see* Fatty, liver
lymph gland 785.6
  tuberculous—*see* Tuberculosis, lymph gland
mammary gland—*see* Hypertrophy, breast
maxillary frenulum 528.5
Meckel's diverticulum (congenital) 751.0
medial meniscus, acquired 717.3
median bar 600.90
  with
    other lower urinary tract symptoms (LUTS)
      600.91
    urinary
      obstruction 600.91
      retention 600.91
mediastinum 519.3
meibomian gland 373.2
meniscus, knee, congenital 755.64
metatarsal head 733.99
metatarsus 733.99
mouth 528.9
mucous membrane
  alveolar process 523.8
  nose 478.19
  turbinate (nasal) 478.0
muscle 728.9
muscular coat, artery NEC 447.8
  carotid 447.8
  renal 447.3
myocardium (*see also* Hypertrophy, cardiac)
  429.3
  idiopathic 425.4
myometrium 621.2
nail 703.8
  congenital 757.5
nasal 478.19
  alae 478.19
  bone 738.0
  cartilage 478.19
  mucous membrane (septum) 478.19
  sinus (*see also* Sinusitis) 473.9

Hypertrophy, hypertrophic—*continued*
nasal—*continued*
  turbinate 478.0
nasopharynx, lymphoid (infectional) (tissue)
  (wall) 478.29
neck, uterus 622.6
nipple 611.1
normal aperture diaphragm (congenital) 756.6
nose (*see also* Hypertrophy, nasal) 478.19
orbit 376.46
organ or site, congenital NEC—*see* Anomaly,
  specified type NEC
osteoarthropathy (pulmonary) 731.2
ovary 620.8
palate (hard) 526.89
  soft 528.9
pancreas (congenital) 751.7
papillae
  anal 569.49
  tongue 529.3
parathyroid (gland) 252.01
parotid gland 527.1
penis 607.89
phallus 607.89
  female (clitoris) 624.2
pharyngeal tonsil 474.12
pharyngitis 472.1
pharynx 478.29
  lymphoid (infectional) (tissue) (wall) 478.29
pituitary (fossa) (gland) 253.8
popliteal fat pad 729.31
preauricular (lymph) gland (Hampstead) 785.6
prepuce (congenital) 605
  female 624.2
prostate (asymptomatic) (early) (recurrent) 600.90
  with
    other lower urinary tract symptoms (LUTS)
      600.91
    urinary
      obstruction 600.91
      retention 600.91
  adenofibromatous 600.20
    with
      other lower urinary tract symptoms
        (LUTS) 600.21
      urinary
        obstruction 600.21
        retention 600.21
  benign 600.00
    with
      other lower urinary tract symptoms
        (LUTS) 600.01
      urinary
        obstruction 600.01
        retention 600.01
  congenital 752.89
psuedoedematous hypodermal 757.0
pseudomuscular 359.1
pylorus (muscle) (sphincter) 537.0
  congenital 750.5
  infantile 750.5
rectal sphincter 569.49
rectum 569.49
renal 593.1
rhinitis (turbinate) 472.0
salivary duct or gland 527.1
  congenital 750.26
scaphoid (tarsal) 733.99
scar 701.4
scrotum 608.89
sella turcica 253.8

Hypertrophy, hypertrophic—*continued*
seminal vesicle 608.89
sigmoid 569.89
skin condition NEC 701.9
spermatic cord 608.89
spinal ligament 724.8
spleen—*see* Splenomegaly
spondylitis (spine) (*see also* Spondylosis) 721.90
stomach 537.89
subaortic stenosis (idiopathic) 425.1
sublingual gland 527.1
  congenital 750.26
submaxillary gland 527.1
suprarenal (gland) 255.8
tendon 727.9
testis 608.89
  congenital 752.89
thymic, thymus (congenital) (gland) 254.0
thyroid (gland) (*see also* Goiter) 240.9
  primary 242.0
  secondary 242.2
toe (congenital) 755.65
  acquired 735.8
tongue 529.8
  congenital 750.15
  frenum 529.8
  papillae (foliate) 529.3
tonsil (faucial) (infective) (lingual) (lymphoid)
  474.11
  and adenoids 474.10
  with
    adenoiditis 474.01
    tonsillitis 474.00
      and adenoiditis 474.02
tunica vaginalis 608.89
turbinate (mucous membrane) 478.0
ureter 593.89
urethra 599.84
uterus 621.2
  puerperal, postpartum 674.8
uvula 528.9
vagina 623.8
vas deferens 608.89
vein 459.89
ventricle, ventricular (heart) (left) (right)—*see
  also* Hypertrophy, cardiac
  congenital 746.89
  due to hypertension (left) (right) (*see also*
    Hypertension, heart) 402.90
    benign 402.10
    malignant 402.00
  right with ventricular septal defect, pulmonary
    stenosis or atresia, and dextraposition of
    aorta 745.2
verumontanum 599.89
vesical 596.8
vocal cord 478.5
vulva 624.3
  stasis (nonfilarial) 624.3
Hypertropia (intermittent) (periodic) 378.31
Hypertyrosinemia 270.2
Hyperuricemia 790.6
Hypervalinemia 270.3
Hyperventilation (tetany) 786.01
hysterical 300.11
psychogenic 306.1
syndrome 306.1
Hyperviscidosis 277.00
Hyperviscosity (of serum) (syndrome) NEC
  273.3
polycythemic 289.0
sclerocythemic 282.8

Hypervitaminosis (dietary) NEC 278.8
A (dietary) 278.2
D (dietary) 278.4
from excessive administration or use of vitamin
  preparations (chronic) 278.8
reaction to sudden overdose 963.5
vitamin A 278.2
  reaction to sudden overdose 963.5
vitamin D 278.4
  reaction to sudden overdose 963.5
vitamin K
  correct substance properly administered 278.8
  overdose or wrong substance given or taken
    964.3
Hypervolemia 276.6
Hypesthesia (*see also* Disturbance, sensation)
  782.0
cornea 371.81
Hyphema (anterior chamber) (ciliary body) (iris)
  364.41
traumatic 921.3
Hyphemia —*see* Hyphema
Hypoacidity, gastric 536.8
psychogenic 306.4
Hypoactive labyrinth (function)—*see*
  Hypofunction, labyrinth
Hypoadrenalism 255.41
tuberculous (*see also* Tuberculosis) 017.6
Hypoadrenocorticism 255.41
pituitary 253.4
Hypoalbuminemia 273.8
Hypoaldosteronism 255.42
Hypoalphalipoproteinemia 272.5
Hypobarism 993.2
Hypobaropathy 993.2
Hypobetalipoproteinemia (familial) 272.5
Hypocalcemia 275.41
cow's milk 775.4
dietary 269.3
neonatal 775.4
phosphate-loading 775.4
Hypocalcification, teeth 520.4
Hypochloremia 276.9
Hypochlorhydria 536.8
neurotic 306.4
psychogenic 306.4
Hypocholesteremia 272.5
Hypochondria (reaction) 300.7
Hypochondriac 300.7
Hypochondriasis 300.7
Hypochromasia blood cells 280.9
Hypochromic anemia 280.9
due to blood loss (chronic) 280.0
  acute 285.1
microcytic 280.9
Hypocoagulability (*see also* Defect, coagulation)
  286.9
Hypocomplementemia 279.8
Hypocythemia (progressive) 284.9
Hypodontia (*see also* Anodontia) 520.0
Hypoeosinophilia 288.59
Hypoesthesia (*see also* Disturbance, sensation)
  782.0
cornea 371.81
tactile 782.0
Hypoestrinism 256.39
Hypoestrogenism 256.39
Hypoferremia 280.9
due to blood loss (chronic) 280.0

Hypofertility
  female 628.9
  male 606.1
Hypofibrinogenemia 286.3
  acquired 286.6
  congenital 286.3
Hypofunction
  adrenal (gland) 255.41
    cortex 255.41
    medulla 255.5
    specified NEC 255.5
  cerebral 331.9
  corticoadrenal NEC 255.41
  intestinal 564.89
  labyrinth (unilateral) 386.53
    with loss of labyrinthine reactivity 386.55
    bilateral 386.54
      with loss of labyrinthine reactivity 386.56
  Leydig cell 257.2
  ovary 256.39
    postablative 256.2
  pituitary (anterior) (gland) (lobe) 253.2
    posterior 253.5
  testicular 257.2
    iatrogenic 257.1
    postablative 257.1
    postirradiation 257.1
    postsurgical 257.1
Hypogammaglobulinemia 279.00
  acquired primary 279.06
  non-sex-linked, congenital 279.06
  sporadic 279.06
  transient of infancy 279.09
Hypogenitalism (congenital) (female) (male)
  752.89
  penis 752.69
Hypoglycemia (spontaneous) 251.2
  coma 251.0
    diabetic 250.3
      due to secondary diabetes 249.3
  diabetic 250.8
    due to secondary diabetes 249.8
  due to insulin 251.0
    therapeutic misadventure 962.3
  familial (idiopathic) 251.2
  following gastrointestinal surgery 579.3
  infantile (idiopathic) 251.2
  in infant of diabetic mother 775.0
  leucine-induced 270.3
  neonatal 775.6
  reactive 251.2
  specified NEC 251.1
Hypoglycemic shock 251.0
  diabetic 250.8
    due to secondary diabetes 249.8
  due to insulin 251.0
  functional (syndrome) 251.1
Hypogonadism
  female 256.39
  gonadotrophic (isolated) 253.4
  hypogonadotropic (isolated) (with anosmia) 253.4
  isolated 253.4
  male 257.2
    hereditary familial (Reifenstein's syndrome)
      259.52
  ovarian (primary) 256.39
  pituitary (secondary) 253.4
  testicular (primary) (secondary) 257.2
Hypohidrosis 705.0
Hypohidrotic ectodermal dysplasia 757.31
Hypoidrosis 705.0

Hypoinsulinemia, postsurgical 251.3
  postpancreatectomy (complete) (partial) 251.3
Hypokalemia 276.8
Hypokinesia 780.99
Hypoleukia splenica 289.4
Hypoleukocytosis 288.50
Hypolipidemia 272.5
Hypolipoproteinemia 272.5
Hypomagnesemia 275.2
  neonatal 775.4
Hypomania, hypomanic reaction (*see also*
    Psychosis, affective) 296.0
  recurrent episode 296.1
  single episode 296.0
Hypomastia (congenital) 611.82
Hypomenorrhea 626.1
Hypometabolism 783.9
Hypomotility
  gastrointestinal tract 536.8
    psychogenic 306.4
  intestine 564.89
    psychogenic 306.4
  stomach 536.8
    psychogenic 306.4
Hyponasality 784.44
Hyponatremia 276.1
Hypo-ovarianism 256.39
Hypo-ovarism 256.39
Hypoparathyroidism (idiopathic) (surgically
    induced) 252.1
  neonatal 775.4
Hypopharyngitis 462
Hypophoria 378.40
Hypophosphatasia 275.3
Hypophosphatemia (acquired) (congenital)
    (familial) 275.3
  renal 275.3
Hypophyseal, hypophysis —*see also* condition
  dwarfism 253.3
  gigantism 253.0
  syndrome 253.8
Hypophyseothalamic syndrome 253.8
Hypopiesis —*see* Hypotension
Hypopigmentation 709.00
  eyelid 374.53
Hypopinealism 259.8
Hypopituitarism (juvenile) (syndrome) 253.2
  due to
    hormone therapy 253.7
    hypophysectomy 253.7
    radiotherapy 253.7
  postablative 253.7
  postpartum hemorrhage 253.2
Hypoplasia, hypoplasis 759.89
  adrenal (gland) 759.1
  alimentary tract 751.8
    lower 751.2
    upper 750.8
  anus, anal (canal) 751.2
  aorta 747.22
  aortic
    arch (tubular) 747.10
    orifice or valve with hypoplasia of ascending
      aorta and defective development of left
      ventricle (with mitral valve atresia) 746.7
  appendix 751.2
  areola 757.6
  arm (*see also* Absence, arm, congenital) 755.20

Hypoplasia, hypoplasis—*continued*
  artery (congenital) (peripheral) NEC 747.60
    brain 747.81
    cerebral 747.81
    coronary 746.85
    gastrointestinal 747.61
    lower limb 747.64
    pulmonary 747.3
    renal 747.62
    retinal 743.58
    specified NEC 747.69
    spinal 747.82
    umbilical 747.5
    upper limb 747.63
  auditory canal 744.29
    causing impairment of hearing 744.02
  biliary duct (common) or passage 751.61
  bladder 753.8
  bone NEC 756.9
    face 756.0
    malar 756.0
    mandible 524.04
      alveolar 524.74
    marrow 284.9
      acquired (secondary) 284.89
      congenital 284.09
      idiopathic 284.9
    maxilla 524.03
      alveolar 524.73
    skull (*see also* Hypoplasia, skull) 756.0
  brain 742.1
    gyri 742.2
    specified part 742.2
  breast (areola) 611.82
  bronchus (tree) 748.3
  cardiac 746.89
    valve—*see* Hypoplasia, heart, valve
    vein 746.89
  carpus (*see also* Absence, carpal, congenital) 755.28
  cartilaginous 756.9
  cecum 751.2
  cementum 520.4
    hereditary 520.5
  cephalic 742.1
  cerebellum 742.2
  cervix (uteri) 752.49
  chin 524.06
  clavicle 755.51
  coccyx 756.19
  colon 751.2
  corpus callosum 742.2
  cricoid cartilage 748.3
  dermal, focal (Goltz) 757.39
  digestive organ(s) or tract NEC 751.8
    lower 751.2
    upper 750.8
  ear 744.29
    auricle 744.23
    lobe 744.29
    middle, except ossicles 744.03
      ossicles 744.04
    ossicles 744.04
  enamel of teeth (neonatal) (postnatal) (prenatal) 520.4
    hereditary 520.5
  endocrine (gland) NEC 759.2
  endometrium 621.8
  epididymis 752.89
  epiglottis 748.3
  erythroid, congenital 284.01

Hypoplasia, hypoplasis—*continued*
  erythropoietic, chronic acquired 284.81
  esophagus 750.3
  Eustachian tube 744.24
  eye (*see also* Microphthalmos) 743.10
    lid 743.62
  face 744.89
    bone(s) 756.0
  fallopian tube 752.19
  femur (*see also* Absence, femur, congenital) 755.34
  fibula (*see also* Absence, fibula, congenital) 755.37
  finger (*see also* Absence, finger, congenital) 755.29
  focal dermal 757.39
  foot 755.31
  gallbladder 751.69
  genitalia, genital organ(s)
    female 752.89
      external 752.49
      internal NEC 752.89
    in adiposogenital dystrophy 253.8
    male 752.89
      penis 752.69
  glottis 748.3
  hair 757.4
  hand 755.21
  heart 746.89
    left (complex) (syndrome) 746.7
    valve NEC 746.89
      pulmonary 746.01
  humerus (*see also* Absence, humerus, congenital) 755.24
  hymen 752.49
  intestine (small) 751.1
    large 751.2
  iris 743.46
  jaw 524.09
  kidney(s) 753.0
  labium (majus) (minus) 752.49
  labyrinth, membranous 744.05
  lacrimal duct (apparatus) 743.65
  larynx 748.3
  leg (*see also* Absence, limb, congenital, lower) 755.30
  limb 755.4
    lower (*see also* Absence, limb, congenital, lower) 755.30
    upper (*see also* Absence, limb, congenital, upper) 755.20
  liver 751.69
  lung (lobe) 748.5
  mammary (areolar) 611.82
  mandibular 524.04
    alveolar 524.74
    unilateral condylar 526.89
  maxillary 524.03
    alveolar 524.73
  medullary 284.9
  megakaryocytic 287.30
  metacarpus (*see also* Absence, metacarpal, congenital) 755.28
  metatarsus (*see also* Absence, metatarsal, congenital) 755.38
  muscle 756.89
    eye 743.69
  myocardium (congenital) (Uhl's anomaly) 746.84
  nail(s) 757.5
  nasolacrimal duct 743.65

Hypoplasia, hypoplasis—*continued*
  nervous system NEC 742.8
  neural 742.8
  nose, nasal 748.1
  ophthalmic (*see also* Microphthalmos) 743.10
  optic nerve 377.43
  organ
    of Corti 744.05
    or site NEC—*see* Anomaly, by site
  osseous meatus (ear) 744.03
  ovary 752.0
  oviduct 752.19
  pancreas 751.7
  parathyroid (gland) 759.2
  parotid gland 750.26
  patella 755.64
  pelvis, pelvic girdle 755.69
  penis 752.69
  peripheral vascular system (congenital) NEC 747.60
    gastrointestinal 747.61
    lower limb 747.64
    renal 747.62
    specified NEC 747.69
    spinal 747.82
    upper limb 747.63
  pituitary (gland) 759.2
  pulmonary 748.5
    arteriovenous 747.3
    artery 747.3
    valve 746.01
  punctum lacrimale 743.65
  radioulnar (*see also* Absence, radius, congenital, with ulna) 755.25
  radius (*see also* Absence, radius, congenital) 755.26
  rectum 751.2
  respiratory system NEC 748.9
  rib 756.3
  sacrum 756.19
  scapula 755.59
  shoulder girdle 755.59
  skin 757.39
  skull (bone) 756.0
    with
      anencephalus 740.0
      encephalocele 742.0
      hydrocephalus 742.3
        with spina bifida (*see also* Spina bifida) 741.0
      microcephalus 742.1
  spinal (cord) (ventral horn cell) 742.59
    vessel 747.82
  spine 756.19
  spleen 759.0
  sternum 756.3
  tarsus (*see also* Absence, tarsal, congenital) 755.38
  testis, testicle 752.89
  thymus (gland) 279.11
  thyroid (gland) 243
    cartilage 748.3
  tibiofibular (*see also* Absence, tibia, congenital, with fibula) 755.35
  toe (*see also* Absence, toe, congenital) 755.39
  tongue 750.16
  trachea (cartilage) (rings) 748.3
  Turner's (tooth) 520.4
  ulna (*see also* Absence, ulna, congenital) 755.27
  umbilical artery 747.5
  ureter 753.29
  uterus 752.3
  vagina 752.49
  vascular (peripheral) NEC (*see also* Hypoplasia, peripheral vascular system) 747.60
    brain 747.81

Hypoplasia, hypoplasis—*continued*
  vein(s) (peripheral) NEC (*see also* Hypoplasia, peripheral vascular system 747.60
    brain 747.81
    cardiac 746.89
    great 747.49
    portal 747.49
    pulmonary 747.49
  vena cava (inferior) (superior) 747.49
  vertebra 756.19
  vulva 752.49
  zonule (ciliary) 743.39
  zygoma 738.12
Hypopotassemia 276.8
Hypoproaccelerinemia (*see also* Defect, coagulation) 286.3
Hypoproconvertinemia (congenital) (*see also* Defect, coagulation) 286.3
Hypoproteinemia (essential) (hypermetabolic) (idiopathic) 273.8
Hypoproteinosis 260
Hypoprothrombinemia (congenital) (hereditary) (idiopathic) (*see also* Defect, coagulation) 286.3
  acquired 286.7
  newborn 776.3
Hypopselaphesia 782.0
Hypopyon (anterior chamber) (eye) 364.05
  iritis 364.05
  ulcer (cornea) 370.04
Hypopyrexia 780.99
Hyporeflex 796.1
Hyporeninemia, extreme 790.99
  in primary aldosteronism 255.10
Hyporesponsive episode 780.09
Hyposecretion
  ACTH 253.4
    ovary 256.39
    postablative 256.2
  salivary gland (any) 527.7
Hyposegmentation of neutrophils, hereditary 288.2
Hyposiderinemia 280.9
Hyposmolality 276.1
  syndrome 276.1
Hyposomatotropism 253.3
Hyposomnia, unspecified (*see also* Insomnia) 780.52
  with sleep apnea, unspecified 780.51
Hypospadias (male) 752.61
  female 753.8
Hypospermatogenesis 606.1
Hyposphagma 372.72
Hyposplenism 289.59
Hypostasis, pulmonary 514
Hypostatic —*see* condition
Hyposthenuria 593.89
Hyposuprarenalism 255.41
Hypo-TBG-nemia 246.8
Hypotension (arterial) (constitutional) 458.9
  chronic 458.1
  iatrogenic 458.29
  maternal, syndrome (following labor and delivery) 669.2
  of hemodialysis 458.21
  orthostatic (chronic) 458.0
    dysautonomic-dyskinetic syndrome 333.0
  permanent idiopathic 458.1
  postoperative 458.29

Hypotension—*continued*
  postural 458.0
  specified type NEC 458.8
  transient 796.3
Hypothermia (accidental) 991.6
  anesthetic 995.89
  associated with low environmental temperature
    991.6
  newborn NEC 778.3
  not associated with low environmental
    temperature 780.65
Hypothymergasia (*see also* Psychosis, affective)
    296.2
  recurrent episode 296.3
  single episode 296.2
Hypothyroidism (acquired) 244.9
  complicating pregnancy, childbirth, or
    puerperium 648.1
  congenital 243
  due to
    ablation 244.1
      radioactive iodine 244.1
      surgical 244.0
    iodine (administration) (ingestion) 244.2
      radioactive 244.1
    irradiation therapy 244.1
    p-aminosalicylic acid (PAS) 244.3
    phenylbutazone 244.3
    resorcinol 244.3
    specified cause NEC 244.8
    surgery 244.0
  goitrous (sporadic) 246.1
  iatrogenic NEC 244.3
  iodine 244.2
  pituitary 244.8
  postablative NEC 244.1
  postsurgical 244.0
  primary 244.9
  secondary NEC 244.8
  specified cause NEC 244.8
  sporadic goitrous 246.1
Hypotonia, hypotonicity, hypotony 781.3
  benign congenital 358.8
  bladder 596.4
  congenital 779.89
    benign 358.8
  eye 360.30
    due to
      fistula 360.32
      ocular disorder NEC 360.33
    following loss of aqueous or vitreous 360.33
    primary 360.31
  infantile muscular (benign) 359.0
  muscle 728.9
  uterus, uterine (contractions)—*see* Inertia,
    uterus
Hypotrichosis 704.09
  congenital 757.4
  lid (congenital) 757.4
    acquired 374.55
  postinfectional NEC 704.09
Hypotropia 378.32
Hypoventilation 786.09
  congenital central alveolar syndrome 327.25
  idiopathic sleep related nonobstructive alveolar
    327.24
  sleep related, in conditions classifiable
    elsewhere 327.26
Hypovitaminosis (*see also* Deficiency, vitamin)
    269.2

Hypovolemia 276.52
  surgical shock 998.0
  traumatic (shock) 958.4
Hypoxemia (*see also* Anoxia) 799.02
  sleep related, in conditions classifiable
    elsewhere 327.26
Hypoxia (*see also* Anoxia) 799.02
  cerebral 348.1
    during or resulting from a procedure 997.01
    newborn 770.88
      mild or moderate 768.6
      severe 768.5
  fetal, affecting newborn 770.88
  intrauterine—*see* Distress, fetal
  myocardial (*see also* Insufficiency, coronary)
    411.89
    arteriosclerotic —*see* Arteriosclerosis,
      coronary
  newborn 770.88
  sleep related 327.24
Hypoxic-ischemic encephalopathy (HIE) 768.70
  mild 768.71
  moderate 768.72
  severe 768.73
Hypsarrhythmia (*see also* Epilepsy) 345.6
Hysteralgia, pregnant uterus 646.8
Hysteria, hysterical 300.10
  anxiety 300.20
  Charcot's gland 300.11
  conversion (any manifestation) 300.11
  dissociative type NEC 300.15
  psychosis, acute 298.1
Hysteroepilepsy 300.11
Hysterotomy, affecting fetus or newborn
    763.89

I

Iatrogenic syndrome of excess cortisol 255.0
IBM (inclusion body myositis) 359.71
Iceland disease (epidemic neuromyasthenia) 049.8
Ichthyosis (congenita) 757.1
  acquired 701.1
  fetalis gravior 757.1
  follicularis 757.1
  hystrix 757.39
  lamellar 757.1
  lingual 528.6
  palmaris and plantaris 757.39
  simplex 757.1
  vera 757.1
  vulgaris 757.1
Ichthyotoxism 988.0
  bacterial (*see also* Poisoning, food) 005.9
Icteroanemia, hemolytic (acquired) 283.9
  congenital (*see also* Spherocytosis) 282.0
Icterus (*see also* Jaundice) 782.4
  catarrhal—*see* Icterus, infectious
  conjunctiva 782.4
    newborn 774.6
  epidemic—*see* Icterus, infectious
  febrilis—*see* Icterus, infectious
  fetus or newborn—*see* Jaundice, fetus or newborn
  gravis (*see also* Necrosis, liver) 570
    complicating pregnancy 646.7
      affecting fetus or newborn 760.8
    fetus or newborn NEC 773.0
    obstetrical 646.7
      affecting fetus or newborn 760.8
  hematogenous (acquired) 283.9
  hemolytic (acquired) 283.9
    congenital (*see also* Spherocytosis) 282.0
  hemorrhagic (acute) 100.0
    leptospiral 100.0
    newborn 776.0
    spirochetal 100.0
  infectious 070.1
    with hepatic coma 070.0
    leptospiral 100.0
    spirochetal 100.0
  intermittens juvenilis 277.4
  malignant (*see also* Necrosis, liver) 570
  neonatorum (*see also* Jaundice, fetus or
    newborn) 774.6
  pernicious (*see also* Necrosis, liver) 570
  spirochetal 100.0
Ictus solaris, solis 992.0
Ideation
  suicidal V62.84
Identity disorder 313.82
  dissociative 300.14
  gender role (child) 302.6
    adult 302.85
  psychosexual (child) 302.6
    adult 302.85
Idioglossia 307.9
Idiopathic —*see* condition
Idiosyncrasy (*see also* Allergy) 995.3
  drug, medicinal substance, and biological—*see*
    Allergy, drug

Idiot, idiocy (congenital) 318.2
  amaurotic (Bielschowsky) (-Jansky) (family)
    (infantile (late)) (juvenile (late))
    (Vogt-Spielmeyer) 330.1
  microcephalic 742.1
  Mongolian 758.0
  oxycephalic 756.0
Id reaction (due to bacteria) 692.89
**IEED (involuntary emotional expression
  disorder)** 310.8
IFIS (intraoperative floppy iris syndrome)
  364.81
IgE asthma 493.0
Ileitis (chronic) (*see also* Enteritis) 558.9
  infectious 009.0
  noninfectious 558.9
  regional (ulcerative) 555.0
    with large intestine 555.2
  segmental 555.0
    with large intestine 555.2
  terminal (ulcerative) 555.0
    with large intestine 555.2
Ileocolitis (*see also* Enteritis) 558.9
  infectious 009.0
  regional 555.2
  ulcerative 556.1
Ileostomy status V44.2
  with complication 569.60
Ileotyphus 002.0
Ileum —*see* condition
Ileus (adynamic) (bowel) (colon) (inhibitory)
  (intestine) (neurogenic) (paralytic) 560.1
  arteriomesenteric duodenal 537.2
  due to gallstone (in intestine) 560.31
  duodenal, chronic 537.2
  following gastrointestinal surgery 997.4
  gallstone 560.31
  mechanical (*see also* Obstruction, intestine) 560.9
  meconium 777.1
    due to cystic fibrosis 277.01
  myxedema 564.89
  postoperative 997.4
  transitory, newborn 777.4
Iliac —*see* condition
Iliotibial band friction syndrome 728.89
Ill, louping 063.1
Illegitimacy V61.6
Illness —*see also* Disease
  factitious 300.19
    with
      combined psychological and physical signs
        and symptoms 300.19
      physical symptoms 300.19
      predominantly
        physical signs and symptoms 300.19
        psychological symptoms 300.16
    chronic (with physical symptoms) 301.51
  heart—*see* Disease, heart
  manic-depressive (*see also* Psychosis, affective)
    296.80
  mental (*see also* Disorder, mental) 300.9
Imbalance 781.2
  autonomic (*see also* Neuropathy, peripheral,
    autonomic) 337.9

Imbalance—*continued*
  electrolyte 276.9
    with
      abortion—*see* Abortion, by type, with
        metabolic disorder
      ectopic pregnancy (*see also* categories
        633.0-633.9) 639.4
      hyperemesis gravidarum (before 22
        completed weeks gestation) 643.1
      molar pregnancy (*see also* categories
        630-632) 639.4
    following
      abortion 639.4
      ectopic or molar pregnancy 639.4
    neonatal, transitory NEC 775.5
  endocrine 259.9
  eye muscle NEC 378.9
    heterophoria—*see* Heterophoria
  glomerulotubular NEC 593.89
  hormone 259.9
  hysterical (*see also* Hysteria) 300.10
  labyrinth NEC 386.50
  posture 729.90
  sympathetic (*see also* Neuropathy, peripheral,
    autonomic) 337.9
Imbecile, imbecility 318.0
  moral 301.7
  old age 290.9
  senile 290.9
  specified IQ—*see* IQ
  unspecified IQ 318.0
Imbedding, intrauterine device 996.32
Imbibition, cholesterol (gallbladder) 575.6
Imerslund (-Gräsbeck) syndrome (anemia due to
  familial selective vitamin B$_{12}$ malabsorption)
  281.1
Iminoacidopathy 270.8
Iminoglycinuria, familial 270.8
Immature —*see also* Immaturity
  personality 301.89
Immaturity 765.1
  extreme 765.0
  fetus or infant light-for-dates—*see*
    Light-for-dates
  lung, fetus or newborn 770.4
  organ or site NEC—*see* Hypoplasia
  pulmonary, fetus or newborn 770.4
  reaction 301.89
  sexual (female) (male) 259.0
Immersion 994.1
  foot 991.4
  hand 991.4
Immobile, immobility
  complete
    due to severe physical disability or frality
      780.72
  intestine 564.89
  joint—*see* Ankylosis
  syndrome (paraplegic) 728.3
Immunization
  ABO
    affecting management of pregnancy 656.2
      fetus or newborn 773.1
  complication—*see* Complications, vaccination
  Rh factor
    affecting management of pregnancy 656.1
      fetus or newborn 773.0
    from transfusion 999.7

Immunodeficiency 279.3
  with
    adenosine-deaminase deficiency 279.2
    defect, predominant
      B-cell 279.00
      T-cell 279.10
    hyperimmunoglobulinemia 279.2
    lymphopenia, hereditary 279.2
    thrombocytopenia and eczema 279.12
    thymic
      aplasia 279.2
      dysplasia 279.2
  autosomal recessive, Swiss-type 279.2
  common variable 279.06
  severe combined (SCID) 279.2
  to Rh factor
    affecting management of pregnancy 656.1
    fetus or newborn 773.0
  X-linked, with increased IgM 279.05
Immunotherapy, prophylactic V07.2
  antineoplastic V58.12
Impaction, impacted
  bowel, colon, rectum 560.30
    with hernia—*see also* Hernia, by site, with
      obstruction
      gangrenous—*see* Hernia, by site, with
        gangrene
    by
      calculus 560.39
      gallstone 560.31
    fecal 560.39
    specified type NEC 560.39
  calculus—*see* Calculus
  cerumen (ear) (external) 380.4
  cuspid 520.6
  dental 520.6
  fecal, feces 560.39
    with hernia—*see also* Hernia, by site, with
      obstruction
      gangrenous—*see* Hernia, by site, with
        gangrene
  fracture—*see* Fracture, by site
  gallbladder—*see* Cholelithiasis
  gallstone(s)—*see* Cholelithiasis
    in intestine (any part) 560.31
  intestine(s) 560.30
    with hernia—*see also* Hernia, by site, with
      obstruction
      gangrenous—*see* Hernia, by site, with
        gangrene
    by
      calculus 560.39
      gallstone 560.31
    fecal 560.39
    specified type NEC 560.39
  intrauterine device (IUD) 996.32
  molar 520.6
  shoulder 660.4
    affecting fetus or newborn 763.1
  tooth, teeth 520.6
  turbinate 733.99
Impaired, impairment (function)
  arm V49.1
    movement, involving
      musculoskeletal system V49.1
      nervous system V49.2
  auditory discrimination 388.43
  back V48.3
  body (entire) V49.89
  cognitive, mild, so stated 331.83
  combined visual hearing V49.85

Impaired, impairment—*continued*
dual sensory V49.85
glucose
  fasting 790.21
  tolerance test (oral) 790.22
hearing (*see also* Deafness) 389.9
  combined with visual impairment V49.85
heart—*see* Disease, heart
kidney (*see also* Disease, renal) 593.9
  disorder resulting from 588.9
   specified NEC 588.89
leg V49.1
  movement, involving
   musculoskeletal system V49.1
   nervous system V49.2
limb V49.1
  movement, involving
   musculoskeletal system V49.1
   nervous system V49.2
liver 573.8
mastication 524.9
mild cognitive, so stated 331.83
mobility
  ear ossicles NEC 385.22
  incostapedial joint 385.22
  malleus 385.21
myocardium, myocardial (*see also*
  Insufficiency, myocardial) 428.0
neuromusculoskeletal NEC V49.89
  back V48.3
  head V48.2
  limb V49.2
  neck V48.3
  spine V48.3
  trunk V48.3
rectal sphincter 787.99
renal (*see also* Disease, renal) 593.9
  disorder resulting from 588.9
   specified NEC 588.89
spine V48.3
vision NEC 369.9
  both eyes NEC 369.3
  combined with hearing impairment V49.85
  moderate 369.74
   both eyes 369.25
    with impairment of lesser eye (specified
     as)
     blind, not further specified 369.15
     low vision, not further specified 369.23
     near-total 369.17
     profound 369.18
     severe 369.24
     total 369.16
   one eye 369.74
    with vision of other eye (specified as)
     near-normal 369.75
     normal 369.76
  near-total 369.64
   both eyes 369.04
    with impairment of lesser eye (specified
     as)
     blind, not further specified 369.02
     total 369.03
   one eye 369.64
    with vision of other eye (specified as)
     near-normal 369.65
     normal 369.66
  one eye 369.60
   with low vision of other eye 369.10

Impaired, impairment—*continued*
vision—*continued*
  profound 369.67
   both eyes 369.08
    with impairment of lesser eye (specified
     as)
     blind, not further specified 369.05
     near-total 369.07
     total 369.06
   one eye 369.67
    with vision of other eye (specified as)
     near-normal 369.68
     normal 369.69
  severe 369.71
   both eyes 369.22
    with impairment of lesser eye (specified as)
     blind, not further specified 369.11
     low vision, not further specified 369.21
     near-total 369.13
     profound 369.14
     total 369.12
   one eye 369.71
    with vision of other eye (specified as)
     near-normal 369.72
     normal 369.73
  total
   both eyes 369.01
   one eye 369.61
    with vision of other eye (specified as)
     near-normal 369.62
     normal 369.63
Impaludism —*see* Malaria
Impediment, speech NEC 784.59
psychogenic 307.9
secondary to organic lesion 784.59
Impending
cerebrovascular accident or attack 435.9
coronary syndrome 411.1
delirium tremens 291.0
myocardial infarction 411.1
Imperception, auditory (acquired) (congenital)
389.9
Imperfect
aeration, lung (newborn) 770.5
closure (congenital)
  alimentary tract NEC 751.8
   lower 751.5
   upper 750.8
  atrioventricular ostium 745.69
  atrium (secundum) 745.5
   primum 745.61
  branchial cleft or sinus 744.41
  choroid 743.59
  cricoid cartilage 748.3
  cusps, heart valve NEC 746.89
   pulmonary 746.09
  ductus
   arteriosus 747.0
   Botalli 747.0
  ear drum 744.29
   causing impairment of hearing 744.03
  endocardial cushion 745.60
  epiglottis 748.3
  esophagus with communication to bronchus or
   trachea 750.3
  Eustachian valve 746.89
  eyelid 743.62
  face, facial (*see also* Cleft, lip) 749.10
  foramen
   Botalli 745.5
   ovale 745.5

Imperfect—*continued*
  closure (congenital)—*continued*
    genitalia, genital organ(s) or system
      female 752.89
        external 752.49
        internal NEC 752.89
        uterus 752.3
      male 752.89
        penis 752.69
    glottis 748.3
    heart valve (cusps) NEC 746.89
    interatrial ostium or septum 745.5
    interauricular ostium or septum 745.5
    interventricular ostium or septum 745.4
    iris 743.46
    kidney 753.3
    larynx 748.3
    lens 743.36
    lip (*see also* Cleft, lip) 749.10
    nasal septum or sinus 748.1
    nose 748.1
    omphalomesenteric duct 751.0
    optic nerve entry 743.57
    organ or site NEC—*see* Anomaly, specified
      type, by site
    ostium
      interatrial 745.5
      interauricular 745.5
      interventricular 745.4
    palate (*see also* Cleft, palate) 749.00
    preauricular sinus 744.46
    retina 743.56
    roof of orbit 742.0
    sclera 743.47
    septum
      aortic 745.0
      aorticopulmonary 745.0
      atrial (secundum) 745.5
        primum 745.61
      between aorta and pulmonary artery 745.0
      heart 745.9
      interatrial (secundum) 745.5
        primum 745.61
      interauricular (secundum) 745.5
        primum 745.61
      interventricular 745.4
        with pulmonary stenosis or atresia,
          dextraposition of aorta, and
          hypertrophy of right ventricle 745.2
        in tetralogy of Fallot 745.2
      nasal 748.1
      ventricular 745.4
        with pulmonary stenosis or atresia,
          dextraposition of aorta, and
          hypertrophy of right ventricle 745.2
        in tetralogy of Fallot 745.2
    skull 756.0
      with
        anencephalus 740.0
        encephalocele 742.0
        hydrocephalus 742.3
          with spina bifida (*see also* Spina bifida)
            741.0
        microcephalus 742.1
      spine (with meningocele) (*see also* Spina
        bifida) 741.90
    thyroid cartilage 748.3
    trachea 748.3
    tympanic membrane 744.29
      causing impairment of hearing 744.03
    uterus (with communication to bladder,
      intestine, or rectum) 752.3

Imperfect—*continued*
  closure (congenital)—*continued*
    uvula 749.02
      with cleft lip (*see also* Cleft, palate, with
        cleft lip) 749.20
    vitelline duct 751.0
  development—*see* Anomaly, by site
  erection 607.84
  fusion—*see* Imperfect, closure
  inflation lung (newborn) 770.5
  intestinal canal 751.5
  poise 729.90
  rotation—*see* Malrotation
  septum, ventricular 745.4
Imperfectly descended testis 752.51
Imperforate (congenital)—*see also* Atresia
  anus 751.2
  bile duct 751.61
  cervix (uteri) 752.49
  esophagus 750.3
  hymen 752.42
  intestine (small) 751.1
    large 751.2
  jejunum 751.1
  pharynx 750.29
  rectum 751.2
  salivary duct 750.23
  urethra 753.6
  urinary meatus 753.6
  vagina 752.49
Impervious (congenital)—*see also* Atresia
  anus 751.2
  bile duct 751.61
  esophagus 750.3
  intestine (small) 751.1
    large 751.5
  rectum 751.2
  urethra 753.6
Impetiginization of other dermatoses 684
Impetigo (any organism) (any site) (bullous)
    (circinate) (contagiosa) (neonatorum)
    (simplex) 684
  Bockhart's (superficial folliculitis) 704.8
  external ear 684 *[380.13]*
  eyelid 684 *[373.5]*
  Fox's (contagiosa) 684
  furfuracea 696.5
  herpetiformis 694.3
    nonobstetrical 694.3
  staphylococcal infection 684
  ulcerative 686.8
  vulgaris 684
Impingement, soft tissue between teeth 524.89
  anterior 524.81
  posterior 524.82
Implant, endometrial 617.9
Implantation
  anomalous—*see also* Anomaly, specified type,
    by site
    ureter 753.4
  cyst
    external area or site (skin) NEC 709.8
    iris 364.61
    vagina 623.8
    vulva 624.8
  dermoid (cyst)
    external area or site (skin) NEC 709.8
    iris 364.61
    vagina 623.8
    vulva 624.8
  placenta, low or marginal—*see* Placenta previa

Impotence (sexual) 607.84
  organic origin NEC 607.84
  psychogenic 302.72
Impoverished blood 285.9
Impression, basilar 756.0
Imprisonment V62.5
Improper
  development, infant 764.9
Improperly tied umbilical cord (causing
  hemorrhage) 772.3
Impulses, obsessional 300.3
Impulsive 799.23
  neurosis 300.3
Impulsiveness 799.23
Inaction, kidney (*see also* Disease, renal) 593.9
Inactive —*see* condition
Inadequate, inadequacy
  aesthetics of dental restoration 525.67
  biologic 301.6
  cardiac and renal—*see* Hypertension, cardiorenal
  constitutional 301.6
  development
    child 783.40
    fetus 764.9
      affecting management of pregnancy 656.5
    genitalia
      after puberty NEC 259.0
      congenital—*see* Hypoplasia, genitalia
    lungs 748.5
    organ or site NEC—*see* Hypoplasia, by site
  dietary 269.9
  distance, interarch 524.28
  education V62.3
  environment
    economic problem V60.2
    household condition NEC V60.1
    poverty V60.2
    unemployment V62.0
  functional 301.6
  household care, due to
    family member
      handicapped or ill V60.4
      temporarily away from home V60.4
        on vacation V60.5
    technical defects in home V60.1
    temporary absence from home of person
      rendering care V60.4
  housing (heating) (space) V60.1
  interarch distance 524.28
  material resources V60.2
  mental (*see also* Retardation, mental) 319
  nervous system 799.29
  personality 301.6
  prenatal care in current pregnancy V23.7
  pulmonary
    function 786.09
      newborn 770.89
    ventilation, newborn 770.89
  respiration 786.09
    newborn 770.89
  sample
    cytology
      anal 796.78
      cervical 795.08
      vaginal 795.18
  social 301.6
Inanition 263.9
  with edema 262
  due to
    deprivation of food 994.2
    malnutrition 263.9
  fever 780.60

Inappropriate secretion
  ACTH 255.0
  antidiuretic hormone (ADH) (excessive) 253.6
    deficiency 253.5
  ectopic hormone NEC 259.3
  pituitary (posterior) 253.6
Inattention after or at birth 995.52
Inborn errors of metabolism —*see* Disorder,
  metabolism
Incarceration, incarcerated
  bubonocele—*see also* Hernia, inguinal, with
    obstruction
    gangrenous—*see* Hernia, inguinal, with
      gangrene
  colon (by hernia)—*see also* Hernia, by site, with
    obstruction
    gangrenous—*see* Hernia, by site, with
      gangrene
  enterocele 552.9
    gangrenous 551.9
  epigastrocele 552.29
    gangrenous 551.29
  epiplocele 552.9
    gangrenous 551.9
  exomphalos 552.1
    gangrenous 551.1
  fallopian tube 620.8
  hernia—*see also* Hernia, by site, with
    obstruction
    gangrenous—*see* Hernia, by site, with
      gangrene
  iris, in wound 871.1
  lens, in wound 871.1
  merocele (*see also* Hernia, femoral, with
    obstruction) 552.00
  Omentum (by hernia)—*see also* Hernia, by site,
    with obstruction
    gangrenous—*see* Hernia, by site, with
      gangrene
  omphalocele 756.72
  rupture (meaning hernia) (*see also* Hernia, by
    site, with obstruction) 552.9
    gangrenous (*see also* Hernia, by site, with
      gangrene) 551.9
  sarcoepiplocele 552.9
    gangrenous 551.9
  sarcoepiplomphalocele 552.1
    with gangrene 551.1
  uterus 621.8
    gravid 654.3
      causing obstructed labor 660.2
        affecting fetus or newborn 763.1
Incident, cerebrovascular (*see also* Disease,
  cerebrovascular, acute) 436
Incineration (entire body) (from fire,
  conflagration, electricity, or lightning)—*see*
  Burn, multiple, specified sites
Incised wound
  external—*see* Wound, open, by site
  internal organs (abdomen, chest, or pelvis)—*see*
    Injury, internal, by site, with open wound
Incision, incisional
  hernia—*see* Hernia, incisional
  surgical, complication—*see* Complications,
    surgical procedures
  traumatic
    external—*see* Wound, open, by site
    internal organs (abdomen, chest or
      pelvis)—*see* Injury, internal, by site, with
      open wound

Inclusion
azurophilic leukocytic 288.2
blennorrhea (neonatal) (newborn) 771.6
cyst—*see* Cyst, skin
gallbladder in liver (congenital) 751.69
Incompatibility
ABO
  affecting management of pregnancy 656.2
  fetus or newborn 773.1
  infusion or transfusion reaction 999.6
blood (group) (Duffy) (E) (K(ell)) (Kidd)
    (Lewis) (M) (N) (P) (S) NEC
  affecting management of pregnancy 656.2
  fetus or newborn 773.2
  infusion or transfusion reaction 999.89
contour of existing restoration of tooth
    with oral health 525.65
marital V61.10
  involving
    divorce V61.03
    estrangement V61.09
Rh (blood group) (factor)
  affecting management of pregnancy 656.1
  fetus or newborn 773.0
  infusion or transfusion reaction 999.7
Rhesus—*see* Incompatibility, Rh
Incompetency, incompetence, incompetent
annular
  aortic (valve) (*see also* Insufficiency, aortic)
      424.1
  mitral (valve)—(*see also* Insufficiency, mitral)
      424.0
  pulmonary valve (heart) (*see also*
      Endocarditis, pulmonary) 424.3
aortic (valve) (*see also* Insufficiency, aortic)
    424.1
  syphilitic 093.22
cardiac (orifice) 530.0
  valve—*see* Endocarditis
cervix, cervical (os) 622.5
  in pregnancy 654.5
    affecting fetus or newborn 761.0
chronotropic 426.89
  with
    autonomic dysfunction 337.9
    ischemic heart disease 414.9
    left ventricular dysfunction 429.89
    sinus node dysfunction 427.81
esophagogastric (junction) (sphincter) 530.0
heart valve, congenital 746.89
mitral (valve)—*see* Insufficiency, mitral
papillary muscle (heart) 429.81
pelvic fundus
  pubocervical tissue 618.81
  rectovaginal tissue 618.82
pulmonary valve (heart) (*see also* Endocarditis,
    pulmonary) 424.3
  congenital 746.09
tricuspid (annular) (rheumatic) (valve) (*see also*
    Endocarditis, tricuspid) 397.0
valvular—*see* Endocarditis
vein, venous (saphenous) (varicose) (*see also*
    Varicose, vein) 454.9
velopharyngeal (closure)
  acquired 528.9
  congenital 750.29
Incomplete —*see also* condition
bladder emptying 788.21
expansion lungs (newborn) 770.5
gestation (liveborn)—*see* Immaturity
rotation—*see* Malrotation

Inconclusive
image test due to excess body fat 793.91
mammogram, mammography 793.82
  due to dense breasts 793.82
Incontinence 788.30
without sensory awareness 788.34
anal sphincter 787.6
continuous leakage 788.37
feces 787.6
  due to hysteria 300.11
  nonorganic origin 307.7
hysterical 300.11
mixed (male) (female) (urge and stress) 788.33
overflow 788.38
paradoxical 788.39
rectal 787.6
specified NEC 788.39
stress (female) 625.6
  male NEC 788.32
urethral sphincter 599.84
urge 788.31
  and stress (male) (female) 788.33
urine 788.30
  active 788.30
  due to
    cognitive impairment 788.91
    severe physical disability 788.91
    immobility 788.91
  functional 788.91
  male 788.30
    stress 788.32
      and urge 788.33
  neurogenic 788.39
  nonorganic origin 307.6
  stress (female) 625.6
    male NEC 788.32
  urge 788.31
    and stress 788.33
Incontinentia pigmenti 757.33
Incoordinate
uterus (action) (contractions) 661.4
  affecting fetus or newborn 763.7
Incoordination
esophageal-pharyngeal (newborn) 787.24
muscular 781.3
papillary muscle 429.81
Increase, increased
abnormal, in development 783.9
androgens (ovarian) 256.1
anticoagulants (antithrombin) (anti-VIIIa)
    (anti-IXa) (anti-Xa) (anti-XIa) 286.5
  postpartum 666.3
cold sense (*see also* Disturbance, sensation)
    782.0
estrogen 256.0
function
  adrenal (cortex) 255.3
    medulla 255.6
  pituitary (anterior) (gland) (lobe) 253.1
    posterior 253.6
heat sense (*see also* Disturbance, sensation) 782.0
intracranial pressure 781.99
  injury at birth 767.8
light reflex of retina 362.13
permeability, capillary 448.9
pressure
  intracranial 781.99
    injury at birth 767.8
  intraocular 365.00
pulsations 785.9
pulse pressure 785.9
sphericity, lens 743.36

Increase, increased—*continued*
  splenic activity 289.4
  venous pressure 459.89
    portal 572.3
Incrustation, cornea, lead or zinc 930.0
Incyclophoria 378.44
Incyclotropia 378.33
Indeterminate sex 752.7
India rubber skin 756.83
Indicanuria 270.2
Indigestion (bilious) (functional) 536.8
  acid 536.8
  catarrhal 536.8
  due to decomposed food NEC 005.9
  fat 579.8
  nervous 306.4
  psychogenic 306.4
Indirect —*see* condition
Indolent bubo NEC 099.8
Induced
  abortion—*see* Abortion, induced
  birth, affecting fetus or newborn 763.89
  delivery—*see* Delivery
  labor—*see* Delivery
Induration, indurated
  brain 348.89
  breast (fibrous) 611.79
    puerperal, postpartum 676.3
  broad ligament 620.8
  chancre 091.0
    anus 091.1
    congenital 090.0
    extragenital NEC 091.2
  corpora cavernosa (penis) (plastic) 607.89
  liver (chronic) 573.8
    acute 573.8
  lung (black) (brown) (chronic) (fibroid) (*see
    also* Fibrosis, lung) 515
    essential brown 275.0 [516.1]
  penile 607.89
  phlebitic—*see* Phlebitis
  skin 782.8
  stomach 537.89
Induratio penis plastica 607.89
Industrial —*see* condition
Inebriety (*see also* Abuse, drugs, nondependent)
    305.0
Inefficiency
  kidney (*see also* Disease, renal) 593.9
  thyroid (acquired) (gland) 244.9
Inelasticity, skin 782.8
Inequality, leg (acquired) (length) 736.81
  congenital 755.30
Inertia
  bladder 596.4
    neurogenic 596.54
      with cauda equina syndrome 344.61
  stomach 536.8
    psychogenic 306.4
  uterus, uterine 661.2
    affecting fetus or newborn 763.7
    primary 661.0
    secondary 661.1
  vesical 596.4
    neurogenic 596.54
      with cauda equina 344.61
Infant —*see also* condition
  excessive crying of 780.92
  fussy (baby) 780.91
  held for adoption V68.89
  newborn—*see* Newborn

Infant—*continued*
  post-term (gestation period over 40 completed
    weeks to 42 completed weeks) 766.21
  prolonged gestation of (period over 42
    completed weeks) 766.22
  syndrome of diabetic mother 775.0
"Infant Hercules" syndrome 255.2
Infantile —*see also* condition
  genitalia, genitals 259.0
    in pregnancy or childbirth NEC 654.4
      affecting fetus or newborn 763.89
      causing obstructed labor 660.2
        affecting fetus or newborn 763.1
  heart 746.9
  kidney 753.3
  lack of care 995.52
  macula degeneration 362.75
  melanodontia 521.05
  os, uterus (*see also* Infantile, genitalia) 259.0
  pelvis 738.6
    with disproportion (fetopelvic) 653.1
      affecting fetus or newborn 763.1
      causing obstructed labor 660.1
        affecting fetus or newborn 763.1
  penis 259.0
  testis 257.2
  uterus (*see also* Infantile, genitalia) 259.0
  vulva 752.49
Infantilism 259.9
  with dwarfism (hypophyseal) 253.3
  Brissaud's (infantile myxedema) 244.9
  celiac 579.0
  Herter's (nontropical sprue) 579.0
  hypophyseal 253.3
  hypothalamic (with obesity) 253.8
  idiopathic 259.9
  intestinal 579.0
  pancreatic 577.8
  pituitary 253.3
  renal 588.0
  sexual (with obesity) 259.0
Infants, healthy liveborn —*see* Newborn
Infarct, infarction
  adrenal (capsule) (gland) 255.41
  amnion 658.8
  anterior (with contiguous portion of
    intraventricular septum) NEC (*see also*
    Infarct, myocardium) 410.1
  appendices epiploicae 557.0
  bowel 557.0
  brain (stem) 434.91
    embolic (*see also* Embolism, brain) 434.11
    healed or old, without residuals V12.54
    iatrogenic 997.02
    postoperative 997.02
    puerperal, postpartum, childbirth 674.0
    thrombotic (*see also* Thrombosis, brain)
      434.01
  breast 611.89
  Brewer's (kidney) 593.81
  cardiac (*see also* Infarct, myocardium) 410.9
  cerebellar (*see also* Infarct, brain) 434.91
    embolic (*see also* Embolism, brain) 434.11
  cerebral (*see also* Infarct, brain) 434.91
    aborted 434.91
    embolic (*see also* Embolism, brain) 434.11
    thrombotic (*see also* Infarct, brain) 434.01
  chorion 658.8
  colon (acute) (agnogenic) (embolic)
    (hemorrhagic) (nonocclusive)
    (nonthrombotic) (occlusive) (segmental)
    (thrombotic) (with gangrene) 557.0

Infarct, infarction—*continued*
coronary artery (*see also* Infarct, myocardium)
  410.9
cortical 434.91
embolic (*see also* Embolism) 444.9
fallopian tube 620.8
gallbladder 575.8
heart (*see also* Infarct, myocardium) 410.9
hepatic 573.4
hypophysis (anterior lobe) 253.8
impending (myocardium) 411.1
intestine (acute) (agnogenic) (embolic)
    (hemorrhagic) (nonocclusive)
    (nonthrombotic) (occlusive) (thrombotic)
    (with gangrene) 557.0
kidney 593.81
liver 573.4
lung (embolic) (thrombotic) 415.19
  with
    abortion—*see* Abortion, by type, with,
      embolism
    ectopic pregnancy (*see also* categories
      633.0-633.9) 639.6
    molar pregnancy (*see also* categories
      630-632) 639.6
  following
    abortion 639.6
    ectopic or molar pregnancy 639.6
  iatrogenic 415.11
  in pregnancy, childbirth, or puerperium—*see*
    Embolism, obstetrical
  postoperative 415.11
  septic 415.12
lymph node or vessel 457.8
medullary (brain)—*see* Infarct, brain
meibomian gland (eyelid) 374.85
mesentery, mesenteric (embolic) (thrombotic)
    (with gangrene) 557.0
midbrain—*see* Infarct, brain
myocardium, myocardial (acute or with a stated
    duration of 8 weeks or less) (with
    hypertension) 410.9

Note—use the following fifth-digit
subclassification with category 410

0 episode unspecified
1 initial episode
2 subsequent episode without recurrence

  with symptoms after 8 weeks from date of
    infarction 414.8
  anterior (wall) (with contiguous portion of
    intraventricular septum) NEC 410.1
  anteroapical (with contiguous portion of
    intraventricular septum) 410.1
  anterolateral (wall) 410.0
  anteroseptal (with contiguous portion of
    intraventricular septum) 410.1
  apical-lateral 410.5
  atrial 410.8
  basal-lateral 410.5
  chronic (with symptoms after 8 weeks from
    date of infarction) 414.8
  diagnosed on ECG, but presenting no
    symptoms 412
  diaphragmatic wall (with contiguous portion
    of intraventricular septum) 410.4
  healed or old, currently presenting no
    symptoms 412
  high lateral 410.5
  impending 411.1

Infarct, infarction—*continued*
  myocardium—*continued*
    inferior (wall) (with contiguous portion of
      intraventricular septum) 410.4
    inferolateral (wall) 410.2
    inferoposterior wall 410.3
    intraoperative 997.1
    lateral wall 410.5
    non-Q wave 410.7
    non-ST elevation (NSTEMI) 410.7
    nontransmural 410.7
    papillary muscle 410.8
    past (diagnosed on ECG or other special
      investigation, but currently presenting no
      symptoms) 412
      with symptoms NEC 414.8
    posterior (strictly) (true) (wall) 410.6
    posterobasal 410.6
    posteroinferior 410.3
    posterolateral 410.5
    postprocedural 997.1
    previous, currently presenting no symptoms
      412
    Q-wave (see also Infarct, myocardium, by
      site) 410.9
    septal 410.8
    specified site NEC 410.8
    ST elevation (STEMI) 410.9
      anterior (wall) 410.1
      anterolateral (wall) 410.0
      inferior (wall) 410.4
      inferolateral (wall) 410.2
      inferoposterior (wall) 410.3
      lateral (wall) 410.5
      posterior (strictly) (true) (wall) 410.6
      specified site NEC 410.8
    subendocardial 410.7
    syphilitic 093.82
  non-ST elevation myocardial infarction
    (NSTEMI) 410.7
  nontransmural 410.7
  omentum 557.0
  ovary 620.8
  pancreas 577.8
  papillary muscle (*see also* Infarct, myocardium)
    410.8
  parathyroid gland 252.8
  pituitary (gland) 253.8
  placenta (complicating pregnancy) 656.7
    affecting fetus or newborn 762.2
  pontine—*see* Infarct, brain
  posterior NEC (*see also* Infarct, myocardium)
    410.6
  prostate 602.8
  pulmonary (artery) (hemorrhagic) (vein) 415.19
    with
      abortion—*see* Abortion, by type, with
        embolism
      ectopic pregnancy (*see also* categories
        633.0-633.9) 639.6
      molar pregnancy (*see also* categories
        630-632) 639.6
    following
      abortion 639.6
      ectopic or molar pregnancy 639.6
    iatrogenic 415.11
    in pregnancy, childbirth, or puerperium—*see*
      Embolism, obstetrical
    postoperative 415.11
    septic 415.12

Infection, infected, infective—*continued*
  dental (pulpal origin) 522.4
  deuteromycetes 117.4
  Dicrocoelium dendriticum 121.8
  Dipetalonema (perstans) 125.4
    streptocerca 125.6
  diphtherial—*see* Diphtheria
  Diphyllobothrium (adult) (latum) (pacificum)
    123.4
    larval 123.5
  Diplogonoporus (grandis) 123.8
  Dipylidium (caninum) 123.8
  Dirofilaria 125.6
  dog tapeworm 123.8
  Dracunculus medinensis 125.7
  Dreschlera 118
    hawaiiensis 117.8
  Ducrey's bacillus (any site) 099.0
  due to or resulting from
    central venous catheter 999.31
    device, implant, or graft (any) (presence
      of)—*see* Complications, infection and
      inflammation, due to (presence of) any
      device, implant, or graft classified to
      996.0-996.5 NEC
    injection, inoculation, infusion, transfusion, or
      vaccination (prophylactic) (therapeutic)
      999.39
    injury NEC—*see* Wound, open, by site,
      complicated
    surgery 998.59
  duodenum 535.6
  ear—*see also* Otitis
    external (*see also* Otitis, externa) 380.10
    inner (*see also* Labyrinthitis) 386.30
    middle —*see* Otitis, media
  Eaton's agent NEC 041.81
  Eberthella typhosa 002.0
  Ebola 078.89
  echinococcosis 122.9
  Echinococcus (*see also* Echinococcus) 122.9
  Echinostoma 121.8
  ECHO virus 079.1
    in diseases classified elsewhere—*see* category
      079
    unspecified nature or site 079.1
  Ehrlichiosis 082.40
    chaffeensis 082.41
    specified type NEC 082.49
  Endamoeba—*see* Infection, ameba
  endocardium (*see also* Endocarditis) 421.0
  endocervix (*see also* Cervicitis) 616.0
  Entamoeba—*see* Infection, ameba
  enteric (*see also* Enteritis, due to, by organism)
    009.0
  Enterobacter aerogenes NEC 041.85
  Enterobacter sakazakii 041.85
  Enterobius vermicularis 127.4
  enterococcus NEC 041.04
  enterovirus NEC 079.89
    central nervous system NEC 048
    enteritis 008.67
    meningitis 047.9
  Entomophthora 117.7
  Epidermophyton—*see* Dermatophytosis
  epidermophytosis—*see* Dermatophytosis
  episiotomy 674.3
  Epstein-Barr virus 075
    chronic 780.79 *[139.8]*
  erysipeloid 027.1
  Erysipelothrix (insidiosa) (rhusiopathiae) 027.1
  erythema infectiosum 057.0

Infection, infected, infective—*continued*
  Escherichia coli NEC 041.4
    enteritis—*see* Enteritis, E. coli
    generalized 038.42
    intestinal—*see* Enteritis, E. coli
  esophagostomy 530.86
  ethmoidal (chronic) (sinus) (*see also* Sinusitis,
    ethmoidal) 473.2
  Eubacterium 041.84
  Eustachian tube (ear) 381.50
    acute 381.51
    chronic 381.52
  exanthema subitum (*see also* Exanthem
    subitum) 058.10
  external auditory canal (meatus) (*see also* Otitis,
    externa) 380.10
  eye NEC 360.00
  eyelid 373.9
    specified NEC 373.8
  fallopian tube (*see also* Salpingo-oophoritis)
    614.2
  fascia 728.89
  Fasciola
    gigantica 121.3
    hepatica 121.3
  Fasciolopsis (buski) 121.4
  fetus (intra-amniotic)—*see* Infection, congenital
  filarial—*see* Infestation, filarial
  finger (skin) 686.9
    abscess (with lymphangitis) 681.00
      pulp 681.01
    cellulitis (with lymphangitis) 681.00
    distal closed space (with lymphangitis) 681.00
    nail 681.02
      fungus 110.1
  fish tapeworm 123.4
    larval 123.5
  flagellate, intestinal 007.9
  fluke—*see* Infestation, fluke
  focal
    teeth (pulpal origin) 522.4
    tonsils 474.00
      and adenoids 474.02
  Fonsecaea
    compactum 117.2
    pedrosoi 117.2
  food (*see also* Poisoning, food) 005.9
  foot (skin) 686.9
    fungus 110.4
  Francisella tularensis (*see also* Tularemia) 021.9
  frontal sinus (chronic) (*see also* Sinusitis,
    frontal) 473.1
  fungus NEC 117.9
    beard 110.0
    body 110.5
    dermatiacious NEC 117.8
    foot 110.4
    groin 110.3
    hand 110.2
    nail 110.1
    pathogenic to compromised host only 118
    perianal (area) 110.3
    scalp 110.0
    scrotum 110.8
    skin 111.9
      foot 110.4
      hand 110.2
    toenails 110.1
    trachea 117.9
  Fusarium 118
  Fusobacterium 041.84
  gallbladder (*see also* Cholecystitis, acute) 575.0

Infection, infected, infective—*continued*
Gardnerella vaginalis 041.89
gas bacillus (*see also* Gas, gangrene) 040.0
gastric (*see also* Gastritis) 535.5
Gastrodiscoides hominis 121.8
gastroenteric (*see also* Enteritis, due to, by
organism) 009.0
gastrointestinal (*see also* Enteritis, due to, by
organism) 009.0
gastrostomy 536.41
generalized NEC (*see also* Septicemia) 038.9
genital organ or tract NEC
female 614.9
with
abortion—*see* Abortion, by type, with sepsis
ectopic pregnancy (*see also* categories
633.0-633.9) 639.0
molar pregnancy (*see also* categories
630-632) 639.0
complicating pregnancy 646.6
affecting fetus or newborn 760.8
following
abortion 639.0
ectopic or molar pregnancy 639.0
puerperal, postpartum, childbirth 670.8
minor or localized 646.6
affecting fetus or newborn 760.8
male 608.4
genitourinary tract NEC 599.0
Ghon tubercle, primary (*see also* Tuberculosis)
010.0
Giardia lamblia 007.1
gingival (chronic) 523.10
acute 523.00
Vincent's 101
glanders 024
Glenosporopsis amazonica 116.2
Gnathostoma spinigerum 128.1
Gongylonema 125.6
gonococcal NEC (*see also* Gonococcus) 098.0
gram-negative bacilli NEC 041.85
anaerobic 041.84
guinea worm 125.7
gum (*see also* Infection, gingival) 523.10
Hantavirus 079.81
heart 429.89
Helicobacter pylori [*H. pylori*] 041.86
helminths NEC 128.9
intestinal 127.9
mixed (types classifiable to more than one
category in 120.0-127.7) 127.8
specified type NEC 127.7
specified type NEC 128.8
Hemophilus influenzae NEC 041.5
generalized 038.41
Herpes (simplex) (*see also* Herpes, simplex)
054.9
congenital 771.2
zoster (*see also* Herpes, zoster) 053.9
eye NEC 053.29
Heterophyes heterophyes 121.6
Histoplasma (*see also* Histoplasmosis) 115.90
capsulatum (*see also* Histoplasmosis,
American) 115.00
duboisii (*see also* Histoplasmosis, African)
115.10
HIV V08
with symptoms, symptomatic 042
hookworm (*see also* Ancylostomiasis) 126.9
human herpesvirus 6 058.81
human herpesvirus 7 058.82
human herpesvirus 8 058.89

Infection, infected, infective—*continued*
human herpesvirus NEC 058.89
human immunodeficiency virus V08
with symptoms, symptomatic 042
human papillomavirus 079.4
hydrocele 603.1
hydronephrosis 591
Hymenolepis 123.6
hypopharynx 478.29
inguinal glands 683
due to soft chancre 099.0
intestine, intestinal (*see also* Enteritis, due to, by
organism) 009.0
intrauterine (*see also* Endometritis) 615.9
complicating delivery 646.6
isospora belli or hominis 007.2
Japanese B encephalitis 062.0
jaw (bone) (acute) (chronic) (lower) (subacute)
(upper) 526.4
joint—*see* Arthritis, infectious or infective
Kaposi's sarcoma-associated herpesvirus 058.89
kidney (cortex) (hematogenous) 590.9
with
abortion—*see* Abortion, by type, with
urinary tract infection
calculus 592.0
ectopic pregnancy (*see also* categories
633.0-633.9) 639.8
molar pregnancy (*see also* categories
630-632) 639.8
complicating pregnancy or puerperium 646.6
affecting fetus or newborn 760.1
following
abortion 639.8
ectopic or molar pregnancy 639.8
pelvis and ureter 590.3
Klebsiella pneumoniae NEC 041.3
knee (skin) NEC 686.9
joint—*see* Arthritis, infectious
Koch's (*see also* Tuberculosis, pulmonary)
011.9
labia (majora) (minora) (*see also* Vulvitis)
616.10
lacrimal
gland (*see also* Dacryoadenitis) 375.00
passages (duct) (sac) (*see also* Dacryocystitis)
375.30
larynx NEC 478.79
leg (skin) NEC 686.9
Leishmania (*see also* Leishmaniasis) 085.9
braziliensis 085.5
donovani 085.0
Ethiopica 085.3
furunculosa 085.1
infantum 085.0
mexicana 085.4
tropica (minor) 085.1
major 085.2
Leptosphaeria senegalensis 117.4
leptospira (*see also* Leptospirosis) 100.9
Australis 100.89
Bataviae 100.89
pyrogenes 100.89
specified type NEC 100.89
leptospirochetal NEC (*see also* Leptospirosis)
100.9
Leptothrix—*see* Actinomycosis
Listeria monocytogenes (listeriosis) 027.0
congenital 771.2
liver fluke—*see* Infestation, fluke, liver
Loa loa 125.2
eyelid 125.2 *[373.6]*

Infection, infected, infective—*continued*
Loboa loboi 116.2
local, skin (staphylococcal) (streptococcal) NEC 686.9
  abscess—*see* Abscess, by site
  cellulitis—*see* Cellulitis, by site
  ulcer (*see also* Ulcer, skin) 707.9
Loefflerella
  mallei 024
  whitmori 025
lung 518.89
  atypical Mycobacterium 031.0
    tuberculous (*see also* Tuberculosis, pulmonary) 011.9
  basilar 518.89
  chronic 518.89
  fungus NEC 117.9
  spirochetal 104.8
  virus—*see* Pneumonia, virus
lymph gland (axillary) (cervical) (inguinal) 683
  mesenteric 289.2
lymphoid tissue, base of tongue or posterior pharynx, NEC 474.00
madurella
  grisea 117.4
  mycetomii 117.4
major
  with
    abortion—*see* Abortion, by type, with sepsis
    ectopic pregnancy (*see also* categories 633.0-633.9) 639.0
    molar pregnancy (*see also* categories 630-632) 639.0
  following
    abortion 639.0
    ectopic or molar pregnancy 639.0
  puerperal, postpartum, childbirth 670.0
malarial—*see* Malaria
Malassezia furfur 111.0
Malleomyces
  mallei 024
  pseudomallei 025
mammary gland 611.0
  puerperal, postpartum 675.2
Mansonella (ozzardi) 125.5
mastoid (suppurative)—*see* Mastoiditis
maxilla, maxillary 526.4
  sinus (chronic) (*see also* Sinusitis, maxillary) 473.0
mediastinum 519.2
medina 125.7
meibomian
  cyst 373.12
  gland 373.12
melioidosis 025
meninges (*see also* Meningitis) 320.9
meningococcal (*see also* condition) 036.9
  brain 036.1
  cerebrospinal 036.0
  endocardium 036.42
  generalized 036.2
  meninges 036.0
  meningococcemia 036.2
  specified site NEC 036.89
mesenteric lymph nodes or glands NEC 289.2
Metagonimus 121.5
metatarsophalangeal 711.97
methicillin
  resistant Staphylococcus aureus (MRSA) 041.12
  susceptible Staphylococcus aureus (MSSA) 041.11

Infection, infected, infective—*continued*
microorganism resistant to drugs—*see* Resistance (to), drugs by microorganisms
Microsporidia 136.8
microsporum, microsporic—*see* Dermatophytosis
Mima polymorpha NEC 041.85
mixed flora NEC 041.89
Monilia (*see also* Candidiasis) 112.9
  neonatal 771.7
monkeypox 059.01
Monosporium apiospermum 117.6
mouth (focus) NEC 528.9
  parasitic 112.0
MRSA (methicillin resistant Staphylococcus aureus) 041.12
MSSA (methicillin susceptible Staphylococcus aureus) 041.11
Mucor 117.7
muscle NEC 728.89
mycelium NEC 117.9
mycetoma
  actinomycotic NEC (*see also* Actinomycosis) 039.9
  mycotic NEC 117.4
Mycobacterium, mycobacterial (*see also* Mycobacterium) 031.9
mycoplasma NEC 041.81
mycotic NEC 117.9
  pathogenic to compromised host only 118
  skin NEC 111.9
  systemic 117.9
myocardium NEC 422.90
nail (chronic) (with lymphangitis) 681.9
  finger 681.02
    fungus 110.1
  ingrowing 703.0
  toe 681.11
    fungus 110.1
nasal sinus (chronic) (*see also* Sinusitis) 473.9
nasopharynx (chronic) 478.29
  acute 460
navel 686.9
  newborn 771.4
Neisserian—*see* Gonococcus
Neotestudina rosatii 117.4
newborn, generalized 771.89
nipple 611.0
  puerperal, postpartum 675.0
    with breast 675.9
      specified type NEC 675.8
Nocardia—*see* Actinomycosis
nose 478.19
nostril 478.19
obstetrical surgical wound 674.3
Oesophagostomum (apiostomum) 127.7
Oestrus ovis 134.0
Oidium albicans (*see also* Candidiasis) 112.9
Onchocerca (volvulus) 125.3
  eye 125.3 *[360.13]*
  eyelid 125.3 *[373.6]*
operation wound 998.59
Opisthorchis (felineus) (tenuicollis) (viverrini) 121.0
orbit 376.00
  chronic 376.10
orthopoxvirus 059.00
  specified NEC 059.09
ovary (*see also* Salpingo-oophoritis) 614.2
Oxyuris vermicularis 127.4
pancreas 577.0
Paracoccidioides brasiliensis 116.1
Paragonimus (westermani) 121.2

Infection, infected, infective—*continued*
  parainfluenza virus 079.89
  parameningococcus NEC 036.9
    with meningitis 036.0
  parapoxvirus 059.10
    specified NEC 059.19
  parasitic NEC 136.9
  paratyphoid 002.9
    Type A 002.1
    Type B 002.2
    Type C 002.3
  paraurethral ducts 597.89
  parotid gland 527.2
  Pasteurella NEC 027.2
    multocida (cat-bite) (dog-bite) 027.2
    pestis (*see also* Plague) 020.9
    pseudotuberculosis 027.2
    septica (cat-bite) (dog-bite) 027.2
    tularensis (*see also* Tularemia) 021.9
  pelvic, female (*see also* Disease, pelvis,
      inflammatory) 614.9
  penis (glans) (retention) NEC 607.2
    herpetic 054.13
  Peptococcus 041.84
  Peptostreptococcus 041.84
  periapical (pulpal origin) 522.4
  peridental 523.30
  perineal wound (obstetrical) 674.3
  periodontal 523.31
  periorbital 376.00
    chronic 376.10
  perirectal 569.49
  perirenal (*see also* Infection, kidney) 590.9
  peritoneal (*see also* Peritonitis) 567.9
  periureteral 593.89
  periurethral 597.89
  Petriellidium boydii 117.6
  pharynx 478.29
    Coxsackie virus 074.0
    phlegmonous 462
    posterior, lymphoid 474.00
  Phialophora
    gougerotii 117.8
    jeanselmei 117.8
    verrucosa 117.2
  Piedraia hortai 111.3
  pinna, acute 380.11
  pinta 103.9
    intermediate 103.1
    late 103.2
    mixed 103.3
    primary 103.0
  pinworm 127.4
  pityrosporum furfur 111.0
  pleuropneumonia-like organisms NEC (PPLO)
      041.81
  pneumococcal NEC 041.2
    generalized (purulent) 038.2
  Pneumococcus NEC 041.2
  postoperative wound 998.59
  posttraumatic NEC 958.3
  postvaccinal 999.39
  poxvirus 059.9
    specified NEC 059.8
  prepuce NEC 607.1
  Propionibacterium 041.84
  prostate (capsule) (*see also* Prostatitis) 601.9
  Proteus (mirabilis) (morganii) (vulgaris) NEC
      041.6
    enteritis 008.3
  protozoal NEC 136.8
    intestinal NEC 007.9

Infection, infected, infective—*continued*
  Pseudomonas NEC 041.7
    mallei 024
    pneumonia 482.1
    pseudomallei 025
  psittacosis 073.9
  puerperal, postpartum (major) 670.0
    minor 646.6
  pulmonary—*see* Infection, lung
  purulent—*see* Abscess
  putrid, generalized—*see* Septicemia
  pyemic—*see* Septicemia
  Pyrenochaeta romeroi 117.4
  Q fever 083.0
  rabies 071
  rectum (sphincter) 569.49
  renal (*see also* Infection, kidney) 590.9
    pelvis and ureter 590.3
  resistant to drugs—*see* Resistance (to), drugs by
      microorganisms
  respiratory 519.8
    chronic 519.8
    influenzal (acute) (upper) 487.1
    lung 518.89
    rhinovirus 460
    syncytial virus 079.6
    upper (acute) (infectious) NEC 465.9
      with flu, grippe, or influenza 487.1
      influenzal 487.1
      multiple sites NEC 465.8
      streptococcal 034.0
      viral NEC 465.9
  respiratory syncytial virus (RSV) 079.6
  resulting from presence of shunt or other
      internal prosthetic device—*see*
      Complications, infection and inflammation,
      due to (presence of) any device, implant, or
      graft classified to 996.0-996.5 NEC
  retroperitoneal 567.39
  retrovirus 079.50
    human immunodeficiency virus type 2
        [HIV-2] 079.53
    human T-cell lymphotrophic virus type I
        [HTLV-I] 079.51
    human T-cell lymphotrophic virus type II
        [HTLV-II] 079.52
    specified NEC 079.59
  Rhinocladium 117.1
  Rhinosporidium (*see*beri) 117.0
  rhinovirus
    in diseases classified elsewhere—*see* category
        079
    unspecified nature or site 079.3
  Rhizopus 117.7
  rickettsial 083.9
  rickettsialpox 083.2
  rubella (*see also* Rubella) 056.9
    congenital 771.0
  Saccharomyces (*see also* Candidiasis) 112.9
  Saksenaea 117.7
  salivary duct or gland (any) 527.2
  Salmonella (aertrycke) (callinarum)
      (choleraesuis) (enteritidis) (suipestifer)
      (typhimurium) 003.9
    with
      arthritis 003.23
      gastroenteritis 003.0
      localized infection 003.20
        specified type NEC 003.29
      meningitis 003.21
      osteomyelitis 003.24
      pneumonia 003.22

Infection, infected, infective—*continued*
  Salmonella—*continued*
    with—*continued*
      septicemia 003.1
      specified manifestation NEC 003.8
    due to food (poisoning) (any serotype) (*see also* Poisoning, food, due to, Salmonella)
    hirschfeldii 002.3
    localized 003.20
      specified type NEC 003.29
    paratyphi 002.9
      A 002.1
      B 002.2
      C 002.3
    schottmuelleri 002.2
    specified type NEC 003.8
    typhi 002.0
    typhosa 002.0
  saprophytic 136.8
  Sarcocystis, lindemanni 136.5
  SARS-associated coronavirus 079.82
  scabies 133.0
  Schistosoma—*see* Infestation, Schistosoma
  Schmorl's bacillus 040.3
  scratch or other superficial injury—*see* Injury, superficial, by site
  scrotum (acute) NEC 608.4
  sealpox 059.12
  secondary, burn or open wound (dislocation) (fracture) 958.3
  seminal vesicle (*see also* Vesiculitis) 608.0
  septic
    generalized—*see* Septicemia
    localized, skin (*see also* Abscess) 682.9
  septicemic—*see* Septicemia
  seroma 998.51
  Serratia (marcescens) 041.85
    generalized 038.44
  sheep liver fluke 121.3
  Shigella 004.9
    boydii 004.2
    dysenteriae 004.0
    Flexneri 004.1
    group
      A 004.0
      B 004.1
      C 004.2
      D 004.3
    Schmitz (-Stutzer) 004.0
    Schmitzii 004.0
    Shiga 004.0
    Sonnei 004.3
    specified type NEC 004.8
  Sin Nombre virus 079.81
  sinus (*see also* Sinusitis) 473.9
    pilonidal 685.1
      with abscess 685.0
    skin NEC 686.9
  Skene's duct or gland (*see also* Urethritis) 597.89
  skin (local) (staphylococcal) (streptococcal) NEC 686.9
    abscess—*see* Abscess, by site
    cellulitis—*see* Cellulitis, by site
    due to fungus 111.9
      specified type NEC 111.8
    mycotic 111.9
      specified type NEC 111.8
    ulcer (*see also* Ulcer, skin) 707.9
  slow virus 046.9
    specified condition NEC 046.8
  Sparganum (mansoni) (proliferum) 123.5

Infection, infected, infective—*continued*
  spermatic cord NEC 608.4
  sphenoidal (chronic) (sinus) (*see also* Sinusitis, sphenoidal) 473.3
  Spherophorus necrophorus 040.3
  spinal cord NEC (*see also* Encephalitis) 323.9
    abscess 324.1
      late effect—*see* category 326
    late effect—*see* category 326
    meninges—*see* Meningitis
    streptococcal 320.2
  Spirillum
    minus or minor 026.0
    morsus muris 026.0
    obermeieri 087.0
  spirochetal NEC 104.9
    lung 104.8
    specified nature or site NEC 104.8
  spleen 289.59
  Sporothrix schenckii 117.1
  Sporotrichum (schenckii) 117.1
  Sporozoa 136.8
  staphylococcal NEC 041.10
    aureus 041.11
      methicillin
        resistant (MRSA) 041.12
        susceptible MSSA 041.11
    food poisoning 005.0
    generalized (purulent) 038.10
      aureus 038.11
        methicillin
          resistant 038.12
          susceptible 038.11
      specified organism NEC 038.19
    pneumonia 482.40
      aureus 482.41
        methicillin
          resistant (MRSA) 482.42
          susceptible (MSSA) 482.41
      MRSA (methicillin resistant staphylococcus aureus) 482.42
      MSSA (methicillin susceptible staphylococcus aureus) 482.41
      specified type NEC 482.49
    septicemia 038.10
      aureus 038.11
        methicillin
          resistant (MRSA) 038.12
          susceptible (MSSA) 038.11
      MRSA (methicillin resistant staphylococcus aureus) 038.12
      MSSA (methicillin susceptible staphylococcus aureus) 038.11
      specified organism NEC 038.19
    specified NEC 041.19
  steatoma 706.2
  Stellantchasmus falcatus 121.6
  Streptobacillus moniliformis 026.1
  streptococcal NEC 041.00
    generalized (purulent) 038.0
    group
      A 041.01
      B 041.02
      C 041.03
      D [enterococcus] 041.04
      G 041.05
    pneumonia—*see* Pneumonia, streptococcal 482.3
    septicemia 038.0
    sore throat 034.0
    specified NEC 041.09

Infection, infected, infective—*continued*
  Streptomyces—*see* Actinomycosis
  streptotrichosis—*see* Actinomycosis
  Strongyloides (stercoralis) 127.2
  stump (amputation) (posttraumatic) (surgical)
    997.62
    traumatic—*see* Amputation, traumatic, by site,
      complicated
  subcutaneous tissue, local NEC 686.9
  submaxillary region 528.9
  suipestifer (*see also* Infection, Salmonella) 003.9
  swimming pool bacillus 031.1
  syphilitic—*see* Syphilis
  systemic—*see* Septicemia
  Taenia—*see* Infestation, Taenia
  Taeniarhynchus saginatus 123.2
  tanapox 059.21
  tapeworm—*see* Infestation, tapeworm
  tendon (sheath) 727.89
  Ternidens diminutus 127.7
  testis (*see also* Orchitis) 604.90
  thigh (skin) 686.9
  threadworm 127.4
  throat 478.29
    pneumococcal 462
    staphylococcal 462
    streptococcal 034.0
    viral NEC (*see also* Pharyngitis) 462
  thumb (skin) 686.9
    abscess (with lymphangitis) 681.00
      pulp 681.01
    cellulitis (with lymphangitis) 681.00
    nail 681.02
  thyroglossal duct 529.8
  toe (skin) 686.9
    abscess (with lymphangitis) 681.10
    cellulitis (with lymphangitis) 681.10
    nail 681.11
      fungus 110.1
  tongue NEC 529.0
    parasitic 112.0
  tonsil (faucial) (lingual) (pharyngeal) 474.00
    acute or subacute 463
    and adenoid 474.02
    tag 474.00
  tooth, teeth 522.4
    periapical (pulpal origin) 522.4
    peridental 523.30
    periodontal 523.31
    pulp 522.0
    socket 526.5
  TORCH - see Infection, congenital NEC
    without active infection 760.2
  Torula histolytica 117.5
  Toxocara (cani) (cati) (felis) 128.0
  Toxoplasma gondii (*see also* Toxoplasmosis) 130.9
  trachea, chronic 491.8
    fungus 117.9
  traumatic NEC 958.3
  trematode NEC 121.9
  trench fever 083.1
  Treponema
    denticola 041.84
    macrodenticum 041.84
    pallidum (*see also* Syphilis) 097.9
  Trichinella (spiralis) 124
  Trichomonas 131.9
    bladder 131.09
    cervix 131.09
    hominis 007.3
    intestine 007.3
    prostate 131.03

Infection, infected, infective—*continued*
  Trichomonas—*continued*
    specified site NEC 131.8
    urethra 131.02
    urogenitalis 131.00
    vagina 131.01
    vulva 131.01
  Trichophyton, trichophytid—*see*
    Dermatophytosis
  Trichosporon (beigelii) cutaneum 111.2
  Trichostrongylus 127.6
  Trichuris (trichiuria) 127.3
  Trombicula (irritans) 133.8
  Trypanosoma (*see also* Trypanosomiasis) 086.9
    cruzi 086.2
  tubal (*see also* Salpingo-oophoritis) 614.2
  tuberculous NEC (*see also* Tuberculosis) 011.9
  tubo-ovarian (*see also* Salpingo-oophoritis)
    614.2
  tunica vaginalis 608.4
  tympanic membrane—*see* Myringitis
  typhoid (abortive) (ambulant) (bacillus) 002.0
  typhus 081.9
    flea-borne (endemic) 081.0
    louse-borne (epidemic) 080
    mite-borne 081.2
    recrudescent 081.1
    tick-borne 082.9
      African 082.1
      North Asian 082.2
  umbilicus (septic) 686.9
    newborn NEC 771.4
  ureter 593.89
  urethra (*see also* Urethritis) 597.80
  urinary (tract) NEC 599.0
    with
      abortion—*see* Abortion, by type, with
        urinary tract infection
      ectopic pregnancy (*see also* categories
        633.0-633.9) 639.8
      molar pregnancy (*see also* categories
        630-632) 639.8
    candidal 112.2
    complicating pregnancy, childbirth, or
      puerperium 646.6
      affecting fetus or newborn 760.1
      asymptomatic 646.5
        affecting fetus or newborn 760.1
    diplococcal (acute) 098.0
      chronic 098.2
    due to Trichomonas (vaginalis) 131.00
    following
      abortion 639.8
      ectopic or molar pregnancy 639.8
    gonococcal (acute) 098.0
      chronic or duration of 2 months or over
        098.2
    newborn 771.82
    trichomonal 131.00
    tuberculous (*see also* Tuberculosis) 016.3
  uterus, uterine (*see also* Endometritis) 615.9
  utriculus masculinus NEC 597.89
  vaccination 999.39
  vagina (granulation tissue) (wall) (*see also*
    Vaginitis) 616.10
  varicella 052.9
  varicose veins—*see* Varicose, veins
  variola 050.9
    major 050.0
    minor 050.1
  vas deferens NEC 608.4
  Veillonella 041.84

Infection, infected, infective—*continued*
verumontanum 597.89
vesical (*see also* Cystitis) 595.9
Vibrio
  cholerae 001.0
    El Tor 001.1
  parahaemolyticus (food poisoning) 005.4
  vulnificus 041.85
Vincent's (gums) (mouth) (tonsil) 101
virus, viral 079.99
  adenovirus
    in diseases classified elsewhere—*see*
      category 079
    unspecified nature or site 079.0
  central nervous system NEC 049.9
    enterovirus 048
      meningitis 047.9
      specified type NEC 047.8
    slow virus 046.9
      specified condition NEC 046.8
  chest 519.8
  conjunctivitis 077.99
    specified type NEC 077.8
  coronavirus 079.89
    SARS-associated 079.82
  Coxsackie (*see also* Infection, Coxsackie) 079.2
  Ebola 065.8
  ECHO
    in diseases classified elsewhere—*see*
      category 079
    unspecified nature or site 079.1
  encephalitis 049.9
    arthropod-borne NEC 064
    tick-borne 063.9
    specified type NEC 063.8
  enteritis NEC (*see also* Enteritis, viral) 008.8
  exanthem NEC 057.9
  Hantavirus 079.81
  human papilloma 079.4
  in diseases classified elsewhere—*see* category 079
  intestine (*see also* Enteritis, viral) 008.8
  lung—*see* Pneumonia, viral
  respiratory syncytial virus (RSV) 079.6
  rhinovirus
    in diseases classified elsewhere—*see*
      category 079
    unspecified nature or site 079.3
  salivary gland disease 078.5
  slow 046.9
    specified condition NEC 046.8
  specified type NEC 079.89
    in diseases classified elsewhere—*see*
      category 079
    unspecified nature or site 079.99
  warts 078.10
    specified NEC 078.19
  yaba monkey tumor 059.22
vulva (*see also* Vulvitis) 616.10
whipworm 127.3
Whitmore's bacillus 025
wound (local) (posttraumatic) NEC 958.3
  with
    dislocation—*see* Dislocation, by site, open
    fracture—*see* Fracture, by site, open
    open wound—*see* Wound, open, by site,
      complicated
  postoperative 998.59
  surgical 998.59
Wuchereria 125.0
  bancrofti 125.0
  malayi 125.1
yaba monkey tumor virus 059.22

Infection, infected, infective—*continued*
  yatapoxvirus 059.20
  yaws—*see* Yaws
  yeast (*see also* Candidiasis) 112.9
  yellow fever (*see also* Fever, yellow) 060.9
  Yersinia pestis (*see also* Plague) 020.9
  Zeis' gland 373.12
  zoonotic bacterial NEC 027.9
  Zopfia senegalensis 117.4
Infective, infectious —*see* condition
Inferiority complex 301.9
  constitutional psychopathic 301.9
Infertility
  female 628.9
    age related 628.8
    associated with
      adhesions, peritubal 614.6 *[628.2]*
      anomaly
        cervical mucus 628.4
        congenital
          cervix 628.4
          fallopian tube 628.2
          uterus 628.3
          vagina 628.4
      anovulation 628.0
      dysmucorrhea 628.4
      endometritis, tuberculous (*see also*
        Tuberculosis) 016.7 *[628.3]*
      Stein-Leventhal syndrome 256.4 *[628.0]*
    due to
      adiposogenital dystrophy 253.8 *[628.1]*
      anterior pituitary disorder NEC 253.4
        [628.1]
        hyperfunction 253.1 *[628.1]*
      cervical anomaly 628.4
      fallopian tube anomaly 628.2
      ovarian failure 256.39 *[628.0]*
      Stein-Leventhal syndrome 256.4 *[628.0]*
      uterine anomaly 628.3
      vaginal anomaly 628.4
    nonimplantation 628.3
    origin
      cervical 628.4
      pituitary-hypothalamus NEC 253.8 *[628.1]*
        anterior pituitary NEC 253.4 *[628.1]*
          hyperfunction NEC 253.1 *[628.1]*
        dwarfism 253.3 *[628.1]*
        panhypopituitarism 253.2 *[628.1]*
      specified NEC 628.8
      tubal (block) (occlusion) (stenosis) 628.2
        adhesions 614.6 *[628.2]*
      uterine 628.3
      vaginal 628.4
    previous, requiring supervision of pregnancy
      V23.0
  male 606.9
    absolute 606.0
    due to
      azoospermia 606.0
      drug therapy 606.8
      extratesticular cause NEC 606.8
      germinal cell
        aplasia 606.0
        desquamation 606.1
      hypospermatogenesis 606.1
      infection 606.8
      obstruction, afferent ducts 606.8
      oligospermia 606.1
      radiation 606.8
      spermatogenic arrest (complete) 606.0
        incomplete 606.1
      systemic disease 606.8

Infestation 134.9
  Acanthocheilonema (perstans) 125.4
    streptocerca 125.6
  Acariasis 133.9
    demodex folliculorum 133.8
    Sarcoptes scabiei 133.0
    trombiculae 133.8
  Agamofilaria streptocerca 125.6
  Ancylostoma, Ankylostoma 126.9
    americanum 126.1
    braziliense 126.2
    canium 126.8
    ceylanicum 126.3
    duodenale 126.0
    new world 126.1
    old world 126.0
  Angiostrongylus cantonensis 128.8
  anisakiasis 127.1
  Anisakis larva 127.1
  arthropod NEC 134.1
  Ascaris lumbricoides 127.0
  Bacillus fusiformis 101
  Balantidium coli 007.0
  beef tapeworm 123.2
  Bothriocephalus (latus) 123.4
    larval 123.5
  broad tapeworm 123.4
    larval 123.5
  Brugia malayi 125.1
  Candiru 136.8
  Capillaria
    hepatica 128.8
    philippinensis 127.5
  cat liver fluke 121.0
  Cercomonas hominis (intestinal) 007.3
  cestodes 123.9
    specified type NEC 123.8
  chigger 133.8
  chigoe 134.1
  Chilomastix 007.8
  Clonorchis (sinensis) (liver) 121.1
  coccidia 007.2
  complicating pregnancy, childbirth, or
      puerperium 647.9
    affecting fetus or newborn 760.8
  Cysticercus cellulosae 123.1
  Demodex folliculorum 133.8
  Dermatobia (hominis) 134.0
  Dibothriocephalus (latus) 123.4
    larval 123.5
  Dicrocoelium dendriticum 121.8
  Diphyllobothrium (adult) (intestinal) (latum)
      (pacificum) 123.4
    larval 123.5
  Diplogonoporus (grandis) 123.8
  Dipylidium (caninum) 123.8
  Distoma hepaticum 121.3
  dog tapeworm 123.8
  Dracunculus medinensis 125.7
  dragon worm 125.7
  dwarf tapeworm 123.6
  Echinococcus (*see also* Echinococcus) 122.9
  Echinostoma ilocanum 121.8
  Embadomonas 007.8
  Endamoeba (histolytica)—*see* Infection, ameba
  Entamoeba (histolytica)—*see* Infection, ameba
  Enterobius vermicularis 127.4
  Epidermophyton—*see* Dermatophytosis
  eyeworm 125.2
  Fasciola
    gigantica 121.3
    hepatica 121.3

Infestation—*continued*
  Fasciolopsis (buski) (small intestine) 121.4
  filarial 125.9
    due to
      Acanthocheilonema (perstans) 125.4
        streptocerca 125.6
      Brugia (Wuchereria) malayi 125.1
      Dracunculus medinensis 125.7
      guinea worms 125.7
      Mansonella (ozzardi) 125.5
      Onchocerca volvulus 125.3
        eye 125.3 *[360.13]*
        eyelid 125.3 *[373.6]*
      Wuchereria (bancrofti) 125.0
        malayi 125.1
    specified type NEC 125.6
  fish tapeworm 123.4
    larval 123.5
  fluke 121.9
    blood NEC (*see also* Schistosomiasis) 120.9
    cat liver 121.0
    intestinal (giant) 121.4
    liver (sheep) 121.3
      cat 121.0
      Chinese 121.1
      clonorchiasis 121.1
      fascioliasis 121.3
      Oriental 121.1
    lung (oriental) 121.2
    sheep liver 121.3
  fly larva 134.0
  Gasterophilus (intestinalis) 134.0
  Gastrodiscoides hominis 121.8
  Giardia lamblia 007.1
  Gnathostoma (spinigerum) 128.1
  Gongylonema 125.6
  guinea worm 125.7
  helminth NEC 128.9
    intestinal 127.9
      mixed (types classifiable to more than one
          category in 120.0-127.7) 127.8
      specified type NEC 127.7
    specified type NEC 128.8
  Heterophyes heterophyes (small intestine) 121.6
  hookworm (*see also* Infestation, ancylostoma)
      126.9
  Hymenolepis (diminuta) (nana) 123.6
  intestinal NEC 129
  leeches (aquatic) (land) 134.2
  Leishmania—*see* Leishmaniasis
  lice (*see also* infestation, pediculus) 132.9
  Linguatulidae, linguatula (pentastoma) (serrata)
      134.1
  Loa loa 125.2
    eyelid 125.2 *[373.6]*
  louse (*see also* Infestation, pediculus) 132.9
    body 132.1
    head 132.0
    pubic 132.2
  maggots 134.0
  Mansonella (ozzardi) 125.5
  medina 125.7
  Metagonimus yokogawai (small intestine) 121.5
  Microfilaria streptocerca 125.3
    eye 125.3 *[360.13]*
    eyelid 125.3 *[373.6]*
  Microsporon furfur 111.0
  microsporum—*see* Dermatophytosis
  mites 133.9
    scabic 133.0
    specified type NEC 133.8

Infestation—*continued*
  Monilia (albicans) (*see also* Candidiasis) 112.9
    vagina 112.1
    vulva 112.1
  mouth 112.0
  Necator americanus 126.1
  nematode (intestinal) 127.9
    Ancylostoma (*see also* Ancylostoma) 126.9
    Ascaris lumbricoides 127.0
    conjunctiva NEC 128.9
    Dioctophyma 128.8
    Enterobius vermicularis 127.4
    Gnathostoma spinigerum 128.1
    Oesophagostomum (apiostomum) 127.7
    Physaloptera 127.4
    specified type NEC 127.7
    Strongyloides stercoralis 127.2
    Ternidens diminutus 127.7
    Trichinella spiralis 124
    Trichostrongylus 127.6
    Trichuris (trichiuria) 127.3
  Oesophagostomum (apiostomum) 127.7
  Oestrus ovis 134.0
  Onchocerca (volvulus) 125.3
    eye 125.3 *[360.13]*
    eyelid 125.3 *[373.6]*
  Opisthorchis (felineus) (tenuicollis) (viverrini)
    121.0
  Oxyuris vermicularis 127.4
  Paragonimus (westermani) 121.2
  parasite, parasitic NEC 136.9
    eyelid 134.9 *[373.6]*
    intestinal 129
    mouth 112.0
    orbit 376.13
    skin 134.9
    tongue 112.0
  pediculus 132.9
    capitis (humanus) (any site) 132.0
    corporis (humanus) (any site) 132.1
    eyelid 132.0 *[373.6]*
    mixed (classifiable to more than one category
      in 132.0-132.2) 132.3
    pubis (any site) 132.2
  phthirus (pubis) (any site) 132.2
    with any infestation classifiable to 132.0 and
      132.1 132.3
  pinworm 127.4
  pork tapeworm (adult) 123.0
  protozoal NEC 136.8
  pubic louse 132.2
  rat tapeworm 123.6
  red bug 133.8
  roundworm (large) NEC 127.0
  sand flea 134.1
  saprophytic NEC 136.8
  Sarcoptes scabiei 133.0
  scabies 133.0
  Schistosoma 120.9
    bovis 120.8
    cercariae 120.3
    hematobium 120.0
    intercalatum 120.8
    japonicum 120.2
    mansoni 120.1
    mattheii 120.8
    specified
      site—*see* Schistosomiasis
      type NEC 120.8
    spindale 120.8
  screw worms 134.0

Infestation—*continued*
  skin NEC 134.9
  Sparganum (mansoni) (proliferum) 123.5
    larval 123.5
  specified type NEC 134.8
  Spirometra larvae 123.5
  Sporozoa NEC 136.8
  Stellantchasmus falcatus 121.6
  Strongyloides 127.2
  Strongylus (gibsoni) 127.7
  Taenia 123.3
    diminuta 123.6
    Echinococcus (*see also* Echinococcus) 122.9
    mediocanellata 123.2
    nana 123.6
    saginata (mediocanellata) 123.2
    solium (intestinal form) 123.0
      larval form 123.1
  Taeniarhynchus saginatus 123.2
  tapeworm 123.9
    beef 123.2
    broad 123.4
      larval 123.5
    dog 123.8
    dwarf 123.6
    fish 123.4
      larval 123.5
    pork 123.0
    rat 123.6
  Ternidens diminutus 127.7
  Tetranychus molestissimus 133.8
  threadworm 127.4
  tongue 112.0
  Toxocara (cani) (cati) (felis) 128.0
  trematode(s) NEC 121.9
  Trichina spiralis 124
  Trichinella spiralis 124
  Trichocephalus 127.3
  Trichomonas 131.9
    bladder 131.09
    cervix 131.09
    intestine 007.3
    prostate 131.03
    specified site NEC 131.8
    urethra (female) (male) 131.02
    urogenital 131.00
    vagina 131.01
    vulva 131.01
  Trichophyton—*see* Dermatophytosis
  Trichostrongylus instabilis 127.6
  Trichuris (trichiuria) 127.3
  Trombicula (irritans) 133.8
  Trypanosoma—*see* Trypanosomiasis
  Tunga penetrans 134.1
  Uncinaria americana 126.1
  whipworm 127.3
  worms NEC 128.9
    intestinal 127.9
  Wuchereria 125.0
    bancrofti 125.0
    malayi 125.1
Infiltrate, infiltration
  with an iron compound 275.0
  amyloid (any site) (generalized) 277.39
  calcareous (muscle) NEC 275.49
    localized—*see* Degeneration, by site
  calcium salt (muscle) 275.49
  chemotherapy, vesicant 999.81
  corneal (*see also* Edema, cornea) 371.20
  eyelid 373.9
  fatty (diffuse) (generalized) 272.8
    localized—*see* Degeneration, by site, fatty

Infiltrate, infiltration—*continued*
  glycogen, glycogenic (*see also* Disease,
      glycogen storage) 271.10
  heart, cardiac
    fatty (*see also* Degeneration, myocardial)
        429.1
    glycogenic 271.0 *[425.7]*
  inflammatory in vitreous 379.29
  kidney (*see also* Disease, renal) 593.9
  leukemic (M9800/3)—*see* Leukemia
  liver 573.8
    fatty—*see* Fatty, liver
    glycogen (*see also* Disease, glycogen storage)
        271.0
  lung (*see also* Infiltrate, pulmonary) 518.3
    eosinophilic 518.3
    x-ray finding only 793.1
  lymphatic (*see also* Leukemia, lymphatic) 204.9
    gland, pigmentary 289.3
  muscle, fatty 728.9
  myelogenous (*see also* Leukemia, myeloid)
      205.9
  myocardium, myocardial
    fatty (*see also* Degeneration, myocardial)
        429.1
    glycogenic 271.0 *[425.7]*
  pulmonary 518.3
    with
      eosinophilia 518.3
      pneumonia—*see* Pneumonia, by type
    x-ray finding only 793.1
  Ranke's primary (*see also* Tuberculosis) 010.0
  skin, lymphocyctic (benign) 709.8
  thymus (gland) (fatty) 254.8
  urine 788.8
  vesicant
    agent NEC 999.82
    chemotherapy 999.81
  vitreous humor 379.29
Infirmity 799.89
  senile 797
Inflammation, inflamed, inflammatory (with
    exudation)
  abducens (nerve) 378.54
  accessory sinus (chronic) (*see also* Sinusitis)
      473.9
  adrenal (gland) 255.8
  alimentary canal—*see* Enteritis
  alveoli (teeth) 526.5
    scorbutic 267
  amnion—*see* Amnionitis
  anal canal 569.49
  antrum (chronic) (*see also* Sinusitis, maxillary)
      473.0
  anus 569.49
  appendix (*see also* Appendicitis) 541
  arachnoid—*see* Meningitis
  areola 611.0
    puerperal, postpartum 675.0
  areolar tissue NEC 686.9
  artery—*see* Arteritis
  auditory meatus (external) (*see also* Otitis,
      externa) 380.10
  Bartholin's gland 616.89
  bile duct or passage 576.1
  bladder (*see also* Cystitis) 595.9
  bleb
    postprocedural 379.60
      stage 1 379.61
      stage 2 379.62
      stage 3 379.63

Inflammation—*continued*
  bone—*see* Osteomyelitis
  bowel (*see also* Enteritis) 558.9
  brain (*see also* Encephalitis) 323.9
    late effect—*see* category 326
    membrane—*see* Meningitis
  breast 611.0
    puerperal, postpartum 675.2
  broad ligament (*see also* Disease, pelvis,
      inflammatory) 614.4
    acute 614.3
  bronchus—*see* Bronchitis
  bursa—*see* Bursitis
  capsule
    liver 573.3
    spleen 289.59
  catarrhal (*see also* Catarrh) 460
    vagina 616.10
  cecum (*see also* Appendicitis) 541
  cerebral (*see also* Encephalitis) 323.9
    late effect—*see* category 326
    membrane—*see* Meningitis
  cerebrospinal (*see also* Meningitis) 322.9
    late effect—*see* category 326
    meningococcal 036.0
    tuberculous (*see also* Tuberculosis) 013.6
  cervix (uteri) (*see also* Cervicitis) 616.0
  chest 519.9
  choroid NEC (*see also* Choroiditis) 363.20
  cicatrix (tissue)—*see* Cicatrix
  colon (*see also* Enteritis) 558.9
    granulomatous 555.1
    newborn 558.9
  connective tissue (diffuse) NEC 728.9
  cornea (*see also* Keratitis) 370.9
    with ulcer (*see also* Ulcer, cornea) 370.00
  corpora cavernosa (penis) 607.2
  cranial nerve—*see* Disorder, nerve, cranial
  diarrhea—*see* Diarrhea
  disc (intervertebral) (space) 722.90
    cervical, cervicothoracic 722.91
    lumbar, lumbosacral 722.93
    thoracic, thoracolumbar 722.93
  Douglas' cul-de-sac or pouch (chronic) (*see also*
      Disease, pelvis, inflammatory) 614.4
    acute 614.3
  due to (presence of) any device, implant, or graft
      classifiable to 996.0-996.5—*see*
      Complications, infection and inflammation,
      due to (presence of) any device, implant, or
      graft classified to 996.0-996.5 NEC
  duodenum 535.6
  dura mater—*see* Meningitis
  ear—*see also* Otitis
    external (*see also* Otitis, externa) 380.10
    inner (*see also* Labyrinthitis) 386.30
    middle—*see* Otitis media
  esophagus 530.10
  ethmoidal (chronic) (sinus) (*see also* Sinusitis,
      ethmoidal) 473.2
  Eustachian tube (catarrhal) 381.50
    acute 381.51
    chronic 381.52
  extrarectal 569.49
  eye 379.99
  eyelid 373.9
    specified NEC 373.8
  fallopian tube (*see also* Salpingo-oophoritis)
      614.2
  fascia 728.9

Inflammation—*continued*
fetal membranes (acute) 658.4
  affecting fetus or newborn 762.7
follicular, pharynx 472.1
frontal (chronic) (sinus) (*see also* Sinusitis, frontal) 473.1
gallbladder (*see also* Cholecystitis, acute) 575.0
gall duct (*see also* Cholecystitis) 575.10
gastrointestinal (*see also* Enteritis) 558.9
genital organ (diffuse) (internal)
  female 614.9
    with
      abortion—*see* Abortion, by type, with sepsis
      ectopic pregnancy (*see also* categories 633.0-633.9) 639.0
      molar pregnancy (*see also* categories 630-632) 639.0
    complicating pregnancy, childbirth, or puerperium 646.6
      affecting fetus or newborn 760.8
    following
      abortion 639.0
      ectopic or molar pregnancy 639.0
  male 608.4
gland (lymph) (*see also* Lymphadenitis) 289.3
glottis (*see also* Laryngitis) 464.00
  with obstruction 464.01
granular, pharynx 472.1
gum 523.10
heart (*see also* Carditis) 429.89
hepatic duct 576.8
hernial sac—*see* Hernia, by site
ileum (*see also* Enteritis) 558.9
  terminal or regional 555.0
  with large intestine 555.2
intervertebral disc 722.90
  cervical, cervicothoracic 722.91
  lumbar, lumbosacral 722.93
  thoracic, thoracolumbar 722.92
intestine (*see also* Enteritis) 558.9
jaw (acute) (bone) (chronic) (lower) (suppurative) (upper) 526.4
jejunum—*see* Enteritis
joint NEC (*see also* Arthritis) 716.9
  sacroiliac 720.2
kidney (*see also* Nephritis) 583.9
knee (joint) 716.66
  tuberculous (active) (*see also* Tuberculosis) 015.2
labium (majus) (minus) (*see also* Vulvitis) 616.10
lacrimal
  gland (*see also* Dacryoadenitis) 375.00
  passages (duct) (sac) (*see also* Dacryocystitis) 375.30
larynx (*see also* Laryngitis) 464.00
  with obstruction 464.01
  diphtheritic 032.3
leg NEC 686.9
lip 528.5
liver (capsule) (*see also* Hepatitis) 573.3
  acute 570
  chronic 571.40
  suppurative 572.0
lung (acute) (*see also* Pneumonia) 486
  chronic (interstitial) 518.89
lymphatic vessel (*see also* Lymphangitis) 457.2
lymph node or gland (*see also* Lymphadenitis) 289.3
mammary gland 611.0
  puerperal, postpartum 675.2

Inflammation—*continued*
maxilla, maxillary 526.4
  sinus (chronic) (*see also* Sinusitis, maxillary) 473.0
membranes of brain or spinal cord—*see* Meningitis
meninges—*see* Meningitis
mouth 528.00
muscle 728.9
myocardium (*see also* Myocarditis) 429.0
nasal sinus (chronic) (*see also* Sinusitis) 473.9
nasopharynx—*see* Nasopharyngitis
navel 686.9
  newborn NEC 771.4
nerve NEC 729.2
nipple 611.0
  puerperal, postpartum 675.0
nose 478.19
  suppurative 472.0
oculomotor nerve 378.51
optic nerve 377.30
orbit (chronic) 376.10
  acute 376.00
  chronic 376.10
ovary (*see also* Salpingo-oophoritis) 614.2
oviduct (*see also* Salpingo-oophoritis) 614.2
pancreas—*see* Pancreatitis
parametrium (chronic) (*see also* Disease, pelvis, inflammatory) 614.4
  acute 614.3
parotid region 686.9
  gland 527.2
pelvis, female (*see also* Disease, pelvis, inflammatory) 614.9
penis (corpora cavernosa) 607.2
perianal 569.49
pericardium (*see also* Pericarditis) 423.9
perineum (female) (male) 686.9
perirectal 569.49
peritoneum (*see also* Peritonitis) 567.9
periuterine (*see also* Disease, pelvis, inflammatory) 614.9
perivesical (*see also* Cystitis) 595.9
petrous bone (*see also* Petrositis) 383.20
pharynx (*see also* Pharyngitis) 462
  follicular 472.1
  granular 472.1
pia mater—*see* Meningitis
pleura—*see* Pleurisy
postmastoidectomy cavity 383.30
  chronic 383.33
pouch, internal ileoanal 569.71
prostate (*see also* Prostatitis) 601.9
rectosigmoid—*see* Rectosigmoiditis
rectum (*see also* Proctitis) 569.49
respiratory, upper (*see also* Infection, respiratory, upper) 465.9
  chronic, due to external agent—*see* Condition, respiratory, chronic, due to, external agent
  due to
    fumes or vapors (chemical) (inhalation) 506.2
    radiation 508.1
retina (*see also* Retinitis) 363.20
retrocecal (*see also* Appendicitis) 541
retroperitoneal (*see also* Peritonitis) 567.9
salivary duct or gland (any) (suppurative) 527.2
scorbutic, alveoli, teeth 267
scrotum 608.4
sigmoid—*see* Enteritis

Inflammation—*continued*
  sinus (*see also* Sinusitis) 473.9
  Skene's duct or gland (*see also* Urethritis)
      597.89
  skin 686.9
  spermatic cord 608.4
  sphenoidal (sinus) (*see also* Sinusitis,
      sphenoidal) 473.3
  spinal
    cord (*see also* Encephalitis) 323.9
      late effect—*see* category 326
    membrane—*see* Meningitis
    nerve—*see* Disorder, nerve
  spine (*see also* Spondylitis) 720.9
  spleen (capsule) 289.59
  stomach—*see* Gastritis
  stricture, rectum 569.49
  subcutaneous tissue NEC 686.9
  suprarenal (gland) 255.8
  synovial (fringe) (membrane)—*see* Bursitis
  tendon (sheath) NEC 726.90
  testis (*see also* Orchitis) 604.90
  thigh 686.9
  throat (*see also* Sore throat) 462
  thymus (gland) 254.8
  thyroid (gland) (*see also* Thyroiditis) 245.9
  tongue 529.0
  tonsil—*see* Tonsillitis
  trachea—*see* Tracheitis
  trochlear nerve 378.53
  tubal (*see also* Salpingo-oophoritis) 614.2
  tuberculous NEC (*see also* Tuberculosis) 011.9
  tubo-ovarian (*see also* Salpingo-oophoritis)
      614.2
  tunica vaginalis 608.4
  tympanic membrane—*see* Myringitis
  umbilicus, umbilical 686.9
    newborn NEC 771.4
  uterine ligament (*see also* Disease, pelvis,
      inflammatory) 614.4
    acute 614.3
  uterus (catarrhal) (*see also* Endometritis) 615.9
  uveal tract (anterior) (*see also* Iridocyclitis)
      364.3
    posterior—*see* Chorioretinitis
    sympathetic 360.11
  vagina (*see also* Vaginitis) 616.10
  vas deferens 608.4
  vein (*see also* Phlebitis) 451.9
    thrombotic 451.9
      cerebral (*see also* Thrombosis, brain) 434.0
      leg 451.2
        deep (vessels) NEC 451.19
        superficial (vessels) 451.0
      lower extremity 451.2
        deep (vessels) NEC 451.19
        superficial (vessels) 451.0
  vocal cord 478.5
  vulva (*see also* Vulvitis) 616.10
Inflation, lung imperfect (newborn) 770.5
Influenza, influenzal 487.1
  with
    bronchitis 487.1
    bronchopneumonia 487.0
    cold (any type) 487.1
    digestive manifestations 487.8
    hemoptysis 487.1
    involvement of
      gastrointestinal tract 487.8
      nervous system 487.8
    laryngitis 487.1

Influenza—*continued*
  with—*continued*
    manifestations NEC 487.8
      respiratory 487.1
        pneumonia 487.0
    pharyngitis 487.1
    pneumonia (any form classifiable to 480-483,
        485-486) 487.0
    respiratory manifestations NEC 487.1
    sinusitis 487.1
    sore throat 487.1
    tonsillitis 487.1
    tracheitis 487.1
    upper respiratory infection (acute) 487.1
  A/H5N1 488.0
  abdominal 487.8
  Asian 487.1
  avian 488.0
  bronchial 487.1
  bronchopneumonia 487.0
  catarrhal 487.1
  due to identified
    avian influenza virus 488.0
    novel H1N1 influenza virus 488.1
  epidemic 487.1
  gastric 487.8
  intestinal 487.8
  laryngitis 487.1
  maternal affecting fetus or newborn 760.2
    manifest influenza in infant 771.2
  novel (2009) H1N1 488.1
  novel A/H1N1 488.1
  pharyngitis 487.1
  pneumonia (any form) 487.0
  respiratory (upper) 487.1
  specified NEC 487.1
  stomach 487.8
  vaccination, prophylactic (against) V04.81
Influenza-like disease 487.1
Infraction, Freiberg's (metatarsal head) 732.5
Infraeruption, teeth 524.34
**Infusion complication, misadventure or
  reaction** —*see* Complication, infusion
Ingestion
  chemical—*see* Table of drugs and chemicals
  drug or medicinal substance
    overdose or wrong substance given or taken
        977.9
      specified drug—*see* Table of drugs and
          chemicals
  foreign body NEC (*see also* Foreign body) 938
Ingrowing
  hair 704.8
  nail (finger) (toe) (infected) 703.0
Inguinal —*see also* condition
  testis 752.51
Inhalation
  carbon monoxide 986
  flame
    mouth 947.0
    lung 947.1
  food or foreign body (*see also* Asphyxia, food or
      foreign body) 933.1
  gas, fumes, or vapor (noxious) 987.9
    specified agent—*see* Table of drugs and
        chemicals
  liquid or vomitus (*see also* Asphyxia, food or
      foreign body) 933.1
  lower respiratory tract NEC 934.9
  meconium (fetus or newborn) 770.11
    with respiratory symptoms 770.12

Inhalation—*continued*
  mucus (*see also* Asphyxia, mucus) 933.1
  oil (causing suffocation) (*see also* Asphyxia,
    food or foreign body) 933.1
  pneumonia—*see* Pneumonia, aspiration
  smoke 987.9
  steam 987.9
  stomach contents or secretions (*see also*
    Asphyxia, food or foreign body) 933.1
    in labor and deliver 668.0
Inhibition, inhibited
  academic as adjustment reaction 309.23
  orgasm
    female 302.73
    male 302.74
  sexual
    desire 302.71
    excitement 302.72
  work as adjustment reaction 309.23
Inhibitor, systemic lupus erythematosus
  (presence of) 286.5
Iniencephalus, iniencephaly 740.2
Injected eye 372.74
Injury 959.9

---

*Note—For abrasion, insect bite (nonvenomous),
blister, or scratch, see Injury, superficial. For
laceration, traumatic rupture, tear, or
penetrating wound of internal organs, such as
heart, lung, liver, kidney, pelvic organs, whether
or not accompanied by open wound in the same
region, see Injury, internal. For nerve injury,
see Injury, nerve. For late effect of injuries
classifiable to 850-854, 860-869, 900-919,
950-959, see Late, effect, injury, by type.*

---

  abdomen, abdominal (viscera)—*see also* Injury,
    internal, abdomen
    muscle or wall 959.12
  acoustic, resulting in deafness 951.5
  adenoid 959.09
  adrenal (gland)—*see* Injury, internal, adrenal
  alveolar (process) 959.09
  ankle (and foot) (and knee) (and leg, except
    thigh) 959.7
  anterior chamber, eye 921.3
  anus 959.19
  aorta (thoracic) 901.0
    abdominal 902.0
  appendix—*see* Injury, internal, appendix
  arm, upper (and shoulder) 959.2
  artery (complicating trauma) (*see also* Injury,
    blood vessel, by site) 904.9
    cerebral or meningeal (*see also* Hemorrhage,
      brain, traumatic, subarachnoid) 852.0
  auditory canal (external) (meatus) 959.09
  auricle, auris, ear 959.09
  axilla 959.2
  back 959.19
  bile duct—*see* Injury, internal, bile duct
  birth—*see also* Birth, injury
    canal NEC, complicating delivery 665.9
  bladder (sphincter)—*see* Injury, internal,
    bladder
  blast (air) (hydraulic) (immersion) (underwater)
    NEC 869.0
    with open wound into cavity NEC 869.1
    abdomen or thorax—*see* Injury, internal, by
      site
    brain—*see* Concussion, brain
  ear (acoustic nerve trauma) 951.5
    with perforation of tympanic
      membrane—*see* Wound, open, ear, drum

Injury—*continued*
  blood vessel NEC 904.9
    abdomen 902.9
      multiple 902.87
      specified NEC 902.89
    aorta (thoracic) 901.0
      abdominal 902.0
    arm NEC 903.9
    axillary 903.00
      artery 903.01
      vein 903.02
    azygos vein 901.89
    basilic vein 903.1
    brachial (artery) (vein) 903.1
    bronchial 901.89
    carotid artery 900.00
      common 900.01
      external 900.02
      internal 900.03
    celiac artery 902.20
      specified branch NEC 902.24
    cephalic vein (arm) 903.1
    colica dextra 902.26
    cystic
      artery 902.24
      vein 902.39
    deep plantar 904.6
    digital (artery) (vein) 903.5
    due to accidental puncture or laceration during
      procedure 998.2
    extremity
      lower 904.8
        multiple 904.7
        specified NEC 904.7
      upper 903.9
        multiple 903.8
        specified NEC 903.8
    femoral
      artery (superficial) 904.1
        above profunda origin 904.0
        common 904.0
      vein 904.2
    gastric
      artery 902.21
      vein 902.39
    head 900.9
      intracranial—*see* Injury, intracranial
      multiple 900.82
      specified NEC 900.89
    hemiazygos vein 901.89
    hepatic
      artery 902.22
      vein 902.11
    hypogastric 902.59
      artery 902.51
      vein 902.52
    ileocolic
      artery 902.26
      vein 902.31
    iliac 902.50
      artery 902.53
      specified branch NEC 902.59
      vein 902.54
    innominate
      artery 901.1
      vein 901.3
    intercostal (artery) (vein) 901.81
    jugular vein (external) 900.81
      internal 900.1
    leg NEC 904.8
    mammary (artery) (vein) 901.82

Injury—*continued*
  blood vessel—*continued*
    mesenteric
      artery 902.20
        inferior 902.27
        specified branch NEC 902.29
        superior (trunk) 902.25
          branches, primary 902.26
      vein 902.39
        inferior 902.32
        superior (and primary subdivisions) 902.31
    neck 900.9
      multiple 900.82
      specified NEC 900.89
    ovarian 902.89
      artery 902.81
      vein 902.82
    palmar artery 903.4
    pelvis 902.9
      multiple 902.87
      specified NEC 902.89
    plantar (deep) (artery) (vein) 904.6
    popliteal 904.40
      artery 904.41
      vein 904.42
    portal 902.33
    pulmonary 901.40
      artery 901.41
      vein 901.42
    radial (artery) (vein) 903.2
    renal 902.40
      artery 902.41
      specified NEC 902.49
      vein 902.42
    saphenous
      artery 904.7
      vein (greater) (lesser) 904.3
    splenic
      artery 902.23
      vein 902.34
    subclavian
      artery 901.1
      vein 901.3
    suprarenal 902.49
    thoracic 901.9
      multiple 901.83
      specified NEC 901.89
    tibial 904.50
      artery 904.50
        anterior 904.51
        posterior 904.53
      vein 904.50
        anterior 904.52
        posterior 904.54
    ulnar (artery) (vein) 903.3
    uterine 902.59
      artery 902.55
      vein 902.56
    vena cava
      inferior 902.10
        specified branches NEC 902.19
      superior 901.2
  brachial plexus 953.4
    newborn 767.6
  brain (traumatic) NEC (*see also* Injury,
    intracranial) 854.0
    due to fracture of skull—see Fracture, skull,
      by site
  breast 959.19
  broad ligament—*see* Injury, internal, broad
    ligament

Injury—*continued*
  bronchus, bronchi—*see* Injury, internal, bronchus
  brow 959.09
  buttock 959.19
  canthus, eye 921.1
  cathode ray 990
  cauda equina 952.4
    with fracture, vertebra—*see* Fracture, vertebra,
      sacrum
  cavernous sinus (*see also* Injury, intracranial)
    854.0
  cecum—*see* Injury, internal, cecum
  celiac ganglion or plexus 954.1
  cerebellum (*see also* Injury, intracranial) 854.0
  cervix (uteri)—*see* Injury, internal, cervix
  cheek 959.09
  chest—*see* Injury, internal, chest
    wall 959.11
  childbirth—*see also* Birth, injury
    maternal NEC 665.9
  chin 959.09
  choroid (eye) 921.3
  clitoris 959.14
  coccyx 959.19
    complicating delivery 665.6
  colon—*see* Injury, internal, colon
  common duct—*see* Injury, internal, common
    duct
  conjunctiva 921.1
    superficial 918.2
  cord
    spermatic—*see* Injury, internal, spermatic
      cord
    spinal—*see* Injury, spinal, by site
  cornea 921.3
    abrasion 918.1
    due to contact lens 371.82
    penetrating—*see* Injury, eyeball, penetrating
    superficial 918.1
      due to contact lens 371.82
  cortex (cerebral) (*see also* Injury, intracranial)
    854.0
    visual 950.3
  costal region 959.11
  costochondral 959.11
  cranial
    bones—*see* Fracture, skull, by site
    cavity (*see also* Injury, intracranial) 854.0
    nerve—*see* Injury, nerve, cranial
  crushing—*see* Crush
  cutaneous sensory nerve
    lower limb 956.4
    upper limb 955.5
  deep tissue—*see* Contusion, by site
    meaning pressure ulcer 707.25
  delivery—*see also* Birth, injury
    maternal NEC 665.9
  Descemet's membrane—*see* Injury, eyeball,
    penetrating
  diaphragm—*see* Injury, internal, diaphragm
  diffuse axonal—*see* Injury, intracranial
  duodenum—*see* Injury, internal, duodenum
  ear (auricle) (canal) (drum) (external) 959.09
  elbow (and forearm) (and wrist) 959.3
  epididymis 959.14
  epigastric region 959.12
  epiglottis 959.09
  epiphyseal, current—*see* Fracture, by site
  esophagus—*see* Injury, internal, esophagus
  Eustachian tube 959.09
  extremity (lower) (upper) NEC 959.8

Injury—*continued*

eye 921.9
  penetrating eyeball—*see* Injury, eyeball,
    penetrating
  superficial 918.9
eyeball 921.3
  penetrating 871.7
    with
      partial loss (of intraocular tissue) 871.12
      prolapse or exposure (of intraocular tissue)
        871.1
      without prolapse 871.0
    foreign body (nonmagnetic) 871.6
      magnetic 871.5
  superficial 918.9
eyebrow 959.09
eyelid(s) 921.1
  laceration—*see* Laceration, eyelid
  superficial 918.0
face (and neck) 959.09
fallopian tube—*see* Injury, internal, fallopian
  tube
finger(s) (nail) 959.5
flank 959.19
foot (and ankle) (and knee) (and leg except
  thigh) 959.7
forceps NEC 767.9
  scalp 767.19
forearm (and elbow) (and wrist) 959.3
forehead 959.09
gallbladder—*see* Injury, internal, gallbladder
gasserian ganglion 951.2
gastrointestinal tract—*see* Injury, internal,
  gastrointestinal tract
genital organ(s)
  with
    abortion—*see* Abortion, by type, with,
      damage to pelvic organs
    ectopic pregnancy (*see also* categories
      633.0-633.9) 639.2
    molar pregnancy (*see also* categories
      630-632) 639.2
  external 959.14
    fracture of corpus cavernosum penis 959.13
  following
    abortion 639.2
    ectopic or molar pregnancy 639.2
  internal—*see* Injury, internal, genital organs
  obstetrical trauma NEC 665.9
    affecting fetus or newborn 763.89
gland
  lacrimal 921.1
    laceration 870.8
  parathyroid 959.09
  salivary 959.09
  thyroid 959.09
globe (eye) (*see also* Injury, eyeball) 921.3
grease gun—*see* Wound, open, by site,
  complicated
groin 959.19
gum 959.09
hand(s) (except fingers) 959.4
head NEC 959.01
  with
    loss of consciousness 850.5
    skull fracture—*see* Fracture, skull, by site
heart—*see* Injury, internal, heart
heel 959.7
hip (and thigh) 959.6
hymen 959.14
hyperextension (cervical) (vertebra) 847.0

Injury—*continued*

ileum—*see* Injury, internal, ileum
iliac region 959.19
infrared rays NEC 990
instrumental (during surgery) 998.2
  birth injury—*see* Birth, injury
  nonsurgical (*see also* Injury, by site) 959.9
  obstetrical 665.9
    affecting fetus or newborn 763.89
    bladder 665.5
    cervix 665.3
    high vaginal 665.4
    perineal NEC 664.9
    urethra 665.5
    uterus 665.5
internal 869.0

Note—*For injury of internal organ(s) by foreign
body entering through a natural orifice (e.g.,
inhaled, ingested, or swallowed)—see Foreign
body, entering through orifice.*

*For internal injury of any of the following sites
with internal injury of any other of the sites—
see Injury, internal, multiple.*

---

with
  fracture
    pelvis—*see* Fracture, pelvis
    specified site, except pelvis—*see* Injury,
      internal, by site
  open wound into cavity 869.1
abdomen, abdominal (viscera) NEC 868.00
  with
    fracture, pelvis—*see* Fracture, pelvis
    open wound into cavity 868.10
  specified site NEC 868.09
    with open wound into cavity 868.19
adrenal (gland) 868.01
  with open wound into cavity 868.11
aorta (thoracic) 901.0
  abdominal 902.0
appendix 863.85
  with open wound into cavity 863.95
bile duct 868.02
  with open wound into cavity 868.12
bladder (sphincter) 867.0
  with
    abortion—*see* Abortion, by type, with,
      damage to pelvic organs
    ectopic pregnancy (*see also* categories
      633.0-633.9) 639.2
    molar pregnancy (*see also* categories
      630-632) 639.2
    open wound into cavity 867.1
  following
    abortion 639.2
    ectopic or molar pregnancy 639.2
  obstetrical trauma 665.5
    affecting fetus or newborn 763.89
blood vessel—*see* Injury, blood vessel, by site
broad ligament 867.6
  with open wound into cavity 867.7
bronchus, bronchi 862.21
  with open wound into cavity 862.31
cecum 863.89
  with open wound into cavity 863.99
cervix (uteri) 867.4
  with
    abortion—*see* Abortion, by type, with
      damage to pelvic organs

Injury—*continued*
  internal—*continued*
    cervix—*continued*
      ectopic pregnancy (*see also* categories
        633.0-633.9) 639.2
      molar pregnancy (*see also* categories
        630-632) 639.2
      open wound into cavity 867.5
      following
        abortion 639.2
        ectopic or molar pregnancy 639.2
      obstetrical trauma 665.3
        affecting fetus or newborn 763.89
    chest (*see also* Injury, internal, intrathoracic
      organs) 862.8
      with open wound into cavity 862.9
    colon 863.40
      with
        open wound into cavity 863.50
        rectum 863.46
          with open wound into cavity 863.56
      ascending (right) 863.41
        with open wound into cavity 863.51
      descending (left) 863.43
        with open wound into cavity 863.53
      multiple sites 863.46
        with open wound into cavity 863.56
      sigmoid 863.44
        with open wound into cavity 863.54
      specified site NEC 863.49
        with open wound into cavity 863.59
      transverse 863.42
        with open wound into cavity 863.52
    common duct 868.02
      with open wound into cavity 868.12
    complicating delivery 665.9
      affecting fetus or newborn 763.89
    diaphragm 862.0
      with open wound into cavity 862.1
    duodenum 863.21
      with open wound into cavity 863.31
    esophagus (intrathoracic) 862.22
      with open wound into cavity 862.32
      cervical region 874.4
        complicated 874.5
    fallopian tube 867.6
      with open wound into cavity 867.7
    gallbladder 868.02
      with open wound into cavity 868.12
    gastrointestinal tract NEC 863.80
      with open wound into cavity 863.90
    genital organ NEC 867.6
      with open wound into cavity 867.7
    heart 861.00
      with open wound into thorax 861.10
    ileum 863.29
      with open wound into cavity 863.39
    intestine NEC 863.89
      with open wound into cavity 863.99
      large NEC 863.40
        with open wound into cavity 863.50
      small NEC 863.20
        with open wound into cavity 863.30
    intra-abdominal (organ) 868.00
      with open wound into cavity 868.10
      multiple sites 868.09
        with open wound into cavity 868.19
      specified site NEC 868.09
        with open wound into cavity 868.19

Injury—*continued*
  internal—*continued*
    intrathoracic organs (multiple) 862.8
      with open wound into cavity 862.9
      diaphragm (only)—*see* Injury, internal,
        diaphragm
      heart (only)—*see* Injury, internal, heart
      lung (only)—*see* Injury, internal, lung
      specified site NEC 862.29
        with open wound into cavity 862.39
    intrauterine (*see also* Injury, internal, uterus)
      867.4
      with open wound into cavity 867.5
    jejunum 863.29
      with open wound into cavity 863.39
    kidney (subcapsular) 866.00
      with
        disruption of parenchyma (complete)
          866.03
          with open wound into cavity 866.13
        hematoma (without rupture of capsule)
          866.01
          with open wound into cavity 866.11
        laceration 866.02
          with open wound into cavity 866.12
        open wound into cavity 866.10
    liver 864.00
      with
        contusion 864.01
          with open wound into cavity 864.11
        hematoma 864.01
          with open wound into cavity 864.11
        laceration 864.05
          with open wound into cavity 864.15
          major (disruption of hepatic
            parenchyma) 864.04
            with open wound into cavity 864.14
          minor (capsule only) 864.02
            with open wound into cavity 864.12
          moderate (involving parenchyma) 864.03
            with open wound into cavity 864.13
          multiple 864.04
          stellate 864.04
            with open wound in cavity 864.14
        open wound into cavity 864.10
    lung 861.20
      with open wound into thorax 861.30
      hemopneumothorax—*see*
        Hemopneumothorax, traumatic
      hemothorax—*see* Hemothorax, traumatic
      pneumohemothorax—*see*
        Pneumohemothorax, traumatic
      pneumothorax—*see* Pneumothorax,
        traumatic
      transfusion related, acute (TRALI) 518.7
    mediastinum 862.29
      with open wound into cavity 862.39
    mesentery 863.89
      with open wound into cavity 863.99
    mesosalpinx 867.6
      with open wound into cavity 867.7
    multiple 869.0

> *Note—Multiple internal injuries of sites
> classifiable to the same three- or four-digit
> category should be classified to that category.
> Multiple injuries classifiable to different
> fourth-digit subdivisions of 861 (heart and lung
> injuries) should be dealt with according to
> coding rules.*

      with open wound into cavity 869.1

Injury—*continued*
  internal—*continued*
    multiple—*continued*
      intra-abdominal organ (sites classifiable to 863-868)
        with
          intrathoracic organ(s) (sites classifiable to 861-862) 869.0
            with open wound into cavity 869.1
          other intra-abdominal organ(s) (sites classifiable to 863-868, except where classifiable to the same three-digit category) 868.09
            with open wound into cavity 868.19
      intrathoracic organ (sites classifiable to 861-862)
        with
          intra-abdominal organ(s) (sites classifiable to 863-868) 869.0
            with open wound into cavity 869.1
          other intrathoracic organ(s) (sites classifiable to 861-862, except where classifiable to the same three-digit category) 862.8
            with open wound into cavity 862.9
    myocardium—*see* Injury, internal, heart
    ovary 867.6
      with open wound into cavity 867.7
    pancreas (multiple sites) 863.84
      with open wound into cavity 863.94
      body 863.82
        with open wound into cavity 863.92
      head 863.81
        with open wound into cavity 863.91
      tail 863.83
        with open wound into cavity 863.93
    pelvis, pelvic (organs) (viscera) 867.8
      with
        fracture, pelvis—*see* Fracture, pelvis
        open wound into cavity 867.9
      specified site NEC 867.6
        with open wound into cavity 867.7
    peritoneum 868.03
      with open wound into cavity 868.13
    pleura 862.29
      with open wound into cavity 862.39
    prostate 867.6
    with open wound into cavity 867.7
    rectum 863.45
      with
        colon 863.46
          with open wound into cavity 863.56
        open wound into cavity 863.55
    retroperitoneum 868.04
      with open wound into cavity 868.14
    round ligament 867.6
      with open wound into cavity 867.7
    seminal vesicle 867.6
      with open wound into cavity 867.7
    spermatic cord 867.6
      with open wound into cavity 867.7
      scrotal—*see* Wound, open, spermatic cord
    spleen 865.00
      with
        disruption of parenchyma (massive) 865.04
          with open wound into cavity 865.14
        hematoma (without rupture of capsule) 865.01
          with open wound into cavity 865.11
        open wound into cavity 865.10

Injury—*continued*
  internal—*continued*
    spleen—*continued*
      with—*continued*
        tear, capsular 865.02
          with open wound into cavity 865.12
          extending into parenchyma 865.03
            with open wound into cavity 865.13
    stomach 863.0
      with open wound into cavity 863.1
    suprarenal gland (multiple) 868.01
      with open wound into cavity 868.11
    thorax, thoracic (cavity) (organs) (multiple) (*see also* Injury, internal, intrathoracic organs) 862.8
      with open wound into cavity 862.9
    thymus (gland) 862.29
      with open wound into cavity 862.39
    trachea (intrathoracic) 862.29
      with open wound into cavity 862.39
      cervical region (*see also* Wound, open, trachea) 874.02
    ureter 867.2
      with open wound into cavity 867.3
    urethra (sphincter) 867.0
      with
        abortion—*see* Abortion, by type, with, damage to pelvic organs
        ectopic pregnancy (*see also* categories 633.0-633.9) 639.2
        molar pregnancy (*see also* categories 630-632) 639.2
        open wound into cavity 867.1
      following
        abortion 639.2
        ectopic or molar pregnancy 639.2
        obstetrical trauma 665.5
          affecting fetus or newborn 763.89
    uterus 867.4
      with
        abortion—*see* Abortion, by type, with, damage to pelvic organs
        ectopic pregnancy (*see also* categories 633.0-633.9) 639.2
        molar pregnancy (*see also* categories 630-632) 639.2
        open wound into cavity 867.5
      following
        abortion 639.2
        ectopic or molar pregnancy 639.2
        obstetrical trauma NEC 665.5
          affecting fetus or newborn 763.89
    vas deferens 867.6
      with open wound into cavity 867.7
    vesical (sphincter) 867.0
      with open wound into cavity 867.1
    viscera (abdominal) (*see also* Injury, internal, multiple) 868.00
      with
        fracture, pelvis—*see* Fracture, pelvis
        open wound into cavity 868.10
        thoracic NEC (*see also* Injury, internal, intrathoracic organs) 862.8
          with open wound into cavity 862.9
  interscapular region 959.19
  intervertebral disc 959.19
  intestine—*see* Injury, internal, intestine
  intra-abdominal (organs) NEC—*see* Injury, internal, intra-abdominal

Injury—*continued*
  intracranial (traumatic) 854.0

Note—Use the following fifth-digit subclassification with categories 851-854:

0 *unspecifidd state of consciousness*
1 *with no loss of consciousness*
2 *with brief [less than one hour] loss of consciousness*
3 *with moderate [1-24 hours] loss of consciousness*
4 *with prolonged [more than 24 hours] loss of consciousness and return to pre-existing conscious level*
5 *with prolonged [more than 24 hours] loss of consciousness, without return to pre-existing conscious level*
Use fifth-digit 5 to designate when a patient is unconscious and dies before regaining consciousness, regardless of the duration of the loss of consciousness
6 *with loss of consciousness of unspecified duration*
9 *with concussion, unspecified*

---

  with
    open intracranial wound 854.1
    skull fracture—*see* Fracture, skull, by site
  contusion 851.8
    with open intracranial wound 851.9
    brain stem 851.4
      with open intracranial wound 851.5
    cerebellum 851.4
      with open intracranial wound 851.5
    cortex (cerebral) 851.0
      with open intracranial wound 851.2
  hematoma—*see* Injury, intracranial, hemorrhage
  hemorrhage 853.0
    with
      laceration—*see* Injury, intracranial, laceration
      open intracranial wound 853.1
    extradural 852.4
      with open intracranial wound 852.5
    subarachnoid 852.0
      with open intracranial wound 852.1
    subdural 852.2
      with open intracranial wound 852.3
  laceration 851.8
    with open intracranial wound 851.9
    brain stem 851.6
      with open intracranial wound 851.7
    cerebellum 851.6
      with open intracranial wound 851.7
    cortex (cerebral) 851.2
      with open intracranial wound 851.3
  intraocular—*see* Injury, eyeball, penetrating
  intrathoracic organs (multiple)—*see* Injury, internal, intrathoracic organs
  intrauterine—*see* Injury, internal, intrauterine
  iris 921.3
    penetrating—*see* Injury, eyeball, penetrating
  jaw 959.09
  jejunum—*see* Injury, internal, jejunum

Injury—*continued*
  joint NEC 959.9
    old or residual 718.80
      ankle 718.87
      elbow 718.82
      foot 718.87
      hand 718.84
      hip 718.85
      knee 718.86
      multiple sites 718.89
      pelvic region 718.85
      shoulder (region) 718.81
      specified site NEC 718.88
      wrist 718.83
  kidney—*see* Injury, internal, kidney
    acute (nontraumatic) 584.9
  knee (and ankle) (and foot) (and leg, except thigh) 959.7
  labium (majus) (minus) 959.14
  labyrinth, ear 959.09
  lacrimal apparatus, gland, or sac 921.1
    laceration 870.8
  larynx 959.09
  late effect—*see* Late, effects (of), injury
  leg except thigh (and ankle) (and foot) (and knee) 959.7
    upper or thigh 959.6
  lens, eye 921.3
    penetrating—*see* Injury, eyeball, penetrating
  lid, eye—*see* Injury, eyelid
  lip 959.09
  liver—*see* Injury, internal, liver
  lobe, parietal—*see* Injury, intracranial
  lumbar (region) 959.19
    plexus 953.5
  lumbosacral (region) 959.19
    plexus 953.5
  lung—*see* Injury, internal, lung
  malar region 959.09
  mastoid region 959.09
  maternal, during pregnancy, affecting fetus or newborn 760.5
  maxilla 959.09
  mediastinum—*see* Injury, internal, mediastinum
  membrane
    brain (*see also* Injury, intracranial) 854.0
    tympanic 959.09
  meningeal artery—*see* Hemorrhage, brain, traumatic, subarachnoid
  meninges (cerebral)—*see* Injury, intracranial
  mesenteric
    artery—*see* Injury, blood vessel, mesenteric, artery
    plexus, inferior 954.1
    vein—*see* Injury, blood vessel, mesenteric, vein
  mesentery—*see* Injury, internal, mesentery
  mesosalpinx—*see* Injury, internal, mesosalpinx
  middle ear 959.09
  midthoracic region 959.11
  mouth 959.09
  multiple (sites not classifiable to the same four-digit category in 959.0-959.7) 959.8
    internal 869.0
      with open wound into cavity 869.1
  musculocutaneous nerve 955.4
  nail
    finger 959.5
    toe 959.7
  nasal (septum) (sinus) 959.09
  nasopharynx 959.09
  neck (and face) 959.09

Injury—*continued*
nerve 957.9
  abducens 951.3
  abducent 951.3
  accessory 951.6
  acoustic 951.5
  ankle and foot 956.9
  anterior crural, femoral 956.1
  arm (*see also* Injury, nerve, upper limb) 955.9
  auditory 951.5
  axillary 955.0
  brachial plexus 953.4
  cervical sympathetic 954.0
  cranial 951.9
    first or olfactory 951.8
    second or optic 950.0
    third or oculomotor 951.0
    fourth or trochlear 951.1
    fifth or trigeminal 951.2
    sixth or abducens 951.3
    seventh or facial 951.4
    eighth, acoustic, or auditory 951.5
    ninth or glossopharyngeal 951.8
    tenth, pneumogastric, or vagus 951.8
    eleventh or accessory 951.6
    twelfth or hypoglossal 951.7
    newborn 767.7
  cutaneous sensory
    lower limb 956.4
    upper limb 955.5
  digital (finger) 955.6
    toe 956.5
  facial 951.4
    newborn 767.5
  femoral 956.1
  finger 955.9
  foot and ankle 956.9
  forearm 955.9
  glossopharyngeal 951.8
  hand and wrist 955.9
  head and neck, superficial 957.0
  hypoglossal 951.7
  involving several parts of body 957.8
  leg (*see also* Injury, nerve, lower limb) 956.9
  lower limb 956.9
    multiple 956.8
    specified site NEC 956.5
  lumbar plexus 953.5
  lumbosacral plexus 953.5
  median 955.1
    forearm 955.1
    wrist and hand 955.1
  multiple (in several parts of body) (sites not
      classifiable to the same three-digit
      category) 957.8
  musculocutaneous 955.4
  musculospiral 955.3
    upper arm 955.3
  oculomotor 951.0
  olfactory 951.8
  optic 950.0
  pelvic girdle 956.9
    multiple sites 956.8
    specified site NEC 956.5
  peripheral 957.9
    multiple (in several regions) (sites not
        classifiable to the same three-digit
        category) 957.8
    specified site NEC 957.1

Injury—*continued*
nerve—*continued*
  peroneal 956.3
    ankle and foot 956.3
    lower leg 956.3
  plantar 956.5
  plexus 957.9
    celiac 954.1
    mesenteric, inferior 954.1
    spinal 953.9
      brachial 953.4
      lumbosacral 953.5
      multiple sites 953.8
    sympathetic NEC 954.1
  pneumogastric 951.8
  radial 955.3
    wrist and hand 955.3
  sacral plexus 953.5
  sciatic 956.0
    thigh 956.0
  shoulder girdle 955.9
    multiple 955.8
    specified site NEC 955.7
  specified site NEC 957.1
  spinal 953.9
    plexus—*see* Injury, nerve, plexus, spinal
    root 953.9
      cervical 953.0
      dorsal 953.1
      lumbar 953.2
      multiple sites 953.8
      sacral 953.3
  splanchnic 954.1
  sympathetic NEC 954.1
    cervical 954.0
  thigh 956.9
  tibial 956.5
    ankle and foot 956.2
    lower leg 956.5
    posterior 956.2
  toe 956.9
  trigeminal 951.2
  trochlear 951.1
  trunk, excluding shoulder and pelvic girdles
      954.9
    specified site NEC 954.8
    sympathetic NEC 954.1
  ulnar 955.2
    forearm 955.2
    wrist (and hand) 955.2
  upper limb 955.9
    multiple 955.8
    specified site NEC 955.7
  vagus 951.8
  wrist and hand 955.9
nervous system, diffuse 957.8
nose (septum) 959.09
obstetrical NEC 665.9
  affecting fetus or newborn 763.89
occipital (region) (scalp) 959.09
  lobe (*see also* Injury, intracranial) 854.0
optic 950.9
  chiasm 950.1
  cortex 950.3
  nerve 950.0
  pathways 950.2
orbit, orbital (region) 921.2
  penetrating 870.3
    with foreign body 870.4
ovary—*see* Injury, internal, ovary
paint-gun—*see* Wound, open, by site,
  complicated

Injury—*continued*
 palate (soft) 959.09
 pancreas—*see* Injury, internal, pancreas
 parathyroid (gland) 959.09
 parietal (region) (scalp) 959.09
  lobe—*see* Injury, intracranial
 pelvic
  floor 959.19
   complicating delivery 664.1
    affecting fetus or newborn 763.89
   joint or ligament, complicating delivery 665.6
    affecting fetus or newborn 763.89
   organs—*see also* Injury, internal, pelvis
    with
     abortion—*see* Abortion, by type, with
      damage to pelvic organs
     ectopic pregnancy (*see also* categories
      633.0-633.9) 639.2
     molar pregnancy (*see also* categories
      633.0-633.9) 639.2
     following
      abortion 639.2
      ectopic or molar pregnancy 639.2
     obstetrical trauma 665.5
      affecting fetus or newborn 763.89
 pelvis 959.19
 penis 959.14
  fracture of corpus cavernosum 959.13
 perineum 959.14
 peritoneum—*see* Injury, internal, peritoneum
 periurethral tissue
  with
   abortion—*see* Abortion, by type, with
    damage to pelvic organs
   ectopic pregnancy (*see also* categories
    633.0-633.9) 639.2
   molar pregnancy (*see also* categories
    630-632) 639.2
   complicating delivery 665.5
    affecting fetus or newborn 763.89
   following
    abortion 639.2
    ectopic or molar pregnancy 639.2
 phalanges
  foot 959.7
  hand 959.5
 pharynx 959.09
 pleura—*see* Injury, internal, pleura
 popliteal space 959.7
 post-cardiac surgery (syndrome) 429.4
 prepuce 959.14
 prostate—*see* Injury, internal, prostate
 pubic region 959.19
 pudenda 959.14
 radiation NEC 990
 radioactive substance or radium NEC 990
 rectovaginal septum 959.14
 rectum—*see* Injury, internal, rectum
 retina 921.3
  penetrating—*see* Injury, eyeball, penetrating
 retroperitoneal—*see* Injury, internal,
  retroperitoneum
 roentgen rays NEC 990
 round ligament—*see* Injury, internal, round
  ligament
 sacral (region) 959.19
  plexus 953.5
 sacroiliac ligament NEC 959.19
 sacrum 959.19
 salivary ducts or glands 959.09

Injury—*continued*
 scalp 959.09
  due to birth trauma 767.19
  fetus or newborn 767.19
 scapular region 959.2
 sclera 921.3
  penetrating—*see* Injury, eyeball, penetrating
  superficial 918.2
 scrotum 959.14
 seminal vesicle—*see* Injury, internal, seminal
  vesicle
 shoulder (and upper arm) 959.2
 sinus
  cavernous (*see also* Injury, intracranial) 854.0
  nasal 959.09
 skeleton NEC, birth injury 767.3
 skin NEC 959.9
 skull—*see* Fracture, skull, by site
 soft tissue (of external sites) (severe)—*see*
  Wound, open, by site
 specified site NEC 959.8
 spermatic cord—*see* Injury, internal, spermatic
  cord
 spinal (cord) 952.9
  with fracture, vertebra—*see* Fracture, vertebra,
   by site, with spinal cord injury
  cervical (C_1-C_4) 952.00
   with
    anterior cord syndrome 952.02
    central cord syndrome 952.03
    complete lesion of cord 952.01
    incomplete lesion NEC 952.04
    posterior cord syndrome 952.04
   C_5-C_7 level 952.05
    with
     anterior cord syndrome 952.07
     central cord syndrome 952.08
     complete lesion of cord 952.06
     incomplete lesion NEC 952.09
     posterior cord syndrome 952.09
     specified type NEC 952.09
    specified type NEC 952.04
  dorsal (D_1-D_6) (T_1-T_6) (thoracic) 952.10
   with
    anterior cord syndrome 952.12
    central cord syndrome 952.13
    complete lesion of cord 952.11
    incomplete lesion NEC 952.14
    posterior cord syndrome 952.14
   D_7-D_{12} level (T_7-T_{12}) 952.15
    with
     anterior cord syndrome 952.17
     central cord syndrome 952.18
     complete lesion of cord 952.16
     incomplete lesion NEC 952.19
     posterior cord syndrome 952.19
     specified type NEC 952.19
    specified type NEC 952.14
  lumbar 952.2
  multiple sites 952.8
  nerve (root) NEC—*see* Injury, nerve, spinal,
   root
  plexus 953.9
   brachial 953.4
   lumbosacral 953.5
   multiple sites 953.8
  sacral 952.3
  thoracic (*see also* Injury, spinal, dorsal)
   952.10
 spleen—*see* Injury, internal, spleen
 stellate ganglion 954.1
 sternal region 959.11

Injury—*continued*
  stomach—*see* Injury, internal, stomach
  subconjunctival 921.1
  subcutaneous 959.9
  subdural—*see* Injury, intracranial
  submaxillary region 959.09
  submental region 959.09
  subungual
    fingers 959.5
    toes 959.7
  superficial 919

Note—Use the following fourth-digit subdivisions with categories 910-919:

.0 *Abrasion or friction burn without mention of infection*
.1 *Abrasion or friction burn, infected*
.2 *Blister without mention of infection*
.3 *Blister, infected*
.4 *Insect bite, nonvenomous, without mention of infection*
.5 *Insect bite, nonvenomous, infected*
.6 *Superficial foreign body (splinter) without major open wound and without mention of infection*
.7 *Superficial foreign body (splinter) without major open wound, infected*
.8 *Other and unspecified superficial injury without mention of infection*
.9 *Other and unspecified superficial injury, infected*

For late effects of superficial injury, see category 906.2.

---

  abdomen, abdominal (muscle) (wall) (and other part(s) of trunk) 911
  ankle (and hip, knee, leg, or thigh) 916
  anus (and other part(s) of trunk) 911
  arm 913
    upper (and shoulder) 912
  auditory canal (external) (meatus) (and other part(s) of face, neck, or scalp, except eye) 910
  axilla (and upper arm) 912
  back (and other part(s) of trunk) 911
  breast (and other part(s) of trunk) 911
  brow (and other part(s) of face, neck or scalp, except eye) 910
  buttock (and other part(s) of trunk) 911
  canthus, eye 918.0
  cheek(s) (and other part(s) of face, neck, or scalp, except eye) 910
  chest wall (and other part(s) of trunk) 911
  chin (and other part(s) of face, neck, or scalp, except eye) 910
  clitoris (and other part(s) of trunk) 911
  conjunctiva 918.2
  cornea 918.1
    due to contact lens 371.82
  costal region (and other part(s) of trunk) 911
  ear(s) (auricle) (canal) (drum) (external) (and other part(s) of face, neck, or scalp, except eye) 910
  elbow (and forearm) (and wrist) 913
  epididymis (and other part(s) of trunk) 911
  epigastric region (and other part(s) of trunk) 911
  epiglottis (and other part(s) of face, neck, or scalp, except eye) 910
  eye(s) (and adnexa) NEC 918.9
  eyelid(s) (and periocular area) 918.0

Injury—*continued*
  superficial—*continued*
    face (any part(s), except eye) (and neck or scalp) 910
    finger(s) (nail) (any) 915
    flank (and other part(s) of trunk) 911
    foot (phalanges) (and toe(s)) 917
    forearm (and elbow) (and wrist) 913
    forehead (and other part(s) of face, neck, or scalp, except eye) 910
    globe (eye) 918.9
    groin (and other part(s) of trunk) 911
    gum(s) (and other part(s) of face, neck, or scalp, except eye) 910
    hand(s) (except fingers alone) 914
    head (and other part(s) of face, neck, or scalp, except eye) 910
    heel (and foot or toe) 917
    hip (and ankle, knee, leg, or thigh) 916
    iliac region (and other part(s) of trunk) 911
    interscapular region (and other part(s) of trunk) 911
    iris 918.9
    knee (and ankle, hip, leg, or thigh) 916
    labium (majus) (minus) (and other part(s) of trunk) 911
    lacrimal (apparatus) (gland) (sac) 918.0
    leg (lower) (upper) (and ankle, hip, knee, or thigh) 916
    lip(s) (and other part(s) of face, neck, or scalp, except eye) 910
    lower extremity (except foot) 916
    lumbar region (and other part(s) of trunk) 911
    malar region (and other part(s) of face, neck, or scalp, except eye) 910
    mastoid region (and other part(s) of face, neck, or scalp, except eye) 910
    midthoracic region (and other part(s) of trunk) 911
    mouth (and other part(s) of face, neck, or scalp, except eye) 910
    multiple sites (not classifiable to the same three-digit category) 919
    nasal (septum) (and other part(s) of face, neck, or scalp, except eye) 910
    neck (and face or scalp, any part(s), except eye) 910
    nose (septum) (and other part(s) of face, neck, or scalp, except eye) 910
    occipital region (and other part(s) of face, neck, or scalp, except eye) 910
    orbital region 918.0
    palate (soft) (and other part(s) of face, neck, or scalp, except eye) 910
    parietal region (and other part(s) of face, neck, or scalp, except eye) 910
    penis (and other part(s) of trunk) 911
    perineum (and other part(s) of trunk) 911
    periocular area 918.0
    pharynx (and other part(s) of face, neck, or scalp, except eye) 910
    popliteal space (and ankle, hip, leg, or thigh) 916
    prepuce (and other part(s) of trunk) 911
    pubic region (and other part(s) of trunk) 911
    pudenda (and other part(s) of trunk) 911
    sacral region (and other part(s) of trunk) 911
    salivary (ducts) (glands) (and other part(s) of face, neck, or scalp, except eye) 910
    scalp (and other part(s) of face or neck, except eye) 910
    scapular region (and upper arm) 912

Injury—*continued*
  superficial—*continued*
    sclera 918.2
    scrotum (and other part(s) of trunk) 911
    shoulder (and upper arm) 912
    skin NEC 919
    specified site(s) NEC 919
    sternal region (and other part(s) of trunk) 911
    subconjunctival 918.2
    subcutaneous NEC 919
    submaxillary region (and other part(s) of face, neck, or scalp, except eye) 910
    submental region (and other part(s) of face, neck, or scalp, except eye) 910
    supraclavicular fossa (and other part(s) of face, neck or scalp, except eye) 910
    supraorbital 918.0
    temple (and other part(s) of face, neck, or scalp, except eye) 910
    temporal region (and other part(s) of face, neck, or scalp, except eye) 910
    testis (and other part(s) of trunk) 911
    thigh (and ankle, hip, knee, or leg) 916
    thorax, thoracic (external) (and other part(s) of trunk) 911
    throat (and other part(s) of face, neck, or scalp, except eye) 910
    thumb(s) (nail) 915
    toe(s) (nail) (subungual) (and foot) 917
    tongue (and other part(s) of face, neck, or scalp, except eye) 910
    tooth, teeth (*see also* Abrasion, dental) 521.20
    trunk (any part(s)) 911
    tunica vaginalis (and other part(s) of trunk) 911
    tympanum, tympanic membrane (and other part(s) of face, neck, or scalp, except eye) 910
    upper extremity NEC 913
    uvula (and other part(s) of face, neck, or scalp, except eye) 910
    vagina (and other part(s) of trunk) 911
    vulva (and other part(s) of trunk) 911
    wrist (and elbow) (and forearm) 913
  supraclavicular fossa 959.19
  supraorbital 959.09
  surgical complication (external or internal site) 998.2
  symphysis pubis 959.19
    complicating delivery 665.6
      affecting fetus or newborn 763.89
  temple 959.09
  temporal region 959.09
  testis 959.14
  thigh (and hip) 959.6
  thorax, thoracic (external) 959.11
    cavity—*see* Injury, internal, thorax
    internal—*see* Injury, internal, intrathoracic organs
  throat 959.09
  thumb(s) (nail) 959.5
  thymus—*see* Injury, internal, thymus
  thyroid (gland) 959.09
  toe (nail) (any) 959.7
  tongue 959.09
  tonsil 959.09
  tooth NEC 873.63
    complicated 873.73
  trachea—*see* Injury, internal, trachea
  trunk 959.19
  tunica vaginalis 959.14
  tympanum, tympanic membrane 959.09

Injury—*continued*
  ultraviolet rays NEC 990
  ureter—*see* Injury, internal, ureter
  urethra (sphincter)—*see* Injury, internal, urethra
  uterus—*see* Injury, internal, uterus
  uvula 959.09
  vagina 959.14
  vascular—*see* Injury, blood vessel
  vas deferens—*see* Injury, internal, vas deferens
  vein (*see also* Injury, blood vessel, by site) 904.9
  vena cava
    inferior 902.10
    superior 901.2
  vesical (sphincter)—*see* Injury, internal, vesical
  viscera (abdominal)—*see* Injury, internal, viscera
    with fracture, pelvis—*see* Fracture, pelvis
  visual 950.9
    cortex 950.3
  vitreous (humor) 871.2
  vulva 959.14
  whiplash (cervical spine) 847.0
  wringer—*see* Crush, by site
  wrist (and elbow) (and forearm) 959.3
  x-ray NEC 990
Inoculation —*see also* Vaccination
  complication or reaction—*see* Complication, vaccination
INPH (idiopathic normal pressure hydrocephalus) 331.5
Insanity, insane (*see also* Psychosis) 298.9
  adolescent (*see also* Schizophrenia) 295.9
  alternating (*see also* Psychosis, affective, circular) 296.7
  confusional 298.9
    acute 293.0
    subacute 293.1
  delusional 298.9
  paralysis, general 094.1
    progressive 094.1
  paresis, general 094.1
  senile 290.20
Insect
  bite—*see* Injury, superficial, by site
  venomous, poisoning by 989.5
Insemination, artificial V26.1
Insensitivity
  adrenocorticotropin hormone (ACTH) 255.41
  androgen 259.50
    complete 259.51
    partial 259.52
Insertion
  cord (umbilical) lateral or velamentous 663.8
    affecting fetus or newborn 762.6
  intrauterine contraceptive device V25.1
  placenta, vicious—*see* Placenta, previa
  subdermal implantable contraceptive V25.5
  velamentous, umbilical cord 663.8
    affecting fetus or newborn 762.6
Insolation 992.0
  meaning sunstroke 992.0
Insomnia, unspecified 780.52
  with sleep apnea, unspecified 780.51
  adjustment 307.41
  alcohol induced 291.82
  behavioral, of childhood V69.5
  drug induced 292.85
  due to
    medical condition classified elsewhere 327.01
    mental disorder 327.02

Insomnia—*continued*
  fatal familial (FFI) 046.72
  idiopathic 307.42
  nonorganic origin 307.41
    persistent (primary) 307.42
    transient 307.41
  organic 327.00
    other 327.09
  paradoxical 307.42
  primary 307.42
  psychophysiological 307.42
  subjective complaint 307.49
Inspiration
  food or foreign body (*see also* Asphyxia, food or
    foreign body) 933.1
  mucus (*see also* Asphyxia, mucus) 933.1
Inspissated bile syndrome, newborn 774.4
Instability
  detrusor 596.59
  emotional (excessive) 301.3
  joint (posttraumatic) 718.80
    ankle 718.87
    elbow 718.82
    foot 718.87
    hand 718.84
    hip 718.85
    knee 718.86
    lumbosacral 724.6
    multiple sites 718.89
    pelvic region 718.85
    sacroiliac 724.6
    shoulder (region) 718.81
    specified site NEC 718.88
    wrist 718.83
  lumbosacral 724.6
  nervous 301.89
  personality (emotional) 301.59
  thyroid, paroxysmal 242.9
  urethral 599.83
  vasomotor 780.2
Insufficiency, insufficient
  accommodation 367.4
  adrenal (gland) (acute) (chronic) 255.41
    medulla 255.5
    primary 255.41
    specified NEC 255.5
  adrenocortical 255.41
  anterior (occlusal) guidance 524.54
  anus 569.49
  aortic (valve) 424.1
    with
      mitral (valve) disease 396.1
        insufficiency, incompetence, or
          regurgitation 396.3
        stenosis or obstruction 396.1
      stenosis or obstruction 424.1
        with mitral (valve) disease 396.8
    congenital 746.4
    rheumatic 395.1
      with
        mitral (valve) disease 396.1
          insufficiency, incompetence, or
            regurgitation 396.3
          stenosis or obstruction 396.1
        stenosis or obstruction 395.2
          with mitral (valve) disease 396.8
    specified cause NEC 424.1
    syphilitic 093.22
  arterial 447.1
    basilar artery 435.0
    carotid artery 435.8

Insufficiency, insufficient—*continued*
  arterial—*continued*
    cerebral 437.1
    coronary (acute or subacute) 411.89
    mesenteric 557.1
    peripheral 443.9
    precerebral 435.9
    vertebral artery 435.1
    vertibrobasilar 435.3
  arteriovenous 459.9
  basilar artery 435.0
  biliary 575.8
  cardiac (*see also* Insufficiency, myocardial)
    428.0
    complicating surgery 997.1
    due to presence of (cardiac) prosthesis 429.4
    postoperative 997.1
      long-term effect of cardiac surgery 429.4
    specified during or due to a procedure 997.1
      long-term effect of cardiac surgery 429.4
  cardiorenal (*see also* Hypertension, cardiorenal)
    404.90
  cardiovascular (*see also* Disease,
    cardiovascular) 429.2
    renal (*see also* Hypertension, cardiorenal)
      404.90
  carotid artery 435.8
  cerebral (vascular) 437.9
  cerebrovascular 437.9
    with transient focal neurological signs and
      symptoms 435.9
    acute 437.1
      with transient focal neurological signs and
        symptoms 435.9
  circulatory NEC 459.9
    fetus or newborn 779.89
  convergence 378.83
  coronary (acute or subacute) 411.89
    chronic or with a stated duration of over 8
      weeks 414.8
  corticoadrenal 255.41
  dietary 269.9
  divergence 378.85
  food 994.2
  gastroesophageal 530.89
  gonadal
    ovary 256.39
    testis 257.2
  gonadotropic hormone secretion 253.4
  heart—*see also* Insufficiency, myocardial
    fetus or newborn 779.89
    valve (*see also* Endocarditis) 424.90
      congenital NEC 746.89
  hepatic 573.8
  idiopathic autonomic 333.0
  interocclusal distance of teeth (ridge) 524.36
  kidney
    acute 593.9
    chronic 585.9
  labyrinth, labyrinthine (function) 386.53
    bilateral 386.54
    unilateral 386.53
  lacrimal 375.15
  liver 573.8
  lung (acute) (*see also* Insufficiency, pulmonary)
    518.82
    following trauma, surgery, or shock 518.5
    newborn 770.89
  mental (congenital) (*see also* Retardation,
    mental) 319
  mesenteric 557.1

Insufficiency, insufficient—*continued*
  mitral (valve) 424.0
    with
      aortic (valve) disease 396.3
        insufficiency, incompetence, or
          regurgitation 396.3
        stenosis or obstruction 396.2
      obstruction or stenosis 394.2
        with aortic valve disease 396.8
    congenital 746.6
    rheumatic 394.1
      with
        aortic (valve) disease 396.3
          insufficiency, incompetence, or
            regurgitation 396.3
          stenosis or obstruction 396.2
        obstruction or stenosis 394.2
          with aortic valve disease 396.8
      active or acute 391.1
        with chorea, rheumatic (Sydenham's)
          392.0
    specified cause, except rheumatic 424.0
  muscle
    heart—*see* Insufficiency, myocardial
  ocular (*see also* Strabismus) 378.9
  myocardial, myocardium (with arteriosclerosis)
    428.0
    with rheumatic fever (conditions classifiable
      to 390)
      active, acute, or subacute 391.2
        with chorea 392.0
      inactive or quiescent (with chorea) 398.0
    congenital 746.89
    due to presence of (cardiac) prosthesis 429.4
    fetus or newborn 779.89
    following cardiac surgery 429.4
    hypertensive (*see also* Hypertension, heart)
      402.91
      benign 402.11
      malignant 402.01
    postoperative 997.1
      long-term effect of cardiac surgery 429.4
    rheumatic 398.0
      active, acute, or subacute 391.2
        with chorea (Sydenham's) 392.0
    syphilitic 093.82
  nourishment 994.2
  organic 799.89
  ovary 256.39
    postablative 256.2
  pancreatic 577.8
  parathyroid (gland) 252.1
  peripheral vascular (arterial) 443.9
  pituitary (anterior) 253.2
    posterior 253.5
  placental—*see* Placenta, insufficiency
  platelets 287.5
  prenatal care in current pregnancy V23.7
  progressive pluriglandular 258.9
  pseudocholinesterase 289.89
  pulmonary (acute) 518.82
    following
      shock 518.5
      surgery 518.5
      trauma 518.5
    newborn 770.89
    valve (*see also* Endocarditis, pulmonary)
      424.3
      congenital 746.09
  pyloric 537.0

Insufficiency, insufficient—*continued*
  renal 593.9
    acute 593.9
    chronic 585.9
    due to a procedure 997.5
  respiratory 786.09
    acute 518.82
      following shock, surgery, or trauma 518.5
    newborn 770.89
  rotation—*see* Malrotation
  suprarenal 255.41
    medulla 255.5
  tarso-orbital fascia, congenital 743.66
  tear film 375.15
  testis 257.2
  thyroid (gland) (acquired)—*see also*
    Hypothyroidism
    congenital 243
  tricuspid (*see also* Endocarditis, tricuspid) 397.0
    congenital 746.89
    syphilitic 093.23
  urethral sphincter 599.84
  valve, valvular (heart) (*see also* Endocarditis)
    424.90
  vascular 459.9
    intestine NEC 557.9
    mesenteric 557.1
    peripheral 443.9
    renal (*see also* Hypertension, kidney) 403.90
  velopharyngeal
    acquired 528.9
    congenital 750.29
  venous (peripheral) 459.81
  ventricular—*see* Insufficiency, myocardial
  vertebral artery 435.1
  vertibrobasilar artery 435.3
  weight gain during pregnancy 646.8
  zinc 269.3
Insufflation
  fallopian
    fertility testing V26.21
    following sterilization reversal V26.22
  meconium 770.11
    with respiratory symptoms 770.12
Insular —*see* condition
Insulinoma (M8151/0)
  malignant (M8151/3)
    pancreas 157.4
    specified site—*see* Neoplasm, by site,
      malignant
    unspecified site 157.4
  pancreas 211.7
  specified site—*see* Neoplasm, by site, benign
  unspecified site 211.7
Insuloma —*see* Insulinoma
Insult
  brain 437.9
    acute 436
    cerebral 437.9
    acute 436
    cerebrovascular 437.9
    acute 436
    vascular NEC 437.9
    acute 436
Insurance examination (certification) V70.3
Intemperance (*see also* Alcoholism) 303.9
Interception of pregnancy (menstrual
  extraction) V25.3
Interference
  balancing side 524.56
  non-working side 524.56

Intermenstrual
bleeding 626.6
 irregular 626.6
 regular 626.5
hemorrhage 626.6
 irregular 626.6
 regular 626.5
ain(s) 625.2
Intermittent— *see* condition
Internal *—see* condition
Interproximal wear 521.10
Interruption
aortic arch 747.11
bundle of His 426.50
fallopian tube (for sterilization) V25.2
phase-shift, sleep cycle 307.45
repeated REM-sleep 307.48
sleep
 due to perceived environmental disturbances
  307.48
 phase-shift, of 24-hour sleep-wake cycle
  307.45
 repeated REM-sleep type 307.48
vas deferens (for sterilization) V25.2
Intersexuality 752.7
Interstitial *—see* condition
Intertrigo 695.89
labialis 528.5
Intervertebral disc *—see* condition
Intestine, intestinal *—see also* condition
flu 487.8
Intolerance
carbohydrate NEC 579.8
cardiovascular exercise, with pain (at rest) (with
 less than ordinary activity) (with ordinary
 activity) V47.2
cold 780.99
disaccharide (hereditary) 271.3
drug
 correct substance properly administered 995.27
 wrong substance given or taken in error 977.9
  specified drug—*see* Table of drugs and
   chemicals
effort 306.2
fat NEC 579.8
foods NEC 579.8
fructose (hereditary) 271.2
glucose (-galactose) (congenital) 271.3
gluten 579.0
lactose (hereditary) (infantile) 271.3
lysine (congenital) 270.7
milk NEC 579.8
protein (familial) 270.7
starch NEC 579.8
sucrose (-isomaltose) (congenital) 271.3
Intoxicated NEC (*see also* Alcoholism) 305.0
Intoxication
acid 276.2
acute
 alcoholic 305.0
  with alcoholism 303.0
  hangover effects 305.0
 caffeine 305.9
 hallucinogenic (*see also* Abuse, drugs,
  nondependent) 305.3
alcohol (acute) 305.0
 with alcoholism 303.0
 hangover effects 305.0
 idiosyncratic 291.4
 pathological 291.4
alimentary canal 558.2
ammonia (hepatic) 572.2

Intoxication— *continued*
caffeine 305.9
chemical—*see also* Table of drugs and
 chemicals
 via placenta or breast milk 760.70
  alcohol 760.71
  anticonvulsants 760.77
  antifungals 760.74
  anti-infective agents 760.74
  antimetabolics 760.78
  cocaine 760.75
  "crack" 760.75
  hallucinogenic agents NEC 760.73
  medicinal agents NEC 760.79
  narcotics 760.72
  obstetric anesthetic or analgesic drug 763.5
  specified agent NEC 760.79
  suspected, affecting management of
   pregnancy 655.5
cocaine, through placenta or breast milk 760.75
delirium
 alcohol 291.0
 drug 292.81
drug 292.89
 with delirium 292.81
 correct substance properly administered (*see*
  also Allergy, drug) 995.27
 newborn 779.4
 obstetric anesthetic or sedation 668.9
  affecting fetus or newborn 763.5
 overdose or wrong substance given or
  taken—*see* Table of drugs and chemicals
 pathologic 292.2
 specific to newborn 779.4
 via placenta or breast milk 760.70
  alcohol 760.71
  anticonvulsants 760.77
  antifungals 760.74
  anti-infective agents 760.74
  antimetabolics 760.78
  cocaine 760.75
  "crack" 760.75
  hallucinogenic agents 760.73
  medicinal agents NEC 760.79
  narcotics 760.72
  obstetric anesthetic or analgesic drug 763.5
  specified agent NEC 760.79
  suspected, affecting management of
   pregnancy 655.5
enteric—*see* Intoxication, intestinal
fetus or newborn, via placenta or breast milk
 760.70
 alcohol 760.71
 anticonvulsants 760.77
 antifungals 760.74
 anti-infective agents 760.74
 antimetabolics 760.78
 cocaine 760.75
 "crack" 760.75
 hallucinogenic agents 760.73
 medicinal agents NEC 760.79
 narcotics 760.72
 obstetric anesthetic or analgesic drug 763.5
 specified agent NEC 760.79
 suspected, affecting management of pregnancy
  655.5
food—*see* Poisoning, food
gastrointestinal 558.2
hallucinogenic (acute) 305.3
hepatocerebral 572.2
idiosyncratic alcohol 291.4

Intoxication—*continued*
 intestinal 569.89
  due to putrefaction of food 005.9
 methyl alcohol (*see also* Alcoholism) 305.0
  with alcoholism 303.0
 non-foodborne due to toxins of Clostridium
  botulinum [*C. botulinum*] —*see* Botulism
 pathologic 291.4
  drug 292.2
 potassium (K) 276.7
 septic
  with
   abortion—*see* Abortion, by type, with sepsis
   ectopic pregnancy (*see also* categories
    633.0-633.9) 639.0
   molar pregnancy (*see also* categories
    630-632) 639.0
   during labor 659.3
   following
    abortion 639.0
    ectopic or molar pregnancy 639.0
   generalized—*see* Septicemia
  puerperal, postpartum, childbirth 670.2
 serum (prophylactic) (therapeutic) 999.5
 uremic—*see* Uremia
 water 276.6
Intracranial —*see* condition
Intrahepatic gallbladder 751.69
Intraligamentous —*see also* condition
 pregnancy—*see* Pregnancy, cornual
Intraocular —*see also* condition
 sepsis 360.00
Intrathoracic —*see also* condition
 kidney 753.3
 stomach—*see* Hernia, diaphragm
Intrauterine contraceptive device
 checking V25.42
 insertion V25.1
 in situ V45.51
 management V25.42
 prescription V25.02
  repeat V25.42
 reinsertion V25.42
 removal V25.42
Intraventricular —*see* condition
Intrinsic deformity —*see* Deformity
Intruded tooth 524.34
Intrusion, repetitive, of sleep (due to
 environmental disturbances) (with atypical
 polysomnographic features) 307.48
Intumescent, lens (eye) NEC 366.9
 senile 366.12
Intussusception (colon) (enteric) (intestine)
 (rectum) 560.0
 appendix 543.9
 congenital 751.5
 fallopian tube 620.8
 ileocecal 560.0
 ileocolic 560.0
 ureter (with obstruction) 593.4
Invagination
 basilar 756.0
 colon or intestine 560.0
Invalid (since birth) 799.89
Invalidism (chronic) 799.89
Inversion
 albumin-globulin (A-G) ratio 273.8
 bladder 596.8
 cecum (*see also* Intussusception) 560.0
 cervix 622.8

Inversion—*continued*
 nipple 611.79
  congenital 757.6
  puerperal, postpartum 676.3
 optic papilla 743.57
 organ or site, congenital NEC—*see* Anomaly,
  specified type NEC
 sleep rhythm 327.39
  nonorganic origin 307.45
 testis (congenital) 752.51
 uterus (postinfectional) (postpartal, old) 621.7
  chronic 621.7
  complicating delivery 665.2
   affecting fetus or newborn 763.89
 vagina—*see* Prolapse, vagina
Investigation
 allergens V72.7
 clinical research (control) (normal comparison)
  (participant) V70.7
Inviability —*see* Immaturity
Involuntary movement, abnormal 781.0
Involution, involutional —*see also* condition
 breast, cystic or fibrocystic 610.1
 depression (*see also* Psychosis, affective) 296.2
  recurrent episode 296.3
  single episode 296.2
 melancholia (*see also* Psychosis, affective) 296.2
  recurrent episode 296.3
  single episode 296.2
 ovary, senile 620.3
 paranoid state (reaction) 297.2
 paraphrenia (climacteric) (menopause) 297.2
 psychosis 298.8
 thymus failure 254.8
IQ
 under 20 318.2
 20-34 318.1
 35-49 318.0
 50-70 317
IRDS 769
Irideremia 743.45
Iridis rubeosis 364.42
 diabetic 250.5 *[364.42]*
 due to secondary diabetes 249.5 *[364.42]*
Iridochoroiditis (panuveitis) 360.12
Iridocyclitis NEC 364.3
 acute 364.00
  primary 364.01
  recurrent 364.02
 chronic 364.10
  in
   lepromatous leprosy 030.0 *[364.11]*
   sarcoidosis 135 *[364.11]*
   tuberculosis (*see also* Tuberculosis) 017.3
    [364.11]
 due to allergy 364.04
 endogenous 364.01
 gonococcal 098.41
 granulomatous 364.10
 herpetic (simplex) 054.44
  zoster 053.22
 hypopyon 364.05
 lens induced 364.23
 nongranulomatous 364.00
 primary 364.01
 recurrent 364.02
 rheumatic 364.10
 secondary 364.04
  infectious 364.03
  noninfectious 364.04

Iridocyclitis—*continued*
  subacute 364.00
    primary 364.01
    recurrent 364.02
  sympathetic 360.11
  syphilitic (secondary) 091.52
  tuberculous (chronic) (*see also* Tuberculosis)
    017.3 *[364.11]*
Iridocyclochoroiditis (panuveitis) 360.12
Iridodialysis 364.76
Iridodonesis 364.89
Iridoplegia (complete) (partial) (reflex) 379.49
Iridoschisis 364.52
Iris —*see* condition
Iritis 364.3
  acute 364.00
    primary 364.01
    recurrent 364.02
  chronic 364.10
    in
      sarcoidosis 135 *[364.11]*
      tuberculosis (*see also* Tuberculosis) 017.3
        [364.11]
  diabetic 250.5 *[364.42]*
  due to secondary diabetes 249.5 *[364.42]*
  due to
    allergy 364.04
    herpes simplex 054.44
    leprosy 030.0 *[364.11]*
  endogenous 364.01
  gonococcal 098.41
  gouty 274.89 *[364.11]*
  granulomatous 364.10
  hypopyon 364.05
  lens induced 364.23
  nongranulomatous 364.00
  papulosa 095.8 *[364.11]*
  primary 364.01
  recurrent 364.02
  rheumatic 364.10
  secondary 364.04
    infectious 364.03
    noninfectious 364.04
  subacute 364.00
    primary 364.01
    recurrent 364.02
  sympathetic 360.11
  syphilitic (secondary) 091.52
    congenital 090.0 *[364.11]*
    late 095.8 *[364.11]*
  tuberculous (*see also* Tuberculosis) 017.3 *[364.11]*
  uratic 274.89 *[364.11]*
Iron
  deficiency anemia 280.9
  metabolism disease 275.0
  storage disease 275.0
Iron-miners' lung 503
Irradiated enamel (tooth, teeth) 521.89
Irradiation
  burn—*see* Burn, by site
  effects, adverse 990
Irreducible, irreducibility —*see* condition
Irregular, irregularity
  action, heart 427.9
  alveolar process 525.8
  bleeding NEC 626.4
  breathing 786.09
  colon 569.89
  contour
    of cornea 743.41
      acquired 371.70
    reconstructed breast 612.0

Irregular, irregularity—*continued*
  dentin in pulp 522.3
  eye movements NEC 379.59
  menstruation (cause unknown) 626.4
  periods 626.4
  prostate 602.9
  pupil 364.75
  respiratory 786.09
  septum (nasal) 470
  shape, organ or site, congenital NEC—*see*
    Distortion
  sleep-wake rhythm (non-24-hour) 327.39
    nonorganic origin 307.45
  vertebra 733.99
Irritability 799.22
  bladder 596.8
    neurogenic 596.54
      with cauda equina syndrome 344.61
  bowel (syndrome) 564.1
  bronchial (*see also* Bronchitis) 490
  cerebral, newborn 779.1
  colon 564.1
    psychogenic 306.4
  duodenum 564.89
  heart (psychogenic) 306.2
  ileum 564.89
  jejunum 564.89
  myocardium 306.2
  nervousness 799.21
  rectum 564.89
  stomach 536.9
    psychogenic 306.4
  sympathetic (nervous system) (*see also*
    Neuropathy, peripheral, autonomic) 337.9
  urethra 599.84
  ventricular (heart) (psychogenic) 306.2
Irritable —(*see also* Irritability) 799.22
Irritation
  anus 569.49
  axillary nerve 353.0
  bladder 596.8
  brachial plexus 353.0
  brain (traumatic) (*see also* Injury, intracranial)
    854.0
    nontraumatic—*see* Encephalitis
  bronchial (*see also* Bronchitis) 490
  cerebral (traumatic) (*see also* Injury,
    intracranial) 854.0
    nontraumatic—*see* Encephalitis
  cervical plexus 353.2
  cervix (*see also* Cervicitis) 616.0
  choroid, sympathetic 360.11
  cranial nerve—*see* Disorder, nerve, cranial
  digestive tract 536.9
    psychogenic 306.4
  gastric 536.9
    psychogenic 306.4
  gastrointestinal (tract) 536.9
    functional 536.9
    psychogenic 306.4
  globe, sympathetic 360.11
  intestinal (bowel) 564.9
  labyrinth 386.50
  lumbosacral plexus 353.1
  meninges (traumatic) (*see also* Injury,
    intracranial) 854.0
    nontraumatic—*see* Meningitis
  myocardium 306.2
  nerve—*see* Disorder, nerve
  nervous 799.21
  nose 478.19
  penis 607.89

Itch *—continued*
  Malabar 110.9
    beard 110.0
    foot 110.4
    scalp 110.0
  meaning scabies 133.0
  Norwegian 133.0
  perianal 698.0
  poultrymen's 133.8
  sarcoptic 133.0
  scrub 134.1
  seven year V61.10
    meaning scabies 133.0
  straw 133.8
  swimmers' 120.3
  washerwoman's 692.4
  water 120.3
  winter 698.8
Itsenko-Cushing syndrome (pituitary
    basophilism) 255.0
Ivemark's syndrome (asplenia with congenital
    heart disease) 759.0
Ivory bones 756.52
Ixodes 134.8
Ixodiasis 134.8

J

Jaccoud's nodular fibrositis, chronic (Jaccoud's syndrome) 714.4
Jackson's
  membrane 751.4
  paralysis or syndrome 344.89
  veil 751.4
Jacksonian
  epilepsy (see also Epilepsy) 345.5
  seizures (focal) (see also Epilepsy) 345.5
Jacob's ulcer (M8090/3)—see Neoplasm, skin, malignant, by site
Jacquet's dermatitis (diaper dermatitis) 691.0
Jadassohn's
  blue nevus (M8780/0)—see Neoplasm, skin, benign
  disease (maculopapular erythroderma) 696.2
  intraepidermal epithelioma (M8096/0)—see Neoplasm, skin, benign
Jadassohn-Lewandowski syndrome (pachyonychia congenita) 757.5
Jadassohn-Pellizari's disease (anetoderma) 701.3
Jadassohn-Tièche nevus (M8780/0)—see Neoplasm, skin, benign
Jaffe-Lichtenstein (-Uehlinger) syndrome 252.01
Jahnke's syndrome (encephalocutaneous angiomatosis) 759.6
Jakob-Creutzfeldt disease (CJD) (syndrome) 046.19
  with dementia
    with behavioral disturbance 046.19 [294.11]
    without behavioral disturbance 046.19 [294.10]
  familial 046.19
  iatrogenic 046.19
  specified NEC 046.19
  sporadic 046.19
  variant (vCJD) 046.11
    with dementia
      with behavioral disturbance 046.11 [294.11]
      without behavioral disturbance 046.11 [294.10]
Jaksch (-Luzet) disease or syndrome (pseudoleukemia infantum) 285.8
Jamaican
  neuropathy 349.82
  paraplegic tropical ataxic-spastic syndrome 349.82
Janet's disease (psychasthenia) 300.89
Janiceps 759.4
Jansky-Bielschowsky amaurotic familial idiocy 330.1
Japanese
  B type encephalitis 062.0
  river fever 081.2
  seven-day fever 100.89
Jaundice (yellow) 782.4
  acholuric (familial) (splenomegalic) (see also Spherocytosis) 282.0
    acquired 283.9
  breast milk 774.39
  catarrhal (acute) 070.1
    with hepatic coma 070.0
    chronic 571.9
    epidemic—see Jaundice, epidemic
  cholestatic (benign) 782.4
  chronic idiopathic 277.4
  epidemic (catarrhal) 070.1

Jaundice—continued
  with hepatic coma 070.0
    leptospiral 100.0
    spirochetal 100.0
  febrile (acute) 070.1
    with hepatic coma 070.0
    leptospiral 100.0
    spirochetal 100.0
  fetus or newborn 774.6
    due to or associated with
      ABO
        antibodies 773.1
        incompatibility, maternal/fetal 773.1
        isoimmunization 773.1
      absence or deficiency of enzyme system for bilirubin conjugation (congenital) 774.39
      blood group incompatibility NEC 773.2
      breast milk inhibitors to conjugation 774.39
      associated with preterm delivery 774.2
      bruising 774.1
      Crigler-Najjar syndrome 277.4 [774.31]
      delayed conjugation 774.30
        associated with preterm delivery 774.2
      development 774.39
      drugs or toxins transmitted from mother 774.1
      G-6-PD deficiency 282.2 [774.0]
      galactosemia 271.1 [774.5]
      Gilbert's syndrome 277.4 [774.31]
      hepatocellular damage 774.4
      hereditary hemolytic anemia (see also Anemia, hemolytic) 282.9 [774.0]
      hypothyroidism, congenital 243 [774.31]
      incompatibility, maternal/fetal NEC 773.2
      infection 774.1
      inspissated bile syndrome 774.4
      isoimmunization NEC 773.2
      mucoviscidosis 277.01 [774.5]
      obliteration of bile duct, congenital 751.61 [774.5]
      polycythemia 774.1
      preterm delivery 774.2
      red cell defect 282.9 [774.0]
      Rh
        antibodies 773.0
        incompatibility, maternal/fetal 773.0
        isoimmunization 773.0
      spherocytosis (congenital) 282.0 [774.0]
      swallowed maternal blood 774.1
    physiological NEC 774.6
  from injection, inoculation, infusion, or transfusion (blood) (plasma) (serum) (other substance) (onset within 8 months after administration)—see Hepatitis, viral
  Gilbert's (familial nonhemolytic) 277.4
  hematogenous 283.9
  hemolytic (acquired) 283.9
    congenital (see also Spherocytosis) 282.0
  hemorrhagic (acute) 100.0
    leptospiral 100.0
    newborn 776.0
    spirochetal 100.0
  hepatocellular 573.8
  homologous (serum)—see Hepatitis, viral
  idiopathic, chronic 277.4
  infectious (acute) (subacute) 070.1
    with hepatic coma 070.0
    leptospiral 100.0
    spirochetal 100.0

Jaundice—*continued*
  leptospiral 100.0
  malignant (*see also* Necrosis, liver) 570
  newborn (physiological) (*see also* Jaundice,
    fetus or newborn) 774.6
  nonhemolytic, congenital familial (Gilbert's)
    277.4
  nuclear, newborn (*see also* Kernicterus of
    newborn) 774.7
  obstructive NEC (*see also* Obstruction, biliary)
    576.8
  postimmunization—*see* Hepatitis, viral
  posttransfusion—*see* Hepatitis, viral
  regurgitation (*see also* Obstruction, biliary)
    576.8
  serum (homologous) (prophylactic)
    (therapeutic)—*see* Hepatitis, viral
  spirochetal (hemorrhagic) 100.0
  symptomatic 782.4
    newborn 774.6
Jaw —*see* condition
Jaw-blinking 374.43
  congenital 742.8
Jaw-winking phenomenon or syndrome 742.8
Jealousy
  alcoholic 291.5
  childhood 313.3
  sibling 313.3
Jejunitis (*see also* Enteritis) 558.9
Jejunostomy status V44.4
Jejunum, jejunal —*see* condition
Jensen's disease 363.05
Jericho boil 085.1
Jerks, myoclonic 333.2
Jervell-Lange-Nielsen syndrome 426.82
Jeune's disease or syndrome (asphyxiating
    thoracic dystrophy) 756.4
Jigger disease 134.1
Job's syndrome (chronic granulomatous disease)
    288.1
Jod-Basedow phenomenon 242.8
Johnson-Stevens disease (erythema multiforme
    exudativum) 695.13
Joint —*see also* condition
  Charcot's 094.0 *[713.5]*
  false 733.82
  flail—*see* Flail, joint
  mice—*see* Loose, body, joint, by site
  sinus to bone 730.9
  von Gies' 095.8
Jordan's anomaly or syndrome 288.2
Josephs-Diamond-Blackfan anemia (congenital
    hypoplastic) 284.01
Joubert syndrome 759.89
Jumpers' knee 727.2
Jungle yellow fever 060.0
Jüngling's disease (sarcoidosis) 135
Junin virus hemorrhagic fever 078.7
Juvenile —*see also* condition
  delinquent 312.9
    group (*see also* Disturbance, conduct) 312.2
    neurotic 312.4

K

Kabuki syndrome 759.89
Kahler (-Bozzolo) disease (multiple myeloma)
   (M9730/3) 203.0
Kakergasia 300.9
Kakke 265.0
Kala-azar (Indian) (infantile) (Mediterranean)
   (Sudanese) 085.0
Kalischer's syndrome (encephalocutaneous
   angiomatosis) 759.6
Kallmann's syndrome (hypogonadotropic
   hypogonadism with anosmia) 253.4
Kanner's syndrome (autism) (*see also*
   Psychosis, childhood) 299.0
Kaolinosis 502
Kaposi's
  disease 757.33
    lichen ruber 696.4
      acuminatus 696.4
      moniliformis 697.8
    xeroderma pigmentosum 757.33
  sarcoma (M9140/3) 176.9
    adipose tissue 176.1
    aponeurosis 176.1
    artery 176.1
    associated herpesvirus infection 058.89
    blood vessel 176.1
    bursa 176.1
    connective tissue 176.1
    external genitalia 176.8
    fascia 176.1
    fatty tissue 176.1
    fibrous tissue 176.1
    gastrointestinal tract NEC 176.3
    ligament 176.1
    lung 176.4
    lymph
      gland(s) 176.5
      node(s) 176.5
    lymphatic(s) NEC 176.1
    muscle (skeletal) 176.1
    oral cavity NEC 176.8
    palate 176.2
    scrotum 176.8
    skin 176.0
    soft tissue 176.1
    specified site NEC 176.8
    subcutaneous tissue 176.1
    synovia 176.1
    tendon (sheath) 176.1
    vein 176.1
    vessel 176.1
    viscera NEC 176.9
    vulva 176.8
  varicelliform eruption 054.0
    vaccinia 999.0
Kartagener's syndrome or triad (sinusitis,
   bronchiectasis, situs inversus) 759.3
Kasabach-Merritt syndrome (capillary
   hemangioma associated with
   thrombocytopenic purpura) 287.39
Kaschin-Beck disease (endemic
   polyarthritis)—*see* Disease, Kaschin-Beck
Kast's syndrome (dyschondroplasia with
   hemangiomas) 756.4
Katatonia (*see also* Schizophrenia) 295.2
Katayama disease or fever 120.2
Kathisophobia 781.0
Kawasaki disease 446.1

Kayser-Fleischer ring (cornea) (pseudosclerosis)
   275.1 *[371.14]*
Kaznelson's syndrome (congenital hypoplastic
   anemia) 284.01
Kearns-Sayre syndrome 277.87
Kedani fever 081.2
Kelis 701.4
Kelly (-Patterson) syndrome (sideropenic
   dysphagia) 280.8
Keloid, cheloid 701.4
  Addison's (morphea) 701.0
  cornea 371.00
  Hawkins' 701.4
  scar 701.4
Keloma 701.4
Kenya fever 082.1
Keratectasia 371.71
  congenital 743.41
Keratinization NEC
  alveolar ridge mucosa
    excessive 528.72
    minimal 528.71
Keratitis (nodular) (nonulcerative) (simple)
   (zonular) NEC 370.9
  with ulceration (*see also* Ulcer, cornea) 370.00
  actinic 370.24
  arborescens 054.42
  areolar 370.22
  bullosa 370.8
  deep—*see* Keratitis, interstitial
  dendritic(a) 054.42
  desiccation 370.34
  diffuse interstitial 370.52
  disciform(is) 054.43
    varicella 052.7 *[370.44]*
  epithelialis vernalis 372.13 *[370.32]*
  exposure 370.34
  filamentary 370.23
  gonococcal (congenital) (prenatal) 098.43
  herpes, herpetic (simplex) NEC 054.43
    zoster 053.21
  hypopyon 370.04
  in
    chickenpox 052.7 *[370.44]*
    exanthema (*see also* Exanthem) 057.9
      [370.44]
    paravaccinia (*see also* Paravaccinia) 051.9
      [370.44]
    smallpox (*see also* Smallpox) 050.9 *[370.44]*
    vernal conjunctivitis 372.13 *[370.32]*
  interstitial (nonsyphilitic) 370.50
    with ulcer (*see also* Ulcer, cornea) 370.00
    diffuse 370.52
    herpes, herpetic (simplex) 054.43
      zoster 053.21
    syphilitic (congenital) (hereditary) 090.3
    tuberculous (*see also* Tuberculosis) 017.3
      [370.59]
  lagophthalmic 370.34
  macular 370.22
  neuroparalytic 370.35
  neurotrophic 370.35
  nummular 370.22
  oyster-shuckers' 370.8
  parenchymatous—*see* Keratitis, interstitial
  petrificans 370.8
  phlyctenular 370.31

Keratitis—*continued*
  postmeasles 055.71
  punctata, punctate 370.21
    leprosa 030.0 *[370.21]*
    profunda 090.3
    superficial (Thygeson's) 370.21
  purulent 370.8
  pustuliformis profunda 090.3
  rosacea 695.3 *[370.49]*
  sclerosing 370.54
  specified type NEC 370.8
  stellate 370.22
  striate 370.22
  superficial 370.20
    with conjunctivitis (*see also*
      Keratoconjunctivitis) 370.40
    punctate (Thygeson's) 370.21
  suppurative 370.8
  syphilitic (congenital) (prenatal) 090.3
  trachomatous 076.1
    late effect 139.1
  tuberculous (phlyctenular) (*see also*
    Tuberculosis) 017.3 *[370.31]*
  ulcerated (*see also* Ulcer, cornea) 370.00
  vesicular 370.8
  welders' 370.24
  xerotic (*see also* Keratomalacia) 371.45
    vitamin A deficiency 264.4
Keratoacanthoma 238.2
Keratocele 371.72
Keratoconjunctivitis (*see also* Keratitis) 370.40
  adenovirus type 8 077.1
  epidemic 077.1
  exposure 370.34
  gonococcal 098.43
  herpetic (simplex) 054.43
    zoster 053.21
  in
    chickenpox 052.7 *[370.44]*
    exanthema (*see also* Exanthem) 057.9
      [370.44]
    paravaccinia (*see also* Paravaccinia) 051.9
      [370.44]
    smallpox (*see also* Smallpox) 050.9 *[370.44]*
  infectious 077.1
  neurotrophic 370.35
  phlyctenular 370.31
  postmeasles 055.71
  shipyard 077.1
  sicca (Sjögren's syndrome) 710.2
    not in Sjögren's syndrome 370.33
  specified type NEC 370.49
  tuberculous (phlyctenular) (*see also*
    Tuberculosis) 017.3 *[370.31]*
Keratoconus 371.60
  acute hydrops 371.62
  congenital 743.41
  stable 371.61
Keratocyst (dental) 526.0
Keratoderma, keratodermia (congenital)
  (palmaris et plantaris) (symmetrical) 757.39
  acquired 701.1
  blennorrhagica 701.1
    gonococcal 098.81
  climacterium 701.1
  eccentrica 757.39
  gonorrheal 098.81
  punctata 701.1
  tylodes, progressive 701.1
Keratodermatocele 371.72

Keratoglobus 371.70
  congenital 743.41
    associated with buphthalmos 743.22
Keratohemia 371.12
Keratoiritis (*see also* Iridocyclitis) 364.3
  syphilitic 090.3
  tuberculous (*see also* Tuberculosis) 017.3
    [364.11]
Keratolysis exfoliativa (congenital) 757.39
  acquired 695.89
  neonatorum 757.39
Keratoma 701.1
  congenital 757.39
  malignum congenitale 757.1
  palmaris et plantaris hereditarium 757.39
  senile 702.0
Keratomalacia 371.45
  vitamin A deficiency 264.4
Keratomegaly 743.41
Keratomycosis 111.1
  nigricans (palmaris) 111.1
Keratopathy 371.40
  band (*see also* Keratitis) 371.43
  bullous (*see also* Keratitis) 371.23
  degenerative (*see also* Degeneration, cornea)
    371.40
  hereditary (*see also* Dystrophy, cornea) 371.50
    discrete colliquative 371.49
Keratoscleritis, tuberculous (*see also*
    Tuberculosis) 017.3 *[370.31]*
Keratosis 701.1
  actinic 702.0
  arsenical 692.4
  blennorrhagica 701.1
    gonococcal 098.81
  congenital (any type) 757.39
  ear (middle) (*see also* Cholesteatoma) 385.30
  female genital (external) 629.89
  follicular, vitamin A deficiency 264.8
  follicularis 757.39
    acquired 701.1
    congenital (acneiformis) (Siemens') 757.39
    spinulosa (decalvans) 757.39
    vitamin A deficiency 264.8
  gonococcal 098.81
  larynx, laryngeal 478.79
  male genital (external) 608.89
  middle ear (*see also* Cholesteatoma) 385.30
  nigricans 701.2
    congenital 757.39
  obturans 380.21
  oral epithelium
    residual ridge mucosa
      excessive 528.72
      minimal 528.71
  palmaris et plantaris (symmetrical) 757.39
  penile 607.89
  pharyngeus 478.29
  pilaris 757.39
    acquired 701.1
  punctata (palmaris et plantaris) 701.1
  scrotal 608.89
  seborrheic 702.19
    inflamed 702.11
  senilis 702.0
  solar 702.0
  suprafollicularis 757.39
  tonsillaris 478.29
  vagina 623.1
  vegetans 757.39
  vitamin A deficiency 264.8
Kerato-uveitis (*see also* Iridocyclitis) 364.3

Keraunoparalysis 994.0
Kerion (celsi) 110.0
Kernicterus of newborn (not due to
  isoimmunization) 774.7
  due to isoimmunization (conditions classifiable
    to 773.0-773.2) 773.4
Ketoacidosis 276.2
  diabetic 250.1
  due to secondary diabetes 249.1
Ketonuria 791.6
  branched-chain, intermittent 270.3
Ketosis 276.2
  diabetic 250.1
  due to secondary diabetes 249.1
Kidney —*see* condition
Kienböck's
  disease 732.3
  adult 732.8
  osteochondrosis 732.3
Kimmelstiel (-Wilson) disease or syndrome
  (intercapillary glomerulosclerosis) 250.4
  [581.81]
  due to secondary diabetes 249.4 *[581.81]*
Kink, kinking
  appendix 543.9
  artery 447.1
  cystic duct, congenital 751.61
  hair (acquired) 704.2
  ileum or intestine (*see also* Obstruction,
    intestine) 560.9
  Lane's (*see also* Obstruction, intestine) 560.9
  organ or site, congenital NEC—*see* Anomaly,
    specified type NEC, by site
  ureter (pelvic junction) 593.3
    congenital 753.20
  vein(s) 459.2
    caval 459.2
    peripheral 459.2
Kinnier Wilson's disease (hepatolenticular
  degeneration) 275.1
Kissing
  osteophytes 721.5
  spine 721.5
  vertebra 721.5
Klauder's syndrome (erythema multiforme
  exudativum) 695.19
Kleb's disease (*see also* Nephritis) 583.9
Klein-Waardenburg syndrome
  (ptosisepicanthus) 270.2
Kleine-Levin syndrome 327.13
Kleptomania 312.32
Klinefelter's syndrome 758.7
Klinger's disease 446.4
Klippel's disease 723.8
Klippel-Feil disease or syndrome (brevicollis)
  756.16
Klippel-Trenaunay syndrome 759.89
Klumpke (-Déjérine) palsy, paralysis (birth)
  (newborn) 767.6
Klüver-Bucy (-Terzian) syndrome 310.0
Knee —*see* condition
Knifegrinders' rot (*see also* Tuberculosis) 011.4
Knock-knee (acquired) 736.41
  congenital 755.64
Knot
  intestinal, syndrome (volvulus) 560.2
  umbilical cord (true) 663.2
    affecting fetus or newborn 762.5
Knots, surfer 919.8
  infected 919.9

Knotting (of)
  hair 704.2
  intestine 560.2
Knuckle pads (Garrod's) 728.79
Köbner's disease (epidermolysis bullosa) 757.39
Koch's
  infection (*see also* Tuberculosis, pulmonary)
    011.9
  relapsing fever 087.9
Koch-Weeks conjunctivitis 372.03
Koenig-Wichman disease (pemphigus) 694.4
Köhler's disease (osteochondrosis) 732.5
  first (osteochondrosis juvenilis) 732.5
  second (Freiburg's infarction, metatarsal head)
    732.5
  patellar 732.4
  tarsal navicular (bone) (osteoarthosis juvenilis)
    732.5
Köhler-Mouchet disease (osteoarthrosis
  juvenilis) 732.5
Köhler-Pellegrini-Stieda disease or syndrome
  (calcification, knee joint) 726.62
Koilonychia 703.8
  congenital 757.5
Kojevnikov's, Kojewnikoff's epilepsy (*see also*
  Epilepsy) 345.7
König's
  disease (osteochondritis dissecans) 732.7
  syndrome 564.89
Koniophthisis (*see also* Tuberculosis) 011.4
Koplik's spots 055.9
Kopp's asthma 254.8
Korean hemorrhagic fever 078.6
Korsakoff (-Wernicke) disease, psychosis, or
  syndrome (nonalcoholic) 294.0
  alcoholic 291.1
Korsakov's disease —*see* Korsakoff's disease
Korsakow's disease —*see* Korsakoff's disease
Kostmann's disease or syndrome (infantile
  genetic agranulocytosis) 288.01
Krabbe's
  disease (leukodystrophy) 330.0
  syndrome
    congenital muscle hypoplasia 756.89
    cutaneocerebral angioma 759.6
Kraepelin-Morel disease (*see also*
  Schizophrenia) 295.9
Kraft-Weber-Dimitri disease 759.6
Kraurosis
  ani 569.49
  penis 607.0
  vagina 623.8
  vulva 624.09
Kreotoxism 005.9
Krukenberg's
  spindle 371.13
  tumor (M8490/6) 198.6
Kufs' disease 330.1
Kugelberg-Welander disease 335.11
Kuhnt-Junius degeneration or disease 362.52
Kulchitsky's cell carcinoma (carcinoid tumor of
  intestine) 259.2
Kümmell's disease or spondylitis 721.7
Kundrat's disease (lymphosarcoma) 200.1
Kunekune —*see* Dermatophytosis
Kunkel syndrome (lupoid hepatitis) 571.49
Kupffer cell sarcoma (M9124/3) 155.0
Kuru 046.0

Kussmaul's
coma (diabetic) 250.3
  due to secondary diabetes 249.3
disease (polyarteritis nodosa) 446.0
respiration (air hunger) 786.09
Kwashiorkor (marasmus type) 260
Kyasanur Forest disease 065.2
Kyphoscoliosis, kyphoscoliotic (acquired) (*see*
  also Scoliosis) 737.30
congenital 756.19
due to radiation 737.33
heart (disease) 416.1
idiopathic 737.30
  infantile
    progressive 737.32
    resolving 737.31
late effect of rickets 268.1 *[737.43]*
specified NEC 737.39
thoracogenic 737.34
tuberculous (*see also* Tuberculosis) 015.0
  [737.43]
Kyphosis, kyphotic (acquired) (postural) 737.10
adolescent postural 737.0
congenital 756.19
dorsalis juvenilis 732.0
due to or associated with
  Charcot-Marie-Tooth disease 356.1 *[737.41]*
  mucopolysaccharidosis 277.5 *[737.41]*
  neurofibromatosis 237.71 *[737.41]*
  osteitis
    deformans 731.0 *[737.41]*
    fibrosa cystica 252.01 *[737.41]*
  osteoporosis (*see also* Osteoporosis) 733.0
    [737.41]
  poliomyelitis (*see also* Poliomyelitis) 138
    [737.41]
  radiation 737.11
  tuberculosis (*see also* Tuberculosis) 015.0
    [737.41]
Kümmell's 721.7
late effect of rickets 268.1 *[737.41]*
Morquio-Brailsford type (spinal) 277.5 *[737.41]*
pelvis 738.6
postlaminectomy 737.12
specified cause NEC 737.19
syphilitic, congenital 090.5 *[737.41]*
tuberculous (*see also* Tuberculosis) 015.0
  [737.41]
Kyrle's disease (hyperkeratosis follicularis in
  cutem penetrans) 701.1

L

Labia, labium —*see* condition
Labiated hymen 752.49
Labile
blood pressure 796.2
emotions, emotionality 301.3
vasomotor system 443.9
Lability, emotional 799.24
Labioglossal paralysis 335.22
Labium leporinum (*see also* Cleft, lip) 749.10
Labor (*see also* Delivery)
with complications—*see* Delivery, complicated
abnormal NEC 661.9
affecting fetus or newborn 763.7
arrested active phase 661.1
affecting fetus or newborn 763.7
desultory 661.2
affecting fetus or newborn 763.7
dyscoordinate 661.4
affecting fetus or newborn 763.7
early onset (22-36 weeks gestation) 644.2
failed
induction 659.1
mechanical 659.0
medical 659.1
surgical 659.0
trial (vaginal delivery) 660.6
false 644.1
forced or induced, affecting fetus or newborn 763.89
hypertonic 661.4
affecting fetus or newborn 763.7
hypotonic 661.2
affecting fetus or newborn 763.7
primary 661.0
affecting fetus or newborn 763.7
secondary 661.1
affecting fetus or newborn 763.7
incoordinate 661.4
affecting fetus or newborn 763.7
irregular 661.2
affecting fetus or newborn 763.7
long—*see* Labor, prolonged
missed (at or near term) 656.4
obstructed NEC 660.9
affecting fetus or newborn 763.1
due to female genital mutilation 660.8
specified cause NEC 660.8
affecting fetus or newborn 763.1
pains, spurious 644.1
precipitate 661.3
affecting fetus or newborn 763.6
premature 644.2
threatened 644.0
prolonged or protracted 662.1
affecting fetus or newborn 763.89
first stage 662.0
affecting fetus or newborn 763.89
second stage 662.2
affecting fetus or newborn 763.89
threatened NEC 644.1
undelivered 644.1
Labored breathing (*see also* Hyperventilation) 786.09

Labyrinthitis (inner ear) (destructive) (latent) 386.30
circumscribed 386.32
diffuse 386.31
focal 386.32
purulent 386.33
serous 386.31
suppurative 386.33
syphilitic 095.8
toxic 386.34
viral 386.35
Laceration —*see also* Wound, open, by site
accidental, complicating surgery 998.2
Achilles tendon 845.09
with open wound 892.2
anus (sphincter) 879.6
with
abortion—*see* Abortion, by type, with damage to pelvic organs
ectopic pregnancy (*see also* categories 633.0-633.9) 639.2
molar pregnancy (*see also* categories 630-632) 639.2
complicated 879.7
complicating delivery (healed) (old) 654.8
with laceration of anal or rectal mucosa 664.3
not associated with third-degree perineal laceration 664.6
following
abortion 639.2
ectopic or molar pregnancy 639.2
nontraumatic, nonpuerperal (healed) (old) 569.43
bladder (urinary)
with
abortion—*see* Abortion, by type, with damage to pelvic organs
ectopic pregnancy (*see also* categories 633.0-633.9) 639.2
molar pregnancy (*see also* categories 630-632) 639.2
following
abortion 639.2
ectopic or molar pregnancy 639.2
obstetrical trauma 665.5
blood vessel—*see* Injury, blood vessel, by site
bowel
with
abortion—*see* Abortion, by type, with damage to pelvic organs
ectopic pregnancy (*see also* categories 633.0-633.9) 639.2
molar pregnancy (*see also* categories 630-632) 639.2
following
abortion 639.2
ectopic or molar pregnancy 639.2
obstetrical trauma 665.5
brain (with hemorrhage) (cerebral) (membrane) 851.8

Laceration—*continued*

Note—Use the following fifth-digit
subclassification with categories 851-854:

0 unspecified state of consciousness
1 with no loss of consciousness
2 with brief [less than one hour] loss of
   consciousness
3 with moderate [1-24 hours] loss of
   consciousness
4 with prolonged [more than 24 hours] loss of
   consciousness and return to pre-existing
   conscious level
5 with prolonged [more than 24 hours] loss of
   consciousness, without return to pre-existing
   conscious level
Use fifth-digit 5 to designate when a patient is
unconscious and dies before regaining
consciousness, regardless of the duration of the
loss of consciousness
6 with loss of consciousness of unspecified
   duration
9 with concussion, unspecified

  with
    open intracranial wound 851.9
    skull fracture—*see* Fracture, skull, by site
  cerebellum 851.6
    with open intracranial wound 851.7
  cortex 851.2
    with open intracranial wound 851.3
    during birth 767.0
  stem 851.6
    with open intracranial wound 851.7
  broad ligament
    with
      abortion—*see* Abortion, by type, with
        damage to pelvic organs
      ectopic pregnancy (*see also* categories
        633.0-633.9) 639.2
      molar pregnancy (*see also* categories
        630-632) 639.2
    following
      abortion 639.2
      ectopic or molar pregnancy 639.2
    nontraumatic 620.6
    obstetrical trauma 665.6
    syndrome (nontraumatic) 620.6
  capsule, joint—*see* Sprain, by site
  cardiac—*see* Laceration, heart
  causing eversion of cervix uteri (old) 622.0
  central, complicating delivery 664.4
  cerebellum—*see* Laceration, brain, cerebellum
  cerebral—*see also* Laceration, brain
    during birth 767.0
  cervix (uteri)
    with
      abortion—*see* Abortion, by type, with
        damage to pelvic organs
      ectopic pregnancy (*see also* categories
        633.0-633.9) 639.2
      molar pregnancy (*see also* categories
        630-632) 639.2
    following
      abortion 639.2
      ectopic or molar pregnancy 639.2
    nonpuerperal, nontraumatic 622.3
    obstetrical trauma (current) 665.3
    old (postpartal) 622.3
    traumatic—*see* Injury, internal, cervix
  chordae heart 429.5

Laceration—*continued*
  complicated 879.9
  cornea—*see* Laceration, eyeball
    superficial 918.1
  cortex (cerebral)—*see* Laceration, brain, cortex
  esophagus 530.89
  eye(s)—*see* Laceration, ocular
  eyeball NEC 871.4
    with prolapse or exposure of intraocular tissue
      871.1
    penetrating—*see* Penetrating wound, eyeball
    specified as without prolapse of intraocular
      tissue 871.0
  eyelid NEC 870.8
    full thickness 870.1
      involving lacrimal passages 870.2
    skin (and periocular area) 870.0
    penetrating—*see* Penetrating wound, orbit
  fourchette
    with
      abortion—*see* Abortion, by type, with
        damage to pelvic organs
      ectopic pregnancy (*see also* categories
        633.0-633.9) 639.2
      molar pregnancy (*see also* categories
        630-632) 639.2
    complicating delivery 664.0
    following
      abortion 639.2
      ectopic or molar pregnancy 639.2
  heart (without penetration of heart chambers)
    861.02
    with
      open wound into thorax 861.12
      penetration of heart chambers 861.03
        with open wound into thorax 861.13
  hernial sac—*see* Hernia, by site
  internal organ (abdomen) (chest) (pelvis)
    NEC—*see* Injury, internal, by site
  kidney (parenchyma) 866.02
    with
      complete disruption of parenchyma (rupture)
        866.03
        with open wound into cavity 866.13
      open wound into cavity 866.12
  labia
    complicating delivery 664.0
  ligament—*see also* Sprain, by site
    with open wound—*see* Wound, open, by site
  liver 864.05
    with open wound into cavity 864.15
    major (disruption of hepatic parenchyma)
      864.04
      with open wound into cavity 864.14
    minor (capsule only) 864.02
      with open wound into cavity 864.12
    moderate (involving parenchyma without
      major disruption) 864.03
      with open wound into cavity 864.13
    multiple 864.04
      with open wound into cavity 864.14
    stellate 864.04
      with open wound into cavity 864.14
  lung 861.22
    with open wound into thorax 861.32
  meninges—*see* Laceration, brain
  meniscus (knee) (*see also* Tear, meniscus) 836.2
    old 717.5
    site other than knee—*see also* Sprain, by site
      old NEC (*see also* Disorder, cartilage,
        articular) 718.0

Laceration—*continued*
  muscle—*see also* Sprain, by site
    with open wound—*see* Wound, open, by site
  myocardium—*see* Laceration, heart
  nerve—*see* Injury, nerve, by site
  ocular NEC (*see also* Laceration, eyeball) 871.4
    adnexa NEC 870.8
      penetrating 870.3
        with foreign body 870.4
  orbit (eye) 870.8
    penetrating 870.3
      with foreign body 870.4
  pelvic
    floor (muscles)
      with
        abortion—*see* Abortion, by type, with
          damage to pelvic organs
        ectopic pregnancy (*see also* categories
          633.0-633.9) 639.2
        molar pregnancy (*see also* categories
          630-632) 639.2
      complicating delivery 664.1
      following
        abortion 639.2
        ectopic or molar pregnancy 639.2
      nonpuerperal 618.7
      old (postpartal) 618.7
    organ NEC
      with
        abortion—*see* Abortion, by type, with
          damage to pelvic organs
        ectopic pregnancy (*see also* categories
          633.0-633.9) 639.2
        molar pregnancy (*see also* categories
          630-632) 639.2
      complicating delivery 665.5
        affecting fetus or newborn 763.89
      following
        abortion 639.2
        ectopic or molar pregnancy 639.2
      obstetrical trauma 665.5
  perineum, perineal (old) (postpartal) 618.7
    with
      abortion—*see* Abortion, by type, with
        damage to pelvic floor
      ectopic pregnancy (*see also* categories
        633.0-633.9) 639.2
      molar pregnancy (*see also* categories
        630-632) 639.2
    complicating delivery 664.4
      first degree 664.0
      second degree 664.1
      third degree 664.2
      fourth degree 664.3
      central 664.4
      involving
        anal sphincter (healed) (old) 654.8
          not associated with third-degree perineal
            laceration 664.6
        fourchette 664.0
        hymen 664.0
        labia 664.0
        pelvic floor 664.1
        perineal muscles 664.1
        rectovaginal septum 664.2
          with anal mucosa 664.3
        skin 664.0
        sphincter (anal) (healed) (old) 654.8
          not associated with third-degree perineal
            laceration 664.6
          with anal mucosa 664.3

Laceration—*continued*
  vagina 664.0
  vaginal muscles 664.1
  vulva 664.0
    secondary 674.2
    following
      abortion 639.2
      ectopic or molar pregnancy 639.2
  male 879.6
    complicated 879.7
  muscles, complicating delivery 664.1
  nonpuerperal, current injury 879.6
    complicated 879.7
  secondary (postpartal) 674.2
  peritoneum
    with
      abortion—*see* Abortion, by type, with
        damage to pelvic organs
      ectopic pregnancy (*see also* categories
        633.0-633.9) 639.2
      molar pregnancy (*see also* categories
        630-632) 639.2
    following
      abortion 639.2
      ectopic or molar pregnancy 639.2
    obstetrical trauma 665.5
  periurethral tissue
    with
      abortion—*see* Abortion, by type, with
        damage to pelvic organs
      ectopic pregnancy (*see also* categories
        633.0-633.9) 639.2
      molar pregnancy (*see also* categories
        630-632) 639.2
    following
      abortion 639.2
      ectopic or molar pregnancy 639.2
    obstetrical trauma 665.5
  rectovaginal (septum)
    with
      abortion—*see* Abortion, by type, with
        damage to pelvic organs
      ectopic pregnancy (*see also* categories
        633.0-633.9) 639.2
      molar pregnancy (*see also* categories
        630-632) 639.2
    complicating delivery 665.4
      with perineum 664.2
        involving anal or rectal mucosa 664.3
    following
      abortion 639.2
      ectopic or molar pregnancy 639.2
    nonpuerperal 623.4
    old (postpartal) 623.4
  spinal cord (meninges)—*see also* Injury, spinal,
    by site
    due to injury at birth 767.4
    fetus or newborn 767.4
  spleen 865.09
    with
      disruption of parenchyma (massive) 865.04
        with open wound into cavity 865.14
      open wound into cavity 865.19
    capsule (without disruption of parenchyma)
      865.02
      with open wound into cavity 865.12
    parenchyma 865.03
      with open wound into cavity 865.13
      massive disruption (rupture) 865.04
        with open wound into cavity 865.14

Laceration—*continued*
  tendon 848.9
    with open wound–*see* Wound, open, by site
    Achilles 845.09
      with open wound 892.2
    lower limb NEC 844.9
      with open wound NEC 894.2
    upper limb NEC 840.9
      with open wound NEC 884.2
  tentorium cerebelli—*see* Laceration, brain,
      cerebellum
  tongue 873.64
    complicated 873.74
  urethra
    with
      abortion—*see* Abortion, by type, with
          damage to pelvic organs
      ectopic pregnancy (*see also* categories
          633.0- 633.9) 639.2
      molar pregnancy (*see also* categories
          630-632) 639.2
    following
      abortion 639.2
      ectopic or molar pregnancy 639.2
    nonpuerperal, nontraumatic 599.84
    obstetrical trauma 665.5
  uterus
    with
      abortion—*see* Abortion, by type, with
          damage to pelvic organs
      ectopic pregnancy (*see also* categories
          633.0-633.9) 639.2
      molar pregnancy (*see also* categories
          630-632) 639.2
    following
      abortion 639.2
      ectopic or molar pregnancy 639.2
    nonpuerperal, nontraumatic 621.8
    obstetrical trauma NEC 665.5
    old (postpartal) 621.8
  vagina
    with
      abortion—*see* Abortion, by type, with
          damage to pelvic organs
      ectopic pregnancy (*see also* categories
          633.0-633.9) 639.2
      molar pregnancy (*see also* categories
          630-632) 639.2
      perineal involvement, complicating delivery
          664.0
    complicating delivery 665.4
      first degree 664.0
      second degree 664.1
      third degree 664.2
      fourth degree 664.3
      high 665.4
      muscles 664.1
      sulcus 665.4
      wall 665.4
    following
      abortion 639.2
      ectopic or molar pregnancy 639.2
    nonpuerperal, nontraumatic 623.4
    old (postpartal) 623.4
  valve, heart—*see* Endocarditis
  vulva
    with
      abortion—*see* Abortion, by type, with
          damage to pelvic organs
      ectopic pregnancy (*see also* categories
          633.0-633.9) 639.2

Laceration—*continued*
    molar pregnancy (*see also* categories
        630-632) 639.2
    complicating delivery 664.0
    following
      abortion 639.2
      ectopic or molar pregnancy 639.2
    nonpuerperal, nontraumatic 624.4
    old (postpartal) 624.4
Lachrymal —*see* condition
Lachrymonasal duct —*see* condition
Lack of
  adequate intermaxillary vertical dimension
      524.36
  appetite (*see also* Anorexia) 783.0
  care
    in home V60.4
    of adult 995.84
    of infant (at or after birth) 995.52
  coordination 781.3
  development—*see also* Hypoplasia
    physiological in childhood 783.40
  education V62.3
  energy 780.79
  financial resources V60.2
  food 994.2
    in environment V60.89
  growth in childhood 783.43
  heating V60.1
  housing (permanent) (temporary) V60.0
    adequate V60.1
  material resources V60.2
  medical attention 799.89
  memory (*see also* Amnesia) 780.93
    mild, following organic brain damage 310.8
  ovulation 628.0
  person able to render necessary care V60.4
  physical exercise V69.0
  physiologic development in childhood 783.40
  posterior occlusal support 524.57
  prenatal care in current pregnancy V23.7
  shelter V60.0
  sleep V69.4
  water 994.3
Lacrimal —*see* condition
Lacrimation, abnormal (*see also* Epiphora) 375.20
Lacrimonasal duct —*see* condition
Lactation, lactating (breast) (puerperal)
    (postpartum)
  defective 676.4
  disorder 676.9
    specified type NEC 676.8
  excessive 676.6
  failed 676.4
  mastitis NEC 675.2
  mother (care and/or examination) V24.1
  nonpuerperal 611.6
  suppressed 676.5
Lacticemia 271.3
  excessive 276.2
Lactosuria 271.3
Lacunar skull 756.0
Laennec's cirrhosis (alcoholic) 571.2
  nonalcoholic 571.5
Lafora's disease 333.2
Lag, lid (nervous) 374.41
Lagleyze-von Hippel disease (retinocerebral
    angiomatosis) 759.6

Lagophthalmos (eyelid) (nervous) 374.20
cicatricial 374.23
keratitis (*see also* Keratitis) 370.34
mechanical 374.22
paralytic 374.21
La grippe —*see* Influenza
Lahore sore 085.1
Lakes, venous (cerebral) 437.8
Laki-Lorand factor deficiency (*see also* Defect,
coagulation) 286.3
Lalling 307.9
Lambliasis 007.1
Lame back 724.5
Lancereaux's diabetes (diabetes mellitus with
marked emaciation) 250.8 *[261]*
due to secondary diabetes 249.8 *[261]*
Landau-Kleffner syndrome 345.8
Landouzy-Déjérine dystrophy
(fascioscapulohumeral atrophy) 359.1
Landry's disease or paralysis 357.0
Landry-Guillain-Barré syndrome 357.0
Lane's
band 751.4
disease 569.89
kink (*see also* Obstruction, intestine) 560.9
Langdon Down's syndrome (mongolism) 758.0
Language abolition 784.69
Lanugo (persistent) 757.4
Laparoscopic surgical procedure converted to
open procedure V64.41
Lardaceous
degeneration (any site) 277.39
disease 277.39
kidney 277.39 *[583.81]*
liver 277.39
Large
baby (regardless of gestational age) 766.1
exceptionally (weight of 4500 grams or more)
766.0
of diabetic mother 775.0
ear 744.22
fetus—*see also* Oversize, fetus
causing disproportion 653.5
with obstructed labor 660.1
for dates
fetus or newborn (regardless of gestational
age) 766.1
affecting management of pregnancy 656.6
exceptionally (weight of 4500 grams or
more) 766.0
physiological cup 743.57
stature 783.9
waxy liver 277.39
white kidney—*see* Nephrosis
Larsen's syndrome (flattened facies and multiple
congenital dislocations) 755.8
Larsen-Johansson disease (juvenile osteopathia
patellae) 732.4
Larva migrans
cutaneous NEC 126.9
ancylostoma 126.9
of Diptera in vitreous 128.0
visceral NEC 128.0
Laryngeal —*see also* condition
syncope 786.2
Laryngismus (acute) (infectious) (stridulous)
478.75
congenital 748.3
diphtheritic 032.3

Laryngitis (acute) (edematous) (fibrinous)
(gangrenous) (infective) (infiltrative)
(malignant) (membranous) (phlegmonous)
(pneumococcal) (pseudomembranous) (septic)
(subglottic) (suppurative) (ulcerative) (viral)
464.00
with
influenza, flu, or grippe 487.1
obstruction 464.01
tracheitis (*see also* Laryngotracheitis) 464.20
with obstruction 464.21
acute 464.20
with obstruction 464.21
chronic 476.1
atrophic 476.0
Borrelia vincentii 101
catarrhal 476.0
chronic 476.0
with tracheitis (chronic) 476.1
due to external agent—*see* Condition,
respiratory, chronic, due to
diphtheritic (membranous) 032.3
due to external agent—*see* Inflammation,
respiratory, upper, due to
H. influenzae 464.00
with obstruction 464.01
Hemophilus influenzae 464.00
with obstruction 464.01
hypertrophic 476.0
influenzal 487.1
pachydermic 478.79
sicca 476.0
spasmodic 478.75
acute 464.00
with obstruction 464.01
streptococcal 034.0
stridulous 478.75
syphilitic 095.8
congenital 090.5
tuberculous (*see also* Tuberculosis, larynx)
012.3
Vincent's 101
Laryngocele (congenital) (ventricular) 748.3
Laryngofissure 478.79
congenital 748.3
Laryngomalacia (congenital) 748.3
Laryngopharyngitis (acute) 465.0
chronic 478.9
due to external agent—*see* Condition,
respiratory, chronic, due to
due to external agent—*see* Inflammation,
respiratory, upper, due to
septic 034.0
Laryngoplegia (*see also* Paralysis, vocal cord)
478.30
Laryngoptosis 478.79
Laryngospasm 478.75
due to external agent—*see* Condition,
respiratory, acute, due to
Laryngostenosis 478.74
congenital 748.3
Laryngotracheitis (acute) (infectional) (viral)
(*see also* Laryngitis) 464.20
with obstruction 464.21
atrophic 476.1
Borrelia vincentii 101
catarrhal 476.1
chronic 476.1
due to external agent—*see* Condition,
respiratory, chronic, due to
diphtheritic (membranous) 032.3

Laryngotracheitis—*continued*
due to external agent—*see* Inflammation,
   respiratory, upper, due to
H. influenzae 464.20
  with obstruction 464.21
hypertrophic 476.1
influenzal 487.1
pachydermic 478.75
sicca 476.1
spasmodic 478.75
  acute 464.20
    with obstruction 464.21
streptococcal 034.0
stridulous 478.75
syphilitic 095.8
  congenital 090.5
tuberculous (*see also* Tuberculosis, larynx)
  012.3
Vincent's 101
Laryngotracheobronchitis (*see also* Bronchitis)
  490
acute 466.0
chronic 491.8
viral 466.0
Laryngotracheobronchopneumonitis —*see*
Pneumonia, broncho-
Larynx, laryngeal —*see* condition
Lasègue's disease (persecution mania) 297.9
Lassa fever 078.89
Lassitude (*see also* Weakness) 780.79
Late —*see also* condition
infant
  post-term (gestation period over 40
    completed weeks to 42 completed
    weeks) 766.21
  prolonged gestation (period over 42
    completed weeks) 766.22
Late effect(s) (of) —*see also* condition
abscess
  intracranial or intraspinal (conditions
    classifiable to 324)–*see* category 326
adverse effect of drug, medicinal or biological
  substance 909.5
allergic reaction 909.9
amputation
  postoperative (late) 997.60
  traumatic (injury classifiable to 885-887 and
    895-897) 905.9
burn (injury classifiable to 948-949) 906.9
  extremities NEC (injury classifiable to 943 or
    945) 906.7
  hand or wrist (injury classifiable to 944)
    906.6
  eye (injury classifiable to 940) 906.5
  face, head, and neck (injury classifiable to
    941) 906.5
  specified site NEC (injury classifiable to 942
    and 946-947) 906.8
cerebrovascular disease (conditions classifiable
  to 430-437) 438.9
  with
    alterations of sensations 438.6
    aphasia 438.11
    apraxia 438.81
    ataxia 438.84
    cognitive deficits 438.0
    disturbances of vision 438.7
    dysarthria 438.13
    dysphagia 438.82
    dysphasia 438.12
    facial droop 438.83

Late effect(s) (of)—*continued*
cerebrovascular disease—*continued*
  with—*continued*
    facial weakness 438.83
    fluency disorder 438.14
    hemiplegia/hemiparesis
      affecting
        dominant side 438.21
        nondominant side 438.22
        unspecified side 438.20
    monoplegia of lower limb
      affecting
        dominant side 438.41
        nondominant side 438.42
        unspecified side 438.40
    monoplegia of upper limb
      affecting
        dominant side 438.31
        nondominant side 438.32
        unspecified side 438.30
    paralytic syndrome NEC
      affecting
        bilateral 438.53
        dominant side 438.51
        nondominant side 438.52
        unspecified side 438.50
    speech and language deficit 438.10
    specified type NEC 438.19
    stuttering 438.14
    vertigo 438.85
  specified type NEC 438.89
childbirth complication(s) 677
complication(s) of
  childbirth 677
  delivery 677
  pregnancy 677
  puerperium 677
  surgical and medical care (conditions
    classifiable to 996-999) 909.3
  trauma (conditions classifiable to 958) 908.6
contusion (injury classifiable to 920-924) 906.3
crushing (injury classifiable to 925-929) 906.4
delivery complication(s) 677
dislocation (injury classifiable to 830-839) 905.6
encephalitis or encephalomyelitis (conditions
  classifiable to 323)—*see* category 326
  in infectious diseases 139.8
  viral (conditions classifiable to 049.8, 049.9,
    062-064) 139.0
external cause NEC (conditions classifiable to
  995) 909.9
certain conditions classifiable to categories
  991-994 909.4
foreign body in orifice (injury classifiable to
  930-939) 908.5
fracture (multiple) (injury classifiable to
  828-829) 905.5
extremity
  lower (injury classifiable to 821-827) 905.4
    neck of femur (injury classifiable to 820)
      905.3
  upper (injury classifiable to 810-819) 905.2
face and skull (injury classifiable to 800-804)
  905.0
skull and face (injury classifiable to 800-804)
  905.0
spine and trunk (injury classifiable to 805 and
  807-809) 905.1
  with spinal cord lesion (injury classifiable to
    806) 907.2

Late effect(s) (of)—*continued*
infection
pyogenic, intracranial—*see* category 326
infectious diseases (conditions classifiable to 001-136) NEC 139.8
injury (injury classifiable to 959) 908.9
blood vessel 908.3
abdomen and pelvis (injury classifiable to 902) 908.4
extremity (injury classifiable to 903-904) 908.3
head and neck (injury classifiable to 900) 908.3
intracranial (injury classifiable to 850-854) 907.0
with skull fracture 905.0
thorax (injury classifiable to 901) 908.4
internal organ NEC (injury classifiable to 867 and 869) 908.2
abdomen (injury classifiable to 863-866 and 868) 908.1
thorax (injury classifiable to 860-862) 908.0
intracranial (injury classifiable to 850-854) 907.0
with skull fracture (injury classifiable to 800-801 and 803-804) 905.0
nerve NEC (injury classifiable to 957) 907.9
cranial (injury classifiable to 950-951) 907.1
peripheral NEC (injury classifiable to 957) 907.9
lower limb and pelvic girdle (injury classifiable to 956) 907.5
upper limb and shoulder girdle (injury classifiable to 955) 907.4
roots and plexus(es), spinal (injury classifiable to 953) 907.3
trunk (injury classifiable to 954) 907.3
pregnancy complication(s) 677
puerperal complication(s) 677
spinal
cord (injury classifiable to 806 and 952) 907.2
nerve root(s) and plexus(es) (injury classifiable to 953) 907.3
superficial (injury classifiable to 910-919) 906.2
tendon (tendon injury classifiable to 840-848, 880-884 with .2, and 890-894 with .2) 905.8
meningitis
bacterial (conditions classifiable to 320)—*see* category 326
unspecified cause (conditions classifiable to 322)—*see* category 326
myelitis (*see also* Late, effect(s) (of), encephalitis)—*see* category 326
parasitic diseases (conditions classifiable to 001-136 NEC) 139.8
phlebitis or thrombophlebitis of intracranial venous sinuses (conditions classifiable to 325)—*see* category 326
poisoning due to drug, medicinal or biological substance (conditions classifiable to 960-979) 909.0
poliomyelitis, acute (conditions classifiable to 045) 138
radiation (conditions classifiable to 990) 909.2
rickets 268.1
sprain and strain without mention of tendon injury (injury classifiable to 840-848, except tendon injury) 905.7
tendon involvement 905.8

Late effect(s) (of)—*continued*
toxic effect of
drug, medicinal or biological substance (conditions classifiable to 960-979) 909.0
nonmedical substance (conditions classifiable to 980-989) 909.1
trachoma (conditions classifiable to 076) 139.1
tuberculosis 137.0
bones and joints (conditions classifiable to 015) 137.3
central nervous system (conditions classifiable to 013) 137.1
genitourinary (conditions classifiable to 016) 137.2
pulmonary (conditions classifiable to 010-012) 137.0
specified organs NEC (conditions classifiable to 014, 017-018) 137.4
viral encephalitis (conditions classifiable to 049.8, 049.9, 062-064) 139.0
wound, open
extremity (injury classifiable to 880-884 and 890-894, except .2) 906.1
tendon (injury classifiable to 880-884 with .2 and 890-894 with .2) 905.8
head, neck, and trunk (injury classifiable to 870-879) 906.0
Latent —*see* condition
Lateral —*see* condition
Laterocession —*see* Lateroversion
Lateroflexion —*see* Lateroversion
Lateroversion
cervix—*see* Lateroversion, uterus
uterus, uterine (cervix) (postinfectional) (postpartal, old) 621.6
congenital 752.3
in pregnancy or childbirth 654.4
affecting fetus or newborn 763.89
Lathyrism 988.2
Launois' syndrome (pituitary gigantism) 253.0
Launois-Bensaude's lipomatosis 272.8
Launois-Cléret syndrome (adiposogenital dystrophy) 253.8
Laurence-Moon-Biedl syndrome (obesity, polydactyly, and mental retardation) 759.89
LAV (disease) (illness) (infection)—*see* Human immunodeficiency virus (disease) (illness) (infection)
LAV/HTLV-III (disease) (illness) (infection)—*see* Human immunodeficiency virus (disease) (illness) (infection)
Lawford's syndrome (encephalocutaneous angiomatosis) 759.6
Lax, laxity —*see also* Relaxation
ligament 728.4
skin (acquired) 701.8
congenital 756.83
Laxative habit (*see also* Abuse, drugs, nondependent) 305.9
Lazy leukocyte syndrome 288.09
LCAD (long chain/very long chain acyl CoA dehydrogenase deficiency, VLCAD) 277.85
LCHAD (long chain 3-hydroxyacyl CoA dehydrogenase deficiency) 277.85
Lead —*see also* condition
exposure (suspected) to V15.86
incrustation of cornea 371.15
poisoning 984.9
specified type of lead—*see* Table of drugs and chemicals
Lead miner's lung 503

Leakage
 amniotic fluid 658.1
  with delayed delivery 658.2
  affecting fetus or newborn 761.1
 bile from drainage tube (T tube) 997.4
 blood (microscopic), fetal, into maternal
  circulation 656.0
  affecting management of pregnancy or
   puerperium 656.0
 device, implant, or graft—*see* Complications,
  mechanical
 spinal fluid at lumbar puncture site 997.09
 urine, continuous 788.37
Leaky heart —*see* Endocarditis
Learning defect, specific NEC
 (strephosymbolia) 315.2
Leather bottle stomach (M8142/3) 151.9
Leber's
 congenital amaurosis 362.76
 optic atrophy (hereditary) 377.16
Lederer's anemia or disease (acquired
 infectious hemolytic anemia) 283.19
Lederer-Brill syndrome (acquired infectious
 hemolytic anemia) 283.19
Leeches (aquatic) (land) 134.2
Left-sided neglect 781.8
Leg —*see* condition
Legal investigation V62.5
Legg (-Calvé) -Perthes disease or syndrome
 (osteochondrosis, femoral capital) 732.1
Legionnaires' disease 482.84
Leigh's disease 330.8
Leiner's disease (exfoliative dermatitis) 695.89
Leiofibromyoma (M8890/0)—*see also*
 Leiomyoma
 uterus (cervix) (corpus) (*see also* Leiomyoma,
  uterus) 218.9
Leiomyoblastoma (M8891/1)—*see* Neoplasm,
 connective tissue, uncertain behavior
Leiomyofibroma (M8890/0)—*see also*
 Neoplasm, connective tissue, benign
 uterus (cervix) (corpus) (*see also* Leiomyoma,
  uterus) 218.9
Leiomyoma (M8890/0)—*see also* Neoplasm,
 connective tissue, benign
 bizarre (M8893/0)—*see* Neoplasm, connective
  tissue, benign
 cellular (M8892/1)—*see* Neoplasm, connective
  tissue, uncertain behavior
 epithelioid (M8891/1)—*see* Neoplasm,
  connective tissue, uncertain behavior
 prostate (polypoid) 600.20
  with
   other lower urinary tract symptoms (LUTS)
    600.21
   urinary
    obstruction 600.21
    retention 600.21
 uterus (cervix) (corpus) 218.9
  interstitial 218.1
  intramural 218.1
  submucous 218.0
  subperitoneal 218.2
  subserous 218.2
  vascular (M8894/0)—*see* Neoplasm,
   connective tissue, benign
Leiomyomatosis (intravascular) (M8890/1)—*see*
 Neoplasm, connective tissue, uncertain
 behavior

Leiomyosarcoma (M8890/3)—*see also*
 Neoplasm, connective tissue, malignant
 epithelioid (M8891/3)—*see* Neoplasm,
  connective tissue, malignant
Leishmaniasis 085.9
 American 085.5
  cutaneous 085.4
  mucocutaneous 085.5
 Asian desert 085.2
 Brazilian 085.5
 cutaneous 085.9
  acute necrotizing 085.2
  American 085.4
  Asian desert 085.2
  diffuse 085.3
  dry form 085.1
  Ethiopian 085.3
  eyelid 085.5 *[373.6]*
  late 085.1
  lepromatous 085.3
  recurrent 085.1
  rural 085.2
  ulcerating 085.1
  urban 085.1
  wet form 085.2
  zoonotic form 085.2
 dermal—*see also* Leishmaniasis, cutaneous
  post kala-azar 085.0
 eyelid 085.5 *[373.6]*
 infantile 085.0
 Mediterranean 085.0
 mucocutaneous (American) 085.5
 naso-oral 085.5
 nasopharyngeal 085.5
 Old World 085.1
 tegumentaria diffusa 085.4
 vaccination, prophylactic (against) V05.2
 visceral (Indian) 085.0
Leishmanoid, dermal —*see also* Leishmaniasis,
 cutaneous
 post kala-azar 085.0
Leloir's disease 695.4
Lemiere syndrome 451.89
Lenegre's disease 426.0
Lengthening, leg 736.81
Lennox-Gastaut syndrome 345.0
 with tonic seizures 345.1
Lennox's syndrome (*see also* Epilepsy) 345.0
Lens —*see* condition
Lenticonus (anterior) (posterior) (congenital)
 743.36
Lenticular degeneration, progressive 275.1
Lentiglobus (posterior) (congenital) 743.36
Lentigo (congenital) 709.09
 juvenile 709.09
 Maligna (M8742/2)—*see also* Neoplasm, skin,
  in situ
 melanoma (M8742/3)—*see* Melanoma
 senile 709.09
Leonine leprosy 030.0
Leontiasis
 ossium 733.3
 syphilitic 095.8
  congenital 090.5
Léopold-Lévi's syndrome (paroxysmal thyroid
 instability) 242.9
Lepore hemoglobin syndrome 282.49
Lepothrix 039.0
Lepra 030.9
 Willan's 696.1
Leprechaunism 259.8

Lepromatous leprosy 030.0
Leprosy 030.9
 anesthetic 030.1
 beriberi 030.1
 borderline (group B) (infiltrated) (neuritic) 030.3
 cornea (*see also* Leprosy, by type) 030.9
  [371.89]
 dimorphous (group B) (infiltrated)
  (lepromatous) (neuritic) (tuberculoid) 030.3
 eyelid 030.0 *[373.4]*
 indeterminate (group I) (macular) (neuritic)
  (uncharacteristic) 030.2
 leonine 030.0
 lepromatous (diffuse) (infiltrated) (macular)
  (neuritic) (nodular) (type L) 030.0
 macular (early) (neuritic) (simple) 030.2
 maculoanesthetic 030.1
 mixed 030.0
 neuro 030.1
 nodular 030.0
 primary neuritic 030.3
 specified type or group NEC 030.8
 tubercular 030.1
 tuberculoid (macular) (maculoanesthetic)
  (major) (minor) (neuritic) (type T) 030.1
Leptocytosis, hereditary 282.49
Leptomeningitis (chronic) (circumscribed)
 (hemorrhagic) (nonsuppurative) (*see also*
 Meningitis) 322.9
 aseptic 047.9
  adenovirus 049.1
  Coxsackie virus 047.0
  ECHO virus 047.1
  enterovirus 047.9
  lymphocytic choriomeningitis 049.0
 epidemic 036.0
 late effect—*see* category 326
 meningococcal 036.0
 pneumococcal 320.1
 syphilitic 094.2
 tuberculous (*see also* Tuberculosis, meninges)
  013.0
Leptomeningopathy (*see also* Meningitis) 322.9
Leptospiral —*see* condition
Leptospirochetal —*see* condition
Leptospirosis 100.9
 autumnalis 100.89
 canicula 100.89
 grippotyphosa 100.89
 hebdomidis 100.89
 icterohemorrhagica 100.0
 nanukayami 100.89
 pomona 100.89
 Weil's disease 100.0
Leptothricosis —*see* Actinomycosis
Leptothrix infestation —*see* Actinomycosis
Leptotricosis —*see* Actinomycosis
Leptus dermatitis 133.8
Léri's pleonosteosis 756.89
Léri-Weill syndrome 756.59
Leriche syndrome (aortic bifurcation occlusion)
 444.0
Lermoyez's syndrome (*see also* Disease,
 Ménière's) 386.00
Lesbianism —*omit code*
 egodystonic 302.0
 problems with 302.0
Lesch-Nyhan syndrome (hypoxanthine-guanine-
 phosphoribosyltransferase deficiency) 277.2

Lesion(s)
 abducens nerve 378.54
 alveolar process 525.8
 anorectal 569.49
 aortic (valve)—*see* Endocarditis, aortic
 auditory nerve 388.5
 basal ganglion 333.90
 bile duct (*see also* Disease, biliary) 576.8
 bladder 596.9
 bone 733.90
 brachial plexus 353.0
 brain 348.89
  congenital 742.9
  vascular (*see also* Lesion, cerebrovascular)
   437.9
   degenerative 437.1
   healed or old without residuals V12.54
   hypertensive 437.2
   late effect—*see* Late effect(s) (of)
    cerebrovascular disease
 buccal 528.9
 calcified—*see* Calcification
 canthus 373.9
 carate—*see* Pinta, lesions
 cardia 537.89
 cardiac—*see also* Disease, heart congenital 746.9
  valvular—*see* Endocarditis
 cauda equina 344.60
  with neurogenic bladder 344.61
 cecum 569.89
 cerebral—*see* Lesion, brain
 cerebrovascular (*see also* Disease,
  cerebrovascular NEC) 437.9
  degenerative 437.1
  healed or old without residuals V12.54
  hypertensive 437.2
  specified type NEC 437.8
 cervical root (nerve) NEC 353.2
 chiasmal 377.54
  associated with
   inflammatory disorders 377.54
   neoplasm NEC 377.52
   pituitary 377.51
   pituitary disorders 377.51
   vascular disorders 377.53
 chorda tympani 351.8
 coin, lung 793.1
 colon 569.89
 congenital—*see* Anomaly
 conjunctiva 372.9
 coronary artery (*see also* Ischemia, heart) 414.9
 cranial nerve 352.9
  first 352.0
  second 377.49
  third
   partial 378.51
   total 378.52
  fourth 378.53
  fifth 350.9
  sixth 378.54
  seventh 351.9
  eighth 388.5
  ninth 352.2
  tenth 352.3
  eleventh 352.4
  twelfth 352.5
 cystic—*see* Cyst
 degenerative—*see* Degeneration
 dermal (skin) 709.9

Lesion(s)—*continued*
  Dieulafoy (hemorrhagic)
    of
      duodenum 537.84
      intestine 569.86
      stomach 537.84
    duodenum 537.89
      with obstruction 537.3
    eyelid 373.9
    gasserian ganglion 350.8
    gastric 537.89
    gastroduodenal 537.89
    gastrointestinal 569.89
    glossopharyngeal nerve 352.2
    heart (organic)—*see also* Disease, heart
      vascular—*see* Disease, cardiovascular
    helix (ear) 709.9
    high grade myelodysplastic syndrome 238.73
    hyperchromic, due to pinta (carate) 103.1
    hyperkeratotic (*see also* Hyperkeratosis) 701.1
    hypoglossal nerve 352.5
    hypopharynx 478.29
    hypothalamic 253.9
    ileocecal coil 569.89
    ileum 569.89
    iliohypogastric nerve 355.79
    ilioinguinal nerve 355.79
    in continuity—*see* Injury, nerve, by site
    inflammatory—*see* Inflammation
    intestine 569.89
    intracerebral—*see* Lesion, brain
    intrachiasmal (optic) (*see also* Lesion, chiasmal)
      377.54
    intracranial, space-occupying NEC 784.2
    joint 719.90
      ankle 719.97
      elbow 719.92
      foot 719.97
      hand 719.94
      hip 719.95
      knee 719.96
      multiple sites 719.99
      pelvic region 719.95
      sacroiliac (old) 724.6
      shoulder (region) 719.91
      specified site NEC 719.98
      wrist 719.93
    keratotic (*see also* Keratosis) 701.1
    kidney (*see also* Disease, renal) 593.9
    laryngeal nerve (recurrent) 352.3
    leonine 030.0
    lip 528.5
    liver 573.8
    low grade myelodysplastic syndrome 238.72
    lumbosacral
      plexus 353.1
      root (nerve) NEC 353.4
    lung 518.89
      coin 793.1
    maxillary sinus 473.0
    mitral—*see* Endocarditis, mitral
    Morel Lavallée — see Hematoma, by site
    motor cortex 348.89
    nerve (*see also* Disorder, nerve) 355.9
    nervous system 349.9
      congenital 742.9

Lesion(s)—*continued*
  nonallopathic NEC 739.9
    in region (of)
      abdomen 739.9
      acromioclavicular 739.7
      cervical, cervicothoracic 739.1
      costochondral 739.8
      costovertebral 739.8
      extremity
        lower 739.6
        upper 739.7
      head 739.0
      hip 739.5
      lower extremity 739.6
      lumbar, lumbosacral 739.3
      occipitocervical 739.0
      pelvic 739.5
      pubic 739.5
      rib cage 739.8
      sacral, sacrococcygeal, sacroiliac 739.4
      sternochondral 739.8
      sternoclavicular 739.7
      thoracic, thoracolumbar 739.2
      upper extremity 739.7
    nose (internal) 478.19
    obstructive—*see* Obstruction
    obturator nerve 355.79
    occlusive
      artery—*see* Embolism, artery
    organ or site NEC—*see* Disease, by site
    osteolytic 733.90
    paramacular, of retina 363.32
    peptic 537.89
    periodontal, due to traumatic occlusion 523.8
    perirectal 569.49
    peritoneum (granulomatous) 568.89
    pigmented (skin) 709.00
    pinta—*see* Pinta, lesions
    polypoid—*see* Polyp
    prechiasmal (optic) (*see also* Lesion, chiasmal)
      377.54
    primary—*see also* Syphilis, primary
      carate 103.0
      pinta 103.0
      yaws 102.0
    pulmonary 518.89
      valve (*see also* Endocarditis, pulmonary)
        424.3
    pylorus 537.89
    radiation NEC 990
    radium NEC 990
    rectosigmoid 569.89
    retina, retinal—*see also* Retinopathy
      vascular 362.17
    retroperitoneal 568.89
    romanus 720.1
    sacroiliac (joint) 724.6
    salivary gland 527.8
      benign lymphoepithelial 527.8
    saphenous nerve 355.79
    secondary—*see* Syphilis, secondary
    sigmoid 569.89
    sinus (accessory) (nasal) (*see also* Sinusitis)
      473.9
    skin 709.9
      suppurative 686.00
    SLAP (superior glenoid labrum) 840.7
    space-occupying, intracranial NEC 784.2

Lesion(s)—*continued*
  spinal cord 336.9
    congenital 742.9
    traumatic (complete) (incomplete)
        (transverse)—*see also* Injury, spinal, by
        site
      with
        broken
          back—*see* Fracture, vertebra, by site,
              with spinal cord injury
          neck—*see* Fracture, vertebra, cervical,
              with spinal cord injury
        fracture, vertebra—*see* Fracture, vertebra,
            by site, with spinal cord injury
  spleen 289.50
  stomach 537.89
  superior glenoid labrum (SLAP) 840.7
  syphilitic—*see* Syphilis
  tertiary—*see* Syphilis, tertiary
  thoracic root (nerve) 353.3
  tonsillar fossa 474.9
  tooth, teeth 525.8
    white spot 521.01
  traumatic NEC (*see also* nature and site of
      injury) 959.9
  tricuspid (valve)—*see* Endocarditis, tricuspid
  trigeminal nerve 350.9
  ulcerated or ulcerative—*see* Ulcer
  uterus NEC 621.9
  vagina 623.8
  vagus nerve 352.3
  valvular—*see* Endocarditis
  vascular 459.9
    affecting central nervous system (*see also*
        Lesion, cerebrovascular) 437.9
    following trauma (*see also* Injury, blood
        vessel, by site) 904.9
    retina 362.17
    traumatic—*see* Injury, blood vessel, by site
    umbilical cord 663.6
      affecting fetus or newborn 762.6
  visual
    cortex NEC (*see also* Disorder, visual, cortex)
        377.73
    pathway NEC (*see also* Disorder, visual,
        pathway) 377.63
  warty—*see* Verruca
  white spot, on teeth 521.01
  x-ray NEC 990
Lethargic —*see* condition
Lethargy 780.79
Letterer-Siwe disease (acute histiocytosis X)
    (M9722/3) 202.5
Leucinosis 270.3
Leucocoria 360.44
Leucosarcoma (M9850/3) 207.8
Leukasmus 270.2
Leukemia, leukemic (congenital) (M9800/3) 208.9

Note—Use the following fifth-digit
subclassification for categories 203-208:

0 without mention of having achieved
    remission, failed remission
1 in remission
2 in relapse

---

  acute NEC (M9801/3) 208.0
  aleukemic NEC (M9804/3) 208.8
    granulocytic (M9864/3) 205.8
  basophilic (M9870/3) 205.1
  blast (cell) (M9801/3) 208.0

Leukemia, leukemic—*continued*
  blastic (M9801/3) 208.0
    granulocytic (M9861/3) 205.0
  chronic NEC (M9803/3) 208.1
  compound (M9810/3) 207.8
  eosinophilic (M9880/3) 205.1
  giant cell (M9910/3) 207.2
  granulocytic (M9860/3) 205.9
    acute (M9861/3) 205.0
    aleukemic (M9864/3) 205.8
    blastic (M9861/3) 205.0
    chronic (M9863/3) 205.1
    subacute (M9862/3) 205.2
    subleukemic (M9864/3) 205.8
  hairy cell (M9940/3) 202.4
  hemoblastic (M9801/3) 208.0
  histiocytic (M9890/3) 206.9
  lymphatic (M9820/3) 204.9
    acute (M9821/3) 204.0
    aleukemic (M9824/3) 204.8
    chronic (M9823/3) 204.1
    subacute (M9822/3) 204.2
    subleukemic (M9824/3) 204.8
  lymphoblastic (M9821/3) 204.0
  lymphocytic (M9820/3) 204.9
    acute (M9821/3) 204.0
    aleukemic (M9824/3) 204.8
    chronic (M9823/3) 204.1
    granular
      large T-cell 204.8
    subacute (M9822/3) 204.2
    subleukemic (M9824/3) 204.8
  lymphogenous (M9820/3)—*see* Leukemia,
      lymphoid
  lymphoid (M9820/3) 204.9
    acute (M9821/3) 204.0
    aleukemic (M9824/3) 204.8
    blastic (M9821/3) 204.0
    chronic (M9823/3) 204.1
    subacute (M9822/3) 204.2
    subleukemic (M9824/3) 204.8
  lymphosarcoma cell (M9850/3) 207.8
  mast cell (M9900/3) 207.8
  megakaryocytic (M9910/3) 207.2
  megakaryocytoid (M9910/3) 207.2
  mixed (cell) (M9810/3) 207.8
  monoblastic (M9891/3) 206.0
  monocytic (Schilling-type) (M9890/3) 206.9
    acute (M9891/3) 206.0
    aleukemic (M9894/3) 206.8
    chronic (M9893/3) 206.1
    Naegeli-type (M9863/3) 205.1
    subacute (M9892/3) 206.2
    subleukemic (M9894/3) 206.8
  monocytoid (M9890/3) 206.9
    acute (M9891/3) 206.0
    aleukemic (M9894/3) 206.8
    chronic (M9893/3) 206.1
    myelogenous (M9863/3) 205.1
    subacute (M9892/3) 206.2
    subleukemic (M9894/3) 206.8
  monomyelocytic (M9860/3)—*see* Leukemia,
      myelomonocytic
  myeloblastic (M9861/3) 205.0
  myelocytic (M9863/3) 205.1
    acute (M9861/3) 205.0
  myelogenous (M9860/3) 205.9
    acute (M9861/3) 205.0
    aleukemic (M9864/3) 205.8
    chronic (M9863/3) 205.1
    monocytoid (M9863/3) 205.1

Leydig cell
carcinoma (M8650/3)
  specified site—*see* Neoplasm, by site,
    malignant
  unspecified site
    female 183.0
    male 186.9
tumor (M8650/1)
  benign (M8650/0)
    specified site—*see* Neoplasm, by site, benign
    unspecified site
      female 220
      male 222.0
  malignant (M8650/3)
    specified site—*see* Neoplasm, by site,
      malignant
    unspecified site
      female 183.0
      male 186.9
  specified site—*see* Neoplasm, by site, uncertain
    behavior
  unspecified site
    female 236.2
    male 236.4
Leydig-Sertoli cell tumor (M8631/0)
specified site—*see* Neoplasm, by site, benign
unspecified site
  female 220
  male 222.0
LGSIL (low grade squamous intraepithelial lesion)
anus 796.73
cervix 795.03
vagina 795.13
Liar, pathologic 301.7
Libman-Sacks disease or syndrome 710.0 *[424.91]*
Lice (infestation) 132.9
body (pediculus corporis) 132.1
crab 132.2
head (pediculus capitis) 132.0
mixed (classifiable to more than one of the
  categories 132.0-132.2) 132.3
pubic (pediculus pubis) 132.2
Lichen 697.9
albus 701.0
annularis 695.89
atrophicus 701.0
corneus obtusus 698.3
myxedematous 701.8
nitidus 697.1
pilaris 757.39
  acquired 701.1
planopilaris 697.0
planus (acute) (chronicus) (hypertrophic)
  (verrucous) 697.0
  morphoeicus 701.0
  sclerosus (et atrophicus) 701.0
ruber 696.4
  acuminatus 696.4
  moniliformis 697.8
  obtusus corneus 698.3
  of Wilson 697.0
  planus 697.0
sclerosus (et atrophicus) 701.0
scrofulosus (primary) (*see also* Tuberculosis)
  017.0
simplex (Vidal's) 698.3
  chronicus 698.3
  circumscriptus 698.3
spinulosus 757.39
  mycotic 117.9
striata 697.8
urticatus 698.2

Lichenification 698.3
nodular 698.3
Lichenoides tuberculosis (primary) (*see also*
Tuberculosis) 017.0
Lichtheim's disease or syndrome (subacute
combined sclerosis with pernicious anemia)
281.0 *[336.2]*
Lien migrans 289.59
Lientery (*see also* Diarrhea) 787.91
infectious 009.2
Life circumstance problem NEC V62.89
Li-Fraumeni cancer syndrome V84.01
Ligament —*see* condition
Light-for-dates (infant) 764.0
with signs of fetal malnutrition 764.1
affecting management of pregnancy 656.5
Light-headedness 780.4
Lightning (effects) (shock) (stroke) (struck by) 994.0
burn—*see* Burn, by site
foot 266.2
Lightwood's disease or syndrome (renal tubular
acidosis) 588.89
Lignac's disease (cystinosis) 270.0
Lignac (-de Toni) (-Fanconi) (-Debré) syndrome
(cystinosis) 270.0
Lignac (-Fanconi) syndrome (cystinosis) 270.0
Ligneous thyroiditis 245.3
Likoff's syndrome (angina in menopausal
women) 413.9
Limb —*see* condition
Limitation of joint motion (*see also* Stiffness,
joint) 719.5
sacroiliac 724.6
Limit dextrinosis 271.0
Limited
cardiac reserve—*see* Disease, heart
duction, eye NEC 378.63
mandibular range of motion 524.52
Lindau's disease (retinocerebral angiomatosis)
759.6
Lindau (-von Hippel) disease (angiomatosis
retinocerebellosa) 759.6
Linea corneae senilis 371.41
Lines
Beau's (transverse furrows on fingernails) 703.8
Harris' 733.91
Hudson-Stähli 371.11
Stähli's 371.11
Lingua
geographical 529.1
nigra (villosa) 529.3
plicata 529.5
  congenital 750.13
tylosis 528.6
Lingual (tongue)—*see also* condition
thyroid 759.2
Linitis (gastric) 535.4
plastica (M8142/3) 151.9
Lioderma essentialis (cum melanosis et
telangiectasia) 757.33
Lip —*see also* condition
biting 528.9
Lipalgia 272.8
Lipedema —*see* Edema
Lipemia (*see also* Hyperlipidemia) 272.4
retina, retinalis 272.3
Lipidosis 272.7
cephalin 272.7
cerebral (infantile) (juvenile) (late) 330.1
cerebroretinal 330.1 *[362.71]*
cerebroside 272.7

Lipidosis—*continued*
  cerebrospinal 272.7
  chemically-induced 272.7
  cholesterol 272.7
  diabetic 250.8 *[272.7]*
    due to secondary diabetes 249.8 *[272.7]*
  dystopic (hereditary) 272.7
  glycolipid 272.7
  hepatosplenomegalic 272.3
  hereditary, dystopic 272.7
  sulfatide 330.0
Lipoadenoma (M8324/0)—*see* Neoplasm, by
    site, benign
Lipoblastoma (M8881/0)—*see* Lipoma, by site
Lipoblastomatosis (M8881/0)—*see* Lipoma, by
    site
Lipochondrodystrophy 277.5
Lipochrome histiocytosis (familial) 288.1
Lipodystrophia progressiva 272.6
Lipodystrophy (progressive) 272.6
  insulin 272.6
  intestinal 040.2
  mesenteric 567.82
Lipofibroma (M8851/0)—*see* Lipoma, by site
Lipoglycoproteinosis 272.8
Lipogranuloma, sclerosing 709.8
Lipogranulomatosis (disseminated) 272.8
  kidney 272.8
Lipoid —*see* condition
  histiocytosis 272.7
    essential 272.7
  nephrosis (*see also* Nephrosis) 581.3
  proteinosis of Urbach 272.8
Lipoidemia (*see also* Hyperlipidemia) 272.4
Lipoidosis (*see also* Lipidosis) 272.7
Lipoma (M8850/0) 214.9
  breast (skin) 214.1
  face 214.0
  fetal (M8881/0)—*see also* Lipoma, by site
    fat cell (M8880/0)—*see* Lipoma, by site
  infiltrating (M8856/0)—*see* Lipoma, by site
  intra-abdominal 214.3
  intramuscular (M8856/0)—*see* Lipoma, by site
  intrathoracic 214.2
  kidney 214.3
  mediastinum 214.2
  muscle 214.8
  peritoneum 214.3
  retroperitoneum 214.3
  skin 214.1
    face 214.0
  spermatic cord 214.4
  spindle cell (M8857/0)—*see* Lipoma, by site
  stomach 214.3
  subcutaneous tissue 214.1
    face 214.0
  thymus 214.2
  thyroid gland 214.2
Lipomatosis (dolorosa) 272.8
  epidural 214.8
  fetal (M8881/0)—*see* Lipoma, by site
  Launois-Bensaude's 272.8
Lipomyohemangioma (M8860/0)
  specified site—*see* Neoplasm, connective tissue,
    benign
  unspecified site 223.0
Lipomyoma (M8860/0)
  specified site—*see* Neoplasm, connective tissue,
    benign
  unspecified site 223.0
Lipomyxoma (M8852/0)—*see* Lipoma, by site

Lipomyxosarcoma (M8852/3)—*see* Neoplasm,
    connective tissue, malignant
Lipophagocytosis 289.89
Lipoproteinemia (alpha) 272.4
  broad-beta 272.2
  floating-beta 272.2
  hyper-pre-beta 272.1
Lipoproteinosis (Rössle-Urbach-Wiethe) 272.8
Liposarcoma (M8850/3)—*see also* Neoplasm,
    connective tissue, malignant
  differentiated type (M8851/3)—*see* Neoplasm,
    connective tissue, malignant
  embryonal (M8852/3)—*see* Neoplasm,
    connective tissue, malignant
  mixed type (M8855/3)—*see* Neoplasm,
    connective tissue, malignant
  myxoid (M8852/3)—*see* Neoplasm, connective
    tissue, malignant
  pleomorphic (M8854/3)—*see* Neoplasm,
    connective tissue, malignant
  round cell (M8853/3)—*see* Neoplasm,
    connective tissue, malignant
  well differentiated type (M8851/3)—*see*
    Neoplasm, connective tissue, malignant
Liposynovitis prepatellaris 272.8
Lipping
  cervix 622.0
  spine (*see also* Spondylosis) 721.90
  vertebra (*see also* Spondylosis) 721.90
Lip pits (mucus), congenital 750.25
Lipschütz disease or ulcer 616.50
Lipuria 791.1
  bilharziasis 120.0
Liquefaction, vitreous humor 379.21
Lisping 307.9
Lissauer's paralysis 094.1
Lissencephalia, lissencephaly 742.2
Listerellose 027.0
Listeriose 027.0
Listeriosis 027.0
  congenital 771.2
  fetal 771.2
  suspected fetal damage affecting management of
    pregnancy 655.4
Listlessness 780.79
Lithemia 790.6
Lithiasis —*see also* Calculus
  hepatic (duct)—*see* Choledocholithiasis
  urinary 592.9
Lithopedion 779.9
  affecting management of pregnancy 656.8
Lithosis (occupational) 502
  with tuberculosis—*see* Tuberculosis, pulmonary
Lithuria 791.9
Litigation V62.5
Little
  league elbow 718.82
  stroke syndrome 435.9
Little's disease —*see* Palsy, cerebral
Littre's
  gland—*see* condition
  hernia—*see* Hernia, Littre's
Littritis (*see also* Urethritis) 597.89
Livedo 782.61
  annularis 782.61
  racemose 782.61
  reticularis 782.61
Live flesh 781.0
Liver —*see also* condition
  donor V59.6

Livida, asphyxia
  newborn 768.6
Living
  alone V60.3
    with handicapped person V60.4
Lloyd's syndrome 258.1
Loa loa 125.2
Loasis 125.2
Lobe, lobar —*see* condition
Lobo's disease or blastomycosis 116.2
Lobomycosis 116.2
Lobotomy syndrome 310.0
Lobstein's disease (brittle bones and blue sclera)
  756.51
Lobster-claw hand 755.58
Lobulation (congenital)—*see also* Anomaly,
  specified type NEC, by site
  kidney, fetal 753.3
  liver, abnormal 751.69
  spleen 759.0
Lobule, lobular —*see* condition
Local, localized —*see* condition
Locked bowel or intestine (*see also* Obstruction,
  intestine) 560.9
Locked twins 660.5
  affecting fetus or newborn 763.1
Locked-in state 344.81
Locking
  joint (*see also* Derangement, joint) 718.90
  knee 717.9
Lockjaw (*see also* Tetanus) 037
Locomotor ataxia (progressive) 094.0
Löffler's
  endocarditis 421.0
  eosinophilia or syndrome 518.3
  pneumonia 518.3
  syndrome (eosinophilic pneumonitis) 518.3
Löfgren's syndrome (sarcoidosis) 135
Loiasis 125.2
  eyelid 125.2 *[373.6]*
Loneliness V62.89
Lone star fever 082.8
Long labor 662.1
  affecting fetus or newborn 763.89
  first stage 662.0
  second stage 662.2
Long-term (current) drug use V58.69
  antibiotics V58.62
  anticoagulants V58.61
  anti-inflammatories, non-steroidal (NSAID)
    V58.64
  antiplatelets/antithrombotics V58.63
  aspirin V58.66
  high-risk medications NEC V58.69
  insulin V58.67
  methadone V58.69
  opiate analgesic V58.69
  pain killers V58.69
    anti-inflammatory non-steroidal (NSAID)
      V58.64
    aspirin V58.66
  steroids V58.65
  tamoxifen V07.51
Longitudinal stripes or grooves, nails 703.8
  congenital 757.5
Loop
  intestine (*see also* Volvulus) 560.2
  intrascleral nerve 379.29
  vascular on papilla (optic) 743.57

Loose —*see also* condition
  body
    in tendon sheath 727.82
    joint 718.10
      ankle 718.17
      elbow 718.12
      foot 718.17
      hand 718.14
      hip 718.15
      knee 717.6
      multiple sites 718.19
      pelvic region 718.15
      prosthetic implant—*see* Complications,
        mechanical
      shoulder (region) 718.11
      specified site NEC 718.18
      wrist 718.13
    cartilage (joint) (*see also* Loose, body, joint)
      718.1
      knee 717.6
    facet (vertebral) 724.9
    prosthetic implant—*see* Complications,
      mechanical
    sesamoid, joint (*see also* Loose, body, joint)
      718.1
    tooth, teeth 525.8
Loosening epiphysis 732.9
Looser (-Debray) -Milkman syndrome
  (osteomalacia with pseudofractures) 268.2
Lop ear (deformity) 744.29
Lorain's disease or syndrome (pituitary
  dwarfism) 253.3
Lorain-Levi syndrome (pituitary dwarfism)
  253.3
Lordosis (acquired) (postural) 737.20
  congenital 754.2
  due to or associated with
    Charcot-Marie-Tooth disease 356.1 *[737.42]*
    mucopolysaccharidosis 277.5 *[737.42]*
    neurofibromatosis 237.71 *[737.42]*
    osteitis
      deformans 731.0 *[737.42]*
      fibrosa cystica 252.01 *[737.42]*
    osteoporosis (*see also* Osteoporosis) 733.00
      [737.42]
    poliomyelitis (*see also* Poliomyelitis) 138
      [737.42]
    tuberculosis (*see also* Tuberculosis) 015.0
      [737.42]
  late effect of rickets 268.1 *[737.42]*
  postlaminectomy 737.21
  postsurgical NEC 737.22
  rachitic 268.1 *[737.42]*
  specified NEC 737.29
  tuberculous (*see also* Tuberculosis) 015.0 *[737.42]*
Loss
  appetite 783.0
    hysterical 300.11
    nonorganic origin 307.59
    psychogenic 307.59
  blood—*see* Hemorrhage
  central vision 368.41
  consciousness 780.09
    transient 780.2
  control, sphincter, rectum 787.6
    nonorganic origin 307.7
  ear ossicle, partial 385.24
  elasticity, skin 782.8
  extremity or member, traumatic, current—*see*
    Amputation, traumatic

Loss —*continued*
  fluid (acute) 276.50
    with
      hypernatremia 276.0
      hyponatremia 276.1
    fetus or newborn 775.5
  hair 704.00
  hearing—*see also* Deafness
    central 389.14
    conductive (air) 389.00
      with sensorineural hearing loss 389.20
        bilateral 389.22
        unilateral 389.21
      bilateral 389.06
      combined types 389.08
      external ear 389.01
      inner ear 389.04
      middle ear 389.03
      multiple types 389.08
      tympanic membrane 389.02
      unilateral 389.05
    mixed conductive and sensorineural 389.20
      bilateral 389.22
      unilateral 389.21
    mixed type 389.20
      bilateral 389.22
      unilateral 389.21
    nerve
      bilateral 389.12
      unilateral 389.13
    neural
      bilateral 389.12
      unilateral 389.13
    noise-induced 388.12
    perceptive NEC (*see also* Loss, hearing,
        sensorineural) 389.10
    sensorineural 389.10
      with conductive hearing loss 389.20
        bilateral 389.22
        unilateral 389.21
      asymmetrical 389.16
      bilateral 389.18
      central 389.14
      neural
        bilateral 389.12
        unilateral 389.13
      sensory
        bilateral 389.11
        unilateral 389.17
      unilateral 389.15
    sensory
      bilateral 389.11
      unilateral 389.17
    specified type NEC 389.8
    sudden NEC 388.2
  height 781.91
  labyrinthine reactivity (unilateral) 386.55
    bilateral 386.56
  memory (*see also* Amnesia) 780.93
    mild, following organic brain damage 310.8
  mind (*see also* Psychosis) 298.9
  occlusal vertical dimension 524.37
  organ or part—*see* Absence, by site, acquired
  sensation 782.0
  sense of
    smell (*see also* Disturbance, sensation) 781.1
    taste (*see also* Disturbance, sensation) 781.1
    touch (*see also* Disturbance, sensation) 781.1
  sight (acquired) (complete) (congenital)—*see*
      Blindness
  spinal fluid
    headache 349.0

Loss —*continued*
  substance of
    bone (*see also* Osteoporosis) 733.00
    cartilage 733.99
    ear 380.32
    vitreous (humor) 379.26
  tooth, teeth
    acquired 525.10
      due to
        caries 525.13
        extraction 525.10
        periodontal disease 525.12
        specified NEC 525.19
        trauma 525.11
  vision, visual (*see also* Blindness) 369.9
    both eyes (*see also* Blindness, both eyes)
        369.3
    complete (*see also* Blindness, both eyes)
        369.00
    one eye 369.8
    sudden 368.11
    transient 368.12
  vitreous 379.26
  voice (*see also* Aphonia) 784.41
  weight (cause unknown) 783.21
Lou Gehrig's disease 335.20
Louis-Bar syndrome (ataxia-telangiectasia) 334.8
Louping ill 063.1
Lousiness —*see* Lice
Low
  back syndrome 724.2
  basal metabolic rate (BMR) 794.7
  birthweight 765.1
    extreme (less than 1000 grams) 765.0
    for gestational age 764.0
    status (*see also* Status, low birth weight)
        V21.30
  bladder compliance 596.52
  blood pressure (*see also* Hypotension) 458.9
    reading (incidental) (isolated) (nonspecific)
        796.3
  cardiac reserve—*see* Disease, heart
  compliance bladder 596.52
  frequency deafness—*see* Disorder, hearing
  function—*see also* Hypofunction
    kidney (*see also* Disease, renal) 593.9
    liver 573.9
  hemoglobin 285.9
  implantation, placenta—*see* Placenta, previa
  insertion, placenta—*see* Placenta, previa
  lying
    kidney 593.0
    organ or site, congenital—*see* Malposition,
        congenital
    placenta—*see* Placenta, previa
  output syndrome (cardiac) (*see also* Failure,
      heart) 428.9
  platelets (blood) (*see also* Thrombocytopenia)
      287.5
  reserve, kidney (*see also* Disease, renal) 593.9
  risk
    human papillomavirus (HPV) DNA test
        positive
      anal 796.79
      cervical 795.09
      vaginal 795.19
  salt syndrome 593.9
  tension glaucoma 365.12
  vision 369.9
    both eyes 369.20
    one eye 369.70

Lowe (-Terrey-MacLachlan) syndrome (oculocerebrorenal dystrophy) 270.8
Lower extremity —*see* condition
Lown (-Ganong)-Levine syndrome (short P-R interval, normal QRS complex, and paroxysmal supraventricular tachycardia) 426.81
LSD reaction (*see also* Abuse, drugs, nondependent) 305.3
L-shaped kidney 753.3
Lucas-Championnière disease (fibrinous bronchitis) 466.0
Lucey-Driscoll syndrome (jaundice due to delayed conjugation) 774.30
Ludwig's
  angina 528.3
  disease (submaxillary cellulitis) 528.3
Lues (venerea), luetic—*see* Syphilis
Luetscher's syndrome (dehydration) 276.51
Lumbago 724.2
  due to displacement, intervertebral disc 722.10
Lumbalgia 724.2
  due to displacement, intervertebral disc 722.10
Lumbar —*see* condition
Lumbarization, vertebra 756.15
Lumbermen's itch 133.8
Lump —*see also* Mass
  abdominal 789.3
  breast 611.72
  chest 786.6
  epigastric 789.3
  head 784.2
  kidney 753.3
  liver 789.1
  lung 786.6
  mediastinal 786.6
  neck 784.2
  nose or sinus 784.2
  pelvic 789.3
  skin 782.2
  substernal 786.6
  throat 784.2
  umbilicus 789.3
Lunacy (*see also* Psychosis) 298.9
Lunatomalacia 732.3
Lung —*see also* condition
  donor V59.8
  drug addict's 417.8
  mainliners' 417.8
  vanishing 492.0
Lupoid (miliary) of Boeck 135
Lupus 710.0
  anticoagulant 289.81
  Cazenave's (erythematosus) 695.4
  discoid (local) 695.4
  disseminated 710.0
  erythematodes (discoid) (local) 695.4
  erythematosus (discoid) (local) 695.4
    disseminated 710.0
    eyelid 373.34
    systemic 710.0
      with
        encephalitis 710.0 *[323.81]*
        lung involvement 710.0 *[517.8]*
      inhibitor (presence of) 286.5
  exedens 017.0
  eyelid (*see also* Tuberculosis) 017.0 *[373.4]*
  Hilliard's 017.0

Lupus—*continued*
  hydralazine
    correct substance properly administered 695.4
    overdose or wrong substance given or taken 972.6
  miliaris disseminatus faciei 017.0
  nephritis 710.0 *[583.81]*
    acute 710.0 *[580.81]*
    chronic 710.0 *[582.81]*
  nontuberculous, not disseminated 695.4
  pernio (Besnier) 135
  tuberculous (*see also* Tuberculosis) 017.0
    eyelid (*see also* Tuberculosis) 017.0 *[373.4]*
  vulgaris 017.0
Luschka's joint disease 721.90
Luteinoma (M8610/0) 220
Lutembacher's disease or syndrome (atrial septal defect with mitral stenosis) 745.5
Luteoma (M8610/0) 220
Lutz-Miescher disease (elastosis perforans serpiginosa) 701.1
Lutz-Splendore-de Almeida disease (Brazilian blastomycosis) 116.1
Luxatio
  bulbi due to birth injury 767.8
  coxae congenita (*see also* Dislocation, hip, congenital) 754.30
  erecta—*see* Dislocation, shoulder
  imperfecta—*see* Sprain, by site
  perinealis—*see* Dislocation, hip
Luxation —*see also* Dislocation, by site
  eyeball 360.81
    due to birth injury 767.8
    lateral 376.36
  genital organs (external) NEC—*see* Wound, open, genital organs
  globe (eye) 360.81
    lateral 376.36
  lacrimal gland (postinfectional) 375.16
  lens (old) (partial) 379.32
    congenital 743.37
      syphilitic 090.49 *[379.32]*
    Marfan's disease 090.49
    spontaneous 379.32
  penis—*see* Wound, open, penis
  scrotum—*see* Wound, open, scrotum
  testis—*see* Wound, open, testis
L-xyloketosuria 271.8
Lycanthropy (*see also* Psychosis) 298.9
Lyell's disease or syndrome (toxic epidermal necrolysis) 695.15
  due to drug
    correct substance properly administered 695.15
    overdose or wrong substance given or taken 977.9
      specified drug—*see* Table of drugs and chemicals
Lyme disease 088.81
Lymph
  gland or node—*see* condition
  scrotum (*see also* Infestation, filarial) 125.9
Lymphadenitis 289.3
  with
    abortion—*see* Abortion, by type, with sepsis
    ectopic pregnancy (*see also* categories 633.0-633.9) 639.0
    molar pregnancy (*see also* categories 630-632) 639.0
  acute 683
    mesenteric 289.2

Lymphadenitis—*continued*
  any site, except mesenteric 289.3
    acute 683
    chronic 289.1
    mesenteric (acute) (chronic) (nonspecific)
      (subacute) 289.2
    subacute 289.1
      mesenteric 289.2
  breast, puerperal, postpartum 675.2
  chancroidal (congenital) 099.0
  chronic 289.1
    mesenteric 289.2
  dermatopathic 695.89
  due to
    anthracosis (occupational) 500
    Brugia (Wuchereria) malayi 125.1
    diphtheria (toxin) 032.89
    lymphogranuloma venereum 099.1
    Wuchereria bancrofti 125.0
  following
    abortion 639.0
    ectopic or molar pregnancy 639.0
  generalized 289.3
  gonorrheal 098.89
  granulomatous 289.1
  infectional 683
  mesenteric (acute) (chronic) (nonspecific)
    (subacute) 289.2
    due to Bacillus typhi 002.0
    tuberculous (*see also* Tuberculosis) 014.8
  mycobacterial 031.8
  purulent 683
  pyogenic 683
  regional 078.3
  septic 683
  streptococcal 683
  subacute, unspecified site 289.1
  suppurative 683
  syphilitic (early) (secondary) 091.4
    late 095.8
  tuberculous—*see* Tuberculosis, lymph gland
  venereal 099.1
Lymphadenoid goiter 245.2
Lymphadenopathy (general) 785.6
  due to toxoplasmosis (acquired) 130.7
  congenital (active) 771.2
Lymphadenopathy-associated virus (disease)
  (illness) (infection)—*see* Human Immunodeficiency virus (disease) (illness) (infection)
Lymphadenosis 785.6
  acute 075
Lymphangiectasis 457.1
  conjunctiva 372.89
  postinfectional 457.1
  scrotum 457.1
Lymphangiectatic elephantiasis , nonfilarial
  457.1
Lymphangioendothelioma (M9170/0) 228.1
  malignant (M9170/3)—*see* Neoplasm,
    connective tissue, malignant
Lymphangioma (M9170/0) 228.1
  capillary (M9171/0) 228.1
  cavernous (M9172/0) 228.1
  cystic (M9173/0) 228.1
  malignant (M9170/3)—*see* Neoplasm,
    connective tissue, malignant
Lymphangiomyoma (M9174/0) 228.1
Lymphangiomyomatosis (M9174/1)—*see*
  Neoplasm, connective tissue, uncertain
  behavior
Lymphangiosarcoma (M9170/3)—*see*
  Neoplasm, connective tissue, malignant

Lymphangitis 457.2
  with
    abortion—*see* Abortion, by type, with sepsis
    abscess—*see* Abscess, by site
    cellulitis—*see* Abscess, by site
    ectopic pregnancy (*see also* categories
      633.0-633.9) 639.0
    molar pregnancy (*see also* categories 630-632)
      639.0
  acute (with abscess or cellulitis) 682.9
    specified site—*see* Abscess, by site
  breast, puerperal, postpartum 675.2
  chancroidal 099.0
  chronic (any site) 457.2
  due to
    Brugia (Wuchereria) malayi 125.1
    Wuchereria bancrofti 125.0
  following
    abortion 639.0
    ectopic or molar pregnancy 639.0
  gangrenous 457.2
  penis
    acute 607.2
    gonococcal (acute) 098.0
      chronic or duration of 2 months or more
        098.2
  puerperal, postpartum, childbirth 670.8
  strumous, tuberculous (*see also* Tuberculosis)
    017.2
  subacute (any site) 457.2
  tuberculous—*see* Tuberculosis, lymph gland
Lymphatic (vessel)—*see* condition
Lymphatism 254.8
  scrofulous (*see also* Tuberculosis) 017.2
Lymphectasia 457.1
Lymphedema (*see also* Elephantiasis) 457.1
  acquired (chronic) 457.1
  chronic hereditary 757.0
  congenital 757.0
  idiopathic hereditary 757.0
  praecox 457.1
  secondary 457.1
  surgical NEC 997.99
    postmastectomy (syndrome) 457.0
Lymph-hemangioma (M9120/0)—*see*
  Hemangioma, by site
Lymphoblastic —*see* condition
Lymphoblastoma (diffuse) (M9630/3) 200.1
  giant follicular (M9690/3) 202.0
  macrofollicular (M9690/3) 202.0
Lymphoblastosis, acute benign 075
Lymphocele 457.8
Lymphocythemia 288.51
Lymphocytic —*see also* condition
  chorioencephalitis (acute) (serous) 049.0
  choriomeningitis (acute) (serous) 049.0
Lymphocytoma (diffuse) (malignant) (M9620/3)
  200.1
Lymphocytomatosis (M9620/3) 200.1
Lymphocytopenia 288.51
Lymphocytosis (symptomatic) 288.61
  infectious (acute) 078.89
Lymphoepithelioma (M8082/3)—*see* Neoplasm,
  by site, malignant
Lymphogranuloma (malignant) (M9650/3) 201.9
  inguinale 099.1
  venereal (any site) 099.1
    with stricture of rectum 099.1
  venereum 099.1

Lymphogranulomatosis (malignant) (M9650/3)
201.9
benign (Boeck's sarcoid) (Schaumann's) 135
Hodgkin's (M9650/3) 201.9
Lymphohistiocytosis, familial hemophagocytic
288.4
Lymphoid —*see* condition
Lympholeukoblastoma (M9850/3) 207.8
Lympholeukosarcoma (M9850/3) 207.8
Lymphoma (malignant) (M9590/3) 202.8

Note—Use the following fifth-digit
subclassification with categories 200-202:

0 *unspecifidd site*
1 *lymph nodes of head, face and neck*
2 *intrathoracic lymph nodes*
3 *intra-abdominal lymph nodes*
4 *lymph nodes of axilla and upper limb*
5 *lymph nodes of inguinal region and*
   lower limb
6 *intrapelvic lymph nodes*
7 *spleen*
8 *lymph nodes of multiple sites*

---

wenign (M9580/0)—*see* Neoplasm, by site, benign
Burkitt's type (lymphoblastic) (undifferentiated)
(M9750/3) 200.2
Castleman's (mediastinal lymph node hyperplasia)
785.6
centroblastic-centrocytic
diffuse (M9614/3) 202.8
follicular (M9692/3) 202.0
centroblastic type (diffuse) (M9632/3) 202.8
follicular (M9697/3) 202.0
centrocytic (M9622/3) 202.8
compound (M9613/3) 200.8
convoluted cell type (lymphoblastic) (M9602/3)
202.8
diffuse NEC (M9590/3) 202.8
large B cell 202.8
follicular (giant) (M9690/3) 202.0
center cell (diffuse) (M9615/3) 202.8
cleaved (diffuse) (M9623/3) 202.8
follicular (M9695/3) 202.0
non-cleaved (diffuse) (M9633/3) 202.8
follicular (M9698/3) 202.0
centroblastic-centrocytic (M9692/3) 202.0
centroblastic type (M9697/3) 202.0
large cell 202.0
lymphocytic
intermediate differentiation (M9694/3) 202.0
poorly differentiated (M9696/3) 202.0
mixed (cell type) (lymphocytic-histiocytic)
(small cell and large cell) (M9691/3) 202.0
germinocytic (M9622/3) 202.8
giant, follicular or follicle (M9690/3) 202.0
histiocytic (diffuse) (M9640/3) 200.0
nodular (M9642/3) 200.0
pleomorphic cell type (M9641/3) 200.0
Hodgkin's (M9650/3) (*see also* Disease,
Hodgkin's) 201.9
immunoblastic (type) (M9612/3) 200.8
large cell (M9640/3) 200.7
anaplastic 200.6
nodular (M9642/3) 202.0
pleomorphic cell type (M9641/3) 200.0
lymphoblastic (diffuse) (M9630/3) 200.1
Burkitt's type (M9750/3) 200.2
convoluted cell type (M9602/3) 202.8

Lymphoma—*continued*
lymphocytic (cell type) (diffuse) (M9620/3) 200.1
with plasmacytoid differentiation, diffuse
(M9611/3) 200.8
intermediate differentiation (diffuse)
(M9621/3) 200.1
follicular (M9694/3) 202.0
nodular (M9694/3) 202.0
nodular (M9690/3) 202.0
poorly differentiated (diffuse) (M9630/3) 200.1
follicular (M9696/3) 202.0
nodular (M9696/3) 202.0
well differentiated (diffuse) (M9620/3) 200.1
follicular (M9693/3) 202.0
nodular (M9693/3) 202.0
lymphocytic-histiocytic, mixed (diffuse)
(M9613/3) 200.8
follicular (M9691/3) 202.0
nodular (M9691/3) 202.0
lymphoplasmacytoid type (M9611/3) 200.8
lymphosarcoma type (M9610/3) 200.1
macrofollicular (M9690/3) 202.0
mantle cell 200.4
marginal zone 200.3
extranodal B-cell 200.3
nodal B-cell 200.3
splenic B-cell 200.3
mixed cell type (diffuse) (M9613/3) 200.8
follicular (M9691/3) 202.0
nodular (M9691/3) 202.0
nodular (M9690/3) 202.0
histiocytic (M9642/3) 200.0
lymphocytic (M9690.3) 202.0
intermediate differentiation (M9694/3) 202.0
poorly differentiated (M9696/3) 202.0
mixed (cell type) (lymphocytic-histiocytic)
(small cell and large cell) (M9691/3) 202.0
non-Hodgkin's type NEC (M9591/3) 202.8
peripheral T-cell 202.7
primary central nervous system 200.5
reticulum cell (type) (M9640/3) 200.0
small cell and large cell, mixed (diffuse)
(M9613/3) 200.8
follicular (M9691/3) 202.0
nodular (9691/3) 202.0
stem cell (type) (M9601/3) 202.8
T-cell 202.1
peripheral 202.7
undifferentiated (cell type) (non-Burkitt's)
(M9600/3) 202.8
Burkitt's type (M9750/3) 200.2
Lymphomatosis (M9590/3)—*see also*
Lymphoma
granulomatous 099.1
Lymphopathia
venereum 099.1
veneris 099.1
Lymphopenia 288.51
familial 279.2
Lymphoreticulosis, benign (of inoculation)
078.3
Lymphorrhea 457.8
Lymphosarcoma (M9610/3) 200.1
diffuse (M9610/3) 200.1
with plasmacytoid differentiation (M9611/3)
200.8
lymphoplasmacytic (M9611/3) 200.8
follicular (giant) (M9690/3) 202.0
lymphoblastic (M9696/3) 202.0
lymphocytic, intermediate differentiation
(M9694/3) 202.0
mixed cell type (M9691/3) 202.0

Lymphosarcoma—*continued*
  giant follicular (M9690/3) 202.0
  Hodgkin's (M9650/3) 201.9
  immunoblastic (M9612/3) 200.8
  lymphoblastic (diffuse) (M9630/3) 200.1
    follicular (M9696/3) 202.0
    nodular (M9696/3) 202.0
  lymphocytic (diffuse) (M9620/3) 200.1
    intermediate differentiation (diffuse)
        (M9621/3) 200.1
      follicular (M9694/3) 202.0
      nodular (M9694/3) 202.0
  mixed cell type (diffuse) (M9613/3) 200.8
    follicular (M9691/3) 202.0
    nodular (M9691/3) 202.0
  nodular (M9690/3) 202.0
    lymphoblastic (M9696/3) 202.0
    lymphocytic, intermediate differentiation
        (M9694/3) 202.0
    mixed cell type (M9691/3) 202.0
  prolymphocytic (M9631/3) 200.1
  reticulum cell (M9640/3) 200.0
Lymphostasis 457.8
Lypemania (*see also* Melancholia) 296.2
Lyssa 071

M

Macacus ear 744.29
Maceration
  fetus (cause not stated) 779.9
  wet feet, tropical (syndrome) 991.4
Machado-Joseph disease 334.8
Machupo virus hemorrhagic fever 078.7
Macleod's syndrome (abnormal transradiancy, one lung) 492.8
Macrocephalia, macrocephaly 756.0
Macrocheilia (congenital) 744.81
Macrochilia (congenital) 744.81
Macrocolon (congenital) 751.3
Macrocornea 743.41
  associated with buphthalmos 743.22
Macrocytic —*see* condition
Macrocytosis 289.89
Macrodactylia, macrodactylism (fingers) (thumbs) 755.57
  toes 755.65
Macrodontia 520.2
Macroencephaly 742.4
Macrogenia 524.05
Macrogenitosomia (female) (male) (praecox) 255.2
Macrogingivae 523.8
Macroglobulinemia (essential) (idiopathic) (monoclonal) (primary) (syndrome) (Waldenström's) 273.3
Macroglossia (congenital) 750.15
  acquired 529.8
Macrognathia, macrognathism (congenital) 524.00
  mandibular 524.02
    alveolar 524.72
  maxillary 524.01
    alveolar 524.71
Macrogyria (congenital) 742.4
Macrohydrocephalus (*see also* Hydrocephalus) 331.4
Macromastia (*see also* Hypertrophy, breast) 611.1
Macrophage activation syndrome 288.4
Macropsia 368.14
Macrosigmoid 564.7
  congenital 751.3
Macrospondylitis, acromegalic 253.0
Macrostomia (congenital) 744.83
Macrotia (external ear) (congenital) 744.22
Macula
  cornea, corneal
    congenital 743.43
      interfering with vision 743.42
    interfering with central vision 371.03
    not interfering with central vision 371.02
  degeneration (*see also* Degeneration, macula) 362.50
    hereditary (*see also* Dystrophy, retina) 362.70
  edema, cystoid 362.53
Maculae ceruleae 132.1
Macules and papules 709.8
Maculopathy, toxic 362.55
Madarosis 374.55
Madelung's
  deformity (radius) 755.54
  disease (lipomatosis) 272.8
  lipomatosis 272.8

Madness (*see also* Psychosis) 298.9
  myxedema (acute) 293.0
    subacute 293.1
Madura
  disease (actinomycotic) 039.9
    mycotic 117.4
  foot (actinomycotic) 039.4
    mycotic 117.4
Maduromycosis (actinomycotic) 039.9
  mycotic 117.4
Maffucci's syndrome (dyschondroplasia with hemangiomas) 756.4
Magenblase syndrome 306.4
Main en griffe (acquired) 736.06
  congenital 755.59
Maintenance
  chemotherapy regimen or treatment V58.11
  dialysis regimen or treatment
    extracorporeal (renal) V56.0
    peritoneal V56.8
    renal V56.0
  drug therapy or regimen
    chemotherapy, antineoplastic V58.11
    immunotherapy, antineoplastic V58.12
  external fixation NEC V54.89
  radiotherapy V58.0
  traction NEC V54.89
Majocchi's
  disease (purpura annularis telangiectodes) 709.1
  granuloma 110.6
Major —*see* condition
Mal
  cerebral (idiopathic) (*see also* Epilepsy) 345.9
  comital (*see also* Epilepsy) 345.9
  de los pintos (*see also* Pinta) 103.9
  de Meleda 757.39
  de mer 994.6
  lie—*see* Presentation, fetal
  perforant (*see also* Ulcer, lower extremity) 707.15
Malabar itch 110.9
  beard 110.0
  foot 110.4
  scalp 110.0
Malabsorption 579.9
  calcium 579.8
  carbohydrate 579.8
  disaccharide 271.3
  drug-induced 579.8
  due to bacterial overgrowth 579.8
  fat 579.8
  folate, congenital 281.2
  galactose 271.1
  glucose-galactose (congenital) 271.3
  intestinal 579.9
  isomaltose 271.3
  lactose (hereditary) 271.3
  methionine 270.4
  monosaccharide 271.8
  postgastrectomy 579.3
  postsurgical 579.3
  protein 579.8
  sucrose (-isomaltose) (congenital) 271.3
  syndrome 579.9
    postgastrectomy 579.3
    postsurgical 579.3

Malacia, bone 268.2
  juvenile (*see also* Rickets) 268.0
  Kienböck's (juvenile) (lunate) (wrist) 732.3
    adult 732.8
Malacoplakia
  bladder 596.8
  colon 569.89
  pelvis (kidney) 593.89
  ureter 593.89
  urethra 599.84
Malacosteon 268.2
  juvenile (*see also* Rickets) 268.0
Maladaptation —*see* Maladjustment
Maladie de Roger 745.4
Maladjustment
  conjugal V61.10
    involving
      divorce V61.03
      estrangement V61.09
  educational V62.3
  family V61.9
    specified circumstance NEC V61.8
  marital V61.10
    involving
      divorce V61.03
      estrangement V61.09
  occupational V62.29
    current military deployment status V62.21
  simple, adult (*see also* Reaction, adjustment)
    309.9
  situational acute (*see also* Reaction, adjustment)
    309.9
  social V62.4
Malaise 780.79
Malakoplakia —*see* Malacoplakia
Malaria, malarial (fever) 084.6
  algid 084.9
  any type, with
    algid malaria 084.9
    blackwater fever 084.8
    fever
      blackwater 084.8
      hemoglobinuric (bilious) 084.8
    hemoglobinuria, malarial 084.8
    hepatitis 084.9 [573.2]
    nephrosis 084.9 [581.81]
    pernicious complication NEC 084.9
      cardiac 084.9
      cerebral 084.9
  cardiac 084.9
  carrier (suspected) of V02.9
  cerebral 084.9
  complicating pregnancy, childbirth, or
    puerperium 647.4
  congenital 771.2
  congestion, congestive 084.6
    brain 084.9
  continued 084.0
  estivo-autumnal 084.0
  falciparum (malignant tertian) 084.0
  hematinuria 084.8
  hematuria 084.8
  hemoglobinuria 084.8
  hemorrhagic 084.6
  induced (therapeutically) 084.7
    accidental—*see* Malaria, by type
  liver 084.9 [573.2]
  malariae (quartan) 084.2
  malignant (tertian) 084.0
  mixed infections 084.5
  monkey 084.4

Malaria, malarial—*continued*
  ovale 084.3
  pernicious, acute 084.0
  Plasmodium, P.
    falciparum 084.0
    malariae 084.2
    ovale 084.3
    vivax 084.1
  quartan 084.2
  quotidian 084.0
  recurrent 084.6
    induced (therapeutically) 084.7
      accidental—*see* Malaria, by type
  remittent 084.6
  specified types NEC 084.4
  spleen 084.6
  subtertian 084.0
  tertian (benign) 084.1
    malignant 084.0
  tropical 084.0
  typhoid 084.6
  vivax (benign tertian) 084.1
Malassez's disease (testicular cyst) 608.89
Malassimilation 579.9
Maldescent, testis 752.51
Maldevelopment —*see also* Anomaly, by site
  brain 742.9
  colon 751.5
  hip (joint) 755.63
    congenital dislocation (*see also* Dislocation,
      hip, congenital) 754.30
  mastoid process 756.0
  middle ear, except ossicles 744.03
    ossicles 744.04
  newborn (not malformation) 764.9
  ossicles, ear 744.04
  spine 756.10
  toe 755.66
Male type pelvis 755.69
  with disproportion (fetopelvic) 653.2
    affecting fetus or newborn 763.1
    causing obstructed labor 660.1
      affecting fetus or newborn 763.1
Malformation (congenital)—*see also* Anomaly
  bone 756.9
  bursa 756.9
  Chiari
    type I 348.4
    type II (*see also* Spina bifida) 741.0
    type III 742.0
    type IV 742.2
  circulatory system NEC 747.9
    specified type NEC 747.89
  cochlea 744.05
  digestive system NEC 751.9
    lower 751.5
    specified type NEC 751.8
    upper 750.9
  eye 743.9
  gum 750.9
  heart NEC 746.9
    specified type NEC 746.89
    valve 746.9
  internal ear 744.05
  joint NEC 755.9
    specified type NEC 755.8
  Mondini's (congenital) (malformation, cochlea)
    744.05
  muscle 756.9
  nervous system (central) 742.9

Malformation—*continued*
pelvic organs or tissues
in pregnancy or childbirth 654.9
affecting fetus or newborn 763.89
causing obstructed labor 660.2
affecting fetus or newborn 763.1
placenta (*see also* Placenta, abnormal) 656.7
respiratory organs 748.9
specified type NEC 748.8
Rieger's 743.44
sense organs NEC 742.9
specified type NEC 742.8
skin 757.9
specified type NEC 757.8
spinal cord 742.9
teeth, tooth NEC 520.9
tendon 756.9
throat 750.9
umbilical cord (complicating delivery) 663.9
affecting fetus or newborn 762.6
umbilicus 759.9
urinary system NEC 753.9
specified type NEC 753.8
venous —*see* Anomaly, vein
Malfunction —*see also* Dysfunction
arterial graft 996.1
cardiac pacemaker 996.01
catheter device—*see* Complications,
mechanical, catheter
colostomy 569.62
valve 569.62
cystostomy 997.5
device, implant, or graft NEC—*see*
Complications, mechanical
enteric stoma 569.62
enterostomy 569.62
esophagostomy 530.87
gastroenteric 536.8
gastrostomy 536.42
ileostomy
valve 569.62
nephrostomy 997.5
pacemaker—*see* Complications, mechanical,
pacemaker
prosthetic device, internal—*see* Complications,
mechanical
tracheostomy 519.02
valve
colostomy 569.62
ileostomy 569.62
vascular graft or shunt 996.1
Malgaigne's fracture (closed) 808.43
open 808.53
Malherbe's
calcifying epithelioma (M8110/0)—*see*
Neoplasm, skin, benign
tumor (M8110/0)—*see* Neoplasm, skin, benign
Malibu disease 919.8
infected 919.9
Malignancy (M8000/3)—*see* Neoplasm, by site,
malignant
Malignant —*see* condition
Malingerer, malingering V65.2
Mallet, finger (acquired) 736.1
congenital 755.59
late effect of rickets 268.1
Malleus 024
Mallory's bodies 034.1
Mallory-Weiss syndrome 530.7

Malnutrition (calorie) 263.9
complicating pregnancy 648.9
degree
first 263.1
second 263.0
third 262
mild 263.1
moderate 263.0
severe 261
protein-calorie 262
fetus 764.2
"light-for-dates" 764.1
following gastrointestinal surgery 579.3
intrauterine or fetal 764.2
fetus or infant "light-for-dates" 764.1
lack of care, or neglect (child) (infant) 995.52
adult 995.84
malignant 260
mild 263.1
moderate 263.0
protein 260
protein-calorie 263.9
severe 262
specified type NEC 263.8
severe 261
protein-calorie NEC 262
Malocclusion (teeth) 524.4
angle's class I 524.21
angle's class II 524.22
angle's class III 524.23
due to
abnormal swallowing 524.59
accessory teeth (causing crowding) 524.31
dentofacial abnormality NEC 524.89
impacted teeth (causing crowding) 520.6
missing teeth 524.30
mouth breathing 524.59
sleep posture 524.59
supernumerary teeth (causing crowding)
524.31
thumb sucking 524.59
tongue, lip, or finger habits 524.59
temporomandibular (joint) 524.69
Malposition
cardiac apex (congenital) 746.87
cervix—*see* Malposition, uterus
congenital
adrenal (gland) 759.1
alimentary tract 751.8
lower 751.5
upper 750.8
aorta 747.21
appendix 751.5
arterial trunk 747.29
artery (peripheral) NEC (*see also* Malposition,
congenital, peripheral vascular system)
747.60
coronary 746.85
pulmonary 747.3
auditory canal 744.29
causing impairment of hearing 744.02
auricle (ear) 744.29
causing impairment of hearing 744.02
cervical 744.43
biliary duct or passage 751.69
bladder (mucosa) 753.8
exteriorized or extroverted 753.5
brachial plexus 742.8
brain tissue 742.4
breast 757.6
bronchus 748.3

Malposition—*continued*
  congenital—*continued*
    cardiac apex 746.87
    cecum 751.5
    clavicle 755.51
    colon 751.5
    digestive organ or tract NEC 751.8
      lower 751.5
      upper 750.8
    ear (auricle) (external) 744.29
      ossicles 744.04
    endocrine (gland) NEC 759.2
    epiglottis 748.3
    Eustachian tube 744.24
    eye 743.8
    facial features 744.89
    fallopian tube 752.19
    finger(s) 755.59
      supernumerary 755.01
    foot 755.67
    gallbladder 751.69
    gastrointestinal tract 751.8
    genitalia, genital organ(s) or tract
      female 752.89
        external 752.49
        internal NEC 752.89
      male 752.89
        penis 752.69
        scrotal transposition 752.81
    glottis 748.3
    hand 755.59
    heart 746.87
      dextrocardia 746.87
        with complete transposition of viscera
          759.3
    hepatic duct 751.69
    hip (joint) (*see also* Dislocation, hip,
      congenital) 754.30
    intestine (large) (small) 751.5
      with anomalous adhesions, fixation, or
        malrotation 751.4
    joint NEC 755.8
    kidney 753.3
    larynx 748.3
    limb 755.8
      lower 755.69
      upper 755.59
    liver 751.69
    lung (lobe) 748.69
    nail(s) 757.5
    nerve 742.8
    nervous system NEC 742.8
    nose, nasal (septum) 748.1
    organ or site NEC—*see* Anomaly, specified
      type NEC, by site
    ovary 752.0
    pancreas 751.7
    parathyroid (gland) 759.2
    patella 755.64
    peripheral vascular system 747.60
      gastrointestinal 747.61
      lower limb 747.64
      renal 747.62
      specified NEC 747.69
      spinal 747.82
      upper limb 747.63
    pituitary (gland) 759.2
    respiratory organ or system NEC 748.9
    rib (cage) 756.3
      supernumerary in cervical region 756.2
    scapula 755.59

Malposition—*continued*
  congenital—*continued*
    shoulder 755.59
    spinal cord 742.59
    spine 756.19
    spleen 759.0
    sternum 756.3
    stomach 750.7
    symphysis pubis 755.69
    testis (undescended) 752.51
    thymus (gland) 759.2
    thyroid (gland) (tissue) 759.2
      cartilage 748.3
    toe(s) 755.66
      supernumerary 755.02
    tongue 750.19
    trachea 748.3
    uterus 752.3
    vein(s) (peripheral) NEC (*see also*
      Malposition, congenital, peripheral
      vascular system) 747.60
      great 747.49
      portal 747.49
      pulmonary 747.49
    vena cava (inferior) (superior) 747.49
  device, implant, or graft—*see* Complications,
    mechanical
  fetus NEC (*see also* Presentation, fetal) 652.9
    with successful version 652.1
    affecting fetus or newborn 763.1
    before labor, affecting fetus or newborn 761.7
    causing obstructed labor 660.0
    in multiple gestation (one fetus or more) 652.6
      with locking 660.5
      causing obstructed labor 660.0
  gallbladder (*see also* Disease, gallbladder) 575.8
  gastrointestinal tract 569.89
    congenital 751.8
  heart (*see also* Malposition, congenital, heart) 746.87
  intestine 569.89
    congenital 751.5
  pelvic organs or tissues
    in pregnancy or childbirth 654.4
      affecting fetus or newborn 763.89
      causing obstructed labor 660.2
        affecting fetus or newborn 763.1
  placenta—*see* Placenta, previa
  stomach 537.89
    congenital 750.7
  tooth, teeth 524.30
    with impaction 520.6
  uterus (acquired) (acute) (adherent) (any degree)
    (asymptomatic) (postinfectional) (postpartal,
    old) 621.6
    anteflexion or anteversion (*see also*
      Anteversion, uterus) 621.6
    congenital 752.3
    flexion 621.6
      lateral (*see also* Lateroversion, uterus) 621.6
    in pregnancy or childbirth 654.4
      affecting fetus or newborn 763.89
      causing obstructed labor 660.2
        affecting fetus or newborn 763.1
    inversion 621.6
    lateral (flexion) (version) (*see also*
      Lateroversion, uterus) 621.6
    lateroflexion (*see also* Lateroversion, uterus)
      621.6
    lateroversion (*see also* Lateroversion, uterus)
      621.6
    retroflexion or retroversion (*see also*
      Retroversion, uterus) 621.6

Malposture 729.90
Malpresentation, fetus (*see also* Presentation, fetal) 652.9
Malrotation
  cecum 751.4
  colon 751.4
  intestine 751.4
  kidney 753.3
MALT (mucosa associated lymphoid tissue) 200.3
Malt workers' lung 495.4
Malta fever (*see also* Brucellosis) 023.9
Maltosuria 271.3
Maltreatment (of)
  adult 995.80
    emotional 995.82
    multiple forms 995.85
    neglect (nutritional) 995.84
    physical 995.81
    psychological 995.82
    sexual 995.83
  child 995.50
    emotional 995.51
    multiple forms 995.59
    neglect (nutritional) 995.52
    psychological 995.51
    physical 995.54
      shaken infant syndrome 995.55
    sexual 995.53
  spouse (*see also* Maltreatment, adult) 995.80
Malum coxae senilis 715.25
Malunion, fracture 733.81
Mammillitis (*see also* Mastitis) 611.0
  puerperal, postpartum 675.2
Mammitis (*see also* Mastitis) 611.0
  puerperal, postpartum 675.2
Mammographic
  calcification 793.89
  calculus 793.89
  microcalcification 793.81
Mammoplasia 611.1
Management
  contraceptive V25.9
    specified type NEC V25.8
  procreative V26.9
    specified type NEC V26.89
Mangled NEC (*see also* nature and site of injury) 959.9
Mania (monopolar) (*see also* Psychosis, affective) 296.0
  alcoholic (acute) (chronic) 291.9
  Bell's—*see* Mania, chronic
  chronic 296.0
    recurrent episode 296.1
    single episode 296.0
  compulsive 300.3
  delirious (acute) 296.0
    recurrent episode 296.1
    single episode 296.0
  epileptic (*see also* Epilepsy) 345.4
  hysterical 300.10
  inhibited 296.89
  puerperal (after delivery) 296.0
    recurrent episode 296.1
    single episode 296.0
  recurrent episode 296.1
  senile 290.8
  single episode 296.0
  stupor 296.89
  stuporous 296.89
  unproductive 296.89

Manic-depressive insanity, psychosis reaction, or syndrome (*see also* Psychosis, affective) 296.80
  circular (alternating) 296.7
    currently
      depressed 296.5
      episode unspecified 296.7
      hypomanic, previously depressed 296.4
      manic 296.4
    mixed 296.6
  depressed (type), depressive 296.2
    atypical 296.82
    recurrent episode 296.3
    single episode 296.2
  hypomanic 296.0
    recurrent episode 296.1
    single episode 296.0
  manic 296.0
    atypical 296.81
    recurrent episode 296.1
    single episode 296.0
  mixed NEC 296.89
  perplexed 296.89
  stuporous 296.89
Manifestations, rheumatoid
  lungs 714.81
  pannus—*see* Arthritis, rheumatoid
  subcutaneous nodules—*see* Arthritis, rheumatoid
Mankowsky's syndrome (familial dysplastic osteopathy) 731.2
Mannoheptulosuria 271.8
Mannosidosis 271.8
Manson's
  disease (schistosomiasis) 120.1
  pyosis (pemphigus contagiosus) 684
  schistosomiasis 120.1
Mansonellosis 125.5
Manual —*see* condition
Maple bark disease 495.6
Maple bark-strippers' lung 495.6
Maple syrup (urine) disease or syndrome 270.3
Marable's syndrome (celiac artery compression) 447.4
Marasmus 261
  brain 331.9
  due to malnutrition 261
  intestinal 569.89
  nutritional 261
  senile 797
  tuberculous NEC (*see also* Tuberculosis) 011.9
Marble
  bones 756.52
  skin 782.61
Marburg disease (virus) 078.89
March
  foot 733.94
  hemoglobinuria 283.2
Marchand multiple nodular hyperplasia (liver) 571.5
Marchesani (-Weill) syndrome (brachymorphism and ectopia lentis) 759.89
Marchiafava (-Bignami) disease or syndrome 341.8
Marchiafava-Micheli syndrome (paroxysmal nocturnal hemoglobinuria) 283.2
Marcus Gunn's syndrome (jaw-winking syndrome) 742.8
Marfan's
  congenital syphilis 090.49
  disease 090.49
  syndrome (arachnodactyly) 759.82
    meaning congenital syphilis 090.49
      with luxation of lens 090.49 *[379.32]*

Marginal
  implantation, placenta—*see* Placenta, previa
  placenta—*see* Placenta, previa
  sinus (hemorrhage) (rupture) 641.2
  affecting fetus or newborn 762.1
Marie's
  cerebellar ataxia 334.2
  syndrome (acromegaly) 253.0
Marie-Bamberger disease or syndrome
  (hypertrophic) (pulmonary) (secondary) 731.2
  idiopathic (acropachyderma) 757.39
  primary (acropachyderma) 757.39
Marie-Charcot-Tooth neuropathic atrophy,
  muscle 356.1
Marie-Strümpell arthritis or disease
  (ankylosing spondylitis) 720.0
Marihuana, marijuana
  abuse (*see also* Abuse, drugs, nondependent) 305.2
  dependence (*see also* Dependence) 304.3
Marion's disease (bladder neck obstruction) 596.0
Marital conflict V61.10
Mark
  port wine 757.32
  raspberry 757.32
  strawberry 757.32
  stretch 701.3
  tattoo 709.09
Maroteaux-Lamy syndrome
  (mucopolysaccharidosis VI) 277.5
Marriage license examination V70.3
Marrow (bone)
  arrest 284.9
  megakaryocytic 287.30
  poor function 289.9
Marseilles fever 082.1
Marsh's disease (exophthalmic goiter) 242.0
Marshall's (hidrotic) ectodermal dysplasia 757.31
Marsh fever (*see also* Malaria) 084.6
Martin's disease 715.27
Martin-Albright syndrome
  (pseudohypoparathyroidism) 275.49
Martorell-Fabre syndrome (pulseless disease)
  446.7
Masculinization, female with adrenal
  hyperplasia 255.2
Masculinovoblastoma (M8670/0) 220
Masochism 302.83
Masons' lung 502
Mass
  abdominal 789.3
  anus 787.99
  bone 733.90
  breast 611.72
  cheek 784.2
  chest 786.6
  cystic—*see* Cyst
  ear 388.8
  epigastric 789.3
  eye 379.92
  female genital organ 625.8
  gum 784.2
  head 784.2
  intracranial 784.2
  joint 719.60
    ankle 719.67
    elbow 719.62
    foot 719.67
    hand 719.64
    hip 719.65
    knee 719.66
    multiple sites 719.69

Mass—*continued*
  joint—*continued*
    pelvic region 719.65
    shoulder (region) 719.61
    specified site NEC 719.68
    wrist 719.63
  kidney (*see also* Disease, kidney) 593.9
  lung 786.6
  lymph node 785.6
  malignant (M8000/3)—*see* Neoplasm, by site,
    malignant
  mediastinal 786.6
  mouth 784.2
  muscle (limb) 729.89
  neck 784.2
  nose or sinus 784.2
  palate 784.2
  pelvis, pelvic 789.3
  penis 607.89
  perineum 625.8
  rectum 787.99
  scrotum 608.89
  skin 782.2
  specified organ NEC—*see* Disease of specified
    organ or site
  splenic 789.2
  substernal 786.6
    thyroid (*see also* Goiter) 240.9
  superficial (localized) 782.2
  testes 608.89
  throat 784.2
  tongue 784.2
  umbilicus 789.3
  uterus 625.8
  vagina 625.8
  vulva 625.8
Massive —*see* condition
Mastalgia 611.71
  psychogenic 307.89
Mast cell
  disease 757.33
    systemic (M9741/3) 202.6
  leukemia (M9900/3) 207.8
  sarcoma (M9742/3) 202.6
  tumor (M9740/1) 238.5
    malignant (M9740/3) 202.6
Masters-Allen syndrome 620.6
Mastitis (acute) (adolescent) (diffuse)
    (interstitial) (lobular) (nonpuerperal)
    (nonsuppurative) (parenchymatous)
    (phlegmonous) (simple) (subacute)
    (suppurative) 611.0
  chronic (cystic) (fibrocystic) 610.1
  cystic 610.1
    Schimmelbusch's type 610.1
  fibrocystic 610.1
  infective 611.0
  lactational 675.2
  lymphangitis 611.0
  neonatal (noninfective) 778.7
    infective 771.5
  periductal 610.4
  plasma cell 610.4
  puerperal, postpartum, (interstitial)
    (nonpurulent) (parenchymatous) 675.2
    purulent 675.1
    stagnation 676.2
  puerperalis 675.2
  retromammary 611.0
    puerperal, postpartum 675.1
  submammary 611.0
    puerperal, postpartum 675.1

Mastocytoma (M9740/1) 238.5
  malignant (M9740/3) 202.6
Mastocytosis 757.33
  malignant (M9741/3) 202.6
  systemic (M9741/3) 202.6
Mastodynia 611.71
  psychogenic 307.89
Mastoid —*see* condition
Mastoidalgia (*see also* Otalgia) 388.70
Mastoiditis (coalescent) (hemorrhagic)
  (pneumococcal) (streptococcal) (suppurative)
  383.9
  acute or subacute 383.00
    with
      Gradenigo's syndrome 383.02
      petrositis 383.02
      specified complication NEC 383.02
      subperiosteal abscess 383.01
  chronic (necrotic) (recurrent) 383.1
  tuberculous (*see also* Tuberculosis) 015.6
Mastopathy, mastopathia 611.9
  chronica cystica 610.1
  diffuse cystic 610.1
  estrogenic 611.89
  ovarian origin 611.89
Mastoplasia 611.1
Masturbation 307.9
Maternal condition, affecting fetus or newborn
  acute yellow atrophy of liver 760.8
  albuminuria 760.1
  anesthesia or analgesia 763.5
  blood loss 762.1
  chorioamnionitis 762.7
  circulatory disease, chronic (conditions
    classifiable to 390-459, 745-747) 760.3
  congenital heart disease (conditions classifiable
    to 745-746) 760.3
  cortical necrosis of kidney 760.1
  death 761.6
  diabetes mellitus 775.0
    manifest diabetes in the infant 775.1
  disease NEC 760.9
    circulatory system, chronic (conditions
      classifiable to 390-459, 745-747) 760.3
    genitourinary system (conditions classifiable
      to 580-599) 760.1
    respiratory (conditions classifiable to 490-519,
      748) 760.3
  eclampsia 760.0
  hemorrhage NEC 762.1
  hepatitis acute, malignant, or subacute 760.8
  hyperemesis (gravidarum) 761.8
  hypertension (arising during pregnancy)
    (conditions classifiable to 642) 760.0
  infection
    disease classifiable to 001-136 760.2
    genital tract NEC 760.8
    urinary tract 760.1
  influenza 760.2
    manifest influenza in the infant 771.2
  injury (conditions classifiable to 800-996) 760.5
  malaria 760.2
    manifest malaria in infant or fetus 771.2
  malnutrition 760.4
  necrosis of liver 760.8
  nephritis (conditions classifiable to 580-583)
    760.1
  nephrosis (conditions classifiable to 581) 760.1

Maternal condition—*continued*
  noxious substance transmitted via breast milk or
    placenta 760.70
    alcohol 760.71
    anticonvulsants 760.77
    antifungals 760.74
    anti-infective agents 760.74
    antimetabolics 760.78
    cocaine 760.75
    "crack" 760.75
    diethylstilbestrol [DES] 760.76
    hallucinogenic agents 760.73
    medicinal agents NEC 760.79
    narcotics 760.72
    obstetric anesthetic or analgesic drug 760.72
    specified agent NEC 760.79
  nutritional disorder (conditions classifiable to
    260-269) 760.4
  operation unrelated to current delivery (*see also*
    Newborn, affected by) 760.64
  pre-eclampsia 760.04
  pyelitis or pyelonephritis, arising during
    pregnancy (conditions classifiable to 590)
    760.1
  renal disease or failure 760.1
  respiratory disease, chronic (conditions
    classifiable to 490-519, 748) 760.3
  rheumatic heart disease (chronic) (conditions
    classifiable to 393-398) 760.3
  rubella (conditions classifiable to 056) 760.2
    manifest rubella in the infant or fetus 771.0
  surgery unrelated to current delivery (*see also*
    Newborn, affected by) 760.6
    to uterus or pelvic organs 760.64
  syphilis (conditions classifiable to 090-097)
    760.2
    manifest syphilis in the infant or fetus 090.0
  thrombophlebitis 760.3
  toxemia (of pregnancy) 760.0
    pre-eclamptic 760.0
  toxoplasmosis (conditions classifiable to 130)
    760.2
    manifest toxoplasmosis in the infant or fetus
      771.2
  transmission of chemical substance through the
    placenta 760.70
    alcohol 760.71
    anticonvulsants 760.77
    antifungals 760.74
    anti-infective agents 760.74
    antimetabolics 760.78
    cocaine 760.75
    "crack" 760.75
    diethylstilbestrol [DES] 760.76
    hallucinogenic agents 760.73
    narcotics 760.72
    specified substance NEC 760.79
  uremia 760.1
  urinary tract conditions (conditions classifiable
    to 580-599) 760.1
  vomiting (pernicious) (persistent) (vicious) 761.8
Maternity —*see* Delivery
Matheiu's disease (leptospiral jaundice) 100.0
Mauclaire's disease or osteochondrosis 732.3
Maxcy's disease 081.0
Maxilla, maxillary —*see* condition
May (-Hegglin) anomaly or syndrome 288.2
Mayaro fever 066.3
Mazoplasia 610.8
MBD (minimal brain dysfunction), child (*see also*
  Hyperkinesia) 314.9

MCAD (medium chain acyl CoA dehydrogenase deficiency) 277.85
McArdle (-Schmid-Pearson) disease or syndrome (glycogenosis V) 271.0
McCune-Albright syndrome (osteitis fibrosa disseminata) 756.59
MCLS (mucocutaneous lymph node syndrome) 446.1
McQuarrie's syndrome (idiopathic familial hypoglycemia) 251.2
Measles (black) (hemorrhagic) (suppressed) 055.9
  with
    encephalitis 055.0
    keratitis 055.71
    keratoconjunctivitis 055.71
    otitis media 055.2
    pneumonia 055.1
  complication 055.8
    specified type NEC 055.79
  encephalitis 055.0
  French 056.9
  German 056.9
  keratitis 055.71
  keratoconjunctivitis 055.71
  liberty 056.9
  otitis media 055.2
  pneumonia 055.1
  specified complications NEC 055.79
  vaccination, prophylactic (against) V04.2
Meatitis, urethral (*see also* Urethritis) 597.89
Meat poisoning —*see* Poisoning, food
Meatus, meatal —*see* condition
Meat-wrappers' asthma 506.9
Meckel's
  diverticulitis 751.0
  diverticulum (displaced) (hypertrophic) 751.0
Meconium
  aspiration 770.11
    with
      pneumonia 770.12
      pneumonitis 770.12
      respiratory symptoms 770.12
    below vocal cords 770.11
      with respiratory symptoms 770.12
    syndrome 770.12
  delayed passage in newborn 777.1
  ileus 777.1
    due to cystic fibrosis 277.01
  in liquor 792.3
    noted during delivery 656.8
  insufflation 770.11
    with respiratory symptoms 770.12
  obstruction
    fetus or newborn 777.1
      in mucoviscidosis 277.01
  passage of 792.3
    noted during delivery 763.84
  peritonitis 777.6
  plug syndrome (newborn) NEC 777.1
  staining 779.84
Median —*see also* condition
  arcuate ligament syndrome 447.4
  bar (prostate) 600.90
    with
      other lower urinary tract symptoms (LUTS) 600.91
      urinary
        obstruction 600.91
        retention 600.91

Median—*continued*
  vesical orifice 600.90
    with
      other lower urinary tract symptoms (LUTS) 600.91
      urinary
        obstruction 600.91
        retention 600.91
  rhomboid glossitis 529.2
Mediastinal shift 793.2
Mediastinitis (acute) (chronic) 519.2
  actinomycotic 039.8
  syphilitic 095.8
  tuberculous (*see also* Tuberculosis) 012.8
Mediastinopericarditis (*see also* Pericarditis) 423.9
  acute 420.90
  chronic 423.8
    rheumatic 393
  rheumatic, chronic 393
Mediastinum, mediastinal —*see* condition
Medical services provided for —*see* Health, services provided because (of)
Medicine poisoning (by overdose) (wrong substance given or taken in error) 977.9
  specified drug or substance—*see* Table of drugs and chemicals
Medin's disease (poliomyelitis) 045.9
Mediterranean
  anemia (with other hemoglobinopathy) 282.49
  disease or syndrome (hemipathic) 282.49
  fever (*see also* Brucellosis) 023.9
    familial 277.31
  kala-azar 085.0
  leishmaniasis 085.0
  tick fever 082.1
Medulla —*see* condition
Medullary
  cystic kidney 753.16
  sponge kidney 753.17
Medullated fibers
  optic (nerve) 743.57
  retina 362.85
Medulloblastoma (M9470/3)
  desmoplastic (M9471/3) 191.6
  specified site—*see* Neoplasm, by site, malignant
  unspecified site 191.6
Medulloepithelioma (M9501/3)—*see also* Neoplasm, by site, malignant
  teratoid (M9502/3)—*see* Neoplasm, by site, malignant
Medullomyoblastoma (M9472/3)
  specified site—*see* Neoplasm, by site, malignant
  unspecified site 191.6
Meekeren-Ehlers-Danlos syndrome 756.83
Megacaryocytic —*see* condition
Megacolon (acquired) (functional) (not Hirschsprung's disease) 564.7
  aganglionic 751.3
  congenital, congenitum 751.3
  Hirschsprung's (disease) 751.3
  psychogenic 306.4
  toxic (*see also* Colitis, ulcerative) 556.9
Megaduodenum 537.3
Megaesophagus (functional) 530.0
  congenital 750.4
Megakaryocytic —*see* condition
Megalencephaly 742.4
Megalerythema (epidermicum) (infectiosum) 057.0
Megalia, cutis et ossium 757.39
Megaloappendix 751.5

Megalocephalus, megalocephaly NEC 756.0
Megalocornea 743.41
  associated with buphthalmos 743.22
Megalocytic anemia 281.9
Megalodactylia (fingers) (thumbs) 755.57
  toes 755.65
Megaloduodenum 751.5
Megaloesophagus (functional) 530.0
  congenital 750.4
Megalogastria (congenital) 750.7
Megalomania 307.9
Megalophthalmos 743.8
Megalopsia 368.14
Megalosplenia (*see also* Splenomegaly) 789.2
Megaloureter 593.89
  congenital 753.22
Megarectum 569.49
Megasigmoid 564.7
  congenital 751.3
Megaureter 593.89
  congenital 753.22
Megrim 346.9
Meibomian
  cyst 373.2
    infected 373.12
  gland—*see* condition
  infarct (eyelid) 374.85
  stye 373.11
Meibomitis 373.12
Meige
  Milroy disease (chronic hereditary edema) 757.0
  syndrome (blepharospasm-oromandibular
    dystonia) 333.82
Melalgia, nutritional 266.2
Melancholia (*see also* Psychosis, affective)
  296.90
  climacteric 296.2
    recurrent episode 296.3
    single episode 296.2
  hypochondriac 300.7
  intermittent 296.2
    recurrent episode 296.3
    single episode 296.2
  involutional 296.2
    recurrent episode 296.3
    single episode 296.2
  menopausal 296.2
    recurrent episode 296.3
    single episode 296.2
  puerperal 296.2
  reactive (from emotional stress, psychological
    trauma) 298.0
  recurrent 296.3
  senile 290.21
  stuporous 296.2
    recurrent episode 296.3
    single episode 296.2
Melanemia 275.0
Melanoameloblastoma (M9363/0)—*see*
  Neoplasm, bone, benign
Melanoblastoma (M8720/3)—*see* Melanoma
Melanoblastosis
  Block-Sulzberger 757.33
  cutis linearis sive systematisata 757.33
Melanocarcinoma (M8720/3)—*see* Melanoma
Melanocytoma, eyeball (M8726/0) 224.0
Melanoderma, melanodermia 709.09
  Addison's (primary adrenal insufficiency) 255.41
Melanodontia, infantile 521.05
Melanodontoclasia 521.05
Melanoepithelioma (M8720/3)—*see* Melanoma

Melanoma (malignant) (M8720/3) 172.9

> *Note—Except where otherwise indicated, the
> morphological varieties of melanoma in the list
> below should be coded by site as for
> "Melanoma (malignant)." Internal sites should
> be coded to malignant neoplasm of those sites.*

  abdominal wall 172.5
  ala nasi 172.3
  amelanotic (M8730/3)—*see* Melanoma, by site
  ankle 172.7
  anus, anal 154.3
    canal 154.2
  arm 172.6
  auditory canal (external) 172.2
  auricle (ear) 172.2
  auricular canal (external) 172.2
  axilla 172.5
  axillary fold 172.5
  back 172.5
  balloon cell (M8722/3)—*see* Melanoma, by site
  benign (M8720/0)—*see* Neoplasm, skin, benign
  breast (female) (male) 172.5
  brow 172.3
  buttock 172.5
  canthus (eye) 172.1
  cheek (external) 172.3
  chest wall 172.5
  chin 172.3
  choroid 190.6
  conjunctiva 190.3
  ear (external) 172.2
  epithelioid cell (M8771/3)—*see also* Melanoma,
    by site
    and spindle cell, mixed (M8775/3)—*see*
      Melanoma, by site
  external meatus (ear) 172.2
  eye 190.9
  eyebrow 172.3
  eyelid (lower) (upper) 172.1
  face NEC 172.3
  female genital organ (external) NEC 184.4
  finger 172.6
  flank 172.5
  foot 172.7
  forearm 172.6
  forehead 172.3
  foreskin 187.1
  gluteal region 172.5
  groin 172.5
  hand 172.6
  heel 172.7
  helix 172.2
  hip 172.7
  in
    giant pigmented nevus (M8761/3)—*see*
      Melanoma, by site
    Hutchinson's melanotic freckle
      (M8742/3)—*see* Melanoma, by site
    junctional nevus (M8740/3)—*see* Melanoma,
      by site
    precancerous melanosis (M8741/3)—*see*
      Melanoma, by site
  in situ—*see* Melanoma, by site
    skin 172.9
  interscapular region 172.5
  iris 190.0
  jaw 172.3
  juvenile (M8770/0)—*see* Neoplasm, skin,
    benign
  knee 172.7

Melanoma—*continued*
labium
majus 184.1
minus 184.2
lacrimal gland 190.2
leg 172.7
lip (lower) (upper) 172.0
liver 197.7
lower limb NEC 172.7
male genital organ (external) NEC 187.9
meatus, acoustic (external) 172.2
meibomian gland 172.1
metastatic
of or from specified site—*see* Melanoma, by site
site not of skin—*see* Neoplasm, by site,
malignant, secondary
to specified site—*see* Neoplasm, by site,
malignant, secondary
unspecified site 172.9
nail 172.9
finger 172.6
toe 172.7
neck 172.4
nodular (M8721/3)—*see* Melanoma, by site
nose, external 172.3
orbit 190.1
penis 187.4
perianal skin 172.5
perineum 172.5
pinna 172.2
popliteal (fossa) (space) 172.7
prepuce 187.1
pubes 172.5
pudendum 184.4
retina 190.5
scalp 172.4
scrotum 187.7
septum nasal (skin) 172.3
shoulder 172.6
skin NEC 172.8
in situ 172.9
spindle cell (M8772/3)—*see also* Melanoma, by
site
type A (M8773/3) 190.0
type B (M8774/3) 190.0
submammary fold 172.5
superficial spreading (M8743/3)—*see*
Melanoma, by site
temple 172.3
thigh 172.7
toe 172.7
trunk NEC 172.5
umbilicus 172.5
upper limb NEC 172.6
vagina vault 184.0
vulva 184.4
Melanoplakia 528.9
Melanosarcoma (M8720/3)—*see also* Melanoma
epithelioid cell (M8771/3)—*see* Melanoma
Melanosis 709.09
addisonian (primary adrenal insufficiency)
255.41
tuberculous (*see also* Tuberculosis) 017.6
adrenal 255.41
colon 569.89
conjunctiva 372.55
congenital 743.49
corii degenerativa 757.33

Melanosis—*continued*
cornea (presenile) (senile) 371.12
congenital 743.43
interfering with vision 743.42
prenatal 743.43
interfering with vision 743.42
eye 372.55
congenital 743.49
jute spinners' 709.09
lenticularis progressiva 757.33
liver 573.8
precancerous (M8741/2)—*see also* Neoplasm,
skin, in situ
malignant melanoma in (M8741/3)—*see* Melanoma
Riehl's 709.09
sclera 379.19
congenital 743.47
suprarenal 255.41
tar 709.09
toxic 709.09
Melanuria 791.9
MELAS syndrome (mitochondrial
encephalopathy, lactic acidosis and stroke-like
episodes) 277.87
Melasma 709.09
adrenal (gland) 255.41
suprarenal (gland) 255.41
Melena 578.1
due to
swallowed maternal blood 777.3
ulcer—*see* Ulcer, by site, with hemorrhage
newborn 772.4
due to swallowed maternal blood 777.3
Meleney's
gangrene (cutaneous) 686.09
ulcer (chronic undermining) 686.09
Melioidosis 025
Melitensis, febris 023.0
Melitococcosis 023.0
Melkersson (-Rosenthal) syndrome 351.8
Mellitus, diabetes —*see* Diabetes
Melorheostosis (bone) (leri) 733.99
Meloschisis 744.83
Melotia 744.29
Membrana
capsularis lentis posterior 743.39
epipapillaris 743.57
Membranacea placenta —*see* Placenta,
abnormal
Membranaceous uterus 621.8
Membrane, membranous —*see also* condition
folds, congenital—*see* Web
Jackson's 751.4
over face (causing asphyxia), fetus or newborn
768.9
premature rupture—*see* Rupture, membranes,
premature
pupillary 364.74
persistent 743.46
retained (complicating delivery) (with
hemorrhage) 666.2
without hemorrhage 667.1
secondary (eye) 366.50
unruptured (causing asphyxia) 768.9
vitreous humor 379.25
Membranitis, fetal 658.4
affecting fetus or newborn 762.7
Memory disturbance, loss or lack (*see also*
Amnesia) 780.93
mild, following organic brain damage 310.8

MEN (multiple endocrine neoplasia) syndrome
- type 1 258.01
- type IIA 258.02
- type IIB 258.03

Menadione (vitamin K) deficiency 269.0
Menarche, precocious 259.1
Mendacity, pathologic 301.7
Mende's syndrome (ptosis-epicanthus) 270.2
Mendelson's syndrome (resulting from a procedure) 997.39
- obstetric 668.0

Ménétrier's disease or syndrome (hypertrophic gastritis) 535.2
Ménière's disease, syndrome, or vertigo 386.00
- cochlear 386.02
- cochleovestibular 386.01
- inactive 386.04
- in remission 386.04
- vestibular 386.03

Meninges, meningeal —*see* condition
Meningioma (M9530/0)—*see also* Neoplasm, meninges, benign
- angioblastic (M9535/0)—*see* Neoplasm, meninges, benign
- angiomatous (M9534/0)—*see* Neoplasm, meninges, benign
- endotheliomatous (M9531/0)—*see* Neoplasm, meninges, benign
- fibroblastic (M9532/0)—*see* Neoplasm, meninges, benign
- fibrous (M9532/0)—*see* Neoplasm, meninges, benign
- hemangioblastic (M9535/0)—*see* Neoplasm, meninges, benign
- hemangiopericytic (M9536/0)—*see* Neoplasm, meninges, benign
- malignant (M9530/3)—*see* Neoplasm, meninges, malignant
- meningiothelial (M9531/0)—*see* Neoplasm, meninges, benign
- meningotheliomatous (M9531/0)—*see* Neoplasm, meninges, benign
- mixed (M9537/0)—*see* Neoplasm, meninges, benign
- multiple (M9530/1) 237.6
- papillary (M9538/1) 237.6
- psammomatous (M9533/0)—*see* Neoplasm, meninges, benign
- syncytial (M9531/0)—*see* Neoplasm, meninges, benign
- transitional (M9537/0)—*see* Neoplasm, meninges, benign

Meningiomatosis (diffuse) (M9530/1) 237.6
Meningism (*see also* Meningismus) 781.6
Meningismus (infectional) (pneumococcal) 781.6
- due to serum or vaccine 997.09 *[321.8]*
- influenzal NEC 487.8

Meningitis (basal) (basic) (basilar) (brain) (cerebral) (cervical) (congestive) (diffuse) (hemorrhagic) (infantile) (membranous) (metastatic) (nonspecific) (pontine) (progressive) (simple) (spinal) (subacute) (sympathetica) (toxic) 322.9
- abacterial NEC (*see also* Meningitis, aseptic) 047.9
- actinomycotic 039.8 *[320.7]*
- adenoviral 049.1
- Aerobacter aerogenes 320.82
- anaerobes (cocci) (gram-negative) (gram-positive) (mixed) (NEC) 320.81
- arbovirus NEC 066.9 *[321.2]*
  - specified type NEC 066.8 *[321.2]*

Meningitis—*continued*
- aseptic (acute) NEC 047.9
  - adenovirus 049.1
  - Coxsackie virus 047.0
  - due to
    - adenovirus 049.1
    - Coxsackie virus 047.0
    - ECHO virus 047.1
    - enterovirus 047.9
    - mumps 072.1
    - poliovirus (*see also* Poliomyelitis) 045.2 *[321.2]*
  - ECHO virus 047.1
  - herpes (simplex) virus 054.72
    - zoster 053.0
  - leptospiral 100.81
  - lymphocytic choriomeningitis 049.0
  - noninfective 322.0
- Bacillus pyocyaneus 320.89
- bacterial NEC 320.9
  - anaerobic 320.81
  - gram-negative 320.82
    - anaerobic 320.81
- Bacteroides (fragilis) (oralis) (melaninogenicus) 320.81
- cancerous (M8000/6) 198.4
- candidal 112.83
- carcinomatous (M8010/6) 198.4
- caseous (*see also* Tuberculosis, meninges) 013.0
- cerebrospinal (acute) (chronic) (diplococcal) (endemic) (epidemic) (fulminant) (infectious) (malignant) (meningococcal) (sporadic) 036.0
  - carrier (suspected) of V02.59
- chronic NEC 322.2
- clear cerebrospinal fluid NEC 322.0
- Clostridium (haemolyticum) (novyi) NEC 320.81
- coccidioidomycosis 114.2
- Coxsackie virus 047.0
- cryptococcal 117.5 *[321.0]*
- diplococcal 036.0
  - gram-negative 036.0
  - gram-positive 320.1
- Diplococcus pneumoniae 320.1
- due to
  - actinomycosis 039.8 *[320.7]*
  - adenovirus 049.1
  - coccidiomycosis 114.2
  - enterovirus 047.9
    - specified NEC 047.8
  - histoplasmosis (*see also* Histoplasmosis) 115.91
  - Listerosis 027.0 *[320.7]*
  - Lyme disease 088.81 *[320.7]*
  - moniliasis 112.83
  - mumps 072.1
  - neurosyphilis 094.2
  - nonbacterial organisms NEC 321.8
  - oidiomycosis 112.83
  - poliovirus (*see also* Poliomyelitis) 045.2 *[321.2]*
  - preventive immunization, inoculation, or vaccination 997.09 *[321.8]*
  - sarcoidosis 135 *[321.4]*
  - sporotrichosis 117.1 *[321.1]*
  - syphilis 094.2
    - acute 091.81
    - congenital 090.42
    - secondary 091.81
  - trypanosomiasis (*see also* Trypanosomiasis) 086.9 *[321.3]*
  - whooping cough 033.9 *[320.7]*
- E. coli 320.82
- ECHO virus 047.1

Meningitis—*continued*
  endothelial-leukocytic, benign, recurrent 047.9
  Enterobacter aerogenes 320.82
  enteroviral 047.9
    specified type NEC 047.8
  enterovirus 047.9
    specified NEC 047.8
  eosinophilic 322.1
  epidemic NEC 036.0
  Escherichia coli (E. coli) 320.82
  Eubacterium 320.81
  fibrinopurulent NEC 320.9
    specified type NEC 320.89
  Friedländer (bacillus) 320.82
  fungal NEC 117.9 *[321.1]*
  Fusobacterium 320.81
  gonococcal 098.82
  gram-negative bacteria NEC 320.82
    anaerobic 320.81
    cocci 036.0
      specified NEC 320.82
  gram-negative cocci NEC 036.0
    specified NEC 320.82
  gram-positive cocci NEC 320.9
  H. influenzae 320.0
  herpes (simplex) virus 054.72
    zoster 053.0
  infectious NEC 320.9
  influenzal 320.0
  Klebsiella pneumoniae 320.82
  late effect—*see* Late, effect, meningitis
  leptospiral (aseptic) 100.81
  Listerella (monocytogenes) 027.0 *[320.7]*
  Listeria monocytogenes 027.0 *[320.7]*
  lymphocytic (acute) (benign) (serous) 049.0
    choriomeningitis virus 049.0
  meningococcal (chronic) 036.0
  Mima polymorpha 320.82
  Mollaret's 047.9
  monilial 112.83
  mumps (virus) 072.1
  mycotic NEC 117.9 *[321.1]*—
  Neisseria 036.0
  neurosyphilis 094.2
  nonbacterial NEC (*see also* Meningitis, aseptic) 047.9
  nonpyogenic NEC 322.0
  oidiomycosis 112.83
  ossificans 349.2
  Peptococcus 320.81
  Peptostreptococcus 320.81
  pneumococcal 320.1
  poliovirus (*see also* Poliomyelitis) 045.2 *[321.2]*
  Proprionibacterium 320.81
  Proteus morganii 320.82
  Pseudomonas (aeruginosa) (pyocyaneus) 320.82
  purulent NEC 320.9
    specified organism NEC 320.89
  pyogenic NEC 320.9
    specified organism NEC 320.89
  Salmonella 003.21
  septic NEC 320.9
    specified organism NEC 320.89
  serosa circumscripta NEC 322.0
  serous NEC (*see also* Meningitis, aseptic) 047.9
    lymphocytic 049.0
    syndrome 348.2
  Serratia (marcescens) 320.82
  specified organism NEC 320.89
  sporadic cerebrospinal 036.0
  sporotrichosis 117.1 *[321.1]*
  staphylococcal 320.3
  sterile 997.09

Meningitis—*continued*
  streptococcal (acute) 320.2
  suppurative 320.9
    specified organism NEC 320.89
  syphilitic 094.2
    acute 091.81
    congenital 090.42
    secondary 091.81
  torula 117.5 *[321.0]*
  traumatic (complication of injury) 958.8
  Treponema (denticola) (macrodenticum) 320.81
  trypanosomiasis 086.1 *[321.3]*
  tuberculous (*see also* Tuberculosis, meninges) 013.0
  typhoid 002.0 *[320.7]*
  Veillonella 320.81
  Vibrio vulnificus 320.82
  viral, virus NEC (*see also* Meningitis, aseptic) 047.9
  Wallgren's (*see also* Meningitis, aseptic) 047.9
Meningocele (congenital) (spinal) (*see also* Spina bifida) 741.9
  acquired (traumatic) 349.2
  cerebral 742.0
  cranial 742.0
Meningocerebritis —*see* Meningoencephalitis
Meningococcemia (acute) (chronic) 036.2
Meningococcus, meningococcal (*see also* condition) 036.9
  adrenalitis, hemorrhagic 036.3
  carditis 036.40
  carrier (suspected) of V02.59
  cerebrospinal fever 036.0
  encephalitis 036.1
  endocarditis 036.42
  exposure to V01.84
  infection NEC 036.9
  meningitis (cerebrospinal) 036.0
  myocarditis 036.43
  optic neuritis 036.81
  pericarditis 036.41
  septicemia (chronic) 036.2
Meningoencephalitis (*see also* Encephalitis) 323.9
  acute NEC 048
  bacterial, purulent, pyogenic, or septic—*see* Meningitis
  chronic NEC 094.1
  diffuse NEC 094.1
  diphasic 063.2
  due to
    actinomycosis 039.8 *[320.7]*
    blastomycosis NEC (*see also* Blastomycosis) 116.0 *[323.41]*
    free-living amebae 136.29
    Listeria monocytogenes 027.0 *[320.7]*
    Lyme disease 088.81 *[320.7]*
    mumps 072.2
    Naegleria (amebae) (gruberi) (organisms) 136.29
    rubella 056.01
    sporotrichosis 117.1 *[321.1]*
    toxoplasmosis (acquired) 130.0
      congenital (active) 771.2 *[323.41]*
    Trypanosoma 086.1 *[323.2]*
  epidemic 036.0
  herpes 054.3
  herpetic 054.3
  H. influenzae 320.0
  infectious (acute) 048
  influenzal 320.0
  late effect—*see* category 326
  Listeria monocytogenes 027.0 *[320.7]*

Meningoencephalitis—*continued*
  lymphocytic (serous) 049.0
  mumps 072.2
  parasitic NEC 123.9 *[323.41]*
  pneumococcal 320.1
  primary amebic 136.29
  rubella 056.01
  serous 048
    lymphocytic 049.0
  specific 094.2
  staphylococcal 320.3
  streptococcal 320.2
  syphilitic 094.2
  toxic NEC 989.9 *[323.71]*
    due to
      carbon tetrachloride (vapor) 987.8 *[323.71]*
      hydroxyquinoline derivatives poisoning
        961.3 *[323.71]*
      lead 984.9 *[323.71]*
      mercury 985.0 *[323.71]*
      thallium 985.8 *[323.71]*
  toxoplasmosis (acquired) 130.0
  trypanosomic 086.1 *[323.2]*
  tuberculous (*see also* Tuberculosis, meninges)
    013.0
  virus NEC 048
Meningoencephalocele 742.0
  syphilitic 094.89
    congenital 090.49
Meningoencephalomyelitis (*see also*
  Meningoencephalitis) 323.9
  acute NEC 048
    disseminated (postinfectious) 136.9 *[323.61]*
      postimmunization or postvaccination 323.51
  due to
    actinomycosis 039.8 *[320.7]*
    torula 117.5 *[323.41]*
    toxoplasma or toxoplasmosis (acquired) 130.0
      congenital (active) 771.2 *[323.41]*
  late effect—*see* category 326
Meningoencephalomyelopathy (*see also*
  Meningoencephalomyelitis) 349.9
Meningoencephalopathy (*see also*
  Meningoencephalitis) 348.39
Meningoencephalopoliomyelitis (*see also*
  Poliomyelitis, bulbar) 045.0
  late effect 138
Meningomyelitis (*see also* Meningoencephalitis)
  323.9
  blastomycotic NEC (*see also* Blastomycosis)
    116.0 *[323.41]*
  due to
    actinomycosis 039.8 *[320.7]*
    blastomycosis (*see also* Blastomycosis) 116.0
      [323.41]
    Meningococcus 036.0
    sporotrichosis 117.1 *[323.41]*
    torula 117.5 *[323.41]*
  late effect—*see* category 326
  lethargic 049.8
  meningococcal 036.0
  syphilitic 094.2
  tuberculous (*see also* Tuberculosis, meninges)
    013.0
Meningomyelocele (*see also* Spina bifida) 741.9
  syphilitic 094.89
Meningomyeloneuritis —*see*
  Meningoencephalitis
Meningoradiculitis —*see* Meningitis
Meningovascular —*see* condition
Meniscocytosis 282.60
Menkes' syndrome —*see* Syndrome, Menkes'

Menolipsis 626.0
Menometrorrhagia 626.2
Menopause, menopausal (symptoms)
  (syndrome) 627.2
  arthritis (any site) NEC 716.3
  artificial 627.4
  bleeding 627.0
  crisis 627.2
  depression (*see also* Psychosis, affective) 296.2
    agitated 296.2
      recurrent episode 296.3
      single episode 296.2
    psychotic 296.2
      recurrent episode 296.3
      single episode 296.2
    recurrent episode 296.3
    single episode 296.2
  melancholia (*see also* Psychosis, affective) 296.2
    recurrent episode 296.3
    single episode 296.2
  paranoid state 297.2
  paraphrenia 297.2
  postsurgical 627.4
  premature 256.31
    postirradiation 256.2
    postsurgical 256.2
  psychoneurosis 627.2
  psychosis NEC 298.8
  surgical 627.4
  toxic polyarthritis NEC 716.39
Menorrhagia (primary) 626.2
  climacteric 627.0
  menopausal 627.0
  postclimacteric 627.1
  postmenopausal 627.1
  preclimacteric 627.0
  premenopausal 627.0
  puberty (menses retained) 626.3
Menorrhalgia 625.3
Menoschesis 626.8
Menostaxis 626.2
Menses, retention 626.8
Menstrual —*see* Menstruation
  cycle, irregular 626.4
  disorders NEC 626.9
  extraction V25.3
  fluid, retained 626.8
  molimen 625.4
  period, normal V65.5
  regulation V25.3
Menstruation
  absent 626.0
  anovulatory 628.0
  delayed 626.8
  difficult 625.3
  disorder 626.9
    psychogenic 306.52
    specified NEC 626.8
  during pregnancy 640.8
  excessive 626.2
  frequent 626.2
  infrequent 626.1
  irregular 626.4
  latent 626.8
  membranous 626.8
  painful (primary) (secondary) 625.3
    psychogenic 306.52
  passage of clots 626.2
  precocious 626.8
  protracted 626.8
  retained 626.8
  retrograde 626.8

Menstruation—*continued*
  scanty 626.1
  suppression 626.8
  vicarious (nasal) 625.8
Mentagra (*see also* Sycosis) 704.8
Mental —*see also* condition
  deficiency (*see also* Retardation, mental) 319
  deterioration (*see also* Psychosis) 298.9
  disorder (*see also* Disorder, mental) 300.9
  exhaustion 300.5
  insufficiency (congenital) (*see also* Retardation, mental) 319
  observation without need for further medical care NEC V71.09
  retardation (*see also* Retardation, mental) 319
  subnormality (*see also* Retardation, mental) 319
    mild 317
    moderate 318.0
    profound 318.2
    severe 318.1
  upset (*see also* Disorder, mental) 300.9
Meralgia paresthetica 355.1
Mercurial —*see* condition
Mercurialism NEC 985.0
Merergasia 300.9
Merkel cell tumor —*see* Carcinoma, Merkel cell
Merocele (*see also* Hernia, femoral) 553.00
Meromelia 755.4
  lower limb 755.30
    intercalary 755.32
      femur 755.34
        tibiofibular (complete) (incomplete) 755.33
      fibula 755.37
      metatarsal(s) 755.38
      tibia 755.36
      tibiofibular 755.35
    terminal (complete) (partial) (transverse) 755.31
      longitudinal 755.32
        metatarsal(s) 755.38
        phalange(s) 755.39
        tarsal(s) 755.38
      transverse 755.31
  upper limb 755.20
    intercalary 755.22
      carpal(s) 755.28
      humeral 755.24
        radioulnar (complete) (incomplete) 755.23
      metacarpal(s) 755.28
      phalange(s) 755.29
      radial 755.26
      radioulnar 755.25
      ulnar 755.27
    terminal (complete) (partial) (transverse) 755.21
      longitudinal 755.22
        carpal(s) 755.28
        metacarpal(s) 755.28
        phalange(s) 755.29
      transverse 755.21
Merosmia 781.1
MERRF syndrome (myoclonus with epilepsy and with ragged red fibers) 277.87
Merycism (*see also* Rumination)—*see also* Vomiting
  psychogenic 307.53
Merzbacher-Pelizaeus disease 330.0
Mesaortitis —*see* Aortitis
Mesarteritis —*see* Arteritis
Mesencephalitis (*see also* Encephalitis) 323.9
  late effect—*see* category 326

Mesenchymoma (M8990/1)—*see also* Neoplasm, connective tissue, uncertain behavior
  benign (M8990/0)—*see* Neoplasm, connective tissue, benign
  malignant (M8990/3)—*see* Neoplasm, connective tissue, malignant
Mesenteritis
  retractile 567.82
  sclerosing 567.82
Mesentery, mesenteric —*see* condition
Mesiodens, mesiodentes 520.1
  causing crowding 524.31
Mesio-occlusion 524.23
Mesocardia (with asplenia) 746.87
Mesocolon —*see* condition
Mesonephroma (malignant) (M9110/3)—*see also* Neoplasm, by site, malignant
  benign (M9110/0)—*see* Neoplasm, by site, benign
Mesophlebitis —*see* Phlebitis
Mesostromal dysgenesis 743.51
Mesothelioma (malignant) (M9050/3)—*see also* Neoplasm, by site, malignant
  benign (M9050/0)—*see* Neoplasm, by site, benign
  biphasic type (M9053/3)—*see also* Neoplasm, by site, malignant
  benign (M9053/0)—*see* Neoplasm, by site, benign
  epithelioid (M9052/3)—*see also* Neoplasm, by site, malignant
  benign (M9052/0)—*see* Neoplasm, by site, benign
  fibrous (M9051/3)—*see also* Neoplasm, by site, malignant
  benign (M9051/0)—*see* Neoplasm, by site, benign
Metabolic syndrome 277.7
Metabolism disorder 277.9
  specified type NEC 277.89
Metagonimiasis 121.5
Metagonimus infestation (small intestine) 121.5
Metal
  pigmentation (skin) 709.00
  polishers' disease 502
Metalliferous miners' lung 503
Metamorphopsia 368.14
Metaplasia
  bone, in skin 709.3
  breast 611.89
  cervix—*omit code*
  endometrium (squamous) 621.8
  esophagus 530.85
  intestinal, of gastric mucosa 537.89
  kidney (pelvis) (squamous) (*see also* Disease, renal) 593.89
  myelogenous 289.89
  myeloid 289.89
    agnogenic 238.76
    megakaryocytic 238.76
  spleen 289.59
  squamous cell
    amnion 658.8
    bladder 596.8
    cervix—*see* condition
    trachea 519.19
    tracheobronchial tree 519.19
    uterus 621.8
      cervix—*see* condition

Microphthalmia (congenital) (*see also*
   Microphthalmos) 743.10
Microphthalmos (congenital) 743.10
   associated with eye and adnexal anomalies NEC
      743.12
   due to toxoplasmosis (congenital) 771.2
   isolated 743.11
   simple 743.11
   syndrome 759.89
Micropsia 368.14
Microsporidiosis 136.8
Microsporon furfur infestation 111.0
Microsporosis (*see also* Dermatophytosis) 110.9
   nigra 111.1
Microstomia (congenital) 744.84
Microthelia 757.6
Microthromboembolism —*see* Embolism
Microtia (congenital) (external ear) 744.23
Microtropia 378.34
Micturition
   disorder NEC 788.69
      psychogenic 306.53
   frequency 788.41
      psychogenic 306.53
   nocturnal 788.43
   painful 788.1
      psychogenic 306.53
Middle
   ear—*see* condition
   lobe (right) syndrome 518.0
Midplane —*see* condition
Miescher's disease 709.3
   cheilitis 351.8
   granulomatosis disciformis 709.3
Miescher-Leder syndrome or granulomatosis
      709.3
Mieten's syndrome 759.89
Migraine (idiopathic) 346.9

> *Note: The following fifth digit subclassification
> is for use with category 346*
>
> 0   *without mention of intractable migraine
>   without mention of status migrainosus*
> 1   *with intractable migraine, so stated, without
>   mention of status migrainosus*
> 2   *without mention of intractable migraine
>   with status migrainosus*
> 3   *with intractable migraine, so stated, with
>   status migrainosus*

   with aura (acute-onset) (without headache)
      (prolonged) (typical) 346.0
   without aura 346.1
      chronic 346.7
      transformed 346.7
   abdominal (syndrome) 346.2
   allergic (histamine) 346.2
   atypical 346.8
   basilar 346.0
   chronic without aura 346.7
   classic(al) 346.0
   common 346.1
   hemiplegic 346.3
      familial 346.3
      sporadic 346.3
   lower-half 339.00
   menstrual 346.4
   menstrually related 346.4
   ophthalmic 346.8
   ophthalmoplegic 346.2
   premenstrual 346.4

Migraine—*continued*
   pure menstrual 346.4
   retinal 346.0
   specified form NEC 346.8
   transformed without aura 346.7
   variant 346.2
Migrant, social V60.0
Migratory, migrating —*see also* condition
   person V60.0
   testis, congenital 752.52
Mikulicz's disease or syndrome (dryness of
      mouth, absent or decreased lacrimation) 527.1
Milian atrophia blanche 701.3
Miliaria (crystallina) (rubra) (tropicalis) 705.1
   apocrine 705.82
Miliary —*see* condition
Milium (*see also* Cyst, sebaceous) 706.2
   colloid 709.3
   eyelid 374.84
Milk
   crust 690.11
   excess secretion 676.6
   fever, female 672
   poisoning 988.8
   retention 676.2
   sickness 988.8
   spots 423.1
Milkers' nodes 051.1
Milk-leg (deep vessels) 671.4
   complicating pregnancy 671.3
   nonpuerperal 451.19
   puerperal, postpartum, childbirth 671.4
Milkman (-Looser) disease or syndrome
      (osteomalacia with pseudofractures) 268.2
Milky urine (*see also* Chyluria) 791.1
Millar's asthma (laryngismus stridulus) 478.75
Millard-Gubler paralysis or syndrome 344.89
Millard-Gubler-Foville paralysis 344.89
Miller-Dieker syndrome 758.33
Miller's disease (osteomalacia) 268.2
Miller Fisher's syndrome 357.0
Milles' syndrome (encephalocutaneous
      angiomatosis) 759.6
Mills' disease 335.29
Millstone makers' asthma or lung 502
Milroy's disease (chronic hereditary edema) 757.0
Miners' —*see also* condition
   asthma 500
   elbow 727.2
   knee 727.2
   lung 500
   nystagmus 300.89
   phthisis (*see also* Tuberculosis) 011.4
   tuberculosis (*see also* Tuberculosis) 011.4
Minkowski-Chauffard syndrome (*see also*
      Spherocytosis) 282.0
Minor —*see* condition
Minor's disease 336.1
Minot's disease (hemorrhagic disease, newborn)
      776.0
Minot-von Willebrand (-Jürgens) disease or
      syndrome (angiohemophilia) 286.4
Minus (and plus) hand (intrinsic) 736.09
Miosis (persistent) (pupil) 379.42
Mirizzi's syndrome (hepatic duct stenosis) (*see
      also* Obstruction, biliary) 576.2
   with calculus, cholelithiasis, or stones—*see*
      Choledocholithiasis
Mirror writing 315.09
   secondary to organic lesion 784.69

Misadventure (prophylactic) (therapeutic) *(see also* Complications) 999.9
administration of insulin 962.3
infusion—*see* Complications, infusion
local applications (of fomentations, plasters, etc.) 999.9
burn or scald—*see* Burn, by site
medical care (early) (late) NEC 999.9
adverse effect of drugs or chemicals—*see* Table of drugs and chemicals
burn or scald—*see* Burn, by site
radiation NEC 990
radiotherapy NEC 990
surgical procedure (early) (late)—*see* Complications, surgical procedure
transfusion—*see* Complications, transfusion
vaccination or other immunological procedure—*see* Complications, vaccination
Misanthropy 301.7
Miscarriage —*see* Abortion, spontaneous
Mischief, malicious, child (*see also* Disturbance, conduct) 312.0
Misdirection
aqueous 365.83
Mismanagement, feeding 783.3
Misplaced, misplacement
kidney (*see also* Disease, renal) 593.0
congenital 753.3
organ or site, congenital NEC—*see* Malposition, congenital
Missed
abortion 632
delivery (at or near term) 656.4
labor (at or near term) 656.4
Misshapen reconstructed breast 612.0
Missing —*see also* Absence
teeth (acquired) 525.10
congenital (*see also* Anodontia) 520.0
due to
caries 525.13
extraction 525.10
periodontal disease 525.12
trauma 525.11
specified NEC 525.19
vertebrae (congenital) 756.13
Misuse of drugs NEC (*see also* Abuse, drug, nondependent) 305.9
Mitchell's disease (erythromelalgia) 443.82
Mite (s)
diarrhea 133.8
grain (itch) 133.8
hair follicle (itch) 133.8
in sputum 133.8
Mitochondrial encephalopathy, lactic acidosis and stroke-like episodes (MELAS syndrome) 277.87
Mitochondrial neurogastrointestinal encephalopathy syndrome (MNGIE) 277.87
Mitral —*see* condition
Mittelschmerz 625.2
Mixed —*see* condition
Mljet disease (mal de Meleda) 757.39
Mobile, mobility
cecum 751.4
coccyx 733.99
excessive—*see* Hypermobility
gallbladder 751.69
kidney 593.0
congenital 753.3
organ or site, congenital NEC—*see* Malposition, congenital
spleen 289.59

Mobitz heart block (atrioventricular) 426.10
type I (Wenckebach's) 426.13
type II 426.12
Möbius'
disease 346.2
syndrome
congenital oculofacial paralysis 352.6
ophthalmoplegic migraine 346.2
Moeller (-Barlow) disease (infantile scurvy) 267
glossitis 529.4
Mohr's syndrome (Types I and II) 759.89
Mola destruens (M9100/1) 236.1
Molarization, premolars 520.2
Molar pregnancy 631
hydatidiform (delivered) (undelivered) 630
Mold (s) in vitreous 117.9
Molding, head (during birth)—*omit code*
Mole (pigmented) (M8720/0)—*see also* Neoplasm, skin, benign
blood 631
Breus' 631
cancerous (M8720/3)—*see* Melanoma
carneous 631
destructive (M9100/1) 236.1
ectopic—*see* Pregnancy, ectopic
fleshy 631
hemorrhagic 631
hydatid, hydatidiform (benign) (complicating pregnancy) (delivered) (undelivered) (*see also* Hydatidiform mole) 630
invasive (M9100/1) 236.1
malignant (M9100/1) 236.1
previous, affecting management of pregnancy V23.1
invasive (hydatidiform) (M9100/1) 236.1
malignant
meaning
malignant hydatidiform mole (M9100/1) 236.1
melanoma (M8720/3)—*see* Melanoma
nonpigmented (M8730/0)—*see* Neoplasm, skin, benign
pregnancy NEC 631
skin (M8720/0)—*see* Neoplasm, skin, benign
tubal—*see* Pregnancy, tubal
vesicular (*see also* Hydatidiform mole) 630
Molimen, molimina (menstrual) 625.4
Mollaret's meningitis 047.9
Mollities (cerebellar) (cerebral) 437.8
ossium 268.2
Molluscum
contagiosum 078.0
epitheliale 078.0
fibrosum (M8851/0)—*see* Lipoma, by site
pendulum (M8851/0)—*see* Lipoma, by site
Mönckeberg's arteriosclerosis, degeneration disease, or sclerosis (*see also* Arteriosclerosis, extremities) 440.20
Monday fever 504
Monday morning dyspnea or asthma 504
Mondini's malformation (cochlea) 744.05
Mondor's disease (thrombophlebitis of breast) 451.89
Mongolian, mongolianism, mongolism mongoloid 758.0
spot 757.33
Monilethrix (congenital) 757.4
Monilia infestation —*see* Candidiasis
Moniliasis —*see also* Candidiasis
neonatal 771.7
vulvovaginitis 112.1
Monkeypox 059.01

Monoarthritis 716.60
  ankle 716.67
  arm 716.62
    lower (and wrist) 716.63
    upper (and elbow) 716.62
  foot (and ankle) 716.67
  forearm (and wrist) 716.63
  hand 716.64
  leg 716.66
    lower 716.66
    upper 716.65
  pelvic region (hip) (thigh) 716.65
  shoulder (region) 716.61
  specified site NEC 716.68
Monoblastic —*see* condition
Monochromatism (cone) (rod) 368.54
Monocytic —*see* condition
Monocytopenia 288.59
Monocytosis (symptomatic) 288.63
Monofixation syndrome 378.34
Monomania (*see also* Psychosis) 298.9
Mononeuritis 355.9
  cranial nerve—*see* Disorder, nerve, cranial
  femoral nerve 355.2
  lateral
    cutaneous nerve of thigh 355.1
    popliteal nerve 355.3
  lower limb 355.8
    specified nerve NEC 355.79
  medial popliteal nerve 355.4
  median nerve 354.1
  multiplex 354.5
  plantar nerve 355.6
  posterior tibial nerve 355.5
  radial nerve 354.3
  sciatic nerve 355.0
  ulnar nerve 354.2
  upper limb 354.9
    specified nerve NEC 354.8
  vestibular 388.5
Mononeuropathy (*see also* Mononeuritis) 355.9
  diabetic NEC 250.6 *[355.9]*
    due to secondary diabetes 249.6 *[355.9]*
    lower limb 250.6 *[355.8]*
      due to secondary diabetes 249.6 *[355.8]*
    upper limb 250.6 *[354.9]*
      due to secondary diabetes 249.6 *[354.9]*
  iliohypogastric nerve 355.79
  ilioinguinal nerve 355.79
  obturator nerve 355.79
  saphenous nerve 355.79
Mononucleosis, infectious 075
  with hepatitis 075 *[573.1]*
Monoplegia 344.5
  brain (current episode) (*see also* Paralysis,
    brain) 437.8
  fetus or newborn 767.8
  cerebral (current episode) (*see also* Paralysis,
    brain) 437.8
  congenital or infantile (cerebral) (spastic)
    (spinal) 343.3
  embolic (current) (*see also* Embolism, brain)
    434.1
    late effect—*see* Late effect(s) (of)
      cerebrovascular disease
  infantile (cerebral) (spastic) (spinal) 343.3

Monoplegia—*continued*
  lower limb 344.30
    affecting
      dominant side 344.31
      nondominant side 344.32
    due to late effect of cerebrovascular accident
      —*see* Late effect(s) (of) cerebrovascular
      accident
  newborn 767.8
  psychogenic 306.0
    specified as conversion reaction 300.11
  thrombotic (current) (*see also* Thrombosis,
    brain) 434.0
    late effect—*see* Late effect(s) (of)
      cerebrovascular disease
  transient 781.4
  upper limb 344.40
    affecting
      dominant side 344.41
      nondominant side 344.42
    due to late effect of cerebrovascular accident
      —*see* Late effect(s) (of) cerebrovascular
      accident
Monorchism, monorchidism 752.89
Monteggia's fracture (closed) 813.03
  open 813.13
Mood swings
  brief compensatory 296.99
  rebound 296.99
Moore's syndrome (*see also* Epilepsy) 345.5
Mooren's ulcer (cornea) 370.07
Mooser-Neill reaction 081.0
Mooser bodies 081.0
Moral
  deficiency 301.7
  imbecility 301.7
Morax-Axenfeld conjunctivitis 372.03
Morbilli (*see also* Measles) 055.9
Morbus
  anglicus, anglorum 268.0
  Beigel 111.2
  caducus (*see also* Epilepsy) 345.9
  caeruleus 746.89
  celiacus 579.0
  comitialis (*see also* Epilepsy) 345.9
  cordis—*see also* Disease, heart
    valvulorum—*see* Endocarditis
  coxae 719.95
    tuberculous (*see also* Tuberculosis) 015.1
  hemorrhagicus neonatorum 776.0
  maculosus neonatorum 772.6
  renum 593.0
  senilis (*see also* Osteoarthrosis) 715.9
Morel-Kraepelin disease (*see also*
  Schizophrenia) 295.9
Morel-Moore syndrome (hyperostosis frontalis
  interna) 733.3
Morel-Morgagni syndrome (hyperostosis
  frontalis interna) 733.3
Morgagni
  cyst, organ, hydatid, or appendage 752.89
  fallopian tube 752.11
  disease or syndrome (hyperostosis frontalis
    interna) 733.3
Morgagni-Adams-Stokes syndrome (syncope
  with heart block) 426.9
Morgagni-Stewart-Morel syndrome
  (hyperostosis frontalis interna) 733.3
Moria (*see also* Psychosis) 298.9
Morning sickness 643.0
Moron 317

Morphea (guttate) (linear) 701.0
Morphine dependence (*see also* Dependence) 304.0
Morphinism (*see also* Dependence) 304.0
Morphinomania (*see also* Dependence) 304.0
Morphoea 701.0
Morquio (-Brailsford) (-Ullrich) disease or syndrome (mucopolysaccharidosis IV) 277.5
kyphosis 277.5
Morris syndrome (testicular feminization) 259.51
Morsus humanus (open wound)—*see also* Wound, open, by site
skin surface intact—*see* Contusion
Mortification (dry) (moist) (*see also* Gangrene) 785.4
Morton's
disease 355.6
foot 355.6
metatarsalgia (syndrome) 355.6
neuralgia 355.6
neuroma 355.6
syndrome (metatarsalgia) (neuralgia) 355.6
toe 355.6
Morvan's disease 336.0
Mosaicism, mosaic (chromosomal) 758.9
autosomal 758.5
sex 758.81
Moschcowitz's syndrome (thrombotic thrombocytopenic purpura) 446.6
Mother yaw 102.0
Motion sickness (from travel, any vehicle) (from roundabouts or swings) 994.6
Mottled teeth (enamel) (endemic) (nonendemic) 520.3
Mottling enamel (endemic) (nonendemic) (teeth) 520.3
Mouchet's disease 732.5
Mould (s) (in vitreous) 117.9
Moulders'
bronchitis 502
tuberculosis (*see also* Tuberculosis) 011.4
Mounier-Kuhn syndrome 748.3
with
acute exacerbation 494.1
bronchiectasis 494.0
with (acute) exacerbation 494.1
acquired 519.19
with bronchiectasis 494.0
with (acute) exacerbation 494.1
Mountain
fever—*see* Fever, mountain
sickness 993.2
with polycythemia, acquired 289.0
acute 289.0
tick fever 066.1
Mouse, joint (*see also* Loose, body, joint) 718.1
knee 717.6
Mouth —*see* condition
Movable
coccyx 724.71
kidney (*see also* Disease, renal) 593.0
congenital 753.3
organ or site, congenital NEC—*see* Malposition, congenital
spleen 289.59
Movement
abnormal (dystonic) (involuntary) 781.0
decreased fetal 655.7
paradoxical facial 374.43
Moya Moya disease 437.5

Mozart's ear 744.29
MRSA (methicillin resistant staphylococcus aureus) 041.12
colonization V02.54
personal history of V12.04
MSSA (methicillin susceptible staphylococcus aureus) 041.11
colonization V02.53
Mucha's disease (acute parapsoriasis varioliformis) 696.2
Mucha-Haberman syndrome (acute parapsoriasis varioliformis) 696.2
Mu-chain disease 273.2
Mucinosis (cutaneous) (papular) 701.8
Mucocele
appendix 543.9
buccal cavity 528.9
gallbladder (*see also* Disease, gallbladder) 575.3
lacrimal sac 375.43
orbit (eye) 376.81
salivary gland (any) 527.6
sinus (accessory) (nasal) 478.19
turbinate (bone) (middle) (nasal) 478.19
uterus 621.8
Mucocutaneous lymph node syndrome (acute) (febrile) (infantile) 446.1
Mucoenteritis 564.9
Mucolipidosis I, II, III 272.7
Mucopolysaccharidosis (types 1-6) 277.5
cardiopathy 277.5 *[425.7]*
Mucormycosis (lung) 117.7
Mucosa associated lymphoid tissue (MALT) 200.3
Mucositis —*see also* Inflammation, by site 528.00
cervix (ulcerative) 616.81
due to
antineoplastic therapy (ulcerative) 528.01
other drugs (ulcerative) 528.02
specified NEC 528.09
gastrointestinal (ulcerative) 538
nasal (ulcerative) 478.11
necroticans agranulocytica (*see also* Agranulocytosis) 288.09
ulcerative 528.00
vagina (ulcerative) 616.81
vulva (ulcerative) 616.81
Mucous —*see also* condition
patches (syphilitic) 091.3
congenital 090.0
Mucoviscidosis 277.00
with meconium obstruction 277.01
Mucus
asphyxia or suffocation (*see also* Asphyxia, mucus) 933.1
newborn 770.18
in stool 792.1
plug, (*see also* Asphyxia, mucus) 933.1
aspiration, of newborn 770.17
tracheobronchial 519.19
newborn 770.18
Muguet 112.0
Mulberry molars 090.5
Müllerian mixed tumor (M8950/3)—*see* Neoplasm, by site, malignant
Multicystic kidney 753.19
Multilobed placenta —*see* Placenta, abnormal
Multinodular prostate 600.10
with
urinary
obstruction 600.11
retention 600.11

Multiparity V61.5
  affecting
    fetus or newborn 763.89
    management of
      labor and delivery 659.4
      pregnancy V23.3
  requiring contraceptive management (*see also*
    Contraception) V25.9
Multipartita placenta —*see* Placenta, abnormal
Multiple, multiplex —*see also* condition
  birth
    affecting fetus or newborn 761.5
    healthy liveborn—*see* Newborn, multiple
  digits (congenital) 755.00
    fingers 755.01
    toes 755.02
  organ or site NEC—*see* Accessory
  personality 300.14
  renal arteries 747.62
Mumps 072.9
  with complication 072.8
    specified type NEC 072.79
  encephalitis 072.2
  hepatitis 072.71
  meningitis (aseptic) 072.1
  meningoencephalitis 072.2
  oophoritis 072.79
  orchitis 072.0
  pancreatitis 072.3
  polyneuropathy 072.72
  vaccination, prophylactic (against) V04.6
Mumu (*see also* Infestation, filarial) 125.9
Münchausen syndrome 301.51
Münchmeyer's disease or syndrome (exostosis
  luxurians) 728.11
Mural —*see* condition
Murmur (cardiac) (heart) (nonorganic) (organic)
  785.2
  abdominal 787.5
  aortic (valve) (*see also* Endocarditis, aortic) 424.1
  benign—*omit code*
  cardiorespiratory 785.2
  diastolic—*see* condition
  Flint (*see also* Endocarditis, aortic) 424.1
  functional—*omit code*
  Graham Steell (pulmonic regurgitation) (*see also*
    Endocarditis, pulmonary) 424.3
  innocent—*omit code*
  insignificant—*omit code*
  midsystolic 785.2
  mitral (valve)—*see* stenosis, mitral
  physiologic—*see* condition
  presystolic, mitral—*see* Insufficiency, mitral
  pulmonic (valve) (*see also* Endocarditis,
    pulmonary) 424.3
  Still's (vibratory)—*omit code*
  systolic (valvular)—*see* condition
  tricuspid (valve)—*see* Endocarditis, tricuspid
  valvular—*see* condition
  vibratory—*omit code*
  undiagnosed 785.2
Murri's disease (intermittent hemoglobinuria)
  283.2
Muscae volitantes 379.24
Muscle, muscular —*see* condition
Musculoneuralgia 729.1
Mushrooming hip 718.95
Mushroom workers' (pickers') lung 495.5
Mutation
  factor V leiden 289.81
  prothrombin gene 289.81

Mutism (*see also* Aphasia) 784.3
  akinetic 784.3
  deaf (acquired) (congenital) 389.7
  hysterical 300.11
  selective (elective) 313.23
    adjustment reaction 309.83
Myà's disease (congenital dilation, colon) 751.3
Myalgia (intercostal) 729.1
  eosinophilia syndrome 710.5
  epidemic 074.1
    cervical 078.89
  psychogenic 307.89
  traumatic NEC 959.9
Myasthenia 358.00
  cordis—*see* Failure, heart
  gravis 358.00
    with exacerbation (acute) 358.01
    in crisis 358.01
    neonatal 775.2
    pseudoparalytica 358.00
  stomach 536.8
    psychogenic 306.4
  syndrome in
    botulism 005.1 *[358.1]*
    diabetes mellitus 250.6 *[358.1]*
      due to secondary diabetes 249.6 *[358.1]*
    hypothyroidism (*see also* Hypothyroidism)
      244.9 *[358.1]*
    malignant neoplasm NEC 199.1 *[358.1]*
    pernicious anemia 281.0 *[358.1]*
    thyrotoxicosis (*see also* Thyrotoxicosis) 242.9
      [358.1]
Myasthenic 728.87
Mycelium infection NEC 117.9
Mycetismus 988.1
Mycetoma (actinomycotic) 039.9
  bone 039.8
    mycotic 117.4
  foot 039.4
    mycotic 117.4
  madurae 039.9
    mycotic 117.4
  maduromycotic 039.9
    mycotic 117.4
  mycotic 117.4
  nocardial 039.9
Mycobacteriosis —*see* Mycobacterium
Mycobacterium, mycobacterial (infection) 031.9
  acid-fast (bacilli) 031.9
  anonymous (*see also* Mycobacterium, atypical)
    031.9
  atypical (acid-fast bacilli) 031.9
    cutaneous 031.1
    pulmonary 031.0
      tuberculous (*see also* Tuberculosis,
        pulmonary) 011.9
    specified site NEC 031.8
  avium 031.0
    intracellulare complex bacteremia (MAC) 031.2
  balnei 031.1
  Battey 031.0
  cutaneous 031.1
  disseminated 031.2
    avium-intracellulare complex (DMAC) 031.2
  fortuitum 031.0
  intracellulare (battey bacillus) 031.0
  kakerifu 031.8
  kansasii 031.0
  kasongo 031.8
  leprae—*see* Leprosy
  luciflavum 031.0

Mycobacterium— *continued*
  marinum 031.1
  pulmonary 031.0
    tuberculous (*see also* Tuberculosis,
      pulmonary) 011.9
  scrofulaceum 031.1
  tuberculosis (human, bovine)—*see also*
    Tuberculosis
  avian type 031.0
  ulcerans 031.1
  xenopi 031.0
Mycosis, mycotic 117.9
  cutaneous NEC 111.9
  ear 111.8 *[380.15]*
  fungoides (M9700/3) 202.1
  mouth 112.0
  pharynx 117.9
  skin NEC 111.9
  stomatitis 112.0
  systemic NEC 117.9
  tonsil 117.9
  vagina, vaginitis 112.1
Mydriasis (persistent) (pupil) 379.43
Myelatelia 742.59
Myelinoclasis, perivascular, acute
    (postinfectious) NEC 136.9 *[323.61]*
  postimmunization or postvaccinal 323.51
Myelinosis, central pontine 341.8
Myelitis (ascending) (cerebellar) (childhood)
    (chronic) (descending) (diffuse) (disseminated)
    (pressure) (progressive) (spinal cord) (subacute)
    (*see also* Encephalitis) 323.9
  acute (transverse) 341.20
    idiopathic 341.22
    in conditions classified elsewhere 341.21
  due to
    infection classified elsewhere 136.9 *[323.42]*
    specified cause NEC 323.82
    vaccination (any) 323.52
    viral diseases classified elsewhere 323.02
  herpes simplex 054.74
  herpes zoster 053.14
  late effect—*see* category 326
  optic neuritis in 341.0
  postchickenpox 052.2
  postimmunization 323.52
  postinfectious 136.9 *[323.63]*
  postvaccinal 323.52
  postvaricella 052.2
  syphilitic (transverse) 094.89
  toxic 989.9 *[323.72]*
  transverse 323.82
    acute 341.20
      idiopathic 341.22
      in conditions classified elsewhere 341.21
    idiopathic 341.22
  tuberculous (*see also* Tuberculosis) 013.6
  virus 049.9
Myeloblastic —*see* condition
Myelocele (*see also* Spina bifida) 741.9
  with hydrocephalus 741.0
Myelocystocele (*see also* Spina bifida) 741.9
Myelocytic —*see* condition
Myelocytoma 205.1
Myelodysplasia (spinal cord) 742.59
  meaning myelodysplastic syndrome—*see*
    Syndrome, myelodysplastic
Myeloencephalitis —*see* Encephalitis

Myelofibrosis 289.83
  with myeloid metaplasia 238.76
  idiopathic (chronic) 238.76
  megakaryocytic 238.79
  primary 238.76
  secondary 289.83
Myelogenous —*see* condition
Myeloid —*see* condition
Myelokathexis 288.09
Myeloleukodystrophy 330.0
Myelolipoma (M8870/0)—*see* Neoplasm, by site,
    benign
Myeloma (multiple) (plasma cell) (plasmacytic)
    (M9730/3) 203.0
  monostotic (M9731/1) 238.6
  solitary (M9731/1) 238.6
Myelomalacia 336.8
Myelomata, multiple (M9730/3) 203.0
Myelomatosis (M9730/3) 203.0
Myelomeningitis —*see* Meningoencephalitis
Myelomeningocele (spinal cord) (*see also* Spina
    bifida) 741.9
  fetal, causing fetopelvic disproportion 653.7
Myelo-osteo-musculodysplasia hereditaria
    756.89
Myelopathic —*see* condition
Myelopathy (spinal cord) 336.9
  cervical 721.1
  diabetic 250.6 *[336.3]*
    due to secondary diabetes 249.6 *[336.3]*
  drug-induced 336.8
  due to or with
    carbon tetrachloride 987.8 *[323.72]*
    degeneration or displacement, intervertebral
      disc 722.70
      cervical, cervicothoracic 722.71
      lumbar, lumbosacral 722.73
      thoracic, thoracolumbar 722.72
    hydroxyquinoline derivatives 961.3 *[323.72]*
    infection—*see* Encephalitis
    intervertebral disc disorder 722.70
      cervical, cervicothoracic 722.71
      lumbar, lumbosacral 722.73
      thoracic, thoracolumbar 722.72
    lead 984.9 *[323.72]*
    mercury 985.0 *[323.72]*
    neoplastic disease (*see also* Neoplasm, by site)
      239.9 *[336.3]*
    pernicious anemia 281.0 *[336.3]*
    spondylosis 721.91
      cervical 721.1
      lumbar, lumbosacral 721.42
      thoracic 721.41
    thallium 985.8 *[323.72]*
  lumbar, lumbosacral 721.42
  necrotic (subacute) 336.1
  radiation-induced 336.8
  spondylogenic NEC 721.91
    cervical 721.1
    lumbar, lumbosacral 721.42
    thoracic 721.41
  thoracic 721.41
  toxic NEC 989.9 *[323.72]*
  transverse (*see also* Myelitis) 323.82
  vascular 336.1
Myelophthisis 284.2
Myeloproliferative disease (M9960/1) 238.79
Myeloradiculitis (*see also* Polyneuropathy) 357.0
Myeloradiculodysplasia (spinal) 742.59
Myelosarcoma (M9930/3) 205.3

Myelosclerosis 289.89
   with myeloid metaplasia (M9961/1) 238.76
   disseminated, of nervous system 340
   megakaryocytic (M9961/1) 238.79
Myelosis (M9860/3) (*see also* Leukemia,
   myeloid) 205.9
   acute (M9861/3) 205.0
   aleukemic (M9864/3) 205.8
   chronic (M9863/3) 205.1
   erythremic (M9840/3) 207.0
      acute (M9841/3) 207.0
   megakaryocytic (M9920/3) 207.2
   nonleukemic (chronic) 288.8
   subacute (M9862/3) 205.2
Myesthenia —*see* Myasthenia
Myiasis (cavernous) 134.0
   orbit 134.0 *[376.13]*
Myoadenoma, prostate 600.20
   with
      other lower urinary tract symptoms (LUTS)
         600.21
      urinary
         obstruction 600.21
         retention 600.21
Myoblastoma
   granular cell (M9580/0)—*see also* Neoplasm,
      connective tissue, benign
   malignant (M9580/3)—*see* Neoplasm,
      connective tissue, malignant
   tongue (M9580/0) 210.1
Myocardial —*see* condition
Myocardiopathy (congestive) (constrictive)
      (familial) (hypertrophic nonobstructive)
      (idiopathic) (infiltrative) (obstructive)
      (primary) (restrictive) (sporadic) 425.4
   alcoholic 425.5
   amyloid 277.39 *[425.7]*
   beriberi 265.0 *[425.7]*
   cobalt-beer 425.5
   due to
      amyloidosis 277.39 *[425.7]*
      beriberi 265.0 *[425.7]*
      cardiac glycogenosis 271.0 *[425.7]*
      Chagas' disease 086.0
      Friedreich's ataxia 334.0 *[425.8]*
      influenza 487.8 *[425.8]*
      mucopolysaccharidosis 277.5 *[425.7]*
      myotonia atrophica 359.21 *[425.8]*
      progressive muscular dystrophy 359.1 *[425.8]*
      sarcoidosis 135 *[425.8]*
   glycogen storage 271.0 *[425.7]*
   hypertrophic obstructive 425.1
   metabolic NEC 277.9 *[425.7]*
   nutritional 269.9 *[425.7]*
   obscure (African) 425.2
   peripartum 674.5
   postpartum 674.5
   secondary 425.9
   thyrotoxic (*see also* Thyrotoxicosis) 242.9
      [425.7]
   toxic NEC 425.9
Myocarditis (fibroid) (interstitial) (old)
      (progressive) (senile) (with arteriosclerosis)
      429.0
   with
      rheumatic fever (conditions classifiable to
         390) 398.0
         active (*see also* Myocarditis, acute,
            rheumatic) 391.2
         inactive or quiescent (with chorea) 398.0

Myocarditis—*continued*
   active (nonrheumatic) 422.90
      rheumatic 391.2
         with chorea (acute) (rheumatic)
            (Sydenham's) 392.0
   acute or subacute (interstitial) 422.90
      due to Streptococcus (beta-hemolytic) 391.2
      idiopathic 422.91
      rheumatic 391.2
         with chorea (acute) (rheumatic)
            (Sydenham's) 392.0
      specified type NEC 422.99
   aseptic of newborn 074.23
   bacterial (acute) 422.92
   chagasic 086.0
   chronic (interstitial) 429.0
   congenital 746.89
   constrictive 425.4
   Coxsackie (virus) 074.23
   diphtheritic 032.82
   due to or in
      Coxsackie (virus) 074.23
      diphtheria 032.82
      epidemic louse-borne typhus 080 *[422.0]*
      influenza 487.8 *[422.0]*
      Lyme disease 088.81 *[422.0]*
      scarlet fever 034.1 *[422.0]*
      toxoplasmosis (acquired) 130.3
      tuberculosis (*see also* Tuberculosis) 017.9
         [422.0]
      typhoid 002.0 *[422.0]*
      typhus NEC 081.9 *[422.0]*
   eosinophilic 422.91
   epidemic of newborn 074.23
   Fiedler's (acute) (isolated) (subacute) 422.91
   giant cell (acute) (subacute) 422.91
   gonococcal 098.85
   granulomatous (idiopathic) (isolated)
      (nonspecific) 422.91
   hypertensive (*see also* Hypertension, heart)
      402.90
   idiopathic 422.91
      granulomatous 422.91
   infective 422.92
   influenzal 487.8 *[422.0]*
   isolated (diffuse) (granulomatous) 422.91
   malignant 422.99
   meningococcal 036.43
   nonrheumatic, active 422.90
   parenchymatous 422.90
   pneumococcal (acute) (subacute) 422.92
   rheumatic (chronic) (inactive) (with chorea)
      398.0
      active or acute 391.2
         with chorea (acute) (rheumatic)
            (Sydenham's) 392.0
   septic 422.92
   specific (giant cell) (productive) 422.91
   staphylococcal (acute) (subacute) 422.92
   suppurative 422.92
   syphilitic (chronic) 093.82
   toxic 422.93
      rheumatic (*see also* Myocarditis, acute
         rheumatic) 391.2
   tuberculous (*see also* Tuberculosis) 017.9
      [422.0]
   typhoid 002.0 *[422.0]*
   valvular—*see* Endocarditis
   viral, except Coxsackie 422.91
      Coxsackie 074.23
      of newborn (Coxsackie) 074.23

Myocardium, myocardial —*see* condition
Myocardosis (*see also* Cardiomyopathy) 425.4
Myoclonia (essential) 333.2
  epileptica 345.1
  Friedrich's 333.2
  massive 333.2
Myoclonic
  epilepsy, familial (progressive) 345.1
  jerks 333.2
Myoclonus (familial essential) (multifocal)
  (simplex) 333.2
  with epilepsy and with ragged red fibers
    (MERRF syndrome) 277.87
  facial 351.8
  massive (infantile) 333.2
  palatal 333.2
  pharyngeal 333.2
Myocytolysis 429.1
Myodiastasis 728.84
Myoendocarditis —*see also* Endocarditis
  acute or subacute 421.9
Myoepithelioma (M8982/0)—*see* Neoplasm, by
  site, benign
Myofascitis (acute) 729.1
  low back 724.2
Myofibroma (M8890/0)—*see also* Neoplasm,
  connective tissue, benign
  uterus (cervix) (corpus) (*see also* Leiomyoma)
    218.9
Myofibromatosis
  infantile 759.89
Myofibrosis 728.2
  heart (*see also* Myocarditis) 429.0
  humeroscapular region 726.2
  scapulohumeral 726.2
Myofibrositis (*see also* Myositis) 729.1
  scapulohumeral 726.2
Myogelosis (occupational) 728.89
Myoglobinuria 791.3
Myoglobulinuria, primary 791.3
Myokymia —*see also* Myoclonus
  facial 351.8
Myolipoma (M8860/0)
  specified site—*see* Neoplasm, connective tissue,
    benign
  unspecified site 223.0
Myoma (M8895/0)—*see also* Neoplasm,
  connective tissue, benign
  cervix (stump) (uterus) (*see also* Leiomyoma)
    218.9
  malignant (M8895/3)—*see* Neoplasm,
    connective tissue, malignant
  prostate 600.20
    with
      other lower urinary tract symptoms (LUTS)
        600.21
      urinary
        obstruction 600.21
        retention 600.21
  uterus (cervix) (corpus) (*see also* Leiomyoma)
    218.9
    in pregnancy or childbirth 654.1
      affecting fetus or newborn 763.89
      causing obstructed labor 660.2
        affecting fetus or newborn 763.1
Myomalacia 728.9
  cordis, heart (*see also* Degeneration,
    myocardial) 429.1
Myometritis (*see also* Endometritis) 615.9
Myometrium —*see* condition
Myonecrosis, clostridial 040.0

Myopathy 359.9
  alcoholic 359.4
  amyloid 277.39 *[359.6]*
  benign congenital 359.0
  central core 359.0
  centronuclear 359.0
  congenital (benign) 359.0
  critical illness 359.81
  distal 359.1
  due to drugs 359.4
  endocrine 259.9 *[359.5]*
    specified type NEC 259.8 *[359.5]*
  extraocular muscles 376.82
  facioscapulohumeral 359.1
  in
    Addison's disease 255.41 *[359.5]*
    amyloidosis 277.39 *[359.6]*
    cretinism 243 *[359.5]*
    Cushing's syndrome 255.0 *[359.5]*
    disseminated lupus erythematosus 710.0 *[359.6]*
    giant cell arteritis 446.5 *[359.6]*
    hyperadrenocorticism NEC 255.3 *[359.5]*
    hyperparathyroidism 252.01 *[359.5]*
    hypopituitarism 253.2 *[359.5]*
    hypothyroidism (*see also* Hypothyroidism)
      244.9 *[359.5]*
    malignant neoplasm NEC (M8000/3) 199.1
      [359.6]
    myxedema (*see also* Myxedema) 244.9 *[359.5]*
    polyarteritis nodosa 446.0 *[359.6]*
    rheumatoid arthritis 714.0 *[359.6]*
    sarcoidosis 135 *[359.6]*
    scleroderma 710.1 *[359.6]*
    Sjögren's disease 710.2 *[359.6]*
    thyrotoxicosis (*see also* Thyrotoxicosis) 242.9
      [359.5]
  inflammatory 359.79
    immune NEC 359.79
    specified NEC 359.79
  intensive care (ICU) 359.81
  limb-girdle 359.1
  myotubular 359.0
  necrotizing, acute 359.81
  nemaline 359.0
  ocular 359.1
  oculopharyngeal 359.1
  of critical illness 359.81
  primary 359.89
  progressive NEC 359.89
  proximal myotonic (PROMM) 359.21
  quadriplegic, acute 359.81
  rod body 359.0
  scapulohumeral 359.1
  specified type NEC 359.89
  toxic 359.4
Myopericarditis (*see also* Pericarditis) 423.9
Myopia (axial) (congenital) (increased curvature
  or refraction, nucleus of lens) 367.1
  degenerative, malignant 360.21
  malignant 360.21
  progressive high (degenerative) 360.21
Myosarcoma (M8895/3)—*see* Neoplasm,
  connective tissue, malignant
Myosis (persistent) 379.42
  stromal (endolymphatic) (M8931/1) 236.0
Myositis 729.1
  clostridial 040.0
  due to posture 729.1
  epidemic 074.1
  fibrosa or fibrous (chronic) 728.2
    Volkmann's (complicating trauma) 958.6

Myositis—*continued*
  inclusion body (IBM) 359.71
  infective 728.0
  interstitial 728.81
  multiple—*see* Polymyositis
  occupational 729.1
  orbital, chronic 376.12
  ossificans 728.12
    circumscribed 728.12
    progressive 728.11
    traumatic 728.12
  progressive fibrosing 728.11
  purulent 728.0
  rheumatic 729.1
  rheumatoid 729.1
  suppurative 728.0
  syphilitic 095.6
  traumatic (old) 729.1
Myospasia impulsiva 307.23
Myotonia (acquisita) (intermittens) 728.85
  atrophica 359.21
  congenita 359.22
    acetazolamide responsive 359.22
    dominant form 359.22
    recessive form 359.22
  drug-induced 359.24
  dystrophica 359.21
  fluctuans 359.29
  levior 359.22
  permanens 359.29
Myotonic pupil 379.46
Myriapodiasis 134.1
Myringitis
  with otitis media—*see* Otitis media
  acute 384.00
    specified type NEC 384.09
  bullosa hemorrhagica 384.01
  bullous 384.01
  chronic 384.1
Mysophobia 300.29
Mytilotoxism 988.0
Myxadenitis labialis 528.5
Myxedema (adult) (idiocy) (infantile) (juvenile)
    (thyroid gland) (*see also* Hypothyroidism)
    244.9
  circumscribed 242.9
  congenital 243
  cutis 701.8
  localized (pretibial) 242.9
  madness (acute) 293.0
    subacute 293.1
  papular 701.8
  pituitary 244.8
  postpartum 674.8
  pretibial 242.9
  primary 244.9
Myxochondrosarcoma (M9220/3)—*see*
    Neoplasm, cartilage, malignant
Myxofibroma (M8811/0)—*see also* Neoplasm,
    connective tissue, benign
  odontogenic (M9320/0) 213.1
  upper jaw (bone) 213.0
Myxofibrosarcoma (M8811/3)—*see* Neoplasm,
    connective tissue, malignant
Myxolipoma (M8852/0) (*see also* Lipoma, by
    site) 214.9
Myxoliposarcoma (M8852/3)—*see* Neoplasm,
    connective tissue, malignant

Myxoma (M8840/0)—*see also* Neoplasm,
    connective tissue, benign
  odontogenic (M9320/0) 213.1
  upper jaw (bone) 213.0
Myxosarcoma (M8840/3)—*see* Neoplasm,
    connective tissue, malignant

N

Naegeli's
disease (hereditary hemorrhagic thrombasthenia) 287.1
leukemia, monocytic (M9863/3) 205.1
syndrome (incontinentia pigmenti) 757.33
Naffziger's syndrome 353.0
Naga sore (*see also* Ulcer, skin) 707.9
Nägele's pelvis 738.6
with disproportion (fetopelvic) 653.0
affecting fetus or newborn 763.1
causing obstructed labor 660.1
affecting fetus or newborn 763.1
Nager-de Reynier syndrome (dysostosis mandibularis) 756.0
Nail —*see also* condition
biting 307.9
patella syndrome (hereditary osteo-onychodysplasia) 756.89
Nanism, nanosomia (*see also* Dwarfism) 259.4
hypophyseal 253.3
pituitary 253.3
renis, renalis 588.0
Nanukayami 100.89
Napkin rash 691.0
Narcissism 301.81
Narcolepsy 347.00
with cataplexy 347.01
in conditions classified elsewhere 347.10
with cataplexy 347.11
Narcosis
carbon dioxide (respiratory) 786.09
due to drug
correct substance properly administered 780.09
overdose or wrong substance given or taken 977.9
specified drug—*see* Table of drugs and chemicals
Narcotism (chronic) (*see also* listing under Dependence) 304.9
acute
correct substance properly administered 349.82
overdose or wrong substance given or taken 967.8
specified drug—*see* Table of drugs and chemicals
NARP syndrome (Neuropathy, ataxia and retinitis pigmentosa) 277.87
Narrow
anterior chamber angle 365.02
pelvis (inlet) (outlet)—*see* Contraction, pelvis
Narrowing
artery NEC 447.1
auditory, internal 433.8
basilar 433.0
with other precerebral artery 433.3
bilateral 433.3
carotid 433.1
with other precerebral artery 433.3
bilateral 433.3
cerebellar 433.8
choroidal 433.8
communicating posterior 433.8
coronary —*see also* Arteriosclerosis, coronary
congenital 746.85
due to syphilis 090.5
hypophyseal 433.8
pontine 433.8

Narrowing—*continued*
precerebral NEC 433.9
multiple or bilateral 433.3
specified NEC 433.8
vertebral 433.2
with other precerebral artery 433.3
bilateral 433.3
auditory canal (external) (*see also* Stricture, ear canal, acquired) 380.50
cerebral arteries 437.0
cicatricial—*see* Cicatrix
congenital—*see* Anomaly, congenital
coronary artery—*see* Narrowing, artery, coronary
ear, middle 385.22
Eustachian tube (*see also* Obstruction, Eustachian tube) 381.60
eyelid 374.46
congenital 743.62
intervertebral disc or space NEC—*see* Degeneration, intervertebral disc
joint space, hip 719.85
larynx 478.74
lids 374.46
congenital 743.62
mesenteric artery (with gangrene) 557.0
palate 524.89
palpebral fissure 374.46
retinal artery 362.13
ureter 593.3
urethra (*see also* Stricture, urethra) 598.9
Narrowness, abnormal, eyelid 743.62
Nasal —*see* condition
Nasolacrimal —*see* condition
Nasopharyngeal —*see also* condition
bursa 478.29
pituitary gland 759.2
torticollis 723.5
Nasopharyngitis (acute) (infective) (subacute) 460
chronic 472.2
due to external agent—*see* Condition, respiratory, chronic, due to
due to external agent—*see* Condition, respiratory, due to
septic 034.0
streptococcal 034.0
suppurative (chronic) 472.2
ulcerative (chronic) 472.2
Nasopharynx, nasopharyngeal —*see* condition
Natal tooth, teeth 520.6
Nausea (*see also* Vomiting) 787.02
epidemic 078.82
gravidarum—*see* Hyperemesis, gravidarum
marina 994.6
with vomiting 787.01
Naval —*see* condition
Neapolitan fever (*see also* Brucellosis) 023.9
Near drowning 994.1
Nearsightedness 367.1
Near-syncope 780.2
Nebécourt's syndrome 253.3
Nebula, cornea (eye) 371.01
congenital 743.43
interfering with vision 743.42
Necator americanus infestation 126.1
Necatoriasis 126.1
Neck —*see* condition
Necrencephalus (*see also* Softening, brain) 437.8

Necrobacillosis 040.3
Necrobiosis 799.89
  brain or cerebral (*see also* Softening, brain) 437.8
  lipoidica 709.3
    diabeticorum 250.8 *[709.3]*
      due to secondary diabetes 249.8 *[709.3]*
Necrodermolysis 695.15
Necrolysis, toxic epidermal 695.15
  due to drug
    correct substance properly administered 695.15
    overdose or wrong substance given or taken
      977.9
      specified drug—*see* Table of drugs and
        chemicals
  Stevens-Johnson syndrome overlap (SJS-TEN
    overlap syndrome) 695.14
Necrophilia 302.89
Necrosis, necrotic
  adrenal (capsule) (gland) 255.8
  antrum, nasal sinus 478.19
  aorta (hyaline) (*see also* Aneurysm, aorta) 441.9
    cystic medial 441.00
      abdominal 441.02
      thoracic 441.01
      thoracoabdominal 441.03
    ruptured 441.5
  arteritis 446.0
  artery 447.5
  aseptic, bone 733.40
    femur (head) (neck) 733.42
      medial condyle 733.43
    humoral head 733.41
    jaw 733.45
    medial femoral condyle 733.43
    specified site NEC 733.49
    talus 733.44
  avascular, bone NEC (*see also* Necrosis, aseptic,
    bone) 733.40
  bladder (aseptic) (sphincter) 596.8
  bone (*see also* Osteomyelitis) 730.1
    acute 730.0
    aseptic or avascular 733.40
      femur (head) (neck) 733.42
        medial condyle 733.43
      humoral head 733.41
      jaw 733.45
      medial femoral condyle 733.43
      specified site NEC 733.49
      talus 733.44
    ethmoid 478.19
    ischemic 733.40
    jaw 526.4
      aseptic 733.45
    marrow 289.89
    Paget's (osteitis deformans) 731.0
    tuberculous—*see* Tuberculosis, bone
  brain (softening) (*see also* Softening, brain) 437.8
  breast (aseptic) (fat) (segmental) 611.3
  bronchus, bronchi 519.19
  central nervous system NEC (*see also*
    Softening, brain) 437.8
  cerebellar (*see also* Softening, brain) 437.8
  cerebral (softening) (*see also* Softening, brain) 437.8
  cerebrospinal (softening) (*see also* Softening,
    brain) 437.8
  colon 557.0
  cornea (*see also* Keratitis) 371.40
  cortical, kidney 583.6
  cystic medial (aorta) 441.00
    abdominal 441.02
    thoracic 441.01
    thoracoabdominal 441.03

Necrosis, necrotic—*continued*
  dental 521.09
    pulp 522.1
  due to swallowing corrosive substance—*see*
    Burn, by site
  ear (ossicle) 385.24
  esophagus 530.89
  ethmoid (bone) 478.19
  eyelid 374.50
  fat, fatty (generalized) (*see also* Degeneration,
    fatty) 272.8
    abdominal wall 567.82
    breast (aseptic) (segmental) 611.3
    intestine 569.89
    localized—*see* Degeneration, by site, fatty
    mesentery 567.82
    omentum 567.82
    pancreas 577.8
    peritoneum 567.82
    skin (subcutaneous) 709.3
      newborn 778.1
  femur (aseptic) (avascular) 733.42
    head 733.42
    medial condyle 733.43
    neck 733.42
  gallbladder (*see also* Cholecystitis, acute) 575.0
  gangrenous 785.4
  gastric 537.89
  glottis 478.79
  heart (myocardium)—*see* Infarct, myocardium
  hepatic (*see also* Necrosis, liver) 570
  hip (aseptic) (avascular) 733.42
  intestine (acute) (hemorrhagic) (massive) 557.0
  ischemic 785.4
  jaw 526.4
    aseptic 733.45
  kidney (bilateral) 583.9
    acute 584.9
    cortical 583.6
      acute 584.6
      with
        abortion—*see* Abortion, by type, with
          renal failure
        ectopic pregnancy (*see also* categories
          633.0-633.9) 639.3
        molar pregnancy (*see also* categories
          630-632) 639.3
      complicating pregnancy 646.2
      affecting fetus or newborn 760.1
      following labor and delivery 669.3
    medullary (papillary) (*see also* Pyelitis) 590.80
      in
        acute renal failure 584.7
        nephritis, nephropathy 583.7
    papillary (*see also* Pyelitis) 590.80
      in
        acute renal failure 584.7
        nephritis, nephropathy 583.7
    tubular 584.5
      with
        abortion—*see* Abortion, by type, with
          renal failure
        ectopic pregnancy (*see also* categories
          633.0-633.9) 639.3
        molar pregnancy (*see also* categories
          630-632) 639.3
      complicating
        abortion 639.3
        ectopic or molar pregnancy 639.3
        pregnancy 646.2
          affecting fetus or newborn 760.1

Necrosis, necrotic—*continued*
kidney—*continued*
tubular—*continued*
following labor and delivery 669.3
traumatic 958.5
larynx 478.79
liver (acute) (congenital) (diffuse) (massive)
(subacute) 570
with
abortion—*see* Abortion, by type, with
specified complication NEC
ectopic pregnancy (*see also* categories
633.0-633.9) 639.8
molar pregnancy (*see also* categories
630-632) 639.8
complicating pregnancy 646.7
affecting fetus or newborn 760.8
following
abortion 639.8
ectopic or molar pregnancy 639.8
obstetrical 646.7
postabortal 639.8
puerperal, postpartum 674.8
toxic 573.3
lung 513.0
lymphatic gland 683
mammary gland 611.3
mastoid (chronic) 383.1
mesentery 557.0
fat 567.82
mitral valve—*see* Insufficiency, mitral
myocardium, myocardial—*see* Infarct,
myocardium
nose (septum) 478.19
omentum 557.0
with mesenteric infarction 557.0
fat 567.82
orbit, orbital 376.10
ossicles, ear (aseptic) 385.24
ovary (*see also* Salpingo-oophoritis) 614.2
pancreas (aseptic) (duct) (fat) 577.8
acute 577.0
infective 577.0
papillary, kidney (*see also* Pyelitis) 590.80
perineum 624.8
peritoneum 557.0
with mesenteric infarction 557.0
fat 567.82
pharynx 462
in granulocytopenia 288.09
phosphorus 983.9
pituitary (gland) (postpartum) (Sheehan) 253.2
placenta (*see also* Placenta, abnormal) 656.7
pneumonia 513.0
pulmonary 513.0
pulp (dental) 522.1
pylorus 537.89
radiation—*see* Necrosis, by site
radium—*see* Necrosis, by site
renal—*see* Necrosis, kidney
sclera 379.19
scrotum 608.89
skin or subcutaneous tissue 709.8
due to burn—*see* Burn, by site
gangrenous 785.4
spine, spinal (column) 730.18
acute 730.18
cord 336.1
spleen 289.59
stomach 537.89
stomatitis 528.1

Necrosis, necrotic—*continued*
subcutaneous fat 709.3
fetus or newborn 778.1
subendocardial—*see* Infarct, myocardium
suprarenal (capsule) (gland) 255.8
teeth, tooth 521.09
testis 608.89
thymus (gland) 254.8
tonsil 474.8
trachea 519.19
tuberculous NEC—*see* Tuberculosis
tubular (acute) (anoxic) (toxic) 584.5
due to a procedure 997.5
umbilical cord, affecting fetus or newborn 762.6
vagina 623.8
vertebra (lumbar) 730.18
acute 730.18
tuberculous (*see also* Tuberculosis) 015.0 *[730.8]*
vesical (aseptic) (bladder) 596.8
vulva 624.8
x-ray—*see* Necrosis, by site
Necrospermia 606.0
Necrotizing angiitis 446.0
Negativism 301.7
Neglect (child) (newborn) NEC 995.52
adult 995.84
after or at birth 995.52
hemispatial 781.8
left-sided 781.8
sensory 781.8
visuospatial 781.8
Negri bodies 071
Neill-Dingwall syndrome (microcephaly and
dwarfism) 759.89
Neisserian infection NEC—*see* Gonococcus
Nematodiasis NEC (*see also* Infestation,
Nematode) 127.9
ancylostoma (*see also* Ancylostomiasis) 126.9
Neoformans cryptococcus infection 117.5
Neonatal —*see also* condition
abstinence syndrome 779.5
adrenoleukodystrophy 277.86
teeth, tooth 520.6
Neonatorum —*see* condition
Neoplasia
anal intraepithelial I [AIN I] (histologically
confirmed) 569.44
anal intraepithelial II [AIN II] (histologically
confirmed) 569.44
anal intraepithelial III [AIN III] 230.6
anal canal 230.5
endometrial intraepithelial [EIN] 621.35
multiple endocrine [MEN]
type I 258.01
type II A 258.02
type II B 258.03
vaginal intraepithelial I [VAIN I] 623.0
vaginal intraepithelial II [VAIN II] 623.0
vaginal intraepithelial III [VAIN III] 233.31
vulvar intraepithelial I [VIN I] 624.01
vulvar intraepithelial II [VIN II] 624.02
vulvar intraepithelial III [VIN III] 233.32

*"N" listing resumes after
"Neoplasm, neoplastic" table...*

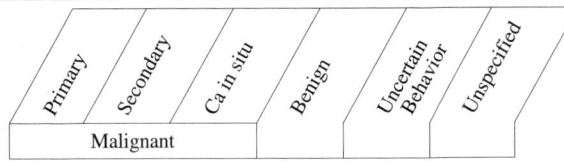

	Malignant				
	Primary	Secondary	Ca in situ	Benign	Uncertain Behavior	Unspecified

Neoplasm, neoplastic	199.1	199.1	234.9	229.9	238.9	239.9

Note—1. The list below gives the code numbers for neoplasms by anatomical site. For each site there are six possible code numbers according to whether the neoplasm in question is malignant, benign, in situ, of uncertain behavior, or of unspecified nature. The description of the neoplasm will often indicate which of the six columns is appropriate; e.g., malignant melanoma of skin, benign fibroadenoma of breast, carcinoma in situ of cervix uteri.

Where such descriptors are not present, the remainder of the Index should be consulted where guidance is given to the appropriate column for each morphological (histological) variety listed; e.g., Mesonephroma—see Neoplasm, malignant; Embryoma—see also Neoplasm, uncertain behavior; Disease, Bowen's—see Neoplasm, skin, in situ. However, the guidance in the Index can be overridden if one of the descriptors mentioned above is present; e.g., malignant adenoma of colon is coded to 153.9 and not to 211.3 as the adjective "malignant" overrides the Index entry "Adenoma—see also Neoplasm, benign."

Note—2. Sites marked with the sign * (e.g., face NEC*) should be classified to malignant neoplasm of skin of these sites if the variety of neoplasm is a squamous cell carcinoma or an epidermoid carcinoma and to benign neoplasm of skin of these sites if the variety of neoplasm is a papilloma (any type).

abdomen, abdominal 195.2	198.89	234.8	229.8	238.8	239.89
cavity. 195.2	198.89	234.8	229.8	238.8	239.89
organ 195.2	198.89	234.8	229.8	238.8	239.89
viscera 195.2	198.89	234.8	229.8	238.8	239.89
wall. 173.5	198.2	232.5	216.5	238.2	239.2
connective tissue 171.5	198.89	—	215.5	238.1	239.2
abdominopelvic 195.8	198.89	234.8	229.8	238.8	239.89
accessory sinus—*see* Neoplasm, sinus					
acoustic nerve 192.0	198.4	—	225.1	237.9	239.7
acromion (process) 170.4	198.5	—	213.4	238.0	239.2
adenoid (pharynx) (tissue) 147.1	198.89	230.0	210.7	235.1	239.0
adipose tissue (*see also* Neoplasm,					
connective tissue) 171.9	198.89	—	215.9	238.1	239.2
adnexa (uterine) 183.9	198.82	233.39	221.8	236.3	239.5
adrenal (cortex) (gland)					
(medulla) 194.0	198.7	234.8	227.0	237.2	239.7
ala nasi (external) 173.3	198.2	232.3	216.3	238.2	239.2
alimentary canal or					
tract NEC 159.9	197.8	230.9	211.9	235.5	239.0
alveolar. 143.9	198.89	230.0	210.4	235.1	239.0
mucosa 143.9	198.89	230.0	210.4	235.1	239.0
lower 143.1	198.89	230.0	210.4	235.1	239.0
upper 143.0	198.89	230.0	210.4	235.1	239.0
ridge or process 170.1	198.5	—	213.1	238.0	239.2
carcinoma 143.9	—	—	—	—	—
lower 143.1	—	—	—	—	—
upper 143.0	—	—	—	—	—
lower 170.1	198.5	—	213.1	238.0	239.2
mucosa 143.9	198.89	230.0	210.4	235.1	239.0
lower 143.1	198.89	230.0	210.4	235.1	239.0
upper 143.0	198.89	230.0	210.4	235.1	239.0
upper 170.0	198.5	—	213.0	238.0	239.2
sulcus. 145.1	198.89	230.0	210.4	235.1	239.0
alveolus. 143.9	198.89	230.0	210.4	235.1	239.0
lower 143.1	198.89	230.0	210.4	235.1	239.0
upper 143.0	198.89	230.0	210.4	235.1	239.0
ampulla of Vater 156.2	197.8	230.8	211.5	235.3	239.0
ankle NEC* 195.5	198.89	232.7	229.8	238.8	239.89
anorectum, anorectal					
(junction) 154.8	197.5	230.7	211.4	235.2	239.0
antecubital fossa or space*. 195.4	198.89	232.6	229.8	238.8	239.89
antrum (Highmore)					
(maxillary) 160.2	197.3	231.8	212.0	235.9	239.1

| | Malignant | | | | | |
	Primary	Secondary	Ca in situ	Benign	Uncertain Behavior	Unspecified
pyloric	151.2	197.8	230.2	211.1	235.2	239.0
tympanicum	160.1	197.3	231.8	212.0	235.9	239.1
anus, anal	154.3	197.5	230.6	211.4	235.5	239.0
canal	154.2	197.5	230.5	211.4	235.5	239.0
contiguous sites with rectosigmoid junction or rectum	154.8	—	—	—	—	—
margin	173.5	198.2	232.5	216.5	238.2	239.2
skin	173.5	198.2	232.5	216.5	238.2	239.2
sphincter	154.2	197.5	230.5	211.4	235.5	239.0
aorta (thoracic)	171.4	198.89	—	215.4	238.1	239.2
abdominal	171.5	198.89	—	215.5	238.1	239.2
aortic body	194.6	198.89	—	227.6	237.3	239.7
aponeurosis	171.9	198.89	—	215.9	238.1	239.2
palmar	171.2	198.89	—	215.2	238.1	239.2
plantar	171.3	198.89	—	215.3	238.1	239.2
appendix	153.5	197.5	230.3	211.3	235.2	239.0
arachnoid (cerebral)	192.1	198.4	—	225.2	237.6	239.7
spinal	192.3	198.4	—	225.4	237.6	239.7
areola (female)	174.0	198.81	233.0	217	238.3	239.3
male	175.0	198.81	233.0	217	238.3	239.3
arm NEC*	195.4	198.89	232.6	229.8	238.8	239.89
artery—*see* Neoplasm, connective tissue						
aryepiglottic fold	148.2	198.89	230.0	210.8	235.1	239.0
hypopharyngeal aspect	148.2	198.89	230.0	210.8	235.1	239.0
laryngeal aspect	161.1	197.3	231.0	212.1	235.6	239.1
marginal zone	148.2	198.89	230.0	210.8	235.1	239.0
arytenoid (cartilage)	161.3	197.3	231.0	212.1	235.6	239.1
fold—*see* Neoplasm, aryepiglottic						
associated with transplanted organ	199.2	—		—	—	—
atlas	170.2	198.5	—	213.2	238.0	239.2
atrium, cardiac	164.1	198.89	—	212.7	238.8	239.89
auditory						
canal (external) (skin)	173.2	198.2	232.2	216.2	238.2	239.2
internal	160.1	197.3	231.8	212.0	235.9	239.1
nerve	192.0	198.4	—	225.1	237.9	239.7
tube	160.1	197.3	231.8	212.0	235.9	239.1
opening	147.2	198.89	230.0	210.7	235.1	239.0
auricle, ear	173.2	198.2	232.2	216.2	238.2	239.2
cartilage	171.0	198.89	—	215.0	238.1	239.2
auricular canal (external)	173.2	198.2	232.2	216.2	238.2	239.2
internal	160.1	197.3	231.8	212.0	235.9	239.1
autonomic nerve or nervous system NEC	171.9	198.89	—	215.9	238.1	239.2
axilla, axillary	195.1	198.89	234.8	229.8	238.8	239.89
fold	173.5	198.2	232.5	216.5	238.2	239.2
back NEC*	195.8	198.89	232.5	229.8	238.8	239.89
Bartholin's gland	184.1	198.82	233.32	221.2	236.3	239.5
basal ganglia	191.0	198.3	—	225.0	237.5	239.6
basis pedunculi	191.7	198.3	—	225.0	237.5	239.6
bile or biliary (tract)	156.9	197.8	230.8	211.5	235.3	239.0
canaliculi (biliferi) (intrahepatic)	155.1	197.8	230.8	211.5	235.3	239.0
canals, interlobular	155.1	197.8	230.8	211.5	235.3	239.0
contiguous sites	156.8	—	—	—	—	—
duct or passage (common) (cyst) (extrahepatic)	156.1	197.8	230.8	211.5	235.3	239.0
contiguous sites with gallbladder	156.8	—	—	—	—	—
interlobular	155.1	197.8	230.8	211.5	235.3	239.0
intrahepatic	155.1	197.8	230.8	211.5	235.3	239.0
and extrahepatic	156.9	197.8	230.8	211.5	235.3	239.0
bladder (urinary)	188.9	198.1	233.7	223.3	236.7	239.4
contiguous sites	188.8	—	—	—	—	—

| | Malignant | | | | |
	Primary	Secondary	Ca in situ	Benign	Uncertain Behavior	Unspecified
dome	188.1	198.1	233.7	223.3	236.7	239.4
neck	188.5	198.1	233.7	223.3	236.7	239.4
orifice	188.9	198.1	233.7	223.3	236.7	239.4
ureteric	188.6	198.1	233.7	223.3	236.7	239.4
urethral	188.5	198.1	233.7	223.3	236.7	239.4
sphincter	188.8	198.1	233.7	223.3	236.7	239.4
trigone	188.0	198.1	233.7	223.3	236.7	239.4
urachus	188.7	—	233.7	223.3	236.7	239.4
wall	188.9	198.1	233.7	223.3	236.7	239.4
anterior	188.3	198.1	233.7	223.3	236.7	239.4
lateral	188.2	198.1	233.7	223.3	236.7	239.4
posterior	188.4	198.1	233.7	223.3	236.7	239.4
blood vessel—*see* Neoplasm, connective tissue						
bone (periosteum)	170.9	198.5	—	213.9	238.0	239.2

Note—*Carcinomas and adenocarcinomas, of any type other than intraosseous or odontogenic, of the sites listed under "Neoplasm, bone" should be considered as constituting metastatic spread from an unspecified primary site and coded to 198.5 for morbidity coding .*

| | Malignant | | | | |
	Primary	Secondary	Ca in situ	Benign	Uncertain Behavior	Unspecified
acetabulum	170.6	198.5	—	213.6	238.0	239.2
acromion (process)	170.4	198.5	—	213.4	238.0	239.2
ankle	170.8	198.5	—	213.8	238.0	239.2
arm NEC	170.4	198.5	—	213.4	238.0	239.2
astragalus	170.8	198.5	—	213.8	238.0	239.2
atlas	170.2	198.5	—	213.2	238.0	239.2
axis	170.2	198.5	—	213.2	238.0	239.2
back NEC	170.2	198.5	—	213.2	238.0	239.2
calcaneus	170.8	198.5	—	213.8	238.0	239.2
calvarium	170.0	198.5	—	213.0	238.0	239.2
carpus (any)	170.5	198.5	—	213.5	238.0	239.2
cartilage NEC	170.9	198.5	—	213.9	238.0	239.2
clavicle	170.3	198.5	—	213.3	238.0	239.2
clivus	170.0	198.5	—	213.0	238.0	239.2
coccygeal vertebra	170.6	198.5	—	213.6	238.0	239.2
coccyx	170.6	198.5	—	213.6	238.0	239.2
costal cartilage	170.3	198.5	—	213.3	238.0	239.2
costovertebral joint	170.3	198.5	—	213.3	238.0	239.2
cranial	170.0	198.5	—	213.0	238.0	239.2
cuboid	170.8	198.5	—	213.8	238.0	239.2
cuneiform	170.9	198.5	—	213.9	238.0	239.2
ankle	170.8	198.5	—	213.8	238.0	239.2
wrist	170.5	198.5	—	213.5	238.0	239.2
digital	170.9	198.5	—	213.9	238.0	239.2
finger	170.5	198.5	—	213.5	238.0	239.2
toe	170.8	198.5	—	213.8	238.0	239.2
elbow	170.4	198.5	—	213.4	238.0	239.2
ethmoid (labyrinth)	170.0	198.5	—	213.0	238.0	239.2
face	170.0	198.5	—	213.0	238.0	239.2
lower jaw	170.1	198.5	—	213.1	238.0	239.2
femur (any part)	170.7	198.5	—	213.7	238.0	239.2
fibula (any part)	170.7	198.5	—	213.7	238.0	239.2
finger (any)	170.5	198.5	—	213.5	238.0	239.2
foot	170.8	198.5	—	213.8	238.0	239.2
forearm	170.4	198.5	—	213.4	238.0	239.2
frontal	170.0	198.5	—	213.0	238.0	239.2
hand	170.5	198.5	—	213.5	238.0	239.2
heel	170.8	198.5	—	213.8	238.0	239.2
hip	170.6	198.5	—	213.6	238.0	239.2
humerus (any part)	170.4	198.5	—	213.4	238.0	239.2
hyoid	170.0	198.5	—	213.0	238.0	239.2
ilium	170.6	198.5	—	213.6	238.0	239.2
innominate	170.6	198.5	—	213.6	238.0	239.2
intervertebral cartilage or disc	170.2	198.5	—	213.2	238.0	239.2

	Malignant			Benign	Uncertain Behavior	Unspecified
	Primary	Secondary	Ca in situ			
ischium.	170.6	198.5	—	213.6	238.0	239.2
jaw (lower).	170.1	198.5	—	213.1	238.0	239.2
upper	170.0	198.5	—	213.0	238.0	239.2
knee	170.7	198.5	—	213.7	238.0	239.2
leg NEC	170.7	198.5	—	213.7	238.0	239.2
limb NEC.	170.9	198.5	—	213.9	238.0	239.2
lower (long bones)	170.7	198.5	—	213.7	238.0	239.2
short bones	170.8	198.5	—	213.8	238.0	239.2
upper (long bones)	170.4	198.5	—	213.4	238.0	239.2
short bones	170.5	198.5	—	213.5	238.0	239.2
long.	170.9	198.5	—	213.9	238.0	239.2
lower limbs NEC.	170.7	198.5	—	213.7	238.0	239.2
upper limbs NEC.	170.4	198.5	—	213.4	238.0	239.2
malar	170.0	198.5	—	213.0	238.0	239.2
mandible	170.1	198.5	—	213.1	238.0	239.2
marrow NEC.	202.9	198.5	—	—	—	238.79
mastoid.	170.0	198.5	—	213.0	238.0	239.2
maxilla, maxillary (superior)	170.0	198.5	—	213.0	238.0	239.2
inferior	170.1	198.5	—	213.1	238.0	239.2
metacarpus (any).	170.5	198.5	—	213.5	238.0	239.2
metatarsus (any)	170.8	198.5	—	213.8	238.0	239.2
navicular (ankle)	170.8	198.5	—	213.8	238.0	239.2
hand	170.5	198.5	—	213.5	238.0	239.2
nose, nasal	170.0	198.5	—	213.0	238.0	239.2
occipital	170.0	198.5	—	213.0	238.0	239.2
orbit	170.0	198.5	—	213.0	238.0	239.2
parietal	170.0	198.5	—	213.0	238.0	239.2
patella	170.8	198.5	—	213.8	238.0	239.2
pelvic	170.6	198.5	—	213.6	238.0	239.2
phalanges.	170.9	198.5	—	213.9	238.0	239.2
foot.	170.8	198.5	—	213.8	238.0	239.2
hand	170.5	198.5	—	213.5	238.0	239.2
pubic	170.6	198.5	—	213.6	238.0	239.2
radius (any part)	170.4	198.5	—	213.4	238.0	239.2
rib.	170.3	198.5	—	213.3	238.0	239.2
sacral vertebra	170.6	198.5	—	213.6	238.0	239.2
sacrum	170.6	198.5	—	213.6	238.0	239.2
scaphoid (of hand)	170.5	198.5	—	213.5	238.0	239.2
of ankle.	170.8	198.5	—	213.8	238.0	239.2
scapula (any part)	170.4	198.5	—	213.4	238.0	239.2
sella turcica.	170.0	198.5	—	213.0	238.0	239.2
short	170.9	198.5	—	213.9	238.0	239.2
lower limb	170.8	198.5	—	213.8	238.0	239.2
upper limb	170.5	198.5	—	213.5	238.0	239.2
shoulder	170.4	198.5	—	213.4	238.0	239.2
skeleton, skeletal NEC.	170.9	198.5	—	213.9	238.0	239.2
skull	170.0	198.5	—	213.0	238.0	239.2
sphenoid	170.0	198.5	—	213.0	238.0	239.2
spine, spinal (column)	170.2	198.5	—	213.2	238.0	239.2
coccyx	170.6	198.5	—	213.6	238.0	239.2
sacrum	170.6	198.5	—	213.6	238.0	239.2
sternum.	170.3	198.5	—	213.3	238.0	239.2
tarsus (any).	170.8	198.5	—	213.8	238.0	239.2
temporal	170.0	198.5	—	213.0	238.0	239.2
thumb.	170.5	198.5	—	213.5	238.0	239.2
tibia (any part)	170.7	198.5	—	213.7	238.0	239.2
toe (any)	170.8	198.5	—	213.8	238.0	239.2
trapezium.	170.5	198.5	—	213.5	238.0	239.2
trapezoid	170.5	198.5	—	213.5	238.0	239.2
turbinate	170.0	198.5	—	213.0	238.0	239.2
ulna (any part)	170.4	198.5	—	213.4	238.0	239.2
unciform	170.5	198.5	—	213.5	238.0	239.2

	Malignant					
	Primary	Secondary	Ca in situ	Benign	Uncertain Behavior	Unspecified
vertebra (column)	170.2	198.5	—	213.2	238.0	239.2
coccyx	170.6	198.5	—	213.6	238.0	239.2
sacrum	170.6	198.5	—	213.6	238.0	239.2
vomer	170.0	198.5	—	213.0	238.0	239.2
wrist	170.5	198.5	—	213.5	238.0	239.2
xiphoid process	170.3	198.5	—	213.3	238.0	239.2
zygomatic	170.0	198.5	—	213.0	238.0	239.2
book-leaf (mouth)	145.8	198.89	230.0	210.4	235.1	239.0
bowel—*see* Neoplasm, intestine						
brachial plexus	171.2	198.89	—	215.2	238.1	239.2
brain NEC	191.9	198.3	—	225.0	237.5	239.6
basal ganglia	191.0	198.3	—	225.0	237.5	239.6
cerebellopontine angle	191.6	198.3	—	225.0	237.5	239.6
cerebellum NOS	191.6	198.3	—	225.0	237.5	239.6
cerebrum	191.0	198.3	—	225.0	237.5	239.6
choroid plexus	191.5	198.3	—	225.0	237.5	239.6
contiguous sites	191.8	—	—	—	—	—
corpus callosum	191.8	198.3	—	225.0	237.5	239.6
corpus striatum	191.0	198.3	—	225.0	237.5	239.6
cortex (cerebral)	191.0	198.3	—	225.0	237.5	239.6
frontal lobe	191.1	198.3	—	225.0	237.5	239.6
globus pallidus	191.0	198.3	—	225.0	237.5	239.6
hippocampus	191.2	198.3	—	225.0	237.5	239.6
hypothalamus	191.0	198.3	—	225.0	237.5	239.6
internal capsule	191.0	198.3	—	225.0	237.5	239.6
medulla oblongata	191.7	198.3	—	225.0	237.5	239.6
meninges	192.1	198.4	—	225.2	237.6	239.7
midbrain	191.7	198.3	—	225.0	237.5	239.6
occipital lobe	191.4	198.3	—	225.0	237.5	239.6
parietal lobe	191.3	198.3	—	225.0	237.5	239.6
peduncle	191.7	198.3	—	225.0	237.5	239.6
pons	191.7	198.3	—	225.0	237.5	239.6
stem	191.7	198.3	—	225.0	237.5	239.6
tapetum	191.8	198.3	—	225.0	237.5	239.6
temporal lobe	191.2	198.3	—	225.0	237.5	239.6
thalamus	191.0	198.3	—	225.0	237.5	239.6
uncus	191.2	198.3	—	225.0	237.5	239.6
ventricle (floor)	191.5	198.3	—	225.0	237.5	239.6
branchial (cleft) (vestiges)	146.8	198.89	230.0	210.6	235.1	239.0
breast (connective tissue) (female) (glandular tissue) (soft parts)	174.9	198.81	233.0	217	238.3	239.3
areola	174.0	198.81	233.0	217	238.3	239.3
male	175.0	198.81	233.0	217	238.3	239.3
axillary tail	174.6	198.81	233.0	217	238.3	239.3
central portion	174.1	198.81	233.0	217	238.3	239.3
contiguous sites	174.8	—	—	—	—	—
ectopic sites	174.8	198.81	233.0	217	238.3	239.3
inner	174.8	198.81	233.0	217	238.3	239.3
lower	174.8	198.81	233.0	217	238.3	239.3
lower-inner quadrant	174.3	198.81	233.0	217	238.3	239.3
lower-outer quadrant	174.5	198.81	233.0	217	238.3	239.3
male	175.9	198.81	233.0	217	238.3	239.3
areola	175.0	198.81	233.0	217	238.3	239.3
ectopic tissue	175.9	198.81	233.0	217	238.3	239.3
nipple	175.0	198.81	233.0	217	238.3	239.3
mastectomy site (skin)	173.5	198.2	—	—	—	—
specified as breast tissue	174.8	198.81	—	—	—	—
midline	174.8	198.81	233.0	217	238.3	239.3
nipple	174.0	198.81	233.0	217	238.3	239.3
male	175.0	198.81	233.0	217	238.3	239.3
outer	174.8	198.81	233.0	217	238.3	239.3
skin	173.5	198.2	232.5	216.5	238.2	239.2

	Malignant					
	Primary	Secondary	Ca in situ	Benign	Uncertain Behavior	Unspecified
tail (axillary)	174.6	198.81	233.0	217	238.3	239.3
upper	174.8	198.81	233.0	217	238.3	239.3
upper-inner quadrant	174.2	198.81	233.0	217	238.3	239.3
upper-outer quadrant	174.4	198.81	233.0	217	238.3	239.3
broad ligament	183.3	198.82	233.39	221.0	236.3	239.5
bronchiogenic, bronchogenic						
(lung)	162.9	197.0	231.2	212.3	235.7	239.1
bronchiole	162.9	197.0	231.2	212.3	235.7	239.1
bronchus	162.9	197.0	231.2	212.3	235.7	239.1
carina	162.2	197.0	231.2	212.3	235.7	239.1
contiguous sites with						
lung or trachea	162.8	—	—	—	—	—
lower lobe of lung	162.5	197.0	231.2	212.3	235.7	239.1
main	162.2	197.0	231.2	212.3	235.7	239.1
middle lobe of lung	162.4	197.0	231.2	212.3	235.7	239.1
upper lobe of lung	162.3	197.0	231.2	212.3	235.7	239.1
brow	173.3	198.2	232.3	216.3	238.2	239.2
buccal (cavity)	145.9	198.89	230.0	210.4	235.1	239.0
commissure	145.0	198.89	230.0	210.4	235.1	239.0
groove (lower) (upper)	145.1	198.89	230.0	210.4	235.1	239.0
mucosa	145.0	198.89	230.0	210.4	235.1	239.0
sulcus (lower) (upper)	145.1	198.89	230.0	210.4	235.1	239.0
bulbourethral gland	189.3	198.1	233.9	223.81	236.99	239.5
bursa—see Neoplasm,						
connective tissue						
buttock NEC*	195.3	198.89	232.5	229.8	238.8	239.89
calf*	195.5	198.89	232.7	229.8	238.8	239.89
calvarium	170.0	198.5	—	213.0	238.0	239.2
calyx, renal	189.1	198.0	233.9	223.1	236.91	239.5
canal						
anal	154.2	197.5	230.5	211.4	235.5	239.0
auditory (external)	173.2	198.2	232.2	216.2	238.2	239.2
auricular (external)	173.2	198.2	232.2	216.2	238.2	239.2
canaliculi, biliary (biliferi)						
(intrahepatic)	155.1	197.8	230.8	211.5	235.3	239.0
canthus (eye) (inner)						
(outer)	173.1	198.2	232.1	216.1	238.2	239.2
capillary—see Neoplasm,						
connective tissue						
caput coli	153.4	197.5	230.3	211.3	235.2	239.0
cardia (gastric)	151.0	197.8	230.2	211.1	235.2	239.0
cardiac orifice (stomach)	151.0	197.8	230.2	211.1	235.2	239.0
cardio-esophageal junction	151.0	197.8	230.2	211.1	235.2	239.0
cardio-esophagus	151.0	197.8	230.2	211.1	235.2	239.0
carina (bronchus)	162.2	197.0	231.2	212.3	235.7	239.1
carotid (artery)	171.0	198.89	—	215.0	238.1	239.2
body	194.5	198.89	—	227.5	237.3	239.7
carpus (any bone)	170.5	198.5	—	213.5	238.0	239.2
cartilage (articular) (joint) NEC—see also						
Neoplasm, bone	170.9	198.5	—	213.9	238.0	239.2
arytenoid	161.3	197.3	231.0	212.1	235.6	239.1
auricular	171.0	198.89	—	215.0	238.1	239.2
bronchi	162.2	197.3	—	212.3	235.7	239.1
connective tissue—see Neoplasm,						
connective tissue						
costal	170.3	198.5	—	213.3	238.0	239.2
cricoid	161.3	197.3	231.0	212.1	235.6	239.1
cuneiform	161.3	197.3	231.0	212.1	235.6	239.1
ear (external)	171.0	198.89	—	215.0	238.1	239.2
ensiform	170.3	198.5	—	213.3	238.0	239.2
epiglottis	161.1	197.3	231.0	212.1	235.6	239.1
anterior surface	146.4	198.89	230.0	210.6	235.1	239.0
eyelid	171.0	198.89	—	215.0	238.1	239.2

	Malignant			Benign	Uncertain Behavior	Unspecified
	Primary	Secondary	Ca in situ			
intervertebral	170.2	198.5	—	213.2	238.0	239.2
larynx, laryngeal	161.3	197.3	231.0	212.1	235.6	239.1
nose, nasal	160.0	197.3	231.8	212.0	235.9	239.1
pinna	171.0	198.89	—	215.0	238.1	239.2
rib	170.3	198.5	—	213.3	238.0	239.2
semilunar (knee)	170.7	198.5	—	213.7	238.0	239.2
thyroid	161.3	197.3	231.0	212.1	235.6	239.1
trachea	162.0	197.3	231.1	212.2	235.7	239.1
cauda equina	192.2	198.3	—	225.3	237.5	239.7
cavity						
buccal	145.9	198.89	230.0	210.4	235.1	239.0
nasal	160.0	197.3	231.8	212.0	235.9	239.1
oral	145.9	198.89	230.0	210.4	235.1	239.0
peritoneal	158.9	197.6	—	211.8	235.4	239.0
tympanic	160.1	197.3	231.8	212.0	235.9	239.1
cecum	153.4	197.5	230.3	211.3	235.2	239.0
central						
nervous system—*see*						
Neoplasm, nervous system						
white matter	191.0	198.3	—	225.0	237.5	239.6
cerebellopontine (angle)	191.6	198.3	—	225.0	237.5	239.6
cerebellum, cerebellar	191.6	198.3	—	225.0	237.5	239.6
cerebrum, cerebral (cortex)						
(hemisphere)						
(white matter)	191.0	198.3	—	225.0	237.5	239.6
meninges	192.1	198.4	—	225.2	237.6	239.7
peduncle	191.7	198.3	—	225.0	237.5	239.6
ventricle (any)	191.5	198.3	—	225.0	237.5	239.6
cervical region	195.0	198.89	234.8	229.8	238.8	239.89
cervix (cervical) (uteri)						
(uterus)	180.9	198.82	233.1	219.0	236.0	239.5
canal	180.0	198.82	233.1	219.0	236.0	239.5
contiguous sites	180.8	—	—	—	—	—
endocervix (canal) (gland)	180.0	198.82	233.1	219.0	236.0	239.5
exocervix	180.1	198.82	233.1	219.0	236.0	239.5
external os	180.1	198.82	233.1	219.0	236.0	239.5
internal os	180.0	198.82	233.1	219.0	236.0	239.5
nabothian gland	180.0	198.82	233.1	219.0	236.0	239.5
squamocolumnar junction	180.8	198.82	233.1	219.0	236.0	239.5
stump	180.8	198.82	233.1	219.0	236.0	239.5
cheek	195.0	198.89	234.8	229.8	238.8	239.89
external	173.3	198.2	232.3	216.3	238.2	239.2
inner aspect	145.0	198.89	230.0	210.4	235.1	239.0
internal	145.0	198.89	230.0	210.4	235.1	239.0
mucosa	145.0	198.89	230.0	210.4	235.1	239.0
chest (wall) NEC	195.1	198.89	234.8	229.8	238.8	239.89
chiasma opticum	192.0	198.4	—	225.1	237.9	239.7
chin	173.3	198.2	232.3	216.3	238.2	239.2
choana	147.3	198.89	230.0	210.7	235.1	239.0
cholangiole	155.1	197.8	230.8	211.5	235.3	239.0
choledochal duct	156.1	197.8	230.8	211.5	235.3	239.0
choroid	190.6	198.4	234.0	224.6	238.8	239.81
plexus	191.5	198.3	—	225.0	237.5	239.6
ciliary body	190.0	198.4	234.0	224.0	238.8	239.89
clavicle	170.3	198.5	—	213.3	238.0	239.2
clitoris	184.3	198.82	233.32	221.2	236.3	239.5
clivus	170.0	198.5	—	213.0	238.0	239.2
cloacogenic zone	154.8	197.5	230.7	211.4	235.5	239.0
coccygeal						
body or glomus	194.6	198.89	—	227.6	237.3	239.7
vertebra	170.6	198.5	—	213.6	238.0	239.2
coccyx	170.6	198.5	—	213.6	238.0	239.2
colon—*see also* Neoplasm,						

	Malignant					
	Primary	Secondary	Ca in situ	Benign	Uncertain Behavior	Unspecified

intestine, large						
and rectum	154.0	197.5	230.4	211.4	235.2	239.0
column, spinal—*see* Neoplasm, spine						
columnella	173.3	198.2	232.3	216.3	238.2	239.2
commissure						
labial, lip	140.6	198.89	230.0	210.4	235.1	239.0
laryngeal	161.0	197.3	231.0	212.1	235.6	239.1
common (bile) duct	156.1	197.8	230.8	211.5	235.3	239.0
concha	173.2	198.2	232.2	216.2	238.2	239.2
nose	160.0	197.3	231.8	212.0	235.9	239.1
conjunctiva	190.3	198.4	234.0	224.3	238.8	239.89
connective tissue NEC	171.9	198.89	—	215.9	238.1	239.2

> Note—For neoplasms of connective tissue (blood vessel, bursa, fasica, ligament, muscle, peripheral nerves, sympathetic and parasympathetic nerves, and ganglia, synovia, tendon, etc.) or of morphological types that indicate connective tissue, code according to the list under "Neoplasm, connective tissue;" for sites that do not appear in this list, code to neoplasm of that site; e.g.: liposarcoma, shoulder 171.2; leiomyosarcoma, stomach 151.9; neurofibroma, chest wall 215.4.
>
> Morphological types that indicate connective tissue appear in their proper palce in the alphabetic index with the instruction "see Neoplasm, connective tissue..."

abdomen	171.5	198.89	—	215.5	238.1	239.2
abdominal wall	171.5	198.89	—	215.5	238.1	239.2
ankle	171.3	198.89	—	215.3	238.1	239.2
antecubital fossa or space	171.2	198.89	—	215.2	238.1	239.2
arm	171.2	198.89	—	215.2	238.1	239.2
auricle (ear).	171.0	198.89	—	215.0	238.1	239.2
axilla	171.4	198.89	—	215.4	238.1	239.2
back	171.7	198.89	—	215.7	238.1	239.2
breast (female) (*see also*						
Neoplasm, breast).	174.9	198.81	233.0	217	238.3	239.3
male	175.9	198.81	233.0	217	238.3	239.3
buttock	171.6	198.89	—	215.6	238.1	239.2
calf	171.3	198.89	—	215.3	238.1	239.2
cervical region	171.0	198.89	—	215.0	238.1	239.2
cheek	171.0	198.89	—	215.0	238.1	239.2
chest (wall).	171.4	198.89	—	215.4	238.1	239.2
chin	171.0	198.89	—	215.0	238.1	239.2
contiguous sites	171.8	—	—	—	—	—
diaphragm	171.4	198.89	—	215.4	238.1	239.2
ear (external).	171.0	198.89	—	215.0	238.1	239.2
elbow	171.2	198.89	—	215.2	238.1	239.2
extrarectal	171.6	198.89	—	215.6	238.1	239.2
extremity	171.8	198.89	—	215.8	238.1	239.2
lower	171.3	198.89	—	215.3	238.1	239.2
upper	171.2	198.89	—	215.2	238.1	239.2
eyelid	171.0	198.89	—	215.0	238.1	239.2
face	171.0	198.89	—	215.0	238.1	239.2
finger	171.2	198.89	—	215.2	238.1	239.2
flank	171.7	198.89	—	215.7	238.1	239.2
foot	171.3	198.89	—	215.3	238.1	239.2
forearm	171.2	198.89	—	215.2	238.1	239.2
forehead	171.0	198.89	—	215.0	238.1	239.2
gastric	171.5	198.89	—	215.5	238.1	—
gastrointestinal	171.5	198.89	—	215.5	238.1	—
gluteal region.	171.6	198.89	—	215.6	238.1	239.2
great vessels NEC	171.4	198.89	—	215.4	238.1	239.2
groin	171.6	198.89	—	215.6	238.1	239.2
hand	171.2	198.89	—	215.2	238.1	239.2
head	171.0	198.89	—	215.0	238.1	239.2
heel	171.3	198.89	—	215.3	238.1	239.2
hip	171.3	198.89	—	215.3	238.1	239.2
hypochondrium.	171.5	198.89	—	215.5	238.1	239.2
iliopsoas muscle	171.6	198.89	—	215.5	238.1	239.2

	Malignant			Benign	Uncertain Behavior	Unspecified
	Primary	Secondary	Ca in situ			
infraclavicular region	171.4	198.89	—	215.4	238.1	239.2
inguinal (canal) (region)	171.6	198.89	—	215.6	238.1	239.2
intestine	171.5	198.89	—	215.5	238.1	—
intrathoracic	171.4	198.89	—	215.4	238.1	239.2
ischorectal fossa	171.6	198.89	—	215.6	238.1	239.2
jaw	143.9	198.89	230.0	210.4	235.1	239.0
knee	171.3	198.89	—	215.3	238.1	239.2
leg	171.3	198.89	—	215.3	238.1	239.2
limb NEC.	171.9	198.89	—	215.8	238.1	239.2
lower	171.3	198.89	—	215.3	238.1	239.2
upper	171.2	198.89	—	215.2	238.1	239.2
nates	171.6	198.89	—	215.6	238.1	239.2
neck	171.0	198.89	—	215.0	238.1	239.2
orbit	190.1	198.4	234.0	224.1	238.8	239.89
pararectal.	171.6	198.89	—	215.6	238.1	239.2
para-urethral	171.6	198.89	—	215.6	238.1	239.2
paravaginal	171.6	198.89	—	215.6	238.1	239.2
pelvis (floor)	171.6	198.89	—	215.6	238.1	239.2
pelvo-abdominal	171.8	198.89	—	215.8	238.1	239.2
perineum	171.6	198.89	—	215.6	238.1	239.2
perirectal (tissue).	171.6	198.89	—	215.6	238.1	239.2
periurethral (tissue)	171.6	198.89	—	215.6	238.1	239.2
popliteal fossa or space	171.3	198.89	—	215.3	238.1	239.2
presacral	171.6	198.89	—	215.6	238.1	239.2
psoas muscle	171.5	198.89	—	215.5	238.1	239.2
pterygoid fossa	171.0	198.89	—	215.0	238.1	239.2
rectovaginal septum						
or wall.	171.6	198.89	—	215.6	238.1	239.2
rectovesical.	171.6	198.89	—	215.6	238.1	239.2
retroperitoneum	158.0	197.6	—	211.8	235.4	239.0
sacrococcygeal region	171.6	198.89	—	215.6	238.1	239.2
scalp	171.0	198.89	—	215.0	238.1	239.2
scapular region	171.4	198.89	—	215.4	238.1	239.2
shoulder	171.2	198.89	—	215.2	238.1	239.2
skin (dermis) NEC	173.9	198.2	232.9	216.9	238.2	239.2
stomach.	171.5	198.89	—	215.5	238.1	—
submental.	171.0	198.89	—	215.0	238.1	239.2
supraclavicular region	171.0	198.89	—	215.0	238.1	239.2
temple	171.0	198.89	—	215.0	238.1	239.2
temporal region.	171.0	198.89	—	215.0	238.1	239.2
thigh	171.3	198.89	—	215.3	238.1	239.2
thoracic (duct) (wall).	171.4	198.89	—	215.4	238.1	239.2
thorax.	171.4	198.89	—	215.4	238.1	239.2
thumb.	171.2	198.89	—	215.2	238.1	239.2
toe	171.3	198.89	—	215.3	238.1	239.2
trunk	171.7	198.89	—	215.7	238.1	239.2
umbilicus	171.5	198.89	—	215.5	238.1	239.2
vesicorectal.	171.6	198.89	—	215.6	238.1	239.2
wrist	171.2	198.89	—	215.2	238.1	239.2
conus medullaris	192.2	198.3	—	225.3	237.5	239.7
cord (true) (vocal)	161.0	197.3	231.0	212.1	235.6	239.1
false	161.1	197.3	231.0	212.1	235.6	239.1
spermatic	187.6	198.82	233.6	222.8	236.6	239.5
spinal (cervical) (lumbar)						
(thoracic)	192.2	198.3	—	225.3	237.5	239.7
cornea (limbus).	190.4	198.4	234.0	224.4	238.8	239.89
corpus						
albicans.	183.0	198.6	233.39	220	236.2	239.5
callosum, brain	191.8	198.3	—	225.0	237.5	239.6
cavernosum.	187.3	198.82	233.5	222.1	236.6	239.5
gastric	151.4	197.8	230.2	211.1	235.2	239.0
penis	187.3	198.82	233.5	222.1	236.6	239.5
striatum, cerebrum	191.0	198.3	—	225.0	237.5	239.6

	Malignant					
	Primary	Secondary	Ca in situ	Benign	Uncertain Behavior	Unspecified
uteri.	182.0	198.82	233.2	219.1	236.0	239.5
isthmus	182.1	198.82	233.2	219.1	236.0	239.5
cortex						
adrenal	194.0	198.7	234.8	227.0	237.2	239.7
cerebral.	191.0	198.3	—	225.0	237.5	239.6
costal cartilage	170.3	198.5	—	213.3	238.0	239.2
costovertebral joint.	170.3	198.5	—	213.3	238.0	239.2
Cowper's gland.	189.3	198.1	233.9	223.81	236.99	239.5
cranial (fossa, any)	191.9	198.3	—	225.0	237.5	239.6
meninges	192.1	198.4	—	225.2	237.6	239.7
nerve (any)	192.0	198.4	—	225.1	237.9	239.7
craniobuccal pouch.	194.3	198.89	234.8	227.3	237.0	239.7
craniopharyngeal (duct)						
(pouch)	194.3	198.89	234.8	227.3	237.0	239.7
cricoid	148.0	198.89	230.0	210.8	235.1	239.0
cartilage	161.3	197.3	231.0	212.1	235.6	239.1
cricopharynx	148.0	198.89	230.0	210.8	235.1	239.0
crypt of Morgagni	154.8	197.5	230.7	211.4	235.2	239.0
crystalline lens	190.0	198.4	234.0	224.0	238.8	239.89
cul-de-sac (Douglas')	158.8	197.6	—	211.8	235.4	239.0
cuneiform cartilage.	161.3	197.3	231.0	212.1	235.6	239.1
cutaneous—*see* Neoplasm, skin						
cutis—*see* Neoplasm, skin						
cystic (bile) duct (common)	156.1	197.8	230.8	211.5	235.3	239.0
dermis—*see* Neoplasm, skin						
diaphragm	171.4	198.89	—	215.4	238.1	239.2
digestive organs, system,						
tube, tract NEC	159.9	197.8	230.9	211.9	235.5	239.0
contiguous sites with						
peritoneum.	159.8	—	—	—	—	—
disc, intervertebral	170.2	198.5	—	213.2	238.0	239.2
disease, generalized	199.0	199.0	234.9	229.9	238.9	199.0
disseminated	199.0	199.0	234.9	229.9	238.9	199.0
Douglas' cul-de-sac or pouch	158.8	197.6	—	211.8	235.4	239.0
duodenojejunal junction	152.8	197.4	230.7	211.2	235.2	239.0
duodenum	152.0	197.4	230.7	211.2	235.2	239.0
dura (cranial) (mater).	192.1	198.4	—	225.2	237.6	239.7
cerebral.	192.1	198.4	—	225.2	237.6	239.7
spinal	192.3	198.4	—	225.4	237.6	239.7
ear (external)	173.2	198.2	232.2	216.2	238.2	239.2
auricle or auris	173.2	198.2	232.2	216.2	238.2	239.2
canal, external	173.2	198.2	232.2	216.2	238.2	239.2
cartilage	171.0	198.89	—	215.0	238.1	239.2
external meatus.	173.2	198.2	232.2	216.2	238.2	239.2
inner	160.1	197.3	231.8	212.0	235.9	239.89
lobule.	173.2	198.2	232.2	216.2	238.2	239.2
middle	160.1	197.3	231.8	212.0	235.9	239.89
contiguous sites with						
accessory sinuses						
or nasal cavities	160.8	—	—	—	—	—
skin	173.2	198.2	232.2	216.2	238.2	239.2
earlobe	173.2	198.2	232.2	216.2	238.2	239.2
ejaculatory duct	187.8	198.82	233.6	222.8	236.6	239.5
elbow NEC*	195.4	198.89	232.6	229.8	238.8	239.89
endocardium	164.1	198.89	—	212.7	238.8	239.89
endocervix (canal) (gland)	180.0	198.82	233.1	219.0	236.0	239.5
endocrine gland NEC	194.9	198.89	—	227.9	237.4	239.7
pluriglandular NEC	194.8	198.89	234.8	227.8	237.4	239.7
endometrium (gland)						
(stroma)	182.0	198.82	233.2	219.1	236.0	239.5
ensiform cartilage	170.3	198.5	—	213.3	238.0	239.2
enteric—*see* Neoplasm, intestine						
ependyma (brain).	191.5	198.3	—	225.0	237.5	239.6

	Malignant			Benign	Uncertain Behavior	Unspecified
	Primary	Secondary	Ca in situ			
epicardium	164.1	198.89	—	212.7	238.8	239.89
epididymis	187.5	198.82	233.6	222.3	236.6	239.5
epidural	192.9	198.4	—	225.9	237.9	239.7
epiglottis	161.1	197.3	231.0	212.1	235.6	239.1
anterior aspect or surface	146.4	198.89	230.0	210.6	235.1	239.0
cartilage	161.3	197.3	231.0	212.1	235.6	239.1
free border (margin)	146.4	198.89	230.0	210.6	235.1	239.0
junctional region	146.5	198.89	230.0	210.6	235.1	239.0
posterior (laryngeal)						
surface	161.1	197.3	231.0	212.1	235.6	239.1
suprahyoid portion	161.1	197.3	231.0	212.1	235.6	239.1
esophagogastric junction	151.0	197.8	230.2	211.1	235.2	239.0
esophagus	150.9	197.8	230.1	211.0	235.5	239.0
abdominal	150.2	197.8	230.1	211.0	235.5	239.0
cervical	150.0	197.8	230.1	211.0	235.5	239.0
contiguous sites	150.8	—	—	—	—	—
distal (third)	150.5	197.8	230.1	211.0	235.5	239.0
lower (third)	150.5	197.8	230.1	211.0	235.5	239.0
middle (third)	150.4	197.8	230.1	211.0	235.5	239.0
proximal (third)	150.3	197.8	230.1	211.0	235.5	239.0
specified part NEC	150.8	197.8	230.1	211.0	235.5	239.0
thoracic	150.1	197.8	230.1	211.0	235.5	239.0
upper (third)	150.3	197.8	230.1	211.0	235.5	239.0
ethmoid (sinus)	160.3	197.3	231.8	212.0	235.9	239.1
bone or labyrinth	170.0	198.5	—	213.0	238.0	239.2
Eustachian tube	160.1	197.3	231.8	212.0	235.9	239.1
exocervix	180.1	198.82	233.1	219.0	236.0	239.5
external						
meatus (ear)	173.2	198.2	232.2	216.2	238.2	239.2
os, cervix uteri	180.1	198.82	233.1	219.0	236.0	239.5
extradural	192.9	198.4	—	225.9	237.9	239.7
extrahepatic (bile) duct	156.1	197.8	230.8	211.5	235.3	239.0
contiguous sites with						
gallbladder	156.8	—	—	—	—	—
extraocular muscle	190.1	198.4	234.0	224.1	238.8	239.89
extrarectal	195.3	198.89	234.8	229.8	238.8	239.89
extremity*	195.8	198.89	232.8	229.8	238.8	239.89
lower*	195.5	198.89	232.7	229.8	238.8	239.89
upper*	195.4	198.89	232.6	229.8	238.8	239.89
eye NEC	190.9	198.4	234.0	224.9	238.8	239.89
contiguous sites	190.8	—	—	—	—	—
specified sites NEC	190.8	198.4	234.0	224.8	238.8	239.89
eyeball	190.0	198.4	234.0	224.0	238.8	239.89
eyebrow	173.3	198.2	232.3	216.3	238.2	239.2
eyelid (lower) (skin) (upper)	173.1	198.2	232.1	216.1	238.2	239.2
cartilage	171.0	198.89	—	215.0	238.1	239.2
face NEC*	195.0	198.89	232.3	229.8	238.8	239.89
fallopian tube (accessory)	183.2	198.82	233.39	221.0	236.3	239.5
falx (cerebelli) (cerebri)	192.1	198.4	—	225.2	237.6	239.7
fascia—see also Neoplasm, connective tissue						
palmar	171.2	198.89	—	215.2	238.1	239.2
plantar	171.3	198.89	—	215.3	238.1	239.2
fatty tissue—see Neoplasm, connective tissue						
fauces, faucial NEC	146.9	198.89	230.0	210.6	235.1	239.0
pillars	146.2	198.89	230.0	210.6	235.1	239.0
tonsil	146.0	198.89	230.0	210.5	235.1	239.0
femur (any part)	170.7	198.5	—	213.7	238.0	239.2
fetal membrane	181	198.82	233.2	219.8	236.1	239.5
fibrous tissue—see Neoplasm, connective tissue						
fibula (any part)	170.7	198.5	—	213.7	238.0	239.2
filum terminale	192.2	198.3	—	225.3	237.5	239.7
finger NEC*	195.4	198.89	232.6	229.8	238.8	239.89
flank NEC*	195.8	198.89	232.5	229.8	238.8	239.89

	Malignant			Benign	Uncertain Behavior	Unspecified
	Primary	Secondary	Ca in situ			
follicle, nabothian	180.0	198.82	233.1	219.0	236.0	239.5
foot NEC*	195.5	198.89	232.7	229.8	238.8	239.89
forearm NEC*	195.4	198.89	232.6	229.8	238.8	239.89
forehead (skin)	173.3	198.2	232.3	216.3	238.2	239.2
foreskin	187.1	198.82	233.5	222.1	236.6	239.5
fornix						
pharyngeal	147.3	198.89	230.0	210.7	235.1	239.0
vagina	184.0	198.82	233.31	221.1	236.3	239.5
fossa (of)						
anterior (cranial)	191.9	198.3	—	225.0	237.5	239.6
cranial	191.9	198.3	—	225.0	237.5	239.6
ischiorectal	195.3	198.89	234.8	229.8	238.8	239.89
middle (cranial)	191.9	198.3	—	225.0	237.5	239.6
pituitary	194.3	198.89	234.8	227.3	237.0	239.7
posterior (cranial)	191.9	198.3	—	225.0	237.5	239.6
pterygoid	171.0	198.89	—	215.0	238.1	239.2
pyriform	148.1	198.89	230.0	210.8	235.1	239.0
Rosenmüller	147.2	198.89	230.0	210.7	235.1	239.0
tonsillar	146.1	198.89	230.0	210.6	235.1	239.0
fourchette	184.4	198.82	233.32	221.2	236.3	239.5
frenulum						
labii—*see* Neoplasm, lip, internal						
linguae	141.3	198.89	230.0	210.1	235.1	239.0
frontal						
bone	170.0	198.5	—	213.0	238.0	239.2
lobe, brain	191.1	198.3	—	225.0	237.5	239.6
meninges	192.1	198.4	—	225.2	237.6	239.7
pole	191.1	198.3	—	225.0	237.5	239.6
sinus	160.4	197.3	231.8	212.0	235.9	239.1
fundus						
stomach	151.3	197.8	230.2	211.1	235.2	239.0
uterus	182.0	198.82	233.2	219.1	236.0	239.5
gall duct (extrahepatic)	156.1	197.8	230.8	211.5	235.3	239.0
intrahepatic	155.1	197.8	230.8	211.5	235.3	239.0
gallbladder	156.0	197.8	230.8	211.5	235.3	239.0
contiguous sites with						
extrahepatic bile ducts	156.8	—	—	—	—	—
ganglia (*see also* Neoplasm,						
connective tissue)	171.9	198.89	—	215.9	238.1	239.2
basal	191.0	198.3	—	225.0	237.5	239.6
ganglion (*see also* Neoplasm,						
connective tissue)	171.9	198.89	—	215.9	238.1	239.2
cranial nerve	192.0	198.4	—	225.1	237.9	239.7
Gartner's duct	184.0	198.82	233.31	221.1	236.3	239.5
gastric—*see* Neoplasm, stomach						
gastrocolic	159.8	197.8	230.9	211.9	235.5	239.0
gastroesophageal junction	151.0	197.8	230.2	211.1	235.2	239.0
gastrointestinal (tract) NEC	159.9	197.8	230.9	211.9	235.5	239.0
generalized	199.0	199.0	234.9	229.9	238.9	199.0
genital organ or tract						
female NEC	184.9	198.82	233.39	221.9	236.3	239.5
contiguous sites	184.8	—	—	—	—	—
specified site NEC	184.8	198.82	233.39	221.8	236.3	239.5
male NEC	187.9	198.82	233.6	222.9	236.6	239.5
contiguous sites	187.8	—	—	—	—	—
specified site NEC	187.8	198.82	233.6	222.8	236.6	239.5
genitourinary tract						
female	184.9	198.82	233.39	221.9	236.3	239.5
male	187.9	198.82	233.6	222.9	236.6	239.5
gingiva (alveolar) (marginal)	143.9	198.89	230.0	210.4	235.1	239.0
lower	143.1	198.89	230.0	210.4	235.1	239.0
mandibular	143.1	198.89	230.0	210.4	235.1	239.0
maxillary	143.0	198.89	230.0	210.4	235.1	239.0

	Malignant			Benign	Uncertain Behavior	Unspecified
	Primary	Secondary	Ca in situ			
upper	143.0	198.89	230.0	210.4	235.1	239.0
gland, glandular (lymphatic) (system)—*see also* Neoplasm, lymph gland						
endocrine NEC	194.9	198.89	—	227.9	237.4	239.7
salivary—*see* Neoplasm, salivary, gland						
glans penis	187.2	198.82	233.5	222.1	236.6	239.5
globus pallidus	191.0	198.3	—	225.0	237.5	239.6
glomus						
coccygeal	194.6	198.89	—	227.6	237.3	239.7
jugularis	194.6	198.89	—	227.6	237.3	239.7
glosso-epiglottic fold(s)	146.4	198.89	230.0	210.6	235.1	239.0
glossopalatine fold	146.2	198.89	230.0	210.6	235.1	239.0
glossopharyngeal sulcus	146.1	198.89	230.0	210.6	235.1	239.0
glottis	161.0	197.3	231.0	212.1	235.6	239.1
gluteal region*	195.3	198.89	232.5	229.8	238.8	239.89
great vessels NEC	171.4	198.89	—	215.4	238.1	239.2
groin NEC*	195.3	198.89	232.5	229.8	238.8	239.89
gum	143.9	198.89	230.0	210.4	235.1	239.0
contiguous sites	143.8	—	—	—	—	—
lower	143.1	198.89	230.0	210.4	235.1	239.0
upper	143.0	198.89	230.0	210.4	235.1	239.0
hand NEC*	195.4	198.89	232.6	229.8	238.8	239.89
head NEC*	195.0	198.89	232.4	229.8	238.8	239.89
heart	164.1	198.89	—	212.7	238.8	239.89
contiguous sites with mediastinum or thymus	164.8	—	—	—	—	—
heel NEC*	195.5	198.89	232.7	229.8	238.8	239.89
helix	173.2	198.2	232.2	216.2	238.2	239.2
hematopoietic, hemopoietic tissue NEC	202.8	198.89	—	—	—	238.79
hemisphere, cerebral	191.0	198.3	—	225.0	237.5	239.6
hemorrhoidal zone	154.2	197.5	230.5	211.4	235.5	239.0
hepatic	155.2	197.7	230.8	211.5	235.3	239.0
duct (bile)	156.1	197.8	230.8	211.5	235.3	239.0
flexure (colon)	153.0	197.5	230.3	211.3	235.2	239.0
primary	155.0	—	—	—	—	—
hilus of lung	162.2	197.0	231.2	212.3	235.7	239.1
hip NEC*	195.5	198.89	232.7	229.8	238.8	239.89
hippocampus, brain	191.2	198.3	—	225.0	237.5	239.6
humerus (any part)	170.4	198.5	—	213.4	238.0	239.2
hymen	184.0	198.82	233.31	221.1	236.3	239.5
hypopharynx, hypopharyngeal NEC	148.9	198.89	230.0	210.8	235.1	239.0
contiguous sites	148.8	—	—	—	—	—
postcricoid region	148.0	198.89	230.0	210.8	235.1	239.0
posterior wall	148.3	198.89	230.0	210.8	235.1	239.0
pyriform fossa (sinus)	148.1	198.89	230.0	210.8	235.1	239.0
specified site NEC	148.8	198.89	230.0	210.8	235.1	239.0
wall	148.9	198.89	230.0	210.8	235.1	239.0
posterior	148.3	198.89	230.0	210.8	235.1	239.0
hypophysis	194.3	198.89	234.8	227.3	237.0	239.7
hypothalamus	191.0	198.3	—	225.0	237.5	239.6
ileocecum, ileocecal (coil, junction, valve)	153.4	197.5	230.3	211.3	235.2	239.0
ileum	152.2	197.4	230.7	211.2	235.2	239.0
ilium	170.6	198.5	—	213.6	238.0	239.2
immunoproliferative NEC	203.8	—	—	—	—	—
infraclavicular (region)*	195.1	198.89	232.5	229.8	238.8	239.89
inguinal (region)*	195.3	198.89	232.5	229.8	238.8	239.89
insula	191.0	198.3	—	225.0	237.5	239.6

	Primary	Secondary	Ca in situ	Benign	Uncertain Behavior	Unspecified
		Malignant				

	Primary	Secondary	Ca in situ	Benign	Uncertain Behavior	Unspecified
insular tissue (pancreas)	157.4	197.8	230.9	211.7	235.5	239.0
brain	191.0	198.3	—	225.0	237.5	239.6
interarytenoid fold	148.2	198.89	230.0	210.8	235.1	239.0
hypopharyngeal aspect	148.2	198.89	230.0	210.8	235.1	239.0
laryngeal aspect	161.1	197.3	231.0	212.1	235.6	239.1
marginal zone	148.2	198.89	230.0	210.8	235.1	239.0
interdental papillae	143.9	198.89	230.0	210.4	235.1	239.0
lower	143.1	198.89	230.0	210.4	235.1	239.0
upper	143.0	198.89	230.0	210.4	235.1	239.0
internal						
capsule	191.0	198.3	—	225.0	237.5	239.6
os (cervix)	180.0	198.82	233.1	219.0	236.0	239.5
intervertebral cartilage						
or disc	170.2	198.5	—	213.2	238.0	239.2
intestine, intestinal	159.0	197.8	230.7	211.9	235.2	239.0
large	153.9	197.5	230.3	211.3	235.2	239.0
appendix	153.5	197.5	230.3	211.3	235.2	239.0
caput coli	153.4	197.5	230.3	211.3	235.2	239.0
cecum	153.4	197.5	230.3	211.3	235.2	239.0
colon	153.9	197.5	230.3	211.3	235.2	239.0
and rectum	154.0	197.5	230.4	211.4	235.2	239.0
ascending	153.6	197.5	230.3	211.3	235.2	239.0
caput	153.4	197.5	230.3	211.3	235.2	239.0
contiguous sites	153.8	—	—	—	—	—
descending	153.2	197.5	230.3	211.3	235.2	239.0
distal	153.2	197.5	230.3	211.3	235.2	239.0
left	153.2	197.5	230.3	211.3	235.2	239.0
pelvic	153.3	197.5	230.3	211.3	235.2	239.0
right	153.6	197.5	230.3	211.3	235.2	239.0
sigmoid (flexure)	153.3	197.5	230.3	211.3	235.2	239.0
transverse	153.1	197.5	230.3	211.3	235.2	239.0
contiguous sites	153.8	—	—	—	—	—
hepatic flexure	153.0	197.5	230.3	211.3	235.2	239.0
ileocecum, ileocecal						
(coil, valve)	153.4	197.5	230.3	211.3	235.2	239.0
sigmoid flexure (lower)						
(upper)	153.3	197.5	230.3	211.3	235.2	239.0
splenic flexure	153.7	197.5	230.3	211.3	235.2	239.0
small	152.9	197.4	230.7	211.2	235.2	239.0
contiguous sites	152.8	—	—	—	—	—
duodenum	152.0	197.4	230.7	211.2	235.2	239.0
ileum	152.2	197.4	230.7	211.2	235.2	239.0
jejunum	152.1	197.4	230.7	211.2	235.2	239.0
tract NEC	159.0	197.8	230.7	211.9	235.2	239.0
intra-abdominal	195.2	198.89	234.8	229.8	238.8	239.89
intracranial NEC	191.9	198.3	—	225.0	237.5	239.6
intrahepatic (bile) duct	155.1	197.8	230.8	211.5	235.3	239.0
intraocular	190.0	198.4	234.0	224.0	238.8	239.89
intraorbital	190.1	198.4	234.0	224.1	238.8	239.89
intrasellar	194.3	198.89	234.8	227.3	237.0	239.7
intrathoracic (cavity)						
(organs NEC)	195.1	198.89	234.8	229.8	238.8	239.89
contiguous sites with respiratory						
organs	165.8	—	—	—	—	—
iris	190.0	198.4	234.0	224.0	238.8	239.89
ischiorectal (fossa)	195.3	198.89	234.8	229.8	238.8	239.89
ischium	170.6	198.5	—	213.6	238.0	239.2
island of Reil	191.0	198.3	—	225.0	237.5	239.6
islands or islets of Langerhans	157.4	197.8	230.9	211.7	235.5	239.0
isthmus uteri	182.1	198.82	233.2	219.1	236.0	239.5
jaw	195.0	198.89	234.8	229.8	238.8	239.89
bone	170.1	198.5	—	213.1	238.0	239.2
carcinoma	143.9	—	—	—	—	—

	Malignant			Benign	Uncertain Behavior	Unspecified
	Primary	Secondary	Ca in situ	Benign	Uncertain Behavior	Unspecified
lower	143.1	—	—	—	—	—
upper	143.0	—	—	—	—	—
lower	170.1	198.5	—	213.1	238.0	239.2
upper	170.0	198.5	—	213.0	238.0	239.2
carcinoma (any type)						
(lower) (upper)	195.0	—	—	—	—	—
skin	173.3	198.2	232.3	216.3	238.2	239.2
soft tissues	143.9	198.89	230.0	210.4	235.1	239.0
lower	143.1	198.89	230.0	210.4	235.1	239.0
upper	143.0	198.89	230.0	210.4	235.1	239.0
jejunum	152.1	197.4	230.7	211.2	235.2	239.0
joint NEC (see also						
Neoplasm, bone)	170.9	198.5	—	213.9	238.0	239.2
acromioclavicular	170.4	198.5	—	213.4	238.0	239.2
bursa or synovial membrane—see						
Neoplasm, connective tissue						
costovertebral	170.3	198.5	—	213.3	238.0	239.2
sternocostal	170.3	198.5	—	213.3	238.0	239.2
temporomandibular	170.1	198.5	—	213.1	238.0	239.2
junction						
anorectal	154.8	197.5	230.7	211.4	235.5	239.0
cardioesophageal	151.0	197.8	230.2	211.1	235.2	239.0
esophagogastric	151.0	197.8	230.2	211.1	235.2	239.0
gastroesophageal	151.0	197.8	230.2	211.1	235.2	239.0
hard and soft palate	145.5	198.89	230.0	210.4	235.1	239.0
ileocecal	153.4	197.5	230.3	211.3	235.2	239.0
pelvirectal	154.0	197.5	230.4	211.4	235.2	239.0
pelviureteric	189.1	198.0	233.9	223.1	236.91	239.5
rectosigmoid	154.0	197.5	230.4	211.4	235.2	239.0
squamocolumnar, of cervix	180.8	198.82	233.1	219.0	236.0	239.5
kidney (parenchyma)	189.0	198.0	233.9	223.0	236.91	239.5
calyx	189.1	198.0	233.9	223.1	236.91	239.5
hilus	189.1	198.0	233.9	223.1	236.91	239.5
pelvis	189.1	198.0	233.9	223.1	236.91	239.5
knee NEC*	195.5	198.89	232.7	229.8	238.8	239.89
labia (skin)	184.4	198.82	233.32	221.2	236.3	239.5
majora	184.1	198.82	233.32	221.2	236.3	239.5
minora	184.2	198.82	233.32	221.2	236.3	239.5
labial—see also Neoplasm, lip						
sulcus (lower) (upper)	145.1	198.89	230.0	210.4	235.1	239.0
labium (skin)	184.4	198.82	233.32	221.2	236.3	239.5
majus	184.1	198.82	233.32	221.2	236.3	239.5
minus	184.2	198.82	233.32	221.2	236.3	239.5
lacrimal						
canaliculi	190.7	198.4	234.0	224.7	238.8	239.89
duct (nasal)	190.7	198.4	234.0	224.7	238.8	239.89
gland	190.2	198.4	234.0	224.2	238.8	239.89
punctum	190.7	198.4	234.0	224.7	238.8	239.89
sac	190.7	198.4	234.0	224.7	238.8	239.89
Langerhans, islands or islets	157.4	197.8	230.9	211.7	235.5	239.0
laryngopharynx	148.9	198.89	230.0	210.8	235.1	239.0
larynx, laryngeal NEC	161.9	197.3	231.0	212.1	235.6	239.1
aryepiglottic fold	161.1	197.3	231.0	212.1	235.6	239.1
cartilage (arytenoid)						
(cricoid) (cuneiform)						
(thyroid)	161.3	197.3	231.0	212.1	235.6	239.1
commissure (anterior)						
(posterior)	161.0	197.3	231.0	212.1	235.6	239.1
contiguous sites	161.8	—	—	—	—	—
extrinsic NEC	161.1	197.3	231.0	212.1	235.6	239.1
meaning hypopharynx	148.9	198.89	230.0	210.8	235.1	239.0
interarytenoid fold	161.1	197.3	231.0	212.1	235.6	239.1
intrinsic	161.0	197.3	231.0	212.1	235.6	239.1

	Malignant			Benign	Uncertain Behavior	Unspecified
	Primary	Secondary	Ca in situ			
ventricular band	161.1	197.3	231.0	212.1	235.6	239.1
leg NEC*	195.5	198.89	232.7	229.8	238.8	239.89
lens, crystalline	190.0	198.4	234.0	224.0	238.8	239.89
lid (lower) (upper)	173.1	198.2	232.1	216.1	238.2	239.2
ligament—*see also* Neoplasm, connective tissue						
broad	183.3	198.82	233.39	221.0	236.3	239.5
Mackenrodt's	183.8	198.82	233.39	221.8	236.3	239.5
non-uterine—*see* Neoplasm, connective tissue						
round	183.5	198.82	—	221.0	236.3	239.5
sacro-uterine	183.4	198.82	—	221.0	236.3	239.5
uterine	183.4	198.82	—	221.0	236.3	239.5
utero-ovarian	183.8	198.82	233.39	221.8	236.3	239.5
uterosacral	183.4	198.82	—	221.0	236.3	239.5
limb*	195.8	198.89	232.8	229.8	238.8	239.89
lower*	195.5	198.89	232.7	229.8	238.8	239.89
upper*	195.4	198.89	232.6	229.8	238.8	239.89
limbus of cornea	190.4	198.4	234.0	224.4	238.8	239.89
lingual NEC (*see also* Neoplasm, tongue)	141.9	198.89	230.0	210.1	235.1	239.0
lingula, lung	162.3	197.0	231.2	212.3	235.7	239.1
lip (external) (lipstick area) (vermillion border)	140.9	198.89	230.0	210.0	235.1	239.0
buccal aspect—*see* Neoplasm, lip, internal						
commissure	140.6	198.89	230.0	210.4	235.1	239.0
contiguous sites	140.8	—	—	—	—	—
with oral cavity or pharynx	149.8	—	—	—	—	—
frenulum—*see* Neoplasm, lip, internal						
inner aspect—*see* Neoplasm, lip, internal						
internal (buccal) (frenulum) (mucosa) (oral)	140.5	198.89	230.0	210.0	235.1	239.0
lower	140.4	198.89	230.0	210.0	235.1	239.0
upper	140.3	198.89	230.0	210.0	235.1	239.0
lower	140.1	198.89	230.0	210.0	235.1	239.0
internal (buccal) (frenulum) (mucosa) (oral)	140.4	198.89	230.0	210.0	235.1	239.0
mucosa—*see* Neoplasm, lip, internal						
oral aspect—*see* Neoplasm, lip, internal						
skin (commissure) (lower) (upper)	173.0	198.2	232.0	216.0	238.2	239.2
upper	140.0	198.89	230.0	210.0	235.1	239.0
internal (buccal) (frenulum) (mucosa) (oral)	140.3	198.89	230.0	210.0	235.1	239.0
liver	155.2	197.7	230.8	211.5	235.3	239.0
primary	155.0	—	—	—	—	—
lobe						
azygos	162.3	197.0	231.2	212.3	235.7	239.1
frontal	191.1	198.3	—	225.0	237.5	239.6
lower	162.5	197.0	231.2	212.3	235.7	239.1
middle	162.4	197.0	231.2	212.3	235.7	239.1
occipital	191.4	198.3	—	225.0	237.5	239.6
parietal	191.3	198.3	—	225.0	237.5	239.6
temporal	191.2	198.3	—	225.0	237.5	239.6
upper	162.3	197.0	231.2	212.3	235.7	239.1
lumbosacral plexus	171.6	198.4	—	215.6	238.1	239.2
lung	162.9	197.0	231.2	212.3	235.7	239.1
azygos lobe	162.3	197.0	231.2	212.3	235.7	239.1
carina	162.2	197.0	231.2	212.3	235.7	239.1
contiguous sites with bronchus or trachea	162.8	—	—	—	—	—
hilus	162.2	197.0	231.2	212.3	235.7	239.1

	Malignant			Benign	Uncertain Behavior	Unspecified
	Primary	Secondary	Ca in situ			
lingula	162.3	197.0	231.2	212.3	235.7	239.1
lobe NEC	162.9	197.0	231.2	212.3	235.7	239.1
lower lobe	162.5	197.0	231.2	212.3	235.7	239.1
main bronchus	162.2	197.0	231.2	212.3	235.7	239.1
middle lobe	162.4	197.0	231.2	212.3	235.7	239.1
upper lobe	162.3	197.0	231.2	212.3	235.7	239.1
lymph, lymphatic						
channel NEC (*see also* Neoplasm, connective tissue)	171.9	198.89	—	215.9	238.1	239.2
gland (secondary)	—	196.9	—	229.0	238.8	239.89
abdominal	—	196.2	—	229.0	238.8	239.89
aortic	—	196.2	—	229.0	238.8	239.89
arm	—	196.3	—	229.0	238.8	239.89
auricular (anterior) (posterior)	—	196.0	—	229.0	238.8	239.89
axilla, axillary	—	196.3	—	229.0	238.8	239.89
brachial	—	196.3	—	229.0	238.8	239.89
bronchial	—	196.1	—	229.0	238.8	239.89
bronchopulmonary	—	196.1	—	229.0	238.8	239.89
celiac	—	196.2	—	229.0	238.8	239.89
cervical	—	196.0	—	229.0	238.8	239.89
cervicofacial	—	196.0	—	229.0	238.8	239.89
Cloquet	—	196.5	—	229.0	238.8	239.89
colic	—	196.2	—	229.0	238.8	239.89
common duct	—	196.2	—	229.0	238.8	239.89
cubital	—	196.3	—	229.0	238.8	239.89
diaphragmatic	—	196.1	—	229.0	238.8	239.89
epigastric, inferior	—	196.6	—	229.0	238.8	239.89
epitrochlear	—	196.3	—	229.0	238.8	239.89
esophageal	—	196.1	—	229.0	238.8	239.89
face	—	196.0	—	229.0	238.8	239.89
femoral	—	196.5	—	229.0	238.8	239.89
gastric	—	196.2	—	229.0	238.8	239.89
groin	—	196.5	—	229.0	238.8	239.89
head	—	196.0	—	229.0	238.8	239.89
hepatic	—	196.2	—	229.0	238.8	239.89
hilar (pulmonary)	—	196.1	—	229.0	238.8	239.89
splenic	—	196.2	—	229.0	238.8	239.89
hypogastric	—	196.6	—	229.0	238.8	239.89
ileocolic	—	196.2	—	229.0	238.8	239.89
iliac	—	196.6	—	229.0	238.8	239.89
infraclavicular	—	196.3	—	229.0	238.8	239.89
inguina, inguinal	—	196.5	—	229.0	238.8	239.89
innominate	—	196.1	—	229.0	238.8	239.89
intercostal	—	196.1	—	229.0	238.8	239.89
intestinal	—	196.2	—	229.0	238.8	239.89
intrabdominal	—	196.2	—	229.0	238.8	239.89
intrapelvic	—	196.6	—	229.0	238.8	239.89
intrathoracic	—	196.1	—	229.0	238.8	239.9
jugular	—	196.0	—	229.0	238.8	239.89
leg	—	196.5	—	229.0	238.8	239.89
limb						
lower	—	196.5	—	229.0	238.8	239.89
upper	—	196.3	—	229.0	238.8	239.89
lower limb	—	196.5	—	229.0	238.8	238.9
lumbar	—	196.2	—	229.0	238.8	239.89
mandibular	—	196.0	—	229.0	238.8	239.89
mediastinal	—	196.1	—	229.0	238.8	239.89
mesenteric (inferior) (superior)	—	196.2	—	229.0	238.8	239.89
midcolic	—	196.2	—	229.0	238.8	239.89
multiple sites in categories 196.0-196.6	—	196.8	—	229.0	238.8	239.89

	Malignant			Benign	Uncertain Behavior	Unspecified
	Primary	Secondary	Ca in situ	Benign	Uncertain Behavior	Unspecified
neck	—	196.0	—	229.0	238.8	239.89
obturator	—	196.6	—	229.0	238.8	239.89
occipital	—	196.0	—	229.0	238.8	239.89
pancreatic	—	196.2	—	229.0	238.8	239.89
para-aortic	—	196.2	—	229.0	238.8	239.89
paracervical	—	196.6	—	229.0	238.8	239.89
parametrial	—	196.6	—	229.0	238.8	239.89
parasternal	—	196.1	—	229.0	238.8	239.89
parotid	—	196.0	—	229.0	238.8	239.89
pectoral	—	196.3	—	229.0	238.8	239.89
pelvic	—	196.6	—	229.0	238.8	239.89
peri-aortic	—	196.2	—	229.0	238.8	239.89
peripancreatic	—	196.2	—	229.0	238.8	239.89
popliteal	—	196.5	—	229.0	238.8	239.89
porta hepatis	—	196.2	—	229.0	238.8	239.89
portal	—	196.2	—	229.0	238.8	239.89
preauricular	—	196.0	—	229.0	238.8	239.89
prelaryngeal	—	196.0	—	229.0	238.8	239.89
presymphysial	—	196.6	—	229.0	238.8	239.89
pretracheal	—	196.0	—	229.0	238.8	239.89
primary (any site) NEC	202.9	—	—	—	—	—
pulmonary (hiler)	—	196.1	—	229.0	238.8	239.89
pyloric	—	196.2	—	229.0	238.8	239.89
retroperitoneal	—	196.2	—	229.0	238.8	239.89
retropharyngeal	—	196.0	—	229.0	238.8	239.89
Rosenmüller's	—	196.5	—	229.0	238.8	239.89
sacral	—	196.6	—	229.0	238.8	239.89
scalene	—	196.0	—	229.0	238.8	239.89
site NEC	—	196.9	—	229.0	238.8	239.89
splenic (hilar)	—	196.2	—	229.0	238.8	239.89
subclavicular	—	196.3	—	229.0	238.8	239.89
subinguinal	—	196.5	—	229.0	238.8	239.89
sublingual	—	196.0	—	229.0	238.8	239.89
submandibular	—	196.0	—	229.0	238.8	239.89
submaxillary	—	196.0	—	229.0	238.8	239.89
submental	—	196.0	—	229.0	238.8	239.89
subscapular	—	196.3	—	229.0	238.8	239.89
supraclavicular	—	196.0	—	229.0	238.8	239.89
thoracic	—	196.1	—	229.0	238.8	239.89
tibial	—	196.5	—	229.0	238.8	239.89
tracheal	—	196.1	—	229.0	238.8	239.89
tracheobronchial	—	196.1	—	229.0	238.8	239.89
upper limb	—	196.3	—	229.0	238.8	239.89
Virchow's	—	196.0	—	229.0	238.8	239.89
node—*see also* Neoplasm, lymph gland						
primary NEC	202.9	—	—	—	—	—
vessel (*see also* Neoplasm, connective tissue)	171.9	198.89	—	215.9	238.1	239.2
Mackenrodt's ligament	183.8	198.82	233.39	221.8	236.3	239.5
malar	170.0	198.5	—	213.0	238.0	239.2
region—*see* Neoplasm, cheek						
mammary gland—*see* Neoplasm, breast						
mandible	170.1	198.5	—	213.1	238.0	239.2
alveolar						
mucosa	143.1	198.89	230.0	210.4	235.1	239.0
ridge or process	170.1	198.5	—	213.1	238.0	239.2
carcinoma	143.1	—	—	—	—	—
carcinoma	143.1	—	—	—	—	—
marrow (bone) NEC	202.9	198.5	—	—	—	238.79
mastectomy site (skin)	173.5	198.2	—	—	—	—
specified as breast tissue	174.8	198.81	—	—	—	—

	Primary	Secondary	Ca in situ	Benign	Uncertain Behavior	Unspecified
		Malignant				
mastoid (air cells) (antrum)						
(cavity)	160.1	197.3	231.8	212.0	235.9	239.1
bone or process.	170.0	198.5	—	213.0	238.0	239.2
maxilla, maxillary (superior)	170.0	198.5	—	213.0	238.0	239.2
alveolar						
mucosa	143.0	198.89	230.0	210.4	235.1	239.0
ridge or process	170.0	198.5	—	213.0	238.0	239.2
carcinoma	143.0	—	—	—	—	—
antrum	160.2	197.3	231.8	212.0	235.9	239.1
carcinoma	143.0	—	—	—	—	—
inferior—see Neoplasm, mandible						
sinus	160.2	197.3	231.8	212.0	235.9	239.1
meatus						
external (ear)	173.2	198.2	232.2	216.2	238.2	239.2
Meckel's diverticulum	152.3	197.4	230.7	211.2	235.2	239.0
mediastinum, mediastinal	164.9	197.1	—	212.5	235.8	239.89
anterior	164.2	197.1	—	212.5	235.8	239.89
contiguous sites with heart						
and thymus	164.8	—	—	—	—	—
posterior	164.3	197.1	—	212.5	235.8	239.89
medulla						
adrenal	194.0	198.7	234.8	227.0	237.2	239.7
oblongata	191.7	198.3	—	225.0	237.5	239.6
meibomian gland	173.1	198.2	232.1	216.1	238.2	239.2
melanoma —see Melanoma						
meninges (brain) (cerebral)						
(cranial) (intracranial)	192.1	198.4	—	225.2	237.6	239.7
spinal (cord)	192.3	198.4	—	225.4	237.6	239.7
meniscus, knee joint						
(lateral) (medial)	170.7	198.5	—	213.7	238.0	239.2
mesentery, mesenteric	158.8	197.6	—	211.8	235.4	239.0
mesoappendix	158.8	197.6	—	211.8	235.4	239.0
mesocolon	158.8	197.6	—	211.8	235.4	239.0
mesopharynx—see Neoplasm, oropharynx						
mesosalpinx	183.3	198.82	233.39	221.0	236.3	239.5
mesovarium	183.3	198.82	233.39	221.0	236.3	239.5
metacarpus (any bone)	170.5	198.5	—	213.5	238.0	239.2
metastatic NEC—see also Neoplasm,						
by site, secondary	—	199.1	—	—	—	—
metatarsus (any bone)	170.8	198.5	—	213.8	238.0	239.2
midbrain	191.7	198.3	—	225.0	237.5	239.6
milk duct—see Neoplasm, breast						
mons						
pubis	184.4	198.82	233.32	221.2	236.3	239.5
veneris	184.4	198.82	233.32	221.2	236.3	239.5
motor tract	192.9	198.4	—	225.9	237.9	239.7
brain	191.9	198.3	—	225.0	237.5	239.6
spinal	192.2	198.3	—	225.3	237.5	239.7
mouth	145.9	198.89	230.0	210.4	235.1	239.0
contiguous sites	145.8	—	—	—	—	—
floor	144.9	198.89	230.0	210.3	235.1	239.0
anterior portion	144.0	198.89	230.0	210.3	235.1	239.0
contiguous sites	144.8	—	—	—	—	—
lateral portion	144.1	198.89	230.0	210.3	235.1	239.0
roof	145.5	198.89	230.0	210.4	235.1	239.0
specified part NEC	145.8	198.89	230.0	210.4	235.1	239.0
vestibule	145.1	198.89	230.0	210.4	235.1	239.0
mucosa						
alveolar (ridge or process)	143.9	198.89	230.0	210.4	235.1	239.0
lower	143.1	198.89	230.0	210.4	235.1	239.0
upper	143.0	198.89	230.0	210.4	235.1	239.0
buccal	145.0	198.89	230.0	210.4	235.1	239.0
cheek	145.0	198.89	230.0	210.4	235.1	239.0

	Malignant					
	Primary	Secondary	Ca in situ	Benign	Uncertain Behavior	Unspecified
lip—*see* Neoplasm, lip, internal						
nasal	160.0	197.3	231.8	212.0	235.9	239.1
oral	145.0	198.89	230.0	210.4	235.1	239.0
Müllerian duct						
female	184.8	198.82	233.39	221.8	236.3	239.5
male	187.8	198.82	233.6	222.8	236.6	239.5
multiple sites NEC	199.0	199.0	234.9	229.9	238.9	199.0
muscle—*see also* Neoplasm, connective tissue						
extraocular	190.1	198.4	234.0	224.1	238.8	239.89
myocardium	164.1	198.89	—	212.7	238.8	239.89
myometrium	182.0	198.82	233.2	219.1	236.0	239.5
myopericardium	164.1	198.89	—	212.7	238.8	239.89
nabothian gland (follicle)	180.0	198.82	233.1	219.0	236.0	239.5
nail	173.9	198.2	232.9	216.9	238.2	239.2
finger	173.6	198.2	232.6	216.6	238.2	239.2
toe	173.7	198.2	232.7	216.7	238.2	239.2
nares, naris (anterior)						
(posterior)	160.0	197.3	231.8	212.0	235.9	239.1
nasal—*see* Neoplasm, nose						
nasolabial groove	173.3	198.2	232.3	216.3	238.2	239.2
nasolacrimal duct	190.7	198.4	234.0	224.7	238.8	239.89
nasopharynx, nasopharyngeal	147.9	198.89	230.0	210.7	235.1	239.0
contiguous sites	147.8	—	—	—	—	—
floor	147.3	198.89	230.0	210.7	235.1	239.0
roof	147.0	198.89	230.0	210.7	235.1	239.0
specified site NEC	147.8	198.89	230.0	210.7	235.1	239.0
wall	147.9	198.89	230.0	210.7	235.1	239.0
anterior	147.3	198.89	230.0	210.7	235.1	239.0
lateral	147.2	198.89	230.0	210.7	235.1	239.0
posterior	147.1	198.89	230.0	210.7	235.1	239.0
superior	147.0	198.89	230.0	210.7	235.1	239.0
nates	173.5	198.2	232.5	216.5	238.2	239.2
neck NEC*	195.0	198.89	234.8	229.8	238.8	239.89
nerve (autonomic) (ganglion) (parasympathetic) (peripheral) (sympathetic)—*see also* Neoplasm, connective tissue						
abducens	192.0	198.4	—	225.1	237.9	239.7
accessory (spinal)	192.0	198.4	—	225.1	237.9	239.7
acoustic	192.0	198.4	—	225.1	237.9	239.7
auditory	192.0	198.4	—	225.1	237.9	239.7
brachial	171.2	198.89	—	215.2	238.1	239.2
cranial (any)	192.0	198.4	—	225.1	237.9	239.7
facial	192.0	198.4	—	225.1	237.9	239.7
femoral	171.3	198.89	—	215.3	238.1	239.2
glossopharyngeal	192.0	198.4	—	225.1	237.9	239.7
hypoglossal	192.0	198.4	—	225.1	237.9	239.7
intercostal	171.4	198.89	—	215.4	238.1	239.2
lumbar	171.7	198.89	—	215.7	238.1	239.2
median	171.2	198.89	—	215.2	238.1	239.2
obturator	171.3	198.89	—	215.3	238.1	239.2
oculomotor	192.0	198.4	—	225.1	237.9	239.7
olfactory	192.0	198.4	—	225.1	237.9	239.7
optic	192.0	198.4	—	225.1	237.9	239.7
peripheral NEC	171.9	198.89	—	215.9	238.1	239.2
radial	171.2	198.89	—	215.2	238.1	239.2
sacral	171.6	198.89	—	215.6	238.1	239.2
sciatic	171.3	198.89	—	215.3	238.1	239.2
spinal NEC	171.9	198.89	—	215.9	238.1	239.2
trigeminal	192.0	198.4	—	225.1	237.9	239.7
trochlear	192.0	198.4	—	225.1	237.9	239.7
ulnar	171.2	198.89	—	215.2	238.1	239.2

	Malignant			Benign	Uncertain Behavior	Unspecified
	Primary	Secondary	Ca in situ			
vagus	192.0	198.4	—	225.1	237.9	239.7
nervous system (central)						
NEC	192.9	198.4	—	225.9	237.9	239.7
autonomic NEC	171.9	198.89	—	215.9	238.1	239.2
brain—*see also* Neoplasm, brain						
membrane or meninges	192.1	198.4	—	225.2	237.6	239.7
contiguous sites	192.8	—	—	—	—	—
parasympathetic NEC	171.9	198.89	—	215.9	238.1	239.2
sympathetic NEC	171.9	198.89	—	215.9	238.1	239.2
nipple (female)	174.0	198.81	233.0	217	238.3	239.3
male	175.0	198.81	233.0	217	238.3	239.3
nose, nasal	195.0	198.89	234.8	229.8	238.8	239.89
ala (external)	173.3	198.2	232.3	216.3	238.2	239.2
bone	170.0	198.5	—	213.0	238.0	239.2
cartilage	160.0	197.3	231.8	212.0	235.9	239.1
cavity	160.0	197.3	231.8	212.0	235.9	239.1
contiguous sites with accessory						
sinuses or middle ear	160.8	—	—	—	—	—
choana	147.3	198.89	230.0	210.7	235.1	239.0
external (skin)	173.3	198.2	232.3	216.3	238.2	239.2
fossa	160.0	197.3	231.8	212.0	235.9	239.1
internal	160.0	197.3	231.8	212.0	235.9	239.1
mucosa	160.0	197.3	231.8	212.0	235.9	239.1
septum	160.0	197.3	231.8	212.0	235.9	239.1
posterior margin	147.3	198.89	230.0	210.7	235.1	239.0
sinus—*see* Neoplasm, sinus						
skin	173.3	198.2	232.3	216.3	238.2	239.2
turbinate (mucosa)	160.0	197.3	231.8	212.0	235.9	239.1
bone	170.0	198.5	—	213.0	238.0	239.2
vestibule	160.0	197.3	231.8	212.0	235.9	239.1
nostril	160.0	197.3	231.8	212.0	235.9	239.1
nucleus pulposus	170.2	198.5	—	213.2	238.0	239.2
occipital						
bone	170.0	198.5	—	213.0	238.0	239.2
lobe or pole, brain	191.4	198.3	—	225.0	237.5	239.6
odontogenic—*see* Neoplasm,						
jaw bone						
oesophagus—*see* Neoplasm,						
esophagus						
olfactory nerve or bulb	192.0	198.4	—	225.1	237.9	239.7
olive (brain)	191.7	198.3	—	225.0	237.5	239.6
omentum	158.8	197.6	—	211.8	235.4	239.0
operculum (brain)	191.0	198.3	—	225.0	237.5	239.6
optic nerve, chiasm, or tract	192.0	198.4	—	225.1	237.9	239.7
oral (cavity)	145.9	198.89	230.0	210.4	235.1	239.0
contiguous sites with lip						
or pharynx	149.8	—	—	—	—	—
ill-defined	149.9	198.89	230.0	210.4	235.1	239.0
mucosa	145.9	198.89	230.0	210.4	235.1	239.0
orbit	190.1	198.4	234.0	224.1	238.8	239.89
bone	170.0	198.5	—	213.0	238.0	239.2
eye	190.1	198.4	234.0	224.1	238.8	239.89
soft parts	190.1	198.4	234.0	224.1	238.8	239.89
organ of Zuckerkandl	194.6	198.89	—	227.6	237.3	239.7
oropharynx	146.9	198.89	230.0	210.6	235.1	239.0
branchial cleft (vestige)	146.8	198.89	230.0	210.6	235.1	239.0
contiguous sites	146.8	—	—	—	—	—
junctional region	146.5	198.89	230.0	210.6	235.1	239.0
lateral wall	146.6	198.89	230.0	210.6	235.1	239.0
pillars of fauces	146.2	198.89	230.0	210.6	235.1	239.0
posterior wall	146.7	198.89	230.0	210.6	235.1	239.0
specified part NEC	146.8	198.89	230.0	210.6	235.1	239.0
vallecula	146.3	198.89	230.0	210.6	235.1	239.0

	Malignant					
	Primary	Secondary	Ca in situ	Benign	Uncertain Behavior	Unspecified
os						
external	180.1	198.82	233.1	219.0	236.0	239.5
internal	180.0	198.82	233.1	219.0	236.0	239.5
ovary	183.0	198.6	233.39	220	236.2	239.5
oviduct	183.2	198.82	233.39	221.0	236.3	239.5
palate	145.5	198.89	230.0	210.4	235.1	239.0
hard	145.2	198.89	230.0	210.4	235.1	239.0
junction of hard and soft palate	145.5	198.89	230.0	210.4	235.1	239.0
soft	145.3	198.89	230.0	210.4	235.1	239.0
nasopharyngeal surface	147.3	198.89	230.0	210.7	235.1	239.0
posterior surface	147.3	198.89	230.0	210.7	235.1	239.0
superior surface	147.3	198.89	230.0	210.7	235.1	239.0
palatoglossal arch	146.2	198.89	230.0	210.6	235.1	239.0
palatopharyngeal arch	146.2	198.89	230.0	210.6	235.1	239.0
pallium	191.0	198.3	—	225.0	237.5	239.6
palpebra	173.1	198.2	232.1	216.1	238.2	239.2
pancreas	157.9	197.8	230.9	211.6	235.5	239.0
body	157.1	197.8	230.9	211.6	235.5	239.0
contiguous sites	157.8	—	—	—	—	—
duct (of Santorini) (of Wirsung)	157.3	197.8	230.9	211.6	235.5	239.0
ectopic tissue	157.8	197.8	230.9	211.6	235.5	239.0
head	157.0	197.8	230.9	211.6	235.5	239.0
islet cells	157.4	197.8	230.9	211.7	235.5	239.0
neck	157.8	197.8	230.9	211.6	235.5	239.0
tail	157.2	197.8	230.9	211.6	235.5	239.0
para-aortic body	194.6	198.89	—	227.6	237.3	239.7
paraganglion NEC	194.6	198.89	—	227.6	237.3	239.7
parametrium	183.4	198.82	—	221.0	236.3	239.5
paranephric	158.0	197.6	—	211.8	235.4	239.0
pararectal	195.3	198.89	—	229.8	238.8	239.89
parasagittal (region)	195.0	198.89	234.8	229.8	238.8	239.89
parasellar	192.9	198.4	—	225.9	237.9	239.7
parathyroid (gland)	194.1	198.89	234.8	227.1	237.4	239.7
paraurethral	195.3	198.89	—	229.8	238.8	239.89
gland	189.4	198.1	233.9	223.89	236.99	239.5
paravaginal	195.3	198.89	—	229.8	238.8	239.89
parenchyma, kidney	189.0	198.0	233.9	223.0	236.91	239.5
parietal bone	170.0	198.5	—	213.0	238.0	239.2
lobe, brain	191.3	198.3	—	225.0	237.5	239.6
paroophoron	183.3	198.82	233.39	221.0	236.3	239.5
parotid (duct) (gland)	142.0	198.89	230.0	210.2	235.0	239.0
parovarium	183.3	198.82	233.39	221.0	236.3	239.5
patella	170.8	198.5	—	213.8	238.0	239.2
peduncle, cerebral	191.7	198.3	—	225.0	237.5	239.6
pelvirectal junction	154.0	197.5	230.4	211.4	235.2	239.0
pelvis, pelvic	195.3	198.89	234.8	229.8	238.8	239.89
bone	170.6	198.5	—	213.6	238.0	239.2
floor	195.3	198.89	234.8	229.8	238.8	239.89
renal	189.1	198.0	233.9	223.1	236.91	239.5
viscera	195.3	198.89	234.8	229.8	238.8	239.89
wall	195.3	198.89	234.8	229.8	238.8	239.89
pelvo-abdominal	195.8	198.89	234.8	229.8	238.8	239.89
penis	187.4	198.82	233.5	222.1	236.6	239.5
body	187.3	198.82	233.5	222.1	236.6	239.5
corpus (cavernosum)	187.3	198.82	233.5	222.1	236.6	239.5
glans	187.2	198.82	233.5	222.1	236.6	239.5
skin NEC	187.4	198.82	233.5	222.1	236.6	239.5
periadrenal (tissue)	158.0	197.6	—	211.8	235.4	239.0
perianal (skin)	173.5	198.2	232.5	216.5	238.2	239.2
pericardium	164.1	198.89	—	212.7	238.8	239.89

	Malignant			Benign	Uncertain Behavior	Unspecified
	Primary	Secondary	Ca in situ			
perinephric	158.0	197.6	—	211.8	235.4	239.0
perineum	195.3	198.89	234.8	229.8	238.8	239.89
periodontal tissue NEC.	143.9	198.89	230.0	210.4	235.1	239.0
periosteum—see Neoplasm, bone						
peripancreatic	158.0	197.6	—	211.8	235.4	239.0
peripheral nerve NEC	171.9	198.89	—	215.9	238.1	239.2
perirectal (tissue)	195.3	198.89	—	229.8	238.8	239.89
perirenal (tissue)	158.0	197.6	—	211.8	235.4	239.0
peritoneum, peritoneal						
(cavity)	158.9	197.6	—	211.8	235.4	239.0
contiguous sites	158.8	—	—	—	—	—
with digestive organs.	159.8	—	—	—	—	—
parietal	158.8	197.6	—	211.8	235.4	239.0
pelvic	158.8	197.6	—	211.8	235.4	239.0
specified part NEC	158.8	197.6	—	211.8	235.4	239.0
peritonsillar (tissue)	195.0	198.89	234.8	229.8	238.8	239.89
periurethral tissue	195.3	198.89	—	229.8	238.8	239.89
phalanges	170.9	198.5	—	213.9	238.0	239.2
foot	170.8	198.5	—	213.8	238.0	239.2
hand	170.5	198.5	—	213.5	238.0	239.2
pharynx, pharyngeal	149.0	198.89	230.0	210.9	235.1	239.0
bursa	147.1	198.89	230.0	210.7	235.1	239.0
fornix	147.3	198.89	230.0	210.7	235.1	239.0
recess	147.2	198.89	230.0	210.7	235.1	239.0
region	149.0	198.89	230.0	210.9	235.1	239.0
tonsil	147.1	198.89	230.0	210.7	235.1	239.0
wall (lateral) (posterior)	149.0	198.89	230.0	210.9	235.1	239.0
pia mater (cerebral) (cranial)	192.1	198.4	—	225.2	237.6	239.7
spinal	192.3	198.4	—	225.4	237.6	239.7
pillars of fauces	146.2	198.89	230.0	210.6	235.1	239.0
pineal (body) (gland)	194.4	198.89	234.8	227.4	237.1	239.7
pinna (ear) NEC	173.2	198.2	232.2	216.2	238.2	239.2
cartilage	171.0	198.89	—	215.0	238.1	239.2
piriform fossa or sinus	148.1	198.89	230.0	210.8	235.1	239.0
pituitary (body) (fossa)						
(gland) (lobe)	194.3	198.89	234.8	227.3	237.0	239.7
placenta	181	198.82	233.2	219.8	236.1	239.5
pleura, pleural (cavity)	163.9	197.2	—	212.4	235.8	239.1
contiguous sites	163.8	—	—	—	—	—
parietal	163.0	197.2	—	212.4	235.8	239.1
visceral	163.1	197.2	—	212.4	235.8	239.1
plexus						
brachial	171.2	198.89	—	215.2	238.1	239.2
cervical	171.0	198.89	—	215.0	238.1	239.2
choroid	191.5	198.3	—	225.0	237.5	239.6
lumbosacral	171.6	198.89	—	215.6	238.1	239.2
sacral	171.6	198.89	—	215.6	238.1	239.2
pluri-endocrine	194.8	198.89	234.8	227.8	237.4	239.7
pole						
frontal	191.1	198.3	—	225.0	237.5	239.6
occipital	191.4	198.3	—	225.0	237.5	239.6
pons (varolii)	191.7	198.3	—	225.0	237.5	239.6
popliteal fossa or space*	195.5	198.89	234.8	229.8	238.8	239.89
postcricoid (region)	148.0	198.89	230.0	210.8	235.1	239.0
posterior fossa (cranial)	191.9	198.3	—	225.0	237.5	239.6
postnasal space	147.9	198.89	230.0	210.7	235.1	239.0
prepuce	187.1	198.82	233.5	222.1	236.6	239.5
prepylorus	151.0	197.8	230.2	211.1	235.2	239.0
presacral (region)	195.3	198.89	—	229.8	238.8	239.89
prostate (gland)	185	198.82	233.4	222.2	236.5	239.5
utricle	189.3	198.1	233.9	223.81	236.99	239.5
pterygoid fossa	171.0	198.89	—	215.0	238.1	239.2
pubic bone	170.6	198.5	—	213.6	238.0	239.2

	Malignant			Benign	Uncertain Behavior	Unspecified
	Primary	Secondary	Ca in situ			
pudenda, pudendum (female)	184.4	198.82	233.32	221.2	236.3	239.5
pulmonary	162.9	197.0	231.2	212.3	235.7	239.1
putamen	191.0	198.3	—	225.0	237.5	239.6
pyloric						
antrum	151.2	197.8	230.2	211.1	235.2	239.0
canal	151.1	197.8	230.2	211.1	235.2	239.0
pylorus	151.1	197.8	230.2	211.1	235.2	239.0
pyramid (brain)	191.7	198.3	—	225.0	237.5	239.6
pyriform fossa or sinus	148.1	198.89	230.0	210.8	235.1	239.0
radius (any part)	170.4	198.5	—	213.4	238.0	239.2
Rathke's pouch	194.3	198.89	234.8	227.3	237.0	239.7
rectosigmoid (colon)						
(junction)	154.0	197.5	230.4	211.4	235.2	239.0
contiguous sites with						
anus or rectum	154.8	—	—	—	—	—
rectouterine pouch	158.8	197.6	—	211.8	235.4	239.0
rectovaginal septum or wall	195.3	198.89	234.8	229.8	238.8	239.89
rectovesical septum	195.3	198.89	234.8	229.8	238.8	239.89
rectum (ampulla)	154.1	197.5	230.4	211.4	235.2	239.0
and colon	154.0	197.5	230.4	211.4	235.2	239.0
contiguous sites with anus or						
rectosigmoid junction	154.8	—	—	—	—	—
renal	189.0	198.0	233.9	223.0	236.91	239.5
calyx	189.1	198.0	233.9	223.1	236.91	239.5
hilus	189.1	198.0	233.9	223.1	236.91	239.5
parenchyma	189.0	198.0	233.9	223.0	236.91	239.5
pelvis	189.1	198.0	233.9	223.1	236.91	239.5
respiratory						
organs or system NEC	165.9	197.3	231.9	212.9	235.9	239.1
contiguous sites with						
intrathoracic organs	165.8	—	—	—	—	—
specified sites NEC	165.8	197.3	231.8	212.8	235.9	239.1
tract NEC	165.9	197.3	231.9	212.9	235.9	239.1
upper	165.0	197.3	231.9	212.9	235.9	239.1
retina	190.5	198.4	234.0	224.5	238.8	239.81
retrobulbar	190.1	198.4	—	224.1	238.8	239.89
retrocecal	158.0	197.6	—	211.8	235.4	239.0
retromolar (area) (triangle)						
(trigone)	145.6	198.89	230.0	210.4	235.1	239.0
retro-orbital	195.0	198.89	234.8	229.8	238.8	239.89
retroperitoneal (space)						
(tissue)	158.0	197.6	—	211.8	235.4	239.0
contiguous sites	158.8	—	—	—	—	—
retroperitoneum	158.0	197.6	—	211.8	235.4	239.0
contiguous sites	158.8	—	—	—	—	—
retropharyngeal	149.0	198.89	230.0	210.9	235.1	239.0
retrovesical (septum)	195.3	198.89	234.8	229.8	238.8	239.89
rhinencephalon	191.0	198.3	—	225.0	237.5	239.6
rib	170.3	198.5	—	213.3	238.0	239.2
Rosenmüller's fossa	147.2	198.89	230.0	210.7	235.1	239.0
round ligament	183.5	198.82	—	221.0	236.3	239.5
sacrococcyx, sacrococcygeal	170.6	198.5	—	213.6	238.0	239.2
region	195.3	198.89	234.8	229.8	238.8	239.89
sacrouterine ligament	183.4	198.82	—	221.0	236.3	239.5
sacrum, sacral (vertebra)	170.6	198.5	—	213.6	238.0	239.2
salivary gland or duct						
(major)	142.9	198.89	230.0	210.2	235.0	239.0
contiguous sites	142.8	—	—	—	—	—
minor NEC	145.9	198.89	230.0	210.4	235.1	239.0
parotid	142.0	198.89	230.0	210.2	235.0	239.0
pluriglandular	142.8	198.89	230.0	210.2	235.0	239.0
sublingual	142.2	198.89	230.0	210.2	235.0	239.0
submandibular	142.1	198.89	230.0	210.2	235.0	239.0

	Malignant			Benign	Uncertain Behavior	Unspecified
	Primary	Secondary	Ca in situ			
submaxillary	142.1	198.89	230.0	210.2	235.0	239.0
salpinx (uterine)	183.2	198.82	233.39	221.0	236.3	239.5
Santorini's duct	157.3	197.8	230.9	211.6	235.5	239.0
scalp	173.4	198.2	232.4	216.4	238.2	239.2
scapula (any part)	170.4	198.5	—	213.4	238.0	239.2
scapular region	195.1	198.89	234.8	229.8	238.8	239.89
scar NEC (*see also*						
Neoplasm, skin)	173.9	198.2	232.9	216.9	238.2	239.2
sciatic nerve	171.3	198.89	—	215.3	238.1	239.2
sclera	190.0	198.4	234.0	224.0	238.8	239.89
scrotum (skin)	187.7	198.82	233.6	222.4	236.6	239.5
sebaceous gland—*see* Neoplasm, skin						
sella turcica	194.3	198.89	234.8	227.3	237.0	239.7
bone	170.0	198.5	—	213.0	238.0	239.2
semilunar cartilage (knee)	170.7	198.5	—	213.7	238.0	239.2
seminal vesicle	187.8	198.82	233.6	222.8	236.6	239.5
septum						
nasal	160.0	197.3	231.8	212.0	235.9	239.1
posterior margin	147.3	198.89	230.0	210.7	235.1	239.0
rectovaginal	195.3	198.89	234.8	229.8	238.8	239.89
rectovesical	195.3	198.89	234.8	229.8	238.8	239.89
urethrovaginal	184.9	198.82	233.39	221.9	236.3	239.5
vesicovaginal	184.9	198.82	233.39	221.9	236.3	239.5
shoulder NEC*	195.4	198.89	232.6	229.8	238.8	239.89
sigmoid flexure (lower)						
(upper)	153.3	197.5	230.3	211.3	235.2	239.0
sinus (accessory)	160.9	197.3	231.8	212.0	235.9	239.1
bone (any)	170.0	198.5	—	213.0	238.0	239.2
contiguous sites with middle ear or						
nasal cavities	160.8	—	—	—	—	—
ethmoidal	160.3	197.3	231.8	212.0	235.9	239.1
frontal	160.4	197.3	231.8	212.0	235.9	239.1
maxillary	160.2	197.3	231.8	212.0	235.9	239.1
nasal, paranasal NEC	160.9	197.3	231.8	212.0	235.9	239.1
pyriform	148.1	198.89	230.0	210.8	235.1	239.0
sphenoidal	160.5	197.3	231.8	212.0	235.9	239.1
skeleton, skeletal NEC	170.9	198.5	—	213.9	238.0	239.2
Skene's gland	189.4	198.1	233.9	223.89	236.99	239.5
skin NEC	173.9	198.2	232.9	216.9	238.2	239.2
abdominal wall	173.5	198.2	232.5	216.5	238.2	239.2
ala nasi	173.3	198.2	232.3	216.3	238.2	239.2
ankle	173.7	198.2	232.7	216.7	238.2	239.2
antecubital space	173.6	198.2	232.6	216.6	238.2	239.2
anus	173.5	198.2	232.5	216.5	238.2	239.2
arm	173.6	198.2	232.6	216.6	238.2	239.2
auditory canal (external)	173.2	198.2	232.2	216.2	238.2	239.2
auricle (ear)	173.2	198.2	232.2	216.2	238.2	239.2
auricular canal (external)	173.2	198.2	232.2	216.2	238.2	239.2
axilla, axillary fold	173.5	198.2	232.5	216.5	238.2	239.2
back	173.5	198.2	232.5	216.5	238.2	239.2
breast	173.5	198.2	232.5	216.5	238.2	239.2
brow	173.3	198.2	232.3	216.3	238.2	239.2
buttock	173.5	198.2	232.5	216.5	238.2	239.2
calf	173.7	198.2	232.7	216.7	238.2	239.2
canthus (eye) (inner)						
(outer)	173.1	198.2	232.1	216.1	238.2	239.2
cervical region	173.4	198.2	232.4	216.4	238.2	239.2
cheek (external)	173.3	198.2	232.3	216.3	238.2	239.2
chest (wall)	173.5	198.2	232.5	216.5	238.2	239.2
chin	173.3	198.2	232.3	216.3	238.2	239.2
clavicular area	173.5	198.2	232.5	216.5	238.2	239.2
clitoris	184.3	198.82	233.32	221.2	236.3	239.5
columnella	173.3	198.2	232.3	216.3	238.2	239.2

	Malignant					
	Primary	Secondary	Ca in situ	Benign	Uncertain Behavior	Unspecified
concha	173.2	198.2	232.2	216.2	238.2	239.2
contiguous sites	173.8	—	—	—	—	—
ear (external).	173.2	198.2	232.2	216.2	238.2	239.2
elbow.	173.6	198.2	232.6	216.6	238.2	239.2
eyebrow	173.3	198.2	232.3	216.3	238.2	239.2
eyelid.	173.1	198.2	232.1	216.1	238.2	239.2
face NEC.	173.3	198.2	232.3	216.3	238.2	239.2
female genital organs						
(external)	184.4	198.82	233.30	221.2	236.3	239.5
clitoris	184.3	198.82	233.32	221.2	236.3	239.5
labium NEC	184.4	198.82	233.32	221.2	236.3	239.5
majus.	184.1	198.82	233.32	221.2	236.3	239.5
minus.	184.2	198.82	233.32	221.2	236.3	239.5
pudendum	184.4	198.82	233.32	221.2	236.3	239.5
vulva	184.4	198.82	233.32	221.2	236.3	239.5
finger.	173.6	198.2	232.6	216.6	238.2	239.2
flank	173.5	198.2	232.5	216.5	238.2	239.2
foot	173.7	198.2	232.7	216.7	238.2	239.2
forearm	173.6	198.2	232.6	216.6	238.2	239.2
forehead	173.3	198.2	232.3	216.3	238.2	239.2
glabella.	173.3	198.2	232.3	216.3	238.2	239.2
gluteal region.	173.5	198.2	232.5	216.5	238.2	239.2
groin	173.5	198.2	232.5	216.5	238.2	239.2
hand	173.6	198.2	232.6	216.6	238.2	239.2
head NEC	173.4	198.2	232.4	216.4	238.2	239.2
heel.	173.7	198.2	232.7	216.7	238.2	239.2
helix	173.2	198.2	232.2	216.2	238.2	239.2
hip	173.7	198.2	232.7	216.7	238.2	239.2
infraclavicular region	173.5	198.2	232.5	216.5	238.2	239.2
inguinal region	173.5	198.2	232.5	216.5	238.2	239.2
jaw	173.3	198.2	232.3	216.3	238.2	239.2
knee	173.7	198.2	232.7	216.7	238.2	239.2
labia						
majora	184.1	198.82	233.32	221.2	236.3	239.5
minora	184.2	198.82	233.32	221.2	236.3	239.5
leg	173.7	198.2	232.7	216.7	238.2	239.2
lid (lower) (upper)	173.1	198.2	232.1	216.1	238.2	239.2
limb NEC.	173.9	198.2	232.9	216.9	238.2	239.5
lower	173.7	198.2	232.7	216.7	238.2	239.2
upper	173.6	198.2	232.6	216.6	238.2	239.2
lip (lower) (upper)	173.0	198.2	232.0	216.0	238.2	239.2
male genital organs.	187.9	198.82	233.6	222.9	236.6	239.5
penis	187.4	198.82	233.5	222.1	236.6	239.5
prepuce	187.1	198.82	233.5	222.1	236.6	239.5
scrotum.	187.7	198.82	233.6	222.4	236.6	239.5
mastectomy site	173.5	198.2	—	—	—	—
specified as breast tissue . . .	174.8	198.81	—	—	—	—
meatus, acoustic (external)	173.2	198.2	232.2	216.2	238.2	239.2
melanoma —*see* Melanoma						
nates	173.5	198.2	232.5	216.5	238.2	239.2
neck	173.4	198.2	232.4	216.4	238.2	239.2
nose (external)	173.3	198.2	232.3	216.3	238.2	239.2
palm	173.6	198.2	232.6	216.6	238.2	239.2
palpebra	173.1	198.2	232.1	216.1	238.2	239.2
penis NEC	187.4	198.82	233.5	222.1	236.6	239.5
perianal.	173.5	198.2	232.5	216.5	238.2	239.2
perineum	173.5	198.2	232.5	216.5	238.2	239.2
pinna	173.2	198.2	232.2	216.2	238.2	239.2
plantar	173.7	198.2	232.7	216.7	238.2	239.2
popliteal fossa or space	173.7	198.2	232.7	216.7	238.2	239.2
prepuce.	187.1	198.82	233.5	222.1	236.6	239.5
pubes	173.5	198.2	232.5	216.5	238.2	239.2
sacrococcygeal region	173.5	198.2	232.5	216.5	238.2	239.2

	Malignant			Benign	Uncertain Behavior	Unspecified
	Primary	Secondary	Ca in situ			
scalp	173.4	198.2	232.4	216.4	238.2	239.2
scapular region	173.5	198.2	232.5	216.5	238.2	239.2
scrotum	187.7	198.82	233.6	222.4	236.6	239.5
shoulder	173.6	198.2	232.6	216.6	238.2	239.2
sole (foot)	173.7	198.2	232.7	216.7	238.2	239.2
specified sites NEC	173.8	198.2	232.8	216.8	232.8	239.2
submammary fold	173.5	198.2	232.5	216.5	238.2	239.2
supraclavicular region	173.4	198.2	232.4	216.4	238.2	239.2
temple	173.3	198.2	232.3	216.3	238.2	239.2
thigh	173.7	198.2	232.7	216.7	238.2	239.2
thoracic wall	173.5	198.2	232.5	216.5	238.2	239.2
thumb	173.6	198.2	232.6	216.6	238.2	239.2
toe	173.7	198.2	232.7	216.7	238.2	239.2
tragus	173.2	198.2	232.2	216.2	238.2	239.2
trunk	173.5	198.2	232.5	216.5	238.2	239.2
umbilicus	173.5	198.2	232.5	216.5	238.2	239.2
vulva	184.4	198.82	233.32	221.2	236.3	239.5
wrist	173.6	198.2	232.6	216.6	238.2	239.2
skull	170.0	198.5	—	213.0	238.0	239.2
soft parts or tissues—see Neoplasm, connective tissue						
specified site NEC	195.8	198.89	234.8	229.8	238.8	239.89
spermatic cord	187.6	198.82	233.6	222.8	236.6	239.5
sphenoid	160.5	197.3	231.8	212.0	235.9	239.1
bone	170.0	198.5	—	213.0	238.0	239.2
sinus	160.5	197.3	231.8	212.0	235.9	239.1
sphincter						
anal	154.2	197.5	230.5	211.4	235.5	239.0
of Oddi	156.1	197.8	230.8	211.5	235.3	239.0
spine, spinal (column)	170.2	198.5	—	213.2	238.0	239.2
bulb	191.7	198.3	—	225.0	237.5	239.6
coccyx	170.6	198.5	—	213.6	238.0	239.2
cord (cervical) (lumbar) (sacral) (thoracic)	192.2	198.3	—	225.3	237.5	239.7
dura mater	192.3	198.4	—	225.4	237.6	239.7
lumbosacral	170.2	198.5	—	213.2	238.0	239.2
membrane	192.3	198.4	—	225.4	237.6	239.7
meninges	192.3	198.4	—	225.4	237.6	239.7
nerve (root)	171.9	198.89	—	215.9	238.1	239.2
pia mater	192.3	198.4	—	225.4	237.6	239.7
root	171.9	198.89	—	215.9	238.1	239.2
sacrum	170.6	198.5	—	213.6	238.0	239.2
spleen, splenic NEC	159.1	197.8	230.9	211.9	235.5	239.0
flexure (colon)	153.7	197.5	230.3	211.3	235.2	239.0
stem, brain	191.7	198.3	—	225.0	237.5	239.6
Stensen's duct	142.0	198.89	230.0	210.2	235.0	239.0
sternum	170.3	198.5	—	213.3	238.0	239.2
stomach	151.9	197.8	230.2	211.1	235.2	239.0
antrum (pyloric)	151.2	197.8	230.2	211.1	235.2	239.0
body	151.4	197.8	230.2	211.1	235.2	239.0
cardia	151.0	197.8	230.2	211.1	235.2	239.0
cardiac orifice	151.0	197.8	230.2	211.1	235.2	239.0
contiguous sites	151.8	—	—	—	—	—
corpus	151.4	197.8	230.2	211.1	235.2	239.0
fundus	151.3	197.8	230.2	211.1	235.2	239.0
greater curvature NEC	151.6	197.8	230.2	211.1	235.2	239.0
lesser curvature NEC	151.5	197.8	230.2	211.1	235.2	239.0
prepylorus	151.1	197.8	230.2	211.1	235.2	239.0
pylorus	151.1	197.8	230.2	211.1	235.2	239.0
wall NEC	151.9	197.8	230.2	211.1	235.2	239.0
anterior NEC	151.8	197.8	230.2	211.1	235.2	239.0
posterior NEC	151.8	197.8	230.2	211.1	235.2	239.0
stroma, endometrial	182.0	198.82	233.2	219.1	236.0	239.5

	Malignant			Benign	Uncertain Behavior	Unspecified
	Primary	Secondary	Ca in situ			
stump, cervical	180.8	198.82	233.1	219.0	236.0	239.5
subcutaneous (nodule) (tissue) NEC—*see* Neoplasm, connective tissue						
subdural	192.1	198.4	—	225.2	237.6	239.7
subglottis, subglottic	161.2	197.3	231.0	212.1	235.6	239.1
sublingual	144.9	198.89	230.0	210.3	235.1	239.0
gland or duct	142.2	198.89	230.0	210.2	235.0	239.0
submandibular gland	142.1	198.89	230.0	210.2	235.0	239.0
submaxillary gland or duct.	142.1	198.89	230.0	210.2	235.0	239.0
submental.	195.0	198.89	234.8	229.8	238.8	239.89
subpleural	162.9	197.0	—	212.3	235.7	239.1
substernal.	164.2	197.1	—	212.5	235.8	239.89
sudoriferous, sudoriparous gland, site unspecified.	173.9	198.2	232.9	216.9	238.2	239.2
specified site—*see* Neoplasm, skin						
supraclavicular region	195.0	198.89	234.8	229.8	238.8	239.89
supraglottis	161.1	197.3	231.0	212.1	235.6	239.1
suprarenal (capsule) (cortex) (gland) (medulla)	194.0	198.7	234.8	227.0	237.2	239.7
suprasellar (region).	191.9	198.3	—	225.0	237.5	239.6
sweat gland (apocrine) (eccrine), site unspecified	173.9	198.2	232.9	216.9	238.2	239.2
specified site—*see* Neoplasm, skin						
sympathetic nerve or nervous system NEC.	171.9	198.89	—	215.9	238.1	239.2
symphysis pubis	170.6	198.5	—	213.6	238.0	239.2
synovial membrane—*see* Neoplasm, connective tissue						
tapetum, brain	191.8	198.3	—	225.0	237.5	239.6
tarsus (any bone)	170.8	198.5	—	213.8	238.0	239.2
temple (skin)	173.3	198.2	232.3	216.3	238.2	239.2
temporal						
bone	170.0	198.5	—	213.0	238.0	239.2
lobe or pole.	191.2	198.3	—	225.0	237.5	239.6
region.	195.0	198.89	234.8	229.8	238.8	239.89
skin.	173.3	198.2	232.3	216.3	238.2	239.2
tendon (sheath)—*see* Neoplasm, connective tissue						
tentorium (cerebelli)	192.1	198.4	—	225.2	237.6	239.7
testis, testes (descended) (scrotal)	186.9	198.82	233.6	222.0	236.4	239.5
ectopic	186.0	198.82	233.6	222.0	236.4	239.5
retained.	186.0	198.82	233.6	222.0	236.4	239.5
undescended	186.0	198.82	233.6	222.0	236.4	239.5
thalamus	191.0	198.3	—	225.0	237.5	239.6
thigh NEC*.	195.5	198.89	234.8	229.8	238.8	239.89
thorax, thoracic (cavity) (organs NEC)	195.1	198.89	234.8	229.8	238.8	239.89
duct.	171.4	198.89	—	215.4	238.1	239.2
wall NEC.	195.1	198.89	234.8	229.8	238.8	239.89
throat	149.0	198.89	230.0	210.9	235.1	239.0
thumb NEC*	195.4	198.89	232.6	229.8	238.8	239.89
thymus (gland)	164.0	198.89	—	212.6	235.8	239.89
contiguous sites with heart and mediastinum	164.8	—	—	—	—	—
thyroglossal duct	193	198.89	234.8	226	237.4	239.7
thyroid (gland)	193	198.89	234.8	226	237.4	239.7
cartilage	161.3	197.3	231.0	212.1	235.6	239.1
tibia (any part)	170.7	198.5	—	213.7	238.0	239.2
toe NEC*.	195.5	198.89	232.7	229.8	238.8	239.89
tongue	141.9	198.89	230.0	210.1	235.1	239.0
anterior (two-thirds) NEC	141.4	198.89	230.0	210.1	235.1	239.0

	Malignant			Benign	Uncertain Behavior	Unspecified
	Primary	Secondary	Ca in situ			
dorsal surface	141.1	198.89	230.0	210.1	235.1	239.0
ventral surface	141.3	198.89	230.0	210.1	235.1	239.0
base (dorsal surface)	141.0	198.89	230.0	210.1	235.1	239.0
border (lateral)	141.2	198.89	230.0	210.1	235.1	239.0
contiguous sites	141.8	—	—	—	—	—
dorsal surface NEC	141.1	198.89	230.0	210.1	235.1	239.0
fixed part NEC	141.0	198.89	230.0	210.1	235.1	239.0
foramen cecum	141.1	198.89	230.0	210.1	235.1	239.0
frenulum linguae	141.3	198.89	230.0	210.1	235.1	239.0
junctional zone	141.5	198.89	230.0	210.1	235.1	239.0
margin (lateral)	141.2	198.89	230.0	210.1	235.1	239.0
midline NEC	141.1	198.89	230.0	210.1	235.1	239.0
mobile part NEC	141.4	198.89	230.0	210.1	235.1	239.0
posterior (third)	141.0	198.89	230.0	210.1	235.1	239.0
root	141.0	198.89	230.0	210.1	235.1	239.0
surface (dorsal)	141.1	198.89	230.0	210.1	235.1	239.0
base	141.0	198.89	230.0	210.1	235.1	239.0
ventral	141.3	198.89	230.0	210.1	235.1	239.0
tip	141.2	198.89	230.0	210.1	235.1	239.0
tonsil	141.6	198.89	230.0	210.1	235.1	239.0
tonsil	146.0	198.89	230.0	210.5	235.1	239.0
fauces, faucial	146.0	198.89	230.0	210.5	235.1	239.0
lingual	141.6	198.89	230.0	210.1	235.1	239.0
palatine	146.0	198.89	230.0	210.5	235.1	239.0
pharyngeal	147.1	198.89	230.0	210.7	235.1	239.0
pillar (anterior) (posterior)	146.2	198.89	230.0	210.6	235.1	239.0
tonsillar fossa	146.1	198.89	230.0	210.6	235.1	239.0
tooth socket NEC	143.9	198.89	230.0	210.4	235.1	239.0
trachea (cartilage) (mucosa)	162.0	197.3	231.1	212.2	235.7	239.1
contiguous sites with bronchus or lung	162.8	—	—	—	—	—
tracheobronchial	162.8	197.3	231.1	212.2	235.7	239.1
contiguous sites with lung	162.8	—	—	—	—	—
tragus	173.2	198.2	232.2	216.2	238.2	239.2
trunk NEC*	195.8	198.89	232.5	229.8	238.8	239.89
tubo-ovarian	183.8	198.82	233.39	221.8	236.3	239.5
tunica vaginalis	187.8	198.82	233.6	222.8	236.6	239.5
turbinate (bone)	170.0	198.5	—	213.0	238.0	239.2
nasal	160.0	197.3	231.8	212.0	235.9	239.1
tympanic cavity	160.1	197.3	231.8	212.0	235.9	239.1
ulna (any part)	170.4	198.5	—	213.4	238.0	239.2
umbilicus, umbilical	173.5	198.2	232.5	216.5	238.2	239.2
uncus, brain	191.2	198.3	—	225.0	237.5	239.6
unknown site or unspecified	199.1	199.1	234.9	229.9	238.9	239.9
urachus	188.7	198.1	233.7	223.3	236.7	239.4
ureter, ureteral	189.2	198.1	233.9	223.2	236.91	239.5
orifice (bladder)	188.6	198.1	233.7	223.3	236.7	239.4
ureter-bladder (junction)	188.6	198.1	233.7	223.3	236.7	239.4
urethra, urethral (gland)	189.3	198.1	233.9	223.81	236.99	239.5
orifice, internal	188.5	198.1	233.7	223.3	236.7	239.4
urethrovaginal (septum)	184.9	198.82	233.39	221.9	236.3	239.5
urinary organ or system NEC	189.9	198.1	233.9	223.9	236.99	239.5
bladder—*see* Neoplasm, bladder						
contiguous sites	189.8	—	—	—	—	—
specified sites NEC	189.8	198.1	233.9	223.89	236.99	239.5
utero-ovarian	183.8	198.82	233.39	221.8	236.3	239.5
ligament	183.3	198.82	—	221.0	236.3	239.5
uterosacral ligament	183.4	198.82	—	221.0	236.3	239.5
uterus, uteri, uterine	179	198.82	233.2	219.9	236.0	239.5
adnexa NEC	183.9	198.82	233.39	221.8	236.3	239.5
contiguous sites	183.8	—	—	—	—	—
body	182.0	198.82	233.2	219.1	236.0	239.5
contiguous sites	182.8	—	—	—	—	—

	Malignant			Benign	Uncertain Behavior	Unspecified
	Primary	Secondary	Ca in situ			
cervix	180.9	198.82	233.1	219.0	236.0	239.5
cornu	182.0	198.82	233.2	219.1	236.0	239.5
corpus	182.0	198.82	233.2	219.1	236.0	239.5
endocervix (canal) (gland)	180.0	198.82	233.1	219.0	236.0	239.5
endometrium	182.0	198.82	233.2	219.1	236.0	239.5
exocervix	180.1	198.82	233.1	219.0	236.0	239.5
external os	180.1	198.82	233.1	219.0	236.0	239.5
fundus	182.0	198.82	233.2	219.1	236.0	239.5
internal os	180.0	198.82	233.1	219.0	236.0	239.5
isthmus	182.1	198.82	233.2	219.1	236.0	239.5
ligament	183.4	198.82	—	221.0	236.3	239.5
broad	183.3	198.82	233.39	221.0	236.3	239.5
round	183.5	198.82	—	221.0	236.3	239.5
lower segment	182.1	198.82	233.2	219.1	236.0	239.5
myometrium	182.0	198.82	233.2	219.1	236.0	239.5
squamocolumnar junction	180.8	198.82	233.1	219.0	236.0	239.5
tube	183.2	198.82	233.39	221.0	236.3	239.5
utricle, prostatic	189.3	198.1	233.9	223.81	236.99	239.5
uveal tract	190.0	198.4	234.0	224.0	238.8	239.89
uvula	145.4	198.89	230.0	210.4	235.1	239.0
vagina, vaginal (fornix)						
(vault) (wall)	184.0	198.82	233.31	221.1	236.3	239.5
vaginovesical	184.9	198.82	233.39	221.9	236.3	239.5
septum	184.9	198.82	233.39	221.9	236.3	239.5
vallecula (epiglottis)	146.3	198.89	230.0	210.6	235.1	239.0
vascular—*see* Neoplasm,						
connective tissue						
vas deferens	187.6	198.82	233.6	222.8	236.6	239.5
Vater's ampulla	156.2	197.8	230.8	211.5	235.3	239.0
vein, venous—*see* Neoplasm,						
connective tissue						
vena cava (abdominal)						
(inferior)	171.5	198.89	—	215.5	238.1	239.2
superior	171.4	198.89	—	215.4	238.1	239.2
ventricle (cerebral) (floor) (fourth)						
(lateral) (third)	191.5	198.3	—	225.0	237.5	239.6
cardiac (left) (right)	164.1	198.89	—	212.7	238.8	239.89
ventricular band of larynx	161.1	197.3	231.0	212.1	235.6	239.1
ventriculus—*see* Neoplasm,						
stomach						
vermillion border—*see*						
Neoplasm, lip						
vermis, cerebellum	191.6	198.3	—	225.0	237.5	239.6
vertebra (column)	170.2	198.5	—	213.2	238.0	239.2
coccyx	170.6	198.5	—	213.6	238.0	239.2
sacrum	170.6	198.5	—	213.6	238.0	239.2
vesical—*see* Neoplasm, bladder						
vesicle, seminal	187.8	198.82	233.6	222.8	236.6	239.5
vesicocervical tissue	184.9	198.82	233.39	221.9	236.3	239.5
vesicorectal	195.3	198.89	234.8	229.8	238.8	239.89
vesicovaginal	184.9	198.82	233.39	221.9	236.3	239.5
septum	184.9	198.82	233.39	221.9	236.3	239.5
vessel (blood)—*see* Neoplasm,						
connective tissue						
vestibular gland, greater	184.1	198.82	233.32	221.2	236.3	239.5
vestibule						
mouth	145.1	198.89	230.0	210.4	235.1	239.0
nose	160.0	197.3	231.8	212.0	235.9	239.1
Virchow's gland	—	196.0	—	229.0	238.8	239.89
viscera NEC	195.8	198.89	234.8	229.8	238.8	239.89
vocal cords (true)	161.0	197.3	231.0	212.1	235.6	239.1
false	161.1	197.3	231.0	212.1	235.6	239.1
vomer	170.0	198.5	—	213.0	238.0	239.2

	Malignant					
	Primary	Secondary	Ca in situ	Benign	Uncertain Behavior	Unspecified
vulva	184.4	198.82	233.32	221.2	236.3	239.5
vulvovaginal gland	184.4	198.82	233.32	221.2	236.3	239.5
Waldeyer's ring	149.1	198.89	230.0	210.9	235.1	239.0
Wharton's duct	142.1	198.89	230.0	210.2	235.0	239.0
white matter (central)						
(cerebral)	191.0	198.3	—	225.0	237.5	239.6
windpipe	162.0	197.3	231.1	212.2	235.7	239.1
Wirsung's duct	157.3	197.8	230.9	211.6	235.5	239.0
wolffian (body) (duct)						
female	184.8	198.82	233.39	221.8	236.3	239.5
male	187.8	198.82	233.6	222.8	236.6	239.5
womb—*see* Neoplasm, uterus						
wrist NEC*	195.4	198.89	232.6	229.8	238.8	239.89
xiphoid process	170.3	198.5	—	213.3	238.0	239.2
Zuckerkandl's organ	194.6	198.89	—	227.6	237.3	239.7

Neovascularization
  choroid 362.16
  ciliary body 364.42
  cornea 370.60
    deep 370.63
    localized 370.61
  iris 364.42
  retina 362.16
  subretinal 362.16
Nephralgia 788.0
Nephritis, nephritic (albuminuric) (azotemic)
    (congenital) (degenerative) (diffuse)
    (disseminated) (epithelial) (familial) (focal)
    (granulomatous) (hemorrhagic) (infantile)
    (nonsuppurative, excretory) (uremic) 583.9
  with
    edema—*see* Nephrosis
    lesion of
      glomerulonephritis
        hypocomplementemic persistent 583.2
          with nephrotic syndrome 581.2
          chronic 582.2
        lobular 583.2
          with nephrotic syndrome 581.2
          chronic 582.2
        membranoproliferative 583.2
          with nephrotic syndrome 581.2
          chronic 582.2
        membranous 583.1
          with nephrotic syndrome 581.1
          chronic 582.1
        mesangiocapillary 583.2
          with nephrotic syndrome 581.2
          chronic 582.2
        mixed membranous and proliferative 583.2
          with nephrotic syndrome 581.2
          chronic 582.2
        proliferative (diffuse) 583.0
          with nephrotic syndrome 581.0
          acute 580.0
          chronic 582.0
        rapidly progressive 583.4
          acute 580.4
          chronic 582.4
      interstitial nephritis (diffuse) (focal) 583.89
        with nephrotic syndrome 581.89
        acute 580.89
        chronic 582.89
      necrotizing glomerulitis 583.4
        acute 580.4
        chronic 582.4
      renal necrosis 583.9
        cortical 583.6
        medullary 583.7
      specified pathology NEC 583.89
        with nephrotic syndrome 581.89
        acute 580.89
        chronic 582.89
    necrosis, renal 583.9
      cortical 583.6
      medullary (papillary) 583.7
    nephrotic syndrome (*see also* Nephrosis) 581.9
    papillary necrosis 583.7
    specified pathology NEC 583.89
  acute 580.9
    extracapillary with epithelial crescents 580.4
    hypertensive (*see also* Hypertension, kidney)
      403.90
    necrotizing 580.4
    poststreptococcal 580.0
    proliferative (diffuse) 580.0

Nephritis, nephritic—*continued*
  acute—*continued*
    rapidly progressive 580.4
    specified pathology NEC 580.89
  amyloid 277.39 *[583.81]*
    chronic 277.39 *[582.81]*
  arteriolar (*see also* Hypertension, kidney)
      403.90
  arteriosclerotic (*see also* Hypertension, kidney)
      403.90
  ascending (*see also* Pyelitis) 590.80
  atrophic 582.9
  basement membrane NEC 583.89
    with
      pulmonary hemorrhage (Goodpasture's
        syndrome) 446.21 *[583.81]*
  calculous, calculus 592.0
  cardiac (*see also* Hypertension, kidney) 403.90
  cardiovascular (*see also* Hypertension, kidney)
      403.90
  chronic 582.9
    arteriosclerotic (*see also* Hypertension,
      kidney) 403.90
    hypertensive (*see also* Hypertension, kidney)
      403.90
  cirrhotic (*see also* Sclerosis, renal) 587
  complicating pregnancy, childbirth, or
      puerperium 646.2
    with hypertension 642.1
      affecting fetus or newborn 760.0
    affecting fetus or newborn 760.1
  croupous 580.9
  desquamative—*see* Nephrosis
  due to
    amyloidosis 277.39 *[583.81]*
      chronic 277.39 *[582.81]*
    arteriosclerosis (*see also* Hypertension,
      kidney) 403.90
    diabetes mellitus 250.4 *[583.81]*
      due to secondary diabetes 249.4 *[583.81]*
      with nephrotic syndrome 250.4 *[581.81]*
        due to secondary diabetes 249.4 *[581.81]*
    diphtheria 032.89 *[580.81]*
    gonococcal infection (acute) 098.19 *[583.81]*
      chronic or duration of 2 months or over
        098.39 *[583.81]*
    gout 274.10
    infectious hepatitis 070.9 *[580.81]*
    mumps 072.79 *[580.81]*
    specified kidney pathology NEC 583.89
      acute 580.89
      chronic 582.89
    streptotrichosis 039.8 *[583.81]*
    subacute bacterial endocarditis 421.0 *[580.81]*
    systemic lupus erythematosus 710.0 *[583.81]*
      chronic 710.0 *[582.81]*
    typhoid fever 002.0 *[580.81]*
  endothelial 582.2
  end stage (chronic) (terminal) NEC 585.6
  epimembranous 581.1
  exudative 583.89
    with nephrotic syndrome 581.89
    acute 580.89
    chronic 582.89
  gonococcal (acute) 098.19 *[583.81]*
    chronic or duration of 2 months or over 098.39
      [583.81]
  gouty 274.10
  hereditary (Alport's syndrome) 759.89
  hydremic—*see* Nephrosis
  hypertensive (*see also* Hypertension, kidney) 403.90

Nephritis, nephritic—*continued*
  hypocomplementemic persistent 583.2
    with nephrotic syndrome 581.2
      chronic 582.2
  immune complex NEC 583.89
  infective (*see also* Pyelitis) 590.80
  interstitial (diffuse) (focal) 583.89
    with nephrotic syndrome 581.89
    acute 580.89
    chronic 582.89
  latent or quiescent—*see* Nephritis, chronic
  lead 984.9
    specified type of lead—*see* Table of drugs and
      chemicals
  lobular 583.2
    with nephrotic syndrome 581.2
      chronic 582.2
  lupus 710.0 [583.81]
    acute 710.0 [580.81]
    chronic 710.0 [582.81]
  membranoproliferative 583.2
    with nephrotic syndrome 581.2
      chronic 582.2
  membranous 583.1
    with nephrotic syndrome 581.1
      chronic 582.1
  mesangiocapillary 583.2
    with nephrotic syndrome 581.2
      chronic 582.2
  minimal change 581.3
  mixed membranous and proliferative 583.2
    with nephrotic syndrome 581.2
      chronic 582.2
  necrotic, necrotizing 583.4
    acute 580.4
    chronic 582.4
  nephrotic—*see* Nephrosis
  old—*see* Nephritis, chronic
  parenchymatous 581.89
  polycystic 753.12
    adult type (APKD) 753.13
    autosomal dominant 753.13
    autosomal recessive 753.14
    childhood type (CPKD) 753.14
    infantile type 753.14
  poststreptococcal 580.0
  pregnancy—*see* Nephritis, complicating
    pregnancy
  proliferative 583.0
    with nephrotic syndrome 581.0
    acute 580.0
    chronic 582.0
  purulent (*see also* Pyelitis) 590.80
  rapidly progressive 583.4
    acute 580.4
    chronic 582.4
  salt-losing or salt-wasting (*see also* Disease,
    renal) 593.9
  saturnine 984.9
    specified type of lead—*see* Table of drugs and
      chemicals
  septic (*see also* Pyelitis) 590.80
  specified pathology NEC 583.89
    acute 580.89
    chronic 582.89
  staphylococcal (*see also* Pyelitis) 590.80
  streptotrichosis 039.8 [583.81]
  subacute (*see also* Nephrosis) 581.9
  suppurative (*see also* Pyelitis) 590.80
  syphilitic (late) 095.4
    congenital 090.5 [583.81]
    early 091.69 [583.81]

Nephritis, nephritic— *continued*
  terminal (chronic) (end-stage) NEC 585.6
  toxic—*see* Nephritis, acute
  tubal, tubular—*see* Nephrosis, tubular
  tuberculous (*see also* Tuberculosis) 016.0 [583.81]
  type II (Ellis)—*see* Nephrosis
  vascular—*see* Hypertension, kidney
  war 580.9
Nephroblastoma (M8960/3) 189.0
  epithelial (M8961/3) 189.0
  mesenchymal (M8962/3) 189.0
Nephrocalcinosis 275.49
Nephrocystitis, pustular (*see also* Pyelitis) 590.80
Nephrolithiasis (congenital) (pelvis) (recurrent)
    592.0
  uric acid 274.11
Nephroma (M8960/3) 189.0
  mesoblastic (M8960/1) 236.9
Nephronephritis (*see also* Nephrosis) 581.9
Nephronopthisis 753.16
Nephropathy (*see also* Nephritis) 583.9
  with
    exudative nephritis 583.89
    interstitial nephritis (diffuse) (focal) 583.89
    medullary necrosis 583.7
    necrosis 583.9
      cortical 583.6
      medullary or papillary 583.7
    papillary necrosis 583.7
    specified lesion or cause NEC 583.89
  analgesic 583.89
    with medullary necrosis, acute 584.7
  arteriolar (*see also* Hypertension, kidney)
    403.90
  arteriosclerotic (*see also* Hypertension, kidney)
    403.90
  complicating pregnancy 646.2
  diabetic 250.4 [583.81]
    due to secondary diabetes 249.4 [583.81]
  gouty 274.10
    specified type NEC 274.19
  hereditary amyloid 277.31
  hypercalcemic 588.89
  hypertensive (*see also* Hypertension, kidney)
    403.90
  hypokalemic (vacuolar) 588.89
  IgA 583.9
  obstructive 593.89
    congenital 753.20
  phenacetin 584.7
  phosphate-losing 588.0
  potassium depletion 588.89
  proliferative (*see also* Nephritis, proliferative) 583.0
  protein-losing 588.89
  salt-losing or salt-wasting (*see also* Disease,
    renal) 593.9
  sickle-cell (*see also* Disease, sickle-cell) 282.60
    [583.81]
  toxic 584.5
  vasomotor 584.5
  water-losing 588.89
Nephroptosis (*see also* Disease, renal) 593.0
  congenital (displaced) 753.3
Nephropyosis (*see also* Abscess, kidney) 590.2
Nephrorrhagia 593.81
Nephrosclerosis (arteriolar) (arteriosclerotic)
    (chronic) (hyaline) (*see also* Hypertension,
    kidney) 403.90
  gouty 274.10
  hyperplastic (arteriolar) (*see also* Hypertension,
    kidney) 403.90
  senile (*see also* Sclerosis, renal) 587

Nephrosis, nephrotic (Epstein's) (syndrome) 581.9
  with
    lesion of
      focal glomerulosclerosis 581.1
      glomerulonephritis
        endothelial 581.2
        hypocomplementemic persistent 581.2
        lobular 581.2
        membranoproliferative 581.2
        membranous 581.1
        mesangiocapillary 581.2
        minimal change 581.3
        mixed membranous and proliferative 581.2
        proliferative 581.0
        segmental hyalinosis 581.1
        specified pathology NEC 581.89
  acute—*see* Nephrosis, tubular
  anoxic—*see* Nephrosis, tubular
  arteriosclerotic (*see also* Hypertension, kidney) 403.90
  chemical—*see* Nephrosis, tubular
  cholemic 572.4
  complicating pregnancy, childbirth, or puerperium—*see* Nephritis, complicating pregnancy
  diabetic 250.4 *[581.81]*
    due to secondary diabetes 249.4 *[581.81]*
  Finnish type (congenital) 759.89
  hemoglobinuric—*see* Nephrosis, tubular
  in
    amyloidosis 277.39 *[581.81]*
    diabetes mellitus 250.4 *[581.81]*
      due to secondary diabetes 249.4 *[581.81]*
    epidemic hemorrhagic fever 078.6
    malaria 084.9 *[581.81]*
    polyarteritis 446.0 *[581.81]*
    systemic lupus erythematosus 710.0 *[581.81]*
  ischemic—*see* Nephrosis, tubular
  lipoid 581.3
  lower nephron—*see* Nephrosis, tubular
  lupoid 710.0 *[581.81]*
  lupus 710.0 *[581.81]*
  malarial 084.9 *[581.81]*
  minimal change 581.3
  necrotizing—*see* Nephrosis, tubular
  osmotic (sucrose) 588.89
  polyarteritic 446.0 *[581.81]*
  radiation 581.9
  specified lesion or cause NEC 581.89
  syphilitic 095.4
  toxic—*see* Nephrosis, tubular
  tubular (acute) 584.5
    due to a procedure 997.5
    radiation 581.9
Nephrosonephritis hemorrhagic (endemic) 078.6
Nephrostomy status V44.6
  with complication 997.5
Nerve —*see* condition
Nerves 799.21
Nervous (*see also* condition) 799.21
  breakdown 300.9
  heart 306.2
  stomach 306.4
  tension 799.21
Nervousness 799.21
Nesidioblastoma (M8150/0)
  pancreas 211.7
  specified site NEC—*see* Neoplasm, by site, benign
  unspecified site 211.7
Netherton's syndrome (ichthyosiform erythroderma) 757.1

Nettle rash 708.8
Nettleship's disease (urticaria pigmentosa) 757.33
Neumann's disease (pemphigus vegetans) 694.4
Neuralgia, neuralgic (acute) (*see also* Neuritis) 729.2
  accessory (nerve) 352.4
  acoustic (nerve) 388.5
  ankle 355.8
  anterior crural 355.8
  anus 787.99
  arm 723.4
  auditory (nerve) 388.5
  axilla 353.0
  bladder 788.1
  brachial 723.4
  brain—*see* Disorder, nerve, cranial
  broad ligament 625.9
  cerebral—*see* Disorder, nerve, cranial
  ciliary 339.00
  cranial nerve—*see also* Disorder, nerve, cranial
    fifth or trigeminal (*see also* Neuralgia, trigeminal) 350.1
  ear 388.71
    middle 352.1
  facial 351.8
  finger 354.9
  flank 355.8
  foot 355.8
  forearm 354.9
  Fothergill's (*see also* Neuralgia, trigeminal) 350.1
    postherpetic 053.12
  glossopharyngeal (nerve) 352.1
  groin 355.8
  hand 354.9
  heel 355.8
  Horton's 339.00
  Hunt's 053.11
  hypoglossal (nerve) 352.5
  iliac region 355.8
  infraorbital (*see also* Neuralgia, trigeminal) 350.1
  inguinal 355.8
  intercostal (nerve) 353.8
    postherpetic 053.19
  jaw 352.1
  kidney 788.0
  knee 355.8
  loin 355.8
  malarial (*see also* Malaria) 084.6
  mastoid 385.89
  maxilla 352.1
  median thenar 354.1
  metatarsal 355.6
  middle ear 352.1
  migrainous 339.00
  Morton's 355.6
  nerve, cranial—*see* Disorder, nerve, cranial
  nose 352.0
  occipital 723.8
  olfactory (nerve) 352.0
  ophthalmic 377.30
    postherpetic 053.19
  optic (nerve) 377.30
  penis 607.9
  perineum 355.8
  pleura 511.0
  postherpetic NEC 053.19
    geniculate ganglion 053.11
    ophthalmic 053.19
    trifacial 053.12
    trigeminal 053.12

Neuralgia, neuralgic—*continued*
pubic region 355.8
radial (nerve) 723.4
rectum 787.99
sacroiliac joint 724.3
sciatic (nerve) 724.3
scrotum 608.9
seminal vesicle 608.9
shoulder 354.9
Sluder's 337.09
specified nerve NEC—*see* Disorder, nerve
spermatic cord 608.9
sphenopalatine (ganglion) 337.09
subscapular (nerve) 723.4
suprascapular (nerve) 723.4
testis 608.89
thenar (median) 354.1
thigh 355.8
tongue 352.5
trifacial (nerve) (*see also* Neuralgia, trigeminal)
    350.1
trigeminal (nerve) 350.1
    postherpetic 053.12
tympanic plexus 388.71
ulnar (nerve) 723.4
vagus (nerve) 352.3
wrist 354.9
writers' 300.89
    organic 333.84
Neurapraxia —*see* Injury, nerve
Neurasthenia 300.5
cardiac 306.2
gastric 306.4
heart 306.2
postfebrile 780.79
postviral 780.79
Neurilemmoma (M9560/0)—*see also* Neoplasm,
    connective tissue, benign
acoustic (nerve) 225.1
malignant (M9560/3)—*see also* Neoplasm,
    connective tissue, malignant
    acoustic (nerve) 192.0
Neurilemmosarcoma (M9560/3)—*see*
    Neoplasm, connective tissue, malignant
Neurilemoma —*see* Neurilemmoma
Neurinoma (M9560/0)—*see* Neurilemmoma
Neurinomatosis (M9560/1)—*see also* Neoplasm,
    connective tissue, uncertain behavior
    centralis 759.5
Neuritis (*see also* Neuralgia) 729.2
abducens (nerve) 378.54
accessory (nerve) 352.4
acoustic (nerve) 388.5
    syphilitic 094.86
alcoholic 357.5
    with psychosis 291.1
amyloid, any site 277.39 *[357.4]*
anterior crural 355.8
arising during pregnancy 646.4
arm 723.4
ascending 355.2
auditory (nerve) 388.5
brachial (nerve) NEC 723.4
    due to displacement, intervertebral disc 722.0
    cervical 723.4
chest (wall) 353.8
costal region 353.8
cranial nerve—*see also* Disorder, nerve, cranial
    first or olfactory 352.0
    second or optic 377.30
    third or oculomotor 378.52
    fourth or trochlear 378.53

Neuritis—*continued*
cranial nerve—*continued*
    fifth or trigeminal (*see also* Neuralgia,
        trigeminal) 350.1
    sixth or abducens 378.54
    seventh or facial 351.8
        newborn 767.5
    eighth or acoustic 388.5
    ninth or glossopharyngeal 352.1
    tenth or vagus 352.3
    eleventh or accessory 352.4
    twelfth or hypoglossal 352.5
Déjérine-Sottas 356.0
diabetic 250.6 *[357.2]*
    due to secondary diabetes 249.6 *[357.2]*
diphtheritic 032.89 *[357.4]*
due to
    beriberi 265.0 *[357.4]*
    displacement, prolapse, protrusion, or rupture
        of intervertebral disc 722.2
        cervical 722.0
        lumbar, lumbosacral 722.10
        thoracic, thoracolumbar 722.11
    herniation, nucleus pulposus 722.2
        cervical 722.0
        lumbar, lumbosacral 722.10
        thoracic, thoracolumbar 722.11
endemic 265.0 *[357.4]*
facial (nerve) 351.8
    newborn 767.5
general—*see* Polyneuropathy
geniculate ganglion 351.1
    due to herpes 053.11
glossopharyngeal (nerve) 352.1
gouty 274.89 *[357.4]*
hypoglossal (nerve) 352.5
ilioinguinal (nerve) 355.8
in diseases classified elsewhere—*see*
    Polyneuropathy, in
infectious (multiple) 357.0
intercostal (nerve) 353.8
interstitial hypertrophic progressive NEC 356.9
leg 355.8
lumbosacral NEC 724.4
median (nerve) 354.1
    thenar 354.1
multiple (acute) (infective) 356.9
    endemic 265.0 *[357.4]*
multiplex endemica 265.0 *[357.4]*
nerve root (*see also* Radiculitis) 729.2
oculomotor (nerve) 378.52
olfactory (nerve) 352.0
optic (nerve) 377.30
    in myelitis 341.0
    meningococcal 036.81
pelvic 355.8
peripheral (nerve)—*see also* Neuropathy,
    peripheral
    complicating pregnancy or puerperium 646.4
    specified nerve NEC—*see* Mononeuritis
pneumogastric (nerve) 352.3
postchickenpox 052.7
postherpetic 053.19
progressive hypertrophic interstitial NEC 356.9
puerperal, postpartum 646.4
radial (nerve) 723.4
retrobulbar 377.32
    syphilitic 094.85
rheumatic (chronic) 729.2
sacral region 355.8
sciatic (nerve) 724.3
    due to displacement of intervertebral disc 722.10

Neuritis—*continued*
  serum 999.5
  specified nerve NEC—*see* Disorder, nerve
  spinal (nerve) 355.9
    root (*see also* Radiculitis) 729.2
  subscapular (nerve) 723.4
  suprascapular (nerve) 723.4
  syphilitic 095.8
  thenar (median) 354.1
  thoracic NEC 724.4
  toxic NEC 357.7
  trochlear (nerve) 378.53
  ulnar (nerve) 723.4
  vagus (nerve) 352.3
Neuroangiomatosis, encephalofacial 759.6
Neuroastrocytoma (M9505/1)—*see* Neoplasm,
  by site, uncertain behavior
Neuro-avitaminosis 269.2
Neuroblastoma (M9500/3)
  olfactory (M9522/3) 160.0
  specified site—*see* Neoplasm, by site, malignant
  unspecified site 194.0
Neurochorioretinitis (*see also* Chorioretinitis)
  363.20
Neurocirculatory asthenia 306.2
Neurocytoma (M9506/0)—*see* Neoplasm, by
  site, benign
Neurodermatitis (circumscribed) (circumscripta)
  (local) 698.3
  atopic 691.8
  diffuse (Brocq) 691.8
  disseminated 691.8
  nodulosa 698.3
Neuroencephalomyelopathy, optic 341.0
Neuroendocrine tumor —see Tumor,
  neuroendocrine
Neuroepithelioma (M9503/3)—*see also*
  Neoplasm, by site, malignant
  olfactory (M9521/3) 160.0
Neurofibroma (M9540/0)—*see also* Neoplasm,
  connective tissue, benign
  melanotic (M9541/0)—*see* Neoplasm,
    connective tissue, benign
  multiple (M9540/1) 237.70
    Type 1 237.71
    Type 2 237.72
  plexiform (M9550/0)—*see* Neoplasm,
    connective tissue, benign
Neurofibromatosis (multiple) (M9540/1) 237.70
  acoustic 237.72
  malignant (M9540/3)—*see* Neoplasm,
    connective tissue, malignant
  Type 1 237.71
  Type 2 237.72
  von Recklinghausen's 237.71
Neurofibrosarcoma (M9540/3)—*see* Neoplasm,
  connective tissue, malignant
Neurogenic —*see also* condition
  bladder (atonic) (automatic) (autonomic)
    (flaccid) (hypertonic) (hypotonic) (inertia)
    (infranuclear) (irritable) (motor) (nonreflex)
    (nuclear) (paralysis) (reflex) (sensory)
    (spastic) (supranuclear) (uninhibited) 596.54
    with cauda equina syndrome 344.61
  bowel 564.81
  heart 306.2
Neuroglioma (M9505/1)—*see* Neoplasm, by site,
  uncertain behavior
Neurolabyrinthitis (of Dix and Hallpike) 386.12
Neurolathyrism 988.2

Neuroleprosy 030.1
Neuroleptic malignant syndrome 333.92
Neurolipomatosis 272.8
Neuroma (M9570/0)—*see also* Neoplasm,
  connective tissue, benign
  acoustic (nerve) (M9560/0) 225.1
  amputation (traumatic)—*see also* Injury, nerve,
    by site
    surgical complication (late) 997.61
  appendix 211.3
  auditory nerve 225.1
  digital 355.6
    toe 355.6
  interdigital (toe) 355.6
  intermetatarsal 355.6
  Morton's 355.6
  multiple 237.70
    Type 1 237.71
    Type 2 237.72
  nonneoplastic 355.9
    arm NEC 354.9
    leg NEC 355.8
    lower extremity NEC 355.8
    specified site NEC—*see* Mononeuritis, by site
    upper extremity NEC 354.9
  optic (nerve) 225.1
  plantar 355.6
  plexiform (M9550/0)—*see* Neoplasm,
    connective tissue, benign
  surgical (nonneoplastic) 355.9
    arm NEC 354.9
    leg NEC 355.8
    lower extremity NEC 355.8
    upper extremity NEC 354.9
  traumatic—*see also* Injury, nerve, by site
    old—*see* Neuroma, nonneoplastic
Neuromyalgia 729.1
Neuromyasthenia (epidemic) 049.8
Neuromyelitis 341.8
  ascending 357.0
  optica 341.0
Neuromyopathy NEC 358.9
Neuromyositis 729.1
Neuronevus (M8725/0)—*see* Neoplasm, skin,
  benign
Neuronitis 357.0
  ascending (acute) 355.2
  vestibular 386.12
Neuroparalytic —*see* condition
Neuropathy, axtaxia and retinitis pigmentosa
  (NARP syndrome) 277.87
Neuropathy, neuropathic (*see also* Disorder,
  nerve) 355.9
  acute motor 357.82
  alcoholic 357.5
    with psychosis 291.1
  arm NEC 354.9
  ataxia and retinitis pigmentosa (NARP
    syndrome) 277.87
  autonomic (peripheral)—*see* Neuropathy,
    peripheral, autonomic
  axillary nerve 353.0
  brachial plexus 353.0
  cervical plexus 353.2
  chronic
    progressive segmentally demyelinating 357.89
    relapsing demyelinating 357.89
  congenital sensory 356.2
  Déjérine-Sottas 356.0

Neurosis, neurotic—*continued*
  mixed NEC 300.89
  musculoskeletal 306.0
  obsessional 300.3
    phobia 300.3
  obsessive-compulsive 300.3
  occupational 300.89
  ocular 306.7
  oral 307.0
  organ (*see also* Disorder, psychosomatic) 306.9
  pharynx 306.1
  phobic 300.20
  posttraumatic (acute) (situational) 309.81
    chronic 309.81
  psychasthenic (type) 300.89
  railroad 300.16
  rectum 306.4
  respiratory 306.1
  rumination 306.4
  senile 300.89
  sexual 302.70
  situational 300.89
  specified type NEC 300.89
  state 300.9
    with depersonalization episode 300.6
  stomach 306.4
  vasomotor 306.2
  visceral 306.4
  war 300.16
Neurospongioblastosis diffusa 759.5
Neurosyphilis (arrested) (early) (inactive) (late)
    (latent) (recurrent) 094.9
  with ataxia (cerebellar) (locomotor) (spastic)
    (spinal) 094.0
  acute meningitis 094.2
  aneurysm 094.89
  arachnoid (adhesive) 094.2
  arteritis (any artery) 094.89
  asymptomatic 094.3
  congenital 090.40
  dura (mater) 094.89
  general paresis 094.1
  gumma 094.9
  hemorrhagic 094.9
  juvenile (asymptomatic) (meningeal) 090.40
  leptomeninges (aseptic) 094.2
  meningeal 094.2
  meninges (adhesive) 094.2
  meningovascular (diffuse) 094.2
  optic atrophy 094.84
  parenchymatous (degenerative) 094.1
  paresis (*see also* Paresis, general) 094.1
  paretic (*see also* Paresis, general) 094.1
  relapse 094.9
  remission in (sustained) 094.9
  serological 094.3
  specified nature or site NEC 094.89
  tabes (dorsalis) 094.0
    juvenile 090.40
  tabetic 094.0
    juvenile 090.40
  taboparesis 094.1
    juvenile 090.40
  thrombosis 094.89
  vascular 094.89
Neurotic (*see also* Neurosis) 300.9
  excoriation 698.4
    psychogenic 306.3
Neurotmesis —*see* Injury, nerve, by site
Neurotoxemia —*see* Toxemia
Neutro-oclusion 524.21

Neutropenia, neutropenic (idiopathic)
    (pernicious) (primary) 288.00
  chronic 288.09
    hypoplastic 288.09
  congenital (nontransient) 288.01
  cyclic 288.02
  drug induced 288.03
  due to infection 288.04
  fever 288.00
  genetic 288.01
  immune 288.09
  infantile 288.01
  malignant 288.09
  neonatal, transitory (isoimmune) (maternal
    transfer) 776.7
  periodic 288.02
  splenic 289.53
  splenomegaly 289.53
  toxic 288.09
Neutrophilia, hereditary giant 288.2
Nevocarcinoma (M8720/3)—*see* Melanoma
Nevus (M8720/0)—*see also* Neoplasm, skin,
    benign

*Note—Except where otherwise indicated, the
varieties of nevus in the list below that are
followed by a morphology code number (M——
-/0) should be coded by site as for "Neoplasm,
skin, benign."*

  acanthotic 702.8
  achromic (M8730/0)
  amelanotic (M8730/0)
  anemic, anemicus 709.09
  angiomatous (M9120/0) (*see also* Hemangioma)
    228.00
  araneus 448.1
  avasculosus 709.09
  balloon cell (M8722/0)
  bathing trunk (M8761/1) 238.2
  blue (M8780/0)
    cellular (M8790/0)
    giant (M8790/0)
    Jadassohn's (M8780/0)
    malignant (M8780/3)—*see* Melanoma
  capillary (M9131/0) (*see also* Hemangioma)
    228.00
  cavernous (M9121/0) (*see also* Hemangioma)
    228.00
  cellular (M8720/0)
    blue (M8790/0)
  comedonicus 757.33
  compound (M8760/0)
  conjunctiva (M8720/0) 224.3
  dermal (M8750/0)
    and epidermal (M8760/0)
  epithelioid cell (and spindle cell) (M8770/0)
  flammeus 757.32
    osteohypertrophic 759.89
  hairy (M8720/0)
  halo (M8723/0)
  hemangiomatous (M9120/0) (*see also*
    Hemangioma) 228.00
  intradermal (M8750/0)
  intraepidermal (M8740/0)
  involuting (M8724/0)
  Jadassohn's (blue) (M8780/0)
  junction, junctional (M8740/0)
    malignant melanoma in (M8740/3)—*see*
      Melanoma
  juvenile (M8770/0)
  lymphatic (M9170/0) 228.1

Nevus—*continued*
  magnocellular (M8726/0)
    specified site—*see* Neoplasm, by site, benign
    unspecified site 224.0
  malignant (M8720/3)—*see* Melanoma
  meaning hemangioma (M9120/0) (*see also*
      Hemangioma) 228.00
  melanotic (pigmented) (M8720/0)
  multiplex 759.5
  nonneoplastic 448.1
  nonpigmented (M8730/0)
  nonvascular (M8720/0)
  oral mucosa, white sponge 750.26
  osteohypertrophic, flammeus 759.89
  papillaris (M8720/0)
  papillomatosus (M8720/0)
  pigmented (M8720/0)
    giant (M8761/1)—*see also* Neoplasm, skin,
        uncertain behavior
      malignant melanoma in (M8761/3)—*see*
          Melanoma
    systematicus 757.33
  pilosus (M8720/0)
  port wine 757.32
  sanguineous 757.32
  sebaceous (senile) 702.8
  senile 448.1
  spider 448.1
  spindle cell (and epithelioid cell) (M8770/0)
  stellar 448.1
  strawberry 757.32
  syringocystadenomatous papilliferous
      (M8406/0)
  unius lateris 757.33
  Unna's 757.32
  vascular 757.32
  verrucous 757.33
  white sponge (oral mucosa) 750.26
Newborn (infant) (liveborn)
  abstinence syndrome 779.5
  affected by
    amniocentesis 760.61
    maternal abuse of drugs (gestational) (via
        placenta) (via breast milk) (see also
        Noxious, substances transmitted through
        placenta or breast milk (affecting fetus or
        newborn)) 760.70
      methamphetamine(s) 760.72
    procedure
      amniocentesis 760.61
      in utero NEC 760.62
      surgical on mother
        during pregnancy NEC 760.63
        previous not associated with pregnancy
            760.64
  apnea 770.81
    obstructive 770.82
    specified NEC 770.82
  breast buds 779.89
  cardiomyopathy 425.4
    congenital 425.3
  convulsion 779.0
  electrolyte imbalance NEC (transitory) 775.5
  fever (environmentally-induced) 778.4
  gestation
    24 completed weeks 765.22
    25-26 completed weeks 765.23
    27-28 completed weeks 765.24
    29-30 completed weeks 765.25
    31-32 completed weeks 765.26
    33-34 completed weeks 765.27

Newborn—*continued*
  gestation—*continued*
    35-36 completed weeks 765.28
    37 or more completed weeks 765.29
    less than 24 completed weeks 765.21
    unspecified completed weeks 765.20
  infection 771.89
    candida 771.7
    mastitis 771.5
    specified NEC 771.89
    urinary tract 771.82
  mastitis 771.5
  multiple NEC
    born in hospital (without mention of cesarean
        delivery or section) V37.00
      with cesarean delivery or section V37.01
    born outside hospital
      hospitalized V37.1
      not hospitalized V37.2
    mates all liveborn
      born in hospital (without mention of
          cesarean delivery or section) V34.00
        with cesarean delivery or section V34.01
      born outside hospital
        hospitalized V34.1
        not hospitalized V34.2
    mates all stillborn
      born in hospital (without mention of
          cesarean delivery or section) V35.00
        with cesarean delivery or section V35.01
      born outside hospital
        hospitalized V35.1
        not hospitalized V35.2
    mates liveborn and stillborn
      born in hospital (without mention of
          cesarean delivery or section) V36.00
        with cesarean delivery or section V36.01
      born outside hospital
        hospitalized V36.1
        not hospitalized V36.2
  omphalitis 771.4
  seizure 779.0
  sepsis 771.81
  single
    born in hospital (without mention of cesarean
        delivery or section) V30.00
      with cesarean delivery or section V30.01
    born outside hospital
      hospitalized V30.1
      not hospitalized V30.2
  specified condition NEC 779.89
  twin NEC
    born in hospital (without mention of cesarean
        delivery or section) V33.00
      with cesarean delivery or section V33.01
    born outside hospital
      hospitalized V33.1
      not hospitalized V33.2
    mate liveborn
      born in hospital V31.0
      born outside hospital
        hospitalized V31.1
        not hospitalized V31.2
    mate stillborn
      born in hospital V32.0
      born outside hospital
        hospitalized V32.1
        not hospitalized V32.2

Newborn—*continued*
  unspecified as to single or multiple birth
    born in hospital (without mention of cesarean
      delivery or section) V39.00
      with cesarean delivery or section V39.01
    born outside hospital
      hospitalized V39.1
      not hospitalized V39.2
    weight check V20.32
Newcastle's conjunctivitis or disease 077.8
Nezelof's syndrome (pure alymphocytosis) 279.13
Niacin (amide) deficiency 265.2
Nicolas-Durand-Favre disease (climatic bubo)
  099.1
Nicolas-Favre disease (climatic bubo) 099.1
Nicotinic acid (amide) deficiency 265.2
Niemann-Pick disease (lipid histiocytosis)
  (splenomegaly) 272.7
Night
  blindness (*see also* Blindness, night) 368.60
    congenital 368.61
    vitamin A deficiency 264.5
  cramps 729.82
  sweats 780.8
  terrors, child 307.46
Nightmare 307.47
  REM-sleep type 307.47
Nipple —*see* condition
Nisbet's chancre 099.0
Nishimoto (-Takeuchi) disease 437.5
Nitritoid crisis or reaction —*see* Crisis, nitritoid
Nitrogen retention, extrarenal 788.99
Nitrosohemoglobinemia 289.89
Njovera 104.0
No
  diagnosis 799.9
  disease (found) V71.9
  room at the inn V65.0
Nocardiasis —*see* Nocardiosis
Nocardiosis 039.9
  with pneumonia 039.1
  lung 039.1
  specified type NEC 039.8
Nocturia 788.43
  psychogenic 306.53
Nocturnal —*see also* condition
  dyspnea (paroxysmal) 786.09
  emissions 608.89
  enuresis 788.36
    psychogenic 307.6
  frequency (micturition) 788.43
    psychogenic 306.53
Nodal rhythm disorder 427.89
Nodding of head 781.0
Node (s)—*see also* Nodule
  Heberden's 715.04
  larynx 478.79
  lymph—*see* condition
  milkers' 051.1
  Osler's 421.0
  rheumatic 729.89
  Schmorl's 722.30
    lumbar, lumbosacral 722.32
    specified region NEC 722.39
    thoracic, thoracolumbar 722.31
  singers' 478.5
  skin NEC 782.2
  tuberculous—*see* Tuberculosis, lymph gland
  vocal cords 478.5
Nodosities, Haygarth's 715.04

Nodule(s), nodular
  actinomycotic (*see also* Actinomycosis) 039.9
  arthritic—*see* Arthritis, nodosa
  breast 793.89
  cutaneous 782.2
  Haygarth's 715.04
  inflammatory—*see* Inflammation
  juxta-articular 102.7
    syphilitic 095.7
    yaws 102.7
  larynx 478.79
  lung, solitary 518.89
    emphysematous 492.8
  milkers' 051.1
  prostate 600.10
    with
      urinary
        obstruction 600.11
        retention 600.11
  retrocardiac 785.9
  rheumatic 729.89
  rheumatoid—*see* Arthritis rheumatoid
  scrotum (inflammatory) 608.4
  singers' 478.5
  skin NEC 782.2
  solitary, lung 518.89
    emphysematous 492.8
  subcutaneous 782.2
  thyroid (gland) (nontoxic) (uninodular) 241.0
    with
      hyperthyroidism 242.1
      thyrotoxicosis 242.1
    toxic or with hyperthyroidism 242.1
  vocal cords 478.5
Noma (gangrenous) (hospital) (infective) 528.1
  auricle (*see also* Gangrene) 785.4
  mouth 528.1
  pudendi (*see also* Vulvitis) 616.10
  vulvae (*see also* Vulvitis) 616.10
Nomadism V60.0
Non-adherence
  artificial skin graft 996.55
  decellularized allodermis graft 996.55
Non-autoimmune hemolytic anemia NEC 283.10
Nonclosure —*see also* Imperfect, closure
  ductus
    arteriosus 747.0
    Botalli 747.0
  Eustachian valve 746.89
  foramen
    Botalli 745.5
    ovale 745.5
Noncompliance with medical treatment V15.81
  renal dialysis V45.12
Nondescent (congenital)—*see also* Malposition,
  congenital
  cecum 751.4
  colon 751.4
  testis 752.51
Nondevelopment
  brain 742.1
    specified part 742.2
  heart 746.89
  organ or site, congenital NEC—*see* Hypoplasia
Nonengagement
  head NEC 652.5
    in labor 660.1
      affecting fetus or newborn 763.1
Nonexanthematous tick fever 066.1
Nonexpansion, lung (newborn) NEC 770.4

Nonfunctioning
cystic duct (*see also* Disease, gallbladder) 575.8
gallbladder (*see also* Disease, gallbladder) 575.8
kidney (*see also* Disease, renal) 593.9
labyrinth 386.58
Nonhealing
stump (surgical) 997.60
wound, surgical 998.83
Nonimplantation of ovum, causing infertility
628.3
Noninsufflation, fallopian tube 628.2
Nonne-Milroy-Meige syndrome (chronic
hereditary edema) 757.0
Nonovulation 628.0
Nonpatent fallopian tube 628.2
Nonpneumatization, lung NEC 770.4
Nonreflex bladder 596.54
with cauda equina 344.61
Nonretention of food —*see also* Vomiting
Nonrotation —*see* Malrotation
Nonsecretion, urine (*see also* Anuria) 788.5
newborn 753.3
Nonunion
fracture 733.82
organ or site, congenital NEC—*see* Imperfect,
closure
symphysis pubis, congenital 755.69
top sacrum, congenital 756.19
Nonviability 765.0
Nonvisualization, gallbladder 793.3
Nonvitalized tooth 522.9
Non-working side interference 524.56
Normal
delivery—*see* category 650
menses V65.5
state (feared complaint unfounded) V65.5
Normoblastosis 289.89
Normocytic anemia (infectional) 285.9
due to blood loss (chronic) 280.0
acute 285.1
Norrie's disease (congenital) (progressive
oculoacousticocerebral degeneration) 743.8
North American blastomycosis 116.0
Norwegian itch 133.0
Nose, nasal —*see* condition
Nosebleed 784.7
Nosomania 298.9
Nosophobia 300.29
Nostalgia 309.89
Notch of iris 743.46
Notched lip, congenital (*see also* Cleft, lip) 749.10
Notching nose, congenital (tip) 748.1
Nothnagel's
syndrome 378.52
vasomotor acroparesthesia 443.89
Novy's relapsing fever (American) 087.1
Noxious
foodstuffs, poisoning by
fish 988.0
fungi 988.1
mushrooms 988.1
plants (food) 988.2
shellfish 988.0
specified type NEC 988.8
toadstool 988.1

Noxious—*continued*
substances transmitted through placenta or
breast milk (affecting fetus or newborn)
760.70
acetretin 760.78
alcohol 760.71
aminopterin 760.78
antiandrogens 760.79
anticonvulsant 760.77
antifungal 760.74
anti-infective agents 760.74
antimetabolic 760.78
atorvastatin 760.78
carbamazepine 760.77
cocaine 760.75
"crack" 760.75
diethylstilbestrol (DES) 760.76
divalproex sodium 760.77
endocrine disrupting chemicals 760.79
estrogens 760.79
etretinate 760.78
fluconazole 760.74
fluvastatin 760.78
hallucinogenic agents NEC 760.73
hormones 760.79
lithium 760.79
lovastatin 760.78
medicinal agents NEC 760.79
methotrexate 760.78
misoprostil 760.79
narcotics 760.72
obstetric anesthetic or analgesic 763.5
phenobarbital 760.77
phenytoin 760.77
pravastatin 760.78
progestins 760.79
retinoic acid 760.78
simvastatin 760.78
solvents 760.79
specified agent NEC 760.79
statins 760.78
suspected, affecting management of pregnancy
655.5
tetracycline 760.74
thalidomide 760.79
trimethadione 760.77
valproate 760.77
valproic acid 760.77
vitamin A 760.78
NPDH (new persistent daily headache) 339.42
Nuchal hitch (arm) 652.8
Nucleus pulposus —*see* condition
Numbness 782.0
Nuns' knee 727.2
Nursemaid's
elbow 832.2
shoulder 831.0
Nutmeg liver 573.8
Nutrition, deficient or insufficient (particular
kind of food) 269.9
due to
insufficient food 994.2
lack of
care (child) (infant) 995.52
adult 995.84
food 994.2
Nyctalopia (*see also* Blindness, night) 368.60
vitamin A deficiency 264.5

Nycturia 788.43
  psychogenic 306.53
Nymphomania 302.89
Nystagmus 379.50
  associated with vestibular system disorders
    379.54
  benign paroxysmal positional 386.11
  central positional 386.2
  congenital 379.51
  deprivation 379.53
  dissociated 379.55
  latent 379.52
  miners' 300.89
  positional
    benign paroxysmal 386.11
    central 386.2
  specified NEC 379.56
  vestibular 379.54
  visual deprivation 379.53

O

Oasthouse urine disease 270.2
Obermeyer's relapsing fever (European) 087.0
Obesity (constitutional) (exogenous) (familial)
    (nutritional) (simple) 278.00
  adrenal 255.8
  complicating pregnancy, childbirth, or the
      puerperium 649.1
  due to hyperalimentation 278.00
  endocrine NEC 259.9
  endogenous 259.9
  Fröhlich's (adiposogenital dystrophy) 253.8
  glandular NEC 259.9
  hypothyroid (see also Hypothyroidism) 244.9
  morbid 278.01
  of pregnancy 649.1
  pituitary 253.8
  severe 278.01
  thyroid (see also Hypothyroidism) 244.9
Oblique —see also condition
  lie before labor, affecting fetus or newborn 761.7
Obliquity, pelvis 738.6
Obliteration
  abdominal aorta 446.7
  appendix (lumen) 543.9
  artery 447.1
  ascending aorta 446.7
  bile ducts 576.8
    with calculus, choledocholithiasis, or
        stones—see Choledocholithiasis
    congenital 751.61
      jaundice from 751.61 [774.5]
  common duct 576.8
    with calculus, choledocholithiasis, or
        stones—see Choledocholithiasis
    congenital 751.61
  cystic duct 575.8
    with calculus, choledocholithiasis, or
        stones—see Choledocholithiasis
  disease, arteriolar 447.1
  endometrium 621.8
  eye, anterior chamber 360.34
  fallopian tube 628.2
  lymphatic vessel 457.1
    postmastectomy 457.0
  organ or site, congenital NEC—see Atresia
  placental blood vessels—see Placenta, abnormal
  supra-aortic branches 446.7
  ureter 593.89
  urethra 599.84
  vein 459.9
  vestibule (oral) 525.8
Observation (for) V71.9
  without need for further medical care V71.9
  accident NEC V71.4
    at work V71.3
  criminal assault V71.6
  deleterious agent ingestion V71.89
  disease V71.9
    cardiovascular V71.7
    heart V71.7
    mental V71.09
    specified condition NEC V71.89
  foreign body ingestion V71.89
  growth and development variations V21.8
  injuries (accidental) V71.4
    inflicted NEC V71.6
      during alleged rape or seduction V71.5

Observation—continued
  malignant neoplasm, suspected V71.1
  postpartum
    immediately after delivery V24.0
    routine follow-up V24.2
  pregnancy
    high-risk V23.9
      specified problem NEC V23.8
    normal (without complication) V22.1
      with nonobstetric complication V22.2
      first V22.0
  rape or seduction, alleged V71.5
    injury during V71.5
  suicide attempt, alleged V71.89
  suspected (undiagnosed) (unproven)
    abuse V71.81
    cardiovascular disease V71.7
    child or wife battering victim V71.6
    concussion (cerebral) V71.6
    condition NEC V71.89
      infant—see Observation, suspected,
        condition, newborn
    maternal and fetal
      amniotic cavity and membrane problem
        V89.01
      cervical shortening V89.05
      fetal anomaly V89.03
      fetal growth problem V89.04
      oligohydramnios V89.01
      other specified problem NEC V89.09
      placental problem V89.02
      polyhydramnios V89.01
    newborn V29.9
      cardiovascular disease V29.8
      congenital anomaly V29.8
      genetic V29.3
      infectious V29.0
      ingestion foreign object V29.8
      injury V29.8
      metabolic V29.3
      neoplasm V29.8
      neurological V29.1
      poison, poisoning V29.8
      respiratory V29.2
      specified NEC V29.8
    exposure
      anthrax V71.82
      biological agent NEC V71.83
      SARS V71.83
    infectious disease not requiring isolation V71.89
    malignant neoplasm V71.1
    mental disorder V71.09
    neglect V71.81
    neoplasm
      benign V71.89
      malignant V71.1
    specified condition NEC V71.89
    tuberculosis V71.2
  tuberculosis, suspected V71.2
Obsession, obsessional 300.3
  ideas and mental images 300.3
  impulses 300.3
  neurosis 300.3
  phobia 300.3
  psychasthenia 300.3
  ruminations 300.3
  state 300.3
  syndrome 300.3

Obsessive-compulsive 300.3
  neurosis 300.3
  personality 301.4
  reaction 300.3
Obstetrical trauma NEC (complicating delivery)
    665.9
  with
    abortion—*see* Abortion, by type, with damage
      to pelvic organs
    ectopic pregnancy (*see also* categories
      633.0-633.9) 639.2
    molar pregnancy (*see also* categories 630-632)
      639.2
  affecting fetus or newborn 763.89
  following
    abortion 639.2
    ectopic or molar pregnancy 639.2
Obstipation (*see also* Constipation) 564.00
  psychogenic 306.4
Obstruction, obstructed, obstructive
  airway NEC 519.8
    with
      allergic alveolitis NEC 495.9
      asthma NEC (*see also* Asthma) 493.9
      bronchiectasis 494.0
        with acute exacerbation 494.1
      bronchitis (*see also* Bronchitis, with,
        obstruction) 491.20
      emphysema NEC 492.8
    chronic 496
      with
        allergic alveolitis NEC 495.5
        asthma NEC (*see also* Asthma) 493.2
        bronchiectasis 494.0
          with acute exacerbation 494.1
        bronchitis (*see also* Bronchitis, chronic,
          obstructive) 491.20
        emphysema NEC 492.8
    due to
      bronchospasm 519.11
      foreign body 934.9
      inhalation of fumes or vapors 506.9
      laryngospasm 478.75
  alimentary canal (*see also* Obstruction,
    intestine) 560.9
  ampulla of Vater 576.2
    with calculus, cholelithiasis, or stones—*see*
      Choledocholithiasis
  aortic (heart) (valve) (*see also* Stenosis, aortic) 424.1
    rheumatic (*see also* Stenosis, aortic,
      rheumatic) 395.0
  aortoiliac 444.0
  aqueduct of Sylvius 331.4
    congenital 742.3
      with spina bifida (*see also* Spina bifida) 741.0
    Arnold-Chiari (*see also* Spina bifida) 741.0
  artery (*see also* Embolism, artery) 444.9
    basilar (complete) (partial) (*see also*
      Occlusion, artery, basilar) 433.0
    carotid (complete) (partial) (*see also*
      Occlusion, artery, carotid) 433.1
    precerebral—*see* Occlusion, artery,
      precerebral NEC
    retinal (central) (*see also* Occlusion, retina)
      362.30
    vertebral (complete) (partial) (*see also*
      Occlusion, artery, vertebral) 433.2
  asthma (chronic) (with obstructive pulmonary
    disease) 493.2
  band (intestinal) 560.81

Obstruction, obstructed—*continued*
  bile duct or passage (*see also* Obstruction,
    biliary) 576.2
    congenital 751.61
      jaundice from 751.61 *[774.5]*
  biliary (duct) (tract) 576.2
    with calculus 574.51
      with cholecystitis (chronic) 574.41
        acute 574.31
    congenital 751.61
      jaundice from 751.61 *[774.5]*
    gallbladder 575.2
      with calculus 574.21
        with cholecystitis (chronic) 574.11
          acute 574.01
  bladder neck (acquired) 596.0
    congenital 753.6
  bowel (*see also* Obstruction, intestine) 560.9
  bronchus 519.19
  canal, ear (*see also* Stricture, ear canal,
    acquired) 380.50
  cardia 537.89
  caval veins (inferior) (superior) 459.2
  cecum (*see also* Obstruction, intestine) 560.9
  circulatory 459.9
  colon (*see also* Obstruction, intestine) 560.9
    sympathicotonic 560.89
  common duct (*see also* Obstruction, biliary)
    576.2
    congenital 751.61
  coronary (*see also* Arteriosclerosis, coronary)
    acute (*see also* Infarct, myocardium) 410.9
      without myocardial infarction 411.81
  cystic duct (*see also* Obstruction, gallbladder)
    575.2
    congenital 751.61
  device, implant, or graft—*see* Complications,
    due to (presence of) any device, implant, or
    graft classified to 996.0-996.5 NEC
  due to foreign body accidentally left in operation
    wound 998.4
  duodenum 537.3
    congenital 751.1
    due to
      compression NEC 537.3
      cyst 537.3
      intrinsic lesion or disease NEC 537.3
      scarring 537.3
      torsion 537.3
      ulcer 532.91
      volvulus 537.3
  ejaculatory duct 608.89
  endocardium 424.90
    arteriosclerotic 424.99
    specified cause, except rheumatic 424.99
  esophagus 530.3
  Eustachian tube (complete) (partial) 381.60
    cartilaginous
      extrinsic 381.63
      intrinsic 381.62
    due to
      cholesteatoma 381.61
      osseous lesion NEC 381.61
      polyp 381.61
    osseous 381.61
  fallopian tube (bilateral) 628.2
  fecal 560.39
    with hernia—*see also* Hernia, by site, with
      obstruction
      gangrenous—*see* Hernia, by site, with
        gangrene

Obstruction, obstructed—*continued*
  foramen of Monro (congenital) 742.3
    with spina bifida (*see also* Spina bifida) 741.0
  foreign body—*see* Foreign body
  gallbladder 575.2
    with calculus, cholelithiasis, or stones 574.21
      with cholecystitis (chronic) 574.11
        acute 574.01
    congenital 751.69
      jaundice from 751.69 *[774.5]*
  gastric outlet 537.0
  gastrointestinal (*see also* Obstruction, intestine) 560.9
  glottis 478.79
  hepatic 573.8
    duct (*see also* Obstruction, biliary) 576.2
      congenital 751.61
  icterus (*see also* Obstruction, biliary) 576.8
    congenital 751.61
  ileocecal coil (*see also* Obstruction, intestine) 560.9
  ileum (*see also* Obstruction, intestine) 560.9
  iliofemoral (artery) 444.81
  internal anastomosis—*see* Complications, mechanical, graft
  intestine (mechanical) (neurogenic) (paroxysmal) (postinfectional) (reflex) 560.9
    with
      adhesions (intestinal) (peritoneal) 560.81
      hernia—*see also* Hernia, by site, with obstruction
        gangrenous—*see* Hernia, by site, with gangrene
    adynamic (*see also* Ileus) 560.1
    by gallstone 560.31
    congenital or infantile (small) 751.1
      large 751.2
    due to
      Ascaris lumbricoides 127.0
      mural thickening 560.89
      procedure 997.4
        involving urinary tract 997.5
    impaction 560.39
    infantile—*see* Obstruction, intestine, congenital
    newborn
      due to
        fecaliths 777.1
        inspissated milk 777.2
        meconium (plug) 777.1
          in mucoviscidosis 277.01
        transitory 777.4
    specified cause NEC 560.89
    transitory, newborn 777.4
    volvulus 560.2
  intracardiac ball valve prosthesis 996.02
  jaundice (*see also* Obstruction, biliary) 576.8
    congenital 751.61
  jejunum (*see also* Obstruction, intestine) 560.9
  kidney 593.89
  labor 660.9
    affecting fetus or newborn 763.1
    by
      bony pelvis (conditions classifiable to 653.0-653.9) 660.1
      deep transverse arrest 660.3
      impacted shoulder 660.4
      locked twins 660.5
      malposition (fetus) (conditions classifiable to 652.0-652.9) 660.0
        head during labor 660.3

Obstruction, obstructed—*continued*
      persistent occipitoposterior position 660.3
      soft tissue, pelvic (conditions classifiable to 654.0-654.9) 660.2
  lacrimal
    canaliculi 375.53
      congenital 743.65
    punctum 375.52
    sac 375.54
  lacrimonasal duct 375.56
    congenital 743.65
    neonatal 375.55
  lacteal, with steatorrhea 579.2
  laryngitis (*see also* Laryngitis) 464.01
  larynx 478.79
    congenital 748.3
  liver 573.8
    cirrhotic (*see also* Cirrhosis, liver) 571.5
  lung 518.89
    with
      asthma—*see* Asthma
      bronchitis (chronic) 491.20
      emphysema NEC 492.8
    airway, chronic 496
    chronic NEC 496
      with
        asthma (chronic) (obstructive) 493.2
    disease, chronic 496
      with
        asthma (chronic) (obstructive) 493.2
      emphysematous 492.8
  lymphatic 457.1
  meconium
    fetus or newborn 777.1
      in mucoviscidosis 277.01
    newborn due to fecaliths 777.1
  mediastinum 519.3
  mitral (rheumatic)—*see* Stenosis, mitral
  nasal 478.19
    duct 375.56
      neonatal 375.55
    sinus—*see* Sinusitis
  nasolacrimal duct 375.56
    congenital 743.65
    neonatal 375.55
  nasopharynx 478.29
  nose 478.19
  organ or site, congenital NEC—*see* Atresia
  pancreatic duct 577.8
  parotid gland 527.8
  pelviureteral junction (*see also* Obstruction, ureter) 593.4
  pharynx 478.29
  portal (circulation) (vein) 452
  prostate 600.90
    with
      other lower urinary tract symptoms (LUTS) 600.91
    urinary
      obstruction 600.91
      retention 600.91
    valve (urinary) 596.0
  pulmonary
    valve (heart) (*see also* Endocarditis, pulmonary) 424.3
    vein, isolated 747.49
  pyemic—*see* Septicemia
  pylorus (acquired) 537.0
    congenital 750.5
    infantile 750.5
  rectosigmoid (*see also* Obstruction, intestine) 560.9

Occlusion—*continued*
breast (duct) 611.89
carotid (artery) (common) (internal)—*see*
Occlusion, artery, carotid
cerebellar (anterior inferior) (artery) (posterior
inferior) (superior) 433.8
cerebral (artery) (*see also* Infarct, brain) 434.9
cerebrovascular (*see also* Infarct, brain) 434.9
diffuse 437.0
cervical canal (*see also* Stricture, cervix) 622.4
by falciparum malaria 084.0
cervix (uteri) (*see also* Stricture, cervix) 622.4
choanal 748.0
choroidal (artery) 433.8
colon (*see also* Obstruction, intestine) 560.9
communicating posterior artery 433.8
coronary (artery) (thrombotic) (*see also* Infarct,
myocardium) 410.9
acute 410.9
without myocardial infarction 411.81
healed or old 412
without myocardial infarction 411.81
cystic duct (*see also* Obstruction, gallbladder)
575.2
congenital 751.69
disto
division I 524.22
division II 524.22
embolic—*see* Embolism
fallopian tube 628.2
congenital 752.19
gallbladder (*see also* Obstruction, gallbladder)
575.2
congenital 751.69
jaundice from 751.69 *[774.5]*
gingiva, traumatic 523.8
hymen 623.3
congenital 752.42
hypophyseal (artery) 433.8
iliac artery 444.81
intestine (*see also* Obstruction, intestine) 560.9
kidney 593.89
lacrimal apparatus—*see* Stenosis, lacrimal
lung 518.89
lymph or lymphatic channel 457.1
mammary duct 611.89
mesenteric artery (embolic) (thrombotic) (with
gangrene) 557.0
nose 478.1
congenital 748.0
organ or site, congenital NEC—*see* Atresia
oviduct 628.2
congenital 752.19
periodontal, traumatic 523.8
peripheral arteries (lower extremity) 444.22
without thrombus or embolus (*see also*
Arteriosclerosis, extremities) 440.20
due to stricture or stenosis 447.1
upper extremity 444.21
without thrombus or embolus (*see also*
Arteriosclerosis, extremities) 440.20
due to stricture or stenosis 447.1
pontine (artery) 433.8
posterior lingual, of mandibular teeth 524.29
precerebral artery—*see* Occlusion, artery,
precerebral NEC
puncta lacrimalia 375.52
pupil 364.74
pylorus (*see also* Stricture, pylorus) 537.0
renal artery 593.81

Occlusion—*continued*
retina, retinal (vascular) 362.30
artery, arterial 362.30
branch 362.32
central (total) 362.31
partial 362.33
transient 362.34
tributary 362.32
vein 362.30
branch 362.36
central (total) 362.35
incipient 362.37
partial 362.37
tributary 362.36
spinal artery 433.8
stent
coronary 996.72
teeth (mandibular) (posterior lingual) 524.29
thoracic duct 457.1
tubal 628.2
ureter (complete) (partial) 593.4
congenital 753.29
urethra (*see also* Stricture, urethra) 598.9
congenital 753.6
uterus 621.8
vagina 623.2
vascular NEC 459.9
vein—*see* Thrombosis
vena cava
inferior 453.2
superior
acute 453.87
chronic 453.77
ventricle (brain) NEC 331.4
vertebral (artery)—*see* Occlusion, artery,
vertebral
vessel (blood) NEC 459.9
vulva 624.8
Occlusio pupillae 364.74
Occupational
problems NEC V62.29
therapy V57.21
Ochlophobia 300.29
Ochronosis (alkaptonuric) (congenital)
(endogenous) 270.2
with chloasma of eyelid 270.2
Ocular muscle —*see also* condition
myopathy 359.1
torticollis 781.93
Oculoauriculovertebral dysplasia 756.0
Oculogyric
crisis or disturbance 378.87
psychogenic 306.7
Oculomotor syndrome 378.81
Oddi's sphincter spasm 576.5
Odelberg's disease (juvenile osteochondrosis)
732.1
Odontalgia 525.9
Odontoameloblastoma (M9311/0) 213.1
upper jaw (bone) 213.0
Odontoclasia 521.05
Odontoclasis 873.63
complicated 873.73
Odontodysplasia, regional 520.4
Odontogenesis imperfecta 520.5
Odontoma (M9280/0) 213.1
ameloblastic (M9311/0) 213.1
upper jaw (bone) 213.0
calcified (M9280/0) 213.1
upper jaw (bone) 213.0

Odontoma—*continued*
  complex (M9282/0) 213.1
    upper jaw (bone) 213.0
  compound (M9281/0) 213.1
    upper jaw (bone) 213.0
  fibroameloblastic (M9290/0) 213.1
    upper jaw (bone) 213.0
  follicular 526.0
    upper jaw (bone) 213.0
Odontomyelitis (closed) (open) 522.0
Odontonecrosis 521.09
Odontorrhagia 525.8
Odontosarcoma, ameloblastic (M9290/3) 170.1
  upper jaw (bone) 170.0
Odynophagia 787.20
Oesophagostomiasis 127.7
Oesophagostomum infestation 127.7
Oestriasis 134.0
Ogilvie's syndrome (sympathicotonic colon
  obstruction) 560.89
Oguchi's disease (retina) 368.61
Ohara's disease (*see also* Tularemia) 021.9
Oidiomycosis (*see also* Candidiasis) 112.9
Oidiomycotic meningitis 112.83
Oidium albicans infection (*see also* Candidiasis)
  112.9
Old age 797
  dementia (of) 290.0
Olfactory —*see* condition
Oligemia 285.9
Oligergasia (*see also* Retardation, mental) 319
Oligoamnios 658.0
  affecting fetus or newborn 761.2
Oligoastrocytoma, mixed (M9382/3)
  specified site—*see* Neoplasm, by site, malignant
  unspecified site 191.9
Oligocythemia 285.9
Oligodendroblastoma (M9460/3)
  specified site—*see* Neoplasm, by site, malignant
  unspecified site 191.9
Oligodendroglioma (M9450/3)
  anaplastic type (M9451/3)
    specified site—*see* Neoplasm, by site, malignant
    unspecified site 191.9
  specified site—*see* Neoplasm, by site, malignant
  unspecified site 191.9
Oligodendroma —*see* Oligodendroglioma
Oligodontia (*see also* Anodontia) 520.0
Oligoencephalon 742.1
Oligohydramnios 658.0
  affecting fetus or newborn 761.2
  due to premature rupture of membranes 658.1
    affecting fetus or newborn 761.2
Oligohydrosis 705.0
Oligomenorrhea 626.1
Oligophrenia (*see also* Retardation, mental) 319
  phenylpyruvic 270.1
Oligospermia 606.1
Oligotrichia 704.09
  congenita 757.4
Oliguria 788.5
  with
    abortion—*see* Abortion, by type, with renal failure
    ectopic pregnancy (*see also* categories
      633.0-633.9) 639.3
    molar pregnancy (*see also* categories 630-632)
      639.3

Oliguria—*continued*
  complicating
    abortion 639.3
    ectopic or molar pregnancy 639.3
    pregnancy 646.2
      with hypertension—*see* Toxemia, of
        pregnancy
    due to a procedure 997.5
    following labor and delivery 669.3
    heart or cardiac—*see* Failure, heart
    puerperal, postpartum 669.3
    specified due to a procedure 997.5
Ollier's disease (chondrodysplasia) 756.4
Omentitis (*see also* Peritonitis) 567.9
Omentocele (*see also* Hernia, omental) 553.8
Omentum, omental —*see* condition
Omphalitis (congenital) (newborn) 771.4
  not of newborn 686.9
  tetanus 771.3
Omphalocele 756.72
Omphalomesenteric duct, persistent 751.0
Omphalorrhagia, newborn 772.3
Omsk hemorrhagic fever 065.1
Onanism 307.9
Onchocerciasis 125.3
  eye 125.3 *[360.13]*
Onchocercosis 125.3
Oncocytoma (M8290/0)—*see* Neoplasm, by site,
  benign
Ondine's curse 348.89
Oneirophrenia (*see also* Schizophrenia) 295.4
Onychauxis 703.8
  congenital 757.5
Onychia (with lymphangitis) 681.9
  dermatophytic 110.1
  finger 681.02
  toe 681.11
Onychitis (with lymphangitis) 681.9
  finger 681.02
  toe 681.11
Onychocryptosis 703.0
Onychodystrophy 703.8
  congenital 757.5
Onychogryphosis 703.8
Onychogryposis 703.8
Onycholysis 703.8
Onychomadesis 703.8
Onychomalacia 703.8
Onychomycosis 110.1
  finger 110.1
  toe 110.1
Onycho-osteodysplasia 756.89
Onychophagy 307.9
Onychoptosis 703.8
Onychorrhexis 703.8
  congenital 757.5
Onychoschizia 703.8
Onychotrophia (*see also* Atrophy, nail) 703.8
O'nyong-nyong fever 066.3
Onyxis (finger) (toe) 703.0
Onyxitis (with lymphangitis) 681.9
  finger 681.02
  toe 681.11
Oocyte (egg) (ovum)
  donor V59.70
    age 35 and over V59.73
      anonymous recipient V59.73
      designated recipient V59.74
    under age 35 V59.71
      anonymous recipient V59.71
      designated recipient V59.72

Oophoritis (cystic) (infectional) (interstitial) (*see also* Salpingo-oophoritis) 614.2
  complicating pregnancy 646.6
  fetal (acute) 752.0
  gonococcal (acute) 098.19
    chronic or duration of 2 months or over 098.39
  tuberculous (*see also* Tuberculosis) 016.6
Opacity, opacities
  cornea 371.00
    central 371.03
    congenital 743.43
      interfering with vision 743.42
    degenerative (*see also* Degeneration, cornea) 371.40
    hereditary (*see also* Dystrophy, cornea) 371.50
    inflammatory (*see also* Keratitis) 370.9
    late effect of trachoma (healed) 139.1
    minor 371.01
    peripheral 371.02
  enamel (fluoride) (nonfluoride) (teeth) 520.3
  lens (*see also* Cataract) 366.9
  snowball 379.22
  vitreous (humor) 379.24
    congenital 743.51
Opalescent dentin (hereditary) 520.5
Open, opening
  abnormal, organ or site, congenital—*see* Imperfect, closure
  angle with
    borderline intraocular pressure 365.01
    cupping of discs 365.01
  bite
    anterior 524.24
    posterior 524.25
  false—*see* Imperfect, closure
  margin on tooth restoration 525.61
  restoration margins 525.61
  wound—*see* Wound, open, by site
Operation
  causing mutilation of fetus 763.89
  destructive, on live fetus, to facilitate birth 763.89
  for delivery, fetus or newborn 763.89
  maternal, unrelated to current delivery, affecting fetus or newborn (*see also* Newborn, affected by) 760.64
Operational fatigue 300.89
Operative —*see* condition
Operculitis (chronic) 523.40
  acute 523.30
Operculum, retina 361.32
  with detachment 361.01
Ophiasis 704.01
Ophthalmia (*see also* Conjunctivitis) 372.30
  actinic rays 370.24
  allergic (acute) 372.05
    chronic 372.14
  blennorrhagic (neonatorum) 098.40
  catarrhal 372.03
  diphtheritic 032.81
  Egyptian 076.1
  electric, electrica 370.24
  gonococcal (neonatorum) 098.40
  metastatic 360.11
  migraine 346.8
  neonatorum, newborn 771.6
    gonococcal 098.40
  nodosa 360.14
  phlyctenular 370.31
    with ulcer (*see also* Ulcer, cornea) 370.00
  sympathetic 360.11
Ophthalmitis —*see* Ophthalmia
Ophthalmocele (congenital) 743.66

Ophthalmoneuromyelitis 341.0
Ophthalmopathy, infiltrative with thyrotoxicosis 242.0
Ophthalmoplegia (*see also* Strabismus) 378.9
  anterior internuclear 378.86
  ataxia-areflexia syndrome 357.0
  bilateral 378.9
  diabetic 250.5 *[378.86]*
    due to secondary diabetes 249.5 *[378.86]*
  exophthalmic 242.0 *[376.22]*
  external 378.55
    progressive 378.72
    total 378.56
  interna(l) (complete) (total) 367.52
  internuclear 378.86
  migraine 346.2
  painful 378.55
  Parinaud's 378.81
  progressive external 378.72
  supranuclear, progressive 333.0
  total (external) 378.56
    internal 367.52
  unilateral 378.9
Opisthognathism 524.00
Opisthorchiasis (felineus) (tenuicollis) (viverrini) 121.0
Opisthotonos, opisthotonus 781.0
Opitz's disease (congestive splenomegaly) 289.51
Opiumism (*see also* Dependence) 304.0
Oppenheim's disease 358.8
Oppenheim-Urbach disease or syndrome (necrobiosis lipoidica diabeticorum) 250.8 *[709.3]*
  due to secondary diabetes 249.8 *[709.3]*
Opsoclonia 379.59
Optic nerve —*see* condition
Orbit —*see* condition
Orchioblastoma (M9071/3) 186.9
Orchitis (nonspecific) (septic) 604.90
  with abscess 604.0
  blennorrhagic (acute) 098.13
    chronic or duration of 2 months or over 098.33
  diphtheritic 032.89 *[604.91]*
  filarial 125.9 *[604.91]*
  gangrenous 604.99
  gonococcal (acute) 098.13
    chronic or duration of 2 months or over 098.33
  mumps 072.0
  parotidea 072.0
  suppurative 604.99
  syphilitic 095.8 *[604.91]*
  tuberculous (*see also* Tuberculosis) 016.5 *[608.81]*
Orf 051.2
Organic —*see also* condition
  heart—*see* Disease, heart
  insufficiency 799.89
Oriental
  bilharziasis 120.2
  schistosomiasis 120.2
  sore 085.1
Orientation
  ego-dystonic sexual 302.0
Orifice —*see* condition
Origin, both great vessels from right ventricle 745.11
Ormond's disease or syndrome 593.4
Ornithosis 073.9
  with
    complication 073.8
      specified NEC 073.7
    pneumonia 073.0
    pneumonitis (lobular) 073.0

Orodigitofacial dysostosis 759.89
Oropouche fever 066.3
Orotaciduria, oroticaciduria (congenital)
  (hereditary) (pyrimidine deficiency) 281.4
Oroya fever 088.0
Orthodontics V58.5
  adjustment V53.4
  aftercare V58.5
  fitting V53.4
Orthopnea 786.02
Orthoptic training V57.4
Os, uterus —*see* condition
Osgood-Schlatter
  disease 732.4
  osteochondrosis 732.4
Osler's
  disease (M9950/1) (polycythemia vera) 238.4
  nodes 421.0
Osler-Rendu disease (familial hemorrhagic
  telangiectasia) 448.0
Osler-Vaquez disease (M9950/1) (polycythemia
  vera) 238.4
Osler-Weber-Rendu syndrome (familial
  hemorrhagic telangiectasia) 448.0
Osmidrosis 705.89
Osseous —*see* condition
Ossification
  artery—*see* Arteriosclerosis
  auricle (ear) 380.39
  bronchus 519.19
  cardiac (*see also* Degeneration, myocardial) 429.1
  cartilage (senile) 733.99
  coronary —*see* Arteriosclerosis, coronary
  diaphragm 728.10
  ear 380.39
    middle (*see also* Otosclerosis) 387.9
  falx cerebri 349.2
  fascia 728.10
  fontanel
    defective or delayed 756.0
    premature 756.0
  heart (*see also* Degeneration, myocardial) 429.1
    valve—*see* Endocarditis
  larynx 478.79
  ligament
    posterior longitudinal 724.8
      cervical 723.7
  meninges (cerebral) 349.2
    spinal 336.8
  multiple, eccentric centers 733.99
  muscle 728.10
    heterotopic, postoperative 728.13
  myocardium, myocardial (*see also*
    Degeneration, myocardial) 429.1
  penis 607.81
  periarticular 728.89
  sclera 379.16
  tendon 727.82
  trachea 519.19
  tympanic membrane (*see also*
    Tympanosclerosis) 385.00
  vitreous (humor) 360.44
Osteitis (*see also* Osteomyelitis) 730.2
  acute 730.0
  alveolar 526.5
  chronic 730.1
  condensans (ilii) 733.5
  deformans (Paget's) 731.0
    due to or associated with malignant neoplasm
      (*see also* Neoplasm, bone, malignant)
      170.9 *[731.1]*

Osteitis—*continued*
  due to yaws 102.6
  fibrosa NEC 733.29
    cystica (generalisata) 252.01
    disseminata 756.59
    osteoplastica 252.01
  fragilitans 756.51
  Garré's (sclerosing) 730.1
  infectious (acute) (subacute) 730.0
    chronic or old 730.1
  jaw (acute) (chronic) (lower) (neonatal)
    (suppurative) (upper) 526.4
  parathyroid 252.01
  petrous bone (*see also* Petrositis) 383.20
  pubis 733.5
  sclerotic, nonsuppurative 730.1
  syphilitic 095.5
  tuberculosa
    cystica (of Jüngling) 135
    multiplex cystoides 135
Osteoarthritica spondylitis (spine) (*see also*
  Spondylosis) 721.90
Osteoarthritis (*see also* Osteoarthrosis) 715.9
  distal interphalangeal 715.9
  hyperplastic 731.2
  interspinalis (*see also* Spondylosis) 721.90
  spine, spinal NEC (*see also* Spondylosis) 721.90
Osteoarthropathy (*see also* Osteoarthrosis) 715.9
  chronic idiopathic hypertrophic 757.39
  familial idiopathic 757.39
  hypertrophic pulmonary 731.2
    secondary 731.2
  idiopathic hypertrophic 757.39
  primary hypertrophic 731.2
  pulmonary hypertrophic 731.2
  secondary hypertrophic 731.2
Osteoarthrosis (degenerative) (hypertrophic)
  (rheumatoid) 715.9

Note—Use the following fifth-digit
subclassification with category 715:

0 site unspecified
1 shoulder region
2 upper arm
3 forearm
4 hand
5 pelvic region and thigh
6 lower leg
7 ankle and foot
8 other specified sites except spine
9 multiple sites

---

  deformans alkaptonurica 270.2
  generalized 715.09
  juvenilis (Köhler's) 732.5
  localized 715.3
    idiopathic 715.1
    primary 715.1
    secondary 715.2
  multiple sites, not specified as generalized 715.89
  polyarticular 715.09
  spine (*see also* Spondylosis) 721.90
  temperomandibular joint 524.69
Osteoblastoma (M9200/0)—*see* Neoplasm, bone,
  benign
Osteochondritis (*see also* Osteochondrosis) 732.9
  dissecans 732.7
    hip 732.7
  ischiopubica 732.1
  multiple 756.59
  syphilitic (congenital) 090.0

Osteochondrodermodysplasia 756.59
Osteochondrodystrophy 277.5
  deformans 277.5
  familial 277.5
  fetalis 756.4
Osteochondrolysis 732.7
Osteochondroma (M9210/0)—*see also*
  Neoplasm, bone, benign
  multiple, congenital 756.4
Osteochondromatosis (M9210/1) 238.0
  synovial 727.82
Osteochondromyxosarcoma (M9180/3)—*see*
  Neoplasm, bone, malignant
Osteochondropathy NEC 732.9
Osteochondrosarcoma (M9180/3)—*see*
  Neoplasm, bone, malignant
Osteochondrosis 732.9
  acetabulum 732.1
  adult spine 732.8
  astragalus 732.5
  Blount's 732.4
  Buchanan's (juvenile osteochondrosis of iliac
    crest) 732.1
  Buchman's (juvenile osteochondrosis) 732.1
  Burns' 732.3
  calcaneus 732.5
  capitular epiphysis (femur) 732.1
  carpal
    lunate (wrist) 732.3
    scaphoid 732.3
  coxae juvenilis 732.1
  deformans juvenilis (coxae) (hip) 732.1
    Scheuermann's 732.0
    spine 732.0
    tibia 732.4
    vertebra 732.0
  Diaz's (astragalus) 732.5
  dissecans (knee) (shoulder) 732.7
  femoral capital epiphysis 732.1
  femur (head) (juvenile) 732.1
  foot (juvenile) 732.5
  Freiberg's (disease) (second metatarsal) 732.5
  Haas' 732.3
  Haglund's (os tibiale externum) 732.5
  hand (juvenile) 732.3
  head of
    femur 732.1
    humerus (juvenile) 732.3
  hip (juvenile) 732.1
  humerus (juvenile) 732.3
  iliac crest (juvenile) 732.1
  ilium (juvenile) 732.1
  ischiopubic synchondrosis 732.1
  Iselin's (osteochondrosis fifth metatarsal) 732.5
  juvenile, juvenilis 732.6
    arm 732.3
    capital femoral epiphysis 732.1
    capitellum humeri 732.3
    capitular epiphysis 732.1
    carpal scaphoid 732.3
    clavicle, sternal epiphysis 732.6
    coxae 732.1
    deformans 732.1
    foot 732.5
    hand 732.3
    hip and pelvis 732.1
    lower extremity, except foot 732.4
    lunate, wrist 732.3
    medial cuneiform bone 732.5
    metatarsal (head) 732.5
    metatarsophalangeal 732.5
    navicular, ankle 732.5

Osteochondrosis—*continued*
  patella 732.4
  primary patellar center (of Köhler) 732.4
  specified site NEC 732.6
  spine 732.0
  tarsal scaphoid 732.5
  tibia (epiphysis) (tuberosity) 732.4
  upper extremity 732.3
  vertebra (body) (Calvé) 732.0
    epiphyseal plates (of Scheuermann) 732.0
  Kienböck's (disease) 732.3
  Köhler's (disease) (navicular, ankle) 732.5
    patellar 732.4
    tarsal navicular 732.5
  Legg-Calvé-Perthes (disease) 732.1
  lower extremity (juvenile) 732.4
  lunate bone 732.3
  Mauclaire's 732.3
  metacarpal heads (of Mauclaire) 732.3
  metatarsal (fifth) (head) (second) 732.5
  navicular, ankle 732.5
  os calcis 732.5
  Osgood-Schlatter 732.4
  os tibiale externum 732.5
  Panner's 732.3
  patella (juvenile) 732.4
  patellar center
    primary (of Köhler) 732.4
    secondary (of Sinding-Larsen) 732.4
  pelvis (juvenile) 732.1
  Pierson's 732.1
  radial head (juvenile) 732.3
  Scheuermann's 732.0
  Sever's (calcaneum) 732.5
  Sinding-Larsen (secondary patellar center) 732.4
  spine (juvenile) 732.0
    adult 732.8
  symphysis pubis (of Pierson) (juvenile) 732.1
  syphilitic (congenital) 090.0
  tarsal (navicular) (scaphoid) 732.5
  tibia (proximal) (tubercle) 732.4
  tuberculous—*see* Tuberculosis, bone
  ulna 732.3
  upper extremity (juvenile) 732.3
  van Neck's (juvenile osteochondrosis) 732.1
  vertebral (juvenile) 732.0
    adult 732.8
Osteoclastoma (M9250/1) 238.0
  malignant (M9250/3)—*see* Neoplasm, bone,
    malignant
Osteocopic pain 733.90
Osteodynia 733.90
Osteodystrophy
  azotemic 588.0
  chronica deformans hypertrophica 731.0
  congenital 756.50
    specified type NEC 756.59
  deformans 731.0
  fibrosa localisata 731.0
  parathyroid 252.01
  renal 588.0
Osteofibroma (M9262/0)—*see* Neoplasm, bone,
  benign
Osteofibrosarcoma (M9182/3)—*see* Neoplasm,
  bone, malignant
Osteogenesis imperfecta 756.51
Osteogenic —*see* condition
Osteoma (M9180/0)—*see also* Neoplasm, bone,
  benign
  osteoid (M9191/0)—*see also* Neoplasm, bone,
    benign
  giant (M9200/0)—*see* Neoplasm, bone, benign

Osteomalacia 268.2
  chronica deformans hypertrophica 731.0
  due to vitamin D deficiency 268.2
  infantile (*see also* Rickets) 268.0
  juvenile (*see also* Rickets) 268.0
  pelvis 268.2
  vitamin D-resistant 275.3
Osteomalacic bone 268.2
Osteomalacosis 268.2
Osteomyelitis (general) (infective) (localized)
    (neonatal) (purulent) (pyogenic) (septic)
    (staphylococcal) (streptococcal) (suppurative)
    (with periostitis) 730.2

---

*Note—Use the following fifth-digit
subclassification with category 730:*

0 site unspecified
1 shoulder region
2 upper arm
3 forearm
4 hand
5 pelvic region and thigh
6 lower leg
7 ankle and foot
8 other specified sites
9 multiple sites

---

  acute or subacute 730.0
  chronic or old 730.1
  due to or associated with
    diabetes mellitus 250.8 *[731.8]*
      due to secondary diabetes 249.8 *[731.8]*
    tuberculosis (*see also* Tuberculosis, bone)
        015.9 *[730.8]*
      limb bones 015.5 *[730.8]*
      specified bones NEC 015.7 *[730.8]*
      spine 015.0 *[730.8]*
    typhoid 002.0 *[730.8]*
  Garré's 730.1
  jaw (acute) (chronic) (lower) (neonatal)
      (suppurative) (upper) 526.4
  nonsuppurating 730.1
  orbital 376.03
  petrous bone (*see also* Petrositis) 383.20
  Salmonella 003.24
  sclerosing, nonsuppurative 730.1
  sicca 730.1
  syphilitic 095.5
    congenital 090.0 *[730.8]*
  tuberculous—*see* Tuberculosis, bone
  typhoid 002.0 *[730.8]*
Osteomyelofibrosis 289.89
Osteomyelosclerosis 289.89
Osteonecrosis 733.40
  meaning osteomyelitis 730.1
Osteo-onycho-arthro dysplasia 756.89
Osteo-onychodysplasia, hereditary 756.89
Osteopathia
  condensans disseminata 756.53
  hyperostotica multiplex infantilis 756.59
  hypertrophica toxica 731.2
  striata 756.4
Osteopathy resulting from poliomyelitis (*see
    also* Poliomyelitis) 045.9 *[730.7]*
  familial dysplastic 731.2
Osteopecilia 756.53
Osteopenia 733.90
  borderline 733.90
Osteoperiostitis (*see also* Osteomyelitis) 730.2
  ossificans toxica 731.2
  toxica ossificans 731.2

Osteopetrosis (familial) 756.52
Osteophyte —*see* Exostosis
Osteophytosis —*see* Exostosis
Osteopoikilosis 756.53
Osteoporosis (generalized) 733.00
  circumscripta 731.0
  disuse 733.03
  drug-induced 733.09
  idiopathic 733.02
  postmenopausal 733.01
  posttraumatic 733.7
  screening V82.81
  senile 733.01
  specified type NEC 733.09
Osteoporosis-osteomalacia syndrome 268.2
Osteopsathyrosis 756.51
Osteoradionecrosis, jaw 526.89
Osteosarcoma (M9180/3)—*see also* Neoplasm,
    bone, malignant
  chondroblastic (M9181/3)—*see* Neoplasm,
      bone, malignant
  fibroblastic (M9182/3)—*see* Neoplasm, bone,
      malignant
  in Paget's disease of bone (M9184/3)—*see*
      Neoplasm, bone, malignant
  juxtacortical (M9190/3)—*see* Neoplasm, bone,
      malignant
  parosteal (M9190/3)—*see* Neoplasm, bone,
      malignant
  telangiectatic (M9183/3)—*see* Neoplasm, bone,
      malignant
Osteosclerosis 756.52
  fragilis (generalisata) 756.52
Osteosclerotic anemia 289.89
Osteosis
  acromegaloid 757.39
  cutis 709.3
  parathyroid 252.01
  renal fibrocystic 588.0
Österreicher-Turner syndrome 756.89
Ostium
  atrioventriculare commune 745.69
  primum (arteriosum) (defect) (persistent) 745.61
  secundum (arteriosum) (defect) (patent)
      (persistent) 745.5
Ostrum-Furst syndrome 756.59
Otalgia 388.70
  otogenic 388.71
  referred 388.72
Othematoma 380.31
Otitic hydrocephalus 348.2
Otitis 382.9
  with effusion 381.4
    purulent 382.4
    secretory 381.4
    serous 381.4
    suppurative 382.4
  acute 382.9
  adhesive (*see also* Adhesions, middle ear)
      385.10
  chronic 382.9
    with effusion 381.3
    mucoid, mucous (simple) 381.20
    purulent 382.3
    secretory 381.3
    serous 381.3
    suppurative 382.3
  diffuse parasitic 136.8
  externa (acute) (diffuse) (hemorrhagica) 380.10
    actinic 380.22
    candidal 112.82

Otitis—*continued*
  chemical 380.22
  chronic 380.23
    mycotic—*see* Otitis, externa, mycotic
    specified type NEC 380.23
  circumscribed 380.10
  contact 380.22
  due to
    erysipelas 035 *[380.13]*
    impetigo 684 *[380.13]*
    seborrheic dermatitis 690.10 *[380.13]*
  eczematoid 380.22
  furuncular 680.0 *[380.13]*
  infective 380.10
    chronic 380.16
  malignant 380.14
  mycotic (chronic) 380.15
    due to
      aspergillosis 117.3 *[380.15]*
      moniliasis 112.82
      otomycosis 111.8 *[380.15]*
  reactive 380.22
  specified type NEC 380.22
  tropical 111.8 *[380.15]*
  insidiosa (*see also* Otosclerosis) 387.9
  interna (*see also* Labyrinthitis) 386.30
  media (hemorrhagic) (staphylococcal)
    (streptococcal) 382.9
  acute 382.9
    with effusion 381.00
    allergic 381.04
      mucoid 381.05
      sanguineous 381.06
      serous 381.04
    catarrhal 381.00
    exudative 381.00
    mucoid 381.02
      allergic 381.05
    necrotizing 382.00
      with spontaneous rupture of ear drum 382.01
      in
        influenza 487.8 *[382.02]*
        measles 055.2
        scarlet fever 034.1 *[382.02]*
    nonsuppurative 381.00
    purulent 382.00
      with spontaneous rupture of ear drum 382.01
    sanguineous 381.03
      allergic 381.06
    secretory 381.01
    seromucinous 381.02
    serous 381.01
      allergic 381.04
    suppurative 382.00
      with spontaneous rupture of ear drum 382.01
      due to
        influenza 487.8 *[382.02]*
        scarlet fever 034.1 *[382.02]*
    transudative 381.00
  adhesive (*see also* Adhesions, middle ear) 385.10
  allergic 381.4
    acute 381.04
      mucoid 381.05
      sanguineous 381.06
      serous 381.04
    chronic 381.3

Otitis—*continued*
  catarrhal 381.4
    acute 381.00
    chronic (simple) 381.10
  chronic 382.9
    with effusion 381.3
    adhesive (*see also* Adhesions, middle ear) 385.10
    allergic 381.3
    atticoantral, suppurative (with posterior or superior marginal perforation of ear drum) 382.2
    benign suppurative (with anterior perforation of ear drum) 382.1
    catarrhal 381.10
    exudative 381.3
    mucinous 381.20
    mucoid, mucous (simple) 381.20
    mucosanguineous 381.29
    nonsuppurative 381.3
    purulent 382.3
    secretory 381.3
    seromucinous 381.3
    serosanguineous 381.19
    serous (simple) 381.10
    suppurative 382.3
      atticoantral (with posterior or superior marginal perforation of ear drum) 382.2
      benign (with anterior perforation of ear drum) 382.1
      tuberculous (*see also* Tuberculosis) 017.4
      tubotympanic 382.1
    transudative 381.3
  exudative 381.4
    acute 381.00
    chronic 381.3
  fibrotic (*see also* Adhesions, middle ear) 385.10
  mucoid, mucous 381.4
    acute 381.02
    chronic (simple) 381.20
  mucosanguineous, chronic 381.29
  nonsuppurative 381.4
    acute 381.00
    chronic 381.3
  postmeasles 055.2
  purulent 382.4
    acute 382.00
      with spontaneous rupture of ear drum 382.01
    chronic 382.3
  sanguineous, acute 381.03
    allergic 381.06
  secretory 381.4
    acute or subacute 381.01
    chronic 381.3
  seromucinous 381.4
    acute or subacute 381.02
    chronic 381.3
  serosanguineous, chronic 381.19
  serous 381.4
    acute or subacute 381.01
    chronic (simple) 381.10
  subacute—*see* Otitis, media, acute
  suppurative 382.4
    acute 382.00
      with spontaneous rupture of ear drum 382.01
    chronic 382.3
      atticoantral 382.2
      benign 382.1

Ovum
  blighted 631
  donor V59.70
    age 35 and over V59.73
      anonymous recipient V59.73
      designated recipient V59.74
    under age 35 V59.71
      anonymous recipient V59.71
      designated recipient V59.72
  dropsical 631
  pathologic 631
Owren's disease or syndrome (parahemophilia)
    (*see also* Defect, coagulation) 286.3
Oxalosis 271.8
Oxaluria 271.8
Ox heart —*see* Hypertrophy, cardiac
OX syndrome 758.6
Oxycephaly, oxycephalic 756.0
  syphilitic, congenital 090.0
Oxyuriasis 127.4
Oxyuris vermicularis (infestation) 127.4
Ozena 472.0

P

Pacemaker syndrome 429.4
Pachyderma, pachydermia 701.8
  laryngis 478.5
  laryngitis 478.79
  larynx (verrucosa) 478.79
Pachydermatitis 701.8
Pachydermatocele (congenital) 757.39
  acquired 701.8
Pachydermatosis 701.8
Pachydermoperiostitis
  secondary 731.2
Pachydermoperiostosis
  primary idiopathic 757.39
  secondary 731.2
Pachymeningitis (adhesive) (basal) (brain)
  (cerebral) (cervical) (chronic) (circumscribed)
  (external) (fibrous) (hemorrhagic)
  (hypertrophic) (internal) (purulent) (spinal)
  (suppurative) (*see also* Meningitis) 322.9
  gonococcal 098.82
Pachyonychia (congenital) 757.5
  acquired 703.8
Pachyperiosteodermia
  primary or idiopathic 757.39
  secondary 731.2
Pachyperiostosis
  primary or idiopathic 757.39
  secondary 731.2
Pacinian tumor (M9507/0)—*see* Neoplasm,
  skin, benign
Pads, knuckle or Garrod's 728.79
Paget's disease (osteitis deformans) 731.0
  with infiltrating duct carcinoma of the breast
    (M8541/3)—*see* Neoplasm, breast,
    malignant
  bone 731.0
    osteosarcoma in (M9184/3)—*see* Neoplasm,
      bone, malignant
  breast (M8540/3) 174.0
  extramammary (M8542/3)—*see also* Neoplasm,
    skin, malignant
    anus 154.3
    skin 173.5
  malignant (M8540/3)
    breast 174.0
    specified site NEC (M8542/3)—*see*
      Neoplasm, skin, malignant
    unspecified site 174.0
  mammary (M8540/3) 174.0
  necrosis of bone 731.0
  nipple (M8540/3) 174.0
  osteitis deformans 731.0
Paget-Schroetter syndrome (intermittent venous
  claudication) 453.89
Pain(s) (*see also* Painful) 780.96
  abdominal 789.0
  acute 338.19
    due to trauma 338.11
    postoperative 338.18
      post-thoracotomy 338.12
  adnexa (uteri) 625.9
  alimentary, due to vascular insufficiency 557.9
  anginoid (*see also* Pain, precordial) 786.51
  anus 569.42
  arch 729.5
  arm 729.5
  axillary 729.5

Pain(s)—*continued*
  back (postural) 724.5
    low 724.2
    psychogenic 307.89
  bile duct 576.9
  bladder 788.99
  bone 733.90
  breast 611.71
    psychogenic 307.89
  broad ligament 625.9
  cancer associated 338.3
  cartilage NEC 733.90
  cecum 789.0
  cervicobrachial 723.3
  chest (central) 786.50
    atypical 786.59
    midsternal 786.51
    musculoskeletal 786.59
    noncardiac 786.59
    substernal 786.51
    wall (anterior) 786.52
  chronic 338.29
    associated with significant psychosocial
      dysfunction 338.4
    due to trauma 338.21
    postoperative 338.28
      post-thoracotomy 338.22
    syndrome 338.4
  coccyx 724.79
  colon 789.0
  common duct 576.9
  coronary—*see* Angina
  costochondral 786.52
  diaphragm 786.52
  due to (presence of) any device, implant, or graft
    classifiable to 996.0-996.5—*see*
    Complications, due to (presence of) any
    device, implant, or graft classified to
    996.0-996.5 NEC
    malignancy (primary) (secondary) 338.3
  ear (*see also* Otalgia) 388.70
  epigastric, epigastrium 789.0
  extremity (lower) (upper) 729.5
  eye 379.91
  face, facial 784.0
    atypical 350.2
    nerve 351.8
  false (labor) 644.1
  female genital organ NEC 625.9
    psychogenic 307.89
  finger 729.5
  flank 789.0
  foot 729.5
  gallbladder 575.9
  gas (intestinal) 787.3
  gastric 536.8
  generalized 780.96
  genital organ
    female 625.9
    male 608.9
    psychogenic 307.89
  groin 789.0
  growing 781.99
  hand 729.5
  head (*see also* Headache) 784.0
  heart (*see also* Pain, precordial) 786.51
  infraorbital (*see also* Neuralgia, trigeminal)
    350.1

Pain(s)—*continued*
  intermenstrual 625.2
  jaw 526.9
  joint 719.40
    ankle 719.47
    elbow 719.42
    foot 719.47
    hand 719.44
    hip 719.45
    knee 719.46
    multiple sites 719.49
    pelvic region 719.45
    psychogenic 307.89
    shoulder (region) 719.41
    specified site NEC 719.48
    wrist 719.43
  kidney 788.0
  labor, false or spurious 644.1
  laryngeal 784.1
  leg 729.5
  limb 729.5
  low back 724.2
  lumbar region 724.2
  mastoid (*see also* Otalgia) 388.70
  maxilla 526.9
  menstrual 625.3
  metacarpophalangeal (joint) 719.44
  metatarsophalangeal (joint) 719.47
  mouth 528.9
  muscle 729.1
    intercostal 786.59
  musculoskeletal (*see also* Pain, by site) 729.1
  nasal 478.19
  nasopharynx 478.29
  neck NEC 723.1
    psychogenic 307.89
  neoplasm related (acute) (chronic) 338.3
  nerve NEC 729.2
  neuromuscular 729.1
  nose 478.19
  ocular 379.91
  ophthalmic 379.91
  orbital region 379.91
  osteocopic 733.90
  ovary 625.9
    psychogenic 307.89
  over heart (*see also* Pain, precordial) 786.51
  ovulation 625.2
  pelvic (female) 625.9
    male NEC 789.0
      psychogenic 307.89
    psychogenic 307.89
  penis 607.9
    psychogenic 307.89
  pericardial (*see also* Pain, precordial) 786.51
  perineum
    female 625.9
    male 608.9
  pharynx 478.29
  pleura, pleural, pleuritic 786.52
  post-operative 338.18
    acute 338.18
    chronic 338.28
  post-thoracotomy 338.12
    acute 338.12
    chronic 338.22
  preauricular 388.70
  precordial (region) 786.51
    psychogenic 307.89
  premenstrual 625.4
  psychogenic 307.80

Pain(s)—*continued*
  cardiovascular system 307.89
  gastrointestinal system 307.89
  genitourinary system 307.89
  heart 307.89
  musculoskeletal system 307.89
  respiratory system 307.89
  skin 306.3
  radicular (spinal) (*see also* Radiculitis) 729.2
  rectum 569.42
  respiration 786.52
  retrosternal 786.51
  rheumatic NEC 729.0
    muscular 729.1
  rib 786.50
  root (spinal) (*see also* Radiculitis) 729.2
  round ligament (stretch) 625.9
  sacroiliac 724.6
  sciatic 724.3
  scrotum 608.9
    psychogenic 307.89
  seminal vesicle 608.9
  sinus 478.19
  skin 782.0
  spermatic cord 608.9
  spinal root (*see also* Radiculitis) 729.2
  stomach 536.8
    psychogenic 307.89
  substernal 786.51
  temporomandibular (joint) 524.62
  temporomaxillary joint 524.62
  testis 608.9
    psychogenic 307.89
  thoracic spine 724.1
    with radicular and visceral pain 724.4
  throat 784.1
  tibia 733.90
  toe 729.5
  tongue 529.6
  tooth 525.9
  total hip replacement 996.77
  total knee replacement 996.77
  trigeminal (*see also* Neuralgia, trigeminal) 350.1
  tumor associated 338.3
  umbilicus 789.0
  ureter 788.0
  urinary (organ) (system) 788.0
  uterus 625.9
    psychogenic 307.89
  vagina 625.9
  vertebrogenic (syndrome) 724.5
  vesical 788.99
  vulva 625.9
  xiphoid 733.90

Painful —*see also* Pain
  arc syndrome 726.19
  coitus
    female 625.0
    male 608.89
      psychogenic 302.76
  ejaculation (semen) 608.89
    psychogenic 302.79
  erection 607.3
  feet syndrome 266.2
  menstruation 625.3
    psychogenic 306.52
  micturition 788.1
  ophthalmoplegia 378.55
  respiration 786.52
  scar NEC 709.2
  urination 788.1
  wire sutures 998.89

Painters' colic 984.9
  specified type of lead—*see* Table of drugs and
    chemicals
Palate —*see* condition
Palatoplegia 528.9
Palatoschisis (*see also* Cleft, palate) 749.00
Palilalia 784.69
Palindromic arthritis (*see also* Rheumatism,
  palindromic) 719.3
Palliative care V66.7
Pallor 782.61
  temporal, optic disc 377.15
Palmar —*see also* condition
  fascia—*see* condition
Palpable
  cecum 569.89
  kidney 593.89
  liver 573.9
  lymph nodes 785.6
  ovary 620.8
  prostate 602.9
  spleen (*see also* Splenomegaly) 789.2
  uterus 625.8
Palpitation (heart) 785.1
  psychogenic 306.2
Palsy (*see also* Paralysis) 344.9
  atrophic diffuse 335.20
  Bell's 351.0
    newborn 767.5
  birth 767.7
  brachial plexus 353.0
    fetus or newborn 767.6
  brain—*see also* Palsy, cerebral
    noncongenital or noninfantile 344.89
    due to vascular lesion—*see* category 438
    late effect—*see* Late effect(s) (of)
      cerebrovascular disease
    syphilitic 094.89
    congenital 090.49
  bulbar (chronic) (progressive) 335.22
    pseudo NEC 335.23
    supranuclear NEC 344.89
  cerebral (congenital) (infantile) (spastic) 343.9
    athetoid 333.71
    diplegic 343.0
      mue to prevhous vascular lesion—*see*
        category 438
      late effect—*see* Late effect(s) (of)
        cerebrovascular disease
    hemiplegic 343.1
    monoplegic 343.3
    noncongenital or noninfantile 437.8
      mue to prevhous vascular lesion—*see*
        category 438
      late effect—*see* Late effect(s) (of)
        cerebrovascular disease
    paraplegic 343.0
    quadriplegic 343.2
    spastic, not congenital or infantile 344.89
    syphilitic 094.89
      congenital 090.49
    tetraplegic 343.2
  cranial nerve—*see also* Disorder, nerve, cranial
    multiple 352.6
  creeping 335.21
  divers' 993.3
  Erb's (birth injury) 767.6
  facial 351.0
    newborn 767.5
  glossopharyngeal 352.2
  Klumpke (-Déjérine) 767.6

Palsy—*continued*
  lead 984.9
    specified type of lead—*see* Table of drugs and
      chemicals
  median nerve (tardy) 354.0
  peroneal nerve (acute) (tardy) 355.3
  progressive supranuclear 333.0
  pseudobulbar NEC 335.23
  radial nerve (acute) 354.3
  seventh nerve 351.0
    newborn 767.5
  shaking (*see also* Parkinsonism) 332.0
  spastic (cerebral) (spinal) 343.9
    hemiplegic 343.1
  specified nerve NEC—*see* Disorder, nerve
  supranuclear NEC 356.8
    progressive 333.0
  ulnar nerve (tardy) 354.2
  wasting 335.21
Paltauf-Sternberg disease 201.9
Paludism —*see* Malaria
Panama fever 084.0
Panaris (with lymphangitis) 681.9
  finger 681.02
  toe 681.11
Panaritium (with lymphangitis) 681.9
  finger 681.02
  toe 681.11
Panarteritis (nodosa) 446.0
  brain or cerebral 437.4
Pancake heart 793.2
  with cor pulmonale (chronic) 416.9
Pancarditis (acute) (chronic) 429.89
  with
    rheumatic fever (active) (acute) (chronic)
      (subacute) 391.8
      inactive or quiescent 398.99
  rheumatic, acute 391.8
    chronic or inactive 398.99
Pancoast's syndrome or tumor (carcinoma,
  pulmonary apex) (M8010/3) 162.3
Pancoast-Tobias syndrome (M8010/3)
  (carcinoma, pulmonary apex) 162.3
Pancolitis 556.6
Pancreas, pancreatic —*see* condition
Pancreatitis 577.0
  acute (edematous) (hemorrhagic) (recurrent) 577.0
  annular 577.0
  apoplectic 577.0
  calcereous 577.0
  chronic (infectious) 577.1
    recurrent 577.1
  cystic 577.2
  fibrous 577.8
  gangrenous 577.0
  hemorrhagic (acute) 577.0
  interstitial (chronic) 577.1
    acute 577.0
  malignant 577.0
  mumps 072.3
  painless 577.1
  recurrent 577.1
  relapsing 577.1
  subacute 577.0
  suppurative 577.0
  syphilitic 095.8
Pancreatolithiasis 577.8
Pancytolysis 289.9
Pancytopenia (acquired) 284.1
  with malformations 284.09
  congenital 284.09

Panencephalitis —*see also* Encephalitis
  subacute, sclerosing 046.2
Panhematopenia 284.81
  congenital 284.09
  constitutional 284.09
  splenic, primary 289.4
Panhemocytopenia 284.81
  congenital 284.09
  constitutional 284.09
Panhypogonadism 257.2
Panhypopituitarism 253.2
  prepubertal 253.3
Panic (attack) (state) 300.01
  reaction to exceptional stress (transient) 308.0
Panmyelopathy, familial constitutional 284.09
Panmyelophthisis 284.2
  acquired (secondary) 284.81
  congenital 284.2
  idiopathic 284.9
Panmyelosis (acute) (M9951/1) 238.79
Panner's disease 732.3
  capitellum humeri 732.3
  head of humerus 732.3
  tarsal navicular (bone) (osteochondrosis) 732.5
Panneuritis endemica 265.0 *[357.4]*
Panniculitis 729.30
  back 724.8
  knee 729.31
  mesenteric 567.82
  neck 723.6
  nodular, nonsuppurative 729.30
  sacral 724.8
  specified site NEC 729.39
Panniculus adiposus (abdominal) 278.1
Pannus (corneal) 370.62
  abdominal (symptomatic) 278.1
  allergic eczematous 370.62
  degenerativus 370.62
  keratic 370.62
  rheumatoid—*see* Arthritis, rheumatoid
  trachomatosus, trachomatous (active) 076.1
    [370.62]
    late effect 139.1
Panophthalmitis 360.02
Panotitis —*see* Otitis media
Pansinusitis (chronic) (hyperplastic)
    (nonpurulent) (purulent) 473.8
  acute 461.8
  due to fungus NEC 117.9
  tuberculous (*see also* Tuberculosis) 012.8
Panuveitis 360.12
  sympathetic 360.11
Panvalvular disease —*see* Endocarditis, mitral
Papageienkrankheit 073.9
Papanicolaou smear
  anus 796.70
    with
      atypical squamous cells
        cannot exclude high grade squamous
          intraepithelial lesion (ASC-H) 796.72
        of undetermined significance (ASC-US)
          796.71
      cytologic evidence of malignancy 796.76
      high grade squamous intraepithelial lesion
        (HGSIL) 796.74
      low grade squamous intraepithelial lesion
        (LGSIL) 796.73
    glandular 796.70
    specified finding NEC 796.79
    unsatisfactory cytology 796.78

Papanicolaou smear—*continued*
  cervix (screening test) V76.2
    as part of gynecological examination V72.31
    for suspected malignant neoplasm V76.2
    no disease found V71.1
    inadequate cytology sample 795.08
    nonspecific abnormal finding 795.00
      with
        atypical squamous cells—changes of
          undetermined significance
          cannot exclude high grade squamous
            intraepithelial lesion (ASC-H)
            795.02
          of undetermined significance (ASC-US)
            795.01
        cytologic evidence of malignancy 795.06
        high grade squamous intraepithelial lesion
          (HGSIL) 795.04
        low grade squamous intraepithelial lesion
          (LGSIL) 795.03
      nonspecific finding NEC 795.09
      satisfactory smear but lacking
        transformation zone 795.07
      to confirm findings of recent normal smear
        following initial abnormal smear V72.32
    unsatisfactory cervical cytology 795.08
    other specified site—*see also* Screening,
      malignant neoplasm
    for suspected malignant neoplasm—*see also*
      Screening, malignant neoplasm
    no disease found V71.1
    nonspecific abnormal finding 796.9
  vagina V76.47
    with
      atypical squamous cells
        cannot exclude high grade squamous
          intraepithelial lesion (ASC-H) 795.12
        of undetermined significance (ASC-US)
          795.11
      cytologic evidence of malignancy 795.16
      high grade squamous intraepithelial lesion
        (HGSIL) 795.14
      low grade squamous intraepithelial lesion
        (LGSIL) 795.13
    abnormal NEC 795.19
    following hysterectomy for malignant
      condition V67.01
    inadequate cytology sample 795.18
    unsatisfactory cytology 795.18
Papilledema 377.00
  associated with
    decreased ocular pressure 377.02
    increased intracranial pressure 377.01
    retinal disorder 377.03
  choked disc 377.00
  infectional 377.00
Papillitis 377.31
  anus 569.49
  chronic lingual 529.4
  necrotizing, kidney 584.7
  optic 377.31
  rectum 569.49
  renal, necrotizing 584.7
  tongue 529.0

Papilloma (M8050/0)—*see also* Neoplasm, by site, benign

> *Note—Except where otherwise indicated, the morphological varieties of papilloma in the list below should be coded by site as for "Neoplasm, benign."*

  acuminatum (female) (male) 078.11
  bladder (urinary) (transitional cell) (M8120/1) 236.7
    benign (M8120/0) 223.3
  choroid plexus (M9390/0) 225.0
    anaplastic type (M9390/3) 191.5
    malignant (M9390/3) 191.5
  ductal (M8503/0)
  dyskeratotic (M8052/0)
  epidermoid (M8052/0)
  hyperkeratotic (M8052/0)
  intracystic (M8504/0)
  intraductal (M8503/0)
  inverted (M8053/0)
  keratotic (M8052/0)
  parakeratotic (M8052/0)
  pinta (primary) 103.0
  renal pelvis (transitional cell) (M8120/1) 236.99
    benign (M8120/0) 223.1
  Schneiderian (M8121/0)
    specified site—*see* Neoplasm, by site, benign
    unspecified site 212.0
  serous surface (M8461/0)
    borderline malignancy (M8461/1)
      specified site—*see* Neoplasm, by site, uncertain behavior
      unspecified site 236.2
    specified site—*see* Neoplasm, by site, benign
    unspecified site 220
  squamous (cell) (M8052/0)
  transitional (cell) (M8120/0)
    bladder (urinary) (M8120/1) 236.7
    inverted type (M8121/1)—*see* Neoplasm, by site, uncertain behavior
    renal pelvis (M8120/1) 236.91
    ureter (M8120/1) 236.91
    ureter (transitional cell) (M8120/1) 236.91
    benign (M8120/0) 223.2
  urothelial (M8120/1)—*see* Neoplasm, by site, uncertain behavior
  verrucous (M8051/0)
  villous (M8261/1)—*see* Neoplasm, by site, uncertain behavior
  yaws, plantar or palmar 102.1
Papillomata, multiple, of yaws 102.1
Papillomatosis (M8060/0)—*see also* Neoplasm, by site, benign
  confluent and reticulate 701.8
  cutaneous 701.8
  ductal, breast 610.1
  Gougerot-Carteaud (confluent reticulate) 701.8
  intraductal (diffuse) (M8505/0)—*see* Neoplasm, by site, benign
  subareolar duct (M8506/0) 217
Papillon-Léage and Psaume syndrome (orodigitofacial dysostosis) 759.89
Papule 709.8
  carate (primary) 103.0
  fibrous, of nose (M8724/0) 216.3
  pinta (primary) 103.0
Papulosis, malignant 447.8
Papyraceous fetus 779.89
  complicating pregnancy 646.0
Paracephalus 759.7

Parachute mitral valve 746.5
Paracoccidioidomycosis 116.1
  mucocutaneous-lymphangitic 116.1
  pulmonary 116.1
  visceral 116.1
Paracoccidiomycosis —*see* Paracoccidioidomycosis
Paracusis 388.40
Paradentosis 523.5
Paradoxical facial movements 374.43
Paraffinoma 999.9
Paraganglioma (M8680/1)
  adrenal (M8700/0) 227.0
    malignant (M8700/3) 194.0
  aortic body (M8691/1) 237.3
    malignant (M8691/3) 194.6
  carotid body (M8692/1) 237.3
    malignant (M8692/3) 194.5
  chromaffin (M8700/0)—*see also* Neoplasm, by site, benign
    malignant (M8700/3)—*see* Neoplasm, by site, malignant
  extra-adrenal (M8693/1)
    malignant (M8693/3)
      specified site—*see* Neoplasm, by site, malignant
      unspecified site 194.6
    specified site—*see* Neoplasm, by site, uncertain behavior
    unspecified site 237.3
  glomus jugulare (M8690/1) 237.3
    malignant (M8690/3) 194.6
  jugular (M8690/1) 237.3
    malignant (M8690/3)
      specified site—*see* Neoplasm, by site, malignant
      unspecified site 194.6
  nonchromaffin (M8693/1)
    malignant (M8693/3)
      specified site—*see* Neoplasm, by site, malignant
      unspecified site 194.6
    specified site—*see* Neoplasm, by site, uncertain behavior
    unspecified site 237.3
  parasympathetic (M8682/1)
    specified site—*see* Neoplasm, by site, uncertain behavior
    unspecified site 237.3
  specified site—*see* Neoplasm, by site, uncertain behavior
  sympathetic (M8681/1)
    specified site—*see* Neoplasm, by site, uncertain behavior
    unspecified site 237.3
  unspecified site 237.3
Parageusia 781.1
  psychogenic 306.7
Paragonimiasis 121.2
Paragranuloma, Hodgkin's (M9660/3) 201.0
Parahemophilia (*see also* Defect, coagulation) 286.3
Parakeratosis 690.8
  psoriasiformis 696.2
  variegata 696.2
Paralysis, paralytic (complete) (incomplete) 344.9
  with
    broken
      back—*see* Fracture, vertebra, by site, with spinal cord injury
      neck—*see* Fracture, vertebra, cervical, with spinal cord injury

Paralysis, paralytic—*continued*
　fracture, vertebra—*see* Fracture, vertebra, by
　　site, with spinal cord injury
　　syphilis 094.89
　abdomen and back muscles 355.9
　abdominal muscles 355.9
　abducens (nerve) 378.54
　abductor 355.9
　　lower extremity 355.8
　　upper extremity 354.9
　accessory nerve 352.4
　accommodation 367.51
　　hysterical 300.11
　acoustic nerve 388.5
　agitans 332.0
　　arteriosclerotic 332.0
　alternating 344.89
　　oculomotor 344.89
　amyotrophic 335.20
　ankle 355.8
　anterior serratus 355.9
　anus (sphincter) 569.49
　apoplectic (current episode) (*see also* Disease,
　　cerebrovascular, acute) 436
　　late effect—*see* Late effect(s) (of)
　　　cerebrovascular disease
　　category 438
　arm 344.40
　　affecting
　　　dominant side 344.41
　　　nondominant side 344.42
　　both 344.2
　　due to old CVA—*see* Category 438
　　hysterical 300.11
　　late effect—*see* Late effect(s) (of)
　　　cerebrovascular disease
　　psychogenic 306.0
　　transient 781.4
　　traumatic NDC (*see also* Injury, nerve,
　　　upper limb) 955.9
　arteriosclerotic (current episode) 437.0
　　late effect—*see* Late effect(s) (of)
　　　cerebrovascular disease
　ascending (spinal), acute 357.0
　associated, nuclear 344.89
　asthenic bulbar 358.00
　ataxic NEC 334.9
　　general 094.1
　athetoid 333.71
　atrophic 356.9
　　infantile, acute (*see also* Poliomyelitis, with
　　　paralysis) 045.1
　　muscle NEC 355.9
　　progressive 335.21
　　spinal (acute) (*see also* Poliomyelitis, with
　　　paralysis) 045.1
　attack (*see also* Disease, cerebrovascular, acute)
　　436
　axillary 353.0
　Babinski-Nageotte's 344.89
　Bell's 351.0
　　newborn 767.5
　Benedikt's 344.89
　birth (injury) 767.7
　　brain 767.0
　　intracranial 767.0
　　spinal cord 767.4
　bladder (sphincter) 596.53
　　neurogenic 596.54
　　　with cauda equina syndrome 344.61
　　puerperal, postpartum, childbirth 665.5

Paralysis, paralytic—*continued*
　sensory 596.54
　　with cauda equina 344.61
　spastic 596.54
　　with cauda equina 344.61
　bowel, colon, or intestine (*see also* Ileus) 560.1
　brachial plexus 353.0
　　due to birth injury 767.6
　　newborn 767.6
　brain
　　congenital—*see* Palsy, cerebral
　　current episode 437.8
　　diplegia 344.2
　　due to previous vascular lesion—*see* category
　　　438
　　hemiplegia 342.9
　　　due to previous vascular lesion—*see*
　　　　category 438
　　　late effect—*see* Late effect(s) (of)
　　　　cerebrovascular disease
　　　infantile—*see* Palsy, cerebral
　　　late effect—*see* Late effect(s) (of)
　　　　cerebrovascular disease
　　monoplegia—*see also* Monoplegia
　　　due to previous vascular lesion—*see*
　　　　category 438
　　　late effect—*see* Late effect(s) (of)
　　　　cerebrovascular disease
　　paraplegia 344.1
　　quadriplegia —*see* Quadriplegia
　　syphilitic, congenital 090.49
　　triplegia 344.89
　bronchi 519.19
　Brown-Séquard's 344.89
　bulbar (chronic) (progressive) 335.22
　　infantile (*see also* Poliomyelitis, bulbar) 045.0
　　poliomyelitic (*see also* Poliomyelitis, bulbar)
　　　045.0
　　pseudo 335.23
　　supranuclear 344.89
　bulbospinal 358.00
　cardiac (*see also* Failure, heart) 428.9
　cerebral
　　current episode 437.8
　　spastic, infantile—*see* Palsy, cerebral
　cerebrocerebellar 437.8
　　diplegic infantile 343.0
　cervical
　　plexus 353.2
　　sympathetic NEC 337.09
　Céstan-Chenais 344.89
　Charcot-Marie-Tooth type 356.1
　childhood—*see* Palsy, cerebral
　Clark's 343.9
　colon (*see also* Ileus) 560.1
　compressed air 993.3
　compression
　　arm NEC 354.9
　　cerebral—*see* Paralysis, brain
　　leg NEC 355.8
　　lower extremity NEC 355.8
　　upper extremity NEC 354.9
　congenital (cerebral) (spastic) (spinal)—*see*
　　Palsy, cerebral
　conjugate movement (of eye) 378.81
　　cortical (nuclear) (supranuclear) 378.81
　convergence 378.83
　cordis (*see also* Failure, heart) 428.9
　cortical (*see also* Paralysis, brain) 437.8
　cranial or cerebral nerve (*see also* Disorder,
　　nerve, cranial) 352.9

Paralysis, paralytic—*continued*
  creeping 335.21
  crossed leg 344.89
  crutch 953.4
  deglutition 784.99
    hysterical 300.11
  dementia 094.1
  descending (spinal) NEC 335.9
  diaphragm (flaccid) 519.4
    due to accidental section of phrenic nerve
      during procedure 998.2
  digestive organs NEC 564.89
  diplegic—*see* Diplegia
  divergence (nuclear) 378.85
  divers' 993.3
  Duchenne's 335.22
  due to intracranial or spinal birth injury—*see*
    Palsy, cerebral
  embolic (current episode) (*see also* Embolism,
    brain) 434.1
    late effect —*see* Late effect(s) (of)
      cerebrovascular disease
  enteric (*see also* Ileus) 560.1
    with hernia—*see* Hernia, by site, with
      obstruction
  Erb's syphilitic spastic spinal 094.89
  Erb (-Duchenne) (birth) (newborn) 767.6
  esophagus 530.89
  essential, infancy (*see also* Poliomyelitis) 045.9
  extremity
    lower —*see* Paralysis, leg
    spastic (hereditary) 343.3
      noncongenital or noninfantile 344.1
    transient (cause unknown) 781.4
    upper —*see* Paralysis, arm
  eye muscle (extrinsic) 378.55
    intrinsic 367.51
  facial (nerve) 351.0
    birth injury 767.5
    congenital 767.5
    following operation NEC 998.2
    newborn 767.5
  familial 359.3
    periodic 359.3
    spastic 334.1
  fauces 478.29
  finger NEC 354.9
  foot NEC 355.8
  gait 781.2
  gastric nerve 352.3
  gaze 378.81
  general 094.1
    ataxic 094.1
    insane 094.1
    juvenile 090.40
    progressive 094.1
    tabetic 094.1
  glossopharyngeal (nerve) 352.2
  glottis (*see also* Paralysis, vocal cord) 478.30
  gluteal 353.4
  Gubler (-Millard) 344.89
  hand 354.9
    hysterical 300.11
    psychogenic 306.0
  heart (*see also* Failure, heart) 428.9
  hemifacial, progressive 349.89
  hemiplegic—*see* Hemiplegia
  hyperkalemic periodic (familial) 359.3
  hypertensive (current episode) 437.8
  hypoglossal (nerve) 352.5
  hypokalemic periodic 359.3

Paralysis, paralytic—*continued*
  Hyrtl's sphincter (rectum) 569.49
  hysterical 300.11
  ileus (*see also* Ileus) 560.1
  infantile (*see also* Poliomyelitis) 045.9
    atrophic acute 045.1
    bulbar 045.0
    cerebral—*see* Palsy, cerebral
    paralytic 045.1
    progressive acute 045.9
    spastic—*see* Palsy, cerebral
    spinal 045.9
  infective (*see also* Poliomyelitis) 045.9
  inferior nuclear 344.9
  insane, general or progressive 094.1
  internuclear 378.86
  interosseous 355.9
  intestine (*see also* Ileus) 560.1
  intracranial (current episode) (*see also* Paralysis,
    brain) 437.8
    due to birth injury 767.0
  iris 379.49
    due to diphtheria (toxin) 032.81 *[379.49]*
  ischemic, Volkmann's (complicating trauma)
    958.6
  isolated sleep, recurrent 327.43
  Jackson's 344.89
  jake 357.7
  Jamaica ginger (jake) 357.7
  juvenile general 090.40
  Klumpke (-Déjérine) (birth) (newborn) 767.6
  labioglossal (laryngeal) (pharyngeal) 335.22
  Landry's 357.0
  laryngeal nerve (recurrent) (superior) (*see also*
    Paralysis, vocal cord) 478.30
  larynx (*see also* Paralysis, vocal cord) 478.30
    due to diphtheria (toxin) 032.3
  late effect
    due to
      birth injury, brain or spinal (cord)—*see*
        Palsy, cerebral
      edema, brain or cerebral—*see* Paralysis,
        brain
      lesion
        cerebrovascular—*see* category 438
        late effect—*see* Late effect(s) (of)
          cerebrovascular disease
        spinal (cord)—*see* Paralysis, spinal
  lateral 335.24
  lead 984.9
    specified type of lead—*see* Table of drugs and
      chemicals
  left side—*see* Hemiplegia
  leg 344.30
    affecting
      dominant side 344.31
      nondominant side 344.32
    both (*see also* Paraplegia) 344.1
    crossed 344.89
    hysterical 300.11
    psychogenic 306.0
    transient or transitory 781.4
    traumatic NEC (*see also* Injury, nerve, lower
      limb) 956.9
  levator palpebrae superioris 374.31
  limb NEC 344.5
    all four—*see* Quadriplegia
    quadriplegia—*see* Quadriplegia
  lip 528.5
  Lissauer's 094.1
  local 355.9

Paralysis, paralytic—*continued*
lower limb—*see also* Paralysis, leg
  both (*see also* Paraplegia) 344.1
lung 518.89
  newborn 770.89
median nerve 354.1
medullary (tegmental) 344.89
mesencephalic NEC 344.89
  tegmental 344.89
middle alternating 344.89
Millard-Gubler-Foville 344.89
monoplegic—*see* Monoplegia
motor NEC 344.9
  cerebral—*see* Paralysis, brain
  spinal—*see* Paralysis, spinal
multiple
  cerebral—*see* Paralysis, brain
  spinal—*see* Paralysis, spinal
muscle (flaccid) 359.9
  due to nerve lesion NEC 355.9
  eye (extrinsic) 378.55
    intrinsic 367.51
    oblique 378.51
  iris sphincter 364.89
  ischemic (complicating trauma) (Volkmann's) 958.6
  pseudohypertrophic 359.1
muscular (atrophic) 359.9
  progressive 335.21
musculocutaneous nerve 354.9
musculospiral 354.9
nerve—*see also* Disorder, nerve
  third or oculomotor (partial) 378.51
    total 378.52
  fourth or trochlear 378.53
  sixth or abducens 378.54
  seventh or facial 351.0
    birth injury 767.5
    due to
      injection NEC 999.9
      operation NEC 997.09
    newborn 767.5
  accessory 352.4
  auditory 388.5
  birth injury 767.7
  cranial or cerebral (*see also* Disorder, nerve, cranial) 352.9
  facial 351.0
    birth injury 767.5
    newborn 767.5
  laryngeal (*see also* Paralysis, vocal cord) 478.30
    newborn 767.7
  phrenic 354.8
    newborn 767.7
  radial 354.3
    birth injury 767.6
    newborn 767.6
  syphilitic 094.89
  traumatic NEC (*see also* Injury, nerve, by site) 957.9
  trigeminal 350.9
  ulnar 354.2
newborn NEC 767.0
normokalemic periodic 359.3
obstetrical, newborn 767.7
ocular 378.9
oculofacial, congenital 352.6
oculomotor (nerve) (partial) 378.51
  alternating 344.89
  external bilateral 378.55
  total 378.52

Paralysis, paralytic—*continued*
olfactory nerve 352.0
palate 528.9
palatopharyngolaryngeal 352.6
paratrigeminal 350.9
periodic (familial) (hyperkalemic) (hypokalemic) (normokalemic) (potassium sensitive) (secondary) 359.3
peripheral
  autonomic nervous system—*see* Neuropathy, peripheral, autonomic
  nerve NEC 355.9
peroneal (nerve) 355.3
pharynx 478.29
phrenic nerve 354.8
plantar nerves 355.6
pneumogastric nerve 352.3
poliomyelitis (current) (*see also* Poliomyelitis, with paralysis) 045.1
  bulbar 045.0
popliteal nerve 355.3
pressure (*see also* Neuropathy, entrapment) 355.9
progressive 335.21
  atrophic 335.21
  bulbar 335.22
  general 094.1
  hemifacial 349.89
  infantile, acute (*see also* Poliomyelitis) 045.9
  multiple 335.20
pseudobulbar 335.23
pseudohypertrophic 359.1
  muscle 359.1
psychogenic 306.0
pupil, pupillary 379.49
quadriceps 355.8
quadriplegic (*see also* Quadriplegia) 344.0
radial nerve 354.3
  birth injury 767.6
rectum (sphincter) 569.49
rectus muscle (eye) 378.55
recurrent
  isolated sleep 327.43
  laryngeal nerve (*see also* Paralysis, vocal cord) 478.30
respiratory (muscle) (system) (tract) 786.09
  center NEC 344.89
    fetus or newborn 770.87
  congenital 768.9
  newborn 768.9
right side—*see* Hemiplegia
Saturday night 354.3
saturnine 984.9
  specified type of lead—*see* Table of drugs and chemicals
sciatic nerve 355.0
secondary—*see* Paralysis, late effect
seizure (cerebral) (current episode) (*see also* Disease, cerebrovascular, acute) 436
  late effect—*see* Late effect(s) (of) cerebrovascular disease
senile NEC 344.9
serratus magnus 355.9
shaking (*see also* Parkinsonism) 332.0
shock (*see also* Disease, cerebrovascular, acute) 436
  late effect—*see* Late effect(s) (of) cerebrovascular disease
shoulder 354.9
soft palate 528.9
spasmodic—*see* Paralysis, spastic

Paralysis, paralytic—*continued*
  spastic 344.9
    cerebral infantile—*see* Palsy, cerebral
    congenital (cerebral)—*see* Palsy, cerebral
    familial 334.1
    hereditary 334.1
    infantile 343.9
    noncongenital or noninfantile, cerebral 344.9
    syphilitic 094.0
      spinal 094.89
  sphincter, bladder (*see also* Paralysis, bladder)
    596.53
  spinal (cord) NEC 344.1
    accessory nerve 352.4
    acute (*see also* Poliomyelitis) 045.9
    ascending acute 357.0
    atrophic (acute) (*see also* Poliomyelitis, with
      paralysis) 045.1
      spastic, syphilitic 094.89
    congenital NEC 343.9
    hemiplegic —*see* Hemiplegia
    hereditary 336.8
    infantile (*see also* Poliomyelitis) 045.9
    late effect NEC 344.89
    monoplegic—*see* Monoplegia
    nerve 355.9
    progressive 335.10
    quadriplegic —*see* Quadriplegia
    spastic NEC 343.9
    traumatic—*see* Injury, spinal, by site
  sternomastoid 352.4
  stomach 536.3
    diabetic 250.6 *[536.3]*
      due to secondary diabetes 249.6 *[536.3]*
    nerve (nondiabetic) 352.3
  stroke (current episode) *see* Infarct, brain
    late effect—*see* Late effect(s) (of)
      cerebrovascular disease
  subscapularis 354.8
  superior nuclear NEC 334.9
  supranuclear 356.8
  sympathetic
    cervical NEC 337.09
    nerve NEC (*see also* Neuropathy, peripheral,
      autonomic) 337.9
    nervous system—*see* Neuropathy, peripheral,
      autonomic
  syndrome 344.9
    specified NEC 344.89
  syphilitic spastic spinal (Erb's) 094.89
  tabetic general 094.1
  thigh 355.8
  throat 478.29
    diphtheritic 032.0
    muscle 478.29
  thrombotic (current episode) (*see also*
    Thrombosis, brain) 434.0
    late effect—*see* Late effect(s) (of)
      cerebrovascular disease
  thumb NEC 354.9
  tick (-bite) 989.5
  Todd's (postepileptic transitory paralysis)
    344.89
  toe 355.6
  tongue 529.8
  transient
    arm or leg NEC 781.4
    traumatic NEC (*see also* Injury, nerve, by site)
      957.9
  trapezius 352.4

Paralysis, paralytic—*continued*
  traumatic, transient NEC (*see also* Injury, nerve,
    by site) 957.9
  trembling (*see also* Parkinsonism) 332.0
  triceps brachii 354.9
  trigeminal nerve 350.9
  trochlear nerve 378.53
  ulnar nerve 354.2
  upper limb —*see also* Paralysis, arm
    both (*see also* Diplegia) 344.2
  uremic—*see* Uremia
  uveoparotitic 135
  uvula 528.9
    hysterical 300.11
    postdiphtheritic 032.0
  vagus nerve 352.3
  vasomotor NEC 337.9
  velum palati 528.9
  vesical (*see also* Paralysis, bladder) 596.53
  vestibular nerve 388.5
  visual field, psychic 368.16
  vocal cord 478.30
    bilateral (partial) 478.33
      complete 478.34
    complete (bilateral) 478.34
    unilateral (partial) 478.31
      complete 478.32
  Volkmann's (complicating trauma) 958.6
  wasting 335.21
  Weber's 344.89
  wrist NEC 354.9
Paramedial orifice, urethrovesical 753.8
Paramenia 626.9
Parametritis (chronic) (*see also* Disease, pelvis,
    inflammatory) 614.4
  acute 614.3
  puerperal, postpartum, childbirth 670.8
Parametrium, parametric —*see* condition
Paramnesia (*see also* Amnesia) 780.93
Paramolar 520.1
  causing crowding 524.31
Paramyloidosis 277.30
Paramyoclonus multiplex 333.2
Paramyotonia 359.29
  congenita (of von Eulenburg) 359.29
Paraneoplastic syndrome —*see* condition
Parangi (*see also* Yaws) 102.9
Paranoia 297.1
  alcoholic 291.5
  querulans 297.8
  senile 290.20
Paranoid
  dementia (*see also* Schizophrenia) 295.3
    praecox (acute) 295.3
    senile 290.20
  personality 301.0
  psychosis 297.9
    alcoholic 291.5
    climacteric 297.2
    drug-induced 292.11
    involutional 297.2
    menopausal 297.2
    protracted reactive 298.4
    psychogenic 298.4
      acute 298.3
    senile 290.20
  reaction (chronic) 297.9
    acute 298.3
  schizophrenia (acute) (*see also* Schizophrenia)
    295.3

Paranoid—*continued*
  state 297.9
    alcohol-induced 291.5
    climacteric 297.2
    drug-induced 292.11
    due to or associated with
      arteriosclerosis (cerebrovascular) 290.42
      presenile brain disease 290.12
      senile brain disease 290.20
    involutional 297.2
    menopausal 297.2
    senile 290.20
    simple 297.0
    specified type NEC 297.8
  tendencies 301.0
  traits 301.0
  trends 301.0
  type, psychopathic personality 301.0
Paraparesis (*see also* Paraplegia) 344.1
Paraphasia 784.3
Paraphilia (*see also* Deviation, sexual) 302.9
Paraphimosis (congenital) 605
  chancroidal 099.0
Paraphrenia, paraphrenic (late) 297.2
  climacteric 297.2
  dementia (*see also* Schizophrenia) 295.3
  involutional 297.2
  menopausal 297.2
  schizophrenia (acute) (*see also* Schizophrenia)
    295.3
Paraplegia 344.1
  with
    broken back—*see* Fracture, vertebra, by site,
      with spinal cord injury
    fracture, vertebra—*see* Fracture, vertebra, by
      site, with spinal cord injury
  ataxic—*see* Degeneration, combined, spinal
    cord
  brain (current episode) (*see also* Paralysis,
    brain) 437.8
  cerebral (current episode) (*see also* Paralysis,
    brain) 437.8
  congenital or infantile (cerebral) (spastic)
    (spinal) 343.0
  cortical—*see* Paralysis, brain
  familial spastic 334.1
  functional (hysterical) 300.11
  hysterical 300.11
  infantile 343.0
  late effect 344.1
  Pott's (*see also* Tuberculosis) 015.0 *[730.88]*
  psychogenic 306.0
  spastic
    Erb's spinal 094.89
    hereditary 334.1
    not infantile or congenital 344.1
  spinal (cord)
    traumatic NEC—*see* Injury, spinal, by site
  syphilitic (spastic) 094.89
  traumatic NEC—*see* Injury, spinal, by site
Paraproteinemia 273.2
  benign (familial) 273.1
  monoclonal 273.1
  secondary to malignant or inflammatory disease
    273.1
Parapsoriasis 696.2
  en plaques 696.2
  guttata 696.2
  lichenoides chronica 696.2
  retiformis 696.2
  varioliformis (acuta) 696.2
Parascarlatina 057.8

Parasitic —*see also* condition
  disease NEC (*see also* Infestation, parasitic)
    136.9
    contact V01.89
    exposure to V01.89
    intestinal NEC 129
    skin NEC 134.9
  stomatitis 112.0
  sycosis 110.0
    beard 110.0
    scalp 110.0
  twin 759.4
Parasitism NEC 136.9
  intestinal NEC 129
  skin NEC 134.9
  specified—*see* Infestation
Parasitophobia 300.29
Parasomnia 307.47
  alcohol induced 291.82
  drug induced 292.85
  nonorganic origin 307.47
  organic 327.40
    in conditions classified elsewhere 327.44
    other 327.49
Paraspadias 752.69
Paraspasm facialis 351.8
Parathyroid gland —*see* condition
Parathyroiditis (autoimmune) 252.1
Parathyroprival tetany 252.1
Paratrachoma 077.0
Paratyphilitis (*see also* Appendicitis) 541
Paratyphoid (fever)—*see* Fever, paratyphoid
Paratyphus —*see* Fever, paratyphoid
Paraurethral duct 753.8
Para-urethritis 597.89
  gonococcal (acute) 098.0
    chronic or duration of 2 months or over 098.2
Paravaccinia NEC 051.9
  milkers' node 051.1
Paravaginitis (*see also* Vaginitis) 616.10
Parencephalitis (*see also* Encephalitis) 323.9
  late effect—*see* category 326
Parergasia 298.9
Paresis (*see also* Paralysis) 344.9
  accommodation 367.51
  bladder (spastic) (sphincter) (*see also* Paralysis,
    bladder) 596.53
    tabetic 094.0
  bowel, colon, or intestine (*see also* Ileus) 560.1
  brain or cerebral—*see* Paralysis, brain
  extrinsic muscle, eye 378.55
  general 094.1
    arrested 094.1
    brain 094.1
    cerebral 094.1
    insane 094.1
    juvenile 090.40
      remission 090.49
    progressive 094.1
    remission (sustained) 094.1
    tabetic 094.1
  heart (*see also* Failure, heart) 428.9
  infantile (*see also* Poliomyelitis) 045.9
  insane 094.1
  juvenile 090.40
  late effect—*see* Paralysis, late effect
  luetic (general) 094.1
  peripheral progressive 356.9
  pseudohypertrophic 359.1
  senile NEC 344.9

Paresis—*continued*
  stomach 536.3
    diabetic 250.6 *[536.3]*
      due to secondary diabetes 249.6 *[536.3]*
  syphilitic (general) 094.1
    congenital 090.40
  transient, limb 781.4
  vesical (sphincter) NEC 596.53
Paresthesia (*see also* Disturbance, sensation)
  782.0
  Berger's (paresthesia of lower limb) 782.0
  Bernhardt 355.1
  Magnan's 782.0
Paretic —*see* condition
Parinaud's
  conjunctivitis 372.02
  oculoglandular syndrome 372.02
  ophthalmoplegia 378.81
  syndrome (paralysis of conjugate upward gaze)
    378.81
Parkes Weber and Dimitri syndrome
  (encephalocutaneous angiomatosis) 759.6
Parkinson's disease, syndrome, or tremor
  —*see* Parkinsonism
Parkinsonism (arteriosclerotic) (idiopathic)
  (primary) 332.0
  associated with orthostatic hypotension
    (idiopathic) (symptomatic) 333.0
  due to drugs 332.1
  neuroleptic-induced 332.1
  secondary 332.1
  syphilitic 094.82
Parodontitis 523.40
Parodontosis 523.5
Paronychia (with lymphangitis) 681.9
  candidal (chronic) 112.3
  chronic 681.9
    candidal 112.3
    finger 681.02
    toe 681.11
  finger 681.02
  toe 681.11
  tuberculous (primary) (*see also* Tuberculosis)
    017.0
Parorexia NEC 307.52
  hysterical 300.11
Parosmia 781.1
  psychogenic 306.7
Parotid gland —*see* condition
Parotiditis (*see also* Parotitis) 527.2
  epidemic 072.9
  infectious 072.9
Parotitis 527.2
  allergic 527.2
  chronic 527.2
  epidemic (*see also* Mumps) 072.9
  infectious (*see also* Mumps) 072.9
  noninfectious 527.2
  nonspecific toxic 527.2
  not mumps 527.2
  postoperative 527.2
  purulent 527.2
  septic 527.2
  suppurative (acute) 527.2
  surgical 527.2
  toxic 527.2
Paroxysmal —*see also* condition
  dyspnea (nocturnal) 786.09
Parrot's disease (syphilitic osteochondritis)
  090.0
Parrot fever 073.9

Parry's disease or syndrome (exophthalmic
  goiter) 242.0
Parry-Romberg syndrome 349.89
Parson's disease (exophthalmic goiter) 242.0
Parsonage-Aldren-Turner syndrome 353.5
Parsonage-Turner syndrome 353.5
Pars planitis 363.21
Particolored infant 757.39
Parturition —*see* Delivery
Parvovirus 079.83
  B19 079.83
  human 079.83
Passage
  false, urethra 599.4
  meconium noted during delivery 763.84
  of sounds or bougies (*see also* Attention to
    artificial opening) V55.9
Passive —*see* condition
Pasteurella septica 027.2
Pasteurellosis (*see also* Infection, Pasteurella)
  027.2
PAT (paroxysmal atrial tachycardia) 427.0
Patau's syndrome (trisomy D_1) 758.1
Patch
  herald 696.3
Patches
  mucous (syphilitic) 091.3
    congenital 090.0
  smokers' (mouth) 528.6
Patellar —*see* condition
Patellofemoral syndrome 719.46
Patent —*see also* Imperfect closure
  atrioventricular ostium 745.69
  canal of Nuck 752.41
  cervix 622.5
    complicating pregnancy 654.5
      affecting fetus or newborn 761.0
  ductus arteriosus or Botalli 747.0
  Eustachian
    tube 381.7
    valve 746.89
  foramen
    Botalli 745.5
    ovale 745.5
  interauricular septum 745.5
  interventricular septum 745.4
  omphalomesenteric duct 751.0
  os (uteri)—*see* Patent, cervix
  ostium secundum 745.5
  urachus 753.7
  vitelline duct 751.0
Paternity testing V70.4
Paterson's syndrome (sideropenic dysphagia)
  280.8
Paterson (-Brown) (-Kelly) syndrome
  (sideropenic dysphagia) 280.8
Paterson-Kelly syndrome or web (sideropenic
  dysphagia) 280.8
Pathologic, pathological —*see also* condition
  asphyxia 799.01
  drunkenness 291.4
  emotionality 301.3
  liar 301.7
  personality 301.9
  resorption, tooth 521.40
    external 521.42
    internal 521.41
    specified NEC 521.49
  sexuality (*see also* Deviation, sexual) 302.9

Pathology (of)—*see also* Disease
  periradicular, associated with previous
    endodontic treatment 526.69
Patterned motor discharges, idiopathic (*see also* Epilepsy) 345.5
Patulous —*see also* Patent
  anus 569.49
  Eustachian tube 381.7
Pause, sinoatrial 427.81
Pavor nocturnus 307.46
Pavy's disease 593.6
Paxton's disease (white piedra) 111.2
Payr's disease or syndrome (splenic flexure syndrome) 569.89
PBA (pseudobulbar affect) 310.8
Pearls
  Elschnig 366.51
  enamel 520.2
Pearl-workers' disease (chronic osteomyelitis) (*see also* Osteomyelitis) 730.1
Pectenitis 569.49
Pectenosis 569.49
Pectoral —*see* condition
Pectus
  carinatum (congenital) 754.82
    acquired 738.3
    rachitic (*see also* Rickets) 268.0
  excavatum (congenital) 754.81
    acquired 738.3
    rachitic (*see also* Rickets) 268.0
  recurvatum (congenital) 754.81
    acquired 738.3
Pedatrophia 261
Pederosis 302.2
Pediculosis (infestation) 132.9
  capitis (head louse) (any site) 132.0
  corporis (body louse) (any site) 132.1
  eyelid 132.0 *[373.6]*
  mixed (classifiable to more than one category in 132.0-132.2) 132.3
  pubis (pubic louse) (any site) 132.2
  vestimenti 132.1
  vulvae 132.2
Pediculus (infestation)—*see* Pediculosis
Pedophilia 302.2
Peg-shaped teeth 520.2
Pel's crisis 094.0
Pel-Ebstein disease —*see* Disease, Hodgkin's
Pelade 704.01
Pelger-Huët anomaly or syndrome (hereditary hyposegmentation) 288.2
Peliosis (rheumatica) 287.0
Pelizaeus-Merzbacher
  disease 330.0
  sclerosis, diffuse cerebral 330.0
Pellagra (alcoholic or with alcoholism) 265.2
  with polyneuropathy 265.2 *[357.4]*
Pellagra-cerebellar-ataxia-renal aminoaciduria syndrome 270.0
Pellegrini's disease (calcification, knee joint) 726.62
Pellegrini (-Stieda) disease or syndrome (calcification, knee joint) 726.62
Pellizzi's syndrome (pineal) 259.8
Pelvic —*see also* condition
  congestion-fibrosis syndrome 625.5
  kidney 753.3
Pelvioectasis 591
Pelviolithiasis 592.0

Pelviperitonitis
  female (*see also* Peritonitis, pelvic, female) 614.5
  male (*see also* Peritonitis) 567.21
Pelvis, pelvic —*see also* condition or type
  infantile 738.6
  Nägele's 738.6
  obliquity 738.6
  Robert's 755.69
Pemphigoid 694.5
  benign, mucous membrane 694.60
    with ocular involvement 694.61
  bullous 694.5
  cicatricial 694.60
    with ocular involvement 694.61
  juvenile 694.2
Pemphigus 694.4
  benign 694.5
    chronic familial 757.39
  Brazilian 694.4
  circinatus 694.0
  congenital, traumatic 757.39
  conjunctiva 694.61
  contagiosus 684
  erythematodes 694.4
  erythematosus 694.4
  foliaceus 694.4
  frambesiodes 694.4
  gangrenous (*see also* Gangrene) 785.4
  malignant 694.4
  neonatorum, newborn 684
  ocular 694.61
  papillaris 694.4
  seborrheic 694.4
  South American 694.4
  syphilitic (congenital) 090.0
  vegetans 694.4
  vulgaris 694.4
  wildfire 694.4
Pendred's syndrome (familial goiter with deaf-mutism) 243
Pendulous
  abdomen 701.9
    in pregnancy or childbirth 654.4
      affecting fetus or newborn 763.89
  breast 611.89
Penetrating wound —*see also* Wound, open, by site
  with internal injury—*see* Injury, internal, by site, with open wound
  eyeball 871.7
    with foreign body (nonmagnetic) 871.6
      magnetic 871.5
  ocular (*see also* Penetrating wound, eyeball) 871.7
    adnexa 870.3
      with foreign body 870.4
    orbit 870.3
      with foreign body 870.4
Penetration, pregnant uterus by instrument
  with
    abortion—*see* Abortion, by type, with damage to pelvic organs
    ectopic pregnancy (*see also* categories 633.0-633.9) 639.2
    molar pregnancy (*see also* categories 630-632) 639.2
  complication of delivery 665.1
    affecting fetus or newborn 763.89
  following
    abortion 639.2
    ectopic or molar pregnancy 639.2

Penfield's syndrome (*see also* Epilepsy) 345.5
Penicilliosis of lung 117.3
Penis —*see* condition
Penitis 607.2
Penta X syndrome 758.81
Pentalogy (of Fallot) 745.2
Pentosuria (benign) (essential) 271.8
Peptic acid disease 536.8
Peregrinating patient V65.2
Perforated —*see* Perforation
Perforation, perforative (nontraumatic)
  antrum (*see also* Sinusitis, maxillary) 473.0
  appendix 540.0
    with peritoneal abscess 540.1
  atrial septum, multiple 745.5
  attic, ear 384.22
    healed 384.81
  bile duct, except cystic (*see also* Disease,
    biliary) 576.3
    cystic 575.4
  bladder (urinary) 596.6
    with
      abortion—*see* Abortion, by type, with
        damage to pelvic organs
      ectopic pregnancy (*see also* categories
        633.0-633.9) 639.2
      molar pregnancy (*see also* categories
        630-632) 639.2
    following
      abortion 639.2
      ectopic or molar pregnancy 639.2
    obstetrical trauma 665.5
  bowel 569.83
    with
      abortion—*see* Abortion, by type, with
        damage to pelvic organs
      ectopic pregnancy (*see also* categories
        633.0-633.9) 639.2
      molar pregnancy (*see also* categories
        630-632) 639.2
    fetus or newborn 777.6
    following
      abortion 639.2
      ectopic or molar pregnancy 639.2
    obstetrical trauma 665.5
  broad ligament
    with
      abortion—*see* Abortion, by type, with
        damage to pelvic organs
      ectopic pregnancy (*see also* categories
        633.0-633.9) 639.2
      molar pregnancy (*see also* categories
        630-632) 639.2
    following
      abortion 639.2
      ectopic or molar pregnancy 639.2
    obstetrical trauma 665.6
  by
    device, implant, or graft—*see* Complications,
      mechanical
    foreign body left accidentally in operation
      wound 998.4
    instrument (any) during a procedure,
      accidental 998.2
  cecum 540.0
    with peritoneal abscess 540.1
  cervix (uteri)—*see also* Injury, internal, cervix
    with
      abortion—*see* Abortion, by type, with
        damage to pelvic organs
      ectopic pregnancy (*see also* categories
        633.0-633.9) 639.2

Perforation, perforative—*continued*
  molar pregnancy (*see also* categories
    630-632) 639.2
  following
    abortion 639.2
    ectopic or molar pregnancy 639.2
    obstetrical trauma 665.3
  colon 569.83
  common duct (bile) 576.3
  cornea (*see also* Ulcer, cornea) 370.00
    due to ulceration 370.06
  cystic duct 575.4
  diverticulum (*see also* Diverticula) 562.10
    small intestine 562.00
  duodenum, duodenal (ulcer)—*see* Ulcer,
    duodenum, with perforation
  ear drum—*see* Perforation, tympanum
  enteritis—*see* Enteritis
  esophagus 530.4
  ethmoidal sinus (*see also* Sinusitis, ethmoidal)
    473.2
  foreign body (external site)—*see also* Wound,
    open, by site, complicated
    internal site, by ingested object—*see* Foreign
      body
  frontal sinus (*see also* Sinusitis, frontal) 473.1
  gallbladder or duct (*see also* Disease,
    gallbladder) 575.4
  gastric (ulcer)—*see* Ulcer, stomach, with
    perforation
  heart valve—*see* Endocarditis
  ileum (*see also* Perforation, intestine) 569.83
  instrumental
    external—*see* Wound, open, by site
    pregnant uterus, complicating delivery 665.9
    surgical (accidental) (blood vessel) (nerve)
      (organ) 998.2
  intestine 569.83
    with
      abortion—*see* Abortion, by type, with
        damage to pelvic organs
      ectopic pregnancy (*see also* categories
        633.0-633.9) 639.2
      molar pregnancy (*see also* categories
        630-632) 639.2
    fetus or newborn 777.6
    obstetrical trauma 665.5
    ulcerative NEC 569.83
  jejunum, jejunal 569.83
    ulcer—*see* Ulcer, gastrojejunal, with
      perforation
  mastoid (antrum) (cell) 383.89
  maxillary sinus (*see also* Sinusitis, maxillary)
    473.0
  membrana tympani—*see* Perforation, tympanum
  nasal
    septum 478.19
      congenital 748.1
      syphilitic 095.8
    sinus (*see also* Sinusitis) 473.9
      congenital 748.1
  palate (hard) 526.89
    soft 528.9
      syphilitic 095.8
    syphilitic 095.8
  palatine vault 526.89
    syphilitic 095.8
      congenital 090.5

Perforation, perforative—*continued*
pelvic
  floor
    with
      abortion—*see* Abortion, by type, with
        damage to pelvic organs
      ectopic pregnancy (*see also* categories
        633.0-633.9) 639.2
      molar pregnancy (*see also* categories
        630-632) 639.2
      obstetrical trauma 664.1
  organ
    with
      abortion—*see* Abortion, by type, with
        damage to pelvic organs
      ectopic pregnancy (*see also* categories
        633.0-633.9) 639.2
      molar pregnancy (*see also* categories
        630-632) 639.2
    following
      abortion 639.2
      ectopic or molar pregnancy 639.2
    obstetrical trauma 665.5
perineum—*see* Laceration, perineum
periurethral tissue
  with
    abortion—*see* Abortion, by type, with
      damage to pelvic organs
    ectopic pregnancy (*see also* categories
      630-632) 639.2
    molar pregnancy (*see also* categories
      630-632) 639.2
pharynx 478.29
pylorus, pyloric (ulcer)—*see* Ulcer, stomach,
  with perforation
rectum 569.49
root canal space 526.61
sigmoid 569.83
sinus (accessory) (chronic) (nasal) (*see also*
  Sinusitis) 473.9
sphenoidal sinus (*see also* Sinusitis, sphenoidal)
  473.3
stomach (due to ulcer)—*see* Ulcer, stomach,
  with perforation
surgical (accidental) (by instrument) (blood
  vessel) (nerve) (organ) 998.2
traumatic
  external—*see* Wound, open, by site
  eye (*see also* Penetrating wound, ocular) 871.7
  internal organ—*see* Injury, internal, by site
  tympanum (membrane) (persistent
    posttraumatic) (postinflammatory) 384.20
    with
      otitis media—*see* Otitis media
    attic 384.22
    central 384.21
    healed 384.81
    marginal NEC 384.23
    multiple 384.24
    pars flaccida 384.22
    total 384.25
    traumatic—*see* Wound, open, ear, drum
typhoid, gastrointestinal 002.0
ulcer—*see* Ulcer, by site, with perforation
ureter 593.89

Perforation, perforative—*continued*
urethra
  with
    abortion—*see* Abortion, by type, with
      damage to pelvic organs
    ectopic pregnancy (*see also* categories
      633.0-633.9) 639.2
    molar pregnancy (*see also* categories
      630-632) 639.2
  following
    abortion 639.2
    ectopic or molar pregnancy 639.2
  obstetrical trauma 665.5
uterus—*see also* Injury, internal, uterus
  with
    abortion—*see* Abortion, by type, with
      damage to pelvic organs
    ectopic pregnancy (*see also* categories
      633.0-633.9) 639.2
    molar pregnancy (*see also* categories
      630-632) 639.2
  by intrauterine contraceptive device 996.32
  following
    abortion 639.2
    ectopic or molar pregnancy 639.2
  obstetrical trauma—*see* Injury, internal,
    uterus, obstetrical trauma
uvula 528.9
  syphilitic 095.8
vagina—*see* Laceration, vagina
viscus NEC 799.89
  traumatic 868.00
    with open wound into cavity 868.10
Periadenitis mucosa necrotica recurrens 528.2
Periangiitis 446.0
Periantritis 535.4
Periappendicitis (acute) (*see also* Appendicitis)
  541
Periarteritis (disseminated) (infectious)
  (necrotizing) (nodosa) 446.0
Periarthritis (joint) 726.90
  Duplay's 726.2
  gonococcal 098.50
  humeroscapularis 726.2
  scapulohumeral 726.2
  shoulder 726.2
  wrist 726.4
Periarthrosis (angioneural)—*see* Periarthritis
Peribronchitis 491.9
  tuberculous (*see also* Tuberculosis) 011.3
Pericapsulitis, adhesive (shoulder) 726.0
Pericarditis (granular) (with decompensation)
  (with effusion) 423.9
  with
    rheumatic fever (conditions classifiable to
      390)
      active (*see also* Pericarditis, rheumatic)
        391.0
      inactive or quiescent 393
  actinomycotic 039.8 *[420.0]*
  acute (nonrheumatic) 420.90
    with chorea (acute) (rheumatic) (Sydenham's)
      392.0
    bacterial 420.99
    benign 420.91
    hemorrhagic 420.90
    idiopathic 420.91
    infective 420.90
    nonspecific 420.91

Pericarditis—*continued*
  rheumatic 391.0
    with chorea (acute) (rheumatic)
      (Sydenham's) 392.0
  sicca 420.90
  viral 420.91
  adhesive or adherent (external) (internal) 423.1
  acute—*see* Pericarditis, acute
    rheumatic (external) (internal) 393
  amebic 006.8 *[420.0]*
  bacterial (acute) (subacute) (with serous or
    seropurulent effusion) 420.99
  calcareous 423.2
  cholesterol (chronic) 423.8
    acute 420.90
  chronic (nonrheumatic) 423.8
    rheumatic 393
  constrictive 423.2
  Coxsackie 074.21
  due to
    actinomycosis 039.8 *[420.0]*
    amebiasis 006.8 *[420.0]*
    Coxsackie (virus) 074.21
    histoplasmosis (*see also* Histoplasmosis)
      115.93
    nocardiosis 039.8 *[420.0]*
    tuberculosis (*see also* Tuberculosis) 017.9
      [420.0]
  fibrinocaseous (*see also* Tuberculosis) 017.9
    [420.0]
  fibrinopurulent 420.99
  fibrinous—*see* Pericarditis, rheumatic
  fibropurulent 420.99
  fibrous 423.1
  gonococcal 098.83
  hemorrhagic 423.0
  idiopathic (acute) 420.91
  infective (acute) 420.90
  meningococcal 036.41
  neoplastic (chronic) 423.8
    acute 420.90
  nonspecific 420.91
  obliterans, obliterating 423.1
  plastic 423.1
  pneumococcal (acute) 420.99
  postinfarction 411.0
  purulent (acute) 420.99
  rheumatic (active) (acute) (with effusion) (with
    pneumonia) 391.0
    with chorea (acute) (rheumatic) (Sydenham's)
      392.0
    chronic or inactive (with chorea) 393
  septic (acute) 420.99
  serofibrinous—*see* Pericarditis, rheumatic
  staphylococcal (acute) 420.99
  streptococcal (acute) 420.99
  suppurative (acute) 420.99
  syphilitic 093.81
  tuberculous (acute) (chronic) (*see also*
    Tuberculosis) 017.9 *[420.0]*
  uremic 585.9 *[420.0]*
  viral (acute) 420.91
Pericardium, pericardial —*see* condition
Pericellulitis (*see also* Cellulitis) 682.9
Pericementitis 523.40
  acute 523.30
  chronic (suppurative) 523.40
Pericholecystitis (*see also* Cholecystitis) 575.10

Perichondritis
  auricle 380.00
    acute 380.01
    chronic 380.02
  bronchus 491.9
  ear (external) 380.00
    acute 380.01
    chronic 380.02
  larynx 478.71
    syphilitic 095.8
    typhoid 002.0 *[478.71]*
  nose 478.19
  pinna 380.00
    acute 380.01
    chronic 380.02
  trachea 478.9
Periclasia 523.5
Pericolitis 569.89
Pericoronitis (chronic) 523.40
  acute 523.33
Pericystitis (*see also* Cystitis) 595.9
Pericytoma (M9150/1)—*see also* Neoplasm,
  connective tissue, uncertain behavior
  benign (M9150/0)—*see* Neoplasm, connective
    tissue, benign
  malignant (M9150/3)—*see* Neoplasm,
    connective tissue, malignant
Peridacryocystitis, acute 375.32
Peridiverticulitis (*see also* Diverticulitis) 562.11
Periduodenitis 535.6
Periendocarditis (*see also* Endocarditis) 424.90
  acute or subacute 421.9
Periepididymitis (*see also* Epididymitis) 604.90
Perifolliculitis (abscedens) 704.8
  capitis, abscedens et suffodiens 704.8
  dissecting, scalp 704.8
  scalp 704.8
  superficial pustular 704.8
Perigastritis (acute) 535.0
Perigastrojejunitis (acute) 535.0
Perihepatitis (acute) 573.3
  chlamydial 099.56
  gonococcal 098.86
Peri-ileitis (subacute) 569.89
Perilabyrinthitis (acute)—*see* Labyrinthitis
Perimeningitis —*see* Meningitis
Perimetritis (*see also* Endometritis) 615.9
Perimetrosalpingitis (*see also*
  Salpingo-oophoritis) 614.2
Perineocele 618.05
Perinephric —*see* condition
Perinephritic —*see* condition
Perinephritis (*see also* Infection, kidney) 590.9
  purulent (*see also* Abscess, kidney) 590.2
Perineum, perineal —*see* condition
Perineuritis NEC 729.2
Periodic —*see also* condition
  disease (familial) 277.31
  edema 995.1
    hereditary 277.6
  fever 277.31
  headache syndrome in child or adolescent 346.2
  limb movement disorder 327.51
  paralysis (familial) 359.3
  peritonitis 277.31
  polyserositis 277.31
  somnolence (*see also* Narcolepsy) 347.00
Periodontal
  cyst 522.8
  pocket 523.8

Periodontitis (chronic) (complex) (compound)
(simplex) 523.40
  acute 523.33
  aggressive 523.30
    generalized 523.32
    localized 523.31
  apical 522.6
    acute (pulpal origin) 522.4
  generalized 523.42
  localized 523.41
Periodontoclasia 523.5
Periodontosis 523.5
Periods —*see also* Menstruation
  heavy 626.2
  irregular 626.4
Perionychia (with lymphangitis) 681.9
  finger 681.02
  toe 681.11
Perioophoritis (*see also* Salpingo-oophoritis) 614.2
Periorchitis (*see also* Orchitis) 604.90
Periosteum, periosteal —*see* condition
Periostitis (circumscribed) (diffuse) (infective) 730.3

Note—Use the following fifth-digit
subclassification with category 730:
0 site unspdcified
1 shoulder region
2 upper arm
3 forearm
4 hand
5 pelvic region and thigh
6 lower leg
7 ankle and foot
8 other specified sites
9 multiple sites

---

  with osteomyelitis (*see also* Osteomyelitis) 730.2
    acute or subacute 730.0
    chronic or old 730.1
  albuminosa, albuminosus 730.3
  alveolar 526.5
  alveolodental 526.5
  dental 526.5
  gonorrheal 098.89
  hyperplastica, generalized 731.2
  jaw (lower) (upper) 526.4
  monomelic 733.99
  orbital 376.02
  syphilitic 095.5
    congenital 090.0 *[730.8]*
    secondary 091.61
  tuberculous (*see also* Tuberculosis, bone) 015.9
    [730.8]
  yaws (early) (hypertrophic) (late) 102.6
Periostosis (*see also* Periostitis) 730.3
  with osteomyelitis (*see also* Osteomyelitis) 730.2
    acute or subacute 730.0
    chronic or old 730.1
  hyperplastic 756.59
Peripartum cardiomyopathy 674.5
Periphlebitis (*see also* Phlebitis) 451.9
  lower extremity 451.2
    deep (vessels) 451.19
    superficial (vessels) 451.0
  portal 572.1
  retina 362.18
  superficial (vessels) 451.0
  tuberculous (*see also* Tuberculosis) 017.9
    retina 017.3 *[362.18]*
Peripneumonia —*see* Pneumonia
Periproctitis 569.49
Periprostatitis (*see also* Prostatitis) 601.9

Perirectal —*see* condition
Perirenal —*see* condition
Perisalpingitis (*see also* Salpingo-oophoritis)
614.2
Perisigmoiditis 569.89
Perisplenitis (infectional) 289.59
Perispondylitis —*see* Spondylitis
Peristalsis reversed or visible 787.4
Peritendinitis (*see also* Tenosynovitis) 726.90
  adhesive (shoulder) 726.0
Perithelioma (M9150/1)—*see* Pericytoma
Peritoneum, peritoneal —*see also* condition
  equilibration test V56.32
Peritonitis (acute) (adhesive) (fibrinous)
(hemorrhagic) (idiopathic) (localized)
(perforative) (primary) (with adhesions) (with
effusion) 567.9
  with or following
    abortion—*see* Abortion, by type, with sepsis
    abscess 567.21
    appendicitis 540.0
      with peritoneal abscess 540.1
    ectopic pregnancy (*see also* categories
      633.0-633.9) 639.0
    molar pregnancy (*see also* categories 630-632)
      639.0
  aseptic 998.7
  bacterial 567.29
    spontaneous 567.23
  bile, biliary 567.81
  chemical 998.7
  chlamydial 099.56
  chronic proliferative 567.89
  congenital NEC 777.6
  diaphragmatic 567.22
  diffuse NEC 567.29
  diphtheritic 032.83
  disseminated NEC 567.29
  due to
    bile 567.81
    foreign
      body or object accidentally left during a
        procedure (instrument) (sponge) (swab)
        998.4
      substance accidentally left during a procedure
        (chemical) (powder) (talc) 998.7
    talc 998.7
    urine 567.89
  fibrinopurulent 567.29
  fibrinous 567.29
  fibrocaseous (*see also* Tuberculosis) 014.0
  fibropurulent 567.29
  general, generalized (acute) 567.21
  gonococcal 098.86
  in infective disease NEC 136.9 *[567.0]*
  meconium (newborn) 777.6
  pancreatic 577.8
  paroxysmal, benign 277.31
  pelvic
    female (acute) 614.5
      chronic NEC 614.7
        with adhesions 614.6
      puerperal, postpartum, childbirth 670.8
    male (acute) 567.21
  periodic (familial) 277.31
  phlegmonous 567.29
  pneumococcal 567.1
  postabortal 639.0
  proliferative, chronic 567.89
  puerperal, postpartum, childbirth 670.8
  purulent 567.29
  septic 567.29

Peritonitis—*continued*
  spontaneous bacterial 567.23
  staphylococcal 567.29
  streptococcal 567.29
  subdiaphragmatic 567.29
  subphrenic 567.29
  suppurative 567.29
  syphilitic 095.2
    congenital 090.0 *[567.0]*
  talc 998.7
  tuberculous (*see also* Tuberculosis) 014.0
  urine 567.89
Peritonsillar —*see* condition
Peritonsillitis 475
Perityphlitis (*see also* Appendicitis) 541
Periureteritis 593.89
Periurethral —*see* condition
Periurethritis (gangrenous) 597.89
Periuterine —*see* condition
Perivaginitis (*see also* Vaginitis) 616.10
Perivasculitis, retinal 362.18
Perivasitis (chronic) 608.4
Periventricular leukomalacia 779.7
Perivesiculitis (seminal) (*see also* Vesiculitis)
    608.0
Perlèche 686.8
  due to
    moniliasis 112.0
    riboflavin deficiency 266.0
Pernicious —*see* condition
Pernio, perniosis 991.5
Persecution
  delusion 297.9
  social V62.4
Perseveration (tonic) 784.69
Persistence, persistent (congenital) 759.89
  anal membrane 751.2
  arteria stapedia 744.04
  atrioventricular canal 745.69
  bloody ejaculate 792.2
  branchial cleft 744.41
  bulbus cordis in left ventricle 745.8
  canal of Cloquet 743.51
  capsule (opaque) 743.51
  cilioretinal artery or vein 743.51
  cloaca 751.5
  communication—*see* Fistula, congenital
  convolutions
    aortic arch 747.21
    fallopian tube 752.19
    oviduct 752.19
    uterine tube 752.19
  double aortic arch 747.21
  ductus
    arteriosus 747.0
    Botalli 747.0
  fetal
    circulation 747.83
    form of cervix (uteri) 752.49
    hemoglobin (hereditary) ("Swiss variety")
      282.7
    pulmonary hypertension 747.83
  foramen
    Botalli 745.5
    ovale 745.5
  Gartner's duct 752.41
  hemoglobin, fetal (hereditary) (HPFH) 282.7
  hyaloid
    artery (generally incomplete) 743.51
    system 743.51

Persistence, persistent—*continued*
  hymen (tag)
    in pregnancy or childbirth 654.8
      causing obstructed labor 660.2
  lanugo 757.4
  left
    posterior cardinal vein 747.49
    root with right arch of aorta 747.21
    superior vena cava 747.49
  Meckel's diverticulum 751.0
  mesonephric duct 752.89
    fallopian tube 752.11
  mucosal disease (middle ear) (with posterior or
    superior marginal perforation of ear drum)
    382.2
  nail(s), anomalous 757.5
  occiput, anterior or posterior 660.3
    fetus or newborn 763.1
  omphalomesenteric duct 751.0
  organ or site NEC—*see* Anomaly, specified
    type NEC
  ostium
    atrioventriculare commune 745.69
    primum 745.61
    secundum 745.5
  ovarian rests in fallopian tube 752.19
  pancreatic tissue in intestinal tract 751.5
  primary (deciduous)
    teeth 520.6
    vitreous hyperplasia 743.51
  pulmonary hypertension 747.83
  pupillary membrane 743.46
    iris 743.46
  Rhesus (Rh) titer 999.7
  right aortic arch 747.21
  sinus
    urogenitalis 752.89
    venosus with imperfect incorporation in right
      auricle 747.49
  thymus (gland) 254.8
    hyperplasia 254.0
  thyroglossal duct 759.2
  thyrolingual duct 759.2
  truncus arteriosus or communis 745.0
  tunica vasculosa lentis 743.39
  umbilical sinus 753.7
  urachus 753.7
  vegetative state 780.03
  vitelline duct 751.0
  wolffian duct 752.89
Person (with)
  admitted for clinical research, as participant or
    control subject V70.7
  affected by
    family member
      currently on deployment (military) V61.01
      returned from deployment (military) (current
        or past conflict) V61.02
  awaiting admission to adequate facility
    elsewhere V63.2
  undergoing social agency investigation V63.8
  concern (normal) about sick person in family
    V61.49
  consulting on behalf of another V65.19
    pediatric
      pre-adoption visit for adoptive parents
        V65.11
      pre-birth visit for expectant parents V65.11
  currently deployed in theater or in support of
    military war, peacekeeping and
    humanitarian operations V62.21

Person—*continued*
  feared
    complaint in whom no diagnosis was made
      V65.5
    condition not demonstrated V65.5
  feigning illness V65.2
  healthy, accompanying sick person V65.0
  history of military war, peacekeeping and
    humanitarian deployment (current or past
    conflict) V62.22
  living (in)
    alone V60.3
    boarding school V60.6
    residence remote from hospital or medical
      care facility V63.0
    residential institution V60.6
    without
      adequate
        financial resources V60.2
        housing (heating) (space) V60.1
      housing (permanent) (temporary) V60.0
      material resources V60.2
      person able to render necessary care V60.4
      shelter V60.0
  medical services in home not available V63.1
  on waiting list V63.2
    undergoing social agency investigation V63.8
  sick or handicapped in family V61.49
  "worried well" V65.5
Personality
  affective 301.10
  aggressive 301.3
  amoral 301.7
  anancastic, anankastic 301.4
  antisocial 301.7
  asocial 301.7
  asthenic 301.6
  avoidant 301.82
  borderline 301.83
  change 310.1
  compulsive 301.4
  cycloid 301.13
  cyclothymic 301.13
  dependent 301.6
  depressive (chronic) 301.12
  disorder, disturbance NEC 301.9
    with
      antisocial disturbance 301.7
      pattern disturbance NEC 301.9
      sociopathic disturbance 301.7
      trait disturbance 301.9
  dual 300.14
  dyssocial 301.7
  eccentric 301.89
    "haltlose" type 301.89
  emotionally unstable 301.59
  epileptoid 301.3
  explosive 301.3
  fanatic 301.0
  histrionic 301.50
  hyperthymic 301.11
  hypomanic 301.11
  hypothymic 301.12
  hysterical 301.50
  immature 301.89
  inadequate 301.6
  labile 301.59
  masochistic 301.89
  morally defective 301.7
  multiple 300.14
  narcissistic 301.81

Personality—*continued*
  obsessional 301.4
  obsessive-compulsive 301.4
  overconscientious 301.4
  paranoid 301.0
  passive (-dependent) 301.6
  passive-aggressive 301.84
  pathologic NEC 301.9
  pattern defect or disturbance 301.9
  pseudosocial 301.7
  psychoinfantile 301.59
  psychoneurotic NEC 301.89
  psychopathic 301.9
    with
      amoral trend 301.7
      antisocial trend 301.7
      asocial trend 301.7
      pathologic sexuality (*see also* Deviation,
        sexual) 302.9
    mixed types 301.9
  schizoid 301.20
    introverted 301.21
    schizotypal 301.22
  type A 301.4
  unstable (emotional) 301.59
Perthes' disease (capital femoral
  osteochondrosis) 732.1
Pertussis (*see also* Whooping cough) 033.9
  vaccination, prophylactic (against) V03.6
Peruvian wart 088.0
Perversion, perverted
  appetite 307.52
    hysterical 300.11
  function
    pineal gland 259.8
    pituitary gland 253.9
      anterior lobe
        deficient 253.2
        excessive 253.1
      posterior lobe 253.6
    placenta—*see* Placenta, abnormal
  sense of smell or taste 781.1
    psychogenic 306.7
  sexual (*see also* Deviation, sexual) 302.9
Pervious, congenital —*see also* Imperfect,
  closure
  ductus arteriosus 747.0
Pes (congenital) (*see also* Talipes) 754.70
  abductus (congenital) 754.60
    acquired 736.79
  acquired NEC 736.79
    planus 734
  adductus (congenital) 754.79
    acquired 736.79
  cavus 754.71
    acquired 736.73
  planovalgus (congenital) 754.69
    acquired 736.79
  planus (acquired) (any degree) 734
    congenital 754.61
    rachitic 268.1
  valgus (congenital) 754.61
    acquired 736.79
  varus (congenital) 754.50
    acquired 736.79
Pest (*see also* Plague) 020.9
Pestis (*see also* Plague) 020.9
  bubonica 020.0
  fulminans 020.0
  minor 020.8
  pneumonica—*see* Plague, pneumonic

Phlebitis—*continued*
  deep (vessels) 451.19
    femoral vein 451.11
    specified vessel NEC 451.19
  due to implanted device—*see* Complications,
    due to (presence of) any device, implant, or
    graft classified to 996.0-996.5 NEC
  during or resulting from a procedure 997.2
  femoral vein (deep) (superficial) 451.11
  femoropopliteal 451.19
  following infusion, perfusion, or transfusion
    999.2
  gouty 274.89 *[451.9]*
  hepatic veins 451.89
  iliac vein 451.81
  iliofemoral 451.11
  intracranial sinus (any) (venous) 325
    late effect—*see* category 326
    nonpyogenic 437.6
      in pregnancy or puerperium 671.5
  jugular vein 451.89
  lateral (venous) sinus—*see* Phlebitis,
    intracranial sinus
  leg 451.2
    deep (vessels) 451.19
      femoral vein 451.11
      specified vessel NEC 451.19
    superficial (vessels) 451.0
      femoral vein 451.11
  longitudinal sinus—*see* Phlebitis, intracranial
    sinus
  lower extremity 451.2
    deep (vessels) 451.19
      femoral vein 451.11
      specified vessel NEC 451.19
    superficial (vessels) 451.0
      femoral vein 451.11
  migrans, migrating (superficial) 453.1
  pelvic
    with
      abortion—*see* Abortion, by type, with sepsis
      ectopic pregnancy (*see also* categories
        633.0-633.9) 639.0
      molar pregnancy (*see also* categories
        630-632) 639.0
    following
      abortion 639.0
      ectopic or molar pregnancy 639.0
    puerperal, postpartum 671.4
  popliteal vein 451.19
  portal (vein) 572.1
  postoperative 997.2
  pregnancy 671.2
    deep 671.3
    specified type NEC 671.5
    superficial 671.2
  puerperal, postpartum, childbirth 671.2
    deep 671.4
    lower extremities 671.2
    pelvis 671.4
    specified site NEC 671.5
    superficial 671.2
  radial vein 451.83
  retina 362.18
  saphenous (great) (long) 451.0
    accessory or small 451.0
  sinus (meninges)—*see* Phlebitis, intracranial
    sinus
  specified site NEC 451.89
  subclavian vein 451.89
  syphilitic 093.89

Phlebitis—*continued*
  tibial vein 451.19
  ulcer, ulcerative 451.9
    leg 451.2
      deep (vessels) 451.19
        femoral vein 451.11
        specified vessel NEC 451.19
      superficial (vessels) 451.0
        femoral vein 451.11
    lower extremity 451.2
      deep (vessels) 451.19
        femoral vein 451.11
        specified vessel NEC 451.19
      superficial (vessels) 451.0
  ulnar vein 451.83
  umbilicus 451.89
  upper extremity—*see* Phlebitis, arm
  uterus (septic) (*see also* Endometritis) 615.9
  varicose (leg) (lower extremity) (*see also*
    Varicose, vein) 454.1
Phlebofibrosis 459.89
Phleboliths 459.89
Phlebosclerosis 459.89
Phlebothrombosis —*see* Thrombosis
Phlebotomus fever 066.0
Phlegm, choked on 933.1
Phlegmasia
  alba dolens (deep vessels) 451.19
    complicating pregnancy 671.3
    nonpuerperal 451.19
    puerperal, postpartum, childbirth 671.4
  cerulea dolens 451.19
Phlegmon (*see also* Abscess) 682.9
  erysipelatous (*see also* Erysipelas) 035
  iliac 682.2
    fossa 540.1
  throat 478.29
Phlegmonous —*see* condition
Phlyctenulosis (allergic) (keratoconjunctivitis)
  (nontuberculous) 370.31
  cornea 370.31
    with ulcer (*see also* Ulcer, cornea) 370.00
  tuberculous (*see also* Tuberculosis) 017.3
    [370.31]
Phobia, phobic (reaction) 300.20
  animal 300.29
  isolated NEC 300.29
  obsessional 300.3
  simple NEC 300.29
  social 300.23
  specified NEC 300.29
  state 300.20
Phocas' disease 610.1
Phocomelia 755.4
  lower limb 755.32
    complete 755.33
    distal 755.35
    proximal 755.34
  upper limb 755.22
    complete 755.23
    distal 755.25
    proximal 755.24
Phoria (*see also* Heterophoria) 378.40
Phosphate-losing tubular disorder 588.0
Phosphatemia 275.3
Phosphaturia 275.3
Photoallergic response 692.72
Photocoproporphyria 277.1
Photodermatitis (sun) 692.72
  light other than sun 692.82
Photokeratitis 370.24

Photo-ophthalmia 370.24
Photophobia 368.13
Photopsia 368.15
Photoretinitis 363.31
Photoretinopathy 363.31
Photosensitiveness (sun) 692.72
  light other than sun 692.82
Photosensitization (sun) skin 692.72
  light other than sun 692.82
Phototoxic response 692.72
Phrenitis 323.9
Phrynoderma 264.8
Phthiriasis (pubis) (any site) 132.2
  with any infestation classifiable to 132.0
    and 132.1 132.3
Phthirus infestation —*see* Phthiriasis
Phthisis (*see also* Tuberculosis) 011.9
  bulbi (infectional) 360.41
  colliers' 011.4
  cornea 371.05
  eyeball (due to infection) 360.41
  millstone makers' 011.4
  miners' 011.4
  potters' 011.4
  sandblasters' 011.4
  stonemasons' 011.4
Phycomycosis 117.7
Physalopteriasis 127.7
Physical therapy NEC V57.1
  breathing exercises V57.0
Physiological cup, optic papilla
  borderline, glaucoma suspect 365.00
  enlarged 377.14
  glaucomatous 377.14
Phytobezoar 938
  intestine 936
  stomach 935.2
Pian (*see also* Yaws) 102.9
Pianoma 102.1
Piarhemia, piarrhemia (*see also* Hyperlipemia)
  272.4
  bilharziasis 120.9
Pica 307.52
  hysterical 300.11
Pick's
  cerebral atrophy 331.11
    with dementia
      with behavioral disturbance 331.11 *[294.11]*
      without behavioral disturbance 331.11
        [294.10]
  disease
    brain 331.11
      dementia in
        with behavioral disturbance 331.11
          [294.11]
        without behavioral disturbance 331.11
          [294.10]
    lipid histiocytosis 272.7
    liver (pericardial pseudocirrhosis of liver)
      423.2
    pericardium (pericardial pseudocirrhosis of
      liver) 423.2
    polyserositis (pericardial pseudocirrhosis of
      liver) 423.2
  syndrome
    heart (pericardial pseudocirrhosis of liver)
      423.2
    liver (pericardial pseudocirrhosis of liver)
      423.2

Pick's—*continued*
  tubular adenoma (M8640/0)
    specified site—*see* Neoplasm, by site, benign
    unspecified site
      female 220
      male 222.0
Pick-Herxheimer syndrome (diffuse idiopathic
  cutaneous atrophy) 701.8
Pick-Niemann disease (lipid histiocytosis) 272.7
Pickwickian syndrome (cardiopulmonary
  obesity) 278.8
Piebaldism, classic 709.09
Piedra 111.2
  beard 111.2
    black 111.3
    white 111.3
  black 111.3
  scalp 111.3
    black 111.3
    white 111.2
  white 111.2
Pierre Marie's syndrome (pulmonary
  hypertrophic osteoarthropathy) 731.2
Pierre Marie-Bamberger syndrome
  (hypertrophic pulmonary osteoarthropathy)
  731.2
Pierre Mauriac's syndrome
  (diabetes-dwarfism-obesity) 258.1
Pierre Robin deformity or syndrome
  (congenital) 756.0
Pierson's disease or osteochondrosis 732.1
Pigeon
  breast or chest (acquired) 738.3
    congenital 754.82
    rachitic (*see also* Rickets) 268.0
  breeders' disease or lung 495.2
  fanciers' disease or lung 495.2
  toe 735.8
Pigmentation (abnormal) 709.00
  anomaly 709.00
    congenital 757.33
    specified NEC 709.09
  conjunctiva 372.55
  cornea 371.10
    anterior 371.11
    posterior 371.13
    stromal 371.12
  lids (congenital) 757.33
    acquired 374.52
  limbus corneae 371.10
  metals 709.00
  optic papilla, congenital 743.57
  retina (congenital) (grouped) (nevoid) 743.53
    acquired 362.74
  scrotum, congenital 757.33
Piles —*see* Hemorrhoids
Pili
  annulati or torti (congenital) 757.4
  incarnati 704.8
Pill roller hand (intrinsic) 736.09
Pilomatrixoma (M8110/0)—*see* Neoplasm, skin,
  benign
Pilonidal —*see* condition
Pimple 709.8
PIN I (prostatic intraepithelial neoplasia I)
  602.3
PIN II (prostatic intraepithelial neoplasia II)
  602.3
PIN III (prostatic intraepithelial neoplasia III)
  233.4
Pinched nerve —*see* Neuropathy, entrapment

Pineal body or gland —*see* condition
Pinealoblastoma (M9362/3) 194.4
Pinealoma (M9360/1) 237.1
    malignant (M9360/3) 194.4
Pineoblastoma (M9362/3) 194.4
Pineocytoma (M9361/1) 237.1
Pinguecula 372.51
Pingueculitis 372.34
Pinhole meatus (*see also* Stricture, urethra) 598.9
Pink
    disease 985.0
    eye 372.03
    puffer 492.8
Pinkus' disease (lichen nitidus) 697.1
Pinpoint
    meatus (*see also* Stricture, urethra) 598.9
    os (uteri) (*see also* Stricture, cervix) 622.4
Pinselhaare (congenital) 757.4
Pinta 103.9
    cardiovascular lesions 103.2
    chancre (primary) 103.0
    erythematous plaques 103.1
    hyperchromic lesions 103.1
    hyperkeratosis 103.1
    lesions 103.9
        cardiovascular 103.2
        hyperchromic 103.1
        intermediate 103.1
        late 103.2
        mixed 103.3
        primary 103.0
        skin (achromic) (cicatricial) (dyschromic)
            103.2
            hyperchromic 103.1
            mixed (achromic and hyperchromic) 103.3
    papule (primary) 103.0
    skin lesions (achromic) (cicatricial)
        (dyschromic) 103.2
        hyperchromic 103.1
        mixed (achromic and hyperchromic) 103.3
    vitiligo 103.0
Pintid 103.0
Pinworms (disease) (infection) (infestation)
    127.4
Piry fever 066.8
Pistol wound —*see* Gunshot wound
Pit, lip (mucus), congenital 750.25
Pitchers' elbow 718.82
Pithecoid pelvis 755.69
    with disproportion (fetopelvic) 653.2
        affecting fetus or newborn 763.1
        causing obstructed labor 660.1
Pithiatism 300.11
Pitted —*see also* Pitting
    teeth 520.4
Pitting (edema) (*see also* Edema) 782.3
    lip 782.3
    nail 703.8
        congenital 757.5
Pituitary gland —*see* condition
Pituitary snuff-takers' disease 495.8
Pityriasis 696.5
    alba 696.5
    capitis 690.11
    circinata (et maculata) 696.3
    Hebra's (exfoliative dermatitis) 695.89
    lichenoides et varioliformis 696.2
    maculata (et circinata) 696.3
    nigra 111.1

Pityriasis— *continued*
    pilaris 757.39
        acquired 701.1
        Hebra's 696.4
    rosea 696.3
    rotunda 696.3
    rubra (Hebra) 695.89
        pilaris 696.4
    sicca 690.18
    simplex 690.18
    specified type NEC 696.5
    streptogenes 696.5
    versicolor 111.0
        scrotal 111.0
Placenta, placental
    ablatio 641.2
        affecting fetus or newborn 762.1
    abnormal, abnormality 656.7
        with hemorrhage 641.8
            affecting fetus or newborn 762.1
        affecting fetus or newborn 762.2
    abruptio 641.2
        affecting fetus or newborn 762.1
    accessory lobe—*see* Placenta, abnormal
    accreta (without hemorrhage) 667.0
        with hemorrhage 666.0
    adherent (without hemorrhage) 667.0
        with hemorrhage 666.0
    apoplexy—*see* Placenta, separation
    battledore—*see* Placenta, abnormal
    bilobate—*see* Placenta, abnormal
    bipartita—*see* Placenta, abnormal
    carneous mole 631
    centralis—*see* Placenta, previa
    circumvallata—*see* Placenta, abnormal
    cyst (amniotic)—*see* Placenta, abnormal
    deficiency—*see* Placenta insufficiency
    degeneration—*see* Placenta, insufficiency
    detachment (partial) (premature) (with
        hemorrhage) 641.2
        affecting fetus or newborn 762.1
    dimidiata—*see* Placenta, abnormal
    disease 656.7
        affecting fetus or newborn 762.2
    duplex—*see* Placenta, abnormal
    dysfunction—*see* Placenta, insufficiency
    fenestrata—*see* Placenta, abnormal
    fibrosis—*see* Placenta, abnormal
    fleshy mole 631
    hematoma—*see* Placenta, abnormal
    hemorrhage NEC—*see* Placenta, separation
    hormone disturbance or malfunction—*see*
        Placenta, abnormal
    hyperplasia—*see* Placenta, abnormal
    increta (without hemorrhage) 667.0
        with hemorrhage 666.0
    infarction 656.7
        affecting fetus or newborn 762.2
    insertion, vicious—*see* Placenta, previa
    insufficiency
        affecting
            fetus or newborn 762.2
            management of pregnancy 656.5
    lateral—*see* Placenta, previa
    low implantation or insertion—*see* Placenta,
        previa
    low-lying—*see* Placenta, previa
    malformation—*see* Placenta, abnormal
    malposition—*see* Placenta, previa
    marginalis, marginata—*see* Placenta, previa

Placenta, placental—*continued*
 marginal sinus (hemorrhage) (rupture) 641.2
  affecting fetus or newborn 762.1
 membranacea—*see* Placenta, abnormal
 multilobed—*see* Placenta, abnormal
 multipartita—*see* Placenta, abnormal
 necrosis—*see* Placenta, abnormal
 percreta (without hemorrhage) 667.0
  with hemorrhage 666.0
 polyp 674.4
 previa (central) (centralis) (complete) (lateral)
   (marginal) (marginalis) (partial) (partialis)
   (total) (with hemorrhage) 641.1
  affecting fetus or newborn 762.0
  noted
   before labor, without hemorrhage (with
     cesarean delivery) 641.0
   during pregnancy (without hemorrhage)
     641.0
  without hemorrhage (before labor and
    delivery) (during pregnancy) 641.0
 retention (with hemorrhage) 666.0
  fragments, complicating puerperium (delayed
    hemorrhage) 666.2
   without hemorrhage 667.1
  postpartum, puerperal 666.2
   without hemorrhage 667.0
 separation (normally implanted) (partial)
   (premature) (with hemorrhage) 641.2
  affecting fetus or newborn 762.1
 septuplex—*see* Placenta, abnormal
 small—*see* Placenta, insufficiency
 softening (premature)—*see* Placenta, abnormal
 spuria—*see* Placenta, abnormal
 succenturiata—*see* Placenta, abnormal
 syphilitic 095.8
 transfusion syndromes 762.3
 transmission of chemical substance—*see*
   Absorption, chemical, through placenta
 trapped (with hemorrhage) 666.0
  without hemorrhage 667.0
 trilobate—*see* Placenta, abnormal
 tripartita—*see* Placenta, abnormal
 triplex—*see* Placenta, abnormal
 varicose vessel—*see* Placenta, abnormal
 vicious insertion—*see* Placenta, previa
Placentitis
 affecting fetus or newborn 762.7
 complicating pregnancy 658.4
Plagiocephaly (skull) 754.0
Plague 020.9
 abortive 020.8
 ambulatory 020.8
 bubonic 020.0
 cellulocutaneous 020.1
 lymphatic gland 020.0
 pneumonic 020.5
  primary 020.3
  secondary 020.4
 pulmonary—*see* Plague, pneumonic
 pulmonic—*see* Plague, pneumonic
 septicemic 020.2
 tonsillar 020.9
  septicemic 020.2
 vaccination, prophylactic (against) V03.3
Planning, family V25.09
 contraception V25.9
 natural
  procreative V26.41
  to avoid pregnancy V25.04
 procreation V26.49
  natural V26.41

Plaque
 artery, arterial—*see* Arteriosclerosis
 calcareous—*see* Calcification
 Hollenhorst's (retinal) 362.33
 tongue 528.6
Plasma cell myeloma 203.0
Plasmacytoma, plasmocytoma (solitary)
   (M9731/1) 238.6
 benign (M9731/0)—*see* Neoplasm, by site,
   benign
 malignant (M9731/3) 203.8
Plasmacytopenia 288.59
Plasmacytosis 288.64
Plaster ulcer (*see also* Ulcer, pressure) 707.00
Plateau iris syndrome 364.82
Platybasia 756.0
Platyonychia (congenital) 757.5
 acquired 703.8
Platypelloid pelvis 738.6
 with disproportion (fetopelvic) 653.2
  affecting fetus or newborn 763.1
  causing obstructed labor 660.1
   affecting fetus or newborn 763.1
 congenital 755.69
Platyspondylia 756.19
Plethora 782.62
 newborn 776.4
Pleura, pleural —*see* condition
Pleuralgia 786.52
Pleurisy (acute) (adhesive) (chronic) (costal)
   (diaphragmatic) (double) (dry) (fetid)
   (fibrinous) (fibrous) (interlobar) (latent) (lung)
   (old) (plastic) (primary) (residual) (sicca)
   (sterile) (subacute) (unresolved) (with
   adherent pleura) 511.0
 with
  effusion (without mention of cause) 511.9
   bacterial, nontuberculous 511.1
   nontuberculous NEC 511.9
    bacterial 511.1
   pneumococcal 511.1
   specified type NEC 511.89
   staphylococcal 511.1
   streptococcal 511.1
   tuberculous (*see also* Tuberculosis, pleura)
     012.0
    primary, progressive 010.1
  influenza, flu, or grippe 487.1
  tuberculosis—*see* Pleurisy, tuberculous
 encysted 511.89
 exudative (*see also* Pleurisy, with effusion)
   511.9
  bacterial, nontuberculous 511.1
 fibrinopurulent 510.9
  with fistula 510.0
 fibropurulent 510.9
  with fistula 510.0
 hemorrhagic 511.89
 influenzal 487.1
 pneumococcal 511.0
  with effusion 511.1
 purulent 510.9
  with fistula 510.0
 septic 510.9
  with fistula 510.0
 serofibrinous (*see also* Pleurisy, with effusion) 511.9
  bacterial, nontuberculous 511.1
 seropurulent 510.9
  with fistula 510.0
 serous (*see also* Pleurisy, with effusion) 511.9
  bacterial, nontuberculous 511.1

Pleurisy—*continued*
staphylococcal 511.0
  with effusion 511.1
streptococcal 511.0
  with effusion 511.1
suppurative 510.9
  with fistula 510.0
traumatic (post) (current) 862.29
  with open wound into cavity 862.39
tuberculous (with effusion) (*see also*
    Tuberculosis, pleura) 012.0
  primary, progressive 010.1
Pleuritis sicca —*see* Pleurisy
Pleurobronchopneumonia (*see also* Pneumonia,
  broncho-) 485
Pleurodynia 786.52
  epidemic 074.1
  viral 074.1
Pleurohepatitis 573.8
Pleuropericarditis (*see also* Pericarditis) 423.9
  acute 420.90
Pleuropneumonia (acute) (bilateral) (double)
    (septic) (*see also* Pneumonia) 486
  chronic (*see also* Fibrosis, lung) 515
Pleurorrhea (*see also* Hydrothorax) 511.89
Plexitis, brachial 353.0
Plica
  knee 727.83
  polonica 132.0
  tonsil 474.8
Plicae dysphonia ventricularis 784.49
Plicated tongue 529.5
  congenital 750.13
Plug
  bronchus NEC 519.19
  meconium (newborn) NEC 777.1
  mucus—*see* Mucus, plug
Plumbism 984.9
  specified type of lead—*see* Table of drugs and
    chemicals
Plummer's disease (toxic nodular goiter) 242.3
Plummer-Vinson syndrome (sideropenic
    dysphagia) 280.8
Pluricarential syndrome of infancy 260
Plurideficiency syndrome of infancy 260
Plus (and minus) hand (intrinsic) 736.09
PMDD (premenstrual dysphoric disorder)
    625.4
PMS 625.4
Pneumathemia —*see* Air, embolism, by type
Pneumatic drill or hammer disease 994.9
Pneumatocele (lung) 518.89
  intracranial 348.89
  tension 492.0
Pneumatosis
  cystoides intestinalis 569.89
  peritonei 568.89
  pulmonum 492.8
Pneumaturia 599.84
Pneumoblastoma (M8981/3)—*see* Neoplasm,
  lung, malignant
Pneumocephalus 348.89
Pneumococcemia 038.2
Pneumococcus, pneumococcal —*see* condition

Pneumoconiosis (due to) (inhalation of) 505
  aluminum 503
  asbestos 501
  bagasse 495.1
  bauxite 503
  beryllium 503
  carbon electrode makers' 503
  coal
    miners' (simple) 500
    workers' (simple) 500
  cotton dust 504
  diatomite fibrosis 502
  dust NEC 504
    inorganic 503
    lime 502
    marble 502
    organic NEC 504
  fumes or vapors (from silo) 506.9
  graphite 503
  hard metal 503
  mica 502
  moldy hay 495.0
  rheumatoid 714.81
  silica NEC 502
    and carbon 500
  silicate NEC 502
  talc 502
Pneumocystis carinii pneumonia 136.3
Pneumocystis jiroveci pneumonia 136.3
Pneumocystosis 136.3
  with pneumonia 136.3
Pneumoenteritis 025
Pneumohemopericardium (*see also* Pericarditis)
    423.9
Pneumohemothorax (*see also* Hemothorax)
    511.89
  traumatic 860.4
    with open wound into thorax 860.5
Pneumohydropericardium (*see also*
    Pericarditis) 423.9
Pneumohydrothorax (*see also* Hydrothorax)
    511.89
Pneumomediastinum 518.1
  congenital 770.2
  fetus or newborn 770.2
Pneumomycosis 117.9
Pneumonia (acute) (Alpenstich) (benign)
    (bilateral) (brain) (cerebral) (circumscribed)
    (congestive) (creeping) (delayed resolution)
    (double) (epidemic) (fever) (flash) (fulminant)
    (fungoid) (granulomatous) (hemorrhagic)
    (incipient) (infantile) (infectious) (infiltration)
    (insular) (intermittent) (latent) (lobe)
    (migratory) (newborn) (organized)
    (overwhelming) (primary) (progressive)
    (pseudolobar) (purulent) (resolved)
    (secondary) (senile) (septic) (suppurative)
    (terminal) (true) (unresolved) (vesicular) 486
  with influenza, flu, or grippe 487.0
  adenoviral 480.0
  adynamic 514
  alba 090.0
  allergic 518.3
  alveolar—*see* Pneumonia, lobar
  anaerobes 482.81
  anthrax 022.1 *[484.5]*
  apex, apical—*see* Pneumonia, lobar
  ascaris 127.0 *[484.8]*

Pneumonia—*continued*
  aspiration 507.0
    due to
      aspiration of microorganisms
        bacterial 482.9
          specified type NEC 482.89
        specified organism NEC 483.8
          bacterial NEC 482.89
        viral 480.9
          specified type NEC 480.8
      food (regurgitated) 507.0
      gastric secretions 507.0
      milk 507.0
      oils, essences 507.1
      solids, liquids NEC 507.8
      vomitus 507.0
    fetal 770.18
      due to
        blood 770.16
        clear amniotic fluid 770.14
        meconium 770.12
        postnatal stomach contents 770.86
    newborn 770.18
      due to
        blood 770.16
        clear amniotic fluid 770.14
        meconium 770.12
        postnatal stomach contents 770.86
  asthenic 514
  atypical (disseminated, focal) (primary) 486
    with influenza 487.0
  bacillus 482.9
    specified type NEC 482.89
  bacterial 482.9
    specified type NEC 482.89
  Bacteroides (fragilis) (oralis) (melaninogenicus)
      482.81
  basal, basic, basilar—*see* Pneumonia, lobar
  bronchiolitis obliterans organized (BOOP) 516.8
  broncho-, bronchial (confluent) (croupous)
      (diffuse) (disseminated) (hemorrhagic)
      (involving lobes) (lobar) (terminal) 485
    with influenza 487.0
    allergic 518.3
    aspiration (*see also* Pneumonia, aspiration)
        507.0
    bacterial 482.9
      specified type NEC 482.89
    capillary 466.19
      with bronchospasm or obstruction 466.19
    chronic (*see also* Fibrosis, lung) 515
    congenital (infective) 770.0
    diplococcal 481
    Eaton's agent 483.0
    Escherichia coli (E. coli) 482.82
    Friedländer's bacillus 482.0
    Hemophilus influenzae 482.2
    hiberno-vernal 083.0 *[484.8]*
    hypostatic 514
    influenzal 487.0
    inhalation (*see also* Pneumonia, aspiration) 507.0
      due to fumes or vapors (chemical) 506.0
    Klebsiella 482.0
    lipid 507.1
      endogenous 516.8
    Mycoplasma (pneumoniae) 483.0
    ornithosis 073.0
    pleuropneumonia-like organisms (PPLO) 483.0
    pneumococcal 481
    Proteus 482.83

Pneumonia—*continued*
  broncho, bronchial—*continued*
    pseudomonas 482.1
    specified organism NEC 483.8
      bacterial NEC 482.89
    staphylococcal 482.40
      aureus 482.41
        methicillin
          resistant (MRSA) 482.42
          susceptible (MSSA) 482.41
      specified type NEC 482.49
    streptococcal—*see* Pneumonia, streptococcal
    typhoid 002.0 *[484.8]*
    viral, virus (*see also* Pneumonia, viral) 480.9
  Butyrivibrio (fibriosolvens) 482.81
  Candida 112.4
  capillary 466.19
    with bronchospasm or obstruction 466.19
  caseous (*see also* Tuberculosis) 011.6
  catarrhal—*see* Pneumonia, broncho-
  central—*see* Pneumonia, lobar
  Chlamydia, chlamydial 483.1
    pneumoniae 483.1
    psittaci 073.0
    specified type NEC 483.1
    trachomatis 483.1
  cholesterol 516.8
  chronic (*see also* Fibrosis, lung) 515
  cirrhotic (chronic) (*see also* Fibrosis, lung) 515
  Clostridium (haemolyticum) (novyi) NEC
      482.81
  confluent—*see* Pneumonia, broncho-
  congenital (infective) 770.0
    aspiration 770.18
  croupous—*see* Pneumonia, lobar
  cytomegalic inclusion 078.5 *[484.1]*
  deglutition (*see also* Pneumonia, aspiration)
      507.0
  desquamative interstitial 516.8
  diffuse—*see* Pneumonia, broncho-
  diplococcal, diplococcus (broncho-) (lobar) 481
  disseminated (focal)—*see* Pneumonia, broncho-
  due to
    adenovirus 480.0
    Bacterium anitratum 482.83
    Chlamydia, chlamydial 483.1
      pneumoniae 483.1
      psittaci 073.0
      specified type NEC 483.1
      trachomatis 483.1
    coccidioidomycosis 114.0
    Diplococcus (pneumoniae) 481
    Eaton's agent 483.0
    Escherichia coli (E. coli) 482.82
    Friedländer's bacillus 482.0
    fumes or vapors (chemical) (inhalation) 506.0
    fungus NEC 117.9 *[484.7]*
      coccidioidomycosis 114.0
    Hemophilus influenzae (H. influenzae) 482.2
    Herellea 482.83
    influenza 487.0
    Klebsiella pneumoniae 482.0
    Mycoplasma (pneumoniae) 483.0
    parainfluenza virus 480.2
    pleuropneumonia-like organism (PPLO) 483.0
    Pneumococcus 481
    Pneumocystis carinii 136.3
    Pneumocystis jiroveci 136.3
    Proteus 482.83
    pseudomonas 482.1
    respiratory syncytial virus 480.1

Pneumonia—*continued*
  due to—*continued*
    rickettsia 083.9 *[484.8]*
    SARS-associated coronavirus 480.3
    specified
      bacteria NEC 482.89
      organism NEC 483.8
      virus NEC 480.8
    Staphylococcus 482.40
      aureus 482.41
        methicillin
          resistant (MRSA) 482.42
          susceptible (MSSA) 482.41
      specified type NEC 482.49
    Streptococcus—*see also* Pneumonia,
      streptococcal
      pneumoniae 481
    virus (*see also* Pneumonia, viral) 480.9
    Eaton's agent 483.0
  embolic, embolism (*see also* Embolism,
    pulmonary) 415.1
  eosinophilic 518.3
  Escherichia coli (E. coli) 482.82
  Eubacterium 482.81
  fibrinous—*see* Pneumonia, lobar
  fibroid (chronic) (*see also* Fibrosis, lung) 515
  fibrous (*see also* Fibrosis, lung) 515
  Friedländer's bacillus 482.0
  Fusobacterium (nucleatum) 482.81
  gangrenous 513.0
  giant cell (*see also* Pneumonia, viral) 480.9
  gram-negative bacteria NEC 482.83
    anaerobic 482.81
  grippal 487.0
  Hemophilus influenzae (bronchial) (lobar) 482.2
  hypostatic (broncho-) (lobar) 514
  in
    actinomycosis 039.1
    anthrax 022.1 *[484.5]*
    aspergillosis 117.3 *[484.6]*
    candidiasis 112.4
    coccidioidomycosis 114.0
    cytomegalic inclusion disease 078.5 *[484.1]*
    histoplasmosis (*see also* Histoplasmosis)
      115.95
    infectious disease NEC 136.9 *[484.8]*
    measles 055.1
    mycosis, systemic NEC 117.9 *[484.7]*
    nocardiasis, nocardiosis 039.1
    ornithosis 073.0
    pneumocystosis 136.3
    psittacosis 073.0
    Q fever 083.0 *[484.8]*
    salmonellosis 003.22
    toxoplasmosis 130.4
    tularemia 021.2
    typhoid (fever) 002.0 *[484.8]*
    varicella 052.1
    whooping cough (*see also* Whooping cough)
      033.9 *[484.3]*
  infective, acquired prenatally 770.0
  influenzal (broncho) (lobar) (virus) 487.0
  inhalation (*see also* Pneumonia, aspiration) 507.0
    fumes or vapors (chemical) 506.0
  interstitial 516.8
    with influenzal 487.0
    acute 136.3
    chronic (*see also* Fibrosis, lung) 515
    desquamative 516.8
    hypostatic 514
    lipoid 507.1
    lymphoid 516.8

Pneumonia—*continued*
  interstitial—*continued*
    plasma cell 136.3
    pseudomonas 482.1
  intrauterine (infective) 770.0
    aspiration 770.18
    blood 770.16
    clear amniotic fluid 770.14
    meconium 770.12
    postnatal stomach contents 770.86
  Klebsiella pneumoniae 482.0
  Legionnaires' 482.84
  lipid, lipoid (exogenous) (interstitial) 507.1
    endogenous 516.8
  lobar (diplococcal) (disseminated) (double)
    (interstitial) (pneumococcal, any type) 481
    with influenza 487.0
    bacterial 482.9
      specified type NEC 482.89
    chronic (*see also* Fibrosis, lung) 515
    Escherichia coli (E. coli) 482.82
    Friedländer's bacillus 482.0
    Hemophilus influenzae (H. influenzae) 482.2
    hypostatic 514
    influenzal 487.0
    Klebsiella 482.0
    ornithosis 073.0
    Proteus 482.83
    pseudomonas 482.1
    psittacosis 073.0
    specified organism NEC 483.8
      bacterial NEC 482.89
    staphylococcal 482.40
      aureus 482.41
        methicillin
          resistant (MRSA) 482.42
          susceptible (MSSA) 482.41
      specified type NEC 482.49
    streptococcal—*see* Pneumonia, streptococcal
    viral, virus (*see also* Pneumonia, viral) 480.9
  lobular (confluent)—*see* Pneumonia, broncho-
  Löffler's 518.3
  massive—*see* Pneumonia, lobar
  meconium aspiration 770.12
  metastatic NEC 038.8 *[484.8]*
  methicillin resistant Staphylococcus aureus
    (MRSA) 482.42
  methicillin susceptible Staphylococcus aureus
    (MSSA) 482.41
  MRSA (methicillin resistant Staphylococcus
    aureus) 482.42
  MSSA (methicillin susceptible Staphylococcus
    aureus) 482.41
  Mycoplasma (pneumoniae) 483.0
  necrotic 513.0
  nitrogen dioxide 506.9
  orthostatic 514
  parainfluenza virus 480.2
  parenchymatous (*see also* Fibrosis, lung) 515
  passive 514
  patchy—*see* Pneumonia, broncho
  Peptococcus 482.81
  Peptostreptococcus 482.81
  plasma cell 136.3
  pleurolobar—*see* Pneumonia, lobar
  pleuropneumonia-like organism (PPLO) 483.0
  pneumococcal (broncho) (lobar) 481
  Pneumocystis (carinii) (jiroveci) 136.3
  postinfectional NEC 136.9 *[484.8]*
  postmeasles 055.1
  postoperative 997.39
  primary atypical 486

Pneumonia—*continued*
  Proprionibacterium 482.81
  Proteus 482.83
  pseudomonas 482.1
  psittacosis 073.0
  radiation 508.0
  respiratory syncytial virus 480.1
  resulting from a procedure 997.39
  rheumatic 390 *[517.1]*
  Salmonella 003.22
  SARS-associated coronavirus 480.3
  segmented, segmental—*see* Pneumonia,
    broncho-
  Serratia (marcescens) 482.83
  specified
    bacteria NEC 482.89
    organism NEC 483.8
    virus NEC 480.8
  spirochetal 104.8 *[484.8]*
  staphylococcal (broncho) (lobar) 482.40
    aureus 482.41
      methicillin
        resistant (MRSA) 482.42
        susceptible (MSSA) 482.41
    specified type NEC 482.49
  static, stasis 514
  streptococcal (broncho) (lobar) NEC 482.30
    Group
      A 482.31
      B 482.32
      specified NEC 482.39
    pneumoniae 481
    specified type NEC 482.39
  Streptococcus pneumoniae 481
  traumatic (complication) (early) (secondary) 958.8
  tuberculous (any) (*see also* Tuberculosis) 011.6
  tularemic 021.2
  TWAR agent 483.1
  varicella 052.1
  Veillonella 482.81
  ventilator associated 997.31
  viral, virus (broncho) (interstitial) (lobar) 480.9
    with influenza, flu, or grippe 487.0
    adenoviral 480.0
    parainfluenza 480.2
    respiratory syncytial 480.1
    SARS-associated coronavirus 480.3
    specified type NEC 480.8
  white (congenital) 090.0
Pneumonic —*see* condition
Pneumonitis (acute) (primary) (*see also*
  Pneumonia) 486
  allergic 495.9
    specified type NEC 495.8
  aspiration 507.0
    due to fumes or gases 506.0
    fetal 770.18
      due to
        blood 770.16
        clear amniotic fluid 770.14
        meconium 770.12
        postnatal stomach contents 770.86
    newborn 770.18
      due to
        blood 770.16
        clear amniotic fluid 770.14
        meconium 770.12
        postnatal stomach contents 770.86
    obstetric 668.0
  chemical 506.0
    due to fumes or gases 506.0
  cholesterol 516.8

Pneumonitis—*continued*
  chronic (*see also* Fibrosis, lung) 515
  congenital rubella 771.0
  crack 506.0
  due to
    crack (cocaine) 506.0
    fumes or vapors 506.0
    inhalation
      food (regurgitated), milk, vomitus 507.0
      oils, essences 507.1
      saliva 507.0
      solids, liquids NEC 507.8
    toxoplasmosis (acquired) 130.4
      congenital (active) 771.2 *[484.8]*
  eosinophilic 518.3
  fetal aspiration 770.18
    due to
      blood 770.16
      clear amniotic fluid 770.14
      meconium 770.12
      postnatal stomach contents 770.86
  hypersensitivity 495.9
  interstitial (chronic) (*see also* Fibrosis, lung) 515
    lymphoid 516.8
  lymphoid, interstitial 516.8
  meconium aspiration 770.12
  postanesthetic
    correct substance properly administered 507.0
    obstetric 668.0
    overdose or wrong substance given 968.4
      specified anesthetic—*see* Table of drugs and
        chemicals
  postoperative 997.3
    obstetric 668.0
  radiation 508.0
  rubella, congenital 771.0
  "ventilation" 495.7
  ventilator associated 997.31
  wood-dust 495.8
Pneumonoconiosis —*see* Pneumoconiosis
Pneumoparotid 527.8
Pneumopathy NEC 518.89
  alveolar 516.9
    specified NEC 516.8
  due to dust NEC 504
  parietoalveolar 516.9
    specified condition NEC 516.8
Pneumopericarditis (*see also* Pericarditis) 423.9
  acute 420.90
Pneumopericardium —*see also* Pericarditis
  congenital 770.2
  fetus or newborn 770.2
  traumatic (post) (*see also* Pneumothorax,
    traumatic) 860.0
    with open wound into thorax 860.1
Pneumoperitoneum 568.89
  fetus or newborn 770.2
Pneumophagia (psychogenic) 306.4
Pneumopleurisy, pneumopleuritis (*see also*
  Pneumonia) 486
Pneumopyopericardium 420.99
Pneumopyothorax (*see also* Pyopneumothorax)
  510.9
  with fistula 510.0
Pneumorrhagia 786.3
  newborn 770.3
  tuberculous (*see also* Tuberculosis, pulmonary)
    011.9
Pneumosiderosis (occupational) 503

Policeman's disease 729.2
Polioencephalitis (acute) (bulbar) (*see also*
   Poliomyelitis, bulbar) 045.0
  inferior 335.22
  influenzal 487.8
  superior hemorrhagic (acute) (Wernicke's)
   265.1
  Wernicke's (superior hemorrhagic) 265.1
Polioencephalomyelitis (acute) (anterior)
  (bulbar) (*see also* Polioencephalitis) 045.0
Polioencephalopathy, superior hemorrhagic
  265.1
  with
   beriberi 265.0
   pellagra 265.2
Poliomeningoencephalitis —*see*
  Meningoencephalitis
Poliomyelitis (acute) (anterior) (epidemic) 045.9

> *Note—Use the following fifth-digit*
> *subclassification with category 045:*
>
> 0 *poliovirus, unspecified type*
> 1 *poliovirus, type I*
> 2 *poliovirus, type II*
> 3 *poliovirus, type III*

  with
   paralysis 045.1
    bulbar 045.0
  abortive 045.2
  ascending 045.9
   progressive 045.9
  bulbar 045.0
  cerebral 045.0
  chronic 335.21
  congenital 771.2
  contact V01.2
  deformities 138
  exposure to V01.2
  late effect 138
  nonepidemic 045.9
  nonparalytic 045.2
  old with deformity 138
  posterior, acute 053.19
  residual 138
  sequelae 138
  spinal, acute 045.9
  syphilitic (chronic) 094.89
  vaccination, prophylactic (against) V04.0
Poliosis (eyebrow) (eyelashes) 704.3
  circumscripta (congenital) 757.4
   acquired 704.3
  congenital 757.4
Pollakiuria 788.41
  psychogenic 306.53
Pollinosis 477.0
Pollitzer's disease (hidradenitis suppurativa)
  705.83
Polyadenitis (*see also* Adenitis) 289.3
  malignant 020.0
Polyalgia 729.99
Polyangiitis (essential) 446.0
Polyarteritis (nodosa) (renal) 446.0
Polyarthralgia 719.49
  psychogenic 306.0

Polyarthritis, polyarthropathy NEC 716.59
  due to or associated with other specified
   conditions—*see* Arthritis, due to or
   associated with
  endemic (*see also* Disease, Kaschin-Beck) 716.0
  inflammatory 714.9
   specified type NEC 714.89
  juvenile (chronic) 714.30
   acute 714.31
  migratory—*see* Fever, rheumatic
  rheumatic 714.0
   fever (acute)—*see* Fever, rheumatic
Polycarential syndrome of infancy 260
Polychondritis (atrophic) (chronic) (relapsing)
  733.99
Polycoria 743.46
Polycystic (congenital) (disease) 759.89
  degeneration, kidney—*see* Polycystic, kidney
  kidney (congenital) 753.12
   adult type (APKD) 753.13
   autosomal dominant 753.13
   autosomal recessive 753.14
   childhood type (CPKD) 753.14
   infantile type 753.14
  liver 751.62
  lung 518.89
   congenital 748.4
  ovary, ovaries 256.4
  spleen 759.0
Polycythemia (primary) (rubra) (vera) (M9950/1)
  238.4
  acquired 289.0
  benign 289.0
   familial 289.6
  due to
   donor twin 776.4
   fall in plasma volume 289.0
   high altitude 289.0
   maternal-fetal transfusion 776.4
   stress 289.0
  emotional 289.0
  erythropoietin 289.0
  familial (benign) 289.6
  Gaisböck's (hypertonica) 289.0
  high altitude 289.0
  hypertonica 289.0
  hypoxemic 289.0
  neonatorum 776.4
  nephrogenous 289.0
  relative 289.0
  secondary 289.0
  spurious 289.0
  stress 289.0
Polycytosis cryptogenica 289.0
Polydactylism, polydactyly 755.00
  fingers 755.01
  toes 755.02
Polydipsia 783.5
Polydystrophic oligophrenia 277.5
Polyembryoma (M9072/3)—*see* Neoplasm, by
  site, malignant
Polygalactia 676.6
Polyglandular
  deficiency 258.9
  dyscrasia 258.9
  dysfunction 258.9
  syndrome 258.8
Polyhydramnios (*see also* Hydramnios) 657
Polymastia 757.6
Polymenorrhea 626.2
Polymicrogyria 742.2

Polymyalgia 725
  arteritica 446.5
  rheumatica 725
Polymyositis (acute) (chronic) (hemorrhagic) 710.4
  with involvement of
    lung 710.4 *[517.8]*
    skin 710.3
  ossificans (generalisata) (progressiva) 728.19
  Wagner's (dermatomyositis) 710.3
Polyneuritis, polyneuritic (*see also*
    Polyneuropathy) 356.9
  alcoholic 357.5
    with psychosis 291.1
  cranialis 352.6
  demyelinating, chronic inflammatory (CIDP)
    357.81
  diabetic 250.6 *[357.2]*
    due to secondary diabetes 249.6 *[357.2]*
    due to lack of vitamin NEC 269.2 *[357.4]*
  endemic 265.0 *[357.4]*
  erythredema 985.0
  febrile 357.0
  hereditary ataxic 356.3
  idiopathic, acute 357.0
  infective (acute) 357.0
  nutritional 269.9 *[357.4]*
  postinfectious 357.0
Polyneuropathy (peripheral) 356.9
  alcoholic 357.5
  amyloid 277.39 *[357.4]*
  arsenical 357.7
  critical illness 357.82
  demyelinating, chronic inflammatory (CIDP)
    357.81
  diabetic 250.6 *[357.2]*
    due to secondary diabetes 249.6 *[357.2]*
  due to
    antitetanus serum 357.6
    arsenic 357.7
    drug or medicinal substance 357.6
      correct substance properly administered 357.6
      overdose or wrong substance given or taken
        977.9
        specified drug—*see* Table of drugs and
          chemicals
    lack of vitamin NEC 269.2 *[357.4]*
    lead 357.7
    organophosphate compounds 357.7
    pellagra 265.2 *[357.4]*
    porphyria 277.1 *[357.4]*
    serum 357.6
    toxic agent NEC 357.7
  hereditary 356.0
  idiopathic 356.9
    progressive 356.4
  in
    amyloidosis 277.39 *[357.4]*
    avitaminosis 269.2 *[357.4]*
      specified NEC 269.1 *[357.4]*
    beriberi 265.0 *[357.4]*
    collagen vascular disease NEC 710.9 *[357.1]*
    deficiency
      B-complex NEC 266.2 *[357.4]*
      vitamin B 266.9 *[357.4]*
      vitamin B$_6$ 266.1 *[357.4]*
    diabetes 250.6 *[357.2]*
      due to secondary diabetes 249.6 *[357.2]*
    diphtheria (*see also* Diphtheria) 032.89 *[357.4]*
    disseminated lupus erythematosus 710.0 *[357.1]*
    herpes zoster 053.13
    hypoglycemia 251.2 *[357.4]*

Polyneuropathy—*continued*
    malignant neoplasm (M8000/3) NEC 199.1
      [357.3]
    mumps 072.72
    pellagra 265.2 *[357.4]*
    polyarteritis nodosa 446.0 *[357.1]*
    porphyria 277.1 *[357.4]*
    rheumatoid arthritis 714.0 *[357.1]*
    sarcoidosis 135 *[357.4]*
    uremia 585.9 *[357.4]*
  lead 357.7
  nutritional 269.9 *[357.4]*
    specified NEC 269.8 *[357.4]*
  postherpetic 053.13
  progressive 356.4
  sensory (hereditary) 356.2
  specified NEC 356.8
Polyonychia 757.5
Polyopia 368.2
  refractive 368.15
Polyorchism, polyorchidism (three testes)
    752.89
Polyorrhymenitis (peritoneal) (*see also*
    Polyserositis) 568.82
  pericardial 423.2
Polyostotic fibrous dysplasia 756.54
Polyotia 744.1
Polyp, polypus

---

*Note—Polyps of organs or sites that do not
appear in the list below should be coded to the
residual category for diseases of the organ or
site concerned.*

---

  accessory sinus 471.8
  adenoid tissue 471.0
  adenomatous (M8210/0)—*see also* Neoplasm,
    by site, benign
    adenocarcinoma in (M8210/3)—*see*
      Neoplasm, by site, malignant
    carcinoma in (M8210/3)—*see* Neoplasm, by
      site, malignant
    multiple (M8221/0)—*see* Neoplasm, by site,
      benign
  antrum 471.8
  anus, anal (canal) (nonadenomatous) 569.0
    adenomatous 211.4
  Bartholin's gland 624.6
  bladder (M8120/1) 236.7
  broad ligament 620.8
  cervix (uteri) 622.7
    adenomatous 219.0
    in pregnancy or childbirth 654.6
      affecting fetus or newborn 763.89
      causing obstructed labor 660.2
    mucous 622.7
    nonneoplastic 622.7
  choanal 471.0
  cholesterol 575.6
  clitoris 624.6
  colon (M8210/0) (*see also* Polyp, adenomatous)
    211.3
  corpus uteri 621.0
  dental 522.0
  ear (middle) 385.30
  endometrium 621.0
  ethmoidal (sinus) 471.8
  fallopian tube 620.8
  female genital organs NEC 624.8
  frontal (sinus) 471.8
  gallbladder 575.6
  gingiva 523.8

Polyp, polypus—*continued*
gum 523.8
labia 624.6
larynx (mucous) 478.4
malignant (M8000/3)—*see* Neoplasm, by site,
   malignant
maxillary (sinus) 471.8
middle ear 385.30
myometrium 621.0
nares
   anterior 471.9
   posterior 471.0
nasal (mucous) 471.9
   cavity 471.0
   septum 471.9
nasopharyngeal 471.0
neoplastic (M8210/0)—*see* Neoplasm, by site,
   benign
nose (mucous) 471.9
oviduct 620.8
paratubal 620.8
pharynx 478.29
   congenital 750.29
placenta, placental 674.4
prostate 600.20
   with
      other lower urinary tract symptoms (LUTS)
         600.21
        urinary
           obstruction 600.21
           retention 600.21
pudenda 624.6
pulp (dental) 522.0
rectosigmoid 211.4
rectum (nonadenomatous) 569.0
   adenomatous 211.4
septum (nasal) 471.9
sinus (accessory) (ethmoidal) (frontal)
   (maxillary) (sphenoidal) 471.8
sphenoidal (sinus) 471.8
stomach (M8210/0) 211.1
tube, fallopian 620.8
turbinate, mucous membrane 471.8
ureter 593.89
urethra 599.3
uterine
   ligament 620.8
   tube 620.8
uterus (body) (corpus) (mucous) 621.0
   in pregnancy or childbirth 654.1
      affecting fetus or newborn 763.89
      causing obstructed labor 660.2
vagina 623.7
vocal cord (mucous) 478.4
vulva 624.6
Polyphagia 783.6
Polypoid —*see* condition
Polyposis —*see also* Polyp
coli (adenomatous) (M8220/0) 211.3
   adenocarcinoma in (M8220/3) 153.9
   carcinoma in (M8220/3) 153.9
familial (M8220/0) 211.3
intestinal (adenomatous) (M8220/0) 211.3
multiple (M8221/0)—*see* Neoplasm, by site,
   benign
Polyradiculitis (acute) 357.0
Polyradiculoneuropathy (acute) (segmentally
   demyelinating) 357.0
Polysarcia 278.00

Polyserositis (peritoneal) 568.82
due to pericarditis 423.2
paroxysmal (familial) 277.31
pericardial 423.2
periodic (familial) 277.31
pleural—*see* Pleurisy
recurrent 277.31
tuberculous (*see also* Tuberculosis,
   polyserositis) 018.9
Polysialia 527.7
Polysplenia syndrome 759.0
Polythelia 757.6
Polytrichia (*see also* Hypertrichosis) 704.1
Polyunguia (congenital) 757.5
acquired 703.8
Polyuria 788.42
Pompe's disease (glycogenosis II) 271.0
Pompholyx 705.81
Poncet's disease (tuberculous rheumatism) (*see
   also* Tuberculosis) 015.9
Pond fracture —*see* Fracture, skull, vault
Ponos 085.0
Pons, pontine —*see* condition
Poor
aesthetics of existing restoration of tooth 525.67
contractions, labor 661.2
   affecting fetus or newborn 763.7
fetal growth NEC 764.9
   affecting management of pregnancy 656.5
incorporation
   artificial skin graft 996.55
   decellularized allodermis graft 996.55
obstetrical history V13.49
   affecting management of current pregnancy V23.49
      pre-term labor V23.41
   pre-term labor V13.41
sucking reflex (newborn) 796.1
vision NEC 369.9
Poradenitis, nostras 099.1
Porencephaly (congenital) (development) (true)
   742.4
acquired 348.0
nondevelopmental 348.0
traumatic (post) 310.2
Porocephaliasis 134.1
Porokeratosis 757.39
disseminated superficial actinic (DSAP) 692.75
Poroma, eccrine (M8402/0)—*see* Neoplasm,
   skin, benign
Porphyria (acute) (congenital) (constitutional)
   (erythropoietic) (familial) (hepatica)
   (idiopathic) (idiosyncratic) (intermittent)
   (latent) (mixed hepatic) (photosensitive)
   (South African genetic) (Swedish) 277.1
acquired 277.1
cutaneatarda
   hereditaria 277.1
   symptomatica 277.1
due to drugs
   correct substance properly administered 277.1
   overdose or wrong substance given or taken 977.9
      specified drug—*see* Table of drugs and
        chemicals
secondary 277.1
toxic NEC 277.1
variegata 277.1
Porphyrinuria (acquired) (congenital)
   (secondary) 277.1
Porphyruria (acquired) (congenital) 277.1
Portal —*see* condition
Port wine nevus or mark 757.32

Posadas-Wernicke disease 114.9
Position
  fetus, abnormal (*see also* Presentation, fetal) 652.9
  teeth, faulty (*see also* Anomaly, position tooth)
    524.30
Positive
  culture (nonspecific) 795.39
    AIDS virus V08
    blood 790.7
    HIV V08
    human immunodeficiency virus V08
    nose 795.39
      Staphylococcus — *see* Carrier (suspected)
        of, Staphylococcus
    skin lesion NEC 795.39
    spinal fluid 792.0
    sputum 795.39
    stool 792.1
    throat 795.39
    urine 791.9
    wound 795.39
  findings, anthrax 795.31
  HIV V08
  human immunodeficiency virus (HIV) V08
  PPD 795.5
  serology
    AIDS virus V08
      inconclusive 795.71
    HIV V08
      inconclusive 795.71
    human immunodeficiency virus V08
      inconclusive 795.71
    syphilis 097.1
      with signs or symptoms—*see* Syphilis, by
        site and stage
      false 795.6
    skin test 795.7
    tuberculin (without active tuberculosis) 795.5
    VDRL 097.1
      with signs or symptoms—*see* Syphilis, by site
        and stage
      false 795.6
    Wassermann reaction 097.1
    false 795.6
Postcardiotomy syndrome 429.4
Postcaval ureter 753.4
Postcholecystectomy syndrome 576.0
Postclimacteric bleeding 627.1
Postcommissurotomy syndrome 429.4
Postconcussional syndrome 310.2
Postcontusional syndrome 310.2
Postcricoid region —*see* condition
Post-dates (pregnancy) —*see* Pregnancy
Postencephalitic —*see also* condition syndrome
  310.8
Posterior —*see* condition
Posterolateral sclerosis (spinal cord)—*see*
  Degeneration, combined
Postexanthematous —*see* condition
Postfebrile —*see* condition
Postgastrectomy dumping syndrome 564.2
Posthemiplegic chorea 344.89
Posthemorrhagic anemia (chronic) 280.0
  acute 285.1
  newborn 776.5
Posthepatitis syndrome 780.79
Postherpetic neuralgia (intercostal) (syndrome)
  (zoster) 053.19
  geniculate ganglion 053.11
  ophthalmica 053.19
  trigeminal 053.12

Posthitis 607.1
Postimmunization complication or reaction
  —*see* Complications, vaccination
Postinfectious —*see* condition
Postinfluenzal syndrome 780.79
Postlaminectomy syndrome 722.80
  cervical, cervicothoracic 722.81
  kyphosis 737.12
  lumbar, lumbosacral 722.83
  thoracic, thoracolumbar 722.82
Postleukotomy syndrome 310.0
Postlobectomy syndrome 310.0
Postmastectomy lymphedema (syndrome) 457.0
Postmaturity, postmature (fetus or newborn)
  (gestation period over 42 completed weeks)
  766.22
  affecting management of pregnancy
    post-term pregnancy 645.1
    prolonged pregnancy 645.2
  syndrome 766.22
Postmeasles —*see also* condition
  complication 055.8
  specified NEC 055.79
Postmenopausal
  endometrium (atrophic) 627.8
    suppurative (*see also* Endometritis) 615.9
  hormone replacement therapy V07.4
  status (age related) (natural) V49.81
Postnasal drip 784.91
Postnatal —*see* condition
Postoperative —*see also* condition
  confusion state 293.9
  psychosis 293.9
  status NEC (*see also* Status (post)) V45.89
Postpancreatectomy hyperglycemia 251.3
Postpartum —*see also* condition
  anemia 648.2
  cardiomyopathy 674.5
  observation
    immediately after delivery V24.0
    routine follow-up V24.2
Postperfusion syndrome NEC 999.89
  bone marrow 996.85
Postpoliomyelitic —*see* condition
Postsurgery status NEC (*see also* Status (post)
  V45.89
Post-term (pregnancy) 645.1
  infant (gestation period over 40 completed
    weeks to 42 completed weeks) 766.21
Post-transplant lymphoproliferative disorder
  (PTLD) 238.77
Posttraumatic —*see* condition
Posttraumatic brain syndrome, nonpsychotic
  310.2
Post-Traumatic Stress Disorder (PTSD) 309.81
Post-typhoid abscess 002.0
Postures, hysterical 300.11
Postvaccinal reaction or complication —*see*
  Complications, vaccination
Postvagotomy syndrome 564.2
Postvalvulotomy syndrome 429.4
Postvasectomy sperm count V25.8
Potain's disease (pulmonary edema) 514
Potain's syndrome (gastrectasis with dyspepsia)
  536.1

Pott's
curvature (spinal) (*see also* Tuberculosis) 015.0
      [737.43]
disease or paraplegia (*see also* Tuberculosis)
      015.0 *[730.88]*
fracture (closed) 824.4
      open 824.5
gangrene 440.24
osteomyelitis (*see also* Tuberculosis) 015.0 *[730.88]*
spinal curvature (*see also* Tuberculosis) 015.0
      [737.43]
tumor, puffy (*see also* Osteomyelitis) 730.2
Potter's
asthma 502
disease 753.0
facies 754.0
lung 502
syndrome (with renal agenesis) 753.0
Pouch
bronchus 748.3
Douglas'—*see* condition
esophagus, esophageal (congenital) 750.4
      acquired 530.6
gastric 537.1
Hartmann's (abnormal sacculation of
      gallbladder neck) 575.8
      of intestine V44.3
         attention to V55.3
pharynx, pharyngeal (congenital) 750.27
Pouchitis 569.71
Poulet's disease 714.2
Poultrymen's itch 133.8
Poverty V60.2
PPE (plamar plantar erythrodysesthesia) 693.0
Prader-Labhart-Willi-Fanconi syndrome
      (hypogenital dystrophy with diabetic
      tendency) 759.81
Prader-Willi syndrome (hypogenital dystrophy
      with diabetic tendency) 759.81
Preachers' voice 784.49
Pre-AIDS —*see* Human immunodeficiency virus
      (disease) (illness) (infection)
Preauricular appendage 744.1
Prebetalipoproteinemia (acquired) (essential)
      (familial) (hereditary) (primary) (secondary)
      272.1
      with chylomicronemia 272.3
Precipitate labor 661.3
      affecting fetus or newborn 763.6
Preclimacteric bleeding 627.0
      menorrhagia 627.0
Precocious
adrenarche 259.1
menarche 259.1
menstruation 626.8
pubarche 259.1
puberty NEC 259.1
sexual development NEC 259.1
thelarche 259.1
Precocity, sexual (constitutional) (cryptogenic)
      (female) (idiopathic) (male) NEC 259.1
      with adrenal hyperplasia 255.2
Precordial pain 786.51
      psychogenic 307.89
Predeciduous teeth 520.2
Prediabetes, prediabetic 790.29
      complicating pregnancy, childbirth, or
         puerperium 648.8
      fetus or newborn 775.89
Predislocation status of hip, at birth (*see also*
      Subluxation, congenital, hip) 754.32

Pre-eclampsia (mild) 642.4
      with pre-existing hypertension 642.7
      affecting fetus or newborn 760.0
      severe 642.5
      superimposed on pre-existing hypertensive
         disease 642.7
Preeruptive color change, teeth, tooth 520.8
Preexcitation 426.7
      atrioventricular conduction 426.7
      ventricular 426.7
Preglaucoma 365.00
Pregnancy (single) (uterine) (without sickness)
      V22.2

---

*Note—Use the following fifth-digit
subclassification with categories 640-649,
651-679:*

0 unspecified as to episode of care
*1 delivered, with or without mention of
      antepartum condition*
*2 delivered, with mention of postpartum
      complication*
3 antepartum condition or complication
4 postpartum condition or complication

---

abdominal (ectopic) 633.00
      affecting fetus or newborn 761.4
      with intrauterine pregnancy 633.01
abnormal NEC 646.9
ampullar—*see* Pregnancy, tubal
broad ligament—*see* Pregnancy, cornual
cervical—*see* Pregnancy, cornual
chemical 631
combined (extrauterine and intrauterine)—*see*
      Pregnancy, cornual
complicated (by) 646.9
      abnormal, abnormality NEC 646.9
         cervix 654.6
         cord (umbilical) 663.9
         glucose tolerance (conditions classifiable to
            790.21-790.29) 648.8
         pelvic organs or tissues NEC 654.9
         pelvis (bony) 653.0
         perineum or vulva 654.8
         placenta, placental (vessel) 656.7
         position
            cervix 654.4
            placenta 641.1
               without hemorrhage 641.0
            uterus 654.4
         size, fetus 653.5
         uterus (congenital) 654.0
      abscess or cellulitis
         bladder 646.6
         genitourinary tract (conditions classifiable to
            590, 595, 597, 599.0, 614.0-614.5,
            614.7-614.9, 615) 646.6
         kidney 646.6
         urinary tract NEC 646.6
      adhesion, pelvic peritoneal 648.9
      air embolism 673.0
      albuminuria 646.2
         with hypertension—*see* Toxemia, of
            pregnancy
      amnionitis 658.4
      amniotic fluid embolism 673.1
      anemia (conditions classifiable to 280-285)
         648.2
      appendicitis 648.9
      atrophy, yellow (acute) (liver) (subacute) 646.7
      bacilluria, asymptomatic 646.5

Pregnancy—*continued*
 complicated by—*continued*
  hemorrhage—*continued*
   due to
    afibrinogenemia or other coagulation
      defect (conditions classifiable to
      286.0-286.9) 641.3
    leiomyoma, uterine 641.8
    marginal sinus (rupture) 641.2
    premature separation, placenta 641.2
    trauma 641.8
   early (before 22 completed weeks gestation)
     640.9
   threatened abortion 640.0
   unavoidable 641.1
  hepatitis (acute) (malignant) (subacute) 646.7
   viral 647.6
  herniation of uterus 654.4
  high head at term 652.5
  hydatidiform mole (delivered) (undelivered)
    630
  hydramnios 657
  hydrocephalic fetus 653.6
  hydrops amnii 657
  hydrorrhea 658.1
  hyperemesis (gravidarum)—*see* Hyperemesis,
    gravidarum
  hypertension—*see* Hypertension, complicating
    pregnancy
  hypertensive heart and chronic kidney disease
    642.2
  hypertensive
   chronic kidney disease 642.2
   heart and chronic kidney disease 642.2
   heart and renal disease 642.2
   heart disease 642.2
   renal disease 642.2
  hyperthyroidism 648.1
  hypothyroidism 648.1
  hysteralgia 646.8
  icterus gravis 646.7
  incarceration, uterus 654.3
  incompetent cervix (os) 654.5
  infection 647.9
   amniotic fluid 658.4
   bladder 646.6
   genital organ (conditions classifiable to
     614.0-614.5, 614.7-614.9, 615) 646.6
   kidney (conditions classifiable to
     590.0-590.9) 646.6
   urinary (tract) 646.6
    asymptomatic 646.5
  infective and parasitic diseases NEC 647.8
  inflammation
   bladder 646.6
   genital organ (conditions classifiable to
     614.0-614.5, 614.7-614.9, 615) 646.6
   urinary tract NEC 646.6
  injury 648.9
   obstetrical NEC 665.9
  insufficient weight gain 646.8
  intrauterine fetal death (near term) NEC 656.4
   early (before 22 completed weeks'
     gestation) 632
  malaria (conditions classifiable to 084) 647.4
  malformation, uterus (congenital) 654.0
  malnutrition (conditions classifiable to
    260-269) 648.9
  malposition
   fetus—*see* Pregnancy, complicated,
     malpresentation
   uterus or cervix 654.4

Pregnancy—*continued*
 complicated by—*continued*
  malpresentation 652.9
   with successful version 652.1
   in multiple gestation 652.6
   specified type NEC 652.8
  marginal sinus hemorrhage or rupture 641.2
  maternal complications from in utero
    procedure 679.0
  maternal drug abuse 648.4
  maternal obesity syndrome 646.1
  menstruation 640.8
  mental disorders (conditions classifiable to
    290-303, 305.0, 305.2-305.9, 306-316,
    317-319) 648.4
  mentum presentation 652.4
  missed
   abortion 632
   delivery (at or near term) 656.4
   labor (at or near term) 656.4
  necrosis
   genital organ or tract (conditions classifiable
     to 614.0-614.5, 614.7-614.9, 615) 646.6
   liver (conditions classifiable to 570) 646.7
   renal, cortical 646.2
  nephritis or nephrosis (conditions classifiable
    to 580-589) 646.2
   with hypertension 642.1
  nephropathy NEC 646.2
  neuritis (peripheral) 646.4
  nutritional deficiency (conditions classifiable
    to 260-269) 648.9
  obesity 649.1
   surgery status 649.2
  oblique lie or presentation 652.3
   with successful version 652.1
  obstetrical trauma NEC 665.9
  oligohydramnios NEC 658.0
  onset of contractions before 37 weeks 644.0
  oversize fetus 653.5
  papyraceous fetus 646.0
  patent cervix 654.5
  pelvic inflammatory disease (conditions
    classifiable to 614.0-614.5, 614.7-614.9,
    615) 646.6
  pelvic peritoneal adhesion 648.9
  placenta, placental
   abnormality 656.7
   abruptio or ablatio 641.2
   detachment 641.2
   disease 656.7
   infarct 656.7
   low implantation 641.1
    without hemorrhage 641.0
   malformation 656.7
   malposition 641.1
    without hemorrhage 641.0
   marginal sinus hemorrhage 641.2
   previa 641.1
    without hemorrhage 641.0
   separation (premature) (undelivered) 641.2
  placentitis 658.4
  polyhydramnios 657
  postmaturity
   post-term 645.1
   prolonged 645.2
  prediabetes 648.8
  pre-eclampsia (mild) 642.4
   severe 642.5
   superimposed on pre-existing hypertensive
     disease 642.7

Pregnancy—*continued*
  complicated by—*continued*
    premature rupture of membranes 658.1
      with delayed delivery 658.2
    previous
      infertility V23.0
      in utero procedure during previous
        pregnancy V23.86
      nonobstetric condition V23.8
      poor obstetrical history V23.49
      premature delivery V23.41
      trophoblastic disease (conditions classifiable
        to 630) V23.1
    prolapse, uterus 654.4
    proteinuria (gestational) 646.2
      with hypertension—*see* Toxemia, of
        pregnancy
    pruritus (neurogenic) 646.8
    psychosis or psychoneurosis 648.4
    ptyalism 646.8
    pyelitis (conditions classifiable to
      590.0-590.9) 646.6
    renal disease or failure NEC 646.2
      with secondary hypertension 642.1
      hypertensive 642.2
    retention, retained dead ovum 631
    retroversion, uterus 654.3
    Rh immunization, incompatibility, or
      sensitization 656.1
    rubella (conditions classifiable to 056) 647.5
    rupture
      amnion (premature) 658.1
        with delayed delivery 658.2
      marginal sinus (hemorrhage) 641.2
      membranes (premature) 658.1
        with delayed delivery 658.2
      uterus (before onset of labor) 665.0
    salivation (excessive) 646.8
    salpingo-oophoritis (conditions classifiable to
      614.0-614.2) 646.6
    septicemia (conditions classifiable to
      038.0-038.9) 647.8
      postpartum 670.2
      puerperal 670.2
    smoking 649.0
    spasms, uterus (abnormal) 646.8
    specified condition NEC 646.8
    spotting 649.5
    spurious labor pains 644.1
    status post
      bariatric surgery 649.2
      gastric banding 649.2
      gastric bypass for obesity 649.2
      obesity surgery 649.2
    superfecundation 651.9
    superfetation 651.9
    syphilis (conditions classifiable to 090-097)
      647.0
    threatened
      abortion 640.0
      premature delivery 644.2
      premature labor 644.0
    thrombophlebitis (superficial) 671.2
      deep 671.3
      septic 670.3
    thrombosis 671.2
      venous (superficial) 671.2
      deep 671.3
    thyroid dysfunction (conditions classifiable to
      240-246) 648.1
    thyroiditis 648.1

Pregnancy—*continued*
  complicated by—*continued*
    thyrotoxicosis 648.1
    tobacco use disorder 649.0
    torsion of uterus 654.4
    toxemia—*see* Toxemia, of pregnancy
    transverse lie or presentation 652.3
      with successful version 652.1
    trauma 648.9
      obstetrical 665.9
    tuberculosis (conditions classifiable to
      010-018) 647.3
    tumor
      cervix 654.6
      ovary 654.4
      pelvic organs or tissue NEC 654.4
      uterus (body) 654.1
        cervix 654.6
      vagina 654.7
      vulva 654.8
    unstable lie 652.0
    uremia—*see* Pregnancy, complicated, renal
      disease
    urethritis 646.6
    vaginitis or vulvitis (conditions classifiable to
      616.1) 646.6
    varicose
      placental vessels 656.7
      veins (legs) 671.0
        perineum 671.1
        vulva 671.1
    varicosity, labia or vulva 671.1
    venereal disease NEC (conditions classifiable
      to 099) 647.2
    venous complication 671.9
    viral disease NEC (conditions classifiable to
      042, 050-055, 057-079, 795.05, 795.15,
      796.75) 647.6
    vomiting (incoercible) (pernicious) (persistent)
      (uncontrollable) (vicious) 643.9
      due to organic disease or other cause 643.8
      early—*see* Hyperemesis, gravidarum
      late (after 22 completed weeks gestation)
        643.2
    young maternal age 659.8
  complications NEC 646.9
  cornual 633.80
    affecting fetus or newborn 761.4
    with intrauterine pregnancy 633.81
  death, maternal NEC 646.9
  delivered—*see* Delivery
  ectopic (ruptured) NEC 633.90
    with intrauterine pregnancy 633.91
    abdominal—*see* Pregnancy, abdominal
    affecting fetus or newborn 761.4
    combined (extrauterine and intrauterine)—*see*
      Pregnancy, cornual
    ovarian—*see* Pregnancy, ovarian
    specified type NEC 633.80
      affecting fetus or newborn 761.4
      with intrauterine pregnancy 633.81
    tubal—*see* Pregnancy, tubal
  examination, pregnancy
    negative result V72.41
    not confirmed V72.40
    positive result V72.42
  extrauterine—*see* Pregnancy, ectopic
  fallopian—*see* Pregnancy, tubal
  false 300.11
    labor (pains) 644.1
  fatigue 646.8

Pregnancy—*continued*
  illegitimate V61.6
  incidental finding V22.2
  in double uterus 654.0
  interstitial—*see* Pregnancy, cornual
  intraligamentous—*see* Pregnancy, cornual
  intramural—*see* Pregnancy, cornual
  intraperitoneal—*see* Pregnancy, abdominal
  isthmian—*see* Pregnancy, tubal
  management affected by
    abnormal, abnormality
      fetus (suspected) 655.9
        specified NEC 655.8
      placenta 656.7
    advanced maternal age NEC 659.6
      multigravida 659.6
      primigravida 659.5
    antibodies (maternal)
      anti-c 656.1
      anti-d 656.1
      anti-e 656.1
      blood group (ABO) 656.2
        Rh(esus) 656.1
    appendicitis 648.9
    bariatric surgery status 649.2
    coagulation defect 649.3
    elderly multigravida 659.6
    elderly primigravida 659.5
    epilepsy 649.4
    fetal (suspected)
      abnormality 655.9
        abdominal 655.8
        acid-base balance 656.8
        cardiovascular 655.8
        facial 655.8
        gastrointestinal 655.8
        genitourinary 655.8
        heart rate or rhythm 659.7
        limb 655.8
        specified NEC 655.8
      acidemia 656.3
      anencephaly 655.0
      aneuploidy 655.1
      bradycardia 659.7
      central nervous system malformation 655.0
      chromosomal abnormalities (conditions
          classifiable to 758.0-758.9) 655.1
      damage from
        drugs 655.5
          obstetric, anesthetic, or sedative 655.5
        environmental toxins 655.8
        intrauterine contraceptive device 655.8
        maternal
          alcohol addiction 655.4
          disease NEC 655.4
          drug use 655.5
          listeriosis 655.4
          rubella 655.3
          toxoplasmosis 655.4
          viral infection 655.3
        radiation 655.6
      death (near term) 656.4
        early (before 22 completed weeks
            gestation) 632
      distress 656.8
      excessive growth 656.6
      growth retardation 656.5
      hereditary disease 655.2
      hydrocephalus 655.0
      intrauterine death 656.4
      poor growth 656.5
      spina bifida (with myelomeningocele) 655.0

Pregnancy—*continued*
  management affected by—*continued*
    fetal-maternal hemorrhage 656.0
    gastric banding status 649.2
    gastric bypass status for obesity 649.2
    hereditary disease in family (possibly)
        affecting fetus 655.2
    incompatibility, blood groups (ABO) 656.2
      rh(esus) 656.1
    insufficient prenatal care V23.7
    intrauterine death 656.4
    isoimmunization (ABO) 656.2
      rh(esus) 656.1
    large-for-dates fetus 656.6
    light-for-dates fetus 656.5
    meconium in liquor 656.8
    mental disorder (conditions classifiable to
        290-303, 305.0, 305.2-305.9, 306-316,
        317-319) 648.4
    multiparity (grand) 659.4
    obesity 649.1
      surgery status 649.2
    poor obstetric history V23.49
      pre-term labor V23.41
    postmaturity
      post-term 645.1
      prolonged 645.2
    post-term pregnancy 645.1
    previous
      abortion V23.2
        habitual 646.3
      cesarean delivery 654.2
      difficult delivery V23.49
      forceps delivery V23.49
      habitual abortions 646.3
      hemorrhage, antepartum or postpartum
          V23.49
      hydatidiform mole V23.1
      infertility V23.0
      in utero procedure during previous
          pregnancy V23.86
      malignancy NEC V23.8
      nonobstetrical conditions V23.8
      premature delivery V23.41
      trophoblastic disease (conditions in 630)
          V23.1
      vesicular mole V23.1
    prolonged pregnancy 645.2
    small-for-dates fetus 656.5
    smoking 649.0
    spotting 649.5
    suspected conditions not found
      amniotic cavity and membrane problem
          V89.01
      cervical shortening V89.05
      fetal anomaly V89.03
      fetal growth problem V89.04
      oligohydramnios V89.01
      other specified problem NEC V89.09
      placental problem V89.02
      polyhydramnios V89.01
    tobacco use disorder 649.0
    venous complication 671.9
    young maternal age 659.8
  maternal death NEC 646.9
  mesometric (mural)—*see* Pregnancy, cornual
  molar 631
    hydatidiform (*see also* Hydatidiform mole)
        630
      previous, affecting management of
          pregnancy V23.1

Pregnancy—*continued*
  molar—*continued*
    previous, affecting management of pregnancy
      V23.49
  multiple NEC 651.9
    with fetal loss and retention of one or more
      fetus(es) 651.6
    affecting fetus or newborn 761.5
    following (elective) fetal reduction 651.7
    specified type NEC 651.8
      with fetal loss and retention of one or more
        fetus(es) 651.6
      following (elective) fetal reduction 651.7
  mural—*see* Pregnancy, cornual
  observation NEC V22.1
    first pregnancy V22.0
    high-risk V23.9
      specified problem NEC V23.8
  ovarian 633.20
    affecting fetus or newborn 761.4
    with intrauterine pregnancy 633.21
  possible, not (yet) confirmed V72.40
  postmature
    post-term 645.1
    prolonged 645.2
  post-term 645.1
  prenatal care only V22.1
    first pregnancy V22.0
    high-risk V23.9
      specified problem NEC V23.8
  prolonged 645.2
  resulting from
    assisted reproductive technology V23.85
    in vitro fertilization V23.85
  quadruplet NEC 651.2
    with fetal loss and retention of one or more
      fetus(es) 651.5
    affecting fetus or newborn 761.5
    following (elective) fetal reduction 651.7
  quintuplet NEC 651.8
    with fetal loss and retention of one or more
      fetus(es) 651.6
    affecting fetus or newborn 761.5
    following (elective) fetal reduction 651.7
  sextuplet NEC 651.8
    with fetal loss and retention of one or more
      fetus(es) 651.6
    affecting fetus or newborn 761.5
    following (elective) fetal reduction 651.7
  spurious 300.11
  superfecundation NEC 651.9
    with fetal loss and retention of one or more
      fetus(es) 651.6
    following (elective) fetal reduction 651.7
  superfetation NEC 651.9
    with fetal loss and retention of one or more
      fetus(es) 651.6
    following (elective) fetal reduction 651.7
  supervision (of) (for)—*see also* Pregnancy,
      management affected by
    elderly
      multigravida V23.82
      primigravida V23.81
    high-risk V23.9
      insufficient prenatal care V23.7
      specified problem NEC V23.8
    multiparity V23.3
    normal NEC V22.1
      first V22.0

Pregnancy—*continued*
  supervision (of)—*continued*
    poor
      obstetric history V23.49
        pre-term labor V23.41
      reproductive history V23.5
    previous
      abortion V23.2
      hydatidiform mole V23.1
      infertility V23.0
      neonatal death V23.5
      stillbirth V23.5
      trophoblastic disease V23.1
      vesicular mole V23.1
    specified problem NEC V23.8
    young
      multigravida V23.84
      primigravida V23.83
  triplet NEC 651.1
    with fetal loss and retention of one or more
      fetus(es) 651.4
    affecting fetus or newborn 761.5
    following (elective) fetal reduction 651.7
  tubal (with rupture) 633.10
    affecting fetus or newborn 761.4
    with intrauterine pregnancy 633.11
  twin NEC 651.0
    with fetal loss and retention of one or more
      fetus(es) 651.3
    affecting fetus or newborn 761.5
    conjoined 678.1
    following (elective) fetal reduction 651.7
  unconfirmed V72.40
  undelivered (no other diagnosis) V22.2
    with false labor 644.1
    high-risk V23.9
      specified problem NEC V23.8
  unwanted NEC V61.7
Pregnant uterus —*see* condition
Preiser's disease (osteoporosis) 733.09
Prekwashiorkor 260
Preleukemia 238.75
Preluxation of hip, congenital (*see also*
    Subluxation, congenital, hip) 754.32
Premature —*see also* condition
  beats (nodal) 427.60
    atrial 427.61
    auricular 427.61
    postoperative 997.1
    specified type NEC 427.69
    supraventricular 427.61
    ventricular 427.69
  birth NEC 765.1
  closure
    cranial suture 756.0
    fontanel 756.0
    foramen ovale 745.8
  contractions 427.60
    atrial 427.61
    auricular 427.61
    auriculoventricular 427.61
    heart (extrasystole) 427.60
    junctional 427.60
    nodal 427.60
    postoperative 997.1
    ventricular 427.69
  ejaculation 302.75
  infant NEC 765.1
    excessive 765.0
    light-for-dates—*see* Light-for-dates

Premature—*continued*
  labor 644.2
    threatened 644.0
  lungs 770.4
  menopause 256.31
  puberty 259.1
  rupture of membranes or amnion 658.1
    affecting fetus or newborn 761.1
    delayed delivery following 658.2
  senility (syndrome) 259.8
  separation, placenta (partial)—*see* Placenta,
    separation
  ventricular systole 427.69
Prematurity NEC 765.1
  extreme 765.0
Premenstrual syndrome 625.4
Premenstrual tension 625.4
Premolarization, cuspids 520.2
Premyeloma 273.1
Prenatal
  care, normal pregnancy V22.1
    first V22.0
  death, cause unknown—*see* Death, fetus
  screening—*see* Antenatal, screening
  teeth 520.6
Prepartum —*see* condition
Preponderance, left or right ventricular 429.3
Prepuce —*see* condition
PRES (posterior reversible encephalopathy
  syndrome) 348.39
Presbycardia 797
  hypertensive (*see also* Hypertension, heart) 402.90
Presbycusis 388.01
Presbyesophagus 530.89
Presbyophrenia 310.1
Presbyopia 367.4
Prescription of contraceptives NEC V25.02
  diaphragm V25.02
  oral (pill) V25.01
    emergency V25.03
    postcoital V25.03
    repeat V25.41
  repeat V25.40
    oral (pill) V25.41
Presenile —*see also* condition
  aging 259.8
  dementia (*see also* Dementia, presenile) 290.10
Presenility 259.8
Presentation, fetal
  abnormal 652.9
    with successful version 652.1
    before labor, affecting fetus or newborn 761.7
    causing obstructed labor 660.0
      affecting fetus or newborn, any, except
        breech 763.1
    in multiple gestation (one or more) 652.6
    specified NEC 652.8
  arm 652.7
    causing obstructed labor 660.0
  breech (buttocks) (complete) (frank) 652.2
    with successful version 652.1
    before labor, affecting fetus or newborn
      761.7
    before labor, affecting fetus or newborn 761.7
  brow 652.4
    causing obstructed labor 660.0
  buttocks 652.2
  chin 652.4
  complete 652.2
  compound 652.8
  cord 663.0

Presentation, fetal—*continued*
  extended head 652.4
  face 652.4
    to pubes 652.8
  footling 652.8
  frank 652.2
  hand, leg, or foot NEC 652.8
  incomplete 652.8
  mentum 652.4
  multiple gestation (one fetus or more) 652.6
  oblique 652.3
    with successful version 652.1
  shoulder 652.8
    affecting fetus or newborn 763.1
  transverse 652.3
    with successful version 652.1
  umbilical cord 663.0
  unstable 652.0
Prespondylolisthesis (congenital) (lumbosacral)
  756.11
Pressure
  area, skin ulcer (*see also* Ulcer, pressure) 707.00
  atrophy, spine 733.99
  birth, fetus or newborn NEC 767.9
  brachial plexus 353.0
  brain 348.4
    injury at birth 767.0
  cerebral—*see* Pressure, brain
  chest 786.59
  cone, tentorial 348.4
    injury at birth 767.0
  funis—*see* Compression, umbilical cord
  hyposystolic (*see also* Hypotension) 458.9
  increased
    intracranial 781.99
      due to
        benign intracranial hypertension 348.2
        hydrocephalus—*see* hydrocephalus
        injury at birth 767.8
    intraocular 365.00
  lumbosacral plexus 353.1
  mediastinum 519.3
  necrosis (chronic) (skin) (*see also* Decubitus)
    707.00
  nerve—*see* Compression, nerve
  paralysis (*see also* Neuropathy, entrapment) 355.9
  pre-ulcer skin changes limited to persistent focal
    erythema (*see also* Ulcer, pressure) 707.21
  sore (chronic) (*see also* Ulcer, pressure) 707.00
  spinal cord 336.9
  ulcer (chronic) (*see also* Ulcer, pressure) 707.00
  umbilical cord—*see* Compression, umbilical cord
  venous, increased 459.89
Pre-syncope 780.2
Preterm infant NEC 765.1
  extreme 765.0
Priapism (penis) 607.3
Prickling sensation (*see also* Disturbance,
  sensation) 782.0
Prickly heat 705.1
Primary —*see* condition
Primigravida, elderly
  affecting
    fetus or newborn 763.89
    management of pregnancy, labor, and delivery
      659.5
Primipara, old
  affecting
    fetus or newborn 763.89
    management of pregnancy, labor, and delivery
      659.5
Primula dermatitis 692.6

Primus varus (bilateral) (metatarsus) 754.52
PRIND (prolonged reversible ischemic
  neurologic deficit) 434.91
  history of personal V12.54
Pringle's disease (tuberous sclerosis) 759.5
Prinzmetal's angina 413.1
Prinzmetal-Massumi syndrome (anterior chest
  wall) 786.52
Prizefighter ear 738.7
Problem (with) V49.9
  academic V62.3
  acculturation V62.4
  adopted child V61.24
  aged
    in-law V61.3
    parent V61.3
    person NEC V61.8
  alcoholism in family V61.41
  anger reaction (*see also* Disturbance, conduct)
    312.0
  behavior, child 312.9
  behavioral V40.9
    specified NEC V40.3
  betting V69.3
  biological child V61.23
  cardiorespiratory NEC V47.2
  care of sick or handicapped person in family or
    household V61.49
  career choice V62.29
  communication V40.1
  conscience regarding medical care V62.6
  delinquency (juvenile) 312.9
  diet, inappropriate V69.1
  digestive NEC V47.3
  ear NEC V41.3
  eating habits, inappropriate V69.1
  economic V60.2
    affecting care V60.9
      specified type NEC V60.89
  educational V62.3
  enuresis, child 307.6
  exercise, lack of V69.0
  eye NEC V41.1
  family V61.9
    specified circumstance NEC V61.8
  fear reaction, child 313.0
  feeding (elderly) (infant) 783.3
    newborn 779.31
    nonorganic 307.59
  fetal, affecting management of pregnancy 656.9
    specified type NEC 656.8
  financial V60.2
  foster child V61.25
  functional V41.9
    specified type NEC V41.8
  gambling V69.3
  genital NEC V47.5
  head V48.9
    deficiency V48.0
    disfigurement V48.6
    mechanical V48.2
    motor V48.2
    movement of V48.2
    sensory V48.4
    specified condition NEC V48.8
  hearing V41.2
  high-risk sexual behavior V69.2
  identity 313.82
  influencing health status NEC V49.89

Problem—*continued*
  internal organ NEC V47.9
    deficiency V47.0
    mechanical or motor V47.1
  interpersonal NEC V62.81
    jealousy, child 313.3
  learning V40.0
  legal V62.5
  life circumstance NEC V62.89
  lifestyle V69.9
    specified NEC V69.8
  limb V49.9
    deficiency V49.0
    disfigurement V49.4
    mechanical V49.1
    motor V49.2
    movement, involving
      musculoskeletal system V49.1
      nervous system V49.2
    sensory V49.3
    specified condition NEC V49.5
  litigation V62.5
  living alone V60.3
  loneliness NEC V62.89
  marital V61.10
    involving
      divorce V61.03
      estrangement V61.09
      psychosexual disorder 302.9
      sexual function V41.7
    relationship V61.10
  mastication V41.6
  medical care, within family V61.49
  mental V40.9
    specified NEC V40.2
  mental hygiene, adult V40.9
  multiparity V61.5
  nail biting, child 307.9
  neck V48.9
    deficiency V48.1
    disfigurement V48.7
    mechanical V48.3
    motor V48.3
    movement V48.3
    sensory V48.5
    specified condition NEC V48.8
  neurological NEC 781.99
  none (feared complaint unfounded) V65.5
  occupational V62.29
  parent-child V61.20
    adopted child V61.24
    biological child V61.23
    foster child V61.25
    relationship V61.20
  partner V61.10
    relationship V61.10
  personal NEC V62.89
    interpersonal conflict NEC V62.81
  personality (*see also* Disorder, personality)
    301.9
  phase of life V62.89
  placenta, affecting management of pregnancy
    656.9
    specified type NEC 656.8
  poverty V60.2
  presence of sick or handicapped person in
    family or household V61.49
  psychiatric 300.9
  psychosocial V62.9
    specified type NEC V62.89
  relational NEC V62.81

Problem—*continued*
  relationship, childhood 313.3
  religious or spiritual belief
    other than medical care V62.89
    regarding medical care V62.6
  self-damaging behavior V69.8
  sexual
    behavior, high-risk V69.2
    function NEC V41.7
  sibling
    relational V61.8
    relationship V61.8
  sight V41.0
  sleep disorder, child 307.40
  sleep, lack of V69.4
  smell V41.5
  speech V40.1
  spite reaction, child (*see also* Disturbance,
    conduct) 312.0
  spoiled child reaction (*see also* Disturbance,
    conduct) 312.1
  substance abuse in family V61.42
  swallowing V41.6
  tantrum, child (*see also* Disturbance, conduct)
    312.1
  taste V41.5
  thumb sucking, child 307.9
  tic (child) 307.21
  trunk V48.9
    deficiency V48.1
    disfigurement V48.7
    mechanical V48.3
    motor V48.3
    movement V48.3
    sensory V48.5
    specified condition NEC V48.8
  unemployment V62.0
  urinary NEC V47.4
  voice production V41.4
Procedure (surgical) not done NEC V64.3
  because of
    contraindication V64.1
    patient's decision V64.2
      for reasons of conscience or religion V62.6
    specified reason NEC V64.3
Procidentia
  anus (sphincter) 569.1
  rectum (sphincter) 569.1
  stomach 537.89
  uteri 618.1
Proctalgia 569.42
  fugax 564.6
  spasmodic 564.6
    psychogenic 307.89
Proctitis 569.49
  amebic 006.8
  chlamydial 099.52
  gonococcal 098.7
  granulomatous 555.1
  idiopathic 556.2
    with ulcerative sigmoiditis 556.3
  tuberculous (*see also* Tuberculosis) 014.8
  ulcerative (chronic) (nonspecific) 556.2
    with ulcerative sigmoiditis 556.3
Proctocele
  female (without uterine prolapse) 618.04
    with uterine prolapse 618.4
      complete 618.3
      incomplete 618.2
  male 569.49
Proctocolitis, idiopathic 556.2
  with ulcerative sigmoiditis 556.3

Proctoptosis 569.1
Proctosigmoiditis 569.89
  ulcerative (chronic) 556.3
Proctospasm 564.6
  psychogenic 306.4
Prodromal-AIDS —*see* Human
    immunodeficiency virus (disease) (illness)
    (infection)
Profichet's disease or syndrome 729.90
Progeria (adultorum) (syndrome) 259.8
Prognathism (mandibular) (maxillary) 524.00
Progonoma (melanotic) (M9363/0)—*see*
    Neoplasm, by site, benign
Progressive —*see* condition
Prolapse, prolapsed
  anus, anal (canal) (sphincter) 569.1
  arm or hand, complicating delivery 652.7
    causing obstructed labor 660.0
      affecting fetus or newborn 763.1
    fetus or newborn 763.1
  bladder (acquired) (mucosa) (sphincter)
    congenital (female) (male) 756.71
    female (*see also* Cystocele, female) 618.01
    male 596.8
  breast implant (prosthetic) 996.54
  cecostomy 569.69
  cecum 569.89
  cervix, cervical (hypertrophied) 618.1
    anterior lip, obstructing labor 660.2
      affecting fetus or newborn 763.1
    congenital 752.49
    postpartal (old) 618.1
    stump 618.84
  ciliary body 871.1
  colon (pedunculated) 569.89
  colostomy 569.69
  conjunctiva 372.73
  cord—*see* Prolapse, umbilical cord
  disc (intervertebral)—*see* Displacement,
    intervertebral disc
  duodenum 537.89
  eye implant (orbital) 996.59
    lens (ocular) 996.53
  fallopian tube 620.4
  fetal extremity, complicating delivery 652.8
    causing obstructed labor 660.0
    fetus or newborn 763.1
  funis—*see* Prolapse, umbilical cord
  gastric (mucosa) 537.89
  genital, female 618.9
    specified NEC 618.89
  globe 360 81
  ileostomy bud 569.69
  intervertebral disc—*see* Displacement,
    intervertebral disc
  intestine (small) 569.89
  iris 364.89
    traumatic 871.1
  kidney (*see also* Disease, renal) 593.0
    congenital 753.3
  laryngeal muscles or ventricle 478.79
  leg, complicating delivery 652.8
    causing obstructed labor 660.0
    fetus or newborn 763.1
  liver 573.8
  meatus urinarius 599.5
  mitral valve 424.0
  ocular lens implant 996.53
  organ or site, congenital NEC—*see* Malposition,
    congenital
  ovary 620.4
  pelvic (floor), female 618.89

Prolapse, prolapsed—*continued*
  perineum, female 618.89
  pregnant uterus 654.4
  rectum (mucosa) (sphincter) 569.1
    due to Trichuris trichiuria 127.3
  spleen 289.59
  stomach 537.89
  umbilical cord
    affecting fetus or newborn 762.4
    complicating delivery 663.0
  ureter 593.89
    with obstruction 593.4
  ureterovesical orifice 593.89
  urethra (acquired) (infected) (mucosa) 599.5
    congenital 753.8
  uterovaginal 618.4
    complete 618.3
    incomplete 618.2
    specified NEC 618.89
  uterus (first degree) (second degree) (third
      degree) (complete) (without vaginal wall
      prolapse) 618.1
    with mention of vaginal wall prolapse—*see*
        Prolapse, uterovaginal
    congenital 752.3
    in pregnancy or childbirth 654.4
      affecting fetus or newborn 763.1
      causing obstructed labor 660.2
        affecting fetus or newborn 763.1
    postpartal (old) 618.1
  uveal 871.1
  vagina (anterior) (posterior) (vault) (wall)
      (without uterine prolapse) 618.00
    with uterine prolapse 618.4
      complete 618.3
      incomplete 618.2
    paravaginal 618.02
    posthysterectomy 618.5
    specified NEC 618.09
  vitreous (humor) 379.26
    traumatic 871.1
  womb—*see* Prolapse, uterus
Prolapsus, female 618.9
Proliferative —*see* condition
Prolinemia 270.8
Prolinuria 270.8
Prolonged, prolongation
  bleeding time (*see also* Defect, coagulation) 790.92
    "idiopathic" (in von Willebrand's disease) 286.4
  coagulation time (*see also* Defect, coagulation)
      790.92
  gestation syndrome 766.22
  labor 662.1
    affecting fetus or newborn 763.89
    first stage 662.0
    second stage 662.2
  PR interval 426.11
  pregnancy 645.2
  prothrombin time (*see also* Defect, coagulation)
      790.92
  QT interval 794.31
    syndrome 426.82
  rupture of membranes (24 hours or more prior to
      onset of labor) 658.2
  uterine contractions in labor 661.4
    affecting fetus or newborn 763.7
Prominauris 744.29
Prominence
  auricle (ear) (congenital) 744.29
    acquired 380.32

Prominence—*continued*
  ischial spine or sacral promontory
    with disproportion (fetopelvic) 653.3
      affecting fetus or newborn 763.1
      causing obstructed labor 660.1
        affecting fetus or newborn 763.1
  nose (congenital) 748.1
    acquired 738.0
PROMM (proximal myotonic myotonia) 359.21
Pronation
  ankle 736.79
  foot 736.79
    congenital 755.67
Prophylactic
  administration of
    agents affecting estrogen receptors and
        estrogen levels NEC V07.59
    anastrozole (Arimidex) V07.52
    antibiotics V07.39
    antitoxin, any V07.2
    antivenin V07.2
    aromatase inhibitors V07.52
    chemotherapeutic agent NEC V07.39
      fluoride V07.31
    diphtheria antitoxin V07.2
    drug V07.39
    estrogen receptor downregulators V07.59
    exemestane (Aromasin) V07.52
    fulvestrant (Faslodex) V07.59
    gamma globulin V07.2
    gonadotropin-releasing hormone (GnRH)
        agonist V07.59
    goserelin acetate (Zoladex) V07.59
    immune sera (gamma globulin) V07.2
    letrozole (Femara) V07.52
    leuprolide acetate (leuprorelin) (Lupron)
        V07.59
    megestrol acetate (Megace) V07.59
    raloxifene (Evista) V07.51
    RhoGAM V07.2
    selective estrogen receptor modulators
        (SERMs) V07.51
    tamoxifen (Nolvadex) V07.51
    tetanus antitoxin V07.2
    toremifene (Fareston) V07.51
  chemotherapy NEC V07.39
    fluoride V07.31
  hormone replacement (postmenopausal) V07.4
  immunotherapy V07.2
  measure V07.9
    specified type NEC V07.8
  medication V07.39
  postmenopausal hormone replacement V07.4
  sterilization V25.2
Proptosis (ocular) (*see also* Exophthalmos)
    376.30
  thyroid 242.0
Propulsion
  eyeball 360.81
Prosecution, anxiety concerning V62.5
Prosopagnosia 368.16
Prostate, prostatic —*see* condition
Prostatism 600.90
  with
    other lower urinary tract symptoms (LUTS) 600.91
    urinary
      obstruction 600.91
      retention 600.91
Prostatitis (congestive) (suppurative) 601.9
  acute 601.0
  cavitary 601.8
  chlamydial 099.54

Prostatitis—*continued*
chronic 601.1
diverticular 601.8
due to Trichomonas (vaginalis) 131.03
fibrous 600.90
with
other lower urinary tract symptoms (LUTS) 600.91
urinary
obstruction 600.91
retention 600.91
gonococcal (acute) 098.12
chronic or duration of 2 months or over 098.32
granulomatous 601.8
hypertrophic 600.00
with
other lower urinary tract symptoms (LUTS) 600.01
urinary
obstruction 600.01
retention 600.01
specified type NEC 601.8
subacute 601.1
trichomonal 131.03
tuberculous (*see also* Tuberculosis) 016.5 *[601.4]*
Prostatocystitis 601.3
Prostatorrhea 602.8
Prostatoseminovesiculitis, trichomonal 131.03
Prostration 780.79
heat 992.5
anhydrotic 992.3
due to
salt (and water) depletion 992.4
water depletion 992.3
nervous 300.5
newborn 779.89
senile 797
Protanomaly 368.51
Protanopia (anomalous trichromat) (complete) (incomplete) 368.51
Protection (against) (from) —*see* Prophylactic
Protein
deficiency 260
malnutrition 260
sickness (prophylactic) (therapeutic) 999.5
Proteinemia 790.99
Proteinosis
alveolar, lung or pulmonary 516.0
lipid 272.8
Proteinosis
lipoid (of Urbach) 272.8
Proteinuria (*see also* Albuminuria) 791.0
Bence-Jones NEC 791.0
gestational 646.2
with hypertension—*see* Toxemia, of pregnancy
orthostatic 593.6
postural 593.6
Proteolysis, pathologic 286.6
Protocoproporphyria 277.1
Protoporphyria (erythrohepatic) (erythropoietic) 277.1
Protrusio acetabuli 718.65
Protrusion
acetabulum (into pelvis) 718.65
device, implant, or graft—*see* Complications, mechanical
ear, congenital 744.29
intervertebral disc—*see* Displacement, intervertebral disc
nucleus pulposus—*see* Displacement, intervertebral disc

Proud flesh 701.5
Prune belly (syndrome) 756.71
Prurigo (ferox) (gravis) (Hebra's) (hebrae) (mitis) (simplex) 698.2
agria 698.3
asthma syndrome 691.8
Besnier's (atopic dermatitis) (infantile eczema) 691.8
eczematodes allergicum 691.8
estivalis (Hutchinson's) 692.72
Hutchinson's 692.72
nodularis 698.3
psychogenic 306.3
Pruritus, pruritic 698.9
ani 698.0
psychogenic 306.3
conditions NEC 698.9
psychogenic 306.3
due to Onchocerca volvulus 125.3
ear 698.9
essential 698.9
genital organ(s) 698.1
psychogenic 306.3
gravidarum 646.8
hiemalis 698.8
neurogenic (any site) 306.3
perianal 698.0
psychogenic (any site) 306.3
scrotum 698.1
psychogenic 306.3
senile, senilis 698.8
Trichomonas 131.9
vulva, vulvae 698.1
psychogenic 306.3
Psammocarcinoma (M8140/3)—*see* Neoplasm, by site, malignant
Pseudarthrosis, pseudoarthrosis (bone) 733.82
joint following fusion V45.4
Pseudoacanthosis
nigricans 701.8
Pseudoaneurysm —*see* Aneurysm
Pseudoangina (pectoris)—*see* Angina
Pseudoangioma 452
Pseudo-Argyll-Robertson pupil 379.45
Pseudoarteriosus 747.89
Pseudoarthrosis —*see* Pseudarthrosis
Pseudoataxia 799.89
Pseudobulbar affect (PBA) 310.8
Pseudobursa 727.89
Pseudocholera 025
Pseudochromidrosis 705.89
Pseudocirrhosis, liver, pericardial 423.2
Pseudocoarctation 747.21
Pseudocowpox 051.1
Pseudocoxalgia 732.1
Pseudocroup 478.75
Pseudocyesis 300.11
Pseudocyst
lung 518.89
pancreas 577.2
retina 361.19
Pseudodementia 300.16
Pseudoelephantiasis neuroarthritica 757.0
Pseudoemphysema 518.89
Pseudoencephalitis
superior (acute) hemorrhagic 265.1
Pseudoerosion cervix, congenital 752.49
Pseudoexfoliation, lens capsule 366.11
Pseudofracture (idiopathic) (multiple) (spontaneous) (symmetrical) 268.2
Pseudoglanders 025

Pseudoglioma 360.44
Pseudogout —*see* Chondrocalcinosis
Pseudohallucination 780.1
Pseudohemianesthesia 782.0
Pseudohemophilia (Bernuth's) (hereditary) (type
    B) 286.4
    type A 287.8
    vascular 287.8
Pseudohermaphroditism 752.7
    with chromosomal anomaly—*see* Anomaly,
        chromosomal
        adrenal 255.2
    female (without adrenocortical disorder) 752.7
        with adrenocortical disorder 255.2
        adrenal 255.2
    male (without gonadal disorder) 752.7
        with
            adrenocortical disorder 255.2
            cleft scrotum 752.7
            feminizing testis 259.51
            gonadal disorder 257.9
            adrenal 255.2
Pseudohole, macula 362.54
Pseudo-Hurler's disease (mucolipidosis III)
    272.7
Pseudohydrocephalus 348.2
Pseudohypertrophic muscular dystrophy
    (Erb's) 359.1
Pseudohypertrophy, muscle 359.1
Pseudohypoparathyroidism 275.49
Psuedopseudohypoparathyroidism 275.49
Pseudoinfluenza 487.1
Pseudoinsomnia 307.49
Pseudoleukemia 288.8
    infantile 285.8
Pseudomembranous —*see* condition
Pseudomeningocele (cerebral) (infective) 349.2
    postprocedural 997.01
    spinal 349.2
Pseudomenstruation 626.8
Pseudomucinous
    cyst (ovary) (M8470/0) 220
    peritoneum 568.89
Pseudomyeloma 273.1
Pseudomyxoma peritonei (M8480/6) 197.6
Pseudoneuritis optic (nerve) 377.24
    papilla 377.24
    congenital 743.57
Pseudoneuroma —*see* Injury, nerve, by site
Pseudo-obstruction
    intestine (chronic) (idiopathic) (intermittent
        secondary) (primary) 564.89
    acute 560.89
Pseudopapilledema 377.24
Pseudoparalysis
    arm or leg 781.4
    atonic, congenital 358.8
Pseudopelade 704.09
Pseudophakia V43.1
Pseudopolycythemia 289.0
Pseudopolyposis, colon 556.4
Pseudoporencephaly 348.0
Pseudopseudohypoparathyroidism 275.49
Pseudopsychosis 300.16
Pseudopterygium 372.52
Pseudoptosis (eyelid) 374.34
Pseudorabies 078.89
Pseudoretinitis, pigmentosa 362.65
Pseudorickets 588.0
    senile (Pozzi's) 731.0
Pseudorubella 057.8

Pseudoscarlatina 057.8
Pseudosclerema 778.1
Pseudosclerosis (brain)
    Jakob's 046.19
    of Westphal (-Strümpell) (hepatolenticular
        degeneration) 275.1
    spastic 046.19
    with dementia
        with behavioral disturbance 046.19 *[294.11]*
        without behavioral disturbance 046.19
            [294.10]
Pseudoseizure 780.39
    non-psychiatric 780.39
    psychiatric 300.11
Pseudotabes 799.89
    diabetic 250.6 *[337.1]*
        due to secondary diabetes 249.6 *[337.1]*
Pseudotetanus (*see also* Convulsions) 780.39
Pseudotetany 781.7
    hysterical 300.11
Pseudothalassemia 285.0
Pseudotrichinosis 710.3
Pseudotruncus arteriosus 747.29
Pseudotuberculosis, pasteurella (infection) 027.2
Pseudotumor
    cerebri 348.2
    orbit (inflammatory) 376.11
Pseudo-Turner's syndrome 759.89
Pseudoxanthoma elasticum 757.39
Psilosis (sprue) (tropical) 579.1
    Monilia 112.89
    nontropical 579.0
    not sprue 704.00
Psittacosis 073.9
Psoitis 728.89
Psora NEC 696.1
Psoriasis 696.1
    any type, except arthropathic 696.1
    arthritic, arthropathic 696.0
    buccal 528.6
    flexural 696.1
    follicularis 696.1
    guttate 696.1
    inverse 696.1
    mouth 528.6
    nummularis 696.1
    psychogenic 316 *[696.1]*
    punctata 696.1
    pustular 696.1
    rupioides 696.1
    vulgaris 696.1
Psorospermiasis 136.4
Psorospermosis 136.4
    follicularis (vegetans) 757.39
Psychalgia 307.80
Psychasthenia 300.89
    compulsive 300.3
    mixed compulsive states 300.3
    obsession 300.3
Psychiatric disorder or problem NEC 300.9
Psychogenic —*see also* condition
    factors associated with physical conditions 316
Psychoneurosis, psychoneurotic (*see also*
    Neurosis) 300.9
    anxiety (state) 300.00
    climacteric 627.2
    compensation 300.16
    compulsion 300.3
    conversion hysteria 300.11
    depersonalization 300.6
    depressive type 300.4

Psychoneurosis, psychoneurotic—*continued*
  dissociative hysteria 300.15
  hypochondriacal 300.7
  hysteria 300.10
    conversion type 300.11
    dissociative type 300.15
  mixed NEC 300.89
  neurasthenic 300.5
  obsessional 300.3
  obsessive-compulsive 300.3
  occupational 300.89
  personality NEC 301.89
  phobia 300.20
  senile NEC 300.89
Psychopathic —*see also* condition
  constitution, posttraumatic 310.2
    with psychosis 293.9
  personality 301.9
    amoral trends 301.7
    antisocial trends 301.7
    asocial trends 301.7
    mixed types 301.7
  state 301.9
Psychopathy, sexual (*see also* Deviation, sexual) 302.9
Psychophysiologic, psychophysiological condition—*see* Reaction, psychophysiologic
Psychose passionelle 297.8
Psychosexual identity disorder 302.6
  adult-life 302.85
  childhood 302.6
Psychosis 298.9
  acute hysterical 298.1
  affecting management of pregnancy, childbirth, or puerperium 648.4
  affective (*see also* Disorder, mood) 296.90
    drug induced 292.84
    due to or associated with physical condition 293.83

Note—Use the following fifth-digit subclassification with categories 296.0-296.6:

0 unspecified
1 mild
2 moderate
3 severe, without mention of psychotic behavior
4 severe, specified as with psychotic behavior
5 in partial or unspecified remission
6 in full remission

---

  involutional 296.2
    recurrent episode 296.3
    single episode 296.2
  manic-depressive 296.80
    circular (alternating) 296.7
      currently depressed 296.5
      currently manic 296.4
    depressed type 296.2
      atypical 296.82
      recurrent episode 296.3
      single episode 296.2
    manic 296.0
      atypical 296.81
      recurrent episode 296.1
      single episode 296.0
    mixed type NEC 296.89
    specified type NEC 296.89
  senile 290.21
  specified type NEC 296.99

Psychosis—*continued*
  alcoholic 291.9
    with
      anxiety 291.89
      delirium tremens 291.0
      delusions 291.5
      dementia 291.2
      hallucinosis 291.3
      jealousy 291.5
      mood disturbance 291.89
      paranoia 291.5
      persisting amnesia 291.1
      sexual dysfunction 291.89
      sleep disturbance 291.89
    amnestic confabulatory 291.1
    delirium tremens 291.0
    hallucinosis 291.3
    Korsakoff's, Korsakov's, Korsakow's 291.1
    paranoid type 291.5
    pathological intoxication 291.4
    polyneuritic 291.1
    specified type NEC 291.89
  alternating (*see also* Psychosis, manic-depressive, circular) 296.7
  anergastic (*see also* Psychosis, organic) 294.9
  arteriosclerotic 290.40
    with
      acute confusional state 290.41
      delirium 290.41
      delusions 290.42
      depressed mood 290.43
    depressed type 290.43
    paranoid type 290.42
    simple type 290.40
    uncomplicated 290.40
  atypical 298.9
    depressive 296.82
    manic 296.81
  borderline (schizophrenia) (*see also* Schizophrenia) 295.5
    of childhood (*see also* Psychosis, childhood) 299.8
    prepubertal 299.8
  brief reactive 298.8
  childhood, with origin specific to 299.9

Note—Use the following fifth-digit subclassification with category 299:

0 current or active state
1 residual state

---

    atypical 299.8
    specified type NEC 299.8
  circular (*see also* Psychosis, manic-depressive, circular) 296.7
  climacteric (*see also* Psychosis, involutional) 298.8
  confusional 298.9
    acute 293.0
    reactive 298.2
    subacute 293.1
  depressive (*see also* Psychosis, affective) 296.2
    atypical 296.82
    involutional 296.2
      recurrent episode 296.3
      single episode 296.2
    psychogenic 298.0
    reactive (emotional stress) (psychological trauma) 298.0
    recurrent episode 296.3
      with hypomania (bipolar II) 296.89
    single episode 296.2

Psychosis—*continued*
disintegrative, childhood (*see also* Psychosis, childhood) 299.1
drug 292.9
  with
    affective syndrome 292.84
    amnestic syndrome 292.83
    anxiety 292.89
    delirium 292.81
      withdrawal 292.0
    delusions 292.11
    dementia 292.82
    depressive state 292.84
    hallucinations 292.12
    hallucinosis 292.12
    mood disorder 292.84
    mood disturbance 292.84
    organic personality syndrome NEC 292.89
    sexual dysfunction 292.89
    sleep disturbance 292.89
    withdrawal syndrome (and delirium) 292.0
  affective syndrome 292.84
  delusions 292.11
  hallucinatory state 292.12
  hallucinosis 292.12
  paranoid state 292.11
  specified type NEC 292.89
  withdrawal syndrome (and delirium) 292.0
due to or associated with physical condition (*see also* Psychosis, organic) 293.9
epileptic NEC 294.8
excitation (psychogenic) (reactive) 298.1
exhaustive (*see also* Reaction, stress, acute) 308.9
hypomanic (*see also* Psychosis, affective) 296.0
  recurrent episode 296.1
  single episode 296.0
hysterical 298.8
  acute 298.1
incipient 298.8
  schizophrenic (*see also* Schizophrenia) 295.5
induced 297.3
infantile (*see also* Psychosis, childhood) 299.0
infective 293.9
  acute 293.0
  subacute 293.1
in
  conditions classified elsewhere
    with
      delusions 293.81
      hallucinations 293.82
  pregnancy, childbirth, or puerperium 648.4
interactional (childhood) (*see also* Psychosis, childhood) 299.1
involutional 298.8
  depressive (*see also* Psychosis, affective) 296.2
    recurrent episode 296.3
    single episode 296.2
  melancholic 296.2
    recurrent episode 296.3
    single episode 296.2
  paranoid state 297.2
  paraphrenia 297.2
Korsakoff's, Korakov's, Korsakow's (nonalcoholic) 294.0
  alcoholic 291.1

Psychosis—*continued*
mania (phase) (*see also* Psychosis, affective) 296.0
  recurrent episode 296.1
  single episode 296.0
manic (*see also* Psychosis, affective) 296.0
  atypical 296.81
  recurrent episode 296.1
  single episode 296.0
manic-depressive 296.80
  circular 296.7
    currently
      depressed 296.5
      manic 296.4
      mixed 296.6
  depressive 296.2
    recurrent episode 296.3
      with hypomania (bipolar II) 296.89
    single episode 296.2
  hypomanic 296.0
    recurrent episode 296.1
    single episode 296.0
  manic 296.0
    atypical 296.81
    recurrent episode 296.1
    single episode 296.0
  mixed NEC 296.89
  perplexed 296.89
  stuporous 296.89
menopausal (*see also* Psychosis, involutional) 298.8
mixed schizophrenic and affective (*see also* Schizophrenia) 295.7
multi-infarct (cerebrovascular) (*see also* Psychosis, arteriosclerotic) 290.40
organic NEC 294.9
  due to or associated with
    addiction
      alcohol (*see also* Psychosis, alcoholic) 291.9
      drug (*see also* Psychosis, drug) 292.9
    alcohol intoxication, acute (*see also* Psychosis, alcoholic) 291.9
    alcoholism (*see also* Psychosis, alcoholic) 291.9
    arteriosclerosis (cerebral) (*see also* Psychosis, arteriosclerotic) 290.40
    cerebrovascular disease
      acute (psychosis) 293.0
      arteriosclerotic (*see also* Psychosis, arteriosclerotic) 290.40
    childbirth—*see* Psychosis, puerperal
    dependence
      alcohol (*see also* Psychosis, alcoholic) 291.9
      drug 292.9
    disease
      alcoholic liver (*see also* Psychosis, alcoholic) 291.9
      brain
        arteriosclerotic (*see also* Psychosis, arteriosclerotic) 290.40
      cerebrovascular
        acute (psychosis) 293.0
        arteriosclerotic (*see also* Psychosis, arteriosclerotic) 290.40
      endocrine or metabolic 293.9
        acute (psychosis) 293.0
        subacute (psychosis) 293.1

Psychosis—*continued*
  organic—*continued*
    due to—*continued*
      disease—*continued*
        Jakob-Creutzfeldt 046.19
          with behavioral disturbance 046.19
            [294.11]
          without behavioral disturbance 046.19
            [294.10]
          familial 046.19
          iatrogenic 046.19
          specified NEC 046.19
          sporadic 046.19
          variant 046.11
            with dementia
              with behavioral disturbance 046.11
                [294.11]
              without behavioral disturbance
                046.11 *[294.10]*
        liver, alcoholic (*see also* Psychosis,
          alcoholic) 291.9
      disorder
        cerebrovascular
          acute (psychosis) 293.0
        endocrine or metabolic 293.9
          acute (psychosis) 293.0
          subacute (psychosis) 293.1
        epilepsy
          with behavioral disturbance 345.9
            [294.11]
          without behavioral disturbance 345.9
            [294.10]
          transient (acute) 293.0
        Huntington's chorea
          with behavioral disturbance 333.4
            [294.11]
          without behavioral disturbance 333.4
            [294.10]
        infection
          brain 293.9
            acute (psychosis) 293.0
            chronic 294.8
            subacute (psychosis) 293.1
          intracranial NEC 293.9
            acute (psychosis) 293.0
            chronic 294.8
            subacute (psychosis) 293.1
        intoxication
          alcoholic (acute) (*see also* Psychosis,
            alcoholic) 291.9
          pathological 291.4
          drug (*see also* Psychosis, drug) 292.9
        ischemia
          cerebrovascular (generalized) (*see also*
            Psychosis, arteriosclerotic) 290.40
        Jakob-Creutzfeldt disease (syndrome)
          046.19
          with behavioral disturbance 046.19
            [294.11]
          without behavioral disturbance 046.19
            [294.10]
          variant 046.11
            with dementia
              with behavioral disturbance 046.11
                [294.11]
              without behavioral disturbance 046.11
                [294.10]
        multiple sclerosis
          with behavioral disturbance 340 *[294.11]*
          without behavioral disturbance 340
            [294.10]

Psychosis—*continued*
  organic—*continued*
    due to—*continued*
      physical condition NEC 293.9
        with
          delusions 293.81
          hallucinations 293.82
      presenility 290.10
      puerperium—*see* Psychosis, puerperal
      sclerosis, multiple
        with behavioral disturbance 340 *[294.11]*
        without behavioral disturbance 340
          [294.10]
      senility 290.20
      status epilepticus
        with behavioral disturbance 345.3
          [294.11]
        without behavioral disturbance 345.3
          [294.10]
      trauma
        brain (birth) (from electrical current)
          (surgical) 293.9
          acute (psychosis) 293.0
          chronic 294.8
          subacute (psychosis) 293.1
      unspecified physical condition 293.9
        with
          delusions 293.81
          hallucinations 293.82
    infective 293.9
      acute (psychosis) 293.0
      subacute 293.1
    posttraumatic 293.9
      acute 293.0
      subacute 293.1
    specified type NEC 294.8
    transient 293.9
      with
        anxiety 293.84
        delusions 293.81
        depression 293.83
        hallucinations 293.82
      depressive type 293.83
      hallucinatory type 293.82
      paranoid type 293.81
      specified type NEC 293.89
  paranoic 297.1
  paranoid (chronic) 297.9
    alcoholic 291.5
    chronic 297.1
    climacteric 297.2
    involutional 297.2
    menopausal 297.2
    protracted reactive 298.4
    psychogenic 298.4
      acute 298.3
    schizophrenic (*see also* Schizophrenia) 295.3
    senile 290.20
  paroxysmal 298.9
    senile 290.20
  polyneuritic, alcoholic 291.1
  postoperative 293.9
  postpartum—*see* Psychosis, puerperal
  prepsychotic (*see also* Schizophrenia) 295.5
  presbyophrenic (type) 290.8
  presenile (*see also* Dementia, presenile) 290.10
  prison 300.16
  psychogenic 298.8
    depressive 298.0
    paranoid 298.4
      acute 298.3

Psychosis—*continued*
  puerperal
    specified type—*see* categories 295-298
    unspecified type 293.89
      acute 293.0
      chronic 293.89
      subacute 293.1
  reactive (emotional stress) (psychological
    trauma) 298.8
    brief 298.8
    confusion 298.2
    depressive 298.0
    excitation 298.1
  schizo-affective (depressed) (excited) (*see also*
    Schizophrenia) 295.7
  schizophrenia, schizophrenic (*see also*
    Schizophrenia) 295.9
    borderline type 295.5
    of childhood (*see also* Psychosis, childhood)
      299.8
    catatonic (excited) (withdrawn) 295.2
    childhood type (*see also* Psychosis, childhood)
      299.9
    hebephrenic 295.1
    incipient 295.5
    latent 295.5
    paranoid 295.3
    prepsychotic 295.5
    prodromal 295.5
    pseudoneurotic 295.5
    pseudopsychopathic 295.5
    schizophreniform 295.4
    simple 295.0
    undifferentiated type 295.9
  schizophreniform 295.4
  senile NEC 290.20
    with
      delusional features 290.20
      depressive features 290.21
    depressed type 290.21
    paranoid type 290.20
    simple deterioration 290.20
    specified type—*see* categories 295-298
  shared 297.3
  situational (reactive) 298.8
  symbiotic (childhood) (*see also* Psychosis,
    childhood) 299.1
  toxic (acute) 293.9
Psychotic (*see also* condition) 298.9
  episode 298.9
  due to or associated with physical conditions
    (*see also* Psychosis, organic) 293.9
Pterygium (eye) 372.40
  central 372.43
  colli 744.5
  double 372.44
  peripheral (stationary) 372.41
  progressive 372.42
  recurrent 372.45
Ptilosis 374.55
PTLD (post-transplant lymphoproliferative
  disorder) 238.77
Ptomaine (poisoning) (*see also* Poisoning, food)
  005.9
Ptosis (adiposa) 374.30
  breast 611.81
  cecum 569.89
  colon 569.89
  congenital (eyelid) 743.61
    specified site NEC—*see* Anomaly, specified
      type NEC

Ptosis—*continued*
  epicanthus syndrome 270.2
  eyelid 374.30
    congenital 743.61
    mechanical 374.33
    myogenic 374.32
    paralytic 374.31
  gastric 537.5
  intestine 569.89
  kidney (*see also* Disease, renal) 593.0
    congenital 753.3
  liver 573.8
  renal (*see also* Disease, renal) 593.0
    congenital 753.3
  splanchnic 569.89
  spleen 289.59
  stomach 537.5
  viscera 569.89
PTSD (Post-Traumatic Stress Disorder) 309.81
Ptyalism 527.7
  hysterical 300.11
  periodic 527.2
  pregnancy 646.8
  psychogenic 306.4
Ptyalolithiasis 527.5
Pubalgia 848.8
Pubarche, precocious 259.1
Pubertas praecox 259.1
Puberty V21.1
  abnormal 259.9
  bleeding 626.3
  delayed 259.0
  precocious (constitutional) (cryptogenic)
    (idiopathic) NEC 259.1
    due to
      adrenal
        cortical hyperfunction 255.2
        hyperplasia 255.2
      cortical hyperfunction 255.2
      ovarian hyperfunction 256.1
        estrogen 256.0
      pineal tumor 259.8
      testicular hyperfunction 257.0
  premature 259.1
    due to
      adrenal cortical hyperfunction 255.2
      pineal tumor 259.8
      pituitary (anterior) hyperfunction 253.1
Puckering, macula 362.56
Pudenda, pudendum —*see* condition
Puente's disease (simple glandular cheilitis)
  528.5
Puerperal
  abscess
    areola 675.1
    Bartholin's gland 646.6
    breast 675.1
    cervix (uteri) 670.8
    fallopian tube 670.8
    genital organ 670.8
    kidney 646.6
    mammary 675.1
    mesosalpinx 670.8
    nabothian 646.6
    nipple 675.0
    ovary, ovarian 670.8
    oviduct 670.8
    parametric 670.8
    para-uterine 670.8
    pelvic 670.8
    perimetric 670

Puerperal—*continued*
  infection—*continued*
    cervix 646.6
    endocervix 646.6
    fallopian tube 670.8
    generalized 670.0
    genital tract (major) 670.0
      minor or localized 646.6
    kidney (bacillus coli) 646.6
    mammary gland 675.2
      with nipple 675.9
        specified type NEC 675.8
    nipple 675.0
      with breast 675.9
        specified type NEC 675.8
    ovary 670.8
    pelvic 670.8
    peritoneum 670.8
    renal 646.6
    tubo-ovarian 670.8
    urinary (tract) NEC 646.6
      asymptomatic 646.5
    uterus, uterine 670.8
    vagina 646.6
  inflammation—*see also* Puerperal, infection
    areola 675.1
    Bartholin's gland 646.6
    breast 675.2
    broad ligament 670.8
    cervix (uteri) 646.6
    fallopian tube 670.8
    genital organs 670.8
      localized 646.6
    mammary gland 675.2
    nipple 675.0
    ovary 670.8
    oviduct 670.8
    pelvis 670.8
    periuterine 670.8
    tubal 670.8
    vagina 646.6
    vein—*see* Puerperal, phlebitis
  inversion, nipple 676.3
  ischemia, cerebral 674.0
  lymphangitis 670.8
    breast 675.2
  malaria (conditions classifiable to 084) 647.4
  malnutrition 648.9
  mammillitis 675.0
  mammitis 675.2
  mania 296.0
    recurrent episode 296.1
    single episode 296.0
  mastitis 675.2
    purulent 675.1
    retromammary 675.1
    submammary 675.1
  melancholia 296.2
    recurrent episode 296.3
    single episode 296.2
  mental disorder (conditions classifiable to
    290-303, 305.0, 305.2-305.9, 306-316,
    317-319) 648.4
  metritis (suppurative) 670.1
    septic 670.2
  metroperitonitis 670.8
  metrorrhagia 666.2
  metrosalpingitis 670.8
  metrovaginitis 670.8
  milk leg 671.4
  monoplegia, cerebral 674.0

Puerperal—*continued*
  necrosis
    kidney, tubular 669.3
    liver (acute) (subacute) (conditions classifiable
      to 570) 674.8
    ovary 670.8
    renal cortex 669.3
  nephritis or nephrosis (conditions classifiable to
    580-589) 646.2
    with hypertension 642.1
  nutritional deficiency (conditions classifiable to
    260-269) 648.9
  occlusion, precerebral artery 674.0
  oliguria 669.3
  oophoritis 670.8
  ovaritis 670.8
  paralysis
    bladder (sphincter) 665.5
    cerebral 674.0
  paralytic stroke 674.0
  parametritis 670.8
  paravaginitis 646.6
  pelviperitonitis 670.8
  perimetritis 670.8
  perimetrosalpingitis 670.8
  perinephritis 646.6
  perioophoritis 670.8
  periphlebitis—*see* Puerperal, phlebitis
  perisalpingitis 670.8
  peritoneal infection 670.8
  peritonitis (pelvic) 670.8
  perivaginitis 646.6
  phlebitis 671.2
    deep 671.4
    intracranial sinus (venous) 671.5
    pelvic 671.4
    specified site NEC 671.5
    superficial 671.2
  phlegmasia alba dolens 671.4
  placental polyp 674.4
  pneumonia, embolic—*see* Puerperal, embolism
  prediabetes 648.8
  pre-eclampsia (mild) 642.4
    with pre-existing hypertension 642.7
    severe 642.5
  psychosis, unspecified (*see also* Psychosis,
    puerperal) 293.89
  pyelitis 646.6
  pyelocystitis 646.6
  pyelohydronephrosis 646.6
  pyelonephritis 646.6
  pyelonephrosis 646.6
  pyemia 670.2
  pyocystitis 646.6
  pyohemia 670.2
  pyometra 670.8
  pyonephritis 646.6
  pyonephrosis 646.6
  pyo-oophoritis 670.8
  pyosalpingitis 670.8
  pyosalpinx 670.8
  pyrexia (of unknown origin) 672
  renal
    disease NEC 646.2
    failure, acute 669.3
  retention
    decidua (fragments) (with delayed
      hemorrhage) 666.2
      without hemorrhage 667.1
    placenta (fragments) (with delayed
      hemorrhage) 666.2
      without hemorrhage 667.1

Purpura—*continued*
 red cell membrane sensitivity 287.2
 rheumatica 287.0
 Schönlein (-Henoch) (allergic) 287.0
 scorbutic 267
 senile 287.2
 simplex 287.2
 symptomatica 287.0
 telangiectasia annularis 709.1
 thrombocytopenic (*see also* Thrombocytopenia)
  287.30
  congenital 287.33
  essential 287.30
  hereditary 287.31
  idiopathic 287.31
  immune 287.31
  neonatal, transitory (*see also*
   Thrombocytopenia, neonatal transitory)
   776.1
  primary 287.30
  puerperal, postpartum 666.3
  thrombotic 446.6
 thrombohemolytic (*see also* Fibrinolysis) 286.6
 thrombopenic (*see also* Thrombocytopenia)
  287.30
  congenital 287.33
  essential 287.30
 thrombotic 446.6
  thrombocytic 446.6
  thrombocytopenic 446.6
 toxic 287.0
 variolosa 050.0
 vascular 287.0
 visceral symptoms 287.0
 Werlhof's (*see also* Purpura, thrombocytopenic)
  287.39
Purpuric spots 782.7
Purulent —*see* condition
Pus
 absorption, general—*see* Septicemia
 in
  stool 792.1
  urine 791.9
 tube (rupture) (*see also* Salpingo-oophoritis)
  614.2
Pustular rash 782.1
Pustule 686.9
 malignant 022.0
 nonmalignant 686.9
Putnam's disease (subacute combined sclerosis
 with pernicious anemia) 281.0 *[336.2]*
Putnam-Dana syndrome (subacute combined
 sclerosis with pernicious anemia) 281.0
 [336.2]
Putrefaction, intestinal 569.89
Putrescent pulp (dental) 522.1
Pyarthritis —*see* Pyarthrosis
Pyarthrosis (*see also* Arthritis, pyogenic) 711.0
 tuberculous—*see* Tuberculosis, joint
Pycnoepilepsy, pycnolepsy (idiopathic) (*see also*
 Epilepsy) 345.0
Pyelectasia 593.89
Pyelectasis 593.89
Pyelitis (congenital) (uremic) 590.80
 with
  abortion—*see* Abortion, by type, with
   specified complication NEC
  contracted kidney 590.00
  ectopic pregnancy (*see also* categories
   633.0-633.9) 639.8

Pyelitis—*continued*
  molar pregnancy (*see also* categories 630-632)
   639.8
 acute 590.10
  with renal medullary necrosis 590.11
 chronic 590.00
  with
   renal medullary necrosis 590.01
 complicating pregnancy, childbirth, or
  puerperium 646.6
  affecting fetus or newborn 760.1
 cystica 590.3
 following
  abortion 639.8
  ectopic or molar pregnancy 639.8
 gonococcal 098.19
  chronic or duration of 2 months or over 098.39
 tuberculous (*see also* Tuberculosis) 016.0 *[590.81]*
Pyelocaliectasis 593.89
Pyelocystitis (*see also* Pyelitis) 590.80
Pyelohydronephrosis 591
Pyelonephritis (*see also* Pyelitis) 590.80
 acute 590.10
  with renal medullary necrosis 590.11
 chronic 590.00
 syphilitic (late) 095.4
 tuberculous (*see also* Tuberculosis) 016.0
  [590.81]
Pyelonephrosis (*see also* Pyelitis) 590.80
 chronic 590.00
Pyelophlebitis 451.89
Pyelo-ureteritis cystica 590.3
Pyemia, pyemic (purulent) (*see also* Septicemia)
 038.9
 abscess—*see* Abscess
 arthritis (*see also* Arthritis, pyogenic) 711.0
 Bacillus coli 038.42
 embolism—(*see also* Septicemia) 415.12
 fever 038.9
 infection 038.9
 joint (*see also* Arthritis, pyogenic) 711.0
 liver 572.1
 meningococcal 036.2
 newborn 771.81
 phlebitis—*see* Phlebitis
 pneumococcal 038.2
 portal 572.1
 postvaccinal 999.39
 puerperal 670.2
 specified organism NEC 038.8
 staphylococcal 038.10
  aureus 038.11
   methicillin
    resistant 038.12
    susceptible 038.11
  specified organism NEC 038.19
 streptococcal 038.0
 tuberculous—*see* Tuberculosis, miliary
Pygopagus 759.4
Pykno-epilepsy, pyknolepsy (idiopathic) (*see
 also* Epilepsy) 345.0
Pyle (-Cohn) disease (craniometaphyseal
 dysplasia) 756.89
Pylephlebitis (suppurative) 572.1
Pylethrombophlebitis 572.1
Pylethrombosis 572.1
Pyloritis (*see also* Gastritis) 535.5
Pylorospasm (reflex) 537.81
 congenital or infantile 750.5
 neurotic 306.4
 newborn 750.5

psychogenic 306.4
Pylorus, pyloric —*see* condition
Pyoarthrosis —*see* Pyarthrosis
Pyocele
mastoid 383.00
sinus (accessory) (nasal) (*see also* Sinusitis)
473.9
turbinate (bone) 473.9
urethra (*see also* Urethritis) 597.0
Pyococcal dermatitis 686.00
Pyococcide, skin 686.00
Pyocolpos (*see also* Vaginitis) 616.10
Pyocyaneus dermatitis 686.09
Pyocystitis (*see also* Cystitis) 595.9
Pyoderma, pyodermia NEC 686.00
gangrenosum 686.01
specified type NEC 686.09
vegetans 686.8
Pyodermatitis 686.00
vegetans 686.8
Pyogenic —*see* condition
Pyohemia —*see* Septicemia
Pyohydronephrosis (*see also* Pyelitis) 590.80
Pyometra 615.9
Pyometritis (*see also* Endometritis) 615.9
Pyometrium (*see also* Endometritis) 615.9
Pyomyositis 728.0
ossificans 728.19
tropical (bungpagga) 040.81
Pyonephritis (*see also* Pyelitis) 590.80
chronic 590.00
Pyonephrosis (congenital) (*see also* Pyelitis)
590.80
acute 590.10
Pyo-oophoritis (*see also* Salpingo-oophoritis)
614.2
Pyo-ovarium (*see also* Salpingo-oophoritis)
614.2
Pyopericarditis 420.99
Pyopericardium 420.99
Pyophlebitis —*see* Phlebitis
Pyopneumopericardium 420.99
Pyopneumothorax (infectional) 510.9
with fistula 510.0
subdiaphragmatic (*see also* Peritonitis) 567.29
subphrenic (*see also* Peritonitis) 567.29
tuberculous (*see also* Tuberculosis, pleura)
012.0
Pyorrhea (alveolar) (alveolaris) 523.40
degenerative 523.5
Pyosalpingitis (*see also* Salpingo-oophoritis) 614.2
Pyosalpinx (*see also* Salpingo-oophoritis) 614.2
Pyosepticemia —*see* Septicemia
Pyosis
Corlett's (impetigo) 684
Manson's (pemphigus contagiosus) 684
Pyothorax 510.9
with fistula 510.0
tuberculous (*see also* Tuberculosis, pleura)
012.0
Pyoureter 593.89
tuberculous (*see also* Tuberculosis) 016.2
Pyramidopallidonigral syndrome 332.0
Pyrexia (of unknown origin) (P.U.O.) 780.60
atmospheric 992.0
during labor 659.2
environmentally-induced
newborn 778.4
heat 992.0
newborn, environmentally-induced 778.4
puerperal 672

Pyroglobulinemia 273.8
Pyromania 312.33
Pyrosis 787.1
Pyrroloporphyria 277.1
Pyuria (bacterial) 791.9

Q

Q fever 083.0
  with pneumonia 083.0 *[484.8]*
Quadricuspid aortic valve 746.89
Quadrilateral fever 083.0
Quadriparesis —*see* Quadriplegia
  meaning muscle weakness 728.87
Quadriplegia 344.00
  with fracture, vertebra (process)—*see* Fracture,
    vertebra, cervical, with spinal cord injury
  brain (current episode) 437.8
  cerebral (current episode) 437.8
  C1-C4
    complete 344.01
    incomplete 344.02
  C5-C7
    complete 344.03
    incomplete 344.04
  congenital or infantile (cerebral) (spastic)
    (spinal) 343.2
  cortical 437.8
  embolic (current episode) (*see also* Embolism,
    brain) 434.1
  functional 780.72
  infantile (cerebral) (spastic) (spinal) 343.2
  newborn NEC 767.0
  specified NEC 344.09
  thrombotic (current episode) (*see also*
    Thrombosis, brain) 434.0
  traumatic—*see* Injury, spinal, cervical
Quadruplet
  affected by maternal complications of pregnancy
    761.5
  healthy liveborn—*see* Newborn, multiple
  pregnancy (complicating delivery) NEC 651.8
    with fetal loss and retention of one or more
      fetus(es) 651.5
    following (elective) fetal reduction 651.7
Quarrelsomeness 301.3
Quartan
  fever 084.2
  malaria (fever) 084.2
Queensland fever 083.0
  coastal 083.0
  seven-day 100.89
Quervain's disease 727.04
  thyroid (subacute granulomatous thyroiditis)
    245.1
Queyrat's erythroplasia (M8080/2)
  specified site—*see* Neoplasm, skin, in situ
  unspecified site 233.5
Quincke's disease or edema —*see* Edema,
  angioneurotic
Quinquaud's disease (acne decalvans) 704.09
Quinsy (gangrenous) 475
Quintan fever 083.1
Quintuplet
  affected by maternal complications of pregnancy
    761.5
  healthy liveborn—*see* Newborn, multiple
  pregnancy (complicating delivery) NEC 651.2
    with fetal loss and retention of one or more
      fetus(es) 651.6
    following (elective) fetal reduction 651.7
Quotidian
  fever 084.0
  malaria (fever) 084.0

R

Rabbia 071
Rabbit fever (*see also* Tularemia) 021.9
Rabies 071
  contact V01.5
  exposure to V01.5
  inoculation V04.5
    reaction—*see* Complications, vaccination
  vaccination, prophylactic (against) V04.5
Rachischisis (*see also* Spina bifida) 741.9
Rachitic —*see also* condition
  deformities of spine 268.1
  pelvis 268.1
    with disproportion (fetopelvic) 653.2
      affecting fetus or newborn 763.1
      causing obstructed labor 660.1
        affecting fetus or newborn 763.1
Rachitis, rachitism —*see also* Rickets
  acute 268.0
  fetalis 756.4
  renalis 588.0
  tarda 268.0
Racket nail 757.5
Radial nerve —*see* condition
Radiation effects or sickness —*see also* Effect,
  adverse, radiation
  cataract 366.46
  dermatitis 692.82
  sunburn (*see also* Sunburn) 692.71
Radiculitis (pressure) (vertebrogenic) 729.2
  accessory nerve 723.4
  anterior crural 724.4
  arm 723.4
  brachial 723.4
  cervical NEC 723.4
  due to displacement of intervertebral disc—*see*
    Neuritis, due to, displacement intervertebral
    disc
  leg 724.4
  lumbar NEC 724.4
  lumbosacral 724.4
  rheumatic 729.2
  syphilitic 094.89
  thoracic (with visceral pain) 724.4
Radiculomyelitis 357.0
  toxic, due to
    Clostridium tetani 037
    Corynebacterium diphtheriae 032.89
Radiculopathy (*see also* Radiculitis) 729.2
Radioactive substances, adverse effect —*see*
  Effect, adverse, radioactive substance
Radiodermal burns (acute) (chronic)
  (occupational)—*see* Burn, by site
Radiodermatitis 692.82
Radionecrosis —*see* Effect, adverse, radiation
Radiotherapy session V58.0
Radium, adverse effect —*see* Effect, adverse,
  radioactive substance
Raeder-Harbitz syndrome (pulseless disease) 446.7
Rage (*see also* Disturbance, conduct) 312.0
  meaning rabies 071
Rag sorters' disease 022.1
Raillietiniasis 123.8
Railroad neurosis 300.16
Railway spine 300.16
Raised —*see* Elevation
Raiva 071
Rake teeth, tooth 524.39
Rales 786.7

Ramifying renal pelvis 753.3
Ramsay Hunt syndrome (herpetic geniculate
  ganglionitis) 053.11
  meaning dyssynergia cerebellaris myoclonica 334.2
Ranke's primary infiltration (*see also*
  Tuberculosis) 010.0
Ranula 527.6
  congenital 750.26
Rape
  adult 995.83
  alleged, observation or examination V71.5
  child 995.53
Rapid
  feeble pulse, due to shock, following injury 958.4
  heart (beat) 785.0
    psychogenic 306.2
  respiration 786.06
    psychogenic 306.1
  second stage (delivery) 661.3
    affecting fetus or newborn 763.6
  time-zone change syndrome 327.35
Rarefaction, bone 733.99
Rash 782.1
  canker 034.1
  diaper 691.0
  drug (internal use) 693.0
    contact 692.3
  ECHO 9 virus 078.89
  enema 692.89
  food (*see also* Allergy, food) 693.1
  heat 705.1
  napkin 691.0
  nettle 708.8
  pustular 782.1
  rose 782.1
    epidemic 056.9
    of infants 057.8
  scarlet 034.1
  serum (prophylactic) (therapeutic) 999.5
  toxic 782.1
  wandering tongue 529.1
Rasmussen's aneurysm (*see also* Tuberculosis)
  011.2
Rat-bite fever 026.9
  due to Streptobacillus moniliformis 026.1
  spirochetal (morsus muris) 026.0
Rathke's pouch tumor (M9350/1) 237.0
Raymond (-Céstan) syndrome 433.8
Raynaud's
  disease or syndrome (paroxysmal digital
    cyanosis) 443.0
  gangrene (symmetric) 443.0 *[785.4]*
  phenomenon (paroxysmal digital cyanosis)
    (secondary) 443.0
RDS 769
Reaction
  acute situational maladjustment (*see also*
    Reaction, adjustment) 309.9
  adaptation (*see also* Reaction, adjustment) 309.9
  adjustment 309.9
    with
      anxious mood 309.24
        with depressed mood 309.28
      conduct disturbance 309.3
        combined with disturbance of emotions 309.4
      depressed mood 309.0
        brief 309.0
          with anxious mood 309.28
        prolonged 309.1
      elective mutism 309.83
      mixed emotions and conduct 309.4

Reaction—*continued*
  adjustment—*continued*
    with—*continued*
      mutism, elective 309.83
      physical symptoms 309.82
      predominant disturbance (of)
        conduct 309.3
        emotions NEC 309.29
          mixed 309.28
        mixed, emotions and conduct 309.4
        specified type NEC 309.89
      specific academic or work inhibition 309.23
      withdrawal 309.83
    depressive 309.0
      with conduct disturbance 309.4
      brief 309.0
      prolonged 309.1
    specified type NEC 309.89
  adverse food NEC 995.7
  affective (*see also* Psychosis, affective) 296.90
    specified type NEC 296.99
  aggressive 301.3
    unsocialized (*see also* Disturbance, conduct)
      312.0
  allergic (*see also* Allergy) 995.3
    drug, medicinal substance, and
      biological—*see* Allergy, drug
    food—*see* Allergy, food
    serum 999.5
  anaphylactic—*see* Shock, anaphylactic
  anesthesia—*see* Anesthesia, complication
  anger 312.0
  antisocial 301.7
  antitoxin (prophylactic) (therapeutic)—*see*
    Complications, vaccination
  anxiety 300.00
  Arthus 995.21
  asthenic 300.5
  compulsive 300.3
  conversion (anesthetic) (autonomic)
    (hyperkinetic) (mixed paralytic)
    (paresthetic) 300.11
  deoxyribonuclease (DNA) (DNase)
    hypersensitivity NEC 287.2
  depressive 300.4
    acute 309.0
    affective (*see also* Psychosis, affective) 296.2
      recurrent episode 296.3
      single episode 296.2
    brief 309.0
    manic (*see also* Psychosis, affective) 296.80
    neurotic 300.4
    psychoneurotic 300.4
    psychotic 298.0
  dissociative 300.15
  drug NEC (*see also* Table of Drugs and
    Chemicals) 995.20
    allergic—*see also* Allergy, drug 995.27
    correct substance properly administered 995.20
    obstetric anesthetic or analgesic NEC 668.9
      affecting fetus or newborn 763.5
      specified drug—*see* Table of drugs and
        chemicals
    overdose or poisoning 977.9
      specified drug—*see* Table of drugs and
        chemicals
    specific to newborn 779.4
    transmitted via placenta or breast milk—*see*
      Absorption, drug, through placenta

Reaction—*continued*
drug—*continued*
withdrawal NEC 292.0
infant of dependent mother 779.5
wrong substance given or taken in error 977.9
specified drug—*see* Table of drugs and chemicals
dyssocial 301.7
dystonic, acute, due to drugs 333.72
erysipeloid 027.1
fear 300.20
child 313.0
fluid loss, cerebrospinal 349.0
food—*see also* Allergy, food
adverse NEC 995.7
anaphylactic shock—*see* Anaphylactic shock, due to food
foreign
body NEC 728.82
in operative wound (inadvertently left) 998.4
due to surgical material intentionally left—*see* Complications, due to (presence of) any device, implant, or graft classified to 996.0-996.5 NEC
substance accidentally left during a procedure (chemical) (powder) (talc) 998.7
body or object (instrument) (sponge) (swab) 998.4
graft-versus-host (GVH) 279.50
grief (acute) (brief) 309.0
prolonged 309.1
gross stress (*see also* Reaction, stress, acute) 308.9
group delinquent (*see also* Disturbance, conduct) 312.2
Herxheimer's 995.0
hyperkinetic (*see also* Hyperkinesia) 314.9
hypochondriacal 300.7
hypoglycemic, due to insulin 251.0
therapeutic misadventure 962.3
hypomanic (*see also* Psychosis, affective) 296.0
recurrent episode 296.1
single episode 296.0
hysterical 300.10
conversion type 300.11
dissociative 300.15
id (bacterial cause) 692.89
immaturity NEC 301.89
aggressive 301.3
emotional instability 301.59
immunization—*see* Complications, vaccination
incompatibility
blood group
ABO 999.6
minor blood group 999.89
Rh (factor) (infusion) (transfusion) 999.7
inflammatory—*see* Infection
infusion—*see* Complications, infusion
inoculation (immune serum)—*see* Complications, vaccination
insulin 995.23
involutional
paranoid 297.2
psychotic (*see also* Psychosis, affective, depressive) 296.2
leukemoid (basophilic) (lymphocytic) (monocytic) (myelocytic) (neutrophilic) 288.62
LSD (*see also* Abuse, drugs, nondependent) 305.3
lumbar puncture 349.0

Reaction—*continued*
manic-depressive (*see also* Psychosis, affective) 296.80
depressed 296.2
recurrent episode 296.3
single episode 296.2
hypomanic 296.0
neurasthenic 300.5
neurogenic (*see also* Neurosis) 300.9
neurotic NEC 300.9
neurotic-depressive 300.4
nitritoid—*see* Crisis, nitritoid
obsessive-compulsive 300.3
organic 293.9
acute 293.0
subacute 293.1
overanxious, child or adolescent 313.0
paranoid (chronic) 297.9
acute 298.3
climacteric 297.2
involutional 297.2
menopausal 297.2
senile 290.20
simple 297.0
passive
aggressive 301.84
dependency 301.6
personality (*see also* Disorder, personality) 301.9
phobic 300.20
postradiation—*see* Effect, adverse, radiation
psychogenic NEC 300.9
psychoneurotic (*see also* Neurosis) 300.9
anxiety 300.00
compulsive 300.3
conversion 300.11
depersonalization 300.6
depressive 300.4
dissociative 300.15
hypochondriacal 300.7
hysterical 300.10
conversion type 300.11
dissociative type 300.15
neurasthenic 300.5
obsessive 300.3
obsessive-compulsive 300.3
phobic 300.20
tension state 300.9
psychophysiologic NEC (*see also* Disorder, psychosomatic) 306.9
cardiovascular 306.2
digestive 306.4
endocrine 306.6
gastrointestinal 306.4
genitourinary 306.50
heart 306.2
hemic 306.8
intestinal (large) (small) 306.4
laryngeal 306.1
lymphatic 306.8
musculoskeletal 306.0
pharyngeal 306.1
respiratory 306.1
skin 306.3
special sense organs 306.7
psychosomatic (*see also* Disorder, psychosomatic) 306.9
psychotic (*see also* Psychosis) 298.9
depressive 298.0
due to or associated with physical condition (*see also* Psychosis, organic) 293.9

Reaction—*continued*
  psychotic—*continued*
    involutional (*see also* Psychosis, affective)
      296.2
      recurrent episode 296.3
      single episode 296.2
  pupillary (myotonic) (tonic) 379.46
  radiation—*see* Effect, adverse, radiation
  runaway—*see also* Disturbance, conduct
    socialized 312.2
    undersocialized, unsocialized 312.1
  scarlet fever toxin—*see* Complications,
    vaccination
  schizophrenic (*see also* Schizophrenia) 295.9
    latent 295.5
  serological for syphilis—*see* Serology for
    syphilis
  serum (prophylactic) (therapeutic) 999.5
    immediate 999.4
  situational (*see also* Reaction, adjustment) 309.9
    acute, to stress 308.3
    adjustment (*see also* Reaction, adjustment) 309.9
  somatization (*see also* Disorder, psychosomatic)
    306.9
  spinal puncture 349.0
  spite, child (*see also* Disturbance, conduct) 312.0
  stress, acute 308.9
    bone or cartilage —*see* Fracture, stress
    with predominant disturbance (of)
      consciousness 308.1
      emotions 308.0
      mixed 308.4
      psychomotor 308.2
      specified type NEC 308.3
  surgical procedure—*see* Complications, surgical
    procedure
  tetanus antitoxin—*see* Complications,
    vaccination
  toxin-antitoxin—*see* Complications, vaccination
  transfusion (blood) (bone marrow)
    (lymphocytes) (allergic)—*see*
    Complications, transfusion
  tuberculin skin test, nonspecific (without active
    tuberculosis) 795.5
    positive (without active tuberculosis) 795.5
  ultraviolet—*see* Effect, adverse, ultraviolet
  undersocialized, unsocialized—*see also*
    Disturbance, conduct
    aggressive (type) 312.0
    unaggressive (type) 312.1
  vaccination (any)—*see* Complications,
    vaccination
  white graft (skin) 996.52
  withdrawing, child or adolescent 313.22
  x-ray—*see* Effect, adverse, x-rays
Reactive depression (*see also* Reaction,
  depressive) 300.4
  neurotic 300.4
  psychoneurotic 300.4
  psychotic 298.0
Rebound tenderness 789.6
Recalcitrant patient V15.81
Recanalization, thrombus —*see* Thrombosis
Recession, receding
  chamber angle (eye) 364.77
  chin 524.06
  gingival (postinfective) (postoperative) 523.20
    generalized 523.25
    localized 523.24
    minimal 523.21
    moderate 523.22
    servere 523.23

Recklinghausen's disease (M9540/1) 237.71
  bones (osteitis fibrosa cystica) 252.01
Recklinghausen-Applebaum disease
  (hemochromatosis) 275.0
Reclus' disease (cystic) 610.1
Recrudescent typhus (fever) 081.1
Recruitment, auditory 388.44
Rectalgia 569.42
Rectitis 569.49
Rectocele
  female (without uterine prolapse) 618.04
    with uterine prolapse 618.4
      complete 618.3
      incomplete 618.2
  in pregnancy or childbirth 654.4
    causing obstructed labor 660.2
      affecting fetus or newborn 763.1
  male 569.49
  vagina, vaginal (outlet) 618.04
Rectosigmoiditis 569.89
  ulcerative (chronic) 556.3
Rectosigmoid junction —*see* condition
Rectourethral —*see* condition
Rectovaginal —*see* condition
Rectovesical —*see* condition
Rectum, rectal —*see* condition
Recurrent —*see* condition
Red bugs 133.8
Red cedar asthma 495.8
Redness
  conjunctiva 379.93
  eye 379.93
  nose 478.19
Reduced ventilatory or vital capacity 794.2
Reduction
  function
    kidney (*see also* Disease, renal) 593.9
    liver 573.8
  ventilatory capacity 794.2
  vital capacity 794.2
Redundant, redundancy
  abdomen 701.9
  anus 751.5
  cardia 537.89
  clitoris 624.2
  colon (congenital) 751.5
  foreskin (congenital) 605
  intestine 751.5
  labia 624.3
  organ or site, congenital NEC—*see* Accessory
  panniculus (abdominal) 278.1
  prepuce (congenital) 605
  pylorus 537.89
  rectum 751.5
  scrotum 608.89
  sigmoid 751.5
  skin (of face) 701.9
    eyelids 374.30
  stomach 537.89
  uvula 528.9
  vagina 623.8
Reduplication —*see* Duplication
Referral
  adoption (agency) V68.89
  nursing care V63.8
  patient without examination or treatment V68.81
  social services V63.8
Reflex —*see also* condition
  blink, deficient 374.45
  hyperactive gag 478.29
  neurogenic bladder NEC 596.54

Reflex—*continued*
    atonic 596.54
        with cauda equina syndrome 344.61
    vasoconstriction 443.9
Reflux 530.81
    acid 530.81
    esophageal 530.81
    esophagitis 530.11
    gastroesophageal 530.81
    mitral—*see* Insufficiency, mitral
    ureteral —*see* Reflux, vesicoureteral
    vasovagal 780.2
    vesicoureteral 593.70
        with
            reflux nephropathy 593.73
                bilateral 593.72
                unilateral 593.71
Reformed gallbladder 576.0
Reforming, artificial openings (*see also*
    Attention to, artificial, opening) V55.9
Refractive error (*see also* Error, refractive) 367.9
Refsum's disease or syndrome (heredopathia
    atactica polyneuritiformis) 356.3
Refusal of
    food 307.59
        hysterical 300.11
    treatment because of, due to
        patient's decision NEC V64.2
        reason of conscience or religion V62.6
Regaud
    tumor (M8082/3)—*see* Neoplasm, nasopharynx,
        malignant
    type carcinoma (M8082/3)—*see* Neoplasm,
        nasopharynx, malignant
Regional —*see* condition
Regulation feeding (elderly) (infant) 783.3
    newborn 779.31
Regurgitated
    food, choked on 933.1
    stomach contents, choked on 933.1
Regurgitation 787.03
    aortic (valve) (*see also* Insufficiency, aortic) 424.1
        congenital 746.4
        syphilitic 093.22
    food—*see also* Vomiting
        with reswallowing—*see* Rumination
        newborn 779.33
    gastric contents—*see* Vomiting
    heart—*see* Endocarditis
    mitral (valve)—*see also* Insufficiency, mitral
        congenital 746.6
    myocardial—*see* Endocarditis
    pulmonary (heart) (valve) (*see also*
        Endocarditis, pulmonary) 424.3
    stomach—*see* Vomiting
    tricuspid—*see* Endocarditis, tricuspid
    valve, valvular—*see* Endocarditis
    vesicoureteral —*see* Reflux, vesicoureteral
Rehabilitation V57.9
    multiple types V57.89
    occupational V57.21
    specified type NEC V57.89
    speech(-language) V57.3
    vocational V57.22
Reichmann's disease or syndrome
    (gastrosuccorrhea) 536.8
Reifenstein's syndrome (hereditary familial
    hypogonadism, male) 259.52
Reilly's syndrome or phenomenon (*see also*
    Neuropathy, peripheral, autonomic) 337.9
Reimann's periodic disease 277.31

Reinsertion, contraceptive device V25.42
Reiter's disease, syndrome, or urethritis 099.3
    [711.1]
Rejection
    food, hysterical 300.11
    transplant 996.80
        bone marrow 996.85
        corneal 996.51
        organ (immune or nonimmune cause) 996.80
            bone marrow 996.85
            heart 996.83
            intestines 996.87
            kidney 996.81
            liver 996.82
            lung 996.84
            pancreas 996.86
            specified NEC 996.89
        skin 996.52
            artificial 996.55
            decellularized allodermis 996.55
Relapsing fever 087.9
    Carter's (Asiatic) 087.0
    Dutton's (West African) 087.1
    Koch's 087.9
    louse-borne (epidemic) 087.0
    Novy's (American) 087.1
    Obermeyer's (European) 087.0
    Spirillum 087.9
    tick-borne (endemic) 087.1
Relaxation
    anus (sphincter) 569.49
        due to hysteria 300.11
    arch (foot) 734
        congenital 754.61
    back ligaments 728.4
    bladder (sphincter) 596.59
    cardio-esophageal 530.89
    cervix (*see also* Incompetency, cervix) 622.5
    diaphragm 519.4
    inguinal rings—*see* Hernia, inguinal
    joint (capsule) (ligament) (paralytic) (*see also*
        Derangement, joint) 718.90
        congenital 755.8
    lumbosacral joint 724.6
    pelvic floor 618.89
    pelvis 618.89
    perineum 618.89
    posture 729.90
    rectum (sphincter) 569.49
    sacroiliac (joint) 724.6
    scrotum 608.89
    urethra (sphincter) 599.84
    uterus (outlet) 618.89
    vagina (outlet) 618.89
    vesical 596.59
Remains
    canal of Cloquet 743.51
    capsule (opaque) 743.51
Remittent fever (malarial) 084.6
Remnant
    canal of Cloquet 743.51
    capsule (opaque) 743.51
    cervix, cervical stump (acquired) (postoperative)
        622.8
    cystic duct, postcholecystectomy 576.0
    fingernail 703.8
        congenital 757.5
    meniscus, knee 717.5
    thyroglossal duct 759.2
    tonsil 474.8
        infected 474.00
    urachus 753.7

Remote effect of cancer —*see* Condition
Removal (of)
  catheter (urinary) (indwelling) V53.6
    from artificial opening—*see* Attention to,
      artificial, opening
    non-vascular V58.82
    vascular V58.81
  cerebral ventricle (communicating) shunt V53.01
  device—*see also* Fitting (of)
    contraceptive V25.42
    fixation
      external V54.89
      internal V54.01
      traction V54.89
  drains V58.49
  dressing
    wound V58.30
      nonsurgical V58.30
      surgical V58.31
  ileostomy V55.2
  Kirschner wire V54.89
  non-vascular catheter V58.82
  pin V54.01
  plaster cast V54.89
  plate (fracture) V54.01
  rod V54.01
  screw V54.01
  splint, external V54.89
  subdermal implantable contraceptive V25.43
  staples V58.32
  sutures V58.32
  traction device, external V54.89
  vascular catheter V58.81
  wound packing V58.30
    nonsurgical V58.30
    surgical V58.31
Ren
  arcuatus 753.3
  mobile, mobilis (*see also* Disease, renal) 593.0
    congenital 753.3
  unguliformis 753.3
Renal —*see also* condition
  glomerulohyalinosis-diabetic syndrome 250.4
    [581.81]
    due to secondary diabetes 249.4 [581.81]
Rendu-Osler-Weber disease or syndrome
  (familial hemorrhagic telangiectasia) 448.0
Reninoma (M8361/1) 236.91
Rénon-Delille syndrome 253.8
Repair
  pelvic floor, previous, in pregnancy or childbirth
    654.4
    affecting fetus or newborn 763.89
  scarred tissue V51.8
Replacement by artificial or mechanical device
  or prosthesis of (*see also* Fitting (of))
  artificial skin V43.83
  bladder V43.5
  blood vessel V43.4
  breast V43.82
  eye globe V43.0
  heart
    with
      assist device V43.21
      fully implantable artificial heart V43.22
    valve V43.3
  intestine V43.89
  joint V43.60
    ankle 43.66
    elbow V43.62
    finger V43.69
    hip (partial) (total) V43.64

Replacement—*continued*
  joint—*continued*
    knee V43.65
    shoulder V43.61
    specified NEC V43.69
    wrist V43.63
  kidney V43.89
  larynx V43.81
  lens V43.1
  limb(s) V43.7
  liver V43.89
  lung V43.89
  organ NEC V43.89
  pancreas V43.89
  skin (artificial) V43.83
  tissue NEC V43.89
Reprogramming
  cardiac pacemaker V53.31
Request for expert evidence V68.2
Reserve, decreased or low
  cardiac—*see* Disease, heart
  kidney (*see also* Disease, renal) 593.9
Residual —*see also* condition
  bladder 596.8
  foreign body—*see* Retention, foreign body
  state, schizophrenic (*see also* Schizophrenia)
    295.6
  urine 788.69
Resistance, resistant (to)

> Note—Use the following subclassification for
> categories V09.5, V09.7, V09.8, V09.9.:
>
> 0 without mention of resistance to multiple
>   drugs
> 1 with resistance to multiple drugs
>
> V09.5 quinolones and fluoroquinolones
> V09.7 antimycobacterial agents
> V09.8 specified drugs NEC
> V09.9 unspecified drugs
>
> 9 multiple sites

  activated protein C 289.81
  drugs by microorganisms V09.90
    Amikacin V09.4
    aminoglycosides V09.4
    Amodiaquine V09.5
    Amoxicillin V09.0
    Ampicillin V09.0
    antimycobacterial agents V09.7
    Azithromycin V09.2
    Azlocillin V09.0
    Aztreonam V09.1
    B-lactam antibiotics V09.1
    Bacampicillin V09.0
    Bacitracin V09.8
    Benznidazole V09.8
    Capreomycin V09.7
    Carbenicillin V09.0
    Cefaclor V09.1
    Cefadroxil V09.1
    Cefamandole V09.1
    Cefatetan V09.1
    Cefazolin V09.1
    Cefixime V09.1
    Cefonicid V09.1
    Cefoperazone V09.1
    Ceforanide V09.1
    Cefotaxime V09.1
    Cefoxitin V09.1
    Ceftazidine V09.1

Resistance, resistant (to)—*continued*
  drugs by microorganisms—*continued*
    Ceftizoxime V09.1
    Ceftriaxone V09.1
    Cefuroxime V09.1
    Cephalexin V09.1
    Cephaloglycin V09.1
    Cephaloridine V09.1
    cephalosporins V09.1
    Cephalothin V09.1
    Cephapirin V09.1
    Cephradine V09.1
    Chloramphenicol V09.8
    Chloraquine V09.5
    Chlorguanide V09.8
    Chlorproguanil V09.8
    Chlortetracycline V09.3
    Cinoxacin V09.5
    Ciprofloxacin V09.5
    Clarithromycin V09.2
    Clindamycin V09.8
    Clioquinol V09.5
    Clofazimine V09.7
    Cloxacillin V09.0
    Cyclacillin V09.0
    Cycloserine V09.7
    Dapsone [DZ] V09.7
    Demeclocycline V09.3
    Dicloxacillin V09.0
    Doxycycline V09.3
    Enoxacin V09.5
    Erythromycin V09.2
    Ethambutol [EMB] V09.7
    Ethionamide [ETA] V09.7
    fluoroquinolones NEC V09.5
    Gentamicin V09.4
    Halofantrine V09.8
    Imipenem V09.1
    Iodoquinol V09.5
    Isoniazid [INH] V09.7
    Kanamycin V09.4
    macrolides V09.2
    Mafenide V09.6
    MDRO (multiple drug resistant organisms) NOS V09.91
    Mefloquine V09.8
    Melassoprol V09.8
    Methacycline V09.3
    Methenamine V09.8
    Methicillin—*see* Infection, methicillin
    Metronidazole V09.8
    Mezlocillin V09.0
    Minocycline V09.3
    multiple drug resistant organisms NOS V09.91
    Nafcillin V09.0
    Nalidixic Acid V09.5
    Natamycin V09.2
    Neomycin V09.4
    Netilmicin V09.4
    Nimorazole V09.8
    Nitrofurantoin V09.8
    Nitrofurtimox V09.8
    Norfloxacin V09.5
    Nystatin V09.2
    Ofloxacin V09.5
    Oleandomycin V09.2
    Oxacillin V09.0
    Oxytetracycline V09.3
    Para-amino salicylic acid [PAS] V09.7
    Paromomycin V09.4
    Penicillin (G)(V)(VK) V09.0
    penicillins V09.0

Resistance, resistant (to)—*continued*
    Pentamidine V09.8
    Piperacillin V09.0
    Primaquine V09.5
    Proguanil V09.8
    Pyrazinamide [PZA] V09.7
    Pyrimethamine/Sulfalene V09.8
    Pyrimethamine/Sulfodoxine V09.8
    Quinacrine V09.5
    Quinidine V09.8
    Quinine V09.8
    quinolones V09.5
    Rifabutin V09.7
    Rifampin [RIF] V09.7
    Rifamycin V09.7
    Rolitetracycline V09.3
    specified drugs NEC V09.8
    Spectinomycin V09.8
    Spiramycin V09.2
    Streptomycin [SM] V09.4
    Sulfacetamide V09.6
    Sulfacytine V90.6
    Sulfadiazine V09.6
    Sulfadoxine V09.6
    Sulfamethoxazole V09.6
    Sulfapyridine V09.6
    Sulfasalizine V09.6
    Sulfasoxazole V09.6
    sulfonamides V09.6
    Sulfoxone V09.7
    Tetracycline V09.3
    tetracyclines V09.3
    Thiamphenicol V09.8
    Ticarcillin V09.0
    Tinidazole V09.8
    Tobramycin V09.4
    Triamphenicol V09.8
    Trimethoprim V09.8
    Vancomycin V09.8
  insulin 277.7
  thyroid hormone 246.8

Resorption
  biliary 576.8
    purulent or putrid (*see also* Cholecystitis) 576.8
  dental (roots) 521.40
    alveoli 525.8
    pathological
      external 521.42
      internal 521.41
      specified NEC 521.49
    septic—*see* Septicemia
  teeth (roots) 521.40
    pathological
      external 521.42
      internal 521.41
      specified NEC 521.49

Respiration
  asymmetrical 786.09
  bronchial 786.09
  Cheyne-Stokes (periodic respiration) 786.04
  decreased, due to shock following injury 958.4
  disorder of 786.00
    psychogenic 306.1
    specified NEC 786.09
  failure 518.81
    acute 518.81
    acute and chronic 518.84
    chronic 518.83
    newborn 770.84

Reticulation, dust (occupational) 504
Reticulocytosis NEC 790.99
Reticuloendotheliosis
  acute infantile (M9722/3) 202.5
  leukemic (M9940/3) 202.4
  malignant (M9720/3) 202.3
  nonlipid (M9722/3) 202.5
Reticulohistiocytoma (giant cell) 277.89
Reticulohistiocytosis, multicentric 272.8
Reticulolymphosarcoma (diffuse) (M9613/3)
    200.8
  follicular (M9691/3) 202.0
  nodular (M9691/3) 202.0
Reticulosarcoma (M9640/3) 200.0
  odular (M9642/3) 200.0
  pleomorphic cell type (M9641/3) 200.0
Reticulosis (skin)
  acute of infancy (M9722/3) 202.5
  familial hemophagocytic 288.4
  histiocytic medullary (M9721/3) 202.3
  lipomelanotic 695.89
  malignant (M9720/3) 202.3
  Sézary's (M9701/3) 202.2
Retina, retinal —*see* condition
Retinitis (*see also* Chorioretinitis) 363.20
  albuminurica 585.9 *[363.10]*
  arteriosclerotic 440.8 *[362.13]*
  central angiospastic 362.41
  Coat's 362.12
  diabetic 250.5 *[362.01]*
    due to secondary diabetes 249.5 *[362.01]*
  disciformis 362.52
  disseminated 363.10
    metastatic 363.14
    neurosyphilitic 094.83
    pigment epitheliopathy 363.15
  exudative 362.12
  focal 363.00
    in histoplasmosis 115.92
      capsulatum 115.02
      duboisii 115.12
    juxtapapillary 363.05
    macular 363.06
    paramacular 363.06
    peripheral 363.08
    posterior pole NEC 363.07
  gravidarum 646.8
  hemorrhagica externa 362.12
  juxtapapillary (Jensen's) 363.05
  luetic—*see* Retinitis, syphilitic
  metastatic 363.14
  pigmentosa 362.74
  proliferans 362.29
  proliferating 362.29
  punctata albescens 362.76
  renal 585.9 *[363.13]*
  syphilitic (secondary) 091.51
    congenital 090.0 *[363.13]*
    early 091.51
    late 095.8 *[363.13]*
  syphilitica, central, recurrent 095.8 *[363.13]*
  tuberculous (*see also* Tuberculous) 017.3 *[363.13]*
Retinoblastoma (M9510/3) 190.5
  differentiated type (M9511/3) 190.5
  undifferentiated type (M9512/3) 190.5
Retinochoroiditis (*see also* Chorioretinitis) 363.20
  central angiospastic 362.41
  disseminated 363.10
    metastatic 363.14
    neurosyphilitic 094.83
    pigment epitheliopathy 363.15
    syphilitic 094.83

Retinochoroiditis—*continued*
  due to toxoplasmosis (acquired) (focal) 130.2
  focal 363.00
    in histoplasmosis 115.92
      capsulatum 115.02
      duboisii 115.12
    juxtapapillary (Jensen's) 363.05
    macular 363.06
    paramacular 363.06
    peripheral 363.08
    posterior pole NEC 363.07
  juxtapapillaris 363.05
  syphilitic (disseminated) 094.83
Retinopathy (background) 362.10
  arteriosclerotic 440.8 *[362.13]*
  atherosclerotic 440.8 *[362.13]*
  central serous 362.41
  circinate 362.10
  Coat's 362.12
  diabetic 250.5 *[362.01]*
    due to secondary diabetes 249.5 *[362.01]*
    nonproliferative 250.5 *[362.03]*
      due to secondary diabetes 249.5 *[362.03]*
      mild 250.5 *[362.04]*
        due to secondary diabetes 249.5 *[362.04]*
      moderate 250.5 *[362.05]*
        due to secondary diabetes 249.5 *[362.05]*
      severe 250.5 *[362.06]*
        due to secondary diabetes 249.5 *[362.06]*
    proliferative 250.5 *[362.02]*
      due to secondary diabetes 249.5 *[362.02]*
  exudative 362.12
  hypertensive 362.11
  of prematurity 362.20
    cicatricial 362.21
    stage
      0 362.22
      1 362.23
      2 362.24
      3 362.25
      4 362.26
      5 362.27
  nonproliferative
    diabetic 250.5 *[362.03]*
      due to secondary diabetes 249.5 *[362.03]*
      mild 250.5 *[362.04]*
        due to secondary diabetes 249.5 *[362.04]*
      moderate 250.5 *[362.05]*
        due to secondary diabetes 249.5 *[362.05]*
      severe 250.5 *[362.06]*
        due to secondary diabetes 249.5 *[362.06]*
  pigmentary, congenital 362.74
  proliferative 362.29
    diabetic 250.5 *[362.02]*
      due to secondary diabetes 249.5 *[362.02]*
    sickle-cell 282.60 *[362.29]*
  solar 363.31
Retinoschisis 361.10
  bullous 361.12
  congenital 743.56
  flat 361.11
  juvenile 362.73
Retractile testis 752.52
Retraction
  cervix *see* Retraction, uterus
  drum (membrane) 384.82
  eyelid 374.41
  finger 736.29
  head 781.0
  lid 374.41
  lung 518.89

Retraction—*continued*
  mediastinum 519.3
  nipple 611.79
    congenital 757.6
    puerperal, postpartum 676.0
  palmar fascia 728.6
  pleura (*see also* Pleurisy) 511.0
  ring, uterus (Bandl's) (pathological) 661.4
    affecting fetus or newborn 763.7
  sternum (congenital) 756.3
    acquired 738.3
    during respiration 786.9
  substernal 738.3
  supraclavicular 738.8
  syndrome (Duane's) 378.71
  uterus 621.6
  valve (heart)—*see* Endocarditis
Retrobulbar —*see* condition
Retrocaval ureter 753.4
Retrocecal —*see also* condition
  appendix (congenital) 751.5
Retrocession —*see* Retroversion
Retrodisplacement —*see* Retroversion
Retroflection, retroflexion —*see* Retroversion
Retrognathia, retrognathism (mandibular)
  (maxillary) 524.06
Retrograde
  ejaculation 608.87
  menstruation 626.8
Retroiliac ureter 753.4
Retroperineal —*see* condition
Retroperitoneal —*see* condition
Retroperitonitis 567.39
Retropharyngeal —*see* condition
Retroplacental —*see* condition
Retroposition —*see* Retroversion
Retrosternal thyroid (congenital) 759.2
Retroversion, retroverted
  cervix *see* Retroversion, uterus
  female NEC (*see also* Retroversion, uterus) 621.6
  iris 364.70
  testis (congenital) 752.51
  uterus, uterine (acquired) (acute) (adherent) (any
    degree) (asymptomatic) (cervix)
    (postinfectional) (postpartal, old) 621.6
    congenital 752.3
    in pregnancy or childbirth 654.3
      affecting fetus or newborn 763.89
      causing obstructed labor 660.2
        affecting fetus or newborn 763.1
Retrusion, premaxilla (developmental) 524.04
Rett's syndrome 330.8
Reverse, reversed
  peristalsis 787.4
Reye's syndrome 331.81
Reye-Sheehan syndrome (postpartum pituitary
  necrosis) 253.2
Rh (factor)
  hemolytic disease 773.0
  incompatibility, immunization, or sensitization
    affecting management of pregnancy 656.1
    fetus or newborn 773.0
    transfusion reaction 999.7
  negative mother, affecting fetus or newborn
    773.0
  titer elevated 999.7
  transfusion reaction 999.7
Rhabdomyolysis (idiopathic) 728.88

Rhabdomyoma (M8900/0)—*see also* Neoplasm,
  connective tissue, benign
  adult (M8904/0)—*see* Neoplasm, connective
    tissue, benign
  fetal (M8903/0)—*see* Neoplasm, connective
    tissue, benign
  glycogenic (M8904/0)—*see* Neoplasm,
    connective tissue, benign
Rhabdomyosarcoma (M8900/3)—*see also*
  Neoplasm connective tissue, malignant
  alveolar (M8920/3)—*see* Neoplasm, connective
    tissue, malignant
  embryonal (M8910/3)—*see* Neoplasm,
    connective tissue malignant
  mixed type (M8902/3)—*see* Neoplasm,
    connective tissue, malignant
  pleomorphic (M8901/3)—*see* Neoplasm,
    connective tissue, malignant
Rhabdosarcoma (M8900/3)—*see*
  Rhabdomyosarcoma
Rhesus (factor) (Rh) incompatibility—*see* Rh,
  incompatibility
Rheumaticosis —*see* Rheumatism
Rheumatism, rheumatic (acute NEC) 729.0
  adherent pericardium 393
  arthritis
    acute or subacute—*see* Fever, rheumatic
    chronic 714.0
      spine 720.0
  articular (chronic) NEC (*see also* Arthritis)
    716.9
    acute or subacute—*see* Fever, rheumatic
  back 724.9
  blennorrhagic 098.59
  carditis—*see* Disease, heart, rheumatic
  cerebral—*see* Fever, rheumatic
  chorea (acute)—*see* Chorea, rheumatic
  chronic NEC 729.0
  coronary arteritis 391.9
    chronic 398.99
  degeneration, myocardium (*see also*
    Degeneration, myocardium, with rheumatic
    fever) 398.0
  desert 114.0
  febrile—*see* Fever, rheumatic
  fever—*see* Fever, rheumatic
  gonococcal 098.59
  gout 274.0
  heart
    disease (*see also* Disease, heart, rheumatic)
      398.90
    failure (chronic) (congestive) (inactive) 398.91
  hemopericardium—*see* Rheumatic, pericarditis
  hydropericardium—*see* Rheumatic, pericarditis
  inflammatory (acute) (chronic) (subacute)—*see*
    Fever, rheumatic
  intercostal 729.0
    meaning Tietze's disease 733.6
  joint (chronic) NEC (*see also* Arthritis) 716.9
    acute—*see* Fever, rheumatic
  mediastinopericarditis—*see* Rheumatic,
    pericarditis
  muscular 729.0
  myocardial degeneration (*see also*
    Degeneration, myocardium, with rheumatic
    fever) 398.0
  myocarditis (chronic) (inactive) (with chorea)
    398.0
    active or acute 391.2
      with chorea (acute) (rheumatic)
        (Sydenham's) 392.0

Rheumatism, rheumatic—*continued*
  myositis 729.1
  neck 724.9
  neuralgic 729.0
  neuritis (acute) (chronic) 729.2
  neuromuscular 729.0
  nodose—*see* Arthritis, nodosa
  nonarticular 729.0
  palindromic 719.30
    ankle 719.37
    elbow 719.32
    foot 719.37
    hand 719.34
    hip 719.35
    knee 719.36
    multiple sites 719.39
    pelvic region 719.35
    shoulder (region) 719.31
    specified site NEC 719.38
    wrist 719.33
  pancarditis, acute 391.8
    with chorea (acute) (rheumatic) (Sydenham's) 392.0
    chronic or inactive 398.99
  pericarditis (active) (acute) (with effusion) (with pneumonia) 391.0
    with chorea (acute) (rheumatic) (Sydenham's) 392.0
    chronic or inactive 393
  pericardium—*see* Rheumatic, pericarditis
  pleuropericarditis—*see* Rheumatic, pericarditis
  pneumonia 390 *[517.1]*
  pneumonitis 390 *[517.1]*
  pneumopericarditis—*see* Rheumatic, pericarditis
  polyarthritis
    acute or subacute—*see* Fever, rheumatic
    chronic 714.0
  polyarticular NEC (*see also* Arthritis) 716.9
  psychogenic 306.0
  radiculitis 729.2
  sciatic 724.3
  septic—*see* Fever, rheumatic
  spine 724.9
  subacute NEC 729.0
  torticollis 723.5
  tuberculous NEC (*see also* Tuberculosis) 015.9
  typhoid fever 002.0
Rheumatoid —*see also* condition
  lungs 714.81
Rhinitis (atrophic) (catarrhal) (chronic) (croupous) (fibrinous) (hyperplastic) (hypertrophic) (membranous) (purulent) (suppurative) (ulcerative) 472.0
  with
    hay fever (*see also* Fever, hay) 477.9
      with asthma (bronchial) 493.0
    sore throat—*see* Nasopharyngitis
  acute 460
  allergic (nonseasonal) (seasonal) (*see also* Fever, hay) 477.9
    due to food 477.1
    with asthma (*see also* Asthma) 493.0
  granulomatous 472.0
  infective 460
  obstructive 472.0
  pneumococcal 460
  syphilitic 095.8
    congenital 090.0
  tuberculous (*see also* Tuberculosis) 012.8
  vasomotor (*see also* Fever, hay) 477.9

Rhinoantritis (chronic) 473.0
  acute 461.0
Rhinodacryolith 375.57
Rhinolalia (aperta) (clausa) (open) 784.43
Rhinolith 478.19
  nasal sinus (*see also* Sinusitis) 473.9
Rhinomegaly 478.19
Rhinopharyngitis (acute) (subacute) (*see also* Nasopharyngitis) 460
  chronic 472.2
  destructive ulcerating 102.5
  mutilans 102.5
Rhinophyma 695.3
Rhinorrhea 478.19
  cerebrospinal (fluid) 349.81
  paroxysmal (*see also* Fever, hay) 477.9
  spasmodic (*see also* Fever, hay) 477.9
Rhinosalpingitis 381.50
  acute 381.51
  chronic 381.52
Rhinoscleroma 040.1
Rhinosporidiosis 117.0
Rhinovirus infection 079.3
Rhizomelic chrondrodysplasia punctata 277.86
Rhizomelique, pseudopolyarthritic 446.5
Rhoads and Bomford anemia (refractory) 238.72
Rhus
  diversiloba dermatitis 692.6
  radicans dermatitis 692.6
  toxicodendron dermatitis 692.6
  venenata dermatitis 692.6
  verniciflua dermatitis 692.6
Rhythm
  atrioventricular nodal 427.89
  disorder 427.9
    coronary sinus 427.89
    ectopic 427.89
    nodal 427.89
  escape 427.89
  heart, abnormal 427.9
    fetus or newborn—*see* Abnormal, heart rate
  idioventricular 426.89
    accelerated 427.89
  nodal 427.89
  sleep, inversion 327.39
    nonorganic origin 307.45
Rhytidosis facialis 701.8
Rib —*see also* condition
  cervical 756.2
Riboflavin deficiency 266.0
Rice bodies (*see also* Loose, body, joint) 718.1
  knee 717.6
Richter's hernia —*see* Hernia, Richter's
Ricinism 988.2
Rickets (active) (acute) (adolescent) (adult) (chest wall) (congenital) (current) (infantile) (intestinal) 268.0
  celiac 579.0
  fetal 756.4
  hemorrhagic 267
  hypophosphatemic with nephrotic-glycosuric dwarfism 270.0
  kidney 588.0
  late effect 268.1
  renal 588.0
  scurvy 267
  vitamin D-resistant 275.3
Rickettsial disease 083.9
  specified type NEC 083.8

Rickettsialpox 083.2
Rickettsiosis NEC 083.9
  specified type NEC 083.8
  tick-borne 082.9
    specified type NEC 082.8
  vesicular 083.2
Ricord's chancre 091.0
Riddoch's syndrome (visual disorientation) 368.16
Rider's
  bone 733.99
  chancre 091.0
Ridge, alveolus —*see also* condition
  edentulous
    atrophy 525.20
      mandible 525.20
        minimal 525.21
        moderate 525.22
        severe 525.23
      maxilla 525.20
        minimal 525.24
        moderate 525.25
        severe 525.26
    flabby 525.20
Ridged ear 744.29
Riedel's
  disease (ligneous thyroiditis) 245.3
  lobe, liver 751.69
  struma (ligneous thyroiditis) 245.3
  thyroiditis (ligneous) 245.3
Rieger's anomaly or syndrome (mesodermal
  dysgenesis, anterior ocular segment) 743.44
Riehl's melanosis 709.09
Rietti-Greppi-Micheli anemia or syndrome 282.49
Rieux's hernia —*see* Hernia, Rieux's
Rift Valley fever 066.3
Riga's disease (cachectic aphthae) 529.0
Riga-Fede disease (cachectic aphthae) 529.0
Riggs' disease (compound periodontitis) 523.40
Right middle lobe syndrome 518.0
Rigid, rigidity —*see also* condition
  abdominal 789.4
  articular, multiple congenital 754.89
  back 724.8
  cervix uteri
    in pregnancy or childbirth 654.6
      affecting fetus or newborn 763.89
      causing obstructed labor 660.2
        affecting fetus or newborn 763.1
  hymen (acquired) (congenital) 623.3
  nuchal 781.6
  pelvic floor
    in pregnancy or childbirth 654.4
      affecting fetus or newborn 763.89
      causing obstructed labor 660.2
        affecting fetus or newborn 763.1
  perineum or vulva
    in pregnancy or childbirth 654.8
      affecting fetus or newborn 763.89
      causing obstructed labor 660.2
        affecting fetus or newborn 763.1
  spine 724.8
  vagina
    in pregnancy or childbirth 654.7
      affecting fetus or newborn 763.89
      causing obstructed labor 660.2
        affecting fetus or newborn 763.1
Rigors 780.99
Riley-Day syndrome (familial dysautonomia) 742.8
RIND (reversible ischemic neurological deficit)
  434.91
  history of personal V12.54

Ring(s)
  aorta 747.21
  Bandl's, complicating delivery 661.4
    affecting fetus or newborn 763.7
  contraction, complicating delivery 661.4
    affecting fetus or newborn 763.7
  esophageal (congenital) 750.3
  Fleischer (-Kayser) (cornea) 275.1 *[371.14]*
  hymenal, tight (acquired) (congenital) 623.3
  Kayser-Fleischer (cornea) 275.1 *[371.14]*
  retraction, uterus, pathological 661.4
    affecting fetus or newborn 763.7
  Schatzki's (esophagus) (congenital) (lower) 750.3
    acquired 530.3
  Soemmering's 366.51
  trachea, abnormal 748.3
  vascular (congenital) 747.21
  Vossius' 921.3
    late effect 366.21
Ringed hair (congenital) 757.4
Ringing in the ear (*see also* Tinnitus) 388.30
Ringworm 110.9
  beard 110.0
  body 110.5
  Burmese 110.9
  corporeal 110.5
  foot 110.4
  groin 110.3
  hand 110.2
  honeycomb 110.0
  nails 110.1
  perianal (area) 110.3
  scalp 110.0
  specified site NEC 110.8
  Tokelau 110.5
Rise, venous pressure 459.89
Risk
  factor —*see* Problem
  falling V15.88
  suicidal 300.9
Ritter's disease (dermatitis exfoliativa
  neonatorum) 695.81
Rivalry, sibling 313.3
Rivalta's disease (cervicofacial actinomycosis)
  039.3
River blindness 125.3 *[360.13]*
Robert's pelvis 755.69
  with disproportion (fetopelvic) 653.0
    affecting fetus or newborn 763.1
    causing obstructed labor 660.1
      affecting fetus or newborn 763.1
Robin's syndrome 756.0
Robinson's (hidrotic) ectodermal dysplasia 757.31
Robles' disease (onchocerciasis) 125.3 *[360.13]*
Rochalimea —*see* Rickettsial disease
Rocky Mountain fever (spotted) 082.0
Rodent ulcer 9M8090/3)—*see also* Neoplasm,
  skin, malignant
  cornea 370.07
Roentgen ray, adverse effect —*see* Effect,
  adverse, x-ray
Roetheln 056.9
Roger's disease (congenital interventricular
  septal defect) 745.4
Rokitansky's
  disease (*see also* Necrosis, liver) 570
  tumor 620.2
Rokitansky-Aschoff sinuses (mucosal
  outpouching of gallbladder) (*see also* Disease,
  gallbladder) 575.8

Rokitansky-Kuster-Hauser syndrome
(congenital absence vagina) 752.49
Rollet's chancre (syphilitic) 091.0
Rolling of head 781.0
Romano-Ward syndrome (prolonged QT
interval syndrome) 426.82
Romanus lesion 720.1
Romberg's disease or syndrome 349.89
Roof, mouth —*see* condition
Rosacea 695.3
acne 695.3
keratitis 695.3 *[370.49]*
Rosary, rachitic 268.0
Rose
cold 477.0
fever 477.0
rash 782.1
epidemic 056.9
of infants 057.8
Rosen-Castleman-Liebow syndrome
(pulmonary proteinosis) 516.0
Rosenbach's erysipelatoid or erysipeloid 027.1
Rosenthal's disease (factor XI deficiency) 286.2
Roseola 057.8
infantum, infantilis (*see also* Exanthem subitum)
058.10
Rossbach's disease (hyperchlorhydria) 536.8
psychogenic 306.4
Rössle-Urbach-Wiethe lipoproteinosis 272.8
Ross river fever 066.3
Rostan's asthma (cardiac) (*see also* Failure,
ventricular, left) 428.1
Rot
Barcoo (*see also* Ulcer, skin) 707.9
knife-grinders' (*see also* Tuberculosis) 011.4
Rot-Bernhardt disease 355.1
Rotation
anomalous, incomplete or insufficient—*see*
Malrotation
cecum (congenital) 751.4
colon (congenital) 751.4
manual, affecting fetus or newborn 763.89
spine, incomplete or insufficient 737.8
tooth, teeth 524.35
vertebra, incomplete or insufficient 737.8
Röteln 056.9
Roth's disease or meralgia 355.1
Roth-Bernhardt disease or syndrome 355.1
Rothmund (-Thomson) syndrome 757.33
Rotor's disease or syndrome (idiopathic
hyperbilirubinemia) 277.4
Rotundum ulcus —*see* Ulcer, stomach
Round
back (with wedging of vertebrae) 737.10
late effect of rickets 268.1
hole, retina 361.31
with detachment 361.01
ulcer (stomach)—*see* Ulcer, stomach
worms (infestation) (large) NEC 127.0
Roussy-Lévy syndrome 334.3
Routine postpartum follow-up V24.2
Roy (-Jutras) syndrome (acropachyderma) 757.39
Rubella (German measles) 056.9
complicating pregnancy, childbirth, or
puerperium 647.5
complication 056.8
neurological 056.00
encephalomyelitis 056.01
specified type NEC 056.09
specified type NEC 056.79

Rubella—*continued*
congenital 771.0
contact V01.4
exposure to V01.4
maternal
with suspected fetal damage affecting
management of pregnancy 655.3
affecting fetus or newborn 760.2
manifest rubella in infant 771.0
specified complications NEC 056.79
vaccination, prophylactic (against) V04.3
Rubeola (measles) (*see also* Measles) 055.9
complicated 055.8
meaning rubella (*see also* Rubella) 056.9
scarlatinosis 057.8
Rubeosis iridis 364.42
diabetica 250.5 *[364.42]*
due to secondary diabetes 249.5 *[364.42]*
Rubinstein-Taybi's syndrome (brachydactylia,
short stature and mental retardation) 759.89
Rud's syndrome (mental deficiency, epilepsy,
and infantilism) 759.89
Rudimentary (congenital)—*see also* Agenesis
arm 755.22
bone 756.9
cervix uteri 752.49
eye (*see also* Microphthalmos) 743.10
fallopian tube 752.19
leg 755.32
lobule of ear 744.21
patella 755.64
respiratory organs in thoracopagus 759.4
tracheal bronchus 748.3
uterine horn 752.3
uterus 752.3
in male 752.7
solid or with cavity 752.3
vagina 752.49
Ruiter-Pompen (-Wyers) syndrome
(angiokeratoma corporis diffusum) 272.7
Ruled out condition (*see also* Observation,
suspected) V71.9
Rumination —*see also* Vomiting
disorder 307.53
neurotic 300.3
obsessional 300.3
psychogenic 307.53
Runaway reaction —*see also* Disturbance,
conduct
socialized 312.2
undersocialized, unsocialized 312.1
Runeberg's disease (progressive pernicious
anemia) 281.0
Runge's syndrome (postmaturity) 766.22
Runny nose 784.99
Rupia 091.3
congenital 090.0
tertiary 095.9
Rupture, ruptured 553.9
abdominal viscera NEC 799.89
obstetrical trauma 665.5
abscess (spontaneous)—*see* Abscess, by site
amnion—*see* Rupture, membranes
aneurysm—*see* Aneurysm
anus (sphincter)—*see* Laceration, anus

Rupture, ruptured—*continued*
aorta, aortic 441.5
  abdominal 441.3
  arch 441.1
  ascending 441.1
  descending 441.5
   abdominal 441.3
   thoracic 441.1
  syphilitic 093.0
  thoracoabdominal 441.6
  thorax, thoracic 441.1
  transverse 441.1
  traumatic (thoracic) 901.0
   abdominal 902.0
  valve or cusp (*see also* Endocarditis, aortic) 424.1
appendix (with peritonitis) 540.0
  traumatic—*see* Injury, internal,
   gastrointestinal tract
  with peritoneal abscess 540.1
arteriovenous fistula, brain (congenital) 430
artery 447.2
  brain (*see also* Hemorrhage, brain) 431
  coronary (*see also* Infarct, myocardium) 410.9
  heart (*see also* Infarct, myocardium) 410.9
  pulmonary 417.8
  traumatic (complication) (*see also* Injury,
   blood vessel, by site) 904.9
bile duct, except cystic (*see also* Disease,
  biliary) 576.3
  cystic 575.4
  traumatic—*see* Injury, internal,
   intra-abdominal
bladder (sphincter) 596.6
  with
   abortion—*see* Abortion, by type, with
    damage to pelvic organs
   ectopic pregnancy (*see also* categories
    633.0-633.9) 639.2
   molar pregnancy (*see also* categories
    630-632) 639.2
  following
   abortion 639.2
   ectopic or molar pregnancy 639.2
  nontraumatic 596.6
  obstetrical trauma 665.5
  spontaneous 596.6
  traumatic—*see* Injury, internal, bladder
blood vessel (*see also* Hemorrhage) 459.0
  brain (*see also* Hemorrhage, brain) 431
  heart (*see also* Infarct, myocardium) 410.9
  traumatic (complication) (*see also* Injury,
   blood vessel, by site) 904.9
bone—*see* Fracture, by site
bowel 569.89
  traumatic—*see* Injury, internal, intestine
Bowman's membrane 371.31
brain
  aneurysm (congenital) (*see also* Hemorrhage,
   subarachnoid) 430
  late effect—*see* Late effect(s) (of)
   cerebrovascular disease
   syphilitic 094.87
  hemorrhagic (*see also* Hemorrhage, brain) 431
  injury at birth 767.0
  syphilitic 094.89
capillaries 448.9
cardiac (*see also* Infarct, myocardium) 410.9
cartilage (articular) (current)—*see also* Sprain,
  by site
  knee—*see* Tear, meniscus
  semilunar—*see* Tear, meniscus

Rupture, ruptured—*continued*
cecum (with peritonitis) 540.0
  traumatic 863.89
   with open wound into cavity 863.99
  with peritoneal abscess 540.1
cerebral aneurysm (congenital) (*see also*
  Hemorrhage, subarachnoid) 430
  late effect—*see* Late effect(s) (of)
   cerebrovascular disease
cervix (uteri)
  with
   abortion—*see* Abortion, by type, with
    damage to pelvic organs
   ectopic pregnancy (*see also* categories
    633.0-633.9) 639.2
   molar pregnancy (*see also* categories
    630-632) 639.2
  following
   abortion 639.2
   ectopic or molar pregnancy 639.2
  obstetrical trauma 665.3
  traumatic—*see* Injury, internal, cervix
chordae tendineae 429.5
choroid (direct) (indirect) (traumatic) 363.63
circle of Willis (*see also* Hemorrhage,
  subarachnoid) 430
  late effect—*see* Late effect(s) (of)
   cerebrovascular disease
colon 569.89
  traumatic—*see* Injury, internal, colon
cornea (traumatic)—*see also* Rupture, eye
  due to ulcer 370.00
coronary (artery) (thrombotic) (*see also* Infarct,
  myocardium) 410.9
corpus luteum (infected) (ovary) 620.1
cyst—*see* Cyst
cystic duct (*see also* Disease, gallbladder) 575.4
Descemet's membrane 371.33
  traumatic—*see* Rupture, eye
diaphragm—*see also* Hernia, diaphragm
  traumatic—*see* Injury, internal, diaphragm
diverticulum
  bladder 596.3
  intestine (large) (*see also* Diverticula) 562.10
   small 562.00
duodenal stump 537.89
duodenum (ulcer)—*see* Ulcer, duodenum, with
  perforation
ear drum (*see also* Perforation, tympanum) 384.20
  with otitis media—*see* Otitis media
  traumatic—*see* Wound, open, ear
esophagus 530.4
  traumatic 862.22
   with open wound into cavity 862.32
   cervical region—*see* Wound, open,
    esophagus
eye (without prolapse of intraocular tissue)
  871.0
  with
   exposure of intraocular tissue 871.1
   partial loss of intraocular tissue 871.2
   prolapse of intraocular tissue 871.1
  due to burn 940.5
fallopian tube 620.8
  due to pregnancy—*see* Pregnancy, tubal
  traumatic—*see* Injury, internal, fallopian tube
fontanel 767.3
free wall (ventricle) (*see also* Infarct,
  myocardium) 410.9
gallbladder or duct (*see also* Disease,
  gallbladder) 575.4
  traumatic—*see* Injury, internal, gallbladder

Rupture, ruptured—*continued*
gastric (*see also* Rupture, stomach) 537.89
  vessel 459.0
globe (eye) (traumatic)—*see* Rupture, eye
graafian follicle (hematoma) 620.0
heart (auricle) (ventricle) (*see also* Infarct,
  myocardium) 410.9
  infectional 422.90
  traumatic—*see* Rupture, myocardium,
    traumatic
hymen 623.8
internal
  organ, traumatic—*see also* Injury, internal, by
    site
    heart—*see* Rupture, myocardium, traumatic
    kidney—*see* Rupture, kidney
    liver—*see* Rupture, liver
    spleen—*see* Rupture, spleen, traumatic
  semilunar cartilage—*see* Tear, meniscus
intervertebral disc—*see* Displacement,
  intervertebral disc
  traumatic (current)—*see* Dislocation, vertebra
intestine 569.89
  traumatic—*see* Injury, internal, intestine
intracranial, birth injury 767.0
iris 364.76
  traumatic—*see* Rupture, eye
joint capsule—*see* Sprain, by site
kidney (traumatic) 866.03
  with open wound into cavity 866.13
  due to birth injury 767.8
  nontraumatic 593.89
lacrimal apparatus (traumatic) 870.2
lens (traumatic) 366.20
ligament—*see also* Sprain, by site
  with open wound—*see* Wound, open, by site
  old (*see also* Disorder, cartilage, articular)
    718.0
liver (traumatic) 864.04
  with open wound into cavity 864.14
  due to birth injury 767.8
  nontraumatic 573.8
lymphatic (node) (vessel) 457.8
marginal sinus (placental) (with hemorrhage)
  641.2
  affecting fetus or newborn 762.1
meaning hernia—*see* Hernia
membrana tympani (*see also* Perforation,
  tympanum) 384.20
  with otitis media—*see* Otitis media
  traumatic—*see* Wound, open, ear
membranes (spontaneous)
  artificial
    delayed delivery following 658.3
      affecting fetus or newborn 761.1
    fetus or newborn 761.1
  delayed delivery following 658.2
    affecting fetus or newborn 761.1
  premature (less than 24 hours prior to onset of
    labor) 658.1
    affecting fetus or newborn 761.1
    delayed delivery following 658.2
      affecting fetus or newborn 761.1
meningeal artery (*see also* Hemorrhage,
  subarachnoid) 430
  late effect—*see* Late effect(s) (of)
    cerebrovascular disease
meniscus (knee)—*see also* Tear, meniscus
  old (*see also* Derangement, meniscus) 717.5
    site other than knee—*see* Disorder, cartilage,
      articular
  site other than knee—*see* Sprain, by site

Rupture, ruptured—*continued*
mesentery 568.89
  traumatic—*see* Injury, internal, mesentery
mitral—*see* Insufficiency, mitral
muscle (traumatic) NEC—*see also* Sprain, by
  site
  with open wound—*see* Wound, open, by site
  nontraumatic 728.83
musculotendinous cuff (nontraumatic)
  (shoulder) 840.4
mycotic aneurysm, causing cerebral hemorrhage
  (*see also* Hemorrhage, subarachnoid) 430
  late effect—*see* Late effect(s) (of)
    cerebrovascular disease
myocardium, myocardial (*see also* Infarct,
  myocardium) 410.9
  traumatic 861.03
    with open wound into thorax 861.13
nontraumatic (meaning hernia) (*see also* Hernia,
  by site) 553.9
  obstructed (*see also* Hernia, by site, with
    obstruction) 552.9
  gangrenous (*see also* Hernia, by site, with
    gangrene) 551.9
operation wound (*see also* Dehiscence) 998.32
  internal 998.31
ovary, ovarian 620.8
  corpus luteum 620.1
  follicle (graafian) 620.0
oviduct 620.8
  due to pregnancy—*see* Pregnancy, tubal
pancreas 577.8
  traumatic—*see* Injury, internal, pancreas
papillary muscle (ventricular) 429.6
pelvic
  floor, complicating delivery 664.1
  organ NEC—*see* Injury, pelvic, organs
penis (traumatic)—*see* Wound, open, penis
perineum 624.8
  during delivery (*see also* Laceration,
    perineum, complicating delivery) 664.4
pharynx (nontraumatic) (spontaneous) 478.29
pregnant uterus (before onset of labor) 665.0
prostate (traumatic)—*see* Injury, internal,
  prostate
pulmonary
  artery 417.8
  valve (heart) (*see also* Endocarditis,
    pulmonary) 424.3
  vein 417.8
  vessel 417.8
pupil, sphincter 364.75
pus tube (*see also* Salpingo-oophoritis) 614.2
pyosalpinx (*see also* Salpingo-oophoritis) 614.2
rectum 569.49
  traumatic—*see* Injury, internal, rectum
retina, retinal (traumatic) (without detachment)
  361.30
  with detachment (*see also* Detachment, retina,
    with retinal defect) 361.00
rotator cuff (capsule) (traumatic) 840.4
  nontraumatic, complete 727.61
sclera 871.0
semilunar cartilage, knee (*see also* Tear,
  meniscus) 836.2
  old (*see also* Derangement, meniscus) 717.5
septum (cardiac) 410.8
sigmoid 569.89
  traumatic—*see* Injury, internal, colon, sigmoid
sinus of Valsalva 747.29

Rupture, ruptured—*continued*
spinal cord—*see also* Injury, spinal, by site
  due to injury at birth 767.4
  fetus or newborn 767.4
  syphilitic 094.89
  traumatic—*see also* Injury, spinal, by site
    with fracture—*see* Fracture, vertebra, by
      site, with spinal cord injury
spleen 289.59
  congenital 767.8
  due to injury at birth 767.8
  malarial 084.9
  nontraumatic 289.59
  spontaneous 289.59
  traumatic 865.04
    with open wound into cavity 865.14
splenic vein 459.0
stomach 537.89
  due to injury at birth 767.8
  traumatic—*see* Injury, internal, stomach
  ulcer—*see* Ulcer, stomach, with perforation
synovium 727.50
  specified site NEC 727.59
tendon (traumatic)—*see also* Sprain, by site
  with open wound—*see* Wound, open, by site
  Achilles 845.09
    nontraumatic 727.67
  ankle 845.09
    nontraumatic 727.68
  biceps (long head) 840.8
    nontraumatic 727.62
  foot 845.10
    interphalangeal (joint) 845.13
    metatarsophalangeal (joint) 845.12
    nontraumatic 727.68
    specified site NEC 845.19
    tarsometatarsal (joint) 845.11
  hand 842.10
    carpometacarpal (joint) 842.11
    interphalangeal (joint) 842.13
    metacarpophalangeal (joint) 842.12
    nontraumatic 727.63
      extensors 727.63
      flexors 727.64
    specified site NEC 842.19
  nontraumatic 727.60
    specified site NEC 727.69
  patellar 844.8
    nontraumatic 727.66
  quadriceps 844.8
    nontraumatic 727.65
  rotator cuff (capsule) 840.4
    nontraumatic, complete 727.61
  wrist 842.00
    carpal (joint) 842.01
    nontraumatic 727.63
      extensors 727.63
      flexors 727.64
    radiocarpal (joint) (ligament) 842.02
    radioulnar (joint), distal 842.09
    specified site NEC 842.09
testis (traumatic) 878.2
  complicated 878.3
  due to syphilis 095.8
thoracic duct 457.8
tonsil 474.8

Rupture, ruptured—*continued*
traumatic
  with open wound—*see* Wound, open, by site
  aorta—*see* Rupture, aorta, traumatic
  ear drum—*see* Wound, open, ear, drum
  external site—*see* Wound, open, by site
  eye 871.2
  globe (eye)—*see* Wound, open, eyeball
  internal organ (abdomen, chest, or
    pelvis)—*see* Injury, internal, by site
    heart—*see* Rupture, myocardium, traumatic
    kidney—*see* Rupture, kidney
    liver—*see* Rupture, liver
    spleen—*see* Rupture, spleen, traumatic
  ligament, muscle, or tendon—*see also* Sprain,
    by site
    with open wound—*see* Wound, open, by site
  meaning hernia—*see* Hernia
tricuspid (heart) (valve)—*see* Endocarditis,
  tricuspid
tube, tubal 620.8
  abscess (*see also* Salpingo-oophoritis) 614.2
  due to pregnancy—*see* Pregnancy, tubal
tympanum, tympanic (membrane) (*see also*
  Perforation, tympanum) 384.20
  with otitis media—*see* Otitis media
  traumatic—*see* Wound, open, ear, drum
umbilical cord 663.8
  fetus or newborn 772.0
ureter (traumatic) (*see also* Injury, internal,
  ureter) 867.2
  nontraumatic 593.89
urethra 599.84
  with
    abortion—*see* Abortion, by type, with
      damage to pelvic organs
    ectopic pregnancy (*see also* categories
      633.0-633.9) 639.2
    molar pregnancy (*see also* categories
      630-632) 639.2
  following
    abortion 639.2
    ectopic or molar pregnancy 639.2
  obstetrical trauma 665.5
  traumatic—*see* Injury, internal urethra
uterosacral ligament 620.8
uterus (traumatic)—*see also* Injury, internal
  uterus
  affecting fetus or newborn 763.89
  during labor 665.1
  nonpuerperal, nontraumatic 621.8
  nontraumatic 621.8
  pregnant (during labor) 665.1
    before labor 665.0
vaginal 878.6
  complicated 878.7
  complicating delivery—*see* Laceration,
    vagina, complicating delivery
valve, valvular (heart)—*see* Endocarditis
varicose vein—*see* Varicose, vein
varix—*see* Varix
vena cava 459.0
ventricle (free wall) (left) (*see also* Infarct,
  myocardium) 410.9
vesical (urinary) 596.6
  traumatic—*see* Injury, internal, bladder
vessel (blood) 459.0
  pulmonary 417.8
viscus 799.89
vulva 878.4
  complicated 878.5
  complicating delivery 664.0

Russell's dwarf (uterine dwarfism and
    craniofacial dysostosis) 759.89
Russell's dysentery 004.8
Russell (-Silver) syndrome (congenital
    hemihypertrophy and short stature) 759.89
Russian spring-summer type encephalitis 063.0
Rust's disease (tuberculous spondylitis) 015.0
    [720.81]
Rustitskii's disease (multiple myeloma)
    (M9730/3) 203.0
Ruysch's disease (Hirschsprung's disease) 751.3
Rytand-Lipsitch syndrome (complete
    atrioventricular block) 426.0

S

Saber
shin 090.5
tibia 090.5
Sac, lacrimal —*see* condition
Saccharomyces infection (*see also* Candidiasis) 112.9
Saccharopinuria 270.7
Saccular —*see* condition
Sacculation
aorta (nonsyphilitic) (*see also* Aneurysm, aorta) 441.9
ruptured 441.5
syphilitic 093.0
bladder 596.3
colon 569.89
intralaryngeal (congenital) (ventricular) 748.3
larynx (congenital) (ventricular) 748.3
organ or site, congenital—*see* Distortion
pregnant uterus, complicating delivery 654.4
affecting fetus or newborn 763.1
causing obstructed labor 660.2
affecting fetus or newborn 763.1
rectosigmoid 569.89
sigmoid 569.89
ureter 593.89
urethra 599.2
vesical 596.3
Sachs (-Tay) disease (amaurotic familial idiocy) 330.1
Sacks-Libman disease 710.0 *[424.91]*
Sacralgia 724.6
Sacralization
fifth lumbar vertebra 756.15
incomplete (vertebra) 756.15
Sacrodynia 724.6
Sacroiliac joint —*see* condition
Sacroiliitis NEC 720.2
Sacrum —*see* condition
Saddle
back 737.8
embolus, aorta 444.0
nose 738.0
congenital 754.0
due to syphilis 090.5
Sadism (sexual) 302.84
Saemisch's ulcer 370.04
Saenger's syndrome 379.46
Sago spleen 277.39
Sailors' skin 692.74
Saint
Anthony's fire (*see also* Erysipelas) 035
Guy's dance—*see* Chorea
Louis-type encephalitis 062.3
triad (*see also* Hernia, diaphragm) 553.3
Vitus' dance—*see* Chorea
Salicylism
correct substance properly administered 535.4
overdose or wrong substance given or taken 965.1
Salivary duct or gland —*see also* condition
virus disease 078.5
Salivation (excessive) (*see also* Ptyalism) 527.7
Salmonella (aertrycke) (choleraesuis) (enteritidis) (gallinarum) (suipestifer) (typhimurium) (*see also* Infection, Salmonella) 003.9
arthritis 003.23
carrier (suspected) of V02.3

Salmonella—*continued*
meningitis 003.21
osteomyelitis 003.24
pneumonia 003.22
septicemia 003.1
typhosa 002.0
carrier (suspected) of V02.1
Salmonellosis 003.0
with pneumonia 003.22
Salpingitis (catarrhal) (fallopian tube) (nodular) (pseudofollicular) (purulent) (septic) (*see also* Salpingo-oophoritis) 614.2
ear 381.50
acute 381.51
chronic 381.52
Eustachian (tube) 381.50
acute 381.51
chronic 381.52
follicularis 614.1
gonococcal (chronic) 098.37
acute 098.17
interstitial, chronic 614.1
isthmica nodosa 614.1
old—*see* Salpingo-oophoritis, chronic
puerperal, postpartum, childbirth 670.8
specific (chronic) 098.37
acute 098.17
tuberculous (acute) (chronic) (*see also* Tuberculosis) 016.6
venereal (chronic) 098.37
acute 098.17
Salpingocele 620.4
Salpingo-oophoritis (catarrhal) (purulent) (ruptured) (septic) (suppurative) 614.2
acute 614.0
with
abortion—*see* Abortion, by type, with sepsis
ectopic pregnancy (*see also* categories 633.0-633.9) 639.0
molar pregnancy (*see also* categories 630-632) 639.0
following
abortion 639.0
ectopic or molar pregnancy 639.0
gonococcal 098.17
puerperal, postpartum, childbirth 670.8
tuberculous (*see also* Tuberculosis) 016.6
chronic 614.1
gonococcal 098.37
tuberculous (*see also* Tuberculosis) 016.6
complicating pregnancy 646.6
affecting fetus or newborn 760.8
gonococcal (chronic) 098.37
acute 098.17
old—*see* Salpingo-oophoritis, chronic
puerperal 670.8
specific—*see* Salpingo-oophoritis, gonococcal
subacute (*see also* Salpingo-oophoritis, acute) 614.0
tuberculous (acute) (chronic) (*see also* Tuberculosis) 016.6
venereal—*see* Salpingo-oophoritis, gonococcal
Salpingo-ovaritis (*see also* Salpingo-oophoritis) 614.2
Salpingoperitonitis (*see also* Salpingo-oophoritis) 614.2

Salt-losing
nephritis (*see also* Disease, renal) 593.9
syndrome (*see also* Disease, renal) 593.9
Salt-rheum (*see also* Eczema) 692.9
Salzmann's nodular dystrophy 371.46
Sampling chorionic villus V28.89
Sampson's cyst or tumor 617.1
Sandblasters'
asthma 502
lung 502
Sander's disease (paranoia) 297.1
Sandfly fever 066.0
Sandhoff's disease 330.1
Sanfilippo's syndrome (mucopolysaccharidosis III) 277.5
Sanger-Brown's ataxia 334.2
San Joaquin Valley fever 114.0
São Paulo fever or typhus 082.0
Saponification, mesenteric 567.89
Sapremia —*see* Septicemia
Sarcocele (benign)
syphilitic 095.8
congenital 090.5
Sarcoepiplocele (*see also* Hernia) 553.9
Sarcoepiplomphalocele (*see also* Hernia, umbilicus) 553.1
Sarcoid (any site) 135
with lung involvement 135 *[517.8]*
Boeck's 135
Darier-Roussy 135
Spiegler-Fendt 686.8
Sarcoidosis 135
cardiac 135 *[425.8]*
lung 135 *[517.8]*
Sarcoma (M8800/3)—*see also* Neoplasm, connective tissue, malignant
alveolar soft part (M9581/3)—*see* Neoplasm, connective tissue, malignant
ameloblastic (M9330/3) 170.1
upper jaw (bone) 170.0
botryoid (M8910/3)—*see* Neoplasm, connective tissue, malignant
botryoides (M8910/3)—*see* Neoplasm, connective tissue, malignant
cerebellar (M9480/3) 191.6
circumscribed (arachnoidal) (M9471/3) 191.6
circumscribed (arachnoidal) cerebellar (M9471/3) 191.6
clear cell, of tendons and aponeuroses (M9044/3)—*see* Neoplasm, connective tissue, malignant
embryonal (M8991/3)—*see* Neoplasm, connective tissue, malignant
endometrial (stromal) (M8930/3) 182.0
isthmus 182.1
endothelial (M9130/3)—*see also* Neoplasm, connective tissue, malignant
bone (M9260/3)—*see* Neoplasm, bone, malignant
epithelioid cell (M8804/3)—*see* Neoplasm, connective tissue, malignant
Ewing's (M9260/3)—*see* Neoplasm, bone, malignant
follicular dendritic cell 202.9
germinoblastic (diffuse) (M9632/3) 202.8
follicular (M9697/3) 202.0
giant cell (M8802/3)—*see also* Neoplasm, connective tissue, malignant
bone (M9250/3)—*see* Neoplasm, bone, malignant

Sarcoma—*continued*
glomoid (M8710/3)—*see* Neoplasm, connective tissue, malignant
granulocytic (M9930/3) 205.3
hemangioendothelial (M9130/3)—*see* Neoplasm, connective tissue, malignant
hemorrhagic, multiple (M9140/3)—*see* Kaposi's, sarcoma
Hodgkin's (M9662/3) 201.2
immunoblastic (M9612/3) 200.8
interdigitating dendritic cell 202.9
Kaposi's (M9140/3)—*see* Kaposi's, sarcoma
Kupffer cell (M9124/3) 155.0
Langerhans cell 202.9
leptomeningeal (M9530/3)—*see* Neoplasm, meninges, malignant
lymphangioendothelial (M9170/3)—*see* Neoplasm, connective tissue, malignant
lymphoblastic (M9630/3) 200.1
lymphocytic (M9620/3) 200.1
mast cell (M9740/3) 202.6
melanotic (M8720/3)—*see* Melanoma
meningeal (M9530/3)—*see* Neoplasm, meninges, malignant
meningothelial (M9530/3)—*see* Neoplasm, meninges, malignant
mesenchymal (M8800/3)—*see also* Neoplasm, connective tissue, malignant
mixed (M8990/3)—*see* Neoplasm, connective tissue, malignant
mesothelial (M9050/3)—*see* Neoplasm, by site, malignant
monstrocellular (M9481/3)
specified site—*see* Neoplasm, by site, malignant
unspecified site 191.9
myeloid (M9930/3) 205.3
neurogenic (M9540/3)—*see* Neoplasm, connective tissue, malignant
odontogenic (M9270/3) 170.1
upper jaw (bone) 170.0
osteoblastic (M9180/3)—*see* Neoplasm, bone, malignant
osteogenic (M9180/3)—*see also* Neoplasm, bone, malignant
juxtacortical (M9190/3)—*see* Neoplasm, bone, malignant
periosteal (M9190/3)—*see* Neoplasm, bone, malignant
periosteal (M8812/3)—*see also* Neoplasm, bone, malignant
osteogenic (M9190/3)—*see* Neoplasm, bone, malignant
plasma cell (M9731/3) 203.8
pleomorphic cell (M8802/3)—*see* Neoplasm, connective tissue, malignant
reticuloendothelial (M9720/3) 202.3
reticulum cell (M9640/3) 200.0
nodular (M9642/3) 200.0
pleomorphic cell type (M9641/3) 200.0
round cell (M8803/3)—*see* Neoplasm, connective tissue, malignant
small cell (M8803/3)—*see* Neoplasm, connective tissue, malignant
spindle cell (M8801/3)—*see* Neoplasm, connective tissue, malignant
stromal (endometrial) (M8930/3) 182.0
isthmus 182.1
synovial (M9040/3)—*see also* Neoplasm, connective tissue, malignant
biphasic type (M9043/3)—*see* Neoplasm, connective tissue, malignant

Sarcoma—*continued*
  epithelioid cell type (M9042/3)—*see*
    Neoplasm, connective tissue, malignant
  spindle cell type (M9041/3)—*see* Neoplasm,
    connective tissue, malignant
Sarcomatosis
  meningeal (M9539/3)—*see* Neoplasm,
    meninges, malignant
  specified site NEC (M8800/3)—*see* Neoplasm,
    connective tissue, malignant
  unspecified site (M8800/6) 171.9
Sarcosinemia 270.8
Sarcosporidiosis 136.5
Satiety, early 780.94
Satisfactory smear but lacking transformation
    zone
  anal 796.77
  cervical 795.07
Saturnine —*see* condition
Saturnism 984.9
  specified type of lead—*see* Table of drugs and
    chemicals
Satyriasis 302.89
Sauriasis —*see* Ichthyosis
Sauriderma 757.39
Sauriosis —*see* Ichthyosis
Savill's disease (epidemic exfoliative dermatitis)
    695.89
SBE (subacute bacterial endocarditis) 421.0
Scabies (any site) 133.0
Scabs 782.8
Scaglietti-Dagnini syndrome (acromegalic
    macrospondylitis) 253.0
Scald, scalded —*see also* Burn, by site
  skin syndrome 695.81
Scalenus anticus (anterior) syndrome 353.0
Scales 782.8
Scalp —*see* condition
Scaphocephaly 756.0
Scaphoiditis, tarsal 732.5
Scapulalgia 733.90
Scapulohumeral myopathy 359.1
Scar, scarring (*see also* Cicatrix) 709.2
  adherent 709.2
  atrophic 709.2
  cervix
    in pregnancy or childbirth 654.6
      affecting fetus or newborn 763.89
      causing obstructed labor 660.2
        affecting fetus or newborn 763.1
  cheloid 701.4
  chorioretinal 363.30
    disseminated 363.35
    macular 363.32
    peripheral 363.34
    posterior pole NEC 363.33
  choroid (*see also* Scar, chorioretinal) 363.30
  compression, pericardial 423.9
  congenital 757.39
  conjunctiva 372.64
  cornea 371.00
    xerophthalmic 264.6
  due to previous cesarean delivery, complicating
    pregnancy or childbirth 654.2
    affecting fetus or newborn 763.89
  duodenal (bulb) (cap) 537.3
  hypertrophic 701.4
  keloid 701.4
  labia 624.4
  lung (base) 518.89

Scar, scarring—*continued*
  macula 363.32
    disseminated 363.35
    peripheral 363.34
  muscle 728.89
  myocardium, myocardial 412
  painful 709.2
  papillary muscle 429.81
  posterior pole NEC 363.33
    macular—*see* Scar, macula
  postnecrotic (hepatic) (liver) 571.9
  psychic V15.49
  retina (*see also* Scar, chorioretinal) 363.30
  trachea 478.9
  uterus 621.8
    in pregnancy or childbirth NEC 654.9
      affecting fetus or newborn 763.89
      due to previous cesarean delivery 654.2
  vulva 624.4
Scarabiasis 134.1
Scarlatina 034.1
  anginosa 034.1
  maligna 034.1
  myocarditis, acute 034.1 *[422.0]*
    old (*see also* Myocarditis) 429.0
  otitis media 034.1 *[382.02]*
  ulcerosa 034.1
Scarlatinella 057.8
Scarlet fever (albuminuria) (angina)
    (convulsions) (lesions of lid) (rash) 034.1
Schamberg's disease, dermatitis, or dermatosis
    (progressive pigmentary dermatosis) 709.09
Schatzki's ring (esophagus) (lower) (congenital)
    750.3
  acquired 530.3
Schaufenster krankheit 413.9
Schaumann's
  benign lymphogranulomatosis 135
  disease (sarcoidosis) 135
  syndrome (sarcoidosis) 135
Scheie's syndrome (mucopolysaccharidosis IS)
    277.5
Schenck's disease (sporotrichosis) 117.1
Scheuermann's disease or osteochondrosis
    732.0
Scheuthauer-Marie-Sainton syndrome
    (cleidocranialis dysostosis) 755.59
Schilder (-Flatau) disease 341.1
Schilling-type monocytic leukemia (M9890/3)
    206.9
**Schimmelbusch's disease, cystic mastitis, or hy-
    perplasia** 610.1
Schirmer's syndrome (encephalocutaneous
    angiomatosis) 759.6
Schistocelia 756.79
Schistoglossia 750.13
Schistosoma infestation —*see* Infestation,
    Schistosoma
Schistosomiasis 120.9
  Asiatic 120.2
  bladder 120.0
  chestermani 120.8
  colon 120.1
  cutaneous 120.3
  due to
    S. hematobium 120.0
    S. japonicum 120.2
    S. mansoni 120.1
    S. mattheii 120.8
  eastern 120.2
  genitourinary tract 120.0

Schistosomiasis—*continued*
  intestinal 120.1
  lung 120.2
  Manson's (intestinal) 120.1
  Oriental 120.2
  pulmonary 120.2
  specified type NEC 120.8
  vesical 120.0
Schizencephaly 742.4
Schizo-affective psychosis (*see also*
    Schizophrenia) 295.7
Schizodontia 520.2
Schizoid personality 301.20
  introverted 301.21
  schizotypal 301.22
Schizophrenia, schizophrenic (reaction) 295.9

> *Note—Use the following fifth-digit subclassification with category 295:*
>
> 0 *unspecified*
> 1 *subchronic*
> 2 *chronic*
> 3 *subchronic with acute exacerbation*
> 4 *chronic with acute exacerbation*
> 5 *in remission*

  acute (attack) NEC 295.8
    episode 295.4
  atypical form 295.8
  borderline 295.5
  catalepsy 295.2
  catatonic (type) (acute) (excited) (withdrawn) 295.2
  childhood (type) (*see also* Psychosis, childhood) 299.9
  chronic NEC 295.6
  coenesthesiopathic 295.8
  cyclic (type) 295.7
  disorganized (type) 295.1
  flexibilitas cerea 295.2
  hebephrenic (type) (acute) 295.1
  incipient 295.5
  latent 295.5
  paranoid (type) (acute) 295.3
  paraphrenic (acute) 295.3
  prepsychotic 295.5
  primary (acute) 295.0
  prodromal 295.5
  pseudoneurotic 295.5
  pseudopsychopathic 295.5
  reaction 295.9
  residual type (state) 295.6
  restzustand 295.6
  schizo-affective (type) (depressed) (excited) 295.7
  schizophreniform type 295.4
  simple (type) (acute) 295.0
  simplex (acute) 295.0
  specified type NEC 295.8
  syndrome of childhood NEC (*see also* Psychosis, childhood) 299.9
  undifferentiated type 295.9
    acute 295.8
    chronic 295.6
Schizothymia 301.20
  introverted 301.21
  schizotypal 301.22
Schlafkrankheit 086.5
Schlatter's tibia (osteochondrosis) 732.4
Schlatter-Osgood disease (osteochondrosis, tibial tubercle) 732.4

Schloffer's tumor (*see also* Peritonitis) 567.29
Schmidt's syndrome
  sphallo-pharyngo-laryngeal hemiplegia 352.6
  thyroid-adrenocortical insufficiency 258.1
  vagoaccessory 352.6
Schmincke
  carcinoma (M8082/3)—*see* Neoplasm, nasopharynx, malignant
  tumor (M8082/3)—*see* Neoplasm, nasopharynx, malignant
Schmitz (-Stutzer) dysentery 004.0
Schmorl's disease or nodes 722.30
  lumbar, lumbosacral 722.32
  specified region NEC 722.39
  thoracic, thoracolumbar 722.31
Schneider's syndrome 047.9
Schneiderian
  carcinoma (M8121/3)
    specified site—*see* Neoplasm, by site, malignant
    unspecified site 160.0
  papilloma (M8121/0)
    specified site—*see* Neoplasm, by site, benign
    unspecified site 212.0
Schnitzler syndrome 273.1
Schoffer's tumor (*see also* Peritonitis) 567.29
Scholte's syndrome (malignant carcinoid) 259.2
Scholz's disease 330.0
Scholz (-Bielschowsky-Henneberg) syndrome 330.0
Schönlein (-Henoch) disease (primary) (purpura) (rheumatic) 287.0
School examination V70.3
  following surgery V67.09
Schottmüller's disease (*see also* Fever, paratyphoid) 002.9
Schroeder's syndrome (endocrine-hypertensive) 255.3
Schüller-Christian disease or syndrome (chronic histiocytosis X) 277.89
Schultz's disease or syndrome (agranulocytosis) 288.09
Schultze's acroparesthesia, simple 443.89
Schwalbe-Ziehen-Oppenheimer disease 333.6
Schwannoma (M9560/0)—*see also* Neoplasm, connective tissue, benign
  malignant (M9560/3)—*see* Neoplasm, connective tissue, malignant
Schwartz (-Jampel) syndrome 359.23
Schwartz-Bartter syndrome (inappropriate secretion of antidiuretic hormone) 253.6
Schweninger-Buzzi disease (macular atrophy) 701.3
Sciatic —*see* condition
Sciatica (infectional) 724.3
  due to
    displacement of intervertebral disc 722.10
    herniation, nucleus pulposus 722.10
  wallet 724.3
Scimitar syndrome (anomalous venous drainage, right lung to inferior vena cava) 747.49
Sclera —*see* condition
Sclerectasia 379.11
Scleredema
  adultorum 710.1
  Buschke's 710.1
  newborn 778.1
Sclerema
  adiposum (newborn) 778.1
  adultorum 710.1
  edematosum (newborn) 778.1
  neonatorum 778.1
  newborn 778.1

Scleriasis —*see* Scleroderma
Scleritis 379.00
　with corneal involvement 379.05
　anterior (annular) (localized) 379.03
　brawny 379.06
　granulomatous 379.09
　posterior 379.07
　specified NEC 379.09
　suppurative 379.09
　syphilitic 095.0
　tuberculous (nodular) (*see also* Tuberculosis)
　　017.3 *[379.09]*
Sclerochoroiditis (*see also* Scleritis) 379.00
Scleroconjunctivitis (*see also* Scleritis) 379.00
Sclerocystic ovary (syndrome) 256.4
Sclerodactylia 701.0
Scleroderma, sclerodermia (acrosclerotic)
　(diffuse) (generalized) (progressive)
　(pulmonary) 710.1
　circumscribed 701.0
　linear 701.0
　localized (linear) 701.0
　newborn 778.1
Sclerokeratitis 379.05
　meaning sclerosing keratitis 370.54
　tuberculous (*see also* Tuberculosis) 017.3
　　[379.09]
Scleroma, trachea 040.1
Scleromalacia
　multiple 731.0
　perforans 379.04
Scleromyxedema 701.8
Scleroperikeratitis 379.05
Sclerose en plaques 340
Sclerosis, sclerotic
　adrenal (gland) 255.8
　Alzheimer's 331.0
　　with dementia—*see* Alzheimer's, demential
　amyotrophic (lateral) 335.20
　annularis fibrosi
　　aortic 424.1
　　mitral 424.0
　aorta, aortic 440.0
　　valve (*see also* Endocarditis, aortic) 424.1
　artery, arterial, arteriolar, arteriovascular—*see*
　　Arteriosclerosis
　ascending multiple 340
　Baló's (concentric) 341.1
　basilar—*see* Sclerosis, brain
　bone (localized) NEC 733.99
　brain (general) (lobular) 348.89
　　Alzheimer's—*see* Alzheimer's dementia
　　artery, arterial 437.0
　　atrophic lobar 331.0
　　　with dementia
　　　　with behavioral disturbance 331.0
　　　　　[294.11]
　　　　without behavioral disturbance 331.0
　　　　　[294.10]
　　diffuse 341.1
　　　familial (chronic) (infantile) 330.0
　　　infantile (chronic) (familial) 330.0
　　　Pelizaeus-Merzbacher type 330.0
　　disseminated 340
　　hereditary 334.2
　　hippocampal 348.81
　　infantile, (degenerative) (diffuse) 330.0
　　insular 340
　　Krabbe's 330.0
　　mesial temporal 348.81
　　miliary 340

Sclerosis, sclerotic—*continued*
　brain—*continued*
　　multiple 340
　　Pelizaeus-Merzbacher 330.0
　　progressive familial 330.0
　　senile 437.0
　　temporal 348.81
　　　mesial 348.81
　　tuberous 759.5
　bulbar, progressive 340
　bundle of His 426.50
　　left 426.3
　　right 426.4
　cardiac—*see* Arteriosclerosis, coronary
　cardiorenal (*see also* Hypertension, cardiorenal)
　　404.90
　cardiovascular (*see also* Disease,
　　cardiovascular) 429.2
　　renal (*see also* Hypertension, cardiorenal)
　　　404.90
　centrolobar, familial 330.0
　cerebellar—*see* Sclerosis, brain
　cerebral—*see* Sclerosis, brain
　cerebrospinal 340
　　disseminated 340
　　multiple 340
　cerebrovascular 437.0
　choroid 363.40
　　diffuse 363.56
　combined (spinal cord)—*see also* Degeneration,
　　combined
　　multiple 340
　concentric, Baló's 341.1
　cornea 370.54
　coronary (artery) —*see* Arteriosclerosis,
　　coronary
　corpus cavernosum
　　female 624.8
　　male 607.89
　Dewitzky's
　　aortic 424.1
　　mitral 424.0
　diffuse NEC 341.1
　disease, heart —*see* Arteriosclerosis, coronary
　disseminated 340
　dorsal 340
　dorsolateral (spinal cord)—*see* Degeneration,
　　combined
　endometrium 621.8
　extrapyramidal 333.90
　eye, nuclear (senile) 366.16
　Friedreich's (spinal cord) 334.0
　funicular (spermatic cord) 608.89
　gastritis 535.4
　general (vascular)—*see* Arteriosclerosis
　gland (lymphatic) 457.8
　hepatic 571.9
　hereditary
　　cerebellar 334.2
　　spinal 334.0
　hippocampal 348.81
　idiopathic cortical (Garré's) (*see also*
　　Osteomyelitis) 730.1
　ilium, piriform 733.5
　insular 340
　　pancreas 251.8
　Islands of Langerhans 251.8
　kidney—*see* Sclerosis, renal
　larynx 478.79

Sclerosis, sclerotic—*continued*
  lateral 335.24
    amyotrophic 335.20
    descending 335.24
    primary 335.24
    spinal 335.24
  liver 571.9
  lobar, atrophic (of brain) 331.0
    with dementia
      with behavioral disturbance 331.0 *[294.11]*
      without behavioral disturbance 331.0 *[294.10]*
  lung (*see also* Fibrosis, lung) 515
  mastoid 383.1
  mesial temporal 348.81
  mitral—*see* Endocarditis, mitral
  Mönckeberg's (medial) (*see also*
    Arteriosclerosis, extremities) 440.20
  multiple (brain stem) (cerebral) (generalized)
    (spinal cord) 340
  myocardium, myocardial —*see*
    Arteriosclerosis, coronary
  nuclear (senile), eye 366.16
  ovary 620.8
  pancreas 577.8
  penis 607.89
  peripheral arteries NEC (*see also*
    Arteriosclerosis, extremities) 440.20
  plaques 340
  pluriglandular 258.8
  polyglandular 258.8
  posterior (spinal cord) (syphilitic) 094.0
  posterolateral (spinal cord)—*see* Degeneration,
    combined
  prepuce 607.89
  primary lateral 335.24
  progressive systemic 710.1
  pulmonary (*see also* Fibrosis, lung) 515
    artery 416.0
    valve (heart) (*see also* Endocarditis,
      pulmonary) 424.3
  renal 587
    with
      cystine storage disease 270.0
      hypertension (*see also* Hypertension,
        kidney) 403.90
      hypertensive heart disease (conditions
        classifiable to 402) (*see also*
        Hypertension, cardiorenal) 404.90
      arteriolar (hyaline) (*see also* Hypertension,
        kidney) 403.90
      hyperplastic (*see also* Hypertension, kidney)
        403.90
  retina (senile) (vascular) 362.17
  rheumatic
    aortic valve 395.9
    mitral valve 394.9
  Schilder's 341.1
  senile—*see* Arteriosclerosis
  spinal (cord) (general) (progressive) (transverse)
    336.8
    ascending 357.0
    combined—*see also* Degeneration, combined
      multiple 340
      syphilitic 094.89
    disseminated 340
    dorsolateral—*see* Degeneration, combined
    hereditary (Friedreich's) (mixed form) 334.0
    lateral (amyotrophic) 335.24
    multiple 340
    posterior (syphilitic) 094.0
  stomach 537.89

Sclerosis, sclerotic—*continued*
  subendocardial, congenital 425.3
  systemic (progressive) 710.1
    with lung involvement 710.1 *[517.2]*
  temporal 348.81
    mesial 348.81
  tricuspid (heart) (valve)—*see* Endocarditis,
    tricuspid
  tuberous (brain) 759.5
  tympanic membrane (*see also*
    Tympanosclerosis) 385.00
  valve, valvular (heart)—*see* Endocarditis
  vascular—*see* Arteriosclerosis
  vein 459.89
Sclerotenonitis 379.07
Sclerotitis (*see also* Scleritis) 379.00
  syphilitic 095.0
  tuberculous (*see also* Tuberculosis) 017.3 *[379.09]*
Scoliosis (acquired) (postural) 737.30
  congenital 754.2
  due to or associated with
    Charcot-Marie-Tooth disease 356.1 *[737.43]*
    mucopolysaccharidosis 277.5 *[737.43]*
    neurofibromatosis 237.71 *[737.43]*
    osteitis
      deformans 731.0 *[737.43]*
      fibrosa cystica 252.01 *[737.43]*
    osteoporosis (*see also* Osteoporosis) 733.00
      [737.43]
    poliomyelitis 138 *[737.43]*
    radiation 737.33
    tuberculosis (*see also* Tuberculosis) 015.0
      [737.43]
  idiopathic 737.30
    infantile
      progressive 737.32
      resolving 737.31
  paralytic 737.39
  rachitic 268.1
  sciatic 724.3
  specified NEC 737.39
  thoracogenic 737.34
  tuberculous (*see also* Tuberculosis) 015.0 *[737.43]*
Scoliotic pelvis 738.6
  with disproportion (fetopelvic) 653.0
    affecting fetus or newborn 763.1
    causing obstructed labor 660.1
      affecting fetus or newborn 763.1
Scorbutus, scorbutic 267
  anemia 281.8
Scotoma (ring) 368.44
  arcuate 368.43
  Bjerrum 368.43
  blind spot area 368.42
  central 368.41
  centrocecal 368.41
  paracecal 368.42
  paracentral 368.41
  scintillating 368.12
  Seidel 368.43
Scratch —*see* Injury, superficial, by site
Scratchy throat 784.99
Screening (for) V82.9
  alcoholism V79.1
  anemia, deficiency NEC V78.1
    iron V78.0
  anomaly, congenital V82.89
  antenatal, of mother V28.9
    alphafetoprotein levels, raised V28.1
    based on amniocentesis V28.2
      chromosomal anomalies V28.0
      raised alphafetoprotein levels V28.1

Screening (for)—*continued*
  hormones in athletes V70.3
  HPV (human papillomavirus) V73.81
  human papillomavirus (HPV) V73.81
  hypercholesterolemia V77.91
  hyperlipidemia V77.91
  hypertension V81.1
  immunity disorder NEC V77.99
  inborn errors of metabolism NEC V77.7
  infection
    bacterial V74.9
      specified type NEC V74.8
    mycotic V75.4
    parasitic NEC V75.8
  infectious disease V75.9
    specified type NEC V75.8
  ingestion of radioactive substance V82.5
  intestinal helminthiasis V75.7
  iron deficiency anemia V78.0
  ischemic heart disease V81.0
  lead poisoning V82.5
  leishmaniasis V75.2
  leprosy V74.2
  leptospirosis V74.8
  leukemia V76.89
  lipoid disorder NEC V77.91
  lymphoma V76.89
  malaria V75.1
  malignant neoplasm (of) V76.9
    bladder V76.3
    blood V76.89
    breast V76.10
      mammogram NEC V76.12
        for high-risk patient V76.11
      specified type NEC V76.19
    cervix V76.2
    colon V76.51
    colorectal V76.51
    hematopoietic system V76.89
    intestine V76.50
      colon V76.51
      small V76.52
    lung V76.0
    lymph (glands) V76.89
    nervous system V76.81
    oral cavity V76.42
    other specified neoplasm NEC V76.89
    ovary V76.46
    prostate V76.44
    rectum V76.41
    respiratory organs V76.0
    skin V76.43
    specified sites NEC V76.49
    testis V76.45
    vagina V76.47
      following hysterectomy for malignant
        condition V67.01
  malnutrition V77.2
  mammogram NEC V76.12
    for high-risk patient V76.11
  maternal postnatal chromosomal anomalies V82.4
  measles V73.2
  mental
    disorder V79.9
      specified type NEC V79.8
    retardation V79.2
  metabolic errors, inborn V77.7
  metabolic disorder NEC V77.99
  mucoviscidosis V77.6
  multiphasic V82.6

Screening (for)—*continued*
  mycosis V75.4
  mycotic infection V75.4
  nephropathy V81.5
  neurological condition NEC V80.09
  nutritional disorder V77.99
    obesity V77.8
  obesity V77.8
  osteoporosis V82.81
  parasitic infection NEC V75.8
  phenylketonuria V77.3
  plague V74.8
  poisoning
    chemical NEC V82.5
    contaminated water supply V82.5
    heavy metal V82.5
  poliomyelitis V73.0
  postnatal chromosomal anomalies, maternal V82.4
  prenatal—*see* Screening, antenatal
  pulmonary tuberculosis V74.1
  radiation exposure V82.5
  renal disease V81.5
  respiratory condition NEC V81.4
  rheumatic disorder NEC V82.2
  rheumatoid arthritis V82.1
  rickettsial disease V75.0
  rubella V73.3
  schistosomiasis V75.5
  senile macular lesions of eye V80.2
  sexually transmitted diseases V74.5
    bacterial V74.5
    spirochetal V74.5
  sickle-cell anemia, disease, or trait V78.2
  skin condition V82.0
  sleeping sickness V75.3
  smallpox V73.1
  special V82.9
    specified condition NEC V82.89
  specified type NEC V82.89
  spirochetal disease V74.9
    sexually transmitted V74.5
    specified type NEC V74.8
  stimulants in athletes V70.3
  syphilis V74.5
  tetanus V74.8
  thyroid disorder V77.0
  trachoma V73.6
  traumatic brain injury V80.01
  trypanosomiasis V75.3
  tuberculosis, pulmonary V74.1
  venereal disease V74.5
  viral encephalitis
    mosquito-borne V73.5
    tick-borne V73.5
  whooping cough V74.8
  worms, intestinal V75.7
  yaws V74.6
  yellow fever V73.4
Scrofula (*see also* Tuberculosis) 017.2
Scrofulide (primary) (*see also* Tuberculosis) 017.0
Scrofuloderma, scrofulodermia (any site)
  (primary) (*see also* Tuberculosis) 017.0
Scrofulosis (universal) (*see also* Tuberculosis)
  017.2
Scrofulosis lichen (primary) (*see also*
  Tuberculosis) 017.0
Scrofulous —*see* condition
Scrotal tongue 529.5
  congenital 750.13
Scrotum —*see* condition
Scurvy (gum) (infantile) (rickets) (scorbutic) 267
Sea-blue histiocyte syndrome 272.7

Seabright-Bantam syndrome
(pseudohypoparathyroidism) 275.49
Sealpox 059.12
Seasickness 994.6
Seatworm 127.4
Sebaceous
cyst (*see also* Cyst, sebaceous) 706.2
gland disease NEC 706.9
Sebocystomatosis 706.2
Seborrhea, seborrheic 706.3
adiposa 706.3
capitis 690.11
congestiva 695.4
corporis 706.3
dermatitis 690.10
infantile 690.12
diathesis in infants 695.89
eczema 690.18
infantile 690.12
keratosis 702.19
inflamed 702.11
nigricans 705.89
sicca 690.18
wart 702.19
inflamed 702.11
Seckel's syndrome 759.89
Seclusion pupil 364.74
Seclusiveness, child 313.22
Secondary —*see also* condition
neoplasm—*see* Neoplasm, by site, malignant,
secondary
Secretan's disease or syndrome (posttraumatic
edema) 782.3
Secretion
antidiuretic hormone, inappropriate (syndrome)
253.6
catecholamine, by pheochromocytoma 255.6
hormone
antidiuretic, inappropriate (syndrome) 253.6
by
carcinoid tumor 259.2
pheochromocytoma 255.6
ectopic NEC 259.3
urinary
excessive 788.42
suppression 788.5
Section
cesarean
affecting fetus or newborn 763.4
post mortem, affecting fetus or newborn 761.6
previous, in pregnancy or childbirth 654.2
affecting fetus or newborn 763.89
nerve, traumatic—*see* Injury, nerve, by site
Seeligmann's syndrome (ichthyosis congenita)
757.1
Segmentation, incomplete (congenital)—*see
also* Fusion
bone NEC 756.9
lumbosacral (joint) 756.15
vertebra 756.15
lumbosacral 756.15
Seizure(s) 780.39
akinetic (idiopathic) (*see also* Epilepsy) 345.0
psychomotor 345.4
apoplexy, apoplectic (*see also* Disease,
cerebrovascular, acute) 436
atonic (*see also* Epilepsy) 345.0
autonomic 300.11
brain or cerebral (*see also* Disease,
cerebrovascular, acute) 436
convulsive (*see also* Convulsions) 780.39

Seizure(s)—*continued*
cortical (focal) (motor) (*see also* Epilepsy) 345.5
disorder (see also Epilepsy) 345.9
due to stroke 438.89
epilepsy, epileptic (cryptogenic) (*see also*
Epilepsy) 345.9
epileptiform, epileptoid 780.39
focal (*see also* Epilepsy) 345.5
febrile (simple) 780.31
atypical 780.32
complex 780.32
complicated 780.32
with status epilepticus 345.3
heart—*see* Disease, heart
hysterical 300.11
Jacksonian (focal) (*see also* Epilepsy) 345.5
motor type 345.5
sensory type 345.5
migraine triggered 346.0
newborn 779.0
paralysis (*see also* Disease, cerebrovascular,
acute) 436
recurrent 345.9
epileptic—*see* Epilepsy
repetitive 780.39
epileptic—*see* Epilepsy
salaam (*see also* Epilepsy) 345.6
uncinate (*see also* Epilepsy) 345.4
Self-mutilation 300.9
Semicoma 780.09
Semiconsciousness 780.09
Seminal
vesicle—*see* condition
vesiculitis (*see also* Vesiculitis) 608.0
Seminoma (M9061/3)
anaplastic type (M9062/3)
specified site—*see* Neoplasm, by site,
malignant
unspecified site 186.9
specified site—*see* Neoplasm, by site, malignant
spermatocytic (M9063/3)
specified site—*see* Neoplasm, by site,
malignant
unspecified site 186.9
unspecified site 186.9
Semliki Forest encephalitis 062.8
Senear-Usher disease or syndrome (pemphigus
erythematosus) 694.4
Senecio jacobae dermatitis 692.6
Senectus 797
Senescence 797
Senile (*see also* condition) 797
cervix (atrophic) 622.8
degenerative atrophy, skin 701.3
endometrium (atrophic) 621.8
fallopian tube (atrophic) 620.3
heart (failure) 797
lung 492.8
ovary (atrophic) 620.3
syndrome 259.8
vagina, vaginitis (atrophic) 627.3
wart 702.0
Senility 797
with
acute confusional state 290.3
delirium 290.3
mental changes 290.9
psychosis NEC (*see also* Psychosis, senile) 290.20
premature (syndrome) 259.8

Sensation
burning (*see also* Disturbance, sensation) 782.0
tongue 529.6
choking 784.99
loss of (*see also* Disturbance, sensation) 782.0
prickling (*see also* Disturbance, sensation) 782.0
tingling (*see also* Disturbance, sensation) 782.0
Sense loss (touch) (*see also* Disturbance, sensation) 782.0
smell 781.1
taste 781.1
Sensibility disturbance NEC (cortical) (deep) (vibratory) (*see also* Disturbance, sensation) 782.0
Sensitive dentine 521.89
Sensitiver Beziehungswahn 297.8
Sensitivity, sensitization —*see also* Allergy
autoerythrocyte 287.2
carotid sinus 337.01
child (excessive) 313.21
cold, autoimmune 283.0
methemoglobin 289.7
suxamethonium 289.89
tuberculin, without clinical or radiological symptoms 795.5
Sensory
extinction 781.8
neglect 781.8
Separation
acromioclavicular—see Dislocation, shoulder
anxiety, abnormal 309.21
apophysis, traumatic—*see* Fracture, by site
choroid 363.70
hemorrhagic 363.72
serous 363.71
costochondral (simple) (traumatic)—*see* Dislocation, costochondral
delayed
umbilical cord 779.83
epiphysis, epiphyseal
nontraumatic 732.9
upper femoral 732.2
traumatic—*see* Fracture, by site
fracture—*see* Fracture, by site
infundibulum cardiac from right ventricle by a partition 746.83
joint (current) (traumatic)—*see* Dislocation, by site
placenta (normally implanted)—*see* Placenta, separation
pubic bone, obstetrical trauma 665.6
retina, retinal (*see also* Detachment, retina) 361.9
layers 362.40
sensory (*see also* Retinoschisis) 361.10
pigment epithelium (exudative) 362.42
hemorrhagic 362.43
sternoclavicular (traumatic)—*see* Dislocation, sternoclavicular
symphysis pubis, obstetrical trauma 665.6
tracheal ring, incomplete (congenital) 748.3
Sepsis (generalized) 995.91
with
abortion—*see* Abortion, by type, with sepsis
acute organ dysfunction 995.92
ectopic pregnancy (*see also* categories 633.0-633.9) 639.0
molar pregnancy (*see also* categories 630-632) 639.0
multiple organ dysfunction (MOD) 995.92
buccal 528.3
complicating labor 659.3
dental (pulpal origin) 522.4

Sepsis—*continued*
female genital organ NEC 614.9
fetus (intrauterine) 771.81
following
abortion 639.0
ectopic or molar pregnancy 639.0
infusion, perfusion, or transfusion 999.39
Friedländer's 038.49
intraocular 360.00
localized
in operation wound 998.59
skin (*see also* Abscess) 682.9
malleus 024
newborn (organism unspecified) NEC 771.81
oral 528.3
puerperal, postpartum, childbirth (pelvic) 670.2
resulting from infusion, injection, transfusion, or vaccination 999.39
severe 995.92
skin, localized (*see also* Abscess) 682.9
umbilical (newborn) (organism unspecified) 771.89
tetanus 771.3
urinary 599.0
meaning sepsis 995.91
meaning urinary tract infection 599.0
Septate —*see also* Septum
Septic —*see also* condition
adenoids 474.01
and tonsils 474.02
arm (with lymphangitis) 682.3
embolus—*see* Embolism
finger (with lymphangitis) 681.00
foot (with lymphangitis) 682.7
gallbladder (*see also* Cholecystitis) 575.8
hand (with lymphangitis) 682.4
joint (*see also* Arthritis, septic) 711.0
kidney (*see also* Infection, kidney) 590.9
leg (with lymphangitis) 682.6
mouth 528.3
nail 681.9
finger 681.02
toe 681.11
shock (endotoxic) 785.52
sore (*see also* Abscess) 682.9
throat 034.0
milk-borne 034.0
streptococcal 034.0
spleen (acute) 289.59
teeth (pulpal origin) 522.4
throat 034.0
thrombus—*see* Thrombosis
toe (with lymphangitis) 681.10
tonsils 474.00
and adenoids 474.02
umbilical cord (newborn) (organism unspecified) 771.89
uterus (*see also* Endometritis) 615.9
Septicemia, septicemic (generalized) (suppurative) 038.9
with
abortion—*see* Abortion, by type, with sepsis
ectopic pregnancy (*see also* categories 633.0-633.9) 639.0
molar pregnancy (*see also* categories 630-632) 639.0
Aerobacter aerogenes 038.49
anaerobic 038.3
anthrax 022.3
Bacillus coli 038.42
Bacteroides 038.3
Clostridium 038.3

Septicemia—*continued*
complicating labor 659.3
cryptogenic 038.9
enteric gram-negative bacilli 038.40
Enterobacter aerogenes 038.49
Erysipelothrix (insidiosa) (rhusiopathiae) 027.1
Escherichia coli 038.42
following
  abortion 639.0
  ectopic or molar pregnancy 639.0
  infusion, injection, transfusion, or vaccination
    999.39
Friedländer's (bacillus) 038.49
gangrenous 038.9
gonococcal 098.89
gram-negative (organism) 038.40
  anaerobic 038.3
Hemophilus influenzae 038.41
herpes (simplex) 054.5
herpetic 054.5
Listeria monocytogenes 027.0
meningeal—*see* Meningitis
meningococcal (chronic) (fulminating) 036.2
methicillin
  resistant Staphylococcus aureus (MRSA) 038.12
  susceptible Staphylococcus aureus (MSSA)
    038.11
MRSA (methicillin resistant Staphylococcus
  aureus) 038.12
MSSA (methicillin susceptible Staphylococcus
  aureus) 038.11
navel, newborn (organism unspecified) 771.89
newborn (organism unspecified) 771.81
plague 020.2
pneumococcal 038.2
postabortal 639.0
postoperative 998.59
Proteus vulgaris 038.49
Pseudomonas (aeruginosa) 038.43
puerperal, postpartum 670.2
Salmonella (aertrycke) (callinarum)
  (choleraesuis) (enteritidis) (suipestifer) 003.1
Serratia 038.44
Shigella (*see also* Dysentery, bacillary) 004.9
specified organism NEC 038.8
staphylococcal 038.10
  aureus 038.11
    methicillin
      resistant (MRSA) 038.12
      susceptible (MSSA) 038.11
  specified organism NEC 038.19
streptococcal (anaerobic) 038.0
suipestifer 003.1
umbilicus, newborn (organism unspecified) 771.89
viral 079.99
Yersinia enterocolitica 038.49
Septum, septate (congenital)—*see also*
  Anomaly, specified type NEC
anal 751.2
aqueduct of Sylvius 742.3
  with spina bifida (*see also* Spina bifida) 741.0
hymen 752.49
uterus (*see also* Double, uterus) 752.2
vagina 752.49
  in pregnancy or childbirth 654.7
    affecting fetus or newborn 763.89
    causing obstructed labor 660.2
      affecting fetus or newborn 763.1

Sequestration
lung (congenital) (extralobar) (intralobar) 748.5
orbit 376.10
pulmonary artery (congenital) 747.3
splenic 289.52
Sequestrum
bone (*see also* Osteomyelitis) 730.1
  jaw 526.4
dental 525.8
jaw bone 526.4
sinus (accessory) (nasal) (*see also* Sinusitis) 473.9
  maxillary 473.0
Sequoiosis asthma 495.8
Serology for syphilis
doubtful
  with signs or symptoms—*see* Syphilis, by site
    and stage
  follow-up of latent syphilis—*see* Syphilis, latent
false positive 795.6
negative, with signs or symptoms—*see* Syphilis,
  by site and stage
positive 097.1
  with signs or symptoms—*see* Syphilis, by site
    and stage
  false 795.6
  follow-up of latent syphilis—*see* Syphilis, latent
  only finding—*see* Syphilis, latent
reactivated 097.1
Seroma (postoperative) (non-infected) 998.13
infected 998.51
post-traumatic 729.91
Seropurulent —*see* condition
Serositis, multiple 569.89
pericardial 423.2
peritoneal 568.82
pleural—*see* Pleurisy
Serotonin syndrome 333.99
Serous —*see* condition
Sertoli cell
adenoma (M8640/0)
  specified site—*see* Neoplasm, by site, benign
  unspecified site
    female 220
    male 222.0
carcinoma (M8640/3)
  specified site—*see* Neoplasm, by site,
    malignant
  unspecified site 186.9
syndrome (germinal aplasia) 606.0
tumor (M8640/0)
  with lipid storage (M8641/0)
    specified site—*see* Neoplasm, by site,
      benign
    unspecified site
      female 220
      male 222.0
  specified site—*see* Neoplasm, by site, benign
  unspecified site
    female 220
    male 222.0
Sertoli-Leydig cell tumor (M8631/0)
specified site—*see* Neoplasm, by site, benign
unspecified site
  female 220
  male 222.0
Serum
allergy, allergic reaction 999.5
  shock 999.4
arthritis 999.5 *[713.6]*
complication or reaction NEC 999.5
disease NEC 999.5

Serum—*continued*
  hepatitis 070.3
  intoxication 999.5
  jaundice (homologous) *see* Hepatitis, viral
  neuritis 999.5
  poisoning NEC 999.5
  rash NEC 999.5
  reaction NEC 999.5
  sickness NEC 999.5
Sesamoiditis 733.99
Seven-day fever 061
  of
    Japan 100.89
    Queensland 100.89
Sever's disease or osteochondrosis (calcaneum) 732.5
Sex chromosome mosaics 758.81
Sex reassignment surgery status (*see also*
  Trans-sexualism) 302.50
Sextuplet
  affected by maternal complications of pregnancy
    761.5
  healthy liveborn—*see* Newborn, multiple
  pregnancy (complicating delivery) NEC 651.8
    with fetal loss and retention of one or more
      fetus(es) 651.6
    following (elective) fetal reduction 651.7
Sexual
  anesthesia 302.72
  deviation (*see also* Deviation, sexual) 302.9
  disorder (*see also* Deviation, sexual) 302.9
  frigidity (female) 302.72
  function, disorder of (psychogenic) 302.70
    specified type NEC 302.79
  immaturity (female) (male) 259.0
  impotence 607.84
    organic origin NEC 607.84
    psychogenic 302.72
  precocity (constitutional) (cryptogenic) (female)
    (idiopathic) (male) NEC 259.1
    with adrenal hyperplasia 255.2
  sadism 302.84
Sexuality, pathological (*see also* Deviation,
  sexual) 302.9
Sézary's disease , reticulosis, or syndrome
  (M9701/3) 202.2
Shadow, lung 793.1
Shaken infant syndrome 995.55
Shaking
  head (tremor) 781.0
  palsy or paralysis (*see also* Parkinsonism) 332.0
Shallowness, acetabulum 736.39
Shaver's disease or syndrome (bauxite
  pneumoconiosis) 503
Shearing
  artificial skin graft 996.55
  decellularized allodermis graft 996.55
Sheath (tendon)—*see* condition
Shedding
  nail 703.8
  teeth, premature, primary (deciduous) 520.6
Sheehan's disease or syndrome (postpartum
  pituitary necrosis) 253.2
Shelf, rectal 569.49
Shell
  shock (current) (*see also* Reaction, stress, acute)
    308.9
    lasting state 300.16
  teeth 520.5
Shield kidney 753.3
Shift, mediastinal 793.2

Shifting
  pacemaker 427.89
  sleep-work schedule (affecting sleep) 327.36
Shiga's
  bacillus 004.0
  dysentery 004.0
Shigella (dysentery) (*see also* Dysentery,
  bacillary) 004.9
  carrier (suspected) of V02.3
Shigellosis (*see also* Dysentery, bacillary) 004.9
Shingles (*see also* Herpes, zoster) 053.9
  eye NEC 053.29
Shin splints 844.9
Shipyard eye or disease 077.1
Shirodkar suture, in pregnancy 654.5
Shock 785.50
  with
    abortion—*see* Abortion, by type, with shock
    ectopic pregnancy (*see also* categories
      633.0-633.9) 639.5
    molar pregnancy (*see also* categories 630-632)
      639.5
  allergic—*see* Shock, anaphylactic
  anaclitic 309.21
  anaphylactic 995.0
    chemical—*see* Table of drugs and chemicals
    correct medicinal substance properly
      administered 995.0
    drug or medicinal substance
      correct substance properly administered
        995.0
      overdose or wrong substance given or taken
        977.9
        specified drug—*see* Table of drugs and
          chemicals
    food—*see* Anaphylactic shock, due to, food
    following sting(s) 989.5
    immunization 999.4
    serum 999.4
  anaphylactoid—*see* Shock, anaphylactic
  anesthetic
    correct substance properly administered 995.4
    overdose or wrong substance given 968.4
      specified anesthetic—*see* Table of drugs and
        chemicals
  birth, fetus or newborn NEC 779.89
  cardiogenic 785.51
  chemical substance—*see* Table of drugs and
    chemicals
  circulatory 785.59
  complicating
    abortion—*see* Abortion, by type, with shock
    ectopic pregnancy (*see also* categories
      633.0-633.9) 639.5
    labor and delivery 669.1
    molar pregnancy (*see also* categories 630-632)
      639.5
  culture 309.29
  due to
    drug 995.0
      correct substance properly administered 995.0
      overdose or wrong substance given or taken
        977.9
        specified drug—*see* Table of drugs and
          chemicals
    food—*see* Anaphylactic shock, due to, food
  during labor and delivery 669.1
  electric 994.8
    from electroshock gun (taser) 994.8
  endotoxic 785.52
    due to surgical procedure 998.0

Shock—*continued*
  following
    abortion 639.5
    ectopic or molar pregnancy 639.5
    injury (immediate) (delayed) 958.4
    labor and delivery 669.1
  gram-negative 785.52
  hematogenic 785.59
  hemorrhagic
    due to
      disease 785.59
      surgery (intraoperative) (postoperative)
        998.0
      trauma 958.4
  hypovolemic NEC 785.59
    surgical 998.0
    traumatic 958.4
  insulin 251.0
    therapeutic misadventure 962.3
  kidney 584.5
    traumatic (following crushing) 958.5
  lightning 994.0
  lung 518.5
  nervous (*see also* Reaction, stress, acute) 308.9
  obstetric 669.1
    with
      abortion—*see* Abortion, by type, with shock
      ectopic pregnancy (*see also* categories
        633.0-633.9) 639.5
      molar pregnancy (*see also* categories
        630-632) 639.5
    following
      abortion 639.5
      ectopic or molar pregnancy 639.5
  paralysis, paralytic (*see also* Disease,
    cerebrovascular, acute) 436
    late effect—*see* Late effect(s) (of)
      cerebrovascular disease
  pleural (surgical) 998.0
    due to trauma 958.4
  postoperative 998.0
    with
      abortion—*see* Abortion, by type, with shock
      ectopic pregnancy (*see also* categories
        633.0-633.9) 639.5
      molar pregnancy (*see also* categories
        630-632) 639.5
    following
      abortion 639.5
      ectopic or molar pregnancy 639.5
  psychic (*see also* Reaction, stress, acute) 308.9
  past history (of) V15.49
  psychogenic (*see also* Reaction, stress, acute)
    308.9
  septic 785.52
    with
      abortion—*see* Abortion, by type, with shock
      ectopic pregnancy (*see also* categories
        633.0-633.9) 639.5
      molar pregnancy (*see also* categories
        630-632) 639.5
    due to
      surgical procedure 998.0
      transfusion NEC 999.89
        bone marrow 996.85
    following
      abortion 639.5
      ectopic or molar pregnancy 639.5
      surgical procedure 998.0
      transfusion NEC 999.89
        bone marrow 996.85

Shock—*continued*
  spinal—*see also* Injury, spinal, by site
    with spinal bone injury—*see* Fracture,
      vertebra, by site, with spinal cord injury
  surgical 998.0
  therapeutic misadventure NEC (*see also*
    Complications) 998.89
  thyroxin 962.7
  toxic 040.82
  transfusion—*see* Complications, transfusion
  traumatic (immediate) (delayed) 958.4
Shoemakers' chest 738.3
Short, shortening, shortness
  Achilles tendon (acquired) 727.81
  arm 736.89
    congenital 755.20
  back 737.9
  bowel syndrome 579.3
  breath 786.05
  cervical, cervix 649.7
    gravid uterus 649.7
    non-gravid uterus 622.5
      acquired 622.5
      congenital 752.49
  chain acyl CoA dehydrogenase deficiency
    (SCAD) 277.85
  common bile duct, congenital 751.69
  cord (umbilical) 663.4
    affecting fetus or newborn 762.6
  cystic duct, congenital 751.69
  esophagus (congenital) 750.4
  femur (acquired) 736.81
    congenital 755.34
  frenulum linguae 750.0
  frenum, lingual 750.0
  hamstrings 727.81
  hip (acquired) 736.39
    congenital 755.63
  leg (acquired) 736.81
    congenital 755.30
  metatarsus (congenital) 754.79
    acquired 736.79
  organ or site, congenital NEC—*see* Distortion
  palate (congenital) 750.26
  P-R interval syndrome 426.81
  radius (acquired) 736.09
    congenital 755.26
  round ligament 629.89
  sleeper 307.49
  stature, constitutional (hereditary) (idiopathic)
    783.43
  tendon 727.81
    Achilles (acquired) 727.81
      congenital 754.79
    congenital 756.89
  thigh (acquired) 736.81
    congenital 755.34
  tibialis anticus 727.81
  umbilical cord 663.4
    affecting fetus or newborn 762.6
  urethra 599.84
  uvula (congenital) 750.26
  vagina 623.8
Shortsightedness 367.1
Shoshin (acute fulminating beriberi) 265.0
Shoulder —*see* condition
Shovel-shaped incisors 520.2
Shower, thromboembolic —*see* Embolism

Shunt (status)
  aortocoronary bypass V45.81
  arterial-venous (dialysis) V45.11
  arteriovenous, pulmonary (acquired) 417.0
    congenital 747.3
    traumatic (complication) 901.40
  cerebral ventricle (communicating) in situ V45.2
  coronary artery bypass V45.81
  surgical, prosthetic, with complications—*see*
      Complications, shunt
  vascular NEC V45.89
Shutdown, renal 586
  with
    abortion—*see* Abortion, by type, with renal
        failure
    ectopic pregnancy (*see also* categories
        633.0-633.9) 639.3
    molar pregnancy (*see also* categories 630-632)
        639.3
  complicating
    abortion 639.3
    ectopic or molar pregnancy 639.3
  following labor and delivery 669.3
Shwachman's syndrome 288.02
Shy-Drager syndrome (orthostatic hypotension
    with multisystem degeneration) 333.0
Sialadenitis (any gland) (chronic) (suppurative)
    527.2
  epidemic—*see* Mumps
Sialadenosis, periodic 527.2
Sialaporia 527.7
Sialectasia 527.8
Sialitis 527.2
Sialoadenitis (*see also* Sialadenitis) 527.2
Sialoangitis 527.2
Sialodochitis (fibrinosa) 527.2
Sialodocholithiasis 527.5
Sialolithiasis 527.5
Sialorrhea (*see also* Ptyalism) 527.7
  periodic 527.2
Sialosis 527.8
  rheumatic 710.2
Siamese twin 759.4
  complicating pregnancy 678.1
Sicard's syndrome 352.6
Sicca syndrome (keratoconjunctivitis) 710.2
Sick 799.9
  cilia syndrome 759.89
  or handicapped person in family V61.49
Sickle-cell
  anemia (*see also* Disease, sickle-cell) 282.60
  disease (*see also* Disease, sickle-cell) 282.60
  hemoglobin
    C disease (without crisis) 282.63
      with
        crisis 282.64
          vaso-occlusive pain 282.64
      D disease (without crisis) 282.68
        with crisis 282.69
      E disease (without crisis) 282.68
        with crisis 282.69
    thalassemia (without crisis) 282.41
      with
        crisis 282.42
          vaso-occlusive pain 282.42
      trait 282.5
Sicklemia (*see also* Disease, sickle-cell) 282.60
  trait 282.5

Sickness
  air (travel) 994.6
  airplane 994.6
  alpine 993.2
  altitude 993.2
  Andes 993.2
  aviators' 993.2
  balloon 993.2
  car 994.6
  compressed air 993.3
  decompression 993.3
  green 280.9
  harvest 100.89
  milk 988.8
  morning 643.0
  motion 994.6
  mountain 993.2
    acute 289.0
  protein (*see also* Complications, vaccination) 999.5
  radiation NEC 990
  roundabout (motion) 994.6
  sea 994.6
  serum NEC 999.5
  sleeping (African) 086.5
    by Trypanosoma 086.5
      gambiense 086.3
      rhodesiense 086.4
    Gambian 086.3
    late effect 139.8
    Rhodesian 086.4
  sweating 078.2
  swing (motion) 994.6
  train (railway) (travel) 994.6
  travel (any vehicle) 994.6
Sick sinus syndrome 427.81
Sideropenia (*see also* Anemia, iron deficiency)
    280.9
Siderosis (lung) (occupational) 503
  cornea 371.15
  eye (bulbi) (vitreous) 360.23
  lens 360.23
Siegal-Cattan-Mamou disease (periodic) 277.31
Siemens' syndrome
  ectodermal dysplasia 757.31
  keratosis follicularis spinulosa (decalvans)
      757.39
Sighing respiration 786.7
Sigmoid
  flexure—*see* condition
  kidney 753.3
Sigmoiditis —*see* Enteritis
Silfverskiöld's syndrome 756.50
Silicosis, sillicotic (complicated) (occupational)
    (simple) 502
  fibrosis, lung (confluent) (massive)
      (occupational) 502
  non-nodular 503
  pulmonum 502
Silicotuberculosis (*see also* Tuberculosis) 011.4
Silo fillers' disease 506.9
Silver's syndrome (congenital hemihypertrophy
    and short stature) 759.89
Silver wire arteries, retina 362.13
Silvestroni-Bianco syndrome (thalassemia
    minima) 282.49
Simian crease 757.2
Simmonds' cachexia or disease (pituitary
    cachexia) 253.2
Simons' disease or syndrome (progressive
    lipodystrophy) 272.6
Simple, simplex —*see* condition

                                        Sleep

Sinding-Larsen disease (juvenile osteopathia patellae) 732.4
Singapore hemorrhagic fever 065.4
Singers' node or nodule 478.5
Single
  atrium 745.69
  coronary artery 746.85
  umbilical artery 747.5
  ventricle 745.3
Singultus 786.8
  epidemicus 078.89
Sinus —*see also* Fistula
  abdominal 569.81
  arrest 426.6
  arrhythmia 427.89
  bradycardia 427.89
    chronic 427.81
  branchial cleft (external) (internal) 744.41
  coccygeal (infected) 685.1
    with abscess 685.0
  dental 522.7
  dermal (congenital) 685.1
    with abscess 685.0
  draining—*see* Fistula
  infected, skin NEC 686.9
  marginal, ruptured or bleeding 641.2
    affecting fetus or newborn 762.1
  pause 426.6
  pericranii 742.0
  pilonidal (infected) (rectum) 685.1
    with abscess 685.0
  preauricular 744.46
  rectovaginal 619.1
  sacrococcygeal (dermoid) (infected) 685.1
    with abscess 685.0
  skin
    infected NEC 686.9
    noninfected—*see* Ulcer, skin
  tachycardia 427.89
  tarsi syndrome 726.79
  testis 608.89
  tract (postinfectional)—*see* Fistula
  urachus 753.7
Sinuses, Rokitansky-Aschoff (*see also* Disease, gallbladder) 575.8
Sinusitis (accessory) (nasal) (hyperplastic) (nonpurulent) (purulent) (chronic) 473.9
  with influenza, flu, or grippe 487.1
  acute 461.9
    ethmoidal 461.2
    frontal 461.1
    maxillary 461.0
    specified type NEC 461.8
    sphenoidal 461.3
  allergic (*see also* Fever, hay) 477.9
  antrum—*see* Sinusitis, maxillary
  due to
    fungus, any sinus 117.9
    high altitude 993.1
  ethmoidal 473.2
    acute 461.2
  frontal 473.1
    acute 461.1
  influenzal 487.1
  maxillary 473.0
    acute 461.0
  specified site NEC 473.8
  sphenoidal 473.3
    acute 461.3
  syphilitic, any sinus 095.8
  tuberculous, any sinus (*see also* Tuberculosis) 012.8

Sinusitis-bronchiectasis-situs inversus (syndrome) (triad) 759.3
Sipple's syndrome (medullary thyroid carcinoma-pheochromocytoma) 258.02
SIRS (systemic inflammatory response syndrome) 995.90
  due to
    infectious process 995.91
      with acute organ dysfunction 995.92
    non-infectious process 995.93
      with acute organ dysfunction 995.94
Sirenomelia 759.89
Siriasis 992.0
Sirkari's disease 085.0
Siti 104.0
Sitophobia 300.29
Situation, psychiatric 300.9
Situational
  disturbance (transient) (*see also* Reaction, adjustment) 309.9
    acute 308.3
  maladjustment, acute (*see also* Reaction, adjustment) 309.9
  reaction (*see also* Reaction, adjustment) 309.9
    acute 308.3
Situs inversus or transversus 759.3
  abdominalis 759.3
  thoracis 759.3
Sixth disease
  due to
    human herpesvirus 6 058.11
    human herpesvirus 7 058.12
Sjögren (-Gougerot) syndrome or disease (keratoconjunctivitis sicca) 710.2
  with lung involvement 710.2 *[517.8]*
Sjögren-Larsson syndrome (ichthyosis congenita) 757.1
SJS-TEN (Stevens-Johnson syndrome-toxic epidermal necrolysis overlap syndrome) 695.14
Skeletal —*see* condition
Skene's gland —*see* condition
Skenitis (*see also* Urethritis) 597.89
  gonorrheal (acute) 098.0
    chronic or duration of 2 months or over 098.2
Skerljevo 104.0
Skevas-Zerfus disease 989.5
Skin —*see also* condition
  donor V59.1
  hidebound 710.9
SLAP lesion (superior glenoid labrum) 840.7
Slate-dressers' lung 502
Slate-miners' lung 502
Sleep
  deprivation V69.4
  disorder 780.50
    with apnea—*see* Apnea, sleep
    child 307.40
    movement, unspecified 780.58
    nonorganic origin 307.40
      specified type NEC 307.49
  disturbance 780.50
    with apnea—*see* Apnea, sleep
    nonorganic origin 307.40
      specified type NEC 307.49
  drunkenness 307.47
  movement disorder, unspecified 780.58
  paroxysmal (*see also* Narcolepsy) 347.00
  related movement disorder, unspecified 780.58

Sleep—*continued*
　rhythm inversion 327.39
　　nonorganic origin 307.45
　walking 307.46
　　hysterical 300.13
Sleeping sickness 086.5
　late effect 139.8
Sleeplessness (*see also* Insomnia) 780.52
　menopausal 627.2
　nonorganic origin 307.41
Slipped, slipping
　epiphysis (postinfectional) 732.9
　　traumatic (old) 732.9
　　　current—*see* Fracture, by site
　　upper femoral (nontraumatic) 732.2
　intervertebral disc—*see* Displacement,
　　intervertebral disc
　ligature, umbilical 772.3
　patella 717.89
　rib 733.99
　sacroiliac joint 724.6
　tendon 727.9
　ulnar nerve, nontraumatic 354.2
　vertebra NEC (*see also* Spondylolisthesis)
　　756.12
Slocumb's syndrome 255.3
Sloughing (multiple) (skin) 686.9
　abscess—*see* Abscess, by site
　appendix 543.9
　bladder 596.8
　fascia 728.9
　graft—*see* Complications, graft
　phagedena (*see also* Gangrene) 785.4
　reattached extremity (*see also* Complications,
　　reattached extremity) 996.90
　rectum 569.49
　scrotum 608.89
　tendon 727.9
　transplanted organ (*see also* Rejection,
　　transplant, organ, by site) 996.80
　ulcer (*see also* Ulcer, skin) 707.9
Slow
　feeding newborn 779.31
　fetal, growth NEC 764.9
　　affecting management of pregnancy 656.5
Slowing
　heart 427.89
　urinary stream 788.62
Sluder's neuralgia or syndrome 337.09
Slurred, slurring, speech 784.59
Small, smallness
　cardiac reserve—*see* Disease, heart
　for dates
　　fetus or newborn 764.0
　　　with malnutrition 764.1
　　　affecting management of pregnancy 656.5
　　infant, term 764.0
　　　with malnutrition 764.1
　　affecting management of pregnancy 656.5
　introitus, vagina 623.3
　kidney, unknown cause 589.9
　　bilateral 589.1
　　unilateral 589.0
　ovary 620.8
　pelvis
　　with disproportion (fetopelvic) 653.1
　　　affecting fetus or newborn 763.1
　　causing obstructed labor 660.1
　　　affecting fetus or newborn 763.1
　placenta—*see* Placenta, insufficiency
　uterus 621.8
　white kidney 582.9

Small-for-dates (*see also* Light-for-dates) 764.0
　affecting management of pregnancy 656.5
Smallpox 050.9
　contact V01.3
　exposure to V01.3
　hemorrhagic (pustular) 050.0
　malignant 050.0
　modified 050.2
　vaccination
　　complications—*see* Complications,
　　　vaccination
　　prophylactic (against) V04.1
Smith's fracture (separation) (closed) 813.41
　open 813.51
Smith-Lemli-Opitz syndrome
　(cerebrohepatorenal syndrome) 759.89
Smith-Magenis syndrome 758.33
Smith-Strang disease (oasthouse urine) 270.2
Smokers'
　bronchitis 491.0
　cough 491.0
　syndrome (*see also* Abuse, drugs,
　　nondependent) 305.1
　throat 472.1
　tongue 528.6
Smoking complicating pregnancy, childbirth, or
　the puerperium 649.0
Smothering spells 786.09
Snaggle teeth, tooth 524.39
Snapping
　finger 727.05
　hip 719.65
　jaw 524.69
　　temporomandibular joint sounds on opening or
　　　closing 524.64
　knee 717.9
　thumb 727.05
Sneddon-Wilkinson disease or syndrome
　(subcorneal pustular dermatosis) 694.1
Sneezing 784.99
　intractable 478.19
Sniffing
　cocaine (*see also* Dependence) 304.2
　ether (*see also* Dependence) 304.6
　glue (airplane) (*see also* Dependence) 304.6
Snoring 786.09
Snow blindness 370.24
Snuffles (nonsyphilitic) 460
　syphilitic (infant) 090.0
Social migrant V60.0
Sodoku 026.0
Soemmering's ring 366.51
Soft —*see also* condition
　enlarged prostate 600.00
　　with
　　　other lower urinary tract symptoms (LUTS)
　　　　600.01
　　urinary
　　　obstruction 600.01
　　　retention 600.01
　nails 703.8
Softening
　bone 268.2
　brain (necrotic) (progressive) 434.9
　　arteriosclerotic 437.0
　　congenital 742.4
　　embolic (*see also* Embolism, brain) 434.1
　　hemorrhagic (*see also* Hemorrhage, brain) 431
　　occlusive 434.9
　　thrombotic (*see also* Thrombosis, brain) 434.0

Spasm, spastic, spasticity—*continued*
   specified as conversion reaction 300.11
   reflex through recurrent laryngeal nerve
     478.75
  habit 307.20
   chronic 307.22
   transient (of childhood) 307.21
  heart—*see* Angina
  hourglass—*see* Contraction, hourglass
  hysterical 300.11
  infantile (*see also* Epilepsy) 345.6
  internal oblique, eye 378.51
  intestinal 564.9
   psychogenic 306.4
  larynx, laryngeal 478.75
   hysterical 300.11
   psychogenic 306.1
    specified as conversion reaction 300.11
  levator palpebrae superioris 333.81
  lightning (*see also* Epilepsy) 345.6
  mobile 781.0
  muscle 728.85
   back 724.8
   psychogenic 306.0
  nerve, trigeminal 350.1
  nervous 306.0
  nodding 307.3
   infantile (*see also* Epilepsy) 345.6
  occupational 300.89
  oculogyric 378.87
  ophthalmic artery 362.30
  orbicularis 781.0
  perineal 625.8
  peroneo-extensor (*see also* Flat, foot) 734
  pharynx (reflex) 478.29
   hysterical 300.11
   psychogenic 306.1
    specified as conversion reaction 300.11
  pregnant uterus, complicating delivery 661.4
  psychogenic 306.0
  pylorus 537.81
   adult hypertrophic 537.0
   congenital or infantile 750.5
   psychogenic 306.4
  rectum (sphincter) 564.6
   psychogenic 306.4
  retinal artery NEC (*see also* Occlusion, retina,
    artery) 362.30
  sacroiliac 724.6
  salaam (infantile) (*see also* Epilepsy) 345.6
  saltatory 781.0
  sigmoid 564.9
   psychogenic 306.4
  sphincter of Oddi (*see also* Disease, gallbladder)
    576.5
  stomach 536.8
   neurotic 306.4
  throat 478.29
   hysterical 300.11
   psychogenic 306.1
    specified as conversion reaction 300.11
  tic 307.20
   chronic 307.22
   transient (of childhood) 307.21
  tongue 529.8
  torsion 333.6
  trigeminal nerve 350.1
   postherpetic 053.12
  ureter 593.89
  urethra (sphincter) 599.84

Spasm, spastic, spasticity—*continued*
  uterus 625.8
   complicating labor 661.4
    affecting fetus or newborn 763.7
  vagina 625.1
   psychogenic 306.51
  vascular NEC 443.9
  vasomotor NEC 443.9
  vein NEC 459.89
  vesical (sphincter, external or internal) 596.8
  viscera 789.0
Spasmodic —*see* condition
Spasmophilia (*see also* Tetany) 781.7
Spasmus nutans 307.3
Spastic —*see also* Spasm
  child 343.9
Spasticity —*see also* Spasm
  cerebral, child 343.9
Speakers' throat 784.49
Specific, specified —*see* condition
Speech
  defect, disorder, disturbance, impediment NEC
    784.59
   psychogenic 307.9
  (language) therapy V57.3
Spells 780.39
  breath-holding 786.9
Spencer's disease (epidemic vomiting) 078.82
Spens' syndrome (syncope with heart block)
    426.9
Spermatic cord —*see* condition
Spermatocele 608.1
  congenital 752.89
Spermatocystitis 608.4
Spermatocytoma (M9063/3)
  specified site—*see* Neoplasm, by site, malignant
  unspecified site 186.9
Spermatorrhea 608.89
Sperm counts
  fertility testing V26.21
  following sterilization reversal V26.22
  postvasectomy V25.8
Sphacelus (*see also* Gangrene) 785.4
Sphenoidal —*see* condition
Sphenoiditis (chronic) (*see also* Sinusitis,
  sphenoidal) 473.3
Sphenopalatine ganglion neuralgia 337.09
Sphericity, increased, lens 743.36
Spherocytosis (congenital) (familial) (hereditary)
    282.0
  hemoglobin disease 287.7
  sickle-cell (disease) 282.60
Spherophakia 743.36
Sphincter —*see* condition
Sphincteritis, sphincter of Oddi (*see also*
  Cholecystitis) 576.8
Sphingolipidosis 272.7
Sphingolipodystrophy 272.7
Sphingomyelinosis 272.7
Spicule tooth 520.2
Spider
  finger 755.59
  nevus 448.1
  vascular 448.1
Spiegler-Fendt sarcoid 686.8
Spielmeyer-Stock disease 330.1
Spielmeyer-Vogt disease 330.1

Spina bifida (aperta) 741.9

> *Note—Use the following fifth-digit subclassification with category 741:*
>
> 0 unspecified region
> 1 cervical region
> 2 dorsal [thoracic] region
> 3 lumbar region

   with hydrocephalus 741.0
   fetal (suspected), affecting management of
      pregnancy 655.0
   occulta 756.17
Spindle, Krukenberg's 371.13
Spine, spinal *—see* condition
Spiradenoma (eccrine) (M8403/0)*—see*
   Neoplasm, skin, benign
Spirillosis NEC (*see also* Fever, relapsing) 087.9
Spirillum minus 026.0
Spirillum obermeieri infection 087.0
Spirochetal *—see* condition
Spirochetosis 104.9
   arthritic, arthritica 104.9 *[711.8]*
   bronchopulmonary 104.8
   icterohemorrhagica 100.0
   lung 104.8
Spitting blood (*see also* Hemoptysis) 786.3
Splanchnomegaly 569.89
Splanchnoptosis 569.89
Spleen, splenic *—see also* condition
   agenesis 759.0
   flexure syndrome 569.89
   neutropenia syndrome 289.53
   sequestration syndrome 289.52
Splenectasis (*see also* Splenomegaly) 789.2
Splenitis (interstitial) (malignant) (nonspecific)
   289.59
   malarial (*see also* Malaria) 084.6
   tuberculous (*see also* Tuberculosis) 017.7
Splenocele 289.59
Splenomegalia *—see* Splenomegaly
Splenomegalic *—see* condition
Splenomegaly 789.2
   Bengal 789.2
   cirrhotic 289.51
   congenital 759.0
   congestive, chronic 289.51
   cryptogenic 789.2
   Egyptian 120.1
   Gaucher's (cerebroside lipidosis) 272.7
   idiopathic 789.2
   malarial (*see also* Malaria) 084.6
   neutropenic 289.53
   Niemann-Pick (lipid histiocytosis) 272.7
   siderotic 289.51
   syphilitic 095.8
      congenital 090.0
   tropical (Bengal) (idiopathic) 789.2
Splenopathy 289.50
Splenopneumonia *—see* Pneumonia
Splenoptosis 289.59
Splinter *—see* Injury, superficial, by site
Split, splitting
   heart sounds 427.89
   lip, congenital (*see also* Cleft, lip) 749.10
   nails 703.8
   urinary stream 788.61
Spoiled child reaction (*see also* Disturbance,
   conduct) 312.1
Spondylarthritis (*see also* Spondylosis) 721.90
Spondylarthrosis (*see also* Spondylosis) 721.90

Spondylitis 720.9
   ankylopoietica 720.0
   ankylosing (chronic) 720.0
   atrophic 720.9
      ligamentous 720.9
   chronic (traumatic) (*see also* Spondylosis) 721.90
   deformans (chronic) (*see also* Spondylosis) 721.90
   gonococcal 098.53
   gouty 274.00
   hypertrophic (*see also* Spondylosis) 721.90
   infectious NEC 720.9
   juvenile (adolescent) 720.0
   Kümmell's 721.7
   Marie-Strümpell (ankylosing) 720.0
   muscularis 720.9
   ossificans ligamentosa 721.6
   osteoarthritica (*see also* Spondylosis) 721.90
   posttraumatic 721.7
   proliferative 720.0
   rheumatoid 720.0
   rhizomelica 720.0
   sacroiliac NEC 720.2
   senescent (*see also* Spondylosis) 721.90
   senile (*see also* Spondylosis) 721.90
   static (*see also* Spondylosis) 721.90
   traumatic (chronic) (*see also* Spondylosis) 721.90
   tuberculous (*see also* Tuberculosis) 015.0 *[720.81]*
   typhosa 002.0 *[720.81]*
Spondyloarthrosis (*see also* Spondylosis) 721.90
Spondylolisthesis (congenital) (lumbosacral)
   756.12
   with disproportion (fetopelvic) 653.3
      affecting fetus or newborn 763.1
      causing obstructed labor 660.1
         affecting fetus or newborn 763.1
   acquired 738.4
   degenerative 738.4
   traumatic 738.4
      acute (lumbar)—*see* Fracture, vertebra,
         lumbar
         site other than lumbosacral—*see* Fracture,
            vertebra, by site
Spondylolysis (congenital) 756.11
   acquired 738.4
   cervical 756.19
   lumbosacral region 756.11
      with disproportion (fetopelvic) 653.3
         affecting fetus or newborn 763.1
         causing obstructed labor 660.1
            affecting fetus or newborn 763.1
Spondylopathy
   inflammatory 720.9
      specified type NEC 720.89
   traumatic 721.7
Spondylose rhizomelique 720.0
Spondylosis 721.90
   with
      disproportion 653.3
         affecting fetus or newborn 763.1
         causing obstructed labor 660.1
            affecting fetus or newborn 763.1
      myelopathy NEC 721.91
   cervical, cervicodorsal 721.0
      with myelopathy 721.1
   inflammatory 720.9
   lumbar, lumbosacral 721.3
      with myelopathy 721.42
   sacral 721.3
      with myelopathy 721.42
   thoracic 721.2
      with myelopathy 721.41
   traumatic 721.7

Sponge
  divers' disease 989.5
  inadvertently left in operation wound 998.4
  kidney (medullary) 753.17
Spongioblastoma (M9422/3)
  multiforme (M9440/3)
    specified site—*see* Neoplasm, by site, malignant
    unspecified site 191.9
  polare (M9423/3)
    specified site—*see* Neoplasm, by site, malignant
    unspecified site 191.9
  primitive polar (M9443/3)
    specified site—*see* Neoplasm, by site, malignant
    unspecified site 191.9
  specified site—*see* Neoplasm, by site, malignant
  unspecified site 191.9
Spongiocytoma (M9400/3)
  specified site—*see* Neoplasm, by site, malignant
  unspecified site 191.9
Spongioneuroblastoma (M9504/3)—*see* Neoplasm, by site, malignant
Spontaneous —*see also* condition
  fracture—*see* Fracture, pathologic
Spoon nail 703.8
  congenital 757.5
Sporadic —*see* condition
Sporotrichosis (bones) (cutaneous) (disseminated) (epidermal) (lymphatic) (lymphocutaneous) (mucous membranes) (pulmonary) (skeletal) (visceral) 117.1
Sporotrichum schenckii infection 117.1
Spots, spotting
  atrophic (skin) 701.3
  Bitôt's (in the young child) 264.1
  café au lait 709.09
  cayenne pepper 448.1
  complicating pregnancy 649.5
  cotton wool (retina) 362.83
  de Morgan's (senile angiomas) 448.1
  Fúchs' black (myopic) 360.21
  intermenstrual
    irregular 626.6
    regular 626.5
  interpalpebral 372.53
  Koplik's 055.9
  liver 709.09
  Mongolian (pigmented) 757.33
  of pregnancy 649.5
  purpuric 782.7
  ruby 448.1
Spotted fever —*see* Fever, spotted
Sprain, strain (joint) (ligament) (muscle) (tendon) 848.9
  abdominal wall (muscle) 848.8
  Achilles tendon 845.09
  acromioclavicular 840.0
  ankle 845.00
    and foot 845.00
  anterior longitudinal, cervical 847.0
  arm 840.9
    upper 840.9
      and shoulder 840.9
  astragalus 845.00
  atlanto-axial 847.0
  atlanto-occipital 847.0
  atlas 847.0
  axis 847.0
  back (*see also* Sprain, spine) 847.9
  breast bone 848.40

Sprain, strain—*continued*
  broad ligament—*see* Injury, internal, broad ligament
  calcaneofibular 845.02
  carpal 842.01
  carpometacarpal 842.11
  cartilage
    costal, without mention of injury to sternum 848.3
      involving sternum 848.42
    ear 848.8
    knee 844.9
      with current tear (*see also* Tear, meniscus) 836.2
    semilunar (knee) 844.8
      with current tear (*see also* Tear, meniscus) 836.2
    septal, nose 848.0
    thyroid region 848.2
    xiphoid 848.49
  cervical, cervicodorsal, cervicothoracic 847.0
  chondrocostal, without mention of injury to sternum 848.3
    involving sternum 848.42
  chondrosternal 848.42
  chronic (joint)—*see* Derangement, joint
  clavicle 840.9
  coccyx 847.4
  collar bone 840.9
  collateral, knee (medial) (tibial) 844.1
    lateral (fibular) 844.0
    recurrent or old 717.89
      lateral 717.81
      medial 717.82
  coracoacromial 840.8
  coracoclavicular 840.1
  coracohumeral 840.2
  coracoid (process) 840.9
  coronary, knee 844.8
  costal cartilage, without mention of injury to sternum 848.3
    involving sternum 848.42
  cricoarytenoid articulation 848.2
  cricothyroid articulation 848.2
  cruciate
    knee 844.2
    old 717.89
      anterior 717.83
      posterior 717.84
  deltoid
    ankle 845.01
    shoulder 840.8
  dorsal (spine) 847.1
  ear cartilage 848.8
  elbow 841.9
    and forearm 841.9
    specified site NEC 841.8
  femur (proximal end) 843.9
    distal end 844.9
  fibula (proximal end) 844.9
    distal end 845.00
  fibulocalcaneal 845.02
  finger(s) 842.10
  foot 845.10
    and ankle 845.00
  forearm 841.9
    and elbow 841.9
    specified site NEC 841.8
  glenoid (shoulder) (*see also* SLAP lesion) 840.8
  hand 842.10

Sprain, strain—*continued*
  hip 843.9
    and thigh 843.9
  humerus (proximal end) 840.9
    distal end 841.9
  iliofemoral 843.0
  infraspinatus 840.3
  innominate
    acetabulum 843.9
    pubic junction 848.5
    sacral junction 846.1
  internal
    collateral, ankle 845.01
    semilunar cartilage 844.8
      with current tear (*see also* Tear, meniscus)
        836.2
      old 717.5
  interphalangeal
    finger 842.13
    toe 845.13
  ischiocapsular 843.1
  jaw (cartilage) (meniscus) 848.1
    old 524.69
  knee 844.9
    and leg 844.9
    old 717.5
      collateral
        lateral 717.81
        medial 717.82
      cruciate
        anterior 717.83
        posterior 717.84
  late effect—*see* Late, effects (of), sprain
  lateral collateral, knee 844.0
    old 717.81
  leg 844.9
    and knee 844.9
  ligamentum teres femoris 843.8
  low back 846.9
  lumbar (spine) 847.2
  lumbosacral 846.0
    chronic or old 724.6
  mandible 848.1
    old 524.69
  maxilla 848.1
  medial collateral, knee 844.1
    old 717.82
  meniscus
    jaw 848.1
      old 524.69
    knee 844.8
      with current tear (*see also* Tear, meniscus)
        836.2
      old 717.5
    mandible 848.1
      old 524.69
    specified site NEC 848.8
  metacarpal 842.10
    distal 842.12
    proximal 842.11
  metacarpophalangeal 842.12
  metatarsal 845.10
  metatarsophalangeal 845.12
  midcarpal 842.19
  midtarsal 845.19
  multiple sites, except fingers alone or toes alone
    848.8
  neck 847.0
  nose (septal cartilage) 848.0
  occiput from atlas 847.0
  old—*see* Derangement, joint

Sprain, strain—*continued*
  orbicular, hip 843.8
  patella(r) 844.8
    old 717.89
  pelvis 848.5
  phalanx
    finger 842.10
    toe 845.10
  radiocarpal 842.02
  radiohumeral 841.2
  radioulnar 841.9
    distal 842.09
  radius, radial (proximal end) 841.9
    and ulna 841.9
      distal 842.09
    collateral 841.0
    distal end 842.00
  recurrent—*see* Sprain, by site
  rib (cage), without mention of injury to sternum
    848.3
    involving sternum 848.42
  rotator cuff (capsule) 840.4
  round ligament—*see also* Injury, internal, round
      ligament
    femur 843.8
  sacral (spine) 847.3
  sacrococcygeal 847.3
  sacroiliac (region) 846.9
    chronic or old 724.6
    ligament 846.1
    specified site NEC 846.8
  sacrospinatus 846.2
  sacrospinous 846.2
  sacrotuberous 846.3
  scaphoid bone, ankle 845.00
  scapula(r) 840.9
  semilunar cartilage (knee) 844.8
    with current tear (*see also* Tear, meniscus)
      836.2
    old 717.5
  septal cartilage (nose) 848.0
  shoulder 840.9
    and arm, upper 840.9
    blade 840.9
  specified site NEC 848.8
  spine 847.9
    cervical 847.0
    coccyx 847.4
    dorsal 847.1
    lumbar 847.2
    lumbosacral 846.0
      chronic or old 724.6
    sacral 847.3
    sacroiliac (*see also* Sprain, sacroiliac) 846.9
      chronic or old 724.6
    thoracic 847.1
  sternoclavicular 848.41
  sternum 848.40
  subglenoid (*see also* SLAP lesion) 840.8
  subscapularis 840.5
  supraspinatus 840.6
  symphysis
    jaw 848.1
      old 524.69
    mandibular 848.1
      old 524.69
    pubis 848.5
  talofibular 845.09
  tarsal 845.10
  tarsometatarsal 845.11
  temporomandibular 848.1
    old 524.69

Sprain, strain—*continued*
  teres
    ligamentum femoris 843.8
    major or minor 840.8
  thigh (proximal end) 843.9
    and hip 843.9
    distal end 844.9
  thoracic (spine) 847.1
  thorax 848.8
  thumb 842.10
  thyroid cartilage or region 848.2
  tibia (proximal end) 844.9
    distal end 845.00
  tibiofibular
    distal 845.03
    superior 844.3
  toe(s) 845.10
  trachea 848.8
  trapezoid 840.8
  ulna, ulnar (proximal end) 841.9
    collateral 841.1
    distal end 842.00
  ulnohumeral 841.3
  vertebrae (*see also* Sprain, spine) 847.9
    cervical, cervicodorsal, cervicothoracic 847.0
  wrist (cuneiform) (scaphoid) (semilunar) 842.00
  xiphoid cartilage 848.49
Sprengel's deformity (congenital) 755.52
Spring fever 309.23
Sprue 579.1
  celiac 579.0
  idiopathic 579.0
  meaning thrush 112.0
  nontropical 579.0
  tropical 579.1
Spur —*see also* Exostosis
  bone 726.91
    calcaneal 726.73
  calcaneal 726.73
  iliac crest 726.5
  nose (septum) 478.19
    bone 726.91
  septal 478.19
Spuria placenta —*see* Placenta, abnormal
Spurway's syndrome (brittle bones and blue
    sclera) 756.51
Sputum, abnormal (amount) (color) (excessive)
    (odor) (purulent) 786.4
  bloody 786.3
Squamous —*see also* condition
  cell metaplasia
    bladder 596.8
    cervix—*see* condition
  epithelium in
    cervical canal (congenital) 752.49
    uterine mucosa (congenital) 752.3
  metaplasia
    bladder 596.8
    cervix—*see* condition
Squashed nose 738.0
  congenital 754.0
Squeeze, divers' 993.3
Squint (*see also* Strabismus) 378.9
  accommodative (*see also* Esotropia) 378.00
  concomitant (*see also* Heterotropia) 378.30
Stab —*see also* Wound, open, by site
  internal organs—*see* Injury, internal, by site,
    with open wound
Staggering gait 781.2
  hysterical 300.11
Staghorn calculus 592.0

Stähl's
  ear 744.29
  pigment line (cornea) 371.11
Stähli's pigment lines (cornea) 371.11
Stain, staining
  meconium 779.84
  port wine 757.32
  tooth, teeth (hard tissues) 521.7
    due to
      accretions 523.6
      deposits (betel) (black) (green) (materia
        alba) (orange) (tobacco) 523.6
      metals (copper) (silver) 521.7
      nicotine 523.6
      pulpal bleeding 521.7
      tobacco 523.6
Stammering 307.0
Standstill
  atrial 426.6
  auricular 426.6
  cardiac (*see also* Arrest, cardiac) 427.5
  sinoatrial 426.6
  sinus 426.6
  ventricular (*see also* Arrest, cardiac) 427.5
Stannosis 503
Stanton's disease (melioidosis) 025
Staphylitis (acute) (catarrhal) (chronic)
    (gangrenous) (membranous) (suppurative)
    (ulcerative) 528.3
Staphylococcemia 038.10
  aureus 038.11
  specified organism NEC 038.19
Staphylococcus, staphylococcal —*see* condition
Staphyloderma (skin) 686.00
Staphyloma 379.11
  anterior, localized 379.14
  ciliary 379.11
  cornea 371.73
  equatorial 379.13
  posterior 379.12
  posticum 379.12
  ring 379.15
  sclera NEC 379.11
Starch eating 307.52
Stargardt's disease 362.75
Starvation (inanition) (due to lack of food) 994.2
  edema 262
  voluntary NEC 307.1
Stasis
  bile (duct) (*see also* Disease, biliary) 576.8
  bronchus (*see also* Bronchitis) 490
  cardiac (*see also* Failure, heart) 428.0
  cecum 564.89
  colon 564.89
  dermatitis (*see also* Varix, with stasis
    dermatitis) 454.1
  duodenal 536.8
  eczema (*see also* Varix, with stasis dermatitis)
    454.1
  edema (*see also* Hypertension, venous) 459.30
  foot 991.4
  gastric 536.3
  ileocecal coil 564.89
  ileum 564.89
  intestinal 564.89
  jejunum 564.89
  kidney 586
  liver 571.9
    cirrhotic—*see* Cirrhosis, liver
  lymphatic 457.8
  pneumonia 514
  portal 571.9

Stasis—*continued*
  pulmonary 514
  rectal 564.89
  renal 586
    tubular 584.5
  stomach 536.3
  ulcer
    with varicose veins 454.0
    without varicose veins 459.81
  urine NEC (*see also* Retention, urine) 788.20
  venous 459.81
State
  affective and paranoid, mixed, organic psychotic
      294.8
  agitated 307.9
    acute reaction to stress 308.2
  anxiety (neurotic) (*see also* Anxiety) 300.00
    specified type NEC 300.09
  apprehension (*see also* Anxiety) 300.00
    specified type NEC 300.09
  climacteric, female 627.2
    following induced menopause 627.4
  clouded
    epileptic (*see also* Epilepsy) 345.9
    paroxysmal (idiopathic) (*see also* Epilepsy)
        345.9
  compulsive (mixed) (with obsession) 300.3
  confusional 298.9
    acute 293.0
      with
        arteriosclerotic dementia 290.41
        presenile brain disease 290.11
        senility 290.3
      alcoholic 291.0
      drug-induced 292.81
    epileptic 293.0
    postoperative 293.9
    reactive (emotional stress) (psychological
        trauma) 298.2
    subacute 293.1
  constitutional psychopathic 301.9
  convulsive (*see also* Convulsions) 780.39
  depressive NEC 311
    induced by drug 292.84
    neurotic 300.4
  dissociative 300.15
  hallucinatory 780.1
    induced by drug 292.12
  hypercoagulable (primary) 289.81
    secondary 289.82
  hyperdynamic beta-adrenergic circulatory
      429.82
  locked-in 344.81
  menopausal 627.2
    artificial 627.4
    following induced menopause 627.4
  neurotic NEC 300.9
    with depersonalization episode 300.6
  obsessional 300.3
  oneiroid (*see also* Schizophrenia) 295.4
  panic 300.01
  paranoid 297.9
    alcohol-induced 291.5
    arteriosclerotic 290.42
    climacteric 297.2
    drug-induced 292.11
    in
      presenile brain disease 290.12
      senile brain disease 290.20
    involutional 297.2
    menopausal 297.2
    senile 290.20

State—*continued*
    simple 297.0
  postleukotomy 310.0
  pregnant (*see also* Pregnancy) V22.2
  psychogenic, twilight 298.2
  psychotic, organic (*see also* Psychosis, organic)
      294.9
    mixed paranoid and affective 294.8
    senile or presenile NEC 290.9
    transient NEC 293.9
      with
        anxiety 293.84
        delusions 293.81
        depression 293.83
        hallucinations 293.82
  residual schizophrenic (*see also* Schizophrenia)
      295.6
  tension (*see also* Anxiety) 300.9
  transient organic psychotic 293.9
    anxiety 293.84
    depressive type 293.83
    hallucinatory type 293.83
    paranoid type 293.81
    specified type NEC 293.89
  twilight
    epileptic 293.0
    psychogenic 298.2
  vegetative (persistent) 780.03
Status (post)
  absence
    epileptic (*see also* Epilepsy) 345.2
    of organ, acquired (postsurgical)—*see*
        Absence, by site, acquired
  administration of tPA (rtPA) in a different
      institution within the last 24 hours prior to
      admission to facility V45.88
  anastomosis of intestine (for bypass) V45.3
  angioplasty, percutaneous transluminal coronary
      V45.82
  anginosus 413.9
  ankle prosthesis V43.66
  aortocoronary bypass or shunt V45.81
  arthrodesis V45.4
  artificially induced condition NEC V45.89
  artificial opening (of) V44.9
    gastrointestinal tract NEC V44.4
    specified site NEC V44.8
    urinary tract NEC V44.6
    vagina V44.7
  aspirator V46.0
  asthmaticus (*see also* Asthma) 493.9
  awaiting organ transplant V49.83
  bariatric surgery V45.86
    complicating pregnancy, childbirth, or the
        puerperium 649.2
  bed confinement V49.84
  breast
    correction V43.82
    implant removal V45.83
    reconstruction V43.82
  cardiac
    device (in situ) V45.00
      defibrillator, automatic implantable V45.02
      pacemaker V45.01
        fitting or adjustment V53.3
      carotid sinus V45.09
        fitting or adjustment V53.3
  carotid sinus stimulator V45.09
  cataract extraction V45.61
  chemotherapy V66.2
    current V58.69
  circumcision, female 629.20

Status—*continued*

clitorectomy (female genital mutilation type I) 629.21

  with excision of labia minora (female genital mutilation type II) 629.22

colonization — *see* Carrier (suspected) of

colostomy V44.3

contraceptive device V45.59

  intrauterine V45.51

  subdermal V45.52

convulsivus idiopathicus (*see also* Epilepsy) 345.3

coronary artery bypass or shunt V45.81

cutting

  female genital 629.20

    specified NEC 629.29

    type I 629.21

    type II 629.22

    type III 629.23

    type IV 629.29

cystostomy V44.50

  appendico-vesicostomy V44.52

  cutaneous-vesicostomy V44.51

  specified type NEC V44.59

defibrillator, automatic implantable cardiac V45.02

delinquent immunization V15.83

dental crowns V45.84

dental fillings V45.84

dental restoration V45.84

dental sealant V49.82

dialysis (hemo) (peritoneal) V45.11

donor V59.9

drug therapy or regimen V67.59

  high-risk medication NEC V67.51

elbow prosthesis V43.62

enterostomy V44.4

epileptic, epilepticus (absence) (grand mal) (*see also* Epilepsy) 345.3

  focal motor 345.7

  partial 345.7

  petit mal 345.2

  psychomotor 345.7

  temporal lobe 345.7

estrogen receptor

  negative [ER-] V86.1

  positive [ER+] V86.0

eye (adnexa) surgery V45.69

female genital

  cutting 629.20

    specified NEC 629.29

    type I 629.21

    type II 629.22

    type III 629.23

    type IV 629.29

  mutilation 629.20

    type IV 629.29

filtering bleb (eye) (postglaucoma) V45.69

  with rupture or complication 997.99

  postcataract extraction (complication) 997.99

finger joint prosthesis V43.69

foster care V60.81

gastric

  banding V45.86

    complicating pregnancy, childbirth, or the puerperium 649.2

  bypass for obesity V45.86

    complicating pregnancy, childbirth, or the puerperium 649.2

gastrostomy V44.1

grand mal 345.3

heart valve prosthesis V43.3

hemodialysis V45.11

Status—*continued*

hip prosthesis (joint) (partial) (total) V43.64

hysterectomy V88.01

  partial with remaining cervical stump V88.02

  total V88.01

ileostomy V44.2

infibulation (female genital mutilation type III) 629.23

insulin pump V45.85

intestinal bypass V45.3

intrauterine contraceptive device V45.51

jejunostomy V44.4

knee joint prosthesis V43.65

lacunaris 437.8

lacunosis 437.8

lapsed immunization schedule V15.83

low birth weight V21.30

  less than 500 grams V21.31

  500-999 grams V21.32

  1000-1499 grams V21.33

  1500-1999 grams V21.34

  2000-2500 grams V21.35

lymphaticus 254.8

malignant neoplasm, ablated or excised—*see* History, malignant neoplasm

marmoratus 333.79

military deployment V62.22

mutilation, female 629.20

  type I 629.21

  type II 629.22

  type III 629.23

  type IV 629.29

nephrostomy V44.6

neuropacemaker NEC V45.89

  brain V45.89

  carotid sinus V45.09

  neurologic NEC V45.89

obesity surgery V45.86

  complicating pregnancy, childbirth, or the puerperium 649.2

organ replacement

  by artificial or mechanical device or prosthesis of

    artery V43.4

    artificial skin V43.83

    bladder V43.5

    blood vessel V43.4

    breast V43.82

    eye globe V43.0

    heart

      assist device V43.21

      fully implantable artificial heart V43.22

      valve V43.3

    intestine V43.89

    joint V43.60

      ankle V43.66

      elbow V43.62

      finger V43.69

      hip (partial) (total) V43.64

      knee V43.65

      shoulder V43.61

      specified NEC 43.69

      wrist V43.63

    kidney V43.89

    larynx V43.81

    lens V43.1

    limb(s) V43.7

    liver V43.89

    lung V43.89

    organ NEC V43.89

    pancreas V43.89

    skin (artificial) V43.83

    tissue NEC V43.89

Status—*continued*
  organ replacement—*continued*
    by artificial—*continued*
      vein V43.4
    by organ transplant (heterologous)
      (homologous)—*see* Status, transplant
  pacemaker
    brain V45.89
    cardiac V45.01
    carotid sinus V45.09
    neurologic NEC V45.89
    specified site NEC V45.89
  percutaneous transluminal coronary angioplasty
    V45.82
  peritoneal dialysis V45.11
  petit mal 345.2
  postcommotio cerebri 310.2
  postmenopausal (age related) (natural) V49.81
  postoperative NEC V45.89
  postpartum NEC V24.2
    care immediately following delivery V24.0
    routine follow-up V24.2
  postsurgical NEC V45.89
  renal dialysis V45.11
    noncompliance V45.12
  respirator (ventilator) V46.11
    encounter
      during
        mechanical failure V46.14
        power failure V46.12
      for weaning V46.13
  reversed jejunal transposition (for bypass) V45.3
  sex reassignment surgery status (*see also*
    Trans-sexualism) 302.50
  shoulder prosthesis V43.61
  shunt
    aortocoronary bypass V45.81
    arteriovenous (for dialysis) V45.11
    cerebrospinal fluid V45.2
    vascular NEC V45.89
      aortocoronary (bypass) V45.81
    ventricular (communicating) (for drainage)
      V45.2
  sterilization
    tubal ligation V26.51
    vasectomy V26.52
  subdermal contraceptive device V45.52
  thymicolymphaticus 254.8
  thymicus 254.8
  thymolymphaticus 254.8
  tooth extraction 525.10
  tracheostomy V44.0
  transplant
    blood vessel V42.89
    bone V42.4
      marrow V42.81
    cornea V42.5
    heart V42.1
      valve V42.2
    intestine V42.84
    kidney V42.0
    liver V42.7
    lung V42.6
    organ V42.9
      removal (due to complication, failure,
        rejection or infection) V45.87
      specified site NEC V42.89
    pancreas V42.83
    peripheral stem cells V42.82
    skin V42.3
    stem cells, peripheral V42.82

Status—*continued*
  transplant—*continued*
    tissue V42.9
      specified type NEC V42.89
    vessel, blood V42.89
  tubal ligation V26.51
  underimmunization V15.83
  ureterostomy V44.6
  urethrostomy V44.6
  vagina, artificial V44.7
  vasectomy V26.52
  vascular shunt NEC V45.89
    aortocoronary (bypass) V45.81
  ventilator (respirator) V46.11
    encounter
      during
        mechanical failure V46.14
        power failure V46.12
      for weaning V46.13
  wheelchair confinement V46.3
  wrist prosthesis V43.63
Stave fracture —*see* Fracture, metacarpus,
  metacarpal bone(s)
Steal
  subclavian artery 435.2
  vertebral artery 435.1
Stealing, solitary, child problem (*see also*
  Disturbance, conduct) 312.1
Steam burn —*see* Burn, by site
Steatocystoma multiplex 706.2
Steatoma (infected) 706.2
  eyelid (cystic) 374.84
    infected 373.13
Steatorrhea (chronic) 579.8
  with lacteal obstruction 579.2
  idiopathic 579.0
    adult 579.0
    infantile 579.0
  pancreatic 579.4
  primary 579.0
  secondary 579.8
  specified cause NEC 579.8
  tropical 579.1
Steatosis 272.8
  heart (*see also* Degeneration, myocardial) 429.1
  kidney 593.89
  liver 571.8
Steele-Richardson (-Olszewski) Syndrome
  333.0
Stein's syndrome (polycystic ovary) 256.4
Stein-Leventhal syndrome (polycystic ovary)
  256.4
Steinbrocker's syndrome (*see also* Neuropathy,
  peripheral, autonomic) 337.9
Steinert's disease 359.21
STEMI (ST elevation myocardial infarction) (*see
  also* Infarct, myocardium, ST elevation) 410.9
Stenocardia (*see also* Angina) 413.9
Stenocephaly 756.0
Stenosis (cicatricial)—*see also* Stricture
  ampulla of Vater 576.2
    with calculus, cholelithiasis, or stones—*see*
      Choledocholithiasis
  anus, anal (canal) (sphincter) 569.2
    congenital 751.2
  aorta (ascending) 747.22
    arch 747.10
    arteriosclerotic 440.0
    calcified 440.0

Stenosis—*continued*
  aortic (valve) 424.1
    with
      mitral (valve)
        insufficiency or incompetence 396.2
        stenosis or obstruction 396.0
    atypical 396.0
    congenital 746.3
    rheumatic 395.0
      with
        insufficiency, incompetency or
          regurgitation 395.2
          with mitral (valve) disease 396.8
        mitral (valve)
          disease (stenosis) 396.0
          insufficiency or incompetence 396.2
          stenosis or obstruction 396.0
    specified cause, except rheumatic 424.1
    syphilitic 093.22
  aqueduct of Sylvius (congenital) 742.3
    with spina bifida (*see also* Spina bifida) 741.0
    acquired 331.4
  artery NEC (*see also* Arteriosclerosis) 447.1
    basilar—*see* Narrowing, artery, basilar
    carotid (common) (internal)—*see* Narrowing,
      artery, carotid
    celiac 447.4
    cerebral 437.0
      due to
        embolism (*see also* Embolism, brain) 434.1
        thrombus (*see also* Thrombosis, brain) 434.0
    extremities 440.20
    precerebral—*see* Narrowing, artery,
      precerebral
    pulmonary (congenital) 747.3
      acquired 417.8
    renal 440.1
    vertebral—*see* Narrowing, artery, vertebral
  bile duct or biliary passage (*see also*
    Obstruction, biliary) 576.2
    congenital 751.61
  bladder neck (acquired) 596.0
    congenital 753.6
  brain 348.89
  bronchus 519.19
    syphilitic 095.8
  cardia (stomach) 537.89
    congenital 750.7
  cardiovascular (*see also* Disease,
    cardiovascular) 429.2
  carotid artery—*see* Narrowing, artery, carotid
  cervix, cervical (canal) 622.4
    congenital 752.49
    in pregnancy or childbirth 654.6
      affecting fetus or newborn 763.89
      causing obstructed labor 660.2
        affecting fetus or newborn 763.1
  colon (*see also* Obstruction, intestine) 560.9
    congenital 751.2
  colostomy 569.62
  common bile duct (*see also* Obstruction, biliary)
    576.2
    congenital 751.61
  coronary (artery) —*see* Arteriosclerosis,
    coronary
  cystic duct (*see also* Obstruction, gallbladder)
    575.2
    congenital 751.61

Stenosis—*continued*
  due to (presence of) any device, implant, or graft
    classifiable to 996.0-996.5—*see*
    Complications, due to (presence of) any
    device, implant, or graft classified to
    996.0-996.5 NEC
  duodenum 537.3
    congenital 751.1
  ejaculatory duct NEC 608.89
  endocervical os—*see* Stenosis, cervix
  enterostomy 569.62
  esophagostomy 530.87
  esophagus 530.3
    congenital 750.3
    syphilitic 095.8
      congenital 090.5
  external ear canal 380.50
    secondary to
      inflammation 380.53
      surgery 380.52
      trauma 380.51
  gallbladder (*see also* Obstruction, gallbladder)
    575.2
  glottis 478.74
  heart valve (acquired)—*see also* Endocarditis
    congenital NEC 746.89
      aortic 746.3
      mitral 746.5
      pulmonary 746.02
      tricuspid 746.1
  hepatic duct (*see also* Obstruction, biliary) 576.2
  hymen 623.3
  hypertrophic subaortic (idiopathic) 425.1
  infundibulum cardiac 746.83
  intestine (*see also* Obstruction, intestine) 560.9
    congenital (small) 751.1
      large 751.2
  lacrimal
    canaliculi 375.53
    duct 375.56
      congenital 743.65
    punctum 375.52
      congenital 743.65
    sac 375.54
      congenital 743.65
  lacrimonasal duct 375.56
    congenital 743.65
    neonatal 375.55
  larynx 478.74
    congenital 748.3
    syphilitic 095.8
      congenital 090.5
  mitral (valve) (chronic) (inactive) 394.0
    with
      aortic (valve)
        disease (insufficiency) 396.1
        insufficiency or incompetence 396.1
        stenosis or obstruction 396.0
      incompetency, insufficiency or regurgitation
        394.2
        with aortic valve disease 396.8
    active or acute 391.1
      with chorea (acute) (rheumatic)
        (Sydenham's) 392.0
    congenital 746.5
    specified cause, except rheumatic 424.0
    syphilitic 093.21
  myocardium, myocardial (*see also*
    Degeneration, myocardial) 429.1
    hypertrophic subaortic (idiopathic) 425.1

Stenosis—*continued*
  nares (anterior) (posterior) 478.19
    congenital 748.0
  nasal duct 375.56
    congenital 743.65
  nasolacrimal duct 375.56
    congenital 743.65
    neonatal 375.55
  organ or site, congenital NEC—*see* Atresia
  papilla of Vater 576.2
    with calculus, cholelithiasis, or stones—*see*
      Choledocholithiasis
  pulmonary (artery) (congenital) 747.3
    with ventricular septal defect, dextraposition
      of aorta and hypertrophy of right ventricle
      745.2
    acquired 417.8
    infundibular 746.83
    in tetralogy of Fallot 745.2
    subvalvular 746.83
    valve (*see also* Endocarditis, pulmonary) 424.3
      congenital 746.02
    vein 747.49
      acquired 417.8
    vessel NEC 417.8
  pulmonic (congenital) 746.02
    infundibular 746.83
    subvalvular 746.83
  pylorus (hypertrophic) 537.0
    adult 537.0
    congenital 750.5
    infantile 750.5
  rectum (sphincter) (*see also* Stricture, rectum) 569.2
  renal artery 440.1
  salivary duct (any) 527.8
  sphincter of Oddi (*see also* Obstruction, biliary) 576.2
  spinal 724.00
    cervical 723.0
    lumbar, lumbosacral 724.02
    nerve (root) NEC 724.9
    specified region NEC 724.09
    thoracic, thoracolumbar 724.01
  stomach, hourglass 537.6
  subaortic 746.81
    hypertrophic (idiopathic) 425.1
  supra (valvular)-aortic 747.22
  trachea 519.19
    congenital 748.3
    syphilitic 095.8
    tuberculous (*see also* Tuberculosis) 012.8
  tracheostomy 519.02
  tricuspid (valve) (*see also* Endocarditis,
    tricuspid) 397.0
    congenital 746.1
    nonrheumatic 424.2
  tubal 628.2
  ureter (*see also* Stricture, ureter) 593.3
    congenital 753.29
  urethra (*see also* Stricture, urethra) 598.9
  vagina 623.2
    congenital 752.49
    in pregnancy or childbirth 654.7
      affecting fetus or newborn 763.89
      causing obstructed labor 660.2
        affecting fetus or newborn 763.1
  valve (cardiac) (heart) (*see also* Endocarditis) 424.90
    congenital NEC 746.89
    aortic 746.3
    mitral 746.5
    pulmonary 746.02
    tricuspid 746.1
    urethra 753.6

Stenosis—*continued*
  valvular (*see also* Endocarditis) 424.90
    congenital NEC 746.89
    urethra 753.6
  vascular graft or shunt 996.1
    atherosclerosis —*see* Arteriosclerosis,
      extremities
    embolism 996.74
    occlusion NEC 996.74
    thrombus 996.74
  vena cava (inferior) (superior) 459.2
    congenital 747.49
  ventricular shunt 996.2
  vulva 624.8
Stercolith (*see also* Fecalith) 560.39
  appendix 543.9
Stercoraceous, stercoral ulcer 569.82
  anus or rectum 569.41
Stereopsis, defective
  with fusion 368.33
  without fusion 368.32
Stereotypies NEC 307.3
Sterility
  female—*see* Infertility, female
  male (*see also* Infertility, male) 606.9
Sterilization, admission for V25.2
  status
    tubal ligation V26.51
    vasectomy V26.52
Sternalgia (*see also* Angina) 413.9
Sternopagus 759.4
Sternum bifidum 756.3
Sternutation 784.99
Steroid
  effects (adverse) (iatrogenic)
    cushingoid
      correct substance properly administered 255.0
      overdose or wrong substance given or taken
        962.0
    diabetes—*see* Diabetes, secondary
      correct substance properly administered 251.8
      overdose or wrong substance given or taken
        962.0
    due to
      correct substance properly administered 255.8
      overdose or wrong substance given or taken
        962.0
    fever
      correct substance properly administered 780.60
      overdose or wrong substance given or taken
        962.0
    withdrawal
      correct substance properly administered 255.41
      overdose or wrong substance given or taken
        962.0
  responder 365.03
Stevens-Johnson disease or syndrome (erythema
  multiforme exudativum) 695.13
  toxic epidermal necrolysis overlap (SJS-TEN
    overlap syndrome) 695.14
Stewart-Morel syndrome (hyperostosis frontalis
  interna) 733.3
Sticker's disease (erythema infectiosum) 057.0
Stickler syndrome 759.89
Sticky eye 372.03
Stieda's disease (calcification, knee joint) 726.62
Stiff
  back 724.8
  neck (*see also* Torticollis) 723.5
Stiff-baby 759.89
Stiff-man syndrome 333.91

Stiffness, joint NEC 719.50
  ankle 719.57
  back 724.8
  elbow 719.52
  finger 719.54
  hip 719.55
  knee 719.56
  multiple sites 719.59
  sacroiliac 724.6
  shoulder 719.51
  specified site NEC 719.58
  spine 724.9
  surgical fusion V45.4
  wrist 719.53
Stigmata, congenital syphilis 090.5
Still's disease or syndrome 714.30
  adult onset 714.2
Still-Felty syndrome (rheumatoid arthritis with
  splenomegaly and leukopenia) 714.1
Stillbirth, stillborn NEC 779.9
Stiller's disease (asthenia) 780.79
Stilling-Türk-Duane syndrome (ocular
  retraction syndrome) 378.71
Stimulation, ovary 256.1
Sting (animal) (bee) (fish) (insect) (jellyfish)
  (Portuguese man-o-war) (wasp) (venomous)
  989.5
  anaphylactic shock or reaction 989.5
  plant 692.6
Stippled epiphyses 756.59
Stitch
  abscess 998.59
  burst (in external operation wound) (*see also*
    Dehiscence) 998.32
    internal 998.31
  in back 724.5
Stojano's (subcostal) syndrome 098.86
Stokes' disease (exophthalmic goiter) 242.0
Stokes-Adams syndrome (syncope with heart
  block) 426.9
Stokvis' (-Talma) disease (enterogenous
  cyanosis) 289.7
Stomach —*see* condition
Stoma malfunction
  colostomy 569.62
  cystostomy 997.5
  enterostomy 569.62
  esophagostomy 530.87
  gastrostomy 536.42
  ileostomy 569.62
  nephrostomy 997.5
  tracheostomy 519.02
  ureterostomy 997.5
Stomatitis 528.00
  angular 528.5
  due to dietary or vitamin deficiency 266.0
  aphthous 528.2
  bovine 059.11
  candidal 112.0
  catarrhal 528.00
  denture 528.9
  diphtheritic (membranous) 032.0
  due to
    dietary deficiency 266.0
    thrush 112.0
    vitamin deficiency 266.0
  epidemic 078.4
  epizootic 078.4
  follicular 528.00
  gangrenous 528.1
  herpetic 054.2

Stomatitis—*continued*
  herpetiformis 528.2
  malignant 528.00
  membranous acute 528.00
  monilial 112.0
  mycotic 112.0
  necrotic 528.1
    ulcerative 101
  necrotizing ulcerative 101
  parasitic 112.0
  septic 528.00
  specified NEC 528.09
  spirochetal 101
  suppurative (acute) 528.00
  ulcerative 528.00
    necrotizing 101
  ulceromembranous 101
  vesicular 528.00
    with exanthem 074.3
  Vincent's 101
Stomatocytosis 282.8
Stomatomycosis 112.0
Stomatorrhagia 528.9
Stone(s) —*see also* Calculus
  bladder 594.1
    diverticulum 594.0
  cystine 270.0
  heart syndrome (*see also* Failure, ventricular,
    left) 428.1
  kidney 592.0
  prostate 602.0
  pulp (dental) 522.2
  renal 592.0
  salivary duct or gland (any) 527.5
  ureter 592.1
  urethra (impacted) 594.2
  urinary (duct) (impacted) (passage) 592.9
    bladder 594.1
      diverticulum 594.0
    lower tract NEC 594.9
    specified site 594.8
  xanthine 277.2
Stonecutters' lung 502
  tuberculous (*see also* Tuberculosis) 011.4
Stonemasons'
  asthma, disease, or lung 502
    tuberculous (*see also* Tuberculosis) 011.4
  phthisis (*see also* Tuberculosis) 011.4
Stoppage
  bowel (*see also* Obstruction, intestine) 560.9
  heart (*see also* Arrest, cardiac) 427.5
  intestine (*see also* Obstruction, intestine) 560.9
  urine NEC (*see also* Retention, urine) 788.20
Storm, thyroid (apathetic) (*see also*
  Thyrotoxicosis) 242.9
Strabismus (alternating) (congenital)
  (nonparalytic) 378.9
  concomitant (*see also* Heterotropia) 378.30
    convergent (*see also* Esotropia) 378.00
    divergent (*see also* Exotropia) 378.10
  convergent (*see also* Esotropia) 378.00
  divergent (*see also* Exotropia) 378.10
  due to adhesions, scars—*see* Strabismus,
    mechanical
  in neuromuscular disorder NEC 378.73
    intermittent 378.20
      vertical 378.31
  latent 378.40
    convergent (esophoria) 378.41
    divergent (exophoria) 378.42
    vertical 378.43

Stricture—*continued*
  renal 440.1
  vertebral—*see* Narrowing, artery, vertebral
  auditory canal (congenital) (external) 744.02
    acquired (*see also* Stricture, ear canal,
      acquired) 380.50
  bile duct or passage (any) (postoperative) (*see
    also* Obstruction, biliary) 576.2
    congenital 751.61
  bladder 596.8
    congenital 753.6
    neck 596.0
      congenital 753.6
  bowel (*see also* Obstruction, intestine) 560.9
  brain 348.89
  bronchus 519.19
    syphilitic 095.8
  cardia (stomach) 537.89
    congenital 750.7
  cardiac—*see* Disease, heart
    orifice (stomach) 537.89
  cardiovascular (*see also* Disease,
    cardiovascular) 429.2
  carotid artery—*see* Narrowing, artery, carotid
  cecum (*see also* Obstruction, intestine) 560.9
  cervix, cervical (canal) 622.4
    congenital 752.49
    in pregnancy or childbirth 654.6
      affecting fetus or newborn 763.89
      causing obstructed labor 660.2
        affecting fetus or newborn 763.1
  colon (*see also* Obstruction, intestine) 560.9
    congenital 751.2
  colostomy 569.62
  common bile duct (*see also* Obstruction, biliary)
    576.2
    congenital 751.61
  coronary (artery) —*see* Arteriosclerosis,
    coronary
    congenital 746.85
  cystic duct (*see also* Obstruction, gallbladder)
    575.2
    congenital 751.61
  cystostomy 997.5
  digestive organs NEC, congenital 751.8
  duodenum 537.3
    congenital 751.1
  ear canal (external) (congenital) 744.02
    acquired 380.50
      secondary to
        inflammation 380.53
        surgery 380.52
        trauma 380.51
  ejaculatory duct 608.85
  enterostomy 569.62
  esophagostomy 530.87
  esophagus (corrosive) (peptic) 530.3
    congenital 750.3
    syphilitic 095.8
      congenital 090.5
  Eustachian tube (*see also* Obstruction,
    Eustachian tube) 381.60
    congenital 744.24
  fallopian tube 628.2
    gonococcal (chronic) 098.37
      acute 098.17
    tuberculous (*see also* Tuberculosis) 016.6
  gallbladder (*see also* Obstruction, gallbladder)
    575.2
    congenital 751.69
  glottis 478.74

Stricture—*continued*
  heart—*see also* Disease, heart
    congenital NEC 746.89
    valve—*see also* Endocarditis
      congenital NEC 746.89
        aortic 746.3
        mitral 746.5
        pulmonary 746.02
        tricuspid 746.1
  hepatic duct (*see also* Obstruction, biliary) 576.2
  hourglass, of stomach 537.6
  hymen 623.3
  hypopharynx 478.29
  intestine (*see also* Obstruction, intestine) 560.9
    congenital (small) 751.1
      large 751.2
    ischemic 557.1
  lacrimal
    canaliculi 375.53
      congenital 743.65
    punctum 375.52
      congenital 743.65
    sac 375.54
      congenital 743.65
  lacrimonasal duct 375.56
    congenital 743.65
    neonatal 375.55
  larynx 478.79
    congenital 748.3
    syphilitic 095.8
      congenital 090.5
  lung 518.89
  meatus
    ear (congenital) 744.02
      acquired (*see also* Stricture, ear canal,
        acquired) 380.50
      osseous (congenital) (ear) 744.03
        acquired (*see also* Stricture, ear canal,
          acquired) 380.50
    urinarius (*see also* Stricture, urethra) 598.9
      congenital 753.6
  mitral (valve) (*see also* Stenosis, mitral) 394.0
    congenital 746.5
    specified cause, except rheumatic 424.0
  myocardium, myocardial (*see also*
    Degeneration, myocardial) 429.1
    hypertrophic subaortic (idiopathic) 425.1
  nares (anterior) (posterior) 478.19
    congenital 748.0
  nasal duct 375.56
    congenital 743.65
    neonatal 375.55
  nasolacrimal duct 375.56
    congenital 743.65
    neonatal 375.55
  nasopharynx 478.29
    syphilitic 095.8
  nephrostomy 997.5
  nose 478.19
    congenital 748.0
  nostril (anterior) (posterior) 478.19
    congenital 748.0
  organ or site, congenital NEC—*see* Atresia
  osseous meatus (congenital) (ear) 744.03
    acquired (*see also* Stricture, ear canal,
      acquired) 380.50
  os uteri (*see also* Stricture, cervix) 622.4
  oviduct—*see* Stricture, fallopian tube
  pelviureteric junction 593.3
  pharynx (dilation) 478.29
  prostate 602.8

Stricture—*continued*
  pulmonary, pulmonic
    artery (congenital) 747.3
      acquired 417.8
      noncongenital 417.8
      infundibulum (congenital) 746.83
    valve (*see also* Endocarditis, pulmonary)
      424.3
        congenital 746.02
    vein (congenital) 747.49
      acquired 417.8
    vessel NEC 417.8
  punctum lacrimale 375.52
    congenital 743.65
  pylorus (hypertrophic) 537.0
    adult 537.0
    congenital 750.5
    infantile 750.5
  rectosigmoid 569.89
  rectum (sphincter) 569.2
    congenital 751.2
    due to
      chemical burn 947.3
      irradiation 569.2
      lymphogranuloma venereum 099.1
    gonococcal 098.7
    inflammatory 099.1
    syphilitic 095.8
    tuberculous (*see also* Tuberculosis) 014.8
  renal artery 440.1
  salivary duct or gland (any) 527.8
  sigmoid (flexure) (*see also* Obstruction,
    intestine) 560.9
  spermatic cord 608.85
  stoma (following) (of)
    colostomy 569.62
    cystostomy 997.5
    enterostomy 569.62
    esophagostomy 530.87
    gastrostomy 536.42
    ileostomy 569.62
    nephrostomy 997.5
    tracheostomy 519.02
    ureterostomy 997.5
  stomach 537.89
    congenital 750.7
    hourglass 537.6
  subaortic 746.81
    hypertrophic (acquired) (idiopathic) 425.1
  subglottic 478.74
  syphilitic NEC 095.8
  tendon (sheath) 727.81
  trachea 519.19
    congenital 748.3
    syphilitic 095.8
    tuberculous (*see also* Tuberculosis) 012.8
  tracheostomy 519.02
  tricuspid (valve) (*see also* Endocarditis,
    tricuspid) 397.0
    congenital 746.1
    nonrheumatic 424.2
  tunica vaginalis 608.85
  ureter (postoperative) 593.3
    congenital 753.29
    tuberculous (*see also* Tuberculosis) 016.2
  ureteropelvic junction 593.3
    congenital 753.21
  ureterovesical orifice 593.3
    congenital 753.22
  urethra (anterior) (meatal) (organic) (posterior)
    (spasmodic) 598.9

Stricture—*continued*
  associated with schistosomiasis (*see also*
    Schistosomiasis) 120.9 *[598.01]*
  congenital (valvular) 753.6
  due to
    infection 598.00
      syphilis 095.8 *[598.01]*
    trauma 598.1
  gonococcal 098.2 *[598.01]*
  gonorrheal 098.2 *[598.01]*
  infective 598.00
  late effect of injury 598.1
  postcatheterization 598.2
  postobstetric 598.1
  postoperative 598.2
  specified cause NEC 598.8
  syphilitic 095.8 *[598.01]*
  traumatic 598.1
  valvular, congenital 753.6
  urinary meatus (*see also* Stricture, urethra)
    598.9
  congenital 753.6
  uterus, uterine 621.5
    os (external) (internal)—see Stricture, cervix
  vagina (outlet) 623.2
    congenital 752.49
  valve (cardiac) (heart) (*see also* Endocarditis)
    424.90
    congenital (cardiac) (heart) NEC 746.89
      aortic 746.3
      mitral 746.5
      pulmonary 746.02
      tricuspid 746.1
    urethra 753.6
  valvular (*see also* Endocarditis) 424.90
  vascular graft or shunt 996.1
    atherosclerosis —*see* Arteriosclerosis,
      extremities
    embolism 996.74
    occlusion NEC 996.74
    thrombus 996.74
  vas deferens 608.85
    congenital 752.89
  vein 459.2
  vena cava (inferior) (superior) NEC 459.2
    congenital 747.49
  ventricular shunt 996.2
  vesicourethral orifice 596.0
    congenital 753.6
  vulva (acquired) 624.8
Stridor 786.1
  congenital (larynx) 748.3
Stridulous —*see* condition
Strippling of nails 703.8
Stroke 434.91
  apoplectic (*see also* Disease, cerebrovascular,
    acute) 436
  brain—*see* Infarct, brain
  embolic 434.11
  epileptic—*see* Epilepsy
  healed or old V12.54
  heart—*see* Disease, heart
  heat 992.0
  hemorrhagic—*see* Hemorrhage, brain
  iatrogenic 997.02
  in evolution 434.91
  ischemic 434.91
  late effect—*see* Late effect(s) (of)
    cerebrovascular disease
  lightning 994.0
  paralytic—*see* Infarct, brain
  postoperative 997.02

Stroke—*continued*
  progressive 435.9
  thrombotic 434.01
Stromatosis, endometrial (M8931/1) 236.0
Strong pulse 785.9
Strongyloides stercoralis infestation 127.2
Strongyloidiasis 127.2
Strongyloidosis 127.2
Strongylus (gibsoni) infestation 127.7
Strophulus (newborn) 779.89
  pruriginosus 698.2
Struck by lightning 994.0
Struma (*see also* Goiter) 240.9
  fibrosa 245.3
  Hashimoto (struma lymphomatosa) 245.2
  lymphomatosa 245.2
  nodosa (simplex) 241.9
    endemic 241.9
    multinodular 241.1
    sporadic 241.9
    toxic or with hyperthyroidism 242.3
      multinodular 242.2
      uninodular 242.1
    toxicosa 242.3
      multinodular 242.2
      uninodular 242.1
    uninodular 241.0
  ovarii (M9090/0) 220
    and carcinoid (M9091/1) 236.2
    malignant (M9090/3) 183.0
  Riedel's (ligneous thyroiditis) 245.3
  scrofulous (*see also* Tuberculosis) 017.2
  tuberculous (*see also* Tuberculosis) 017.2
    abscess 017.2
    adenitis 017.2
    lymphangitis 017.2
    ulcer 017.2
Strumipriva cachexia (*see also* Hypothyroidism)
  244.9
Strümpell-Marie disease or spine (ankylosing
  spondylitis) 720.0
Strümpell-Westphal pseudosclerosis
  (hepatolenticular degeneration) 275.1
Stuart's disease (congenital factor X deficiency)
  (*see also* Defect, coagulation) 286.3
Stuart-Prower factor deficiency (congenital
  factor X deficiency) (*see also* Defect,
  coagulation) 286.3
Students' elbow 727.2
Stuffy nose 478.19
Stump —*see also* Amputation
  cervix, cervical (healed) 622.8
Stupor 780.09
  catatonic (*see also* Schizophrenia) 295.2
  circular (*see also* Psychosis, manic-depressive,
    circular) 296.7
  manic 296.89
  manic-depressive (*see also* Psychosis, affective)
    296.89
  mental (anergic) (delusional) 298.9
  psychogenic 298.8
  reaction to exceptional stress (transient) 308.2
  traumatic NEC—*see also* Injury, intracranial
    with spinal (cord)
      lesion—*see* Injury, spinal, by site
      shock—*see* Injury, spinal, by site
Sturge (-Weber) (-Dimitri) disease or syndrome
  (encephalocutaneous angiomatosis) 759.6
Sturge-Kalischer-Weber syndrome
  (encephalocutaneous angiomatosis) 759.6

Stuttering 307.0
  due to late effect of cerebrovascular disease (see
    also Late effect(s) (of) cerebrovascular
    disease) 438.14
Sty, stye 373.11
  external 373.11
  internal 373.12
  meibomian 373.12
Subacidity, gastric 536.8
  psychogenic 306.4
Subacute —*see* condition
Subarachnoid —*see* condition
Subclavian steal syndrome 435.2
Subcortical —*see* condition
Subcostal syndrome 098.86
  nerve compression 354.8
Subcutaneous, subcuticular —*see* condition
Subdelirium 293.1
Subdural —*see* condition
Subendocardium —*see* condition
Subependymoma (M9383/1) 237.5
Suberosis 495.3
Subglossitis —*see* Glossitis
Subhemophilia 286.0
Subinvolution (uterus) 621.1
  breast (postlactational) (postpartum) 611.89
  chronic 621.1
  puerperal, postpartum 674.8
Sublingual —*see* condition
Sublinguitis 527.2
Subluxation —*see also* Dislocation, by site
  congenital NEC—*see also* Malposition,
    congenital
    hip (unilateral) 754.32
      with dislocation of other hip 754.35
      bilateral 754.33
    joint
      lower limb 755.69
      shoulder 755.59
      upper limb 755.59
    lower limb (joint) 755.69
    shoulder (joint) 755.59
    upper limb (joint) 755.59
  lens 379.32
    anterior 379.33
    posterior 379.34
  radial head 832.2
  rotary, cervical region of spine—*see* Fracture,
    vertebra, cervical
Submaxillary —*see* condition
Submersion (fatal) (nonfatal) 994.1
Submissiveness (undue), in child 313.0
Submucous —*see* condition
Subnormal, subnormality
  accommodation (*see also* Disorder,
    accommodation) 367.9
  mental (*see also* Retardation, mental) 319
    mild 317
    moderate 318.0
    profound 318.2
    severe 318.1
  temperature (accidental) 991.6
    not associated with low environmental
      temperature 780.99
Subphrenic —*see* condition
Subscapular nerve —*see* condition
Subseptus uterus 752.3
Subsiding appendicitis 542
Substance abuse in family V61.42
Substernal thyroid (*see also* Goiter) 240.9
  congenital 759.2

Substitution disorder 300.11
Subtentorial —*see* condition
Subtertian
  fever 084.0
  malaria (fever) 084.0
Subthyroidism (acquired) (*see also*
  Hypothyroidism) 244.9
  congenital 243
Succenturiata placenta —*see* Placenta,
  abnormal
Succussion sounds, chest 786.7
Sucking thumb, child 307.9
Sudamen 705.1
Sudamina 705.1
Sudanese kala-azar 085.0
Sudden
  death, cause unknown (less than 24 hours) 798.1
    cardiac (SCD)
      family history of V17.41
      personal history of, successfully resuscitated
        V12.53
    during childbirth 669.9
    infant 798.0
    puerperal, postpartum 674.9
  hearing loss NEC 388.2
  heart failure (*see also* Failure, heart) 428.9
  infant death syndrome 798.0
Sudeck's atrophy, disease, or syndrome 733.7
SUDS (Sudden unexplained death) 798.2
Suffocation (*see also* Asphyxia) 799.01
  by
    bed clothes 994.7
    bunny bag 994.7
    cave-in 994.7
    constriction 994.7
    drowning 994.1
    inhalation
      food or foreign body (*see also* Asphyxia,
        food or foreign body) 933.1
      oil or gasoline (*see also* Asphyxia, food or
        foreign body) 933.1
    overlying 994.7
    plastic bag 994.7
    pressure 994.7
    strangulation 994.7
  during birth 768.1
  mechanical 994.7
Sugar
  blood
    high 790.29
    low 251.2
  in urine 791.5
Suicide, suicidal (attempted)
  by poisoning—*see* Table of drugs and chemicals
  ideation V62.84
  risk 300.9
  tendencies 300.9
  trauma NEC (*see also* nature and site of injury)
    959.9
Suipestifer infection (*see also* Infection,
  Salmonella) 003.9
Sulfatidosis 330.0
Sulfhemoglobinemia, sulphemoglobinemia
  (acquired) (congenital) 289.7
Sumatran mite fever 081.2
Summer —*see* condition
Sunburn 692.71
  dermatitis 692.71

Sunburn—*continued*
  due to
    other ultraviolet radiation 692.82
    tanning bed 692.82
  first degree 692.71
  second degree 692.76
  third degree 692.77
SUNCT (Short-lasting Unilateral Neuralgiform
  headache with Conjunctival injection and
  Tearing) 339.05
Sunken
  acetabulum 718.85
  fontanels 756.0
Sunstroke 992.0
Superfecundation 651.9
  with fetal loss and retention of one or more
    fetus(es) 651.6
  following (elective) fetal reduction 651.7
Superfetation 651.9
  with fetal loss and retention of one or more
    fetus(es) 651.6
  following (elective) fetal reduction 651.7
Supernumerary (congenital)
  aortic cusps 746.89
  auditory ossicles 744.04
  bone 756.9
  breast 757.6
  carpal bones 755.56
  cusps, heart valve NEC 746.89
    mitral 746.5
    pulmonary 746.09
  digit(s) 755.00
    finger 755.01
    toe 755.02
  ear (lobule) 744.1
  fallopian tube 752.19
  finger 755.01
  hymen 752.49
  kidney 753.3
  lacrimal glands 743.64
  lacrimonasal duct 743.65
  lobule (ear) 744.1
  mitral cusps 746.5
  muscle 756.82
  nipples 757.6
  organ or site NEC—*see* Accessory
  ossicles, auditory 744.04
  ovary 752.0
  oviduct 752.19
  pulmonic cusps 746.09
  rib 756.3
    cervical or first 756.2
      syndrome 756.2
  roots (of teeth) 520.2
  spinal vertebra 756.19
  spleen 759.0
  tarsal bones 755.67
  teeth 520.1
    causing crowding 524.31
  testis 752.89
  thumb 755.01
  toe 755.02
  uterus 752.2
  vagina 752.49
  vertebra 756.19
Supervision (of)
  contraceptive method previously prescribed V25.40
    intrauterine device V25.42
    oral contraceptive (pill) V25.41
    specified type NEC V25.49
    subdermal implantable contraceptive V25.43

Supervision—*continued*
  dietary (for) V65.3
    allergy (food) V65.3
    colitis V65.3
    diabetes mellitus V65.3
    food allergy intolerance V65.3
    gastritis V65.3
    hypercholesterolemia V65.3
    hypoglycemia V65.3
    intolerance (food) V65.3
    obesity V65.3
    specified NEC V65.3
  lactation V24.1
  newborn health
    8 to 28 days old V20.32
    under 8 days old V20.31
  pregnancy—*see* Pregnancy, supervision of
Supplemental teeth 520.1
  causing crowding 524.31
Suppression
  binocular vision 368.31
  lactation 676.5
  menstruation 626.8
  ovarian secretion 256.39
  renal 586
  urinary secretion 788.5
  urine 788.5
Suppuration, suppurative —*see also* condition
  accessory sinus (chronic) (*see also* Sinusitis) 473.9
  adrenal gland 255.8
  antrum (chronic) (*see also* Sinusitis, maxillary) 473.0
  bladder (*see also* Cystitis) 595.89
  bowel 569.89
  brain 324.0
    late effect 326
  breast 611.0
    puerperal, postpartum 675.1
  dental periosteum 526.5
  diffuse (skin) 686.00
  ear (middle) (*see also* Otitis media) 382.4
    external (*see also* Otitis, externa) 380.10
    internal 386.33
  ethmoidal (sinus) (chronic) (*see also* Sinusitis, ethmoidal) 473.2
  fallopian tube (*see also* Salpingo-oophoritis) 614.2
  frontal (sinus) (chronic) (*see also* Sinusitis, frontal) 473.1
  gallbladder (*see also* Cholecystitis, acute) 575.0
  gum 523.30
  hernial sac—*see* Hernia, by site
  intestine 569.89
  joint (*see also* Arthritis, suppurative) 711.0
  labyrinthine 386.33
  lung 513.0
  mammary gland 611.0
    puerperal, postpartum 675.1
  maxilla, maxillary 526.4
    sinus (chronic) (*see also* Sinusitis, maxillary) 473.0
  muscle 728.0
  nasal sinus (chronic) (*see also* Sinusitis) 473.9
  pancreas 577.0
  parotid gland 527.2
  pelvis, pelvic
    female (*see also* Disease, pelvis, inflammatory) 614.4
      acute 614.3
    male (*see also* Peritonitis) 567.21

Suppuration, suppurative—*continued*
  pericranial (*see also* Osteomyelitis) 730.2
  salivary duct or gland (any) 527.2
  sinus (nasal) (*see also* Sinusitis) 473.9
  sphenoidal (sinus) (chronic) (*see also* Sinusitis, sphenoidal) 473.3
  thymus (gland) 254.1
  thyroid (gland) 245.0
  tonsil 474.8
  uterus (*see also* Endometritis) 615.9
  vagina 616.10
  wound—*see also* Wound, open, by site, complicated
    dislocation—*see* Dislocation, by site, compound
    fracture—*see* Fracture, by site, open
    scratch or other superficial injury—*see* Injury, superficial, by site
Supraeruption, teeth 524.34
Supraglottitis 464.50
  with obstruction 464.51
Suprapubic drainage 596.8
Suprarenal (gland)—*see* condition
Suprascapular nerve —*see* condition
Suprasellar —*see* condition
Supraspinatus syndrome 726.10
Surfer knots 919.8
  infected 919.9
Surgery
  cosmetic NEC V50.1
    breast reconstruction following mastectomy V51.0
    following healed injury or operation V51.8
    hair transplant V50.0
  elective V50.9
    breast
      augmentation or reduction V50.1
      reconstruction following mastectomy V51.0
    circumcision, ritual or routine (in absence of medical indication) V50.2
    cosmetic NEC V50.1
    ear piercing V50.3
    face-lift V50.1
    following healed injury or operation V51.8
    hair transplant V50.0
  not done because of
    contraindication V64.1
    patient's decision V64.2
    specified reason NEC V64.3
  plastic
    breast
      augmentation or reduction V50.1
      reconstruction following mastectomy V51.0
    cosmetic V50.1
    face-lift V50.1
    following healed injury or operation V51.8
    repair of scarred tissue (following healed injury or operation) V51.8
    specified type NEC V50.8
  previous, in pregnancy or childbirth
    cervix 654.6
      affecting fetus or newborn (*see also* Newborn, affected by) 760.63
      causing obstructed labor 660.2
        affecting fetus or newborn 763.1
    pelvic soft tissues NEC 654.9
      affecting fetus or newborn (*see also* Newborn, affected by) 760.63
      causing obstructed labor 660.2
        affecting fetus or newborn 763.1
    perineum or vulva 654.8

Surgery—*continued*
  previous, in pregnancy or childbirth—*continued*
    uterus NEC 654.9
      affecting fetus or newborn (*see also*
        Newborn, affected by) 760.63
      causing obstructed labor 660.2
        affecting fetus or newborn 763.1
      due to previous cesarean delivery 654.2
      vagina 654.7
Surgical
  abortion—*see* Abortion, legal
  emphysema 998.81
  kidney (*see also* Pyelitis) 590.80
  operation NEC 799.9
  procedures, complication or misadventure—*see*
    Complications, surgical procedure
  shock 998.0
Survey
  fetal anatomic V28.81
Susceptibility
  genetic
    to
      MEN (multiple endocrine neoplasia) V84.81
      neoplasia
        multiple endocrine [MEN] V84.81
      neoplasm
        malignant, of
          breast V84.01
          endometrium V84.04
          other V84.09
          ovary V84.02
          prostate V84.03
        specified disease NEC V84.89
Suspected condition, ruled out (*see also*
  Observation, suspected) V71.9
  specified condition NEC V71.89
Suspended uterus, in pregnancy or childbirth
  654.4
  affecting fetus or newborn 763.89
  causing obstructed labor 660.2
    affecting fetus or newborn 763.1
Sutton's disease 709.09
Sutton and Gull's disease (arteriolar
  nephrosclerosis) (*see also* Hypertension,
  kidney) 403.90
Suture
  burst (in external operation wound) (*see also*
    Dehiscence) 998.32
    internal 998.31
  inadvertently left in operation wound 998.4
  removal V58.32
  Shirodkar, in pregnancy (with or without
    cervical incompetence) 654.5
Swab inadvertently left in operation wound
  998.4
Swallowed, swallowing
  difficulty (*see also* Dysphagia) 787.20
  foreign body NEC (*see also* Foreign body) 938
Swamp fever 100.89
Swan neck hand (intrinsic) 736.09
Sweat (s), sweating
  disease or sickness 078.2
  excessive (*see also* Hyperhidrosis) 780.8
  fetid 705.89
  fever 078.2
  gland disease 705.9
    specified type NEC 705.89
  miliary 078.2
  night 780.8
Sweeley-Klionsky disease (angiokeratoma
  corporis diffusum) 272.7

Sweet's syndrome (acute febrile neutrophilic
  dermatosis) 695.89
Swelling 782.3
  abdominal (not referable to specific organ)
    789.3
  adrenal gland, cloudy 255.8
  ankle 719.07
  anus 787.99
  arm 729.81
  breast 611.72
  Calabar 125.2
  cervical gland 785.6
  cheek 784.2
  chest 786.6
  ear 388.8
  epigastric 789.3
  extremity (lower) (upper) 729.81
  eye 379.92
  female genital organ 625.8
  finger 729.81
  foot 729.81
  glands 785.6
  gum 784.2
  hand 729.81
  head 784.2
  inflammatory—*see* Inflammation
  joint (*see also* Effusion, joint) 719.0
    tuberculous—*see* Tuberculosis, joint
  kidney, cloudy 593.89
  leg 729.81
  limb 729.81
  liver 573.8
  lung 786.6
  lymph nodes 785.6
  mediastinal 786.6
  mouth 784.2
  muscle (limb) 729.81
  neck 784.2
  nose or sinus 784.2
  palate 784.2
  pelvis 789.3
  penis 607.83
  perineum 625.8
  rectum 787.99
  scrotum 608.86
  skin 782.2
  splenic (*see also* Splenomegaly) 789.2
  substernal 786.6
  superficial, localized (skin) 782.2
  testicle 608.86
  throat 784.2
  toe 729.81
  tongue 784.2
  tubular (*see also* Disease, renal) 593.9
  umbilicus 789.3
  uterus 625.8
  vagina 625.8
  vulva 625.8
  wandering, due to Gnathostoma (spinigerum)
    128.1
  white—*see* Tuberculosis, arthritis
Swift's disease 985.0
Swimmers'
  ear (acute) 380.12
  itch 120.3
Swimming in the head 780.4
Swollen —*see also* Swelling
  glands 785.6
Swyer-James syndrome (unilateral hyperlucent
  lung) 492.8
Swyer's syndrome (XY pure gonadal
  dysgenesis) 752.7

Sycosis 704.8
  barbae (not parasitic) 704.8
  contagiosa 110.0
  lupoid 704.8
  mycotic 110.0
  parasitic 110.0
  vulgaris 704.8
Sydenham's chorea —*see* Chorea, Sydenham's
Sylvatic yellow fever 060.0
Sylvest's disease (epidemic pleurodynia) 074.1
Symblepharon 372.63
  congenital 743.62
Symonds' syndrome 348.2
Sympathetic —*see* condition
Sympatheticotonia (*see also* Neuropathy,
    peripheral, autonomic) 337.9
Sympathicoblastoma (M9500/3)
  specified site—*see* Neoplasm, by site, malignant
  unspecified site 194.0
Sympathicogonioma (M9500/3)—*see*
    Sympathicoblastoma
Sympathoblastoma (M9500/3)—*see*
    Sympathicoblastoma
Sympathogonioma (M9500/3)—*see*
    Sympathicoblastoma
Symphalangy (*see also* Syndactylism) 755.10
Symptoms, specified (general) NEC 780.99
  abdomen NEC 789.9
  bone NEC 733.90
  breast NEC 611.79
  cardiac NEC 785.9
  cardiovascular NEC 785.9
  chest NEC 786.9
  development NEC 783.9
  digestive system NEC 787.99
  emotional state NEC 799.29
  eye NEC 379.99
  gastrointestinal tract NEC 787.99
  genital organs NEC
    female 625.9
    male 608.9
  head and neck NEC 784.99
  heart NEC 785.9
  joint NEC 719.60
    ankle 719.67
    elbow 719.62
    foot 719.67
    hand 719.64
    hip 719.65
    knee 719.66
    multiple sites 719.69
    pelvic region 719.65
    shoulder (region) 719.61
    specified site NEC 719.68
    wrist 719.63
  larynx NEC 784.99
  limbs NEC 729.89
  lymphatic system NEC 785.9
  menopausal 627.2
  metabolism NEC 783.9
  mouth NEC 528.9
  muscle NEC 728.9
  musculoskeletal NEC 781.99
    limbs NEC 729.89
  nervous system NEC 781.99
  neurotic NEC 300.9
  nutrition, metabolism, and development NEC 783.9
  pelvis NEC 789.9
    female 625.9
  peritoneum NEC 789.9
  respiratory system NEC 786.9

Symptoms, specified—*continued*
  skin and integument NEC 782.9
  subcutaneous tissue NEC 782.9
  throat NEC 784.99
  tonsil NEC 784.99
  urinary system NEC 788.99
  vascular NEC 785.9
Sympus 759.89
Synarthrosis 719.80
  ankle 719.87
  elbow 719.82
  foot 719.87
  hand 719.84
  hip 719.85
  knee 719.86
  multiple sites 719.89
  pelvic region 719.85
  shoulder (region) 719.81
  specified site NEC 719.88
  wrist 719.83
Syncephalus 759.4
Synchondrosis 756.9
  abnormal (congenital) 756.9
  ischiopubic (van Neck's) 732.1
Synchysis (senile) (vitreous humor) 379.21
  scintillans 379.22
Syncope (near) (pre-) 780.2
  anginosa 413.9
  bradycardia 427.89
  cardiac 780.2
  carotid sinus 337.01
  complicating delivery 669.2
  due to lumbar puncture 349.0
  fatal 798.1
  heart 780.2
  heat 992.1
  laryngeal 786.2
  tussive 786.2
  vasoconstriction 780.2
  vasodepressor 780.2
  vasomotor 780.2
  vasovagal 780.2
Syncytial infarct —*see* Placenta, abnormal
Syndactylism, syndactyly (multiple sites) 755.10
  fingers (without fusion of bone) 755.11
    with fusion of bone 755.12
  toes (without fusion of bone) 755.13
    with fusion of bone 755.14
Syndrome —*see also* Disease
  5q minus 238.74
  abdominal
    acute 789.0
    migraine 346.2
    muscle deficiency 756.79
  Abercrombie's (amyloid degeneration) 277.39
  abnormal innervation 374.43
  abstinence
    alcohol 291.81
    drug 292.0
    neonatal 779.5
  Abt-Letterer-Siwe (acute histiocytosis X)
    (M9722/3) 202.5
  Achard-Thiers (adrenogenital) 255.2
  acid pulmonary aspiration 997.39
    obstetric (Mendelson's) 668.0
  acquired immune deficiency 042
  acquired immunodeficiency 042
  acrocephalosyndactylism 755.55
  acute abdominal 789.0
  acute chest 517.3
  acute coronary 411.1

Syndrome—*continued*
Adair-Dighton (brittle bones and blue sclera, deafness) 756.51
Adams-Stokes (-Morgagni) (syncope with heart block) 426.9
addisonian 255.41
Adie (-Holmes) (pupil) 379.46
adiposogenital 253.8
adrenal
  hemorrhage 036.3
  meningococcic 036.3
adrenocortical 255.3
adrenogenital (acquired) (congenital) 255.2
  feminizing 255.2
  iatrogenic 760.79
  virilism (acquired) (congenital) 255.2
affective organic NEC 293.89
  drug-induced 292.84
afferent loop NEC 537.89
African macroglobulinemia 273.3
Ahumada-Del Castillo (nonpuerperal galactorrhea and amenorrhea) 253.1
air blast concussion—*see* Injury, internal, by site
Alagille 759.89
Albright (-Martin) (pseudohypoparathyroidism) 275.49
Albright-McCune-Sternberg (osteitis fibrosa disseminata) 756.59
alcohol withdrawal 291.81
Alder's (leukocyte granulation anomaly) 288.2
Aldrich (-Wiskott) (eczema-thrombocytopenia) 279.12
Alibert-Bazin (mycosis, fungoides) (M9700/3) 202.1
Alice in Wonderland 293.89
alien hand 781.8
Allen-Masters 620.6
Alligator baby (ichthyosis congenita) 757.1
Alport's (hereditary hematuria-nephropathy-deafness) 759.89
Alvarez (transient cerebral ischemia) 435.9
alveolar capillary block 516.3
Alzheimer's 331.0
  with dementia—*see* Alzheimer's, dementia
amnestic (confabulatory) 294.0
  alcohol-induced persisting 291.1
  drug-induced 292.83
  posttraumatic 294.0
amotivational 292.89
amyostatic 275.1
amyotrophic lateral sclerosis 335.20
androgen insensitivity 259.51
  partial 259.52
Angelman 759.89
angina (*see also* Angina) 413.9
ankyloglossia superior 750.0
anterior
  chest wall 786.52
  compartment (tibial) 958.8
  spinal artery 433.8
    compression 721.1
  tibial (compartment) 958.8
antibody deficiency 279.00
  agammaglobulinemic 279.00
  congenital 279.04
  hypogammaglobulinemic 279.00
anticardiolipin antibody 289.81
antimongolism 758.39
antiphospholipid antibody 289.81
Anton (-Babinski) (hemiasomatognosia) 307.9
anxiety (*see also* Anxiety) 300.00
  organic 293.84

Syndrome—*continued*
aortic
  arch 446.7
  bifurcation (occlusion) 444.0
  ring 747.21
Apert's (acrocephalosyndactyly) 755.55
Apert-Gallais (adrenogenital) 255.2
aphasia-apraxia-alexia 784.69
apical ballooning 429.83
"approximate answers" 300.16
arcuate ligament (-celiac axis) 447.4
arcus aortae 446.7
arc-welders' 370.24
argentaffin, argintaffinoma 259.2
Argonz-Del Castillo (nonpuerperal galactorrhea and amenorrhea) 253.1
Argyll Robertson's (syphilitic) 094.89
  nonsyphilitic 379.45
arm-shoulder (*see also* Neuropathy, peripheral, autonomic) 337.9
Armenian 277.31
Arnold-Chiari (*see also* Spina bifida) 741.0
  type I 348.4
  type II 741.0
  type III 742.0
  type IV 742.2
Arrillaga-Ayerza (pulmonary artery sclerosis with pulmonary hypertension) 416.0
arteriomesenteric duodenum occlusion 537.89
arteriovenous steal 996.73
arteritis, young female (obliterative brachiocephalic) 446.7
aseptic meningitis—*see* Meningitis, aseptic
Asherman's 621.5
Asperger's 299.8
asphyctic (*see also* Anxiety) 300.00
aspiration, of newborn (massive) 770.18
  meconium 770.12
ataxia-telangiectasia 334.8
Audry's (acropachyderma) 757.39
auriculotemporal 350.8
autoimmune lymphoproliferative (ALPS) 279.41
autosomal—*see also* Abnormal, autosomes NEC
  deletion 758.39
    5p 758.31
    22q11.2 758.32
Avellis' 344.89
Axenfeld's 743.44
Ayerza (-Arrillaga) (pulmonary artery sclerosis with pulmonary hypertension) 416.0
Baader's (erythema multiforme exudativum) 695.19
Baastrup's 721.5
Babinski (-Vaquez) (cardiovascular syphilis) 093.89
Babinski-Fröhlich (adiposogenital dystrophy) 253.8
Babinski-Nageotte 344.89
Bagratuni's (temporal arteritis) 446.5
Bakwin-Krida (craniometaphyseal dysplasia) 756.89
Balint's (psychic paralysis of visual disorientation) 368.16
Ballantyne (-Runge) (postmaturity) 766.22
ballooning posterior leaflet 424.0
Banti's—*see* Cirrhosis, liver
Bard-Pic's (carcinoma, head of pancreas) 157.0
Bardet-Biedl (obesity, polydactyly, and mental retardation) 759.89
Barlow's (mitral valve prolapse) 424.0
Barlow (-Möller) (infantile scurvy) 267

Syndrome—*continued*
  Baron Munchausen's 301.51
  Barré-Guillain 357.0
  Barré-Liéou (posterior cervical sympathetic)
    723.2
  Barrett's (chronic peptic ulcer of esophagus)
    530.85
  Bársony-Polgár (corkscrew esophagus) 530.5
  Bársony-Teschendorf (corkscrew esophagus)
    530.5
  Barth 759.89
  Bartter's (secondary hyperaldosteronism with
    juxtaglomerular hyperplasia) 255.13
  basal cell nevus 759.89
  Basedow's (exophthalmic goiter) 242.0
  basilar artery 435.0
  basofrontal 377.04
  Bassen-Kornzweig (abetalipoproteinemia) 272.5
  Batten-Steinert 359.21
  battered
    adult 995.81
    baby or child 995.54
    spouse 995.81
  Baumgarten-Cruveilhier (cirrhosis of liver)
    571.5
  Beals 759.82
  Bearn-Kunkel (-Slater) (lupoid hepatitis) 571.49
  Beau's (*see also* Degeneration, myocardial) 429.1
  Bechterew-Strümpell-Marie (ankylosing
    spondylitis) 720.0
  Beck's (anterior spinal artery occlusion) 433.8
  Beckwith (-Wiedemann) 759.89
  Behçet's 136.1
  Bekhterev-Strümpell-Marie (ankylosing
    spondylitis) 720.0
  Benedikt's 344.89
  Béquez César (-Steinbrinck-Chédiak-Higashi)
    (congenital gigantism of peroxidase
    granules) 288.2
  Bernard-Horner (*see also* Neuropathy,
    peripheral, autonomic) 337.9
  Bernard-Sergent (acute adrenocortical
    insufficiency) 255.41
  Bernhardt-Roth 355.1
  Bernheim's (*see also* Failure, heart) 428.0
  Bertolotti's (sacralization of fifth lumbar
    vertebra) 756.15
  Besnier-Boeck-Schaumann (sarcoidosis) 135
  Bianchi's (aphasia-apraxia-alexia syndrome)
    784.69
  Biedl-Bardet (obesity, polydactyly, and mental
    retardation) 759.89
  Biemond's (obesity, polydactyly, and mental
    retardation) 759.89
  big spleen 289.4
  bilateral polycystic ovarian 256.4
  Bing-Horton's 339.00
  Biörck (-Thorson) (malignant carcinoid) 259.2
  Birt-Hogg-Dube 759.89
  Blackfan-Diamond (congenital hypoplastic
    anemia) 284.01
  black lung 500
  black widow spider bite 989.5
  bladder neck (*see also* Incontinence, urine)
    788.30
  blast (concussion)—*see* Blast, injury
  blind loop (postoperative) 579.2
  Bloch-Siemens (incontinentia pigmenti) 757.33
  Bloch-Sulzberger (incontinentia pigmenti) 757.33
  Bloom (-Machacek) (-Torre) 757.39
  Blount-Barber (tibia vara) 732.4

Syndrome—*continued*
  blue
    bloater 491.20
    with
      acute bronchitis 491.22
      exacerbation (acute) 491.21
    diaper 270.0
    drum 381.02
    sclera 756.51
    toe 445.02
  Boder-Sedgwick (ataxia-telangiectasia) 334.8
  Boerhaave's (spontaneous esophageal rupture)
    530.4
  Bonnevie-Ullrich 758.6
  Bonnier's 386.19
  Borjeson-Forssman-Lehmann 759.89
  Bouillaud's (rheumatic heart disease) 391.9
  Bourneville (-Pringle) (tuberous sclerosis) 759.5
  Bouveret (-Hoffmann) (paroxysmal tachycardia)
    427.2
  brachial plexus 353.0
  Brachman-de Lange (Amsterdam dwarf, mental
    retardation, and brachycephaly) 759.89
  bradycardia-tachycardia 427.81
  Brailsford-Morquio (dystrophy)
    (mucopolysaccharidosis IV) 277.5
  brain (acute) (chronic) (nonpsychotic) (organic)
    (with behavioral reaction) (with neurotic
    reaction) 310.9
    with
      presenile brain disease (*see also* Dementia,
        presenile) 290.10
      psychosis, psychotic reaction (*see also*
        Psychosis, organic) 294.9
    chronic alcoholic 291.2
    congenital (*see also* Retardation, mental) 319
    postcontusional 310.2
    posttraumatic
      nonpsychotic 310.2
      psychotic 293.9
        acute 293.0
        chronic (*see also* Psychosis, organic) 294.8
        subacute 293.1
    psycho-organic (*see also* Syndrome,
      psycho-organic) 310.9
    psychotic (*see also* Psychosis, organic) 294.9
    senile (*see also* Dementia, senile) 290.0
  branchial arch 744.41
  Brandt's (acrodermatitis enteropathica) 686.8
  Brennemann's 289.2
  Briquet's 300.81
  Brissaud-Meige (infantile myxedema) 244.9
  broad ligament laceration 620.6
  Brock's (atelectasis due to enlarged lymph
    nodes) 518.0
  broken heart 429.83
  Brown's tendon sheath 378.61
  Brown-Séquard 344.89
  brown spot 756.59
  Brugada 746.89
  Brugsch's (acropachyderma) 757.39
  bubbly lung 770.7
  Buchem's (hyperostosis corticalis) 733.3
  Budd-Chiari (hepatic vein thrombosis) 453.0
  Büdinger-Ludloff-Läwen 717.89
  bulbar 335.22
    lateral (*see also* Disease, cerebrovascular,
      acute) 436

Syndrome—*continued*
Bullis fever 082.8
bundle of Kent (anomalous atrioventricular
  excitation) 426.7
Bürger-Grütz (essential familial hyperlipemia)
  272.3
Burke's (pancreatic insufficiency and chronic
  neutropenia) 577.8
Burnett's (milk-alkali) 275.42
Burnier's (hypophyseal dwarfism) 253.3
burning feet 266.2
Bywaters' 958.5
Caffey's (infantile cortical hyperostosis) 756.59
Calvé-Legg-Perthes (osteochondrosis, femoral
  capital) 732.1
Caplan (-Colinet) syndrome 714.81
capsular thrombosis (*see also* Thrombosis,
  brain) 434.0
carbohydrate-deficient glycoprotein (CDGS) 271.8
carcinogenic thrombophlebitis 453.1
carcinoid 259.2
cardiac asthma (*see also* Failure, ventricular,
  left) 428.1
cardiacos negros 416.0
cardiofaciocutaneous 759.89
cardiopulmonary obesity 278.8
cardiorenal (*see also* Hypertension, cardiorenal)
  404.90
cardiorespiratory distress (idiopathic), newborn
  769
cardiovascular renal (*see also* Hypertension,
  cardiorenal) 404.90
cardiovasorenal 272.7
Carini's (ichthyosis congenita) 757.1
carotid
  artery (internal) 435.8
  body or sinus 337.01
carpal tunnel 354.0
Carpenter's 759.89
Cassidy (-Scholte) (malignant carcinoid) 259.2
cat-cry 758.31
cauda equina 344.60
causalgia 355.9
  lower limb 355.71
  upper limb 354.4
cavernous sinus 437.6
celiac 579.0
  artery compression 447.4
  axis 447.4
central pain 338.0
cerebellomedullary malformation (*see also*
  Spina bifida) 741.0
cerebral gigantism 253.0
cerebrohepatorenal 759.89
cervical (root) (spine) NEC 723.8
  disc 722.71
  posterior, sympathetic 723.2
  rib 353.0
  sympathetic paralysis 337.09
  traumatic (acute) NEC 847.0
cervicobrachial (diffuse) 723.3
cervicocranial 723.2
cervicodorsal outlet 353.2
Céstan's 344.89
Céstan (-Raymond) 433.8
Céstan-Chenais 344.89
chancriform 114.1
Charcot's (intermittent claudication) 443.9
  angina cruris 443.9
  due to atherosclerosis 440.21
Charcot-Marie-Tooth 356.1

Syndrome—*continued*
Charcot-Weiss-Baker 337.01
CHARGE association 759.89
Cheadle (-Möller) (-Barlow) (infantile scurvy)
  267
Chédiak-Higashi (-Steinbrinck) (congenital
  gigantism of peroxidase granules) 288.2
chest wall 786.52
Chiari's (hepatic vein thrombosis) 453.0
Chiari-Frommel 676.6
chiasmatic 368.41
Chilaiditi's (subphrenic displacement, colon)
  751.4
chondroectodermal dysplasia 756.55
chorea-athetosis-agitans 275.1
Christian's (chronic histiocytosis X) 277.89
chromosome 4 short arm deletion 758.39
chronic pain 338.4
Churg-Strauss 446.4
Clarke-Hadfield (pancreatic infantilism) 577.8
Claude's 352.6
Claude Bernard-Horner (*see also* Neuropathy,
  peripheral, autonomic) 337.9
Clérambault's
  automatism 348.89
  erotomania 297.8
Clifford's (postmaturity) 766.22
climacteric 627.2
Clouston's (hidrotic ectodermal dysplasia)
  757.31
clumsiness 315.4
Cockayne's (microencephaly and dwarfism)
  759.89
Cockayne-Weber (epidermolysis bullosa)
  757.39
Coffin-Lowry 759.89
Cogan's (nonsyphilitic interstitial keratitis)
  370.52
cold injury (newborn) 778.2
Collet (-Sicard) 352.6
combined immunity deficiency 279.2
compartment(al) (anterior) (deep) (posterior) 958.8
  nontraumatic
    abdomen 729.73
    arm 729.71
    buttock 729.72
    fingers 729.71
    foot 729.72
    forearm 729.71
    hand 729.71
    hip 729.72
    leg 729.72
    lower extremity 729.72
    shoulder 729.71
    specified site NEC 729.79
    thigh 729.72
    toes 729.72
    upper extremity 729.71
    wrist 729.71
  post-surgical (see also Syndrome,
    compartment, non-traumatic) 998.89
  traumatic 958.90
    abdomen 958.93
    arm 958.91
    buttock 958.92
    fingers 958.91
    foot 958.92
    forearm 958.91
    hand 958.91
    hip 958.92
    leg 958.92
    lower extremity 958.92

Syndrome—*continued*
  double whammy 360.81
  Down's (mongolism) 758.0
  Dresbach's (elliptocytosis) 282.1
  Dressler's (postmyocardial infarction) 411.0
    hemoglobinuria 283.2
    postcardiotomy 429.4
  drug withdrawal, infant, of dependent mother
    779.5
  dry skin 701.1
    eye 375.15
  DSAP (disseminated superficial actinic
    porokeratosis) 692.75
  Duane's (retraction) 378.71
  Duane-Stilling-Türk (ocular retraction
    syndrome) 378.71
  Dubin-Johnson (constitutional
    hyperbilirubinemia) 277.4
  Dubin-Sprinz (constitutional
    hyperbilirubinemia) 277.4
  Duchenne's 335.22
  due to abnormality
    autosomal NEC (*see also* Abnormal,
      autosomes NEC) 758.5
      13 758.1
      18 758.2
      21 or 22 758.0
      D₁ 758.1
      E₃ 758.2
      G 758.0
    chromosomal 758.89
      sex 758.81
  dumping 564.2
    nonsurgical 536.8
  Duplay's 726.2
  Dupré's (meningism) 781.6
  Dyke-Young (acquired macrocytic hemolytic
    anemia) 283.9
  dyspraxia 315.4
  dystocia, dystrophia 654.9
  Eagle-Barrett 756.71
  Eales' 362.18
  Eaton-Lambert (*see also* Neoplasm, by site,
    malignant) 199.1 *[358.1]*
  Ebstein's (downward displacement, tricuspid
    valve into right ventricle) 746.2
  ectopic ACTH secretion 255.0
  eczema-thrombocytopenia 279.12
  Eddowes' (brittle bones and blue sclera) 756.51
  Edwards' 758.2
  efferent loop 537.89
  effort (aviators') (psychogenic) 306.2
  Ehlers-Danlos 756.83
  Eisenmenger's (ventricular septal defect) 745.4
  Ekbom's (restless legs) 333.94
  Ekman's (brittle bones and blue sclera) 756.51
  electric feet 266.2
  Elephant man 237.71
  Ellison-Zollinger (gastric hypersecretion with
    pancreatic islet cell tumor) 251.5
  Ellis-van Creveld (chondroectodermal
    dysplasia) 756.55
  embryonic fixation 270.2
  empty sella (turcica) 253.8
  endocrine-hypertensive 255.3
  Engel-von Recklinghausen (osteitis fibrosa
    cystica) 252.01
  enteroarticular 099.3
  entrapment—*see* Neuropathy, entrapment
  eosinophilia myalgia 710.5
  epidemic vomiting 078.82

Syndrome—*continued*
  Epstein's—*see* Nephrosis
  Erb (-Oppenheim) -Goldflam 358.00
  Erdheim-Chester 277.89
  Erdheim's (acromegalic macrospondylitis) 253.0
  Erlacher-Blount (tibia vara) 732.4
  erythrocyte fragmentation 283.19
  euthyroid sick 790.94
  Evans' (thrombocytopenic purpura) 287.32
  excess cortisol, iatrogenic 255.0
  exhaustion 300.5
  extrapyramidal 333.90
  eyelid-malar-mandible 756.0
  eye retraction 378.71
  Faber's (achlorhydric anemia) 280.9
  Fabry (-Anderson) (angiokeratoma corporis
    diffusum) 272.7
  facet 724.8
  Fallot's 745.2
  falx (*see also* Hemorrhage, brain) 431
  familial eczema-thrombocytopenia 279.12
  Fanconi's (anemia) (congenital pancytopenia)
    284.09
  Fanconi (-de Toni) (-Debré) (cystinosis) 270.0
  Farber (-Uzman) (disseminated
    lipogranulomatosis) 272.8
  fatigue NEC 300.5
    chronic 780.71
  faulty bowel habit (idiopathic megacolon) 564.7
  FDH (focal dermal hypoplasia) 757.39
  fecal reservoir 560.39
  Feil-Klippel (brevicollis) 756.16
  Felty's (rheumatoid arthritis with splenomegaly
    and leukopenia) 714.1
  fertile eunuch 257.2
  fetal alcohol 760.71
    late effect 760.71
  fibrillation-flutter 427.32
  fibrositis (periarticular) 729.0
  Fiedler's (acute isolated myocarditis) 422.91
  Fiessinger-Leroy (-Reiter) 099.3
  Fiessinger-Rendu (erythema multiforme
    exudativum) 695.19
  first arch 756.0
  fish odor 270.8
  Fisher's 357.0
  Fitz's (acute hemorrhagic pancreatitis) 577.0
  Fitz-Hugh and Curtis 098.86
    due to
      Chlamydia trachomatis 099.56
      Neisseria gonorrhoeae (gonococcal
        peritonitis) 098.86
  Flajani (-Basedow) (exophthalmic goiter) 242.0
  flat back
    acquired 737.29
    postprocedural 738.5
  floppy
    infant 781.99
    iris 364.81
    valve (mitral) 424.0
  flush 259.2
  Foix-Alajouanine 336.1
  Fong's (hereditary osteo-onychodysplasia)
    756.89
  foramen magnum 348.4
  Forbes-Albright (nonpuerperal amenorrhea and
    lactation associated with pituitary tumor)
    253.1
  Foster-Kennedy 377.04
  Foville's (peduncular) 344.89
  Fragile X 759.83

Syndrome—*continued*

Morgagni (-Stewart-Morel) (hyperostosis frontalis interna) 733.3

Morgagni-Adams-Stokes (syncope with heart block) 426.9

Morquio (-Brailsford) (-Ullrich) (mucopolysaccharidosis IV) 277.5

Morris (testicular feminization) 259.51

Morton's (foot) (metatarsalgia) (metatarsal neuralgia) (neuralgia) (neuroma) (toe) 355.6

Moschcowitz (-Singer-Symmers) (thrombotic thrombocytopenic purpura) 446.6

Mounier-Kuhn 748.3
 with
  acute exacerbation 494.1
  bronchiectasis 494.0
   with (acute) exacerbation 494.1
 acquired 519.19
  with bronchiectasis 494.0
   with (acute) exacerbation 494.1

Mucha-Haberman (acute parapsoriasis varioliformis) 696.2

mucocutaneous lymph node (acute) (febrile) (infantile) (MCLS) 446.1

multiple
 deficiency 260
 endocrine neoplasia [MEN]
  type I 258.01
  type IIA 258.02
  type IIB 258.03
 operations 301.51

Munchausen's 301.51

Münchmeyer's (exostosis luxurians) 728.11

Murchison-Sanderson—*see* Disease, Hodgkin's

myasthenic—*see* Myasthenia, syndrome

myelodysplastic 238.75
 with 5q deletion 238.74
 high grade with 5q deletion 238.73
 therapy-related 289.83

myeloproliferative (chronic) (M9960/1) 238.79

myofascial pain NEC 729.1

Naffziger's 353.0

Nager-de Reynier (dysostosis mandibularis) 756.0

nail-patella (hereditary osteo-onychodysplasia) 756.89

NARP (neuropathy, ataxia and retinitis pigmentosa) 277.87

Nebécourt's 253.3

Neill-Dingwall (microencephaly and dwarfism) 759.89

nephrotic (*see also* Nephrosis) 581.9
 diabetic 250.4 *[581.81]*
  due to secondary diabetes 249.4 *[581.81]*

Netherton's (ichthyosiform erythroderma) 757.1

neurocutaneous 759.6

neuroleptic malignant 333.92

Nezelof's (pure alymphocytosis) 279.13

Niemann-Pick (lipid histiocytosis) 272.7

Nonne-Milroy-Meige (chronic hereditary edema) 757.0

nonsense 300.16

Noonan's 759.89

Nothnagel's
 ophthalmoplegia-cerebellar ataxia 378.52
 vasomotor acroparesthesia 443.89

nucleus ambiguous-hypoglossal 352.6

OAV (oculoauriculovertebral dysplasia) 756.0

obsessional 300.3

oculocutaneous 364.24

oculomotor 378.81

Syndrome—*continued*

oculourethroarticular 099.3

Ogilvie's (sympathicotonic colon obstruction) 560.89

ophthalmoplegia-cerebellar ataxia 378.52

Oppenheim-Urbach (necrobiosis lipoidica diabeticorum) 250.8 *[709.3]*
 due to secondary diabetes 249.8 *[709.3]*

oral-facial-digital 759.89

organic
 affective NEC 293.83
  drug-induced 292.84
 anxiety 293.84
 delusional 293.81
  alcohol-induced 291.5
  drug-induced 292.11
  due to or associated with
   arteriosclerosis 290.42
   presenile brain disease 290.12
   senility 290.20
 depressive 293.83
  drug-induced 292.84
  due to or associated with
   arteriosclerosis 290.43
   presenile brain disease 290.13
   senile brain disease 290.21
 hallucinosis 293.82
  drug-induced 292.84

organic affective 293.83
 induced by drug 292.84

organic personality 310.1
 induced by drug 292.89

Ormond's 593.4

orodigitofacial 759.89

orthostatic hypotensive-dysautonomic-dyskinetic 333.0

Osler-Weber-Rendu (familial hemorrhagic telangiectasia) 448.0

osteodermopathic hyperostosis 757.39

osteoporosis-osteomalacia 268.2

Österreicher-Turner (hereditary osteo-onychodysplasia) 756.89

os trigonum 755.69

Ostrum-Furst 756.59

otolith 386.19

otopalatodigital 759.89

outlet (thoracic) 353.0

ovarian remnant 620.8

Owren's (*see also* Defect, coagulation) 286.3

OX 758.6

pacemaker 429.4

Paget-Schroetter (intermittent venous claudication) 453.89

pain—*see also* Pain
 central 338.0
 chronic 338.4
 complex regional 355.9
  type I 337.20
   lower limb 337.22
   specified site NEC 337.29
   upper limb 337.21
  type II
   lower limb 355.71
   upper limb 354.4
 myelopathic 338.0
 thalamic (hypersthetic) 338.0

painful
 apicocostal vertebral (M8010/3) 162.3
 arc 726.19
 bruising 287.2
 feet 266.2

Syndrome—*continued*
Pancoast's (carcinoma, pulmonary apex)
  (M8010/3) 162.3
panhypopituitary (postpartum) 253.2
papillary muscle 429.81
  with myocardial infarction 410.8
Papillon-Léage and Psaume (orodigitofacial
  dysostosis) 759.89
parabiotic (transfusion)
  donor (twin) 772.0
  recipient (twin) 776.4
paralysis agitans 332.0
paralytic 344.9
  specified type NEC 344.89
Paraneoplastic —*see* condition
Parinaud's (paralysis of conjugate upward gaze)
  378.81
  oculoglandular 372.02
Parkes Weber and Dimitri (encephalocutaneous
  angiomatosis) 759.6
Parkinson's (*see* also Parkinsonism) 332.0
parkinsonian (*see* also Parkinsonism) 332.0
Parry's (exophthalmic goiter) 242.0
Parry-Romberg 349.89
Parsonage-Aldren-Turner 353.5
Parsonage-Turner 353.5
Patau's (trisomy D_1) 758.1
patella clunk 719.66
patellofemoral 719.46
Paterson (-Brown) (-Kelly) (sideropenic
  dysphagia) 280.8
Payr's (splenic flexure syndrome) 569.89
pectoral girdle 447.8
pectoralis minor 447.8
Pelger-Huët (hereditary hyposegmentation)
  288.2
pellagra-cerebellar ataxia-renal aminoaciduria
  270.0
Pellegrini-Stieda 726.62
pellagroid 265.2
Pellizzi's (pineal) 259.8
pelvic congestion (-fibrosis) 625.5
Pendred's (familial goiter with deaf-mutism)
  243
Penfield's (*see* also Epilepsy) 345.5
Penta X 758.81
peptic ulcer—*see* Ulcer, peptic 533.9
perabduction 447.8
periodic 277.31
periurethral fibrosis 593.4
persistent fetal circulation 747.83
Petges-Cléjat (poikilodermatomyositis) 710.3
Peutz-Jeghers 759.6
Pfeiffer (acrocephalosyndactyly) 755.55
phantom limb 353.6
pharyngeal pouch 279.11
Pick's (pericardial pseudocirrhosis of liver)
  423.2
  heart 423.2
  liver 423.2
Pick-Herxheimer (diffuse idiopathic cutaneous
  atrophy) 701.8
Pickwickian (cardiopulmonary obesity) 278.8
PIE (pulmonary infiltration with eosinophilia)
  518.3
Pierre Marie-Bamberger (hypertrophic
  pulmonary osteoarthropathy) 731.2
Pierre Mauriac's (diabetes-dwarfism-obesity)
  258.1
Pierre Robin 756.0
pigment dispersion, iris 364.53

Syndrome—*continued*
pineal 259.8
pink puffer 492.8
pituitary 253.0
placental
  dysfunction 762.2
  insufficiency 762.2
  transfusion 762.3
plantar fascia 728.71
plateau iris 364.82
plica knee 727.83
Plummer-Vinson (sideropenic dysphagia) 280.8
pluricarential of infancy 260
plurideficiency of infancy 260
pluriglandular (compensatory) 258.8
polycarential of infancy 260
polyglandular 258.8
polysplenia 759.0
pontine 433.8
popliteal
  artery entrapment 447.8
  web 756.89
postartificial menopause 627.4
postcardiac injury
  postcardiotomy 429.4
  postmyocardial infarction 411.0
postcardiotomy 429.4
postcholecystectomy 576.0
postcommissurotomy 429.4
postconcussional 310.2
postcontusional 310.2
postencephalitic 310.8
posterior
  cervical sympathetic 723.2
  fossa compression 348.4
  inferior cerebellar artery (*see* also Disease,
    cerebrovascular, acute) 436
  reversible encephalopathy (PRES) 348.39
postgastrectomy (dumping) 564.2
post-gastric surgery 564.2
posthepatitis 780.79
postherpetic (neuralgia) (zoster) 053.19
  geniculate ganglion 053.11
  ophthalmica 053.19
postimmunization—*see* Complications,
  vaccination
postinfarction 411.0
postinfluenza (asthenia) 780.79
postirradiation 990
postlaminectomy 722.80
  cervical, cervicothoracic 722.81
  lumbar, lumbosacral 722.83
  thoracic, thoracolumbar 722.82
postleukotomy 310.0
postlobotomy 310.0
postmastectomy lymphedema 457.0
postmature (of newborn) 766.22
postmyocardial infarction 411.0
postoperative NEC 998.9
  blind loop 579.2
postpartum panhypopituitary 253.2
postperfusion NEC 999.89
  bone marrow 996.85
postpericardiotomy 429.4
postphlebitic (asymptomatic) 459.10
  with
    complications NEC 459.19
    inflammation 459.12
      and ulcer 459.13
    stasis dermatitis 459.12
      with ulcer 459.13

Syndrome—*continued*
twin-to-twin transfusion 762.3
  recipient twin 776.4
Uehlinger's (acrochyderma) 757.39
Ullrich (-Bonnevie) (-Turner) 758.6
Ullrich-Feichtiger 759.89
underwater blast injury (abdominal) (*see also*
  Injury, internal, abdomen) 868.00
universal joint, cervix 620.6
Unverricht (-Lundborg) 345.1
Unverricht-Wagner (dermatomyositis) 710.3
upward gaze 378.81
Urbach-Oppenheim (necrobiosis lipoidica
  diabeticorum) 250.8 *[709.3]*
  due to secondary diabetes 249.8 *[709.3]*
Urbach-Wiethe (lipoid proteinosis) 272.8
uremia, chronic 585.9
urethral 597.81
urethro-oculoarticular 099.3
urethro-oculosynovial 099.3
urohepatic 572.4
uveocutaneous 364.24
uveomeningeal, uveomeningitis 363.22
vagohypoglossal 352.6
vagovagal 780.2
van Buchem's (hyperostosis corticalis) 733.3
van der Hoeve's (brittle bones and blue sclera,
  deafness) 756.51
van der Hoeve-Halbertsma-Waardenburg
  (ptosis-epicanthus) 270.2
van der Hoeve-Waardenburg-Gualdi
  (ptosis-epicanthus) 270.2
van Neck-Odelberg (juvenile osteochondrosis)
  732.1
vanishing twin 651.33
vascular splanchnic 557.0
vasomotor 443.9
vasovagal 780.2
VATER 759.89
Velo-cardio-facial 758.32
vena cava (inferior) (superior) (obstruction)
  459.2
Verbiest's (claudicatio intermittens spinalis)
  435.1
Vernet's 352.6
vertebral
  artery 435.1
    compression 721.1
  lumbar 724.4
  steal 435.1
vertebrogenic (pain) 724.5
vertiginous NEC 386.9
video display tube 723.8
Villaret's 352.6
Vinson-Plummer (sideropenic dysphagia) 280.8
virilizing adrenocortical hyperplasia, congenital
  255.2
virus, viral 079.99
visceral larval migrans 128.0
visual disorientation 368.16
vitamin B$_6$ deficiency 266.1
vitreous touch 997.99
Vogt's (corpus striatum) 333.71
Vogt-Koyanagi 364.24
Volkmann's 958.6
von Bechterew-Strümpell (ankylosing
  spondylitis) 720.0
von Graefe's 378.72
von Hippel-Lindau (angiomatosis
  retinocerebellosa) 759.6

Syndrome—*continued*
von Schroetter's (intermittent venous
  claudication) 453.89
von Willebrand (-Jürgens) (angiohemophilia)
  286.4
Waardenburg-Klein (ptosis epicanthus) 270.2
Wagner (-Unverricht) (dermatomyositis) 710.3
Waldenström's (macroglobulinemia) 273.3
Waldenström-Kjellberg (sideropenic dysphagia)
  280.8
Wallenberg's (posterior inferior cerebellar
  artery) (*see also* Disease, cerebrovascular,
  acute) 436
Waterhouse (-Friderichsen) 036.3
water retention 276.6
Weber's 344.89
Weber-Christian (nodular nonsuppurative
  panniculitis) 729.30
Weber-Cockayne (epidermolysis bullosa)
  757.39
Weber-Dimitri (encephalocutaneous
  angiomatosis) 759.6
Weber-Gubler 344.89
Weber-Leyden 344.89
Weber-Osler (familial hemorrhagic
  telangiectasia) 448.0
Wegener's (necrotizing respiratory
  granulomatosis) 446.4
Weill-Marchesani (brachymorphism and ectopia
  lentis) 759.89
Weingarten's (tropical eosinophilia) 518.3
Weiss-Baker (carotid sinus syncope) 337.01
Weissenbach-Thibierge (cutaneous systemic
  sclerosis) 710.1
Werdnig-Hoffmann 335.0
Werlhof-Wichmann (*see also* Purpura,
  thrombocytopenic) 287.39
Wermer's (polyendocrine adenomatosis) 258.01
Werner's (progeria adultorum) 259.8
Wernicke's (nonalcoholic) (superior
  hemorrhagic polioencephalitis) 265.1
Wernicke-Korsakoff (nonalcoholic) 294.0
  alcoholic 291.1
Westphal-Strümpell (hepatolenticular
  degeneration) 275.1
wet
  brain (alcoholic) 303.9
  feet (maceration) (tropical) 991.4
  lung
    adult 518.5
    newborn 770.6
whiplash 847.0
Whipple's (intestinal lipodystrophy) 040.2
"whistling face" (craniocarpotarsal dystrophy)
  759.89
Widal (-Abrami) (acquired hemolytic jaundice)
  283.9
Wilkie's 557.1
Wilkinson-Sneddon (subcorneal pustular
  dermatosis) 694.1
Willan-Plumbe (psoriasis) 696.1
Willebrand (-Jürgens) (angiohemophilia) 286.4
Willi-Prader (hypogenital dystrophy with
  diabetic tendency) 759.81
Wilson's (hepatolenticular degeneration) 275.1
Wilson-Mikity 770.7
Wiskott-Aldrich (eczema-thrombocytopenia)
  279.12

Syndrome—*continued*
  withdrawal
    alcohol 291.81
    drug 292.0
      infant of dependent mother 779.5
  Woakes' (ethmoiditis) 471.1
  Wolff-Parkinson-White (anomalous
      atrioventricular excitation) 426.7
  Wright's (hyperabduction) 447.8
  X
    cardiac 413.9
    dysmetabolic 277.7
  xiphoidalgia 733.99
  XO 758.6
  XXX 758.81
  XXXXY 758.81
  XXY 758.7
  yellow vernix (placental dysfunction) 762.2
  Zahorsky's 074.0
  Zellweger 277.86
  Zieve's (jaundice, hyperlipemia and hemolytic
      anemia) 571.1
  Zollinger-Ellison (gastric hypersecretion with
      pancreatic islet cell tumor) 251.5
  Zuelzer-Ogden (nutritional megaloblastic
      anemia) 281.2
Synechia (iris) (pupil) 364.70
  anterior 364.72
    peripheral 364.73
  intrauterine (traumatic) 621.5
  posterior 364.71
  vulvae, congenital 752.49
Synesthesia (*see also* Disturbance, sensation)
      782.0
Synodontia 520.2
Synophthalmus 759.89
Synorchidism 752.89
Synorchism 752.89
Synostosis (congenital) 756.59
  astragaloscaphoid 755.67
  radioulnar 755.53
  talonavicular (bar) 755.67
  tarsal 755.67
Synovial —*see* condition
Synovioma (M9040/3)—*see also* Neoplasm,
    connective tissue, malignant
  benign (M9040/3)—*see* Neoplasm, connective
    tissue, benign
Synoviosarcoma (M9040/3)—*see* Neoplasm,
    connective tissue, malignant
Synovitis (*see also* Tenosynovitis) 727.00
  chronic crepitant, wrist 727.2
  due to crystals—*see* Arthritis, due to crystals
  gonococcal 098.51
  gouty 274.00
  specified NEC 727.09
  syphilitic 095.7
    congenital 090.0
  traumatic, current—*see* Sprain, by site
  tuberculous—*see* Tuberculosis, synovitis
  villonodular 719.20
    ankle 719.27
    elbow 719.22
    foot 719.27
    hand 719.24
    hip 719.25
    knee 719.26
    multiple sites 719.29
    pelvic region 719.25
    shoulder (region) 719.21
    specified site NEC 719.28
    wrist 719.23

Syphilide 091.3
  congenital 090.0
  newborn 090.0
  tubercular 095.8
    congenital 090.0
Syphilis, syphilitic (acquired) 097.9
  with lung involvement 095.1
  abdomen (late) 095.2
  acoustic nerve 094.86
  adenopathy (secondary) 091.4
  adrenal (gland) 095.8
    with cortical hypofunction 095.8
  age under 2 years NEC (*see also* Syphilis,
      congenital) 090.9
  acquired 097.9
  alopecia (secondary) 091.82
  anemia 095.8
  aneurysm (artery) (ruptured) 093.89
    aorta 093.0
    central nervous system 094.89
    congenital 090.5
  anus 095.8
    primary 091.1
    secondary 091.3
  aorta, aortic (arch) (abdominal) (insufficiency)
      (pulmonary) (regurgitation) (stenosis)
      (thoracic) 093.89
    aneurysm 093.0
  arachnoid (adhesive) 094.2
  artery 093.89
    cerebral 094.89
    spinal 094.89
  arthropathy (neurogenic) (tabetic) 094.0 *[713.5]*
  asymptomatic—*see* Syphilis, latent
  ataxia, locomotor (progressive) 094.0
  atrophoderma maculatum 091.3
  auricular fibrillation 093.89
  Bell's palsy 094.89
  bladder 095.8
  bone 095.5
    secondary 091.61
  brain 094.89
  breast 095.8
  bronchus 095.8
  bubo 091.0
  bulbar palsy 094.89
  bursa (late) 095.7
  cardiac decompensation 093.89
  cardiovascular (early) (late) (primary)
      (secondary) (tertiary) 093.9
    specified type and site NEC 093.89
  causing death under 2 years of age (*see also*
      Syphilis, congenital) 090.9
    stated to be acquired NEC 097.9
  central nervous system (any site) (early) (late)
      (latent) (primary) (recurrent) (relapse)
      (secondary) (tertiary) 094.9
    with
      ataxia 094.0
      paralysis, general 094.1
        juvenile 090.40
      paresis (general) 094.1
        juvenile 090.40
      tabes (dorsalis) 094.0
        juvenile 090.40
      taboparesis 094.1
        juvenile 090.40
    aneurysm (ruptured) 094.87
    congenital 090.40
    juvenile 090.40
    remission in (sustained) 094.9

Syphilis, syphilitic—*continued*
  serology doubtful, negative, or positive 094.9
    specified nature or site NEC 094.89
    vascular 094.89
  cerebral 094.89
    meningovascular 094.2
    nerves 094.89
    sclerosis 094.89
    thrombosis 094.89
  cerebrospinal 094.89
    tabetic 094.0
  cerebrovascular 094.89
  cervix 095.8
  chancre (multiple) 091.0
    extragenital 091.2
    Rollet's 091.0
  Charcot's joint 094.0 *[713.5]*
  choked disc 094.89 *[377.00]*
  chorioretinitis 091.51
    congenital 090.0 *[363.13]*
    late 094.83
  choroiditis 091.51
    congenital 090.0 *[363.13]*
    late 094.83
    prenatal 090.0 *[363.13]*
  choroidoretinitis (secondary) 091.51
    congenital 090.0 *[363.13]*
    late 094.83
  ciliary body (secondary) 091.52
    late 095.8 *[364.11]*
  colon (late) 095.8
  combined sclerosis 094.89
  complicating pregnancy, childbirth or
    puerperium 647.0
    affecting fetus or newborn 760.2
  condyloma (latum) 091.3
  congenital 090.9
    with
      encephalitis 090.41
      paresis (general) 090.40
      tabes (dorsalis) 090.40
      taboparesis 090.40
    chorioretinitis, choroiditis 090.0 *[363.13]*
    early or less than 2 years after birth NEC 090.2
      with manifestations 090.0
      latent (without manifestations) 090.1
        negative spinal fluid test 090.1
        serology, positive 090.1
      symptomatic 090.0
    interstitial keratitis 090.3
    juvenile neurosyphilis 090.40
    late or 2 years or more after birth NEC 090.7
      chorioretinitis, choroiditis 090.5 *[363.13]*
      interstitial keratitis 090.3
      juvenile neurosyphilis NEC 090.40
      latent (without manifestations) 090.6
        negative spinal fluid test 090.6
        serology, positive 090.6
      symptomatic or with manifestations NEC
        090.5
        interstitial keratitis 090.3
  conjugal 097.9
    tabes 094.0
  conjunctiva 095.8 *[372.10]*
  contact V01.6
  cord, bladder 094.0
  cornea, late 095.8 *[370.59]*
  coronary (artery) 093.89
    sclerosis 093.89
  coryza 095.8
    congenital 090.0

Syphilis, syphilitic—*continued*
  cranial nerve 094.89
  cutaneous—*see* Syphilis, skin
  dacryocystitis 095.8
  degeneration, spinal cord 094.89
  d'emblée 095.8
  dementia 094.1
    paralytica 094.1
      juvenilis 090.40
  destruction of bone 095.5
  dilatation, aorta 093.0
  due to blood transfusion 097.9
  dura mater 094.89
  ear 095.8
    inner 095.8
      nerve (eighth) 094.86
      neurorecurrence 094.86
  early NEC 091.0
    cardiovascular 093.9
    central nervous system 094.9
      paresis 094.1
      tabes 094.0
    latent (without manifestations) (less than 2
      years after infection) 092.9
      negative spinal fluid test 092.9
      serological relapse following treatment
        092.0
      serology positive 092.9
    paresis 094.1
    relapse (treated, untreated) 091.7
    skin 091.3
    symptomatic NEC 091.89
      extragenital chancre 091.2
      primary, except extragenital chancre 091.0
      secondary (*see also* Syphilis, secondary)
        091.3
        relapse (treated, untreated) 091.7
      tabes 094.0
    ulcer 091.3
  eighth nerve 094.86
  endemic, nonvenereal 104.0
  endocarditis 093.20
    aortic 093.22
    mitral 093.21
    pulmonary 093.24
    tricuspid 093.23
  epididymis (late) 095.8
  epiglottis 095.8
  epiphysitis (congenital) 090.0
  esophagus 095.8
  Eustachian tube 095.8
  exposure to V01.6
  eye 095.8 *[363.13]*
    neuromuscular mechanism 094.85
  eyelid 095.8 *[373.5]*
    with gumma 095.8 *[373.5]*
    ptosis 094.89
  fallopian tube 095.8
  fracture 095.5
  gallbladder (late) 095.8
  gastric 095.8
    crisis 094.0
    polyposis 095.8
  general 097.9
    paralysis 094.1
      juvenile 090.40
  genital (primary) 091.0
  glaucoma 095.8
  gumma (late) NEC 095.9
    cardiovascular system 093.9
    central nervous system 094.9

Syphilis, syphilitic—*continued*
  congenital 090.5
  heart or artery 093.89
  heart 093.89
    block 093.89
    decompensation 093.89
    disease 093.89
    failure 093.89
    valve (*see also* Syphilis, endocarditis) 093.20
  hemianesthesia 094.89
  hemianopsia 095.8
  hemiparesis 094.89
  hemiplegia 094.89
  hepatic artery 093.89
  hepatitis 095.3
  hepatomegaly 095.3
    congenital 090.0
  hereditaria tarda (*see also* Syphilis, congenital, late) 090.7
  hereditary (*see also* Syphilis, congenital) 090.9
    interstitial keratitis 090.3
  Hutchinson's teeth 090.5
  hyalitis 095.8
  inactive—*see* Syphilis, latent
  infantum NEC (*see also* Syphilis, congenital) 090.9
  inherited—*see* Syphilis, congenital
  internal ear 095.8
  intestine (late) 095.8
  iris, iritis (secondary) 091.52
    late 095.8 *[364.11]*
  joint (late) 095.8
  keratitis (congenital) (early) (interstitial) (late) (parenchymatous) (punctata profunda) 090.3
  kidney 095.4
  lacrimal apparatus 095.8
  laryngeal paralysis 095.8
  larynx 095.8
  late 097.0
    cardiovascular 093.9
    central nervous system 094.9
    latent or 2 years or more after infection (without manifestations) 096
      negative spinal fluid test 096
      serology positive 096
    paresis 094.1
    specified site NEC 095.8
    symptomatic or with symptoms 095.9
    tabes 094.0
  latent 097.1
    central nervous system 094.9
    date of infection unspecified 097.1
    early or less than 2 years after infection 092.9
    late or 2 years or more after infection 096
    serology
      doubtful
        follow-up of latent syphilis 097.1
          central nervous system 094.9
          date of infection unspecified 097.1
          early or less than 2 years after infection 092.9
          late or 2 years or more after infection 096
      positive, only finding 097.1
        date of infection unspecified 097.1
        early or less than 2 years after infection 097.1
        late or 2 years or more after infection 097.1
  lens 095.8
  leukoderma 091.3
    late 095.8

Syphilis, syphilitic—*continued*
  lienis 095.8
  lip 091.3
    chancre 091.2
    late 095.8
    primary 091.2
  Lissauer's paralysis 094.1
  liver 095.3
    secondary 091.62
  locomotor ataxia 094.0
  lung 095.1
  lymphadenitis (secondary) 091.4
  lymph gland (early) (secondary) 091.4
    late 095.8
  macular atrophy of skin 091.3
    striated 095.8
  maternal, affecting fetus or newborn 760.2
    manifest syphilis in newborn—*see* Syphilis, congenital
  mediastinum (late) 095.8
  meninges (adhesive) (basilar) (brain) (spinal cord) 094.2
  meningitis 094.2
    acute 091.81
    congenital 090.42
  meningoencephalitis 094.2
  meningovascular 094.2
    congenital 090.49
  mesarteritis 093.89
    brain 094.89
    spine 094.89
  middle ear 095.8
  mitral stenosis 093.21
  monoplegia 094.89
  mouth (secondary) 091.3
    late 095.8
  mucocutaneous 091.3
    late 095.8
  mucous
    membrane 091.3
      late 095.8
    patches 091.3
      congenital 090.0
  mulberry molars 090.5
  muscle 095.6
  myocardium 093.82
  myositis 095.6
  nasal sinus 095.8
  neonatorum NEC (*see also* Syphilis, congenital) 090.9
  nerve palsy (any cranial nerve) 094.89
  nervous system, central 094.9
  neuritis 095.8
    acoustic nerve 094.86
  neurorecidive of retina 094.83
  neuroretinitis 094.85
  newborn (*see also* Syphilis, congenital) 090.9
  nodular superficial 095.8
  nonvenereal, endemic 104.0
  nose 095.8
    saddle back deformity 090.5
    septum 095.8
      perforated 095.8
  occlusive arterial disease 093.89
  ophthalmic 095.8 *[363.13]*
  ophthalmoplegia 094.89
  optic nerve (atrophy) (neuritis) (papilla) 094.84
  orbit (late) 095.8
  orchitis 095.8
  organic 097.9
  osseous (late) 095.5

Syphilis, syphilitic—*continued*
osteochondritis (congenital) 090.0
osteoporosis 095.5
ovary 095.8
oviduct 095.8
palate 095.8
  gumma 095.8
  perforated 090.5
pancreas (late) 095.8
pancreatitis 095.8
paralysis 094.89
  general 094.1
  juvenile 090.40
paraplegia 094.89
paresis (general) 094.1
  juvenile 090.40
paresthesia 094.89
Parkinson's disease or syndrome 094.82
paroxysmal tachycardia 093.89
pemphigus (congenital) 090.0
penis 091.0
  chancre 091.0
  late 095.8
pericardium 093.81
perichondritis, larynx 095.8
periosteum 095.5
  congenital 090.0
  early 091.61
  secondary 091.61
peripheral nerve 095.8
petrous bone (late) 095.5
pharynx 095.8
  secondary 091.3
pituitary (gland) 095.8
placenta 095.8
pleura (late) 095.8
pneumonia, white 090.0
pontine (lesion) 094.89
portal vein 093.89
primary NEC 091.2
  anal 091.1
  and secondary (*see also* Syphilis, secondary) 091.9
  cardiovascular 093.9
  central nervous system 094.9
  extragenital chancre NEC 091.2
  fingers 091.2
  genital 091.0
  lip 091.2
  specified site NEC 091.2
  tonsils 091.2
prostate 095.8
psychosis (intracranial gumma) 094.89
ptosis (eyelid) 094.89
pulmonary (late) 095.1
  artery 093.89
pulmonum 095.1
pyelonephritis 095.4
recently acquired, symptomatic NEC 091.89
rectum 095.8
respiratory tract 095.8
retina
  late 094.83
  neurorecidive 094.83
retrobulbar neuritis 094.85
salpingitis 095.8
sclera (late) 095.0
sclerosis
  cerebral 094.89
  coronary 093.89
  multiple 094.89

Syphilis, syphilitic—*continued*
  subacute 094.89
scotoma (central) 095.8
scrotum 095.8
secondary (and primary) 091.9
  adenopathy 091.4
  anus 091.3
  bone 091.61
  cardiovascular 093.9
  central nervous system 094.9
  chorioretinitis, choroiditis 091.51
  hepatitis 091.62
  liver 091.62
  lymphadenitis 091.4
  meningitis, acute 091.81
  mouth 091.3
  mucous membranes 091.3
  periosteum 091.61
  periostitis 091.61
  pharynx 091.3
  relapse (treated) (untreated) 091.7
  skin 091.3
  specified form NEC 091.89
  tonsil 091.3
  ulcer 091.3
  viscera 091.69
  vulva 091.3
seminal vesicle (late) 095.8
seronegative
  with signs or symptoms—*see* Syphilis, by site and stage
seropositive
  with signs or symptoms—*see* Syphilis, by site and stage
  follow-up of latent syphilis—*see* Syphilis, latent
  only finding—*see* Syphilis, latent
seventh nerve (paralysis) 094.89
sinus 095.8
sinusitis 095.8
skeletal system 095.5
skin (early) (secondary) (with ulceration) 091.3
  late or tertiary 095.8
small intestine 095.8
spastic spinal paralysis 094.0
spermatic cord (late) 095.8
spinal (cord) 094.89
  with
    paresis 094.1
    tabes 094.0
spleen 095.8
splenomegaly 095.8
spondylitis 095.5
staphyloma 095.8
stigmata (congenital) 090.5
stomach 095.8
synovium (late) 095.7
tabes dorsalis (early) (late) 094.0
  juvenile 090.40
tabetic type 094.0
  juvenile 090.40
taboparesis 094.1
  juvenile 090.40
tachycardia 093.89
tendon (late) 095.7
tertiary 097.0
  with symptoms 095.8
  cardiovascular 093.9
  central nervous system 094.9
  multiple NEC 095.8
  specified site NEC 095.8

Syphilis, syphilitic—*continued*
 testis 095.8
 thorax 095.8
 throat 095.8
 thymus (gland) 095.8
 thyroid (late) 095.8
 tongue 095.8
 tonsil (lingual) 095.8
  primary 091.2
  secondary 091.3
 trachea 095.8
 tricuspid valve 093.23
 tumor, brain 094.89
 tunica vaginalis (late) 095.8
 ulcer (any site) (early) (secondary) 091.3
  late 095.9
   perforating 095.9
    foot 094.0
 urethra (stricture) 095.8
 urogenital 095.8
 uterus 095.8
 uveal tract (secondary) 091.50
  late 095.8 *[363.13]*
 uveitis (secondary) 091.50
  late 095.8 *[363.13]*
 uvula (late) 095.8
  perforated 095.8
 vagina 091.0
  late 095.8
 valvulitis NEC 093.20
 vascular 093.89
  brain or cerebral 094.89
 vein 093.89
  cerebral 094.89
 ventriculi 095.8
 vesicae urinariae 095.8
 viscera (abdominal) 095.2
  secondary 091.69
 vitreous (hemorrhage) (opacities) 095.8
 vulva 091.0
  late 095.8
  secondary 091.3
Syphiloma 095.9
 cardiovascular system 093.9
 central nervous system 094.9
 circulatory system 093.9
 congenital 090.5
Syphilophobia 300.29
Syringadenoma (M8400/0)—*see also* Neoplasm, skin, benign
 papillary (M8406/0)—*see* Neoplasm, skin, benign
Syringobulbia 336.0
Syringocarcinoma (M8400/3)—*see* Neoplasm, skin, malignant
Syringocystadenoma (M8400/0)—*see also* Neoplasm, skin, benign
 papillary (M8406/0)—*see* Neoplasm, skin, benign
Syringocystoma (M8407/0)—*see* Neoplasm, skin, benign
Syringoma (M8407/0)—*see also* Neoplasm, skin, benign
 chondroid (M8940/0)—*see* Neoplasm, by site, benign
Syringomyelia 336.0
Syringomyelitis 323.9
 late effect—*see* category 326
Syringomyelocele (*see also* Spina bifida) 741.9
Syringopontia 336.0

System, systemic —*see also* condition
 disease, combined—*see* Degeneration, combined
 fibrosclerosing syndrome 710.8
 inflammatory response syndrome (SIRS) 995.90
  due to
   infectious process 995.91
    with acute organ dysfunction 995.92
   non-infectious process 995.93
    with acute organ dysfunction 995.94
 lupus erythematosus 710.0
  inhibitor 286.5

T

Tab —*see* Tag
Tabacism 989.8
Tabacosis 989.8
Tabardillo 080
  flea-borne 081.0
  louse-borne 080
Tabes, tabetic
  with
    central nervous system syphilis 094.0
    Charcot's joint 094.0 *[713.5]*
    cord bladder 094.0
    crisis, viscera (any) 094.0
    paralysis, general 094.1
    paresis (general) 094.1
    perforating ulcer 094.0
  arthropathy 094.0 *[713.5]*
  bladder 094.0
  bone 094.0
  cerebrospinal 094.0
  congenital 090.40
  conjugal 094.0
  dorsalis 094.0
    neurosyphilis 094.0
  early 094.0
  juvenile 090.40
  latent 094.0
  mesenterica (*see also* Tuberculosis) 014.8
  paralysis insane, general 094.1
  peripheral (nonsyphilitic) 799.89
  spasmodic 094.0
    not dorsal or dorsalis 343.9
  syphilis (cerebrospinal) 094.0
Taboparalysis 094.1
Taboparesis (remission) 094.1
  with
    Charcot's joint 094.1 *[713.5]*
    cord bladder 094.1
    perforating ulcer 094.1
  juvenile 090.40
Tache noir 923.20
Tachyalimentation 579.3
Tachyarrhythmia, tachyrhythmia —*see also*
  Tachycardia
  paroxysmal with sinus bradycardia 427.81
Tachycardia 785.0
  atrial 427.89
  auricular 427.89
  AV nodal re-entry (re-entrant) 427.89
  newborn 779.82
  nodal 427.89
  nonparoxysmal atrioventricular 426.89
  nonparoxysmal atrioventricular (nodal) 426.89
  nonsustained 427.2
  paroxysmal 427.2
    with sinus bradycardia 427.81
    atrial (PAT) 427.0
      psychogenic 316 *[427.0]*
    atrioventricular (AV) 427.0
      psychogenic 316 *[427.0]*
    essential 427.2
    junctional ectopic 427.0
    nodal 427.0
    psychogenic 316 *[427.2]*
      atrial 316 *[427.0]*
      supraventricular 316 *[427.0]*
      ventricular 316 *[427.1]*

Tachycardia—*continued*
  supraventricular 427.0
    psychogenic 316 *[427.0]*
  ventricular 427.1
    psychogenic 316 *[427.1]*
  postoperative 997.1
  psychogenic 306.2
  sick sinus 427.81
  sinoauricular 427.89
  sinus 427.89
  supraventricular 427.89
  sustained 427.2
    supraventricular 427.0
    ventricular 427.1
  ventricular (paroxysmal) 427.1
    psychogenic 316 *[427.1]*
Tachygastria 536.8
Tachypnea 786.06
  hysterical 300.11
  newborn (idiopathic) (transitory) 770.6
  psychogenic 306.1
  transitory, of newborn 770.6
Taenia (infection) (infestation) (*see also*
  Infestation, taenia) 123.3
  diminuta 123.6
  echinococcal infestation (*see also*
    Echinococcus) 122.9
  nana 123.6
  saginata infestation 123.2
  solium (intestinal form) 123.0
    larval form 123.1
Taeniasis (intestine) (*see also* Infestation, Taenia)
  123.3
  saginata 123.2
  solium 123.0
Taenzer's disease 757.4
Tag (hypertrophied skin) (infected) 701.9
  adenoid 474.8
  anus 455.9
  endocardial (*see also* Endocarditis) 424.90
  hemorrhoidal 455.9
  hymen 623.8
  perineal 624.8
  preauricular 744.1
  rectum 455.9
  sentinel 455.9
  skin 701.9
    accessory 757.39
    anus 455.9
    congenital 757.39
    preauricular 744.1
    rectum 455.9
  tonsil 474.8
  urethra, urethral 599.84
  vulva 624.8
Tahyna fever 062.5
Takayasu (-Onishi) disease or syndrome
  (pulseless disease) 446.7
Takotsubo syndrome 429.83
Talc granuloma 728.82
  in operation wound 998.7
Talcosis 502
Talipes (congenital) 754.70
  acquired NEC 736.79
    planus 734
  asymmetric 754.79
    acquired 736.79

Talipes—*continued*
  calcaneovalgus 754.62
    acquired 736.76
  calcaneovarus 754.59
    acquired 736.76
  calcaneus 754.79
    acquired 736.76
  cavovarus 754.59
    acquired 736.75
  cavus 754.71
    acquired 736.73
  equinovalgus 754.69
    acquired 736.72
  equinovarus 754.51
    acquired 736.71
  equinus 754.79
    acquired, NEC 736.72
  percavus 754.71
    acquired 736.73
  planovalgus 754.69
    acquired 736.79
  planus (acquired) (any degree) 734
    congenital 754.61
    due to rickets 268.1
  valgus 754.60
    acquired 736.79
  varus 754.50
    acquired 736.79
Talma's disease 728.85
Talon noir 924.20
  hand 923.20
  heel 924.20
  toe 924.3
Tamponade heart (Rose's) (*see also*
    Pericarditis) 423.3
Tanapox 059.21
Tangier disease (familial high-density
    lipoprotein deficiency) 272.5
Tank ear 380.12
Tantrum (childhood) (*see also* Disturbance,
    conduct) 312.1
Tapeworm (infection) (infestation) (*see also*
    Infestation, tapeworm) 123.9
Tapia's syndrome 352.6
Tarantism 297.8
Target-oval cell anemia 282.49
Tarlov's cyst 355.9
Tarral-Besnier disease (pityriasis rubra pilaris)
    696.4
Tarsalgia 729.2
Tarsal tunnel syndrome 355.5
Tarsitis (eyelid) 373.00
  syphilitic 095.8 *[373.00]*
  tuberculous (*see also* Tuberculosis) 017.0 *[373.4]*
Tartar (teeth) 523.6
Tattoo (mark) 709.09
Taurodontism 520.2
Taussig-Bing defect, heart, or syndrome
    (transposition, aorta and overriding pulmonary
    artery) 745.11
Tay's choroiditis 363.41
Tay-Sachs
  amaurotic familial idiocy 330.1
  disease 330.1
Taybi's syndrome (otopalatodigital) 759.89
Taylor's
  disease (diffuse idiopathic cutaneous atrophy) 701.8
  syndrome 625.5
TBI (traumatic brain injury) (see also Injury,
    intracranial) 854.0
  with skull fracture —see Fracture, skull, by site

Tear, torn (traumatic)—*see also* Wound, open,
    by site
  anus, anal (sphincter) 863.89
    with open wound in cavity 863.99
    complicating delivery (healed) (old) 654.8
      with mucosa 664.3
      not associated with third-degree perineal
        laceration 664.6
    nontraumatic, nonpuerperal (healed) (old)
      569.43
  articular cartilage, old (*see also* Disorder,
      cartilage, articular) 718.0
  bladder
    with
      abortion—*see* Abortion, by type, with
        damage to pelvic organs
      ectopic pregnancy (*see also* categories
        633.0-633.9) 639.2
      molar pregnancy (*see also* categories
        630-632) 639.2
    following
      abortion 639.2
      ectopic or molar pregnancy 639.2
    obstetrical trauma 665.5
  bowel
    with
      abortion—*see* Abortion, by type, with
        damage to pelvic organs
      ectopic pregnancy (*see also* categories
        633.0-633.9) 639.2
      molar pregnancy (*see also* categories
        630-632) 639.2
    following
      abortion 639.2
      ectopic or molar pregnancy 639.2
    obstetrical trauma 665.5
  broad ligament
    with
      abortion—*see* Abortion, by type, with
        damage to pelvic organs
      ectopic pregnancy (*see also* categories
        633.0-633.9) 639.2
      molar pregnancy (*see also* categories
        630-632) 639.2
    following
      abortion 639.2
      ectopic or molar pregnancy 639.2
    obstetrical trauma 665.6
  bucket handle (knee) (meniscus)—*see* Tear,
    meniscus
  capsule
    joint—*see* Sprain, by site
    spleen—*see* Laceration, spleen, capsule
  cartilage—*see also* Sprain, by site
    articular, old (*see also* Disorder, cartilage,
      articular) 718.0
    knee—*see* Tear, meniscus
    semilunar (knee) (current injury)—*see* Tear,
      meniscus
  cervix
    with
      abortion—*see* Abortion, by type, with
        damage to pelvic organs
      ectopic pregnancy (*see also* categories
        633.0-633.9) 639.2
      molar pregnancy (*see also* categories
        630-632) 639.2
    following
      abortion 639.2
      ectopic or molar pregnancy 639.2
    obstetrical trauma (current) 665.3
    old 622.3

Tear, torn—*continued*
dural 349.31
  accidental puncture or laceration during a
    procedure 349.31
  incidental (inadvertent) 349.31
  nontraumatic NEC 349.39
internal organ (abdomen, chest, or pelvis)—*see*
  Injury, internal, by site
ligament—*see also* Sprain, by site
  with open wound—*see* Wound, open by site
meniscus (knee) (current injury) 836.2
  bucket handle 836.0
    old 717.0
  lateral 836.1
    anterior horn 836.1
      old 717.42
    bucket handle 836.1
      old 717.41
    old 717.40
    posterior horn 836.1
      old 717.43
    specified site NEC 836.1
      old 717.49
  medial 836.0
    anterior horn 836.0
      old 717.1
    bucket handle 836.0
      old 717.0
    old 717.3
    posterior horn 836.0
      old 717.2
  old NEC 717.5
  site other than knee—*see* Sprain, by site
muscle—*see also* Sprain, by site
  with open wound—*see* Wound, open by site
pelvic
  floor, complicating delivery 664.1
  organ NEC
    with
      abortion—*see* Abortion, by type, with
        damage to pelvic organs
      ectopic pregnancy (*see also* categories
        633.0-633.9) 639.2
      molar pregnancy (*see also* categories
        630-632) 639.2
    following
      abortion 639.2
      ectopic or molar pregnancy 639.2
    obstetrical trauma 665.5
perineum—*see also* Laceration, perineum
  obstetrical trauma 665.5
periurethral tissue
  with
    abortion—*see* Abortion, by type, with
      damage to pelvic organs
    ectopic pregnancy (*see also* categories
      633.0-633.9) 639.2
    molar pregnancy (*see also* categories
      630-632) 639.2
  following
    abortion 639.2
    ectopic or molar pregnancy 639.2
  obstetrical trauma 665.5
rectovaginal septum—*see* Laceration,
  rectovaginal septum
retina, retinal (recent) (with detachment) 361.00
  without detachment 361.30
  dialysis (juvenile) (with detachment) 361.04
  giant (with detachment) 361.03
  horseshoe (without detachment) 361.32
  multiple (with detachment) 361.02
    without detachment 361.33

Tear, torn—*continued*
old
  delimited (partial) 361.06
  partial 361.06
  total or subtotal 361.07
partial (without detachment)
  giant 361.03
  multiple defects 361.02
  old (delimited) 361.06
  single defect 361.01
round hole (without detachment) 361.31
single defect (with detachment) 361.01
total or subtotal (recent) 361.05
  old 361.07
rotator cuff (traumatic) 840.4
  current injury 840.4
  degenerative 726.10
  nontraumatic 727.61
semilunar cartilage, knee (*see also* Tear,
  meniscus) 836.2
  old 717.5
tendon—*see also* Sprain, by site
  with open wound—*see* Wound, open by site
tentorial, at birth 767.0
umbilical cord
  affecting fetus or newborn 772.0
  complicating delivery 663.8
urethra
  with
    abortion—*see* Abortion, by type, with
      damage to pelvic organs
    ectopic pregnancy (*see also* categories
      633.0-633.9) 639.2
    molar pregnancy (*see also* categories
      630-632) 639.2
  following
    abortion 639.2
    ectopic or molar pregnancy 639.2
  obstetrical trauma 665.5
uterus—*see* Injury, internal, uterus
vagina—*see* Laceration, vagina
vessel, from catheter 998.2
vulva, complicating delivery 664.0
Tear stone 375.57
Teeth, tooth —*see also* condition
grinding 306.8
prenatal 520.6
Teething 520.7
syndrome 520.7
Tegmental syndrome 344.89
Telangiectasia, telangiectasis (verrucous) 448.9
ataxic (cerebellar) 334.8
familial 448.0
hemorrhagic, hereditary (congenital) (senile) 448.0
hereditary hemorrhagic 448.0
retina 362.15
spider 448.1
Telecanthus (congenital) 743.63
Telescoped bowel or intestine (*see also*
  Intussusception) 560.0
Teletherapy, adverse effect NEC 990
Telogen effluvium 704.02
Temperature
body, high (of unknown origin) (*see also*
  Pyrexia) 780.60
cold, trauma from 991.9
  newborn 778.2
  specified effect NEC 991.8
high
  body (of unknown origin) (*see also* Pyrexia)
    780.60
  trauma from—*see* Heat

Temper tantrum (childhood) (*see also* Disturbance, conduct) 312.1
Temple —*see* condition
Temporal —*see also* condition
  lobe syndrome 310.0
Temporomandibular joint-pain-dysfunction syndrome 524.60
Temporosphenoidal —*see* condition
Tendency
  bleeding (*see also* Defect, coagulation) 286.9
  homosexual, ego-dystonic 302.0
  paranoid 301.0
  suicide 300.9
Tenderness
  abdominal (generalized) (localized) 789.6
  rebound 789.6
  skin 782.0
Tendinitis, tendonitis (*see also* Tenosynovitis) 726.90
  Achilles 726.71
  adhesive 726.90
    shoulder 726.0
  calcific 727.82
    shoulder 726.11
  gluteal 726.5
  patellar 726.64
  peroneal 726.79
  pes anserinus 726.61
  psoas 726.5
  tibialis (anterior) (posterior) 726.72
  trochanteric 726.5
Tendon —*see* condition
Tendosynovitis —*see* Tenosynovitis
Tendovaginitis —*see* Tenosynovitis
Tenesmus 787.99
  rectal 787.99
  vesical 788.99
Tenia —*see* Taenia
Teniasis —*see* Taeniasis
Tennis elbow 726.32
Tenonitis —*see also* Tenosynovitis
  eye (capsule) 376.04
Tenontosynovitis —*see* Tenosynovitis
Tenontothecitis —*see* Tenosynovitis
Tenophyte 727.9
Tenosynovitis (*see also* Synovitis) 727.00
  adhesive 726.90
    shoulder 726.0
  ankle 727.06
  bicipital (calcifying) 726.12
  buttock 727.09
  due to crystals—*see* Arthritis, due to crystals
  elbow 727.09
  finger 727.05
  foot 727.06
  gonococcal 098.51
  hand 727.05
  hip 727.09
  knee 727.09
  radial styloid 727.04
  shoulder 726.10
    adhesive 726.0
  specified NEC 727.09
  spine 720.1
  supraspinatus 726.10
  toe 727.06
  tuberculous—*see* Tuberculosis, tenosynovitis
  wrist 727.05
Tenovaginitis —*see* Tenosynovitis
Tension
  arterial, high (*see also* Hypertension) 401.9
    without diagnosis of hypertension 796.2

Tension—*continued*
  headache 307.81
  intraocular (elevated) 365.00
  nervous 799.21
  ocular (elevated) 365.00
  pneumothorax 512.0
    iatrogenic 512.1
    postoperative 512.1
    spontaneous 512.0
  premenstrual 625.4
  state 300.9
Tentorium —*see* condition
Teratencephalus 759.89
Teratism 759.7
Teratoblastoma (malignant) (M9080/3)—*see* Neoplasm, by site, malignant
Teratocarcinoma (M9081/3)—*see also* Neoplasm, by site, malignant
  liver 155.0
Teratoma (solid) (M9080/1)—*see also* Neoplasm, by site, uncertain behavior
  adult (cystic) (M9080/0)—*see* Neoplasm, by site, benign
  and embryonal carcinoma, mixed (M9081/3)—*see* Neoplasm, by site, malignant
  benign (M9080/0)—*see* Neoplasm, by site, benign
  combined with choriocarcinoma (M9101/3)—*see* Neoplasm, by site, malignant
  cystic (adult) (M9080/0)—*see* Neoplasm, by site, benign
  differentiated type (M9080/0)—*see* Neoplasm, by site, benign
  embryonal (M9080/3)—*see also* Neoplasm, by site, malignant
    liver 155.0
  fetal
    sacral, causing fetopelvic disproportion 653.7
  immature (M9080/3)—*see* Neoplasm, by site, malignant
  liver (M9080/3) 155.0
    adult, benign, cystic, differentiated type or mature (M9080/0) 211.5
  malignant (M9080/3)—*see also* Neoplasm, by site, malignant
    anaplastic type (M9082/3)—*see* Neoplasm, by site, malignant
    intermediate type (M9083/3)—*see* Neoplasm, by site, malignant
    liver (M9080/3) 155.0
    trophoblastic (M9102/3)
      specified site—*see* Neoplasm, by site, malignant
      unspecified site 186.9
    undifferentiated type (M9082/3)—*see* Neoplasm, by site, malignant
  mature (M9080/0)—*see* Neoplasm, by site, benign
    malignant (M9080/3) —*see* Neoplasm, by site, malignant
  ovary (M9080/0) 220
    embryonal, immature, or malignant (M9080/3) 183.0
  suprasellar (M9080/3)—*see* Neoplasm, by site, malignant
  testis (M9080/3) 186.9
    adult, benign, cystic, differentiated type or mature (M9080/0) 222.0
    undescended 186.0
Terminal care V66.7

Termination
  anomalous—*see also* Malposition, congenital
    portal vein 747.49
    right pulmonary vein 747.42
  pregnancy (legal) (therapeutic) (*see* Abortion,
    legal) 635.9
    fetus NEC 779.6
    illegal (*see also* Abortion, illegal) 636.9
Ternidens diminutus infestation 127.7
Terrors, night (child) 307.46
Terry's syndrome (*see also* Retinopathy of
  prematurity) 362.21
Tertiary —*see* condition
Tessellated fundus, retina (tigroid) 362.89
Test(s)
  adequacy
    hemodialysis V56.31
    peritoneal dialysis V56.32
  AIDS virus V72.69
  allergen V72.7
  bacterial disease NEC (*see also* Screening, by
    name of disease) V74.9
  basal metabolic rate V72.69
  blood
    alcohol V70.4
    drug V70.4
      for therapeutic drug monitoring V58.83
      for routine general physical examination
        V72.62
      prior to treatment or procedure V72.63
    typing V72.86
      Rh typing V72.86
  developmental, infant or child V20.2
  Dick V74.8
  fertility V26.21
  genetic
    female V26.32
    for genetic disease carrier status
      female V26.31
      male V26.34
    male V26.39
  hearing V72.19
    following failed hearing screening V72.11
    routine, for infant and child V20.2
  HIV V72.69
  human immunodeficiency virus V72.69
  immunity status V72.61
  Kveim V82.89
  laboratory V72.60
    for medicolegal reason V70.4
    ordered as part of a routine general medical
      examination V72.62
    pre-operative V72.63
    pre-procedural V72.63
    specified NEC V72.69
  male partner of habitual aborter V26.35
  Mantoux (for tuberculosis) V74.1
  mycotic organism V75.4
  nuchal translucency V28.89
  parasitic agent NEC V75.8
  paternity V70.4
  peritoneal equilibration V56.32
  pregnancy
    negative result V72.41
    positive result V72.42
      first pregnancy V72.42
    unconfirmed V72.40
  preoperative V72.84
    cardiovascular V72.81
    respiratory V72.82
    specified NEC V72.83

Test(s)—*continued*
  procreative management NEC V26.29
    genetic disease carrier status
      female V26.31
      male V26.34
  Rh typing V72.86
  sarcoidosis V82.89
  Schick V74.3
  Schultz-Charlton V74.8
  skin, diagnostic
    allergy V72.7
    bacterial agent NEC (*see also* Screening, by
      name of disease) V74.9
    Dick V74.8
    hypersensitivity V72.7
    Kveim V82.89
    Mantoux V74.1
    mycotic organism V75.4
    parasitic agent NEC V75.8
    sarcoidosis V82.89
    Schick V74.3
    Schultz-Charlton V74.8
    tuberculin V74.1
  specified type NEC V72.85
  tuberculin V74.1
  vision V72.0
    routine, for infant and child V20.2
  Wassermann
    positive (*see also* Serology for syphilis,
      positive) 097.1
    false 795.6
Testicle, testicular, testis —*see also* condition
  feminization (syndrome) 259.51
Tetanus, tetanic (cephalic) (convulsions) 037
  with
    abortion—*see* Abortion, by type, with sepsis
    ectopic pregnancy (*see also* categories
      633.0-633.9) 639.0
    molar pregnancy (*see* categories 630-632) 639.0
  following
    abortion 639.0
    ectopic or molar pregnancy 639.0
  inoculation V03.7
    reaction (due to serum)—*see* Complications,
      vaccination
  neonatorum 771.3
  puerperal, postpartum, childbirth 670.8
Tetany, tetanic 781.7
  alkalosis 276.3
  associated with rickets 268.0
  convulsions 781.7
    hysterical 300.11
  functional (hysterical) 300.11
  hyperkinetic 781.7
    hysterical 300.11
  hyperpnea 786.01
    hysterical 300.11
    psychogenic 306.1
  hyperventilation 786.01
    hysterical 300.11
    psychogenic 306.1
  hypocalcemic, neonatal 775.4
    hysterical 300.11
  neonatal 775.4
  parathyroid (gland) 252.1
  parathyroprival 252.1
  postoperative 252.1
  postthyroidectomy 252.1
  pseudotetany 781.7
    hysterical 300.11
  psychogenic 306.1
    specified as conversion reaction 300.11

Tetralogy of Fallot 745.2
Tetraplegia —*see* Quadriplegia
Thailand hemorrhagic fever 065.4
Thalassanemia 282.49
Thalassemia (alpha) (beta) (disease) (Hb-C)
  (Hb-D) (Hb-E) (Hb-H) (Hb-I) (high fetal
  gene) (high fetal hemoglobin) (intermedia)
  (major) (minima) (minor) (mixed) (trait) (with
  other hemoglobinopathy) 282.49
  Hb-S (without crisis) 282.41
    with
      crisis 282.42
      vaso-occlusive pain 282.42
    sickle-cell (without crisis) 282.41
    with
      crisis 282.42
      vaso-occlusive pain 282.42
Thalassemic variants 282.49
Thaysen-Gee disease (nontropical sprue) 579.0
Thecoma (M8600/0) 220
  malignant (M8600/3) 183.0
Thelarche, precocious 259.1
Thelitis 611.0
  puerperal, postpartum 675.0
Therapeutic —*see* condition
Therapy V57.9
  blood transfusion, without reported diagnosis
    V58.2
  breathing V57.0
  chemotherapy, antineoplastic V58.11
    fluoride V07.31
    prophylactic NEC V07.39
  dialysis (intermittent) (treatment)
    extracorporeal V56.0
    peritoneal V56.8
    renal V56.0
    specified type NEC V56.8
  exercise NEC V57.1
    breathing V57.0
  extracorporeal dialysis (renal) V56.0
  fluoride prophylaxis V07.31
  hemodialysis V56.0
  hormone replacement (postmenopausal) V07.4
  immunotherapy, antineoplastic V58.12
  long term oxygen therapy V46.2
  occupational V57.21
  orthoptic V57.4
  orthotic V57.81
  peritoneal dialysis V56.8
  physical NEC V57.1
  postmenopausal hormone replacement V07.4
  radiation V58.0
  speech (-language) V57.3
  vocational V57.22
Thermalgesia 782.0
Thermalgia 782.0
Thermanalgesia 782.0
Thermanesthesia 782.0
Thermic —*see* condition
Thermography (abnormal) 793.99
  breast 793.89
Thermoplegia 992.0
Thesaurismosis
  amyloid 277.39
  bilirubin 277.4
  calcium 275.40
  cystine 270.0
  glycogen (*see also* Disease, glycogen storage)
    271.0
  kerasin 272.7

Thesaurismosis— *continued*
  lipoid 272.7
  melanin 255.41
  phosphatide 272.7
  urate 274.9
Thiaminic deficiency 265.1
  with beriberi 265.0
Thibierge-Weissenbach syndrome (cutaneous
  systemic sclerosis) 710.1
Thickened endometrium 793.5
Thickening
  bone 733.99
    extremity 733.99
  breast 611.79
  hymen 623.3
  larynx 478.79
  nail 703.8
    congenital 757.5
  periosteal 733.99
  pleura (*see also* Pleurisy) 511.0
  skin 782.8
  subepiglottic 478.79
  tongue 529.8
  valve, heart—*see* Endocarditis
Thiele syndrome 724.6
Thigh —*see* condition
Thinning vertebra (*see also* Osteoporosis) 733.00
Thirst, excessive 783.5
  due to deprivation of water 994.3
Thomsen's disease 359.22
Thomson's disease (congenital poikiloderma) 757.33
Thoracic —*see also* condition
  kidney 753.3
  outlet syndrome 353.0
  stomach—*see* Hernia, diaphragm
Thoracogastroschisis (congenital) 759.89
Thoracopagus 759.4
Thoracoschisis 756.3
Thorax —*see* condition
Thorn's syndrome (*see also* Disease, renal) 593.9
Thornwaldt's, Tornwaldt's
  bursitis (pharyngeal) 478.29
  cyst 478.26
  disease (pharyngeal bursitis) 478.29
Thoracoscopic surgical procedure converted to
  open procedure V64.42
Thorson-Biörck syndrome (malignant
  carcinoid) 259.2
Threadworm (infection) (infestation) 127.4
Threatened
  abortion or miscarriage 640.0
    with subsequent abortion (*see also* Abortion,
      spontaneous) 634.9
    affecting fetus 762.1
  labor 644.1
    affecting fetus or newborn 761.8
    premature 644.0
  miscarriage 640.0
    affecting fetus 762.1
  premature
    delivery 644.2
      affecting fetus or newborn 761.8
    labor 644.0
      before 22 completed weeks gestation 640.0
Three-day fever 066.0
Threshers' lung 495.0
Thrix annulata (congenital) 757.4
Throat —*see* condition
Thrombasthenia (Glanzmann's) (hemorrhagic)
  (hereditary) 287.1

Thromboangiitis 443.1
  obliterans (general) 443.1
    cerebral 437.1
    vessels
      brain 437.1
      spinal cord 437.1
Thromboarteritis —*see* Arteritis
Thromboasthenia (Glanzmann's) (hemorrhagic)
    (hereditary) 287.1
Thrombocytasthenia (Glanzmann's) 287.1
Thrombocythemia (primary) (M9962/1) 238.71
  essential 238.71
  hemorrhagic 238.71
  idiopathic (hemorrhagic) (M9962/1) 238.71
Thrombocytopathy (dystrophic) (granulopenic)
    287.1
Thrombocytopenia, thrombocytopenic 287.5
  with
    absent radii (TAR) syndrome 287.33
    giant hemangioma 287.39
  amegakaryocytic, congenital 287.33
  congenital 287.33
  cyclic 287.39
  dilutional 287.4
  due to
    drugs 287.4
    extracorporeal circulation of blood 287.4
    massive blood transfusion 287.4
    platelet alloimmunization 287.4
  essential 287.30
  fetal 678.0
  heparin-induced (HIT) 289.84
  hereditary 287.33
  Kasabach-Merritt 287.39
  neonatal, transitory 776.1
    due to
      exchange transfusion 776.1
      idiopathic maternal thrombocytopenia 776.1
      isoimmunization 776.1
  primary 287.30
  puerperal, postpartum 666.3
  purpura (*see also* Purpura, thrombocytopenic)
      287.30
    thrombotic 446.6
  secondary 287.4
  sex-linked 287.39
Thrombocytosis 238.71
  essential 238.71
  primary 238.71
Thromboembolism —*see* Embolism
Thrombopathy (Bernard-Soulier) 287.1
  constitutional 286.4
  Willebrand-Jürgens (angiohemophilia) 286.4
Thrombopenia (*see also* Thrombocytopenia) 287.5
Thrombophlebitis 451.9
  antecubital vein 451.82
  antepartum (superficial) 671.2
    affecting fetus or newborn 760.3
    deep 671.3
  arm 451.89
    deep 451.83
    superficial 451.82
  breast, superficial 451.89
  cavernous (venous) sinus—*see*
      Thrombophlebitis, intracranial venous sinus
  cephalic vein 451.82
  cerebral (sinus) (vein) 325
    late effect—*see* category 326
    nonpyogenic 437.6
      in pregnancy or puerperium 671.5
      late effect—*see* Late effect(s) (of)
        cerebrovascular disease

Thrombophlebitis—*continued*
  due to implanted device—*see* Complications,
      due to (presence of) any device, implant, or
      graft classified to 996.0-996.5 NEC
  during or resulting from a procedure NEC 997.2
  femoral 451.11
  femoropopliteal 451.19
  following infusion, perfusion, or transfusion
      999.2
  hepatic (vein) 451.89
  idiopathic, recurrent 453.1
  iliac vein 451.81
  iliofemoral 451.11
  intracranial venous sinus (any) 325
    late effect—*see* category 326
    nonpyogenic 437.6
      in pregnancy or puerperium 671.5
      late effect—*see* Late effect(s) (of)
        cerebrovascular disease
  jugular vein 451.89
  lateral (venous) sinus—*see* Thrombophlebitis,
      intracranial venous sinus
  leg 451.2
    deep (vessels) 451.19
      femoral vein 451.11
      specified vessel NEC 451.19
    superficial (vessels) 451.0
      femoral vein 451.11
  longitudinal (venous) sinus—*see*
      Thrombophlebitis, intracranial venous sinus
  lower extremity 451.2
    deep (vessels) 451.19
      femoral vein 451.11
      specified vessel NEC 451.19
    superficial (vessels) 451.0
  migrans, migrating 453.1
  pelvic
    with
      abortion—*see* Abortion, by type, with sepsis
      ectopic pregnancy (*see also* categories
        633.0-633.9) 639.0
      molar pregnancy (*see also* categories
        630-632) 639.0
    following
      abortion 639.0
      ectopic or molar pregnancy 639.0
    puerperal 671.4
  popliteal vein 451.19
  portal (vein) 572.1
  postoperative 997.2
  pregnancy (superficial) 671.2
    affecting fetus or newborn 760.3
    deep 671.3
  puerperal, postpartum, childbirth (extremities)
      (superficial) 671.2
    deep 671.4
    pelvic 671.4
    septic 670.3
    specified site NEC 671.5
  radial vein 451.83
  saphenous (greater) (lesser) 451.0
  sinus (intracranial)—*see* Thrombophlebitis,
      intracranial venous sinus
  specified site NEC 451.89
  tibial vein 451.19
Thrombosis, thrombotic (marantic) (multiple)
    (progressive) (vein) (vessel) 453.9
  with childbirth or during the puerperium—*see*
      Thrombosis, puerperal, postpartum
  antepartum—*see* Thrombosis, pregnancy

Thrombosis, thrombotic—*continued*
  aorta, aortic 444.1
    abdominal 444.0
    bifurcation 444.0
    saddle 444.0
    terminal 444.0
    thoracic 444.1
    valve—*see* Endocarditis, aortic
  apoplexy (*see also* Thrombosis, brain) 434.0
    late effect—*see* Late effect(s) (of)
      cerebrovascular disease
  appendix, septic—*see* Appendicitis, acute
  arteriolar-capillary platelet, disseminated 446.6
  artery, arteries (postinfectional) 444.9
    auditory, internal 433.8
    basilar (*see also* Occlusion, artery, basilar)
      433.0
    carotid (common) (internal) (*see also*
      Occlusion, artery, carotid) 433.1
      with other precerebral artery 433.3
    cerebellar (anterior inferior) (posterior
      inferior) (superior) 433.8
    cerebral (*see also* Thrombosis, brain) 434.0
    choroidal (anterior) 433.8
    communicating posterior 433.8
    coronary (*see also* Infarct, myocardium) 410.9
      due to syphilis 093.89
      healed or specified as old 412
      without myocardial infarction 411.81
    extremities 444.22
      lower 444.22
      upper 444.21
    femoral 444.22
    hepatic 444.89
    hypophyseal 433.8
    meningeal, anterior or posterior 433.8
    mesenteric (with gangrene) 557.0
    ophthalmic (*see also* Occlusion, retina) 362.30
    pontine 433.8
    popliteal 444.22
    precerebral—*see* Occlusion, artery,
      precerebral NEC
    pulmonary 415.19
      iatrogenic 415.11
      personal history of V12.51
      postoperative 415.11
      septic 415.12
    renal 593.81
    retinal (*see also* Occlusion, retina) 362.30
    specified site NEC 444.89
    spinal, anterior or posterior 433.8
    traumatic (complication) (early) (*see also*
      Injury, blood vessel, by site) 904.9
    vertebral (*see also* Occlusion, artery,
      vertebral) 433.2
      with other precerebral artery 433.3
  atrial (endocardial) 424.90
    due to syphilis 093.89
    without endocarditis 429.89
  auricular (*see also* Infarct, myocardium) 410.9
  axillary (acute) (vein) 453.84
    chronic 453.74
    personal history of V12.51
  basilar (artery) (*see also* Occlusion, artery,
    basilar) 433.0
  bland NEC 453.9
  brain (artery) (stem) 434.0
    due to syphilis 094.89
    iatrogenic 997.02
    late effect—*see* Late effect(s) (of)
      cerebrovascular disease
    postoperative 997.02

Thrombosis, thrombotic—*continued*
  brain—*continued*
    puerperal, postpartum, childbirth 674.0
    sinus (*see also* Thrombosis, intracranial
      venous sinus) 325
  capillary 448.9
    arteriolar, generalized 446.6
  cardiac (*see also* Infarct, myocardium) 410.9
    due to syphilis 093.89
    healed or specified as old 412
    valve—*see* Endocarditis
  carotid (artery) (common) (internal) (*see also*
    Occlusion, artery, carotid) 433.1
    with other precerebral artery 433.3
  cavernous sinus (venous)—*see* Thrombosis,
    intracranial venous sinus
  cerebellar artery (anterior inferior) (posterior
    inferior) (superior) 433.8
    late effect—*see* Late effect(s) (of)
      cerebrovascular disease
  cerebral (arteries) (*see also* Thrombosis, brain)
    434.0
    late effect—*see* Late effect(s) (of)
      cerebrovascular disease
  coronary (artery) (*see also* Infarct, myocardium)
    410.9
    due to syphilis 093.89
    healed or specified as old 412
    without myocardial infarction 411.81
  corpus cavernosum 607.82
  cortical (*see also* Thrombosis, brain) 434.0
  due to (presence of) any device, implant, or graft
    classifiable to 996.0-996.5—*see*
    Complications, due to (presence of) any
    device, implant, or graft classified to
    996.0-996.5 NEC
  effort 453.89
  endocardial—*see* Infarct, myocardium
  eye (*see also* Occlusion, retina) 362.30
  femoral (vein) 453.6
    with inflammation or phlebitis 451.11
    artery 444.22
    deep 453.41
    personal history of V12.51
  genital organ, male 608.83
  heart (chamber) (*see also* Infarct, myocardium)
    410.9
  hepatic (vein) 453.0
    artery 444.89
    infectional or septic 572.1
  iliac (vein) 453.89
    with inflammation or phlebitis 451.81
    artery (common) (external) (internal) 444.81
    personal history of V12.51
  inflammation, vein—*see* Thrombophlebitis
  internal carotid artery (*see also* Occlusion,
    artery, carotid) 433.1
    with other precerebral artery 433.3
  intestine (with gangrene) 557.0
  intracranial (*see also* Thrombosis, brain) 434.0
    venous sinus (any) 325
      nonpyogenic origin 437.6
      in pregnancy or puerperium 671.5
  intramural (*see also* Infarct, myocardium) 410.9
    without
      cardiac condition 429.89
      coronary artery disease 429.89
      myocardial infarction 429.89
      healed or specified as old 412

Thrombosis, thrombotic—*continued*
jugular (bulb)
 external
  acute 453.89
  chronic 453.79
 internal
  acute 453.86
  chronic 453.76
kidney 593.81
 artery 593.81
lateral sinus (venous)—*see* Thrombosis,
  intracranial venous sinus
leg (see also Thrombosis, lower extremity)
  453.6
 with inflammation or phlebitis—*see*
   Thrombophlebitis
 deep (vessels) 453.40
  acute 453.40
   lower (distal) 453.42
   upper (proximal) 453.41
  chronic 453.50
   lower (distal) 453.52
   upper (proximal) 453.51
 personal history of V12.51
 superficial (vessels) 453.6
liver (venous) 453.0
 artery 444.89
 infectional or septic 572.1
 portal vein 452
longitudinal sinus (venous)—*see* Thrombosis,
  intracranial venous sinus
lower extremity (superficial) 453.6
 deep vessels 453.40
  acute 453.40
   calf 453.42
   distal (lower leg) 453.42
   femoral 453.41
   iliac 453.41
   lower leg 453.42
   peroneal 453.42
   popliteal 453.41
   proximal (upper leg) 453.41
   thigh 453.41
   tibial 453.42
  chronic 453.50
   calf 453.52
   distal (lower leg) 453.52
   femoral 453.51
   iliac 453.51
   lower leg 453.52
   peroneal 453.52
   popliteal 453.51
   proximal (upper leg) 453.51
   thigh 453.51
   tibial 453.52
 personal history of V12.51
 saphenous (greater) (lesser) 453.6
 superficial 453.6
lung 415.19
 iatrogenic 415.11
 personal history of V12.51
 postoperative 415.11
 septic 415.12
marantic, dural sinus 437.6
meninges (brain) (*see also* Thrombosis, brain)
  434.0
mesenteric (artery) (with gangrene) 557.0
 vein (inferior) (superior) 557.0
mitral—*see* Insufficiency, mitral

Thrombosis, thrombotic—*continued*
mural (heart chamber) (*see also* Infarct,
  myocardium) 410.9
 without
  cardiac condition 429.89
  coronary artery disease 429.89
  myocardial infarction 429.89
 due to syphilis 093.89
 following myocardial infarction 429.79
 healed or specified as old 412
omentum (with gangrene) 557.0
ophthalmic (artery) (*see also* Occlusion, retina)
  362.30
pampiniform plexus (male) 608.83
 female 620.8
parietal (*see also* Infarct, myocardium) 410.9
penis, penile 607.82
peripheral arteries 444.22
 lower 444.22
 upper 444.21
platelet 446.6
portal 452
 due to syphilis 093.89
 infectional or septic 572.1
precerebral artery—*see also* Occlusion, artery,
  precerebral NEC
pregnancy 671.2
 deep (vein) 671.3
 superficial (vein) 671.2
puerperal, postpartum, childbirth 671.2
 brain (artery) 674.0
  venous 671.5
 cardiac 674.8
 cerebral (artery) 674.0
  venous 671.5
 deep (vein) 671.4
 intracranial sinus (nonpyogenic) (venous)
   671.5
 pelvic 671.4
 pulmonary (artery) 673.2
 specified site NEC 671.5
 superficial 671.2
pulmonary (artery) (vein) 415.19
 iatrogenic 415.11
 personal history of V12.51
 postoperative 415.11
 septic 415.12
radial vein 451.83
renal (artery) 593.81
 vein 453.3
resulting from presence of shunt or other
   internal prosthetic device—*see*
   Complications, due to (presence of) any
   device, implant, or graft classified to
   996.0-996.5 NEC
retina, retinal (artery) 362.30
 arterial branch 362.32
 central 362.31
 partial 362.33
 vein
  central 362.35
  tributary (branch) 362.36
saphenous vein (greater) (lesser) 453.6
scrotum 608.83
seminal vesicle 608.83
sigmoid (venous) sinus (*see* Thrombosis,
  intracranial venous sinus) 325
silent NEC 453.9
sinus, intracranial (venous) (any) (*see also*
  Thrombosis, intracranial venous sinus) 325

Thrombosis, thrombotic—*continued*
softening, brain (*see also* Thrombosis, brain) 434.0
specified site NEC (acute) 453.89
  chronic 453.79
spermatic cord 608.83
spinal cord 336.1
  due to syphilis 094.89
  in pregnancy or puerperium 671.5
  pyogenic origin 324.1
    late effect—*see* category 326
spleen, splenic 289.59
  artery 444.89
testis 608.83
traumatic (complication) (early) (*see also* Injury, blood vessel, by site) 904.9
tricuspid—*see* Endocarditis, tricuspid
tumor—*see* Neoplasm, by site
tunica vaginalis 608.83
umbilical cord (vessels) 663.6
  affecting fetus or newborn 762.6
upper extremity 453.83
  acute 453.83
    deep 453.82
    superficial 453.81
  chronic 453.73
    deep 453.72
    superficial 453.71
vas deferens 608.83
vein
  antecubital
    acute 453.81
    chronic 453.71
  axillary
    acute 453.84
    chronic 453.74
  basilic
    acute 453.81
    chronic 453.71
  brachial
    acute 453.82
    chronic 453.72
  brachiocephalic (innominate)
    acute 453.87
    chronic 453.77
  cephalic
    acute 453.81
    chronic 453.71
  deep 453.40
    personal history of V12.51
  internal jugular
    acute 453.86
    chronic 453.76
  lower extremity—*see* Thrombosis, lower extremity
  personal history of V12.51
  radial
    acute 453.82
    chronic 453.72
  saphenous (greater) (lesser) 453.6
  specified site NEC
    acute 453.89
    chronic 453.79
  subclavian
    acute 453.85
    chronic 453.75
  superior vena cava
    acute 453.87
    chronic 453.77
  thoracic
    acute 453.87
    chronic 453.77

Thrombosis, thrombotic—*continued*
vein—*continued*
  ulnar
    acute 453.82
    chronic 453.72
  upper extremity - see Thrombosis, upper extremity
  vena cava
    inferior 453.2
    personal history of V12.51
    superior
      acute 453.87
      chronic 453.77
Thrombus —*see* Thrombosis
Thrush 112.0
  newborn 771.7
Thumb —*see also* condition
  gamekeeper's 842.12
  sucking (child problem) 307.9
Thygeson's superficial punctate keratitis 370.21
Thymergasia (*see also* Psychosis, affective) 296.80
Thymitis 254.8
Thymoma (benign) (M8580/0) 212.6
  malignant (M8580/3) 164.0
Thymus, thymic (gland)—*see* condition
Thyrocele (*see also* Goiter) 240.9
Thyroglossal —*see also* condition
  cyst 759.2
  duct, persistent 759.2
Thyroid (body) (gland)—*see also* condition
  hormone resistance 246.8
  lingual 759.2
Thyroiditis 245.9
  acute (pyogenic) (suppurative) 245.0
    nonsuppurative 245.0
  autoimmune 245.2
  chronic (nonspecific) (sclerosing) 245.8
    fibrous 245.3
    lymphadenoid 245.2
    lymphocytic 245.2
    lymphoid 245.2
  complicating pregnancy, childbirth, or puerperium 648.1
  de Quervain's (subacute granulomatous) 245.1
  fibrous (chronic) 245.3
  giant (cell) (follicular) 245.1
  granulomatous (de Quervain's) (subacute) 245.1
  Hashimoto's (struma lymphomatosa) 245.2
  iatrogenic 245.4
  invasive (fibrous) 245.3
  ligneous 245.3
  lymphocytic (chronic) 245.2
  lymphoid 245.2
  lymphomatous 245.2
  pseudotuberculous 245.1
  pyogenic 245.0
  radiation 245.4
  Riedel's (ligneous) 245.3
  subacute 245.1
  suppurative 245.0
  tuberculous (*see also* Tuberculosis) 017.5
  viral 245.1
  woody 245.3
Thyrolingual duct, persistent 759.2
Thyromegaly 240.9
Thyrotoxic
  crisis or storm (*see also* Thyrotoxicosis) 242.9
  heart failure (*see also* Thyrotoxicosis) 242.9 *[425.7]*

Thyrotoxicosis 242.9

Note—Use the following fifth-digit
subclassification with category 242:

0 without mention of thyrotoxic crisis or storm
1 with mention of thyrotoxic crisis or storm

with
  goiter (diffuse) 242.0
    adenomatous 242.3
      multinodular 242.2
      uninodular 242.1
    nodular 242.3
      multinodular 242.2
      uninodular 242.1
  infiltrative
    dermopathy 242.0
    ophthalmopathy 242.0
  thyroid acropachy 242.0
complicating pregnancy, childbirth, or
  puerperium 648.1
due to
  ectopic thyroid nodule 242.4
  ingestion of (excessive) thyroid material 242.8
  specified cause NEC 242.8
factitia 242.8
heart 242.9 [425.7]
neonatal (transient) 775.3
TIA (transient ischemic attack) 435.9
with transient neurologic deficit 435.9
late effect—see Late effect(s) (of)
  cerebrovascular disease
Tibia vara 732.4
Tic 307.20
breathing 307.20
child problem 307.21
compulsive 307.22
convulsive 307.20
degenerative (generalized) (localized) 333.3
  facial 351.8
douloureux (see also Neuralgia, trigeminal)
  350.1
  atypical 350.2
habit 307.20
  chronic (motor or vocal) 307.22
  transient (of childhood) 307.21
lid 307.20
  transient (of childhood) 307.21
motor-verbal 307.23
occupational 300.89
orbicularis 307.20
  transient (of childhood) 307.21
organic origin 333.3
postchoreic—see Chorea
psychogenic 307.20
  compulsive 307.22
salaam 781.0
spasm 307.20
  chronic (motor or vocal) 307.22
  transient (of childhood) 307.21
Tick (-borne) fever NEC 066.1
American mountain 066.1
Colorado 066.1
hemorrhagic NEC 065.3
  Crimean 065.0
  Kyasanur Forest 065.2
  Omsk 065.1
mountain 066.1
nonexanthematous 066.1

Tick-bite fever NEC 066.1
African 087.1
Colorado (virus) 066.1
Rocky Mountain 082.0
Tick paralysis 989.5
Tics and spasms, compulsive 307.22
Tietze's disease or syndrome 733.6
Tight, tightness
anus 564.89
chest 786.59
fascia (lata) 728.9
foreskin (congenital) 605
hymen 623.3
introitus (acquired) (congenital) 623.3
rectal sphincter 564.89
tendon 727.81
  Achilles (heel) 727.81
urethral sphincter 598.9
Tilting vertebra 737.9
Timidity, child 313.21
Tinea (intersecta) (tarsi) 110.9
amiantacea 110.0
asbestina 110.0
barbae 110.0
beard 110.0
black dot 110.0
blanca 111.2
capitis 110.0
corporis 110.5
cruris 110.3
decalvans 704.09
flava 111.0
foot 110.4
furfuracea 111.0
imbricata (Tokelau) 110.5
lepothrix 039.0
manuum 110.2
microsporic (see also Dermatophytosis) 110.9
nigra 111.1
nodosa 111.2
pedis 110.4
scalp 110.0
specified site NEC 110.8
sycosis 110.0
tonsurans 110.0
trichophytic (see also Dermatophytosis) 110.9
unguium 110.1
versicolor 111.0
Tingling sensation (see also Disturbance,
  sensation) 782.0
Tin-miners' lung 503
Tinnitus (aurium) 388.30
audible 388.32
objective 388.32
subjective 388.31
Tipped, teeth 524.33
Tipping
pelvis 738.6
  with disproportion (fetopelvic) 653.0
    affecting fetus or newborn 763.1
    causing obstructed labor 660.1
      affecting fetus or newborn 763.1
teeth 524.33
Tiredness 780.79
Tissue —see condition
Tobacco
abuse (affecting health) NEC (see also Abuse,
  drugs, nondependent) 305.1
heart 989.8
use disorder complicating pregnancy, childbirth,
  or the puerperium 649.0

Tobias' syndrome (carcinoma, pulmonary apex)
  (M8010/3) 162.3
Tocopherol deficiency 269.1
Todd's
  cirrhosis—*see* Cirrhosis, biliary
  paralysis (postepileptic transitory paralysis)
    344.89
Toe —*see* condition
Toilet, artificial opening (*see also* Attention to,
  artificial, opening) V55.9
Tokelau ringworm 110.5
Tollwut 071
Tolosa-Hunt syndrome 378.55
Tommaselli's disease
  correct substance properly administered 599.70
  overdose or wrong substance given or taken 961.4
Tongue —*see also* condition
  worms 134.1
Tongue tie 750.0
Toni-Fanconi syndrome (cystinosis) 270.0
Tonic pupil 379.46
Tonsil —*see* condition
Tonsillitis (acute) (catarrhal) (croupous)
  (follicular) (gangrenous) (infective) (lacunar)
  (lingual) (malignant) (membranous)
  (phlegmonous) (pneumococcal)
  (pseudomembranous) (purulent) (septic)
  (staphylococcal) (subacute) (suppurative)
  (toxic) (ulcerative) (vesicular) (viral) 463
  with influenza, flu, or grippe 487.1
  chronic 474.00
  diphtheritic (membranous) 032.0
  hypertrophic 474.00
  influenzal 487.1
  parenchymatous 475
  streptococcal 034.0
  tuberculous (*see also* Tuberculosis) 012.8
  Vincent's 101
Tonsillopharyngitis 465.8
Tooth, teeth —*see* condition
Toothache 525.9
Topagnosis 782.0
Tophi (gouty) 274.03
  ear 274.81
  heart 274.82
  specified site NEC 274.82
TORCH infection (—see also Infection,
  congenital) 760.2
Torn —*see* Tear, torn
Tornwaldt's bursitis (disease) (pharyngeal
  bursitis) 478.29
  cyst 478.26
Torpid liver 573.9
Torsion
  accessory tube 620.5
  adnexa (female) 620.5
  aorta (congenital) 747.29
    acquired 447.1
  appendix
    epididymis 608.24
    testis 608.23
  bile duct 576.8
    with calculus, choledocholithiasis or
      stones—*see* Choledocholithiasis
    congenital 751.69
  bowel, colon, or intestine 560.2
  cervix (*see* Malposition, uterus)
  duodenum 537.3
  dystonia—*see* Dystonia, torsion

Torsion—*continued*
  epididymis 608.24
    appendix 608.24
  fallopian tube 620.5
  gallbladder (*see also* Disease, gallbladder) 575.8
    congenital 751.69
  gastric 537.89
  hydatid of Morgagni (female) 620.5
  kidney (pedicle) 593.89
  Meckel's diverticulum (congenital) 751.0
  mesentery 560.2
  omentum 560.2
  organ or site, congenital NEC—*see* Anomaly,
    specified type NEC
  ovary (pedicle) 620.5
    congenital 752.0
  oviduct 620.5
  penis 607.89
    congenital 752.69
  renal 593.89
  spasm—*see* Dystonia, torsion
  spermatic cord 608.22
    extravaginal 608.21
    intravaginal 608.22
  spleen 289.59
  testicle, testis 608.20
    appendix 608.23
  tibia 736.89
  umbilical cord—*see* Compression, umbilical
    cord
  uterus (*see also* Malposition, uterus) 621.6
Torticollis (intermittent) (spastic) 723.5
  congenital 754.1
    sternomastoid 754.1
  due to birth injury 767.8
  hysterical 300.11
  ocular 781.93
  psychogenic 306.0
    specified as conversion reaction 300.11
  rheumatic 723.5
  rheumatoid 714.0
  spasmodic 333.83
  traumatic, current NEC 847.0
Tortuous
  artery 447.1
  fallopian tube 752.19
  organ or site, congenital NEC—*see* Distortion
  renal vessel, congenital 747.62
  retina vessel (congenital) 743.58
    acquired 362.17
  ureter 593.4
  urethra 599.84
  vein—*see* Varicose, vein
Torula, torular (infection) 117.5
  histolytica 117.5
  lung 117.5
Torulosis 117.5
Torus
  fracture
    fibula 823.41
      with tibia 823.42
    humerus 812.49
    radius (alone) 813.45
      with ulna 813.47
    tibia 823.40
      with fibula 823.42
    ulna (alone) 813.46
      with radius 813.47
  mandibularis 526.81
  palatinus 526.81
Touch, vitreous 997.99

Touraine's syndrome (hereditary
  osteo-onychodysplasia) 756.89
Touraine-Solente-Golé syndrome
  (acropachyderma) 757.39
Tourette's disease (motor-verbal tic) 307.23
Tower skull 756.0
  with exophthalmos 756.0
Toxemia 799.89
  with abortion—*see* Abortion, by type, with toxemia
  bacterial—*see* Septicemia
  biliary (*see also* Disease, biliary) 576.8
  burn—*see* Burn, by site
  congenital NEC 779.89
  eclamptic 642.6
    with pre-existing hypertension 642.7
  erysipelatous (*see also* Erysipelas) 035
  fatigue 799.89
  fetus or newborn NEC 779.89
  food (*see also* Poisoning, food) 005.9
  gastric 537.89
  gastrointestinal 558.2
  intestinal 558.2
  kidney (*see also* Disease, renal) 593.9
  lung 518.89
  malarial NEC (*see also* Malaria) 084.6
  maternal (of pregnancy), affecting fetus or
    newborn 760.0
  myocardial—*see* Myocarditis, toxic
  of pregnancy (mild) (pre-eclamptic) 642.4
    with
      convulsions 642.6
      pre-existing hypertension 642.7
    affecting fetus or newborn 760.0
    severe 642.5
  pre-eclamptic—*see* Toxemia, of pregnancy
  puerperal, postpartum—*see* Toxemia, of
    pregnancy
  pulmonary 518.89
  renal (*see also* Disease, renal) 593.9
  septic (*see also* Septicemia) 038.9
  small intestine 558.2
  staphylococcal 038.10
    aureus 038.11
    due to food 005.0
    specified organism NEC 038.19
  stasis 799.89
  stomach 537.89
  uremic (*see also* Uremia) 586
  urinary 586
Toxemica cerebropathia psychica
  (nonalcoholic) 294.0
  alcoholic 291.1
Toxic (poisoning)—*see also* condition
  from drug or poison—*see* Table of drugs and
    chemicals
  oil syndrome 710.5
  shock syndrome 040.82
  thyroid (gland) (*see also* Thyrotoxicosis) 242.9
Toxicemia —*see* Toxemia
Toxicity
  dilantin
    asymptomatic 796.0
    symptomatic—*see* Table of Drugs and Chemicals
  drug
    asymptomatic 796.0
    symptomatic—*see* Table of Drugs and Chemicals
  fava bean 282.2
  from drug or poison
    asymptomatic 796.0
    symptomatic—*see* Table of Drugs and
      Chemicals

Toxicosis (*see also* Toxemia) 799.89
  capillary, hemorrhagic 287.0
Toxinfection 799.89
  gastrointestinal 558.2
Toxocariasis 128.0
Toxoplasma infection, generalized 130.9
Toxoplasmosis (acquired) 130.9
  with pneumonia 130.4
  congenital, active 771.2
  disseminated (multisystemic) 130.8
  maternal
    with suspected damage to fetus affecting
      management of pregnancy 655.4
    affecting fetus or newborn 760.2
      manifest toxoplasmosis in fetus or newborn
        771.2
  multiple sites 130.8
  multisystemic disseminated 130.8
  specified site NEC 130.7
Trabeculation, bladder 596.8
Trachea —*see* condition
Tracheitis (acute)(catarrhal)(infantile)
  (membranous) (plastic) (pneumococcal)
  (septic) (suppurative) (viral) 464.10
  with
    bronchitis 490
      acute or subacute 466.0
      chronic 491.8
      tuberculosis—*see* Tuberculosis, pulmonary
    laryngitis (acute) 464.20
      with obstruction 464.21
      chronic 476.1
      tuberculous (*see also* Tuberculosis, larynx) 012.3
    obstruction 464.11
  chronic 491.8
    with
      bronchitis (chronic) 491.8
      laryngitis (chronic) 476.1
    due to external agent—*see* Condition,
      respiratory, chronic, due to
  diphtheritic (membranous) 032.3
  due to external agent—*see* Inflammation,
    respiratory, upper, due to
  edematous 464.11
  influenzal 487.1
  streptococcal 034.0
  syphilitic 095.8
  tuberculous (*see also* Tuberculosis) 012.8
Trachelitis (nonvenereal) (*see also* Cervicitis) 616.0
  trichomonal 131.09
Tracheobronchial —*see* condition
Tracheobronchitis (*see also* Bronchitis) 490
  acute or subacute 466.0
    with bronchospasm or obstruction 466.0
  chronic 491.8
  influenzal 487.1
  senile 491.8
Tracheobronchomegaly (congenital) 748.3
  with bronchiectasis 494.0
    with (acute) exacerbation 494.1
  acquired 519.19
    with bronchiectasis 494.0
      with (acute) exacerbation 494.1
Tracheobronchopneumonitis —*see* Pneumonia,
  broncho
Tracheocele (external) (internal) 519.19
  congenital 748.3
Tracheomalacia 519.19
  congenital 748.3

Tracheopharyngitis (acute) 465.8
  chronic 478.9
    due to external agent—*see* Condition,
      respiratory, chronic, due to
    due to external agent—*see* Inflammation,
      respiratory, upper, due to
Tracheostenosis 519.19
  congenital 748.3
Tracheostomy
  attention to V55.0
  complication 519.00
  granuloma 519.09
  hemorrhage 519.09
  infection 519.01
  malfunctioning 519.02
  obstruction 519.09
  sepsis 519.01
  status V44.0
  stenosis 519.02
Trachoma, trachomatous 076.9
  active (stage) 076.1
  contraction of conjunctiva 076.1
  dubium 076.0
  healed or late effect 139.1
  initial (stage) 076.0
  Türck's (chronic catarrhal laryngitis) 476.0
Trachyphonia 784.49
Training
  insulin pump V65.46
  orthoptic V57.4
  orthotic V57.81
Train sickness 994.6
Trait
  hemoglobin
    abnormal NEC 282.7
      with thalassemia 282.49
    C (*see also* Disease, hemoglobin, C) 282.7
      with elliptocytosis 282.7
    S (Hb-S) 282.5
  Lepore 282.49
    with other abnormal hemoglobin NEC 282.49
  paranoid 301.0
  sickle-cell 282.5
    with
      elliptocytosis 282.5
      spherocytosis 282.5
Traits, paranoid 301.0
Tramp V60.0
Trance 780.09
  hysterical 300.13
Transaminasemia 790.4
Transfusion, blood
  donor V59.01
    stem cells V59.02
  fetal twin to twin 678.0
  incompatible
    ABO 999.6
    minor blood group 999.89
  reaction or complication—*see* Complications,
    transfusion
  related acute lung injury (TRALI) 518.7
  syndrome
    fetomaternal 772.0
    twin-to-twin
      blood loss (donor twin) 772.0
      recipient twin 776.4
    twin to twin fetal 678.0
  without reported diagnosis V58.2
Transient —*see also* condition
  alteration of awareness 780.02
  blindness 368.12
  deafness (ischemic) 388.02

Transient—*continued*
  global amnesia 437.7
  hyperglycemia (post-procedural) 790.29
  hypoglycemia (post-procedural) 251.2
  person (homeless) NEC V60.0
Transitional, lumbosacral joint of vertebra
    756.19
Translocation
  autosomes NEC 758.5
    13-15 758.1
    16-18 758.2
    21 or 22 758.0
    balanced in normal individual 758.4
    D₁ 758.1
    E₃ 758.2
    G 758.0
  balanced autosomal in normal individual 758.4
  chromosomes NEC 758.89
  Down's syndrome 758.0
Translucency, iris 364.53
Transmission of chemical substances through
    the placenta (affecting fetus or newborn)
    760.70
  alcohol 760.71
  anticonvulsants 760.77
  antifungals 760.74
  anti-infective agents 760.74
  antimetabolics 760.78
  cocaine 760.75
  "crack" 760.75
  diethylstilbestrol [DES] 760.76
  hallucinogenic agents 760.73
  medicinal agents NEC 760.79
  narcotics 760.72
  obstetric anesthetic or analgesic drug 763.5
  specified agent NEC 760.79
  suspected, affecting management of pregnancy
    655.5
Transplant(ed)
  bone V42.4
    marrow V42.81
  complication—*see also* Complications, due to
    (presence of) any device, implant, or graft
    classified to 996.0-996.5 NEC
  bone marrow 996.85
  corneal graft NEC 996.79
    infection or inflammation 996.69
    reaction 996.51
    rejection 996.51
  organ (failure) (immune or nonimmune cause)
    (infection) (rejection) 996.80
    bone marrow 996.85
    heart 996.83
    intestines 996.87
    kidney 996.81
    liver 996.82
    lung 996.84
    pancreas 996.86
    specified NEC 996.89
  previously removed due to complication,
    failure, rejection or infection V45.87
  removal status V45.87
  skin NEC 996.79
    infection or inflammation 996.69
    rejection 996.52
      artificial 996.55
      decellularized allodermis 996.55
  cornea V42.5
  hair V50.0
  heart V42.1
    valve V42.2

Transplant(ed)—*continued*
  intestine V42.84
  kidney V42.0
  liver V42.7
  lung V42.6
  organ V42.9
    specified NEC V42.89
  pancreas V42.83
  peripheral stem cells V42.82
  skin V42.3
  stem cells, peripheral V42.82
  tissue V42.9
    specified NEC V42.89
Transplants, ovarian, endometrial 617.1
Transposed —*see* Transposition
Transposition (congenital)—*see also*
  Malposition, congenital
  abdominal viscera 759.3
  aorta (dextra) 745.11
  appendix 751.5
  arterial trunk 745.10
  colon 751.5
  great vessels (complete) 745.10
    both originating from right ventricle 745.11
    corrected 745.12
    double outlet right ventricle 745.11
    incomplete 745.11
    partial 745.11
    specified type NEC 745.19
  heart 746.87
    with complete transposition of viscera 759.3
  intestine (large) (small) 751.5
  pulmonary veins 747.49
  reversed jejunal (for bypass) (status) V45.3
  scrotal 752.81
  stomach 750.7
    with general transposition of viscera 759.3
  teeth, tooth 524.30
  vessels (complete) 745.10
    partial 745.11
  viscera (abdominal) (thoracic) 759.3
Trans-sexualism 302.50
  with
    asexual history 302.51
    heterosexual history 302.53
    homosexual history 302.52
Transverse —*see also* condition
  arrest (deep), in labor 660.3
  affecting fetus or newborn 763.1
  lie 652.3
    before labor, affecting fetus or newborn 761.7
    causing obstructed labor 660.0
      affecting fetus or newborn 763.1
    during labor, affecting fetus or newborn 763.1
Transvestism, transvestitism (transvestic
  fetishism) 302.3
Trapped placenta (with hemorrhage) 666.0
  without hemorrhage 667.0
Trauma, traumatism (*see also* Injury, by site)
  959.9
  birth—*see* Birth, injury NEC
  causing hemorrhage of pregnancy or delivery
    641.8
  complicating
    abortion—*see* Abortion, by type, with damage
      to pelvic organs
    ectopic pregnancy (*see also* categories
      633.0-633.9) 639.2
    molar pregnancy (*see also* categories 630-632)
      639.2
  during delivery NEC 665.9

Trauma—*continued*
  following
    abortion 639.2
    ectopic or molar pregnancy 639.2
  maternal, during pregnancy, affecting fetus or
    newborn 760.5
  neuroma—*see* Injury, nerve, by site
  previous major, affecting management of
    pregnancy, childbirth, or puerperium V23.8
  psychic (current)—*see also* Reaction,
    adjustment
    previous (history) V15.49
  psychologic, previous (affecting health) V15.49
  transient paralysis—*see* Injury, nerve, by site
Traumatic —*see also* condition
  brain injury (TBI) (see also Injury, intracranial)
    854.0
    with skull fracture - see Fracture, skull, by site
Treacher Collins' syndrome (incomplete facial
  dysostosis) 756.0
Treitz's hernia —*see* Hernia, Treitz's
Trematode infestation NEC 121.9
Trematodiasis NEC 121.9
Trembles 988.8
Trembling paralysis (*see also* Parkinsonism)
  332.0
Tremor 781.0
  essential (benign) 333.1
  familial 333.1
  flapping (liver) 572.8
  hereditary 333.1
  hysterical 300.11
  intention 333.1
  medication-induced postural 333.1
  mercurial 985.0
  muscle 728.85
  Parkinson's (*see also* Parkinsonism) 332.0
  psychogenic 306.0
    specified as conversion reaction 300.11
  senilis 797
  specified type NEC 333.1
Trench
  fever 083.1
  foot 991.4
  mouth 101
  nephritis—*see* Nephritis, acute
Treponema pallidum infection (*see also*
  Syphilis) 097.9
Treponematosis 102.9
  due to
    T. pallidum—*see* Syphilis
    T. pertenue (yaws) (*see also* Yaws) 102.9
Triad
  Kartagener's 759.3
  Reiter's (complete) (incomplete) 099.3
  Saint's (*see also* Hernia, diaphragm) 553.3
Trichiasis 704.2
  cicatricial 704.2
  eyelid 374.05
    with entropion (*see also* Entropion) 374.00
Trichinella spiralis (infection) (infestation) 124
Trichinelliasis 124
Trichinellosis 124
Trichiniasis 124
Trichinosis 124
Trichobezoar 938
  intestine 936
  stomach 935.2
Trichocephaliasis 127.3
Trichocephalosis 127.3
Trichocephalus infestation 127.3

Trichoclasis 704.2
Trichoepithelioma (M8100/0)—*see also*
  Neoplasm, skin, benign
  breast 217
  genital organ NEC—*see* Neoplasm, by site,
    benign
  malignant (M8100/3)—*see* Neoplasm, skin,
    malignant
Trichofolliculoma (M8101/0)—*see* Neoplasm,
  skin, benign
Tricholemmoma (M8102/0)—*see* Neoplasm,
  skin, benign
Trichomatosis 704.2
Trichomoniasis 131.9
  bladder 131.09
  cervix 131.09
  intestinal 007.3
  prostate 131.03
  seminal vesicle 131.09
  specified site NEC 131.8
  urethra 131.02
  urogenitalis 131.00
  vagina 131.01
  vulva 131.01
  vulvovaginal 131.01
Trichomycosis 039.0
  axillaris 039.0
  nodosa 111.2
  nodularis 111.2
  rubra 039.0
Trichonocardiosis (axillaris) (palmellina) 039.0
Trichonodosis 704.2
Trichophytid, trichophyton infection (*see also*
  Dermatophytosis) 110.9
Trichophytide —*see* Dermatophytosis
Trichophytobezoar 938
  intestine 936
  stomach 935.2
Trichophytosis —*see* Dermatophytosis
Trichoptilosis 704.2
Trichorrhexis (nodosa) 704.2
Trichosporosis nodosa 111.2
Trichostasis spinulosa (congenital) 757.4
Trichostrongyliasis (small intestine) 127.6
Trichostrongylosis 127.6
Trichostrongylus (instabilis) infection 127.6
Trichotillomania 312.39
Trichromat, anomalous (congenital) 368.59
Trichromatopsia, anomalous (congenital)
  368.59
Trichuriasis 127.3
Trichuris trichiuria (any site) (infection)
  (infestation) 127.3
Tricuspid (valve)—*see* condition
Trifid —*see also* Accessory
  kidney (pelvis) 753.3
  tongue 750.13
Trigeminal neuralgia (*see also* Neuralgia,
  trigeminal) 350.1
Trigeminoencephaloangiomatosis 759.6
Trigeminy 427.89
  postoperative 997.1
Trigger finger (acquired) 727.03
  congenital 756.89
Trigonitis (bladder) (chronic)
  (pseudomembranous) 595.3
  tuberculous (*see also* Tuberculosis) 016.1
Trigonocephaly 756.0
Trihexosidosis 272.7
Trilobate placenta —*see* Placenta, abnormal
Trilocular heart 745.8

Trimethylaminuria 270.8
Tripartita placenta —*see* Placenta, abnormal
Triple —*see also* Accessory
  kidneys 753.3
  uteri 752.2
  X female 758.81
Triplegia 344.89
  congenital or infantile 343.8
Triplet
  affected by maternal complications of pregnancy
    761.5
  healthy liveborn—*see* Newborn, multiple
  pregnancy (complicating delivery) NEC 651.1
    with fetal loss and retention of one or more
      fetus(es) 651.4
    following (elective) fetal reduction 651.7
Triplex placenta —*see* Placenta, abnormal
Triplication —*see* Accessory
Trismus 781.0
  neonatorum 771.3
  newborn 771.3
Trisomy (syndrome) NEC 758.5
  13 (partial) 758.1
  16-18 758.2
  18 (partial) 758.2
  21 (partial) 758.0
  22 758.0
  autosomes NEC 758.5
  D_1 758.1
  E_3 758.2
  G (group) 758.0
  group D_1 758.1
  group E 758.2
  group G 758.0
Tritanomaly 368.53
Tritanopia 368.53
Troisier-Hanot-Chauffard syndrome (bronze
  diabetes) 275.0
Trombidiosis 133.8
Trophedema (hereditary) 757.0
  congenital 757.0
Trophoblastic disease (*see also* Hydatidiform
  mole) 630
  previous, affecting management of pregnancy
    V23.1
Tropholymphedema 757.0
Trophoneurosis NEC 356.9
  arm NEC 354.9
  disseminated 710.1
  facial 349.89
  leg NEC 355.8
  lower extremity NEC 355.8
  upper extremity NEC 354.9
Tropical —*see also* condition
  maceration feet (syndrome) 991.4
  wet foot (syndrome) 991.4
Trouble —*see also* Disease
  bowel 569.9
  heart—*see* Disease, heart
  intestine 569.9
  kidney (*see also* Disease, renal) 593.9
  nervous 799.21
  sinus (*see also* Sinusitis) 473.9
Trousseau's syndrome (thrombophlebitis
  migrans) 453.1
Truancy, childhood —*see also* Disturbance,
  conduct
  socialized 312.2
  undersocialized, unsocialized 312.1

Truncus
  arteriosus (persistent) 745.0
  common 745.0
  communis 745.0
Trunk —*see* condition
Trychophytide —*see* Dermatophytosis
Trypanosoma infestation —*see*
    Trypanosomiasis
Trypanosomiasis 086.9
  with meningoencephalitis 086.9 *[323.2]*
  African 086.5
    due to Trypanosoma 086.5
      gambiense 086.3
      rhodesiense 086.4
  American 086.2
    with
      heart involvement 086.0
      other organ involvement 086.1
    without mention of organ involvement 086.2
  Brazilian—*see* Trypanosomiasis, American
  Chagas'—*see* Trypanosomiasis, American
  due to Trypanosoma
    cruzi—*see* Trypanosomiasis, American
    gambiense 086.3
    rhodesiense 086.4
  gambiensis, Gambian 086.3
  North American—*see* Trypanosomiasis,
    American
  rhodesiensis, Rhodesian 086.4
  South American—*see* Trypanosomiasis,
    American
T-shaped incisors 520.2
Tsutsugamushi fever 081.2
Tube, tubal, tubular —*see also* condition
  ligation, admission for V25.2
Tubercle —*see also* Tuberculosis
  brain, solitary 013.2
  Darwin's 744.29
  epithelioid noncaseating 135
  Ghon, primary infection 010.0
Tuberculid, tuberculide (indurating) (lichenoid)
    (miliary) (papulonecrotic) (primary) (skin)
    (subcutaneous) (*see also* Tuberculosis) 017.0
Tuberculoma —*see also* Tuberculosis
  brain (any part) 013.2
  meninges (cerebral) (spinal) 013.1
  spinal cord 013.4

Tuberculosis, tubercular, tuberculous
    (calcification) (calcified) (caseous)
    (chromogenic acid-fast bacilli) (congenital)
    (degeneration) (disease) (fibrocaseous)
    (fistula) (gangrene) (interstitial) (isolated
    circumscribed lesions) (necrosis)
    (parenchymatous) (ulcerative) 011.9

> *Note—Use the following fifth-digit
> subclassification with categories 010-018:*
>
> *0 unspecified*
> *1 bacteriological or histological examination
>   not done*
> *2 bacteriological or histological examination
>   unknown (at present)*
> *3 tubercle bacilli found (in sputum) by
>   microscopy*
> *4 tubercle bacilli not found (in sputum) by
>   microscopy, but found by bacterial culture*
> *5 tubercle bacilli not found by bacteriological
>   examination, but tuberculosis confirmed
>   histologically*
> *6 tubercle bacilli not found by bacteriological or
>   histological examination, but tuberculosis
>   confirmed by other methods [inoculation of
>   animals]*
>
> *For tuberculous conditions specified as late
> effects or sequelae, see category 137.*

abdomen 014.8
  lymph gland 014.8
abscess 011.9
  arm 017.9
  bone (*see also* Osteomyelitis, due to,
      tuberculosis) 015.9 *[730.8]*
    hip 015.1 *[730.85]*
    knee 015.2 *[730.86]*
    sacrum 015.0 *[730.88]*
    specified site NEC 015.7 *[730.88]*
    spinal 015.0 *[730.88]*
    vertebra 015.0 *[730.88]*
  brain 013.3
  breast 017.9
  Cowper's gland 016.5
  dura (mater) 013.8
    brain 013.3
    spinal cord 013.5
  epidural 013.8
    brain 013.3
    spinal cord 013.5
  frontal sinus—*see* Tuberculosis, sinus
  genital organs NEC 016.9
    female 016.7
    male 016.5
  genitourinary NEC 016.9
  gland (lymphatic)—*see* Tuberculosis, lymph
      gland
  hip 015.1
  iliopsoas 015.0 *[730.88]*
  intestine 014.8
  ischiorectal 014.8
  joint 015.9
    hip 015.1
    knee 015.2
    specified joint NEC 015.8
    vertebral 015.0 *[730.88]*
  kidney 016.0 *[590.81]*
  knee 015.2
  lumbar 015.0 *[730.88]*

Tuberculosis, tubercular—*continued*
  lung 011.2
    primary, progressive 010.8
  meninges (cerebral) (spinal) 013.0
  pelvic 016.9
    female 016.7
    male 016.5
  perianal 014.8
    fistula 014.8
  perinephritic 016.0 *[590.81]*
  perineum 017.9
  perirectal 014.8
  psoas 015.0 *[730.88]*
  rectum 014.8
  retropharyngeal 012.8
  sacrum 015.0 *[730.88]*
  scrofulous 017.2
  scrotum 016.5
  skin 017.0
    primary 017.0
  spinal cord 013.5
  spine or vertebra (column) 015.0 *[730.88]*
  strumous 017.2
  subdiaphragmatic 014.8
  testis 016.5
  thigh 017.9
  urinary 016.3
    kidney 016.0 *[590.81]*
  uterus 016.7
  accessory sinus—*see* Tuberculosis, sinus
  Addison's disease 017.6
  adenitis (*see also* Tuberculosis, lymph gland) 017.2
  adenoids 012.8
  adenopathy (*see also* Tuberculosis, lymph gland) 017.2
    tracheobronchial 012.1
      primary progressive 010.8
  adherent pericardium 017.9 *[420.0]*
  adnexa (uteri) 016.7
  adrenal (capsule) (gland) 017.6
  air passage NEC 012.8
  alimentary canal 014.8
  anemia 017.9
  ankle (joint) 015.8
    bone 015.5 *[730.87]*
  anus 014.8
  apex (*see also* Tuberculosis, pulmonary) 011.9
  apical (*see also* Tuberculosis, pulmonary) 011.9
  appendicitis 014.8
  appendix 014.8
  arachnoid 013.0
  artery 017.9
  arthritis (chronic) (synovial) 015.9 *[711.40]*
    ankle 015.8 *[730.87]*
    hip 015.1 *[711.45]*
    knee 015.2 *[711.46]*
    specified site NEC 015.8 *[711.48]*
    spine or vertebra (column) 015.0 *[720.81]*
    wrist 015.8 *[730.83]*
  articular—*see* Tuberculosis, joint
  ascites 014.0
  asthma (*see also* Tuberculosis, pulmonary) 011.9
  axilla, axillary 017.2
    gland 017.2
  bilateral (*see also* Tuberculosis, pulmonary) 011.9
  bladder 016.1

Tuberculosis, tubercular—*continued*
  bone (*see also* Osteomyelitis, due to, tuberculosis) 015.9 *[730.8]*
    hip 015.1 *[730.85]*
    knee 015.2 *[730.86]*
    limb NEC 015.5 *[730.88]*
    sacrum 015.0 *[730.88]*
    specified site NEC 015.7 *[730.88]*
    spinal or vertebral column 015.0 *[730.88]*
  bowel 014.8
    miliary 018.9
  brain 013.2
  breast 017.9
  broad ligament 016.7
  bronchi, bronchial, bronchus 011.3
    ectasia, ectasis 011.5
    fistula 011.3
      primary, progressive 010.8
    gland 012.1
      primary, progressive 010.8
    isolated 012.2
    lymph gland or node 012.1
      primary, progressive 010.8
  bronchiectasis 011.5
  bronchitis 011.3
  bronchopleural 012.0
  bronchopneumonia, bronchopneumonic 011.6
  bronchorrhagia 011.3
  bronchotracheal 011.3
    isolated 012.2
  bronchus—*see* Tuberculosis, bronchi
  bronze disease (Addison's) 017.6
  buccal cavity 017.9
  bulbourethral gland 016.5
  bursa (*see also* Tuberculosis, joint) 015.9
  cachexia NEC (*see also* Tuberculosis, pulmonary) 011.9
  cardiomyopathy 017.9 *[425.8]*
  caries (*see also* Tuberculosis, bone) 015.9 *[730.8]*
  cartilage (*see also* Tuberculosis, bone) 015.9 *[730.8]*
    intervertebral 015.0 *[730.88]*
  catarrhal (*see also* Tuberculosis, pulmonary) 011.9
  cecum 014.8
  cellular tissue (primary) 017.0
  cellulitis (primary) 017.0
  central nervous system 013.9
    specified site NEC 013.8
  cerebellum (current) 013.2
  cerebral (current) 013.2
    meninges 013.0
  cerebrospinal 013.6
    meninges 013.0
  cerebrum (current) 013.2
  cervical 017.2
    gland 017.2
    lymph nodes 017.2
  cervicitis (uteri) 016.7
  cervix 016.7
  chest (*see also* Tuberculosis, pulmonary) 011.9

Tuberculosis, tubercular—*continued*
childhood type or first infection 010.0
choroid 017.3 *[363.13]*
choroiditis 017.3 *[363.13]*
ciliary body 017.3 *[364.11]*
colitis 014.8
colliers' 011.4
colliquativa (primary) 017.0
colon 014.8
  ulceration 014.8
complex, primary 010.0
complicating pregnancy, childbirth, or
  puerperium 647.3
  affecting fetus or newborn 760.2
congenital 771.2
conjunctiva 017.3 *[370.31]*
connective tissue 017.9
  bone—*see* Tuberculosis, bone
contact V01.1
converter (tuberculin skin test) (without disease)
  795.5
cornea (ulcer) 017.3 *[370.31]*
Cowper's gland 016.5
coxae 015.1 *[730.85]*
coxalgia 015.1 *[730.85]*
cul-de-sac of Douglas 014.8
curvature, spine 015.0 *[737.40]*
cutis (colliquativa) (primary) 017.0
cyst, ovary 016.6
cystitis 016.1
dacryocystitis 017.3 *[375.32]*
dactylitis 015.5
diarrhea 014.8
diffuse (*see also* Tuberculosis, miliary) 018.9
  lung—*see* Tuberculosis, pulmonary
  meninges 013.0
digestive tract 014.8
disseminated (*see also* Tuberculosis, miliary)
  018.9
  meninges 013.0
duodenum 014.8
dura (mater) 013.9
  abscess 013.8
    cerebral 013.3
    spinal 013.5
dysentery 014.8
ear (inner) (middle) 017.4
  bone 015.6
  external (primary) 017.0
  skin (primary) 017.0
elbow 015.8
emphysema—*see* Tuberculosis, pulmonary
empyema 012.0
encephalitis 013.6
endarteritis 017.9
endocarditis (any valve) 017.9 *[424.91]*
endocardium (any valve) 017.9 *[424.91]*
endocrine glands NEC 017.9
endometrium 016.7
enteric, enterica 014.8
enteritis 014.8
enterocolitis 014.8
epididymis 016.4
epididymitis 016.4
epidural abscess 013.8
  brain 013.3
  spinal cord 013.5
epiglottis 012.3
episcleritis 017.3 *[379.00]*
erythema (induratum) (nodosum) (primary)
  017.1

Tuberculosis, tubercular—*continued*
esophagus 017.8
Eustachian tube 017.4
exposure to V01.1
exudative 012.0
  primary, progressive 010.1
eye 017.3
eyelid (primary) 017.0
  lupus 017.0 *[373.4]*
fallopian tube 016.6
fascia 017.9
fauces 012.8
finger 017.9
first infection 010.0
fistula, perirectal 014.8
Florida 011.6
foot 017.9
funnel pelvis 137.3
gallbladder 017.9
galloping (*see also* Tuberculosis, pulmonary)
  011.9
ganglionic 015.9
gastritis 017.9
gastrocolic fistula 014.8
gastroenteritis 014.8
gastrointestinal tract 014.8
general, generalized 018.9
  acute 018.0
  chronic 018.8
genital organs NEC 016.9
  female 016.7
  male 016.5
genitourinary NEC 016.9
genu 015.2
glandulae suprarenalis 017.6
glandular, general 017.2
glottis 012.3
grinders' 011.4
groin 017.2
gum 017.9
hand 017.9
heart 017.9 *[425.8]*
hematogenous—*see* Tuberculosis, miliary
hemoptysis (*see also* Tuberculosis, pulmonary)
  011.9
hemorrhage NEC (*see also* Tuberculosis,
  pulmonary) 011.9
hemothorax 012.0
hepatitis 017.9
hilar lymph nodes 012.1
  primary, progressive 010.8
hip (disease) (joint) 015.1
  bone 015.1 *[730.85]*
hydrocephalus 013.8
hydropneumothorax 012.0
hydrothorax 012.0
hypoadrenalism 017.6
hypopharynx 012.8
ileocecal (hyperplastic) 014.8
ileocolitis 014.8
ileum 014.8
iliac spine (superior) 015.0 *[730.88]*
incipient NEC (*see also* Tuberculosis,
  pulmonary) 011.9
indurativa (primary) 017.1
infantile 010.0
infection NEC 011.9
  without clinical manifestation 010.0
infraclavicular gland 017.2
inguinal gland 017.2
inguinalis 017.2

Tuberculosis, tubercular—*continued*
intestine (any part) 014.8
iris 017.3 *[364.11]*
iritis 017.3 *[364.11]*
ischiorectal 014.8
jaw 015.7 *[730.88]*
jejunum 014.8
joint 015.9
  hip 015.1
  knee 015.2
  specified site NEC 015.8
  vertebral 015.0 *[730.88]*
keratitis 017.3 *[370.31]*
  interstitial 017.3 *[370.59]*
keratoconjunctivitis 017.3 *[370.31]*
kidney 016.0
knee (joint) 015.2
kyphoscoliosis 015.0 *[737.43]*
kyphosis 015.0 *[737.41]*
lacrimal apparatus, gland 017.3
laryngitis 012.3
larynx 012.3
leptomeninges, leptomeningitis (cerebral)
    (spinal) 013.0
lichenoides (primary) 017.0
linguae 017.9
lip 017.9
liver 017.9
lordosis 015.0 *[737.42]*
lung—*see* Tuberculosis, pulmonary
luposa 017.0
  eyelid 017.0 *[373.4]*
lymphadenitis—*see* Tuberculosis, lymph gland
lymphangitis—*see* Tuberculosis, lymph gland
lymphatic (gland) (vessel)—*see* Tuberculosis,
    lymph gland
lymph gland or node (peripheral) 017.2
  abdomen 014.8
  bronchial 012.1
    primary, progressive 010.8
  cervical 017.2
  hilar 012.1
    primary, progressive 010.8
  intrathoracic 012.1
    primary, progressive 010.8
  mediastinal 012.1
    primary, progressive 010.8
  mesenteric 014.8
  peripheral 017.2
  retroperitoneal 014.8
  tracheobronchial 012.1
    primary, progressive 010.8
malignant NEC (*see also* Tuberculosis,
    pulmonary) 011.9
mammary gland 017.9
marasmus NEC (*see also* Tuberculosis,
    pulmonary) 011.9
mastoiditis 015.6
maternal, affecting fetus or newborn 760.2
mediastinal (lymph) gland or node 012.1
    primary, progressive 010.8
mediastinitis 012.8
    primary, progressive 010.8
mediastinopericarditis 017.9 *[420.0]*
mediastinum 012.8
    primary, progressive 010.8
medulla 013.9
  brain 013.2
  spinal cord 013.4
melanosis, Addisonian 017.6
membrane, brain 013.0

Tuberculosis, tubercular—*continued*
meninges (cerebral) (spinal) 013.0
meningitis (basilar) (brain) (cerebral)
    (cerebrospinal) (spinal) 013.0
meningoencephalitis 013.0
mesentery, mesenteric 014.8
  lymph gland or node 014.8
miliary (any site) 018.9
  acute 018.0
  chronic 018.8
  specified type NEC 018.8
millstone makers' 011.4
miners' 011.4
moulders' 011.4
mouth 017.9
multiple 018.9
  acute 018.0
  chronic 018.8
muscle 017.9
myelitis 013.6
myocarditis 017.9 *[422.0]*
myocardium 017.9 *[422.0]*
nasal (passage) (sinus) 012.8
nasopharynx 012.8
neck gland 017.2
nephritis 016.0 *[583.81]*
nerve 017.9
nose (septum) 012.8
ocular 017.3
old NEC 137.0
  without residuals V12.01
omentum 014.8
oophoritis (acute) (chronic) 016.6
optic 017.3 *[377.39]*
  nerve trunk 017.3 *[377.39]*
  papilla, papillae 017.3 *[377.39]*
orbit 017.3
orchitis 016.5 *[608.81]*
organ, specified NEC 017.9
orificialis (primary) 017.0
osseous (*see also* Tuberculosis, bone) 015.9
    [730.8]
osteitis (*see also* Tuberculosis, bone) 015.9
    [730.8]
osteomyelitis (*see also* Tuberculosis, bone)
    015.9 *[730.8]*
otitis (media) 017.4
ovaritis (acute) (chronic) 016.6
ovary (acute) (chronic) 016.6
oviducts (acute) (chronic) 016.6
pachymeningitis 013.0
palate (soft) 017.9
pancreas 017.9
papulonecrotic (primary) 017.0
parathyroid glands 017.9
paronychia (primary) 017.0
parotid gland or region 017.9
pelvic organ NEC 016.9
  female 016.7
  male 016.5
pelvis (bony) 015.7 *[730.85]*
penis 016.5
peribronchitis 011.3
pericarditis 017.9 *[420.0]*
pericardium 017.9 *[420.0]*
perichondritis, larynx 012.3
perineum 017.9
periostitis (*see also* Tuberculosis, bone) 015.9
    [730.8]

Tuberculosis, tubercular—*continued*
  periphlebitis 017.9
    eye vessel 017.3 *[362.18]*
    retina 017.3 *[362.18]*
  perirectal fistula 014.8
  peritoneal gland 014.8
  peritoneum 014.0
  peritonitis 014.0
  pernicious NEC (*see also* Tuberculosis,
      pulmonary) 011.9
  pharyngitis 012.8
  pharynx 012.8
  phlyctenulosis (conjunctiva) 017.3 *[370.31]*
  phthisis NEC (*see also* Tuberculosis,
      pulmonary) 011.9
  pituitary gland 017.9
  placenta 016.7
  pleura, pleural, pleurisy, pleuritis (fibrinous)
      (obliterative) (purulent) (simple plastic)
      (with effusion) 012.0
    primary, progressive 010.1
  pneumonia, pneumonic 011.6
  pneumothorax 011.7
  polyserositis 018.9
    acute 018.0
    chronic 018.8
  potters' 011.4
  prepuce 016.5
  primary 010.9
    complex 010.0
    complicated 010.8
      with pleurisy or effusion 010.1
    progressive 010.8
      with pleurisy or effusion 010.1
    skin 017.0
  proctitis 014.8
  prostate 016.5 *[601.4]*
  prostatitis 016.5 *[601.4]*
  pulmonaris (*see also* Tuberculosis, pulmonary)
      011.9
  pulmonary (artery) (incipient) (malignant)
      (multiple round foci) (pernicious)
      (reinfection stage) 011.9
    cavitated or with cavitation 011.2
      primary, progressive 010.8
    childhood type or first infection 010.0
    chromogenic acid-fast bacilli 795.39
    fibrosis or fibrotic 011.4
    infiltrative 011.0
      primary, progressive 010.9
    nodular 011.1
    specified NEC 011.8
    sputum positive only 795.39
    status following surgical collapse of lung NEC
      011.9
  pyelitis 016.0 *[590.81]*
  pyelonephritis 016.0 *[590.81]*
  pyemia—*see* Tuberculosis, miliary
  pyonephrosis 016.0
  pyopneumothorax 012.0
  pyothorax 012.0
  rectum (with abscess) 014.8
    fistula 014.8
  reinfection stage (*see also* Tuberculosis,
      pulmonary) 011.9
  renal 016.0
  renis 016.0
  reproductive organ 016.7
  respiratory NEC (*see also* Tuberculosis,
      pulmonary) 011.9
    specified site NEC 012.8

Tuberculosis, tubercular—*continued*
  retina 017.3 *[363.13]*
  retroperitoneal (lymph gland or node) 014.8
    gland 014.8
  retropharyngeal abscess 012.8
  rheumatism 015.9
  rhinitis 012.8
  sacroiliac (joint) 015.8
  sacrum 015.0 *[730.88]*
  salivary gland 017.9
  salpingitis (acute) (chronic) 016.6
  sandblasters' 011.4
  sclera 017.3 *[379.09]*
  scoliosis 015.0 *[737.43]*
  scrofulous 017.2
  scrotum 016.5
  seminal tract or vesicle 016.5 *[608.81]*
  senile NEC (*see also* Tuberculosis, pulmonary)
      011.9
  septic NEC (*see also* Tuberculosis, miliary)
      018.9
  shoulder 015.8
    blade 015.7 *[730.8]*
  sigmoid 014.8
  sinus (accessory) (nasal) 012.8
    bone 015.7 *[730.88]*
    epididymis 016.4
  skeletal NEC (*see also* Osteomyelitis, due to
      tuberculosis) 015.9 *[730.8]*
  skin (any site) (primary) 017.0
  small intestine 014.8
  soft palate 017.9
  spermatic cord 016.5
  spinal
    column 015.0 *[730.88]*
    cord 013.4
    disease 015.0 *[730.88]*
    medulla 013.4
    membrane 013.0
    meninges 013.0
  spine 015.0 *[730.88]*
  spleen 017.7
  splenitis 017.7
  spondylitis 015.0 *[720.81]*
  spontaneous pneumothorax—*see* Tuberculosis,
      pulmonary
  sternoclavicular joint 015.8
  stomach 017.9
  stonemasons' 011.4
  struma 017.2
  subcutaneous tissue (cellular) (primary) 017.0
  subcutis (primary) 017.0
  subdeltoid bursa 017.9
  submaxillary 017.9
    region 017.9
  supraclavicular gland 017.2
  suprarenal (capsule) (gland) 017.6
  swelling, joint (*see also* Tuberculosis, joint)
      015.9
  symphysis pubis 015.7 *[730.88]*
  synovitis 015.9 *[727.01]*
    hip 015.1 *[727.01]*
    knee 015.2 *[727.01]*
    specified site NEC 015.8 *[727.01]*
    spine or vertebra 015.0 *[727.01]*
  systemic—*see* Tuberculosis, miliary
  tarsitis (eyelid) 017.0 *[373.4]*
    ankle (bone) 015.5 *[730.87]*
  tendon (sheath)—*see* Tuberculosis,
      tenosynovitis

Tuberculosis, tubercular—*continued*
  tenosynovitis 015.9 *[727.01]*
    hip 015.1 *[727.01]*
    knee 015.2 *[727.01]*
    specified site NEC 015.8 *[727.01]*
    spine or vertebra 015.0 *[727.01]*
  testis 016.5 *[608.81]*
  throat 012.8
  thymus gland 017.9
  thyroid gland 017.5
  toe 017.9
  tongue 017.9
  tonsil (lingual) 012.8
  tonsillitis 012.8
  trachea, tracheal 012.8
    gland 012.1
      primary, progressive 010.8
      isolated 012.2
  tracheobronchial 011.3
    glandular 012.1
      primary, progressive 010.8
      isolated 012.2
    lymph gland or node 012.1
      primary, progressive 010.8
  tubal 016.6
  tunica vaginalis 016.5
  typhlitis 014.8
  ulcer (primary) (skin) 017.0
    bowel or intestine 014.8
    specified site NEC—*see* Tuberculosis, by site
    unspecified site—*see* Tuberculosis, pulmonary
  ureter 016.2
  urethra, urethral 016.3
  urinary organ or tract 016.3
    kidney 016.0
  uterus 016.7
  uveal tract 017.3 *[363.13]*
  uvula 017.9
  vaccination, prophylactic (against) V03.2
  vagina 016.7
  vas deferens 016.5
  vein 017.9
  verruca (primary) 017.0
  verrucosa (cutis) (primary) 017.0
  vertebra (column) 015.0 *[730.88]*
  vesiculitis 016.5 *[608.81]*
  viscera NEC 014.8
  vulva 016.7 *[616.51]*
  wrist (joint) 015.8
    bone 015.5 *[730.83]*
Tuberculum
  auriculae 744.29
  occlusal 520.2
  paramolare 520.2
Tuberosity
  jaw, excessive 524.07
  maxillary, entire 524.07
Tuberous sclerosis (brain) 759.5
Tubo-ovarian —*see* condition
Tuboplasty, after previous sterilization V26.0
Tubotympanitis 381.10
Tularemia 021.9
  with
    conjunctivitis 021.3
    pneumonia 021.2
  bronchopneumonic 021.2
  conjunctivitis 021.3
  cryptogenic 021.1
  disseminated 021.8
  enteric 021.1
  generalized 021.8

Tularemia—*continued*
  glandular 021.8
  intestinal 021.1
  oculoglandular 021.3
  ophthalmic 021.3
  pneumonia 021.2
  pulmonary 021.2
  specified NEC 021.8
  typhoidal 021.1
  ulceroglandular 021.0
  vaccination, prophylactic (against) V03.4
Tularensis conjunctivitis 021.3
Tumefaction —*see also* Swelling
  liver (*see also* Hypertrophy, liver) 789.1
Tumor (M8000/1)—*see also* Neoplasm, by site,
  unspecified nature
  Abrikossov's (M9580/0)—*see also* Neoplasm,
    connective tissue, benign
    malignant (M9580/3)—*see* Neoplasm,
      connective tissue, malignant
  acinar cell (M8550/1)—*see* Neoplasm, by site,
    uncertain behavior
  acinic cell (M8550/1)—*see* Neoplasm, by site,
    uncertain behavior
  adenomatoid (M9054/0)—*see also* Neoplasm,
    by site, benign
    odontogenic (M9300/0) 213.1
      upper jaw (bone) 213.0
  adnexal (skin) (M8390/0)—*see* Neoplasm, skin,
    benign
  adrenal
    cortical (benign) (M8370/0) 227.0
      malignant (M8370/3) 194.0
    rest (M8671/0)—*see* Neoplasm, by site,
      benign
  alpha cell (M8152/0)
    malignant (M8152/3)
      pancreas 157.4
      specified site NEC—*see* Neoplasm, by site,
        malignant
      unspecified site 157.4
    pancreas 211.7
    specified site NEC—*see* Neoplasm, by site,
      benign
    unspecified site 211.7
  aneurysmal (*see also* Aneurysm) 442.9
  aortic body (M8691/1) 237.3
    malignant (M8691/3) 194.6
  argentaffin (M8241/1)—*see* Neoplasm, by site,
    uncertain behavior
  basal cell (M8090/1)—*see also* Neoplasm, skin,
    uncertain behavior
  benign (M8000/0)—*see* Neoplasm, by site,
    benign
  beta cell (M8151/0)
    malignant (M8151/3)
      pancreas 157.4
      specified site—*see* Neoplasm, by site,
        malignant
      unspecified site 157.4
    pancreas 211.7
    specified site NEC—*see* Neoplasm, by site,
      benign
    unspecified site 211.7
  blood—*see* Hematoma
  brenner (M9000/0) 220
    borderline malignancy (M9000/1) 236.2
    malignant (M9000/3) 183.0
    proliferating (M9000/1) 236.2
  Brooke's (M8100/0)—*see* Neoplasm, skin,
    benign

Tumor—*continued*
  brown fat (M8880/0)—*see* Lipoma, by site
  Burkitt's (M9750/3) 200.2
  calcifying epithelial odontogenic (M9340/0)
    213.1
    upper jaw (bone) 213.0
  carcinoid (M8240/1) 209.60
    benign 209.60
      appendix 209.51
      ascending colon 209.53
      bronchus 209.61
      cecum 209.52
      colon 209.50
      descending colon 209.55
      duodenum 209.41
      foregut 209.65
      hindgut 209.67
      ileum 209.43
      jejunum 209.42
      kidney 209.64
      large intestine 209.50
      lung 209.61
      midgut 209.66
      rectum 209.57
      sigmoid colon 209.56
      small intestine 209.40
      specified NEC 209.69
      stomach 209.63
      thymus 209.62
      transverse colon 209.54
    malignant (of) 209.20
      appendix 209.11
      ascending colon 209.13
      bronchus 209.21
      cecum 209.12
      colon 209.10
      descending colon 209.15
      duodenum 209.01
      foregut 209.25
      hindgut 209.27
      ileum 209.03
      jejunum 209.02
      kidney 209.24
      large intestine 209.10
      lung 209.21
      midgut 209.26
      rectum 209.17
      sigmoid colon 209.16
      small intestine 209.00
      specified NEC 209.29
      stomach 209.23
      thymus 209.22
      transverse colon 209.14
    secondary—see Tumor, neuroendocrine,
      secondary
  carotid body (M8692/1) 237.3
    malignant (M8692/3) 194.5
  Castleman's (mediastinal lymph node
    hyperplasia) 785.6
  cells (M8001/1)—*see also* Neoplasm, by site,
    unspecified nature
    benign (M8001/0)—*see* Neoplasm, by site,
      benign
    malignant (M8001/3)—*see* Neoplasm, by site,
      malignant
    uncertain whether benign or malignant
      (M8001/1)—*see* Neoplasm, by site,
      uncertain nature

Tumor—*continued*
  cervix
    in pregnancy or childbirth 654.6
      affecting fetus or newborn 763.89
      causing obstructed labor 660.2
        affecting fetus or newborn 763.1
  chondromatous giant cell (M9230/0)—*see*
    Neoplasm, bone, benign
  chromaffin (M8700/0)—*see also* Neoplasm, by
    site, benign
    malignant (M8700/3)—*see* Neoplasm, by site,
      malignant
  Cock's peculiar 706.2
  Codman's (benign chondroblastoma)
    (M9230/0)—*see* Neoplasm, bone, benign
  dentigerous, mixed (M9282/0) 213.1
    upper jaw (bone) 213.0
  dermoid (M9084/0)—*see* Neoplasm, by site,
    benign
    with malignant transformation (M9084/3)
      183.0
  desmoid (extra-abdominal) (M8821/1)—*see*
    also Neoplasm, connective tissue, uncertain
    behavior
    abdominal (M8822/1)—*see* Neoplasm,
      connective tissue, uncertain behavior
  embryonal (mixed) (M9080/1)—*see also*
    Neoplasm, by site, uncertain behavior
    liver (M9080/3) 155.0
  endodermal sinus (M9071/3)
    specified site—*see* Neoplasm, by site,
      malignant
    unspecified site
      female 183.0
      male 186.9
  epithelial
    benign (M8010/0)—*see* Neoplasm, by site,
      benign
    malignant (M8010/3)—*see* Neoplasm, by site,
      malignant
  Ewing's (M9260/3)—*see* Neoplasm, bone,
    malignant
  fatty—*see* Lipoma
  fetal, causing disproportion 653.7
    causing obstructed labor 660.1
  fibroid (M8890/0)—*see* Leiomyoma
  G cell (M8153/1)
    malignant (M8153/3)
      pancreas 157.4
      specified site NEC—*see* Neoplasm, by site,
        malignant
      unspecified site 157.4
    specified site—*see* Neoplasm, by site,
      uncertain behavior
    unspecified site 235.5
  giant cell (type) (M8003/1)—*see also*
    Neoplasm, by site, unspecified nature
    bone (M9250/1) 238.0
      malignant (M9250/3)—*see* Neoplasm, bone,
        malignant
    chondromatous (M9230/0)—*see* Neoplasm,
      bone, benign
    malignant (M8003/3)—*see* Neoplasm, by site,
      malignant
    peripheral (gingiva) 523.8
    soft parts (M9251/1)—*see also* Neoplasm,
      connective tissue, uncertain behavior
      malignant (M9251/3)—*see* Neoplasm,
        connective tissue, malignant
    tendon sheath 727.02

Tumor—*continued*
  glomus (M8711/0)—*see also* Hemangioma, by
    site
    jugulare (M8690/1) 237.3
      malignant (M8690/3) 194.6
  gonadal stromal (M8590/1)—*see* Neoplasm, by
    site, uncertain behavior
  granular cell (M9580/0)—*see also* Neoplasm,
    connective tissue, benign
    malignant (M9580/3)—*see* Neoplasm,
      connective tissue, malignant
  granulosa cell (M8620/1) 236.2
    malignant (M8620/3) 183.0
  granulosa cell-theca cell (M8621/1) 236.2
    malignant (M8621/3) 183.0
  Grawitz's (hypernephroma) (M8312/3) 189.0
  hazard-crile (M8350/3) 193
  hemorrhoidal—*see* Hemorrhoids
  hilar cell (M8660/0) 220
  hurthle cell (benign) (M8290/0) 226
    malignant (M8290/3) 193
  hydatid (*see also* Echinococcus) 122.9
  hypernephroid (M8311/1)—*see also* Neoplasm,
    by site, uncertain behavior
  interstitial cell (M8650/1)—*see also* Neoplasm,
    by site, uncertain behavior
    benign (M8650/0)—*see* Neoplasm, by site,
      benign
    malignant (M8650/3)—*see* Neoplasm, by site,
      malignant
  islet cell (M8150/0)
    malignant (M8150/3)
      pancreas 157.4
      specified site—*see* Neoplasm, by site,
        malignant
      unspecified site 157.4
    pancreas 211.7
    specified site NEC—*see* Neoplasm, by site,
      benign
    unspecified site 211.7
  juxtaglomerular (M8361/1) 236.91
  Krukenberg's (M8490/6) 198.6
  Leydig cell (M8650/1)
    benign (M8650/0)
      specified site—*see* Neoplasm, by site,
        benign
      unspecified site
        female 220
        male 220.0
    malignant (M8650/3)
      specified site—*see* Neoplasm, by site,
        malignant
      unspecified site
        female 183.0
        male 186.9
    specified site—*see* Neoplasm, by site,
      uncertain behavior
    unspecified site
      female 236.2
      male 236.4
  lipid cell, ovary (M8670/0) 220
  lipoid cell, ovary (M8670/0) 220
  lymphomatous, benign (M9590/0)—*see also*
    Neoplasm, by site, benign
  lysis syndrome (following antineoplastic drug
    therapy) (spontaneous) 277.88
  Malherbe's (M8110/0)—*see* Neoplasm, skin,
    benign

Tumor—*continued*
  malignant (M8000/3)—*see also* Neoplasm, by
    site, malignant
    fusiform cell (type) (M8004/3)—*see*
      Neoplasm, by site, malignant
    giant cell (type) (M8003/3)—*see* Neoplasm,
      by site, malignant
    mixed NEC (M8940/3)—*see* Neoplasm, by
      site, malignant
    small cell (type) (M8002/3)—*see* Neoplasm,
      by site, malignant
    spindle cell (type) (M8004/3)—*see* Neoplasm,
      by site, malignant
  mast cell (M9740/1) 238.5
    malignant (M9740/3) 202.6
  melanotic, neuroectodermal (M9363/0)—*see*
    Neoplasm, by site, benign
  Merkel cell—*see* Carcinoma, Merkel cell
  mesenchymal
    malignant (M8800/3)—*see* Neoplasm,
      connective tissue, malignant
    mixed (M8990/1)—*see* Neoplasm, connective
      tissue, uncertain behavior
  mesodermal, mixed (M8951/3)—*see also*
    Neoplasm, by site, malignant
    liver 155.0
  mesonephric (M9110/1)—*see also* Neoplasm,
    by site, uncertain behavior
    malignant (M9110/3)—*see* Neoplasm, by site,
      malignant
  metastatic
    from specified site (M8000/3)—*see*
      Neoplasm, by site, malignant
    to specified site (M8000/6)—*see* Neoplasm,
      by site, malignant, secondary
  mixed NEC (M8940/0)—*see also* Neoplasm, by
    site, benign
    malignant (M8940/3)—*see* Neoplasm, by site,
      malignant
  mucocarcinoid, malignant (M8243/3)—*see*
    Neoplasm, by site, malignant
  mucoepidermoid (M8430/1)—*see* Neoplasm, by
    site, uncertain behavior
  Müllerian, mixed (M8950/3)—*see* Neoplasm,
    by site, malignant
  myoepithelial (M8982/0)—*see* Neoplasm, by
    site, benign
  neuroendocrine 209.60
    malignant poorly differentiated 209.30
    secondary 209.70
      bone 209.73
      distant lymph nodes 209.71
      liver 209.72
      peritoneum 209.74
      site specified NEC 209.79
  neurogenic olfactory (M9520/3) 160.0
  nonencapsulated sclerosing (M8350/3) 193
  odontogenic (M9270/1) 238.0
    adenomatoid (M9300/0) 213.1
      upper jaw (bone) 213.0
    benign (M9270/0) 213.1
      upper jaw (bone) 213.0
    calcifying epithelial (M9340/0) 213.1
      upper jaw (bone) 213.0
    malignant (M9270/3) 170.1
      upper jaw (bone) 170.0
    squamous (M9312/0) 213.1
      upper jaw (bone) 213.0
  ovarian stromal (M8590/1) 236.2

Tumor—*continued*
  ovary
    in pregnancy or childbirth 654.4
      affecting fetus or newborn 763.89
      causing obstructed labor 660.2
        affecting fetus or newborn 763.1
  pacinian (M9507/0)—*see* Neoplasm, skin,
    benign
  Pancoast's (M8010/3) 162.3
  papillary—*see* Papilloma
  pelvic, in pregnancy or childbirth 654.9
    affecting fetus or newborn 763.89
    causing obstructed labor 660.2
      affecting fetus or newborn 763.1
  phantom 300.11
  plasma cell (M9731/1) 238.6
    benign (M9731/0)—*see* Neoplasm, by site,
      benign
    malignant (M9731/3) 203.8
  polyvesicular vitelline (M9071/3)
    specified site—*see* Neoplasm, by site,
      malignant
    unspecified site
      female 183.0
      male 186.9
  Pott's puffy (*see also* Osteomyelitis) 730.2
  Rathke's pouch (M9350/1) 237.0
  regaud's (M8082/3)—*see* Neoplasm,
    nasopharynx, malignant
  rete cell (M8140/0) 222.0
  retinal anlage (M9363/0)—*see* Neoplasm, by
    site, benign
  Rokitansky's 620.2
  salivary gland type, mixed (M8940/0)—*see also*
    Neoplasm, by site, benign
    malignant (M8940/3)—*see* Neoplasm, by site,
      malignant
  Sampson's 617.1
  Schloffer's (*see also* Peritonitis) 567.29
  Schmincke (M8082/3)—*see* Neoplasm,
    nasopharynx, malignant
  sebaceous (*see also* Cyst, sebaceous) 706.2
  secondary (M8000/6)—*see* Neoplasm, by site,
    secondary
    carcinoid — *see* Tumor, neuroendocrine,
      secondary
    neuroendocrine — *see* Tumor,
      neuroendocrine, secondary
  Sertoli cell (M8640/0)
    with lipid storage (M8641/0)
      specified site—*see* Neoplasm, by site,
        benign
      unspecified site
        female 220
        male 222.0
    specified site—*see* Neoplasm, by site, benign
    unspecified site
      female 220
      male 222.0
  Sertoli-Leydig cell (M8631/0)
    specified site—*see* Neoplasm, by site, benign
    unspecified site
      female 220
      male 222.0
  sex cord (-stromal) (M8590/1)—*see* Neoplasm,
    by site, uncertain behavior
  skin appendage (M8390/0)—*see* Neoplasm,
    skin, benign

Tumor—*continued*
  soft tissue
    benign (M8800/0)—*see* Neoplasm, connective
      tissue, benign
    malignant (M8800/3)—*see* Neoplasm,
      connective tissue, malignant
  sternomastoid 754.1
  stromal
    abdomen
      benign 215.5
      malignant NEC 171.5
      uncertain behavior 238.1
    digestive system 238.1
      benign 215.5
      malignant NEC 171.5
      uncertain behavior 238.1
    gastric 238.1
      benign 215.5
      malignant NEC 171.5
      uncertain behavior 238.1
    gastrointestinal 238.1
      benign 215.5
      malignant NEC 171.5
      uncertain behavior 238.1
    intestine (small) 238.1
      benign 215.5
      malignant 152.9
      uncertain behavior 238.1
    stomach 238.1
      benign 215.5
      malignant 151.9
      uncertain behavior 238.1
  superior sulcus (lung) (pulmonary) (syndrome)
    (M8010/3) 162.3
  suprasulcus (M8010/3) 162.3
  sweat gland (M8400/1)—*see also* Neoplasm,
    skin, uncertain behavior
    benign (M8400/0)—*see* Neoplasm, skin,
      benign
    malignant (M8400/3)—*see* Neoplasm, skin,
      malignant
  syphilitic brain 094.89
    congenital 090.49
  testicular stromal (M8590/1) 236.4
  theca cell (M8600/0) 220
  theca cell-granulosa cell (M8621/1) 236.2
  theca-lutein (M8610/0) 220
  turban (M8200/0) 216.4
  uterus
    in pregnancy or childbirth 654.1
      affecting fetus or newborn 763.89
      causing obstructed labor 660.2
        affecting fetus or newborn 763.1
  vagina
    in pregnancy or childbirth 654.7
      affecting fetus or newborn 763.89
      causing obstructed labor 660.2
        affecting fetus or newborn 763.1
  varicose (*see also* Varicose, vein) 454.9
  von Recklinghausen's (M9540/1) 237.71
  vulva
    in pregnancy or childbirth 654.8
      affecting fetus or newborn 763.89
      causing obstructed labor 660.2
        affecting fetus or newborn 763.1
  Warthin's (salivary gland) (M8561/0) 210.2
  white—*see also* Tuberculosis, arthritis
  White-Darier 757.39
  Wilms' (nephroblastoma) (M8960/3) 189.0

U

Uehlinger's syndrome (acropachyderma) 757.39
Uhl's anomaly or disease (hypoplasia of
    myocardium, right ventricle) 746.84
**Ulcer, ulcerated, ulcerating, ulceration, ulcer-
    ative** 707.9
  with gangrene 707.9 *[785.4]*
  abdomen (wall) (*see also* Ulcer, skin) 707.8
  ala, nose 478.19
  alveolar process 526.5
  amebic (intestine) 006.9
    skin 006.6
  anastomotic—*see* Ulcer, gastrojejunal
  anorectal 569.41
  antral—*see* Ulcer, stomach
  anus (sphincter) (solitary) 569.41
    varicose—*see* Varicose, ulcer, anus
  aorta —*see* Aneurysm
  aphthous (oral) (recurrent) 528.2
    genital organ(s)
      female 616.50
      male 608.89
    mouth 528.2
  arm (*see also* Ulcer, skin) 707.8
  arteriosclerotic plaque—*see* Arteriosclerosis, by
    site
  artery NEC 447.2
    without rupture 447.8
  atrophic NEC—*see* Ulcer, skin
  Barrett's (chronic peptic ulcer of esophagus)
    530.85
  bile duct 576.8
  bladder (solitary) (sphincter) 596.8
    bilharzial (*see also* Schistosomiasis) 120.9
      [595.4]
    submucosal (*see also* Cystitis) 595.1
    tuberculous (*see also* Tuberculosis) 016.1
  bleeding NEC—*see* Ulcer, peptic, with
    hemorrhage
  bone 730.9
  bowel (*see also* Ulcer, intestine) 569.82
  breast 611.0
  bronchitis 491.8
  bronchus 519.19
  buccal (cavity) (traumatic) 528.9
  burn (acute)—*see* Ulcer, duodenum
  Buruli 031.1
  buttock (*see also* Ulcer, skin) 707.8
    decubitus (*see also* Ulcer, pressure) 707.00
  cancerous (M8000/3)—*see* Neoplasm, by site,
    malignant
  cardia—*see* Ulcer, stomach
  cardio-esophageal (peptic) 530.20
    with bleeding 530.21
  cecum (*see also* Ulcer, intestine) 569.82
  cervix (uteri) (trophic) 622.0
    with mention of cervicitis 616.0
  chancroidal 099.0
  chest (wall) (*see also* Ulcer, skin) 707.8
  Chiclero 085.4
  chin (pyogenic) (*see also* Ulcer, skin) 707.8
  chronic (cause unknown)—*see also* Ulcer, skin
    penis 607.89
  Cochin-China 085.1
  colitis —*see* Colitis, ulcerative
  colon (*see also* Ulcer, intestine) 569.82
  conjunctiva (acute) (postinfectional) 372.00

Ulcer, ulcerated, ulcerating—*continued*
  cornea (infectional) 370.00
    with perforation 370.06
    annular 370.02
    catarrhal 370.01
    central 370.03
    dendritic 054.42
    marginal 370.01
    mycotic 370.05
    phlyctenular, tuberculous (*see also*
      Tuberculosis) 017.3 *[370.31]*
    ring 370.02
    rodent 370.07
    serpent, serpiginous 370.04
    superficial marginal 370.01
    tuberculous (*see also* Tuberculosis) 017.3
      [370.31]
  corpus cavernosum (chronic) 607.89
  crural—*see* Ulcer, lower extremity
  Curling's—*see* Ulcer, duodenum
  Cushing's—*see* Ulcer, peptic
  cystitis (interstitial) 595.1
  decubitus (unspecified site) (*see also* Ulcer,
    pressure) 707.00
    with gangrene 707.00 *[785.4]*
    ankle 707.06
    back
      lower 707.03
      upper 707.02
    buttock 707.05
    coccyx 707.03
    elbow 707.01
    head 707.09
    heel 707.07
    hip 707.04
    other site 707.09
    sacrum 707.03
    shoulder blades 707.02
  dendritic 054.42
  diabetes, diabetic (mellitus) 250.8 *[707.9]*
    due to secondary diabetes 249.8 *[707.9]*
    lower limb 250.8 *[707.10]*
      due to secondary diabetes 249.8 *[707.10]*
      ankle 250.8 *[707.13]*
        due to secondary diabetes 249.8 *[707.13]*
      calf 250.8 *[707.12]*
        due to secondary diabetes 249.8 *[707.12]*
      foot 250.8 *[707.15]*
        due to secondary diabetes 249.8 *[707.15]*
      heel 250.8 *[707.14]*
        due to secondary diabetes 249.8 *[707.14]*
      knee 250.8 *[707.19]*
        due to secondary diabetes 249.8 *[707.19]*
      specified site NEC 250.8 *[707.19]*
        due to secondary diabetes 249.8 *[707.19]*
      thigh 250.8 *[707.11]*
        due to secondary diabetes 249.8 *[707.11]*
      toes 250.8 *[707.15]*
        due to secondary diabetes 249.8 *[707.15]*
    specified site NEC 250.8 *[707.8]*
      due to secondary diabetes 249.8 *[707.8]*
  Dieulafoy—*see* Lesion, Dieulafoy
  due to
    infection NEC—*see* Ulcer, skin
    radiation, radium—*see* Ulcer, by site
    trophic disturbance (any region)—*see* Ulcer,
      skin
    x-ray—*see* Ulcer, by site

Ulcer, ulcerated, ulcerating—*continued*
  duodenum, duodenal (eroded) (peptic) 532.9

> *Note—Use the following fifth-digit*
> *subclassification with categories 531-534:*
>
> *0   without mention of obstruction*
> *1   with obstruction*

  with
    hemorrhage (chronic) 532.4
      and perforation 532.6
    perforation (chronic) 532.5
      and hemorrhage 532.6
  acute 532.3
    with
      hemorrhage 532.0
        and perforation 532.2
      perforation 532.1
        and hemorrhage 532.2
  bleeding (recurrent)—*see* Ulcer, duodenum,
    with hemorrhage
  chronic 532.7
    with
      hemorrhage 532.4
        and perforation 532.6
      perforation 532.5
        and hemorrhage 532.6
  penetrating—*see* Ulcer, duodenum, with
    perforation
  perforating—*see* Ulcer, duodenum, with
    perforation
  dysenteric NEC 009.0
  elusive 595.1
  endocarditis (any valve) (acute) (chronic)
    (subacute) 421.0
  enteritis —*see* Colitis, ulcerative
  enterocolitis 556.0
  epiglottis 478.79
  esophagus (peptic) 530.20
    with bleeding 530.21
    due to ingestion
      aspirin 530.20
      chemicals 530.20
      medicinal agents 530.20
    fungal 530.20
    infectional 530.20
    varicose (*see also* Varix, esophagus) 456.1
      bleeding (*see also* Varix, esophagus,
        bleeding) 456.0
  eye NEC 360.00
    dendritic 054.42
  eyelid (region) 373.01
  face (*see also* Ulcer, skin) 707.8
  fauces 478.29
  Fenwick (-Hunner) (solitary) (*see also* Cystitis)
    595.1
  fistulous NEC—*see* Ulcer, skin
  foot (indolent) (*see also* Ulcer, lower extremity)
    707.15
    perforating 707.15
      leprous 030.1
      syphilitic 094.0
    trophic 707.15
    varicose 454.0
      inflamed or infected 454.2
  frambesial, initial or primary 102.0
  gallbladder or duct 575.8
  gall duct 576.8
  gangrenous (*see also* Gangrene) 785.4
  gastric—*see* Ulcer, stomach
  gastrocolic—*see* Ulcer, gastrojejunal

Ulcer, ulcerated, ulcerating—*continued*
  gastroduodenal—*see* Ulcer, peptic
  gastroesophageal—*see* Ulcer, stomach
  gastrohepatic—*see* Ulcer, stomach
  gastrointestinal—*see* Ulcer, gastrojejunal
  gastrojejunal (eroded) (peptic) 534.9

> *Note—Use the following fifth-digit*
> *subclassification with categories 531-534:*
>
> *0   without mention of obstruction*
> *1   with obstruction*

  with
    hemorrhage (chronic) 534.4
      and perforation 534.6
    perforation 534.5
      and hemorrhage 534.6
  acute 534.3
    with
      hemorrhage 534.0
        and perforation 534.2
      perforation 534.1
        and hemorrhage 534.2
  bleeding (recurrent)—*see* Ulcer, gastrojejunal,
    with hemorrhage
  chronic 534.7
    with
      hemorrhage 534.4
        and perforation 534.6
      perforation 534.5
        and hemorrhage 534.6
  penetrating—*see* Ulcer, gastrojejunal, with
    perforation
  perforating—*see* Ulcer, gastrojejunal, with
    perforation
  gastrojejunocolic—*see* Ulcer, gastrojejunal
  genital organ
    female 629.89
    male 608.89
  gingiva 523.8
  gingivitis 523.10
  glottis 478.79
  granuloma of pudenda 099.2
  groin (*see also* Ulcer, skin) 707.8
  gum 523.8
  gumma, due to yaws 102.4
  hand (*see also* Ulcer, skin) 707.8
  hard palate 528.9
  heel (*see also* Ulcer, lower extremity) 707.14
    decubitus (*see also* Ulcer, pressure) 707.07
  hemorrhoids 455.8
    external 455.5
    internal 455.2
  hip (*see also* Ulcer, skin) 707.8
    decubitus (*see also* Ulcer, pressure) 707.04
  Hunner's 595.1
  hypopharynx 478.29
  hypopyon (chronic) (subacute) 370.04
  hypostaticum—*see* Ulcer, varicose
  ileocolitis 556.1
  ileum (*see also* Ulcer, intestine) 569.82
  intestine, intestinal 569.82
    with perforation 569.83
    amebic 006.9
    duodenal—*see* Ulcer, duodenum
    granulocytopenic (with hemorrhage) 288.09
    marginal 569.82
    perforating 569.83
    small, primary 569.82
    stercoraceous 569.82
    stercoral 569.82

Ulcer, ulcerated, ulcerating—*continued*
  tuberculous (*see also* Tuberculosis) 014.8
  typhoid (fever) 002.0
  varicose 456.8
  ischemic 707.9
    lower extremity (*see also* Ulcer, lower
      extremity) 707.10
      ankle 707.13
      calf 707.12
      foot 707.15
      heel 707.14
      knee 707.19
      specified site NEC 707.19
      thigh 707.11
      toes 707.15
  jejunum, jejunal—*see* Ulcer, gastrojejunal
  keratitis (*see also* Ulcer, cornea) 370.00
  knee—*see* Ulcer, lower extremity
  labium (majus) (minus) 616.50
  laryngitis (*see also* Laryngitis) 464.00
    with obstruction 464.01
  larynx (aphthous) (contact) 478.79
    diphtheritic 032.3
  leg—*see* Ulcer, lower extremity
  lip 528.5
  Lipschütz's 616.50
  lower extremity (atrophic) (chronic)
    (neurogenic) (perforating) (pyogenic)
    (trophic) (tropical) 707.10
    with gangrene (*see also* Ulcer, lower
      extremity) 707.10 *[785.4]*
      arteriosclerotic 440.24
    ankle 707.13
      arteriosclerotic 440.23
      with gangrene 440.24
    calf 707.12
    decubitus (*see also* Ulcer, pressure) 707.00
      with gangrene 707.00 *[785.4]*
      ankle 707.06
      buttock 707.05
      heel 707.07
      hip 707.04
    foot 707.15
    heel 707.14
    knee 707.19
    specified site NEC 707.19
    thigh 707.11
    toes 707.15
    varicose 454.0
      inflamed or infected 454.2
  luetic—*see* Ulcer, syphilitic
  lung 518.89
    tuberculous (*see also* Tuberculosis) 011.2
  malignant (M8000/3)—*see* Neoplasm, by site,
    malignant
  marginal NEC—*see* Ulcer, gastrojejunal
  meatus (urinarius) 597.89
  Meckel's diverticulum 751.0
  Meleney's (chronic undermining) 686.09
  Mooren's (cornea) 370.07
  mouth (traumatic) 528.9
  mycobacterial (skin) 031.1
  nasopharynx 478.29
  navel cord (newborn) 771.4
  neck (*see also* Ulcer, skin) 707.8
    uterus 622.0
  neurogenic NEC—*see* Ulcer, skin

Ulcer, ulcerated, ulcerating—*continued*
  nose, nasal (infectional) (passage) 478.19
    septum 478.19
      varicose 456.8
    skin—*see* Ulcer, skin
    spirochetal NEC 104.8
  oral mucosa (traumatic) 528.9
  palate (soft) 528.9
  penetrating NEC—*see* Ulcer, peptic, with
    perforation
  penis (chronic) 607.89
  peptic (site unspecified) 533.9

> *Note*—*Use the following fifth-digit*
> *subclassification with categories 531-534:*
>
> *0 without mention of obstruction*
> *1 with obstruction*

    with
      hemorrhage 533.4
        and perforation 533.6
      perforation (chronic) 533.5
        and hemorrhage 533.6
    acute 533.3
      with
        hemorrhage 533.0
          and perforation 533.2
        perforation 533.1
          and hemorrhage 533.2
    bleeding (recurrent)—*see* Ulcer, peptic, with
      hemorrhage
    chronic 533.7
      with
        hemorrhage 533.4
          and perforation 533.6
        perforation 533.5
          and hemorrhage 533.6
    penetrating—*see* Ulcer, peptic, with
      perforation
  perforating NEC (*see also* Ulcer, peptic, with
    perforation) 533.5
    skin 707.9
  perineum (*see also* Ulcer, skin) 707.8
  peritonsillar 474.8
  phagedenic (tropical) NEC—*see* Ulcer, skin
  pharynx 478.29
  phlebitis—*see* Phlebitis
  plaster (*see also* Ulcer, pressure) 707.00
  popliteal space—*see* Ulcer, lower extremity
  postpyloric—*see* Ulcer, duodenum
  prepuce 607.89
  prepyloric—*see* Ulcer, stomach
  pressure 707.00
    with
      abrasion, blister, partial thickness skin loss
        involving epidermis and/or dermis
        707.22
      full thickness skin loss involving damage or
        necrosis of subcutaneous tissue 707.23
      gangrene 707.00 [785.4]
      necrosis of soft tissues through to underlying
        muscle, tendon, or bone 707.24
    ankle 707.06
    back
      lower 707.03
      upper 707.02
    buttock 707.05
    coccyx 707.03
    elbow 707.01
    head 707.09
    healed — omit code
    healing — code to Ulcer, pressure, by stage

Ulcer, ulcerated, ulcerating—*continued*
 heel 707.07
 hip 707.04
 other site 707.09
 sacrum 707.03
 shoulder blades 707.02
 stage
  I (healing) 707.21
  II (healing) 707.22
  III (healing) 707.23
  IV (healing) 707.24
  unspecified (healing) 707.20
 unstageable 707.25
 primary of intestine 569.82
  with perforation 569.83
 proctitis 556.2
  with ulcerative sigmoiditis 556.3
 prostate 601.8
 pseudopeptic—*see* Ulcer, peptic
 pyloric—*see* Ulcer, stomach
 rectosigmoid 569.82
  with perforation 569.83
 rectum (sphincter) (solitary) 569.41
  stercoraceous, stercoral 569.41
  varicose—*see* Varicose, ulcer, anus
 retina (*see also* Chorioretinitis) 363.20
 rodent (M8090/3)—*see also* Neoplasm, skin,
   malignant
  cornea 370.07
 round—*see* Ulcer, stomach
 sacrum (region) (*see also* Ulcer, skin) 707.8
 Saemisch's 370.04
 scalp (*see also* Ulcer, skin) 707.8
 sclera 379.09
 scrofulous (*see also* Tuberculosis) 017.2
 scrotum 608.89
  tuberculous (*see also* Tuberculosis) 016.5
  varicose 456.4
 seminal vesicle 608.89
 sigmoid 569.82
  with perforation 569.83
 skin (atrophic) (chronic) (neurogenic)
   (non-healing) (perforating) (pyogenic)
   (trophic) 707.9
  with gangrene 707.9 *[785.4]*
  amebic 006.6
  decubitus (*see also* Ulcer, pressure) 707.00
   with gangrene 707.00 *[785.4]*
  in granulocytopenia 288.09
  lower extremity (*see also* Ulcer, lower
    extremity) 707.10
   with gangrene 707.10 *[785.4]*
    arteriosclerotic 440.24
   ankle 707.13
   arteriosclerotic 440.23
    with gangrene 440.24
   calf 707.12
   foot 707.15
   heel 707.14
   knee 707.19
   specified site NEC 707.19
   thigh 707.11
   toes 707.15
  mycobacterial 031.1
  syphilitic (early) (secondary) 091.3
  tuberculous (primary) (*see also* Tuberculosis)
    017.0
  varicose—*see* Ulcer, varicose
 sloughing NEC—*see* Ulcer, skin
 soft palate 528.9
 solitary, anus or rectum (sphincter) 569.41

Ulcer, ulcerated, ulcerating—*continued*
 sore throat 462
  streptococcal 034.0
 spermatic cord 608.89
 spine (tuberculous) 015.0 *[730.88]*
 stasis (leg) (venous) 454.0
  with varicose veins 454.0
  inflamed or infected 454.2
  without varicose veins 459.81
 stercoral, stercoraceous 569.82
  with perforation 569.83
  anus or rectum 569.41
 stoma, stomal—*see* Ulcer, gastrojejunal
 stomach (eroded) (peptic) (round) 531.9

> Note—*Use the following fifth-digit
> subclassification with categories 531-534:*
>
> 0 *without mention of obstruction*
> 1 *with obstruction*

  with
   hemorrhage 531.4
    and perforation 531.6
   perforation (chronic) 531.5
    and hemorrhage 531.6
  acute 531.3
   with
    hemorrhage 531.0
     and perforation 531.2
    perforation 531.1
     and hemorrhage 531.2
  bleeding (recurrent)—*see* Ulcer, stomach,
    with hemorrhage
  chronic 531.7
   with
    hemorrhage 531.4
     and perforation 531.6
    perforation 531.5
     and hemorrhage 531.6
  penetrating—*see* Ulcer, stomach, with
    perforation
  perforating—*see* Ulcer, stomach, with
    perforation
 stomatitis 528.00
 stress—*see* Ulcer, peptic
 strumous (tuberculous) (*see also* Tuberculosis)
   017.2
 submental (*see also* Ulcer, skin) 707.8
 submucosal, bladder 595.1
 syphilitic (any site) (early) (secondary) 091.3
  late 095.9
  perforating 095.9
   foot 094.0
 testis 608.89
 thigh—*see* Ulcer, lower extremity
 throat 478.29
  diphtheritic 032.0
 toe—*see* Ulcer, lower extremity
 tongue (traumatic) 529.0
 tonsil 474.8
  diphtheritic 032.0
 trachea 519.19
 trophic—*see* Ulcer, skin
 tropical NEC (*see also* Ulcer, skin) 707.9
 tuberculous—*see* Tuberculosis, ulcer
 tunica vaginalis 608.89
 turbinate 730.9
 typhoid (fever) 002.0
  perforating 002.0
 umbilicus (newborn) 771.4
 unspecified site NEC—*see* Ulcer, skin

Ulcer, ulcerated, ulcerating—*continued*
  urethra (meatus) (*see also* Urethritis) 597.89
  uterus 621.8
    cervix 622.0
      with mention of cervicitis 616.0
    neck 622.0
      with mention of cervicitis 616.0
  vagina 616.89
  valve, heart 421.0
  varicose (lower extremity, any part) 454.0
    anus—*see* Varicose, ulcer, anus
    broad ligament 456.5
    esophagus (*see also* Varix, esophagus) 456.1
      bleeding (*see also* Varix, esophagus,
        bleeding) 456.0
    inflamed or infected 454.2
    nasal septum 456.8
    perineum 456.6
    rectum—*see* Varicose, ulcer, anus
    scrotum 456.4
    specified site NEC 456.8
    sublingual 456.3
    vulva 456.6
  vas deferens 608.89
  vesical (*see also* Ulcer, bladder) 596.8
  vulva (acute) (infectional) 616.50
    Behçet's syndrome 136.1 *[616.51]*
    herpetic 054.12
    tuberculous 016.7 *[616.51]*
  vulvobuccal, recurring 616.50
  x-ray—*see* Ulcer, by site
  yaws 102.4
Ulcerosa scarlatina 034.1
Ulcus —*see also* Ulcer
  cutis tuberculosum (*see also* Tuberculosis)
    017.0
  duodeni—*see* Ulcer, duodenum
  durum 091.0
    extragenital 091.2
  gastrojejunale—*see* Ulcer, gastrojejunal
  hypostaticum—*see* Ulcer, varicose
  molle (cutis) (skin) 099.0
  serpens cornea (pneumococcal) 370.04
  ventriculi—*see* Ulcer, stomach
Ulegyria 742.4
Ulerythema
  acneiforma 701.8
  centrifugum 695.4
  ophryogenes 757.4
Ullrich (-Bonnevie) (-Turner) syndrome 758.6
Ullrich-Feichtiger syndrome 759.89
Ulnar —*see* condition
Ulorrhagia 523.8
Ulorrhea 523.8
Umbilicus, umbilical —*see also* condition
  cord necrosis, affecting fetus or newborn 762.6
Unacceptable
  existing dental restoration
    contours 525.65
    morphology 525.65
Unavailability of medical facilities (at) V63.9
  due to
    investigation by social service agency V63.8
    lack of services at home V63.1
    remoteness from facility V63.0
    waiting list V63.2
  home V63.1
  outpatient clinic V63.0
  specified reason NEC V63.8
Uncinaria americana infestation 126.1
Uncinariasis (*see also* Ancylostomiasis) 126.9
Unconscious, unconsciousness 780.09

Underdevelopment —*see also* Undeveloped
  sexual 259.0
Underfill, endodontic 526.63
Undernourishment 269.9
Undernutrition 269.9
Under observation —*see* Observation
Underweight 783.22
  for gestational age—*see* Light-for-dates
Underwood's disease (sclerema neonatorum)
  778.1
Undescended —*see also* Malposition, congenital
  cecum 751.4
  colon 751.4
  testis 752.51
Undetermined diagnosis or cause 799.9
Undeveloped, undevelopment —*see also*
    Hypoplasia
  brain (congenital) 742.1
  cerebral (congenital) 742.1
  fetus or newborn 764.9
  heart 746.89
  lung 748.5
  testis 257.2
  uterus 259.0
Undiagnosed (disease) 799.9
Undulant fever (*see also* Brucellosis) 023.9
Unemployment, anxiety concerning V62.0
Unequal leg (acquired) (length) 736.81
  congenital 755.30
Unerupted teeth, tooth 520.6
Unextracted dental root 525.3
Unguis incarnatus 703.0
Unicornis uterus 752.3
Unicorporeus uterus 752.3
Uniformis uterus 752.3
Unilateral —*see also* condition
  development, breast 611.89
  organ or site, congenital NEC—*see* Agenesis
  vagina 752.49
Unilateralis uterus 752.3
Unilocular heart 745.8
Uninhibited (neurogenic) bladder 596.54
  with cauda equina syndrome 344.61
  neurogenic—*see* Neurogenic, bladder 596.54
Union, abnormal —*see also* Fusion
  divided tendon 727.89
  larynx and trachea 748.3
Universal
  joint, cervix 620.6
  mesentery 751.4
Unknown
  cause of death 799.9
  diagnosis 799.9
Unna's disease (seborrheic dermatitis) 690.10
Unresponsiveness, adrenocorticotropin
    (ACTH) 255.41
Unsoundness of mind (*see also* Psychosis) 298.9
Unspecified cause of death 799.9
Unsatisfactory
  cytology smear
    anal 796.78
    cervical 795.08
    vaginal 795.18
  restoration, tooth (existing) 525.60
    specified NEC 525.69
Unstable
  back NEC 724.9
  colon 569.89
  joint—*see* Instability, joint

Unstable—*continued*
  lie 652.0
    affecting fetus or newborn (before labor) 761.7
    causing obstructed labor 660.0
      affecting fetus or newborn 763.1
  lumbosacral joint (congenital) 756.19
    acquired 724.6
  sacroiliac 724.6
  spine NEC 724.9
Untruthfulness, child problem (*see also*
    Disturbance, conduct) 312.0
Unverricht (-Lundborg) disease, syndrome, or
    epilepsy 345.1
Unverricht-Wagner syndrome
    (dermatomyositis) 710.3
Upper respiratory —*see* condition
Upset
  gastric 536.8
    psychogenic 306.4
  gastrointestinal 536.8
    psychogenic 306.4
    virus (*see also* Enteritis, viral) 008.8
  intestinal (large) (small) 564.9
    psychogenic 306.4
  menstruation 626.9
  mental 300.9
  stomach 536.8
    psychogenic 306.4
Urachus —*see also* condition
  patent 753.7
  persistent 753.7
Uratic arthritis 274.00
Urbach's lipoid proteinosis 272.8
Urbach-Oppenheim disease or syndrome
    (necrobiosis lipoidica diabeticorum) 250.8
    [709.3]
    due to secondary diabetes 249.8 *[709.3]*
Urbach-Wiethe disease or syndrome (lipoid
    proteinosis) 272.8
Urban yellow fever 060.1
Urea, blood, high —*see* Uremia
Uremia, uremic (absorption) (amaurosis)
    (amblyopia) (aphasia) (apoplexy) (coma)
    (delirium) (dementia) (dropsy) (dyspnea)
    (fever) (intoxication) (mania) (paralysis)
    (poisoning) (toxemia) (vomiting) 586
  with
    abortion—*see* Abortion, by type, with renal
      failure
    ectopic pregnancy (*see also* categories
      633.0-633.9) 639.3
    hypertension (*see also* Hypertension, kidney)
      403.91
    molar pregnancy (*see also* categories 630-632)
      639.3
  chronic 585.9
  complicating
    abortion 639.3
    ectopic or molar pregnancy 639.3
    hypertension (*see also* Hypertension, kidney)
      403.91
    labor and delivery 669.3
  congenital 779.89
  extrarenal 788.99
  hypertensive (chronic) (*see also* Hypertension,
    kidney) 403.91
  maternal NEC, affecting fetus or newborn 760.1
  neuropathy 585.9 *[357.4]*
  pericarditis 585.9 *[420.0]*
  prerenal 788.99
  pyelitic (*see also* Pyelitis) 590.80

Ureter, ureteral —*see* condition
Ureteralgia 788.0
Ureterectasis 593.89
Ureteritis 593.89
  cystica 590.3
  due to calculus 592.1
  gonococcal (acute) 098.19
    chronic or duration of 2 months or over 098.39
  nonspecific 593.89
Ureterocele (acquired) 593.89
  congenital 753.23
Ureterolith 592.1
Ureterolithiasis 592.1
Ureterostomy status V44.6
  with complication 997.5
Urethra, urethral —*see* condition
Urethralgia 788.99
Urethritis (abacterial) (acute) (allergic) (anterior)
    (chronic) (nonvenereal) (posterior) (recurrent)
    (simple) (subacute) (ulcerative)
    (undifferentiated) 597.80
  diplococcal (acute) 098.0
    chronic or duration of 2 months or over 098.2
  due to Trichomonas (vaginalis) 131.02
  gonococcal (acute) 098.0
    chronic or duration of 2 months or over 098.2
  nongonococcal (sexually transmitted) 099.40
    Chlamydia trachomatis 099.41
    Reiter's 099.3
    specified organism NEC 099.49
  nonspecific (sexually transmitted) (*see also*
    Urethritis, nongonococcal) 099.40
  not sexually transmitted 597.80
  Reiter's 099.3
  trichomonal or due to Trichomonas (vaginalis)
    131.02
  tuberculous (*see also* Tuberculosis) 016.3
  venereal NEC (*see also* Urethritis,
    nongonococcal) 099.40
Urethrocele
  female 618.03
    with uterine prolapse 618.4
      complete 618.3
      incomplete 618.2
  male 599.5
Urethrolithiasis 594.2
Urethro-oculoarticular syndrome 099.3
Urethro-oculosynovial syndrome 099.3
Urethrorectal —*see* condition
Urethrorrhagia 599.84
Urethrorrhea 788.7
Urethrostomy status V44.6
  with complication 997.5
Urethrotrigonitis 595.3
Urethrovaginal —*see* condition
Urhidrosis, uridrosis 705.89
Uric acid
  diathesis 274.9
  in blood 790.6
Uricacidemia 790.6
Uricemia 790.6
Uricosuria 791.9
Urination
  frequent 788.41
  painful 788.1
  urgency 788.63
Urine, urinary —*see also* condition
  abnormality NEC 788.69
  blood in (*see also* Hematuria) 599.70
  discharge, excessive 788.42

Urine, urinary—*continued*
  enuresis 788.30
    nonorganic origin 307.6
  extravasation 788.8
  frequency 788.41
  hesitancy 788.64
  incontinence 788.30
    active 788.30
    female 788.30
      stress 625.6
        and urge 788.33
    male 788.30
      stress 788.32
        and urge 788.33
    mixed (stress and urge) 788.33
    neurogenic 788.39
    nonorganic origin 307.6
    overflow 788.38
    stress (female) 625.6
      male NEC 788.32
  intermittent stream 788.61
  pus in 791.9
  retention or stasis NEC 788.20
    bladder, incomplete emptying 788.21
    psychogenic 306.53
    specified NEC 788.29
  secretion
    deficient 788.5
    excessive 788.42
    frequency 788.41
  strain 788.65
  stream
    intermittent 788.61
    slowing 788.62
    splitting 788.61
    weak 788.62
  urgency 788.63
Urinemia —*see* Uremia
Urinoma NEC 599.9
  bladder 596.8
  kidney 593.89
  renal 593.89
  ureter 593.89
  urethra 599.84
Uroarthritis, infectious 099.3
Urodialysis 788.5
Urolithiasis 592.9
Uronephrosis 593.89
Uropathy 599.9
  obstructive 599.60
Urosepsis 599.0
  meaning sepsis 995.91
  meaning urinary tract infection 599.0
Urticaria 708.9
  with angioneurotic edema 995.1
    hereditary 277.6
  allergic 708.0
  cholinergic 708.5
  chronic 708.8
  cold, familial 708.2
  dermatographic 708.3
  due to
    cold or heat 708.2
    drugs 708.0
    food 708.0
    inhalants 708.0
    plants 708.8
    serum 999.5
  factitial 708.3
  giant 995.1
    hereditary 277.6

Urticaria—*continued*
  gigantea 995.1
    hereditary 277.6
  idiopathic 708.1
  larynx 995.1
    hereditary 277.6
  neonatorum 778.8
  nonallergic 708.1
  papulosa (Hebra) 698.2
  perstans hemorrhagica 757.39
  pigmentosa 757.33
  recurrent periodic 708.8
  serum 999.5
  solare 692.72
  specified type NEC 708.8
  thermal (cold) (heat) 708.2
  vibratory 708.4
Urticarioides acarodermatitis 133.9
Use of
  methadone 304.00
  nonprescribed drugs (*see also* Abuse, drugs,
    nondependent) 305.9
  patent medicines (*see also* Abuse, drugs,
    nondependent) 305.9
Usher-Senear disease (pemphigus
  erythematosus) 694.4
Uta 085.5
Uterine size-date discrepancy 649.6
Uteromegaly 621.2
Uterovaginal —*see* condition
Uterovesical —*see* condition
Uterus —*see* condition
Utriculitis (utriculus prostaticus) 597.89
Uveal —*see* condition
Uveitis (anterior) (*see also* Iridocyclitis) 364.3
  acute or subacute 364.00
    due to or associated with
      gonococcal infection 098.41
      herpes (simplex) 054.44
        zoster 053.22
    primary 364.01
    recurrent 364.02
    secondary (noninfectious) 364.04
      infectious 364.03
  allergic 360.11
  chronic 364.10
    due to or associated with
      sarcoidosis 135 *[364.11]*
      tuberculosis (*see also* Tuberculosis) 017.3
        [364.11]
  due to
    operation 360.11
    toxoplasmosis (acquired) 130.2
      congenital (active) 771.2
  granulomatous 364.10
  heterochromic 364.21
  lens-induced 364.23
  nongranulomatous 364.00
  posterior 363.20
    disseminated—*see* Chorioretinitis,
      disseminated
    focal—*see* Chorioretinitis, focal
  recurrent 364.02
  sympathetic 360.11
  syphilitic (secondary) 091.50
    congenital 090.0 *[363.13]*
    late 095.8 *[363.13]*
  tuberculous (*see also* Tuberculosis) 017.3
    [364.11]
Uveoencephalitis 363.22
Uveokeratitis (*see also* Iridocyclitis) 364.3

V

Vaginitis—*continued*
　gonococcal (acute) 098.0
　　chronic or duration of 2 months or over 098.2
　granuloma 099.2
　Monilia 112.1
　mycotic 112.1
　pinworm 127.4 *[616.11]*
　postirradiation 616.10
　postmenopausal atrophic 627.3
　senile (atrophic) 627.3
　syphilitic (early) 091.0
　　late 095.8
　trichomonal 131.01
　tuberculous (*see also* Tuberculosis) 016.7
　venereal NEC 099.8
Vaginosis —*see* Vaginitis
Vagotonia 352.3
Vagrancy V60.0
VAIN I (vaginal intraepithelial neoplasia I)
　623.0
VAIN II (vaginal intraepithelial neoplasia II)
　623.0
VAIN III (vaginal intraepithelial neoplasia III)
　233.31
Vallecula —*see* condition
Valley fever 114.0
Valsuani's disease (progressive pernicious
　anemia, puerperal) 648.2
Valve, valvular (formation)—*see also* condition
　cerebral ventricle (communicating) in situ V45.2
　cervix, internal os 752.49
　colon 751.5
　congenital NEC—*see* Atresia
　formation, congenital NEC—*see* Atresia
　heart defect—*see* Anomaly, heart, valve
　ureter 753.29
　　pelvic junction 753.21
　　vesical orifice 753.22
　urethra 753.6
Valvulitis (chronic) (*see also* Endocarditis)
　424.90
　rheumatic (chronic) (inactive) (with chorea)
　　397.9
　　active or acute (aortic) (mitral) (pulmonary)
　　　(tricuspid) 391.1
　syphilitic NEC 093.20
　　aortic 093.22
　　mitral 093.21
　　pulmonary 093.24
　　tricuspid 093.23
Valvulopathy —*see* Endocarditis
van Bogaert's leukoencephalitis (sclerosing)
　(subacute) 046.2
van Bogaert-Nijssen (-Peiffer) disease 330.0
van Buchem's syndrome (hyperostosis
　corticalis) 733.3
Vancomycin (glycopeptide)
　intermediate staphylococcus aureus
　　(VISA/GISA) V09.8
　resistant
　　enterococcus (VRE) V09.8
　　staphylococcus aureus (VRSA/GRSA) V09.8
van Creveld-von Gierke disease (glycogenosis
　I) 271.0
van den Bergh's disease (enterogenous cyanosis)
　289.7
van der Hoeve's syndrome (brittle bones and
　blue sclera, deafness) 756.51
**van der Hoeve-Halbertsma-Waardenburg
　syndrome** (ptosis-epicanthus) 270.2

**van der Hoeve-Waardenburg-Gualdi syn-
　drome** (ptosis epicanthus) 270.2
Vanillism 692.89
Vanishing lung 492.0
Vanishing twin 651.33
van Neck (-Odelberg) disease or syndrome
　(juvenile osteochondrosis) 732.1
Vapor asphyxia or suffocation NEC 987.9
　specified agent—*see* Table of drugs and
　　chemicals
Vaquez's disease (M9950/1) 238.4
Vaquez-Osler disease (polycythemia vera)
　(M9950/1) 238.4
Variance, lethal ball, prosthetic heart valve
　996.02
Variants, thalassemic 282.49
Variations in hair color 704.3
Varicella 052.9
　with
　　complication 052.8
　　　specified NEC 052.7
　　pneumonia 052.1
　exposure to V01.71
　vaccination and inoculation (prophylactic)
　　V05.4
Varices —*see* Varix
Varicocele (scrotum) (thrombosed) 456.4
　ovary 456.5
　perineum 456.6
　spermatic cord (ulcerated) 456.4
Varicose
　aneurysm (ruptured) (*see also* Aneurysm) 442.9
　dermatitis (lower extremity)—*see* Varicose,
　　vein, inflamed or infected
　eczema—*see* Varicose, vein
　phlebitis—*see* Varicose, vein, inflamed or
　　infected
　placental vessel—*see* Placenta, abnormal
　tumor—*see* Varicose, vein
　ulcer (lower extremity, any part) 454.0
　　anus 455.8
　　　external 455.5
　　　internal 455.2
　　esophagus (*see also* Varix, esophagus) 456.1
　　　bleeding (*see also* Varix, esophagus,
　　　　bleeding) 456.0
　　inflamed or infected 454.2
　　nasal septum 456.8
　　perineum 456.6
　　rectum—*see* Varicose, ulcer, anus
　　scrotum 456.4
　　specified site NEC 456.8
　　vein (lower extremity) (ruptured) (*see also*
　　　Varix) 454.9
　　with
　　　complications NEC 454.8
　　　edema 454.8
　　　inflammation or infection 454.1
　　　　ulcerated 454.2
　　　pain 454.8
　　　stasis dermatitis 454.1
　　　　with ulcer 454.2
　　　swelling 454.8
　　　ulcer 454.0
　　　　inflamed or infected 454.2
　　anus—*see* Hemorrhoids
　　broad ligament 456.5
　　congenital (peripheral) NEC 747.60
　　　gastrointestinal 747.61
　　　lower limb 747.64
　　　renal 747.62

Varicose—*continued*
  specified NEC 747.69
  upper limb 747.63
  esophagus (ulcerated) (*see also* Varix,
    esophagus) 456.1
    bleeding (*see also* Varix, esophagus,
      bleeding) 456.0
  inflamed or infected 454.1
    with ulcer 454.2
  in pregnancy or puerperium 671.0
    vulva or perineum 671.1
  nasal septum (with ulcer) 456.8
  pelvis 456.5
  perineum 456.6
    in pregnancy, childbirth, or puerperium
      671.1
  rectum—*see* Hemorrhoids
  scrotum (ulcerated) 456.4
  specified site NEC 456.8
  sublingual 456.3
  ulcerated 454.0
    inflamed or infected 454.2
  umbilical cord, affecting fetus or newborn
    762.6
  urethra 456.8
  vulva 456.6
    in pregnancy, childbirth, or puerperium
      671.1
  vessel—*see also* Varix
  placenta—*see* Placenta, abnormal
Varicosis, varicosities, varicosity (*see also*
  Varix) 454.9
Variola 050.9
  hemorrhagic (pustular) 050.0
  major 050.0
  minor 050.1
  modified 050.2
Varioloid 050.2
Variolosa, purpura 050.0
Varix (lower extremity) (ruptured) 454.9
  with
    complications NEC 454.8
    edema 454.8
    inflammation or infection 454.1
      with ulcer 454.2
    pain 454.8
    stasis dermatitis 454.1
      with ulcer 454.2
    swelling 454.8
    ulcer 454.0
      with inflammation or infection 454.2
  aneurysmal (*see also* Aneurysm) 442.9
  anus—*see* Hemorrhoids
  arteriovenous (congenital) (peripheral) NEC
    747.60
    gastrointestinal 747.61
    lower limb 747.64
    renal 747.62
    specified NEC 747.69
    spinal 747.82
    upper limb 747.63
  bladder 456.5
  broad ligament 456.5
  congenital (peripheral) NEC 747.60
  esophagus (ulcerated) 456.1
    bleeding 456.0
    in
      cirrhosis of liver 571.5 *[456.20]*
      portal hypertension 572.3 *[456.20]*
    congenital 747.69

Varix—*continued*
  in
    cirrhosis of liver 571.5 *[456.21]*
      with bleeding 571.5 *[456.20]*
    portal hypertension 572.3 *[456.21]*
      with bleeding 572.3 *[456.20]*
  gastric 456.8
  inflamed or infected 454.1
    ulcerated 454.2
  in pregnancy or puerperium 671.0
    perineum 671.1
    vulva 671.1
  labia (majora) 456.6
  orbit 456.8
    congenital 747.69
  ovary 456.5
  papillary 448.1
  pelvis 456.5
  perineum 456.6
    in pregnancy or puerperium 671.1
  pharynx 456.8
  placenta—*see* Placenta, abnormal
  prostate 456.8
  rectum—*see* Hemorrhoids
  renal papilla 456.8
  retina 362.17
  scrotum (ulcerated) 456.4
  sigmoid colon 456.8
  specified site NEC 456.8
  spinal (cord) (vessels) 456.8
  spleen, splenic (vein) (with phlebolith) 456.8
  sublingual 456.3
  ulcerated 454.0
    inflamed or infected 454.2
  umbilical cord, affecting fetus or newborn 762.6
  uterine ligament 456.5
  vocal cord 456.8
  vulva 456.6
    in pregnancy, childbirth, or puerperium 671.1
Vasa previa 663.5
  affecting fetus or newborn 762.6
  hemorrhage from, affecting fetus or newborn 772.0
Vascular —*see also* condition
  loop on papilla (optic) 743.57
  sheathing, retina 362.13
  spasm 443.9
  spider 448.1
Vascularity, pulmonary, congenital 747.3
Vascularization
  choroid 362.16
  cornea 370.60
    deep 370.63
    localized 370.61
  retina 362.16
  subretinal 362.16
Vasculitis 447.6
  allergic 287.0
  cryoglobulinemic 273.2
  disseminated 447.6
  kidney 447.8
  leukocytoclastic 446.29
  nodular 695.2
  retinal 362.18
  rheumatic—*see* Fever, rheumatic
Vasculopathy
  cardiac allograft 996.83
Vas deferens —*see* condition
Vas deferentitis 608.4
Vasectomy, admission for V25.2

Vasitis 608.4
nodosa 608.4
scrotum 608.4
spermatic cord 608.4
testis 608.4
tuberculous (*see also* Tuberculosis) 016.5
tunica vaginalis 608.4
vas deferens 608.4
Vasodilation 443.9
Vasomotor —*see* condition
Vasoplasty, after previous sterilization V26.0
Vasoplegia, splanchnic (*see also* Neuropathy,
peripheral, autonomic) 337.9
Vasospasm 443.9
cerebral (artery) 435.9
with transient neurologic deficit 435.9
coronary 413.1
nerve
arm NEC 354.9
autonomic 337.9
brachial plexus 353.0
cervical plexus 353.2
leg NEC 355.8
lower extremity NEC 355.8
peripheral NEC 355.9
spinal NEC 355.9
sympathetic 337.9
upper extremity NEC 354.9
peripheral NEC 443.9
retina (artery) (*see also* Occlusion, retinal,
artery) 362.30
Vasospastic —*see* condition
Vasovagal attack (paroxysmal) 780.2
psychogenic 306.2
Vater's ampulla —*see* condition
VATER syndrome 759.89
vCJD (variant Creutzfeldt-Jakob disease) 046.11
Vegetation, vegetative
adenoid (nasal fossa) 474.2
consciousness (persistent) 780.03
endocarditis (acute) (any valve) (chronic)
(subacute) 421.0
heart (mycotic) (valve) 421.0
state (persistent) 780.03
Veil
Jackson's 751.4
over face (causing asphyxia) 768.9
Vein, venous —*see* condition
Veldt sore (*see also* Ulcer, skin) 707.9
Velo-cardio-facial syndrome 758.32
Velpeau's hernia —*see* Hernia, femoral
Venereal
balanitis NEC 099.8
bubo 099.1
disease 099.9
specified nature or type NEC 099.8
granuloma inguinale 099.2
lymphogranuloma (Durand-Nicolas-Favre), any
site 099.1
salpingitis 098.37
urethritis (*see also* Urethritis, nongonococcal)
099.40
vaginitis NEC 099.8
warts 078.11
Vengefulness, in child (*see also* Disturbance,
conduct) 312.0
Venofibrosis 459.89
Venom, venomous
bite or sting (animal or insect) 989.5
poisoning 989.5
Venous —*see* condition

Ventouse delivery NEC 669.5
affecting fetus or newborn 763.3
Ventral —*see* condition
Ventricle, ventricular —*see also* condition
escape 427.69
standstill (*see also* Arrest, cardiac) 427.5
Ventriculitis, cerebral (*see also* Meningitis)
322.9
Ventriculostomy status V45.2
Verbiest's syndrome (claudicatio intermittens
spinalis) 435.1
Vernet's syndrome 352.6
Verneuil's disease (syphilitic bursitis) 095.7
Verruca (filiformis) 078.10
acuminata (any site) 078.11
necrogenica (primary) (*see also* Tuberculosis)
017.0
peruana 088.0
peruviana 088.0
plana (juvenilis) 078.19
plantaris 078.12
seborrheica 702.19
inflamed 702.11
senilis 702.0
tuberculosa (primary) (*see also* Tuberculosis)
017.0
venereal 078.11
viral 078.10
specified NEC 078.19
vulgaris 078.10
Verrucosities (*see also* Verruca) 078.10
Verrucous endocarditis (acute) (any valve)
(chronic) (subacute) 710.0 *[424.91]*
nonbacterial 710.0 *[424.91]*
Verruga
peruana 088.0
peruviana 088.0
Verse's disease (calcinosis intervertebralis)
275.49 *[722.90]*
Version
before labor, affecting fetus or newborn 761.7
cephalic (correcting previous malposition) 652.1
affecting fetus or newborn 763.1
cervix (*see* Version, uterus)
uterus (postinfectional) (postpartal, old) (*see
also* Malposition, uterus) 621.6
forward—*see* Anteversion, uterus
lateral—*see* Lateroversion, uterus
Vertebra, vertebral —*see* condition
Vertigo 780.4
auditory 386.19
aural 386.19
benign paroxysmal positional 386.11
central origin 386.2
cerebral 386.2
Dix and Hallpike (epidemic) 386.12
endemic paralytic 078.81
epidemic 078.81
Dix and Hallpike 386.12
Gerlier's 078.81
Pedersen's 386.12
vestibular neuronitis 386.12
epileptic—*see* Epilepsy
Gerlier's (epidemic) 078.81
hysterical 300.11
labyrinthine 386.10
laryngeal 786.2
malignant positional 386.2
Ménière's (*see also* Disease, Ménière's) 386.00
menopausal 627.2
otogenic 386.19

Vertigo—*continued*
  paralytic 078.81
  paroxysmal positional, benign 386.11
  Pedersen's (epidemic) 386.12
  peripheral 386.10
    specified type NEC 386.19
  positional
    benign paroxysmal 386.11
    malignant 386.2
Verumontanitis (chronic) (*see also* Urethritis)
    597.89
Vesania (*see also* Psychosis) 298.9
Vesical —*see* condition
Vesicle
  cutaneous 709.8
  seminal—*see* condition
  skin 709.8
Vesicocolic —*see* condition
Vesicoperineal —*see* condition
Vesicorectal —*see* condition
Vesicourethrorectal —*see* condition
Vesicovaginal —*see* condition
Vesicular —*see* condition
Vesiculitis (seminal) 608.0
  amebic 006.8
  gonorrheal (acute) 098.14
    chronic or duration of 2 months or over 098.34
  trichomonal 131.09
  tuberculous (*see also* Tuberculosis) 016.5
    [608.81]
Vestibulitis (ear) (*see also* Labyrinthitis) 386.30
  nose (external) 478.19
  vulvar 625.71
Vestibulopathy, acute peripheral (recurrent)
    386.12
Vestige, vestigial —*see also* Persistence
  branchial 744.41
  structures in vitreous 743.51
Vibriosis NEC 027.9
Vidal's disease (lichen simplex chronicus) 698.3
Video display tube syndrome 723.8
Vienna type encephalitis 049.8
Villaret's syndrome 352.6
Villous —*see* condition
VIN I (vulvar intraepithelial neoplasia I) 624.01
VIN II (vulvar intraepithelial neoplasia II) 624.02
VIN III (vulvar intraepithelial neoplasia III)
    233.32
Vincent's
  angina 101
  bronchitis 101
  disease 101
  gingivitis 101
  infection (any site) 101
  laryngitis 101
  stomatitis 101
  tonsillitis 101
Vinson-Plummer syndrome (sideropenic
    dysphagia) 280.8
Viosterol deficiency (*see also* Deficiency,
    calciferol) 268.9
Virchow's disease 733.99
Viremia 790.8
Virilism (adrenal) (female) NEC 255.2
  with
    3-beta-hydroxysteroid dehydrogenase defect
      255.2
    11-hydroxylase defect 255.2
    21-hydroxylase defect 255.2

Virilism—*continued*
  adrenal
    hyperplasia 255.2
    insufficiency (congenital) 255.2
  cortical hyperfunction 255.2
Virilization (female) (suprarenal) (*see also*
    Virilism) 255.2
  isosexual 256.4
Virulent bubo 099.0
Virus, viral —*see also* condition
  infection NEC (*see also* Infection, viral) 079.99
  septicemia 079.99
  yaba monkey tumor 059.22
VISA (vancomycin intermediate staphylococcus
    aureus) V09.8
Viscera, visceral —*see* condition
Visceroptosis 569.89
Visible peristalsis 787.4
Vision, visual
  binocular, suppression 368.31
  blurred, blurring 368.8
    hysterical 300.11
  defect, defective (*see also* Impaired, vision)
    369.9
  disorientation (syndrome) 368.16
  disturbance NEC (*see also* Disturbance, vision)
    368.9
  hysterical 300.11
  examination V72.0
  field, limitation 368.40
  fusion, with defective steropsis 368.33
  hallucinations 368.16
  halos 368.16
  loss 369.9
    both eyes (*see also* Blindness, both eyes)
      369.3
    complete (*see also* Blindness, both eyes)
      369.00
    one eye 369.8
    sudden 368.16
  low (both eyes) 369.20
    one eye (other eye normal) (*see also* Impaired,
      vision) 369.70
      blindness, other eye 369.10
  perception, simultaneous without fusion 368.32
  tunnel 368.45
Vitality, lack or want of 780.79
  newborn 779.89
Vitamin deficiency NEC (*see also* Deficiency,
    vitamin) 269.2
Vitelline duct, persistent 751.0
Vitiligo 709.01
  due to pinta (carate) 103.2
  eyelid 374.53
  vulva 624.8
Vitium cordis —*see* Disease, heart
Vitreous —*see also* condition
  touch syndrome 997.99
VLCAD (long chain/very long chain acyl CoA
    dehydrogenase deficiency, LCAD) 277.85
Vocal cord —*see* condition
Vocational rehabilitation V57.22
Vogt's (Cecile) disease or syndrome 333.7
Vogt-Koyanagi syndrome 364.24
Vogt-Spielmeyer disease (amaurotic familial
    idiocy) 330.1
Voice
  change (*see also* Dysphonia) 784.49
  loss (*see also* Aphonia) 784.41
Volhard-Fahr disease (malignant
    nephrosclerosis) 403.00

Volhynian fever 083.1
Volkmann's ischemic contracture or paralysis (complicating trauma) 958.6
Voluntary starvation 307.1
Volvulus (bowel) (colon) (intestine) 560.2
  with
    hernia—*see also* Hernia, by site, with
      obstruction
      gangrenous—*see* Hernia, by site, with
        gangrene
    perforation 560.2
  congenital 751.5
  duodenum 537.3
  fallopian tube 620.5
  oviduct 620.5
  stomach (due to absence of gastrocolic
    ligament) 537.89
Vomiting 787.03
  with nausea 787.01
  allergic 535.4
  asphyxia 933.1
  bilious (cause unknown) 787.04
    following gastrointestinal surgery 564.3
    newborn 779.32
  blood (*see also* Hematemesis) 578.0
  causing asphyxia, choking, or suffocation (*see
    also* Asphyxia, food) 933.1
  cyclical 536.2
    associated with migraine 346.2
    psychogenic 306.4
  epidemic 078.82
  fecal matter 569.87
  following gastrointestinal surgery 564.3
  functional 536.8
    psychogenic 306.4
  habit 536.2
  hysterical 300.11
  nervous 306.4
  neurotic 306.4
  newborn 779.33
    bilious 779.32
  of or complicating pregnancy 643.9
    due to
      organic disease 643.8
      specific cause NEC 643.8
    early—*see* Hyperemesis, gravidarum
    late (after 22 completed weeks of gestation)
      643.2
  pernicious or persistent 536.2
    complicating pregnancy—*see* Hyperemesis,
      gravidarum
    psychogenic 306.4
  physiological 787.03
    bilious 787.04
  psychic 306.4
  psychogenic 307.54
  stercoral 569.89
  uncontrollable 536.2
    psychogenic 306.4
  uremic—*see* Uremia
  winter 078.82
von Bechterew (-Strumpell) disease or syndrome
  (ankylosing spondylitis) 720.0
von Bezold's abscess 383.01
von Economo's disease (encephalitis lethargica)
  049.8
von Eulenburg's disease (congenital
  paramyotonia) 359.29
von Gierke's disease (glycogenosis I) 271.0
von Gies' joint 095.8
von Graefe's disease or syndrome 378.72

von Hippel (-Lindau) disease or syndrome
  (retinocerebral angiomatosis) 759.6
von Jaksch's anemia or disease
  (pseudoleukemia infantum) 285.8
von Recklinghausen's
  disease or syndrome (nerves) (skin) (M9540/1)
    237.71
  bones (osteitis fibrosa cystica) 252.01
  tumor (M9540/1) 237.71
von Recklinghausen-Applebaum disease
  (hemochromatosis) 275.0
von Schroetter's syndrome (intermittent venous
  claudication) 453.89
von Willebrand (-Jürgens) (-Minot) disease or
  syndrome (angiohemophilia) 286.4
von Zambusch's disease (lichen sclerosus et
  atrophicus) 701.0
Voorhoeve's disease or dyschondroplasia 756.4
Vossius' ring 921.3
  late effect 366.21
Voyeurism 302.82
VRE (vancomycin resistant enterococcus) V09.8
Vrolik's disease (osteogenesis imperfecta) 756.51
VRSA (vancomycin resistant staphylococcus
  aureus) V09.8
Vulva —*see* condition
Vulvismus 625.1
Vulvitis (acute) (allergic) (chronic) (gangrenous)
  (hypertrophic) (intertriginous) 616.10
  with
    abortion—*see* Abortion, by type, with sepsis
    ectopic pregnancy (*see also* categories
      633.0-633.9) 639.0
    molar pregnancy (*see also* categories 630-632)
      639.0
  adhesive, congenital 752.49
  blennorrhagic (acute) 098.0
    chronic or duration of 2 months or over 098.2
  chlamydial 099.53
  complicating pregnancy or puerperium 646.6
  due to Ducrey's bacillus 099.0
  following
    abortion 639.0
    ectopic or molar pregnancy 639.0
  gonococcal (acute) 098.0
    chronic or duration of 2 months or over 098.2
  herpetic 054.11
  leukoplakic 624.09
  monilial 112.1
  puerperal, postpartum, childbirth 646.6
  syphilitic (early) 091.0
    late 095.8
  trichomonal 131.01
Vulvodynia 625.70
  specified NEC 625.79
Vulvorectal —*see* condition
Vulvovaginitis (*see also* Vulvitis) 616.10
  amebic 006.8
  chlamydial 099.53
  gonococcal (acute) 098.0
    chronic or duration of 2 months or over 098.2
  herpetic 054.11
  monilial 112.1
  trichomonal (Trichomonas vaginalis) 131.01

W

Willebrand (-Jürgens) syndrome or thrombopathy (angiohemophilia) 286.4
Willi-Prader syndrome (hypogenital dystrophy with diabetic tendency) 759.81
Willis' disease (diabetes mellitus) (*see also* Diabetes) 250.0
due to secondary diabetes 249.0
Wilms' tumor or neoplasm (nephroblastoma) (M8960/3) 189.0
Wilson's
disease or syndrome (hepatolenticular degeneration) 275.1
hepatolenticular degeneration 275.1
lichen ruber 697.0
Wilson-Brocq disease (dermatitis exfoliativa) 695.89
Wilson-Mikity syndrome 770.7
Window —*see also* Imperfect, closure
aorticopulmonary 745.0
Winged scapula 736.89
Winter —*see also* condition
vomiting disease 078.82
Wise's disease 696.2
Wiskott-Aldrich syndrome (eczema-thrombocytopenia) 279.12
Withdrawal symptoms, syndrome
alcohol 291.81
delirium (acute) 291.0
chronic 291.1
newborn 760.71
drug or narcotic 292.0
newborn, infant of dependent mother 779.5
steroid NEC
correct substance properly administered 255.41
overdose or wrong substance given or taken 962.0
Withdrawing reaction, child or adolescent 313.22
Witts' anemia (achlorhydric anemia) 280.9
Witzelsucht 301.9
Woakes' syndrome (ethmoiditis) 471.1
Wohlfart-Kugelberg-Welander disease 335.11
Woillez's disease (acute idiopathic pulmonary congestion) 518.5
Wolff-Parkinson-White syndrome (anomalous atrioventricular excitation) 426.7
Wolhynian fever 083.1
Wolman's disease (primary familial xanthomatosis) 272.7
Wood asthma 495.8
Woolly, wooly hair (congenital) (nevus) 757.4
Wool-sorters' disease 022.1
Word
blindness (congenital) (developmental) 315.01
secondary to organic lesion 784.61
deafness (secondary to organic lesion) 784.69
developmental 315.31
Worm (s) (colic) (fever) (infection) (infestation) (*see also* Infestation) 128.9
guinea 125.7
in intestine NEC 127.9
Worm-eaten soles 102.3
Worn out (*see also* Exhaustion) 780.79
artificial heart valve 996.02
cardiac defibrillator V53.32
cardiac pacemaker lead or battery V53.31
joint prosthesis (see also Complications, mechanical, device NEC, prosthetic NEC, joint) 996.46
"Worried well" V65.5

Wound, open (by cutting or piercing instrument) (by firearms) (cut) (dissection) (incised) (laceration) (penetration) (perforating) (puncture) (with initial hemorrhage, not internal) 879.8

Note—For fracture with open wound, see Fracture. For laceration, traumatic rupture, tear or penetrating wound of internal organs, such as heart, lung, liver, kidney, pelvic organs, etc., whether or not accompanied by open wound or fracture in the same region, see Injury, internal. For contused wound, see Contusion. For crush injury, see Crush. For abrasion, insect bite (nonvenomous), blister, or scratch, see Injury, superficial.

Complicated includes wounds with:
delayed healing
delayed treatment
foreign body
primary infection

For late effect of open wound, see Late, effect, wound, open, by site.

---

abdomen, abdominal (external) (muscle) 879.2
complicated 879.3
wall (anterior) 879.2
complicated 879.3
lateral 879.4
complicated 879.5
alveolar (process) 873.62
complicated 873.72
ankle 891.0
with tendon involvement 891.2
complicated 891.1
anterior chamber, eye (*see also* Wound, open, intraocular) 871.9
anus 879.6
complicated 879.7
arm 884.0
with tendon involvement 884.2
complicated 884.1
forearm 881.00
with tendon involvement 881.20
complicated 881.10
multiple sites—*see* Wound, open, multiple, upper limb
upper 880.03
with tendon involvement 880.23
complicated 880.13
multiple sites (with axillary or shoulder regions) 880.09
with tendon involvement 880.29
complicated 880.19
artery—*see* Injury, blood vessel, by site
auditory
canal (external) (meatus) 872.02
complicated 872.12
ossicles (incus) (malleus) (stapes) 872.62
complicated 872.72
auricle, ear 872.01
complicated 872.11
axilla 880.02
with tendon involvement 880.22
complicated 880.12
with tendon involvement 880.29
involving other sites of upper arm 880.09
complicated 880.19
back 876.0
complicated 876.1

Wound, open—*continued*
 bladder—*see* Injury, internal, bladder
 blood vessel—*see* Injury, blood vessel, by site
 brain—*see* Injury, intracranial, with open
  intracranial wound
 breast 879.0
  complicated 879.1
 brow 873.42
  complicated 873.52
 buccal mucosa 873.61
  complicated 873.71
 buttock 877.0
  complicated 877.1
 calf 891.0
  with tendon involvement 891.2
  complicated 891.1
 canaliculus lacrimalis 870.8
  with laceration of eyelid 870.2
 canthus, eye 870.8
  laceration—*see* Laceration, eyelid
 cavernous sinus—*see* Injury, intracranial
 cerebellum—*see* Injury, intracranial
 cervical esophagus 874.4
  complicated 874.5
 cervix—*see* Injury, internal, cervix
 cheek(s) (external) 873.41
  complicated 873.51
  internal 873.61
   complicated 873.71
 chest (wall) (external) 875.0
  complicated 875.1
 chin 873.44
  complicated 873.54
 choroid 363.63
 ciliary body (eye) (*see also* Wound, open,
  intraocular) 871.9
 clitoris 878.8
  complicated 878.9
 cochlea 872.64
  complicated 872.74
 complicated 879.9
 conjunctiva—*see* Wound, open, intraocular
 cornea (nonpenetrating) (*see also* Wound, open,
  intraocular) 871.9
 costal region 875.0
  complicated 875.1
 Descemet's membrane (*see also* Wound, open,
  intraocular) 871.9
 digit(s)
  foot 893.0
   with tendon involvement 893.2
   complicated 893.1
  hand 883.0
   with tendon involvement 883.2
   complicated 883.1
 drumhead, ear 872.61
  complicated 872.71
 ear 872.8
  canal 872.02
   complicated 872.12
  complicated 872.9
  drum 872.61
   complicated 872.71
  external 872.00
   complicated 872.10
  multiple sites 872.69
   complicated 872.79
  ossicles (incus) (malleus) (stapes) 872.62
   complicated 872.72
  specified part NEC 872.69
   complicated 872.79

Wound, open—*continued*
 elbow 881.01
  with tendon involvement 881.21
  complicated 881.11
 epididymis 878.2
  complicated 878.3
 epigastric region 879.2
  complicated 879.3
 epiglottis 874.01
  complicated 874.11
 esophagus (cervical) 874.4
  complicated 874.5
  thoracic—*see* Injury, internal, esophagus
 Eustachian tube 872.63
  complicated 872.73
 extremity
  lower (multiple) NEC 894.0
   with tendon involvement 894.2
   complicated 894.1
  upper (multiple) NEC 884.0
   with tendon involvement 884.2
   complicated 884.1
 eye(s) (globe)—*see* Wound, open, intraocular
 eyeball NEC 871.9
  laceration (*see also* Laceration, eyeball) 871.4
  penetrating (*see also* Penetrating wound,
   eyeball) 871.7
 eyebrow 873.42
  complicated 873.52
 eyelid NEC 870.8
  laceration—*see* Laceration, eyelid
 face 873.40
  complicated 873.50
  multiple sites 873.49
   complicated 873.59
  specified part NEC 873.49
   complicated 873.59
 fallopian tube—*see* Injury, internal, fallopian
  tube
 finger(s) (nail) (subungual) 883.0
  with tendon involvement 883.2
  complicated 883.1
 flank 879.4
  complicated 879.5
 foot (any part except toe(s) alone) 892.0
  with tendon involvement 892.2
  complicated 892.1
 forearm 881.00
  with tendon involvement 881.20
  complicated 881.10
 forehead 873.42
  complicated 873.52
 genital organs (external) NEC 878.8
  complicated 878.9
  internal—*see* Injury, internal, by site
 globe (eye) (*see also* Wound, open, eyeball)
  871.9
 groin 879.4
  complicated 879.5
 gum(s) 873.62
  complicated 873.72
 hand (except finger(s) alone) 882.0
  with tendon involvement 882.2
  complicated 882.1
 head NEC 873.8
  with intracranial injury—*see* Injury,
   intracranial
  due to or associated with skull fracture—*see*
   Fracture, skull
  complicated 873.9
  scalp—*see* Wound, open, scalp

Wound, open—*continued*
heel 892.0
  with tendon involvement 892.2
  complicated 892.1
high-velocity (grease gun)—*see* Wound, open,
  complicated, by site
hip 890.0
  with tendon involvement 890.2
  complicated 890.1
hymen 878.6
  complicated 878.7
hypochondrium 879.4
  complicated 879.5
hypogastric region 879.2
  complicated 879.3
iliac (region) 879.4
  complicated 879.5
incidental to
  dislocation—*see* Dislocation, open, by site
  fracture—*see* Fracture, open, by site
  intracranial injury—*see* Injury, intracranial,
    with open intracranial wound
  nerve injury—*see* Injury, nerve, by site
inguinal region 879.4
  complicated 879.5
instep 892.0
  with tendon involvement 892.2
  complicated 892.1
interscapular region 876.0
  complicated 876.1
intracranial—*see* Injury, intracranial, with open
  intracranial wound
intraocular 871.9
  with
    partial loss (of intraocular tissue) 871.2
    prolapse or exposure (of intraocular tissue)
      871.1
  laceration (*see also* Laceration, eyeball) 871.4
  penetrating 871.7
    with foreign body (nonmagnetic) 871.6
      magnetic 871.5
  without prolapse (of intraocular tissue) 871.0
iris (*see also* Wound, open, eyeball) 871.9
jaw (fracture not involved) 873.44
  with fracture—*see* Fracture, jaw
  complicated 873.54
knee 891.0
  with tendon involvement 891.2
  complicated 891.1
labium (majus) (minus) 878.4
  complicated 878.5
lacrimal apparatus, gland, or sac 870.8
  with laceration of eyelid 870.2
larynx 874.01
  with trachea 874.00
    complicated 874.10
  complicated 874.11
leg (multiple) 891.0
  with tendon involvement 891.2
  complicated 891.1
  lower 891.0
    with tendon involvement 891.2
    complicated 891.1
  thigh 890.0
    with tendon involvement 890.2
    complicated 890.1
  upper 890.0
    with tendon involvement 890.2
    complicated 890.1
lens (eye) (alone) (*see also* Cataract, traumatic)
  366.20

Wound, open—*continued*
  with involvement of other eye structures—*see*
    Wound, open, eyeball
limb
  lower (multiple) NEC 894.0
    with tendon involvement 894.2
    complicated 894.1
  upper (multiple) NEC 884.0
    with tendon involvement 884.2
    complicated 884.1
lip 873.43
  complicated 873.53
loin 876.0
  complicated 876.1
lumbar region 876.0
  complicated 876.1
malar region 873.41
  complicated 873.51
mastoid region 873.49
  complicated 873.59
mediastinum—*see* Injury, internal, mediastinum
midthoracic region 875.0
  complicated 875.1
mouth 873.60
  complicated 873.70
  floor 873.64
    complicated 873.74
  multiple sites 873.69
    complicated 873.79
  specified site NEC 873.69
    complicated 873.79
multiple, unspecified site(s) 879.8

> *Note—Multiple open wounds of sites
> classifiable to the same four-digit category
> should be classified to that category unless they
> are in different limbs.*
>
> *Multiple open wounds of sites classifiable to
> different four-digit categories, or to different
> limbs, should be coded separately.*

  complicated 879.9
  lower limb(s) (one or both) (sites classifiable
    to more than one three-digit category in
    890 to 893) 894.0
    with tendon involvement 894.2
    complicated 894.1
  upper limb(s) (one or both) (sites classifiable
    to more than one three-digit category in
    880 to 883) 884.0
    with tendon involvement 884.2
    complicated 884.1
muscle—*see* Sprain, by site
nail
  finger(s) 883.0
    complicated 883.1
  thumb 883.0
    complicated 883.1
  toe(s) 893.0
    complicated 893.1
nape (neck) 874.8
  complicated 874.9
  specified part NEC 874.8
    complicated 874.9
nasal—*see also* Wound, open, nose
  cavity 873.22
    complicated 873.32
  septum 873.21
    complicated 873.31
  sinuses 873.23
    complicated 873.33

Wound, open—*continued*
  complicated 893.1
  tongue 873.64
    complicated 873.74
  tonsil—*see* Wound, open, neck
  trachea (cervical region) 874.02
    with larynx 874.00
      complicated 874.10
    complicated 874.12
    intrathoracic—*see* Injury, internal, trachea
  trunk (multiple) NEC 879.6
    complicated 879.7
    specified site NEC 879.6
      complicated 879.7
  tunica vaginalis 878.2
    complicated 878.3
  tympanic membrane 872.61
    complicated 872.71
  tympanum 872.61
    complicated 872.71
  umbilical region 879.2
    complicated 879.3
  ureter—*see* Injury, internal, ureter
  urethra—*see* Injury, internal, urethra
  uterus—*see* Injury, internal, uterus
  uvula 873.69
    complicated 873.79
  vagina 878.6
    complicated 878.7
  vas deferens—*see* Injury, internal, vas deferens
  vitreous (humor) 871.2
  vulva 878.4
    complicated 878.5
  wrist 881.02
    with tendon involvement 881.22
    complicated 881.12
Wright's syndrome (hyperabduction) 447.8
  pneumonia 390 *[517.1]*
Wringer injury —*see* Crush injury, by site
Wrinkling of skin 701.8
Wrist —*see also* condition
  drop (acquired) 736.05
Wrong drug (given in error) NEC 977.9
  specified drug or substance—*see* Table of drugs
    and chemicals
Wry neck —*see also* Torticollis
  congenital 754.1
Wuchereria infestation 125.0
  bancrofti 125.0
  Brugia malayi 125.1
  malayi 125.1
Wuchereriasis 125.0
Wuchereriosis 125.0
Wuchernde struma langhans (M8332/3) 193

X

Y

Yaba monkey tumor virus 059.22
Yawning 786.09
  psychogenic 306.1
Yaws 102.9
  bone or joint lesions 102.6
  butter 102.1
  chancre 102.0
  cutaneous, less than five years after infection
    102.2
  early (cutaneous) (macular) (maculopapular)
    (micropapular) (papular) 102.2
    frambeside 102.2
    skin lesions NEC 102.2
  eyelid 102.9 *[373.4]*
  ganglion 102.6
  gangosis, gangosa 102.5
  gumma, gummata 102.4
    bone 102.6
  gummatous
    frambeside 102.4
    osteitis 102.6
    periostitis 102.6
  hydrarthrosis 102.6
  hyperkeratosis (early) (late) (palmar) (plantar)
    102.3
  initial lesions 102.0
  joint lesions 102.6
  juxta-articular nodules 102.7
  late nodular (ulcerated) 102.4
  latent (without clinical manifestations) (with
    positive serology) 102.8
  mother 102.0
  mucosal 102.7
  multiple papillomata 102.1
  nodular, late (ulcerated) 102.4
  osteitis 102.6
  papilloma, papillomata (palmar) (plantar) 102.1
  periostitis (hypertrophic) 102.6
  ulcers 102.4
  wet crab 102.1
Yeast infection (*see also* Candidiasis) 112.9
Yellow
  atrophy (liver) 570
    chronic 571.8
    resulting from administration of blood,
      plasma, serum, or other biological
      substance (within 8 months of
      administration)—*see* Hepatitis, viral
  fever—*see* Fever, yellow
  jack (*see also* Fever, yellow) 060.9
  jaundice (*see also* Jaundice) 782.4
Yersinia septica 027.8

Z

Zagari's disease (xerostomia) 527.7
Zahorsky's disease (exanthema subitum) (*see
  also* Exanthem subitum) 058.10
  syndrome (herpangina) 074.0
Zellweger syndrome 277.86
Zenker's diverticulum (esophagus) 530.6
Ziehen-Oppenheim disease 333.6
Zieve's syndrome (jaundice, hyperlipemia, and
  hemolytic anemia) 571.1
Zika fever 066.3
Zollinger-Ellison syndrome (gastric
  hypersecretion with pancreatic islet cell
  tumor) 251.5
Zona (*see also* Herpes, zoster) 053.9
Zoophilia (erotica) 302.1
Zoophobia 300.29
Zoster (herpes) (*see also* Herpes, zoster) 053.9
Zuelzer (-Ogden) anemia or syndrome
  (nutritional megaloblastic anemia) 281.2
Zygodactyly (*see also* Syndactylism) 755.10
Zygomycosis 117.7
Zymotic —*see* condition

SECTION 2

ALPHABETIC INDEX TO POISONING AND EXTERNAL CAUSES OF ADVERSE EFFECTS OF DRUGS AND OTHER CHEMICAL SUBSTANCES

TABLE OF DRUGS AND CHEMICALS

This table contains a classification of drugs and other chemical substances to identify poisoning states and external causes of adverse effects.

Each of the listed substances in the table is assigned a code according to the poisoning classification (960–989). These codes are used when there is a statement of poisoning, overdose, wrong substance given or taken, or intoxication.

The table also contains a listing of external causes of adverse effects. An adverse effect is a pathologic manifestation due to ingestion or exposure to drugs or other chemical substances (e.g., dermatitis, hypersensitivity reaction, aspirin gastritis). The adverse effect is to be identified by the appropriate code found in Section 1, Index to Diseases and Injuries. An external cause code can then be used to identify the circumstances involved. The table headings pertaining to external causes are defined below:

> **Accidental poisoning (E850–E869)**—accidental overdose of drug, wrong substance given or taken, drug taken inadvertently, accidents in the usage of drugs and biologicals in medical and surgical procedures, and to show external causes of poisonings classifiable to 980–989.

> **Therapeutic use (E930–E949)**—a correct substance properly administered in therapeutic or prophylactic dosage as the external cause of adverse effects.

> **Suicide attempt (E950–E952)**—instances in which self–inflicted injuries or poisonings are involved.

> **Assault (E961–E962)**—injury or poisoning inflicted by another person with the intent to injure or kill.

> **Undetermined (E980–E982)**—to be used when the intent of the poisoning or injury cannot be determined whether it was intentional or accidental.

The American Hospital Formulary Service list numbers are included in the table to help classify new drugs not identified in the table by name. The AHFS list numbers are keyed to the continually revised American Hospital Formulary Service (AHFS).* These listings are found in the table under the main term **Drug**.

Excluded from the table are radium and other radioactive substances. The classification of adverse effects and complications pertaining to these substances will be found in Section 1, Index to Diseases and Injuries, and Section 3, Index to External Causes of Injuries.

Although certain substances are indexed with one or more subentries, the majority are listed according to one use or state. It is recognized that many substances may be used in various ways, in medicine and in industry, and may cause adverse effects whatever the state of the agent (solid, liquid, or fumes arising from a liquid). In cases in which the reported data indicates a use or state not in the table, or which is clearly different from the one listed, an attempt should be made to classify the substance in the form which most nearly expresses the reported facts.

*American Hospital Formulary Service, 2 vol. (Washington, DC: American Society of Hospital Pharmacists, 1959)

Substance	Poisoning	Accident	Therapeutic Use	Suicide Attempt	Assault	Undetermined
			External Cause (E-Code)			
1–propanol	980.3	E860.4	—	E950.9	E962.1	E980.9
2–propanol	980.2	E860.3	—	E950.9	E962.1	E980.9
2, 4–D (dichlorophenoxyacetic acid)	989.4	E863.5	—	E950.6	E962.1	E980.7
2, 4–toluene diisocyanate	983.0	E864.0	—	E950.7	E962.1	E980.6
2, 4, 5–T (trichlorophenoxyacetic acid)	989.2	E863.5	—	E950.6	E962.1	E980.7
14–hydroxydihydromorphinone	965.09	E850.2	E935.2	E950.0	E962.0	E980.0
ABOB	961.7	E857	E931.7	E950.4	E962.0	E980.4
Abrus (seed)	988.2	E865.3	—	E950.9	E962.1	E980.9
Absinthe	980.0	E860.1	—	E950.9	E962.1	E980.9
beverage	980.0	E860.0	—	E950.9	E962.1	E980.9
Acenocoumarin, acenocoumarol	964.2	E858.2	E934.2	E950.4	E962.0	E980.4
Acepromazine	969.1	E853.0	E939.1	E950.3	E962.0	E980.3
Acetal	982.8	E862.4	—	E950.9	E962.1	E980.9
Acetaldehyde (vapor)	987.8	E869.8	—	E952.8	E962.2	E982.8
liquid	989.89	E866.8	—	E950.9	E962.1	E980.9
Acetaminophen	965.4	E850.4	E935.4	E950.0	E962.0	E980.0
Acetaminosalol	965.1	E850.3	E935.3	E950.0	E962.0	E980.0
Acetanilid(e)	965.4	E850.4	E935.4	E950.0	E962.0	E980.0
Acetarsol, acetarsone	961.1	E857	E931.1	E950.4	E962.0	E980.4
Acetazolamide	974.2	E858.5	E944.2	E950.4	E962.0	E980.4
Acetic						
acid	983.1	E864.1	—	E950.7	E962.1	E980.6
with sodium acetate (ointment)	976.3	E858.7	E946.3	E950.4	E962.0	E980.4
irrigating solution	974.5	E858.5	E944.5	E950.4	E962.0	E980.4
lotion	976.2	E858.7	E946.2	E950.4	E962.0	E980.4
anhydride	983.1	E864.1	—	E950.7	E962.1	E980.6
ether (vapor)	982.8	E862.4	—	E950.9	E962.1	E980.9
Acetohexamide	962.3	E858.0	E932.3	E950.4	E962.0	E980.4
Acetomenaphthone	964.3	E858.2	E934.3	E950.4	E962.0	E980.4
Acetomorphine	965.01	E850.0	E935.0	E950.0	E962.0	E980.0
Acetone (oils) (vapor)	982.8	E862.4	—	E950.9	E962.1	E980.9
Acetophenazine (maleate)	969.1	E853.0	E939.1	E950.3	E962.0	E980.3
Acetophenetidin	965.4	E850.4	E935.4	E950.0	E962.0	E980.0
Acetophenone	982.0	E862.4	—	E950.9	E962.1	E980.9
Acetorphine	965.09	E850.2	E935.2	E950.0	E962.0	E980.0
Acetosulfone (sodium)	961.8	E857	E931.8	E950.4	E962.0	E980.4
Acetrizoate (sodium)	977.8	E858.8	E947.8	E950.4	E962.0	E980.4
Acetylcarbromal	967.3	E852.2	E937.3	E950.2	E962.0	E980.2
Acetylcholine (chloride)	971.0	E855.3	E941.0	E950.4	E962.0	E980.4
Acetylcysteine	975.5	E858.6	E945.5	E950.4	E962.0	E980.4
Acetyldigitoxin	972.1	E858.3	E942.1	E950.4	E962.0	E980.4
Acetyldihydrocodeine	965.09	E850.2	E935.2	E950.0	E962.0	E980.0
Acetyldihydrocodeinone	965.09	E850.2	E935.2	E950.0	E962.0	E980.0
Acetylene (gas) (industrial)	987.1	E868.1	—	E951.8	E962.2	E981.8
incomplete combustion of — *see* Carbon monoxide, fuel, utility						
tetrachloride (vapor)	982.3	E862.4	—	E950.9	E962.1	E980.9
Acetyliodosalicylic acid	965.1	E850.3	E935.3	E950.0	E962.0	E980.0
Acetylphenylhydrazine	965.8	E850.8	E935.8	E950.0	E962.0	E980.0
Acetylsalicylic acid	965.1	E850.3	E935.3	E950.0	E962.0	E980.0
Achromycin	960.4	E856	E930.4	E950.4	E962.0	E980.4
ophthalmic preparation	976.5	E858.7	E946.5	E950.4	E962.0	E980.4
topical NEC	976.0	E858.7	E946.0	E950.4	E962.0	E980.4
Acidifying agents	963.2	E858.1	E933.2	E950.4	E962.0	E980.4
Acids (corrosive) NEC	983.1	E864.1	—	E950.7	E962.1	E980.6
Aconite (wild)	988.2	E865.4	—	E950.9	E962.1	E980.9
Aconitine (liniment)	976.8	E858.7	E946.8	E950.4	E962.0	E980.4
Aconitum ferox	988.2	E865.4	—	E950.9	E962.1	E980.9
Acridine	983.0	E864.0	—	E950.7	E962.1	E980.6
vapor	987.8	E869.8	—	E952.8	E962.2	E982.8

Substance	Poisoning	Accident	Therapeutic Use	Suicide Attempt	Assault	Undetermined
			External Cause (E-Code)			
Acriflavine	961.9	E857	E931.9	E950.4	E962.0	E980.4
Acrisorcin.	976.0	E858.7	E946.0	E950.4	E962.0	E980.4
Acrolein (gas)	987.8	E869.8	—	E952.8	E962.2	E982.8
liquid	989.89	E866.8	—	E950.9	E962.1	E980.9
Actaea spicata	988.2	E865.4	—	E950.9	E962.1	E980.9
Acterol	961.5	E857	E931.5	E950.4	E962.0	E980.4
ACTH	962.4	E858.0	E932.4	E950.4	E962.0	E980.4
Acthar	962.4	E858.0	E932.4	E950.4	E962.0	E980.4
Actinomycin (C) (D)	960.7	E856	E930.7	E950.4	E962.0	E980.4
Adalin (acetyl).	967.3	E852.2	E937.3	E950.2	E962.0	E980.2
Adenosine (phosphate)	977.8	E858.8	E947.8	E950.4	E962.0	E980.4
Adhesives.	989.89	E866.6	—	E950.9	E962.1	E980.9
ADH.	962.5	E858.0	E932.5	E950.4	E962.0	E980.4
Adicillin	960.0	E856	E930.0	E950.4	E962.0	E980.4
Adiphenine	975.1	E855.6	E945.1	E950.4	E962.0	E980.4
Adjunct, pharmaceutical	977.4	E858.8	E947.4	E950.4	E962.0	E980.4
Adrenal (extract, cortex or medulla) (glucocorticoids) (hormones) (mineralocorticoids)	962.0	E858.0	E932.0	E950.4	E962.0	E980.4
ENT agent.	976.6	E858.7	E946.6	E950.4	E962.0	E980.4
ophthalmic preparation.	976.5	E858.7	E946.5	E950.4	E962.0	E980.4
topical NEC	976.0	E858.7	E946.0	E950.4	E962.0	E980.4
Adrenalin	971.2	E855.5	E941.2	E950.4	E962.0	E980.4
Adrenergic blocking agents.	971.3	E855.6	E941.3	E950.4	E962.0	E980.4
Adrenergics	971.2	E855.5	E941.2	E950.4	E962.0	E980.4
Adrenochrome (derivatives).	972.8	E858.3	E942.8	E950.4	E962.0	E980.4
Adrenocorticotropic hormone	962.4	E858.0	E932.4	E950.4	E962.0	E980.4
Adrenocorticotropin.	962.4	E858.0	E932.4	E950.4	E962.0	E980.4
Adriamycin	960.7	E856	E930.7	E950.4	E962.0	E980.4
Aerosol spray — see Sprays						
Aerosporin	960.8	E856	E930.8	E950.4	E962.0	E980.4
ENT agent.	976.6	E858.7	E946.6	E950.4	E962.0	E980.4
ophthalmic preparation.	976.5	E858.7	E946.5	E950.4	E962.0	E980.4
topical NEC	976.0	E858.7	E946.0	E950.4	E962.0	E980.4
Aethusa cynapium	988.2	E865.4	—	E950.9	E962.1	E980.9
Afghanistan black	969.6	E854.1	E939.6	E950.3	E962.0	E980.3
Aflatoxin	989.7	E865.9	—	E950.9	E962.1	E980.9
African boxwood	988.2	E865.4	—	E950.9	E962.1	E980.9
Agar (–agar).	973.3	E858.4	E943.3	E950.4	E962.0	E980.4
Agricultural agent NEC	989.89	E863.9	—	E950.6	E962.1	E980.7
Agrypnal	967.0	E851	E937.0	E950.1	E962.0	E980.1
Air contaminant(s), source or type not specified	987.9	E869.9	—	E952.9	E962.2	E982.9
specified type — see specific substance						
Akee.	988.2	E865.4	—	E950.9	E962.1	E980.9
Akrinol	976.0	E858.7	E946.0	E950.4	E962.0	E980.4
Alantolactone	961.6	E857	E931.6	E950.4	E962.0	E980.4
Albamycin	960.8	E856	E930.8	E950.4	E962.0	E980.4
Albumin (normal human serum).	964.7	E858.2	E934.7	E950.4	E962.0	E980.4
Albuterol	975.7	E858.6	E945.7	E950.4	E962.0	E980.4
Alcohol.	980.9	E860.9	—	E950.9	E962.1	E980.9
absolute.	980.0	E860.1	—	E950.9	E962.1	E980.9
beverage	980.0	E860.0	E947.8	E950.9	E962.1	E980.9
amyl	980.3	E860.4	—	E950.9	E962.1	E980.9
antifreeze	980.1	E860.2	—	E950.9	E962.1	E980.9
butyl	980.3	E860.4	—	E950.9	E962.1	E980.9
dehydrated.	980.0	E860.1	—	E950.9	E962.1	E980.9
beverage	980.0	E860.0	E947.8	E950.9	E962.1	E980.9
denatured	980.0	E860.1	—	E950.9	E962.1	E980.9
deterrents	977.3	E858.8	E947.3	E950.4	E962.0	E980.4
diagnostic (gastric function).	977.8	E858.8	E947.8	E950.4	E962.0	E980.4

Substance	Poisoning	Accident	Therapeutic Use	Suicide Attempt	Assault	Undetermined
			External Cause (E-Code)			
ethyl	980.0	E860.1	—	E950.9	E962.1	E980.9
beverage	980.0	E860.0	E947.8	E950.9	E962.1	E980.9
grain	980.0	E860.1	—	E950.9	E962.1	E980.9
beverage	980.0	E860.0	E947.8	E950.9	E962.1	E980.9
industrial	980.9	E860.9	—	E950.9	E962.1	E980.9
isopropyl	980.2	E860.3	—	E950.9	E962.1	E980.9
methyl	980.1	E860.2	—	E950.9	E962.1	E980.9
preparation for consumption	980.0	E860.0	E947.8	E950.9	E962.1	E980.9
propyl	980.3	E860.4	—	E950.9	E962.1	E980.9
secondary	980.2	E860.3	—	E950.9	E962.1	E980.9
radiator	980.1	E860.2	—	E950.9	E962.1	E980.9
rubbing	980.2	E860.3	—	E950.9	E962.1	E980.9
specified type NEC	980.8	E860.8	—	E950.9	E962.1	E980.9
surgical	980.9	E860.9	—	E950.9	E962.1	E980.9
vapor (from any type of alcohol)	987.8	E869.8	—	E952.8	E962.2	E982.8
wood	980.1	E860.2	—	E950.9	E962.1	E980.9
Alcuronium chloride	975.2	E858.6	E945.2	E950.4	E962.0	E980.4
Aldactone	974.4	E858.5	E944.4	E950.4	E962.0	E980.4
Aldicarb	989.3	E863.2	—	E950.6	E962.1	E980.7
Aldomet	972.6	E858.3	E942.6	E950.4	E962.0	E980.4
Aldosterone	962.0	E858.0	E932.0	E950.4	E962.0	E980.4
Aldrin (dust)	989.2	E863.0	—	E950.6	E962.1	E980.7
Algeldrate	973.0	E858.4	E943.0	E950.4	E962.0	E980.4
Alidase	963.4	E858.1	E933.4	E950.4	E962.0	E980.4
Aliphatic thiocyanates	989.0	E866.8	—	E950.9	E962.1	E980.9
Alkaline antiseptic solution (aromatic)	976.6	E858.7	E946.6	E950.4	E962.0	E980.4
Alkalinizing agents (medicinal)	963.3	E858.1	E933.3	E950.4	E962.0	E980.4
Alkalis, caustic	983.2	E864.2	—	E950.7	E962.1	E980.6
Alkalizing agents (medicinal)	963.3	E858.1	E933.3	E950.4	E962.0	E980.4
Alka–seltzer	965.1	E850.3	E935.3	E950.0	E962.0	E980.0
Alkavervir	972.6	E858.3	E942.6	E950.4	E962.0	E980.4
Allegron	969.05	E854.0	E939.0	E950.3	E962.0	E980.3
Alleve *see* Naproxen						
Allobarbital, allobarbitone	967.0	E851	E937.0	E950.1	E962.0	E980.1
Allopurinol	974.7	E858.5	E944.7	E950.4	E962.0	E980.4
Allylestrenol	962.2	E858.0	E932.2	E950.4	E962.0	E980.4
Allylisopropylacetylurea	967.8	E852.8	E937.8	E950.2	E962.0	E980.2
Allylisopropylmalonylurea	967.0	E851	E937.0	E950.1	E962.0	E980.1
Allyltribromide	967.3	E852.2	E937.3	E950.2	E962.0	E980.2
Aloe, aloes, aloin	973.1	E858.4	E943.1	E950.4	E962.0	E980.4
Alosetron	973.8	E858.4	E943.8	E950.4	E962.0	E980.4
Aloxidone	966.0	E855.0	E936.0	E950.4	E962.0	E980.4
Aloxiprin	965.1	E850.3	E935.3	E950.0	E962.0	E980.0
Alpha amylase	963.4	E858.1	E933.4	E950.4	E962.0	E980.4
Alpha-1 blockers	971.3	E855.6	E941.3	E950.4	E962.0	E980.4
Alpha tocopherol	963.5	E858.1	E933.5	E950.4	E962.0	E980.4
Alphaprodine (hydrochloride)	965.09	E850.2	E935.2	E950.0	E962.0	E980.0
Alseroxylon	972.6	E858.3	E942.6	E950.4	E962.0	E980.4
Alum (ammonium) (potassium)	983.2	E864.2	—	E950.7	E962.1	E980.6
medicinal (astringent) NEC	976.2	E858.7	E946.2	E950.4	E962.0	E980.4
Aluminium, aluminum (gel) (hydroxide)	973.0	E858.4	E943.0	E950.4	E962.0	E980.4
acetate solution	976.2	E858.7	E946.2	E950.4	E962.0	E980.4
aspirin	965.1	E850.3	E935.3	E950.0	E962.0	E980.0
carbonate	973.0	E858.4	E943.0	E950.4	E962.0	E980.4
glycinate	973.0	E858.4	E943.0	E950.4	E962.0	E980.4
nicotinate	972.2	E858.3	E942.2	E950.4	E962.0	E980.4
ointment (surgical) (topical)	976.3	E858.7	E946.3	E950.4	E962.0	E980.4
phosphate	973.0	E858.4	E943.0	E950.4	E962.0	E980.4
subacetate	976.2	E858.7	E946.2	E950.4	E962.0	E980.4
topical NEC	976.3	E858.7	E946.3	E950.4	E962.0	E980.4

Substance	Poisoning	Accident	Therapeutic Use	Suicide Attempt	Assault	Undetermined
			External Cause (E-Code)			
Alurate	967.0	E851	E937.0	E950.1	E962.0	E980.1
Alverine (citrate)	975.1	E858.6	E945.1	E950.4	E962.0	E980.4
Alvodine	965.09	E850.2	E935.2	E950.0	E962.0	E980.0
Amanita phalloides	988.1	E865.5	—	E950.9	E962.1	E980.9
Amantadine (hydrochloride)	966.4	E855.0	E936.4	E950.4	E962.0	E980.4
Ambazone.	961.9	E857	E931.9	E950.4	E962.0	E980.4
Ambenonium	971.0	E855.3	E941.0	E950.4	E962.0	E980.4
Ambutonium bromide	971.1	E855.4	E941.1	E950.4	E962.0	E980.4
Ametazole.	977.8	E858.8	E947.8	E950.4	E962.0	E980.4
Amethocaine (infiltration) (topical)	968.5	E855.2	E938.5	E950.4	E962.0	E980.4
nerve block (peripheral) (plexus).	968.6	E855.2	E938.6	E950.4	E962.0	E980.4
spinal	968.7	E855.2	E938.7	E950.4	E962.0	E980.4
Amethopterin	963.1	E858.1	E933.1	E950.4	E962.0	E980.4
Amfepramone	977.0	E858.8	E947.0	E950.4	E962.0	E980.4
Amidon.	965.02	E850.1	E935.1	E950.0	E962.0	E980.0
Amidopyrine.	965.5	E850.5	E935.5	E950.0	E962.0	E980.0
Aminacrine	976.0	E858.7	E946.0	E950.4	E962.0	E980.4
Aminitrozole.	961.5	E857	E931.5	E950.4	E962.0	E980.4
Aminoacetic acid	974.5	E858.5	E944.5	E950.4	E962.0	E980.4
Amino acids	974.5	E858.5	E944.5	E950.4	E962.0	E980.4
Aminocaproic acid	964.4	E858.2	E934.4	E950.4	E962.0	E980.4
Aminoethylisothiourium	963.8	E858.1	E933.8	E950.4	E962.0	E980.4
Aminoglutethimide	966.3	E855.0	E936.3	E950.4	E962.0	E980.4
Aminometradine	974.3	E858.5	E944.3	E950.4	E962.0	E980.4
Aminopentamide	971.1	E855.4	E941.1	E950.4	E962.0	E980.4
Aminophenazone	965.5	E850.5	E935.5	E950.0	E962.0	E980.0
Aminophenol	983.0	E864.0	—	E950.7	E962.1	E980.6
Aminophenylpyridone	969.5	E853.8	E939.5	E950.3	E962.0	E980.3
Aminophyllin	975.7	E858.6	E945.7	E950.4	E962.0	E980.4
Aminopterin	963.1	E858.1	E933.1	E950.4	E962.0	E980.4
Aminopyrine.	965.5	E850.5	E935.5	E950.0	E962.0	E980.0
Aminosalicylic acid	961.8	E857	E931.8	E950.4	E962.0	E980.4
Amiphenazole	970.1	E854.3	E940.1	E950.4	E962.0	E980.4
Amiquinsin	972.6	E858.3	E942.6	E950.4	E962.0	E980.4
Amisometradine	974.3	E858.5	E944.3	E950.4	E962.0	E980.4
Amitriptyline	969.05	E854.0	E939.0	E950.3	E962.0	E980.3
Ammonia (fumes) (gas) (vapor)	987.8	E869.8	—	E952.8	E962.2	E982.8
liquid (household) NEC	983.2	E861.4	—	E950.7	E962.1	E980.6
spirit, aromatic	970.8	E854.3	E940.8	E950.4	E962.0	E980.4
Ammoniated mercury	976.0	E858.7	E946.0	E950.4	E962.0	E980.4
Ammonium						
carbonate	983.2	E864.2	—	E950.7	E962.1	E980.6
chloride (acidifying agent)	963.2	E858.1	E933.2	E950.4	E962.0	E980.4
expectorant	975.5	E858.6	E945.5	E950.4	E962.0	E980.4
compounds (household) NEC	983.2	E861.4	—	E950.7	E962.1	E980.6
fumes (any usage)	987.8	E869.8	—	E952.8	E962.2	E982.8
industrial.	983.2	E864.2	—	E950.7	E962.1	E980.6
ichthyosulfonate	976.4	E858.7	E946.4	E950.4	E962.0	E980.4
mandelate	961.9	E857	E931.9	E950.4	E962.0	E980.4
Amobarbital	967.0	E851	E937.0	E950.1	E962.0	E980.1
Amodiaquin(e)	961.4	E857	E931.4	E950.4	E962.0	E980.4
Amopyroquin(e)	961.4	E857	E931.4	E950.4	E962.0	E980.4
Amphenidone	969.5	E853.8	E939.5	E950.3	E962.0	E980.3
Amphetamine	969.72	E854.2	E939.7	E950.3	E962.0	E980.3
Amphomycin	960.8	E856	E930.8	E950.4	E962.0	E980.4
Amphotericin B	960.1	E856	E930.1	E950.4	E962.0	E980.4
topical	976.0	E858.7	E946.0	E950.4	E962.0	E980.4
Ampicillin.	960.0	E856	E930.0	E950.4	E962.0	E980.4
Amprotropine	971.1	E855.4	E941.1	E950.4	E962.0	E980.4
Amygdalin	977.8	E858.8	E947.8	E950.4	E962.0	E980.4
Amyl						

Substance	Poisoning	Accident	Therapeutic Use	Suicide Attempt	Assault	Undetermined
				External Cause (E-Code)		
acetate (vapor)	982.8	E862.4	—	E950.9	E962.1	E980.9
alcohol	980.3	E860.4	—	E950.9	E962.1	E980.9
nitrite (medicinal)	972.4	E858.3	E942.4	E950.4	E962.0	E980.4
Amylase (alpha)	963.4	E858.1	E933.4	E950.4	E962.0	E980.4
Amylene hydrate	980.8	E860.8	—	E950.9	E962.1	E980.9
Amylobarbitone	967.0	E851	E937.0	E950.1	E962.0	E980.1
Amylocaine	968.9	E855.2	E938.9	E950.4	E962.0	E980.4
infiltration (subcutaneous)	968.5	E855.2	E938.5	E950.4	E962.0	E980.4
nerve block (peripheral) (plexus)	968.6	E855.2	E938.6	E950.4	E962.0	E980.4
spinal	968.7	E855.2	E938.7	E950.4	E962.0	E980.4
topical (surface)	968.5	E855.2	E938.5	E950.4	E962.0	E980.4
Amytal (sodium)	967.0	E851	E937.0	E950.1	E962.0	E980.1
Analeptics	970.0	E854.3	E940.0	E950.4	E962.0	E980.4
Analgesics	965.9	E850.9	E935.9	E950.0	E962.0	E980.0
aromatic NEC	965.4	E850.4	E935.4	E950.0	E962.0	E980.0
non–narcotic NEC	965.7	E850.7	E935.7	E950.0	E962.0	E980.0
specified NEC	965.8	E850.8	E935.8	E950.0	E962.0	E980.0
Anamirta cocculus	988.2	E865.3	—	E950.9	E962.1	E980.9
Ancillin	960.0	E856	E930.0	E950.4	E962.0	E980.4
Androgens (anabolic congeners)	962.1	E858.0	E932.1	E950.4	E962.0	E980.4
Androstalone	962.1	E858.0	E932.1	E950.4	E962.0	E980.4
Androsterone	962.1	E858.0	E932.1	E950.4	E962.0	E980.4
Anemone pulsatilla	988.2	E865.4	—	E950.9	E962.1	E980.9
Anesthesia, anesthetic (general) NEC	968.4	E855.1	E938.4	E950.4	E962.0	E980.4
block (nerve) (plexus)	968.6	E855.2	E938.6	E950.4	E962.0	E980.4
gaseous NEC	968.2	E855.1	E938.2	E950.4	E962.0	E980.4
halogenated hydrocarbon derivatives NEC	968.2	E855.1	E938.2	E950.4	E962.0	E980.4
infiltration (intradermal) (subcutaneous) (submucosal)	968.5	E855.2	E938.5	E950.4	E962.0	E980.4
intravenous	968.3	E855.1	E938.3	E950.4	E962.0	E980.4
local NEC	968.9	E855.2	E938.9	E950.4	E962.0	E980.4
nerve blocking (peripheral) (plexus)	968.6	E855.2	E938.6	E950.4	E962.0	E980.4
rectal NEC	968.3	E855.1	E938.3	E950.4	E962.0	E980.4
spinal	968.7	E855.2	E938.7	E950.4	E962.0	E980.4
surface	968.5	E855.2	E938.5	E950.4	E962.0	E980.4
topical	968.5	E855.2	E938.5	E950.4	E962.0	E980.4
Aneurine	963.5	E858.1	E933.5	E950.4	E962.0	E980.4
Angio–Conray	977.8	E858.8	E947.8	E950.4	E962.0	E980.4
Anginine see Glyceryl trinitrate						
Angiotensin	971.2	E855.5	E941.2	E950.4	E962.0	E980.4
Anhydrohydroxyprogesterone	962.2	E858.0	E932.2	E950.4	E962.0	E980.4
Anhydron	974.3	E858.5	E944.3	E950.4	E962.0	E980.4
Anileridine	965.09	E850.2	E935.2	E950.0	E962.0	E980.0
Aniline (dye) (liquid)	983.0	E864.0	—	E950.7	E962.1	E980.6
analgesic	965.4	E850.4	E935.4	E950.0	E962.0	E980.0
derivatives, therapeutic NEC	965.4	E850.4	E935.4	E950.0	E962.0	E980.0
vapor	987.8	E869.8	—	E952.8	E962.2	E982.8
Anisindione	964.2	E858.2	E934.2	E950.4	E962.0	E980.4
Anisotropine	971.1	E855.4	E941.1	E950.4	E962.0	E980.4
Anorexic agents	977.0	E858.8	E947.0	E950.4	E962.0	E980.4
Ant (bite) (sting)	989.5	E905.5	—	E950.9	E962.1	E980.9
Antabuse	977.3	E858.8	E947.3	E950.4	E962.0	E980.4
Antacids	973.0	E858.4	E943.0	E950.4	E962.0	E980.4
Antazoline	963.0	E858.1	E933.0	E950.4	E962.0	E980.4
Anthelmintics	961.6	E857	E931.6	E950.4	E962.0	E980.4
Anthralin	976.4	E858.7	E946.4	E950.4	E962.0	E980.4
Anthramycin	960.7	E856	E930.7	E950.4	E962.0	E980.4
Antiadrenergics	971.3	E855.6	E941.3	E950.4	E962.0	E980.4
Antiallergic agents	963.0	E858.1	E933.0	E950.4	E962.0	E980.4

TABLE OF DRUGS AND CHEMICALS

Substance	Poisoning	Accident	Therapeutic Use	Suicide Attempt	Assault	Undetermined
		External Cause (E-Code)				
Antianemic agents NEC	964.1	E858.2	E934.1	E950.4	E962.0	E980.4
Antiaris toxicaria	988.2	E865.4	—	E950.9	E962.1	E980.9
Antiarteriosclerotic agents	972.2	E858.3	E942.2	E950.4	E962.0	E980.4
Antiasthmatics	975.7	E858.6	E945.7	E950.4	E962.0	E980.4
Antibiotics	960.9	E856	E930.9	E950.4	E962.0	E980.4
antifungal	960.1	E856	E930.1	E950.4	E962.0	E980.4
antimycobacterial	960.6	E856	E930.6	E950.4	E962.0	E980.4
antineoplastic	960.7	E856	E930.7	E950.4	E962.0	E980.4
cephalosporin (group)	960.5	E856	E930.5	E950.4	E962.0	E980.4
chloramphenicol (group)	960.2	E856	E930.2	E950.4	E962.0	E980.4
macrolides	960.3	E856	E930.3	E950.4	E962.0	E980.4
specified NEC	960.8	E856	E930.8	E950.4	E962.0	E980.4
tetracycline (group)	960.4	E856	E930.4	E950.4	E962.0	E980.4
Anticancer agents NEC	963.1	E858.1	E933.1	E950.4	E962.0	E980.4
antibiotics	960.7	E856	E930.7	E950.4	E962.0	E980.4
Anticholinergics	971.1	E855.4	E941.1	E950.4	E962.0	E980.4
Anticholinesterase (organophosphorus) (reversible)	971.0	E855.3	E941.0	E950.4	E962.0	E980.4
Anticoagulants	964.2	E858.2	E934.2	E950.4	E962.0	E980.4
antagonists	964.5	E858.2	E934.5	E950.4	E962.0	E980.4
Anti–common cold agents NEC	975.6	E858.6	E945.6	E950.4	E962.0	E980.4
Anticonvulsants NEC	966.3	E855.0	E936.3	E950.4	E962.0	E980.4
Antidepressants	969.00	E854.0	E939.0	E950.3	E962.0	E980.3
monoamine oxidase inhibitors (MAOI)	969.01	E854.0	E939.0	E950.3	E962.0	E980.3
specified type NEC	969.09	E854.0	E939.0	E950.3	E962.0	E980.3
SSNRI (selective serotonin and norepinephrine reuptake inhibitors)	969.02	E854.0	E939.0	E950.3	E962.0	E980.3
SSRI (selective serotonin reuptake inhibitors)	969.03	E854.0	E939.0	E950.3	E962.0	E980.3
tetracyclic	969.04	E854.0	E939.0	E950.3	E962.0	E980.3
tricyclic	969.05	E854.0	E939.0	E950.3	E962.0	E980.3
Antidiabetic agents	962.3	E858.0	E932.3	E950.4	E962.0	E980.4
Antidiarrheal agents	973.5	E858.4	E943.5	E950.4	E962.0	E980.4
Antidiuretic hormone	962.5	E858.0	E932.5	E950.4	E962.0	E980.4
Antidotes NEC	977.2	E858.8	E947.2	E950.4	E962.0	E980.4
Antiemetic agents	963.0	E858.1	E933.0	E950.4	E962.0	E980.4
Antiepilepsy agent NEC	966.3	E855.0	E936.3	E950.4	E962.0	E980.4
Antifertility pills	962.2	E858.0	E932.2	E950.4	E962.0	E980.4
Antiflatulents	973.8	E858.4	E943.8	E950.4	E962.0	E980.4
Antifreeze	989.89	E866.8	—	E950.9	E962.1	E980.9
alcohol	980.1	E860.2	—	E950.9	E962.1	E980.9
ethylene glycol	982.8	E862.4	—	E950.9	E962.1	E980.9
Antifungals (nonmedicinal) (sprays)	989.4	E863.6	—	E950.6	E962.1	E980.7
medicinal NEC	961.9	E857	E931.9	E950.4	E962.0	E980.4
antibiotic	960.1	E856	E930.1	E950.4	E962.0	E980.4
topical	976.0	E858.7	E946.0	E950.4	E962.0	E980.4
Antigastric secretion agents	973.0	E858.4	E943.0	E950.4	E962.0	E980.4
Antihelmintics	961.6	E857	E931.6	E950.4	E962.0	E980.4
Antihemophilic factor (human)	964.7	E858.2	E934.7	E950.4	E962.0	E980.4
Antihistamine	963.0	E858.1	E933.0	E950.4	E962.0	E980.4
Antihypertensive agents NEC	972.6	E858.3	E942.6	E950.4	E962.0	E980.4
Anti–infectives NEC	961.9	E857	E931.9	E950.4	E962.0	E980.4
antibiotics	960.9	E856	E930.9	E950.4	E962.0	E980.4
specified NEC	960.8	E856	E930.8	E950.4	E962.0	E980.4
antihelmintic	961.6	E857	E931.6	E950.4	E962.0	E980.4
antimalarial	961.4	E857	E931.4	E950.4	E962.0	E980.4
antimycobacterial NEC	961.8	E857	E931.8	E950.4	E962.0	E980.4
antibiotics	960.6	E856	E930.6	E950.4	E962.0	E980.4
antiprotozoal NEC	961.5	E857	E931.5	E950.4	E962.0	E980.4
blood	961.4	E857	E931.4	E950.4	E962.0	E980.4
antiviral	961.7	E857	E931.7	E950.4	E962.0	E980.4
arsenical	961.1	E857	E931.1	E950.4	E962.0	E980.4

1499

Substance	Poisoning	Accident	Therapeutic Use	Suicide Attempt	Assault	Undetermined
			External Cause (E-Code)			
ENT agents	976.6	E858.7	E946.6	E950.4	E962.0	E980.4
heavy metals NEC	961.2	E857	E931.2	E950.4	E962.0	E980.4
local	976.0	E858.7	E946.0	E950.4	E962.0	E980.4
ophthalmic preparation	976.5	E858.7	E946.5	E950.4	E962.0	E980.4
topical NEC	976.0	E858.7	E946.0	E950.4	E962.0	E980.4
Anti–inflammatory agents (topical)	976.0	E858.7	E946.0	E950.4	E962.0	E980.4
Antiknock (tetraethyl lead)	984.1	E862.1	—	E950.9	E962.1	E980.9
Antilipemics	972.2	E858.3	E942.2	E950.4	E962.0	E980.4
Antimalarials	961.4	E857	E931.4	E950.4	E962.0	E980.4
Antimony (compounds) (vapor) NEC	985.4	E866.2	—	E950.9	E962.1	E980.9
anti–infectives	961.2	E857	E931.2	E950.4	E962.0	E980.4
pesticides (vapor)	985.4	E863.4	—	E950.6	E962.2	E980.7
potassium tartrate	961.2	E857	E931.2	E950.4	E962.0	E980.4
tartrated	961.2	E857	E931.2	E950.4	E962.0	E980.4
Antimuscarinic agents	971.1	E855.4	E941.1	E950.4	E962.0	E980.4
Antimycobacterials NEC	961.8	E857	E931.8	E950.4	E962.0	E980.4
antibiotics	960.6	E856	E930.6	E950.4	E962.0	E980.4
Antineoplastic agents	963.1	E858.1	E933.1	E950.4	E962.0	E980.4
antibiotics	960.7	E856	E930.7	E950.4	E962.0	E980.4
Anti–Parkinsonism agents	966.4	E855.0	E936.4	E950.4	E962.0	E980.4
Antiphlogistics	965.69	E850.6	E935.6	E950.0	E962.0	E980.0
Antiprotozoals NEC	961.5	E857	E931.5	E950.4	E962.0	E980.4
blood	961.4	E857	E931.4	E950.4	E962.0	E980.4
Antipruritics (local)	976.1	E858.7	E946.1	E950.4	E962.0	E980.4
Antipsychotic agents NEC	969.3	E853.8	E939.3	E950.3	E962.0	E980.3
Antipyretics	965.9	E850.9	E935.9	E950.0	E962.0	E980.0
specified NEC	965.8	E850.8	E935.8	E950.0	E962.0	E980.0
Antipyrine	965.5	E850.5	E935.5	E950.0	E962.0	E980.0
Antirabies serum (equine)	979.9	E858.8	E949.9	E950.4	E962.0	E980.4
Antirheumatics	965.69	E850.6	E935.6	E950.0	E962.0	E980.0
Antiseborrheics	976.4	E858.7	E946.4	E950.4	E962.0	E980.4
Antiseptics (external) (medicinal)	976.0	E858.7	E946.0	E950.4	E962.0	E980.4
Antistine	963.0	E858.1	E933.0	E950.4	E962.0	E980.4
Antithyroid agents	962.8	E858.0	E932.8	E950.4	E962.0	E980.4
Antitoxin, any	979.9	E858.8	E949.9	E950.4	E962.0	E980.4
Antituberculars	961.8	E857	E931.8	E950.4	E962.0	E980.4
antibiotics	960.6	E856	E930.6	E950.4	E962.0	E980.4
Antitussives	975.4	E858.6	E945.5	E950.4	E962.0	E980.4
Antivaricose agents (sclerosing)	972.7	E858.3	E942.7	E950.4	E962.0	E980.4
Antivenin (crotaline) (spider–bite)	979.9	E858.8	E949.9	E950.4	E962.0	E980.4
Antivert	963.0	E858.1	E933.0	E950.4	E962.0	E980.4
Antivirals NEC	961.7	E857	E931.7	E950.4	E962.0	E980.4
Ant poisons — see Pesticides						
Antrol	989.4	E863.4	—	E950.6	E962.1	E980.7
fungicide	989.4	E863.6	—	E950.6	E962.1	E980.7
Apomorphine hydrochloride (emetic)	973.6	E858.4	E943.6	E950.4	E962.0	E980.4
Appetite depressants, central	977.0	E858.8	E947.0	E950.4	E962.0	E980.4
Apresoline	972.6	E858.3	E942.6	E950.4	E962.0	E980.4
Aprobarbital, aprobarbitone	967.0	E851	E937.0	E950.1	E962.0	E980.1
Apronalide	967.8	E852.8	E937.8	E950.2	E962.0	E980.2
Aqua fortis	983.1	E864.1	—	E950.7	E962.1	E980.6
Arachis oil (topical)	976.3	E858.7	E946.3	E950.4	E962.0	E980.4
cathartic	973.2	E858.4	E943.2	E950.4	E962.0	E980.4
Aralen	961.4	E857	E931.4	E950.4	E962.0	E980.4
Arginine salts	974.5	E858.5	E944.5	E950.4	E962.0	E980.4
Argyrol	976.0	E858.7	E946.0	E950.4	E962.0	E980.4
ENT agent	976.6	E858.7	E946.6	E950.4	E962.0	E980.4
ophthalmic preparation	976.5	E858.7	E946.5	E950.4	E962.0	E980.4
Aristocort	962.0	E858.0	E932.0	E950.4	E962.0	E980.4
ENT agent	976.6	E858.7	E946.6	E950.4	E962.0	E980.4

Substance	Poisoning	Accident	Therapeutic Use	Suicide Attempt	Assault	Undetermined
			External Cause (E-Code)			
ophthalmic preparation	976.5	E858.7	E946.5	E950.4	E962.0	E980.4
topical NEC	976.0	E858.7	E946.0	E950.4	E962.0	E980.4
Aromatics, corrosive	983.0	E864.0	—	E950.7	E962.1	E980.6
disinfectants	983.0	E861.4	—	E950.7	E962.1	E980.6
Arsenate of lead (insecticide)	985.1	E863.4	—	E950.8	E962.1	E980.8
herbicide	985.1	E863.5	—	E950.8	E962.1	E980.8
Arsenic, arsenicals (compounds) (dust)						
(fumes) (vapor) NEC	985.1	E866.3	—	E950.8	E962.1	E980.8
anti–infectives	961.1	E857	E931.1	E950.4	E962.0	E980.4
pesticide (dust) (fumes)	985.1	E863.4	—	E950.8	E962.1	E980.8
Arsine (gas)	985.1	E866.3	—	E950.8	E962.1	E980.8
Arsphenamine (silver)	961.1	E857	E931.1	E950.4	E962.0	E980.4
Arsthinol	961.1	E857	E931.1	E950.4	E962.0	E980.4
Artane	971.1	E855.4	E941.1	E950.4	E962.0	E980.4
Arthropod (venomous) NEC	989.5	E905.5	—	E950.9	E962.1	E980.9
Asbestos	989.81	E866.8	—	E950.9	E962.1	E980.9
Ascaridole	961.6	E857	E931.6	E950.4	E962.0	E980.4
Ascorbic acid	963.5	E858.1	E933.5	E950.4	E962.0	E980.4
Asiaticoside	976.0	E858.7	E946.0	E950.4	E962.0	E980.4
Aspidium (oleoresin)	961.6	E857	E931.6	E950.4	E962.0	E980.4
Aspirin	965.1	E850.3	E935.3	E950.0	E962.0	E980.0
Astringents (local)	976.2	E858.7	E946.2	E950.4	E962.0	E980.4
Atabrine	961.3	E857	E931.3	E950.4	E962.0	E980.4
Ataractics	969.5	E853.8	E939.5	E950.3	E962.0	E980.3
Atonia drug, intestinal	973.3	E858.4	E943.3	E950.4	E962.0	E980.4
Atophan	974.7	E858.5	E944.7	E950.4	E962.0	E980.4
Atropine	971.1	E855.4	E941.1	E950.4	E962.0	E980.4
Attapulgite	973.5	E858.4	E943.5	E950.4	E962.0	E980.4
Attenuvax	979.4	E858.8	E949.4	E950.4	E962.0	E980.4
Aureomycin	960.4	E856	E930.4	E950.4	E962.0	E980.4
ophthalmic preparation	976.5	E858.7	E946.5	E950.4	E962.0	E980.4
topical NEC	976.0	E858.7	E946.0	E950.4	E962.0	E980.4
Aurothioglucose	965.69	E850.6	E935.6	E950.0	E962.0	E980.0
Aurothioglycanide	965.69	E850.6	E935.6	E950.0	E962.0	E980.0
Aurothiomalate	965.69	E850.6	E935.6	E950.0	E962.0	E980.0
Automobile fuel	981	E862.1	—	E950.9	E962.1	E980.9
Autonomic nervous system agents NEC . . .	971.9	E855.9	E941.9	E950.4	E962.0	E980.4
Avlosulfon	961.8	E857	E931.8	E950.4	E962.0	E980.4
Avomine	967.8	E852.8	E937.8	E950.2	E962.0	E980.2
Azacyclonol	969.5	E853.8	E939.5	E950.3	E962.0	E980.3
Azapetine	971.3	E855.6	E941.3	E950.4	E962.0	E980.4
Azaribine	963.1	E858.1	E933.1	E950.4	E962.0	E980.4
Azaserine	960.7	E856	E930.7	E950.4	E962.0	E980.4
Azathioprine	963.1	E858.1	E933.1	E950.4	E962.0	E980.4
Azosulfamide	961.0	E857	E931.0	E950.4	E962.0	E980.4
Azulfidine	961.0	E857	E931.0	E950.4	E962.0	E980.4
Azuresin	977.8	E858.8	E947.8	E950.4	E962.0	E980.4
Bacimycin	976.0	E858.7	E946.0	E950.4	E962.0	E980.4
ophthalmic preparation	976.5	E858.7	E946.5	E950.4	E962.0	E980.4
Bacitracin	960.8	E856	E930.8	E950.4	E962.0	E980.4
ENT agent	976.6	E858.7	E946.6	E950.4	E962.0	E980.4
ophthalmic preparation	976.5	E858.7	E946.5	E950.4	E962.0	E980.4
topical NEC	976.0	E858.7	E946.0	E950.4	E962.0	E980.4
Baking soda	963.3	E858.1	E933.3	E950.4	E962.0	E980.4
BAL	963.8	E858.1	E933.8	E950.4	E962.0	E980.4
Bamethan (sulfate)	972.5	E858.3	E942.5	E950.4	E962.0	E980.4
Bamipine	963.0	E858.1	E933.0	E950.4	E962.0	E980.4
Baneberry	988.2	E865.4	—	E950.9	E962.1	E980.9
Banewort	988.2	E865.4	—	E950.9	E962.1	E980.9
Barbenyl	967.0	E851	E937.0	E950.1	E962.0	E980.1
Barbital, barbitone	967.0	E851	E937.0	E950.1	E962.0	E980.1

Substance	Poisoning	Accident	Therapeutic Use	Suicide Attempt	Assault	Undetermined
			External Cause (E-Code)			
Barbiturates, barbituric acid	967.0	E851	E937.0	E950.1	E962.0	E980.1
anesthetic (intravenous)	968.3	E855.1	E938.3	E950.4	E962.0	E980.4
Barium (carbonate) (chloride) (sulfate)	985.8	E866.4	—	E950.9	E962.1	E980.9
diagnostic agent	977.8	E858.8	E947.8	E950.4	E962.0	E980.4
pesticide.	985.8	E863.4	—	E950.6	E962.1	E980.7
rodenticide	985.8	E863.7	—	E950.6	E962.1	E980.7
Barrier cream	976.3	E858.7	E946.3	E950.4	E962.0	E980.4
Battery acid or fluid	983.1	E864.1	—	E950.7	E962.1	E980.6
Bay rum	980.8	E860.8	—	E950.9	E962.1	E980.9
BCG vaccine	978.0	E858.8	E948.0	E950.4	E962.0	E980.4
Bearsfoot	988.2	E865.4	—	E950.9	E962.1	E980.9
Beclamide	966.3	E855.0	E936.3	E950.4	E962.0	E980.4
Bee (sting) (venom)	989.5	E905.3	—	E950.9	E962.1	E980.9
Belladonna (alkaloids)	971.1	E855.4	E941.1	E950.4	E962.0	E980.4
Bemegride	970.0	E854.3	E940.0	E950.4	E962.0	E980.4
Benactyzine	969.8	E855.8	E939.8	E950.3	E962.0	E980.3
Benadryl	963.0	E858.1	E933.0	E950.4	E962.0	E980.4
Bendrofluazide	974.3	E858.5	E944.3	E950.4	E962.0	E980.4
Bendroflumethiazide	974.3	E858.5	E944.3	E950.4	E962.0	E980.4
Benemid	974.7	E858.5	E944.7	E950.4	E962.0	E980.4
Benethamine penicillin G	960.0	E856	E930.0	E950.4	E962.0	E980.4
Benisone	976.0	E858.7	E946.0	E950.4	E962.0	E980.4
Benoquin	976.8	E858.7	E946.8	E950.4	E962.0	E980.4
Benoxinate	968.5	E855.2	E938.5	E950.4	E962.0	E980.4
Bentonite	976.3	E858.7	E946.3	E950.4	E962.0	E980.4
Benzalkonium (chloride)	976.0	E858.7	E946.0	E950.4	E962.0	E980.4
ophthalmic preparation	976.5	E858.7	E946.5	E950.4	E962.0	E980.4
Benzamidosalicylate (calcium)	961.8	E857	E931.8	E950.4	E962.0	E980.4
Benzathine penicillin	960.0	E856	E930.0	E950.4	E962.0	E980.4
Benzcarbimine	963.1	E858.1	E933.1	E950.4	E962.0	E980.4
Benzedrex	971.2	E855.5	E941.2	E950.4	E962.0	E980.4
Benzedrine (amphetamine)	969.72	E854.2	E939.7	E950.3	E962.0	E980.3
Benzene (acetyl) (dimethyl) (methyl) (solvent) (vapor)	982.0	E862.4	—	E950.9	E962.1	E980.9
hexachloride (gamma) (insecticide) (vapor)	989.2	E863.0	—	E950.6	E962.1	E980.7
Benzethonium	976.0	E858.7	E946.0	E950.4	E962.0	E980.4
Benzhexol (chloride)	966.4	E855.0	E936.4	E950.4	E962.0	E980.4
Benzilonium	971.1	E855.4	E941.1	E950.4	E962.0	E980.4
Benzin(e) — see Ligroin						
Benziodarone	972.4	E858.3	E942.4	E950.4	E962.0	E980.4
Benzocaine	968.5	E855.2	E938.5	E950.4	E962.0	E980.4
Benzodiapin	969.4	E853.2	E939.4	E950.3	E962.0	E980.3
Benzodiazepines (tranquilizers) NEC	969.4	E853.2	E939.4	E950.3	E962.0	E980.3
Benzoic acid (with salicylic acid) (anti–infective)	976.0	E858.7	E946.0	E950.4	E962.0	E980.4
Benzoin	976.3	E858.7	E946.3	E950.4	E962.0	E980.4
Benzol (vapor)	982.0	E862.4	—	E950.9	E962.1	E980.9
Benzomorphan	965.09	E850.2	E935.2	E950.0	E962.0	E980.0
Benzonatate	975.4	E858.6	E945.4	E950.4	E962.0	E980.4
Benzothiadiazides	974.3	E858.5	E944.3	E950.4	E962.0	E980.4
Benzoylpas	961.8	E857	E931.8	E950.4	E962.0	E980.4
Benzperidol	969.5	E853.8	E939.5	E950.3	E962.0	E980.3
Benzphetamine	977.0	E858.8	E947.0	E950.4	E962.0	E980.4
Benzpyrinium	971.0	E855.3	E941.0	E950.4	E962.0	E980.4
Benzquinamide	963.0	E858.1	E933.0	E950.4	E962.0	E980.4
Benzthiazide	974.3	E858.5	E944.3	E950.4	E962.0	E980.4
Benztropine	971.1	E855.4	E941.1	E950.4	E962.0	E980.4
Benzyl acetate	982.8	E862.4	—	E950.9	E962.1	E980.9

Substance	Poisoning	Accident	Therapeutic Use	Suicide Attempt	Assault	Undetermined
			External Cause (E-Code)			

benzoate (anti–infective)	976.0	E858.7	E946.0	E950.4	E962.0	E980.4
morphine	965.09	E850.2	E935.2	E950.0	E962.0	E980.0
penicillin	960.0	E856	E930.0	E950.4	E962.0	E980.4
Bephenium hydroxynapthoate	961.6	E857	E931.6	E950.4	E962.0	E980.4
Bergamot oil	989.89	E866.8	—	E950.9	E962.1	E980.9
Berries, poisonous	988.2	E865.3	—	E950.9	E962.1	E980.9
Beryllium (compounds) (fumes)	985.3	E866.4	—	E950.9	E962.1	E980.9
Beta–carotene	976.3	E858.7	E946.3	E950.4	E962.0	E980.4
Beta–Chlor	967.1	E852.0	E937.1	E950.2	E962.0	E980.2
Betamethasone	962.0	E858.0	E932.0	E950.4	E962.0	E980.4
topical	976.0	E858.7	E946.0	E950.4	E962.0	E980.4
Betazole	977.8	E858.8	E947.8	E950.4	E962.0	E980.4
Bethanechol	971.0	E855.3	E941.0	E950.4	E962.0	E980.4
Bethanidine	972.6	E858.3	E942.6	E950.4	E962.0	E980.4
Betula oil	976.3	E858.7	E946.3	E950.4	E962.0	E980.4
Bhang	969.6	E854.1	E939.6	E950.3	E962.0	E980.3
Bialamicol	961.5	E857	E931.5	E950.4	E962.0	E980.4
Bichloride of mercury — *see* Mercury, chloride						
Bichromates (calcium) (crystals) (potassium) (sodium)	983.9	E864.3	—	E950.7	E962.1	E980.6
fumes	987.8	E869.8	—	E952.8	E962.2	E982.8
Biguanide derivatives, oral	962.3	E858.0	E932.3	E950.4	E962.0	E980.4
Biligrafin	977.8	E858.8	E947.8	E950.4	E962.0	E980.4
Bilopaque	977.8	E858.8	E947.8	E950.4	E962.0	E980.4
Bioflavonoids	972.8	E858.3	E942.8	E950.4	E962.0	E980.4
Biological substance NEC	979.9	E858.8	E949.9	E950.4	E962.0	E980.4
Biperiden	966.4	E855.0	E936.4	E950.4	E962.0	E980.4
Bisacodyl	973.1	E858.4	E943.1	E950.4	E962.0	E980.4
Bishydroxycoumarin	964.2	E858.2	E934.2	E950.4	E962.0	E980.4
Bismarsen	961.1	E857	E931.1	E950.4	E962.0	E980.4
Bismuth (compounds) NEC	985.8	E866.4	—	E950.9	E962.1	E980.9
anti–infectives	961.2	E857	E931.2	E950.4	E962.0	E980.4
subcarbonate	973.5	E858.4	E943.5	E950.4	E962.0	E980.4
sulfarsphenamine	961.1	E857	E931.1	E950.4	E962.0	E980.4
Bisphosphonates						
intravenous	963.1	E858.1	E933.7	E950.4	E962.0	E980.4
oral	963.1	E858.1	E933.6	E950.4	E962.0	E980.4
Bithionol	961.6	E857	E931.6	E950.4	E962.0	E980.4
Bitter almond oil	989.0	E866.8	—	E950.9	E962.1	E980.9
Bittersweet	988.2	E865.4	—	E950.9	E962.1	E980.9
Black						
flag	989.4	E863.4	—	E950.6	E962.1	E980.7
henbane	988.2	E865.4	—	E950.9	E962.1	E980.9
leaf (40)	989.4	E863.4	—	E950.6	E962.1	E980.7
widow spider (bite)	989.5	E905.1	—	E950.9	E962.1	E980.9
antivenin	979.9	E858.8	E949.9	E950.4	E962.0	E980.4
Blast furnace gas (carbon monoxide from) . .	986	E868.8	—	E952.1	E962.2	E982.1
Bleach NEC	983.9	E864.3	—	E950.7	E962.1	E980.6
Bleaching solutions	983.9	E864.3	—	E950.7	E962.1	E980.6
Bleomycin (sulfate)	960.7	E856	E930.7	E950.4	E962.0	E980.4
Blockain	968.9	E855.2	E938.9	E950.4	E962.0	E980.4
infiltration (subcutaneous)	968.5	E855.2	E938.5	E950.4	E962.0	E980.4
nerve block (peripheral) (plexus)	968.6	E855.2	E938.6	E950.4	E962.0	E980.4
topical (surface)	968.5	E855.2	E938.5	E950.4	E962.0	E980.4
Blood (derivatives) (natural) (plasma)						
(whole)	964.7	E858.2	E934.7	E950.4	E962.0	E980.4
affecting agent	964.9	E858.2	E934.9	E950.4	E962.0	E980.4
specified NEC	964.8	E858.2	E934.8	E950.4	E962.0	E980.4
substitute (macromolecular)	964.8	E858.2	E934.8	E950.4	E962.0	E980.4
Blue velvet	965.09	E850.2	E935.2	E950.0	E962.0	E980.0

TABLE OF DRUGS AND CHEMICALS

Substance	Poisoning	Accident	Therapeutic Use	Suicide Attempt	Assault	Undetermined
				External Cause (E-Code)		
Bone meal	989.89	E866.5	—	E950.9	E962.1	E980.9
Bonine	963.0	E858.1	E933.0	E950.4	E962.0	E980.4
Boracic acid	976.0	E858.7	E946.0	E950.4	E962.0	E980.4
ENT agent	976.6	E858.7	E946.6	E950.4	E962.0	E980.4
ophthalmic preparation	976.5	E858.7	E946.5	E950.4	E962.0	E980.4
Borate (cleanser) (sodium)	989.6	E861.3	—	E950.9	E962.1	E980.9
Borax (cleanser)	989.6	E861.3	—	E950.9	E962.1	E980.9
Boric acid	976.0	E858.7	E946.0	E950.4	E962.0	E980.4
ENT agent	976.6	E858.7	E946.6	E950.4	E962.0	E980.4
ophthalmic preparation	976.5	E858.7	E946.5	E950.4	E962.0	E980.4
Boron hydride NEC	989.89	E866.8	—	E950.9	E962.1	E980.9
fumes or gas	987.8	E869.8	—	E952.8	E962.2	E982.8
Botox	975.3	E858.6	E945.3	E950.4	E962.0	E980.4
Brake fluid vapor	987.8	E869.8	—	E952.8	E962.2	E982.8
Brass (compounds) (fumes)	985.8	E866.4	—	E950.9	E962.1	E980.9
Brasso	981	E861.3	—	E950.9	E962.1	E980.9
Bretylium (tosylate)	972.6	E858.3	E942.6	E950.4	E962.0	E980.4
Brevital (sodium)	968.3	E855.1	E938.3	E950.4	E962.0	E980.4
British antilewisite	963.8	E858.1	E933.8	E950.4	E962.0	E980.4
Bromal (hydrate)	967.3	E852.2	E937.3	E950.2	E962.0	E980.2
Bromelains	963.4	E858.1	E933.4	E950.4	E962.0	E980.4
Bromides NEC	967.3	E852.2	E937.3	E950.2	E962.0	E980.2
Bromine (vapor)	987.8	E869.8	—	E952.8	E962.2	E982.8
compounds (medicinal)	967.3	E852.2	E937.3	E950.2	E962.0	E980.2
Bromisovalum	967.3	E852.2	E937.3	E950.2	E962.0	E980.2
Bromobenzyl cyanide	987.5	E869.3	—	E952.8	E962.2	E982.8
Bromodiphenhydramine	963.0	E858.1	E933.0	E950.4	E962.0	E980.4
Bromoform	967.3	E852.2	E937.3	E950.2	E962.0	E980.2
Bromophenol blue reagent	977.8	E858.8	E947.8	E950.4	E962.0	E980.4
Bromosalicylhydroxamic acid	961.8	E857	E931.8	E950.4	E962.0	E980.4
Bromo–seltzer	965.4	E850.4	E935.4	E950.0	E962.0	E980.0
Brompheniramine	963.0	E858.1	E933.0	E950.4	E962.0	E980.4
Bromural	967.3	E852.2	E937.3	E950.2	E962.0	E980.2
Brown spider (bite) (venom)	989.5	E905.1	—	E950.9	E962.1	E980.9
Brucia	988.2	E865.3	—	E950.9	E962.1	E980.9
Brucine	989.1	E863.7	—	E950.6	E962.1	E980.7
Brunswick green — see Copper						
Bruten — see Ibuprofen						
Bryonia (alba) (dioica)	988.2	E865.4	—	E950.9	E962.1	E980.9
Buclizine	969.5	E853.8	E939.5	E950.3	E962.0	E980.3
Bufferin	965.1	E850.3	E935.3	E950.0	E962.0	E980.0
Bufotenine	969.6	E854.1	E939.6	E950.3	E962.0	E980.3
Buphenine	971.2	E855.5	E941.2	E950.4	E962.0	E980.4
Bupivacaine	968.9	E855.2	E938.9	E950.4	E962.0	E980.4
infiltration (subcutaneous)	968.5	E855.2	E938.5	E950.4	E962.0	E980.4
nerve block (peripheral) (plexus)	968.6	E855.2	E938.6	E950.4	E962.0	E980.4
Busulfan	963.1	E858.1	E933.1	E950.4	E962.0	E980.4
Butabarbital (sodium)	967.0	E851	E937.0	E950.1	E962.0	E980.1
Butabarbitone	967.0	E851	E937.0	E950.1	E962.0	E980.1
Butabarpal	967.0	E851	E937.0	E950.1	E962.0	E980.1
Butacaine	968.5	E855.2	E938.5	E950.4	E962.0	E980.4
Butallylonal	967.0	E851	E937.0	E950.1	E962.0	E980.1
Butane (distributed in mobile container)	987.0	E868.0	—	E951.1	E962.2	E981.1
distributed through pipes	987.0	E867	—	E951.0	E962.2	E981.0
incomplete combustion of — see Carbon monoxide, butane						
Butanol	980.3	E860.4	—	E950.9	E962.1	E980.9
Butanone	982.8	E862.4	—	E950.9	E962.1	E980.9
Butaperazine	969.1	E853.0	E939.1	E950.3	E962.0	E980.3
Butazolidin	965.5	E850.5	E935.5	E950.0	E962.0	E980.0

1504

Substance	Poisoning	Accident	Therapeutic Use	Suicide Attempt	Assault	Undetermined
			External Cause (E-Code)			
Butethal	967.0	E851	E937.0	E950.1	E962.0	E980.1
Butethamate	971.1	E855.4	E941.1	E950.4	E962.0	E980.4
Buthalitone (sodium)	968.3	E855.1	E938.3	E950.4	E962.0	E980.4
Butisol (sodium)	967.0	E851	E937.0	E950.1	E962.0	E980.1
Butobarbital, butobarbitone	967.0	E851	E937.0	E950.1	E962.0	E980.1
Butriptyline	969.05	E854.0	E939.0	E950.3	E962.0	E980.3
Buttercups	988.2	E865.4	—	E950.9	E962.1	E980.9
Butter of antimony — *see* Antimony						
Butyl						
acetate (secondary)	982.8	E862.4	—	E950.9	E962.1	E980.9
alcohol	980.3	E860.4	—	E950.9	E962.1	E980.9
carbinol	980.8	E860.8	—	E950.9	E962.1	E980.9
carbitol	982.8	E862.4	—	E950.9	E962.1	E980.9
cellosolve	982.8	E862.4	—	E950.9	E962.1	E980.9
chloral (hydrate)	967.1	E852.0	E937.1	E950.2	E962.0	E980.2
formate	982.8	E862.4	—	E950.9	E962.1	E980.9
scopolammonium bromide	971.1	E855.4	E941.1	E950.4	E962.0	E980.4
Butyn	968.5	E855.2	E938.5	E950.4	E962.0	E980.4
Butyrophenone (–based tranquilizers)	969.2	E853.1	E939.2	E950.3	E962.0	E980.3
Cacodyl, cacodylic acid — *see* Arsenic						
Cactinomycin	960.7	E856	E930.7	E950.4	E962.0	E980.4
Cade oil	976.4	E858.7	E946.4	E950.4	E962.0	E980.4
Cadmium (chloride) (compounds) (dust) (fumes) (oxide)	985.5	E866.4	—	E950.9	E962.1	E980.9
sulfide (medicinal) NEC	976.4	E858.7	E946.4	E950.4	E962.0	E980.4
Caffeine	969.71	E854.2	E939.7	E950.3	E962.0	E980.3
Calabar bean	988.2	E865.4	—	E950.9	E962.1	E980.9
Caladium seguinium	988.2	E865.4	—	E950.9	E962.1	E980.9
Calamine (liniment) (lotion)	976.3	E858.7	E946.3	E950.4	E962.0	E980.4
Calciferol	963.5	E858.1	E933.5	E950.4	E962.0	E980.4
Calcium (salts) NEC	974.5	E858.5	E944.5	E950.4	E962.0	E980.4
acetylsalicylate	965.1	E850.3	E935.3	E950.0	E962.0	E980.0
benzamidosalicylate	961.8	E857	E931.8	E950.4	E962.0	E980.4
carbaspirin	965.1	E850.3	E935.3	E950.0	E962.0	E980.0
carbamide (citrated)	977.3	E858.8	E947.3	E950.4	E962.0	E980.4
carbonate (antacid)	973.0	E858.4	E943.0	E950.4	E962.0	E980.4
cyanide (citrated)	977.3	E858.8	E947.3	E950.4	E962.0	E980.4
dioctyl sulfosuccinate	973.2	E858.4	E943.2	E950.4	E962.0	E980.4
disodium edathamil	963.8	E858.1	E933.8	E950.4	E962.0	E980.4
disodium edetate	963.8	E858.1	E933.8	E950.4	E962.0	E980.4
EDTA	963.8	E858.1	E933.8	E950.4	E962.0	E980.4
hydrate, hydroxide	983.2	E864.2	—	E950.7	E962.1	E980.6
mandelate	961.9	E857	E931.9	E950.4	E962.0	E980.4
oxide	983.2	E864.2	—	E950.7	E962.1	E980.6
Calomel — *see* Mercury, chloride						
Caloric agents NEC	974.5	E858.5	E944.5	E950.4	E962.0	E980.4
Calusterone	963.1	E858.1	E933.1	E950.4	E962.0	E980.4
Camoquin	961.4	E857	E931.4	E950.4	E962.0	E980.4
Camphor (oil)	976.1	E858.7	E946.1	E950.4	E962.0	E980.4
Candeptin	976.0	E858.7	E946.0	E950.4	E962.0	E980.4
Candicidin	976.0	E858.7	E946.0	E950.4	E962.0	E980.4
Cannabinols	969.6	E854.1	E939.6	E950.3	E962.0	E980.3
Cannabis (derivatives) (indica) (sativa)	969.6	E854.1	E939.6	E950.3	E962.0	E980.3
Canned heat	980.1	E860.2	—	E950.9	E962.1	E980.9
Cantharides, cantharidin, cantharis	976.8	E858.7	E946.8	E950.4	E962.0	E980.4
Capillary agents	972.8	E858.3	E942.8	E950.4	E962.0	E980.4
Capreomycin	960.6	E856	E930.6	E950.4	E962.0	E980.4
Captodiame, captodiamine	969.5	E853.8	E939.5	E950.3	E962.0	E980.3
Caramiphen (hydrochloride)	971.1	E855.4	E941.1	E950.4	E962.0	E980.4
Carbachol	971.0	E855.3	E941.0	E950.4	E962.0	E980.4
Carbacrylamine resins	974.5	E858.5	E944.5	E950.4	E962.0	E980.4

Substance	Poisoning	Accident	Therapeutic Use	Suicide Attempt	Assault	Undetermined
			External Cause (E-Code)			
Carbamate (sedative)	967.8	E852.8	E937.8	E950.2	E962.0	E980.2
herbicide	989.3	E863.5	—	E950.6	E962.1	E980.7
insecticide	989.3	E863.2	—	E950.6	E962.1	E980.7
Carbamazepine	966.3	E855.0	E936.3	E950.4	E962.0	E980.4
Carbamic esters	967.8	E852.8	E937.8	E950.2	E962.0	E980.2
Carbamide	974.4	E858.5	E944.4	E950.4	E962.0	E980.4
topical	976.8	E858.7	E946.8	E950.4	E962.0	E980.4
Carbamylcholine chloride	971.0	E855.3	E941.0	E950.4	E962.0	E980.4
Carbarsone	961.1	E857	E931.1	E950.4	E962.0	E980.4
Carbaryl	989.3	E863.2	—	E950.6	E962.1	E980.7
Carbaspirin	965.1	E850.3	E935.3	E950.0	E962.0	E980.0
Carbazochrome	972.8	E858.3	E942.8	E950.4	E962.0	E980.4
Carbenicillin	960.0	E856	E930.0	E950.4	E962.0	E980.4
Carbenoxolone	973.8	E858.4	E943.8	E950.4	E962.0	E980.4
Carbetapentane	975.4	E858.6	E945.4	E950.4	E962.0	E980.4
Carbimazole	962.8	E858.0	E932.8	E950.4	E962.0	E980.4
Carbinol	980.1	E860.2	—	E950.9	E962.1	E980.9
Carbinoxamine	963.0	E858.1	E933.0	E950.4	E962.0	E980.4
Carbitol	982.8	E862.4	—	E950.9	E962.1	E980.9
Carbocaine	968.9	E855.2	E938.9	E950.4	E962.0	E980.4
infiltration (subcutaneous)	968.5	E855.2	E938.5	E950.4	E962.0	E980.4
nerve block (peripheral) (plexus)	968.6	E855.2	E938.6	E950.4	E962.0	E980.4
topical (surface)	968.5	E855.2	E938.5	E950.4	E962.0	E980.4
Carbol–fuchsin solution	976.0	E858.7	E946.0	E950.4	E962.0	E980.4
Carbolic acid (*see also* Phenol)	983.0	E864.0	—	E950.7	E962.1	E980.6
Carbomycin	960.8	E856	E930.8	E950.4	E962.0	E980.4
Carbon						
bisulfide (liquid) (vapor)	982.2	E862.4	—	E950.9	E962.1	E980.9
dioxide (gas)	987.8	E869.8	—	E952.8	E962.2	E982.8
disulfide (liquid) (vapor)	982.2	E862.4	—	E950.9	E962.1	E980.9
monoxide (from incomplete combustion of) (in) NEC	986	E868.9	—	E952.1	E962.2	E982.1
blast furnace gas	986	E868.8	—	E952.1	E962.2	E982.1
butane (distributed in mobile container)	986	E868.0	—	E951.1	E962.2	E981.1
distributed through pipes	986	E867	—	E951.0	E962.2	E981.0
charcoal fumes	986	E868.3	—	E952.1	E962.2	E982.1
coal						
gas (piped)	986	E867	—	E951.0	E962.2	E981.0
solid (in domestic stoves, fireplaces)	986	E868.3	—	E952.1	E962.2	E982.1
coke (in domestic stoves, fireplaces)	986	E868.3	—	E952.1	E962.2	E982.1
exhaust gas (motor) not in transit	986	E868.2	—	E952.0	E962.2	E982.0
combustion engine, any not in watercraft	986	E868.2	—	E952.0	E962.2	E982.0
farm tractor, not in transit	986	E868.2	—	E952.0	E962.2	E982.0
gas engine	986	E868.2	—	E952.0	E962.2	E982.0
motor pump	986	E868.2	—	E952.0	E962.2	E982.0
motor vehicle, not in transit	986	E868.2	—	E952.0	E962.2	E982.0
fuel (in domestic use)	986	E868.3	—	E952.1	E962.2	E982.1
gas (piped)	986	E867	—	E951.0	E962.2	E981.0
in mobile container	986	E868.0	—	E951.1	E962.2	E981.1
utility	986	E868.1	—	E951.8	E962.2	E981.1
in mobile container	986	E868.0	—	E951.1	E962.2	E981.1
piped (natural)	986	E867	—	E951.0	E962.2	E981.0
illuminating gas	986	E868.1	—	E951.8	E962.2	E981.8
industrial fuels or gases, any	986	E868.8	—	E952.1	E962.2	E982.1
kerosene (in domestic stoves, fireplaces)	986	E868.3	—	E952.1	E962.2	E982.1
kiln gas or vapor	986	E868.8	—	E952.1	E962.2	E982.1

Substance	Poisoning	Accident	Therapeutic Use	Suicide Attempt	Assault	Undetermined
			External Cause (E-Code)			
motor exhaust gas, not in transit	986	E868.2	—	E952.0	E962.2	E982.0
piped gas (manufactured) (natural)	986	E867	—	E951.0	E962.2	E981.0
producer gas	986	E868.8	—	E952.1	E962.2	E982.1
propane (distributed in mobile container)	986	E868.0	—	E951.1	E962.2	E981.1
distributed through pipes	986	E867	—	E951.0	E962.2	E981.0
specified source NEC	986	E868.8	—	E952.1	E962.2	E982.1
stove gas	986	E868.1	—	E951.8	E962.2	E981.8
piped	986	E867	—	E951.0	E962.2	E981.0
utility gas	986	E868.1	—	E951.8	E962.2	E981.8
piped	986	E867	—	E951.0	E962.2	E981.0
water gas	986	E868.1	—	E951.8	E962.2	E981.8
wood (in domestic stoves, fireplaces)	986	E868.3	—	E952.1	E962.2	E982.1
tetrachloride (vapor) NEC	987.8	E869.8	—	E952.8	E962.2	E982.8
liquid (cleansing agent) NEC	982.1	E861.3	—	E950.9	E962.1	E980.9
solvent	982.1	E862.4	—	E950.9	E962.1	E980.9
Carbonic acid (gas)	987.8	E869.8	—	E952.8	E962.2	E982.8
anhydrase inhibitors	974.2	E858.5	E944.2	E950.4	E962.0	E980.4
Carbowax	976.3	E858.7	E946.3	E950.4	E962.0	E980.4
Carbrital	967.0	E851	E937.0	E950.1	E962.0	E980.1
Carbromal (derivatives)	967.3	E852.2	E937.3	E950.2	E962.0	E980.2
Cardiac						
depressants	972.0	E858.3	E942.0	E950.4	E962.0	E980.4
rhythm regulators	972.0	E858.3	E942.0	E950.4	E962.0	E980.4
Cardiografin	977.8	E858.8	E947.8	E950.4	E962.0	E980.4
Cardio–green	977.8	E858.8	E947.8	E950.4	E962.0	E980.4
Cardiotonic glycosides	972.1	E858.3	E942.1	E950.4	E962.0	E980.4
Cardiovascular agents NEC	972.9	E858.3	E942.9	E950.4	E962.0	E980.4
Cardrase	974.2	E858.5	E944.2	E950.4	E962.0	E980.4
Carfusin	976.0	E858.7	E946.0	E950.4	E962.0	E980.4
Carisoprodol	968.0	E855.1	E938.0	E950.4	E962.0	E980.4
Carmustine	963.1	E858.1	E933.1	E950.4	E962.0	E980.4
Carotene	963.5	E858.1	E933.5	E950.4	E962.0	E980.4
Carphenazine (maleate)	969.1	E853.0	E939.1	E950.3	E962.0	E980.3
Carter's Little Pills	973.1	E858.4	E943.1	E950.4	E962.0	E980.4
Cascara (sagrada)	973.1	E858.4	E943.1	E950.4	E962.0	E980.4
Cassava	988.2	E865.4	—	E950.9	E962.1	E980.9
Castellani's paint	976.0	E858.7	E946.0	E950.4	E962.0	E980.4
Castor						
bean	988.2	E865.3	—	E950.9	E962.1	E980.9
oil	973.1	E858.4	E943.1	E950.4	E962.0	E980.4
Caterpillar (sting)	989.5	E905.5	—	E950.9	E962.1	E980.9
Catha (edulis)	970.8	E854.3	E940.8	E950.4	E962.0	E980.4
Cathartics NEC	973.3	E858.4	E943.3	E950.4	E962.0	E980.4
contact	973.1	E858.4	E943.1	E950.4	E962.0	E980.4
emollient	973.2	E858.4	E943.2	E950.4	E962.0	E980.4
intestinal irritants	973.1	E858.4	E943.1	E950.4	E962.0	E980.4
saline	973.3	E858.4	E943.3	E950.4	E962.0	E980.4
Cathomycin	960.8	E856	E930.8	E950.4	E962.0	E980.4
Caustic(s)	983.9	E864.4	—	E950.7	E962.1	E980.6
alkali	983.2	E864.2	—	E950.7	E962.1	E980.6
hydroxide	983.2	E864.2	—	E950.7	E962.1	E980.6
potash	983.2	E864.2	—	E950.7	E962.1	E980.6
soda	983.2	E864.2	—	E950.7	E962.1	E980.6
specified NEC	983.9	E864.3	—	E950.7	E962.1	E980.6
Ceepryn	976.0	E858.7	E946.0	E950.4	E962.0	E980.4
ENT agent	976.6	E858.7	E946.6	E950.4	E962.0	E980.4
lozenges	976.6	E858.7	E946.6	E950.4	E962.0	E980.4
Celestone	962.0	E858.0	E932.0	E950.4	E962.0	E980.4
topical	976.0	E858.7	E946.0	E950.4	E962.0	E980.4
Cellosolve	982.8	E862.4	—	E950.9	E962.1	E980.9

Substance	Poisoning	Accident	Therapeutic Use	Suicide Attempt	Assault	Undetermined
			External Cause (E-Code)			
Cell stimulants and proliferants	976.8	E858.7	E946.8	E950.4	E962.0	E980.4
Cellulose derivatives, cathartic	973.3	E858.4	E943.3	E950.4	E962.0	E980.4
nitrates (topical)	976.3	E858.7	E946.3	E950.4	E962.0	E980.4
Centipede (bite)	989.5	E905.4	—	E950.9	E962.1	E980.9
Central nervous system						
depressants.	968.4	E855.1	E938.4	E950.4	E962.0	E980.4
anesthetic (general) NEC	968.4	E855.1	E938.4	E950.4	E962.0	E980.4
gases NEC	968.2	E855.1	E938.2	E950.4	E962.0	E980.4
intravenous	968.3	E855.1	E938.3	E950.4	E962.0	E980.4
barbiturates.	967.0	E851	E937.0	E950.1	E962.0	E980.1
bromides.	967.3	E852.2	E937.3	E950.2	E962.0	E980.2
cannabis sativa	969.6	E854.1	E939.6	E950.3	E962.0	E980.3
chloral hydrate	967.1	E852.0	E937.1	E950.2	E962.0	E980.2
hallucinogenics	969.6	E854.1	E939.6	E950.3	E962.0	E980.3
hypnotics	967.9	E852.9	E937.9	E950.2	E962.0	E980.2
specified NEC.	967.8	E852.8	E937.8	E950.2	E962.0	E980.2
muscle relaxants.	968.0	E855.1	E938.0	E950.4	E962.0	E980.4
paraldehyde	967.2	E852.1	E937.2	E950.2	E962.0	E980.2
sedatives	967.9	E852.9	E937.9	E950.2	E962.0	E980.2
mixed NEC.	967.6	E852.5	E937.6	E950.2	E962.0	E980.2
specified NEC.	967.8	E852.8	E937.8	E950.2	E962.0	E980.2
muscle-tone depressants	968.0	E855.1	E938.0	E950.4	E962.0	E980.4
stimulants	970.9	E854.3	E940.9	E950.4	E962.0	E980.4
amphetamines.	969.72	E854.2	E939.7	E950.3	E962.0	E980.3
analeptics	970.0	E854.3	E940.0	E950.4	E962.0	E980.4
antidepressants	969.00	E854.0	E939.0	E950.3	E962.0	E980.3
opiate antagonists	970.1	E854.3	E940.1	E950.4	E962.0	E980.4
specified NEC	970.8	E854.3	E940.8	E950.4	E962.0	E980.4
Cephalexin	960.5	E856	E930.5	E950.4	E962.0	E980.4
Cephaloglycin	960.5	E856	E930.5	E950.4	E962.0	E980.4
Cephaloridine	960.5	E856	E930.5	E950.4	E962.0	E980.4
Cephalosporins NEC	960.5	E856	E930.5	E950.4	E962.0	E980.4
N (adicillin)	960.0	E856	E930.0	E950.4	E962.0	E980.4
Cephalothin (sodium)	960.5	E856	E930.5	E950.4	E962.0	E980.4
Cerbera (odallam)	988.2	E865.4	—	E950.9	E962.1	E980.9
Cerberin	972.1	E858.3	E942.1	E950.4	E962.0	E980.4
Cerebral stimulants	970.9	E854.3	E940.9	E950.4	E962.0	E980.4
psychotherapeutic	969.79	E854.2	E939.7	E950.3	E962.0	E980.3
specified NEC	970.8	E854.3	E940.8	E950.4	E962.0	E980.4
Cetalkonium (chloride)	976.0	E858.7	E946.0	E950.4	E962.0	E980.4
Cetoxime	963.0	E858.1	E933.0	E950.4	E962.0	E980.4
Cetrimide	976.2	E858.7	E946.2	E950.4	E962.0	E980.4
Cetylpyridinium	976.0	E858.7	E946.0	E950.4	E962.0	E980.4
ENT agent.	976.6	E858.7	E946.6	E950.4	E962.0	E980.4
lozenges.	976.6	E858.7	E946.6	E950.4	E962.0	E980.4
Cevadilla — see Sabadilla						
Cevitamic acid	963.5	E858.1	E933.5	E950.4	E962.0	E980.4
Chalk, precipitated	973.0	E858.4	E943.0	E950.4	E962.0	E980.4
Charcoal						
fumes (carbon monoxide).	986	E868.3	—	E952.1	E962.2	E982.1
industrial.	986	E868.8	—	E952.1	E962.2	E982.1
medicinal (activated).	973.0	E858.4	E943.0	E950.4	E962.0	E980.4
Chelating agents NEC.	977.2	E858.8	E947.2	E950.4	E962.0	E980.4
Chelidonium majus	988.2	E865.4	—	E950.9	E962.1	E980.9
Chemical substance	989.9	E866.9	—	E950.9	E962.1	E980.9
specified NEC	989.89	E866.8	—	E950.9	E962.1	E980.9
Chemotherapy, antineoplastic	963.1	E858.1	E933.1	E950.4	E962.0	E980.4
Chenopodium (oil)	961.6	E857	E931.6	E950.4	E962.0	E980.4
Cherry laurel	988.2	E865.4	—	E950.9	E962.1	E980.9
Chiniofon.	961.3	E857	E931.3	E950.4	E962.0	E980.4

Substance	Poisoning	Accident	Therapeutic Use	Suicide Attempt	Assault	Undetermined
			External Cause (E-Code)			

Chlophedianol 975.4	E858.6	E945.4	E950.4	E962.0	E980.4	
Chloral (betaine) (formamide) (hydrate) . . . 967.1	E852.0	E937.1	E950.2	E962.0	E980.2	
Chloralamide 967.1	E852.0	E937.1	E950.2	E962.0	E980.2	
Chlorambucil 963.1	E858.1	E933.1	E950.4	E962.0	E980.4	
Chloramphenicol 960.2	E856	E930.2	E950.4	E962.0	E980.4	
ENT agent. 976.6	E858.7	E946.6	E950.4	E962.0	E980.4	
ophthalmic preparation 976.5	E858.7	E946.5	E950.4	E962.0	E980.4	
topical NEC 976.0	E858.7	E946.0	E950.4	E962.0	E980.4	
Chlorate(s) (potassium) (sodium) NEC 983.9	E864.3	—	E950.7	E962.1	E980.6	
herbicides 989.4	E863.5	—	E950.6	E962.1	E980.7	
Chlorcyclizine 963.0	E858.1	E933.0	E950.4	E962.0	E980.4	
Chlordan(e) (dust) 989.2	E863.0	—	E950.6	E962.1	E980.7	
Chlordantoin. 976.0	E858.7	E946.0	E950.4	E962.0	E980.4	
Chlordiazepoxide 969.4	E853.2	E939.4	E950.3	E962.0	E980.3	
Chloresium 976.8	E858.7	E946.8	E950.4	E962.0	E980.4	
Chlorethiazol 967.1	E852.0	E937.1	E950.2	E962.0	E980.2	
Chlorethyl — *see* Ethyl, chloride						
Chloretone 967.1	E852.0	E937.1	E950.2	E962.0	E980.2	
Chlorex. 982.3	E862.4	—	E950.9	E962.1	E980.9	
Chlorhexadol 967.1	E852.0	E937.1	E950.2	E962.0	E980.2	
Chlorhexidine (hydrochloride). 976.0	E858.7	E946.0	E950.4	E962.0	E980.4	
Chlorhydroxyquinolin 976.0	E858.7	E946.0	E950.4	E962.0	E980.4	
Chloride of lime (bleach) 983.9	E864.3	—	E950.7	E962.1	E980.6	
Chlorinated						
camphene 989.2	E863.0	—	E950.6	E962.1	E980.7	
diphenyl. 989.89	E866.8	—	E950.9	E962.1	E980.9	
hydrocarbons NEC 989.2	E863.0	—	E950.6	E962.1	E980.7	
solvent. 982.3	E862.4	—	E950.9	E962.1	E980.9	
lime (bleach). 983.9	E864.3	—	E950.7	E962.1	E980.6	
naphthalene — *see* Naphthalene						
pesticides NEC 989.2	E863.0	—	E950.6	E962.1	E980.7	
soda — *see* Sodium, hypochlorite						
Chlorine (fumes) (gas). 987.6	E869.8	—	E952.8	E962.2	E982.8	
bleach. 983.9	E864.3	—	E950.7	E962.1	E980.6	
compounds NEC 983.9	E864.3	—	E950.7	E962.1	E980.6	
disinfectant 983.9	E861.4	—	E950.7	E962.1	E980.6	
releasing agents NEC 983.9	E864.3	—	E950.7	E962.1	E980.6	
Chlorisondamine 972.3	E858.3	E942.3	E950.4	E962.0	E980.4	
Chlormadinone. 962.2	E858.0	E932.2	E950.4	E962.0	E980.4	
Chlormerodrin 974.0	E858.5	E944.0	E950.4	E962.0	E980.4	
Chlormethiazole 967.1	E852.0	E937.1	E950.2	E962.0	E980.2	
Chlormethylenecycline. 960.4	E856	E930.4	E950.4	E962.0	E980.4	
Chlormezanone. 969.5	E853.8	E939.5	E950.3	E962.0	E980.3	
Chloroacetophenone. 987.5	E869.3	—	E952.8	E962.2	E982.8	
Chloroaniline 983.0	E864.0	—	E950.7	E962.1	E980.6	
Chlorobenzene, chlorobenzol 982.0	E862.4	—	E950.9	E962.1	E980.9	
Chlorobutanol 967.1	E852.0	E937.1	E950.2	E962.0	E980.2	
Chlorodinitrobenzene 983.0	E864.0	—	E950.7	E962.1	E980.6	
dust or vapor. 987.8	E869.8	—	E952.8	E962.2	E982.8	
Chloroethane — *see* Ethyl, chloride						
Chloroform (fumes) (vapor) 987.8	E869.8	—	E952.8	E962.2	E982.8	
anesthetic (gas). 968.2	E855.1	E938.2	E950.4	E962.0	E980.4	
liquid NEC 968.4	E855.1	E938.4	E950.4	E962.0	E980.4	
solvent. 982.3	E862.4	—	E950.9	E962.1	E980.9	
Chloroguanide 961.4	E857	E931.4	E950.4	E962.0	E980.4	
Chloromycetin 960.2	E856	E930.2	E950.4	E962.0	E980.4	
ENT agent. 976.6	E858.7	E946.6	E950.4	E962.0	E980.4	
ophthalmic preparation. 976.5	E858.7	E946.5	E950.4	E962.0	E980.4	
otic solution 976.6	E858.7	E946.6	E950.4	E962.0	E980.4	
topical NEC 976.0	E858.7	E946.0	E950.4	E962.0	E980.4	
Chloronitrobenzene 983.0	E864.0	—	E950.7	E962.1	E980.6	

TABLE OF DRUGS AND CHEMICALS

Substance	Poisoning	Accident	Therapeutic Use	Suicide Attempt	Assault	Undetermined
			External Cause (E-Code)			
dust or vapor	987.8	E869.8	—	E952.8	E962.2	E982.8
Chlorophenol	983.0	E864.0	—	E950.7	E962.1	E980.6
Chlorophenothane	989.2	E863.0	—	E950.6	E962.1	E980.7
Chlorophyll (derivatives)	976.8	E858.7	E946.8	E950.4	E962.0	E980.4
Chloropicrin (fumes)	987.8	E869.8	—	E952.8	E962.2	E982.8
fumigant	989.4	E863.8	—	E950.6	E962.1	E980.7
fungicide	989.4	E863.6	—	E950.6	E962.1	E980.7
pesticide (fumes)	989.4	E863.4	—	E950.6	E962.1	E980.7
Chloroprocaine	968.9	E855.2	E938.9	E950.4	E962.0	E980.4
infiltration (subcutaneous)	968.5	E855.2	E938.5	E950.4	E962.0	E980.4
nerve block (peripheral) (plexus)	968.6	E855.2	E938.6	E950.4	E962.0	E980.4
Chloroptic	976.5	E858.7	E946.5	E950.4	E962.0	E980.4
Chloropurine	963.1	E858.1	E933.1	E950.4	E962.0	E980.4
Chloroquine (hydrochloride) (phosphate)	961.4	E857	E931.4	E950.4	E962.0	E980.4
Chlorothen	963.0	E858.1	E933.0	E950.4	E962.0	E980.4
Chlorothiazide	974.3	E858.5	E944.3	E950.4	E962.0	E980.4
Chlorotrianisene	962.2	E858.0	E932.2	E950.4	E962.0	E980.4
Chlorovinyldichloroarsine	985.1	E866.3	—	E950.8	E962.1	E980.8
Chloroxylenol	976.0	E858.7	E946.0	E950.4	E962.0	E980.4
Chlorphenesin (carbamate)	968.0	E855.1	E938.0	E950.4	E962.0	E980.4
topical (antifungal)	976.0	E858.7	E946.0	E950.4	E962.0	E980.4
Chlorpheniramine	963.0	E858.1	E933.0	E950.4	E962.0	E980.4
Chlorophenoxamine	966.4	E855.0	E936.4	E950.4	E962.0	E980.4
Chlorophentermine	977.0	E858.8	E947.0	E950.4	E962.0	E980.4
Chlorproguanil	961.4	E857	E931.4	E950.4	E962.0	E980.4
Chlorpromazine	969.1	E853.0	E939.1	E950.3	E962.0	E980.3
Chlorpropamide	962.3	E858.0	E932.3	E950.4	E962.0	E980.4
Chlorprothixene	969.3	E853.8	E939.3	E950.3	E962.0	E980.3
Chlorquinaldol	976.0	E858.7	E946.0	E950.4	E962.0	E980.4
Chlortetracycline	960.4	E856	E930.4	E950.4	E962.0	E980.4
Chlorthalidone	974.4	E858.5	E944.4	E950.4	E962.0	E980.4
Chlortrianisene	962.2	E858.0	E932.2	E950.4	E962.0	E980.4
Chlor–Trimeton	963.0	E858.1	E933.0	E950.4	E962.0	E980.4
Chlorzoxazone	968.0	E855.1	E938.0	E950.4	E962.0	E980.4
Choke damp	987.8	E869.8	—	E952.8	E962.2	E982.8
Cholebrine	977.8	E858.8	E947.8	E950.4	E962.0	E980.4
Cholera vaccine	978.2	E858.8	E948.2	E950.4	E962.0	E980.4
Cholesterol–lowering agents	972.2	E858.3	E942.2	E950.4	E962.0	E980.4
Cholestyramine (resin)	972.2	E858.3	E942.2	E950.4	E962.0	E980.4
Cholic acid	973.4	E858.4	E943.4	E950.4	E962.0	E980.4
Choline						
dihydrogen citrate	977.1	E858.8	E947.1	E950.4	E962.0	E980.4
salicylate	965.1	E850.3	E935.3	E950.0	E962.0	E980.0
theophyllinate	974.1	E858.5	E944.1	E950.4	E962.0	E980.4
Cholinergics	971.0	E855.3	E941.0	E950.4	E962.0	E980.4
Cholografin	977.8	E858.8	E947.8	E950.4	E962.0	E980.4
Chorionic gonadotropin	962.4	E858.0	E932.4	E950.4	E962.0	E980.4
Chromates	983.9	E864.3	—	E950.7	E962.1	E980.6
dust or mist	987.8	E869.8	—	E952.8	E962.2	E982.8
lead	984.0	E866.0	—	E950.9	E962.1	E980.9
paint	984.0	E861.5	—	E950.9	E962.1	E980.9
Chromic acid	983.9	E864.3	—	E950.7	E962.1	E980.6
dust or mist	987.8	E869.8	—	E952.8	E962.2	E982.8
Chromium	985.6	E866.4	—	E950.9	E962.1	E980.9
compounds — see Chromates						
Chromonar	972.4	E858.3	E942.4	E950.4	E962.0	E980.4
Chromyl chloride	983.9	E864.3	—	E950.7	E962.1	E980.6
Chrysarobin (ointment)	976.4	E858.7	E946.4	E950.4	E962.0	E980.4
Chrysazin	973.1	E858.4	E943.1	E950.4	E962.0	E980.4
Chymar	963.4	E858.1	E933.4	E950.4	E962.0	E980.4

Substance	Poisoning	Accident	Therapeutic Use	Suicide Attempt	Assault	Undetermined
			External Cause (E-Code)			
ophthalmic preparation 976.5	E858.7	E946.5	E950.4	E962.0	E980.4
Chymotrypsin 963.4	E858.1	E933.4	E950.4	E962.0	E980.4
ophthalmic preparation 976.5	E858.7	E946.5	E950.4	E962.0	E980.4
Cicuta maculata or virosa 988.2	E865.4	—	E950.9	E962.1	E980.9
Cigarette lighter fluid 981	E862.1	—	E950.9	E962.1	E980.9
Cinchocaine (spinal) 968.7	E855.2	E938.7	E950.4	E962.0	E980.4
topical (surface) 968.5	E855.2	E938.5	E950.4	E962.0	E980.4
Cinchona 961.4	E857	E931.4	E950.4	E962.0	E980.4
Cinchonine alkaloids 961.4	E857	E931.4	E950.4	E962.0	E980.4
Cinchophen 974.7	E858.5	E944.7	E950.4	E962.0	E980.4
Cinnarizine 963.0	E858.1	E933.0	E950.4	E962.0	E980.4
Citanest 968.9	E855.2	E938.9	E950.4	E962.0	E980.4
infiltration (subcutaneous) 968.5	E855.2	E938.5	E950.4	E962.0	E980.4
nerve block (peripheral) (plexus) 968.6	E855.2	E938.6	E950.4	E962.0	E980.4
Citric acid 989.89	E866.8	—	E950.9	E962.1	E980.9
Citrovorum factor 964.1	E858.2	E934.1	E950.4	E962.0	E980.4
Claviceps purpurea 988.2	E865.4	—	E950.9	E962.1	E980.9
Cleaner, cleansing agent NEC 989.89	E861.3	—	E950.9	E962.1	E980.9
of paint or varnish 982.8	E862.9	—	E950.9	E962.1	E980.9
Clematis vitalba 988.2	E865.4	—	E950.9	E962.1	E980.9
Clemizole 963.0	E858.1	E933.0	E950.4	E962.0	E980.4
penicillin 960.0	E856	E930.0	E950.4	E962.0	E980.4
Clidinium 971.1	E855.4	E941.1	E950.4	E962.0	E980.4
Clindamycin 960.8	E856	E930.8	E950.4	E962.0	E980.4
Cliradon 965.09	E850.2	E935.2	E950.0	E962.0	E980.0
Clocortolone 962.0	E858.0	E932.0	E950.4	E962.0	E980.4
Clofedanol 975.4	E858.6	E945.4	E950.4	E962.0	E980.4
Clofibrate 972.2	E858.3	E942.2	E950.4	E962.0	E980.4
Clomethiazole 967.1	E852.0	E937.1	E950.2	E962.0	E980.2
Clomiphene 977.8	E858.8	E947.8	E950.4	E962.0	E980.4
Clonazepam 969.4	E853.2	E939.4	E950.3	E962.0	E980.3
Clonidine 972.6	E858.3	E942.6	E950.4	E962.0	E980.4
Clopamide 974.3	E858.5	E944.3	E950.4	E962.0	E980.4
Clorazepate 969.4	E853.2	E939.4	E950.3	E962.0	E980.3
Clorexolone 974.4	E858.5	E944.4	E950.4	E962.0	E980.4
Clorox (bleach) 983.9	E864.3	—	E950.7	E962.1	E980.6
Clortermine 977.0	E858.8	E947.0	E950.4	E962.0	E980.4
Clotrimazole 976.0	E858.7	E946.0	E950.4	E962.0	E980.4
Cloxacillin 960.0	E856	E930.0	E950.4	E962.0	E980.4
Coagulants NEC 964.5	E858.2	E934.5	E950.4	E962.0	E980.4
Coal (carbon monoxide from) — *see also*					
Carbon, monoxide, coal					
oil — *see* Kerosene					
tar NEC 983.0	E864.0	—	E950.7	E962.1	E980.6
fumes 987.8	E869.8	—	E952.8	E962.2	E982.8
medicinal (ointment) 976.4	E858.7	E946.4	E950.4	E962.0	E980.4
analgesics NEC 965.5	E850.5	E935.5	E950.0	E962.0	E980.0
naphtha (solvent) 981	E862.0	—	E950.9	E962.1	E980.9
Cobalt (fumes) (industrial) 985.8	E866.4	—	E950.9	E962.1	E980.9
Cobra (venom) 989.5	E905.0	—	E950.9	E962.1	E980.9
Coca (leaf) 970.8	E854.3	E940.8	E950.4	E962.0	E980.4
Cocaine (hydrochloride) (salt) 970.8	E854.3	E940.8	E950.4	E962.0	E980.4
topical anesthetic 968.5	E855.2	E938.5	E950.4	E962.0	E980.4
Coccidioidin 977.8	E858.8	E947.8	E950.4	E962.0	E980.4
Cocculus indicus 988.2	E865.3	—	E950.9	E962.1	E980.9
Cochineal 989.89	E866.8	—	E950.9	E962.1	E980.9
medicinal products 977.4	E858.8	E947.4	E950.4	E962.0	E980.4
Codeine 965.09	E850.2	E935.2	E950.0	E962.0	E980.0
Coffee 989.89	E866.8	—	E950.9	E962.1	E980.9
Cogentin 971.1	E855.4	E941.1	E950.4	E962.0	E980.4
Coke fumes or gas (carbon monoxide) 986	E868.3	—	E952.1	E962.2	E982.1

Substance	Poisoning	Accident	Therapeutic Use	Suicide Attempt	Assault	Undetermined
			External Cause (E-Code)			
industrial use.	986	E868.8	—	E952.1	E962.2	E982.1
Colace	973.2	E858.4	E943.2	E950.4	E962.0	E980.4
Colchicine.	974.7	E858.5	E944.7	E950.4	E962.0	E980.4
Colchicum	988.2	E865.3	—	E950.9	E962.1	E980.9
Cold cream	976.3	E858.7	E946.3	E950.4	E962.0	E980.4
Colestipol	972.2	E858.3	E942.2	E950.4	E962.0	E980.4
Colistimethate	960.8	E856	E930.8	E950.4	E962.0	E980.4
Colistin	960.8	E856	E930.8	E950.4	E962.0	E980.4
Collagen	977.8	E866.8	E947.8	E950.9	E962.1	E980.9
Collagenase	976.8	E858.7	E946.8	E950.4	E962.0	E980.4
Collodion (flexible)	976.3	E858.7	E946.3	E950.4	E962.0	E980.4
Colocynth	973.1	E858.4	E943.1	E950.4	E962.0	E980.4
Coloring matter — *see* Dye(s)						
Combustion gas — *see* Carbon, monoxide						
Compazine	969.1	E853.0	E939.1	E950.3	E962.0	E980.3
Compound						
42 (warfarin)	989.4	E863.7	—	E950.6	E962.1	E980.7
269 (endrin)	989.2	E863.0	—	E950.6	E962.1	E980.7
497 (dieldrin)	989.2	E863.0	—	E950.6	E962.1	E980.7
1080 (sodium fluoroacetate)	989.4	E863.7	—	E950.6	E962.1	E980.7
3422 (parathion)	989.3	E863.1	—	E950.6	E962.1	E980.7
3911 (phorate)	989.3	E863.1	—	E950.6	E962.1	E980.7
3956 (toxaphene)	989.2	E863.0	—	E950.6	E962.1	E980.7
4049 (malathion)	989.3	E863.1	—	E950.6	E962.1	E980.7
4124 (dicapthon)	989.4	E863.4	—	E950.6	E962.1	E980.7
E (cortisone)	962.0	E858.0	E932.0	E950.4	E962.0	E980.4
F (hydrocortisone)	962.0	E858.0	E932.0	E950.4	E962.0	E980.4
Congo red	977.8	E858.8	E947.8	E950.4	E962.0	E980.4
Coniine, conine	965.7	E850.7	E935.7	E950.0	E962.0	E980.0
Conium (maculatum)	988.2	E865.4	—	E950.9	E962.1	E980.9
Conjugated estrogens (equine)	962.2	E858.0	E932.2	E950.4	E962.0	E980.4
Contac	975.6	E858.6	E945.6	E950.4	E962.0	E980.4
Contact lens solution	976.5	E858.7	E946.5	E950.4	E962.0	E980.4
Contraceptives (oral)	962.2	E858.0	E932.2	E950.4	E962.0	E980.4
vaginal	976.8	E858.7	E946.8	E950.4	E962.0	E980.4
Contrast media (roentgenographic)	977.8	E858.8	E947.8	E950.4	E962.0	E980.4
Convallaria majalis	988.2	E865.4	—	E950.9	E962.1	E980.9
Copper (dust) (fumes) (salts) NEC . .	985.8	E866.4	—.	E950.9	E962.1	E980.9
arsenate, arsenite	985.1	E866.3	—	E950.8	E962.1	E980.8
insecticide	985.1	E863.4	—	E950.8	E962.1	E980.8
emetic	973.6	E858.4	E943.6	E950.4	E962.0	E980.4
fungicide	985.8	E863.6	—	E950.6	E962.1	E980.7
insecticide	985.8	E863.4	—	E950.6	E962.1	E980.7
oleate	976.0	E858.7	E946.0	E950.4	E962.0	E980.4
sulfate	983.9	E864.3	—	E950.7	E962.1	E980.6
fungicide	983.9	E863.6	—	E950.7	E962.1	E980.6
cupric	973.6	E858.4	E943.6	E950.4	E962.0	E980.4
cuprous	983.9	E864.3	—	E950.7	E962.1	E980.6
Copperhead snake (bite) (venom)	989.5	E905.0	—	E950.9	E962.1	E980.9
Coral (sting)	989.5	E905.6	—	E950.9	E962.1	E980.9
snake (bite) (venom)	989.5	E905.0	—	E950.9	E962.1	E980.9
Cordran	976.0	E858.7	E946.0	E950.4	E962.0	E980.4
Corn cures	976.4	E858.7	E946.4	E950.4	E962.0	E980.4
Cornhusker's lotion	976.3	E858.7	E946.3	E950.4	E962.0	E980.4
Corn starch	976.3	E858.7	E946.3	E950.4	E962.0	E980.4
Corrosive	983.9	E864.4	—	E950.7	E962.1	E980.6
acids NEC	983.1	E864.1	—	E950.7	E962.1	E980.6
aromatics	983.0	E864.0	—	E950.7	E962.1	E980.6
disinfectant	983.0	E861.4	—	E950.7	E962.1	E980.6
fumes NEC	987.9	E869.9	—	E952.9	E962.2	E982.9

Substance	Poisoning	Accident	Therapeutic Use	Suicide Attempt	Assault	Undetermined
				External Cause (E-Code)		
specified NEC 983.9		E864.3	—	E950.7	E962.1	E980.6
sublimate — *see* Mercury, chloride						
Cortate 962.0		E858.0	E932.0	E950.4	E962.0	E980.4
Cort–Dome 962.0		E858.0	E932.0	E950.4	E962.0	E980.4
ENT agent. 976.6		E858.7	E946.6	E950.4	E962.0	E980.4
ophthalmic preparation. 976.5		E858.7	E946.5	E950.4	E962.0	E980.4
topical NEC 976.0		E858.7	E946.0	E950.4	E962.0	E980.4
Cortef 962.0		E858.0	E932.0	E950.4	E962.0	E980.4
ENT agent. 976.6		E858.7	E946.6	E950.4	E962.0	E980.4
ophthalmic preparation. 976.5		E858.7	E946.5	E950.4	E962.0	E980.4
topical NEC 976.0		E858.7	E946.0	E950.4	E962.0	E980.4
Corticosteroids (fluorinated) 962.0		E858.0	E932.0	E950.4	E962.0	E980.4
ENT agent. 976.6		E858.7	E946.6	E950.4	E962.0	E980.4
ophthalmic preparation. 976.5		E858.7	E946.5	E950.4	E962.0	E980.4
topical NEC 976.0		E858.7	E946.0	E950.4	E962.0	E980.4
Corticotropin 962.4		E858.0	E932.4	E950.4	E962.0	E980.4
Cortisol 962.0		E858.0	E932.0	E950.4	E962.0	E980.4
ENT agent. 976.6		E858.7	E946.6	E950.4	E962.0	E980.4
ophthalmic preparation. 976.5		E858.7	E946.5	E950.4	E962.0	E980.4
topical NEC 976.0		E858.7	E946.0	E950.4	E962.0	E980.4
Cortisone derivatives (acetate) 962.0		E858.0	E932.0	E950.4	E962.0	E980.4
ENT agent. 976.6		E858.7	E946.6	E950.4	E962.0	E980.4
ophthalmic preparation. 976.5		E858.7	E946.5	E950.4	E962.0	E980.4
topical NEC 976.0		E858.7	E946.0	E950.4	E962.0	E980.4
Cortogen 962.0		E858.0	E932.0	E950.4	E962.0	E980.4
ENT agent. 976.6		E858.7	E946.6	E950.4	E962.0	E980.4
ophthalmic preparation. 976.5		E858.7	E946.5	E950.4	E962.0	E980.4
Cortone. 962.0		E858.0	E932.0	E950.4	E962.0	E980.4
ENT agent. 976.6		E858.7	E946.6	E950.4	E962.0	E980.4
ophthalmic preparation. 976.5		E858.7	E946.5	E950.4	E962.0	E980.4
Cortril 962.0		E858.0	E932.0	E950.4	E962.0	E980.4
ENT agent. 976.6		E858.7	E946.6	E950.4	E962.0	E980.4
ophthalmic preparation. 976.5		E858.7	E946.5	E950.4	E962.0	E980.4
topical NEC 976.0		E858.7	E946.0	E950.4	E962.0	E980.4
Cosmetics. 989.89		E866.7	—	E950.9	E962.1	E980.9
Cosyntropin 977.8		E858.8	E947.8	E950.4	E962.0	E980.4
Cotarnine 964.5		E858.2	E934.5	E950.4	E962.0	E980.4
Cotton*seed* oil 976.3		E858.7	E946.3	E950.4	E962.0	E980.4
Cough mixtures (antitussives). 975.4		E858.6	E945.4	E950.4	E962.0	E980.4
containing opiates. 965.09		E850.2	E935.2	E950.0	E962.0	E980.0
expectorants 975.5		E858.6	E945.5	E950.4	E962.0	E980.4
Coumadin 964.2		E858.2	E934.2	E950.4	E962.0	E980.4
rodenticide. 989.4		E863.7	—	E950.6	E962.1	E980.7
Coumarin 964.2		E858.2	E934.2	E950.4	E962.0	E980.4
Coumetarol 964.2		E858.2	E934.2	E950.4	E962.0	E980.4
Cowbane 988.2		E865.4	—	E950.9	E962.1	E980.9
Cozyme. 963.5		E858.1	E933.5	E950.4	E962.0	E980.4
Crack. 970.8		E854.3	E940.8	E950.4	E962.0	E980.4
Creolin 983.0		E864.0	—	E950.7	E962.1	E980.6
disinfectant 983.0		E861.4	—	E950.7	E962.1	E980.6
Creosol (compound). 983.0		E864.0	—	E950.7	E962.1	E980.6
Creosote (beechwood) (coal tar). 983.0		E864.0	—	E950.7	E962.1	E980.6
medicinal (expectorant) 975.5		E858.6	E945.5	E950.4	E962.0	E980.4
syrup 975.5		E858.6	E945.5	E950.4	E962.0	E980.4
Cresol 983.0		E864.0	—	E950.7	E962.1	E980.6
disinfectant 983.0		E861.4	—	E950.7	E962.1	E980.6
Cresylic acid 983.0		E864.0	—	E950.7	E962.1	E980.6
Cropropamide 965.7		E850.7	E935.7	E950.0	E962.0	E980.0
with crotethamide. 970.0		E854.3	E940.0	E950.4	E962.0	E980.4
Crotamiton 976.0		E858.7	E946.0	E950.4	E962.0	E980.4
Crotethamide 965.7		E850.7	E935.7	E950.0	E962.0	E980.0

TABLE OF DRUGS AND CHEMICALS

Substance	Poisoning	Accident	Therapeutic Use	Suicide Attempt	Assault	Undetermined
			External Cause (E-Code)			
with cropropamide	970.0	E854.3	E940.0	E950.4	E962.0	E980.4
Croton (oil)	973.1	E858.4	E943.1	E950.4	E962.0	E980.4
chloral	967.1	E852.0	E937.1	E950.2	E962.0	E980.2
Crude oil	981	E862.1	—	E950.9	E962.1	E980.9
Cryogenine	965.8	E850.8	E935.8	E950.0	E962.0	E980.0
Cryolite (pesticide)	989.4	E863.4	—	E950.6	E962.1	E980.7
Cryptenamine	972.6	E858.3	E942.6	E950.4	E962.0	E980.4
Crystal violet	976.0	E858.7	E946.0	E950.4	E962.0	E980.4
Cuckoopint	988.2	E865.4	—	E950.9	E962.1	E980.9
Cumetharol	964.2	E858.2	E934.2	E950.4	E962.0	E980.4
Cupric sulfate	973.6	E858.4	E943.6	E950.4	E962.0	E980.4
Cuprous sulfate	983.9	E864.3	—	E950.7	E962.1	E980.6
Curare, curarine	975.2	E858.6	E945.2	E950.4	E962.0	E980.4
Cyanic acid — *see* Cyanide(s)						
Cyanide(s) (compounds) (hydrogen) (potassium) (sodium) NEC	989.0	E866.8	—	E950.9	E962.1	E980.9
dust or gas (inhalation) NEC	987.7	E869.8	—	E952.8	E962.2	E982.8
fumigant	989.0	E863.8	—	E950.6	E962.1	E980.7
mercuric — *see* Mercury						
pesticide (dust) (fumes)	989.0	E863.4	—	E950.6	E962.1	E980.7
Cyanocobalamin	964.1	E858.2	E934.1	E950.4	E962.0	E980.4
Cyanogen (chloride) (gas) NEC	987.8	E869.8	—	E952.8	E962.2	E982.8
Cyclaine	968.5	E855.2	E938.5	E950.4	E962.0	E980.4
Cyclamen europaeum	988.2	E865.4	—	E950.9	E962.1	E980.9
Cyclandelate	972.5	E858.3	E942.5	E950.4	E962.0	E980.4
Cyclazocine	965.09	E850.2	E935.2	E950.0	E962.0	E980.0
Cyclizine	963.0	E858.1	E933.0	E950.4	E962.0	E980.4
Cyclobarbital, cyclobarbitone	967.0	E851	E937.0	E950.1	E962.0	E980.1
Cycloguanil	961.4	E857	E931.4	E950.4	E962.0	E980.4
Cyclohexane	982.0	E862.4	—	E950.9	E962.1	E980.9
Cyclohexanol	980.8	E860.8	—	E950.9	E962.1	E980.9
Cyclohexanone	982.8	E862.4	—	E950.9	E962.1	E980.9
Cyclomethycaine	968.5	E855.2	E938.5	E950.4	E962.0	E980.4
Cyclopentamine	971.2	E855.5	E941.2	E950.4	E962.0	E980.4
Cyclopenthiazide	974.3	E858.5	E944.3	E950.4	E962.0	E980.4
Cyclopentolate	971.1	E855.4	E941.1	E950.4	E962.0	E980.4
Cyclophosphamide	963.1	E858.1	E933.1	E950.4	E962.0	E980.4
Cyclopropane	968.2	E855.1	E938.2	E950.4	E962.0	E980.4
Cycloserine	960.6	E856	E930.6	E950.4	E962.0	E980.4
Cyclothiazide	974.3	E858.5	E944.3	E950.4	E962.0	E980.4
Cycrimine	966.4	E855.0	E936.4	E950.4	E962.0	E980.4
Cymarin	972.1	E858.3	E942.1	E950.4	E962.0	E980.4
Cyproheptadine	963.0	E858.1	E933.0	E950.4	E962.0	E980.4
Cyprolidol	969.09	E854.0	E939.0	E950.3	E962.0	E980.3
Cytarabine	963.1	E858.1	E933.1	E950.4	E962.0	E980.4
Cytisus						
laburnum	988.2	E865.4	—	E950.9	E962.1	E980.9
scoparius	988.2	E865.4	—	E950.9	E962.1	E980.9
Cytomel	962.7	E858.0	E932.7	E950.4	E962.0	E980.4
Cytosine (antineoplastic)	963.1	E858.1	E933.1	E950.4	E962.0	E980.4
Cytoxan	963.1	E858.1	E933.1	E950.4	E962.0	E980.4
Dacarbazine	963.1	E858.1	E933.1	E950.4	E962.0	E980.4
Dactinomycin	960.7	E856	E930.7	E950.4	E962.0	E980.4
DADPS	961.8	E857	E931.8	E950.4	E962.0	E980.4
Dakin's solution (external)	976.0	E858.7	E946.0	E950.4	E962.0	E980.4
Dalmane	969.4	E853.2	E939.4	E950.3	E962.0	E980.3
DAM	977.2	E858.8	E947.2	E950.4	E962.0	E980.4
Danilone	964.2	E858.2	E934.2	E950.4	E962.0	E980.4
Danthron	973.1	E858.4	E943.1	E950.4	E962.0	E980.4
Dantrolene	975.2	E858.6	E945.2	E950.4	E962.0	E980.4

Substance	Poisoning	Accident	Therapeutic Use	Suicide Attempt	Assault	Undetermined
			External Cause (E-Code)			
Daphne (gnidium) (mezereum)	988.2	E865.4	—	E950.9	E962.1	E980.9
berry	988.2	E865.3	—	E950.9	E962.1	E980.9
Dapsone	961.8	E857	E931.8	E950.4	E962.0	E980.4
Daraprim	961.4	E857	E931.4	E950.4	E962.0	E980.4
Darnel	988.2	E865.3	—	E950.9	E962.1	E980.9
Darvon	965.8	E850.8	E935.8	E950.0	E962.0	E980.0
Daunorubicin	960.7	E856	E930.7	E950.4	E962.0	E980.4
DBI	962.3	E858.0	E932.3	E950.4	E962.0	E980.4
D–Con (rodenticide)	989.4	E863.7	—	E950.6	E962.1	E980.7
DDS	961.8	E857	E931.8	E950.4	E962.0	E980.4
DDT	989.2	E863.0	—	E950.6	E962.1	E980.7
Deadly nightshade	988.2	E865.4	—	E950.9	E962.1	E980.9
berry	988.2	E865.3	—	E950.9	E962.1	E980.9
Deanol	969.79	E854.2	E939.7	E950.3	E962.0	E980.3
Debrisoquine	972.6	E858.3	E942.6	E950.4	E962.0	E980.4
Decaborane	989.89	E866.8	—	E950.9	E962.1	E980.9
fumes	987.8	E869.8	—	E952.8	E962.2	E982.8
Decadron	962.0	E858.0	E932.0	E950.4	E962.0	E980.4
ENT agent	976.6	E858.7	E946.6	E950.4	E962.0	E980.4
ophthalmic preparation	976.5	E858.7	E946.5	E950.4	E962.0	E980.4
topical NEC	976.0	E858.7	E946.0	E950.4	E962.0	E980.4
Decahydronaphthalene	982.0	E862.4	—	E950.9	E962.1	E980.9
Decalin	982.0	E862.4	—	E950.9	E962.1	E980.9
Decamethonium	975.2	E858.6	E945.2	E950.4	E962.0	E980.4
Decholin	973.4	E858.4	E943.4	E950.4	E962.0	E980.4
sodium (diagnostic)	977.8	E858.8	E947.8	E950.4	E962.0	E980.4
Declomycin	960.4	E856	E930.4	E950.4	E962.0	E980.4
Deferoxamine	963.8	E858.1	E933.8	E950.4	E962.0	E980.4
Dehydrocholic acid	973.4	E858.4	E943.4	E950.4	E962.0	E980.4
DeKalin	982.0	E862.4	—	E950.9	E962.1	E980.9
Delalutin	962.2	E858.0	E932.2	E950.4	E962.0	E980.4
Delphinium	988.2	E865.3	—	E950.9	E962.1	E980.9
Deltasone	962.0	E858.0	E932.0	E950.4	E962.0	E980.4
Deltra	962.0	E858.0	E932.0	E950.4	E962.0	E980.4
Delvinal	967.0	E851	E937.0	E950.1	E962.0	E980.1
Demecarium (bromide)	971.0	E855.3	E941.0	E950.4	E962.0	E980.4
Demeclocycline	960.4	E856	E930.4	E950.4	E962.0	E980.4
Demecolcine	963.1	E858.1	E933.1	E950.4	E962.0	E980.4
Demelanizing agents	976.8	E858.7	E946.8	E950.4	E962.0	E980.4
Demerol	965.09	E850.2	E935.2	E950.0	E962.0	E980.0
Demethylchlortetracycline	960.4	E856	E930.4	E950.4	E962.0	E980.4
Demethyltetracycline	960.4	E856	E930.4	E950.4	E962.0	E980.4
Demeton	989.3	E863.1	—	E950.6	E962.1	E980.7
Demulcents	976.3	E858.7	E946.3	E950.4	E962.0	E980.4
Demulen	962.2	E858.0	E932.2	E950.4	E962.0	E980.4
Denatured alcohol	980.0	E860.1	—	E950.9	E962.1	E980.9
Dendrid	976.5	E858.7	E946.5	E950.4	E962.0	E980.4
Dental agents, topical	976.7	E858.7	E946.7	E950.4	E962.0	E980.4
Deodorant spray (feminine hygiene)	976.8	E858.7	E946.8	E950.4	E962.0	E980.4
Deoxyribonuclease	963.4	E858.1	E933.4	E950.4	E962.0	E980.4
Depressants						
appetite, central	977.0	E858.8	E947.0	E950.4	E962.0	E980.4
cardiac	972.0	E858.3	E942.0	E950.4	E962.0	E980.4
central nervous system (anesthetic)	968.4	E855.1	E938.4	E950.4	E962.0	E980.4
psychotherapeutic	969.5	E853.9	E939.5	E950.3	E962.0	E980.3
Dequalinium	976.0	E858.7	E946.0	E950.4	E962.0	E980.4
Dermolate	976.2	E858.7	E946.2	E950.4	E962.0	E980.4
DES	962.2	E858.0	E932.2	E950.4	E962.0	E980.4
Desenex	976.0	E858.7	E946.0	E950.4	E962.0	E980.4
Deserpidine	972.6	E858.3	E942.6	E950.4	E962.0	E980.4
Desipramine	969.05	E854.0	E939.0	E950.3	E962.0	E980.3

Substance	Poisoning	Accident	Therapeutic Use	Suicide Attempt	Assault	Undetermined
			External Cause (E-Code)			
Deslanoside	972.1	E858.3	E942.1	E950.4	E962.0	E980.4
Desocodeine	965.09	E850.2	E935.2	E950.0	E962.0	E980.0
Desomorphine	965.09	E850.2	E935.2	E950.0	E962.0	E980.0
Desonide	976.0	E858.7	E946.0	E950.4	E962.0	E980.4
Desoxycorticosterone derivatives	962.0	E858.0	E932.0	E950.4	E962.0	E980.4
Desoxyephedrine	969.72	E854.2	E939.7	E950.3	E962.0	E980.3
DET	969.6	E854.1	E939.6	E950.3	E962.0	E980.3
Detergents (ingested) (synthetic)	989.6	E861.0	—	E950.9	E962.1	E980.9
external medication	976.2	E858.7	E946.2	E950.4	E962.0	E980.4
Deterrent, alcohol	977.3	E858.8	E947.3	E950.4	E962.0	E980.4
Detrothyronine	962.7	E858.0	E932.7	E950.4	E962.0	E980.4
Dettol (external medication)	976.0	E858.7	E946.0	E950.4	E962.0	E980.4
Dexamethasone	962.0	E858.0	E932.0	E950.4	E962.0	E980.4
ENT agent	976.6	E858.7	E946.6	E950.4	E962.0	E980.4
ophthalmic preparation	976.5	E858.7	E946.5	E950.4	E962.0	E980.4
topical NEC	976.0	E858.7	E946.0	E950.4	E962.0	E980.4
Dexamphetamine	969.72	E854.2	E939.7	E950.3	E962.0	E980.3
Dexedrine	969.72	E854.2	E939.7	E950.3	E962.0	E980.3
Dexpanthenol	963.5	E858.1	E933.5	E950.4	E962.0	E980.4
Dextran	964.8	E858.2	E934.8	E950.4	E962.0	E980.4
Dextriferron	964.0	E858.2	E934.0	E950.4	E962.0	E980.4
Dextroamphetamine	969.72	E854.2	E939.7	E950.3	E962.0	E980.3
Dextro calcium pantothenate	963.5	E858.1	E933.5	E950.4	E962.0	E980.4
Dextromethorphan	975.4	E858.6	E945.4	E950.4	E962.0	E980.4
Dextromoramide	965.09	E850.2	E935.2	E950.0	E962.0	E980.0
Dextro pantothenyl alcohol	963.5	E858.1	E933.5	E950.4	E962.0	E980.4
topical	976.8	E858.7	E946.8	E950.4	E962.0	E980.4
Dextropropoxyphene (hydrochloride)	965.8	E850.8	E935.8	E950.0	E962.0	E980.0
Dextrorphan	965.09	E850.2	E935.2	E950.0	E962.0	E980.0
Dextrose NEC	974.5	E858.5	E944.5	E950.4	E962.0	E980.4
Dextrothyroxin	962.7	E858.0	E932.7	E950.4	E962.0	E980.4
DFP	971.0	E855.3	E941.0	E950.4	E962.0	E980.4
DHE–45	972.9	E858.3	E942.9	E950.4	E962.0	E980.4
Diabinese	962.3	E858.0	E932.3	E950.4	E962.0	E980.4
Diacetyl monoxime	977.2	E858.8	E947.2	E950.4	E962.0	E980.4
Diacetylmorphine	965.01	E850.0	E935.0	E950.0	E962.0	E980.0
Diagnostic agents	977.8	E858.8	E947.8	E950.4	E962.0	E980.4
Dial (soap)	976.2	E858.7	E946.2	E950.4	E962.0	E980.4
sedative	967.0	E851	E937.0	E950.1	E962.0	E980.1
Diallylbarbituric acid	967.0	E851	E937.0	E950.1	E962.0	E980.1
Diaminodiphenylsulfone	961.8	E857	E931.8	E950.4	E962.0	E980.4
Diamorphine	965.01	E850.0	E935.0	E950.0	E962.0	E980.0
Diamox	974.2	E858.5	E944.2	E950.4	E962.0	E980.4
Diamthazole	976.0	E858.7	E946.0	E950.4	E962.0	E980.4
Diaphenylsulfone	961.8	E857	E931.8	E950.4	E962.0	E980.4
Diasone (sodium)	961.8	E857	E931.8	E950.4	E962.0	E980.4
Diazepam	969.4	E853.2	E939.4	E950.3	E962.0	E980.3
Diazinon	989.3	E863.1	—	E950.6	E962.1	E980.7
Diazomethane (gas)	987.8	E869.8	—	E952.8	E962.2	E982.8
Diazoxide	972.5	E858.3	E942.5	E950.4	E962.0	E980.4
Dibenamine	971.3	E855.6	E941.3	E950.4	E962.0	E980.4
Dibenzheptropine	963.0	E858.1	E933.0	E950.4	E962.0	E980.4
Dibenzyline	971.3	E855.6	E941.3	E950.4	E962.0	E980.4
Diborane (gas)	987.8	E869.8	—	E952.8	E962.2	E982.8
Dibromomannitol	963.1	E858.1	E933.1	E950.4	E962.0	E980.4
Dibucaine (spinal)	968.7	E855.2	E938.7	E950.4	E962.0	E980.4
topical (surface)	968.5	E855.2	E938.5	E950.4	E962.0	E980.4
Dibunate sodium	975.4	E858.6	E945.4	E950.4	E962.0	E980.4
Dibutoline	971.1	E855.4	E941.1	E950.4	E962.0	E980.4
Dicapthon	989.4	E863.4	—	E950.6	E962.1	E980.7

TABLE OF DRUGS AND CHEMICALS

Substance	Poisoning	Accident	Therapeutic Use	Suicide Attempt	Assault	Undetermined
				External Cause (E-Code)		
Dichloralphenazone 967.1	E852.0	E937.1	E950.2	E962.0	E980.2
Dichlorodifluoromethane 987.4	E869.2	—	E952.8	E962.2	E982.8
Dichloroethane 982.3	E862.4	—	E950.9	E962.1	E980.9
Dichloroethylene 982.3	E862.4	—	E950.9	E962.1	E980.9
Dichloroethyl sulfide 987.8	E869.8	—	E952.8	E962.2	E982.8
Dichlorohydrin 982.3	E862.4	—	E950.9	E962.1	E980.9
Dichloromethane (solvent) (vapor) 982.3	E862.4	—	E950.9	E962.1	E980.9
Dichlorophen(e) 961.6	E857	E931.6	E950.4	E962.0	E980.4
Dichlorphenamide 974.2	E858.5	E944.2	E950.4	E962.0	E980.4
Dichlorvos 989.3	E863.1	—	E950.6	E962.1	E980.7
Diclofenac sodium 965.69	E850.6	E935.6	E950.0	E962.0	E980.0
Dicoumarin, dicumarol 964.2	E858.2	E934.2	E950.4	E962.0	E980.4
Dicyanogen (gas) 987.8	E869.8	—	E952.8	E962.2	E982.8
Dicyclomine 971.1	E855.4	E941.1	E950.4	E962.0	E980.4
Dieldrin (vapor) 989.2	E863.0	—	E950.6	E962.1	E980.7
Dienestrol 962.2	E858.0	E932.2	E950.4	E962.0	E980.4
Dietetics 977.0	E858.8	E947.0	E950.4	E962.0	E980.4
Diethazine 966.4	E855.0	E936.4	E950.4	E962.0	E980.4
Diethyl					
barbituric acid 967.0	E851	E937.0	E950.1	E962.0	E980.1
carbamazine 961.6	E857	E931.6	E950.4	E962.0	E980.4
carbinol 980.8	E860.8	—	E950.9	E962.1	E980.9
carbonate 982.8	E862.4	—	E950.9	E962.1	E980.9
ether (vapor) — see Ether(s)					
propion 977.0	E858.8	E947.0	E950.4	E962.0	E980.4
stilbestrol 962.2	E858.0	E932.2	E950.4	E962.0	E980.4
Diethylene					
dioxide 982.8	E862.4	—	E950.9	E962.1	E980.9
glycol (monoacetate) (monoethyl ether) . . . 982.8	E862.4	—	E950.9	E962.1	E980.9
Diethylsulfone–diethylmethane 967.8	E852.8	E937.8	E950.2	E962.0	E980.2
Difencloxazine 965.09	E850.2	E935.2	E950.0	E962.0	E980.0
Diffusin 963.4	E858.1	E933.4	E950.4	E962.0	E980.4
Diflos 971.0	E855.3	E941.0	E950.4	E962.0	E980.4
Digestants 973.4	E858.4	E943.4	E950.4	E962.0	E980.4
Digitalin(e) 972.1	E858.3	E942.1	E950.4	E962.0	E980.4
Digitalis glycosides 972.1	E858.3	E942.1	E950.4	E962.0	E980.4
Digitoxin 972.1	E858.3	E942.1	E950.4	E962.0	E980.4
Digoxin 972.1	E858.3	E942.1	E950.4	E962.0	E980.4
Dihydrocodeine 965.09	E850.2	E935.2	E950.0	E962.0	E980.0
Dihydrocodeinone 965.09	E850.2	E935.2	E950.0	E962.0	E980.0
Dihydroergocristine 972.9	E858.3	E942.9	E950.4	E962.0	E980.4
Dihydroergotamine 972.9	E858.3	E942.9	E950.4	E962.0	E980.4
Dihydroergotoxine 972.9	E858.3	E942.9	E950.4	E962.0	E980.4
Dihydrohydroxycodeinone 965.09	E850.2	E935.2	E950.0	E962.0	E980.0
Dihydrohydroxymorphinone 965.09	E850.2	E935.2	E950.0	E962.0	E980.0
Dihydroisocodeine 965.09	E850.2	E935.2	E950.0	E962.0	E980.0
Dihydromorphine 965.09	E850.2	E935.2	E950.0	E962.0	E980.0
Dihydromorphinone 965.09	E850.2	E935.2	E950.0	E962.0	E980.0
Dihydrostreptomycin 960.6	E856	E930.6	E950.4	E962.0	E980.4
Dihydrotachysterol 962.6	E858.0	E932.6	E950.4	E962.0	E980.4
Dihydroxyanthraquinone 973.1	E858.4	E943.1	E950.4	E962.0	E980.4
Dihydroxycodeinone 965.09	E850.2	E935.2	E950.0	E962.0	E980.0
Diiodohydroxyquin . . . . : 961.3	E857	E931.3	E950.4	E962.0	E980.4
topical 976.0	E858.7	E946.0	E950.4	E962.0	E980.4
Diiodohydroxyquinoline 961.3	E857	E931.3	E950.4	E962.0	E980.4
Dilantin 966.1	E855.0	E936.1	E950.4	E962.0	E980.4
Dilaudid 965.09	E850.2	E935.2	E950.0	E962.0	E980.0
Diloxanide 961.5	E857	E931.5	E950.4	E962.0	E980.4
Dimefline 970.0	E854.3	E940.0	E950.4	E962.0	E980.4
Dimenhydrinate 963.0	E858.1	E933.0	E950.4	E962.0	E980.4
Dimercaprol 963.8	E858.1	E933.8	E950.4	E962.0	E980.4

Substance	Poisoning	Accident	Therapeutic Use	Suicide Attempt	Assault	Undetermined
			External Cause (E-Code)			
Dimercaptopropanol	963.8	E858.1	E933.8	E950.4	E962.0	E980.4
Dimetane	963.0	E858.1	E933.0	E950.4	E962.0	E980.4
Dimethicone	976.3	E858.7	E946.3	E950.4	E962.0	E980.4
Dimethindene	963.0	E858.1	E933.0	E950.4	E962.0	E980.4
Dimethisoquin	968.5	E855.2	E938.5	E950.4	E962.0	E980.4
Dimethisterone	962.2	E858.0	E932.2	E950.4	E962.0	E980.4
Dimethoxanate	975.4	E858.6	E945.4	E950.4	E962.0	E980.4
Dimethyl						
arsine, arsinic acid — *see* Arsenic						
carbinol	980.2	E860.3	—	E950.9	E962.1	E980.9
diguanide	962.3	E858.0	E932.3	E950.4	E962.0	E980.4
ketone	982.8	E862.4	—	E950.9	E962.1	E980.9
vapor	987.8	E869.8	—	E952.8	E962.2	E982.8
meperidine	965.09	E850.2	E935.2	E950.0	E962.0	E980.0
parathion	989.3	E863.1	—	E950.6	E962.1	E980.7
polysiloxane	973.8	E858.4	E943.8	E950.4	E962.0	E980.4
sulfate (fumes)	987.8	E869.8	—	E952.8	E962.2	E982.8
liquid	983.9	E864.3	—	E950.7	E962.1	E980.6
sulfoxide NEC	982.8	E862.4	—	E950.9	E962.1	E980.9
medicinal	976.4	E858.7	E946.4	E950.4	E962.0	E980.4
triptamine	969.6	E854.1	E939.6	E950.3	E962.0	E980.3
tubocurarine	975.2	E858.6	E945.2	E950.4	E962.0	E980.4
Dindevan	964.2	E858.2	E934.2	E950.4	E962.0	E980.4
Dinitro (–ortho–) cresol (herbicide) (spray)	989.4	E863.5	—	E950.6	E962.1	E980.7
insecticide	989.4	E863.4	—	E950.6	E962.1	E980.7
Dinitrobenzene	983.0	E864.0	—	E950.7	E962.1	E980.6
vapor	987.8	E869.8	—	E952.8	E962.2	E982.8
Dinitro–orthocresol (herbicide)	989.4	E863.5	—	E950.6	E962.1	E980.7
insecticide	989.4	E863.4	—	E950.6	E962.1	E980.7
Dinitrophenol (herbicide) (spray)	989.4	E863.5	—	E950.6	E962.1	E980.7
insecticide	989.4	E863.4	—	E950.6	E962.1	E980.7
Dinoprost	975.0	E858.6	E945.0	E950.4	E962.0	E980.4
Dioctyl sulfosuccinate (calcium) (sodium)	973.2	E858.4	E943.2	E950.4	E962.0	E980.4
Diodoquin	961.3	E857	E931.3	E950.4	E962.0	E980.4
Dione derivatives NEC	966.3	E855.0	E936.3	E950.4	E962.0	E980.4
Dionin	965.09	E850.2	E935.2	E950.0	E962.0	E980.0
Dioxane	982.8	E862.4	—	E950.9	E962.1	E980.9
Dioxin — *see* herbicide						
Dioxyline	972.5	E858.3	E942.5	E950.4	E962.0	E980.4
Dipentene	982.8	E862.4	—	E950.9	E962.1	E980.9
Diphemanil	971.1	E855.4	E941.1	E950.4	E962.0	E980.4
Diphenadione	964.2	E858.2	E934.2	E950.4	E962.0	E980.4
Diphenhydramine	963.0	E858.1	E933.0	E950.4	E962.0	E980.4
Diphenidol	963.0	E858.1	E933.0	E950.4	E962.0	E980.4
Diphenoxylate	973.5	E858.4	E943.5	E950.4	E962.0	E980.4
Diphenylchloroarsine	985.1	E866.3	—	E950.8	E962.1	E980.8
Diphenylhydantoin (sodium)	966.1	E855.0	E936.1	E950.4	E962.0	E980.4
Diphenylpyraline	963.0	E858.1	E933.0	E950.4	E962.0	E980.4
Diphtheria						
antitoxin	979.9	E858.8	E949.9	E950.4	E962.0	E980.4
toxoid	978.5	E858.8	E948.5	E950.4	E962.0	E980.4
with tetanus toxoid	978.9	E858.8	E948.9	E950.4	E962.0	E980.4
with pertussis component	978.6	E858.8	E948.6	E950.4	E962.0	E980.4
vaccine	978.5	E858.8	E948.5	E950.4	E962.0	E980.4
Dipipanone	965.09	E850.2	E935.2	E950.0	E962.0	E980.0
Diplovax	979.5	E858.8	E949.5	E950.4	E962.0	E980.4
Diprophylline	975.1	E858.6	E945.1	E950.4	E962.0	E980.4
Dipyridamole	972.4	E858.3	E942.4	E950.4	E962.0	E980.4
Dipyrone	965.5	E850.5	E935.5	E950.0	E962.0	E980.0
Diquat	989.4	E863.5	—	E950.6	E962.1	E980.7

Substance	Poisoning	Accident	Therapeutic Use	Suicide Attempt	Assault	Undetermined
			External Cause (E-Code)			
Disinfectant NEC.	983.9	E861.4	—	E950.7	E962.1	E980.6
alkaline	983.2	E861.4	—	E950.7	E962.1	E980.6
aromatic.	983.0	E861.4	—	E950.7	E962.1	E980.6
Disipal	966.4	E855.0	E936.4	E950.4	E962.0	E980.4
Disodium edetate.	963.8	E858.1	E933.8	E950.4	E962.0	E980.4
Disulfamide	974.4	E858.5	E944.4	E950.4	E962.0	E980.4
Disulfanilamide	961.0	E857	E931.0	E950.4	E962.0	E980.4
Disulfiram.	977.3	E858.8	E947.3	E950.4	E962.0	E980.4
Dithiazanine.	961.6	E857	E931.6	E950.4	E962.0	E980.4
Dithioglycerol	963.8	E858.1	E933.8	E950.4	E962.0	E980.4
Dithranol	976.4	E858.7	E946.4	E950.4	E962.0	E980.4
Diucardin	974.3	E858.5	E944.3	E950.4	E962.0	E980.4
Diupres.	974.3	E858.5	E944.3	E950.4	E962.0	E980.4
Diuretics NEC.	974.4	E858.5	E944.4	E950.4	E962.0	E980.4
carbonic acid anhydrase inhibitors	974.2	E858.5	E944.2	E950.4	E962.0	E980.4
mercurial	974.0	E858.5	E944.0	E950.4	E962.0	E980.4
osmotic	974.4	E858.5	E944.4	E950.4	E962.0	E980.4
purine derivatives	974.1	E858.5	E944.1	E950.4	E962.0	E980.4
saluretic.	974.3	E858.5	E944.3	E950.4	E962.0	E980.4
Diuril.	974.3	E858.5	E944.3	E950.4	E962.0	E980.4
Divinyl ether	968.2	E855.1	E938.2	E950.4	E962.0	E980.4
D–lysergic acid diethylamide	969.6	E854.1	E939.6	E950.3	E962.0	E980.3
DMCT	960.4	E856	E930.4	E950.4	E962.0	E980.4
DMSO	982.8	E862.4	—	E950.9	E962.1	E980.9
DMT.	969.6	E854.1	E939.6	E950.3	E962.0	E980.3
DNOC	989.4	E863.5	—	E950.6	E962.1	E980.7
DOCA	962.0	E858.0	E932.0	E950.4	E962.0	E980.4
Dolophine.	965.02	E850.1	E935.1	E950.0	E962.0	E980.0
Doloxene	965.8	E850.8	E935.8	E950.0	E962.0	E980.0
DOM.	969.6	E854.1	E939.6	E950.3	E962.0	E980.3
Domestic gas — see Gas, utility						
Domiphen (bromide) (lozenges)	976.6	E858.7	E946.6	E950.4	E962.0	E980.4
Dopa (levo)	966.4	E855.0	E936.4	E950.4	E962.0	E980.4
Dopamine	971.2	E855.5	E941.2	E950.4	E962.0	E980.4
Doriden.	967.5	E852.4	E937.5	E950.2	E962.0	E980.2
Dormiral	967.0	E851	E937.0	E950.1	E962.0	E980.1
Dormison	967.8	E852.8	E937.8	E950.2	E962.0	E980.2
Dornase.	963.4	E858.1	E933.4	E950.4	E962.0	E980.4
Dorsacaine	968.5	E855.2	E938.5	E950.4	E962.0	E980.4
Dothiepin hydrochloride	969.05	E854.0	E939.0	E950.3	E962.0	E980.3
Doxapram.	970.0	E854.3	E940.0	E950.4	E962.0	E980.4
Doxepin	969.05	E854.0	E939.0	E950.3	E962.0	E980.3
Doxorubicin	960.7	E856	E930.7	E950.4	E962.0	E980.4
Doxycycline	960.4	E856	E930.4	E950.4	E962.0	E980.4
Doxylamine	963.0	E858.1	E933.0	E950.4	E962.0	E980.4
Dramamine	963.0	E858.1	E933.0	E950.4	E962.0	E980.4
Drano (drain cleaner)	983.2	E864.2	—	E950.7	E962.1	E980.6
Dromoran	965.09	E850.2	E935.2	E950.0	E962.0	E980.0
Dromostanolone	962.1	E858.0	E932.1	E950.4	E962.0	E980.4
Droperidol.	969.2	E853.1	E939.2	E950.3	E962.0	E980.3
Drotrecogin alfa	964.2	E858.2	E934.2	E950.4	E962.0	E980.4
Drug.	977.9	E858.9	E947.9	E950.5	E962.0	E980.5
specified NEC	977.8	E858.8	E947.8	E950.4	E962.0	E980.4
AHFS List						
4:00 antihistamine drugs	963.0	E858.1	E933.0	E950.4	E962.0	E980.4
8:04 amebacides	961.5	E857	E931.5	E950.4	E962.0	E980.4
arsenical anti–infectives.	961.1	E857	E931.1	E950.4	E962.0	E980.4
quinoline derivatives	961.3	E857	E931.3	E950.4	E962.0	E980.4
8:08 anthelmintics.	961.6	E857	E931.6	E950.4	E962.0	E980.4
quinoline derivatives	961.3	E857	E931.3	E950.4	E962.0	E980.4
8:12.04 antifungal antibiotics	960.1	E856	E930.1	E950.4	E962.0	E980.4

Substance	Poisoning	Accident	Therapeutic Use	Suicide Attempt	Assault	Undetermined
			External Cause (E-Code)			
8:12.06 cephalosporins	960.5	E856	E930.5	E950.4	E962.0	E980.4
8:12.08 chloramphenicol	960.2	E856	E930.2	E950.4	E962.0	E980.4
8:12.12 erythromycins	960.3	E856	E930.3	E950.4	E962.0	E980.4
8:12.16 penicillins	960.0	E856	E930.0	E950.4	E962.0	E980.4
8:12.20 streptomycins	960.6	E856	E930.6	E950.4	E962.0	E980.4
8:12.24 tetracyclines	960.4	E856	E930.4	E950.4	E962.0	E980.4
8:12.28 other antibiotics	960.8	E856	E930.8	E950.4	E962.0	E980.4
antimycobacterial	960.6	E856	E930.6	E950.4	E962.0	E980.4
macrolides	960.3	E856	E930.3	E950.4	E962.0	E980.4
8:16 antituberculars	961.8	E857	E931.8	E950.4	E962.0	E980.4
antibiotics	960.6	E856	E930.6	E950.4	E962.0	E980.4
8:18 antivirals	961.7	E857	E931.7	E950.4	E962.0	E980.4
8:20 plasmodicides (antimalarials)	961.4	E857	E931.4	E950.4	E962.0	E980.4
8:24 sulfonamides	961.0	E857	E931.0	E950.4	E962.0	E980.4
8:26 sulfones	961.8	E857	E931.8	E950.4	E962.0	E980.4
8:28 treponemicides	961.2	E857	E931.2	E950.4	E962.0	E980.4
8:32 trichomonacides	961.5	E857	E931.5	E950.4	E962.0	E980.4
quinoline derivatives	961.3	E857	E931.3	E950.4	E962.0	E980.4
nitrofuran derivatives	961.9	E857	E931.9	E950.4	E962.0	E980.4
8:36 urinary germicides	961.9	E857	E931.9	E950.4	E962.0	E980.4
quinoline derivatives	961.3	E857	E931.3	E950.4	E962.0	E980.4
8:40 other anti–infectives	961.9	E857	E931.9	E950.4	E962.0	E980.4
10:00 antineoplastic agents	963.1	E858.1	E933.1	E950.4	E962.0	E980.4
antibiotics	960.7	E856	E930.7	E950.4	E962.0	E980.4
progestogens	962.2	E858.0	E932.2	E950.4	E962.0	E980.4
12:04 parasympathomimetic (cholinergic) agents	971.0	E855.3	E941.0	E950.4	E962.0	E980.4
12:08 parasympatholytic (cholinergic –blocking) agents	971.1	E855.4	E941.1	E950.4	E962.0	E980.4
12:12 Sympathomimetic (adrenergic) agents	971.2	E855.5	E941.2	E950.4	E962.0	E980.4
12:16 sympatholytic (adrenergic– blocking) agents	971.3	E855.6	E941.3	E950.4	E962.0	E980.4
12:20 skeletal muscle relaxants central nervous system muscle-tone depressants	968.0	E855.1	E938.0	E950.4	E962.0	E980.4
myoneural blocking agents	975.2	E858.6	E945.2	E950.4	E962.0	E980.4
16:00 blood derivatives	964.7	E858.2	E934.7	E950.4	E962.0	E980.4
20:04 antianemia drugs	964.1	E858.2	E934.1	E950.4	E962.0	E980.4
20:04.04 iron preparations	964.0	E858.2	E934.0	E950.4	E962.0	E980.4
20:04.08 liver and stomach preparations	964.1	E858.2	E934.1	E950.4	E962.0	E980.4
20:12.04 anticoagulants	964.2	E858.2	E934.2	E950.4	E962.0	E980.4
20:12.08 antiheparin agents	964.5	E858.2	E934.5	E950.4	E962.0	E980.4
20:12.12 coagulants	964.5	E858.2	E934.5	E950.4	E962.0	E980.4
20:12.16 hemostatics NEC	964.5	E858.2	E934.5	E950.4	E962.0	E980.4
capillary active drugs	972.8	E858.3	E942.8	E950.4	E962.0	E980.4
24:04 cardiac drugs	972.9	E858.3	E942.9	E950.4	E962.0	E980.4
cardiotonic agents	972.1	E858.3	E942.1	E950.4	E962.0	E980.4
rhythm regulators	972.0	E858.3	E942.0	E950.4	E962.0	E980.4
24:06 antilipemic agents	972.2	E858.3	E942.2	E950.4	E962.0	E980.4
thyroid derivatives	962.7	E858.0	E932.7	E950.4	E962.0	E980.4
24:08 hypotensive agents	972.6	E858.3	E942.6	E950.4	E962.0	E980.4
adrenergic blocking agents	971.3	E855.6	E941.3	E950.4	E962.0	E980.4
ganglion blocking agents	972.3	E858.3	E942.3	E950.4	E962.0	E980.4
vasodilators	972.5	E858.3	E942.5	E950.4	E962.0	E980.4
24:12 vasodilating agents NEC	972.5	E858.3	E942.5	E950.4	E962.0	E980.4
coronary	972.4	E858.3	E942.4	E950.4	E962.0	E980.4
nicotinic acid derivatives	972.2	E858.3	E942.2	E950.4	E962.0	E980.4
24:16 sclerosing agents	972.7	E858.3	E942.7	E950.4	E962.0	E980.4
28:04 general anesthetics	968.4	E855.1	E938.4	E950.4	E962.0	E980.4

Substance	Poisoning	Accident	Therapeutic Use	Suicide Attempt	Assault	Undetermined
			External Cause (E-Code)			
gaseous anesthetics	968.2	E855.1	E938.2	E950.4	E962.0	E980.4
halothane	968.1	E855.1	E938.1	E950.4	E962.0	E980.4
intravenous anesthetics	968.3	E855.1	E938.3	E950.4	E962.0	E980.4
28:08 analgesics and antipyretics	965.9	E850.9	E935.9	E950.0	E962.0	E980.0
antirheumatics	965.69	E850.6	E935.6	E950.0	E962.0	E980.0
aromatic analgesics	965.4	E850.4	E935.4	E950.0	E962.0	E980.0
non–narcotic NEC	965.7	E850.7	E935.7	E950.0	E962.0	E980.0
opium alkaloids	965.00	E850.2	E935.2	E950.0	E962.0	E980.0
heroin	965.01	E850.0	E935.0	E950.0	E962.0	E980.0
methadone	965.02	E850.1	E935.1	E950.0	E962.0	E980.0
specified type NEC	965.09	E850.2	E935.2	E950.0	E962.0	E980.0
pyrazole derivatives	965.5	E850.5	E935.5	E950.0	E962.0	E980.0
salicylates	965.1	E850.3	E935.3	E950.0	E962.0	E980.0
specified NEC	965.8	E850.8	E935.8	E950.0	E962.0	E980.0
28:10 narcotic antagonists	970.1	E854.3	E940.1	E950.4	E962.0	E980.4
28:12 anticonvulsants	966.3	E855.0	E936.3	E950.4	E962.0	E980.4
barbiturates	967.0	E851	E937.0	E950.1	E962.0	E980.1
benzodiazepine–based tranquilizers	969.4	E853.2	E939.4	E950.3	E962.0	E980.3
bromides	967.3	E852.2	E937.3	E950.2	E962.0	E980.2
hydantoin derivatives	966.1	E855.0	E936.1	E950.4	E962.0	E980.4
oxazolidine (derivatives)	966.0	E855.0	E936.0	E950.4	E962.0	E980.4
succinimides	966.2	E855.0	E936.2	E950.4	E962.0	E980.4
28:16.04 anti-depressants	969.00	E854.0	E939.0	E950.3	E962.0	E980.3
28:16.08 tranquilizers	969.5	E853.9	E939.5	E950.3	E962.0	E980.3
benzodiazepine–based	969.4	E853.2	E939.4	E950.3	E962.0	E980.3
butyrophenone–based	969.2	E853.1	E939.2	E950.3	E962.0	E980.3
major NEC	969.3	E853.8	E939.3	E950.3	E962.0	E980.3
phenothiazine–based	969.1	E853.0	E939.1	E950.3	E962.0	E980.3
28:16.12 other psychotherapeutic agents	969.8	E855.8	E939.8	E950.3	E962.0	E980.3
28:20 respiratory and cerebral stimulants	970.9	E854.3	E940.9	E950.4	E962.0	E980.4
analeptics	970.0	E854.3	E940.0	E950.4	E962.0	E980.4
anorexigenic agents	977.0	E858.8	E947.0	E950.4	E962.0	E980.4
psychostimulants	969.70	E854.2	E939.7	E950.3	E962.0	E980.3
specified NEC	970.8	E854.3	E940.8	E950.4	E962.0	E980.4
28:24 sedatives and hypnotics	967.9	E852.9	E937.9	E950.2	E962.0	E980.2
barbiturates	967.0	E851	E937.0	E950.1	E962.0	E980.1
benzodiazepine–based tranquilizers	969.4	E853.2	E939.4	E950.3	E962.0	E980.3
chloral hydrate (group)	967.1	E852.0	E937.1	E950.2	E962.0	E980.2
glutethamide group	967.5	E852.4	E937.5	E950.2	E962.0	E980.2
intravenous anesthetics	968.3	E855.1	E938.3	E950.4	E962.0	E980.4
methaqualone (compounds)	967.4	E852.3	E937.4	E950.2	E962.0	E980.2
paraldehyde	967.2	E852.1	E937.2	E950.2	E962.0	E980.2
phenothiazine–based tranquilizers	969.1	E853.0	E939.1	E950.3	E962.0	E980.3
specified NEC	967.8	E852.8	E937.8	E950.2	E962.0	E980.2
thiobarbiturates	968.3	E855.1	E938.3	E950.4	E962.0	E980.4
tranquilizer NEC	969.5	E853.9	E939.5	E950.3	E962.0	E980.3
36:04 to 36:88 diagnostic agents	977.8	E858.8	E947.8	E950.4	E962.0	E980.4
40:00 electrolyte, caloric, and water balance agents NEC	974.5	E858.5	E944.5	E950.4	E962.0	E980.4
40:04 acidifying agents	963.2	E858.1	E933.2	E950.4	E962.0	E980.4
40:08 alkalinizing agents	963.3	E858.1	E933.3	E950.4	E962.0	E980.4
40:10 ammonia detoxicants	974.5	E858.5	E944.5	E950.4	E962.0	E980.4
40:12 replacement solutions	974.5	E858.5	E944.5	E950.4	E962.0	E980.4
plasma expanders	964.8	E858.2	E934.8	E950.4	E962.0	E980.4
40:16 sodium–removing resins	974.5	E858.5	E944.5	E950.4	E962.0	E980.4
40:18 potassium–removing resins	974.5	E858.5	E944.5	E950.4	E962.0	E980.4
40:20 caloric agents	974.5	E858.5	E944.5	E950.4	E962.0	E980.4
40:24 salt and sugar substitutes	974.5	E858.5	E944.5	E950.4	E962.0	E980.4
40:28 diuretics NEC	974.4	E858.5	E944.4	E950.4	E962.0	E980.4
carbonic acid anhydrase inhibitors	974.2	E858.5	E944.2	E950.4	E962.0	E980.4

Substance	Poisoning	Accident	Therapeutic Use	Suicide Attempt	Assault	Undetermined
			External Cause (E-Code)			
mercurials 974.0	E858.5	E944.0	E950.4	E962.0	E980.4
purine derivatives 974.1	E858.5	E944.1	E950.4	E962.0	E980.4
saluretics. 974.3	E858.5	E944.3	E950.4	E962.0	E980.4
thiazides 974.3	E858.5	E944.3	E950.4	E962.1	E980.4
40:36 irrigating solutions 974.5	E858.5	E944.5	E950.4	E962.0	E980.4
40:40 uricosuric agents. 974.7	E858.5	E944.7	E950.4	E962.0	E980.4
44:00 enzymes 963.4	E858.1	E933.4	E950.4	E962.0	E980.4
fibrinolysis–affecting agents 964.4	E858.2	E934.4	E950.4	E962.0	E980.4
gastric agents 973.4	E858.4	E943.4	E950.4	E962.0	E980.4
48:00 expectorants and cough preparations					
antihistamine agents 963.0	E858.1	E933.0	E950.4	E962.0	E980.4
antitussives. 975.4	E858.6	E945.4	E950.4	E962.0	E980.4
codeine derivatives. 965.09	E850.2	E935.2	E950.0	E962.0	E980.0
expectorants 975.5	E858.6	E945.5	E950.4	E962.0	E980.4
narcotic agents NEC 965.09	E850.2	E935.2	E950.0	E962.0	E980.0
52:04 anti–infectives (EENT)					
ENT agent 976.6	E858.7	E946.6	E950.4	E962.0	E980.4
ophthalmic preparation 976.5	E858.7	E946.5	E950.4	E962.0	E980.4
52:04.04 antibiotics (EENT)					
ENT agent 976.6	E858.7	E946.6	E950.4	E962.0	E980.4
ophthalmic preparation 976.5	E858.7	E946.5	E950.4	E962.0	E980.4
52:04.06 antivirals (EENT)					
ENT agent 976.6	E858.7	E946.6	E950.4	E962.0	E980.4
ophthalmic preparation 976.5	E858.7	E946.5	E950.4	E962.0	E980.4
52:04.08 sulfonamides (EENT)					
ENT agent 976.6	E858.7	E946.6	E950.4	E962.0	E980.4
ophthalmic preparation 976.5	E858.7	E946.5	E950.4	E962.0	E980.4
52:04.12 miscellaneous anti–infectives (EENT)					
ENT agent 976.6	E858.7	E946.6	E950.4	E962.0	E980.4
ophthalmic preparation 976.5	E858.7	E946.5	E950.4	E962.0	E980.4
52:08 anti–inflammatory agents (EENT)					
ENT agent 976.6	E858.7	E946.6	E950.4	E962.0	E980.4
ophthalmic preparation 976.5	E858.7	E946.5	E950.4	E962.0	E980.4
52:10 carbonic anhydrase inhibitors 974.2	E858.5	E944.2	E950.4	E962.0	E980.4
52:12 contact lens solutions. 976.5	E858.7	E946.5	E950.4	E962.0	E980.4
52:16 local anesthetics (EENT) 968.5	E855.2	E938.5	E950.4	E962.0	E980.4
52:20 miotics. 971.0	E855.3	E941.0	E950.4	E962.0	E980.4
52:24 mydriatics					
adrenergics. 971.2	E855.5	E941.2	E950.4	E962.0	E980.4
anticholinergics 971.1	E855.4	E941.1	E950.4	E962.0	E980.4
antimuscarinics 971.1	E855.4	E941.1	E950.4	E962.0	E980.4
parasympatholytics. 971.1	E855.4	E941.1	E950.4	E962.0	E980.4
spasmolytics 971.1	E855.4	E941.1	E950.4	E962.0	E980.4
sympathomimetics 971.2	E855.5	E941.2	E950.4	E962.0	E980.4
52:28 mouth washes and gargles. 976.6	E858.7	E946.6	E950.4	E962.0	E980.4
52:32 vasoconstrictors (EENT) 971.2	E855.5	E941.2	E950.4	E962.0	E980.4
52:36 unclassified agents (EENT)					
ENT agent 976.6	E858.7	E946.6	E950.4	E962.0	E980.4
ophthalmic preparation 976.5	E858.7	E946.5	E950.4	E962.0	E980.4
56:04 antacids and adsorbents 973.0	E858.4	E943.0	E950.4	E962.0	E980.4
56:08 antidiarrhea agents 973.5	E858.4	E943.5	E950.4	E962.0	E980.4
56:10 antiflatulents 973.8	E858.4	E943.8	E950.4	E962.0	E980.4
56:12 cathartics NEC 973.3	E858.4	E943.3	E950.4	E962.0	E980.4
emollients 973.2	E858.4	E943.2	E950.4	E962.0	E980.4
irritants 973.1	E858.4	E943.1	E950.4	E962.0	E980.4
56:16 digestants 973.4	E858.4	E943.4	E950.4	E962.0	E980.4
56:20 emetics and antiemetics					
antiemetics 963.0	E858.1	E933.0	E950.4	E962.0	E980.4
emetics 973.6	E858.4	E943.6	E950.4	E962.0	E980.4
56:24 lipotropic agents. 977.1	E858.8	E947.1	E950.4	E962.0	E980.4

Substance	Poisoning	Accident	Therapeutic Use	Suicide Attempt	Assault	Undetermined
		External Cause (E-Code)				
56:40 miscellaneous G.I. drugs	973.8	E858.4	E943.8	E950.4	E962.0	E980.4
60:00 gold compounds	965.69	E850.6	E935.6	E950.0	E962.0	E980.0
64:00 heavy metal antagonists	963.8	E858.1	E933.8	E950.4	E962.0	E980.4
68:04 adrenals	962.0	E858.0	E932.0	E950.4	E962.0	E980.4
68:08 androgens	962.1	E858.0	E932.1	E950.4	E962.0	E980.4
68:12 contraceptives, oral	962.2	E858.0	E932.2	E950.4	E962.0	E980.4
68:16 estrogens	962.2	E858.0	E932.2	E950.4	E962.0	E980.4
68:18 gonadotropins	962.4	E858.0	E932.4	E950.4	E962.0	E980.4
68:20 insulins and antidiabetic agents	962.3	E858.0	E932.3	E950.4	E962.0	E980.4
68:20.08 insulins	962.3	E858.0	E932.3	E950.4	E962.0	E980.4
68:24 parathyroid	962.6	E858.0	E932.6	E950.4	E962.0	E980.4
68:28 pituitary (posterior)	962.5	E858.0	E932.5	E950.4	E962.0	E980.4
anterior	962.4	E858.0	E932.4	E950.4	E962.0	E980.4
68:32 progestogens	962.2	E858.0	E932.2	E950.4	E962.0	E980.4
68:34 other corpus luteum hormones NEC	962.2	E858.0	E932.2	E950.4	E962.0	E980.4
68:36 thyroid and antithyroid						
antithyroid	962.8	E858.0	E932.8	E950.4	E962.0	E980.4
thyroid (derivatives)	962.7	E858.0	E932.7	E950.4	E962.0	E980.4
72:00 local anesthetics NEC	968.9	E855.2	E938.9	E950.4	E962.0	E980.4
topical (surface)	968.5	E855.2	E938.5	E950.4	E962.0	E980.4
infiltration (intradermal) (subcutaneous) (submucosal)	968.5	E855.2	E938.5	E950.4	E962.0	E980.4
nerve blocking (peripheral) (plexus) (regional)	968.6	E855.2	E938.6	E950.4	E962.0	E980.4
spinal	968.7	E855.2	E938.7	E950.4	E962.0	E980.4
76:00 oxytocics	975.0	E858.6	E945.0	E950.4	E962.0	E980.4
78:00 radioactive agents	990	—	—	—	—	—
80:04 serums NEC	979.9	E858.8	E949.9	E950.4	E962.0	E980.4
immune gamma globulin (human)	964.6	E858.2	E934.6	E950.4	E962.0	E980.4
80:08 toxoids NEC	978.8	E858.8	E948.8	E950.4	E962.0	E980.4
diphtheria	978.5	E858.8	E948.5	E950.4	E962.0	E980.4
and tetanus	978.9	E858.8	E948.9	E950.4	E962.0	E980.4
with pertussis component	978.6	E858.8	E948.6	E950.4	E962.0	E980.4
tetanus	978.4	E858.8	E948.4	E950.4	E962.0	E980.4
and diphtheria	978.9	E858.8	E948.9	E950.4	E962.0	E980.4
with pertussis component	978.6	E858.8	E948.6	E950.4	E962.0	E980.4
80:12 vaccines	979.9	E858.8	E949.9	E950.4	E962.0	E980.4
bacterial NEC	978.8	E858.8	E948.8	E950.4	E962.0	E980.4
with						
other bacterial components	978.9	E858.8	E948.9	E950.4	E962.0	E980.4
pertussis component	978.6	E858.8	E948.6	E950.4	E962.0	E980.4
viral and rickettsial components	979.7	E858.8	E949.7	E950.4	E962.0	E980.4
rickettsial NEC	979.6	E858.8	E949.6	E950.4	E962.0	E980.4
with						
bacterial component	979.7	E858.8	E949.7	E950.4	E962.0	E980.4
pertussis component	978.6	E858.8	E948.6	E950.4	E962.0	E980.4
viral component	979.7	E858.8	E949.7	E950.4	E962.0	E980.4
viral NEC	979.6	E858.8	E949.6	E950.4	E962.0	E980.4
with						
bacterial component	979.7	E858.8	E949.7	E950.4	E962.0	E980.4
pertussis component	978.6	E858.8	E948.6	E950.4	E962.0	E980.4
rickettsial component	979.7	E858.8	E949.7	E950.4	E962.0	E980.4
84:04.04 antibiotics (skin and mucous membrane)	976.0	E858.7	E946.0	E950.4	E962.0	E980.4
84:04.08 fungicides (skin and mucous membrane)	976.0	E858.7	E946.0	E950.4	E962.0	E980.4
84:04.12 scabicides and pediculicides (skin and mucous membrane)	976.0	E858.7	E946.0	E950.4	E962.0	E980.4

Substance	Poisoning	Accident	Therapeutic Use	Suicide Attempt	Assault	Undetermined
			External Cause (E-Code)			
84:04.16 miscellaneous local anti–infectives (skin and mucous membrane)	976.0	E858.7	E946.0	E950.4	E962.0	E980.4
84:06 anti–inflammatory agents (skin and mucous membrane)	976.0	E858.7	E946.0	E950.4	E962.0	E980.4
84:08 antipruritics and local anesthetics antipruritics	976.1	E858.7	E946.1	E950.4	E962.0	E980.4
local anesthetics	968.5	E855.2	E938.5	E950.4	E962.0	E980.4
84:12 astringents	976.2	E858.7	E946.2	E950.4	E962.0	E980.4
84:16 cell stimulants and proliferants	976.8	E858.7	E946.8	E950.4	E962.0	E980.4
84:20 detergents	976.2	E858.7	E946.2	E950.4	E962.0	E980.4
84:24 emollients, demulcents, and protectants	976.3	E858.7	E946.3	E950.4	E962.0	E980.4
84:28 keratolytic agents	976.4	E858.7	E946.4	E950.4	E962.0	E980.4
84:32 keratoplastic agents	976.4	E858.7	E946.4	E950.4	E962.0	E980.4
84:36 miscellaneous agents (skin and mucous membrane)	976.8	E858.7	E946.8	E950.4	E962.0	E980.4
86:00 spasmolytic agents	975.1	E858.6	E945.1	E950.4	E962.0	E980.4
antiasthmatics	975.7	E858.6	E945.7	E950.4	E962.0	E980.4
papaverine	972.5	E858.3	E942.5	E950.4	E962.0	E980.4
theophylline	974.1	E858.5	E944.1	E950.4	E962.0	E980.4
88:04 vitamin A	963.5	E858.1	E933.5	E950.4	E962.0	E980.4
88:08 vitamin B complex	963.5	E858.1	E933.5	E950.4	E962.0	E980.4
hematopoietic vitamin	964.1	E858.2	E934.1	E950.4	E962.0	E980.4
nicotinic acid derivatives	972.2	E858.3	E942.2	E950.4	E962.0	E980.4
88:12 vitamin C	963.5	E858.1	E933.5	E950.4	E962.0	E980.4
88:16 vitamin D	963.5	E858.1	E933.5	E950.4	E962.0	E980.4
88:20 vitamin E	963.5	E858.1	E933.5	E950.4	E962.0	E980.4
88:24 vitamin K activity	964.3	E858.2	E934.3	E950.4	E962.0	E980.4
88:28 multivitamin preparations	963.5	E858.1	E933.5	E950.4	E962.0	E980.4
92:00 unclassified therapeutic agents	977.8	E858.8	E947.8	E950.4	E962.0	E980.4
Duboisine	971.1	E855.4	E941.1	E950.4	E962.0	E980.4
Dulcolax	973.1	E858.4	E943.1	E950.4	E962.0	E980.4
Duponol (C) (EP)	976.2	E858.7	E946.2	E950.4	E962.0	E980.4
Durabolin	962.1	E858.0	E932.1	E950.4	E962.0	E980.4
Dyclone	968.5	E855.2	E938.5	E950.4	E962.0	E980.4
Dyclonine	968.5	E855.2	E938.5	E950.4	E962.0	E980.4
Dydrogesterone	962.2	E858.0	E932.2	E950.4	E962.0	E980.4
Dyes NEC	989.89	E866.8	—	E950.9	E962.1	E980.9
diagnostic agents	977.8	E858.8	E947.8	E950.4	E962.0	E980.4
pharmaceutical NEC	977.4	E858.8	E947.4	E950.4	E962.0	E980.4
Dyfols	971.0	E855.3	E941.0	E950.4	E962.0	E980.4
Dymelor	962.3	E858.0	E932.3	E950.4	E962.0	E980.4
Dynamite	989.89	E866.8	—	E950.9	E962.1	E980.9
fumes	987.8	E869.8	—	E952.8	E962.2	E982.8
Dyphylline	975.1	E858.6	E945.1	E950.4	E962.0	E980.4
Ear preparations	976.6	E858.7	E946.6	E950.4	E962.0	E980.4
Echothiopate, ecothiopate	971.0	E855.3	E941.0	E950.4	E962.0	E980.4
Ecstasy	969.72	E854.2	E939.7	E950.3	E962.0	E980.3
Ectylurea	967.8	E852.8	E937.8	E950.2	E962.0	E980.2
Edathamil disodium	963.8	E858.1	E933.8	E950.4	E962.0	E980.4
Edecrin	974.4	E858.5	E944.4	E950.4	E962.0	E980.4
Edetate, disodium (calcium)	963.8	E858.1	E933.8	E950.4	E962.0	E980.4
Edrophonium	971.0	E855.3	E941.0	E950.4	E962.0	E980.4
Elase	976.8	E858.7	E946.8	E950.4	E962.0	E980.4
Elaterium	973.1	E858.4	E943.1	E950.4	E962.0	E980.4
Elder	988.2	E865.4	—	E950.9	E962.1	E980.9
berry (unripe)	988.2	E865.3	—	E950.9	E962.1	E980.9
Electrolytes NEC	974.5	E858.5	E944.5	E950.4	E962.0	E980.4
Electrolytic agent NEC	974.5	E858.5	E944.5	E950.4	E962.0	E980.4

Substance	Poisoning	Accident	Therapeutic Use	Suicide Attempt	Assault	Undetermined
		External Cause (E-Code)				
Embramine	963.0	E858.1	E933.0	E950.4	E962.0	E980.4
Emetics	973.6	E858.4	E943.6	E950.4	E962.0	E980.4
Emetine (hydrochloride)	961.5	E857	E931.5	E950.4	E962.0	E980.4
Emollients	976.3	E858.7	E946.3	E950.4	E962.0	E980.4
Emylcamate	969.5	E853.8	E939.5	E950.3	E962.0	E980.3
Encyprate	969.09	E854.0	E939.0	E950.3	E962.0	E980.3
Endocaine	968.5	E855.2	E938.5	E950.4	E962.0	E980.4
Endrin	989.2	E863.0	—	E950.6	E962.1	E980.7
Enflurane	968.2	E855.1	E938.2	E950.4	E962.0	E980.4
Enovid	962.2	E858.0	E932.2	E950.4	E962.0	E980.4
ENT preparations (anti–infectives)	976.6	E858.7	E946.6	E950.4	E962.0	E980.4
Enzodase	963.4	E858.1	E933.4	E950.4	E962.0	E980.4
Enzymes NEC	963.4	E858.1	E933.4	E950.4	E962.0	E980.4
Epanutin	966.1	E855.0	E936.1	E950.4	E962.0	E980.4
Ephedra (tincture)	971.2	E855.5	E941.2	E950.4	E962.0	E980.4
Ephedrine	971.2	E855.5	E941.2	E950.4	E962.0	E980.4
Epiestriol	962.2	E858.0	E932.2	E950.4	E962.0	E980.4
Epilim — *see* Sodium valproate						
Epinephrine	971.2	E855.5	E941.2	E950.4	E962.0	E980.4
Epsom salt	973.3	E858.4	E943.3	E950.4	E962.0	E980.4
Equanil	969.5	E853.8	E939.5	E950.3	E962.0	E980.3
Equisetum (diuretic)	974.4	E858.5	E944.4	E950.4	E962.0	E980.4
Ergometrine	975.0	E858.6	E945.0	E950.4	E962.0	E980.4
Ergonovine	975.0	E858.6	E945.0	E950.4	E962.0	E980.4
Ergot NEC	988.2	E865.4	—	E950.9	E962.1	E980.9
medicinal (alkaloids)	975.0	E858.6	E945.0	E950.4	E962.0	E980.4
Ergotamine (tartrate) (for migraine) NEC	972.9	E858.3	E942.9	E950.4	E962.0	E980.4
Ergotrate	975.0	E858.6	E945.0	E950.4	E962.0	E980.4
Erythrityl tetranitrate	972.4	E858.3	E942.4	E950.4	E962.0	E980.4
Erythrol tetranitrate	972.4	E858.3	E942.4	E950.4	E962.0	E980.4
Erythromycin	960.3	E856	E930.3	E950.4	E962.0	E980.4
ophthalmic preparation	976.5	E858.7	E946.5	E950.4	E962.0	E980.4
topical NEC	976.0	E858.7	E946.0	E950.4	E962.0	E980.4
Eserine	971.0	E855.3	E941.0	E950.4	E962.0	E980.4
Eskabarb	967.0	E851	E937.0	E950.1	E962.0	E980.1
Eskalith	969.8	E855.8	E939.8	E950.3	E962.0	E980.3
Estradiol (cypionate) (dipropionate) (valerate)	962.2	E858.0	E932.2	E950.4	E962.0	E980.4
Estriol	962.2	E858.0	E932.2	E950.4	E962.0	E980.4
Estrogens (with progestogens)	962.2	E858.0	E932.2	E950.4	E962.0	E980.4
Estrone	962.2	E858.0	E932.2	E950.4	E962.0	E980.4
Etafedrine	971.2	E855.5	E941.2	E950.4	E962.0	E980.4
Ethacrynate sodium	974.4	E858.5	E944.4	E950.4	E962.0	E980.4
Ethacrynic acid	974.4	E858.5	E944.4	E950.4	E962.0	E980.4
Ethambutol	961.8	E857	E931.8	E950.4	E962.0	E980.4
Ethamide	974.2	E858.5	E944.2	E950.4	E962.0	E980.4
Ethamivan	970.0	E854.3	E940.0	E950.4	E962.0	E980.4
Ethamsylate	964.5	E858.2	E934.5	E950.4	E962.0	E980.4
Ethanol	980.0	E860.1	—	E950.9	E962.1	E980.9
beverage	980.0	E860.0	—	E950.9	E962.1	E980.9
Ethchlorvynol	967.8	E852.8	E937.8	E950.2	E962.0	E980.2
Ethebenecid	974.7	E858.5	E944.7	E950.4	E962.0	E980.4
Ether(s) (diethyl) (ethyl) (vapor)	987.8	E869.8	—	E952.8	E962.2	E982.8
anesthetic	968.2	E855.1	E938.2	E950.4	E962.0	E980.4
petroleum — *see* Ligroin						
solvent	982.8	E862.4	—	E950.9	E962.1	E980.9
Ethidine chloride (vapor)	987.8	E869.8	—	E952.8	E962.2	E982.8
liquid (solvent)	982.3	E862.4	—	E950.9	E962.1	E980.9
Ethinamate	967.8	E852.8	E937.8	E950.2	E962.0	E980.2
Ethinylestradiol	962.2	E858.0	E932.2	E950.4	E962.0	E980.4
Ethionamide	961.8	E857	E931.8	E950.4	E962.0	E980.4

TABLE OF DRUGS AND CHEMICALS

Substance	Poisoning	Accident	Therapeutic Use	Suicide Attempt	Assault	Undetermined
			External Cause (E-Code)			
Ethisterone	962.2	E858.0	E932.2	E950.4	E962.0	E980.4
Ethobral	967.0	E851	E937.0	E950.1	E962.0	E980.1
Ethocaine (infiltration) (topical)	968.5	E855.2	E938.5	E950.4	E962.0	E980.4
nerve block (peripheral) (plexus)	968.6	E855.2	E938.6	E950.4	E962.0	E980.4
spinal	968.7	E855.2	E938.7	E950.4	E962.0	E980.4
Ethoheptazine (citrate)	965.7	E850.7	E935.7	E950.0	E962.0	E980.0
Ethopropazine	966.4	E855.0	E936.4	E950.4	E962.0	E980.4
Ethosuximide	966.2	E855.0	E936.2	E950.4	E962.0	E980.4
Ethotoin	966.1	E855.0	E936.1	E950.4	E962.0	E980.4
Ethoxazene	961.9	E857	E931.9	E950.4	E962.0	E980.4
Ethoxzolamide	974.2	E858.5	E944.2	E950.4	E962.0	E980.4
Ethyl						
acetate (vapor)	982.8	E862.4	—	E950.9	E962.1	E980.9
alcohol	980.0	E860.1	—	E950.9	E962.1	E980.9
beverage	980.0	E860.0	—	E950.9	E962.1	E980.9
aldehyde (vapor)	987.8	E869.8	—	E952.8	E962.2	E982.8
liquid	989.89	E866.8	—	E950.9	E962.1	E980.9
aminobenzoate	968.5	E855.2	E938.5	E950.4	E962.0	E980.4
biscoumacetate	964.2	E858.2	E934.2	E950.4	E962.0	E980.4
bromide (anesthetic)	968.2	E855.1	E938.2	E950.4	E962.0	E980.4
carbamate (antineoplastic)	963.1	E858.1	E933.1	E950.4	E962.0	E980.4
carbinol	980.3	E860.4	—	E950.9	E962.1	E980.9
chaulmoograte	961.8	E857	E931.8	E950.4	E962.0	E980.4
chloride (vapor)	987.8	E869.8	—	E952.8	E962.2	E982.8
anesthetic (local)	968.5	E855.2	E938.5	E950.4	E962.0	E980.4
inhaled	968.2	E855.1	E938.2	E950.4	E962.0	E980.4
solvent	982.3	E862.4	—	E950.9	E962.1	E980.9
estranol	962.1	E858.0	E932.1	E950.4	E962.0	E980.4
ether — *see* Ether(s)						
formate (solvent) NEC	982.8	E862.4	—	E950.9	E962.1	E980.9
iodoacetate	987.5	E869.3	—	E952.8	E962.2	E982.8
lactate (solvent) NEC	982.8	E862.4	—	E950.9	E962.1	E980.9
methylcarbinol	980.8	E860.8	—	E950.9	E962.1	E980.9
morphine	965.09	E850.2	E935.2	E950.0	E962.0	E980.0
Ethylene (gas)	987.1	E869.8	—	E952.8	E962.2	E982.8
anesthetic (general)	968.2	E855.1	E938.2	E950.4	E962.0	E980.4
chlorohydrin (vapor)	982.3	E862.4	—	E950.9	E962.1	E980.9
dichloride (vapor)	982.3	E862.4	—	E950.9	E962.1	E980.9
glycol(s) (any) (vapor)	982.8	E862.4	—	E950.9	E962.1	E980.9
Ethylidene						
chloride NEC	982.3	E862.4	—	E950.9	E962.1	E980.9
diethyl ether	982.8	E862.4	—	E950.9	E962.1	E980.9
Ethynodiol	962.2	E858.0	E932.2	E950.4	E962.0	E980.4
Etidocaine	968.9	E855.2	E938.9	E950.4	E962.0	E980.4
infiltration (subcutaneous)	968.5	E855.2	E938.5	E950.4	E962.0	E980.4
nerve (peripheral) (plexus)	968.6	E855.2	E938.6	E950.4	E962.0	E980.4
Etilfen	967.0	E851	E937.0	E950.1	E962.0	E980.1
Etomide	965.7	E850.7	E935.7	E950.0	E962.0	E980.0
Etorphine	965.09	E850.2	E935.2	E950.0	E962.0	E980.0
Etoval	967.0	E851	E937.0	E950.1	E962.0	E980.1
Etryptamine	969.01	E854.0	E939.0	E950.3	E962.0	E980.3
Eucaine	968.5	E855.2	E938.5	E950.4	E962.0	E980.4
Eucalyptus (oil) NEC	975.5	E858.6	E945.5	E950.4	E962.0	E980.4
Eucatropine	971.1	E855.4	E941.1	E950.4	E962.0	E980.4
Eucodal	965.09	E850.2	E935.2	E950.0	E962.0	E980.0
Euneryl	967.0	E851	E937.0	E950.1	E962.0	E980.1
Euphthalmine	971.1	E855.4	E941.1	E950.4	E962.0	E980.4
Eurax	976.0	E858.7	E946.0	E950.4	E962.0	E980.4
Euresol	976.4	E858.7	E946.4	E950.4	E962.0	E980.4
Euthroid	962.7	E858.0	E932.7	E950.4	E962.0	E980.4

Substance	Poisoning	Accident	Therapeutic Use	Suicide Attempt	Assault	Undetermined
			External Cause (E-Code)			
Evans blue 977.8	E858.8	E947.8	E950.4	E962.0	E980.4
Evipal 967.0	E851	E937.0	E950.1	E962.0	E980.1
sodium 968.3	E855.1	E938.3	E950.4	E962.0	E980.4
Evipan 967.0	E851	E937.0	E950.1	E962.0	E980.1
sodium 968.3	E855.1	E938.3	E950.4	E962.0	E980.4
Exalgin 965.4	E850.4	E935.4	E950.0	E962.0	E980.0
Excipients, pharmaceutical 977.4	E858.8	E947.4	E950.4	E962.0	E980.4
Exhaust gas — *see* Carbon, monoxide					
Ex–Lax (phenolphthalein) 973.1	E858.4	E943.1	E950.4	E962.0	E980.4
Expectorants 975.5	E858.6	E945.5	E950.4	E962.0	E980.4
External medications (skin) (mucous					
membrane) 976.9	E858.7	E946.9	E950.4	E962.0	E980.4
dental agent 976.7	E858.7	E946.7	E950.4	E962.0	E980.4
ENT agent 976.6	E858.7	E946.6	E950.4	E962.0	E980.4
ophthalmic preparation 976.5	E858.7	E946.5	E950.4	E962.0	E980.4
specified NEC 976.8	E858.7	E946.8	E950.4	E962.0	E980.4
Eye agents (anti–infective) 976.5	E858.7	E946.5	E950.4	E962.0	E980.4
Factor IX complex (human) 964.5	E858.2	E934.5	E950.4	E962.0	E980.4
Fecal softeners 973.2	E858.4	E943.2	E950.4	E962.0	E980.4
Fenbutrazate 977.0	E858.8	E947.0	E950.4	E962.0	E980.4
Fencamfamin 970.8	E854.3	E940.8	E950.4	E962.0	E980.4
Fenfluramine 977.0	E858.8	E947.0	E950.4	E962.0	E980.4
Fenoprofen 965.61	E850.6	E935.6	E950.0	E962.0	E980.0
Fentanyl 965.09	E850.2	E935.2	E950.0	E962.0	E980.0
Fentazin 969.1	E853.0	E939.1	E950.3	E962.0	E980.3
Fenticlor, fentichlor 976.0	E858.7	E946.0	E950.4	E962.0	E980.4
Fer de lance (bite) (venom) 989.5	E905.0	—	E950.9	E962.1	E980.9
Ferric — *see* Iron					
Ferrocholinate 964.0	E858.2	E934.0	E950.4	E962.0	E980.4
Ferrous fumerate, gluconate, lactate, salt					
NEC, sulfate (medicinal) 964.0	E858.2	E934.0	E950.4	E962.0	E980.4
Ferrum — *see* Iron					
Fertilizers NEC 989.89	E866.5	—	E950.9	E962.1	E980.4
with herbicide mixture 989.4	E863.5	—	E950.6	E962.1	E980.7
Fibrinogen (human) 964.7	E858.2	E934.7	E950.4	E962.0	E980.4
Fibrinolysin 964.4	E858.2	E934.4	E950.4	E962.0	E980.4
Fibrinolysis–affecting agents 964.4	E858.2	E934.4	E950.4	E962.0	E980.4
Filix mas 961.6	E857	E931.6	E950.4	E962.0	E980.4
Fiorinal 965.1	E850.3	E935.3	E950.0	E962.0	E980.0
Fire damp 987.1	E869.8	—	E952.8	E962.2	E982.8
Fish, nonbacterial or noxious 988.0	E865.2	—	E950.9	E962.1	E980.9
shell 988.0	E865.1	—	E950.9	E962.1	E980.9
Flagyl 961.5	E857	E931.5	E950.4	E962.0	E980.4
Flavoxate 975.1	E858.6	E945.1	E950.4	E962.0	E980.4
Flaxedil 975.2	E858.6	E945.2	E950.4	E962.0	E980.4
Flaxseed (medicinal) 976.3	E858.7	E946.3	E950.4	E962.0	E980.4
Flomax 971.3	E855.6	E941.3	E950.4	E962.0	E980.4
Florantyrone 973.4	E858.4	E943.4	E950.4	E962.0	E980.4
Floraquin 961.3	E857	E931.3	E950.4	E962.0	E980.4
Florinef 962.0	E858.0	E932.0	E950.4	E962.0	E980.4
ENT agent 976.6	E858.7	E946.6	E950.4	E962.0	E980.4
ophthalmic preparation 976.5	E858.7	E946.5	E950.4	E962.0	E980.4
topical NEC 976.0	E858.7	E946.0	E950.4	E962.0	E980.4
Flowers of sulfur 976.4	E858.7	E946.4	E950.4	E962.0	E980.4
Floxuridine 963.1	E858.1	E933.1	E950.4	E962.0	E980.4
Flucytosine 961.9	E857	E931.9	E950.4	E962.0	E980.4
Fludrocortisone 962.0	E858.0	E932.0	E950.4	E962.0	E980.4
ENT agent 976.6	E858.7	E946.6	E950.4	E962.0	E980.4
ophthalmic preparation 976.5	E858.7	E946.5	E950.4	E962.0	E980.4
topical NEC 976.0	E858.7	E946.0	E950.4	E962.0	E980.4
Flumethasone 976.0	E858.7	E946.0	E950.4	E962.0	E980.4

Substance	Poisoning	Accident	Therapeutic Use	Suicide Attempt	Assault	Undetermined
			External Cause (E-Code)			
Flumethiazide	974.3	E858.5	E944.3	E950.4	E962.0	E980.4
Flumidin	961.7	E857	E931.7	E950.4	E962.0	E980.4
Flunitrazepam	969.4	E853.2	E939.4	E950.3	E962.0	E980.3
Fluocinolone	976.0	E858.7	E946.0	E950.4	E962.0	E980.4
Fluocortolone	962.0	E858.0	E932.0	E950.4	E962.0	E980.4
Fluohydrocortisone	962.0	E858.0	E932.0	E950.4	E962.0	E980.4
ENT agent	976.6	E858.7	E946.6	E950.4	E962.0	E980.4
ophthalmic preparation	976.5	E858.7	E946.5	E950.4	E962.0	E980.4
topical NEC	976.0	E858.7	E946.0	E950.4	E962.0	E980.4
Fluonid	976.0	E858.7	E946.0	E950.4	E962.0	E980.4
Fluopromazine	969.1	E853.0	E939.1	E950.3	E962.0	E980.3
Fluoracetate	989.4	E863.7	—	E950.6	E962.1	E980.7
Fluorescein (sodium)	977.8	E858.8	E947.8	E950.4	E962.0	E980.4
Fluoride(s) (pesticides) (sodium) NEC	989.4	E863.4	—	E950.6	E962.1	E980.7
hydrogen — see Hydrofluoric acid						
medicinal	976.7	E858.7	E946.7	E950.4	E962.0	E980.4
not pesticide NEC	983.9	E864.4	—	E950.7	E962.1	E980.6
stannous	976.7	E858.7	E946.7	E950.4	E962.0	E980.4
Fluorinated corticosteroids	962.0	E858.0	E932.0	E950.4	E962.0	E980.4
Fluorine (compounds) (gas)	987.8	E869.8	—	E952.8	E962.2	E982.8
salt — see Fluoride(s)						
Fluoristan	976.7	E858.7	E946.7	E950.4	E962.0	E980.4
Fluoroacetate	989.4	E863.7	—	E950.6	E962.1	E980.7
Fluorodeoxyuridine	963.1	E858.1	E933.1	E950.4	E962.0	E980.4
Fluorometholone (topical) NEC	976.0	E858.7	E946.0	E950.4	E962.0	E980.4
ophthalmic preparation	976.5	E858.7	E946.5	E950.4	E962.0	E980.4
Fluorouracil	963.1	E858.1	E933.1	E950.4	E962.0	E980.4
Fluothane	968.1	E855.1	E938.1	E950.4	E962.0	E980.4
Fluoxetine hydrochloride	969.03	E854.0	E939.0	E950.3	E962.0	E980.3
Fluoxymesterone	962.1	E858.0	E932.1	E950.4	E962.0	E980.4
Fluphenazine	969.1	E853.0	E939.1	E950.3	E962.0	E980.3
Fluprednisolone	962.0	E858.0	E932.0	E950.4	E962.0	E980.4
Flurandrenolide	976.0	E858.7	E946.0	E950.4	E962.0	E980.4
Flurazepam (hydrochloride)	969.4	E853.2	E939.4	E950.3	E962.0	E980.3
Flurbiprofen	965.61	E850.6	E935.6	E950.0	E962.0	E980.0
Flurobate	976.0	E858.7	E946.0	E950.4	E962.0	E980.4
Flurothyl	969.8	E855.8	E939.8	E950.3	E962.0	E980.3
Fluroxene	968.2	E855.1	E938.2	E950.4	E962.0	E980.4
Folacin	964.1	E858.2	E934.1	E950.4	E962.0	E980.4
Folic acid	964.1	E858.2	E934.1	E950.4	E962.0	E980.4
Follicle stimulating hormone	962.4	E858.0	E932.4	E950.4	E962.0	E980.4
Food, foodstuffs, nonbacterial or noxious	988.9	E865.9	—	E950.9	E962.1	E980.9
berries, seeds	988.2	E865.3	—	E950.9	E962.1	E980.9
fish	988.0	E865.2	—	E950.9	E962.1	E980.9
mushrooms	988.1	E865.5	—	E950.9	E962.1	E980.9
plants	988.2	E865.9	—	E950.9	E962.1	E980.9
specified type NEC	988.2	E865.4	—	E950.9	E962.1	E980.9
shellfish	988.0	E865.1	—	E950.9	E962.1	E980.9
specified NEC	988.8	E865.8	—	E950.9	E962.1	E980.9
Fool's parsley	988.2	E865.4	—	E950.9	E962.1	E980.9
Formaldehyde (solution)	989.89	E861.4	—	E950.9	E962.1	E980.9
fungicide	989.4	E863.6	—	E950.6	E962.1	E980.7
gas or vapor	987.8	E869.8	—	E952.8	E962.2	E982.8
Formalin	989.89	E861.4	—	E950.9	E962.1	E980.9
fungicide	989.4	E863.6	—	E950.6	E962.1	E980.7
vapor	987.8	E869.8	—	E952.8	E962.2	E982.8
Formic acid	983.1	E864.1	—	E950.7	E962.1	E980.6
vapor	987.8	E869.8	—	E952.8	E962.2	E982.8
Fowler's solution	985.1	E866.3	—	E950.8	E962.1	E980.8
Foxglove	988.2	E865.4	—	E950.9	E962.1	E980.9

Substance	Poisoning	Accident	Therapeutic Use	Suicide Attempt	Assault	Undetermined
			External Cause (E-Code)			
Fox green 977.8	E858.8	E947.8	E950.4	E962.0	E980.4
Framycetin 960.8	E856	E930.8	E950.4	E962.0	E980.4
Frangula (extract). 973.1	E858.4	E943.1	E950.4	E962.0	E980.4
Frei antigen 977.8	E858.8	E947.8	E950.4	E962.0	E980.4
Freons 987.4	E869.2	—	E952.8	E962.2	E982.8
Fructose 974.5	E858.5	E944.5	E950.4	E962.0	E980.4
Frusemide 974.4	E858.5	E944.4	E950.4	E962.0	E980.4
FSH 962.4	E858.0	E932.4	E950.4	E962.0	E980.4
Fuel					
automobile. 981	E862.1	—	E950.9	E962.1	E980.9
exhaust gas, not in transit 986	E868.2	—	E952.0	E962.2	E982.0
vapor NEC 987.1	E869.8	—	E952.8	E962.2	E982.8
gas (domestic use) — *see also* Carbon, monoxide, fuel					
utility 987.1	E868.1	—	E951.8	E962.2	E981.8
incomplete combustion of — *see* Carbon, monoxide, fuel, utility					
in mobile container. 987.0	E868.0	—	E951.1	E962.2	E981.1
piped (natural). 987.1	E867	—	E951.0	E962.2	E981.0
industrial, incomplete combustion 986	E868.3	—	E952.1	E962.2	E982.1
Fugillin 960.8	E856	E930.8	E950.4	E962.0	E980.4
Fulminate of mercury 985.0	E866.1	—	E950.9	E962.1	E980.9
Fulvicin. 960.1	E856	E930.1	E950.4	E962.0	E980.4
Fumadil. 960.8	E856	E930.8	E950.4	E962.0	E980.4
Fumagillin 960.8	E856	E930.8	E950.4	E962.0	E980.4
Fumes (from) 987.9	E869.9	—	E952.9	E962.2	E982.9
carbon monoxide — *see* Carbon, monoxide					
charcoal (domestic use) 986	E868.3	—	E952.1	E962.2	E982.1
chloroform — *see* Chloroform					
coke (in domestic stoves, fireplaces) 986	E868.3	—	E952.1	E962.2	E982.1
corrosive NEC 987.8	E869.8	—	E952.8	E962.2	E982.8
ether — *see* Ether(s)					
freons 987.4	E869.2	—	E952.8	E962.2	E982.8
hydrocarbons 987.1	E869.8	—	E952.8	E962.2	E982.8
petroleum (liquefied) 987.0	E868.0	—	E951.1	E962.2	E981.1
distributed through pipes (pure or mixed with air) 987.0	E867	—	E951.0	E962.2	E981.0
lead — *see* Lead					
metals — *see* specified metal					
nitrogen dioxide 987.2	E869.0	—	E952.8	E962.2	E982.8
pesticides — *see* Pesticides					
petroleum (liquefied) 987.0	E868.0	—	E951.1	E962.2	E981.1
distributed through pipes (pure or mixed with air) 987.0	E867	—	E951.0	E962.2	E981.0
polyester 987.8	E869.8	—	E952.8	E962.2	E982.8
specified source, other (*see also* substance specified) 987.8	E869.8	—	E952.8	E962.2	E982.8
sulfur dioxide 987.3	E869.1	—	E952.8	E962.2	E982.8
Fumigants 989.4	E863.8	—	E950.6	E962.1	E980.7
Fungi, noxious, used as food 988.1	E865.5	—	E950.9	E962.1	E980.9
Fungicides (*see also* Antifungals) 989.4	E863.6	—	E950.6	E962.1	E980.7
Fungizone. 960.1	E856	E930.1	E950.4	E962.0	E980.4
topical 976.0	E858.7	E946.0	E950.4	E962.0	E980.4
Furacin 976.0	E858.7	E946.0	E950.4	E962.0	E980.4
Furadantin. 961.9	E857	E931.9	E950.4	E962.0	E980.4
Furazolidone. 961.9	E857	E931.9	E950.4	E962.0	E980.4
Furnace (coal burning) (domestic), gas from 986	E868.3	—	E952.1	E962.2	E982.1
industrial 986	E868.8	—	E952.1	E962.2	E982.1
Furniture polish 989.89	E861.2	—	E950.9	E962.1	E980.9
Furosemide 974.4	E858.5	E944.4	E950.4	E962.0	E980.4

Substance	Poisoning	Accident	Therapeutic Use	Suicide Attempt	Assault	Undetermined
			External Cause (E-Code)			
Furoxone 961.9	E857	E931.9	E950.4	E962.0	E980.4	
Fusel oil (amyl) (butyl) (propyl). 980.3	E860.4	—	E950.9	E962.1	E980.9	
Fusidic acid 960.8	E856	E930.8	E950.4	E962.0	E980.4	
Gallamine 975.2	E858.6	E945.2	E950.4	E962.0	E980.4	
Gallotannic acid 976.2	E858.7	E946.2	E950.4	E962.0	E980.4	
Gamboge 973.1	E858.4	E943.1	E950.4	E962.0	E980.4	
Gamimune 964.6	E858.2	E934.6	E950.4	E962.0	E980.4	
Gamma–benzene hexachloride (vapor) 989.2	E863.0	—	E950.6	E962.1	E980.7	
Gamma globulin 964.6	E858.2	E934.6	E950.4	E962.0	E980.4	
Gamma Hydroxy Butyrate (GHB) 968.4	E855.1	E938.4	E950.4	E962.0	E980.4	
Gamulin 964.6	E858.2	E934.6	E950.4	E962.0	E980.4	
Ganglionic blocking agents. 972.3	E858.3	E942.3	E950.4	E962.0	E980.4	
Ganja. 969.6	E854.1	E939.6	E950.3	E962.0	E980.3	
Garamycin 960.8	E856	E930.8	E950.4	E962.0	E980.4	
ophthalmic preparation 976.5	E858.7	E946.5	E950.4	E962.0	E980.4	
topical NEC 976.0	E858.7	E946.0	E950.4	E962.0	E980.4	
Gardenal 967.0	E851	E937.0	E950.1	E962.0	E980.1	
Gardepanyl 967.0	E851	E937.0	E950.1	E962.0	E980.1	
Gas 987.9	E869.9	—	E952.9	E962.2	E982.9	
acetylene 987.1	E868.1	—	E951.8	E962.2	E981.8	
incomplete combustion of — see Carbon, monoxide, fuel, utility						
air contaminants, source or type not specified 987.9	E869.9	—	E952.9	E962.2	E982.9	
anesthetic (general) NEC 968.2	E855.1	E938.2	E950.4	E962.0	E980.4	
blast furnace 986	E868.8	—	E952.1	E962.2	E982.1	
butane — see Butane						
carbon monoxide — see Carbon, monoxide						
chlorine 987.6	E869.8	—	E952.8	E962.2	E982.8	
coal — see Carbon, monoxide, coal						
cyanide 987.7	E869.8	—	E952.8	E962.2	E982.8	
dicyanogen. 987.8	E869.8	—	E952.8	E962.2	E982.8	
domestic — see Gas, utility						
exhaust — see Carbon, monoxide, exhaust gas						
from wood– or coal–burning stove or fireplace 986	E868.3	—	E952.1	E962.2	E982.1	
fuel (domestic use) — see also Carbon, monoxide, fuel						
industrial use 986	E868.8	—	E952.1	E962.2	E982.1	
utility 987.1	E868.1	—	E951.8	E962.2	E981.8	
incomplete combustion of — see Carbon, monoxide, fuel, utility						
in mobile container. 987.0	E868.0	—	E951.1	E962.2	E981.1	
piped (natural). 987.1	E867	—	E951.0	E962.2	E981.0	
garage 986	E868.2	—	E952.0	E962.2	E982.0	
hydrocarbon NEC 987.1	E869.8	—	E952.8	E962.2	E982.8	
incomplete combustion of — see Carbon, monoxide, fuel, utility						
liquefied (mobile container) 987.0	E868.0	—	E951.1	E962.2	E981.1	
piped 987.0	E867	—	E951.0	E962.2	E981.0	
hydrocyanic acid 987.7	E869.8	—	E952.8	E962.2	E982.8	
illuminating — see Gas, utility						
incomplete combustion, any — see Carbon, monoxide						
kiln. 986	E868.8	—	E952.1	E962.2	E982.1	
lacrimogenic 987.5	E869.3	—	E952.8	E962.2	E982.8	
marsh. 987.1	E869.8	—	E952.8	E962.2	E982.8	
motor exhaust, not in transit 986	E868.8	—	E952.1	E962.2	E982.1	
mustard — see Mustard, gas						
natural 987.1	E867	—	E951.0	E962.2	E981.0	

Substance	Poisoning	Accident	Therapeutic Use	Suicide Attempt	Assault	Undetermined
			External Cause (E-Code)			
nerve (war)	987.9	E869.9	—	E952.9	E962.2	E982.9
oils	981	E862.1	—	E950.9	E962.1	E980.9
petroleum (liquefied) (distributed in mobile containers)	987.0	E868.0	—	E951.1	E962.2	E981.1
piped (pure or mixed with air)	987.0	E867	—	E951.1	E962.2	E981.1
piped (manufactured) (natural) NEC	987.1	E867	—	E951.0	E962.2	E981.0
producer	986	E868.8	—	E952.1	E962.2	E982.1
propane — see Propane						
refrigerant (freon)	987.4	E869.2	—	E952.8	E962.2	E982.8
not freon	987.9	E869.9	—	E952.9	E962.2	E982.9
sewer	987.8	E869.8	—	E952.8	E962.2	E982.8
specified source NEC (see also substance specified)	987.8	E869.8	—	E952.8	E962.2	E982.8
stove — see Gas, utility						
tear	987.5	E869.3	—	E952.8	E962.2	E982.8
utility (for cooking, heating, or lighting) (piped) NEC	987.1	E868.1	—	E951.8	E962.2	E981.8
incomplete combustion of — see Carbon, monoxide, fuel, utility						
in mobile container	987.0	E868.0	—	E951.1	E962.2	E981.1
piped (natural)	987.1	E867	—	E951.0	E962.2	E981.0
water	987.1	E868.1	—	E951.8	E962.2	E981.8
incomplete combustion of — see Carbon, monoxide, fuel, utility						
Gaseous substance — see Gas						
Gasoline, gasolene	981	E862.1	—	E950.9	E962.1	E980.9
vapor	987.1	E869.8	—	E952.8	E962.2	E982.8
Gastric enzymes	973.4	E858.4	E943.4	E950.4	E962.0	E980.4
Gastrografin	977.8	E858.8	E947.8	E950.4	E962.0	E980.4
Gastrointestinal agents	973.9	E858.4	E943.9	E950.4	E962.0	E980.4
specified NEC	973.8	E858.4	E943.8	E950.4	E962.0	E980.4
Gaultheria procumbens	988.2	E865.4	—	E950.9	E962.1	E980.9
Gelatin (intravenous)	964.8	E858.2	E934.8	E950.4	E962.0	E980.4
absorbable (sponge)	964.5	E858.2	E934.5	E950.4	E962.0	E980.4
Gelfilm	976.8	E858.7	E946.8	E950.4	E962.0	E980.4
Gelfoam	964.5	E858.2	E934.5	E950.4	E962.0	E980.4
Gelsemine	970.8	E854.3	E940.8	E950.4	E962.0	E980.4
Gelsemium (sempervirens)	988.2	E865.4	—	E950.9	E962.1	E980.9
Gemonil	967.0	E851	E937.0	E950.1	E962.0	E980.1
Gentamicin	960.8	E856	E930.8	E950.4	E962.0	E980.4
ophthalmic preparation	976.5	E858.7	E946.5	E950.4	E962.0	E980.4
topical NEC	976.0	E858.7	E946.0	E950.4	E962.0	E980.4
Gentian violet	976.0	E858.7	E946.0	E950.4	E962.0	E980.4
Gexane	976.0	E858.7	E946.0	E950.4	E962.0	E980.4
Gila monster (venom)	989.5	E905.0	—	E950.9	E962.1	E980.9
Ginger, Jamaica	989.89	E866.8	—	E950.9	E962.1	E980.9
Gitalin	972.1	E858.3	E942.1	E950.4	E962.0	E980.4
Gitoxin	972.1	E858.3	E942.1	E950.4	E962.0	E980.4
Glandular extract (medicinal) NEC	977.9	E858.9	E947.9	E950.5	E962.0	E980.5
Glaucarubin	961.5	E857	E931.5	E950.4	E962.0	E980.4
Globin zinc insulin	962.3	E858.0	E932.3	E950.4	E962.0	E980.4
Glucagon	962.3	E858.0	E932.3	E950.4	E962.0	E980.4
Glucochloral	967.1	E852.0	E937.1	E950.2	E962.0	E980.2
Glucocorticoids	962.0	E858.0	E932.0	E950.4	E962.0	E980.4
Glucose	974.5	E858.5	E944.5	E950.4	E962.0	E980.4
oxidase reagent	977.8	E858.8	E947.8	E950.4	E962.0	E980.4
Glucosulfone sodium	961.8	E857	E931.8	E950.4	E962.0	E980.4
Glue(s)	989.89	E866.6	—	E950.9	E962.1	E980.9
Glutamic acid (hydrochloride)	973.4	E858.4	E943.4	E950.4	E962.0	E980.4
Glutaraldehyde	989.89	E861.4	—	E950.9	E962.1	E980.9
Glutathione	963.8	E858.1	E933.8	E950.4	E962.0	E980.4

Substance	Poisoning	Accident	Therapeutic Use	Suicide Attempt	Assault	Undetermined
			External Cause (E-Code)			
Glutethimide (group)	967.5	E852.4	E937.5	E950.2	E962.0	E980.2
Glycerin (lotion)	976.3	E858.7	E946.3	E950.4	E962.0	E980.4
Glycerol (topical)	976.3	E858.7	E946.3	E950.4	E962.0	E980.4
Glyceryl						
guaiacolate	975.5	E858.6	E945.5	E950.4	E962.0	E980.4
triacetate (topical)	976.0	E858.7	E946.0	E950.4	E962.0	E980.4
trinitrate	972.4	E858.3	E942.4	E950.4	E962.0	E980.4
Glycine	974.5	E858.5	E944.5	E950.4	E962.0	E980.4
Glycobiarsol	961.1	E857	E931.1	E950.4	E962.0	E980.4
Glycols (ether)	982.8	E862.4	—	E950.9	E962.1	E980.9
Glycopyrrolate	971.1	E855.4	E941.1	E950.4	E962.0	E980.4
Glymidine	962.3	E858.0	E932.3	E950.4	E962.0	E980.4
Gold (compounds) (salts)	965.69	E850.6	E935.6	E950.0	E962.0	E980.0
Golden sulfide of antimony	985.4	E866.2	—	E950.9	E962.1	E980.9
Goldylocks	988.2	E865.4	—	E950.9	E962.1	E980.9
Gonadal tissue extract	962.9	E858.0	E932.9	E950.4	E962.0	E980.4
female	962.2	E858.0	E932.2	E950.4	E962.0	E980.4
male	962.1	E858.0	E932.1	E950.4	E962.0	E980.4
Gonadotropin	962.4	E858.0	E932.4	E950.4	E962.0	E980.4
Grain alcohol	980.0	E860.1	—	E950.9	E962.1	E980.9
beverage	980.0	E860.0	—	E950.9	E962.1	E980.9
Gramicidin	960.8	E856	E930.8	E950.4	E962.0	E980.4
Gratiola officinalis	988.2	E865.4	—	E950.9	E962.1	E980.9
Grease	989.89	E866.8	—	E950.9	E962.1	E980.9
Green hellebore	988.2	E865.4	—	E950.9	E962.1	E980.9
Green soap	976.2	E858.7	E946.2	E950.4	E962.0	E980.4
Grifulvin	960.1	E856	E930.1	E950.4	E962.0	E980.4
Griseofulvin	960.1	E856	E930.1	E950.4	E962.0	E980.4
Growth hormone	962.4	E858.0	E932.4	E950.4	E962.0	E980.4
Guaiacol	975.5	E858.6	E945.5	E950.4	E962.0	E980.4
Guaiac reagent	977.8	E858.8	E947.8	E950.4	E962.0	E980.4
Guaifenesin	975.5	E858.6	E945.5	E950.4	E962.0	E980.4
Guaiphenesin	975.5	E858.6	E945.5	E950.4	E962.0	E980.4
Guanatol	961.4	E857	E931.4	E950.4	E962.0	E980.4
Guanethidine	972.6	E858.3	E942.6	E950.4	E962.0	E980.4
Guano	989.89	E866.5	—	E950.9	E962.1	E980.9
Guanochlor	972.6	E858.3	E942.6	E950.4	E962.0	E980.4
Guanoctine	972.6	E858.3	E942.6	E950.4	E962.0	E980.4
Guanoxan	972.6	E858.3	E942.6	E950.4	E962.0	E980.4
Hair treatment agent NEC	976.4	E858.7	E946.4	E950.4	E962.0	E980.4
Halcinonide	976.0	E858.7	E946.0	E950.4	E962.0	E980.4
Halethazole	976.0	E858.7	E946.0	E950.4	E962.0	E980.4
Hallucinogens	969.6	E854.1	E939.6	E950.3	E962.0	E980.3
Haloperidol	969.2	E853.1	E939.2	E950.3	E962.0	E980.3
Haloprogin	976.0	E858.7	E946.0	E950.4	E962.0	E980.4
Halotex	976.0	E858.7	E946.0	E950.4	E962.0	E980.4
Halothane	968.1	E855.1	E938.1	E950.4	E962.0	E980.4
Halquinols	976.0	E858.7	E946.0	E950.4	E962.0	E980.4
Hand sanitizer	976.0	E858.7	E946.0	E950.4	E962.0	E980.4
Harmonyl	972.6	E858.3	E942.6	E950.4	E962.0	E980.4
Hartmann's solution	974.5	E858.5	E944.5	E950.4	E962.0	E980.4
Hashish	969.6	E854.1	E939.6	E950.3	E962.0	E980.3
Hawaiian wood rose seeds	969.6	E854.1	E939.6	E950.3	E962.0	E980.3
Headache cures, drugs, powders NEC	977.9	E858.9	E947.9	E950.5	E962.0	E980.9
Heavenly Blue (morning glory)	969.6	E854.1	E939.6	E950.3	E962.0	E980.3
Heavy metal						
antagonists	963.8	E858.1	E933.8	E950.4	E962.0	E980.4
anti–infectives	961.2	E857	E931.2	E950.4	E962.0	E980.4
Hedaquinium	976.0	E858.7	E946.0	E950.4	E962.0	E980.4
Hedge hyssop	988.2	E865.4	—	E950.9	E962.1	E980.9

Substance	Poisoning	Accident	Therapeutic Use	Suicide Attempt	Assault	Undetermined
			External Cause (E-Code)			
Heet	976.8	E858.7	E946.8	E950.4	E962.0	E980.4
Helenin	961.6	E857	E931.6	E950.4	E962.0	E980.4
Hellebore (black) (green) (white)	988.2	E865.4	—	E950.9	E962.1	E980.9
Hemlock	988.2	E865.4	—	E950.9	E962.1	E980.9
Hemostatics	964.5	E858.2	E934.5	E950.4	E962.0	E980.4
capillary active drugs	972.8	E858.3	E942.8	E950.4	E962.0	E980.4
Henbane	988.2	E865.4	—	E950.9	E962.1	E980.9
Heparin (sodium)	964.2	E858.2	E934.2	E950.4	E962.0	E980.4
Heptabarbital, heptabarbitone	967.0	E851	E937.0	E950.1	E962.0	E980.1
Heptachlor	989.2	E863.0	—	E950.6	E962.1	E980.7
Heptalgin	965.09	E850.2	E935.2	E950.0	E962.0	E980.0
Herbicides	989.4	E863.5	—	E950.6	E962.1	E980.7
Heroin	965.01	E850.0	E935.0	E950.0	E962.0	E980.0
Herplex	976.5	E858.7	E946.5	E950.4	E962.0	E980.4
HES	964.8	E858.2	E934.8	E950.4	E962.0	E980.4
Hetastarch	964.8	E858.2	E934.8	E950.4	E962.0	E980.4
Hexachlorocyclohexane	989.2	E863.0	—	E950.6	E962.1	E980.7
Hexachlorophene	976.2	E858.7	E946.2	E950.4	E962.0	E980.4
Hexadimethrine (bromide)	964.5	E858.2	E934.5	E950.4	E962.0	E980.4
Hexafluorenium	975.2	E858.6	E945.2	E950.4	E962.0	E980.4
Hexa–germ	976.2	E858.7	E946.2	E950.4	E962.0	E980.4
Hexahydrophenol	980.8	E860.8	—	E950.9	E962.1	E980.9
Hexalin	980.8	E860.8	—	E950.9	E962.1	E980.9
Hexamethonium	972.3	E858.3	E942.3	E950.4	E962.0	E980.4
Hexamethyleneamine	961.9	E857	E931.9	E950.4	E962.0	E980.4
Hexamine	961.9	E857	E931.9	E950.4	E962.0	E980.4
Hexanone	982.8	E862.4	—	E950.9	E962.1	E980.9
Hexapropymate	967.8	E852.8	E937.8	E950.2	E962.0	E980.2
Hexestrol	962.2	E858.0	E932.2	E950.4	E962.0	E980.4
Hexethal (sodium)	967.0	E851	E937.0	E950.1	E962.0	E980.1
Hexetidine	976.0	E858.7	E946.0	E950.4	E962.0	E980.4
Hexobarbital, hexabarbitone	967.0	E851	E937.0	E950.1	E962.0	E980.1
sodium (anesthetic)	968.3	E855.1	E938.3	E950.4	E962.0	E980.4
soluble	968.3	E855.1	E938.3	E950.4	E962.0	E980.4
Hexocyclium	971.1	E855.4	E941.1	E950.4	E962.0	E980.4
Hexoestrol	962.2	E858.0	E932.2	E950.4	E962.0	E980.4
Hexone	982.8	E862.4	—	E950.9	E962.1	E980.9
Hexylcaine	968.5	E855.2	E938.5	E950.4	E962.0	E980.4
Hexylresorcinol	961.6	E857	E931.6	E950.4	E962.0	E980.4
Hinkle's pills	973.1	E858.4	E943.1	E950.4	E962.0	E980.4
Histalog	977.8	E858.8	E947.8	E950.4	E962.0	E980.4
Histamine (phosphate)	972.5	E858.3	E942.5	E950.4	E962.0	E980.4
Histoplasmin	977.8	E858.8	E947.8	E950.4	E962.0	E980.4
Holly berries	988.2	E865.3	—	E950.9	E962.1	E980.9
Homatropine	971.1	E855.4	E941.1	E950.4	E962.0	E980.4
Homo–tet	964.6	E858.2	E934.6	E950.4	E962.0	E980.4
Hormones (synthetic substitute) NEC	962.9	E858.0	E932.9	E950.4	E962.0	E980.4
adrenal cortical steroids	962.0	E858.0	E932.0	E950.4	E962.0	E980.4
antidiabetic agents	962.3	E858.0	E932.3	E950.4	E962.0	E980.4
follicle stimulating	962.4	E858.0	E932.4	E950.4	E962.0	E980.4
gonadotropic	962.4	E858.0	E932.4	E950.4	E962.0	E980.4
growth	962.4	E858.0	E932.4	E950.4	E962.0	E980.4
ovarian (substitutes)	962.2	E858.0	E932.2	E950.4	E962.0	E980.4
parathyroid (derivatives)	962.6	E858.0	E932.6	E950.4	E962.0	E980.4
pituitary (posterior)	962.5	E858.0	E932.5	E950.4	E962.0	E980.4
anterior	962.4	E858.0	E932.4	E950.4	E962.0	E980.4
thyroid (derivative)	962.7	E858.0	E932.7	E950.4	E962.0	E980.4
Hornet (sting)	989.5	E905.3	—	E950.9	E962.1	E980.9
Horticulture agent NEC	989.4	E863.9	—	E950.6	E962.1	E980.7
Hyaluronidase	963.4	E858.1	E933.4	E950.4	E962.0	E980.4
Hyazyme	963.4	E858.1	E933.4	E950.4	E962.0	E980.4

Substance	Poisoning	Accident	Therapeutic Use	Suicide Attempt	Assault	Undetermined
			External Cause (E-Code)			
Hycodan	965.09	E850.2	E935.2	E950.0	E962.0	E980.0
Hydantoin derivatives	966.1	E855.0	E936.1	E950.4	E962.0	E980.4
Hydeltra	962.0	E858.0	E932.0	E950.4	E962.0	E980.4
Hydergine	971.3	E855.6	E941.3	E950.4	E962.0	E980.4
Hydrabamine penicillin	960.0	E856	E930.0	E950.4	E962.0	E980.4
Hydralazine, hydrallazine	972.6	E858.3	E942.6	E950.4	E962.0	E980.4
Hydrargaphen	976.0	E858.7	E946.0	E950.4	E962.0	E980.4
Hydrazine	983.9	E864.3	—	E950.7	E962.1	E980.6
Hydriodic acid	975.5	E858.6	E945.5	E950.4	E962.0	E980.4
Hydrocarbon gas	987.1	E869.8	—	E952.8	E962.2	E982.8
incomplete combustion of — see						
Carbon, monoxide, fuel, utility						
liquefied (mobile container)	987.0	E868.0	—	E951.1	E962.2	E981.1
piped (natural)	987.0	E867	—	E951.0	E962.2	E981.0
Hydrochloric acid (liquid)	983.1	E864.1	—	E950.7	E962.1	E980.6
medicinal	973.4	E858.4	E943.4	E950.4	E962.0	E980.4
vapor	987.8	E869.8	—	E952.8	E962.2	E982.8
Hydrochlorothiazide	974.3	E858.5	E944.3	E950.4	E962.0	E980.4
Hydrocodone	965.09	E850.2	E935.2	E950.0	E962.0	E980.0
Hydrocortisone	962.0	E858.0	E932.0	E950.4	E962.0	E980.4
ENT agent	976.6	E858.7	E946.6	E950.4	E962.0	E980.4
ophthalmic preparation	976.5	E858.7	E946.5	E950.4	E962.0	E980.4
topical NEC	976.0	E858.7	E946.0	E950.4	E962.0	E980.4
Hydrocortone	962.0	E858.0	E932.0	E950.4	E962.0	E980.4
ENT agent	976.6	E858.7	E946.6	E950.4	E962.0	E980.4
ophthalmic preparation	976.5	E858.7	E946.5	E950.4	E962.0	E980.4
topical NEC	976.0	E858.7	E946.0	E950.4	E962.0	E980.4
Hydrocyanic acid — see Cyanide(s)						
Hydroflumethiazide	974.3	E858.5	E944.3	E950.4	E962.0	E980.4
Hydrofluoric acid (liquid)	983.1	E864.1	—	E950.7	E962.1	E980.6
vapor	987.8	E869.8	—	E952.8	E962.2	E982.8
Hydrogen	987.8	E869.8	—	E952.8	E962.2	E982.8
arsenide	985.1	E866.3	—	E950.8	E962.1	E980.8
arseniureted	985.1	E866.3	—	E950.8	E962.1	E980.8
cyanide (salts)	989.0	E866.8	—	E950.9	E962.1	E980.9
gas	987.7	E869.8	—	E952.8	E962.2	E982.8
fluoride (liquid)	983.1	E864.1	—	E950.7	E962.1	E980.6
vapor	987.8	E869.8	—	E952.8	E962.2	E982.8
peroxide (solution)	976.6	E858.7	E946.6	E950.4	E962.0	E980.4
phosphureted	987.8	E869.8	—	E952.8	E962.2	E982.8
sulfide (gas)	987.8	E869.8	—	E952.8	E962.2	E982.8
arseniureted	985.1	E866.3	—	E950.8	E962.1	E980.8
sulfureted	987.8	E869.8	—	E952.8	E962.2	E982.8
Hydromorphinol	965.09	E850.2	E935.2	E950.0	E962.0	E980.0
Hydromorphinone	965.09	E850.2	E935.2	E950.0	E962.0	E980.0
Hydromorphone	965.09	E850.2	E935.2	E950.0	E962.0	E980.0
Hydromox	974.3	E858.5	E944.3	E950.4	E962.0	E980.4
Hydrophilic lotion	976.3	E858.7	E946.3	E950.4	E962.0	E980.4
Hydroquinone	983.0	E864.0	—	E950.7	E962.1	E980.6
vapor	987.8	E869.8	—	E952.8	E962.2	E982.8
Hydrosulfuric acid (gas)	987.8	E869.8	—	E952.8	E962.2	E982.8
Hydrous wool fat (lotion)	976.3	E858.7	E946.3	E950.4	E962.0	E980.4
Hydroxide, caustic	983.2	E864.2	—	E950.7	E962.1	E980.6
Hydroxocobalamin	964.1	E858.2	E934.1	E950.4	E962.0	E980.4
Hydroxyamphetamine	971.2	E855.5	E941.2	E950.4	E962.0	E980.4
Hydroxychloroquine	961.4	E857	E931.4	E950.4	E962.0	E980.4
Hydroxydihydrocodeinone	965.09	E850.2	E935.2	E950.0	E962.0	E980.0
Hydroxyethyl starch	964.8	E858.2	E934.8	E950.4	E962.0	E980.4
Hydroxyphenamate	969.5	E853.8	E939.5	E950.3	E962.0	E980.3
Hydroxyphenylbutazone	965.5	E850.5	E935.5	E950.0	E962.0	E980.0

Substance	Poisoning	Accident	Therapeutic Use	Suicide Attempt	Assault	Undetermined
			External Cause (E-Code)			
Hydroxyprogesterone 962.2	E858.0	E932.2	E950.4	E962.0	E980.4
Hydroxyquinoline derivatives 961.3	E857	E931.3	E950.4	E962.0	E980.4
Hydroxystilbamidine 961.5	E857	E931.5	E950.4	E962.0	E980.4
Hydroxyurea. 963.1	E858.1	E933.1	E950.4	E962.0	E980.4
Hydroxyzine. 969.5	E853.8	E939.5	E950.3	E962.0	E980.3
Hyoscine (hydrobromide) 971.1	E855.4	E941.1	E950.4	E962.0	E980.4
Hyoscyamine 971.1	E855.4	E941.1	E950.4	E962.0	E980.4
Hyoscyamus (albus) (niger) 988.2	E865.4	—	E950.9	E962.1	E980.9
Hypaque 977.8	E858.8	E947.8	E950.4	E962.0	E980.4
Hypertussis 964.6	E858.2	E934.6	E950.4	E962.0	E980.4
Hypnotics NEC 967.9	E852.9	E937.9	E950.2	E962.0	E980.2
Hypochlorites — see Sodium, hypochlorite					
Hypotensive agents NEC. 972.6	E858.3	E942.6	E950.4	E962.0	E980.4
Ibufenac 965.69	E850.6	E935.6	E950.0	E962.0	E980.0
ibuprofen 965.61	E850.6	E935.6	E950.0	E962.0	E980.0
ICG 977.8	E858.8	E947.8	E950.4	E962.0	E980.4
Ichthammol 976.4	E858.7	E946.4	E950.4	E962.0	E980.4
Ichthyol. 976.4	E858.7	E946.4	E950.4	E962.0	E980.4
Idoxuridine 976.5	E858.7	E946.5	E950.4	E962.0	E980.4
IDU 976.5	E858.7	E946.5	E950.4	E962.0	E980.4
Iletin 962.3	E858.0	E932.3	E950.4	E962.0	E980.4
Ilex 988.2	E865.4	—	E950.9	E962.1	E980.9
Illuminating gas — see Gas, utility					
Ilopan 963.5	E858.1	E933.5	E950.4	E962.0	E980.4
Ilotycin 960.3	E856	E930.3	E950.4	E962.0	E980.4
ophthalmic preparation. 976.5	E858.7	E946.5	E950.4	E962.0	E980.4
topical NEC 976.0	E858.7	E946.0	E950.4	E962.0	E980.4
Imipramine 969.05	E854.0	E939.0	E950.3	E962.0	E980.3
Immu–G 964.6	E858.2	E934.6	E950.4	E962.0	E980.4
Immuglobin 964.6	E858.2	E934.6	E950.4	E962.0	E980.4
Immune serum globulin 964.6	E858.2	E934.6	E950.4	E962.0	E980.4
Immunosuppressive agents 963.1	E858.1	E933.1	E950.4	E962.0	E980.4
Immu–tetanus 964.6	E858.2	E934.6	E950.4	E962.0	E980.4
Indandione (derivatives) 964.2	E858.2	E934.2	E950.4	E962.0	E980.4
Inderal 972.0	E858.3	E942.0	E950.4	E962.0	E980.4
Indian					
hemp 969.6	E854.1	E939.6	E950.3	E962.0	E980.3
tobacco 988.2	E865.4	—	E950.9	E962.1	E980.9
Indigo carmine. 977.8	E858.8	E947.8	E950.4	E962.0	E980.4
Indocin 965.69	E850.6	E935.6	E950.0	E962.0	E980.0
Indocyanine green 977.8	E858.8	E947.8	E950.4	E962.0	E980.4
Indomethacin 965.69	E850.6	E935.6	E950.0	E962.0	E980.0
Industrial					
alcohol 980.9	E860.9	—	E950.9	E962.1	E980.9
fumes. 987.8	E869.8	—	E952.8	E962.2	E982.8
solvents (fumes) (vapors). 982.8	E862.9	—	E950.9	E962.1	E980.9
Influenza vaccine. 979.6	E858.8	E949.6	E950.4	E962.0	E982.8
Ingested substances NEC 989.9	E866.9	—	E950.9	E962.1	E980.9
INH (isoniazid) 961.8	E857	E931.8	E950.4	E962.0	E980.4
Inhalation, gas (noxious) — see Gas					
Ink. 989.89	E866.8	—	E950.9	E962.1	E980.9
Innovar. 967.6	E852.5	E937.6	E950.2	E962.0	E980.2
Inositol niacinate 972.2	E858.3	E942.2	E950.4	E962.0	E980.4
Inproquone 963.1	E858.1	E933.1	E950.4	E962.0	E980.4
Insect (sting), venomous 989.5	E905.5	—	E950.9	E962.1	E980.9
Insecticides (see also Pesticides) 989.4	E863.4	—	E950.6	E962.1	E980.7
chlorinated. 989.2	E863.0	—	E950.6	E962.1	E980.7
mixtures. 989.4	E863.3	—	E950.6	E962.1	E980.7
organochlorine (compounds) 989.2	E863.0	—	E950.6	E962.1	E980.7
organophosphorus (compounds) 989.3	E863.1	—	E950.6	E962.1	E980.7
Insular tissue extract 962.3	E858.0	E932.3	E950.4	E962.0	E980.4

Substance	Poisoning	Accident	Therapeutic Use	Suicide Attempt	Assault	Undetermined
			External Cause (E-Code)			
Insulin (amorphous) (globin) (isophane) (Lente) (NPH) (protamine) (Semilente) (Ultralente) (zinc)	962.3	E858.0	E932.3	E950.4	E962.0	E980.4
Intranarcon	968.3	E855.1	E938.3	E950.4	E962.0	E980.4
Inulin.	977.8	E858.8	E947.8	E950.4	E962.0	E980.4
Invert sugar	974.5	E858.5	E944.5	E950.4	E962.0	E980.4
Inza—*see* Naproxen						
Iodide NEC (*see also* Iodine)	976.0	E858.7	E946.0	E950.4	E962.0	E980.4
mercury (ointment)	976.0	E858.7	E946.0	E950.4	E962.0	E980.4
methylate	976.0	E858.7	E946.0	E950.4	E962.0	E980.4
potassium (expectorant) NEC	975.5	E858.6	E945.5	E950.4	E962.0	E980.4
Iodinated glycerol	975.5	E858.6	E945.5	E950.4	E962.0	E980.4
Iodine (antiseptic, external) (tincture)						
NEC	976.0	E858.7	E946.0	E950.4	E962.0	E980.4
diagnostic	977.8	E858.8	E947.8	E950.4	E962.0	E980.4
for thyroid conditions (antithyroid)	962.8	E858.0	E932.8	E950.4	E962.0	E980.4
vapor	987.8	E869.8	—	E952.8	E962.2	E982.8
Iodized oil	977.8	E858.8	E947.8	E950.4	E962.0	E980.4
Iodobismitol	961.2	E857	E931.2	E950.4	E962.0	E980.4
Iodochlorhydroxyquin	961.3	E857	E931.3	E950.4	E962.0	E980.4
topical	976.0	E858.7	E946.0	E950.4	E962.0	E980.4
Iodoform	976.0	E858.7	E946.0	E950.4	E962.0	E980.4
Iodopanoic acid	977.8	E858.8	E947.8	E950.4	E962.0	E980.4
Iodophthalein	977.8	E858.8	E947.8	E950.4	E962.0	E980.4
Ion exchange resins	974.5	E858.5	E944.5	E950.4	E962.0	E980.4
Iopanoic acid	977.8	E858.8	E947.8	E950.4	E962.0	E980.4
Iophendylate	977.8	E858.8	E947.8	E950.4	E962.0	E980.4
Iothiouracil	962.8	E858.0	E932.8	E950.4	E962.0	E980.4
Ipecac	973.6	E858.4	E943.6	E950.4	E962.0	E980.4
Ipecacuanha	973.6	E858.4	E943.6	E950.4	E962.0	E980.4
Ipodate	977.8	E858.8	E947.8	E950.4	E962.0	E980.4
Ipral	967.0	E851	E937.0	E950.1	E962.0	E980.1
Ipratropium	975.1	E858.6	E945.1	E950.4	E962.0	E980.4
Iproniazid	969.01	E854.0	E939.0	E950.3	E962.0	E980.3
Iron (compounds) (medicinal)						
(preparations)	964.0	E858.2	E934.0	E950.4	E962.0	E980.4
dextran	964.0	E858.2	E934.0	E950.4	E962.0	E980.4
nonmedicinal (dust) (fumes) NEC	985.8	E866.4	—	E950.9	E962.1	E980.9
Irritant drug	977.9	E858.9	E947.9	E950.5	E962.0	E980.5
Ismelin	972.6	E858.3	E942.6	E950.4	E962.0	E980.4
Isoamyl nitrite	972.4	E858.3	E942.4	E950.4	E962.0	E980.4
Isobutyl acetate	982.8	E862.4	—	E950.9	E962.1	E980.9
Isocarboxazid	969.01	E854.0	E939.0	E950.3	E962.0	E980.3
Isoephedrine	971.2	E855.5	E941.2	E950.4	E962.0	E980.4
Isoetharine	971.2	E855.5	E941.2	E950.4	E962.0	E980.4
Isofluorophate	971.0	E855.3	E941.0	E950.4	E962.0	E980.4
Isoniazid (INH)	961.8	E857	E931.8	E950.4	E962.0	E980.4
Isopentaquine	961.4	E857	E931.4	E950.4	E962.0	E980.4
Isophane insulin	962.3	E858.0	E932.3	E950.4	E962.0	E980.4
Isopregnenone	962.2	E858.0	E932.2	E950.4	E962.0	E980.4
Isoprenaline	971.2	E855.5	E941.2	E950.4	E962.0	E980.4
Isopropamide	971.1	E855.4	E941.1	E950.4	E962.0	E980.4
Isopropanol	980.2	E860.3	—	E950.9	E962.1	E980.9
topical (germicide)	976.0	E858.7	E946.0	E950.4	E962.0	E980.4
Isopropyl						
acetate	982.8	E862.4	—	E950.9	E962.1	E980.9
alcohol	980.2	E860.3	—	E950.9	E962.1	E980.9
topical (germicide)	976.0	E858.7	E946.0	E950.4	E962.0	E980.4
ether	982.8	E862.4	—	E950.9	E962.1	E980.9
Isoproterenol	971.2	E855.5	E941.2	E950.4	E962.0	E980.4

Substance	Poisoning	Accident	Therapeutic Use	Suicide Attempt	Assault	Undetermined
				External Cause (E-Code)		
Isosorbide dinitrate 972.4	E858.3	E942.4	E950.4	E962.0	E980.4
Isothipendyl 963.0	E858.1	E933.0	E950.4	E962.0	E980.4
Isoxazolyl penicillin. 960.0	E856	E930.0	E950.4	E962.0	E980.4
Isoxsuprine hydrochloride 972.5	E858.3	E942.5	E950.4	E962.0	E980.4
I–thyroxine sodium 962.7	E858.0	E932.7	E950.4	E962.0	E980.4
Jaborandi (pilocarpus) (extract) 971.0	E855.3	E941.0	E950.4	E962.0	E980.4
Jalap 973.1	E858.4	E943.1	E950.4	E962.0	E980.4
Jamaica					
dogwood (bark). 965.7	E850.7	E935.7	E950.0	E962.0	E980.0
ginger. 989.89	E866.8	—	E950.9	E962.1	E980.9
Jatropha. 988.2	E865.4	—	E950.9	E962.1	E980.9
curcas. 988.2	E865.3	—	E950.9	E962.1	E980.9
Jectofer. 964.0	E858.2	E934.0	E950.4	E962.0	E980.4
Jellyfish (sting). 989.5	E905.6	—	E950.9	E962.1	E980.9
Jequirity (bean) 988.2	E865.3	—	E950.9	E962.1	E980.9
Jimson weed. 988.2	E865.4	—	E950.9	E962.1	E980.9
seeds 988.2	E865.3	—	E950.9	E962.1	E980.9
Juniper tar (oil) (ointment) 976.4	E858.7	E946.4	E950.4	E962.0	E980.4
Kallikrein 972.5	E858.3	E942.5	E950.4	E962.0	E980.4
Kanamycin 960.6	E856	E930.6	E950.4	E962.0	E980.4
Kantrex 960.6	E856	E930.6	E950.4	E962.0	E980.4
Kaolin 973.5	E858.4	E943.5	E950.4	E962.0	E980.4
Karaya (gum) 973.3	E858.4	E943.3	E950.4	E962.0	E980.4
Kemithal 968.3	E855.1	E938.3	E950.4	E962.0	E980.4
Kenacort 962.0	E858.0	E932.0	E950.4	E962.0	E980.4
Keratolytics 976.4	E858.7	E946.4	E950.4	E962.0	E980.4
Keratoplastics 976.4	E858.7	E946.4	E950.4	E962.0	E980.4
Kerosene, kerosine (fuel) (solvent) NEC . . . 981	E862.1	—	E950.9	E962.1	E980.9
insecticide. 981	E863.4	—	E950.6	E962.1	E980.7
vapor 987.1	E869.8	—	E952.8	E962.2	E982.8
Ketamine 968.3	E855.1	E938.3	E950.4	E962.0	E980.4
Ketobemidone 965.09	E850.2	E935.2	E950.0	E962.0	E980.0
Ketols 982.8	E862.4	—	E950.9	E962.1	E980.9
Ketone oils 982.8	E862.4	—	E950.9	E962.1	E980.9
Ketoprofen 965.61	E850.6	E935.6	E950.0	E962.0	E980.0
Kiln gas or vapor (carbon monoxide) 986	E868.8	—	E952.1	E962.2	E982.1
Konsyl 973.3	E858.4	E943.3	E950.4	E962.0	E980.4
Kosam seed 988.2	E865.3	—	E950.9	E962.1	E980.9
Krait (venom) 989.5	E905.0	—	E950.9	E962.1	E980.9
Kwell (insecticide) 989.2	E863.0	—	E950.6	E962.1	E980.7
anti–infective (topical) 976.0	E858.7	E946.0	E950.4	E962.0	E980.4
Laburnum (flowers) (seeds) 988.2	E865.3	—	E950.9	E962.1	E980.9
leaves. 988.2	E865.4	—	E950.9	E962.1	E980.9
Lacquers 989.89	E861.6	—	E950.9	E962.1	E980.9
Lacrimogenic gas. 987.5	E869.3	—	E952.8	E962.2	E982.8
Lactic acid 983.1	E864.1	—	E950.7	E962.1	E980.6
Lactobacillus acidophilus 973.5	E858.4	E943.5	E950.4	E962.0	E980.4
Lactoflavin 963.5	E858.1	E933.5	E950.4	E962.0	E980.4
Lactuca (virosa) (extract) 967.8	E852.8	E937.8	E950.2	E962.0	E980.2
Lactucarium 967.8	E852.8	E937.8	E950.2	E962.0	E980.2
Laevulose. 974.5	E858.5	E944.5	E950.4	E962.0	E980.4
Lanatoside(C) 972.1	E858.3	E942.1	E950.4	E962.0	E980.4
Lanolin (lotion) 976.3	E858.7	E946.3	E950.4	E962.0	E980.4
Largactil 969.1	E853.0	E939.1	E950.3	E962.0	E980.3
Larkspur 988.2	E865.3	—	E950.9	E962.1	E980.9
Laroxyl 969.05	E854.0	E939.0	E950.3	E962.0	E980.3
Lasix 974.4	E858.5	E944.4	E950.4	E962.0	E980.4
Latex 989.82	E866.8	—	E950.9	E962.1	E980.9
Lathyrus (seed). 988.2	E865.3	—	E950.9	E962.1	E980.9
Laudanum. 965.09	E850.2	E935.2	E950.0	E962.0	E980.0
Laudexium 975.2	E858.6	E945.2	E950.4	E962.0	E980.4

Substance	Poisoning	Accident	Therapeutic Use	Suicide Attempt	Assault	Undetermined
			External Cause (E-Code)			
Laurel, black or cherry	988.2	E865.4	—	E950.9	E962.1	E980.9
Laurolinium	976.0	E858.7	E946.0	E950.4	E962.0	E980.4
Lauryl sulfoacetate	976.2	E858.7	E946.2	E950.4	E962.0	E980.4
Laxatives NEC	973.3	E858.4	E943.3	E950.4	E962.0	E980.4
emollient	973.2	E858.4	E943.2	E950.4	E962.0	E980.4
L–dopa	966.4	E855.0	E936.4	E950.4	E962.0	E980.4
L Tryptophan—*see* amino acid						
Lead (dust) (fumes) (vapor) NEC	984.9	E866.0	—	E950.9	E962.1	E980.9
acetate (dust)	984.1	E866.0	—	E950.9	E962.1	E980.9
anti–infectives	961.2	E857	E931.2	E950.4	E962.0	E980.4
antiknock compound (tetraethyl)	984.1	E862.1	—	E950.9	E962.1	E980.9
arsenate, arsenite (dust) (insecticide)						
(vapor)	985.1	E863.4	—	E950.8	E962.1	E980.8
herbicide	985.1	E863.5	—	E950.8	E962.1	E980.8
carbonate	984.0	E866.0	—	E950.9	E962.1	E980.9
paint	984.0	E861.5	—	E950.9	E962.1	E980.9
chromate	984.0	E866.0	—	E950.9	E962.1	E980.9
paint	984.0	E861.5	—	E950.9	E962.1	E980.9
dioxide	984.0	E866.0	—	E950.9	E962.1	E980.9
inorganic (compound)	984.0	E866.0	—	E950.9	E962.1	E980.9
paint	984.0	E861.5	—	E950.9	E962.1	E980.9
iodine	984.0	E866.0	—	E950.9	E962.1	E980.9
pigment (paint)	984.0	E861.5	—	E950.9	E962.1	E980.9
monoxide (dust)	984.0	E866.0	—	E950.9	E962.1	E980.9
paint	984.0	E861.5	—	E950.9	E962.1	E980.9
organic	984.1	E866.0	—	E950.9	E962.1	E980.9
oxide	984.0	E866.0	—	E950.9	E962.1	E980.9
paint	984.0	E861.5	—	E950.9	E962.1	E980.9
paint	984.0	E861.5	—	E950.9	E962.1	E980.9
salts	984.0	E866.0	—	E950.9	E962.1	E980.9
specified compound NEC	984.8	E866.0	—	E950.9	E962.1	E980.9
tetra–ethyl	984.1	E862.1	—	E950.9	E962.1	E980.9
Lebanese red	969.6	E854.1	E939.6	E950.3	E962.0	E980.3
Lente Iletin (insulin)	962.3	E858.0	E932.3	E950.4	E962.0	E980.4
Leptazol	970.0	E854.3	E940.0	E950.4	E962.0	E980.4
Leritine	965.09	E850.2	E935.2	E950.0	E962.0	E980.0
Letter	962.7	E858.0	E932.7	E950.4	E962.0	E980.4
Lettuce opium	967.8	E852.8	E937.8	E950.2	E962.0	E980.2
Leucovorin (factor)	964.1	E858.2	E934.1	E950.4	E962.0	E980.4
Leukeran	963.1	E858.1	E933.1	E950.4	E962.0	E980.4
Levalbuterol	975.7	E858.6	E945.7	E950.4	E962.0	E980.4
Levallorphan	970.1	E854.3	E940.1	E950.4	E962.0	E980.4
Levanil	967.8	E852.8	E937.8	E950.2	E962.0	E980.2
Levarterenol	971.2	E855.5	E941.2	E950.4	E962.0	E980.4
Levodopa	966.4	E855.0	E936.4	E950.4	E962.0	E980.4
Levo–dromoran	965.09	E850.2	E935.2	E950.0	E962.0	E980.0
Levoid	962.7	E858.0	E932.7	E950.4	E962.0	E980.4
Levo–iso–methadone	965.02	E850.1	E935.1	E950.0	E962.0	E980.0
Levomepromazine	967.8	E852.8	E937.8	E950.2	E962.0	E980.2
Levoprome	967.8	E852.8	E937.8	E950.2	E962.0	E980.2
Levopropoxyphene	975.4	E858.6	E945.4	E950.4	E962.0	E980.4
Levorphan, levophanol	965.09	E850.2	E935.2	E950.0	E962.0	E980.0
Levothyroxine (sodium)	962.7	E858.0	E932.7	E950.4	E962.0	E980.4
Levsin	971.1	E855.4	E941.1	E950.4	E962.0	E980.4
Levulose	974.5	E858.5	E944.5	E950.4	E962.0	E980.4
Lewisite (gas)	985.1	E866.3	—	E950.8	E962.1	E980.8
Librium	969.4	E853.2	E939.4	E950.3	E962.0	E980.3
Lidex	976.0	E858.7	E946.0	E950.4	E962.0	E980.4
Lidocaine (infiltration) (topical)	968.5	E855.2	E938.5	E950.4	E962.0	E980.4
nerve block (peripheral) (plexus)	968.6	E855.2	E938.6	E950.4	E962.0	E980.4

Substance	Poisoning	Accident	Therapeutic Use	Suicide Attempt	Assault	Undetermined
			External Cause (E-Code)			
spinal	968.7	E855.2	E938.7	E950.4	E962.0	E980.4
Lighter fluid	981	E862.1	—	E950.9	E962.1	E980.9
Lignocaine (infiltration) (topical)	968.5	E855.2	E938.5	E950.4	E962.0	E980.4
nerve block (peripheral) (plexus)	968.6	E855.2	E938.6	E950.4	E962.0	E980.4
spinal	968.7	E855.2	E938.7	E950.4	E962.0	E980.4
Ligroin(e) (solvent)	981	E862.0	—	E950.9	E962.1	E980.9
vapor	987.1	E869.8	—	E952.8	E962.2	E982.8
Ligustrum vulgare	988.2	E865.3	—	E950.9	E962.1	E980.9
Lily of the valley	988.2	E865.4	—	E950.9	E962.1	E980.9
Lime (chloride)	983.2	E864.2	—	E950.7	E962.1	E980.6
solution, sulferated	976.4	E858.7	E946.4	E950.4	E962.0	E980.4
Limonene	982.8	E862.4	—	E950.9	E962.1	E980.9
Lincomycin	960.8	E856	E930.8	E950.4	E962.0	E980.4
Lindane (insecticide) (vapor)	989.2	E863.0	—	E950.6	E962.1	E980.7
anti–infective (topical)	976.0	E858.7	E946.0	E950.4	E962.0	E980.4
Liniments NEC	976.9	E858.7	E946.9	E950.4	E962.0	E980.4
Linoleic acid	972.2	E858.3	E942.2	E950.4	E962.0	E980.4
Liothyronine	962.7	E858.0	E932.7	E950.4	E962.0	E980.4
Liotrix	962.7	E858.0	E932.7	E950.4	E962.0	E980.4
Lipancreatin	973.4	E858.4	E943.4	E950.4	E962.0	E980.4
Lipo–Lutin	962.2	E858.0	E932.2	E950.4	E962.0	E980.4
Lipotropic agents	977.1	E858.8	E947.1	E950.4	E962.0	E980.4
Liquefied petroleum gases	987.0	E868.0	—	E951.1	E962.2	E981.1
piped (pure or mixed with air)	987.0	E867	—	E951.0	E962.2	E981.0
Liquid petrolatum	973.2	E858.4	E943.2	E950.4	E962.0	E980.4
substance	989.9	E866.9	—	E950.9	E962.1	E980.9
specified NEC	989.89	E866.8	—	E950.9	E962.1	E980.9
Lirugen	979.4	E858.8	E949.4	E950.4	E962.0	E980.4
Lithane	969.8	E855.8	E939.8	E950.3	E962.0	E980.3
Lithium	985.8	E866.4	—	E950.9	E962.1	E980.9
carbonate	969.8	E855.8	E939.8	E950.3	E962.0	E980.3
Lithonate	969.8	E855.8	E939.8	E950.3	E962.0	E980.3
Liver (extract) (injection) (preparations)	964.1	E858.2	E934.1	E950.4	E962.0	E980.4
Lizard (bite) (venom)	989.5	E905.0	—	E950.9	E962.1	E980.9
LMD	964.8	E858.2	E934.8	E950.4	E962.0	E980.4
Lobelia	988.2	E865.4	—	E950.9	E962.1	E980.9
Lobeline	970.0	E854.3	E940.0	E950.4	E962.0	E980.4
Locorten	976.0	E858.7	E946.0	E950.4	E962.0	E980.4
Lolium temulentum	988.2	E865.3	—	E950.9	E962.1	E980.9
Lomotil	973.5	E858.4	E943.5	E950.4	E962.0	E980.4
Lomustine	963.1	E858.1	E933.1	E950.4	E962.0	E980.4
Lophophora williamsii	969.6	E854.1	E939.6	E950.3	E962.0	E980.3
Lorazepam	969.4	E853.2	E939.4	E950.3	E962.0	E980.3
Lotions NEC	976.9	E858.7	E946.9	E950.4	E962.0	E980.4
Lotronex	973.8	E858.4	E943.8	E950.4	E962.0	E980.4
Lotusate	967.0	E851	E937.0	E950.1	E962.0	E980.1
Lowila	976.2	E858.7	E946.2	E950.4	E962.0	E980.4
Loxapine	969.3	E853.8	E939.3	E950.3	E962.0	E980.3
Lozenges (throat)	976.6	E858.7	E946.6	E950.4	E962.0	E980.4
LSD (25)	969.6	E854.1	E939.6	E950.3	E962.0	E980.3
Lubricating oil NEC	981	E862.2	—	E950.9	E962.1	E980.9
Lucanthone	961.6	E857	E931.6	E950.4	E962.0	E980.4
Luminal	967.0	E851	E937.0	E950.1	E962.0	E980.1
Lung irritant (gas) NEC	987.9	E869.9	—	E952.9	E962.2	E982.9
Lutocylol	962.2	E858.0	E932.2	E950.4	E962.0	E980.4
Lutromone	962.2	E858.0	E932.2	E950.4	E962.0	E980.4
Lututrin	975.0	E858.6	E945.0	E950.4	E962.0	E980.4
Lye (concentrated)	983.2	E864.2	—	E950.7	E962.1	E980.6
Lygranum (skin test)	977.8	E858.8	E947.8	E950.4	E962.0	E980.4
Lymecycline	960.4	E856	E930.4	E950.4	E962.0	E980.4
Lymphogranuloma venereum antigen	977.8	E858.8	E947.8	E950.4	E962.0	E980.4

TABLE OF DRUGS AND CHEMICALS

Substance	Poisoning	Accident	Therapeutic Use	Suicide Attempt	Assault	Undetermined
			External Cause (E-Code)			
Lynestrenol	962.2	E858.0	E932.2	E950.4	E962.0	E980.4
Lyovac Sodium Edecrin	974.4	E858.5	E944.4	E950.4	E962.0	E980.4
Lypressin	962.5	E858.0	E932.5	E950.4	E962.0	E980.4
Lysergic acid (amide) (diethylamide)	969.6	E854.1	E939.6	E950.3	E962.0	E980.3
Lysergide	969.6	E854.1	E939.6	E950.3	E962.0	E980.3
Lysine vasopressin	962.5	E858.0	E932.5	E950.4	E962.0	E980.4
Lysol	983.0	E864.0	—	E950.7	E962.1	E980.6
Lytta (vitatta)	976.8	E858.7	E946.8	E950.4	E962.0	E980.4
Mace	987.5	E869.3	—	E952.8	E962.2	E982.8
Macrolides (antibiotics)	960.3	E856	E930.3	E950.4	E962.0	E980.4
Mafenide	976.0	E858.7	E946.0	E950.4	E962.0	E980.4
Magaldrate	973.0	E858.4	E943.0	E950.4	E962.0	E980.4
Magic mushroom	969.6	E854.1	E939.6	E950.3	E962.0	E980.3
Magnamycin	960.8	E856	E930.8	E950.4	E962.0	E980.4
Magnesia magma	973.0	E858.4	E943.0	E950.4	E962.0	E980.4
Magnesium (compounds) (fumes) NEC	985.8	E866.4	—	E950.9	E962.1	E980.9
antacid	973.0	E858.4	E943.0	E950.4	E962.0	E980.4
carbonate	973.0	E858.4	E943.0	E950.4	E962.0	E980.4
cathartic	973.3	E858.4	E943.3	E950.4	E962.0	E980.4
citrate	973.3	E858.4	E943.3	E950.4	E962.0	E980.4
hydroxide	973.0	E858.4	E943.0	E950.4	E962.0	E980.4
oxide	973.0	E858.4	E943.0	E950.4	E962.0	E980.4
sulfate (oral)	973.3	E858.4	E943.3	E950.4	E962.0	E980.4
intravenous	966.3	E855.0	E936.3	E950.4	E962.0	E980.4
trisilicate	973.0	E858.4	E943.0	E950.4	E962.0	E980.4
Malathion (insecticide)	989.3	E863.1	—	E950.6	E962.1	E980.7
Male fern (oleoresin)	961.6	E857	E931.6	E950.4	E962.0	E980.4
Mandelic acid	961.9	E857	E931.9	E950.4	E962.0	E980.4
Manganese compounds (fumes) NEC	985.2	E866.4	—	E950.9	E962.1	E980.9
Mannitol (diuretic) (medicinal) NEC	974.4	E858.5	E944.4	E950.4	E962.0	E980.4
hexanitrate	972.4	E858.3	E942.4	E950.4	E962.0	E980.4
mustard	963.1	E858.1	E933.1	E950.4	E962.0	E980.4
Mannomustine	963.1	E858.1	E933.1	E950.4	E962.0	E980.4
MAO inhibitors	969.01	E854.0	E939.0	E950.3	E962.0	E980.3
Mapharsen	961.1	E857	E931.1	E950.4	E962.0	E980.4
Marcaine	968.9	E855.2	E938.9	E950.4	E962.0	E980.4
infiltration (subcutaneous)	968.5	E855.2	E938.5	E950.4	E962.0	E980.4
nerve block (peripheral) (plexus)	968.6	E855.2	E938.6	E950.4	E962.0	E980.4
Marezine	963.0	E858.1	E933.0	E950.4	E962.0	E980.4
Marihuana, marijuana (derivatives)	969.6	E854.1	E939.6	E950.3	E962.0	E980.3
Marine animals or plants (sting)	989.5	E905.6	—	E950.9	E962.1	E980.9
Marplan	969.01	E854.0	E939.0	E950.3	E962.0	E980.3
Marsh gas	987.1	E869.8	—	E952.8	E962.2	E982.8
Marsilid	969.01	E854.0	E939.0	E950.3	E962.0	E980.3
Matulane	963.1	E858.1	E933.1	E950.4	E962.0	E980.4
Mazindol	977.0	E858.8	E947.0	E950.4	E962.0	E980.4
MDMA	969.72	E854.2	E939.7	E950.3	E962.0	E980.3
Meadow saffron	988.2	E865.3	—	E950.9	E962.1	E980.9
Measles vaccine	979.4	E858.8	E949.4	E950.4	E962.0	E980.4
Meat, noxious or nonbacterial	988.8	E865.0	—	E950.9	E962.1	E980.9
Mebanazine	969.01	E854.0	E939.0	E950.3	E962.0	E980.3
Mebaral	967.0	E851	E937.0	E950.1	E962.0	E980.1
Mebendazole	961.6	E857	E931.6	E950.4	E962.0	E980.4
Mebeverine	975.1	E858.6	E945.1	E950.4	E962.0	E980.4
Mebhydroline	963.0	E858.1	E933.0	E950.4	E962.0	E980.4
Mebrophenhydramine	963.0	E858.1	E933.0	E950.4	E962.0	E980.4
Mebutamate	969.5	E853.8	E939.5	E950.3	E962.0	E980.3
Mecamylamine (chloride)	972.3	E858.3	E942.3	E950.4	E962.0	E980.4
Mechlorethamine hydrochloride	963.1	E858.1	E933.1	E950.4	E962.0	E980.4
Meclizene (hydrochloride)	963.0	E858.1	E933.0	E950.4	E962.0	E980.4

Substance	Poisoning	External Cause (E-Code)				
		Accident	Therapeutic Use	Suicide Attempt	Assault	Undetermined
Meclofenoxate	970.0	E854.3	E940.0	E950.4	E962.0	E980.4
Meclozine (hydrochloride)	963.0	E858.1	E933.0	E950.4	E962.0	E980.4
Medazepam	969.4	E853.2	E939.4	E950.3	E962.0	E980.3
Medicine, medicinal substance	977.9	E858.9	E947.9	E950.5	E962.0	E980.5
specified NEC	977.8	E858.8	E947.8	E950.4	E962.0	E980.4
Medinal	967.0	E851	E937.0	E950.1	E962.0	E980.1
Medomin	967.0	E851	E937.0	E950.1	E962.0	E980.1
Medroxyprogesterone	962.2	E858.0	E932.2	E950.4	E962.0	E980.4
Medrysone	976.5	E858.7	E946.5	E950.4	E962.0	E980.4
Mefenamic acid	965.7	E850.7	E935.7	E950.0	E962.0	E980.0
Megahallucinogen	969.6	E854.1	E939.6	E950.3	E962.0	E980.3
Megestrol	962.2	E858.0	E932.2	E950.4	E962.0	E980.4
Meglumine	977.8	E858.8	E947.8	E950.4	E962.0	E980.4
Meladinin	976.3	E858.7	E946.3	E950.4	E962.0	E980.4
Melanizing agents	976.3	E858.7	E946.3	E950.4	E962.0	E980.4
Melarsoprol	961.1	E857	E931.1	E950.4	E962.0	E980.4
Melia azedarach	988.2	E865.3	—	E950.9	E962.1	E980.9
Mellaril	969.1	E853.0	E939.1	E950.3	E962.0	E980.3
Meloxine	976.3	E858.7	E946.3	E950.4	E962.0	E980.4
Melphalan	963.1	E858.1	E933.1	E950.4	E962.0	E980.4
Menadiol sodium diphosphate	964.3	E858.2	E934.3	E950.4	E962.0	E980.4
Menadione (sodium bisulfate)	964.3	E858.2	E934.3	E950.4	E962.0	E980.4
Menaphthone	964.3	E858.2	E934.3	E950.4	E962.0	E980.4
Meningococcal vaccine	978.8	E858.8	E948.8	E950.4	E962.0	E980.4
Menningovax–C	978.8	E858.8	E948.8	E950.4	E962.0	E980.4
Menotropins	962.4	E858.0	E932.4	E950.4	E962.0	E980.4
Menthol NEC	976.1	E858.7	E946.1	E950.4	E962.0	E980.4
Mepacrine	961.3	E857	E931.3	E950.4	E962.0	E980.4
Meparfynol	967.8	E852.8	E937.8	E950.2	E962.0	E980.2
Mepazine	969.1	E853.0	E939.1	E950.3	E962.0	E980.3
Mepenzolate	971.1	E855.4	E941.1	E950.4	E962.0	E980.4
Meperidine	965.09	E850.2	E935.2	E950.0	E962.0	E980.0
Mephenamin(e)	966.4	E855.0	E936.4	E950.4	E962.0	E980.4
Mephenesin (carbamate)	968.0	E855.1	E938.0	E950.4	E962.0	E980.4
Mephenoxalone	969.5	E853.8	E939.5	E950.3	E962.0	E980.3
Mephentermine	971.2	E855.5	E941.2	E950.4	E962.0	E980.4
Mephenytoin	966.1	E855.0	E936.1	E950.4	E962.0	E980.4
Mephobarbital	967.0	E851	E937.0	E950.1	E962.0	E980.1
Mepiperphenidol	971.1	E855.4	E941.1	E950.4	E962.0	E980.4
Mepivacaine	968.9	E855.2	E938.9	E950.4	E962.0	E980.4
infiltration (subcutaneous)	968.5	E855.2	E938.5	E950.4	E962.0	E980.4
nerve block (peripheral) (plexus)	968.6	E855.2	E938.6	E950.4	E962.0	E980.4
topical (surface)	968.5	E855.2	E938.5	E950.4	E962.0	E980.4
Meprednisone	962.0	E858.0	E932.0	E950.4	E962.0	E980.4
Meprobam	969.5	E853.8	E939.5	E950.3	E962.0	E980.3
Meprobamate	969.5	E853.8	E939.5	E950.3	E962.0	E980.3
Mepyramine (maleate)	963.0	E858.1	E933.0	E950.4	E962.0	E980.4
Meralluride	974.0	E858.5	E944.0	E950.4	E962.0	E980.4
Merbaphen	974.0	E858.5	E944.0	E950.4	E962.0	E980.4
Merbromin	976.0	E858.7	E946.0	E950.4	E962.0	E980.4
Mercaptomerin	974.0	E858.5	E944.0	E950.4	E962.0	E980.4
Mercaptopurine	963.1	E858.1	E933.1	E950.4	E962.0	E980.4
Mercumatilin	974.0	E858.5	E944.0	E950.4	E962.0	E980.4
Mercuramide	974.0	E858.5	E944.0	E950.4	E962.0	E980.4
Mercuranin	976.0	E858.7	E946.0	E950.4	E962.0	E980.4
Mercurochrome	976.0	E858.7	E946.0	E950.4	E962.0	E980.4
Mercury, mercuric, mercurous (compounds) (cyanide) (fumes) (nonmedicinal) (vapor) NEC	985.0	E866.1	—	E950.9	E962.1	E980.9
ammoniated	976.0	E858.7	E946.0	E950.4	E962.0	E980.4
anti–infective	961.2	E857	E931.2	E950.4	E962.0	E980.4

TABLE OF DRUGS AND CHEMICALS

Substance	Poisoning	Accident	Therapeutic Use	Suicide Attempt	Assault	Undetermined
			External Cause (E-Code)			
topical 976.0	E858.7	E946.0	E950.4	E962.0	E980.4
chloride (antiseptic) NEC 976.0	E858.7	E946.0	E950.4	E962.0	E980.4
fungicide 985.0	E863.6	—	E950.6	E962.1	E980.7
diuretic compounds 974.0	E858.5	E944.0	E950.4	E962.0	E980.4
fungicide 985.0	E863.6	—	E950.6	E962.1	E980.7
organic (fungicide) 985.0	E863.6	—	E950.6	E962.1	E980.7
Merethoxylline 974.0	E858.5	E944.0	E950.4	E962.0	E980.4
Mersalyl 974.0	E858.5	E944.0	E950.4	E962.0	E980.4
Merthiolate (topical) 976.0	E858.7	E946.0	E950.4	E962.0	E980.4
ophthalmic preparation 976.5	E858.7	E946.5	E950.4	E962.0	E980.4
Meruvax 979.4	E858.8	E949.4	E950.4	E962.0	E980.4
Mescal buttons 969.6	E854.1	E939.6	E950.3	E962.0	E980.3
Mescaline (salts) 969.6	E854.1	E939.6	E950.3	E962.0	E980.3
Mesoridazine besylate 969.1	E853.0	E939.1	E950.3	E962.0	E980.3
Mestanolone 962.1	E858.0	E932.1	E950.4	E962.0	E980.4
Mestranol 962.2	E858.0	E932.2	E950.4	E962.0	E980.4
Metacresylacetate 976.0	E858.7	E946.0	E950.4	E962.0	E980.4
Metaldehyde (snail killer) NEC 989.4	E863.4	—	E950.6	E962.1	E980.7
Metals (heavy) (nonmedicinal) NEC 985.9	E866.4	—	E950.9	E962.1	E980.9
dust, fumes, or vapor NEC 985.9	E866.4	—	E950.9	E962.1	E980.9
light NEC 985.9	E866.4	—	E950.9	E962.1	E980.9
dust, fumes, or vapor NEC 985.9	E866.4	—	E950.9	E962.1	E980.9
pesticides (dust) (vapor) 985.9	E863.4	—	E950.6	E962.1	E980.7
Metamucil 973.3	E858.4	E943.3	E950.4	E962.0	E980.4
Metaphen 976.0	E858.7	E946.0	E950.4	E962.0	E980.4
Metaproterenol 975.1	E858.6	E945.1	E950.4	E962.0	E980.4
Metaraminol 972.8	E858.3	E942.8	E950.4	E962.0	E980.4
Metaxalone 968.0	E855.1	E938.0	E950.4	E962.0	E980.4
Metformin 962.3	E858.0	E932.3	E950.4	E962.0	E980.4
Methacycline 960.4	E856	E930.4	E950.4	E962.0	E980.4
Methadone 965.02	E850.1	E935.1	E950.0	E962.0	E980.0
Methallenestril 962.2	E858.0	E932.2	E950.4	E962.0	E980.4
Methamphetamine 969.72	E854.2	E939.7	E950.3	E962.0	E980.3
Methandienone 962.1	E858.0	E932.1	E950.4	E962.0	E980.4
Methandriol 962.1	E858.0	E932.1	E950.4	E962.0	E980.4
Methandrostenolone 962.1	E858.0	E932.1	E950.4	E962.0	E980.4
Methane gas 987.1	E869.8	—	E952.8	E962.2	E982.8
Methanol 980.1	E860.2	—	E950.9	E962.1	E980.9
vapor 987.8	E869.8	—	E952.8	E962.2	E982.8
Methantheline 971.1	E855.4	E941.1	E950.4	E962.0	E980.4
Methaphenilene 963.0	E858.1	E933.0	E950.4	E962.0	E980.4
Methapyrilene 963.0	E858.1	E933.0	E950.4	E962.0	E980.4
Methaqualone (compounds) 967.4	E852.3	E937.4	E950.2	E962.0	E980.2
Metharbital, metharbitone 967.0	E851	E937.0	E950.1	E962.0	E980.1
Methazolamide 974.2	E858.5	E944.2	E950.4	E962.0	E980.4
Methdilazine 963.0	E858.1	E933.0	E950.4	E962.0	E980.4
Methedrine 969.72	E854.2	E939.7	E950.3	E962.0	E980.3
Methenamine (mandelate) 961.9	E857	E931.9	E950.4	E962.0	E980.4
Methenolone 962.1	E858.0	E932.1	E950.4	E962.0	E980.4
Methergine 975.0	E858.6	E945.0	E950.4	E962.0	E980.4
Methiacil 962.8	E858.0	E932.8	E950.4	E962.0	E980.4
Methicillin (sodium) 960.0	E856	E930.0	E950.4	E962.0	E980.4
Methimazole 962.8	E858.0	E932.8	E950.4	E962.0	E980.4
Methionine 977.1	E858.8	E947.1	E950.4	E962.0	E980.4
Methisazone 961.7	E857	E931.7	E950.4	E962.0	E980.4
Methitural 967.0	E851	E937.0	E950.1	E962.0	E980.1
Methixene 971.1	E855.4	E941.1	E950.4	E962.0	E980.4
Methobarbital, methobarbitone 967.0	E851	E937.0	E950.1	E962.0	E980.1
Methocarbamol 968.0	E855.1	E938.0	E950.4	E962.0	E980.4
Methohexital, methohexitone (sodium) 968.3	E855.1	E938.3	E950.4	E962.0	E980.4

TABLE OF DRUGS AND CHEMICALS

Substance	Poisoning	Accident	Therapeutic Use	Suicide Attempt	Assault	Undetermined
			External Cause (E-Code)			
Methoin	966.1	E855.0	E936.1	E950.4	E962.0	E980.4
Methopholine	965.7	E850.7	E935.7	E950.0	E962.0	E980.0
Methorate	975.4	E858.6	E945.4	E950.4	E962.0	E980.4
Methoserpidine	972.6	E858.3	E942.6	E950.4	E962.0	E980.4
Methotrexate	963.1	E858.1	E933.1	E950.4	E962.0	E980.4
Methotrimeprazine	967.8	E852.8	E937.8	E950.2	E962.0	E980.2
Methoxa–Dome	976.3	E858.7	E946.3	E950.4	E962.0	E980.4
Methoxamine	971.2	E855.5	E941.2	E950.4	E962.0	E980.4
Methoxsalen	976.3	E858.7	E946.3	E950.4	E962.0	E980.4
Methoxybenzyl penicillin	960.0	E856	E930.0	E950.4	E962.0	E980.4
Methoxychlor	989.2	E863.0	—	E950.6	E962.1	E980.7
Methoxyflurane	968.2	E855.1	E938.2	E950.4	E962.0	E980.4
Methoxyphenamine	971.2	E855.5	E941.2	E950.4	E962.0	E980.4
Methoxypromazine	969.1	E853.0	E939.1	E950.3	E962.0	E980.3
Methoxypsoralen	976.3	E858.7	E946.3	E950.4	E962.0	E980.4
Methscopolamine (bromide)	971.1	E855.4	E941.1	E950.4	E962.0	E980.4
Methsuximide	966.2	E855.0	E936.2	E950.4	E962.0	E980.4
Methyclothiazide	974.3	E858.5	E944.3	E950.4	E962.0	E980.4
Methyl						
acetate	982.8	E862.4	—	E950.9	E962.1	E980.9
acetone	982.8	E862.4	—	E950.9	E962.1	E980.9
alcohol	980.1	E860.2	—	E950.9	E962.1	E980.9
amphetamine	969.72	E854.2	E939.7	E950.3	E962.0	E980.3
androstanolone	962.1	E858.0	E932.1	E950.4	E962.0	E980.4
atropine	971.1	E855.4	E941.1	E950.4	E962.0	E980.4
benzene	982.0	E862.4	—	E950.9	E962.1	E980.9
bromide (gas)	987.8	E869.8	—	E952.8	E962.2	E982.8
fumigant	987.8	E863.8	—	E950.6	E962.2	E980.7
butanol	980.8	E860.8	—	E950.9	E962.1	E980.9
carbinol	980.1	E860.2	—	E950.9	E962.1	E980.9
cellosolve	982.8	E862.4	—	E950.9	E962.1	E980.9
cellulose	973.3	E858.4	E943.3	E950.4	E962.0	E980.4
chloride (gas)	987.8	E869.8	—	E952.8	E962.2	E982.8
cyclohexane	982.8	E862.4	—	E950.9	E962.1	E980.9
cyclohexanone	982.8	E862.4	—	E950.9	E962.1	E980.9
dihydromorphinone	965.09	E850.2	E935.2	E950.0	E962.0	E980.0
ergometrine	975.0	E858.6	E945.0	E950.4	E962.0	E980.4
ergonovine	975.0	E858.6	E945.0	E950.4	E962.0	E980.4
ethyl ketone	982.8	E862.4	—	E950.9	E962.1	E980.9
hydrazine	983.9	E864.3	—	E950.7	E962.1	E980.6
isobutyl ketone	982.8	E862.4	—	E950.9	E962.1	E980.9
morphine NEC	965.09	E850.2	E935.2	E950.0	E962.0	E980.0
parafynol	967.8	E852.8	E937.8	E950.2	E962.0	E980.2
parathion	989.3	E863.1	—	E950.6	E962.1	E980.7
pentynol NEC	967.8	E852.8	E937.8	E950.2	E962.0	E980.2
peridol	969.2	E853.1	E939.2	E950.3	E962.0	E980.3
phenidate	969.73	E854.2	E939.7	E950.3	E962.0	E980.3
prednisolone	962.0	E858.0	E932.0	E950.4	E962.0	E980.4
ENT agent	976.6	E858.7	E946.6	E950.4	E962.0	E980.4
ophthalmic preparation	976.5	E858.7	E946.5	E950.4	E962.0	E980.4
topical NEC	976.0	E858.7	E946.0	E950.4	E962.0	E980.4
propylcarbinol	980.8	E860.8	—	E950.9	E962.1	E980.9
rosaniline NEC	976.0	E858.7	E946.0	E950.4	E962.0	E980.4
salicylate NEC	976.3	E858.7	E946.3	E950.4	E962.0	E980.4
sulfate (fumes)	987.8	E869.8	—	E952.8	E962.2	E982.8
liquid	983.9	E864.3	—	E950.7	E962.1	E980.6
sulfonal	967.8	E852.8	E937.8	E950.2	E962.0	E980.2
testosterone	962.1	E858.0	E932.1	E950.4	E962.0	E980.4
thiouracil	962.8	E858.0	E932.8	E950.4	E962.0	E980.4
Methylated spirit	980.0	E860.1	—	E950.9	E962.1	E980.9
Methyldopa	972.6	E858.3	E942.6	E950.4	E962.0	E980.4

Substance	Poisoning	Accident	Therapeutic Use	Suicide Attempt	Assault	Undetermined
			External Cause (E-Code)			
Methylene						
blue	961.9	E857	E931.9	E950.4	E962.0	E980.4
chloride or dichloride (solvent) NEC	982.3	E862.4	—	E950.9	E962.1	E980.9
Methylhexabital	967.0	E851	E937.0	E950.1	E962.0	E980.1
Methylparaben (ophthalmic)	976.5	E858.7	E946.5	E950.4	E962.0	E980.4
Methyprylon	967.5	E852.4	E937.5	E950.2	E962.0	E980.2
Methysergide	971.3	E855.6	E941.3	E950.4	E962.0	E980.4
Metoclopramide	963.0	E858.1	E933.0	E950.4	E962.0	E980.4
Metofoline	965.7	E850.7	E935.7	E950.0	E962.0	E980.0
Metopon	965.09	E850.2	E935.2	E950.0	E962.0	E980.0
Metronidazole	961.5	E857	E931.5	E950.4	E962.0	E980.4
Metycaine	968.9	E855.2	E938.9	E950.4	E962.0	E980.4
infiltration (subcutaneous)	968.5	E855.2	E938.5	E950.4	E962.0	E980.4
nerve block (peripheral) (plexus)	968.6	E855.2	E938.6	E950.4	E962.0	E980.4
topical (surface)	968.5	E855.2	E938.5	E950.4	E962.0	E980.4
Metyrapone	977.8	E858.8	E947.8	E950.4	E962.0	E980.4
Mevinphos	989.3	E863.1	—	E950.6	E962.1	E980.7
Mezereon (berries)	988.2	E865.3	—	E950.9	E962.1	E980.9
Micatin	976.0	E858.7	E946.0	E950.4	E962.0	E980.4
Miconazole	976.0	E858.7	E946.0	E950.4	E962.0	E980.4
Midol	965.1	E850.3	E935.3	E950.0	E962.0	E980.0
Mifepristone	962.9	E858.0	E932.9	E950.4	E962.0	E980.4
Milk of magnesia	973.0	E858.4	E943.0	E950.4	E962.0	E980.4
Millipede (tropical) (venomous)	989.5	E905.4	—	E950.9	E962.1	E980.9
Miltown	969.5	E853.8	E939.5	E950.3	E962.0	E980.3
Mineral						
oil (medicinal)	973.2	E858.4	E943.2	E950.4	E962.0	E980.4
nonmedicinal	981	E862.1	—	E950.9	E962.1	E980.9
topical	976.3	E858.7	E946.3	E950.4	E962.0	E980.4
salts NEC	974.6	E858.5	E944.6	E950.4	E962.0	E980.4
spirits	981	E862.0	—	E950.9	E962.1	E980.9
Minocycline	960.4	E856	E930.4	E950.4	E962.0	E980.4
Mithramycin (antineoplastic)	960.7	E856	E930.7	E950.4	E962.0	E980.4
Mitobronitol	963.1	E858.1	E933.1	E950.4	E962.0	E980.4
Mitomycin (antineoplastic)	960.7	E856	E930.7	E950.4	E962.0	E980.4
Mitotane	963.1	E858.1	E933.1	E950.4	E962.0	E980.4
Moderil	972.6	E858.3	E942.6	E950.4	E962.0	E980.4
Mogadon—*see* Nitrazepam						
Molindone	969.3	E853.8	E939.3	E950.3	E962.0	E980.3
Monistat	976.0	E858.7	E946.0	E950.4	E962.0	E980.4
Monkshood	988.2	E865.4	—	E950.9	E962.1	E980.9
Monoamine oxidase inhibitors	969.01	E854.0	E939.0	E950.3	E962.0	E980.3
Monochlorobenzene	982.0	E862.4	—	E950.9	E962.1	E980.9
Monosodium glutamate	989.89	E866.8	—	E950.9	E962.1	E980.9
Monoxide, carbon — *see* Carbon, monoxide						
Moperone	969.2	E853.1	E939.2	E950.3	E962.0	E980.3
Morning glory seeds	969.6	E854.1	E939.6	E950.3	E962.0	E980.3
Moroxydine (hydrochloride)	961.7	E857	E931.7	E950.4	E962.0	E980.4
Morphazinamide	961.8	E857	E931.8	E950.4	E962.0	E980.4
Morphinans	965.09	E850.2	E935.2	E950.0	E962.0	E980.0
Morphine NEC	965.09	E850.2	E935.2	E950.0	E962.0	E980.0
antagonists	970.1	E854.3	E940.1	E950.4	E962.0	E980.4
Morpholinylethylmorphine	965.09	E850.2	E935.2	E950.0	E962.0	E980.0
Morrhuate sodium	972.7	E858.3	E942.7	E950.4	E962.0	E980.4
Moth balls (*see also* Pesticides)	989.4	E863.4	—	E950.6	E962.1	E980.7
naphthalene	983.0	E863.4	—	E950.7	E962.1	E980.6
Motor exhaust gas — *see* Carbon, monoxide, exhaust gas						
Mouth wash	976.6	E858.7	E946.6	E950.4	E962.0	E980.4
Mucolytic agent	975.5	E858.6	E945.5	E950.4	E962.0	E980.4

Substance	Poisoning	Accident	Therapeutic Use	Suicide Attempt	Assault	Undetermined
			External Cause (E-Code)			
Mucomyst.	975.5	E858.6	E945.5	E950.4	E962.0	E980.4
Mucous membrane agents (external)	976.9	E858.7	E946.9	E950.4	E962.0	E980.4
specified NEC	976.8	E858.7	E946.8	E950.4	E962.0	E980.4
Mumps						
immune globulin (human)	964.6	E858.2	E934.6	E950.4	E962.0	E980.4
skin test antigen	977.8	E858.8	E947.8	E950.4	E962.0	E980.4
vaccine	979.6	E858.8	E949.6	E950.4	E962.0	E980.4
Mumpsvax	979.6	E858.8	E949.6	E950.4	E962.0	E980.4
Muriatic acid — *see* Hydrochloric acid						
Muscarine.	971.0	E855.3	E941.0	E950.4	E962.0	E980.4
Muscle affecting agents NEC	975.3	E858.6	E945.3	E950.4	E962.0	E980.4
oxytocic.	975.0	E858.6	E945.0	E950.4	E962.0	E980.4
relaxants.	975.3	E858.6	E945.3	E950.4	E962.0	E980.4
central nervous system	968.0	E855.1	E938.0	E950.4	E962.0	E980.4
skeletal	975.2	E858.6	E945.2	E950.4	E962.0	E980.4
smooth	975.1	E858.6	E945.1	E950.4	E962.0	E980.4
Mushrooms, noxious	988.1	E865.5	—	E950.9	E962.1	E980.9
Mussel, noxious	988.0	E865.1	—	E950.9	E962.1	E980.9
Mustard (emetic)	973.6	E858.4	E943.6	E950.4	E962.0	E980.4
gas	987.8	E869.8	—	E952.8	E962.2	E982.8
nitrogen	963.1	E858.1	E933.1	E950.4	E962.0	E980.4
Mustine.	963.1	E858.1	E933.1	E950.4	E962.0	E980.4
M–vac	979.4	E858.8	E949.4	E950.4	E962.0	E980.4
Mycifradin	960.8	E856	E930.8	E950.4	E962.0	E980.4
topical	976.0	E858.7	E946.0	E950.4	E962.0	E980.4
Mycitracin	960.8	E856	E930.8	E950.4	E962.0	E980.4
ophthalmic preparation	976.5	E858.7	E946.5	E950.4	E962.0	E980.4
Mycostatin	960.1	E856	E930.1	E950.4	E962.0	E980.4
topical	976.0	E858.7	E946.0	E950.4	E962.0	E980.4
Mydriacyl	971.1	E855.4	E941.1	E950.4	E962.0	E980.4
Myelobromal	963.1	E858.1	E933.1	E950.4	E962.0	E980.4
Myleran.	963.1	E858.1	E933.1	E950.4	E962.0	E980.4
Myochrysin(e)	965.69	E850.6	E935.6	E950.0	E962.0	E980.0
Myoneural blocking agents	975.2	E858.6	E945.2	E950.4	E962.0	E980.4
Myristica fragrans	988.2	E865.3	—	E950.9	E962.1	E980.9
Myristicin	988.2	E865.3	—	E950.9	E962.1	E980.9
Mysoline	966.3	E855.0	E936.3	E950.4	E962.0	E980.4
Nafcillin (sodium)	960.0	E856	E930.0	E950.4	E962.0	E980.4
Nail polish remover	982.8	E862.4	—	E950.9	E962.1	E980.9
Nalidixic acid	961.9	E857	E931.9	E950.4	E962.0	E980.4
Nalorphine	970.1	E854.3	E940.1	E950.4	E962.0	E980.4
Naloxone	970.1	E854.3	E940.1	E950.4	E962.0	E980.4
Nandrolone (decanoate) (phenproprioate) . . .	962.1	E858.0	E932.1	E950.4	E962.0	E980.4
Naphazoline	971.2	E855.5	E941.2	E950.4	E962.0	E980.4
Naphtha (painter's) (petroleum)	981	E862.0	—	E950.9	E962.1	E980.9
solvent	981	E862.0	—	E950.9	E962.1	E980.9
vapor	987.1	E869.8	—	E952.8	E962.2	E982.8
Naphthalene (chlorinated)	983.0	E864.0	—	E950.7	E962.1	E980.6
insecticide or moth repellent	983.0	E863.4	—	E950.7	E962.1	E980.6
vapor	987.8	E869.8	—	E952.8	E962.2	E982.8
Naphthol	983.0	E864.0	—	E950.7	E962.1	E980.6
Naphthylamine	983.0	E864.0	—	E950.7	E962.1	E980.6
Naprosyn—*see* Naproxen						
Naproxen	965.61	E850.6	E935.6	E950.0	E962.0	E980.0
Narcotic (drug).	967.9	E852.9	E937.9	E950.2	E962.0	E980.2
analgesic NEC	965.8	E850.8	E935.8	E950.0	E962.0	E980.0
antagonist	970.1	E854.3	E940.1	E950.4	E962.0	E980.4
specified NEC	967.8	E852.8	E937.8	E950.2	E962.0	E980.2
Narcotine	975.4	E858.6	E945.4	E950.4	E962.0	E980.4
Nardil	969.01	E854.0	E939.0	E950.3	E962.0	E980.3
Natrium cyanide — *see* Cyanide(s)						

Substance	Poisoning	Accident	Therapeutic Use	Suicide Attempt	Assault	Undetermined
			External Cause (E-Code)			
Natural						
blood (product)	964.7	E858.2	E934.7	E950.4	E962.0	E980.4
gas (piped)	987.1	E867	—	E951.0	E962.2	E981.0
incomplete combustion	986	E867	—	E951.0	E962.2	E981.0
Nealbarbital, nealbarbitone	967.0	E851	E937.0	E950.1	E962.0	E980.1
Nectadon	975.4	E858.6	E945.4	E950.4	E962.0	E980.4
Nematocyst (sting)	989.5	E905.6	—	E950.9	E962.1	E980.9
Nembutal	967.0	E851	E937.0	E950.1	E962.0	E980.1
Neoarsphenamine	961.1	E857	E931.1	E950.4	E962.0	E980.4
Neocinchophen	974.7	E858.5	E944.7	E950.4	E962.0	E980.4
Neomycin	960.8	E856	E930.8	E950.4	E962.0	E980.4
ENT agent	976.6	E858.7	E946.6	E950.4	E962.0	E980.4
ophthalmic preparation	976.5	E858.7	E946.5	E950.4	E962.0	E980.4
topical NEC	976.0	E858.7	E946.0	E950.4	E962.0	E980.4
Neonal	967.0	E851	E937.0	E950.1	E962.0	E980.1
Neoprontosil	961.0	E857	E931.0	E950.4	E962.0	E980.4
Neosalvarsan	961.1	E857	E931.1	E950.4	E962.0	E980.4
Neosilversalvarsan	961.1	E857	E931.1	E950.4	E962.0	E980.4
Neosporin	960.8	E856	E930.8	E950.4	E962.0	E980.4
ENT agent	976.6	E858.7	E946.6	E950.4	E962.0	E980.4
ophthalmic preparation	976.5	E858.7	E946.5	E950.4	E962.0	E980.4
topical NEC	976.0	E858.7	E946.0	E950.4	E962.0	E980.4
Neostigmine	971.0	E855.3	E941.0	E950.4	E962.0	E980.4
Neraval	967.0	E851	E937.0	E950.1	E962.0	E980.1
Neravan	967.0	E851	E937.0	E950.1	E962.0	E980.1
Nerium oleander	988.2	E865.4	—	E950.9	E962.1	E980.9
Nerve gases (war)	987.9	E869.9	—	E952.9	E962.2	E982.9
Nesacaine	968.9	E855.2	E938.9	E950.4	E962.0	E980.4
infiltration (subcutaneous)	968.5	E855.2	E938.5	E950.4	E962.0	E980.4
nerve block (peripheral) (plexus)	968.6	E855.2	E938.6	E950.4	E962.0	E980.4
Neurobarb	967.0	E851	E937.0	E950.1	E962.0	E980.1
Neuroleptics NEC	969.3	E853.8	E939.3	E950.3	E962.0	E980.3
Neuroprotective agent	977.8	E858.8	E947.8	E950.4	E962.0	E980.4
Neutral spirits	980.0	E860.1	—	E950.9	E962.1	E980.9
beverage	980.0	E860.0	—	E950.9	E962.1	E980.9
Niacin, niacinamide	972.2	E858.3	E942.2	E950.4	E962.0	E980.4
Nialamide	969.01	E854.0	E939.0	E950.3	E962.0	E980.3
Nickle (carbonyl) (compounds) (fumes) (tetracarbonyl) (vapor)	985.8	E866.4	—	E950.9	E962.1	E980.9
Niclosamide	961.6	E857	E931.6	E950.4	E962.0	E980.4
Nicomorphine	965.09	E850.2	E935.2	E950.0	E962.0	E980.0
Nicotinamide	972.2	E858.3	E942.2	E950.4	E962.0	E980.4
Nicotine (insecticide) (spray) (sulfate) NEC	989.4	E863.4	—	E950.6	E962.1	E980.7
not insecticide	989.89	E866.8	—	E950.9	E962.1	E980.9
Nicotinic acid (derivatives)	972.2	E858.3	E942.2	E950.4	E962.0	E980.4
Nicotinyl alcohol	972.2	E858.3	E942.2	E950.4	E962.0	E980.4
Nicoumalone	964.2	E858.2	E934.2	E950.4	E962.0	E980.4
Nifenazone	965.5	E850.5	E935.5	E950.0	E962.0	E980.0
Nifuraldezone	961.9	E857	E931.9	E950.4	E962.0	E980.4
Nightshade (deadly)	988.2	E865.4	—	E950.9	E962.1	E980.9
Nikethamide	970.0	E854.3	E940.0	E950.4	E962.0	E980.4
Nilstat	960.1	E856	E930.1	E950.4	E962.0	E980.4
topical	976.0	E858.7	E946.0	E950.4	E962.0	E980.4
Nimodipine	977.8	E858.8	E947.8	E950.4	E962.0	E980.4
Niridazole	961.6	E857	E931.6	E950.4	E962.0	E980.4
Nisentil	965.09	E850.2	E935.2	E950.0	E962.0	E980.0
Nitrates	972.4	E858.3	E942.4	E950.4	E962.0	E980.4
Nitrazepam	969.4	E853.2	E939.4	E950.3	E962.0	E980.3
Nitric						
acid (liquid)	983.1	E864.1	—	E950.7	E962.1	E980.6

Substance	Poisoning	Accident	Therapeutic Use	Suicide Attempt	Assault	Undetermined
			External Cause (E-Code)			
vapor 987.8	E869.8	—	E952.8	E962.2	E982.8	
oxide (gas). 987.2	E869.0	—	E952.8	E962.2	E982.8	
Nitrite, amyl (medicinal) (vapor) 972.4	E858.3	E942.4	E950.4	E962.0	E980.4	
Nitroaniline 983.0	E864.0	—	E950.7	E962.1	E980.6	
vapor 987.8	E869.8	—	E952.8	E962.2	E982.8	
Nitrobenzene, nitrobenzol 983.0	E864.0	—	E950.7	E962.1	E980.6	
vapor 987.8	E869.8	—	E952.8	E962.2	E982.8	
Nitrocellulose 976.3	E858.7	E946.3	E950.4	E962.0	E980.4	
Nitrofuran derivatives 961.9	E857	E931.9	E950.4	E962.0	E980.4	
Nitrofurantoin 961.9	E857	E931.9	E950.4	E962.0	E980.4	
Nitrofurazone 976.0	E858.7	E946.0	E950.4	E962.0	E980.4	
Nitrogen (dioxide) (gas) (oxide). 987.2	E869.0	—	E952.8	E962.2	E982.8	
mustard (antineoplastic) 963.1	E858.1	E933.1	E950.4	E962.0	E980.4	
Nitroglycerin, nitroglycerol (medicinal) . . . 972.4	E858.3	E942.4	E950.4	E962.0	E980.4	
nonmedicinal 989.89	E866.8	—	E950.9	E962.1	E980.9	
fumes 987.8	E869.8	—	E952.8	E962.2	E982.8	
Nitrohydrochloric acid. 983.1	E864.1	—	E950.7	E962.1	E980.6	
Nitromersol 976.0	E858.7	E946.0	E950.4	E962.0	E980.4	
Nitronaphthalene 983.0	E864.0	—	E950.7	E962.2	E980.6	
Nitrophenol 983.0	E864.0	—	E950.7	E962.2	E980.6	
Nitrothiazol 961.6	E857	E931.6	E950.4	E962.0	E980.4	
Nitrotoluene, nitrotoluol 983.0	E864.0	—	E950.7	E962.1	E980.6	
vapor 987.8	E869.8	—	E952.8	E962.2	E982.8	
Nitrous 968.2	E855.1	E938.2	E950.4	E962.0	E980.4	
acid (liquid) 983.1	E864.1	—	E950.7	E962.1	E980.6	
fumes 987.2	E869.0	—	E952.8	E962.2	E982.8	
oxide (anesthetic) NEC 968.2	E855.1	E938.2	E950.4	E962.0	E980.4	
Nitrozone 976.0	E858.7	E946.0	E950.4	E962.0	E980.4	
Noctec 967.1	E852.0	E937.1	E950.2	E962.0	E980.2	
Noludar. 967.5	E852.4	E937.5	E950.2	E962.0	E980.2	
Noptil 967.0	E851	E937.0	E950.1	E962.0	E980.1	
Noradrenalin. 971.2	E855.5	E941.2	E950.4	E962.0	E980.4	
Noramidopyrine 965.5	E850.5	E935.5	E950.0	E962.0	E980.0	
Norepinephrine. 971.2	E855.5	E941.2	E950.4	E962.0	E980.4	
Norethandrolone 962.1	E858.0	E932.1	E950.4	E962.0	E980.4	
Norethindrone 962.2	E858.0	E932.2	E950.4	E962.0	E980.4	
Norethisterone 962.2	E858.0	E932.2	E950.4	E962.0	E980.4	
Norethynodrel 962.2	E858.0	E932.2	E950.4	E962.0	E980.4	
Norlestrin 962.2	E858.0	E932.2	E950.4	E962.0	E980.4	
Norlutin. 962.2	E858.0	E932.2	E950.4	E962.0	E980.4	
Normison—*see* Benzodiazepines						
Normorphine. 965.09	E850.2	E935.2	E950.0	E962.0	E980.0	
Nortriptyline. 969.05	E854.0	E939.0	E950.3	E962.0	E980.3	
Noscapine. 975.4	E858.6	E945.4	E950.4	E962.0	E980.4	
Nose preparations 976.6	E858.7	E946.6	E950.4	E962.0	E980.4	
Novobiocin 960.8	E856	E930.8	E950.4	E962.0	E980.4	
Novocain (infiltration) (topical) 968.5	E855.2	E938.5	E950.4	E962.0	E980.4	
nerve block (peripheral) (plexus). 968.6	E855.2	E938.6	E950.4	E962.0	E980.4	
spinal 968.7	E855.2	E938.7	E950.4	E962.0	E980.4	
Noxythiolin 961.9	E857	E931.9	E950.4	E962.0	E980.4	
NPH Iletin (insulin). 962.3	E858.0	E932.3	E950.4	E962.0	E980.4	
Numorphan 965.09	E850.2	E935.2	E950.0	E962.0	E980.0	
Nunol 967.0	E851	E937.0	E950.1	E962.0	E980.1	
Nupercaine (spinal anesthetic) 968.7	E855.2	E938.7	E950.4	E962.0	E980.4	
topical (surface) 968.5	E855.2	E938.5	E950.4	E962.0	E980.4	
Nutmeg oil (liniment) 976.3	E858.7	E946.3	E950.4	E962.0	E980.4	
Nux vomica 989.1	E863.7	—	E950.6	E962.1	E980.7	
Nydrazid 961.8	E857	E931.8	E950.4	E962.0	E980.4	
Nylidrin. 971.2	E855.5	E941.2	E950.4	E962.0	E980.4	
Nystatin 960.1	E856	E930.1	E950.4	E962.0	E980.4	
topical 976.0	E858.7	E946.0	E950.4	E962.0	E980.4	

Substance	Poisoning	Accident	Therapeutic Use	Suicide Attempt	Assault	Undetermined
			External Cause (E-Code)			
Nytol	963.0	E858.1	E933.0	E950.4	E962.0	E980.4
Oblivion	967.8	E852.8	E937.8	E950.2	E962.0	E980.2
Octyl nitrite	972.4	E858.3	E942.4	E950.4	E962.0	E980.4
Oestradiol (cypionate) (dipropionate)						
(valerate)	962.2	E858.0	E932.2	E950.4	E962.0	E980.4
Oestriol	962.2	E858.0	E932.2	E950.4	E962.0	E980.4
Oestrone	962.2	E858.0	E932.2	E950.4	E962.0	E980.4
Oil (of) NEC	989.89	E866.8	—	E950.9	E962.1	E980.9
bitter almond	989.0	E866.8	—	E950.9	E962.1	E980.9
camphor	976.1	E858.7	E946.1	E950.4	E962.0	E980.4
colors	989.89	E861.6	—	E950.9	E962.1	E980.9
fumes	987.8	E869.8	—	E952.8	E962.2	E982.8
lubricating	981	E862.2	—	E950.9	E962.1	E980.9
specified source, other — *see* substance						
specified						
vitriol (liquid)	983.1	E864.1	—	E950.7	E962.1	E980.6
fumes	987.8	E869.8	—	E952.8	E962.2	E982.8
wintergreen (bitter) NEC	976.3	E858.7	E946.3	E950.4	E962.0	E980.4
Ointments NEC	976.9	E858.7	E946.9	E950.4	E962.0	E980.4
Oleander	988.2	E865.4	—	E950.9	E962.1	E980.9
Oleandomycin	960.3	E856	E930.3	E950.4	E962.0	E980.4
Oleovitamin A	963.5	E858.1	E933.5	E950.4	E962.0	E980.4
Oleum ricini	973.1	E858.4	E943.1	E950.4	E962.0	E980.4
Olive oil (medicinal) NEC	973.2	E858.4	E943.2	E950.4	E962.0	E980.4
OMPA	989.3	E863.1	—	E950.6	E962.1	E980.7
Oncovin	963.1	E858.1	E933.1	E950.4	E962.0	E980.4
Ophthaine	968.5	E855.2	E938.5	E950.4	E962.0	E980.4
Ophthetic	968.5	E855.2	E938.5	E950.4	E962.0	E980.4
Opiates, opioids, opium NEC	965.00	E850.2	E935.2	E950.0	E962.0	E980.0
antagonists	970.1	E854.3	E940.1	E950.4	E962.0	E980.4
Oracon	962.2	E858.0	E932.2	E950.4	E962.0	E980.4
Oragrafin	977.8	E858.8	E947.8	E950.4	E962.0	E980.4
Oral contraceptives	962.2	E858.0	E932.2	E950.4	E962.0	E980.4
Orciprenaline	975.1	E858.6	E945.1	E950.4	E962.0	E980.4
Organidin	975.5	E858.6	E945.5	E950.4	E962.0	E980.4
Organophosphates	989.3	E863.1	—	E950.6	E962.1	E980.7
Orimune	979.5	E858.8	E949.5	E950.4	E962.0	E980.4
Orinase	962.3	E858.0	E932.3	E950.4	E962.0	E980.4
Orphenadrine	966.4	E855.0	E936.4	E950.4	E962.0	E980.4
Ortal (sodium)	967.0	E851	E937.0	E950.1	E962.0	E980.1
Orthoboric acid	976.0	E858.7	E946.0	E950.4	E962.0	E980.4
ENT agent	976.6	E858.7	E946.6	E950.4	E962.0	E980.4
ophthalmic preparation	976.5	E858.7	E946.5	E950.4	E962.0	E980.4
Orthocaine	968.5	E855.2	E938.5	E950.4	E962.0	E980.4
Ortho–Novum	962.2	E858.0	E932.2	E950.4	E962.0	E980.4
Orthotolidine (reagent)	977.8	E858.8	E947.8	E950.4	E962.0	E980.4
Osmic acid (liquid)	983.1	E864.1	—	E950.7	E962.1	E980.6
fumes	987.8	E869.8	—	E952.8	E962.2	E982.8
Osmotic diuretics	974.4	E858.5	E944.4	E950.4	E962.0	E980.4
Ouabain	972.1	E858.3	E942.1	E950.4	E962.0	E980.4
Ovarian hormones (synthetic substitutes)	962.2	E858.0	E932.2	E950.4	E962.0	E980.4
Ovral	962.2	E858.0	E932.2	E950.4	E962.0	E980.4
Ovulation suppressants	962.2	E858.0	E932.2	E950.4	E962.0	E980.4
Ovulen	962.2	E858.0	E932.2	E950.4	E962.0	E980.4
Oxacillin (sodium)	960.0	E856	E930.0	E950.4	E962.0	E980.4
Oxalic acid	983.1	E864.1	—	E950.7	E962.1	E980.6
Oxanamide	969.5	E853.8	E939.5	E950.3	E962.0	E980.3
Oxandrolone	962.1	E858.0	E932.1	E950.4	E962.0	E980.4
Oxaprozin	965.61	E850.6	E935.6	E950.0	E962.0	E980.0
Oxazepam	969.4	E853.2	E939.4	E950.3	E962.0	E980.3

Substance	Poisoning	Accident	Therapeutic Use	Suicide Attempt	Assault	Undetermined
			External Cause (E-Code)			
Oxazolidine derivatives	966.0	E855.0	E936.0	E950.4	E962.0	E980.4
Ox bile extract	973.4	E858.4	E943.4	E950.4	E962.0	E980.4
Oxedrine	971.2	E855.5	E941.2	E950.4	E962.0	E980.4
Oxeladin	975.4	E858.6	E945.4	E950.4	E962.0	E980.4
Oxethazaine NEC	968.5	E855.2	E938.5	E950.4	E962.0	E980.4
Oxidizing agents NEC	983.9	E864.3	—	E950.7	E962.1	E980.6
Oxolinic acid	961.3	E857	E931.3	E950.4	E962.0	E980.4
Oxophenarsine	961.1	E857	E931.1	E950.4	E962.0	E980.4
Oxsoralen	976.3	E858.7	E946.3	E950.4	E962.0	E980.4
Oxtriphylline	975.7	E858.6	E945.7	E950.4	E962.0	E980.4
Oxybuprocaine	968.5	E855.2	E938.5	E950.4	E962.0	E980.4
Oxybutynin	975.1	E858.6	E945.1	E950.4	E962.0	E980.4
Oxycodone	965.09	E850.2	E935.2	E950.0	E962.0	E980.0
Oxygen	987.8	E869.8	—	E952.8	E962.2	E982.8
Oxylone	976.0	E858.7	E946.0	E950.4	E962.0	E980.4
ophthalmic preparation	976.5	E858.7	E946.5	E950.4	E962.0	E980.4
Oxymesterone	962.1	E858.0	E932.1	E950.4	E962.0	E980.4
Oxymetazoline	971.2	E855.5	E941.2	E950.4	E962.0	E980.4
Oxymetholone	962.1	E858.0	E932.1	E950.4	E962.0	E980.4
Oxymorphone	965.09	E850.2	E935.2	E950.0	E962.0	E980.0
Oxypertine	969.0	E854.0	E939.0	E950.3	E962.0	E980.3
Oxyphenbutazone	965.5	E850.5	E935.5	E950.0	E962.0	E980.0
Oxyphencyclimine	971.1	E855.4	E941.1	E950.4	E962.0	E980.4
Oxyphenisatin	973.1	E858.4	E943.1	E950.4	E962.0	E980.4
Oxyphenonium	971.1	E855.4	E941.1	E950.4	E962.0	E980.4
Oxyquinoline	961.3	E857	E931.3	E950.4	E962.0	E980.4
Oxytetracycline	960.4	E856	E930.4	E950.4	E962.0	E980.4
Oxytocics	975.0	E858.6	E945.0	E950.4	E962.0	E980.4
Oxytocin	975.0	E858.6	E945.0	E950.4	E962.0	E980.4
Ozone	987.8	E869.8	—	E952.8	E962.2	E982.8
PABA	976.3	E858.7	E946.3	E950.4	E962.0	E980.4
Packed red cells	964.7	E858.2	E934.7	E950.4	E962.0	E980.4
Paint NEC	989.89	E861.6	—	E950.9	E962.1	E980.9
cleaner	982.8	E862.9	—	E950.9	E962.1	E980.9
fumes NEC	987.8	E869.8	—	E952.8	E962.1	E982.8
lead (fumes)	984.0	E861.5	—	E950.9	E962.1	E980.9
solvent NEC	982.8	E862.9	—	E950.9	E962.1	E980.9
stripper	982.8	E862.9	—	E950.9	E962.1	E980.9
Palfium	965.09	E850.2	E935.2	E950.0	E962.0	E980.0
Palivizumab	979.9	E858.8	E949.6	E950.4	E962.0	E980.4
Paludrine	961.4	E857	E931.4	E950.4	E962.0	E980.4
PAM	977.2	E855.8	E947.2	E950.4	E962.0	E980.4
Pamaquine (naphthoate)	961.4	E857	E931.4	E950.4	E962.0	E980.4
Pamprin	965.1	E850.3	E935.3	E950.0	E962.0	E980.0
Panadol	965.4	E850.4	E935.4	E950.0	E962.0	E980.0
Pancreatic dornase (mucolytic)	963.4	E858.1	E933.4	E950.4	E962.0	E980.4
Pancreatin	973.4	E858.4	E943.4	E950.4	E962.0	E980.4
Pancrelipase	973.4	E858.4	E943.4	E950.4	E962.0	E980.4
Pangamic acid	963.5	E858.1	E933.5	E950.4	E962.0	E980.4
Panthenol	963.5	E858.1	E933.5	E950.4	E962.0	E980.4
topical	976.8	E858.7	E946.8	E950.4	E962.0	E980.4
Pantopaque	977.8	E858.8	E947.8	E950.4	E962.0	E980.4
Pantopon	965.00	E850.2	E935.2	E950.0	E962.0	E980.0
Pantothenic acid	963.5	E858.1	E933.5	E950.4	E962.0	E980.4
Panwarfin	964.2	E858.2	E934.2	E950.4	E962.0	E980.4
Papain	973.4	E858.4	E943.4	E950.4	E962.0	E980.4
Papaverine	972.5	E858.3	E942.5	E950.4	E962.0	E980.4
Para–aminobenzoic acid	976.3	E858.7	E946.3	E950.4	E962.0	E980.4
Para–aminophenol derivatives	965.4	E850.4	E935.4	E950.0	E962.0	E980.0
Para–aminosalicylic acid (derivatives)	961.8	E857	E931.8	E950.4	E962.0	E980.4
Paracetaldehyde (medicinal)	967.2	E852.1	E937.2	E950.2	E962.0	E980.2

TABLE OF DRUGS AND CHEMICALS

Substance	Poisoning	Accident	Therapeutic Use	Suicide Attempt	Assault	Undetermined
			External Cause (E-Code)			
Paracetamol	965.4	E850.4	E935.4	E950.0	E962.0	E980.0
Paracodin	965.09	E850.2	E935.2	E950.0	E962.0	E980.0
Paradione	966.0	E855.0	E936.0	E950.4	E962.0	E980.4
Paraffin(s) (wax)	981	E862.3	—	E950.9	E962.1	E980.9
liquid (medicinal)	973.2	E858.4	E943.2	E950.4	E962.0	E980.4
nonmedicinal (oil)	981	E962.1	—	E950.9	E962.1	E980.9
Paraldehyde (medicinal)	967.2	E852.1	E937.2	E950.2	E962.0	E980.2
Paramethadione	966.0	E855.0	E936.0	E950.4	E962.0	E980.4
Paramethasone	962.0	E858.0	E932.0	E950.4	E962.0	E980.4
Paraquat	989.4	E863.5	—	E950.6	E962.1	E980.7
Parasympatholytics	971.1	E855.4	E941.1	E950.4	E962.0	E980.4
Parasympathomimetics	971.0	E855.3	E941.0	E950.4	E962.0	E980.4
Parathion	989.3	E863.1	—	E950.6	E962.1	E980.7
Parathormone	962.6	E858.0	E932.6	E950.4	E962.0	E980.4
Parathyroid (derivatives)	962.6	E858.0	E932.6	E950.4	E962.0	E980.4
Paratyphoid vaccine	978.1	E858.8	E948.1	E950.4	E962.0	E980.4
Paredrine	971.2	E855.5	E941.2	E950.4	E962.0	E980.4
Paregoric	965.00	E850.2	E935.2	E950.0	E962.0	E980.0
Pargyline	972.3	E858.3	E942.3	E950.4	E962.0	E980.4
Paris green	985.1	E866.3	—	E950.8	E962.1	E980.8
insecticide	985.1	E863.4	—	E950.8	E962.1	E980.8
Parnate	969.01	E854.0	E939.0	E950.3	E962.0	E980.3
Paromomycin	960.8	E856	E930.8	E950.4	E962.0	E980.4
Paroxypropione	963.1	E858.1	E933.1	E950.4	E962.0	E980.4
Parzone	965.09	E850.2	E935.2	E950.0	E962.0	E980.0
PAS	961.8	E857	E931.8	E950.4	E962.0	E980.4
PCBs	981	E862.3	—	E950.9	E962.1	E980.9
PCP (pentachlorophenol)	989.4	E863.6	—	E950.6	E962.1	E980.7
herbicide	989.4	E863.5	—	E950.6	E962.1	E980.7
insecticide	989.4	E863.4	—	E950.6	E962.1	E980.7
phencyclidine	968.3	E855.1	E938.3	E950.4	E962.0	E980.4
Peach kernel oil (emulsion)	973.2	E858.4	E943.2	E950.4	E962.0	E980.4
Peanut oil (emulsion) NEC	973.2	E858.4	E943.2	E950.4	E962.0	E980.4
topical	976.3	E858.7	E946.3	E950.4	E962.0	E980.4
Pearly Gates (morning glory seeds)	969.6	E854.1	E939.6	E950.3	E962.0	E980.3
Pecazine	969.1	E853.0	E939.1	E950.3	E962.0	E980.3
Pecilocin	960.1	E856	E930.1	E950.4	E962.0	E980.4
Pectin (with kaolin) NEC	973.5	E858.4	E943.5	E950.4	E962.0	E980.4
Pelletierine tannate	961.6	E857	E931.6	E950.4	E962.0	E980.4
Pemoline	969.79	E854.2	E939.7	E950.3	E962.0	E980.3
Pempidine	972.3	E858.3	E942.3	E950.4	E962.0	E980.4
Penamecillin	960.0	E856	E930.0	E950.4	E962.0	E980.4
Penethamate hydriodide	960.0	E856	E930.0	E950.4	E962.0	E980.4
Penicillamine	963.8	E858.1	E933.8	E950.4	E962.0	E980.4
Penicillin (any type)	960.0	E856	E930.0	E950.4	E962.0	E980.4
Penicillinase	963.4	E858.1	E933.4	E950.4	E962.0	E980.4
Pentachlorophenol (fungicide)	989.4	E863.6	—	E950.6	E962.1	E980.7
herbicide	989.4	E863.5	—	E950.6	E962.1	E980.7
insecticide	989.4	E863.4	—	E950.6	E962.1	E980.7
Pentaerythritol	972.4	E858.3	E942.4	E950.4	E962.0	E980.4
chloral	967.1	E852.0	E937.1	E950.2	E962.0	E980.2
tetranitrate NEC	972.4	E858.3	E942.4	E950.4	E962.0	E980.4
Pentagastrin	977.8	E858.8	E947.8	E950.4	E962.0	E980.4
Pentalin	982.3	E862.4	—	E950.9	E962.1	E980.9
Pentamethonium (bromide)	972.3	E858.3	E942.3	E950.4	E962.0	E980.4
Pentamidine	961.5	E857	E931.5	E950.4	E962.0	E980.4
Pentanol	980.8	E860.8	—	E950.9	E962.1	E980.9
Pentaquine	961.4	E857	E931.4	E950.4	E962.0	E980.4
Pentazocine	965.8	E850.8	E935.8	E950.0	E962.0	E980.0
Penthienate	971.1	E855.4	E941.1	E950.4	E962.0	E980.4

1550

TABLE OF DRUGS AND CHEMICALS

Substance	Poisoning	Accident	Therapeutic Use	Suicide Attempt	Assault	Undetermined
			External Cause (E-Code)			
Pentobarbital, pentobarbitone (sodium)	967.0	E851	E937.0	E950.1	E962.0	E980.1
Pentolinium (tartrate)	972.3	E858.3	E942.3	E950.4	E962.0	E980.4
Pentothal	968.3	E855.1	E938.3	E950.4	E962.0	E980.4
Pentylenetetrazol	970.0	E854.3	E940.0	E950.4	E962.0	E980.4
Pentylsalicylamide	961.8	E857	E931.8	E950.4	E962.0	E980.4
Pepsin	973.4	E858.4	E943.4	E950.4	E962.0	E980.4
Peptavlon	977.8	E858.8	E947.8	E950.4	E962.0	E980.4
Percaine (spinal)	968.7	E855.2	E938.7	E950.4	E962.0	E980.4
topical (surface)	968.5	E855.2	E938.5	E950.4	E962.0	E980.4
Perchloroethylene (vapor)	982.3	E862.4	—	E950.9	E962.1	E980.9
medicinal	961.6	E857	E931.6	E950.4	E962.0	E980.4
Percodan	965.09	E850.2	E935.2	E950.0	E962.0	E980.0
Percogesic	965.09	E850.2	E935.2	E950.0	E962.0	E980.0
Percorten	962.0	E858.0	E932.0	E950.4	E962.0	E980.4
Pergonal	962.4	E858.0	E932.4	E950.4	E962.0	E980.4
Perhexiline	972.4	E858.3	E942.4	E950.4	E962.0	E980.4
Periactin	963.0	E858.1	E933.0	E950.4	E962.0	E980.4
Periclor	967.1	E852.0	E937.1	E950.2	E962.0	E980.2
Pericyazine	969.1	E853.0	E939.1	E950.3	E962.0	E980.3
Peritrate	972.4	E858.3	E942.4	E950.4	E962.0	E980.4
Permanganates NEC	983.9	E864.3	—	E950.7	E962.1	E980.6
potassium (topical)	976.0	E858.7	E946.0	E950.4	E962.0	E980.4
Pernocton	967.0	E851	E937.0	E950.1	E962.0	E980.1
Pernoston	967.0	E851	E937.0	E950.1	E962.0	E980.1
Peronin(e)	965.09	E850.2	E935.2	E950.0	E962.0	E980.0
Perphenazine	969.1	E853.0	E939.1	E950.3	E962.0	E980.3
Pertofrane	969.05	E854	E939.0	E950.3	E962.0	E980.3
Pertussis						
immune serum (human)	964.6	E858.2	E934.6	E950.4	E962.0	E980.4
vaccine (with diphtheria toxoid) (with tetanus toxoid)	978.6	E858.8	E948.6	E950.4	E962.0	E980.4
Peruvian balsam	976.8	E858.7	E946.8	E950.4	E962.0	E980.4
Pesticides (dust) (fumes) (vapor)	989.4	E863.4	—	E950.6	E962.1	E980.7
arsenic	985.1	E863.4	—	E950.8	E962.1	E980.8
chlorinated	989.2	E863.0	—	E950.6	E962.1	E980.7
cyanide	989.0	E863.4	—	E950.6	E962.1	E980.7
kerosene	981	E863.4	—	E950.6	E962.1	E980.7
mixture (of compounds)	989.4	E863.3	—	E950.6	E962.1	E980.7
naphthalene	983.0	E863.4	—	E950.7	E962.1	E980.6
organochlorine (compounds)	989.2	E863.0	—	E950.6	E962.1	E980.7
petroleum (distillate) (products) NEC	981	E863.4	—	E950.6	E962.1	E980.7
specified ingredient NEC	989.4	E863.4	—	E950.6	E962.1	E980.7
strychnine	989.1	E863.4	—	E950.6	E962.1	E980.7
thallium	985.8	E863.7	—	E950.6	E962.1	E980.7
Pethidine (hydrochloride)	965.09	E850.2	E935.2	E950.0	E962.0	E980.0
Petrichloral	967.1	E852.0	E937.1	E950.2	E962.0	E980.2
Petrol	981	E862.1	—	E950.9	E962.1	E980.9
vapor	987.1	E869.8	—	E952.8	E962.2	E982.8
Petrolatum (jelly) (ointment)	976.3	E858.7	E946.3	E950.4	E962.0	E980.4
hydrophilic	976.3	E858.7	E946.3	E950.4	E962.0	E980.4
liquid	973.2	E858.4	E943.2	E950.4	E962.0	E980.4
topical	976.3	E858.7	E946.3	E950.4	E962.0	E980.4
nonmedicinal	981	E862.1	—	E950.9	E962.1	E980.9
Petroleum (cleaners) (fuels) (products) NEC	981	E862.1	—	E950.9	E962.1	E980.9
benzin(e) — *see* Ligroin						
ether — *see* Ligroin						
jelly — *see* Petrolatum						
naphtha — *see* Ligroin						
pesticide	981	E863.4	—	E950.6	E962.1	E980.7

1551

Substance	Poisoning	Accident	Therapeutic Use	Suicide Attempt	Assault	Undetermined
			External Cause (E-Code)			
solids	981	E862.3	—	E950.9	E962.1	E980.9
solvents	981	E862.0	—	E950.9	E962.1	E980.9
vapor	987.1	E869.8	—	E952.8	E962.2	E982.8
Peyote	969.6	E854.1	E939.6	E950.3	E962.0	E980.3
Phanodorm, phanodorn	967.0	E851	E937.0	E950.1	E962.0	E980.1
Phanquinone, phanquone	961.5	E857	E931.5	E950.4	E962.0	E980.4
Pharmaceutical excipient or adjunct	977.4	E858.8	E947.4	E950.4	E962.0	E980.4
Phenacemide	966.3	E855.0	E936.3	E950.4	E962.0	E980.4
Phenacetin	965.4	E850.4	E935.4	E950.0	E962.0	E980.0
Phenadoxone	965.09	E850.2	E935.2	E950.0	E962.0	E980.0
Phenaglycodol	969.5	E853.8	E939.5	E950.3	E962.0	E980.3
Phenantoin	966.1	E855.0	E936.1	E950.4	E962.0	E980.4
Phenaphthazine reagent	977.8	E858.8	E947.8	E950.4	E962.0	E980.4
Phenazocine	965.09	E850.2	E935.2	E950.0	E962.0	E980.0
Phenazone	965.5	E850.5	E935.5	E950.0	E962.0	E980.0
Phenazopyridine	976.1	E858.7	E946.1	E950.4	E962.0	E980.4
Phenbenicillin	960.0	E856	E930.0	E950.4	E962.0	E980.4
Phenbutrazate	977.0	E858.8	E947.0	E950.4	E962.0	E980.4
Phencyclidine	968.3	E855.1	E938.3	E950.4	E962.0	E980.4
Phendimetrazine	977.0	E858.8	E947.0	E950.4	E962.0	E980.4
Phenelzine	969.01	E854.0	E939.0	E950.3	E962.0	E980.3
Phenergan	967.8	E852.8	E937.8	E950.2	E962.0	E980.2
Phenethicillin (potassium)	960.0	E856	E930.0	E950.4	E962.0	E980.4
Phenetsal	965.1	E850.3	E935.3	E950.0	E962.0	E980.0
Pheneturide	966.3	E855.0	E936.3	E950.4	E962.0	E980.4
Phenformin	962.3	E858.0	E932.3	E950.4	E962.0	E980.4
Phenglutarimide	971.1	E855.4	E941.1	E950.4	E962.0	E980.4
Phenicarbazide	965.8	E850.8	E935.8	E950.0	E962.0	E980.0
Phenindamine (tartrate)	963.0	E858.1	E933.0	E950.4	E962.0	E980.4
Phenindione	964.2	E858.2	E934.2	E950.4	E962.0	E980.4
Pheniprazine	969.01	E854.0	E939.0	E950.3	E962.0	E980.3
Pheniramine (maleate)	963.0	E858.1	E933.0	E950.4	E962.0	E980.4
Phenmetrazine	977.0	E858.8	E947.0	E950.4	E962.0	E980.4
Phenobal	967.0	E851	E937.0	E950.1	E962.0	E980.1
Phenobarbital	967.0	E851	E937.0	E950.1	E962.0	E980.1
Phenobarbitone	967.0	E851	E937.0	E950.1	E962.0	E980.1
Phenoctide	976.0	E858.7	E946.0	E950.4	E962.0	E980.4
Phenol (derivatives) NEC	983.0	E864.0	—	E950.7	E962.1	E980.6
disinfectant	983.0	E864.0	—	E950.7	E962.1	E980.6
pesticide	989.4	E863.4	—	E950.6	E962.1	E980.7
red	977.8	E858.8	E947.8	E950.4	E962.0	E980.4
Phenolphthalein	973.1	E858.4	E943.1	E950.4	E962.0	E980.4
Phenolsulfonphthalein	977.8	E858.8	E947.8	E950.4	E962.0	E980.4
Phenomorphan	965.09	E850.2	E935.2	E950.0	E962.0	E980.0
Phenonyl	967.0	E851	E937.0	E950.1	E962.0	E980.1
Phenoperidine	965.09	E850.2	E935.2	E950.0	E962.0	E980.0
Phenoquin	974.7	E858.5	E944.7	E950.4	E962.0	E980.4
Phenothiazines (tranquilizers) NEC	969.1	E853.0	E939.1	E950.3	E962.0	E980.3
insecticide	989.3	E863.4	—	E950.6	E962.1	E980.7
Phenoxybenzamine	971.3	E855.6	E941.3	E950.4	E962.0	E980.4
Phenoxymethyl penicillin	960.0	E856	E930.0	E950.4	E962.0	E980.4
Phenprocoumon	964.2	E858.2	E934.2	E950.4	E962.0	E980.4
Phensuximide	966.2	E855.0	E936.2	E950.4	E962.0	E980.4
Phentermine	977.0	E858.8	E947.0	E950.4	E962.0	E980.4
Phentolamine	971.3	E855.6	E941.3	E950.4	E962.0	E980.4
Phenyl						
butazone	965.5	E850.5	E935.5	E950.0	E962.0	E980.0
enediamine	983.0	E864.0	—	E950.7	E962.1	E980.6
hydrazine	983.0	E864.0	—	E950.7	E962.1	E980.6
antineoplastic	963.1	E858.1	E933.1	E950.4	E962.0	E980.4

Substance	Poisoning	Accident	Therapeutic Use	Suicide Attempt	Assault	Undetermined
		External Cause (E-Code)				
mercuric compounds — *see* Mercury						
salicylate	976.3	E858.7	E946.3	E950.4	E962.0	E980.4
Phenylephrin	971.2	E855.5	E941.2	E950.4	E962.0	E980.4
Phenylethybiguanide	962.3	E858.0	E932.3	E950.4	E962.0	E980.4
Phenylpropanolamine	971.2	E855.5	E941.2	E950.4	E962.0	E980.4
Phenylsulfthion	989.3	E863.1	—	E950.6	E962.1	E980.7
Phenyramidol, phenyramidon	965.7	E850.7	E935.7	E950.0	E962.0	E980.0
Phenytoin	966.1	E855.0	E936.1	E950.4	E962.0	E980.4
pHisoHex	976.2	E858.7	E946.2	E950.4	E962.0	E980.4
Pholcodine	965.09	E850.2	E935.2	E950.0	E962.0	E980.0
Phorate	989.3	E863.1	—	E950.6	E962.1	E980.7
Phosdrin	989.3	E863.1	—	E950.6	E962.1	E980.7
Phosgene (gas)	987.8	E869.8	—	E952.8	E962.2	E982.8
Phosphate (tricresyl)	989.89	E866.8	—	E950.9	E962.1	E980.9
organic	989.3	E863.1	—	E950.6	E962.1	E980.7
solvent	982.8	E862.4	—	E950.9	E926.1	E980.9
Phosphine	987.8	E869.8	—	E952.8	E962.2	E982.8
fumigant	987.8	E863.8	—	E950.6	E962.2	E980.7
Phospholine	971.0	E855.3	E941.0	E950.4	E962.0	E980.4
Phosphoric acid	983.1	E864.1	—	E950.7	E962.1	E980.6
Phosphorus (compounds) NEC	983.9	E864.3	—	E950.7	E962.1	E980.6
rodenticide	983.9	E863.7	—	E950.7	E962.1	E980.6
Phthalimidogluarimide	967.8	E852.8	E937.8	E950.2	E962.0	E980.2
Phthalylsulfathiazole	961.0	E857	E931.0	E950.4	E962.0	E980.4
Phylloquinone	964.3	E858.2	E934.3	E950.4	E962.0	E980.4
Physeptone	965.02	E850.1	E935.1	E950.0	E962.0	E980.0
Physostigma venenosum	988.2	E865.4	—	E950.9	E962.1	E980.9
Physostigmine	971.0	E855.3	E941.0	E950.4	E962.0	E980.4
Phytolacca decandra	988.2	E865.4	—	E950.9	E962.1	E980.9
Phytomenadione	964.3	E858.2	E934.3	E950.4	E962.0	E980.4
Phytonadione	964.3	E858.2	E934.3	E950.4	E962.0	E980.4
Picric (acid)	983.0	E864.0	—	E950.7	E962.1	E980.6
Picrotoxin	970.0	E854.3	E940.0	E950.4	E962.0	E980.4
Pilocarpine	971.0	E855.3	E941.0	E950.4	E962.0	E980.4
Pilocarpus (jaborandi) extract	971.0	E855.3	E941.0	E950.4	E962.0	E980.4
Pimaricin	960.1	E856	E930.1	E950.4	E962.0	E980.4
Piminodine	965.09	E850.2	E935.2	E950.0	E962.0	E980.0
Pine oil, pinesol (disinfectant)	983.9	E861.4	—	E950.7	E962.1	E980.6
Pinkroot	961.6	E857	E931.6	E950.4	E962.0	E980.4
Pipadone	965.09	E850.2	E935.2	E950.0	E962.0	E980.0
Pipamazine	963.0	E858.1	E933.0	E950.4	E962.0	E980.4
Pipazethate	975.4	E858.6	E945.4	E950.4	E962.0	E980.4
Pipenzolate	971.1	E855.4	E941.1	E950.4	E962.0	E980.4
Piperacetazine	969.1	E853.0	E939.1	E950.3	E962.0	E980.3
Piperazine NEC	961.6	E857	E931.6	E950.4	E962.0	E980.4
estrone sulfate	962.2	E858.0	E932.2	E950.4	E962.0	E980.4
Piper cubeba	988.2	E865.4	—	E950.9	E962.1	E980.9
Piperidione	975.4	E858.6	E945.4	E950.4	E962.0	E980.4
Piperidolate	971.1	E855.4	E941.1	E950.4	E962.0	E980.4
Piperocaine	968.9	E855.2	E938.9	E950.4	E962.0	E980.4
infiltration (subcutaneous)	968.5	E855.2	E938.5	E950.4	E962.0	E980.4
nerve block (peripheral) (plexus)	968.6	E855.2	E938.6	E950.4	E962.0	E980.4
topical (surface)	968.5	E855.2	E938.5	E950.4	E962.0	E980.4
Pipobroman	963.1	E858.1	E933.1	E950.4	E962.0	E980.4
Pipradrol	970.8	E854.3	E940.8	E950.4	E962.0	E980.4
Piscidia (bark) (erythrina)	965.7	E850.7	E935.7	E950.0	E962.0	E980.0
Pitch	983.0	E864.0	—	E950.7	E962.1	E980.6
Pitkin's solution	968.7	E855.2	E938.7	E950.4	E962.0	E980.4
Pitocin	975.0	E858.6	E945.0	E950.4	E962.0	E980.4
Pitressin (tannate)	962.5	E858.0	E932.5	E950.4	E962.0	E980.4
Pituitary extracts (posterior)	962.5	E858.0	E932.5	E950.4	E962.0	E980.4

TABLE OF DRUGS AND CHEMICALS

Substance	Poisoning	Accident	Therapeutic Use	Suicide Attempt	Assault	Undetermined
			External Cause (E-Code)			
anterior	962.4	E858.0	E932.4	E950.4	E962.0	E980.4
Pituitrin	962.5	E858.0	E932.5	E950.4	E962.0	E980.4
Placental extract	962.9	E858.0	E932.9	E950.4	E962.0	E980.4
Placidyl	967.8	E852.8	E937.8	E950.2	E962.0	E980.2
Plague vaccine	978.3	E858.8	E948.3	E950.4	E962.0	E980.4
Plant foods or fertilizers NEC	989.89	E866.5	—	E950.9	E962.1	E980.9
mixed with herbicides	989.4	E863.5	—	E950.6	E962.1	E980.7
Plants, noxious, used as food	988.2	E865.9	—	E950.9	E962.1	E980.9
berries and seeds	988.2	E865.3	—	E950.9	E962.1	E980.9
specified type NEC	988.2	E865.4	—	E950.9	E962.1	E980.9
Plasma (blood)	964.7	E858.2	E934.7	E950.4	E962.0	E980.4
expanders	964.8	E858.2	E934.8	E950.4	E962.0	E980.4
Plasmanate	964.7	E858.2	E934.7	E950.4	E962.0	E980.4
Plegicil	969.1	E853.0	E939.1	E950.3	E962.0	E980.3
Podophyllin	976.4	E858.7	E946.4	E950.4	E962.0	E980.4
Podophyllum resin	976.4	E858.7	E946.4	E950.4	E962.0	E980.4
Poison NEC	989.9	E866.9	—	E950.9	E962.1	E980.9
Poisonous berries	988.2	E865.3	—	E950.9	E962.1	E980.9
Pokeweed (any part)	988.2	E865.4	—	E950.9	E962.1	E980.9
Poldine	971.1	E855.4	E941.1	E950.4	E962.0	E980.4
Poliomyelitis vaccine	979.5	E858.8	E949.5	E950.4	E962.0	E980.4
Poliovirus vaccine	979.5	E858.8	E949.5	E950.4	E962.0	E980.4
Polish (car) (floor) (furniture) (metal) (silver)	989.89	E861.2	—	E950.9	E962.1	E980.9
abrasive	989.89	E861.3	—	E950.9	E962.1	E980.9
porcelain	989.89	E861.3	—	E950.9	E962.1	E980.9
Poloxalkol	973.2	E858.4	E943.2	E950.4	E962.0	E980.4
Polyaminostyrene resins	974.5	E858.5	E944.5	E950.4	E962.0	E980.4
Polychlorinated biphenyl—see PCBs						
Polycycline	960.4	E856	E930.4	E950.4	E962.0	E980.4
Polyester resin hardener	982.8	E862.4	—	E950.9	E962.1	E980.9
fumes	987.8	E869.8	—	E952.8	E962.2	E982.8
Polyestradiol (phosphate)	962.2	E858.0	E932.2	E950.4	E962.0	E980.4
Polyethanolamine alkyl sulfate	976.2	E858.7	E946.2	E950.4	E962.0	E980.4
Polyethylene glycol	976.3	E858.7	E946.3	E950.4	E962.0	E980.4
Polyferose	964.0	E858.2	E934.0	E950.4	E962.0	E980.4
Polymyxin B	960.8	E856	E930.8	E950.4	E962.0	E980.4
ENT agent	976.6	E858.7	E946.6	E950.4	E962.0	E980.4
ophthalmic preparation	976.5	E858.7	E946.5	E950.4	E962.0	E980.4
topical NEC	976.0	E858.7	E946.0	E950.4	E962.0	E980.4
Polynoxylin(e)	976.0	E858.7	E946.0	E950.4	E962.0	E980.4
Polyoxymethyleneurea	976.0	E858.7	E946.0	E950.4	E962.0	E980.4
Polytetrafluoroethylene (inhaled)	987.8	E869.8	—	E952.8	E962.2	E982.8
Polythiazide	974.3	E858.5	E944.3	E950.4	E962.0	E980.4
Polyvinylpyrrolidone	964.8	E858.2	E934.8	E950.4	E962.0	E980.4
Pontocaine (hydrochloride) (infiltration) (topical)	968.5	E855.2	E938.5	E950.4	E962.0	E980.4
nerve block (peripheral) (plexus)	968.6	E855.2	E938.6	E950.4	E962.0	E980.4
spinal	968.7	E855.2	E938.7	E950.4	E962.0	E980.4
Pot	969.6	E854.1	E939.6	E950.3	E962.0	E980.3
Potash (caustic)	983.2	E864.2	—	E950.7	E962.1	E980.6
Potassic saline injection (lactated)	974.5	E858.5	E944.5	E950.4	E962.0	E980.4
Potassium (salts) NEC	974.5	E858.5	E944.5	E950.4	E962.0	E980.4
aminosalicylate	961.8	E857	E931.8	E950.4	E962.0	E980.4
arsenite (solution)	985.1	E866.3	—	E950.8	E962.1	E980.8
bichromate	983.9	E864.3	—	E950.7	E962.1	E980.6
bisulfate	983.9	E864.3	—	E950.7	E962.1	E980.6
bromide (medicinal) NEC	967.3	E852.2	E937.3	E950.2	E962.0	E980.2
carbonate	983.2	E864.2	—	E950.7	E962.1	E980.6
chlorate NEC	983.9	E864.3	—	E950.7	E962.1	E980.6

Substance	Poisoning	Accident	Therapeutic Use	Suicide Attempt	Assault	Undetermined
				External Cause (E-Code)		
cyanide — *see* Cyanide						
hydroxide	983.2	E864.2	—	E950.7	E962.1	E980.6
iodide (expectorant) NEC.	975.5	E858.6	E945.5	E950.4	E962.0	E980.4
nitrate.	989.89	E866.8	—	E950.9	E962.1	E980.9
oxalate	983.9	E864.3	—	E950.7	E962.1	E980.6
perchlorate NEC	977.8	E858.8	E947.8	E950.4	E962.0	E980.4
antithyroid	962.8	E858.0	E932.8	E950.4	E962.0	E980.4
permanganate.	976.0	E858.7	E946.0	E950.4	E962.0	E980.4
nonmedicinal	983.9	E864.3	—	E950.7	E962.1	E980.6
Povidone–iodine (anti–infective) NEC	976.0	E858.7	E946.0	E950.4	E962.0	E980.4
Practolol	972.0	E858.3	E942.0	E950.4	E962.0	E980.4
Pralidoxime (chloride).	977.2	E858.8	E947.2	E950.4	E962.0	E980.4
Pramoxine.	968.5	E855.2	E938.5	E950.4	E962.0	E980.4
Prazosin	972.6	E858.3	E942.6	E950.4	E962.0	E980.4
Prednisolone.	962.0	E858.0	E932.0	E950.4	E962.0	E980.4
ENT agent.	976.6	E858.7	E946.6	E950.4	E962.0	E980.4
ophthalmic preparation.	976.5	E858.7	E946.5	E950.4	E962.0	E980.4
topical NEC	976.0	E858.7	E946.0	E950.4	E962.0	E980.4
Prednisone	962.0	E858.0	E932.0	E950.4	E962.0	E980.4
Pregnanediol.	962.2	E858.0	E932.2	E950.4	E962.0	E980.4
Pregneninolone.	962.2	E858.0	E932.2	E950.4	E962.0	E980.4
Preludin.	977.0	E858.8	E947.0	E950.4	E962.0	E980.4
Premarin	962.2	E858.0	E932.2	E950.4	E962.0	E980.4
Prenylamine.	972.4	E858.3	E942.4	E950.4	E962.0	E980.4
Preparation H	976.8	E858.7	E946.8	E950.4	E962.0	E980.4
Preservatives.	989.89	E866.8	—	E950.9	E962.1	E980.9
Pride of China.	988.2	E865.3	—	E950.9	E962.1	E980.9
Prilocaine.	968.9	E855.2	E938.9	E950.4	E962.0	E980.4
infiltration (subcutaneous)	968.5	E855.2	E938.5	E950.4	E962.0	E980.4
nerve block (peripheral) (plexus).	968.6	E855.2	E938.6	E950.4	E962.0	E980.4
Primaquine	961.4	E857	E931.4	E950.4	E962.0	E980.4
Primidone.	966.3	E855.0	E936.3	E950.4	E962.0	E980.4
Primula (veris).	988.2	E865.4	—	E950.9	E962.1	E980.9
Prinadol.	965.09	E850.2	E935.2	E950.0	E962.0	E980.0
Priscol, Priscoline	971.3	E855.6	E941.3	E950.4	E962.0	E980.4
Privet.	988.2	E865.4	—	E950.9	E962.1	E980.9
Privine	971.2	E855.5	E941.2	E950.4	E962.0	E980.4
Pro–Banthine	971.1	E855.4	E941.1	E950.4	E962.0	E980.4
Probarbital	967.0	E851	E937.0	E950.1	E962.0	E980.1
Probenecid	974.7	E858.5	E944.7	E950.4	E962.0	E980.4
Procainamide (hydrochloride).	972.0	E858.3	E942.0	E950.4	E962.0	E980.4
Procaine (hydrochloride) (infiltration) (topical)	968.5	E855.2	E938.5	E950.4	E962.0	E980.4
nerve block (peripheral) (plexus).	968.6	E855.2	E938.6	E950.4	E962.0	E980.4
penicillin G	960.0	E856	E930.0	E950.4	E962.0	E980.4
spinal.	968.7	E855.2	E938.7	E950.4	E962.0	E980.4
Procalmidol	969.5	E853.8	E939.5	E950.3	E962.0	E980.3
Procarbazine.	963.1	E858.1	E933.1	E950.4	E962.0	E980.4
Prochlorperazine.	969.1	E853.0	E939.1	E950.3	E962.0	E980.3
Procyclidine.	966.4	E855.0	E936.4	E950.4	E962.0	E980.4
Producer gas.	986	E868.8	—	E952.1	E962.2	E982.1
Profenamine.	966.4	E855.0	E936.4	E950.4	E962.0	E980.4
Profenil.	975.1	E858.6	E945.1	E950.4	E962.0	E980.4
Progesterones	962.2	E858.0	E932.2	E950.4	E962.0	E980.4
Progestin	962.2	E858.0	E932.2	E950.4	E962.0	E980.4
Progestogens (with estrogens).	962.2	E858.0	E932.2	E950.4	E962.0	E980.4
Progestone.	962.2	E858.0	E932.2	E950.4	E962.0	E980.4
Proguanil	961.4	E857	E931.4	E950.4	E962.0	E980.4
Prolactin	962.4	E858.0	E932.4	E950.4	E962.0	E980.4
Proloid.	962.7	E858.0	E932.7	E950.4	E962.0	E980.4
Proluton	962.2	E858.0	E932.2	E950.4	E962.0	E980.4

Substance	Poisoning	Accident	Therapeutic Use	Suicide Attempt	Assault	Undetermined
			External Cause (E-Code)			
Promacetin	961.8	E857	E931.8	E950.4	E962.0	E980.4
Promazine	969.1	E853.0	E939.1	E950.3	E962.0	E980.3
Promedol	965.09	E850.2	E935.2	E950.0	E962.0	E980.0
Promethazine	967.8	E852.8	E937.8	E950.2	E962.0	E980.2
Promin	961.8	E857	E931.8	E950.4	E962.0	E980.4
Pronestyl (hydrochloride)	972.0	E858.3	E942.0	E950.4	E962.0	E980.4
Pronetalol, pronethalol	972.0	E858.3	E942.0	E950.4	E962.0	E980.4
Prontosil	961.0	E857	E931.0	E950.4	E962.0	E980.4
Propamidine isethionate	961.5	E857	E931.5	E950.4	E962.0	E980.4
Propanal (medicinal)	967.8	E852.8	E937.8	E950.2	E962.0	E980.2
Propane (gas) (distributed in mobile container)	987.0	E868.0	—	E951.1	E962.2	E981.1
distributed through pipes	987.0	E867	—	E951.0	E962.2	E981.0
incomplete combustion of – *see* Carbon monoxide, Propane						
Propanidid	968.3	E855.1	E938.3	E950.4	E962.0	E980.4
Propanol	980.3	E860.4	—	E950.9	E962.1	E980.9
Propantheline	971.1	E855.4	E941.1	E950.4	E962.0	E980.4
Proparacaine	968.5	E855.2	E938.5	E950.4	E962.0	E980.4
Propatyl nitrate	972.4	E858.3	E942.4	E950.4	E962.0	E980.4
Propicillin	960.0	E856	E930.0	E950.4	E962.0	E980.4
Propiolactone (vapor)	987.8	E869.8	—	E952.8	E962.2	E982.8
Propiomazine	967.8	E852.8	E937.8	E950.2	E962.0	E980.2
Propionaldehyde (medicinal)	967.8	E852.8	E937.8	E950.2	E962.0	E980.2
Propionate compound	976.0	E858.7	E946.0	E950.4	E962.0	E980.4
Propion gel	976.0	E858.7	E946.0	E950.4	E962.0	E980.4
Propitocaine	968.9	E855.2	E938.9	E950.4	E962.0	E980.4
infiltration (subcutaneous)	968.5	E855.2	E938.5	E950.4	E962.0	E980.4
nerve block (peripheral) (plexus)	968.6	E855.2	E938.6	E950.4	E962.0	E980.4
Propoxur	989.3	E863.2	—	E950.6	E962.1	E980.7
Propoxycaine	968.9	E855.2	E938.9	E950.4	E962.0	E980.4
infiltration (subcutaneous)	968.5	E855.2	E938.5	E950.4	E962.0	E980.4
nerve block (peripheral) (plexus)	968.6	E855.2	E938.6	E950.4	E962.0	E980.4
topical (surface)	968.5	E855.2	E938.5	E950.4	E962.0	E980.4
Propoxyphene (hydrochloride)	965.8	E850.8	E935.8	E950.0	E962.0	E980.0
Propranolol	972.0	E858.3	E942.0	E950.4	E962.0	E980.4
Propyl						
alcohol	980.3	E860.4	—	E950.9	E962.1	E980.9
carbinol	980.3	E860.4	—	E950.9	E962.1	E980.9
hexadrine	971.2	E855.5	E941.2	E950.4	E962.0	E980.4
iodone	977.8	E858.8	E947.8	E950.4	E962.0	E980.4
thiouracil	962.8	E858.0	E932.8	E950.4	E962.0	E980.4
Propylene	987.1	E869.8	—	E952.8	E962.2	E982.8
Propylparaben (ophthalmic)	976.5	E858.7	E946.5	E950.4	E962.0	E980.4
Proscillaridin	972.1	E858.3	E942.1	E950.4	E962.0	E980.4
Prostaglandins	975.0	E858.6	E945.0	E950.4	E962.0	E980.4
Prostigmin	971.0	E855.3	E941.0	E950.4	E962.0	E980.4
Protamine (sulfate)	964.5	E858.2	E934.5	E950.4	E962.0	E980.4
zinc insulin	962.3	E858.0	E932.3	E950.4	E962.0	E980.4
Protectants (topical)	976.3	E858.7	E946.3	E950.4	E962.0	E980.4
Protein hydrolysate	974.5	E858.5	E944.5	E950.4	E962.0	E980.4
Prothiaden—*see* Dothiepin hydrochloride						
Prothionamide	961.8	E857	E931.8	E950.4	E962.0	E980.4
Prothipendyl	969.5	E853.8	E939.5	E950.3	E962.0	E980.3
Protokylol	971.2	E855.5	E941.2	E950.4	E962.0	E980.4
Protopam	977.2	E858.8	E947.2	E950.4	E962.0	E980.4
Protoveratrine(s) (A) (B)	972.6	E858.3	E942.6	E950.4	E962.0	E980.4
Protriptyline	969.05	E854.0	E939.0	E950.3	E962.0	E980.3
Provera	962.2	E858.0	E932.2	E950.4	E962.0	E980.4
Provitamin A	963.5	E858.1	E933.5	E950.4	E962.0	E980.4

Substance	Poisoning	Accident	Therapeutic Use	Suicide Attempt	Assault	Undetermined
			External Cause (E-Code)			
Proxymetacaine 968.5	E855.2	E938.5	E950.4	E962.0	E980.4
Proxyphylline 975.1	E858.6	E945.1	E950.4	E962.0	E980.4
Prozac—*see* Fluoxetine hydrochloride					
Prunus					
laurocerasus 988.2	E865.4	—	E950.9	E962.1	E980.9
virginiana 988.2	E865.4	—	E950.9	E962.1	E980.9
Prussic acid 989.0	E866.8	—	E950.9	E962.1	E980.9
vapor 987.7	E869.8	—	E952.8	E962.2	E982.8
Pseudoephedrine 971.2	E855.5	E941.2	E950.4	E962.0	E980.4
Psilocin. 969.6	E854.1	E939.6	E950.3	E962.0	E980.3
Psilocybin. 969.6	E854.1	E939.6	E950.3	E962.0	E980.3
PSP 977.8	E858.8	E947.8	E950.4	E962.0	E980.4
Psychedelic agents 969.6	E854.1	E939.6	E950.3	E962.0	E980.3
Psychodysleptics 969.6	E854.1	E939.6	E950.3	E962.0	E980.3
Psychostimulants 969.70	E854.2	E939.7	E950.3	E962.0	E980.3
Psychotherapeutic agents. 969.9	E855.9	E939.9	E950.3	E962.0	E980.3
antidepressants 969.00	E854.0	E939.0	E950.3	E962.0	E980.3
specified NEC 969.8	E855.8	E939.8	E950.3	E962.0	E980.3
tranquilizers NEC 969.5	E853.9	E939.5	E950.3	E962.0	E980.3
Psychotomimetic agents 969.6	E854.1	E939.6	E950.3	E962.0	E980.3
Psychotropic agents 969.9	E854.8	E939.9	E950.3	E962.0	E980.3
specified NEC 969.8	E854.8	E939.8	E950.3	E962.0	E980.3
Psyllium 973.3	E858.4	E943.3	E950.4	E962.0	E980.4
Pteroylglutamic acid 964.1	E858.2	E934.1	E950.4	E962.0	E980.4
Pteroyltriglutamate 963.1	E858.1	E933.1	E950.4	E962.0	E980.4
PTFE. 987.8	E869.8	—	E952.8	E962.2	E982.8
Pulsatilla 988.2	E865.4	—	E950.9	E962.1	E980.9
Purex (bleach) 983.9	E864.3	—	E950.7	E962.1	E980.6
Purine diuretics 974.1	E858.5	E944.1	E950.4	E962.0	E980.4
Purinethol 963.1	E858.1	E933.1	E950.4	E962.0	E980.4
PVP 964.8	E858.2	E934.8	E950.4	E962.0	E980.4
Pyrabital 965.7	E850.7	E935.7	E950.0	E962.0	E980.0
Pyramidon. 965.5	E850.5	E935.5	E950.0	E962.0	E980.0
Pyrantel (pamoate) 961.6	E857	E931.6	E950.4	E962.0	E980.4
Pyrathiazine 963.0	E858.1	E933.0	E950.4	E962.0	E980.4
Pyrazinamide 961.8	E857	E931.8	E950.4	E962.0	E980.4
Pyrazinoic acid (amide) 961.8	E857	E931.8	E950.4	E962.0	E980.4
Pyrazole (derivatives) 965.5	E850.5	E935.5	E950.0	E962.0	E980.0
Pyrazolone (analgesics) 965.5	E850.5	E935.5	E950.0	E962.0	E980.0
Pyrethrins, pyrethrum 989.4	E863.4	—	E950.6	E962.1	E980.7
Pyribenzamine 963.0	E858.1	E933.0	E950.4	E962.0	E980.4
Pyridine (liquid) (vapor) 982.0	E862.4	—	E950.9	E962.1	E980.9
aldoxime chloride 977.2	E858.8	E947.2	E950.4	E962.0	E980.4
Pyridium 976.1	E858.7	E946.1	E950.4	E962.0	E980.4
Pyridostigmine 971.0	E855.3	E941.0	E950.4	E962.0	E980.4
Pyridoxine. 963.5	E858.1	E933.5	E950.4	E962.0	E980.4
Pyrilamine 963.0	E858.1	E933.0	E950.4	E962.0	E980.4
Pyrimethamine 961.4	E857	E931.4	E950.4	E962.0	E980.4
Pyrogallic acid 983.0	E864.0	—	E950.7	E962.1	E980.6
Pyroxylin 976.3	E858.7	E946.3	E950.4	E962.0	E980.4
Pyrrobutamine 963.0	E858.1	E933.0	E950.4	E962.0	E980.4
Pyrrocaine 968.5	E855.2	E938.5	E950.4	E962.0	E980.4
Pyrvinium (pamoate) 961.6	E857	E931.6	E950.4	E962.0	E980.4
PZI 962.3	E858.0	E932.3	E950.4	E962.0	E980.4
Quaalude 967.4	E852.3	E937.4	E950.2	E962.0	E980.2
Quaternary ammonium derivatives 971.1	E855.4	E941.1	E950.4	E962.0	E980.4
Quicklime. 983.2	E864.2	—	E950.7	E962.1	E980.6
Quinacrine 961.3	E857	E931.3	E950.4	E962.0	E980.4
Quinaglute 972.0	E858.3	E942.0	E950.4	E962.0	E980.4
Quinalbarbitone 967.0	E851	E937.0	E950.1	E962.0	E980.1
Quinestradiol 962.2	E858.0	E932.2	E950.4	E962.0	E980.4

Substance	Poisoning	Accident	Therapeutic Use	Suicide Attempt	Assault	Undetermined
			External Cause (E-Code)			
Quinethazone 974.3	E858.5	E944.3	E950.4	E962.0	E980.4	
Quinidine (gluconate) (polygalacturonate)						
(salts) (sulfate) 972.0	E858.3	E942.0	E950.4	E962.0	E980.4	
Quinine 961.4	E857	E931.4	E950.4	E962.0	E980.4	
Quiniobine 961.3	E857	E931.3	E950.4	E962.0	E980.4	
Quinolines 961.3	E857	E931.3	E950.4	E962.0	E980.4	
Quotane 968.5	E855.2	E938.5	E950.4	E962.0	E980.4	
Rabies						
immune globulin (human) 964.6	E858.2	E934.6	E950.4	E962.0	E980.4	
vaccine 979.1	E858.8	E949.1	E950.4	E962.0	E980.4	
Racemoramide 965.09	E850.2	E935.2	E950.0	E962.0	E980.0	
Racemorphan 965.09	E850.2	E935.2	E950.0	E962.0	E980.0	
Radiator alcohol 980.1	E860.2	—	E950.9	E962.1	E980.9	
Radio–opaque (drugs) (materials) 977.8	E858.8	E947.8	E950.4	E962.0	E980.4	
Ranunculus 988.2	E865.4	—	E950.9	E962.1	E980.9	
Rat poison 989.4	E863.7	—	E950.6	E962.1	E980.7	
Rattlesnake (venom) 989.5	E905.0	—	E950.9	E962.1	E980.9	
Raudixin 972.6	E858.3	E942.6	E950.4	E962.0	E980.4	
Rautensin 972.6	E858.3	E942.6	E950.4	E962.0	E980.4	
Rautina 972.6	E858.3	E942.6	E950.4	E962.0	E980.4	
Rautotal 972.6	E858.3	E942.6	E950.4	E962.0	E980.4	
Rauwiloid 972.6	E858.3	E942.6	E950.4	E962.0	E980.4	
Rauwoldin 972.6	E858.3	E942.6	E950.4	E962.0	E980.4	
Rauwolfia (alkaloids) 972.6	E858.3	E942.6	E950.4	E962.0	E980.4	
Realgar 985.1	E866.3	—	E950.8	E962.1	E980.8	
Red cells, packed 964.7	E858.2	E934.7	E950.4	E962.0	E980.4	
Reducing agents, industrial NEC 983.9	E864.3	—	E950.7	E962.1	E980.6	
Refrigerant gas (freon) 987.4	E869.2	—	E952.8	E962.2	E982.8	
not freon 987.9	E869.9	—	E952.9	E962.2	E982.9	
Regroton 974.4	E858.5	E944.4	E950.4	E962.0	E980.4	
Rela 968.0	E855.1	E938.0	E950.4	E962.0	E980.4	
Relaxants, skeletal muscle (autonomic) . . . 975.2	E858.6	E945.2	E950.4	E962.0	E980.4	
central nervous system 968.0	E855.1	E938.0	E950.4	E962.0	E980.4	
Renese 974.3	E858.5	E944.3	E950.4	E962.0	E980.4	
Renografin 977.8	E858.8	E947.8	E950.4	E962.0	E980.4	
Replacement solutions 974.5	E858.5	E944.5	E950.4	E962.0	E980.4	
Rescinnamine 972.6	E858.3	E942.6	E950.4	E962.0	E980.4	
Reserpine 972.6	E858.3	E942.6	E950.4	E962.0	E980.4	
Resorcin, resorcinol 976.4	E858.7	E946.4	E950.4	E962.0	E980.4	
Respaire 975.5	E858.6	E945.5	E950.4	E962.0	E980.4	
Respiratory agents NEC 975.8	E858.6	E945.8	E950.4	E962.0	E980.4	
Retinoic acid 976.8	E858.7	E946.8	E950.4	E962.0	E980.4	
Retinol 963.5	E858.1	E933.5	E950.4	E962.0	E980.4	
Rh₀ (D) immune globulin (human) 964.6	E858.2	E934.6	E950.4	E962.0	E980.4	
Rhodine 965.1	E850.3	E935.3	E950.0	E962.0	E980.0	
RhoGAM 964.6	E858.2	E934.6	E950.4	E962.0	E980.4	
Riboflavin 963.5	E858.1	E933.5	E950.4	E962.0	E980.4	
Ricin 989.89	E866.8	—	E950.9	E962.1	E980.9	
Ricinus communis 988.2	E865.3	—	E950.9	E962.1	E980.9	
Rickettsial vaccine NEC 979.6	E858.8	E949.6	E950.4	E962.0	E980.4	
with viral and bacterial vaccine 979.7	E858.8	E949.7	E950.4	E962.0	E980.4	
Rifampin 960.6	E856	E930.6	E950.4	E962.0	E980.4	
Rimifon 961.8	E857	E931.8	E950.4	E962.0	E980.4	
Ringer's injection (lactated) 974.5	E858.5	E944.5	E950.4	E962.0	E980.4	
Ristocetin 960.8	E856	E930.8	E950.4	E962.0	E980.4	
Ritalin 969.73	E854.2	E939.7	E950.3	E962.0	E980.3	
Roach killers — *see* Pesticides						
Rocky Mountain spotted fever vaccine 979.6	E858.8	E949.6	E950.4	E962.0	E980.4	
Rodenticides 989.4	E863.7	—	E950.6	E962.1	E980.7	
Rohypnol 969.4	E853.2	E939.4	E950.3	E962.0	E980.3	

Substance	Poisoning	Accident	Therapeutic Use	Suicide Attempt	Assault	Undetermined
			External Cause (E-Code)			
Rolaids	973.0	E858.4	E943.0	E950.4	E962.0	E980.4
Rolitetracycline	960.4	E856	E930.4	E950.4	E962.0	E980.4
Romilar	975.4	E858.6	E945.4	E950.4	E962.0	E980.4
Rose water ointment	976.3	E858.7	E946.3	E950.4	E962.0	E980.4
Rotenone	989.4	E863.7	—	E950.6	E962.1	E980.7
Rotoxamine	963.0	E858.1	E933.0	E950.4	E962.0	E980.4
Rough–on–rats	989.4	E863.7	—	E950.6	E962.1	E980.7
Rubbing alcohol	980.2	E860.3	—	E950.9	E962.1	E980.9
Rubella virus vaccine	979.4	E858.8	E949.4	E950.4	E962.0	E980.4
Rubelogen	979.4	E858.8	E949.4	E950.4	E962.0	E980.4
Rubeovax	979.4	E858.8	E949.4	E950.4	E962.0	E980.4
Rubidomycin	960.7	E856	E930.7	E950.4	E962.0	E980.4
Rue	988.2	E965.4	—	E950.9	E962.1	E980.9
RU486	962.9	E858.0	E932.9	E950.4	E962.0	E980.4
Ruta	988.2	E865.4	—	E950.9	E962.1	E980.9
Sabadilla (medicinal)	976.0	E858.7	E946.0	E950.4	E962.0	E980.4
pesticide	989.4	E863.4	—	E950.6	E962.1	E980.7
Sabin oral vaccine	979.5	E858.8	E949.5	E950.4	E962.0	E980.4
Saccharated iron oxide	964.0	E858.2	E934.0	E950.4	E962.0	E980.4
Saccharin	974.5	E858.5	E944.5	E950.4	E962.0	E980.4
Safflower oil	972.2	E858.3	E942.2	E950.4	E962.0	E980.4
Salbutamol sulfate	975.7	E858.6	E945.7	E950.4	E962.0	E980.4
Salicylamide	965.1	E850.3	E935.3	E950.0	E962.0	E980.0
Salicylate(s)	965.1	E850.3	E935.3	E950.0	E962.0	E980.0
methyl	976.3	E858.7	E946.3	E950.4	E962.0	E980.4
theobromine calcium	974.1	E858.5	E944.1	E950.4	E962.0	E980.4
Salicylazosulfapyridine	961.0	E857	E931.0	E950.4	E962.0	E980.4
Salicylhydroxamic acid	976.0	E858.7	E946.0	E950.4	E962.0	E980.4
Salicylic acid (keratolytic) NEC	976.4	E858.7	E946.4	E950.4	E962.0	E980.4
congeners	965.1	E850.3	E935.3	E950.0	E962.0	E980.0
salts	965.1	E850.3	E935.3	E950.0	E962.0	E980.0
Saliniazid	961.8	E857	E931.8	E950.4	E962.0	E980.4
Salol	976.3	E858.7	E946.3	E950.4	E962.0	E980.4
Salt (substitute) NEC	974.5	E858.5	E944.5	E950.4	E962.0	E980.4
Saluretics	974.3	E858.5	E944.3	E950.4	E962.0	E980.4
Saluron	974.3	E858.5	E944.3	E950.4	E962.0	E980.4
Salvarsan 606 (neosilver) (silver)	961.1	E857	E931.1	E950.4	E962.0	E980.4
Sambucus canadensis	988.2	E865.4	—	E950.9	E962.1	E980.9
berry	988.2	E865.3	—	E950.9	E962.1	E980.9
Sandril	972.6	E858.3	E942.6	E950.4	E962.0	E980.4
Sanguinaria canadensis	988.2	E865.4	—	E950.9	E962.1	E980.9
Saniflush (cleaner)	983.9	E861.3	—	E950.7	E962.1	E980.6
Santonin	961.6	E857	E931.6	E950.4	E962.0	E980.4
Santyl	976.8	E858.7	E946.8	E950.4	E962.0	E980.4
Sarkomycin	960.7	E856	E930.7	E950.4	E962.0	E980.4
Saroten	969.05	E854.0	E939.0	E950.3	E962.0	E980.3
Saturnine – see Lead						
Savin (oil)	976.4	E858.7	E946.4	E950.4	E962.0	E980.4
Scammony	973.1	E858.4	E943.1	E950.4	E962.0	E980.4
Scarlet red	976.8	E858.7	E946.8	E950.4	E962.0	E980.4
Scheele's green	985.1	E866.3	—	E950.8	E962.1	E980.8
insecticide	985.1	E863.4	—	E950.8	E962.1	E980.8
Schradan	989.3	E863.1	—	E950.6	E962.1	E980.7
Schweinfurt (h) green	985.1	E866.3	—	E950.8	E962.1	E980.8
insecticide	985.1	E863.4	—	E950.8	E962.1	E980.8
Scilla — see Squill						
Sclerosing agents	972.7	E858.3	E942.7	E950.4	E962.0	E980.4
Scopolamine	971.1	E855.4	E941.1	E950.4	E962.0	E980.4
Scouring powder	989.89	E861.3	—	E950.9	E962.1	E980.9
Sea						
anemone (sting)	989.5	E905.6	—	E950.9	E962.1	E980.9

Substance	Poisoning	Accident	Therapeutic Use	Suicide Attempt	Assault	Undetermined
			External Cause (E-Code)			
cucumber (sting)	989.5	E905.6	—	E950.9	E962.1	E980.9
snake (bite) (venom)	989.5	E905.0	—	E950.9	E962.1	E980.9
urchin spine (puncture)	989.5	E905.6	—	E950.9	E962.1	E980.9
Secbutabarbital	967.0	E851	E937.0	E950.1	E962.0	E980.1
Secbutabaritone	967.0	E851	E937.0	E950.1	E962.0	E980.1
Secobarbital	967.0	E851	E937.0	E950.1	E962.0	E980.1
Seconal	967.0	E851	E937.0	E950.1	E962.0	E980.1
Secretin	977.8	E858.8	E947.8	E950.4	E962.0	E980.4
Sedatives, nonbarbiturate	967.9	E852.9	E937.9	E950.2	E962.0	E980.2
specified NEC	967.8	E852.8	E937.8	E950.2	E962.0	E980.2
Sedormid	967.8	E852.8	E937.8	E950.2	E962.0	E980.2
Seed (plant)	988.2	E865.3	—	E950.9	E962.1	E980.9
disinfectant or dressing	989.89	E866.5	—	E950.9	E962.1	E980.9
Selective serotonin and norepinephrine reuptake inhibitors (SSNRI)	969.02	E854.0	E939.0	E950.3	E962.0	E980.3
Selective serotonin reuptake inhibitors (SSRI)	969.03	E854.0	E939.0	E950.3	E962.0	E980.3
Selenium (fumes) NEC	985.8	E866.4	—	E950.9	E962.1	E980.9
disulfide or sulfide	976.4	E858.7	E946.4	E950.4	E962.0	E980.4
Selsun	976.4	E858.7	E946.4	E950.4	E962.0	E980.4
Senna	973.1	E858.4	E943.1	E950.4	E962.0	E980.4
Septisol	976.2	E858.7	E946.2	E950.4	E962.0	E980.4
Serax	969.4	E853.2	E939.4	E950.3	E962.0	E980.3
Serenesil	967.8	E852.8	E937.8	E950.2	E962.0	E980.2
Serenium (hydrochloride)	961.9	E857	E931.9	E950.4	E962.0	E980.4
Serepax—*see* Oxazepam						
Sernyl	968.3	E855.1	E938.3	E950.4	E962.0	E980.4
Serotonin	977.8	E858.8	E947.8	E950.4	E962.0	E980.4
Serpasil	972.6	E858.3	E942.6	E950.4	E962.0	E980.4
Sewer gas	987.8	E869.8	—	E952.8	E962.2	E982.8
Shampoo	989.6	E861.0	—	E950.9	E962.1	E980.9
Shellfish, nonbacterial or noxious	988.0	E865.1	—	E950.9	E962.1	E980.9
Silicones NEC	989.83	E866.8	E947.8	E950.9	E962.1	E980.9
Silvadene	976.0	E858.7	E946.0	E950.4	E962.0	E980.4
Silver (compound) (medicinal) NEC	976.0	E858.7	E946.0	E950.4	E962.0	E980.4
anti–infectives	976.0	E858.7	E946.0	E950.4	E962.0	E980.4
arsphenamine	961.1	E857	E931.1	E950.4	E962.0	E980.4
nitrate	976.0	E858.7	E946.0	E950.4	E962.0	E980.4
ophthalmic preparation	976.5	E858.7	E946.5	E950.4	E962.0	E980.4
toughened (keratolytic)	976.4	E858.7	E946.4	E950.4	E962.0	E980.4
nonmedicinal (dust)	985.8	E866.4	—	E950.9	E962.1	E980.9
protein (mild) (strong)	976.0	E858.7	E946.0	E950.4	E962.0	E980.4
salvarsan	961.1	E857	E931.1	E950.4	E962.0	E980.4
Simethicone	973.8	E858.4	E943.8	E950.4	E962.0	E980.4
Sinequan	969.05	E854.0	E939.0	E950.3	E962.0	E980.3
Singoserp	972.6	E858.3	E942.6	E950.4	E962.0	E980.4
Sintrom	964.2	E858.2	E934.2	E950.4	E962.0	E980.4
Sitosterols	972.2	E858.3	E942.2	E950.4	E962.0	E980.4
Skeletal muscle relaxants	975.2	E858.6	E945.2	E950.4	E962.0	E980.4
Skin						
agents (external)	976.9	E858.7	E946.9	E950.4	E962.0	E980.4
specified NEC	976.8	E858.7	E946.8	E950.4	E962.0	E980.4
test antigen	977.8	E858.8	E947.8	E950.4	E962.0	E980.4
Sleep–eze	963.0	E858.1	E933.0	E950.4	E962.0	E980.4
Sleeping draught (drug) (pill) (tablet)	967.9	E852.9	E937.9	E950.2	E962.0	E980.2
Smallpox vaccine	979.0	E858.8	E949.0	E950.4	E962.0	E980.4
Smelter fumes NEC	985.9	E866.4	—	E950.9	E962.1	E980.9
Smog	987.3	E869.1	—	E952.8	E962.2	E982.8
Smoke NEC	987.9	E869.9	—	E952.9	E962.2	E982.9
Smooth muscle relaxant	975.1	E858.6	E945.1	E950.4	E962.0	E980.4
Snail killer	989.4	E863.4	—	E950.6	E962.1	E980.7

Substance	Poisoning	Accident	Therapeutic Use	Suicide Attempt	Assault	Undetermined
			External Cause (E-Code)			
Snake (bite) (venom)	989.5	E905.0	—	E950.9	E962.1	E980.9
Snuff	989.89	E866.8	—	E950.9	E962.1	E980.9
Soap (powder) (product)	989.6	E861.1	—	E950.9	E962.1	E980.9
medicinal, soft	976.2	E858.7	E946.2	E950.4	E962.0	E980.4
Soda (caustic)	983.2	E864.2	—	E950.7	E962.1	E980.6
bicarb	963.3	E858.1	E933.3	E950.4	E962.0	E980.4
chlorinated — Sodium, hypochlorite						
Sodium						
acetosulfone	961.8	E857	E931.8	E950.4	E962.0	E980.4
acetrizoate	977.8	E858.8	E947.8	E950.4	E962.0	E980.4
amytal	967.0	E851	E937.0	E950.1	E962.0	E980.1
arsenate — see Arsenic						
bicarbonate	963.3	E858.1	E933.3	E950.4	E962.0	E980.4
bichromate	983.9	E864.3	—	E950.7	E962.1	E980.6
biphosphate	963.2	E858.1	E933.2	E950.4	E962.0	E980.4
bisulfate	983.9	E864.3	—	E950.7	E962.1	E980.6
borate (cleanser)	989.6	E861.3	—	E950.9	E962.1	E980.9
bromide NEC	967.3	E852.2	E937.3	E950.2	E962.0	E980.2
cacodylate (nonmedicinal) NEC . . .	978.8	E858.8	E948.8	E950.4	E962.0	E980.4
anti–infective	961.1	E857	E931.1	E950.4	E962.0	E980.4
herbicide	989.4	E863.5	—	E950.6	E962.1	E980.7
calcium edetate	963.8	E858.1	E933.8	E950.4	E962.0	E980.4
carbonate NEC	983.2	E864.2	—	E950.7	E962.1	E980.6
chlorate NEC	983.9	E864.3	—	E950.7	E962.1	E980.6
herbicide	983.9	E863.5	—	E950.7	E962.1	E980.6
chloride NEC	974.5	E858.5	E944.5	E950.4	E962.0	E980.4
chromate	983.9	E864.3	—	E950.7	E962.1	E980.6
citrate	963.3	E858.1	E933.3	E950.4	E962.0	E980.4
cyanide — see Cyanide(s)						
cyclamate	974.5	E858.5	E944.5	E950.4	E962.0	E980.4
diatrizoate	977.8	E858.8	E947.8	E950.4	E962.0	E980.4
dibunate	975.4	E858.6	E945.4	E950.4	E962.0	E980.4
dioctyl sulfosuccinate	973.2	E858.4	E943.2	E950.4	E962.0	E980.4
edetate	963.8	E858.1	E933.8	E950.4	E962.0	E980.4
ethacrynate	974.4	E858.5	E944.4	E950.4	E962.0	E980.4
fluoracetate (dust) (rodenticide)	989.4	E863.7	—	E950.6	E962.1	E980.7
fluoride — see Fluoride(s)						
free salt	974.5	E858.5	E944.5	E950.4	E962.0	E980.4
glucosulfone	961.8	E857	E931.8	E950.4	E962.0	E980.4
hydroxide	983.2	E864.2	—	E950.7	E962.1	E980.6
hypochlorite (bleach) NEC	983.9	E864.3	—	E950.7	E962.1	E980.6
disinfectant	983.9	E861.4	—	E950.7	E962.1	E980.6
medicinal (anti–infective) (external)	976.0	E858.7	E946.0	E950.4	E962.0	E980.4
vapor	987.8	E869.8	—	E952.8	E962.2	E982.8
hyposulfite	976.0	E858.7	E946.0	E950.4	E962.0	E980.4
indigotindisulfonate	977.8	E858.8	E947.8	E950.4	E962.0	E980.4
iodide	977.8	E858.8	E947.8	E950.4	E962.0	E980.4
iothalamate	977.8	E858.8	E947.8	E950.4	E962.0	E980.4
iron edetate	964.0	E858.2	E934.0	E950.4	E962.0	E980.4
lactate	963.3	E858.1	E933.3	E950.4	E962.0	E980.4
lauryl sulfate	976.2	E858.7	E946.2	E950.4	E962.0	E980.4
L–triiodothyronine	962.7	E858.0	E932.7	E950.4	E962.0	E980.4
metrizoate	977.8	E858.8	E947.8	E950.4	E962.0	E980.4
monofluoracetate (dust) (rodenticide)	989.4	E863.7	—	E950.6	E962.1	E980.7
morrhuate	972.7	E858.3	E942.7	E950.4	E962.0	E980.4
nafcillin	960.0	E856	E930.0	E950.4	E962.0	E980.4
nitrate (oxidizing agent)	983.9	E864.3	—	E950.7	E962.1	E980.6
nitrite (medicinal)	972.4	E858.3	E942.4	E950.4	E962.0	E980.4
nitroferricyanide	972.6	E858.3	E942.6	E950.4	E962.0	E980.4
nitroprusside	972.6	E858.3	E942.6	E950.4	E962.0	E980.4
para–aminohippurate	977.8	E858.8	E947.8	E950.4	E962.0	E980.4

TABLE OF DRUGS AND CHEMICALS

Substance	Poisoning	Accident	Therapeutic Use	Suicide Attempt	Assault	Undetermined
			External Cause (E-Code)			
perborate (non-medicinal) NEC	989.89	E866.8	—	E950.9	E962.1	E980.9
medicinal	976.6	E858.7	E946.6	E950.4	E962.0	E980.4
soap	989.6	E861.1	—	E950.9	E962.1	E980.9
percarbonate — see Sodium, perborate						
phosphate	973.3	E858.4	E943.3	E950.4	E962.0	E980.4
polystyrene sulfonate	974.5	E858.5	E944.5	E950.4	E962.0	E980.4
propionate	976.0	E858.7	E946.0	E950.4	E962.0	E980.4
psylliate	972.7	E858.3	E942.7	E950.4	E962.0	E980.4
removing resins	974.5	E858.5	E944.5	E950.4	E962.0	E980.4
salicylate	965.1	E850.3	E935.3	E950.0	E962.0	E980.0
sulfate	973.3	E858.4	E943.3	E950.4	E962.0	E980.4
sulfoxone	961.8	E857	E931.8	E950.4	E962.0	E980.4
tetradecyl sulfate	972.7	E858.3	E942.7	E950.4	E962.0	E980.4
thiopental	968.3	E855.1	E938.3	E950.4	E962.0	E980.4
thiosalicylate	965.1	E850.3	E935.3	E950.0	E962.0	E980.0
thiosulfate	976.0	E858.7	E946.0	E950.4	E962.0	E980.4
tolbutamide	977.8	E858.8	E947.8	E950.4	E962.0	E980.4
tyropanoate	977.8	E858.8	E947.8	E950.4	E962.0	E980.4
valproate	966.3	E855.0	E936.3	E950.4	E962.0	E980.4
Solanine	977.8	E858.8	E947.8	E950.4	E962.0	E980.4
Solanum dulcamara	988.2	E865.4	—	E950.9	E962.1	E980.9
Solapsone	961.8	E857	E931.8	E950.4	E962.0	E980.4
Solasulfone	961.8	E857	E931.8	E950.4	E962.0	E980.4
Soldering fluid	983.1	E864.1	—	E950.7	E962.1	E980.6
Solid substance	989.9	E866.9	—	E950.9	E962.1	E980.9
specified NEC	989.9	E866.8	—	E950.9	E962.1	E980.9
Solvents, industrial	982.8	E862.9	—	E950.9	E962.1	E980.9
naphtha	981	E862.0	—	E950.9	E962.1	E980.9
petroleum	981	E862.0	—	E950.9	E962.1	E980.9
specified NEC	982.8	E862.4	—	E950.9	E962.1	E980.9
Soma	968.0	E855.1	E938.0	E950.4	E962.0	E980.4
Somatotropin	962.4	E858.0	E932.4	E950.4	E962.0	E980.4
Sominex	963.0	E858.1	E933.0	E950.4	E962.0	E980.4
Somnos	967.1	E852.0	E937.1	E950.2	E962.0	E980.2
Somonal	967.0	E851	E937.0	E950.1	E962.0	E980.1
Soneryl	967.0	E851	E937.0	E950.1	E962.0	E980.1
Soothing syrup	977.9	E858.9	E947.9	E950.5	E962.0	E980.5
Sopor	967.4	E852.3	E937.4	E950.2	E962.0	E980.2
Soporific drug	967.9	E852.9	E937.9	E950.2	E962.0	E980.2
specified type NEC	967.8	E852.8	E937.8	E950.2	E962.0	E980.2
Sorbitol NEC	977.4	E858.8	E947.4	E950.4	E962.0	E980.4
Sotradecol	972.7	E858.3	E942.7	E950.4	E962.0	E980.4
Spacoline	975.1	E858.6	E945.1	E950.4	E962.0	E980.4
Spanish fly	976.8	E858.7	E946.8	E950.4	E962.0	E980.4
Sparine	969.1	E853.0	E939.1	E950.3	E962.0	E980.3
Sparteine	975.0	E858.6	E945.0	E950.4	E962.0	E980.4
Spasmolytics	975.1	E858.6	E945.1	E950.4	E962.0	E980.4
anticholinergics	971.1	E855.4	E941.1	E950.4	E962.0	E980.4
Spectinomycin	960.8	E856	E930.8	E950.4	E962.0	E980.4
Speed	969.72	E854.2	E939.7	E950.3	E962.0	E980.3
Spermicides	976.8	E858.7	E946.8	E950.4	E962.0	E980.4
Spider (bite) (venom)	989.5	E905.1	—	E950.9	E962.1	E980.9
antivenin	979.9	E858.8	E949.9	E950.4	E962.0	E980.4
Spigelia (root)	961.6	E857	E931.6	E950.4	E962.0	E980.4
Spiperone	969.2	E853.1	E939.2	E950.3	E962.0	E980.3
Spiramycin	960.3	E856	E930.3	E950.4	E962.0	E980.4
Spirilene	969.5	E853.8	E939.5	E950.3	E962.0	E980.3
Spirit(s) (neutral) NEC	980.0	E860.1	—	E950.9	E962.1	E980.9
beverage	980.0	E860.0	—	E950.9	E962.1	E980.9
industrial	980.9	E860.9	—	E950.9	E962.1	E980.9

TABLE OF DRUGS AND CHEMICALS

Substance	Poisoning	Accident	Therapeutic Use	Suicide Attempt	Assault	Undetermined
			External Cause (E-Code)			
mineral 981	E862.0	—	E950.9	E962.1	E980.9
of salt — *see* Hydrochloric acid						
surgical 980.9	E860.9	—	E950.9	E962.1	E980.9
Spironolactone 974.4	E858.5	E944.4	E950.4	E962.0	E980.4
Sponge, absorbable (gelatin) 964.5	E858.2	E934.5	E950.4	E962.0	E980.4
Sporostacin 976.0	E858.7	E946.0	E950.4	E962.0	E980.4
Sprays (aerosol) 989.89	E866.8	—	E950.9	E962.1	E980.9
cosmetic. 989.89	E866.7	—	E950.9	E962.1	E980.9
medicinal NEC 977.9	E858.9	E947.9	E950.5	E962.0	E980.5
pesticides — *see* Pesticides						
specified content — *see* substance						
specified						
Spurge flax 988.2	E865.4	—	E950.9	E962.1	E980.9
Spurges. 988.2	E865.4	—	E950.9	E962.1	E980.9
Squill (expectorant) NEC 975.5	E858.6	E945.5	E950.4	E962.0	E980.4
rat poison 989.4	E863.7	—	E950.6	E962.1	E980.7
Squirting cucumber (cathartic) 973.1	E858.4	E943.1	E950.4	E962.0	E980.4
SSNRI (selective serotonin and						
norepinephrine reuptake inhibitors) 969.02	E854.0	E939.0	E950.3	E962.0	E980.3
SSRI (selective serotonin reuptake inhibitors) . 969.03	E854.0	E939.0	E950.3	E962.0	E980.3
Stains 989.89	E866.8	—	E950.9	E962.1	E980.9
Stannous — *see also* Tin						
fluoride 976.7	E858.7	E946.7	E950.4	E962.0	E980.4
Stanolone 962.1	E858.0	E932.1	E950.4	E962.0	E980.4
Stanozolol 962.1	E853.0	E932.1	E950.4	E962.0	E980.4
Staphisagria or stavesacre (pediculicide) . . . 976.0	E858.7	E946.0	E950.4	E962.0	E980.4
Stelazine 969.1	E853.0	E939.1	E950.3	E962.0	E980.3
Stemetil. 969.1	E853.0	E939.1	E950.3	E962.0	E980.3
Sterculia (cathartic) (gum) 973.3	E858.4	E943.3	E950.4	E962.0	E980.4
Sternutator gas 987.8	E869.8	—	E952.8	E962.2	E982.8
Steroids NEC 962.0	E858.0	E932.0	E950.4	E962.0	E980.4
ENT agent. 976.6	E858.7	E946.6	E950.4	E962.0	E980.4
ophthalmic preparation 976.5	E858.7	E946.5	E950.4	E962.0	E980.4
topical NEC 976.0	E858.7	E946.0	E950.4	E962.0	E980.4
Stibine 985.8	E866.4	—	E950.9	E962.1	E980.9
Stibophen 961.2	E857	E931.2	E950.4	E962.0	E980.4
Stilbamide, stilbamidine 961.5	E857	E931.5	E950.4	E962.0	E980.4
Stilbestrol 962.2	E858.0	E932.2	E950.4	E962.0	E980.4
Stimulants (central nervous system) 970.9	E854.3	E940.9	E950.4	E962.0	E980.4
analeptics 970.0	E854.3	E940.0	E950.4	E962.0	E980.4
opiate antagonist 970.1	E854.3	E940.1	E950.4	E962.0	E980.4
psychotherapeutic NEC 969.09	E854.0	E939.0	E950.3	E962.0	E980.3
specified NEC 970.8	E854.3	E940.8	E950.4	E962.0	E980.4
Storage batteries (acid) (cells) 983.1	E864.1	—	E950.7	E962.1	E980.6
Stovaine 968.9	E855.2	E938.9	E950.4	E962.0	E980.4
infiltration (subcutaneous) 968.5	E855.2	E938.5	E950.4	E962.0	E980.4
nerve block (peripheral) (plexus). 968.6	E855.2	E938.6	E950.5	E962.0	E980.4
spinal. 968.7	E855.2	E938.7	E950.4	E962.0	E980.4
topical (surface) 968.5	E855.2	E938.5	E950.4	E962.0	E980.4
Stovarsal 961.1	E857	E931.1	E950.4	E962.0	E980.4
Stove gas — *see* Gas, utility						
Stoxil. 976.5	E858.7	E946.5	E950.4	E962.0	E980.4
STP 969.6	E854.1	E939.6	E950.3	E962.0	E980.3
Stramonium (medicinal) NEC. 971.1	E855.4	E941.1	E950.4	E962.0	E980.4
natural state 988.2	E865.4	—	E950.9	E962.1	E980.9
Streptodornase 964.4	E858.2	E934.4	E950.4	E962.0	E980.4
Streptoduocin 960.6	E856	E930.6	E950.4	E962.0	E980.4
Streptokinase 964.4	E858.2	E934.4	E950.4	E962.0	E980.4
Streptomycin 960.6	E856	E930.6	E950.4	E962.0	E980.4
Streptozocin 960.7	E856	E930.7	E950.4	E962.0	E980.4
Stripper (paint) (solvent). 982.8	E862.9	—	E950.9	E962.1	E980.9

TABLE OF DRUGS AND CHEMICALS

Substance	Poisoning	Accident	Therapeutic Use	Suicide Attempt	Assault	Undetermined
			External Cause (E-Code)			
Strobane	989.2	E863.0	—	E950.6	E962.1	E980.7
Strophanthin	972.1	E858.3	E942.1	E950.4	E962.0	E980.4
Strophanthus hispidus or kombe	988.2	E865.4	—	E950.9	E962.1	E980.9
Strychnine (rodenticide) (salts)	989.1	E863.7	—	E950.6	E962.1	E980.7
medicinal NEC	970.8	E854.3	E940.8	E950.4	E962.0	E980.4
Strychnos (ignatii) — see Strychnine						
Styramate	968.0	E855.1	E938.0	E950.4	E962.0	E980.4
Styrene	983.0	E864.0	—	E950.7	E962.1	E980.6
Succinimide (anticonvulsant)	966.2	E855.0	E936.2	E950.4	E962.0	E980.4
mercuric — see Mercury						
Succinylcholine	975.2	E858.6	E945.2	E950.4	E962.0	E980.4
Succinylsulfathiazole	961.0	E857	E931.0	E950.4	E962.0	E980.4
Sucrose	974.5	E858.5	E944.5	E950.4	E962.0	E980.4
Sulfacetamide	961.0	E857	E931.0	E950.4	E962.0	E980.4
ophthalmic preparation	976.5	E858.7	E946.5	E950.4	E962.0	E980.4
Sulfachlorpyridazine	961.0	E857	E931.0	E950.4	E962.0	E980.4
Sulfacytine	961.0	E857	E931.0	E950.4	E962.0	E980.4
Sulfadiazine	961.0	E857	E931.0	E950.4	E962.0	E980.4
silver (topical)	976.0	E858.7	E946.0	E950.4	E962.0	E980.4
Sulfadimethoxine	961.0	E857	E931.0	E950.4	E962.0	E980.4
Sulfadimidine	961.0	E857	E931.0	E950.4	E962.0	E980.4
Sulfaethidole	961.0	E857	E931.0	E950.4	E962.0	E980.4
Sulfafurazole	961.0	E857	E931.0	E950.4	E962.0	E980.4
Sulfaguanidine	961.0	E857	E931.0	E950.4	E962.0	E980.4
Sulfamerazine	961.0	E857	E931.0	E950.4	E962.0	E980.4
Sulfameter	961.0	E857	E931.0	E950.4	E962.0	E980.4
Sulfamethizole	961.0	E857	E931.0	E950.4	E962.0	E980.4
Sulfamethoxazole	961.0	E857	E931.0	E950.4	E962.0	E980.4
Sulfamethoxydiazine	961.0	E857	E931.0	E950.4	E962.0	E980.4
Sulfamethoxypyridazine	961.0	E857	E931.0	E950.4	E962.0	E980.4
Sulfamethylthiazole	961.0	E857	E931.0	E950.4	E962.0	E980.4
Sulfamylon	976.0	E858.7	E946.0	E950.4	E962.0	E980.4
Sulfan blue (diagnostic dye)	977.8	E858.8	E947.8	E950.4	E962.0	E980.4
Sulfanilamide	961.0	E857	E931.0	E950.4	E962.0	E980.4
Sulfanilylguanidine	961.0	E857	E931.0	E950.4	E962.0	E980.4
Sulfaphenazole	961.0	E857	E931.0	E950.4	E962.0	E980.4
Sulfaphenylthiazole	961.0	E857	E931.0	E950.4	E962.0	E980.4
Sulfaproxyline	961.0	E857	E931.0	E950.4	E962.0	E980.4
Sulfapyridine	961.0	E857	E931.0	E950.4	E962.0	E980.4
Sulfapyrimidine	961.0	E857	E931.0	E950.4	E962.0	E980.4
Sulfarsphenamine	961.1	E857	E931.1	E950.4	E962.0	E980.4
Sulfasalazine	961.0	E857	E931.0	E950.4	E962.0	E980.4
Sulfasomizole	961.0	E857	E931.0	E950.4	E962.0	E980.4
Sulfasuxidine	961.0	E857	E931.0	E950.4	E962.0	E980.4
Sulfinpyrazone	974.7	E858.5	E944.7	E950.4	E962.0	E980.4
Sulfisoxazole	961.0	E857	E931.0	E950.4	E962.0	E980.4
ophthalmic preparation	976.5	E858.7	E946.5	E950.4	E962.0	E980.4
Sulfomyxin	960.8	E856	E930.8	E950.4	E962.0	E980.4
Sulfonal	967.8	E852.8	E937.8	E950.2	E962.0	E980.2
Sulfonamides (mixtures)	961.0	E857	E931.0	E950.4	E962.0	E980.4
Sulfones	961.8	E857	E931.8	E950.4	E962.0	E980.4
Sulfonethylmethane	967.8	E852.8	E937.8	E950.2	E962.0	E980.2
Sulfonmethane	967.8	E852.8	E937.8	E950.2	E962.0	E980.2
Sulfonphthal, sulfonphthol	977.8	E858.8	E947.8	E950.4	E962.0	E980.4
Sulfonylurea derivatives, oral	962.3	E858.0	E932.3	E950.4	E962.0	E980.4
Sulfoxone	961.8	E857	E931.8	E950.4	E962.0	E980.4
Sulfur, sulfureted, sulfuric, sulfurous, sulfuryl (compounds) NEC	989.89	E866.8	—	E950.9	E962.1	E980.9
acid	983.1	E864.1	—	E950.7	E962.1	E980.6
dioxide	987.3	E869.1	—	E952.8	E962.2	E982.8

Substance	Poisoning	Accident	Therapeutic Use	Suicide Attempt	Assault	Undetermined
			External Cause (E-Code)			
ether — *see* Ether(s)						
hydrogen	987.8	E869.8	—	E952.8	E962.2	E982.8
medicinal (keratolytic) (ointment) NEC	976.4	E858.7	E946.4	E950.4	E962.0	E980.4
pesticide (vapor)	989.4	E863.4	—	E950.6	E962.1	E980.7
vapor NEC	987.8	E869.8	—	E952.8	E962.2	E982.8
Sulkowitch's reagent	977.8	E858.8	E947.8	E950.4	E962.0	E980.4
Sulph — *see also* Sulf–						
Sulphadione	961.8	E857	E931.8	E950.4	E962.0	E980.4
Sulthiame, sultiame	966.3	E855.0	E936.3	E950.4	E962.0	E980.4
Superinone	975.5	E858.6	E945.5	E950.4	E962.0	E980.4
Suramin	961.5	E857	E931.5	E950.4	E962.0	E980.4
Surfacaine	968.5	E855.2	E938.5	E950.4	E962.0	E980.4
Surital	968.3	E855.1	E938.3	E950.4	E962.0	E980.4
Sutilains	976.8	E858.7	E946.8	E950.4	E962.0	E980.4
Suxamethonium (bromide) (chloride)						
(iodide)	975.2	E858.6	E945.2	E950.4	E962.0	E980.4
Suxethonium (bromide)	975.2	E858.6	E945.2	E950.4	E962.0	E980.4
Sweet oil (birch)	976.3	E858.7	E946.3	E950.4	E962.0	E980.4
Sym–dichloroethyl ether	982.3	E862.4	—	E950.9	E962.1	E980.9
Sympatholytics	971.3	E855.6	E941.3	E950.4	E962.0	E980.4
Sympathomimetics	971.2	E855.5	E941.2	E950.4	E962.0	E980.4
Synagis	979.6	E858.8	E949.6	E950.4	E962.0	E980.4
Synalar	976.0	E858.7	E946.0	E950.4	E962.0	E980.4
Synthroid	962.7	E858.0	E932.7	E950.4	E962.0	E980.4
Syntocinon	975.0	E858.6	E945.0	E950.4	E962.0	E950.4
Syrosingopine	972.6	E858.3	E942.6	E950.4	E962.0	E980.4
Systemic agents (primarily)	963.9	E858.1	E933.9	E950.4	E962.0	E980.4
specified NEC	963.8	E858.1	E933.8	E950.4	E962.0	E980.4
Tablets (*see also* specified substance)	977.9	E858.9	E947.9	E950.5	E962.0	E980.5
Tace	962.2	E858.0	E932.2	E950.4	E962.0	E980.4
Tacrine	971.0	E855.3	E941.0	E950.4	E962.0	E980.4
Talbutal	967.0	E851	E937.0	E950.1	E962.0	E980.1
Talc	976.3	E858.7	E946.3	E950.4	E962.0	E980.4
Talcum	976.3	E858.7	E946.3	E950.4	E962.0	E980.4
Tamsulosin	971.3	E855.6	E941.3	E950.4	E962.0	E980.4
Tandearil, tanderil	965.5	E850.5	E935.5	E950.0	E962.0	E980.0
Tannic acid	983.1	E864.1	—	E950.7	E962.1	E980.6
medicinal (astringent)	976.2	E858.7	E946.2	E950.4	E962.0	E980.4
Tannin — *see* Tannic acid						
Tansy	988.2	E865.4	—	E950.9	E962.1	E980.9
TAO	960.3	E856	E930.3	E950.4	E962.0	E980.4
Tapazole	962.8	E858.0	E932.8	E950.4	E962.0	E980.4
Tar NEC	983.0	E864.0	—	E950.7	E962.1	E980.6
camphor — *see* Naphthalene						
fumes	987.8	E869.8	—	E952.8	E962.2	E982.8
Taractan	969.3	E853.8	E939.3	E950.3	E962.0	E980.3
Tarantula (venomous)	989.5	E905.1	—	E950.9	E962.1	E980.9
Tartar emetic (anti–infective)	961.2	E857	E931.2	E950.4	E962.0	E980.4
Tartaric acid	983.1	E864.1	—	E950.7	E962.1	E980.6
Tartrated antimony (anti–infective)	961.2	E857	E931.2	E950.4	E962.0	E980.4
TCA — *see* Trichloroacetic acid						
TDI	983.0	E864.0	—	E950.7	E962.1	E980.6
vapor	987.8	E869.8	—	E952.8	E962.2	E982.8
Tear gas	987.5	E869.3	—	E952.8	E962.2	E982.8
Teclothiazide	974.3	E858.5	E944.3	E950.4	E962.0	E980.4
Tegretol	966.3	E855.0	E936.3	E950.4	E962.0	E980.4
Telepaque	977.8	E858.8	E947.8	E950.4	E962.0	E980.4
Tellurium	985.8	E866.4	—	E950.9	E962.1	E980.9
fumes	985.8	E866.4	—	E950.9	E962.1	E980.9
TEM	963.1	E858.1	E933.1	E950.4	E962.0	E980.4
Temazepan—*see* Benzodiazepines						

Substance	Poisoning	Accident	Therapeutic Use	Suicide Attempt	Assault	Undetermined
			External Cause (E-Code)			
TEPA	963.1	E858.1	E933.1	E950.4	E962.0	E980.4
TEPP	989.3	E863.1	—	E950.6	E962.1	E980.7
Terbutaline	971.2	E855.5	E941.2	E950.4	E962.0	E980.4
Teroxalene	961.6	E857	E931.6	E950.4	E962.0	E980.4
Terpin hydrate	975.5	E858.6	E945.5	E950.4	E962.0	E980.4
Terramycin	960.4	E856	E930.4	E950.4	E962.0	E980.4
Tessalon	975.4	E858.6	E945.4	E950.4	E962.0	E980.4
Testosterone	962.1	E858.0	E932.1	E950.4	E962.0	E980.4
Tetanus (vaccine)	978.4	E858.8	E948.4	E950.4	E962.0	E980.4
antitoxin	979.9	E858.8	E949.9	E950.4	E962.0	E980.4
immune globulin (human)	964.6	E858.2	E934.6	E950.4	E962.0	E980.4
toxoid	978.4	E858.8	E948.4	E950.4	E962.0	E980.4
with diphtheria toxoid	978.9	E858.8	E948.9	E950.4	E962.0	E980.4
with pertussis	978.6	E858.8	E948.6	E950.4	E962.0	E980.4
Tetrabenazine	969.5	E853.8	E939.5	E950.3	E962.0	E980.3
Tetracaine (infiltration) (topical)	968.5	E855.2	E938.5	E950.4	E962.0	E980.4
nerve block (peripheral) (plexus)	968.6	E855.2	E938.6	E950.4	E962.0	E980.4
spinal	968.7	E855.2	E938.7	E950.4	E962.0	E980.4
Tetrachlorethylene—*see* Tetrachloroethylene						
Tetrachlormethiazide	974.3	E858.5	E944.3	E950.4	E962.0	E980.4
Tetrachloroethane (liquid) (vapor)	982.3	E862.4	—	E950.9	E962.1	E980.9
paint or varnish	982.3	E861.6	—	E950.9	E962.1	E980.9
Tetrachloroethylene (liquid) (vapor)	982.3	E862.4	—	E950.9	E962.1	E980.9
medicinal	961.6	E857	E931.6	E950.4	E962.0	E980.4
Tetrachloromethane — *see* Carbon, tetrachloride						
Tetracycline	960.4	E856	E930.4	E950.4	E962.0	E980.4
ophthalmic preparation	976.5	E858.7	E946.5	E950.4	E962.0	E980.4
topical NEC	976.0	E858.7	E946.0	E950.4	E962.0	E980.4
Tetraethylammonium chloride	972.3	E858.3	E942.3	E950.4	E962.0	E980.4
Tetraethyl lead (antiknock compound)	984.1	E862.1	—	E950.9	E962.1	E980.9
Tetraethyl pyrophosphate	989.3	E863.1	—	E950.6	E962.1	E980.7
Tetraethylthiuram disulfide	977.3	E858.8	E947.3	E950.4	E962.0	E980.4
Tetrahydroaminoacridine	971.0	E855.3	E941.0	E950.4	E962.0	E980.4
Tetrahydrocannabinol	969.6	E854.1	E939.6	E950.3	E962.0	E980.3
Tetrahydronaphthalene	982.0	E862.4	—	E950.9	E962.1	E980.9
Tetrahydrozoline	971.2	E855.5	E941.2	E950.4	E962.0	E980.4
Tetralin	982.0	E862.4	—	E950.9	E962.1	E980.9
Tetramethylthiuram (disulfide) NEC	989.4	E863.6	—	E950.6	E962.1	E980.7
medicinal	976.2	E858.7	E946.2	E950.4	E962.0	E980.4
Tetronal	967.8	E852.8	E937.8	E950.2	E962.0	E980.2
Tetryl	983.0	E864.0	—	E950.7	E962.1	E980.6
Thalidomide	967.8	E852.8	E937.8	E950.2	E962.0	E980.2
Thallium (compounds) (dust) NEC	985.8	E866.4	—	E950.9	E962.1	E980.9
pesticide (rodenticide)	985.8	E863.7	—	E950.6	E962.1	E980.7
THC	969.6	E854.1	E939.6	E950.3	E962.0	E980.3
Thebacon	965.09	E850.2	E935.2	E950.0	E962.0	E980.0
Thebaine	965.09	E850.2	E935.2	E950.0	E962.0	E980.0
Theobromine (calcium salicylate)	974.1	E858.5	E944.1	E950.4	E962.0	E980.4
Theophylline (diuretic)	974.1	E858.5	E944.1	E950.4	E962.0	E980.4
ethylenediamine	975.7	E858.6	E945.7	E950.4	E962.0	E980.4
Thiabendazole	961.6	E857	E931.6	E950.4	E962.0	E980.4
Thialbarbital, thialbarbitone	968.3	E855.1	E938.3	E950.4	E962.0	E980.4
Thiamine	963.5	E858.1	E933.5	E950.4	E962.0	E980.4
Thiamylal (sodium)	968.3	E855.1	E938.3	E950.4	E962.0	E980.4
Thiazesim	969.09	E854.0	E939.0	E950.3	E962.0	E980.3
Thiazides (diuretics)	974.3	E858.5	E944.3	E950.4	E962.0	E980.4
Thiethylperazine	963.0	E858.1	E933.0	E950.4	E962.0	E980.4
Thimerosal (topical)	976.0	E858.7	E946.0	E950.4	E962.0	E980.4
ophthalmic preparation	976.5	E858.7	E946.5	E950.4	E962.0	E980.4

Substance	Poisoning	Accident	Therapeutic Use	Suicide Attempt	Assault	Undetermined
			External Cause (E-Code)			
Thioacetazone	961.8	E857	E931.8	E950.4	E962.0	E980.4
Thiobarbiturates	968.3	E855.1	E938.3	E950.4	E962.0	E980.4
Thiobismol	961.2	E857	E931.2	E950.4	E962.0	E980.4
Thiocarbamide	962.8	E858.0	E932.8	E950.4	E962.0	E980.4
Thiocarbarsone	961.1	E857	E931.1	E950.4	E962.0	E980.4
Thiocarlide	961.8	E857	E931.8	E950.4	E962.0	E980.4
Thioguanine	963.1	E858.1	E933.1	E950.4	E962.0	E980.4
Thiomercaptomerin	974.0	E858.5	E944.0	E950.4	E962.0	E980.4
Thiomerin	974.0	E858.5	E944.0	E950.4	E962.0	E980.4
Thiopental, thiopentone (sodium)	968.3	E855.1	E938.3	E950.4	E962.0	E980.4
Thiopropazate	969.1	E853.0	E939.1	E950.3	E962.0	E980.3
Thioproperazine	969.1	E853.0	E939.1	E950.3	E962.0	E980.3
Thioridazine	969.1	E853.0	E939.1	E950.3	E962.0	E980.3
Thio–TEPA, thiotepa	963.1	E858.1	E933.1	E950.4	E962.0	E980.4
Thiothixene	969.3	E853.8	E939.3	E950.3	E962.0	E980.3
Thiouracil	962.8	E858.0	E932.8	E950.4	E962.0	E980.4
Thiourea	962.8	E858.0	E932.8	E950.4	E962.0	E980.4
Thiphenamil	971.1	E855.4	E941.1	E950.4	E962.0	E980.4
Thiram NEC	989.4	E863.6	—	E950.6	E962.1	E980.7
medicinal	976.2	E858.7	E946.2	E950.4	E962.0	E980.4
Thonzylamine	963.0	E858.1	E933.0	E950.4	E962.0	E980.4
Thorazine	969.1	E853.0	E939.1	E950.3	E962.0	E980.3
Thornapple	988.2	E865.4	—	E950.9	E962.1	E980.9
Throat preparation (lozenges) NEC	976.6	E858.7	E946.6	E950.4	E962.0	E980.4
Thrombin	964.5	E858.2	E934.5	E950.4	E962.0	E980.4
Thrombolysin	964.4	E858.2	E934.4	E950.4	E962.0	E980.4
Thymol	983.0	E864.0	—	E950.7	E962.1	E980.6
Thymus extract	962.9	E858.0	E932.9	E950.4	E962.0	E980.4
Thyroglobulin	962.7	E858.0	E932.7	E950.4	E962.0	E980.4
Thyroid (derivatives) (extract)	962.7	E858.0	E932.7	E950.4	E962.0	E980.4
Thyrolar	962.7	E858.0	E932.7	E950.4	E962.0	E980.4
Thyrothrophin, thyrotropin	977.8	E858.8	E947.8	E950.4	E962.0	E980.4
Thyroxin(e)	962.7	E858.0	E932.7	E950.4	E962.0	E980.4
Tigan	963.0	E858.1	E933.0	E950.4	E962.0	E980.4
Tigloidine	968.0	E855.1	E938.0	E950.4	E962.0	E980.4
Tin (chloride) (dust) (oxide) NEC	985.8	E866.4	—	E950.9	E962.1	E980.9
anti–infectives	961.2	E857	E931.2	E950.4	E962.0	E980.4
Tinactin	976.0	E858.7	E946.0	E950.4	E962.0	E980.4
Tincture, iodine — see Iodine						
Tindal	969.1	E853.0	E939.1	E950.3	E962.0	E980.3
Titanium (compounds) (vapor)	985.8	E866.4	—	E950.9	E962.1	E980.9
ointment	976.3	E858.7	E946.3	E950.4	E962.0	E980.4
Titroid	962.7	E858.0	E932.7	E950.4	E962.0	E980.4
TMTD — see Tetramethylthiuram disulfide						
TNT	989.89	E866.8	—	E950.9	E962.1	E980.9
fumes	987.8	E869.8	—	E952.8	E962.2	E982.8
Toadstool	988.1	E865.5	—	E950.9	E962.1	E980.9
Tobacco NEC	989.84	E866.8	—	E950.9	E962.1	E980.9
Indian	988.2	E865.4	—	E950.9	E962.1	E980.9
smoke, second-hand	987.8	E869.4	—	—	—	—
Tocopherol	963.5	E858.1	E933.5	E950.4	E962.0	E980.4
Tocosamine	975.0	E858.6	E945.0	E950.4	E962.0	E980.4
Tofranil	969.05	E854.0	E939.0	E950.3	E962.0	E980.3
Toilet deodorizer	989.8	E866.8	—	E950.9	E962.1	E980.9
Tolazamide	962.3	E858.0	E932.3	E950.4	E962.0	E980.4
Tolazoline	971.3	E855.6	E941.3	E950.4	E962.0	E980.4
Tolbutamide	962.3	E858.0	E932.3	E950.4	E962.0	E980.4
sodium	977.8	E858.8	E947.8	E950.4	E962.0	E980.4
Tolmetin	965.69	E850.6	E935.6	E950.0	E962.0	E980.0
Tolnaftate	976.0	E858.7	E946.0	E950.4	E962.0	E980.4
Tolpropamine	976.1	E858.7	E946.1	E950.4	E962.0	E980.4

Substance	Poisoning	Accident	Therapeutic Use	Suicide Attempt	Assault	Undetermined
			External Cause (E-Code)			
Tolserol	968.0	E855.1	E938.0	E950.4	E962.0	E980.4
Toluene (liquid) (vapor)	982.0	E862.4	—	E950.9	E962.1	E980.9
diisocyanate	983.0	E864.0	—	E950.7	E962.1	E980.6
Toluidine	983.0	E864.0	—	E950.7	E962.1	E980.6
vapor	987.8	E869.8	—	E952.8	E962.2	E982.8
Toluol (liquid) (vapor)	982.0	E862.4	—	E950.9	E962.1	E980.9
Tolylene–2,4–diisocyanate	983.0	E864.0	—	E950.7	E962.1	E980.6
Tonics, cardiac	972.1	E858.3	E942.1	E950.4	E962.0	E980.4
Toxaphene (dust) (spray)	989.2	E863.0	—	E950.6	E962.1	E980.7
Toxoids NEC	978.8	E858.8	E948.8	E950.4	E962.0	E980.4
Tractor fuel NEC	981	E862.1	—	E950.9	E962.1	E980.9
Tragacanth	973.3	E858.4	E943.3	E950.4	E962.0	E980.4
Tramazoline	971.2	E855.5	E941.2	E950.4	E962.0	E980.4
Tranquilizers	969.5	E853.9	E939.5	E950.3	E962.0	E980.3
benzodiazepine–based	969.4	E853.2	E939.4	E950.3	E962.0	E980.3
butyrophenone–based	969.2	E853.1	E939.2	E950.3	E962.0	E980.3
major NEC	969.3	E853.8	E939.3	E950.3	E962.0	E980.3
phenothiazine–based	969.1	E853.0	E939.1	E950.3	E962.0	E980.3
specified NEC	969.5	E853.8	E939.5	E950.3	E962.0	E980.3
Trantoin	961.9	E857	E931.9	E950.4	E962.0	E980.4
Tranxene	969.4	E853.2	E939.4	E950.3	E962.0	E980.3
Tranylcypromine (sulfate)	969.01	E854.0	E939.0	E950.3	E962.0	E980.3
Trasentine	975.1	E858.6	E945.1	E950.4	E962.0	E980.4
Travert	974.5	E858.5	E944.5	E950.4	E962.0	E980.4
Trecator	961.8	E857	E931.8	E950.4	E962.0	E980.4
Tretinoin	976.8	E858.7	E946.8	E950.4	E962.0	E980.4
Triacetin	976.0	E858.7	E946.0	E950.4	E962.0	E980.4
Triacetyloleandomycin	960.3	E856	E930.3	E950.4	E962.0	E980.4
Triamcinolone	962.0	E858.0	E932.0	E950.4	E962.0	E980.4
ENT agent	976.6	E858.7	E946.6	E950.4	E962.0	E980.4
ophthalmic preparation	976.5	E858.7	E946.5	E950.4	E962.0	E980.4
topical NEC	976.0	E858.7	E946.0	E950.4	E962.0	E980.4
Triamterene	974.4	E858.5	E944.4	E950.4	E962.0	E980.4
Triaziquone	963.1	E858.1	E933.1	E950.4	E962.0	E980.4
Tribromacetaldehyde	967.3	E852.2	E937.3	E950.2	E962.0	E980.2
Tribromoethanol	968.2	E855.1	E938.2	E950.4	E962.0	E980.4
Tribromomethane	967.3	E852.2	E937.3	E950.2	E962.0	E980.2
Trichlorethane	982.3	E862.4	—	E950.9	E962.1	E980.9
Trichlormethiazide	974.3	E858.5	E944.3	E950.4	E962.0	E980.4
Trichloroacetic acid	983.1	E864.1	—	E950.7	E962.1	E980.6
medicinal (keratolytic)	976.4	E858.7	E946.4	E950.4	E962.0	E980.4
Trichloroethanol	967.1	E852.0	E937.1	E950.2	E962.0	E980.2
Trichloroethylene (liquid) (vapor)	982.3	E862.4	—	E950.9	E962.1	E980.9
anesthetic (gas)	968.2	E855.1	E938.2	E950.4	E962.0	E980.4
Trichloroethyl phosphate	967.1	E852.0	E937.1	E950.2	E962.0	E980.2
Trichlorofluoromethane NEC	987.4	E869.2	—	E952.8	E962.2	E982.8
Trichlorotriethylamine	963.1	E858.1	E933.1	E950.4	E962.0	E980.4
Trichomonacides NEC	961.5	E857	E931.5	E950.4	E962.0	E980.4
Trichomycin	960.1	E856	E930.1	E950.4	E962.0	E980.4
Triclofos	967.1	E852.0	E937.1	E950.2	E962.0	E980.2
Tricresyl phosphate	989.89	E866.8	—	E950.9	E962.1	E980.9
solvent	982.8	E862.4	—	E950.9	E962.1	E980.9
Tricyclamol	966.4	E855.0	E936.4	E950.4	E962.0	E980.4
Tridesilon	976.0	E858.7	E946.0	E950.4	E962.0	E980.4
Tridihexethyl	971.1	E855.4	E941.1	E950.4	E962.0	E980.4
Tridione	966.0	E855.0	E936.0	E950.4	E962.0	E980.4
Triethanolamine NEC	983.2	E864.2	—	E950.7	E962.1	E980.6
detergent	983.2	E861.0	—	E950.7	E962.1	E980.6
trinitrate	972.4	E858.3	E942.4	E950.4	E962.0	E980.4
Triethanomelamine	963.1	E858.1	E933.1	E950.4	E962.0	E980.4

Substance	Poisoning	Accident	Therapeutic Use	Suicide Attempt	Assault	Undetermined
			External Cause (E-Code)			
Triethylene melamine	963.1	E858.1	E933.1	E950.4	E962.0	E980.4
Triethylenephosphoramide	963.1	E858.1	E933.1	E950.4	E962.0	E980.4
Triethylenethiophosphoramide	963.1	E858.1	E933.1	E950.4	E962.0	E980.4
Trifluoperazine	969.1	E853.0	E939.1	E950.3	E962.0	E980.3
Trifluperidol	969.2	E853.1	E939.2	E950.3	E962.0	E980.3
Triflupromazine	969.1	E853.0	E939.1	E950.3	E962.0	E980.3
Trihexyphenidyl	971.1	E855.4	E941.1	E950.4	E962.0	E980.4
Triiodothyronine	962.7	E858.0	E932.7	E950.4	E962.0	E980.4
Trilene	968.2	E855.1	E938.2	E950.4	E962.0	E980.4
Trimeprazine	963.0	E858.1	E933.0	E950.4	E962.0	E980.4
Trimetazidine	972.4	E858.3	E942.4	E950.4	E962.0	E980.4
Trimethadione	966.0	E855.0	E936.0	E950.4	E962.0	E980.4
Trimethaphan	972.3	E858.3	E942.3	E950.4	E962.0	E980.4
Trimethidinium	972.3	E858.3	E942.3	E950.4	E962.0	E980.4
Trimethobenzamide	963.0	E858.1	E933.0	E950.4	E962.0	E980.4
Trimethylcarbinol	980.8	E860.8	—	E950.9	E962.1	E980.9
Trimethylpsoralen	976.3	E858.7	E946.3	E950.4	E962.0	E980.4
Trimeton	963.0	E858.1	E933.0	E950.4	E962.0	E980.4
Trimipramine	969.05	E854.0	E939.0	E950.3	E962.0	E980.3
Trimustine	963.1	E858.1	E933.1	E950.4	E962.0	E980.4
Trinitrin	972.4	E858.3	E942.4	E950.4	E962.0	E980.4
Trinitrophenol	983.0	E864.0	—	E950.7	E962.1	E980.6
Trinitrotoluene	989.89	E866.8	—	E950.9	E962.1	E980.9
fumes	987.8	E869.8	—	E952.8	E962.2	E982.8
Trional	967.8	E852.8	E937.8	E950.2	E962.0	E980.2
Trioxide of arsenic — see Arsenic						
Trioxsalen	976.3	E858.7	E946.3	E950.4	E962.0	E980.4
Tripelennamine	963.0	E858.1	E933.0	E950.4	E962.0	E980.4
Triperidol	969.2	E853.1	E939.2	E950.3	E962.0	E980.3
Triprolidine	963.0	E858.1	E933.0	E950.4	E962.0	E980.4
Trisoralen	976.3	E858.7	E946.3	E950.4	E962.0	E980.4
Troleandomycin	960.3	E856	E930.3	E950.4	E962.0	E980.4
Trolnitrate (phosphate)	972.4	E858.3	E942.4	E950.4	E962.0	E980.4
Trometamol	963.3	E858.1	E933.3	E950.4	E962.0	E980.4
Tromethamine	963.3	E858.1	E933.3	E950.4	E962.0	E980.4
Tronothane	968.5	E855.2	E938.5	E950.4	E962.0	E980.4
Tropicamide	971.1	E855.4	E941.1	E950.4	E962.0	E980.4
Troxidone	966.0	E855.0	E936.0	E950.4	E962.0	E980.4
Tryparsamide	961.1	E857	E931.1	E950.4	E962.0	E980.4
Trypsin	963.4	E858.1	E933.4	E950.4	E962.0	E980.4
Tryptizol	969.05	E854.0	E939.0	E950.3	E962.0	E980.3
Tuaminoheptane	971.2	E855.5	E941.2	E950.4	E962.0	E980.4
Tuberculin (old)	977.8	E858.8	E947.8	E950.4	E962.0	E980.4
Tubocurare	975.2	E858.6	E945.2	E950.4	E962.0	E980.4
Tubocurarine	975.2	E858.6	E945.2	E950.4	E962.0	E980.4
Turkish green	969.6	E854.1	E939.6	E950.3	E962.0	E980.3
Turpentine (spirits of) (liquid) (vapor)	982.8	E862.4	—	E950.9	E962.1	E980.9
Tybamate	969.5	E853.8	E939.5	E950.3	E962.0	E980.3
Tyloxapol	975.5	E858.6	E945.5	E950.4	E962.0	E980.4
Tymazoline	971.2	E855.5	E941.2	E950.4	E962.0	E980.4
Typhoid vaccine	978.1	E858.8	E948.1	E950.4	E962.0	E980.4
Typhus vaccine	979.2	E858.8	E949.2	E950.4	E962.0	E980.4
Tyrothricin	976.0	E858.7	E946.0	E950.4	E962.0	E980.4
ENT agent	976.6	E858.7	E946.6	E950.4	E962.0	E980.4
ophthalmic preparation	976.5	E858.7	E946.5	E950.4	E962.0	E980.4
Undecenoic acid	976.0	E858.7	E946.0	E950.4	E962.0	E980.4
Undecylenic acid	976.0	E858.7	E946.0	E950.4	E962.0	E980.4
Unna's boot	976.3	E858.7	E946.3	E950.4	E962.0	E980.4
Uracil mustard	963.1	E858.1	E933.1	E950.4	E962.0	E980.4
Uramustine	963.1	E858.1	E933.1	E950.4	E962.0	E980.4
Urari	975.2	E858.6	E945.2	E950.4	E962.0	E980.4

Substance	Poisoning	Accident	Therapeutic Use	Suicide Attempt	Assault	Undetermined
			External Cause (E-Code)			
Urea 974.4	E858.5	E944.4	E950.4	E962.0	E980.4
topical 976.8	E858.7	E946.8	E950.4	E962.0	E980.4
Urethan(e) (antineoplastic) 963.1	E858.1	E933.1	E950.4	E962.0	E980.4
Urginea (maritima) (scilla) — see Squill					
Uric acid metabolism agents NEC. 974.7	E858.5	E944.7	E950.4	E962.0	E980.4
Urokinase. 964.4	E858.2	E934.4	E950.4	E962.0	E980.4
Urokon 977.8	E858.8	E947.8	E950.4	E962.0	E980.4
Urotropin 961.9	E857	E931.9	E950.4	E962.0	E980.4
Urtica 988.2	E865.4	—	E950.9	E962.1	E980.9
Utility gas — see Gas, utility					
Vaccine NEC 979.9	E858.8	E949.9	E950.4	E962.0	E980.4
bacterial NEC 978.8	E858.8	E948.8	E950.4	E962.0	E980.4
with					
other bacterial component 978.9	E858.8	E948.9	E950.4	E962.0	E980.4
pertussis component 978.6	E858.8	E948.6	E950.4	E962.0	E980.4
viral–rickettsial component. 979.7	E858.8	E949.7	E950.4	E962.0	E980.4
mixed NEC. 978.9	E858.8	E948.9	E950.4	E962.0	E980.4
BCG 978.0	E858.8	E948.0	E950.4	E962.0	E980.4
cholera 978.2	E858.8	E948.2	E950.4	E962.0	E980.4
diphtheria 978.5	E858.8	E948.5	E950.4	E962.0	E980.4
influenza 979.6	E858.8	E949.6	E950.4	E962.0	E980.4
measles 979.4	E858.8	E949.4	E950.4	E962.0	E980.4
meningococcal 978.8	E858.8	E948.8	E950.4	E962.0	E980.4
mumps 979.6	E858.8	E949.6	E950.4	E962.0	E980.4
paratyphoid 978.1	E858.8	E948.1	E950.4	E962.0	E980.4
pertussis (with diphtheria toxoid) (with tetanus toxoid). 978.6	E858.8	E948.6	E950.4	E962.0	E980.4
plague 978.3	E858.8	E948.3	E950.4	E962.0	E980.4
poliomyelitis 979.5	E858.8	E949.5	E950.4	E962.0	E980.4
poliovirus 979.5	E858.8	E949.5	E950.4	E962.0	E980.4
rabies 979.1	E858.8	E949.1	E950.4	E962.0	E980.4
respiratory syncytial virus 979.6	E858.8	E949.6	E950.4	E962.0	E980.4
rickettsial NEC 979.6	E858.8	E949.6	E950.4	E962.0	E980.4
with					
bacterial component 979.7	E858.8	E949.7	E950.4	E962.0	E980.4
pertussis component 978.6	E858.8	E948.6	E950.4	E962.0	E980.4
viral component 979.7	E858.8	E949.7	E950.4	E962.0	E980.4
Rocky Mountain spotted fever. 979.6	E858.8	E949.6	E950.4	E962.0	E980.4
rotavirus. 979.6	E858.8	E949.6	E950.4	E962.0	E980.4
rubella virus 979.4	E858.8	E949.4	E950.4	E962.0	E980.4
sabin oral 979.5	E858.8	E949.5	E950.4	E962.0	E980.4
smallpox 979.0	E858.8	E949.0	E950.4	E962.0	E980.4
tetanus 978.4	E858.8	E948.4	E950.4	E962.0	E980.4
typhoid 978.1	E858.8	E948.1	E950.4	E962.0	E980.4
typhus 979.2	E858.8	E949.2	E950.4	E962.0	E980.4
viral NEC 979.6	E858.8	E949.6	E950.4	E962.0	E980.4
with					
bacterial component 979.7	E858.8	E949.7	E950.4	E962.0	E980.4
pertussis component 978.6	E858.8	E948.6	E950.4	E962.0	E980.4
rickettsial component 979.7	E858.8	E949.7	E950.4	E962.0	E980.4
yellow fever 979.3	E858.8	E949.3	E950.4	E962.0	E980.4
Vaccinia immune globulin (human) 964.6	E858.2	E934.6	E950.4	E962.0	E980.4
Vaginal contraceptives 976.8	E858.7	E946.8	E950.4	E962.0	E980.4
Valethamate 971.1	E855.4	E941.1	E950.4	E962.0	E980.4
Valisone 976.0	E858.7	E946.0	E950.4	E962.0	E980.4
Valium 969.4	E853.2	E939.4	E950.3	E962.0	E980.3
Valmid 967.8	E852.8	E937.8	E950.2	E962.0	E980.2
Vanadium 985.8	E866.4	—	E950.9	E962.1	E980.9
Vancomycin 960.8	E856	E930.8	E950.4	E962.0	E980.4
Vapor (see also Gas) 987.9	E869.9	—	E952.9	E962.2	E982.9

Substance	Poisoning	Accident	Therapeutic Use	Suicide Attempt	Assault	Undetermined
			External Cause (E-Code)			
kiln (carbon monoxide)	986	E868.8	—	E952.1	E962.2	E982.1
lead — *see* Lead						
specified source NEC (*see also*						
specific substance)	987.8	E869.8	—	E952.8	E962.2	E982.8
Varidase	964.4	E858.2	E934.4	E950.4	E962.0	E980.4
Varnish	989.89	E861.6	—	E950.9	E962.1	E980.9
cleaner	982.8	E862.9	—	E950.9	E962.1	E980.9
Vaseline	976.3	E858.7	E946.3	E950.4	E962.0	E980.4
Vasodilan	972.5	E858.3	E942.5	E950.4	E962.0	E980.4
Vasodilators NEC.	972.5	E858.3	E942.5	E950.4	E962.0	E980.0
coronary.	972.4	E858.3	E942.4	E950.4	E962.0	E980.4
Vasopressin	962.5	E858.0	E932.5	E950.4	E962.0	E980.4
Vasopressor drugs	962.5	E858.0	E932.5	E950.4	E962.0	E980.4
Venom, venomous (bite) (sting)	989.5	E905.9	—	E950.9	E962.1	E980.9
arthropod NEC	989.5	E905.5	—	E950.9	E962.1	E980.9
bee	989.5	E905.3	—	E950.9	E962.1	E980.9
centipede	989.5	E905.4	—	E950.9	E962.1	E980.9
hornet.	989.5	E905.3	—	E950.9	E962.1	E980.9
lizard	989.5	E905.0	—	E950.9	E962.1	E980.9
marine animals or plants	989.5	E905.6	—	E950.9	E962.1	E980.9
millipede (topical).	989.5	E905.4	—	E950.9	E962.1	E980.9
plant NEC.	989.5	E905.7	—	E950.9	E962.1	E980.9
marine.	989.5	E905.6	—	E950.9	E962.1	E980.9
scorpion	989.5	E905.2	—	E950.9	E962.1	E980.9
snake	989.5	E905.0	—	E950.9	E962.1	E980.9
specified NEC	989.5	E905.8	—	E950.9	E962.1	E980.9
spider	989.5	E905.1	—	E950.9	E962.1	E980.9
wasp	989.5	E905.3	—	E950.9	E962.1	E980.9
Ventolin—*see* Salbutamol sulfate						
Veramon	967.0	E851	E937.0	E950.1	E962.0	E980.1
Veratrum						
album.	988.2	E865.4	—	E950.9	E962.1	E980.9
alkaloids.	972.6	E858.3	E942.6	E950.4	E962.0	E980.4
viride	988.2	E865.4	—	E950.9	E962.1	E980.9
Verdigris (*see also* Copper).	985.8	E866.4	—	E950.9	E962.1	E980.9
Veronal	967.0	E851	E937.0	E950.1	E962.0	E980.1
Veroxil	961.6	E857	E931.6	E950.4	E962.0	E980.4
Versidyne	965.7	E850.7	E935.7	E950.0	E962.0	E980.0
Viagra	972.5	E858.3	E942.5	E950.4	E962.0	E980.4
Vienna						
green	985.1	E866.3	—	E950.8	E962.1	E980.8
insecticide	985.1	E863.4	—	E950.6	E962.1	E980.7
red	989.89	E866.8	—	E950.9	E962.1	E980.9
pharmaceutical dye	977.4	E858.8	E947.4	E950.4	E962.0	E980.4
Vinbarbital, vinbarbitone.	967.0	E851	E937.0	E950.1	E962.0	E980.1
Vinblastine	963.1	E858.1	E933.1	E950.4	E962.0	E980.4
Vincristine	963.1	E858.1	E933.1	E950.4	E962.0	E980.4
Vinesthene, vinethene	968.2	E855.1	E938.2	E950.4	E962.0	E980.4
Vinyl						
bital	967.0	E851	E937.0	E950.1	E962.0	E980.1
ether	968.2	E855.1	E938.2	E950.4	E962.0	E980.4
Vioform.	961.3	E857	E931.3	E950.4	E962.0	E980.4
topical	976.0	E858.7	E946.0	E950.4	E962.0	E980.4
Viomycin	960.6	E856	E930.6	E950.4	E962.0	E980.4
Viosterol	963.5	E858.1	E933.5	E950.4	E962.0	E980.4
Viper (venom)	989.5	E905.0	—	E950.9	E962.1	E980.9
Viprynium (embonate).	961.6	E857	E931.6	E950.4	E962.0	E980.4
Virugon.	961.7	E857	E931.7	E950.4	E962.0	E980.4
Visine	976.5	E858.7	E946.5	E950.4	E962.0	E980.4
Vitamins NEC	963.5	E858.1	E933.5	E950.4	E962.0	E980.4
B_{12}.	964.1	E858.2	E934.1	E950.4	E962.0	E980.4

Substance	Poisoning	Accident	Therapeutic Use	Suicide Attempt	Assault	Undetermined
			External Cause (E-Code)			
hematopoietic	964.1	E858.2	E934.1	E950.4	E962.0	E980.4
K	964.3	E858.2	E934.3	E950.4	E962.0	E980.4
Vleminckx's solution	976.4	E858.7	E946.4	E950.4	E962.0	E980.4
Voltaren—*see* Diclofenac sodium						
Warfarin (potassium) (sodium)	964.2	E858.2	E934.2	E950.4	E962.0	E980.4
rodenticide	989.4	E863.7	—	E950.6	E962.1	E980.7
Wasp (sting)	989.5	E905.3	—	E950.9	E962.1	E980.9
Water						
balance agents NEC	974.5	E858.5	E944.5	E950.4	E962.0	E980.4
gas	987.1	E868.1	—	E951.8	E962.2	E981.8
incomplete combustion of — *see* Carbon, monoxide, fuel, utility						
hemlock	988.2	E865.4	—	E950.9	E962.1	E980.9
moccasin (venom)	989.5	E905.0	—	E950.9	E962.1	E980.9
Wax (paraffin) (petroleum)	981	E862.3	—	E950.9	E962.1	E980.9
automobile	989.89	E861.2	—	E950.9	E962.1	E980.9
floor	981	E862.0	—	E950.9	E962.1	E980.9
Weed killers NEC	989.4	E863.5	—	E950.6	E962.1	E980.7
Welldorm	967.1	E852.0	E937.1	E950.2	E962.0	E980.2
White						
arsenic — *see* Arsenic						
hellebore	988.2	E865.4	—	E950.9	E962.1	E980.9
lotion (keratolytic)	976.4	E858.7	E946.4	E950.4	E962.0	E980.4
spirit	981	E862.0	—	E950.9	E962.1	E980.9
Whitewashes	989.89	E861.6	—	E950.9	E962.1	E980.9
Whole blood	964.7	E858.2	E934.7	E950.4	E962.0	E980.4
Wild						
black cherry	988.2	E865.4	—	E950.9	E962.1	E980.9
poisonous plants NEC	988.2	E865.4	—	E950.9	E962.1	E980.9
Window cleaning fluid	989.89	E861.3	—	E950.9	E962.1	E980.9
Wintergreen (oil)	976.3	E858.7	E946.3	E950.4	E962.0	E980.4
Witch hazel	976.2	E858.7	E946.2	E950.4	E962.0	E980.4
Wood						
alcohol	980.1	E860.2	—	E950.9	E962.1	E980.9
spirit	980.1	E860.2	—	E950.9	E962.1	E980.9
Woorali	975.2	E858.6	E945.2	E950.4	E962.0	E980.4
Wormseed, American	961.6	E857	E931.6	E950.4	E962.0	E980.4
Xanthine diuretics	974.1	E858.5	E944.1	E950.4	E962.0	E980.4
Xanthocillin	960.0	E856	E930.0	E950.4	E962.0	E980.4
Xanthotoxin	976.3	E858.7	E946.3	E950.4	E962.0	E980.4
Xigris	964.2	E858.2	E934.2	E950.4	E962.0	E980.4
Xylene (liquid) (vapor)	982.0	E862.4	—	E950.9	E962.1	E980.9
Xylocaine (infiltration) (topical)	968.5	E855.2	E938.5	E950.4	E962.0	E980.4
nerve block (peripheral) (plexus)	968.6	E855.2	E938.6	E950.4	E962.0	E980.4
spinal	968.7	E855.2	E938.7	E950.4	E962.0	E980.4
Xylol (liquid) (vapor)	982.0	E862.4	—	E950.9	E962.1	E980.9
Xylometazoline	971.2	E855.5	E941.2	E950.4	E962.0	E980.4
Yellow						
fever vaccine	979.3	E858.8	E949.3	E950.4	E962.0	E980.4
jasmine	988.2	E865.4	—	E950.9	E962.1	E980.9
Yew	988.2	E865.4	—	E950.9	E962.1	E980.9
Zactane	965.7	E850.7	E935.7	E950.0	E962.0	E980.0
Zaroxolyn	974.3	E858.5	E944.3	E950.4	E962.0	E980.4
Zephiran (topical)	976.0	E858.7	E946.0	E950.4	E962.0	E980.4
ophthalmic preparation	976.5	E858.7	E946.5	E950.4	E962.0	E980.4
Zerone	980.1	E860.2	—	E950.9	E962.1	E980.9
Zinc (compounds) (fumes) (salts)						
(vapor) NEC	985.8	E866.4	—	E950.9	E962.1	E980.9
anti–infectives	976.0	E858.7	E946.0	E950.4	E962.0	E980.4
antivaricose	972.7	E858.3	E942.7	E950.4	E962.0	E980.4

Substance	Poisoning	Accident	Therapeutic Use	Suicide Attempt	Assault	Undetermined
		External Cause (E-Code)				
bacitracin 976.0		E858.7	E946.0	E950.4	E962.0	E980.4
chloride 976.2		E858.7	E946.2	E950.4	E962.0	E980.4
gelatin 976.3		E858.7	E946.3	E950.4	E962.0	E980.4
oxide 976.3		E858.7	E946.3	E950.4	E962.0	E980.4
peroxide 976.0		E858.7	E946.0	E950.4	E962.0	E980.4
pesticides 985.8		E863.4	—	E950.6	E962.1	E980.7
phosphide (rodenticide) 985.8		E863.7	—	E950.6	E962.1	E980.7
stearate 976.3		E858.7	E946.3	E950.4	E962.0	E980.4
sulfate (antivaricose) 972.7		E858.3	E942.7	E950.4	E962.0	E980.4
ENT agent 976.6		E858.7	E946.6	E950.4	E962.0	E980.4
ophthalmic solution 976.5		E858.7	E946.5	E950.4	E962.0	E980.4
topical NEC 976.0		E858.7	E946.0	E950.4	E962.0	E980.4
undecylenate 976.0		E858.7	E946.0	E950.4	E962.0	E980.4
Zovant 964.2		E858.2	E934.2	E950.4	E962.0	E980.4
Zoxazolamine 968.0		E855.1	E938.0	E950.4	E962.0	E980.4
Zygadenus (venenosus) 988.2		E865.4	—	E950.9	E962.1	E980.9

TABLE OF DRUGS AND CHEMICALS

Substance	Poisoning	Accident	Therapeutic Use	Suicide Attempt	Assault	Undetermined
		External Cause (E-Code)				

SECTION 3

ALPHABETIC INDEX TO EXTERNAL CAUSES OF INJURY AND POISONING (E CODE)

This section contains the index to the codes which classify environmental events, circumstances, and other conditions as the cause of injury and other adverse effects. Where a code from the section Supplementary Classification of External Causes of Injury and Poisoning (E800-E998) is applicable, it is intended that the E code shall be used in addition to a code from the main body of the classification, Chapters 1-17.

The alphabetic index to the E codes is organized by main terms which describe the *accident, circumstance, event,* or specific *agent* which caused the injury or other adverse effect.

> *Note—Transport accidents (E800-E848) include accidents involving:*
> *aircraft and space craft (E840-E845)*
> *watercraft (E830-E838)*
> *motor vehicle (E810-E825)*
> *railway (E800-E807)*
> *other road vehicles (E826-E829)*
>
> *For definitions and examples related to transport accidents—see Volume 1, pages 571-585.*
>
> *The fourth-digit subdivisions for use with categories E800-E848 to identify the injured person are found on pages 1447-1451.*
>
> *For identifying the place in which an accident or poisoning occurred (circumstances classifiable to categories E850-E869 and E880-E928)— see the listing in this section under "Accident, occurring."*

See the Table of Drugs and Chemicals (Section 2 of this volume) for identifying the specific agent involved in drug overdose or a wrong substance given or taken in error, and for intoxication or poisoning by a drug or other chemical substance.

The specific adverse effect, reaction, or localized toxic effect to a correct drug or substance properly administered in therapeutic or prophylactic dosage should be classified according to the nature of the adverse effect (e.g.: allergy, dermatitis, tachycardia) listed in Section 1 of this volume.

A

Abandonment
causing exposure to weather conditions—*see*
Exposure
child, with intent to injure or kill E968.4
helpless person, infant, newborn E904.0
with intent to injure or kill E968.4
Abortion, criminal, injury to child E968.8
Abuse, (alleged) (suspected)
adult
by
child E967.4
ex-partner E967.3
ex-spouse E967.3
father E967.0
grandchild E967.7
grandparent E967.6
mother E967.2
non-related caregiver E967.8
other relative E967.7
other specified person(s) E967.1
partner E967.3
sibling E967.5
spouse E967.3
stepfather E967.0
stepmother E967.2
unspecified person E967.9
child
by
boyfriend of parent or guardian E967.0
child E967.4
father E967.0
female partner of parent or guardian
E967.2
girlfriend of parent or guardian E967.2
grandchild E967.7
grandparent E967.6
male partner of parent or guardian E967.0
mother E967.2
non-related caregiver E967.8
other relative E967.7
other specified person(s) E967.1
sibling E967.5
stepfather E967.0
stepmother E967.2
unspecified person E967.9
Accident (to) E928.9
aircraft (in transit) (powered) E841
at landing, take-off E840
due to, caused by cataclysm—*see* categories
E908, E909
late effect of E929.1
unpowered (*see also* Collision, aircraft,
unpowered) E842
while alighting, boarding E843
amphibious vehicle
on
land—*see* Accident, motor vehicle
water—*see* Accident, watercraft
animal, ridden NEC E828
animal-drawn vehicle NEC E827
balloon (*see also* Collision, aircraft,
unpowered) E842
caused by, due to
abrasive wheel (metalworking) E919.3
animal NEC E906.9
being ridden (in sport or transport) E828
avalanche NEC E909.2
band saw E919.4
bench saw E919.4

Accident—*continued*
bore, earth-drilling or mining (land) (seabed)
E919.1
bulldozer E919.7
cataclysmic
earth surface movement or eruption E909.9
storm E908.9
chain
hoist E919.2
agricultural operations E919.0
mining operations E919.1
saw E920.1
circular saw E919.4
cold (excessive) (*see also* Cold, exposure to)
E901.9
combine E919.0
conflagration—*see* Conflagration
corrosive liquid, substance NEC E924.1
cotton gin E919.8
crane E919.2
agricultural operations E919.0
mining operations E919.1
cutting or piercing instrument (*see also* Cut)
E920.9
dairy equipment E919.8
derrick E919.2
agricultural operations E919.0
mining operations E919.1
drill E920.1
earth (land) (seabed) E919.1
hand (powered) E920.1
not powered E920.4
metalworking E919.3
woodworking E919.4
earth(-)
drilling machine E919.1
moving machine E919.7
scraping machine E919.7
electric
current (*see also* Electric shock) E925.9
motor—*see also* Accident, machine, by
type of machine
current (of)—*see* Electric shock
elevator (building) (grain) E919.2
agricultural operations E919.0
mining operations E919.1
environmental factors NEC E928.9
excavating machine E919.7
explosive material (*see also* Explosion)
E923.9
farm machine E919.0
fire, flames—*see also* Fire
conflagration—*see* Conflagration
firearm missile—*see* Shooting
forging (metalworking) machine E919.3
forklift (truck) E919.2
agricultural operations E919.0
mining operations E919.1
gas turbine E919.5
harvester E919.0
hay derrick, mower, or rake E919.0
heat (excessive) (*see also* Heat) E900.9
hoist (*see also* Accident, caused by, due to,
lift) E919.2
chain—*see* Accident, caused by, due to,
chain
shaft E919.1

Accident—*continued*
  hot
    liquid E924.0
      caustic or corrosive E924.1
    object (not producing fire or flames)
      E924.8
    substance E924.9
      caustic or corrosive E924.1
      liquid (metal) NEC E924.0
      specified type NEC E924.8
  human bite E928.3
  ignition—*see* Ignition
  internal combustion engine E919.5
  landslide NEC E909.2
  lathe (metalworking) E919.3
    turnings E920.8
    woodworking E919.4
  lift, lifting (appliances) E919.2
    agricultural operations E919.0
    mining operations E919.1
    shaft E919.1
  lightning NEC E907
  machine, machinery—*see also* Accident,
    machine
    drilling, metal E919.3
    manufacturing, for manufacture of
      beverages E919.8
      clothing E919.8
      foodstuffs E919.8
      paper E919.8
      textiles E919.8
    milling, metal E919.3
    moulding E919.4
    power press, metal E919.3
    printing E919.8
    rolling mill, metal E919.3
    sawing, metal E919.3
    specified type NEC E919.8
    spinning E919.8
    weaving E919.8
  natural factor NEC E928.9
  overhead plane E919.4
  plane E920.4
    overhead E919.4
  powered
    hand tool NEC E920.1
    saw E919.4
      hand E920.1
  printing machine E919.8
  pulley (block) E919.2
    agricultural operations E919.0
    mining operations E919.1
    transmission E919.6
  radial saw E919.4
  radiation—*see* Radiation
  reaper E919.0
  road scraper E919.7
    when in transport under its own
      power—*see* categories E810—E825
  roller coaster E919.8
  sander E919.4
  saw E920.4
    band E919.4
    bench E919.4
    chain E920.1
    circular E919.4
    hand E920.4
      powered E920.1
    powered, except hand E919.4
    radial E919.4
  sawing machine, metal E919.3

Accident—*continued*
  shaft
    hoist E919.1
    lift E919.1
    transmission E919.6
  shears E920.4
    hand E920.4
      powered E920.1
    mechanical E919.3
  shovel E920.4
    steam E919.7
  spinning machine E919.8
  steam—*see also* Burning, steam
    engine E919.5
    shovel E919.7
  thresher E919.0
  thunderbolt NEC E907
  tractor E919.0
    when in transport under its own
      power—*see* categories E810-E825
  transmission belt, cable, chain, gear, pinion,
    pulley, shaft E919.6
  turbine (gas) (water driven) E919.5
  under-cutter E919.1
  weaving machine E919.8
  winch E919.2
    agricultural operations E919.0
    mining operations E919.1
  diving E883.0
    with insufficient air supply E913.2
  glider (hang) (*see also* Collision, aircraft,
    unpowered) E842
  hovercraft
    on
      land—*see* Accident, motor vehicle
      water—*see* Accident, watercraft
  ice yacht (*see also* Accident, vehicle NEC)
    E848
  in
    medical, surgical procedure
      as, or due to misadventure—*see*
        Misadventure
      causing an abnormal reaction or later
        complication without mention of
        misadventure—*see* Reaction, abnormal
  kite carrying a person (*see also* Collision,
    aircraft, unpowered) E842
  land yacht (*see also* Accident, vehicle NEC)
    E848
  late effect of—*see* Late effect
  launching pad E845
  machine, machinery (*see also* Accident,
    caused by, due to, by specific type of
    machine) E919.9
    agricultural including animal-powered
      E919.0
    earth-drilling E919.1
    earth moving or scraping E919.7
    excavating E919.7
    involving transport under own power on
      highway or transport vehicle—*see*
      categories E810-E825, E840-E845
    lifting (appliances) E919.2
    metalworking E919.3
    mining E919.1
    prime movers, except electric motors E919.5
      electric motors—*see* Accident, machine, by
        specific type of machine
    recreational E919.8
    specified type NEC E919.8

Accident—*continued*

transmission E919.6

watercraft (deck) (engine room) (galley) (laundry) (loading) E836

woodworking or forming E919.4

motor vehicle (on public highway) (traffic) E819

due to cataclysm—*see* categories E908, E909

involving

collision (*see also* Collision, motor vehicle) E812

nontraffic, not on public highway—*see* categories E820-E825

not involving collision—*see* categories E816-E819

nonmotor vehicle NEC E829

nonroad—*see* Accident, vehicle NEC

road, except pedal cycle, animal-drawn vehicle, or animal being ridden E829

nonroad vehicle NEC—*see* Accident, vehicle NEC

not elsewhere classifiable involving

cable car (not on rails) E847

on rails E829

coal car in mine E846

hand truck—*see* Accident, vehicle NEC

logging car E846

sled(ge), meaning snow or ice vehicle E848

tram, mine or quarry E846

truck

mine or quarry E846

self-propelled, industrial E846

station baggage E846

tub, mine or quarry E846

vehicle NEC E848

snow and ice E848

used only on industrial premises E846

wheelbarrow E848

occurring (at) (in)

apartment E849.0

baseball field, diamond E849.4

construction site, any E849.3

dock E849.8

yard E849.3

dormitory E849.7

factory (building) (premises) E849.3

farm E849.1

buildings E849.1

house E849.0

football field E849.4

forest E849.8

garage (place of work) E849.3

private (home) E849.0

gravel pit E849.2

gymnasium E849.4

highway E849.5

home (private) (residential) E849.0

institutional E849.7

hospital E849.7

hotel E849.6

house (private) (residential) E849.0

movie E849.6

public E849.6

institution, residential E849.7

jail E849.7

mine E849.2

motel E849.6

movie house E849.6

office (building) E849.6

Accident—*continued*

orphanage E849.7

park (public) E849.4

mobile home E849.8

trailer E849.8

parking lot or place E849.8

place

industrial NEC E849.3

parking E849.8

public E849.8

specified place NEC E849.5

recreational NEC E849.4

sport NEC E849.4

playground (park) (school) E849.4

prison E849.6

public building NEC E849.6

quarry E849.2

railway

line NEC E849.8

yard E849.3

residence

home (private) E849.0

resort (beach) (lake) (mountain) (seashore) (vacation) E849.4

restaurant E849.6

sand pit E849.2

school (building) (private) (public) (state) E849.6

reform E849.7

riding E849.4

seashore E849.8

resort E849.4

shop (place of work) E849.3

commercial E849.6

skating rink E849.4

sports palace E849.4

stadium E849.4

store E849.6

street E849.5

swimming pool (public) E849.4

private home or garden E849.0

tennis court E849.4

theatre, theater E849.6

trailer court E849.8

tunnel E849.8

under construction E849.2

warehouse E849.3

yard

dock E849.3

industrial E849.3

private (home) E849.0

railway E849.3

off-road type motor vehicle (not on public highway) NEC E821

on public highway—*see* categories E810-E819

pedal cycle E826

railway E807

due to cataclysm—*see* categories E908, E909

involving

avalanche E909.2

burning by engine, locomotive, train (*see also* Explosion, railway engine) E803

collision (*see also* Collision, railway) E800

derailment (*see also* Derailment, railway) E802

explosion (*see also* Explosion, railway engine) E803

fall (*see also* Fall, from, railway rolling stock) E804

Activity—*continued*
floor mopping and cleaning E013.4
food preparation and clean up E015.0
football (American) NOS E007.0
  flag E007.1
  tackle E007.0
  touch E007.1
four square E007.8
free weights E010.2
frisbee (ultimate) E008.3
furniture
  building E012.2
  finishing E012.2
  repair E012.2
game playing (electronic)
  using
    interactive device E011.1
    keyboard or other stationary device E011.0
gardening E016.1
golf E006.2
grass drills E009.5
grilling and smoking food E015.1
grooming and shearing an animal E019.2
guerilla drills E009.5
gymnastics (rhythmic) E005.2
handball E008.2
handcrafts NEC E012.9
hand held interactive electronic device E011.1
hang gliding E004.4
hiking (on level or elevated terrain) E001.0
hockey (ice) E003.1
  field E007.4
horseback riding E006.1
household maintenance NEC E013.9
ice NEC E003.9
  dancing E003.0
  hockey E003.1
  skating E003.0
inline roller skating E006.0
ironing E013.3
judo E008.4
jumping (off) NEC E004.9
  BASE (Building, Antenna, Span, Earth) E004.2
  bungee E004.3
  jacks E009.1
  rope E006.5
jumping jacks E009.1
jumping rope E006.5
karate E008.4
kayaking (in calm and turbulent water) E002.5
keyboarding (computer) E011.0
kickball E007.8
knitting E012.0
lacrosse E007.4
land maintenance NEC E016.9
landscaping E016.1
laundry E013.1
machines (exercise) primarily for cardiorespiratory conditioning E009.0
maintenance
  building E016.9
  household NEC E013.9
  land E016.9
  property E016.9
marching (on level or elevated terrain) E001.0
martial arts E008.4
microwave oven E015.2
mopping (floor) E013.4
mountain climbing E004.0
milking an animal E019.1

Activity—*continued*
muscle strengthening
  exercises (non-machine) NEC E010.9
  machines E010.0
musical keyboard (electronic) playing E018.0
nordic skiing E003.3
obstacle course E009.4
oven (microwave) E015.2
packing up and unpacking in moving to a new residence E013.5
parasailing E002.9
percussion instrument playing NEC E018.1
personal
  bathing and showering E013.0
  hygiene NEC E013.8
  showering E013.0
physical
  games generally associated with school recess, summer camp and children 007.8
  training NEC E009.9
piano playing E018.0
pilates E010.3
platform diving E002.1
playing musical instrument
  brass instrument E018.3
  drum E018.1
  musical keyboard (electronic) E018.0
  percussion instrument NEC E018.1
  piano E018.0
  string instrument E018.2
  wind instrument E018.3
property maintenance NEC E016.9
pruning (garden and lawn) E016.1
pull-ups E010.1
push-ups E010.1
racquetball E008.2
rafting (in calm and turbulent water) E002.5
raking (leaves) E016.0
rappelling E004.1
refereeing a sports activity E029.0
residential relocation E013.5
rhythmic
  gymnastics E005.2
  movement NEC E005.9
riding
  horseback E006.1
  rollercoaster E017.0
rock climbing E004.0
rollercoaster riding E017.0
roller skating (inline) E006.0
rough housing and horseplay E029.2
rowing (in calm and turbulent water) E002.5
rugby E007.2
running E001.1
SCUBA diving E002.4
sewing E012.1
shoveling E016.0
  dirt E016.0
  snow E016.0
showering (personal) E013.0
sit-ups E010.1
skateboarding E006.0
skating (ice) E003.0
  roller E006.0
skiing (alpine) (downhill) E003.2
  cross country E003.3
  nordic E003.3
sledding (snow) E003.2
smoking and grilling food E015.1
snorkeling E002.4

Assault (homicidal) (by) (in) E968.9
  acid E961
    swallowed E962.1
  air gun E968.6
  BB gun E968.6
  bite NEC E968.8
    of human being E968.7
  bomb ((placed in) car or house) E965.8
    antipersonnel E965.5
    letter E965.7
    petrol E965.7
  brawl (hand) (fists) (foot) E960.0
  burning, burns (by fire) E968.0
    acid E961
      swallowed E962.1
    caustic, corrosive substance E961
      swallowed E962.1
    chemical from swallowing caustic, corrosive
      substance NEC E962.1
    hot liquid E968.3
    scalding E968.3
    vitriol E961
      swallowed E962.1
  caustic, corrosive substance E961
    swallowed E962.1
  cut, any part of body E966
  dagger E966
  drowning E964
  explosive(s) E965.9
    bomb (see also Assault, bomb) E965.8
    dynamite E965.8
  fight (hand) (fists) (foot) E960.0
    with weapon E968.9
      blunt or thrown E968.2
      cutting or piercing E966
      firearm—see Shooting, homicide
  fire E968.0
  firearm(s)—see Shooting, homicide
  garrotting E963
  gunshot (wound)—see Shooting, homicide
  hanging E963
  injury NEC E968.9
  knife E966
  late effect of E969
  ligature E963
  poisoning E962.9
    drugs or medicinals E962.0
    gas(es) or vapors, except drugs and
      medicinals E962.2
    solid or liquid substances, except drugs and
      medicinals E962.1
  puncture, any part of body E966
  pushing
    before moving object, train, vehicle E968.5
    from high place E968.1
  rape E960.1
  scalding E968.3
  shooting—see Shooting, homicide
  sodomy E960.1
  stab, any part of body E966
  strangulation E963
  submersion E964
  suffocation E963
  transport vehicle E968.5
  violence NEC E968.9
  vitriol E961
    swallowed E962.1
  weapon E968.9
    blunt or thrown E968.2
    cutting or piercing E966
    firearm—see Shooting, homicide

Assault—continued
  wound E968.9
    cutting E966
    gunshot—see Shooting, homicide
    knife E966
    piercing E966
    puncture E966
    stab E966
Attack by animal NEC E906.9
Avalanche E909.2
  falling on or hitting
    motor vehicle (in motion) (on public
      highway) E909.2
    railway train E909.2
Aviators' disease E902.1

B

Barotitis, barodontalgia, barosinusitis,
  barotrauma (otitic) (sinus)—see Effects of,
  air pressure
Battered
  baby or child (syndrome)—see Abuse, child;
    category E967
  person other than baby or child—see Assault
Bayonet wound (see also Cut, by bayonet)
  E920.3
  in
    legal intervention E974
    terrorism E979.8
    war operations E995.2
Bean in nose E912
Bed set on fire NEC E898.0
Beheading (by guillotine)
  homicide E966
  legal execution E978
Bending, injury in E927.8
Bends E902.0
Bite
  animal (nonvenomous) NEC E906.5
    venomous NEC E905.9
  arthropod (nonvenomous) NEC E906.4
    venomous—see Sting
  black widow spider E905.1
  cat E906.3
  centipede E905.4
  cobra E905.0
  copperhead snake E905.0
  coral snake E905.0
  dog E906.0
  fer de lance E905.0
  gila monster E905.0
  human being
    accidental E928.3
    assault E968.7
  insect (nonvenomous) E906.4
    venomous—see Sting
  krait E905.0
  late effect of—see Late effect
  lizard E906.2
    venomous E905.0
  mamba E905.0
  marine animal
    nonvenomous E906.3
      snake E906.2
    venomous E905.6
      snake E905.0
  millipede E906.4
    venomous E905.4
  moray eel E906.3

Bite —*continued*
rat E906.1
rattlesnake E905.0
rodent, except rat E906.3
serpent—*see* Bite, snake
shark E906.3
snake (venomous) E905.0
nonvenomous E906.2
sea E905.0
spider E905.1
nonvenomous E906.4
tarantula (venomous) E905.1
venomous NEC E905.9
by specific animal—*see* category E905
viper E905.0
water moccasin E905.0
Blast (air)
from nuclear explosion E996
in
terrorism E979.2
from nuclear explosion E979.5
underwater E979.0
war operations E993.9
from nuclear explosion (see also War
operations, injury due to, nuclear
weapons) E996.0
underwater E992.9
underwater E992
Blizzard E908.3
Blow E928.9
by law-enforcing agent, police (on duty) E975
with blunt object (baton) (nightstick) (stave)
(truncheon) E973
Blowing up (*see also* Explosion) E923.9
Brawl (hand) (fists) (foot) E960.0
Breakage (accidental)
cable of cable car not on rails E847
ladder (causing fall) E881.0
part (any) of
animal-drawn vehicle E827
ladder (causing fall) E881.0
motor vehicle
in motion (on public highway) E818
not on public highway E825
nonmotor road vehicle, except animal-drawn
vehicle or pedal cycle E829
off-road type motor vehicle (not on public
highway) NEC E821
on public highway E818
pedal cycle E826
scaffolding (causing fall) E881.1
snow vehicle, motor-driven (not on public
highway) E820
on public highway E818
vehicle NEC—*see* Accident, vehicle
Broken
glass
fall on E888.0
injury by E920.8
power line (causing electric shock) E925.1
Bumping against, into (accidentally)
object (moving) E917.9
caused by crowd E917.1
with subsequent fall E917.6
furniture E917.3
with subsequent fall E917.7
in
running water E917.2
sports E917.0
with subsequent fall E917.5

Bumping against, into—*continued*
stationary E917.4
with subsequent fall E917.8
person(s) E917.9
with fall E886.9
in sports E886.0
as, or caused by, a crowd E917.1
with subsequent fall E917.6
in sports E917.0
with fall E886.0
Burning, burns (accidental) (by) (from) (on)
E899
acid (any kind) E924.1
swallowed—*see* Table of drugs and
chemicals
airgun E928.7
bedclothes (*see also* Fire, specified NEC)
E898.0
blowlamp (*see also* Fire, specified NEC)
E898.1
blowtorch (*see also* Fire, specified NEC)
E898.1
boat, ship, watercraft—*see* categories E830,
E831, E837
bonfire (controlled) E897
uncontrolled E892
candle (*see also* Fire, specified NEC) E898.1
caustic liquid, substance E924.1
swallowed—*see* Table of drugs and
chemicals
chemical E924.1
from swallowing caustic, corrosive
substance—*see* Table of drugs and
chemicals
in
terrorism E979.7
war operations E997.2
cigar(s) or cigarette(s) (*see also* Fire, specified
NEC) E898.1
clothes, clothing, nightdress—*see* Ignition,
clothes
with conflagration—*see* Conflagration
conflagration—*see* Conflagration
corrosive liquid, substance E924.1
swallowed—*see* Table of drugs and
chemicals
electric current (*see also* Electric shock)
E925.9
fire, flames (*see also* Fire) E899
firearm E928.7
flare, Verey pistol E922.8
heat
from appliance (electrical) E924.8
in local application or packing during
medical or surgical procedure E873.5
homicide (attempt) (*see also* Assault, burning)
E968.0
hot
liquid E924.0
caustic or corrosive E924.1
object (not producing fire or flames) E924.8
substance E924.9
caustic or corrosive E924.1
liquid (metal) NEC E924.0
specified type NEC E924.8
tap water E924.2
ignition—*see also* Ignition
clothes, clothing, nightdress—*see also*
Ignition, clothes
with conflagration—*see* Conflagration

Burning, burns—*continued*
  highly inflammable material (benzine) (fat)
    (gasoline) (kerosine) (paraffin) (petrol)
    E894
  inflicted by other person
    stated as
      homicidal, intentional (*see also* Assault,
        burning) E968.0
      undetermined whether accidental or
        intentional (*see also* Burn, stated as
        undetermined whether accidental or
        intentional) E988.1
  internal, from swallowed caustic, corrosive
    liquid, substance—*see* Table of drugs and
    chemicals
  in
    from nuclear explosion E996
    petrol bomb E990.0
    terrorism E979.3
      from nuclear explosion E979.5
      petrol bomb E979.3
    war operations (from fire-producing device
      or conventional weapon) E990.9
      from nuclear explosion (see also War
        operations, injury due to, nuclear
        weapons) E996.2
      incendiary bomb E990.0
      petrol bomb E990.0
  lamp (*see also* Fire, specified NEC) E898.1
  late effect of NEC E929.4
  lighter (cigar) (cigarette) (*see also* Fire,
    specified NEC) E898.1
  lightning E907
  liquid (boiling) (hot) (molten) E924.0
    caustic, corrosive (external) E924.1
      swallowed—*see* Table of drugs and
        chemicals
  local application of externally applied
    substance in medical or surgical care
    E873.5
  machinery—*see* Accident, machine
  matches (*see also* Fire, specified NEC) E898.1
  medicament, externally applied E873.5
  metal, molten E924.8
  object (hot) E924.8
    producing fire or flames—*see* Fire
  oven (electric) (gas) E924.8
  pipe (smoking) (*see also* Fire, specified NEC)
    E898.1
  radiation—*see* Radiation
  railway engine, locomotive, train (*see also*
    Explosion, railway engine) E803
  self-inflicted (unspecified whether accidental
    or intentional) E988.1
    caustic or corrosive substance NEC E988.7
    stated as intentional, purposeful E958.1
      caustic or corrosive substance NEC E958.7
    stated as undetermined whether accidental or
      intentional E988.1
      caustic or corrosive substance NEC E988.7
  steam E924.0
    pipe E924.8
  substance (hot) E924.9
    boiling or molten E924.0
    caustic, corrosive (external) E924.1
      swallowed—*see* Table of drugs and
        chemicals
  suicidal (attempt) NEC E958.1
    caustic substance E958.7
    late effect of E959
  tanning bed E926.2

Burning, burns—*continued*
  therapeutic misadventure
    overdose of radiation E873.2
  torch, welding (*see also* Fire, specified NEC)
    E898.1
  trash fire (*see also* Burning, bonfire) E897
  vapor E924.0
  vitriol E924.1
  x-rays E926.3
    in medical, surgical procedure—*see*
      Misadventure, failure, in dosage,
      radiation
Butted by animal E906.8

C

Cachexia, lead or saturnine E866.0
  from pesticide NEC (*see also* Table of drugs
    and chemicals) E863.4
Caisson disease E902.2
Capital punishment (any means) E978
Car sickness E903
Casualty (not due to war) NEC E928.9
  terrorism E979.8
  war (*see also* War operations) E995.9
Cat
  bite E906.3
  scratch E906.8
Cataclysmic (any injury)
  earth surface movement or eruption E909.9
    specified type NEC E909.8
  storm or flood resulting from storm E908.9
    specified type NEC E909.8
Catching fire —*see* Ignition
Caught
  between
    objects (moving) (stationary and moving)
      E918
    and machinery—*see* Accident, machine
  by cable car, not on rails E847
  in
    machinery (moving parts of)—*see* Accident,
      machine
    object E918
Cave-in (causing asphyxia, suffocation (by
  pressure)) (*see also* Suffocation, due to,
  cave-in) E913.3
Cave-in—*continued*
  with injury other than asphyxia or suffocation
    E916
    with asphyxia or suffocation (*see also*
      Suffocation, due to, cave-in) E913.3
  struck or crushed by E916
    with asphyxia or suffocation (*see also*
      Suffocation, due to, cave-in) E913.3
Change(s) in air pressure—*see also* Effects of,
  air pressure
  sudden, in aircraft (ascent) (descent) (causing
    aeroneurosis or aviators' disease) E902.1
Chilblains E901.0
  due to manmade conditions E901.1
Choking (on) (any object except food or
  vomitus) E912
  apple E911
  bone E911
  food, any type (regurgitated) E911
  mucus or phlegm E912
  seed E911
Civil insurrection —*see* War operations
Cloudburst E908.8

Cold, exposure to (accidental) (excessive)
(extreme) (place) E901.9
causing chilblains or immersion foot E901.0
due to
  manmade conditions E901.1
  specified cause NEC E901.8
  weather (conditions) E901.0
late effect of NEC E929.5
self-inflicted (undetermined whether accidental
  or intentional) E988.3
suicidal E958.3
suicide E958.3
Colic, lead, painters', or saturnine —*see*
category E866
Collapse
building E916
  burning (uncontrolled fire) E891.8
    in terrorism E979.3
    private E890.8
dam E909.3
due to heat—*see* Heat
machinery—*see* Accident, machine
man-made structure E909.3
postoperative NEC E878.9
structure, burning NEC E891.8
  burning (uncontrolled fire)
    in terrorism E979.3
Collision (accidental)

Note—In the case of collisions between different
types of vehicles, persons and objects, priority in
classification is in the following order:

  Aircraft
  Watercraft
  Motor vehicle
  Railway vehicle
  Pedal Cycle
  Animal-drawn vehicle
  Animal being ridden
  Streetcar or other nonmotor road vehicle
  Other vehicle
  Pedestrian or person using pedestrian
    conveyance
  Object (except where falling from or set in
    motion by vehicle etc. listed above)

In the listing below, the combinations are listed
only under the vehicle etc. having priority. For
definitions, *see* E code introduction.

---

aircraft (with object or vehicle) (fixed)
  (movable) (moving) E841
  with
    person (while landing, taking off) (without
      accident to aircraft) E844
    powered (in transit) (with unpowered
      aircraft) E841
    while landing, taking off E840
    unpowered E842
    while landing, taking off E840
animal being ridden (in sport or transport)
  E828
  and
    animal (being ridden) (herded)
      (unattended) E828
    nonmotor road vehicle, except pedal cycle
      or animal-drawn vehicle E828
    object (fallen) (fixed) (movable) (moving)
      not falling from or set in motion by
      vehicle of higher priority E828
    pedestrian (conveyance or vehicle) E828

Collision—*continued*
animal-drawn vehicle E827
  and
    animal (being ridden) (herded)
      (unattended) E827
    nonmotor road vehicle, except pedal cycle
      E827
    object (fallen) (fixed) (movable) (moving)
      not falling from or set in motion by
      vehicle of higher priority E827
    pedestrian (conveyance or vehicle) E827
    streetcar E827
motor vehicle (on public highway) (traffic
  accident) E812
after leaving, running off, public highway
  (without antecedent collision) (without
  re-entry) E816
with antecedent collision on public
  highway—*see* categories E810-E815
with re-entrance collision with another
  motor vehicle E811
and
  abutment (bridge) (overpass) E815
  animal (herded) (unattended) E815
    carrying person, property E813
  animal-drawn vehicle E813
  another motor vehicle (abandoned)
    (disabled) (parked) (stalled) (stopped)
    E812
    with, involving re-entrance (on same
      roadway) (across median strip) E811
  any object, person, or vehicle off the
    public highway resulting from a
    noncollision motor vehicle nontraffic
    accident E816
  avalanche, fallen or not moving E815
    falling E909
  boundary fence E815
  culvert E815
  fallen
    stone E815
    tree E815
  falling E909.2
  guard post or guard rail E815
  inter-highway divider E815
  landslide, fallen or not moving E815
    moving E909
  machinery (road) E815
  moving E909.2
  nonmotor road vehicle NEC E813
  object (any object, person, or vehicle off
    the public highway resulting from a
    noncollision motor vehicle nontraffic
    accident) E815
    off, normally not on, public highway
      resulting from a noncollision motor
      vehicle traffic accident E816
  pedal cycle E813
  pedestrian (conveyance) E814
  person (using pedestrian conveyance) E814
  post or pole (lamp) (light) (signal)
    (telephone) (utility) E815
  railway rolling stock, train, vehicle E810
  safety island E815
  street car E813
  traffic signal, sign, or marker (temporary)
    E815
  tree E815
  tricycle E813
  wall of cut made for road E815

Collision—*continued*
  due to cataclysm—*see* categories E908, E909
  not on public highway, nontraffic accident E822
  and
    animal (carrying person, property) (herded) (unattended) E822
    animal-drawn vehicle E822
    another motor vehicle (moving), except off-road motor vehicle E822
      stationary E823
    avalanche, fallen, not moving E823
      moving E909
    landslide, fallen, not moving E823
      moving E909
    nonmotor vehicle (moving) E822
      stationary E823
    object (fallen) (normally) (fixed) (movable but not in motion) (stationary) E823
      moving, except when falling from, set in motion by, aircraft or cataclysm E822
    pedal cycle (moving) E822
      stationary E823
    pedestrian (conveyance) E822
    person (using pedestrian conveyance) E822
    railway rolling stock, train, vehicle (moving) E822
      stationary E823
    road vehicle (any) (moving) E822
      stationary E823
    tricycle (moving) E822
      stationary E823
    moving E909.2
  off-road type motor vehicle (not on public highway) E821
  and
    animal (being ridden) (-drawn vehicle) E821
    another off-road motor vehicle, except snow vehicle E821
    other motor vehicle, not on public highway E821
    other object or vehicle NEC, fixed or movable, not set in motion by aircraft, motor vehicle on highway, or snow vehicle, motor-driven E821
    pedal cycle E821
    pedestrian (conveyance) E821
    railway train E821
  on public highway—*see* Collision, motor vehicle
  pedal cycle E826
  and
    animal (carrying person, property) (herded) (unherded) E826
    animal-drawn vehicle E826
    another pedal cycle E826
    nonmotor road vehicle E826
    object (fallen) (fixed) (movable) (moving) not falling from or set in motion by aircraft, motor vehicle, or railway train NEC E826
    pedestrian (conveyance) E826
    person (using pedestrian conveyance) E826
    street car E826

Collision—*continued*
  pedestrian(s) (conveyance) E917.9
    with fall E886.9
      in sports E886.0
    and
      crowd, human stampede E917.1
        with subsequent fall E917.6
      furniture E917.3
        with subsequent fall E917.7
      machinery—*see* Accident, machine
      object (fallen) (moving) not falling from or set in motion by any vehicle classifiable to E800-E848, E917.9
      caused by a crowd E917.1
        with subsequent fall E917.6
      furniture E917.3
        with subsequent fall E917.7
      in
        running water E917.2
          with drowning or submersion—*see* Submersion
        sports E917.0
          with subsequent fall E917.5
        stationary E917.4
          with subsequent fall E917.8
      vehicle, nonmotor, nonroad E848
    in
      running water E917.2
        with drowning or submersion—*see* Submersion
      sports E917.0
        with fall E886.0
  person(s) (using pedestrian conveyance) (*see also* Collision, pedestrian) E917.9
  railway (rolling stock) (train) (vehicle) (with (subsequent) derailment, explosion, fall or fire) E800
    with antecedent derailment E802
    and
      animal (carrying person) (herded) (unattended) E801
      another railway train or vehicle E800
      buffers E801
      fallen tree on railway E801
      farm machinery, nonmotor (in transport) (stationary) E801
      gates E801
      nonmotor vehicle E801
      object (fallen) (fixed) (movable) (moving) not falling from, set in motion by, aircraft or motor vehicle NEC E801
      pedal cycle E801
      pedestrian (conveyance) E805
      person (using pedestrian conveyance) E805
      platform E801
      rock on railway E801
      street car E801
  snow vehicle, motor-driven (not on public highway) E820
  and
    animal (being ridden) (-drawn vehicle) E820
    another off-road motor vehicle E820
    other motor vehicle, not on public highway E820
    other object or vehicle NEC, fixed or movable, not set in motion by aircraft or motor vehicle on highway E820
    pedal cycle E820
    pedestrian (conveyance) E820
    railway train E820

Collision—*continued*
  on public highway—*see* Collision, motor
    vehicle
  street car(s) E829
    and
      animal, herded, not being ridden,
        unattended E829
      nonmotor road vehicle NEC E829
      object (fallen) (fixed) (movable) (moving)
        not falling from or set in motion by
        aircraft, animal-drawn vehicle, animal
        being ridden, motor vehicle, pedal
        cycle, or railway train E829
      pedestrian (conveyance) E829
      person (using pedestrian conveyance) E829
  vehicle
    animal-drawn—*see* Collision, animal-drawn
      vehicle
    motor—*see* Collision, motor vehicle
    nonmotor
      nonroad E848
        and
          another nonmotor, nonroad vehicle
            E848
          object (fallen) (fixed) (movable)
            (moving) not falling from or set in
            motion by aircraft, animal-drawn
            vehicle, animal being ridden, motor
            vehicle, nonmotor road vehicle,
            pedal cycle, railway train, or
            streetcar E848
    road, except animal being ridden,
      animal-drawn vehicle, or pedal cycle
      E829
      and
        animal, herded, not being ridden,
          unattended E829
        another nonmotor road vehicle, except
          animal being ridden, animal-drawn
          vehicle, or pedal cycle E829
        object (fallen) (fixed) (movable)
          (moving) not falling from or set in
          motion by, aircraft, animal-drawn
          vehicle, animal being ridden, motor
          vehicle, pedal cycle, or railway
          train E829
        pedestrian (conveyance) E829
        person (using pedestrian conveyance)
          E829
        vehicle, nonmotor, nonroad E829
  watercraft E838
    and
      person swimming or water skiing E838
    causing
      drowning, submersion E830
      injury except drowning, submersion E831
Combustion, spontaneous —*see* Ignition
Complication of medical or surgical
  procedure or treatment
  as an abnormal reaction—*see* Reaction,
    abnormal
  delayed, without mention of
    misadventure—*see* Reaction, abnormal
  due to misadventure—*see* Misadventure
Compression
  divers' squeeze E902.2
  trachea by
    food E911
    foreign body, except food E912

Conflagration
  building or structure, except private dwelling
    (barn) (church) (convalescent or residential
    home) (factory) (farm outbuilding)
    (hospital) (hotel) (institution) (educational)
    (dormitory) (residential) (school) (shop)
    (store) (theatre) E891.9
    with or causing (injury due to)
      accident or injury NEC E891.9
        specified circumstance NEC E891.8
      burns, burning E891.3
      carbon monoxide E891.2
      fumes E891.2
        polyvinylchloride (PVC) or similar
          material E891.1
      smoke E891.2
    causing explosion E891.0
  in terrorism E979.3
  not in building or structure E892
  private dwelling (apartment) (boarding house)
    (camping place) (caravan) (farmhouse)
    (home (private)) (house) (lodging house)
    (private garage) (rooming house)
    (tenement) E890.9
    with or causing (injury due to)
      accident or injury NEC E890.9
        specified circumstance NEC E890.8
      burns, burning E890.3
      carbon monoxide E890.2
      fumes E890.2
        polyvinylchloride (PVC) or similar
          material E890.1
      smoke E890.2
    causing explosion E890.0
Constriction, external
  caused by
    hair E928.4
    other object E928.5
Contact with
  dry ice E901.1
  liquid air, hydrogen, nitrogen E901.1
Cramp(s)
  Heat—*see* Heat
  swimmers (*see also* category E910) E910.2
    not in recreation or sport E910.3
Cranking (car) (truck) (bus) (engine), injury
  by E917.9
Crash
  aircraft (in transit) (powered) E841
    at landing, take-off E840
    in
      terrorism E979.1
      war operations E994.9
    on runway NEC E840
    stated as
      homicidal E968.8
      suicidal E958.6
      undetermined whether accidental or
        intentional E988.6
    unpowered E842
  glider E842
  motor vehicle—*see also* Accident, motor
    vehicle
    homicidal E968.5
    suicidal E958.5
    undetermined whether accidental or
      intentional E988.5

Crushed (accidentally) E928.9
between
  boat(s), ship(s), watercraft (and dock or pier)
    (without accident to watercraft) E838
    after accident to, or collision, watercraft
      E831
  objects (moving) (stationary and moving)
    E918
by
  avalanche NEC E909.2
  boat, ship, watercraft after accident to,
    collision, watercraft E831
  cave-in E916
    with asphyxiation or suffocation (*see also*
      Suffocation, due to, cave-in) E913.3
  crowd, human stampede E917.1
  falling
    aircraft (*see also* Accident, aircraft) E841
      in
        terrorism E979.1
        war operations E994.8
    earth, material E916
      with asphyxiation or suffocation (*see
        also* Suffocation, due to, cave-in)
        E913.3
    object E916
      on ship, watercraft E838
      while loading, unloading watercraft E838
    firearm E928.7
  landslide NEC E909.2
  lifeboat after abandoning ship E831
  machinery—*see* Accident, machine
  railway rolling stock, train, vehicle (part of)
    E805
  slide trigger mechanism, scope or other part
    of gun E928.7
  street car E829
  vehicle NEC—*see* Accident, vehicle NEC
in
  machinery—*see* Accident, machine
  object E918
  transport accident—*see* categories
    E800-E848
late effect of NEC E929.9
Cut, cutting (any part of body) (accidental)
  E920.9
by
  arrow E920.8
  axe E920.4
  bayonet (*see also* Bayonet wound) E920.3
    in war operations E995.2
  blender E920.2
  broken glass E920.8
    following fall E888.0
  can opener E920.4
    powered E920.2
  chisel E920.4
  circular saw E919.4
  cutting or piercing instrument—*see also*
    category E920
    following fall E888.0
    late effect of E929.8
  dagger E920.3
  dart E920.8
  drill—*see* Accident, caused by drill
  edge of stiff paper E920.8
  electric
    beater E920.2
    fan E920.2
    knife E920.2
    mixer E920.2

Cut, cutting—*continued*
  firearm component E928.7
  fork E920.4
  garden fork E920.4
  hand saw or tool (not powered) E920.4
    powered E920.1
  hedge clipper E920.4
    powered E920.1
  hoe E920.4
  ice pick E920.4
  knife E920.3
    electric E920.2
    in war operations E995.2
  lathe turnings E920.8
  lawn mower E920.4
    powered E920.0
    riding E919.8
  machine—*see* Accident, machine
  meat
    grinder E919.8
    slicer E919.8
  nails E920.8
  needle E920.4
    hypodermic E920.5
  object, edged, pointed, sharp—*see* category
    E920
    following fall E888.0
  paper cutter E920.4
  piercing instrument—*see also* category E920
    late effect of E929.8
  pitchfork E920.4
  powered
    can opener E920.2
    garden cultivator E920.1
      riding E919.8
    hand saw E920.1
    hand tool NEC E920.1
    hedge clipper E920.1
    household appliance or implement E920.2
    lawn mower (hand) E920.0
      riding E919.8
    rivet gun E920.1
    staple gun E920.1
  rake E920.4
  saw
    circular E919.4
    hand E920.4
  scissors E920.4
  screwdriver E920.4
  sewing machine (electric) (powered) E920.2
    not powered E920.4
  shears E920.4
  shovel E920.4
  slide trigger mechanism, scope or other part
    of gun E928.7
  spade E920.4
  splinters E920.8
  sword E920.3
    in war operations E995.2
  tin can lid E920.8
  wood slivers E920.8
homicide (attempt) E966
inflicted by other person
  stated as
    intentional, homicidal E966
    undetermined whether accidental or
      intentional E986
late effect of NEC E929.8
legal
  execution E978
  intervention E974

Cut, cutting—*continued*
self-inflicted (unspecified whether accidental
or intentional) E986
stated as intentional, purposeful E956
stated as undetermined whether accidental or
intentional E986
suicidal (attempt) E956
terrorism E979.8
war operations E995.2
Cyclone E908.1

D

**Death due to injury occurring one year or
more previous** —*see* Late effect
Decapitation (accidental circumstances) NEC
E928.9
homicidal E966
legal execution (by guillotine) E978
Deprivation —*see also* Privation
homicidal intent E968.4
Derailment (accidental)
railway (rolling stock) (train) (vehicle) (with
subsequent collision) E802
with
collision (antecedent) (*see also* Collision,
railway) E800
Derailment (accidental)—*continued*
explosion (subsequent) (without antecedent
collision) E802
antecedent collision E803
fall (without collision (antecedent)) E802
fire (without collision (antecedent)) E802
street car E829
Descent
parachute (voluntary) (without accident to
aircraft) E844
due to accident to aircraft—*see* categories
E840-E842
Desertion
child, with intent to injure or kill E968.4
helpless person, infant, newborn E904.0
with intent to injure or kill E968.4
Destitution —*see* Privation
Dirty bomb (*see also* War operations, injury
due to, nuclear weapons) E996.9
Disability, late effect or sequela of injury
—*see Late effect*
Disease
Andes E902.0
aviators' E902.1
caisson E902.2
range E902.0
Divers' disease, palsy, paralysis, squeeze
E902.0
Dog bite E906.0
Dragged by
cable car (not on rails) E847
on rails E829
motor vehicle (on highway) E814
not on highway, nontraffic accident E825
street car E829
Drinking poison (accidental) —*see* Table of
drugs and chemicals
Drowning —*see* Submersion
Dust in eye E914\

E

Earth falling (on) (with asphyxia or suffocation
(by pressure)) (*see also* Suffocation, due to,
cave-in) E913.3
as, or due to, a cataclysm (involving any
transport vehicle)—*see* categories E908,
E909
not due to cataclysmic action E913.3
motor vehicle (in motion) (on public
highway) E818
not on public highway E825
nonmotor road vehicle NEC E829
pedal cycle E826
railway rolling stock, train, vehicle E806
street car E829
struck or crushed by E916
with asphyxiation or suffocation E913.3
with injury other than asphyxia,
suffocation E916
Earthquake (any injury) E909.0
Effect(s) (adverse) of
air pressure E902.9
at high altitude E902.9
in aircraft E902.1
residence or prolonged visit (causing
conditions classifiable to E902.0)
E902.0
due to
diving E902.2
specified cause NEC E902.8
in aircraft E902.1
cold, excessive (exposure to) (*see also* Cold,
exposure to) E901.9
heat (excessive) (*see also* Heat) E900.9
hot
place—*see* Heat
weather E900.0
insulation—*see* Heat
late—*see* Late effect of
motion E903
nuclear explosion or weapon
in
terrorism E979.5
war operations (*see also* War operations,
injury due to, nuclear weapons) E996.9
radiation—*see* Radiation
terrorism, secondary E979.9
travel E903
Electric shock, electrocution (accidental) (from
exposed wire, faulty appliance, high voltage
cable, live rail, open socket) (by) (in) E925.9
appliance or wiring
domestic E925.0
factory E925.2
farm (building) E925.8
house E925.0
home E925.0
industrial (conductor) (control apparatus)
(transformer) E925.2
outdoors E925.8
public building E925.8
residential institution E925.8
school E925.8
specified place NEC E925.8
caused by other person
stated as
intentional, homicidal E968.8
undetermined whether accidental or
intentional E988.4

Explosion—*continued*
  of mine E923.8
  in
    terrorism
      at sea or in harbor E979.0
      land E979.2
      marine E979.0
    war operations
      after cessation of hostilities E998.0
      at sea or in harbor E992.2
      land E993.8
        after cessation of hostilities E998.0
        injury by fragments from E991.4
      marine E992.2
  own weapons
  in
    terrorism (*see also* Suicide) E979.2
    war operations E993.7
      injury by fragments from E991.9
        antipersonnel bomb E991.3
  pressure
    cooker E921.8
    gas tank (in machinery) E921.1
    vessel (in machinery) E921.9
      on transport vehicle—*see* categories
        E800-E848
      specified type NEC E921.8
  propane E923.2
  railway engine, locomotive, train (boiler) (with
    subsequent collision, derailment, fall) E803
    with
      collision (antecedent) (*see also* Collision,
        railway) E800
      derailment (antecedent) E802
      fire (without antecedent collision or
        derailment) E803
  secondary fire resulting from—*see* Fire
  self-inflicted (unspecified whether accidental
    or intentional) E985.5
    stated as intentional, purposeful E955.5
  shell (artillery) E923.8
  in
    terrorism E979.2
    war operations E993.2
      injury by fragments from E991.4
  stated as undetermined whether caused
    accidentally or purposely inflicted E985.5
  steam or water lines (in machinery) E921.0
  suicide (attempted) E955.5
  terrorism—*see* Terrorism, explosion
  torpedo E923.8
  in
    terrorism E979.0
    war operations E992.0
  transport accident—*see* categories E800-E848
  war operations—*see* War operations, explosion
  watercraft (boiler) E837
    causing drowning, submersion (after jumping
      from watercraft) E830
Exposure (weather) (conditions) (rain) (wind)
  E904.3
  with homicidal intent E968.4

Exposure—*continued*
  environmental
    to
      algae bloom E928.6
      blue-green algae bloom E928.6
      brown tide E928.6
      cyanobacteria bloom E928.6
      Florida red tide E928.6
      harmful algae
        and toxins E928.6
        bloom E928.6
      pfiesteria piscicida E928.6
      red tide E928.6
  excessive E904.3
    cold (*see also* Cold, exposure to) E901.9
      self-inflicted—*see* Cold, exposure to,
        self-inflicted
    heat (*see also* Heat) E900.9
  fire—*see* Fire
  helpless person, infant, newborn due to
    abandonment or neglect E904.0
  noise E928.1
  prolonged in deep-freeze unit or refrigerator
    E901.1
  radiation—*see* Radiation
  resulting from transport accident—*see*
    categories E800-E848
  smoke from, due to
    fire—*see* Fire
    tobacco, second-hand E869.4
  vibration E928.2
External cause status E000.9
  civilian
    done for
      financial or other compensation E000.0
      pay or income E000.0
  for income E000.0
  hobby or leisure E000.8
  off duty military E000.8
  military E000.1
    off duty E000.8
  recreation E000.8
  specified NEC E000.8
  sport not for income E000.8
  student E000.8
  volunteer E000.8

F

Fall, falling (accidental) E888.9
  building E916
    burning E891.8
    private E890.8
  down
    escalator E880.0
    ladder E881.0
      in boat, ship, watercraft E833
    staircase E880.9
    stairs, steps—*see* Fall, from, stairs
  earth (with asphyxia or suffocation (by
    pressure)) (*see also* Earth, falling) E913.3
  from, off
    aircraft (at landing, take-off) (in-transit)
      (while alighting, boarding) E843
      resulting from accident to aircraft—*see*
        categories E840-E842
    animal (in sport or transport) E828
    animal-drawn vehicle E827

Fall, falling—*continued*
- balcony E882
- bed E884.4
- bicycle E826
- boat, ship, watercraft (into water) E832
  - after accident to, collision, fire on E830
    - and subsequently struck by (part of) boat E831
    - and subsequently struck by (part of) boat E838
  - burning, crushed, sinking E830
    - and subsequently struck by (part of) boat E831
- bridge E882
- building E882
  - burning (uncontrolled fire) E891.8
    - in terrorism E979.3
    - private E890.8
- bunk in boat, ship, watercraft E834
  - due to accident to watercraft E831
- cable car (not on rails) E847
  - on rails E829
- car—*see* Fall from motor vehicle
- chair E884.2
- cliff E884.1
- commode E884.6
- curb (sidewalk) E880.1
- elevation aboard ship E834
  - due to accident to ship E831
- embankment E884.9
- escalator E880.0
- fire escape E882
- flagpole E882
- furniture NEC E884.5
- gangplank (into water) (*see also* Fall, from, boat) E832
  - to deck, dock E834
- hammock on ship E834
  - due to accident to watercraft E831
- haystack E884.9
- heelies E885.1
- high place NEC E884.9
  - stated as undetermined whether accidental or intentional—*see* Jumping, from, high place
- horse (in sport or transport) E828
- in-line skates E885.1
- ladder E881.0
  - in boat, ship, watercraft E833
  - due to accident to watercraft E831
- machinery—*see also* accident, machine
  - not in operation E884.9
- motor vehicle (in motion) (on public highway) E818
  - not on public highway E825
    - stationary, except while alighting, boarding, entering, leaving E884.9
    - while alighting, boarding, entering, leaving E824
  - stationary, except while alighting, boarding, entering, leaving E884.9
  - while alighting, boarding, entering, leaving, except off-road type motor vehicle E817
    - off-road type—*see* Fall, from, off-road type motor vehicle
- nonmotor road vehicle (while alighting, boarding) NEC E829
  - stationary, except while alighting, boarding, entering, leaving E884.9

Fall, falling—*continued*
- off road type motor vehicle (not on public highway) NEC E821
- on public highway E818
  - while alighting, boarding, entering, leaving E817
- snow vehicle—*see* Fall from snow vehicle, motor-driven
- one
  - deck to another on ship E834
    - due to accident to ship E831
  - level to another NEC E884.9
    - boat, ship, or watercraft E834
    - due to accident to watercraft E831
- pedal cycle E826
- playground equipment E884.0
- railway rolling stock, train, vehicle (while alighting, boarding) E804
  - with
    - collision (*see also* Collision, railway) E800
    - derailment (*see also* Derailment, railway) E802
    - explosion (*see also* Explosion, railway engine) E803
- rigging (aboard ship) E834
  - due to accident to watercraft E831
- roller skates E885.1
- scaffolding E881.1
- scooter (nonmotorized) E885.0
- sidewalk (curb) E880.1
  - moving E885.9
- skateboard E885.2
- skis E885.3
- snowboard E885.4
- snow vehicle, motor-driven (not on public highway) E820
  - on public highway E818
    - while alighting, boarding, entering, leaving E817
- stairs, steps E880.9
  - boat, ship, watercraft E833
    - due to accident to watercraft E831
  - motor bus, motor vehicle—*see* Fall, from, motor vehicle, while alighting, boarding
  - street car E829
- stationary vehicle NEC E884.9
- stepladder E881.0
- street car (while boarding, alighting) E829
  - stationary, except while boarding or alighting E884.9
- structure NEC E882
  - burning (uncontrolled fire) E891.8
    - in terrorism E979.3
- table E884.9
- toilet E884.6
- tower E882
- tree E884.9
- turret E882
- vehicle NEC—*see also* Accident, vehicle NEC
  - stationary E884.9
- viaduct E882
- wall E882
- wheelchair E884.3
- wheelies E885.1
- window E882

Fall, falling—*continued*
in, on
  aircraft (at landing, take-off) (in-transit)
    E843
    resulting from accident to aircraft—*see*
      categories E840-E842
  boat, ship, watercraft E835
    due to accident to watercraft E831
    one level to another NEC E834
    on ladder, stairs E833
  cutting or piercing instrument or machine
    E888.0
  deck (of boat, ship, watercraft) E835
    due to accident to watercraft E831
  escalator E880.0
  gangplank E835
  glass, broken E888.0
  knife E888.0
  ladder E881.0
    in boat, ship, watercraft E833
    due to accident to watercraft E831
  object
    edged, pointed or sharp E888.0
    other E888.1
  pitchfork E888.0
  railway rolling stock, train, vehicle (while
    alighting, boarding) E804
    with
      collision (*see also* Collision, railway)
        E800
      derailment (*see also* Derailment, railway)
        E802
      explosion (*see also* Explosion, railway
        engine) E803
  scaffolding E881.1
  scissors E888.0
  staircase, stairs, steps (*see also* Fall, from,
    stairs) E880.9
  street car E829
  water transport (*see also* Fall, in, boat) E835
into
  cavity E883.9
  dock E883.9
    from boat, ship, watercraft (*see also* Fall,
      from, boat) E832
  hold (of ship) E834
    due to accident to watercraft E831
  hole E883.9
  manhole E883.2
  moving part of machinery—*see* Accident,
    machine
  opening in surface NEC E883.9
  pit E883.9
  quarry E883.9
  shaft E883.9
  storm drain E883.2
  tank E883.9
  water (with drowning or submersion) E910.9
  well E883.1
late effect of NEC E929.3
object (*see also* Hit by, object, falling) E916
other E888.8
over
  animal E885.9
  cliff E884.1
  embankment E884.9
  small object E885.9
overboard (*see also* Fall, from, boat) E832
resulting in striking against object E888.1
  sharp E888.0
rock E916

Fall, falling—*continued*
same level NEC E888.9
  aircraft (any kind) E843
    resulting from accident to aircraft—*see*
      categories E840-E842
  boat, ship, watercraft E835
    due to accident to, collision, watercraft E831
  from
    collision, pushing, shoving, by or with
      other person(s) E886.9
    as, or caused by, a crowd E917.6
    in sports E886.0
    in-line skates E885.1
    roller skates E885.1
    scooter (nonmotorized) E885.0
    skateboard E885.2
    skis E885.3
    slipping, stumbling, tripping E885.9
    snowboard E885.4
  snowslide E916
    as avalanche E909.2
  stone E916
  through
    hatch (on ship) E834
    due to accident to watercraft E831
    roof E882
    window E882
  timber E916
  while alighting from, boarding, entering,
    leaving
  aircraft (any kind) E843
  motor bus, motor vehicle—*see* Fall, from,
    motor vehicle, while alighting, boarding
  nonmotor road vehicle NEC E829
  railway train E804
  street car E829
Fallen on by
animal (horse) (not being ridden) E906.8
being ridden (in sport or transport) E828
Fell or jumped from high place, so stated
  —*see Jumping, from, high place*
Felo-de-se (*see also* Suicide) E958.9
Fever
heat—*see* Heat
thermic—*see* Heat
Fight (hand) (fist) (foot) (*see also* Assault,
  fight) E960.0
Fire (accidental) (caused by great heat from
  appliance (electrical), hot object or hot
  substance) (secondary, resulting from
  explosion) E899
conflagration—*see* Conflagration
controlled, normal (in brazier, fireplace,
  furnace, or stove) (charcoal) (coal) (coke)
  (electric) (gas) (wood)
  bonfire E897
  brazier, not in building or structure E897
  in building or structure, except private
    dwelling (barn) (church) (convalescent or
    residential home) (factory) (farm
    outbuilding) (hospital) (hotel) (institution
    (educational) (dormitory) (residential))
    (private garage) (school) (shop) (store)
    (theatre) E896
  in private dwelling (apartment) (boarding
    house) (camping place) (caravan)
    (farmhouse) (home (private)) (house)
    (lodging house) (rooming house)
    (tenement) E895
  not in building or structure E897
  trash E897

Foreign body—*continued*
  eye (any part) E914
  eyelid E914
  hairball (stomach) (with obstruction) E915
  ingestion—*see* Foreign body, alimentary canal
  inhalation—*see* Foreign body, aspiration
  intestine (causing injury or obstruction) E915
  iris E914
  lacrimal apparatus E914
  larynx—*see* Foreign body, air passage
  late effect of NEC E929.8
  lung—*see* Foreign body, air passage
  mouth—*see* Foreign body, alimentary canal,
    mouth
  nasal passage—*see* Foreign body, air passage,
    nose
  nose—*see* Foreign body, air passage, nose
  ocular muscle E914
  operation wound (left in)—*see* Misadventure,
    foreign object
  orbit E914
  pharynx—*see* Foreign body, alimentary canal,
    pharynx
  rectum (causing injury or obstruction) E915
  stomach (hairball) (causing injury or
    obstruction) E915
  tear ducts or glands E914
  trachea—*see* Foreign body, air passage
  urethra (causing injury or obstruction) E915
  vagina (causing injury or obstruction) E915
Found dead, injured
  from exposure (to)—*see* Exposure
  on
    public highway E819
    railway right of way E807
Fracture (circumstances unknown or
    unspecified) E887
  due to specified external means—*see* manner
    of accident
  late effect of NEC E929.3
  occurring in water transport NEC E835
Freezing —*see* Cold, exposure to
Frostbite E901.0
  due to manmade conditions E901.1
Frozen —*see* Cold, exposure to

G

Garrotting, homicidal (attempted) E963
Gored E906.8
Gunshot wound (*see also* Shooting) E922.9

H

Hailstones, injury by E904.3
Hairball (stomach) (with obstruction) E915
Hanged himself (*see also* Hanging,
    self-inflicted) E983.0
Hang gliding E842
Hanging (accidental) E913.8
  caused by other person
    in accidental circumstances E913.8
    stated as
      intentional, homicidal E963
      undetermined whether accidental or
        intentional E983.0
  homicide (attempt) E963
  in bed or cradle E913.0
  legal execution E978

Hanging—*continued*
  self-inflicted (unspecified whether accidental
    or intentional) E983.0
    in accidental circumstances E913.8
    stated as intentional, purposeful E953.0
  stated as undetermined whether accidental or
    intentional E983.0
  suicidal (attempt) E953.0
Heat (apoplexy) (collapse) (cramps) (effects of)
    (excessive) (exhaustion) (fever) (prostration)
    (stroke) E900.9
  due to
    manmade conditions (listed in E900.1,
      except boat, ship, watercraft) E900.1
    weather (conditions) E900.0
  from
    electric heating apparatus causing burning E924.8
    nuclear explosion
      in
        terrorism E979.5
        war operations (see also War operations,
          injury due to, nuclear weapons)
          E996.2
  generated in, boiler, engine, evaporator, fire
    room of boat, ship, watercraft E838
  inappropriate in local application or packing in
    medical or surgical procedure E873.5
  late effect of NEC E989
Hemorrhage
  delayed following medical or surgical
    treatment without mention of
    misadventure—*see* Reaction, abnormal
  during medical or surgical treatment as
    misadventure—*see* Misadventure, cut
High
  altitude, effects E902.9
  level of radioactivity, effects—*see* Radiation
  pressure effects—*see also* Effects of, air
    pressure
    from rapid descent in water (causing caisson
      or divers' disease, palsy, or paralysis)
      E902.2
  temperature, effects—*see* Heat
Hit, hitting (accidental) by
  aircraft (propeller) (without accident to
    aircraft) E844
    unpowered E842
  avalanche E909.2
  being thrown against object in or part of
    motor vehicle (in motion) (on public
      highway) E818
    not on public highway E825
    nonmotor road vehicle NEC E829
    street car E829
  boat, ship, watercraft
    after fall from watercraft E838
    damaged, involved in accident E831
    while swimming, water skiing E838
  bullet (*see also* Shooting) E922.9
    from air gun E922.4
    in
      terrorism E979.4
      war operations E991.2
        rubber E991.0
  flare, Very pistol (*see also* Shooting) E922.8
  hailstones E904.3
  landslide E909.2
  law-enforcing agent (on duty) E975
    with blunt object (baton) (night stick) (stave)
      (truncheon) E973
  machine—*see* Accident, machine

Hit, hitting—*continued*
missile
  firearm (*see also* Shooting) E922.9
  in
    terrorism—*see* Terrorism, missle
    war operations—*see* War operations,
      missile
  motor vehicle (on public highway) (traffic
    accident) E814
  not on public highway, nontraffic accident
    E822
  nonmotor road vehicle NEC E829
object
  falling E916
    from, in, on
      aircraft E844
        due to accident to aircraft—*see*
          categories E840-E842
        unpowered E842
      boat, ship, watercraft E838
        due to accident to watercraft E831
      building E916
        burning E891.8
          in terrorism E979.3
          private E890.8
      cataclysmic
        earth surface movement or eruption
          E909.9
        storm E908.9
      cave-in E916
        with asphyxiation or suffocation (*see
          also* Suffocation, due to, cave-in)
          E913.3
      earthquake E909.0
      motor vehicle (in motion) (on public
        highway) E818
        not on public highway E825
        stationary E916
      nonmotor road vehicle NEC E829
      pedal cycle E826
      railway rolling stock, train, vehicle E806
      street car E829
      structure, burning NEC E891.8
      vehicle, stationary E916
  moving NEC—*see* Striking against, object
  projected NEC—*see* Striking against, object
  set in motion by
    compressed air or gas, spring, striking,
      throwing—*see* Striking against, object
    explosion—*see* Explosion
  thrown into, on, or towards
    motor vehicle (in motion) (on public
      highway) E818
    not on public highway E825
    nonmotor road vehicle NEC E829
    pedal cycle E826
    street car E829
  off-road type motor vehicle (not on public
    highway) E821
    on public highway E814
  other person(s) E917.9
    with blunt or thrown object E917.9
      in sports E917.0
        with subsequent fall E917.5
      intentionally, homicidal E968.2
    as, or caused by, a crowd E917.1
      with subsequent fall E917.6
      in sports E917.0
  pedal cycle E826

Hit, hitting—*continued*
police (on duty) E975
  with blunt object (baton) (nightstick) (stave)
    (truncheon) E973
railway, rolling stock, train, vehicle (part of)
  E805
shot—*see* Shooting
snow vehicle, motor-driven (not on public
  highway) E820
  on public highway E814
street car E829
vehicle NEC—*see* Accident, vehicle NEC
Homicide, homicidal (attempt) (justifiable) (*see
  also* Assault) E968.9
Hot
liquid, object, substance, accident caused
  by—*see also* Accident, caused by, hot, by
  type of substance
late effect of E929.8
place, effects—*see* Heat
weather, effects E900.0
Humidity, causing problem E904.3
Hunger E904.1
resulting from
  abandonment or neglect E904.0
  transport accident—*see* categories
    E800-E848
Hurricane (any injury) E908.0
Hypobarism, hypobaropathy —*see* Effects of,
  air pressure
Hypothermia —*see* Cold, exposure to

I

Ictus
caloris—*see* Heat
solaris E900.0
Ignition (accidental)
anesthetic gas in operating theatre E923.2
bedclothes
  with
    conflagration—*see* Conflagration
    ignition (of)
      clothing—*see* Ignition, clothes
      highly inflammable material (benzine)
        (fat) (gasoline) (kerosene) (paraffin)
        (petrol) E894
benzine E894
clothes, clothing (from controlled fire) (in
  building) E893.9
  with conflagration—*see* Conflagration
  from
    bonfire E893.2
    highly inflammable material E894
    sources or material as listed in E893.8
    trash fire E893.2
    uncontrolled fire—*see* Conflagration
  in
    private dwelling E893.0
    specified building or structure, except
      private dwelling E893.1
    not in building or structure E893.2
explosive material—*see* Explosion
fat E894
gasoline E894
kerosene E894
material
  explosive—*see* Explosion
  highly inflammable E894
    with conflagration—*see* Conflagration
    with explosion E923.2

Ignition—*continued*
nightdress—*see* Ignition, clothes
paraffin E894
petrol E894
Immersion —*see* Submersion
Implantation of quills of porcupine E906.8
Inanition (from) E904.9
hunger—*see* Lack of, food
resulting from homicidal intent E968.4
thirst—*see* Lack of, water
Inattention after, at birth E904.0
homicidal, infanticidal intent E968.4
Infanticide (*see also* Assault)
Ingestion
foreign body (causing injury) (with
obstruction)—*see* Foreign body, alimentary
canal
poisonous substance NEC—*see* Table of drugs
and chemicals
Inhalation
excessively cold substance, manmade E901.1
foreign body—*see* Foreign body, aspiration
liquid air, hydrogen, nitrogen E901.1
mucus, not of newborn (with asphyxia,
obstruction respiratory passage,
suffocation) E912
phlegm (with asphyxia, obstruction respiratory
passage, suffocation) E912
poisonous gas—*see* Table of drugs and chemicals
smoke from, due to
fire —*see* Fire
tobacco, second-hand E869.4
vomitus (with asphyxia, obstruction respiratory
passage, suffocation) E911
Injury, injured (accidental(ly)) NEC E928.9
by, caused by, from
air rifle (B-B gun) E922.4
animal (not being ridden) NEC E906.9
being ridden (in sport or transport) E828
assault (*see also* Assault) E968.9
avalanche E909.2
bayonet (*see also* Bayonet wound) E920.3
being thrown against some part of, or object
in
motor vehicle (in motion) (on public
highway) E818
not on public highway E825
nonmotor road vehicle NEC E829
off-road motor vehicle NEC E821
railway train E806
snow vehicle, motor-driven E820
street car E829
bending E927.8
bite, human E928.3
broken glass E920.8
bullet—*see* Shooting
cave-in (*see also* Suffocation, due to,
cave-in) E913.3
without asphyxiation or suffocation E916
cloudburst E908.8
component of firearm or air gun E928.7
cutting or piercing instrument (*see also* Cut)
E920.9
cyclone E908.1
earth surface movement or eruption E909.9
earthquake E909.0
electric current (*see also* Electric shock)
E925.9
explosion (*see also* Explosion) E923.9
of gun part E928.7
fire—*see* Fire

Injury, injured—*continued*
by —*continued*
flare, Very pistol E922.8
flood E908.2
foreign body—*see* Foreign body
gun recoil E928.7
hailstones E904.3
hurricane E908.0
landslide E909.2
law-enforcing agent, police, in course of
legal intervention—*see* Legal intervention
lightning E907
live rail or live wire—*see* Electric shock
machinery—*see also* Accident, machine
aircraft, without accident to aircraft E844
boat, ship, watercraft (deck) (engine room)
(galley) (laundry) (loading) E836
mechanism of firearm or air gun E928.7
missile
explosive E923.8
firearm—*see* Shooting
in
terrorism—*see* Terrorism, missile
war operations—*see* War operations,
missile
moving part of motor vehicle (in motion)
(on public highway) E818
not on public highway, nontraffic accident
E825
while alighting, boarding, entering,
leaving—*see* Fall, from, motor vehicle,
while alighting, boarding
nail E920.8
needle (sewing) E920.4
hypodermic E920.5
noise E928.1
object
fallen on
motor vehicle (in motion) (on public
highway) E818
not on public highway E825
falling—*see* Hit by, object, falling
paintball gun E922.5
radiation—*see* Radiation
railway rolling stock, train, vehicle (part of)
E805
door or window E806
recoil of firearm E928.7
rotating propeller, aircraft E844
rough landing of off-road type motor vehicle
(after leaving ground or rough terrain)
E821
snow vehicle E820
saber (*see also* Wound, saber) E920.3
shot—*see* Shooting
sound waves E928.1
splinter or sliver, wood E920.8
storm E908.9
straining E927.8
street car (door) E829
suicide (attempt) E958.9
sword E920.3
terrorism—*see* Terrorism
third rail—*see* Electric shock
thunderbolt E907
tidal wave E909.4
caused by storm E908.0
tornado E908.1
torrential rain E908.2
twisting E927.8
vehicle NEC—*see* Accident, vehicle NEC
vibration E928.2

Injury, injured—*continued*
by —*continued*
volcanic eruption E909.1
weapon burst, in war operations E993.9
weightlessness (in spacecraft, real or
simulated) E928.0
wood splinter or sliver E920.8
due to
civil insurrection—*see* War operations
occurring after cessation of hostilities
E998.9
terrorism—*see* Terrorism
war operations—*see* War operations
occurring after cessation of hostilities
E998.9
weapon of mass destruction [WMD] E997.3
homicidal (*see also* Assault) E968.9
in, on
civil insurrection—*see* War operations
fight E960.0
parachute descent (voluntary) (without
accident to aircraft) E844
with accident to aircraft—*see* categories
E840-E842
public highway E819
railway right of way E807
terrorism—*see* Terrorism
war operations—*see* War operations
inflicted (by)
in course of arrest (attempted), suppression
of disturbance, maintenance of order, by
law-enforcing agents—*see* Legal
intervention
law-enforcing agent (on duty)—*see* Legal
intervention
other person
stated as
accidental E928.9
homicidal, intentional—*see* Assault
undetermined whether accidental or
intentional—*see* Injury, stated as
undetermined
police (on duty)—*see* Legal intervention
late effect of E929.9
purposely (inflicted) by other person(s)—*see*
Assault
self-inflicted (unspecified whether accidental
or intentional) E988.9
stated as
accidental E928.9
intentionally, purposely E958.9
specified cause NEC E928.8
stated as
undetermined whether accidentally or
purposely inflicted (by) E988.9
cut (any part of body) E986
cutting or piercing instrument (classifiable
to E920) E986
drowning E984
explosive(s) (missile) E985.5
falling from high place E987.9
manmade structure, except residential E987.1
natural site E987.2
residential premises E987.0
hanging E983.0
knife E986
late effect of E989
puncture (any part of body) E986
shooting—*see* Shooting, stated as undetermined
whether accidental or intentional
specified means NEC E988.8

Injury, injured—*continued*
stab (any part of body) E986
strangulation—*see* Suffocation, stated as
undetermined whether accidental or
intentional
submersion E984
suffocation—*see* Suffocation, stated as
undetermined whether accidental or
intentional
to child due to criminal abortion E968.8
Insufficient nourishment —*see also* Lack of,
food
homicidal intent E968.4
Insulation, effects —*see* Heat
Interruption of respiration by
food lodged in esophagus E911
foreign body, except food, in esophagus E912
Intervention, legal —*see* Legal intervention
Intoxication, drug or poison —*see* Table of
drugs and chemicals
Irradiation —*see* Radiation

J

Jammed (accidentally)
between objects (moving) (stationary and
moving) E918
in object E918
Jumped or fell from high place, so stated
—*see* Jumping, from, high place, stated as
in undetermined circumstances
Jumping
before train, vehicle or other moving object
(unspecified whether accidental or
intentional) E988.0
stated as
intentional, purposeful E958.0
suicidal (attempt) E958.0
from
aircraft
by parachute (voluntarily) (without
accident to aircraft) E844
due to accident to aircraft—*see* categories
E840-E842
boat, ship, watercraft (into water)
after accident to, fire on, watercraft E830
and subsequently struck by (part of) boat
E831
burning, crushed, sinking E830
and subsequently struck by (part of) boat
E831
voluntarily, without accident (to boat) with
injury other than drowning or
submersion E883.0
building—*see also* Jumping, from, high
place
burning (uncontrolled fire) E891.8
in terrorism E979.3
private E890.8
cable car (not on rails) E847
on rails E829
high place
in accidental circumstances or in
sport—*see* categories E880-E884
stated as
with intent to injure self E957.9
man-made structures NEC E957.1
natural sites E957.2
residential premises E957.0

Jumping—*continued*

in undetermined circumstances E987.9
man-made structures NEC E987.1
natural sites E987.2
residential premises E987.0
suicidal (attempt) E957.9
man-made structures NEC E957.1
natural sites E957.1
residential premises E957.0
motor vehicle (in motion) (on public highway)—*see* Fall, from, motor vehicle
nonmotor road vehicle NEC E829
street car E829
structure—*see also* Jumping, from, high place
burning NEC (uncontrolled fire) E891.8
in terrorism E979.3
into water
with injury other than drowning or submersion E883.0
drowning or submersion—*see* Submersion
from, off, watercraft—*see* Jumping, from, boat

Justifiable homicide —*see* Assault

K

Kicked by

animal E906.8
person(s) (accidentally) E917.9
with intent to injure or kill E960.0
as, or caused by a crowd E917.1
with subsequent fall E917.6
in fight E960.0
in sports E917.0
with subsequent fall E917.5

Kicking against

object (moving) E917.9
in sports E917.0
with subsequent fall E917.5
stationary E917.4
with subsequent fall E917.8
person—*see* Striking against, person

Killed, killing (accidentally) NEC (*see also* Injury) E928.9

in
action—*see* War operations
brawl, fight (hand) (fists) (foot) E960.0
by weapon—*see also* Assault
cutting, piercing E966
firearm—*see* Shooting, homicide
self
stated as
accident E928.9
suicide—*see* Suicide
unspecified whether accidental or suicidal E988.9

Knocked down (accidentally) (by) NEC E928.9

animal (not being ridden) E906.8
being ridden (in sport or transport) E828
blast from explosion (*see also* Explosion) E923.9
crowd, human stampede E917.6
late effect of—*see* Late effect
person (accidentally) E917.9
in brawl, fight E960.0
in sports E917.5
transport vehicle—*see* vehicle involved under Hit by
while boxing E917.5

L

Laceration NEC E928.9

Lack of

air (refrigerator or closed place), suffocation by E913.2
care (helpless person) (infant) (newborn) E904.0
homicidal intent E968.4
food except as result of transport accident E904.1
helpless person, infant, newborn due to abandonment or neglect E904.0
water except as result of transport accident E904.2
helpless person, infant, newborn due to abandonment or neglect E904.0

Landslide E909.2

falling on, hitting
motor vehicle (any) (in motion) (on or off public highway) E909.2
railway rolling stock, train, vehicle E909.2

Late effect of

accident NEC (accident classifiable to E928.9) E929.9
specified NEC (accident classifiable to E910-E928.8) E929.8
assault E969
fall, accidental (accident classifiable to E880-E888) E929.3
fire, accident caused by (accident classifiable to E890-E899) E929.4
homicide, attempt (any means) E969
injury due to terrorism E999.1
injury undetermined whether accidentally or purposely inflicted (injury classifiable to E980-E988) E989
legal intervention (injury classifiable to E970-E976) E977
medical or surgical procedure, test or therapy
as, or resulting in, or from
abnormal or delayed reaction or complication—*see* Reaction, abnormal
misadventure—*see* Misadventure
motor vehicle accident (accident classifiable to E810-E825) E929.0
natural or environmental factor, accident due to (accident classifiable to E900-E909) E929.5
poisoning, accidental (accident classifiable to E850-E858, E860-E869) E929.2
suicide, attempt (any means) E959
transport accident NEC (accident classifiable to E800-E807, E826-E838, E840-E848) E929.1
war operations, injury due to (injury classifiable to E990-E998) E999.0

Launching pad accident E845

Legal

execution, any method E978
intervention (by) (injury from) E976
baton E973
bayonet E974
blow E975
blunt object (baton) (nightstick) (stave) (truncheon) E973
cutting or piercing instrument E974
dynamite E971
execution, any method E973
explosive(s) (shell) E971
firearms(s) E970

Legal—*continued*
  gas (asphyxiation) (poisoning) (tear) E972
  grenade E971
  late effect of E977
  machine gun E970
  manhandling E975
  mortar bomb E971
  nightstick E973
  revolver E970
  rifle E970
  specified means NEC E975
  stabbing E974
  stave E973
  truncheon E973
Lifting, injury in E927.8
Lightning (shock) (stroke) (struck by) E907
Liquid (noncorrosive) in eye E914
  corrosive E924.1
Loss of control
  motor vehicle (on public highway) (without
    antecedent collision) E816
    with
      antecedent collision on public highway
        —*see* Collision, motor vehicle
      involving any object, person or vehicle
        not on public highway E816
      on public highway—*see* Collision, motor
        vehicle
    not on public highway, nontraffic accident
      E825
      with antecedent collision—*see* Collision,
        motor vehicle, not on public highway
    off-road type motor vehicle (not on public
      highway) E821
      on public highway—*see* Loss of control,
        motor vehicle
    snow vehicle, motor-driven (not on public
      highway) E820
      on public highway—*see* Loss of control,
        motor vehicle
Lost at sea E832
  with accident to watercraft E830
  in war operations E995.8
Low
  pressure, effects—*see* Effects of, air pressure
  temperature, effects—*see* Cold, exposure to
**Lying before train, vehicle or other moving
  object** (unspecified whether accidental or
  intentional) E988.0
  stated as intentional, purposeful, suicidal
    (attempt) E958.0
Lynching (*see also* Assault) E968.9

M

**Malfunction, atomic power plant in water
  transport** E838
Mangled (accidentally) NEC E928.9
Manhandling (in brawl, fight) E960.0
  legal intervention E975
Manslaughter (nonaccidental)—*see* Assault
Marble in nose E912
Mauled by animal E906.8
Medical procedure, complication of
  delayed or as an abnormal reaction without
    mention of misadventure—*see* Reaction,
    abnormal
  due to or as a result of misadventure—*see*
    Misadventure
Melting of fittings and furniture in burning
  in terrorism E979.3

Minamata disease E865.2
Misadventure(s) to patient(s) during surgical or
  medical care E876.9
  contaminated blood, fluid, drug or biological
    substance (presence of agents and toxins
    as listed in E875) E875.9
    administered (by) NEC E875.9
      infusion E875.0
      injection E875.1
      specified means NEC E875.2
      transfusion E875.0
      vaccination E875.1
  cut, cutting, puncture, perforation or
    hemorrhage (accidental) (inadvertent)
    (inappropriate) (during) E870.9
    aspiration of fluid or tissue (by puncture or
      catheterization, except heart) E870.5
    biopsy E870.8
      needle (aspirating) E870.5
    blood sampling E870.5
    catheterization E870.5
      heart E870.6
    dialysis (kidney) E870.2
    endoscopic examination E870.4
    enema E870.7
    infusion E870.1
    injection E870.3
    lumbar puncture E870.5
    needle biopsy E870.5
    paracentesis, abdominal E870.5
    perfusion E870.2
    specified procedure NEC E870.8
    surgical operation E870.0
    thoracentesis E870.5
    transfusion E870.1
    vaccination E870.3
  excessive amount of blood or other fluid
    during transfusion or infusion E873.0
  failure
    in dosage E873.9
      electroshock therapy E873.4
      inappropriate temperature (too hot or too
        cold) in local application and packing
        E873.5
      infusion
        excessive amount of fluid E873.0
        incorrect dilution of fluid E873.1
      insulin-shock therapy E873.4
      nonadministration of necessary drug or
        medicinal E873.6
      overdose—*see also* Overdose
        radiation, in therapy E873.2
      radiation
        inadvertent exposure of patient (receiving
          radiation for test or therapy) E873.3
        not receiving radiation for test or
          therapy—*see* Radiation
        overdose E873.2
      specified procedure NEC 873.8
      transfusion
        excessive amount of blood E873.0
    mechanical, of instrument or apparatus
      (during procedure) E874.9
      aspiration of fluid or tissue (by puncture or
        catheterization, except of heart) E874.4
      biopsy E874.8
        needle (aspirating) E874.4
      blood sampling E874.4
      catheterization E874.4
        heart E874.5
      dialysis (kidney) E874.2

Misadventure(s)—*continued*
  endoscopic examination E874.3
  enema E874.8
  infusion E874.1
  injection E874.8
  lumbar puncture E874.4
  needle biopsy E874.4
  paracentesis, abdominal E874.4
  perfusion E874.2
  specified procedure NEC E874.8
  surgical operation E874.0
  thoracentesis E874.4
  transfusion E874.1
  vaccination E874.8
  sterile precautions (during procedure) E872.9
  aspiration of fluid or tissue (by puncture or
    catheterization, except heart) E872.5
  biopsy E872.8
    needle (aspirating) E872.5
  blood sampling E872.5
  catheterization E872.5
    heart E872.6
  dialysis (kidney) E872.2
  endoscopic examination E872.4
  enema E872.8
  infusion E872.1
  injection E872.3
  lumbar puncture E872.5
  needle biopsy E872.5
  paracentesis, abdominal E872.5
  perfusion E872.2
  removal of catheter or packing E872.8
  specified procedure NEC E872.8
  surgical operation E872.0
  thoracentesis E872.5
  transfusion E872.1
  vaccination E872.3
  suture or ligature during surgical procedure
    E876.2
  to introduce or to remove tube or instrument
    E876.4
  foreign object left in body—*see*
    Misadventure, foreign object
  foreign object left in body (during procedure)
    E871.9
  aspiration of fluid or tissue (by puncture or
    catheterization, except heart) E871.5
  biopsy E871.8
    needle (aspirating) E871.5
  blood sampling E871.5
  catheterization E871.5
    heart E871.6
  dialysis (kidney) E871.2
  endoscopic examination E871.4
  enema E871.8
  infusion E871.1
  injection E871.3
  lumbar puncture E871.5
  needle biopsy E871.5
  paracentesis, abdominal E871.5
  perfusion E871.2
  removal of catheter or packing E871.7
  specified procedure NEC E871.8
  surgical operation E871.0
  thoracentesis E871.5
  transfusion E871.1
  vaccination E871.3
  hemorrhage—*see* Misadventure, cut
  inadvertent exposure of patient to radiation
    (being received for test or therapy) E873.3

Misadventure(s)—*continued*
  inappropriate
    temperature (too hot or too cold) in local
      application or packing E873.5
  infusion—*see also* Misadventure, by specific
    type, infusion
    excessive amount of fluid E873.0
    incorrect dilution of fluid E873.1
    wrong fluid E876.1
  mismatched blood in transfusion E876.0
  nonadministration of necessary drug or
    medicinal E873.6
  overdose—*see also* Overdose
    radiation, in therapy E873.2
  perforation—*see* Misadventure, cut
  performance of correct operation (procedure)
    on wrong
    body part E876.7
    side E876.7
    site E876.7
  performance of operation (procedure)
    intended for another patient E876.6
    on patient not scheduled for surgery E876.6
    on wrong patient E876.6
  performance of wrong operation on correct
    patient E876.5
  puncture—*see* Misadventure, cut
  specified type NEC E876.8
    failure
      suture or ligature during surgical operation
        E876.2
      to introduce or to remove tube or
        instrument E876.4
        foreign object left in body E871.9
    infusion of wrong fluid E876.1
    transfusion of mismatched blood E876.0
    wrong
      fluid in infusion E876.1
      placement of endotracheal tube during
        anesthetic procedure E876.3
  transfusion—*see also* Misadventure, by
    specific type, transfusion
    excessive amount of blood E873.0
    mismatched blood E876.0
  wrong
    device implanted into correct surgical site
      E876.5
    procedure (operation) performed on the
      correct patient E876.5
    drug given in error—*see* Table of drugs and
      chemicals
    fluid in infusion E876.1
    placement of endotracheal tube during
      anesthetic procedure E876.3
Motion (effects) E903
  sickness E903
Mountain sickness E902.0
**Mucus aspiration or inhalation, not of
  newborn** (with asphyxia, obstruction
  respiratory passage, suffocation) E912
Mudslide of cataclysmic nature E909.2
Murder (attempt) (*see also* Assault) E968.9

N

Nail, injury by E920.8
Needlestick (sewing needle) E920.4
  hypodermic E920.5
Neglect —*see also* Privation
  criminal E968.4
  homicidal intent E968.4

Noise (causing injury) (pollution) E928.1
Nuclear weapon (see also War operations, injury due to, nuclear weapons) E996.9

O

Object
  falling
    from, in, on, hitting
      aircraft E844
        due to accident to aircraft—see categories E840-E842
      machinery—see also Accident, machine
        not in operation E916
      motor vehicle (in motion) (on public highway) E818
        not on public highway E825
        stationary E916
      nonmotor road vehicle NEC E829
      pedal cycle E826
      person E916
      railway rolling stock, train, vehicle E806
      street car E829
      watercraft E838
        due to accident to watercraft E831
  set in motion by
    accidental explosion of pressure vessel—see category E921
    firearm—see category E922
    machine(ry)—see Accident, machine
    transport vehicle—see categories E800-E848
  thrown from, in, on, towards
    aircraft E844
    cable car (not on rails) E847
      on rails E829
    motor vehicle (in motion) (on public highway) E818
      not on public highway E825
    nonmotor road vehicle NEC E829
    pedal cycle E826
    street car E829
    vehicle NEC—see Accident, vehicle NEC
Obstruction
  air passages, larynx, respiratory passages
    by
      external means NEC—see Suffocation
      food, any type (regurgitated) (vomited) E911
      material or object, except food E912
      mucus E912
      phlegm E912
      vomitus E911
  digestive tract, except mouth or pharynx
    by
      food, any type E915
      foreign body (any) E915
  esophagus
    food E911
    foreign body, except food E912
    without asphyxia or obstruction of respiratory passage E915
  mouth or pharynx
    by
      food, any type E911
      material or object, except food E912
  respiration—see Obstruction, air passages
Oil in eye E914
Overdose
  anesthetic (drug)—see Table of drugs and chemicals
  drug—see Table of drugs and chemicals

Overexertion E927.9
  from
    lifting E927.8
    maintaining prolonged positions E927.1
      holding E927.1
      sitting E927.1
      standing E927.1
    prolonged static position E927.1
    pulling E927.8
    pushing E927.8
    sudden strenuous movement E927.0
Overexposure (accidental) (to)
  cold (see also Cold, exposure to) E901.9
    due to manmade conditions E901.1
  heat (see also Heat) E900.9
  radiation—see Radiation
  radioactivity—see Radiation
  sun, except sunburn E900.0
  weather—see Exposure
  wind—see Exposure
Overheated (see also Heat) E900.9
Overlaid E913.0
Overturning (accidental)
  animal-drawn vehicle E827
  boat, ship, watercraft
    causing
      drowning, submersion E830
      injury except drowning, submersion E831
  machinery—see Accident, machine
  motor vehicle (see also Loss of control, motor vehicle) E816
    with antecedent collision on public highway—see Collision, motor vehicle
    not on public highway, nontraffic accident E825
      with antecedent collision—see Collision, motor vehicle, not on public highway
  nonmotor road vehicle NEC E829
  off-road type motor vehicle—see Loss of control, off-road type motor vehicle
  pedal cycle E826
  railway rolling stock, train, vehicle (see also Derailment, railway) E802
  street car E829
  vehicle NEC—see Accident, vehicle NEC

P

Palsy, divers' E902.2
Parachuting (voluntary) (without accident to aircraft) E844
  due to accident to aircraft—see categories E840-E842
Paralysis
  divers' E902.2
  lead or saturnine E866.0
    from pesticide NEC E863.4
Pecked by bird E906.8
Performance of correct operation (procedure) on wrong
  body part E876.7
  side E876.7
  site E876.7
Performance of operation (procedure)
  intended for another patient E876.6
  on patient not scheduled for surgery E876.6
  on wrong patient E876.6
Performance of wrong operation on correct patient E876.5

Phlegm aspiration or inhalation (with asphyxia, obstruction respiratory passage, suffocation) E912
Piercing (*see also* Cut) E920.9
  by slide trigger mechanism, scope or other part of gun E928.7
Pinched
  between objects (moving) (stationary and moving) E918
  by slide trigger mechanism, scope or other part of gun E928.7
  in object E918
Pinned under
  machine(ry)—*see* Accident, machine
Place of occurrence of accident —*see* Accident (to), occurring (at) (in)
Plumbism E866.0
  from insecticide NEC E863.4
Poisoning (accidental) (by)—*see also* Table of drugs and chemicals
  carbon monoxide
  generated by
    aircraft in transit E844
    motor vehicle
      in motion (on public highway) E818
      not on public highway E825
    watercraft (in transit) (not in transit) E838
  caused by injection of poisons or toxins into or through skin by plant thorns, spines, or other mechanism E905.7
    marine or sea plants E905.6
  fumes or smoke due to
    conflagration—*see* Conflagration
    explosion or fire—*see* Fire
    ignition—*see* Ignition
  gas
    in legal intervention E972
    legal execution, by E978
    on watercraft E838
    used as anesthetic—*see* Table of drugs and chemicals
  in
    terrorism (chemical weapons) E979.7
    war operations E997.2
  late effect of—*see* Late effect
  legal
    execution E978
    intervention
      by gas E972
Pressure, external, causing asphyxia, suffocation (*see also* Suffocation) E913.9
Privation E904.9
  food (*see also* Lack of, food) E904.1
  helpless person, infant, newborn due to abandonment or neglect E904.0
  late effect of NEC E929.5
  resulting from transport accident—*see* categories E800-E848
  water (*see also* Lack of, water) E904.2
Projected objects, striking against or struck by —*see* Striking against, object
Prolonged stay in
  high altitude (causing conditions as listed in E902.0) E902.0
  weightless environment E928.0
Prostration
  heat—*see* Heat
Pulling, injury in E927.8

Puncture, puncturing (*see also* Cut) E920.9
  by
    plant thorns or spines E920.8
    toxic reaction E905.7
      marine or sea plants E905.6
    sea-urchin spine E905.6
Pushing (injury in) (overexertion) E927.8
  by other person(s) (accidental) E917.9
    as, or caused by, a crowd, human stampede E917.1
      with subsequent fall E917.6
    before moving vehicle or object
      stated as
        intentional, homicidal E968.5
        undetermined whether accidental or intentional E988.8
  from
    high place
      in accidental circumstances—*see* categories E880-E884
      stated as
        intentional, homicidal E968.1
        undetermined whether accidental or intentional E987.9
        man-made structure, except residential E987.1
        natural site E987.2
        residential E987.0
    motor vehicle (*see also* Fall, from, motor vehicle) E818
      stated as
        intentional, homicidal E968.5
        undetermined whether accidental or intentional E988.8
    in sports E917.0
      with fall E886.0
    with fall E886.9
      in sports E886.0

R

Radiation (exposure to) E926.9
  abnormal reaction to medical test or therapy E879.2
  arc lamps E926.2
  atomic power plant (malfunction) NEC E926.9
    in water transport E838
  electromagnetic, ionizing E926.3
  gamma rays E926.3
  in
    terrorism (from or following nuclear explosion) (direct) (secondary) E979.5
      laser E979.8
    war operations (see also War operations, injury due to, nuclear weapons) E996.3
      laser(s) E997.0
    water transport E838
  inadvertent exposure of patient (receiving test or therapy) E873.3
  infrared (heaters and lamps) E926.1
    excessive heat E900.1
  ionized, ionizing (particles, artificially accelerated) E926.8
    electromagnetic E926.3
  isotopes, radioactive—*see* Radiation, radioactive isotopes

Radiation—*continued*
  laser(s) E926.4
    in
      terrorism E979.8
      war operations E997.0
    misadventure in medical care—*see*
      Misadventure, failure, in dosage,
      radiation
  late effect of NEC E929.8
    excessive heat from—*see* Heat
  light sources (visible) (ultraviolet) E926.2
  misadventure in medical or surgical
    procedure—*see* Misadventure, failure, in
    dosage, radiation
  overdose (in medical or surgical procedure)
    E873.2
  radar E926.0
  radioactive isotopes E926.5
    atomic power plant malfunction E926.5
      in water transport E838
    misadventure in medical or surgical
      treatment—*see* Misadventure, failure, in
      dosage, radiation
  radiobiologicals—*see* Radiation, radioactive
    isotopes
  radiofrequency E926.0
  radiopharmaceuticals—*see* Radiation,
    radioactive isotopes
  radium NEC E926.9
  sun E926.2
    excessive heat from E900.0
  tanning bed E926.2
  welding arc or torch E926.2
    excessive heat from E900.1
  x-rays (hard) (soft) E926.3
    misadventure in medical or surgical
      treatment—*see* Misadventure, failure, in
      dosage, radiation
Rape E960.1
Reaction —abnormal to or following(medical or
    surgical procedure) E879.9
  amputation (of limbs) E878.5
  anastomosis (arteriovenous) (blood vessel)
    (gastrojejunal) (skin) (tendon) (natural,
    artificial material, tissue) E878.2
    external stoma, creation of E878.3
  aspiration (of fluid) E879.4
    tissue E879.8
  biopsy E879.8
  blood
    sampling E879.7
    transfusion
      procedure E879.8
  bypass—*see* Reaction, abnormal, anastomosis
  catheterization
    cardiac E879.0
    urinary E879.6
  colostomy E878.3
  cystostomy E878.3
  dialysis (kidney) E879.1
  drugs or biologicals—*see* Table of drugs and
    chemicals
  duodenostomy E878.3
  electroshock therapy E879.3
  formation of external stoma E878.3
  gastrostomy E878.3
  graft—*see* Reaction, abnormal, anastomosis
  hypothermia E879.8

Reaction—*continued*
  implant, implantation (of)
    artificial
      internal device (cardiac pacemaker)
        (electrodes in brain) (heart valve
        prosthesis) (orthopedic) E878.1
      material or tissue (for anastomosis or
        bypass) E878.2
        with creation of external stoma E878.3
    natural tissues (for anastomosis or bypass)
      E878.2
      as transplantation—*see* Reaction, abnormal,
        transplant
      with creation of external stoma E878.3
  infusion
    procedure E879.8
  injection
    procedure E879.8
  insertion of gastric or duodenal sound E879.5
  insulin-shock therapy E879.3
  lumbar puncture E879.4
  perfusion E879.1
  procedures other than surgical operation (*see
    also* Reaction, abnormal, by specific type
    of procedure) E879.9
    specified procedure NEC E879.8
  radiological procedure or therapy E879.2
  removal of organ (partial) (total) NEC E878.6
    with
      anastomosis, bypass or graft E878.2
      formation of external stoma E878.3
      implant of artificial internal device E878.1
      transplant(ation)
        partial organ E878.4
        whole organ E878.0
  sampling
    blood E879.7
    fluid NEC E879.4
    tissue E879.8
  shock therapy E879.3
  surgical operation (*see also* Reaction,
    abnormal, by specified type of operation)
    E878.9
    restorative NEC E878.4
      with
        anastomosis, bypass or graft E878.2
        formation of external stoma E878.3
        implant(ation)—*see* Reaction, abnormal,
          implant
        transplant(ation)—*see* Reaction,
          abnormal, transplant
      specified operation NEC E878.8
  thoracentesis E879.4
  transfusion
    procedure E879.8
  transplant, transplantation (heart) (kidney)
    (liver) E878.0
    partial organ E878.4
  ureterostomy E878.3
  vaccination E879.8
Reduction in
  atmospheric pressure—*see also* Effects of, air
    pressure
    while surfacing from
      deep water diving causing caisson or
        divers' disease, palsy or paralysis
        E902.2
      underground E902.8
Residual (effect)—*see* Late effect

Rock falling on or hitting (accidentally)
  motor vehicle (in motion) (on public highway)
    E818
    not on public highway E825
  nonmotor road vehicle NEC E829
  pedal cycle E826
  person E916
  railway rolling stock, train, vehicle E806
Running off, away
  animal (being ridden) (in sport or transport)
    E828
    not being ridden E906.8
  animal-drawn vehicle E827
  rails, railway (*see also* Derailment) E802
  roadway
    motor vehicle (without antecedent collision)
      E816
      nontraffic accident E825
      with antecedent collision—*see* Collision,
        motor vehicle, not on public highway
    with
      antecedent collision—*see* Collision motor
        vehicle
      subsequent collision
        involving any object, person or vehicle
          not on public highway E816
          on public highway E811
    nonmotor road vehicle NEC E829
    pedal cycle E826
Run over (accidentally) (by)
  animal (not being ridden) E906.8
    being ridden (in sport or transport) E828
  animal-drawn vehicle E827
  machinery—*see* Accident, machine
  motor vehicle (on public highway)—*see* Hit
    by, motor vehicle
  nonmotor road vehicle NEC E829
  railway train E805
  street car E829
  vehicle NEC E848

S

Saturnism E866.0
  from insecticide NEC E863.4
Scald, scalding (accidental) (by) (from) (in)
    E924.0
  acid—*see* Scald, caustic
  boiling tap water E924.2
  caustic or corrosive liquid, substance E924.1
    swallowed—*see* Table of drugs and
      chemicals
  homicide (attempt)—*see* Assault, burning
  inflicted by other person
    stated as
      intentional or homicidal E968.3
      undetermined whether accidental or
        intentional E988.2
  late effect of NEC E929.8
  liquid (boiling) (hot) E924.0
  local application of externally applied
    substance in medical or surgical care
    E873.5
  molten metal E924.0
  self-inflicted (unspecified whether accidental
    or intentional) E988.2
    stated as intentional, purposeful E958.2
  stated as undetermined whether accidental or
    intentional E988.2
  steam E924.0

Scald, scalding—*continued*
  tap water (boiling) E924.2
  transport accident—*see* categories E800-E848
  vapor E924.0
Scratch, cat E906.8
Sea
  sickness E903
Self-mutilation —*see* Suicide
Sequelai (of)
  in
    terrorism E999.1
    war operations E999.0
Shock
  anaphylactic (*see also* Table of drugs and
    chemicals) E947.9
    due to
      bite (venomous)—*see* Bite, venomous NEC
      sting—*see* Sting
  electric (*see also* Electric shock) E925.9
  from electric appliance or current (*see also*
    Electric shock) E925.9
Shooting, shot (accidental(ly)) E922.9
  air gun E922.4
  BB gun E922.4
  hand gun (pistol) (revolver) E922.0
  himself (*see also* Shooting, self-inflicted)
    E985.4
    hand gun (pistol) (revolver) E985.0
    military firearm, except hand gun E985.3
      hand gun (pistol) (revolver) E985.0
    rifle (hunting) E985.2
      military E985.3
    shotgun (automatic) E985.1
    specified firearm NEC E985.4
    Verey pistol E985.4
  homicide (attempt) E965.4
    air gun E968.6
    BB gun E968.6
    hand gun (pistol) (revolver) E965.0
    military firearm, except hand gun E965.3
      hand gun (pistol) (revolver) E965.0
    paintball gun E965.4
    rifle (hunting) E965.2
      military E965.3
    shotgun (automatic) E965.1
    specified firearm NEC E965.4
    Verey pistol E965.4
  inflicted by other person
    in accidental circumstances E922.9
      hand gun (pistol) (revolver) E922.0
      military firearm, except hand gun E922.3
        hand gun (pistol) (revolver) E922.0
      rifle (hunting) E922.2
        military E922.3
      shotgun (automatic) E922.1
      specified firearm NEC E922.8
      Verey pistol E922.8
    stated as
      intentional, homicidal E965.4
        hand gun (pistol) (revolver) E965.0
        military firearm, except hand gun E965.3
          hand gun (pistol) (revolver) E965.0
        paintball gun E965.4
        rifle (hunting) E965.2
          military E965.3
        shotgun (automatic) E965.1
        specified firearm E965.4
        Verey pistol E965.4

Shooting, shot—*continued*
    undetermined whether accidental or
        intentional E985.4
        air gun E985.6
        BB gun E985.6
        hand gun (pistol) (revolver) E985.0
        military firearm, except hand gun E985.3
          hand gun (pistol) (revolver) E985.0
        paintball gun E985.7
        rifle (hunting) E985.2
        shotgun (automatic) E985.1
        specified firearm NEC E985.4
        Verey pistol E985.4
  in
    terrorism—*see* Terrorism, shooting
    war operations—*see* War operations,
      shooting
  legal
    execution E978
    intervention E970
  military firearm, except hand gun E922.3
    hand gun (pistol) (revolver) E922.0
  paintball gun E922.5
  rifle (hunting) 922.2
    military E922.3
  self-inflicted (unspecified whether accidental
    or intentional) E985.4
    air gun E985.6
    BB gun E985.6
    hand gun (pistol) (revolver) E985.0
    military firearm, except hand gun E985.3
      hand gun (pistol) (revolver) E985.0
    paintball gun E985.7
    rifle (hunting) E985.2
      military E985.3
    shotgun (automatic) E985.1
    specified firearm NEC E985.4
  stated as
    accidental E922.9
      hand gun (pistol) (revolver) E922.0
      military firearm, except hand gun E922.3
        hand gun (pistol) (revolver) E922.0
      paintball gun E922.5
      rifle (hunting) E922.2
        military E922.3
      shotgun (automatic) E922.1
      specified firearm NEC E922.8
      Verey pistol E922.8
    intentional, purposeful E955.4
      hand gun (pistol) (revolver) E955.0
      military firearm, except hand gun E955.3
        hand gun (pistol) (revolver) E955.0
      paintball gun E955.7
      rifle (hunting) E955.2
        military E955.3
      shotgun (automatic) E955.1
      specified firearm NEC E955.4
      Verey pistol E955.4
  shotgun (automatic) E922.1
  specified firearm NEC E922.8
  stated as undetermined whether accidental or
    intentional E985.4
    hand gun (pistol) (revolver) E985.0
    military firearm, except hand gun E985.3
      hand gun (pistol) (revolver) E985.0
    paintball gun E985.7
    rifle (hunting) E985.2
      military E985.3
    shotgun (automatic) E985.1
    specified firearm NEC E985.4
    Verey pistol E985.4

Shooting, shot—*continued*
  suicidal (attempt) E955.4
    air gun E955.6
    BB gun E955.6
    hand gun (pistol) (revolver) E955.0
    military firearm, except hand gun E955.3
      hand gun (pistol) (revolver) E955.0
    paintball gun E955.7
    rifle (hunting) E955.2
      military E955.3
    shotgun (automatic) E955.1
    specified firearm NEC E955.4
    Verey pistol E955.4
  Verey pistol E922.8
Shoving (accidentally) by other person (*see also*
  Pushing by other person) E917.9
Sickness
  air E903
  alpine E902.0
  car E903
  motion E903
  mountain E902.0
  sea E903
  travel E903
Sinking (accidental)
  boat, ship, watercraft (causing drowning,
    submersion) E830
  causing injury except drowning, submersion
    E831
Siriasis E900.0
Skydiving E844
Slashed wrists (*see also* Cut, self-inflicted)
  E986
Slipping (accidental)
  on
    deck (of boat, ship, watercraft) (icy) (oily)
      (wet) E835
    ice E885.9
    ladder of ship E833
      due to accident to watercraft E831
    mud E885.9
    oil E885.9
    snow E885.9
    stairs of ship E833
      due to accident to watercraft E831
    surface
      slippery E885.9
      wet E885.9
Sliver, wood, injury by E920.8
Smothering, smothered (*see also* Suffocation)
  E913.9
**Smouldering building or structure in
  terrorism** E979.3
Sodomy (assault) E960.1
Solid substance in eye (any part) or adnexa
  E914
Sound waves (causing injury) E928.1
Splinter, injury by E920.8
Stab, stabbing E966
  accidental—*see* Cut
Starvation E904.1
  helpless person, infant, newborn—*see* Lack of
    food
  homicidal intent E968.4
  late effect of NEC E929.5
  resulting from accident connected with
    transport—*see* categories E800-E848

Stepped on
by
  animal (not being ridden) E906.8
    being ridden (in sport or transport) E828
  crowd E917.1
  person E917.9
    in sports E917.0
  in sports E917.0
Stepping on
object (moving) E917.9
  in sports E917.0
    with subsequent fall E917.5
  stationary E917.4
    with subsequent fall E917.8
person E917.9
  as, or caused by a crowd E917.1
    with subsequent fall E917.6
  in sports E917.0
Sting E905.9
ant E905.5
bee E905.3
caterpillar E905.5
coral E905.6
hornet E905.3
insect NEC E905.5
jelly fish E905.6
marine animal or plant E905.6
nematocysts E905.6
scorpion E905.2
sea anemone E905.6
sea cucumber E905.6
wasp E905.3
yellow jacket E905.3
Storm E908.9
specified type NEC E908.8
Straining, injury in E927.8
Strangling —*see* Suffocation
Strangulation —*see* Suffocation
Strenuous movements (in recreational or other
  activities) E927.8
Striking against
bottom (when jumping or diving into water)
  E883.0
object (moving) E917.9
  caused by crowd E917.1
    with subsequent fall E917.6
  furniture E917.3
    with subsequent fall E917.7
  in
    running water E917.2
      with drowning or submersion—*see*
        Submersion
    sports E917.0
      with subsequent fall E917.5
    stationary E917.4
      with subsequent fall E917.8
  person(s) E917.9
    with fall E886.9
    in sports E886.0
    as, or caused by, a crowd E917.1
      with subsequent fall E917.6
    in sports E917.0
      with fall E886.0
Stroke
heat—*see* Heat
lightning E907

Struck by —*see also* Hit by
bullet
  in
    terrorism E979.4
    war operation E991.2
      rubber E991.0
lightning E907
missile
  in terrorism—*see* Terrorism, missile
object
  falling
    from, in, on
      building
        burning (uncontrolled fire)
          in terrorism E979.3
thunderbolt E907
Stumbling over animal, carpet, curb, rug or
  (small) object (with fall) E885.9
without fall—*see* Striking against, object
Submersion (accidental) E910.8
boat, ship, watercraft (causing drowning,
  submersion) E830
  causing injury except drowning, submersion
    E831
by other person
  in accidental circumstances—*see* category
    E910
  intentional, homicidal E964
  stated as undetermined whether accidental or
    intentional E984
due to
  accident
    machinery—*see* Accident, machine
    to boat, ship, watercraft E830
    transport—*see* categories E800-E848
  avalanche E909.2
  cataclysmic
    earth surface movement or eruption E909.9
    storm E908.9
  cloudburst E908.8
  cyclone E908.1
  fall
    from
      boat, ship, watercraft (not involved in
        accident) E832
      burning, crushed E830
      involved in accident, collision E830
      gangplank (into water) E832
      overboard NEC E832
  flood E908.2
  hurricane E908.0
  jumping into water E910.8
    from boat, ship, watercraft
      burning, crushed, sinking E830
      involved in accident, collision E830
      not involved in accident, for swim
        E910.2
    in recreational activity (without diving
      equipment) E910.2
      with or using diving equipment E910.1
    to rescue another person E910.3
  homicide (attempt) E964
  in
    bathtub E910.4
    specified activity, not sport, transport or
      recreational E910.3
    sport or recreational activity (without diving
      equipment) E910.2
      with or using diving equipment E910.1
      water skiing E910.0
    swimming pool NEC E910.8

Submersion—*continued*
  terrorism E979.8
  war operations E995.4
    intentional E995.3
  water transport E832
    due to accident to boat, ship, watercraft
      E830
  landslide E909.2
    overturning boat, ship, watercraft E909.2
    sinking boat, ship, watercraft E909.2
    submersion boat, ship, watercraft E909.2
  tidal wave E909.4
    caused by storm E908.0
  torrential rain E908.2
  late effect of NEC E929.8
  quenching tank E910.8
  self-inflicted (unspecified whether accidental
    or intentional) E984
    in accidental circumstances—*see* category
      E910
    stated as intentional, purposeful E954
  stated as undetermined whether accidental or
    intentional E984
  suicidal (attempted) E954
  while
    attempting rescue of another person E910.3
    engaged in
      marine salvage E910.3
      underwater construction or repairs E910.3
    fishing, not from boat E910.2
    hunting, not from boat E910.2
    ice skating E910.2
    pearl diving E910.3
    placing fishing nets E910.3
    playing in water E910.2
    scuba diving E910.1
      nonrecreational E910.3
    skin diving E910.1
    snorkel diving E910.2
    spear fishing underwater E910.1
    surfboarding E910.2
    swimming (swimming pool) E910.2
    wading (in water) E910.2
    water skiing E910.0
Sucked
  into
    jet (aircraft) E844
Suffocation (accidental) (by external means) (by
    pressure) (mechanical) E913.9
  caused by other person
    in accidental circumstances—*see* category
      E913
    stated as
      intentional, homicidal E963
      undetermined whether accidental or
        intentional E983.9
      by, in
        hanging E983.0
        plastic bag E983.1
        specified means NEC E983.3
  due to, by
    avalanche E909.2
    bedclothes E913.0
    bib E913.0
    blanket E913.0
    cave-in E913.3
      caused by cataclysmic earth surface
        movement or eruption E909.9
    conflagration—*see* Conflagration
    explosion—*see* Explosion
    falling earth, other substance E913.3

Suffocation—*continued*
  fire—*see* Fire
  food, any type (ingestion) (inhalation)
    (regurgitated) (vomited) E911
  foreign body, except food (ingestion)
    (inhalation) E912
  ignition—*see* Ignition
  landslide E909.2
  machine(ry)—*see* Accident, machine
  material, object except food entering by nose
    or mouth, ingested, inhaled E912
  mucus (aspiration) (inhalation), not of
    newborn E912
  phlegm (aspiration) (inhalation) E912
  pillow E913.0
  plastic bag—*see* Suffocation, in, plastic bag
  sheet (plastic) E913.0
  specified means NEC E913.8
  vomitus (aspiration) (inhalation) E911
  homicidal (attempt) E963
    in war operations E995.3
  in
    airtight enclosed place E913.2
    baby carriage E913.0
    bed E913.0
    closed place E913.2
    cot, cradle E913.0
    perambulator E913.0
    plastic bag (in accidental circumstances)
      E913.1
      homicidal, purposely inflicted by other
        person E963
      self-inflicted (unspecified whether
        accidental or intentional) E983.1
        in accidental circumstances E913.1
        intentional, suicidal E953.1
      stated as undetermined whether
        accidentally or purposely inflicted
        E983.1
      suicidal, purposely self-inflicted E953.1
    refrigerator E913.2
    war operations E995.3
  self-inflicted—*see also* Suffocation, stated as
    undetermined whether accidental or
    intentional E953.9
    in accidental circumstances—*see* category
      E913
    stated as intentional, purposeful—*see*
      Suicide, suffocation
  stated as undetermined whether accidental or
    intentional E983.9
    by, in
      hanging E983.0
      plastic bag E983.1
      specified means NEC E983.8
  suicidal—*see* Suicide, suffocation
Suicide, suicidal (attempted) (by) E958.9
  burning, burns E958.1
  caustic substance E958.7
    poisoning E950.7
    swallowed E950.7
  cold, extreme E958.3
  cut (any part of body) E956
  cutting or piercing instrument (classifiable to
    E920) E956
  drowning E954
  electrocution E958.4
  explosive(s) (classifiable to E923) E955.5
  fire E958.1
  firearm (classifiable to E922)—*see* Shooting,
    suicidal

Suicide, suicidal—*continued*
  hanging E953.0
  jumping
    before moving object, train, vehicle E958.0
    from high place—*see* Jumping, from, high
      place, stated as, suicidal
  knife E956
  late effect of E959
  motor vehicle, crashing of E958.5
  poisoning—*see* Table of drugs and chemicals
  puncture (any part of body) E956
  scald E958.2
  shooting—*see* Shooting, suicidal
  specified means NEC E958.8
  stab (any part of body) E956
  strangulation—*see* Suicide, suffocation
  submersion E954
  suffocation E953.9
    by, in
      hanging E953.0
      plastic bag E953.1
      specified means NEC E953.8
  wound NEC E958.9
Sunburn E926.2
Sunstroke E900.0
Supersonic waves (causing injury) E928.1
Surgical procedure, complication of
  delayed or as an abnormal reaction without
    mention of misadventure—*see* Reaction,
    abnormal
  due to or as a result of misadventure—*see*
    Misadventure
Swallowed, swallowing
  foreign body—*see* Foreign body, alimentary
    canal
  poison—*see* Table of drugs and chemicals
  substance
    caustic—*see* Table of drugs and chemicals
    corrosive—*see* Table of drugs and chemicals
    poisonous—*see* Table of drugs and
      chemicals
Swimmers cramp (*see also* category E910)
  E910.2
  not in recreation or sport E910.3
Syndrome, battered
  baby or child—*see* Abuse, child
  wife—*see* Assault

T

Tackle in sport E886.0
Terrorism (injury) (by) (in) E979.8
  air blast E979.2
  aircraft burned, destroyed, exploded, shot
    down E979.1
    used as a weapon E979.1
  anthrax E979.6
  asphyxia from
    chemical (weapons) E979.7
    fire, conflagration (caused by fire-producing
      device) E979.3
      from nuclear explosion E979.5
    gas or fumes E979.7
  bayonet E979.8
  biological agents E979.6
  blast (air) (effects) E979.2
    from nuclear explosion E979.5
    underwater E979.0

Terrorism—*continued*
  bomb (antipersonnel) (mortor) (explosion)
    (fragments) E979.2
  bullet(s) (from carbine, machine gun, pistol,
    rifle, shotgun) E979.4
  burn from
    chemical E979.7
    fire, conflagration (caused by fire-producing
      device) E979.3
    from nuclear explosion E979.5
    gas E979.7
  burning aircraft E979.1
  chemical E979.7
  cholera E979.6
  conflagration E979.3
  crushed by falling aircraft E979.1
  depth charge E979.0
  destruction of aircraft E979.1
  disability, as seqelae one year or more after
    injury E999.1
  drowning E979.8
  effect
    of nuclear weapon (direct) (secondary)
      E979.5
    secondary NEC E979.9
  sequelae E999.1
  explosion (artillery shell) (breech-block)
    (cannon block) E979.2
    aircraft E979.1
    bomb (antipersonnel) (mortar) E979.2
      nuclear (atom) (hydrogen) E979.5
    depth-charge E979.0
    grenade E979.2
    injury by fragments from E979.2
    land-mine E979.2
    marine weapon E979.0
    mine (land) E979.2
      at sea or in harbor E979.0
      marine E979.0
    missile (explosive) NEC E979.2
    munitions (dump) (factory) E979.2
    nuclear (weapon) E979.5
      other direct and secondary effects of
        E979.5
    sea-based artillery shell E979.0
    torpedo E979.0
  exposure to ionizing radiation from nuclear
    explosion E979.5
  falling aircraft E979.1
  fire or fire-producing device E979.3
  firearms E979.4
  fireball effects from nuclear explosion E979.5
  fragments from artillery shell, bomb NEC,
    grenade, guided missile, land-mine, rocket,
    shell, shrapnel E979.2
  gas or fumes E979.7
  grenade (explosion) (fragments) E979.2
  guided missile (explosion) (fragments) E979.2
    nuclear E979.5
  heat from nuclear explosion E979.5
  hot substances E979.3
  hydrogen cyanide E979.7
  land-mine (explosion) (fragments) E979.2
  laser(s) E979.8
  late effect of E999.1
  lewisite E979.7
  lung irritant (chemical) (fumes) (gas) E979.7
  marine mine E979.0

Terrorism—*continued*
  mine E979.2
    at sea E979.0
    in harbor E979.0
    land (explosion) (fragments) E979.2
    marine E979.0
  missile (explosion) (fragments) (guided)
    E979.2
    marine E979.0
    nuclear E979.5
  mortar bomb (explosion) (fragments) E979.2
  mustard gas E979.7
  nerve gas E979.7
  nuclear weapons E979.5
  pellets (shotgun) E979.4
  petrol bomb E979.3
  piercing object E979.8
  phosgene E979.7
  poisoning (chemical) (fumes) (gas) E979.7
  radiation, ionizing from nuclear explosion
    E979.5
  rocket (explosion) (fragments) E979.2
  saber, sabre E979.8
  sarin E979.7
  screening smoke E979.7
  sequelae effect (of) E999.1
  shell (aircraft) (artillery) (cannon) (land-based)
    (explosion) (fragments) E979.2
    sea-based E979.0
  shooting E979.4
    bullet(s) E979.4
    pellet(s) (rifle) (shotgun) E979.4
  shrapnel E979.2
  smallpox E979.7
  stabbing object(s) E979.8
  submersion E979.8
  torpedo E979.0
  underwater blast E979.0
  vesicant (chemical) (fumes) (gas) E979.7
  weapon burst E979.2
Thermic fever E900.9
Thermoplegia E900.9
Thirst —*see also* Lack of water
  resulting from accident connected with
    transport—*see* categories E800-E848
Thrown (accidently)
  against object in or part of vehicle
    by motion of vehicle
      aircraft E844
      boat, ship, watercraft E838
      motor vehicle (on public highway) E818
        not on public highway E825
        off-road type (not on public highway)
          E821
          on public highway E818
        snow vehicle E820
          on public highway E818
      nonmotor road vehicle NEC E829
      railway rolling stock, train, vehicle E806
      street car E829
  from
    animal (being ridden) (in sport or transport)
      E828
    high place, homicide (attempt) E968.1
    machinery—*see* Accident, machine
    vehicle NEC—*see* Accident, vehicle NEC
    off—*see* Thrown, from
  overboard (by motion of boat, ship, watercraft)
    E832
    by accident to boat, ship, watercraft E830
Thunderbolt NEC E907

Tidal wave (any injury) E909.4
  caused by storm E908.0
Took
  overdose of drug—*see* Table of drugs and
    chemicals
  poison—*see* Table of drugs and chemicals
Tornado (any injury) E908.1
Torrential rain (any injury) E908.2
Traffic accident NEC E819
Trampled by animal E906.8
  being ridden (in sport or transport) E828
Trapped (accidentally)
  between
    objects (moving) (stationary and moving)
      E918
  by
    door of
      elevator E918
      motor vehicle (on public highway) (while
        alighting, boarding)—*see* Fall, from,
        motor vehicle, while alighting
      railway train (underground) E806
      street car E829
      subway train E806
    in object E918
Trauma
  cumulative
    from
      repetitive
        impact E927.4
        motion or movements E927.3
    sudden from strenuous movements E927.0
Travel (effects) E903
  sickness E903
Tree
  falling on or hitting E916
    motor vehicle (in motion) (on public
      highway) E818
      not on public highway E825
      nonmotor road vehicle NEC E829
      pedal cycle E826
    person E916
    railway rolling stock, train, vehicle E806
    street car E829
Trench foot E901.0
Tripping over animal, carpet, curb, rug, or
  small object (with fall) E885.9
  without fall—*see* Striking against, object
Tsunami E909.4
Twisting, injury in E927.8

V

Violence, nonaccidental (*see also* Assault)
  E968.9
Volcanic eruption (any injury) E909.1
Vomitus in air passages (with asphyxia,
  obstruction or suffocation) E911

W

War operations (during hostilities) (injury) (by)
  (in) E995.9
  after cessation of hostilities, injury due to
    E998.9
  air blast E993.9
  aircraft burned, destroyed, exploded, shot
    down E994

War operations—*continued*
asphyxia from
  chemical E997.2
  fire, conflagration (caused by fire-producing
    device or conventional weapon) E990.9
  from nuclear explosion (see also War
    operations, injury due to, nuclear
    weapons) E996.8
    incendiary bomb E990.0
    petrol bomb E990.0
  fumes E997.2
  gas E997.2
baton (nightstick) E995.1
battle wound NEC E995.8
bayonet E995.2
biological warfare agents E997.1
blast (air) (effects) E993.9
  from nuclear explosion (see also War
    operations, injury due to, nuclear
    weapons) E996.1
  underwater E992.9
bomb (mortar) (explosion) E993.2
  after cessation of hostilities E998.1
  fragments, injury by E991.4
    antipersonnel E991.3
bullet(s) (from carbine, machine gun, pistol,
    rifle, shotgun) E991.2
  rubber E991.0
burn from
  chemical E997.2
  fire, conflagration (caused by fire-producing
    device or conventional weapon) E990.9
  from
    conventional weapon E990.3
    flamethrower E990.1
    incendiary bomb E990.0
    incendiary bullet E990.2
    nuclear explosion E996.2
    petrol bomb E990.0
  gas E997.2
burning aircraft E994.3
chemical E997.2
chlorine E997.2
conventional warfare, specified form NEC
    E995.8
crushing by falling aircraft E994.8
depth charge E992.1
destruction of aircraft E994.9
detonation of own munitions (ammunition)
    (artillery) (mortars), unintentional E993.6
disability as sequela one year or more after
    injury E999.0
discharge of own munitions launch device
    (autocannons) (automatic grenade
    launchers) (missile launchers) (small arms),
    unintentional E993.7
drowning E995.4
effect, nuclear weapon (see also War
    operations, injury due to, nuclear weapons)
    E996.9
explosion (breech block) (cannon shell)
    E993.9
  after cessation of hostilities
    bomb placed in war E998.1
    mine placed in war E998.0
  aircraft E994.1
  due to
    enemy fire or explosives E994.0
    own onboard explosives E994.1
  artillery shell E993.2

War operations—*continued*
bomb (mortar) E993.2
  aerial E993.0
  atom (see also War operations, injury due
    to, nuclear weapons) E996.9
  hydrogen (see also War operations, injury
    due to, nuclear weapons) E996.9
  injury by fragments from E991.4
    antipersonnel E991.3
  nuclear (see also War operations, injury
    due to, nuclear weapons) E996.9
depth charge E992.1
  injury by fragments from E991.4
    antipersonnel E991.3
marine weapon NEC E992.8
mine
  at sea or in harbor E992.2
  land E993.8
    injury by fragments from E991.4
  marine E992.2
missle, guided E993.1
mortar E993.2
munitions (accidental) (being used in war)
    (dump) (factory) E993.9
  own E993.7
    launch device (autocannons) (automatic
      grenade launchers) (missile launchers)
      (small arms) E993.7
nuclear (weapon) (see also War operations,
    injury due to, nuclear weapons) E996.9
own weapons (accidental) E993.7
  injury by fragments from E991.9
    antipersonnel E991.3
sea-based artillery shell E992.3
specified NEC E993.8
torpedo E992.0
exposure to ionizing radiation from nuclear
    explosion (see also War operations, injury
    due to, nuclear weapons) E996.3
falling aircraft E994.8
fire or fire-producing device E990.9
  flamethrower E990.1
  incendiary bomb E990.0
  incendiary bullet E990.2
  indirectly caused from conventional weapon
    E990.3
  petrol bomb E990.0
fireball effects from nuclear explosion E996.2
fragments from
  antipersonnel bomb E991.3
  artillery shell E991.4
  bomb NEC E991.4
  grenade E991.4
  guided missile E991.4
  land mine E991.4
  rocket E991.4
  shell E991.4
  shrapnel E991.9
fumes E997.2
gas E997.2
grenade (explosion) E993.8
  fragments, injury by E991.4
guided missile (explosion) E993.1
  fragments, injury by E991.4
  nuclear (see also War operations, injury due
    to, nuclear weapons) E996.9
heat from nuclear explosion E996.2
injury due to
  aerial bomb E993.0
  air blast E993.9
  aircraft shot down E994.0

War operations—*continued*
  mine
    after cessation of hostilities E998.0
    at sea E992.2
    in harbor E992.2
    land (explosion) E993.8
      fragments, injury by E991.4
    marine E992.2
    missile (guided) (explosion) E993.1
      fragments, injury by E991.4
    marine E992.8
    nuclear (*see also* War operations, injury due
      to, nuclear weapons) E996.9
  mortar bomb (explosion) E993.2
    fragments, injury by E991.4
  mustard gas E997.2
  nerve gas E997.2
  phosgene E997.2
  piercing object E995.2
  poisoning (chemical) (fumes) (gas) E997.2
  radiation, ionizing from nuclear explosion (*see
    also* War operations, injury due to, nuclear
    weapons) E996.3
  rocket (explosion) E993.8
    fragments, injury by E991.4
  saber, sabre E995.2
  screening smoke E997.8
  shell (aircraft) (artillery) (cannon) (land based)
    (explosion) E993.2
    fragments, injury by E991.4
    sea-based E992.3
  shooting E991.2
    after cessation of hostilities E998.8
    bullet(s) E991.2
      rubber E991.0
    pellet(s) (rifle) E991.1
  shrapnel E991.9
  stave E995.2
  strike by blunt object (baton) (nightstick)
    (stave) E995.1
  submersion E995.4
    intentional E995.3
  sword E995.2
  torpedo E992.0
  unconventional warfare, except by nuclear
    weapon E997.9
    biological (warfare) E997.1
    gas, fumes, chemicals E997.2
    laser(s) E997.0
    specified type NEC E997.8
  underwater blast E992.9
  vesicant (chemical) (fumes) (gas) E997.2
  weapon burst E993.9
Washed
  away by flood—*see* Flood
  away by tidal wave—*see* Tidal wave
  off road by storm (transport vehicle) E908.9
  overboard E832
Weapon of mass destruction [WMD] E997.3
Weather exposure —*see also* Exposure
  cold E901.0
  hot E900.0
Weightlessness (causing injury) (effects of) (in
  spacecraft, real or simulated) E928.0
Wound (accidental) NEC (*see also* Injury)
  E928.9
  battle (*see also* War operation) E995.9
  bayonet E920.3
  in
    legal intervention E974
    war operations E995.2

Wound—*continued*
  gunshot—*see* Shooting
  incised—*see* Cut
  saber, sabre E920.3
    in war operations E995.2
Wrong
  body part, performance of correct operation
    (procedure) on E876.7
  device implanted into correct surgical site
    E876.5
  patient, performance of operation (procedure)
    on E876.6
  procedure (operation) performed on correct
    patient E876.5
  side, performance of correct operation
    (procedure) on E876.7
  site, performance of correct operation
    (procedure) on E876.7

RAILWAY ACCIDENTS (E800–E807)

The following fourth-digit subdivisions are for use with categories E800-E807 to identify the injured person.

.0 Railway employee

Any person who by virtue of his employment in connection with a railway, whether by the railway company or not, is at increased risk of involvement in a railway accident, such as:

catering staff on train	postal staff on train
driver	railway fireman
guard	shunter
porter	sleeping car attendant

.1 Passenger on railway

Any authorized person traveling on a train, except a railway employee

Excludes: intending passenger waiting at station (.8)
unauthorized rider on railway vehicle (.8)

.2 Pedestrian

See definition (r), Vol. 1, E code introduction

.3 Pedal cyclist

See definition (p), Vol. 1, E code introduction

.8 Other specified person

Intending passenger waiting at station

Unauthorized rider on railway vehicle

.9 Unspecified person

MOTOR VEHICLE TRAFFIC AND NONTRAFFIC ACCIDENTS
(E810–825)

The following fourth–digit subdivisions are for use with categories E810–E819 and E820–E825 to identify the injured person:

.0 Driver of motor vehicle other than motorcycle

See definition (l), Vol. 1, E code introduction

.1 Passenger in motor vehicle other than motorcycle

See definition (l), Vol. 1, E code introduction

.2 Motorcyclist

See definition (l), Vol. 1, E code introduction

.3 Passenger on motorcycle

See definition (l), Vol. 1, E code introduction

.4 Occupant of streetcar

.5 Rider of animal; occupant of animal–drawn vehicle

.6 Pedal cyclist

See definition (p), Vol. 1, E code introduction

.7 Pedestrian

See definition (r), Vol. 1, E code introduction

.8 Other specified person

Occupant of vehicle other than above

Person in railway train involved in accident

Unauthorized rider of motor vehicle

.9 Unspecified person

OTHER ROAD VEHICLE ACCIDENTS (E826–E829)

(animal–drawn vehicle, streetcar, pedal cycle, and other nonmotor road vehicle accidents)

The following fourth–digit subdivisions are for use with categories E826–E829 to identify the injured person:

.0 Pedestrian

See definition (r), Vol. 1, E code introduction

.1 Pedal cyclist (does not apply to codes E827, E828, E829)

See definition (p), Vol. 1, E code introduction

.2 Rider of animal (does not apply to code E829)

.3 Occupant of animal–drawn vehicle (does not apply to codes E828, E829)

.4 Occupant of streetcar

.8 Other specified person

.9 Unspecified person

WATER TRANSPORT ACCIDENTS (E830–E838)

The following fourth–digit subdivisions are for use with categories E830–E838 to identify the injured person:

.0 Occupant of small boat, unpowered

.1 Occupant of small boat, powered

See definition (t), Vol. 1, E code introduction

Excludes: water skier (.4)

.2 Occupant of other watercraft — crew

Persons:

> engaged in operation of watercraft

> providing passenger services [cabin attendants, ship's physician, catering personnel]

> working on ship during voyage in other capacity [musician in band, operators of shops and beauty parlors]

.3 Occupant of other watercraft — other than crew

Passenger

Occupant of lifeboat, other than crew, after abandoning ship

.4 Water skier

.5 Swimmer

.6 Dockers, stevedores

Longshoreman employed on the dock in loading and unloading ships

.8 Other specified person

Immigration and custom officials on board ship

Person:
accompanying passenger or member of crew
visiting boat

Pilot (guiding ship into port)

.9 Unspecified person

AIR AND SPACE TRANSPORT ACCIDENTS (E840–E845)

The following fourth–digit subdivisions are for use with categories E840–E845 to identify the injured person:

.0 Occupant of spacecraft

.1 Occupant of military aircraft, any

Crew in military aircraft [air force] [army] [national guard] [navy]

Passenger (civilian) (military) in military aircraft [air force] [army] [national guard] [navy]

Troops in military aircraft [air force] [army] [national guard] [navy]

Excludes: occupants of aircraft operated under jurisdiction of police departments (.5) parachutist (.7).

.2 Crew of commercial aircraft (powered) in surface to surface transport

.3 Other occupant of commercial aircraft (powered) in surface to surface transport

Flight personnel:
not part of crew
on familiarization flight

Passenger on aircraft (powered) NOS

.4 Occupant of commercial aircraft (powered) in surface to air transport

Occupant [crew] [passenger] of aircraft (powered) engaged in activities, such as:
aerial spraying (crops) (fire retardants)
air drops of emergency supplies
air drops of parachutists, except from military craft
crop dusting
lowering of construction material [bridge or telephone pole]
sky writing

.5 Occupant of other powered aircraft

Occupant [crew] [passenger] of aircraft (powered) engaged in activities, such as:
aerobatic flying
aircraft racing
rescue operation
storm surveillance
traffic surveillance

Occupant of private plane NOS

.6 Occupant of unpowered aircraft, except parachutist

Occupant of aircraft classifiable to E842

.7 Parachutist (military) (other)

Person making voluntary descent

Excludes: person making descent after accident to aircraft (.1–.6)

.8 Ground crew, airline employee

Persons employed at airfields (civil) (military) or launching pads, not occupants of aircraft

.9 Other person

008.63   **Norwalk virus**
Add inclusion term

008.65   **Calicivirus**
Revise code title

035   **Erysipelas**
Revise exclusion term

037   **Tetanus**
Revise exclusion term

041.3   **Klebsiella pneumoniae**
Revise code title

041.86   **Helicobacter pylor98i [H. pylori]**
Revise code title

046.1   **Jakob-Creutzfeldt disease**
Add "Use additional" notes

078.89   **Other specified diseases due to viruses**
Delete inclusion term

190   **Malignant neoplasm of eye**
Add exclusion terms

196   **Secondary and unspecified malignant neoplasm of lymph nodes**
Add exclusion term

197   **Secondary malignant neoplasm of respiratory and digestive systems**
Add exclusion terms

198   **Secondary malignant neoplasm of other specified sites**
Add exclusion term

199   **Malignant neoplasm without specification of site**
Add and revise exclusion terms

199.2   **Malignant neoplasm associated with transplanted organ**
Revise "Use additional" note

202.0   **Nodular lymphoma**
Revise inclusion term

202.1   **Mycosis fungoides**
Add exclusion term

209   **Neuroendocrine tumors**
Add and revise exclusion terms

209.30   **Malignant poorly differentiated neuroendocrine carcinoma, any site**
Add exclusion term

209.31   **Merkel cell carcinoma of the face**
New code

209.32   **Merkel cell carcinoma of the scalp and neck**
New code

209.33   **Merkel cell carcinoma of the upper limb**
New code

209.34   **Merkel cell carcinoma of the lower limb**
New code

209.35   **Merkel cell carcinoma of the trunk**
New code

209.36   **Merkel cell carcinoma of other sites**
New code

209.7   **Secondary neuroendocrine tumors**
New subcategory

209.70   **Secondary neuroendocrine tumor, unspecified site**
New code

209.71   **Secondary neuroendocrine tumor of distant lymph nodes**
New code

209.72   **Secondary neuroendocrine tumor of liver**
New code

209.73   **Secondary neuroendocrine tumor of bone**
New code

209.74   **Secondary neuroendocrine tumor of peritoneum**
New code

209.75   **Secondary Merkel cell carcinoma**
New code

209.79   **Secondary neuroendocrine tumor of other sites**
New code

238.72   **Low grade myelodysplastic syndrome lesions**
Add inclusion term

238.73   **High grade myelodysplastic syndrome lesions**
Delete inclusion term

239.81   **Retina and choroid**
New code

239.89   **Other specified sites**
New code

251.3   **Postsurgical hypoinsulinemia**
Add "Use additional" note and exclusion terms

269.8   **Other nutritional deficiency**
Revise exclusion term

270   **Disorders of amino-acid transport and metabolism**
Revise exclusion term

272.2   **Mixed hyperlipidemia**
Add inclusion terms

272.4   **Other and unspecified hyperlipidemia**
Delete inclusion term

274.00   **Gouty arthropathy, unspecified**
New code

274.01   **Acute gouty arthropathy**
New code

274.02   **Chronic gouty arthropathy without mention of tophus (tophi)**
New code

274.03   **Chronic gouty arthropathy with tophus (tophi)**
New code

274.82   **Gouty tophi of other sites**
Add exclusion terms

277.2   **Other disorders of purine and pyrimidine metabolism**
Revise exclusion term

277.88   **Tumor lysis syndrome**
New code

279.4   **Autoimmune disease, not elsewhere classified**
Delete inclusion term

279.41   **Autoimmune lymphoproliferative syndrome**
New code

279.49 **Autoimmune disease, not elsewhere classified**
New code

279.5 **Graft-versus-host disease**
Revise terms

285.2 **Anemia of chronic disease**
Revise inclusion term

285.22 **Anemia in neoplastic disease**
Add exclusion term

285.3 **Antineoplastic chemotherapy induced anemia**
New code

290.0 **Senile dementia, uncomplicated**
Revise exclusion term

294.1 **Dementia in conditions classified elsewhere**
Revise "Code first" note

294.8 **Other persistent mental disorders due to conditions classified elsewhere**
Revise exclusion term

305 **Nondependent abuse of drugs**
Delete 5th digit notation

307.0 **Stuttering**
Add and revise exclusion terms

310.1 **Personality change due to conditions classified elsewhere**
Add exclusion terms

310.8 **Other specified nonpsychotic mental disorders following organic brain damage**
Add exclusion term

331.7 **Cerebral degeneration in diseases classified elsewhere**
Revise exclusion term

331.83 **Mild cognitive impairment, so stated**
Add exclusion term

333.2 **Myoclonus**
Revise inclusion terms and add exclusion terms

345 **Epilepsy and recurrent seizures**
Add fifth digit "1" descriptions; add exclusion terms

345.1 **Generalized convulsive epilepsy**
Add inclusion terms

348.8 **Other conditions of brain**
Delete inclusion terms

348.81 **Temporal sclerosis**
New code

348.89 **Other conditions of brain**
New code

359.22 **Myotonia congenita**
Add inclusion term

359.29 **Other specified myotonic disorder**
Delete inclusion term

359.7 **Inflammatory and immune myopathies, NEC**
New subcategory

359.71 **Inclusion body myositis**
New code

359.79 **Other inflammatory and immune myopathies, NEC**
New code

372.06 **Acute chemical conjunctivitis**
New code

372.34 **Pingueculitis**
Add exclusion term

372.51 **Pinguecula**
Add exclusion term

403 **Hypertensive chronic kidney disease**
Revise exclusion term

413.9 **Other and unspecified angina pectoris**
Add "Use additional" note

415.1 **Pulmonary embolism and infarction**
Add exclusion terms

416.2 **Chronic pulmonary embolism**
New code

438.13 **Dysarthria**
New code

438.14 **Fluency disorder**
New code

445.81 **Kidney**
Revise "Use additional" note

453 **Other venous embolism and thrombosis**
Delete exclusion term

453.2 **Of inferior vena cava**
Revise code title

453.4 **Acute venous embolism and thrombosis of deep vessels of lower extremity**
Revise code title

453.40 **Acute venous embolism and thrombosis of unspecified deep vessels of lower extremity**
Revise code title

453.41 **Acute venous embolism and thrombosis of deep vessels of proximal lower extremity**
Revise code title

453.42 **Acute venous embolism and thrombosis of deep vessels of distal lower extremity**
Revise code title

453.5 **Chronic venous embolism and thrombosis of deep vessels of lower extremity**
New subcategory

453.50 **Chronic venous embolism and thrombosis of unspecified deep vessels of lower extremity**
New code

453.51 **Chronic venous embolism and thrombosis of deep vessels of proximal lower extremity**
New code

453.52 **Chronic venous embolism and thrombosis of deep vessels of distal lower extremity**
New code

453.6 **Venous embolism and thrombosis of superficial vessels of lower extremity**
New code

453.7 **Chronic venous embolism and thrombosis of other specified vessels**
New subcategory

453.71 **Chronic venous embolism and thrombosis of superficial veins of upper extremity**
New code

453.72 **Chronic venous embolism and thrombosis of deep veins of upper extremity**
New code

453.73 Chronic venous embolism and thrombosis of upper extremity, unspecified
New code

453.74 Chronic venous embolism and thrombosis of axillary veins
New code

453.75 Chronic venous embolism and thrombosis of subclavian veins
New code

453.76 Chronic venous embolism and thrombosis of internal jugular veins
New code

453.77 Chronic venous embolism and thrombosis of other thoracic veins
New code

453.79 Chronic venous embolism and thrombosis of other specified veins
New code

453.8 Acute venous embolism and thrombosis of other specified veins
Revise code title

453.81 Acute venous embolism and thrombosis of superficial veins of upper extremity
New code

453.82 Acute venous embolism and thrombosis of deep veins of upper extremity
New code

453.83 Acute venous embolism and thrombosis of upper extremity, unspecified
New code

453.84 Acute venous embolism and thrombosis of axillary veins
New code

453.85 Acute venous embolism and thrombosis of subclavian veins
New code

453.86 Acute venous embolism and thrombosis of internal jugular veins
New code

453.87 Acute venous embolism and thrombosis of other thoracic veins
New code

453.89 Acute venous embolism and thrombosis of other specified veins
New code

487 Influenza
Add inclusion term; revise exclusion terms

488 Influenza due to certain identified influenza viruses
Revise code title, revise exclusion term

488.0 Influenza due to identified avian influenza virus
New code

488.1 Influenza due to identified novel H1N1 influenza virus
New code

536.2 Persistent vomiting
Add exclusion terms

567 Peritonitis and retroperitoneal infections
Revise exclusion term

569.7 Complications of intestinal pouch
New subcategory

569.71 Pouchitis
New code

569.79 Other complications of intestinal pouch
New code

569.87 Vomiting of fecal matter
New code

572.2 Hepatic encephalopathy
Revise code title; revise inclusion terms

584 Acute kidney failure
Revise code title; add inclusion term

584.5 Acute kidney failure with lesion of tubular necrosis
Revise code title

584.6 Acute kidney failure with lesion of renal cortical necrosis
Revise code title

584.7 Acute kidney failure with lesion of renal medullary [papillary] necrosis
Revise code title

584.8 Acute kidney failure with other specified pathological lesion in kidney
Revise code title

584.9 Acute kidney failure, unspecified
Revise code title

587 Renal sclerosis, unspecified
Revise exclusion terms

611.82 Hypoplasia of breast
Add exclusion term

614 Inflammatory disease of ovary, fallopian tube, pelvic cellular tissue, and peritoneum
Revise exclusion term

615 Inflammatory diseases of uterus, except cervix
Revise exclusion terms

621.3 Endometrial hyperplasia
Delete inclusion terms

621.30 Endometrial hyperplasia, unspecified
Add inclusion terms

621.31 Simple endometrial hyperplasia without atypia
Add exclusion term

621.32 Complex endometrial hyperplasia without atypia
Add exclusion term

621.33 Endometrial hyperplasia with atypia
Add exclusion term

621.34 Benign endometrial hyperplasia
New code

621.35 Endometrial intraepithelial neoplasia [EIN]
New code

624 Noninflammatory disorders of vulva and perineum
Revise exclusion term

639.3 Kidney failure
Revise code title

646.6 Infections of genitourinary tract in pregnancy
Revise exclusion term

649.3   **Coagulation defects complicating pregnancy, childbirth, or the puerperium**
Revise description and "Use additional code" note

669.3   **Acute kidney failure following labor and delivery**
Revise code title

670   **Major puerperal infection**
Inclusion terms deleted

670.0   **Major puerperal infection, unspecified**
Subcategory revised

670.1   **Puerperal endometritis**
New subcategory

670.2   **Puerperal sepsis**
New subcategory

670.3   **Puerperal septic thrombophlebitis**
New subcategory

670.8   **Other major puerperal infection**
New subcategory

671   **Venous complications in pregnancy and the puerperium**
Exclusion terms added

671.2   **Superficial thrombophlebitis**
Inclusion terms added

671.3   **Deep phlebothrombosis, antepartum**
"Use additional" notes added

671.4   **Deep phlebothrombosis, postpartum**
"Use additional" notes added

671.9   **Unspecified venous complication**
Inclusion terms added

707.03   **Lower back**
Inclusion term added

712   **Crystal arthropathies**
Exclusion term revised

713.0   **Arthropathy associated with other endocrine and metabolic disorders**
Exclusion term revised

727.01   **Synovitis and tenosynovitis in diseases classified elsewhere**
Exclusion term revised

733.1   **Pathologic fracture**
Inclusion term added

756.72   **Omphalocele**
New code

756.73   **Gastroschisis**
New code

756.79   **Other congenital anomalies of abdominal wall**
Inclusion terms deleted

757.6   **Specified congenital anomalies of breast**
Subcategory title revised, exclusion term added

762.3   **Placental transfusion syndromes**
"Use additional code" note revised

768.5   **Severe birth asphyxia**
Exclusion term revised

768.6   **Mild or moderate birth asphyxia**
Exclusion term revised

768.70   **Hypoxic-ischemic encephalopathy, unspecified**
New code

768.71   **Mild hypoxic-ischemic encephalopathy**
New code

768.72   **Moderate hypoxic-ischemic encephalopathy**
New code

768.73   **Severe hypoxic-ischemic encephalopathy**
New code

772   **Fetal and neonatal hemorrhage**
Exclusion term added

772.0   **Fetal blood loss affecting newborn**
Code title revised

776   **Hematological disorders of newborn**
Inclusion term revised

776.9   **Unspecified hematological disorder specific to newborn**
Code title revised

777.5   **Necrotizing enterocolitis in newborn**
Inclusion term deleted

777.51   **Stage I necrotizing enterocolitis in newborn**
Inclusion terms added

779.3   **Disorder of stomach function and feeding problems in newborn**
Subcategory title revised

779.31   **Feeding problems in newborn**
New code

779.32   **Bilious vomiting in newborn**
New code

779.33   **Other vomiting in newborn**
New code

779.34   **Failure to thrive in newborn**
New code

780.0   **Alteration of consciousness**
Exclusion terms added

780.93   **Memory loss**
Exclusion terms added and revised

783.3   **Feeding difficulties and mismanagement**
Exclusion term revised

783.41   **Failure to thrive**
Exclusion term added

784.4   **Voice and resonance disorders**
Subcategory title revised

784.40   **Voice disturbance and resonance disorder, unspecified**
Code title revised

784.42   **Dysphonia**
New code

784.43   **Hypernasality**
New code

784.44   **Hyponasality**
New code

784.49   **Other voice and resonance disorders**
Code title revised

784.5   **Other speech disturbance**
Inclusion terms deleted, exclusion term added

784.51   **Dysarthria**
New code

784.59   **Other speech disturbance**
New code

787.0   **Nausea and vomiting**
Exclusion terms revised

787.04   **Bilious emesis**
New code

789.0   **Abdominal pain**
Inclusion terms and exclusion term deleted

789.7   **Colic**
New code

790.01   **Precipitous drop in hematocrit**
Inclusion term added

793   **Nonspecific (abnormal) findings on radiological and other examination of body structure**
Category title revised

793.82   **Inconclusive mammogram**
New code

793.89   **Other (abnormal) findings on radiological examination of breast**
Code title revised

795.0   **Abnormal Papanicolaou smear of cervix and cervical HPV**
Code title revised

795.39   **Other nonspecific positive culture findings**
Exclusion term added

796.7   **Abnormal cytologic smear of anus and anal HPV**
Exclusion term revised

799.2   **Signs and symptoms involving emotional state**
Subcategory revised

799.21   **Nervousness**
New code

799.22   **Irritability**
New code

799.23   **Impulsiveness**
New code

799.24   **Emotional lability**
New code

799.25   **Demoralization and apathy**
New code

799.29   **Other signs and symptoms involving emotional state**
New code

799.82   **Apparent life threatening event in infant**
New code

813.45   **Torus fracture of radius (alone)**
Code title revised

813.46   **Torus fracture of ulna (alone)**
New code

813.47   **Torus fracture of radius and ulna**
New code

832   **Dislocation of elbow**
5th digit instructions revised

832.2   **Nursemaid's elbow**
New code

854   **Intracranial injury of other and unspecified nature**
Inclusion terms revised and added

945.0   **Unspecified degree**
Fifth digits revised

945.1   **Erythema [first degree]**
Fifth digits revised

945.2   **Blisters, epidermal loss [second degree]**
Fifth digits revised

945.3   **Full-thickness skin loss [third degree NOS]**
Fifth digits revised

945.4   **Deep necrosis of underlying tissues [deep third degree] without mention of loss of a body part**
Fifth digits revised

945.5   **Deep necrosis of underlying tissues [deep third degree] with loss of a body part**
Fifth digits revised

969.0   **Antidepressants**
Inclusion terms deleted

969.00   **Antidepressant, unspecified**
New code

969.01   **Monoamine oxidase inhibitors**
New code

969.02   **Selective serotonin and norepinephrine reuptake inhibitors**
New code

969.03   **Selective serotonin reuptake inhibitors**
New code

969.04   **Tetracyclic antidepressants**
New code

969.05   **Tricyclic antidepressants**
New code

969.09   **Other antidepressants**
New code

969.7   **Psychostimulants**
Inclusion terms deleted

969.70   **Psychostimulant, unspecified**
New code

969.71   **Caffeine**
New code

969.72   **Amphetamines**
New code

969.73   **Methylphenidate**
New code

969.79   **Other psychostimulants**
New code

974.1   **Purine derivative diuretics**
Exclusion term revised

995.24   **Failed moderate sedation during procedure**
New code

995.92   **Severe sepsis**
"Use additional code" note revised

995.94   **Systemic inflammatory response syndrome due to non-infectious process with acute organ dysfunction**
"Use additional code" note revised

996.43   **Broken prosthetic joint implant**
Code title revised

996.47   **Other mechanical complication of prosthetic joint implant**
Inclusion term added

996.7   **Other complications of internal (biological) (synthetic) prosthetic device, implant, and graft**
Inclusion term added

997.31   **Ventilator associated pneumonia**
Inclusion term added

997.4   **Digestive system complications**
Exclusion terms added

997.5   **Urinary complications**
Inclusion term added

999.6 ABO incompatibility reaction
Exclusion term added

V07.52 Prophylactic use of aromatase inhibitors
Inclusion term revised

V10 Personal history of malignant neoplasm
"Code first" note deleted

V10.0 Gastrointestinal tract
Exclusion terms added

V10.1 Trachea, bronchus, and lung
Exclusion terms added

V10.8 Personal history of malignant neoplasm of other sites
Exclusion terms added

V10.9 Other and unspecified personal history of malignant neoplasm
Code title revised

V10.90 Personal history of unspecified malignant neoplasm
New code

V10.91 Personal history of malignant neuroendocrine tumor
New code

V12.54 Transient ischemic attack (TIA), and cerebral infarction without residual deficits
Exclusion term added

V15.06 Allergy to insects and arachnids
Code title revised

V15.52 History of traumatic brain injury
New code

V15.80 History of failed moderate sedation
New code

V15.83 Underimmunization status
New code

V15.84 Contact with and (suspected) exposure to asbestos
Code title revised

V15.85 Contact with and (suspected) exposure to potentially hazardous body fluids
Code title revised

V15.86 Contact with and (suspected) exposure to lead
Code title revised

V20.2 Routine infant or child health check
Inclusion terms revised, and exclusion terms added

V20.3 Newborn health supervision
New subcategory

V20.31 Health supervision for newborn under 8 days old
New code

V20.32 Health supervision for newborn 8 to 28 days old
New code

V23.86 Pregnancy with history of in utero procedure during previous pregnancy
Exclusion term revised

V26.42 Encounter for fertility preservation counseling
New code

V26.82 Encounter for fertility preservation procedure
New code

V45.71 Acquired absence of breast and nipple
Exclusion term added

V53.5 Other gastrointestinal appliance and device
Subcategory title revised

V53.50 Fitting and adjustment of intestinal appliance and device
New code

V53.51 Fitting and adjustment of gastric lap band
New code

V53.59 Fitting and adjustment of other gastrointestinal appliance and device
New code

V54.1 Aftercare for healing traumatic fracture
Exclusion term added

V54.2 Aftercare for healing pathologic fracture
Exclusion term added

V57.3 Speech-language therapy
Code title revised

V60.81 Foster care (status)
New code

V60.89 Other specified housing or economic circumstances
New code

V61.01 Family disruption due to family member on military deployment
Exclusion term added

V61.07 Family disruption due to death of family member
New code

V61.08 Family disruption due to other extended absence of family member
New code

V61.23 Counseling for parent-biological child problem
New code

V61.24 Counseling for parent-adopted child problem
New code

V61.25 Counseling for parent (guardian)-foster child problem
New code

V61.29 Other parent-child problems
Revise code title

V61.42 Substance abuse in family
New code

V62.82 Bereavement, uncomplicated
Exclusion term added

V65.11 Pediatric pre-birth visit for expectant parent(s)
Revise code title

V70.0 Routine general medical examination at a health care facility
Revise and add exclusion terms

V72 Special investigations and examinations
Revise and add exclusion terms

V72.5 Radiological examination, not elsewhere classified
Revise and add exclusion terms

V72.6 Laboratory examination
Add inclusion term, delete exclusion term

V72.60 Laboratory examination, unspecified New code	**E002.4 Underwater diving and snorkeling** New code
V72.61 Antibody response examination New code	**E002.5 Rowing, canoeing, kayaking, rafting and tubing** New code
V72.62 Laboratory examination ordered as part of a routine general medical examination New code	**E002.6 Water skiing and wake boarding** New code
V72.63 Pre-procedural laboratory examination New code	**E002.7 Surfing, windsurfing and boogie boarding** New code
V72.69 Other laboratory examination New code	**E002.8 Water sliding** New code
V72.8 Other specified examinations Exclusion term added	**E002.9 Other activity involving water and watercraft** New code
V72.83 Other specified preoperative examination Inclusion term added	**E003 Activities involving ice and snow** New category
V80.01 Traumatic brain injury New code	**E003.0 Ice skating** New code
V80.09 Other neurological conditions New code	**E003.1 Ice hockey** New code
V87.32 Contact with and (suspected) exposure to algae bloom New code	**E003.2 Snow (alpine) (downhill) skiing, snow boarding, sledding, tobogganing and snow tubing** New code
V87.43 Personal history of estrogen therapy New code	**E003.3 Cross country skiing** New code
V87.44 Personal history of inhaled steroid therapy New code	**E003.9 Other activity involving ice and snow** New code
V87.45 Personal history of systemic steroid therapy New code	**E004 Activities involving climbing, rappelling and jumping off** New category
V87.46 Personal history of immunosuppression therapy New code	**E004.0 Mountain climbing, rock climbing and wall climbing** New code
E000 External cause status New category	**E004.1 Rappelling** New code
E000.0 Civilian activity done for income or pay New code	**E004.2 BASE jumping** New code
E000.1 Military activity New code	**E004.3 Bungee jumping** New code
E000.8 Other external cause status New code	**E004.4 Hang gliding** New code
E000.9 Unspecified external cause status New code	**E004.9 Other activity involving climbing, rappelling and jumping off** New code
E001 Activities involving walking and running New category	**E005 Activities involving dancing and other rhythmic movement** New category
E001.0 Walking, marching and hiking New code	**E005.0 Dancing** New code
E001.1 Running New code	**E005.1 Yoga** New code
E002 Activities involving water and water craft New category	**E005.2 Gymnastics** New code
E002.0 Swimming New code	**E005.3 Trampoline** New code
E002.1 Springboard and platform diving New code	**E005.4 Cheerleading** New code
E002.2 Water polo New code	**E005.9 Other activity involving dancing and other rhythmic movements** New code
E002.3 Water aerobics and water exercise New code	**E006 Activities involving other sports and athletics played individually** New category

E006.0 Roller skating (inline) and skateboarding
New code

E006.1 Horseback riding
New code

E006.2 Golf
New code

E006.3 Bowling
New code

E006.4 Bike riding
New code

E006.5 Jumping rope
New code

E006.6 Non-running track and field events
New code

E006.9 Other activity involving other sports and athletics played individually
New code

E007 Activities involving other sports and athletics played as a team or group
New category

E007.0 American tackle football
New code

E007.1 American flag or touch football
New code

E007.2 Rugby
New code

E007.3 Baseball
New code

E007.4 Lacrosse and field hockey
New code

E007.5 Soccer
New code

E007.6 Basketball
New code

E007.7 Volleyball (beach) (court)
New code

E007.8 Physical games generally associated with school recess, summer camp and children
New code

E007.9 Other activity involving other sports and athletics played as a team or group
New code

E008 Activities involving other specified sports and athletics
New category

E008.0 Boxing
New code

E008.1 Wrestling
New code

E008.2 Racquet and hand sports
New code

E008.3 Frisbee
New code

E008.4 Martial arts
New code

E008.9 Other specified sports and athletics activity
New code

E009 Activity involving other cardiorespiratory exercise
New category

E009.0 Exercise machines primarily for cardiorespiratory conditioning
New code

E009.1 Calisthenics
New code

E009.2 Aerobic and step exercise
New code

E009.3 Circuit training
New code

E009.4 Obstacle course
New code

E009.5 Grass drills
New code

E009.9 Other activity involving other cardiorespiratory exercise
New code

E010 Activity involving other muscle strengthening exercises
New category

E010.0 Exercise machines primarily for muscle strengthening
New code

E010.1 Push-ups, pull-ups, sit-ups
New code

E010.2 Free weights
New code

E010.3 Pilates
New code

E010.9 Other activity involving other muscle strengthening exercises
New code

E011 Activities involving computer technology and electronic devices
New category

E011.0 Computer keyboarding
New code

E011.1 Hand held interactive electronic device
New code

E011.9 Other activity involving computer technology and electronic devices
New code

E012 Activities involving arts and handcrafts
New category

E012.0 Knitting and crocheting
New code

E012.1 Sewing
New code

E012.2 Furniture building and finishing
New code

E012.9 Activity involving other arts and handcrafts
New code

E013 Activities involving personal hygiene and household maintenance
New category

E013.0 Personal bathing and showering
New code

E013.1 Laundry
New code

E013.2 Vacuuming
New code

E013.3 Ironing
New code

E013.4 Floor mopping and cleaning
New code

E013.5 Residential relocation
New code

E013.8 Other personal hygiene activity
New code

E013.9 Other household maintenance
New code

E014 Activities involving person providing caregiving
New category

E014.0 Caregiving involving bathing
New code

E014.1 Caregiving involving lifting
New code

E014.9 Other activity involving person providing caregiving
New code

E015 Activities involving food preparation, cooking and grilling
New category

E015.0 Food preparation and clean up
New code

E015.1 Grilling and smoking food
New code

E015.2 Cooking and baking
New code

E015.9 Other activity involving cooking and grilling
New code

E016 Activities involving property and land maintenance, building and construction
New category

E016.0 Digging, shoveling and raking
New code

E016.1 Gardening and landscaping
New code

E016.2 Building and construction
New code

E016.9 Other activity involving property and land maintenance, building and construction
New code

E017 Activities involving roller coasters and other types of external motion
New category

E017.0 Rollercoaster riding
New code

E017.9 Other activity involving external motion
New code

E018 Activities involving playing musical instrument
New category

E018.0 Piano playing
New code

E018.1 Drum and other percussion instrument playing
New code

E018.2 String instrument playing
New code

E018.3 Wind and brass instrument playing
New code

E019 Activities involving animal care
New category

E019.0 Walking an animal
New code

E019.1 Milking an animal
New code

E019.2 Grooming and shearing an animal
New code

E019.9 Other activity involving animal care
New code

E029 Other activity
New category

E029.0 Refereeing a sports activity
New code

E029.1 Spectator at an event
New code

E029.2 Rough housing and horseplay
New code

E029.9 Other activity
New code

E030 Unspecified activity
New category

E876.5 Performance of wrong operation (procedure) on correct patient
Revise code

E876.6 Performance of operation (procedure) on patient not scheduled for surgery
New code

E876.7 Performance of correct operation (procedure) on wrong side/body part
New code

E918 Caught accidentally in or between objects
Exclusion term added

E919 Accidents caused by machinery
Exclusion term added

E920 Accidents caused by cutting and piercing instruments or objects
Exclusion term added

E922 Accident caused by firearm and air gun missile
Exclusion term added

E923 Accident caused by explosive material
Exclusion term added

E927 Overexertion and strenuous and repetitive movements or loads
"Use additional code" note added

E928.7 Mechanism or component of firearm and air gun
New code

E990.0 From gasoline bomb
Inclusion term added

E990.1 From flamethrower
New code

E990.2 From incendiary bullet
New code

E990.3 From fire caused indirectly from conventional weapon
New code

E991 Injury due to war operations by bullets and fragments
Exclusion terms added

E991.4 Fragments from munitions
New code

E991.5 Fragments from person-borne improvised explosive device [IED]
New code

E991.6 Fragments from vehicle-borne improvised explosive device [IED]
New code

E991.7 Fragments from other improvised explosive device [IED]
New code

E991.8 Fragments from weapons
New code

E991.9 Other and unspecified fragments
Delete and revise inclusion terms

E992 Injury due to war operations by explosion of marine weapons
Delete inclusion terms

E992.0 Torpedo
New code

E992.1 Depth charge
New code

E992.2 Marine mines
New code

E992.3 Sea-based artillery shell
New code

E992.8 Other by other marine weapons
New code

E992.9 Unspecified marine weapon
New code

E993 Injury due to war operations by other explosion
Delete inclusion terms, add exclusion terms

E993.0 Aerial bomb
New code

E993.1 Guided missile
New code

E993.2 Mortar
New code

E993.3 Person-borne improvised explosive device [IED]
New code

E993.4 Vehicle-borne improvised explosive device [IED]
New code

E993.5 Other improvised explosive device [IED]
New code

E993.6 Unintentional detonation of own munitions
New code

E993.7 Unintentional discharge of own munitions launch device
New code

E993.8 Other specified explosion
New code

E993.9 Unspecified explosion
New code

E994 Injury due to war operations by destruction of aircraft
Delete inclusion terms

E994.0 Destruction of aircraft due to enemy fire or explosives
New code

E994.1 Unintentional destruction of aircraft due to own onboard explosives
New code

E994.2 Destruction of aircraft due to collision with other aircraft
New code

E994.3 Destruction of aircraft due to onboard fire
New code

E994.8 Other destruction of aircraft
New code

E994.9 Unspecified destruction of aircraft
New code

E995 Injury due to war operations by other and unspecified forms of conventional warfare
Delete inclusion terms

E995.0 Unarmed hand-to-hand combat
New code

E995.1 Struck by blunt object
New code

E995.2 Piercing object
New code

E995.3 Intentional restriction of air and airway
New code

E995.4 Unintentional drowning due to inability to surface or obtain air
New code

E995.8 Other forms of conventional warfare
New code

E995.9 Unspecified form of conventional warfare
New code

E996 Injury due to war operations by nuclear weapons
Delete inclusion terms, add exclusion terms

E996.0 Direct blast effect of nuclear weapon
New code

E996.1 Indirect blast effect of nuclear weapon
New code

E996.2 Thermal radiation effect of nuclear weapon
New code

E996.3 Nuclear radiation effects
New code

E996.8 Other effects of nuclear weapons
New code

E996.9 Unspecified effect of nuclear weapon
New code

E997.3 Weapon of mass destruction [WMD], unspecified
New code

E998.0 Explosion of mines
New code

E998.1 Explosion of bombs
New code

E998.8 Injury due to other war operations but occurring after cessation of hostilities
New code

E998.9 Injury due to unspecified war operations but occurring after cessation of hostilities
New code